血管医学
Braunwald心脏病学姊妹篇

Vascular Medicine: A Companion to
Braunwald's Heart Disease

第3版 THIRD EDITION

中文精要·英文影印版

◎ 主编

[美] 马克·A. 克雷格（Mark A. Creager）

[美] 约书亚·A. 贝克曼（Joshua A. Beckman）

[美] 约瑟夫·洛斯卡尔佐（Joseph Loscalzo）

◎ 编译

舒　畅　编译委员会主任委员

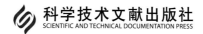

科学技术文献出版社
SCIENTIFIC AND TECHNICAL DOCUMENTATION PRESS

·北京·

图书在版编目（CIP）数据

血管医学：Braunwald心脏病学姊妹篇：第3版/（美）马克·A.克雷格（Mark A. Creager），（美）约书亚·A.贝克曼（Joshua A. Beckman），（美）约瑟夫·洛斯卡尔佐（Joseph Loscalzo）主编；舒畅编译.—北京：科学技术文献出版社，2023.6

书名原文：Vascular Medicine: A Companion to Braunwald's Heart Disease（THIRD EDITION）

ISBN 978-7-5189-9607-0

Ⅰ.①血… Ⅱ.①马… ②约… ③约… ④舒… Ⅲ.①血管疾病—诊疗 Ⅳ.①R543

中国版本图书馆CIP数据核字（2022）第177219号

著作权合同登记号 图字：01-2022-5272

中文简体字版权专有权归科学技术文献出版社所有

Elsevier (Singapore) Pte Ltd.
3 Killiney Road,
#08-01 Winsland House I,
Singapore 239519
Tel: (65) 6349-0200; Fax: (65) 6733-1817

血管医学：Braunwald心脏病学姊妹篇（第3版）

策划编辑：张 蓉　　　责任编辑：张 蓉 危文慧　　　责任校对：张永霞　　　责任出版：张志平

出 版 者	科学技术文献出版社
地　　址	北京市复兴路15号　邮编　100038
编 务 部	（010）58882938，58882087（传真）
发 行 部	（010）58882868，58882870（传真）
邮 购 部	（010）58882873
官方网址	www.stdp.com.cn
发 行 者	科学技术文献出版社发行　全国各地新华书店经销
印 刷 者	北京地大彩印有限公司
版　　次	2023 年 6 月第 1 版　2023 年 6 月第 1 次印刷
开　　本	889 × 1194　1/16
字　　数	1800 千
印　　张	70.25
书　　号	ISBN 978-7-5189-9607-0
定　　价	698.00 元

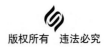

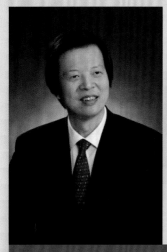

舒 畅

美国斯坦福大学医学院血管外科博士后，一级主任医师、教授，中国医学科学院阜外医院血管外科中心主任、二病区主任，中南大学血管病研究所所长，中南大学湘雅二医院血管中心主任

【社会任职】

现任国家血管外科质控专家组组长，国家心血管病专家委员会血管外科专业委员会主任委员，中国医疗器械行业协会临床试验分会主任委员，以及中国医师协会血管外科医师分会副会长等职务。

【所获荣誉】

擅长主动脉疾病、外周血管疾病的诊治，主刀主动脉手术5000余台，并在海外16个国家进行手术演示170余台，有印度尼西亚、泰国行医资质。以第一完成人获中华医学科技奖一等奖，北京市科技进步奖一等奖，湖南省科技进步奖一等奖、三等奖各一项。发明的主动脉弓部裙边支架和C-Skirt（以名字ChangShu命名）主动脉弓部支架系统已通过国家药品监督管理局绿色通道审批并已在全国30多家医疗中心完成或正在进行多中心研究。被评为全国卫生系统先进工作者及第九届国家卫生健康突出贡献中青年专家；是血管外科专业首届"金柳叶刀奖"获得者和首届湘雅名医；还被评为美国中华医学基金会杰出教授、阿根廷心胸血管外科学会荣誉委员等。

【学术成果】

主持国家自然科学基金重大国际合作、北京市重点科技计划、中国医学科学院医学与健康科技创新工程、"揭榜挂帅"等多项科研课题。主持撰写5项中国血管外科专家共识，主持卫生部医疗服务与质量安全报告血管外科部分撰写工作。参与国家病历首页信息修订工作，成果向全国推行。参编或主编全国医学统编教材、专著等20余部。以第一/通讯作者发表论文199篇，其中，SCI收录论文112篇，中文核心期刊收录论文71篇。

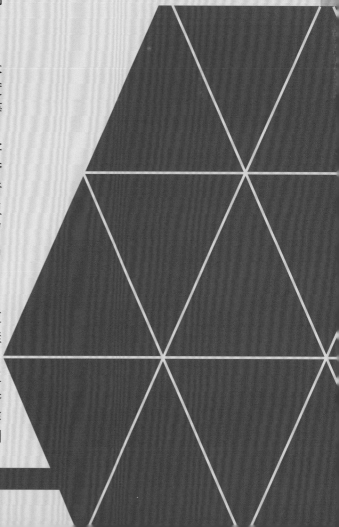

Victor Aboyans, MD, PhD
Professor, Department of Cardiology
Dupuytren University Hospital
Limoges, France

Cherrie Z. Abraham, MD
Associate Professor of Surgery
Division of Vascular and
    Endovascular Surgery
Oregon Health & Sciences University
Portland, Oregon

Aaron W. Aday, MD
Division of Cardiovascular Medicine
Vanderbilt University Medical Center
Nashville, Tennessee

Olamide Alabi, MD
Assistant Professor of Surgery
Division of Vascular and Endovascular Therapy
Emory University
Atlanta, Georgia

George A. Alba, MD
Instructor in Medicine
Division of Pulmonary and Critical Care
Department of Medicine
Massachusetts General Hospital
Boston, Massachusetts

Mark J. Alberts, MD
Chief of Neurology
Department of Neurology
Hartford Hospital;
Physician-in-Chief
Ayer Neuroscience Institute
Hartford HealthCare
Hartford, Connecticut

George J. Arnaoutakis, MD
Assistant Professor
Division of Thoracic and Cardiovascular Surgery
University of Florida College of Medicine
Gainesville, Florida

Elisabeth M. Battinelli, MD, PhD
Assistant Professor
Department of Hematology
Brigham and Women's Hospital
Boston, Massachusetts

Joseph E. Bavaria, MD, PhD
Brooke Roberts-William M. Measey Professor
    of Surgery

Vice-Chief, Division of Cardiovascular Surgery
Director, Thoracic Aortic Surgery Program
Co-Director, Transcatheter Valve Program
Hospital of the University of Pennsylvania
Philadelphia, Pennsylvania

Joshua A. Beckman, MD, MS
Director, Section of Vascular Medicine
Cardiovascular Division
Vanderbilt University Medical Center;
Professor of Medicine
Vanderbilt University
Nashville, Tennessee

Michael Belkin, MD
Division Chief
Professor of Surgery
Harvard Medical School;
Vascular and Endovascular Surgery
Brigham and Women's Hospital
Boston, Massachusetts

Francine Blei, MD, MBA
Professor
Department of Pediatrics
Northwell Health/Lenox Hill Hospital
New York, New York

Peter Blume, DPM
Assistant Clinical Professor of Surgery
Orthopedics and Rehabilitation
Yale University School of Medicine;
Director of Limb Preservation
Department of Orthopedics and Rehabilitation
Yale-New Haven Hospital
New Haven, Connecticut

Marc P. Bonaca, MD, MPH
Director of Vascular Research
Associate Professor
University of Colorado School of Medicine
Executive Director
CPC Clinical Research
Aurora, Colorado

Evan L. Brittain, MD, MSCI
Division of Cardiovascular Medicine and Vanderbilt
    Translational and Clinical Cardiovascular
    Research Center
Vanderbilt University Medical Center
Nashville, Tennessee

Marc Carrier, MD, MSc
Professor of Medicine

University of Ottawa
Ottawa, Ontario, Canada

Brett J. Carroll, MD
Instructor in Medicine
Harvard Medical School;
Director, Section of Vascular Medicine
Division of Cardiovascular Medicine
Beth Israel Deaconess Medical Center
Boston, Massachusetts

Armando Ugo Cavallo, MD
Diagnostic and Interventional Radiology
Policlinico "Tor Vergata"
Rome, Italy;
Departments of Medicine and Radiology
University Hospitals, Harrington & Vascular Institute
Cleveland, Ohio

Stephen Y. Chan, MD, PhD
Director, Center for Pulmonary Vascular Biology and
    Medicine
Department of Medicine
University of Pittsburgh
Pittsburgh, Pennsylvania

Jayer Chung, MD, MSc
Assistant Professor
Division of Vascular Surgery and Endovascular Therapy
Michael E. DeBakey Department of Surgery
Baylor College of Medicine
Houston, Texas

Maria C. Cid, MD
Senior Consultant
Department of Autoimmune Diseases
Clinical Institute of Medicine and Dermatology
Hospital Clinic;
Associate Professor
University of Barcelona;
Senior Group Leader
Institut d'Investigacions Biomèdiques August Pi i Sunyer
    (IDIBAPS)
Barcelona, Spain

Benjamin D. Colvard, MD
Resident Physician
Department of Surgery
Division of Vascular and Endovascular Surgery
Stanford University
Stanford, California

Christopher J. Cooper, MD
Dean, College of Medicine and Life Sciences
Executive Vice President of Clinical Affairs
University of Toledo
Toledo, Ohio

Mark A. Creager, MD
Director, Heart and Vascular Center
Dartmouth-Hitchcock Medical Center;
Professor of Medicine and Surgery
Geisel School of Medicine at Dartmouth

Lebanon, New Hampshire

Michael H. Criqui, MD, MPH
Distinguished Professor
Division of Preventive Medicine
Department of Family Medicine and Public Health
University of California, San Diego
La Jolla, California

Mary Cushman, MD, MSc
Professor of Medicine
Larner College of Medicine at the University
    of Vermont
Burlington, Vermont

Michael D. Dake, MD
Professor of Cardiothoracic Surgery
Stanford University School of Medicine
Director, Catheterization Angiography Laboratory
Stanford University Medical Center
Stanford, California

Annie L. Darves-Bornoz, MD
Resident Physician
Department of Urology
Vanderbilt University
Nashville, Tennessee

Mark D.P. Davis, MD
Professor
Department of Dermatology
Mayo Clinic
Rochester, Minnesota

Steven M. Dean, DO, FSVM, RPVI
Clinical Professor of Medicine
Department of Cardiovascular Medicine
Ohio State University Wexner Medical Center
Columbus, Ohio

Robert T. Eberhardt, MD
Associate Professor of Medicine
Department of Medicine
Boston University School of Medicine;
Director of Vascular Medical Services
Department of Cardiovascular Medicine
Boston Medical Center
Boston, Massachusetts

Matthew S. Edwards, MD
Richard H. Dean Professor and Chair
Department of Vascular and Endovascular
    Surgery
Wake Forest University School
    of Medicine
Winston-Salem, North Carolina

Alfonso Eirin, MD
Assistant Professor of Medicine
Division of Nephrology and Hypertension
Mayo Clinic
Rochester, Minnesota

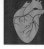

Alik Farber, MD
Chief, Division of Vascular and Endovascular
  Surgery
Boston Medical Center;
Professor of Surgery and Radiology
Boston University School of Medicine
Boston, Massachusetts

Marc Fisher, MD
Neurologist
Department of Neurology
Beth Israel Deaconess Medical Center
Boston, Massachusetts

Nicholas A. Flavahan, PhD
Professor
Department of Anesthesiology and Critical Care
  Medicine
Johns Hopkins University
Baltimore, Maryland

Kevin G. Friedman, MD
Assistant Professor
Harvard Medical School;
Department of Pediatric Cardiology
Boston Children's Hospital
Boston, MA

Marie Gerhard-Herman, MD
Associate Professor
Department of Medicine
Harvard Medical School;
Vascular Diagnostic Laboratory
Cardiovascular Division
Brigham and Women's Hospital
Boston, Massachusetts

Peter Gloviczki, MD
Joe M. and Ruth Roberts Professor of Surgery, Emeritus
Mayo Clinic College of Medicine;
Chair Emeritus
Division of Vascular and Endovascular Surgery
Mayo Clinic
Rochester, Minnesota

Samuel Z. Goldhaber, MD
Professor of Medicine
Harvard Medical School;
Director, Thrombosis Research Group
Interim Chief, Division of Cardiovascular Medicine
Section Head, Vascular Medicine
Brigham and Women's Hospital
Boston, Massachusetts

Larry B. Goldstein, MD, FAAN, FANA, FAHA
Ruth L. Works Professor and Chairman
Department of Neurology
University of Kentucky;
Co-Director
Kentucky Neuroscience Institute
Lexington, Kentucky

Heather L. Gornik, MD, MHS
Associate Professor of Medicine

Case Western Reserve University;
Co-Director, Vascular Center
Harrington Heart and Vascular Institute
University Hospitals
Cleveland, Ohio

Daniel M. Greif, MD
Associate Professor
Departments of Medicine and Genetics
Yale University School of Medicine
New Haven, Connecticut

Kathy K. Griendling, PhD
Professor of Medicine
Department of Medicine
Division of Cardiology
Emory University
Atlanta, Georgia

Naomi M. Hamburg, MD, MSc
Chief, Vascular Biology Section
Joseph Vita Professor of Cardiovascular
  Medicine
Boston University Medical Center
Boston, Massachusetts

Stanislav Henkin, MD, MPH
Assistant Professor of Medicine
Geisel School of Medicine at Dartmouth;
Heart and Vascular Center
Dartmouth-Hitchcock Medical Center
Lebanon, New Hampshire

Lula L. Hilenski, PhD
Assistant Professor
Department of Medicine
Division of Cardiology
Emory University
Atlanta, Georgia

Arjun Jayaraj, MD, MPH, RPVI
Vascular Surgeon
RANE Center for Venous and Lymphatic
  Diseases
St. Dominic Hospital
Jackson, Mississippi

Senthil Jayarajan, MD, MS
Staff Vascular Surgeon
Vascular Specialists of Minnesota
Minneapolis Heart Institute
Minneapolis, Minnesota

Douglas W. Jones, MD
Assistant Professor
Department of Vascular and Endovascular
  Surgery
Boston University Medical School
Boston Medical Center
Boston, Massachusetts

Enjae Jung, MD
Assistant Professor of Surgery

Division of Vascular and Endovascular
  Surgery
Oregon Health & Science University
Portland, Oregon

Inamul Kabir, PhD
Postdoctoral Fellow
Departments of Medicine and Genetics
Yale University School of Medicine
New Haven, Connecticut

Kirk A. Keegan, MD, MPH
Assistant Professor
Department of Urology
Vanderbilt University
Nashville, Tennessee

Tanaz A. Kermani, MD, MS
Director, Vasculitis Program
Associate Clinical Professor
Department of Rheumatology
University of California Los Angeles
Los Angeles, California

Matthew C. Koopmann, MD
Vascular Surgeon, Operative Care Division
Portland VA Medical Center;
Assistant Professor, Division of Vascular
  Surgery
Oregon Health & Science University
Portland, Oregon

Matthew J. Koster, MD
Assistant Professor of Medicine
Division of Rheumatology
Department of Internal Medicine
Mayo Clinic
Rochester, Minnesota

Christopher M. Kramer, MD
Ruth C. Heede Professor of Cardiology, Professor
  of Radiology
Departments of Medicine and
  Radiology
University of Virginia Health System
Charlottesville, Virginia

Gregory J. Landry, MD
Professor and Chief
Division of Vascular Surgery
Oregon Health & Science University
Portland, Oregon

Jane A. Leopold, MD
Associate Professor of Medicine
Harvard Medical School;
Division of Cardiovascular Medicine
Brigham and Women's Hospital
Boston, Massachusetts

Lilach O. Lerman, MD, PhD
Professor of Medicine and Physiology
Division of Nephrology and Hypertension

Mayo Clinic
Rochester, Minnesota

Peter Libby, MD
Professor of Medicine
Harvard Medical School;
Cardiovascular Division
Brigham and Women's Hospital
Boston, Massachusetts

Joseph Loscalzo, MD, PhD
Hersey Professor of the Theory and Practice of Medicine
Harvard Medical School;
Chairman and Physician-in-Chief
Soma Weiss, MD, Distinguished Chair in Medicine
Department of Medicine
Brigham and Women's Hospital
Boston, Massachusetts

Christine E. Lotto, MD
Department of Vascular and Endovascular Surgery
Brigham and Women's Hospital
Boston, Massachusetts

Lars Maegdefessel, MD, PhD
Technical University Munich
Vascular and Endovascular Surgery
Klinikum rechts der Isar
Munich, Bavaria, Germany

Bharti Manwani, MD, PhD
Department of Neurology
University of Texas Health Science Center at Houston
Houston, Texas

Bradley A. Maron, MD
Division of Cardiovascular Medicine
Brigham and Women's Hospital;
Department of Cardiology
Boston VA Healthcare System
Boston, Massachusetts

Carlos Mena-Hurtado, MD
Assistant Professor
Department of Medicine
Section of Cardiovascular Medicine
Yale University School of Medicine
New Haven, Connecticut

Matthew T. Menard, MD
Co-Director of Endovascular Surgery
Division of Vascular and Endovascular Surgery
Brigham and Women's Hospital
Boston, Massachusetts

Peter A. Merkel, MD, MPH
Chief of Rheumatology
Department of Medicine
Professor
Department of Medicine and Departments of
  Biostatistics, Epidemiology, and Informatics
University of Pennsylvania
Philadelphia, Pennsylvania

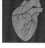

Paul A. Monach, MD, PhD
Chief, Rheumatology Section
Boston VA Healthcare System
Division of Rheumatology, Immunology,
    and Allergy
Brigham and Women's Hospital
Boston, Massachusetts

Gregory L. Moneta, MD
Professor of Surgery
Division of Vascular and Endovascular Surgery
Oregon Health & Science University
Portland, Oregon

Jane W. Newburger, MD, MPH
Associate Cardiologist-in-Chief for Academic Affairs
Boston Children's Hospital;
Commonwealth Professor of Pediatrics
Harvard Medical School
Boston, Massachusetts

Aglaia Ntokou, PhD
Postdoctoral Associate
Departments of Medicine and Genetics
Yale University School of Medicine
New Haven, Connecticut

Patrick T. O'Gara, MD
Professor of Medicine
Harvard Medical School;
Senior Physician
Cardiovascular Division
Brigham and Women's Hospital
Boston, Massachusetts

Jeffrey W. Olin, DO
Professor of Medicine
Director, Vascular Medicine
Zena and Michael A. Wiener Cardiovascular
    Institute
Icahn School of Medicine at Mount Sinai
New York, New York

David F. Penson, MD, MPH
Professor
Department of Urology
Director
Center for Surgical Quality and Outcomes
    Research
Vanderbilt University
Nashville, Tennessee

Gregory Piazza, MD, MS
Assistant Professor of Medicine
Harvard Medical School;
Staff Physician
Cardiovascular Division
Department of Medicine
Brigham and Women's Hospital
Boston, Massachusetts

Amy West Pollak, MD, MS
Assistant Professor
Department of Cardiovascular Medicine

Mayo Clinic, Florida
Jacksonville, Florida

Richard J. Powell, MD
Professor of Surgery
Department of Surgery
Dartmouth-Hitchcock Medical Center
Lebanon, New Hampshire

Uwe Raaz, MD
Molecular and Translational Vascular
    Medicine
Department of Cardiology and Pneumology
University Heart Center Göttingen
Göttingen, Germany

Sanjay Rajagopalan, MD, FACC, FAHA
Chief, Division of Cardiovascular Medicine
Department of Cardiology
Harrington Heart and Vascular Institute;
Director, Case Cardiovascular Research
    Institute
Department of Cardiology;
Professor of Internal Medicine
Case Western Reserve University
Cleveland, Ohio

Stanley G. Rockson, MD
Allan and Tina Neill Professor of Lymphatic Research
    and Medicine
Division of Cardiovascular Medicine
Stanford University School of Medicine
Stanford, California

Thom W. Rooke, MD
Krehbiel Professor of Vascular Medicine
Vascular Center
Mayo Clinic
Rochester, Minnesota

Rishi A. Roy, MD
Department of Surgery
Division of Vascular and Endovascular
    Surgery
Baptist Medical Center
Jackson, Mississippi

Fatima Zahra Saddouk, PhD
Postdoctoral Associate
Departments of Medicine and Genetics
Yale University School of Medicine
New Haven, Connecticut

Julio C. Sartori-Valinotti, MD
Department of Dermatology
Mayo Clinic College of Medicine
Rochester, Minnesota

Alexander H. Shannon, MD
Department of Surgery
University of Virginia
Charlottesville, Virginia

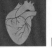

Aditya Sharma, MBBS, FSVM
Associate Professor of Medicine
Department of Cardiovascular Medicine
University of Virginia School of Medicine
Charlottesville, Virginia

Roger F.J. Shepherd, MB, BCh
Assistant Professor of Medicine
Department of Cardiovascular Medicine
Mayo Clinic College of Medicine
Rochester, Minnesota

Piotr Sobieszczyk, MD, RVT
Instructor in Medicine
Harvard Medical School;
Attending Physician
Cardiovascular Division
Vascular Medicine Section
Brigham and Women's Hospital
Boston, Massachusetts

Joshua M. Spin, MD, PhD
Clinical Assistant Professor
Department of Cardiovascular
    Medicine
Stanford University School of Medicine;
VA Palo Alto Health Care System
Palo Alto, California

David H. Stone, MD
Associate Professor of Surgery
Section of Vascular Surgery
Dartmouth-Hitchcock Medical Center
Lebanon, New Hampshire

Bjoern D. Suckow, MD, MS
Assistant Professor of Surgery
Section of Vascular Surgery
Dartmouth-Hitchcock Medical Center
Lebanon, New Hampshire

Bauer E. Sumpio, MD, PhD
Professor
Surgery and Radiology
Yale University School of Medicine;
Chief, Vascular Surgery
Director, Vascular Center
Program Director, Vascular Surgery
Yale-New Haven Medical Center
New Haven, Connecticut

Stephen C. Textor, MD
Professor of Medicine
Division of Nephrology and
    Hypertension
Mayo Clinic
Rochester, Minnesota

Rahul B. Thomas, MD
Cardiology Imaging Fellow

Department of Cardiology
University Hospitals
Cleveland, Ohio

Robert Thompson, MD
Professor of Surgery
Department of Surgery
Washington University School of Medicine
St. Louis, Missouri

Philip S. Tsao, PhD
Professor of Medicine
School of Medicine
Stanford University
Palo Alto, California

Gilbert R. Upchurch, Jr., MD
Woodward Professor and Chairman
Department of Surgery
University of Florida
Gainesville, Florida

Meg VanNostrand, MD
Neurologist
Department of Neurology
Beth Israel Deaconess Medical Center
Boston, Massachusetts

Kenneth J. Warrington, MD
Professor of Medicine
Department of Rheumatology/Internal Medicine
Mayo Clinic
Rochester, Minnesota

Suman Wasan, MD, MS, RVT
Professor
Department of Medicine
University of Oklahoma Health Sciences Center
Oklahoma City, Oklahoma

Christopher J. White, MD
Chairman and Professor of Medicine
Department of Cardiovascular Diseases
Ochsner Clinical School of the University of Queensland,
    Ochsner Medical Institutions
New Orleans, Louisiana

Khendi T. White Solaru, MD
Assistant Professor of Medicine
Case Western Reserve University;
Staff, Cardiovascular Medicine
Harrington Heart and Vascular Institute
University Hospitals
Cleveland, Ohio

Nikolaos Zacharias, MD
Clinical Assistant Professor of Surgery
Section of Vascular Surgery
Dartmouth-Hitchcock Medical Center
Lebanon, New Hampshire

编译委员会名单

　　随着人口老龄化和糖尿病发病率的升高，冠状动脉以外的其他血管疾病已成为严重且快速增加的健康问题。越来越多的外周血管疾病，包括肢体动脉、肾动脉、中枢神经系统动脉、内脏动脉、肺动脉及各类静脉疾病的发病率升高，这一现象对临床医师提出了很大的挑战。不同脏器相关的血管疾病都可引起相应的临床表现，从较轻的偶发不适到危及生命的急危重症。

　　幸运的是，随着现代临床影像学技术的快速发展，我们对于血管疾病的病理生理学及诊断有了很好的了解，对于血管疾病的治疗也日趋高效。基于导管的血管腔内治疗、外科手术治疗和药物治疗都取得了重大进步。血管疾病影响非常多的器官和系统，其治疗牵涉面广，可能需要如血管外科、介入放射科、影像科、泌尿外科、神经内科、神经外科、血液科等相关领域的专家共同讨论，决定治疗方案。其他医学领域很少需要如此庞大数量的学科专家来协作以保证高效的治疗效果。

　　由于在过去 10 年间，治疗血管疾病所需要的知识总量增加太过迅速，我们需要一本能贯穿从学习阶段到指导实践阶段的优质血管疾病教科书。Creager 医师、Beckman 医师和 Loscalzo 医师结合他们丰富的血管疾病知识和临床经验，共同编撰了本册血管医学教科书。本书还特邀众多经验丰富的编者参与撰写了极具深度和广度的内容，相信本书对于从事血管疾病治疗的临床医师、基础研究工作者及医学生具有很高的参考价值。

　　第三版相对于之前的版本做了很多修改。与 6 年前的第二版相比，本书介绍了很多领域内的重要进展。除外原有章节的大幅修改，本书还增加了 7 个新的章节、200 余张图片和 75 个表格。本书将成为血管疾病领域内的标准参考书籍。此外，我们也非常荣幸地介绍，本书成为了心血管医学领域内的著名教科书 *Braunwald's Heart Disease: A Textbook of Cardiovascular Medicine* 的姊妹篇。

Eugene Brauwald, MD

Douglas P. Zipes, MD

Peter Libby, MD

Robert O. Bonow, MD

Douglas L. Mann, MD

Gordon F. Tomaselli, MD

血管与血管互相连接，血液在各个器官之间流动……它们是人类生命的源泉，就像江河灌溉农田一样滋养整个机体，赋予人类身体和生命。

——Hippocrates

生命的悲剧常来源于动脉。

——William Osler

　　血管疾病是西方国家最主要的致死和致残原因之一。美国约有 2500 万人因动脉硬化和血管血栓形成获得相关的后遗症，还有很多人因血管痉挛、血管炎、慢性静脉功能不全和淋巴水肿等血管疾病长期不适甚至残疾。血管生理领域内的重大发现提高了我们对血管疾病的认识和理解。血管影像学技术的进步、血管腔内治疗等治疗手段的迅速发展为血管疾病的治疗提供了充足的动力。血管医学是一门重要且充满活力的学科，同时它涉及很多实验室的成果向临床的转化研究，从而使患者从基础研究的成果中迅速获益。

　　Vascular Medicine: A Companion to Braunwald's Heart Disease（*THIRD EDITION*）是一本整合了从血管生理到各种血管疾病的全面、系统的教科书。本书重点介绍了血管生理领域内的新发现，且所有的临床章节都包含了最新诊断方法和治疗方法的发展。本书还提供了专家咨询网站的查找方式，从而可进一步为读者提供图片、视频和其他各种资料。

　　和之前的版本一脉相承，本书由血管生理的重要规律、血管系统评估原则及血管疾病的细节讨论等几个部分组成。每章的作者都是该领域内的著名专家。血管生理的规律在第一部分（血管生物学）讲述，这部分内容包括血管胚胎学和血管新生、血管内皮、血管平滑肌、正常血管止血机制和血管药理学。第二部分（血管病理生理学）的章节有动脉粥样硬化的病理生理学、血管炎的病理生理学、血栓形成的病理生理学，以及新增加的章节——主动脉瘤的病理生理学、心血管系统纤维化的病理生理学和评估。第三部分（血管检查相关原则）讲解了血管疾病患者的检查工具，并从病史采集与体格检查、非创伤性检查（磁共振血管成像、CT 血管成像）、基于导管的周围血管造影术等血管检查方法做了全面的介绍。第四到第十部分主要讲述血管疾病，包括外周动脉疾病、主

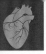

动脉夹层、主动脉瘤等，并对这些血管疾病的流行病学、病理生理学、临床评估和药物治疗、腔内治疗、外科治疗等内容均进行了更新，还专门用一章介绍了比较特殊的疾病——血管源性勃起功能障碍。

第十一部分（血管炎）阐述了所有血管炎的临床表现、评估及治疗，其中包括大血管血管炎、中小血管血管炎、血栓闭塞性脉管炎、川崎病等。第十二部分（急性肢体缺血）介绍了急性动脉闭塞和动脉粥样硬化栓塞。第十三部分（血管痉挛及其他相关血管疾病）介绍了血管痉挛性疾病如雷诺现象，以及温度相关性血管疾病如肢端发绀、红斑性肢痛、冻疮等。

静脉血栓栓塞性疾病主要在第十四部分介绍，包括静脉血栓栓塞性疾病的流行病学、临床评估、治疗、预后及肺栓塞的诊疗要点等。第十五部分主要介绍慢性静脉疾病的诊断和治疗，包括静脉曲张、慢性静脉功能不全。第十六部分介绍肺高压，包括原发性肺动脉高压和非肺动脉高压性肺高压。淋巴水肿的治疗在第十七部分（淋巴疾病）。最后一部分介绍了其他重要的血管疾病，包括纤维肌发育不良、血管感染、下肢溃疡、血管损伤、压迫综合征、血管瘤、血管畸形等，还有新的章节介绍关于血管疾病的皮肤表现。

从事血管疾病治疗的医务人员，包括实习医师、心血管疾病医师、血管外科医师、介入放射科医师等均可从本书中获益。我们也希望本书对于医学生有比较重要的教育意义。希望通过阅读本书，读者能掌握血管生理及血管疾病等知识，并在临床实践中灵活运用。血管系统分布于全身所有器官，通过学习本书，读者也能够全面地理解血管疾病与全身各个系统之间的联系，从而能够从全局来理解血管疾病，这样也能为血管疾病患者提供合理的诊断和治疗对策。

Mark A. Creager, MD

Joshua A. Beckman, MD, MS

Joseph Loscalzo, MD, PhD

原书致谢

我们特别感谢助理编辑 Diana Doheny 和 Stephanie Tribuna 的工作！

原书献词

献给我们的妻子、孩子和孙子孙女！

Vascular Medicine: A Companion to Braunwald's Heart Disease 是西方医学著名教材 *Braunwald's Heart Disease: A Textbook of Cardiovascular Medicine* 的姊妹篇，此版为第三版，由来自美国 Dartmouth-Hitchcock 医学中心的 Mark A. Creager 教授、哈佛大学医学院 Brigham and Women 医院的 Joseph Loscalzo 教授和 Vanderbilt 大学医学中心的 Joshua A. Beckman 教授三位心血管病专业领域的专家作为共同主编编写。本书从全身血管系统的胚胎发生，生理机制（包括分子机制等），各种血管疾病的病理机制、临床诊断、最新治疗方法及其进展等方面，非常全面和系统地介绍了作为医学学科里的一门重要分支"血管医学"的知识，是一本不可多得的全面且重点突出的医学教材。对于在校医学生，培训阶段的住院医师，血管外科、心血管内科、心血管外科等专科培训阶段的医师和高年资的心血管专科医师，以及研究血管疾病发病机制和新的治疗方法的科研人员来说都很适用。

本书由中国医学科学院阜外医院血管外科中心舒畅教授组织全国各大医院从事心脏和血管外科的专家进行详细的编译工作，创新性地将英文内容结合自身的丰富临床经验于每个章节前撰写了提纲挈领的导读内容，既保留原书的全部英文内容，将其原汁原味地呈现给读者，又结合了国内各位专家的丰富血管医学知识及实践经验，从而向读者提供更具参考意义的内容。舒畅教授是我带的第一位血管外科专业博士，他勤奋好学、勇于创新，是我国血管外科界的杰出专家。尤其在主动脉疾病的微创治疗领域，他在近10年来为亚洲、欧洲、南美洲地区的16个国家的160多位主动脉疾病患者进行了成功的手术治疗，称得上是站在国际血管外科领域最前沿的医师。他在国内致力于主动脉疾病微创治疗的标准化术式和质量控制，为提高我国主动脉微创治疗的整体质量做出了艰苦的努力；他开创性地使用了多项新的诊治技术；创新性地设计和牵头研发出了多款拥有自主知识产权的主动脉疾病微创治疗器械；在国际上不遗余力地推广我国血管外科的主动脉微创治疗经验，对五大洲数十个国家的500余名血管外科医师进行了专科培训。舒畅教授牵头组织我国数十位血管外科和心脏外科的专家共同精心打造了本书的编译版本。我相信，凭借他们对本书的精确理解

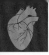

和结合自身专业领域内的丰富经验必将给读者带来一道血管医学知识的盛宴。

回望过去50余年，我国血管医学发展从无到有，从弱到强，从基础到高精尖，凝结了我国老一辈专家和现在年富力强的医者们的艰辛努力；展望未来，我们需要更好地培养我们血管医学事业的接班人，通过学习和借鉴先进国家血管医学的基础和临床的经验，结合我国的国情，把我们的接力棒高效平稳地交到下一代医者手中，为健康中国和国际卫生健康事业助力！

汪忠镐

心血管疾病已成为危害我国人民生命和健康的"头号杀手"。血管疾病首当其冲，近年来的发病率也日渐升高。认识血管疾病的生理学和病理学基础，辨明血管疾病的发病机制，掌握血管疾病的经典治疗和创新治疗的方法是医务工作者必需的知识储备。对于临床诊治血管疾病的专科医师和研究血管疾病及诊治方法的医学科学工作者而言，更是必备的理论和技能。我们很荣幸能够将这本世界著名心血管病教材的影印版《血管医学：Braunwald 心脏病学的姊妹篇（第 3 版）》带给中国广大从事血管医学工作和研究的医师、医学生和科技工作者。本书从血管的发育、生理学、病理学等最为基础的内容开始介绍，到目前最前沿的血管外科学、腔内血管治疗学、血管影像学、免疫学、遗传学等领域深入浅出，抽丝剥茧地将每一个血管医学相关的知识点进行透彻的剖析。此外，全书插入了大量精美的分子作用机制图，具有代表性的临床影像图及生动易懂的手绘外科手术图等，可帮助读者更容易理解其内容。本书的中文编译团队由国内相关领域内的著名专家组成，在仔细阅读各章节内容的基础之上，结合其丰富的临床和基础科研经验对每个章节的内容进行了提纲挈领的概括。希望读者在理解原著的基础上能够有效地结合和借鉴中国专家的经验。

中国的血管医学从无到有，从弱到强，经历了无数先辈医学科学工作者的刻苦钻研和深厚积淀。即便处于优良基础之上，我们仍然不能忘记回眸英文原著，"西学东渐""取长补短"，才能更好地完善血管医学知识体系和血管医学的诊治创新工作。

最后，衷心感谢为本书付出辛勤劳动的医学专家和出版社的编辑同道。不妥之处请各位读者批评指正！

舒畅

PART I Biology of Blood Vessels

1 **Vascular Embryology and Angiogenesis 5**
Aglaia Ntokou, Inamul Kabir, Fatima Zahra Saddouk, and Daniel M. Greif

2 **The Endothelium 23**
Jane A. Leopold

3 **Vascular Smooth Muscle 41**
Lula L. Hilenski and Kathy K. Griendling

4 **Normal Mechanisms of Vascular Hemostasis 75**
Elisabeth M. Battinelli and Joseph Loscalzo

5 **Vascular Pharmacology 83**
Nicholas A. Flavahan

PART II Pathobiology of Blood Vessels

6 **Pathobiology of Atherosclerosis 115**
Peter Libby

7 **Pathobiology of Aortic Aneurysms 133**
Uwe Raaz, Joshua M. Spin, Lars Maegdefessel, and Philip S. Tsao

8 **Pathobiology of Thrombosis 143**
Elisabeth M. Battinelli, Jane A. Leopold, and Joseph Loscalzo

9 **Pathobiology and Assessment of Cardiovascular Fibrosis 151**
Evan L. Brittain and Bradley A. Maron

10 **Pathobiology of Vasculitis 163**
Paul A. Monach

PART III Principles of Vascular Examination

11 **The History and Physical Examination 173**
Joshua A. Beckman and Mark A. Creager

12 **Vascular Laboratory Testing 185**
Marie Gerhard-Herman and Mark A. Creager

13 **Magnetic Resonance Imaging 205**
Amy West Pollak and Christopher M. Kramer

14 **Computed Tomographic Angiography 223**
Rahul B. Thomas, Armando Ugo Cavallo, and Sanjay Rajagopalan

15 **Catheter-Based Peripheral Angiography 243**
Christopher J. White

PART IV Peripheral Artery Disease

16 **The Epidemiology of Peripheral Artery Disease 257**
Victor Aboyans and Michael H. Criqui

17 **Pathophysiology of Peripheral Artery Disease 279**
Naomi M. Hamburg and Mark A. Creager

18 **Peripheral Artery Disease: Clinical Evaluation 289**
Joshua A. Beckman and Mark A. Creager

19 **Medical Treatment of Peripheral Artery Disease 303**
Marc P. Bonaca and Mark A. Creager

20 **Endovascular Treatment of Peripheral Artery Disease 327**
Christopher J. White

21 **Reconstructive Surgery for Peripheral Artery Disease 339**
Matthew T. Menard, Christine E. Lotto, and Michael Belkin

PART V Renal Artery Disease

22 **Pathophysiology of Renal Artery Disease 363**
Alfonso Eirin, Lilach O. Lerman, and Stephen C. Textor

23 **Clinical Evaluation of Renal Artery Disease 377**
Jeffrey W. Olin

24 **Treatment of Renal Artery Disease 391**
Christopher J. Cooper and Matthew S. Edwards

PART VI Mesenteric Vascular Disease

25 **Epidemiology and Pathophysiology of Mesenteric Vascular Disease 405**
Olamide Alabi, Matthew C. Koopmann, and Gregory L. Moneta

26 **Clinical Evaluation and Treatment of Mesenteric Vascular Disease 415**
Enjae Jung, Cherrie Abraham, Gregory J. Landry, and Gregory L. Moneta

PART VII Vasculogenic Erectile Dysfunction

27 **Vasculogenic Erectile Dysfunction 431**
Annie L. Darves-Bornoz, Kirk A. Keegan, and David F. Penson

PART VIII Cerebrovascular Ischemia

28 **Epidemiology of Cerebrovascular Disease 445**
Larry B. Goldstein

29 **Clinical Presentation and Diagnosis of Cerebrovascular Disease 463**
Mark J. Alberts

30 **Prevention and Treatment of Stroke 481**
Marc Fisher, Bharti Manwani, and Meg VanNostrand

31 **Carotid Artery Revascularization 501**
Richard J. Powell and Nikolaos Zacharias

PART IX Aortic Dissection

32 **Pathophysiology, Clinical Evaluation, and Medical Management of Aortic Dissection 511**
Brett J. Carroll, Bradley A. Maron, and Patrick T. O'Gara

33 **Surgical Therapy for Aortic Dissection** 535
George J. Arnaoutakis and Joseph E. Bavaria

34 **Endovascular Therapy for Aortic Dissection** 553
Benjamin D. Colvard and Michael D. Dake

PART X Aortic Aneurysm

35 **Epidemiology and Prognosis of Aortic Aneurysms** 569
Aaron W. Aday and Joshua A. Beckman

36 **Clinical Evaluation of Aortic Aneurysms** 583
Joshua A. Beckman and Mark A. Creager

37 **Surgical Treatment of Abdominal Aortic Aneurysms** 595
Bjoern D. Suckow and David H. Stone

38 **Endovascular Therapy for Abdominal Aortic Aneurysm** 617
Alexander H. Shannon, Rishi A. Roy, and Gilbert R. Upchurch, Jr.

PART XI Vasculitis

39 **Overview of Vasculitis** 637
Peter A. Merkel

40 **Large Vessel Vasculitis** 655
Peter A. Merkel and Maria C. Cid

41 **Medium and Small Vessel Vasculitis** 673
Matthew J. Koster, Kenneth J. Warrington, and Tanaz A. Kermani

42 **Thromboangiitis Obliterans (Buerger Disease)** 695
Gregory Piazza and Jeffrey W. Olin

43 **Kawasaki Disease** 709
Kevin G. Friedman and Jane W. Newburger

PART XII Acute Limb Ischemia

44 **Acute Arterial Occlusion** 725
Piotr Sobieszczyk

45 **Atheroembolism** 745
Roger F.J. Shepherd

PART XIII Vasospasm and Other Related Vascular Diseases

46 **Raynaud Phenomenon** 765
Stanislav Henkin and Mark A. Creager

47 **Acrocyanosis** 783
Robert T. Eberhardt

48 **Erythromelalgia** 789
Julio C. Sartori-Valinotti, Mark D.P. Davis, and Thom W. Rooke

49 **Pernio (Chilblains)** 801
Jeffrey W. Olin

PART XIV Venous Thromboembolic Disease

50 **Epidemiology of Venous Thromboembolic Disease** 811
Marc Carrier and Mary Cushman

51 **Clinical Evaluation of Venous Thromboembolism** 819
Brett J. Carroll and Gregory Piazza

52 **Management of Venous Thromboembolism** 835
Samuel Z. Goldhaber and Gregory Piazza

PART XV Chronic Venous Disorders

53 **Varicose Veins** 855
Aditya Sharma and Suman Wasan

54 **Chronic Venous Insufficiency** 873
Arjun Jayaraj and Peter Gloviczki

PART XVI Pulmonary Hypertension

55 **Pulmonary Arterial Hypertension** 897
Stephen Y. Chan and Joseph Loscalzo

56 **Pulmonary Hypertension in Patients With Nonpulmonary Arterial Hypertension** 929
Bradley A. Maron, George A. Alba, and Joseph Loscalzo

PART XVII Lymphatic Disorders

57 **Diseases of the Lymphatic Circulation** 947
Stanley G. Rockson

PART XVIII Miscellaneous

58 **Fibromuscular Dysplasia** 965
Khendi T. White Solaru and Heather L. Gornik

59 **Vascular Infections** 985
Jayer Chung

60 **Dermatological Manifestations of Vascular Disease** 1009
Steven M. Dean

61 **Lower Extremity Ulceration** 1023
Bauer E. Sumpio, Peter Blume, and Carlos Mena-Hurtado

62 **Vascular Trauma** 1039
Douglas W. Jones and Alik Farber

63 **Vascular Compression Syndromes** 1055
Senthil Jayarajan and Robert Thompson

64 **Peripheral Vascular Anomalies, Malformations, and Vascular Tumors** 1071
Francine Blei

第一部分　血管生物学

第1章　血管胚胎学和血管新生 ……………………………………………3

第2章　血管内皮 ……………………………… 21

第3章　血管平滑肌 ……………………………… 39

第4章　正常血管止血机制 ……………………………… 73

第5章　血管药理学 ……………………………… 81

第二部分　血管病理生理学

第6章　动脉粥样硬化的病理生理学 ………………………113

第7章　主动脉瘤的病理生理学 ……………………………131

第8章　血栓形成的病理生理学 ……………………………141

第9章　心血管系统纤维化的病理生理学和评估 …………149

第10章　血管炎的病理生理学 ……………………………161

第三部分　血管检查相关原则

第11章　病史采集与体格检查 ……………………………171

第12章　血管相关实验室检查 ……………………………183

第13章　磁共振血管成像 ……………………………203

第14章　CT血管成像 ……………………………221

第15章　基于导管的周围血管造影术 ……………………241

第四部分　外周动脉疾病

第16章　外周动脉疾病流行病学 …………………………255

第17章　外周动脉疾病的病理生理学 ……………………277

第18章　外周动脉疾病的临床评估 ………………………287

第19章　外周动脉疾病的内科治疗 ………………………301

第20章　外周动脉疾病的腔内治疗 ………………………325

第21章　外周动脉疾病的重建手术 ………………………337

第五部分　肾动脉疾病

第22章　肾动脉疾病的病理生理学 ………………………361

第23章　肾动脉疾病的临床评估 ················ 375
第24章　肾动脉狭窄的治疗 ···················· 389

第六部分　肠系膜血管疾病

第25章　肠系膜血管疾病的流行病学和病理生理学 ··········· 403
第26章　肠系膜血管疾病的临床评估和治疗 ············· 413

第七部分　血管源性勃起功能障碍

第27章　血管源性勃起功能障碍 ················· 429

第八部分　脑血管缺血

第28章　脑血管疾病的流行病学 ················· 443
第29章　脑血管疾病的临床表现和诊断 ············· 461
第30章　脑卒中的预防和治疗 ·················· 479
第31章　颈动脉血管重建 ····················· 499

第九部分　主动脉夹层

第32章　主动脉夹层的病理生理学、临床评估和药物治疗 ········ 509
第33章　主动脉夹层的手术治疗 ················· 533
第34章　主动脉夹层的腔内治疗 ················· 551

第十部分　主动脉瘤

第35章　主动脉瘤的流行病学与预后 ··············· 567
第36章　主动脉瘤的临床评估 ·················· 581
第37章　腹主动脉瘤的手术治疗 ················· 593
第38章　腹主动脉瘤的腔内修复术 ················ 615

第十一部分　血管炎

第39章　血管炎概述 ························ 635
第40章　大血管血管炎 ······················ 653
第41章　中小血管血管炎 ····················· 671
第42章　血栓闭塞性脉管炎 ···················· 693
第43章　川崎病 ·························· 707

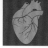

第十二部分　急性肢体缺血

第44章　急性动脉闭塞 ··· 723

第45章　动脉粥样硬化栓塞 ·· 743

第十三部分　血管痉挛及其他相关血管疾病

第46章　雷诺现象 ··· 763

第47章　肢端发绀 ··· 781

第48章　红斑性肢痛症 ·· 787

第49章　冻疮 ··· 799

第十四部分　静脉血栓栓塞性疾病

第50章　静脉血栓栓塞性疾病的流行病学 ························ 809

第51章　静脉血栓栓塞性疾病的临床评估 ························ 817

第52章　静脉血栓栓塞性疾病的管理 ···························· 833

第十五部分　慢性静脉疾病

第53章　静脉曲张 ··· 853

第54章　慢性静脉功能不全 ·· 871

第十六部分　肺高压

第55章　肺动脉高压 ··· 895

第56章　非肺动脉高压性肺高压 ··································· 927

第十七部分　淋巴疾病

第57章　淋巴系统疾病 ·· 945

第十八部分　其他杂类血管疾病

第58章　纤维肌发育不良 ·· 963

第59章　血管感染 ··· 983

第60章　血管疾病的皮肤表现 ····································· 1007

第61章　下肢溃疡 ··· 1021

第62章　血管损伤 ··· 1037

第63章　各类血管压迫综合征 ····································· 1053

第64章　各类血管发育异常疾病：血管瘤和血管畸形 ·········· 1069

BRAUNWALD'S HEART DISEASE FAMILY OF BOOKS

BRAUNWALD'S HEART DISEASE COMPANIONS

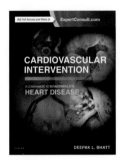

BHATT
Cardiovascular Intervention

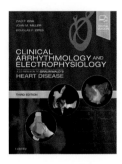

ISSA, MILLER, AND ZIPES
Clinical Arrhythmology and Electrophysiology

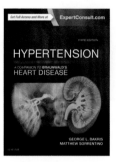

BAKRIS AND SORRENTINO
Hypertension

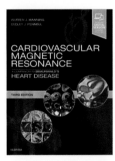

MANNING AND PENNELL
Cardiovascular Magnetic Resonance

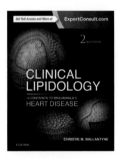

BALLANTYNE
Clinical Lipidology

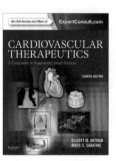

ANTMAN AND SABATINE
Cardiovascular Therapeutics

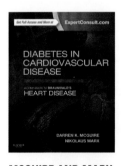

MCGUIRE AND MARX
Diabetes in Cardiovascular Disease

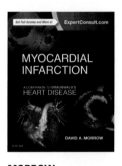

MORROW
Myocardial Infarction

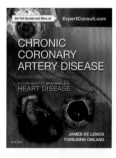

DE LEMOS AND OMLAND
Chronic Coronary Artery Disease

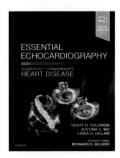

SOLOMON, WU, AND GILLAM
Essential Echocardiography

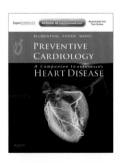

BLUMENTHAL, FOODY, AND WONG
Preventive Cardiology

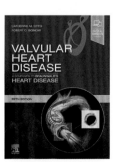

OTTO AND BONOW
Valvular Heart Disease

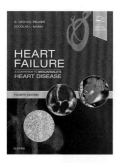

FELKER AND MANN
Heart Failure

Coming Soon
KIRKLIN
Mechanical Circulatory Support

BRAUNWALD'S HEART DISEASE REVIEW AND ASSESSMENT

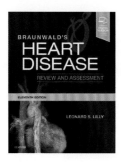

LILLY
Braunwald's Heart Disease Review and Assessment

BRAUNWALD'S HEART DISEASE IMAGING COMPANIONS

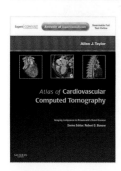

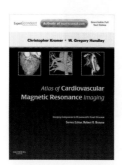

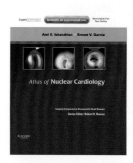

TAYLOR
Atlas of Cardiovascular Computed Tomography

KRAMER AND HUNDLEY
Atlas of Cardiovascular Magnetic Resonance Imaging

ISKANDRIAN AND GARCIA
Atlas of Nuclear Cardiology

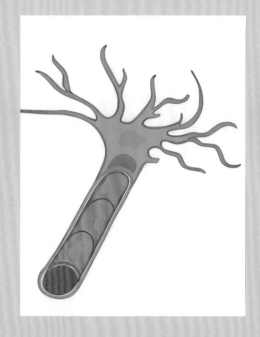

PART I

第一部分

Biology of
Blood Vessels

血管生物学

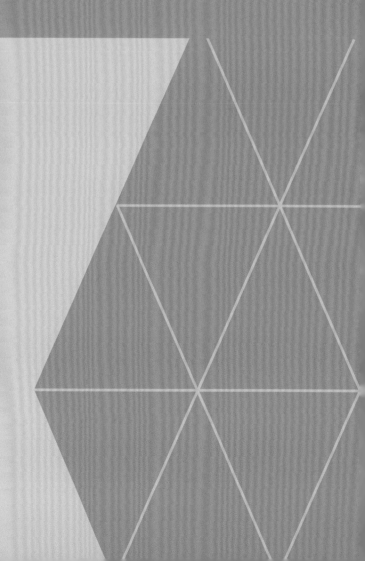

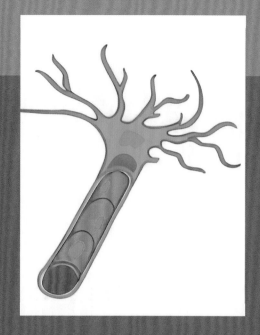

中文导读

第1章
血管胚胎学和血管新生

　　本章介绍了循环系统在胚胎形态和功能发育时期的关键分子和细胞的发育过程，并介绍了以上诸多机制中的信号转导机制。需要特别指出的是，血管内皮在血管的结构和功能上起的作用十分重要，本章就早期内皮细胞的排列、分化及与之相关的早期血管管腔的形成、分支、代谢，以及淋巴管的形成等做了详细描述。接下来介绍了血管中膜的组成，重点是中膜层的血管平滑肌细胞及其分化和功能。此后介绍了血管外膜的组成，包括血管的细胞外基质层、外膜干细胞和巨噬细胞等。了解血管各层的组成成分，生理结构，分子、细胞层面的功能和属性对于更好地理解血管疾病的发病机制，并以此为基础发现探索新的治疗方法和药物等具有至关重要的作用。

舒　畅

Vascular Embryology and Angiogenesis

Aglaia Ntokou, Inamul Kabir, Fatima Zahra Saddouk, and Daniel M. Greif

In simple terms, the cardiovascular system consists of a sophisticated pump (i.e., the heart) and a remarkable array of tubes (i.e., the blood and lymphatic vessels). Arteries and arterioles (the efferent blood vessels in relation to the heart) deliver oxygen, nutrients, paracrine hormones, blood and immune cells, and many other products to the capillaries, small-caliber, thin-walled vascular tubes. These substances are then transported through the capillary wall into the extravascular tissues, where they participate in critical physiological processes. In turn, waste products are transported from the extravascular space back into the blood capillaries and returned by the venules and veins (the afferent vessels) to the heart. Alternatively, approximately 10% of the fluid returned to the heart courses via the lymphatic system to the large veins. To develop normally, the embryo requires the delivery of nutrients and removal of waste products beginning early in development, and, indeed, the cardiovascular system functions early during morphogenesis.

The fields of vascular embryology and angiogenesis have been revolutionized through experimentation with model organisms. In particular, this chapter focuses on key studies using common vascular developmental models, including the mouse, zebrafish, chick, and chick-quail transplants, each of which has its advantages. Among mammals, the most powerful genetic-engineering tools and the greatest breadth of mutants are readily available in the mouse. Furthermore, the mouse is a good model of many aspects of human vascular development, and, in particular, the vasculature of the mouse retina is a powerful model as it develops postnatally and is visible externally. The zebrafish is a transparent organism that develops rapidly with a well-described pattern of cardiovascular morphogenesis and sophisticated genetic manipulations that are readily available. The chick egg is large with a yolk sac vasculature that is easily visualized and develops rapidly. And finally, the coupling of chick-quail transplants with species-specific antibodies allows for cell tracing experiments. The combination of studies with these powerful model systems, as well as others, has yielded key insights into human vascular embryology and angiogenesis.

Although blood vessels are composed of three tissue layers, the vast majority of the vascular-development literature has focused on the morphogenesis of the intima, or inner, layer. This intima consists of a single layer of flat endothelial cells (ECs) that line the vessel lumen and are elongated in the direction of flow. Moving radially outward, the next layer is the media consisting of layers of circumferentially oriented vascular smooth muscle cells (VSMCs) and extracellular matrix (ECM) components, including elastin and collagen. In smaller vessels, such as capillaries, the mural cells consist of pericytes instead of VSMCs.

Finally, the outermost layer of the vessel wall is the adventitia, a collection of loose connective tissue, fibroblasts, macrophages, cells expressing stem-cell markers, and small vessels, known as the vasa vasorum, that perfuse the cells of larger arteries.

This chapter summarizes many of the key molecular and cellular processes and underlying signals in the morphogenesis of the different layers of the blood vessel wall and of the circulatory system in general. Specifically, for intimal development, it concentrates on early EC patterning, specification and differentiation, lumen formation, branching, metabolism, and lymphatic vessel morphogenesis. In the second section, the development of the tunica media is divided into subsections examining the components of the media, VSMC origins, smooth muscle cell (SMC) differentiation, and patterning of the developing VSMC layers and the ECM. Finally, the chapter concludes with a succinct summary of morphogenesis of the adventitia, adventitial stem cells, and macrophages. Understanding these fundamental vascular developmental processes is important from a pathophysiological and therapeutic standpoint because many diseases almost certainly involve the recapitulation of developmental programs. For instance, in many vascular disorders, mature VSMCs dedifferentiate and exhibit increased rates of proliferation, migration, and ECM synthesis through a process termed *phenotypic switching*.[1]

TUNICA INTIMA: ENDOTHELIUM

Early Development

Development begins with the fertilization of the ovum by the sperm. Chromosomes of the ovum and sperm fuse, and then a mitotic period ensues. The early 16- to 32-cell embryo, or *morula*, consists of a sphere of cells with an inner core termed the *inner cell mass*. The first segregation of the inner cell mass generates the *hypoblast* and *epiblast*. The hypoblast gives rise to the *extraembryonic yolk sac* and the epiblast to the *amnion* and the three germ layers of the embryo, known as the *endoderm*, *mesoderm*, and *ectoderm*. The epiblast is divided into these layers in the process of gastrulation when many of the embryonic epiblast cells invaginate through the cranial-caudal primitive streak and become the mesoderm and endoderm, while the cells that remain in the embryonic epiblast become the ectoderm. Most of the cardiovascular system derives from the mesoderm, including the initial ECs, which are first observed during gastrulation. A notable exception to the mesodermal origin is the SMCs of the aortic arch and cranial vessels, which instead derive from the neural crest cells of the ectoderm.[2]

Although ECs are thought to derive exclusively from mesodermal origins, the other germ layers may play an important role in regulating the differentiation of the mesodermal cells to an EC fate. In a classic study of quail-chick intracelomic grafts, host ECs invaded limb bud grafts, whereas in internal organ grafts, EC precursors derived from the graft itself.[3] Thus the authors hypothesized that the endoderm (i.e., from internal organ grafts) stimulates the emergence of ECs from associated mesoderm, whereas the ectoderm (i.e., from the limb bud grafts) may have an inhibitory influence.[3] Yet, the endoderm does not appear to be absolutely required for the initial formation of EC precursors.[4,5]

The initial primitive vascular system is formed prior to the first cardiac contraction, and the early development of ECs involves the interplay of multiple signaling pathways.[6,7] This early vasculature develops through vasculogenesis, a two-step process in which mesodermal cells differentiate into angioblasts in situ, which, in turn, subsequently coalesce into blood vessels.[8] Early in this process, many EC progenitors apparently pass through a bipotential hemangioblast stage in which they can give rise to endothelial or hematopoietic cells. Fibroblast growth factor (FGF) 2 and bone morphogenetic protein (BMP) 4 signaling are required for mesoderm specification and its differentiation toward endothelial and hematopoietic cell fates.[7] In addition, Indian hedgehog is secreted by the yolk sac visceral endoderm during vasculogenesis and promotes the differentiation of posterior epiblast cells into both endothelial and hematopoietic cells.[9,10] The visceral endoderm also secretes vascular endothelial growth factor (VEGF), which is widely implicated in EC biology. The ligand VEGF-A signals predominantly through receptor VEGFR2, and Vegfr2-null embryos lack blood vessel islands and vasculogenesis and die in utero.[11] Importantly, most genes that specify an EC fate contain binding sites for the E-twenty-six (ETS) family of transcription factors, and ETS variant 2 regulates the differentiation of mesodermal progenitors toward an EC fate.[12,13]

Following the formation of the initial vascular plexus, more capillaries are generated through sprouting and nonsprouting angiogenesis, and the vascular system is refined through pruning and regression.[14] In the most well studied form of angiogenesis, existing blood vessels sprout new vessels, usually into areas of low perfusion, through a process involving proteolytic degradation of surrounding ECM, EC proliferation and migration, lumen formation, and EC maturation.

Nonsprouting angiogenesis is often initiated by EC proliferation, which results in lumen widening.[14] The lumen then splits through transcapillary ECM pillars or fusion and splitting of capillaries to generate more vessels.[14] In addition, the developing vascular tree is fine-tuned by the pruning of small vessels. Although not involved in the construction of the initial vascular plan, flow is an important factor in shaping the maturation of the vascular system, determining which vessels mature and which regress. For instance, unperfused vessels will regress.

Arterial and Venous Endothelial Cell Differentiation

Classically, it was thought that arterial and venous blood vessel identity was established as a result of oxygenation and hemodynamic factors, such as blood pressure, shear stress, and the direction of flow. However, over the past two decades, it has become increasingly evident that arterial-specific and venous-specific markers are segregated to the proper vessels quite early in the program of vascular morphogenesis. For instance, ephrinB2, a transmembrane ligand, and one of its receptors, the EphB4 tyrosine kinase, are expressed in the mouse embryo in an arterial-specific and relatively venous-specific manner, respectively, prior to the onset of angiogenesis (Fig. 1.1).[15–18] EphrinB2 and EphB4 are each required for normal angiogenesis of both arteries and veins.[16,17] However, in mice homozygous for a tau-lacZ knock-in into the ephrinB2 or EphB4 locus (which renders the mouse null for the gene of interest), lacZ staining is restricted to arteries or veins, respectively.[16,17] This result indicates that neither of these signaling partners is required for the arterial and venous specification of ECs.

Furthermore, even before initial ephrinB2 and EphB4 expression and prior to the first heartbeat, Notch pathway members, delta C and gridlock, mark presumptive ECs in the zebrafish.[19–21] The zebrafish gene deltaC is a homologue of the Notch ligand gene Delta, and gridlock (grl) encodes a basic helix-loop-helix protein that is a member of the Hairy-related transcription factor family and is downstream of Notch. The lateral plate mesoderm (LPM) contains artery and vein precursors,[22] and prior to vessel formation, the grl gene is expressed as two bilateral stripes in the LPM.[21] Subsequently, gridlock expression is limited to the trunk artery (dorsal aorta) and excluded from the trunk vein (cardinal vein).[21] Lineage-tracking experiments of the zebrafish LPM

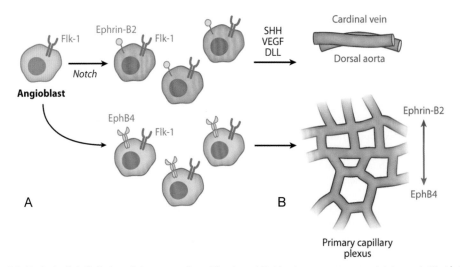

Fig. 1.1 Endothelial Cell Arterial-venous Specification. (A) Notch promotes arterial fate of Flk-1+ (i.e., VEGFR2+) angioblasts. (B) In the embryo, angioblasts aggregate directly into the dorsal aorta or cardinal vein, a process mediated by vascular endothelial growth factor *(VEGF)*, Sonic hedgehog *(SHH)*, and Notch signaling via the delta-like ligand *(DLL)*. In the yolk sac, angioblasts fuse to form the vascular plexus with expression of arterial *(Ephrin-B2)* and venous *(EphB4)* markers. (Redrawn with permission from Chung AS, Ferrara N. Developmental and pathological angiogenesis. *Annu Rev Cell Dev Biol.* 2011;27:563–584.)

suggest that by the 7- to 12-somite stage, an individual angioblast is destined to contribute in a mutually exclusive fashion to the arterial or venous system.[20]

In addition to being an early marker of arterial ECs, the Notch pathway is a key component of a signaling cascade that regulates arterial EC fate (see Fig. 1.1).[18] In zebrafish, downregulating the Notch pathway through genetic means or injection of mRNA encoding a dominant-negative Suppressor of Hairless, a known intermediary in the Notch pathway, results in reduced ephrinB2 expression with loss of regions of the dorsal aorta.[20,23] Reciprocally, contiguous regions of the cardinal vein expand and EphB4 expression increases.[20] By contrast, activation of the Notch pathway results in reduced expression of flt4, a marker of venous cell identity, without an effect on arterial marker expression or dorsal aorta size, suggesting that Notch is not sufficient to induce arterial EC fate.[20,23] Further studies demonstrated that Sonic hedgehog (SHH) is upstream of VEGF, and VEGF-A binds to VEGFR2 and its coreceptor neuropilin 1 (NRP1), leading to activation of Notch signaling.[24,25] The specific expression of NRP1 and NRP2 in arteries and veins, respectively, is established prior to blood flow.[26] Importantly, the fate of venous ECs is mediated primarily by the chicken ovalbumin upstream promoter-transcription factor II (COUP-TFII).[7] Deletion of the gene encoding COUP-TFII in ECs leads to veins expressing NRP1 and Notch signaling molecules.[27] Taken together, these results suggest that the SHH-VEGF-Notch axis is necessary for arterial EC differentiation and that venous identity is not simply a default pathway in the absence of Notch signaling but is actively maintained by COUP-TFII.

A study of the origins of the coronary vascular endothelium highlights the plasticity of ECs during early mouse development.[28] This study suggests that ECs sprout from the sinus venosus, the structure which returns blood to the embryonic heart, and dedifferentiate as they migrate over and through the myocardium.[28] ECs that invade the myocardium differentiate into the coronary arterial and capillary ECs, whereas those that remain on surface of the heart will redifferentiate into the coronary veins.[28]

Endothelial Tip and Stalk Cell Specification in Sprouting Angiogenesis

Tubular structures are essential for diverse physiological processes, and the proper construction of these tubes is critical. Tube morphogenesis requires the coordinated migration and growth of cells that comprise the tubes, and the intricate modulation of the biology of these cells invariably uses sensors that detect external stimuli.[29] This information is then integrated and translated into a biological response. Important examples of such biological sensors include the growth cones of neurons and the terminal cells of the *Drosophila* tracheal system. Both of these sensors have long dynamic filopodia that sense and respond to external guidance cues and are critical in determining the ultimate pattern of their respective tubular structures.

Similarly, endothelial tip cells are located at the end of angiogenic sprouts and are polarized with long filopodia that play both a sensory and motor role (Fig. 1.2).[29,30] In a classic study published approximately 40 years ago, Ausprunk and Folkman reported that on the day after V2 carcinoma implantation into the rabbit cornea, ECs of the host limbal vessels display surface projections that resemble "regenerating ECs,"[31] consistent with what is now classified as tip cell filopodia. Tip cells are highly migratory leading cells, are rarely proliferative, and are enriched in platelet-derived growth factor (PDGF)-B, VEGFR-2, the Notch ligand delta-like ligand 4 (DLL4), and apelin.[29,32] Proximal to tip cells are stalk cells which also express VEGFR-2 but, unlike tip cells, are highly proliferative (see Fig. 1.2).[29,32] During the initiation of sprouting angiogenesis, endothelial tip cells develop initial projections prior to stalk cell proliferation.[31]

The mouse retina model has been widely used in studies of angiogenesis and is an excellent model for studying different aspects of blood vessel development: the retinal vasculature is visible externally and develops postnatally through a stereotyped sequence of well-described steps. In addition, at most time points, the retina simultaneously includes sprouting at the vascular front and remodeling at the core. The VEGF pathway is critical for guiding angiogenic sprouts, and in the retina, the expression of the ligand VEGF-A is limited to astrocytes with the highest levels at the leading edge of the front of the extending EC plexus,[29] suggesting that the astrocytes lay down a road map for the ECs to follow.[33] VEGF-A signals through VEGFR-2 on tip and stalk cells. Interestingly, the proper distribution of VEGF-A is required for tip cell filopodia extension and tip cell migration, whereas the absolute concentration, but not the gradient, of VEGF-A appears to be critical for stalk cell proliferation.[29]

VEGF induces DLL4 expression, and Notch pathway-mediated lateral inhibition is critical for assigning ECs in sprouting angiogenesis to tip and stalk positions (Fig. 1.3).[30] DLL4 is specifically expressed in arterial and capillary ECs, and in development, DLL4 is enriched in tip cells, whereas Notch activity is greatest in stalk cells.[30,34,35] Attenuation

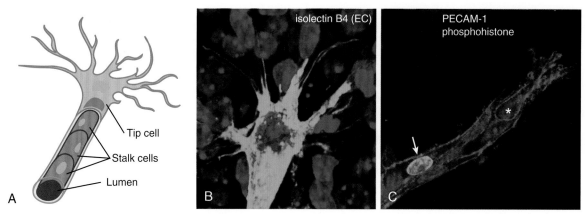

Fig. 1.2 Endothelial Tip and Stalk Cells. (A) Graphic illustration of tip and stalk cells of an endothelial sprout. (B) Endothelial tip cell with filopodia from a mouse retina stained to mark endothelial cells *(EC) (isolectin B4, green)* and nuclei *(blue)*. (C) Vascular sprout labeled with markers for ECs *(PECAM-1, red)*, mitosis *(phosphohistone, green)* and nuclei *(blue)*. Arrow indicates a mitotic stalk cell nucleus; asterisk indicates tip cell nucleus. (Redrawn with permission from Gerhardt H, Golding M, Fruttiger M, et al. VEGF guides angiogenic sprouting utilizing endothelial tip cell filopodia. *J Cell Biol.* 2003;161:1163–1177.)

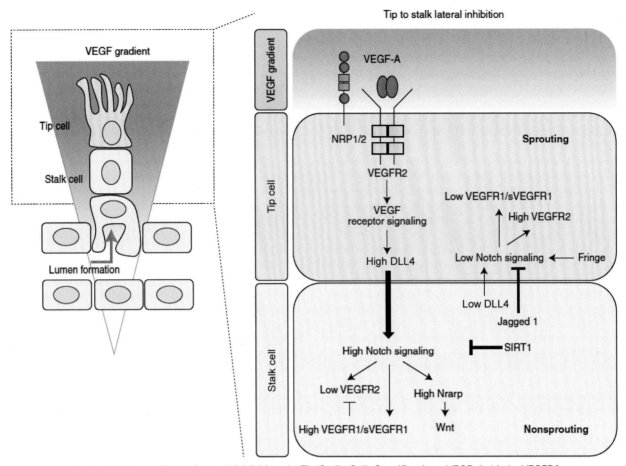

Fig. 1.3 Notch-mediated Lateral Inhibition in Tip/Stalk Cell Specification. VEGF-A binds VEGFR2, expressed at the endothelial cell surface, and neuropilin *(NRP)* modulates the VEGF signaling output. VEGF stimulation upregulates DLL4 in tip cells, which in turn, activates Notch signaling in the stalk, suppressing the tip cell phenotype. Notch signaling activation reduces VEGFR2 expression and increases levels of VEGFR1 and soluble VEGFR1 *(sVEGFR1)*, as well as that of Notch target genes (e.g., Notch-regulated ankyrin repeat protein *[Nrarp]*). In contrast, the tip cell has low Notch signaling, facilitating elevated expression of VEGFR2 and NRP but low VEGFR1. In contrast to DLL4, the Jagged1 ligand is expressed by stalk cells. Jagged1 antagonizes DLL4-Notch signaling in the sprouting front when the Notch receptor is modified by the glycosyltransferase Fringe, thereby enhancing differential Notch activity between tip and stalk cells. The duration and amplitude of the Notch signal are modulated by the histone deacetylase SIRT1. (Redrawn with permission from Blanco R, Gerhardt H. VEGF and Notch in tip and stalk cell selection. *Cold Spring Harb Perspect Med.* 2013;3:a006569.)

of Notch activity through genetic (i.e., $Dll4^{(+/-)}$) or pharmacological (i.e., γ-secretase inhibitors) approaches results in increased capillary sprouting and branching, filopodia formation, and tip cell marker expression.[30,36]

In addition to DLL4, Jagged1 is another Notch ligand that is involved in regulating tip and stalk cell fate in a related but contrasting manner. Stalk cells express higher levels of Jagged1, and Jagged1 levels are inversely proportional to the amount of EC sprouting.[30] Interestingly, Jagged1 antagonizes DLL4-Notch signaling, reducing overall EC Notch activity.[30] Thus high stalk expression of Jagged1 enhances the differential Notch activity in stalk (high activity) versus tip (low activity) cells by competitively inhibiting against DLL4-mediated Notch activity in adjacent tip cells.[30]

Mosaic analyses indicate that competition between cells (in this case for Notch activity) is critical in determining the division of labor in sprouting angiogenesis. Genetic mosaic analysis involves the mixing of at least two populations of genetically distinct cells frequently in the early embryo and, subsequently, comparing the contribution of each cell population to a specific structure or process. Notably, mosaic

analysis usually is complementary to experiments with total knockouts and often can, in fact, be more informative as complete removal of a gene may impair interpretation by grossly distorting the tissue architecture or eliminating competition between cells that harbor differing levels of a gene product.

Experiments using mosaic analysis of Notch pathway mutants in a *wild-type* background indicate that the Notch pathway acts in a cell autonomous fashion to limit the number of tip cells. In comparison to *wild-type* ECs in the mouse retina, ECs that are genetically engineered to have reduced or no *Notch1* receptor expression are enriched in the tip cell population.[34] In addition, mosaic studies of Notch signaling components in the developing zebrafish intersegmental vessels (ISVs) are informative. The ISVs traverse between the somites from the dorsal aorta to the dorsal longitudinal anastomotic vessel (DLAV) and are widely used in investigation of blood vessel development. The ISV has been classified as consisting of three (or four) cells in distinct positions: a base cell that contributes to the dorsal aortic cell, a connector cell that courses through the somites, and the most dorsal cell that contributes to the DLAV.[37,38] LPM angioblasts contribute to the ECs of all the trunk

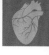

vasculature, including the dorsal aorta, posterior cardinal vein, ISVs, DLAV, and the subintestinal venous vessels. Precursors destined for the ISVs and DLAV initially migrate to the midline dorsal aorta and then between somites to their ultimate positions.[37,38] Siekmann and Lawson generated mosaic zebrafish by transplanting into early *wild-type* embryos marked cells from embryos either lacking the key Notch signaling component recombining protein suppressor of hairless (Rbpsuh) or expressing an activated form of Notch.[38] Interestingly, *rbpsuh*-deficient cells were excluded from the dorsal aorta and enriched in the DLAV position.[38] In turn, transplanted cells harboring activated Notch mutations were excluded from the DLAV in mosaics and instead preferentially localized to the base cell and dorsal aorta positions.[38]

Taken together, the findings indicate that in sprouting angiogenesis, ECs compete for the tip position through Notch-mediated lateral inhibition of neighboring cells (see Fig. 1.3).[30] High levels of DLL4 and Jagged1 are expressed on tip and stalk cells, respectively, resulting in high relative Notch activity in stalk cells and thereby promoting distinct tip and stalk cell identity. Furthermore, in the developing retina, the expression of DLL4 is regulated by VEGF-A, which is secreted by astrocytes in response to hypoxia.

Molecular Determinants of Branching

The pattern of many branched structures such as the vasculature is critical for function, and diverse branched structures use similar signaling pathways to generate their specific patterns. A number of well-studied systems, such as the *Drosophila* trachea, mammalian lung, ureteric bud (UB), and the vasculature, consist of hierarchical tubes, progressing from larger to smaller diameter, that transport important gas and/or fluid constituents. The molecular strategies underlying the morphogenesis of these patterns often includes receptor tyrosine kinase–mediated signaling, as well as fine-tuning with inhibitors of these signaling pathways.[39,40]

Similar to its key role in *Drosophila* tracheogenesis, the FGF pathway is essential for determining branch patterning in the mammalian lung. In the mouse, the trachea and lung bronchi bud from the epithelium of the gut wall at approximately E9.5,[41] and, subsequently, three distinct branching subroutines are repeated in various combinations to generate a highly stereotyped, complex treelike structure[42] that facilitates gas exchange. In early embryogenesis, the visceral mesenchyme adjacent to the heart expresses FGF10, and FGF10 binds endodermal FGFR2b.[39] *Fgf10* null mice lack lungs and have a blind trachea,[43] and similarly, *Fgfr2b*$^{(-/-)}$ mice form underdeveloped lungs that undergo apoptosis.[44] As an additional level of regulation, the inhibitor of FGFR signaling, sprouty, is a key component of an FGF-induced negative feedback loop in the lung. In response to FGF10, FGFR2b induces sprouty2 tyrosine phosphorylation and activation, and active sprouty2 inhibits signaling downstream of FGFR2b.[39] In addition, carefully regulated levels of the morphogens SHH and BMP4 modulate the branching of lung airways.[39]

As with the lung, generation of the metanephric kidney requires signals conveyed through epithelial receptor tyrosine kinase. The metanephric mesenchyme secretes glial-derived neurotrophic factor (GDNF), which activates the receptor tyrosine kinase RET and its membrane-anchored coreceptor Gdnf family receptor α 1 (GFRα1), thereby inducing the UB to evaginate from the nephric duct.[45,46] These components are required for UB branching, because UB outgrowth fails in mice null for *Gdnf*, *Gfrα1*, or *Ret*.[45] Furthermore, *Ret* is frequently mutated in humans with renal agenesis.[47] In addition, FGFR2b is also highly expressed on UB epithelium and FGFR2b-mediated signaling regulates UB branching.[39] FGF7 and FGF10 are expressed in mesenchymal tissue surrounding the UB, and FGFR2b binds with comparable affinity to these ligands.[39] Similar to lung development, BMP4-mediated signaling modulates the branching of the renal system.[39]

The most well-studied molecular determinants of vascular branching are the VEGF family of ligands (VEGF-A, -B, -C, and -D) and endothelial receptor tyrosine kinases (VEGFR1, 2, and 3).[48] VEGF is a potent EC mitogen, motogen, and vascular permeability factor, and the level of VEGF is strictly regulated in development, because VEGF heterozygous mice die at approximately E11.5 with impaired angiogenesis and blood island formation.[49,50] During embryogenesis, VEGFRs are expressed in proliferating ECs and the ligands in adjacent tissues. For instance, the secretion of VEGF by the ventricular neuroectoderm is thought to induce capillary ingrowth from the perineural vascular plexus.[51] Mice null for *Vegfr2* or *Vegfr1* die at approximately E9.0 with *Vegfr2*$^{(-/-)}$ mice lacking yolk-sac blood islands and vasculogenesis,[11] and *Vegfr1*$^{(-/-)}$ mice displaying disorganized vascular channels and blood islands.[52] Although VEGFR3 expression eventually restricts to lymphatic ECs, its broad vascular endothelial expression early in development is critical for embryonic morphogenesis. Indeed, *Vegfr3*-null mice undergo vasculogenesis and angiogenesis; however, the lumens of large vessels are defective, resulting in pericardial effusion and cardiovascular failure by E9.5.[53] Low oxygen levels induce vascular EC branching through hypoxia inducible factor-1 alpha–mediated expression of VEGFR2.[54] VEGFR1 largely functions as a negative regulator of VEGF signaling by sequestering VEGF-A. The affinity of VEGFR1 for VEGF-A is higher than that of VEGFR2, and VEGFR1 kinase domain mutants are viable.[55]

Although not as well studied as the role of the VEGF pathway in vessel branching, other signaling pathways, such as those mediated by FGF, Notch, and other guidance factors, are also likely to play important roles. For instance, EC-specific deletion of *Fgfr1* on a global *Fgfr3*-null background attenuates branching of the skin vasculature.[56] In addition, transgenic FGF expression in myocardium augmented coronary artery branching and blood flow, whereas expression of a dominant-negative FGFR1 in retinal-pigmented epithelium reduced the density and branching of retinal vessels.[39] The role of the Notch pathway is discussed earlier in the section of endothelial tip and stalk cells. Finally, the maturation of branches to a more stable state that is resistant to pruning is thought to largely be regulated by signaling pathways that modulate EC branch coverage by mural cells. Interestingly, two of the most important such pathways involve receptor tyrosine kinases such as the angiopoietin-Tie and the PDGF ligand-receptor pathways.

Vascular Lumenization

ECs at the tip of newly formed branches do not create lumens, but as the vasculature matures, formation of a lumen is an essential step in generating tubes that can transport products. Angioblasts initially migrate and coalesce to form a solid cord that is subsequently hollowed out to generate a lumen through a mechanism that is controversial. Approximately 100 years ago, researchers first suggested that vascular lumenization in the embryo occurs through an intracellular process involving vacuole formation.[57] Seventy years later, Folkman and Haudenschild developed the first method for long-term culture of ECs, and bovine or human ECs cultured in the presence of tumor-conditioned medium were shown to form lumenized tubes.[58] In this and similar in vitro approaches, an individual cell forms CDC42$^+$ pinocytic vacuoles that coalesce, extend longitudinally, and then join the vacuole of neighboring ECs to progressively generate an extended lumen.[58-60] Subsequently, a study using two-photon high-resolution time-lapse microscopy suggested that the lumens of zebrafish ISVs are generated through a similar mechanism of endothelial intracellular vacuole coalescence followed by intercellular vacuole fusion.[61]

More recently, however, a number of studies have called this intracellular vacuole coalescence model into question and, instead, support an alternate model in which the lumen is generated extracellularly.[62] One such investigation[63] suggests that in contrast to what has been thought previously,[37,38] ECs are not arranged serially along the longitudinal axis of the zebrafish ISV but, instead, overlap one another substantially; the circumference of an ISV at a given longitudinal position usually traverses multiple cells. If the lumen of a vessel were derived intracellularly in a unicellular tube, then the tube would be "seamless" (as in the terminal cells of the *Drosophila* airways)[64] and have intercellular junctions only at the proximal and distal ends of the cells. However, in the 30-hour postfertilization zebrafish, the junctional proteins zona occludens 1 (ZO-1) and VE-cadherin are coexpressed, often in two medial "stripes" along the longitudinal axis of the ISV, suggesting that ECs align and overlap along extended regions of the ISV.[63] Thus the lumen is exclusively an extracellular structure developmentally (i.e., between adjacent cells, and not within the cytoplasm of a single cell).

EC polarization is a prerequisite for lumen formation, and the Par3 complex, VE-cadherin, and microtubule dynamics play a critical role in establishing polarity.[65] Endothelial-specific deletion of the gene encoding integrin β1 reduces levels of Par3 and leads to a multilayered endothelium with cuboidal-shaped ECs and frequent occlusion of mid-sized vascular lumens.[65] VE-cadherin is a transmembrane EC-specific cell adhesion molecule that fosters homotypic interactions between neighboring ECs, and in vascular cords, VE-cadherin is distributed broadly in the apical membrane.[62] *VE-cadherin* deletion is lethal in the embryonic mouse, because the development of *VE-cadherin*[(−/−)] embryonic vessels arrests at the cord stage and does not proceed to lumenization.[62,66,67] Under normal conditions, during polarization, junctions form at the lateral regions of the apical membrane as VE-cadherin translocates to these regions, which also harbor ZO-1.[62] VE-cadherin is required for the apical accumulation of de-adhesive molecules, such as the highly glycosylated podocalyxin/gp135, which likely contributes to lumen formation through cell-cell repulsion. In addition to anchoring neighboring ECs, VE-cadherin also is linked through β-catenin, plakogobin, and α-catenin to the F-actin cytoskeleton.[62] In reparative angiogenesis of ischemic hindlimbs, the RAS homolog R-RAS activates AKT and stabilizes microtubules, augmenting lumen formation.[68] VEGF-A treatment also activates AKT but, in contrast, does not induce microtubule stabilization or lumenogenesis.[68] Mechanistically, R-RAS distributes activated AKT along microtubule fibers, all the way to the (+) end, whereas VEGF-A induces perinuclear localization of activated AKT.[68]

Although establishing polarity of the ECs is a critical step, it is not sufficient to induce lumen formation. Indeed, in *Vegfa*[(+/−)] mice, ECs of the dorsal aorta polarize but this vessel does not develop a lumen.[67] VEGF-A activates Rho-associated protein kinases (ROCKs), which induce nonmuscle myosin II light chain phosphorylation, thereby enhancing the recruitment of nonmuscle myosin to the apical membrane.[67] Actomyosin complexes at the apical surface are thought to play an important role in pulling the apical membranes of neighboring cells apart, thus generating an extracellular lumen.[65]

Another important component of the process of EC cord lumenization is the dynamic dissolution and formation of inter-EC junctions. EGFL7 is an EC-derived secreted protein that promotes EC motility and is required for tube formation.[69] The knockdown of Egfl7 in zebrafish impairs angioblasts from dissolving their junctions, thus preventing them from separating, which is required for tube formation.[69] Interestingly, the excessive cell-cell junctions in migratory angioblasts may explain the delayed migration of these cells in endodermless zebrafish.[4]

Metabolism

Although ECs line the vessel lumen and are thereby in contact with sufficient oxygen for oxidative respiration, surprisingly, up to 85% of their adenosine triphosphate (ATP) is generated from glycolysis.[70] Of note, ECs have a low mitochondrial content, and when glucose is unlimited, high glycolytic flux can produce more ATP than oxidative metabolism in a shorter time, which is critical for rapid EC sprouting.[71] Furthermore, VEGF enhances the kinetics of glycolysis by increasing levels of phosphofructokinase-2/fructose-2,6-bisphosphatase3 (PFKFB3).[70] PFKFB3 catalyzes the synthesis of fructose-2-6-bisphosphate, which, in turn, allosterically activates 6-phosphofructo-1-kinase, a rate-limiting glycolytic enzyme. EC expression of another key glycolytic enzyme, hexokinase, is regulated by FGF-mediated signaling, and EC deletion of this enzyme impairs lymphatic EC branching and migration.[56] In addition to the rapid kinetics, anaerobic glycolysis has other potential advantages for ECs, including preserving oxygen levels for transfer to perivascular cells and priming ECs for growth into hypoxic regions.[71]

The enzyme PFKFB3 is essential for tip EC phenotype. Lamellipodia are thin structures which lack mitochondria, whereas PFKFB3 is present in membrane ruffles of lamellipodia in migrating ECs.[70] Silencing of Pfkfb3 in ECs diminishes proliferation, lamellipodia formation, sprouting, and directional migration.[70] Moreover, tamoxifen-induced neonatal *VE-cadherin-CreER*[T2], *Pfkfb3*[(flox/flox)] mice have impaired retinal vascularization.[70] The importance of this pathway is emphasized by studies with both EC spheroids and zebrafish, indicating that PFKB3 trumps Notch activity in regard to specifying tip cell fate.[70]

In addition to glycolysis, fatty acid oxidation (FAO) is another metabolic process that is critical for angiogenesis. A key enzyme controlling FAO rates is carnitine palmitoyltransferase 1 (CPT1), which imports fatty acids (FAs) into the mitochondria, where they are oxidized to acetyl coenzyme A for the Krebs cycle.[72] CPT1a is essential for EC proliferation and thus sprouting, but not for EC migration.[72] FA-derived carbons are incorporated into aspartate (a nucleotide precursor), uridine monophosphate (a precursor of pyrimidine nucleoside triphosphate), and DNA, and EC silencing of CPT1a depletes stores of aspartate and deoxyribonucleoside trisphosphates.[72] This DNA synthesis through FAO is a specialized characteristic of ECs and fibroblasts.[72]

Lymphatic Vessel Development

Complementing the veins, the lymphatic system plays a critical role in transporting lymph (i.e., fluid, macromolecules, and cells) from the interstitial space to the subclavian veins and thereby back to heart. Lymphatic capillaries are highly permeable by virtue of their structure: a single layer of discontinuous lymphatic endothelial cells (LECs) without mural cells or basement membrane. Lymph drains from lymphatic capillaries into precollector vessels and then into collecting lymphatic vessels, which have valves, continuous inter-EC junctions, basement membrane, and an SMC layer. These collecting vessels drain into the right lymphatic trunk or thoracic duct and then into the right or left subclavian vein, respectively.

Based on her experiments more than 100 years ago, Florence Sabin proposed the "centrifugal model" in which lymphatic sacs derive from veins, and vessels sprouting from these sacs give rise to the lymphatic vasculature.[73,74] Subsequently, histological, marker, and lineage studies yielded findings supportive of Sabin's model.[75] The homeobox transcription factor SOX18 (sex determining region Y box 18) is a molecular switch that turns on the differentiation of venous ECs to a lymphatic EC fate,[76] and mutations in *SOX18* underlie lymphatic abnormalities in the human disorder hypotrichosis lymphedema telangectasia.[77] SOX18 induces expression of a number of lymphatic markers, including the homeobox gene *Prox1*,[76] which is absolutely required to initiate lymphatic vessel morphogenesis.[75] Lymphatic development begins in the lateral parts of the cardinal veins with EC expression of *Sox18*, followed by *Prox1* expression, and subsequently these SOX18+PROX1+ ECs sprout laterally and form lymph sacs.[75] The peripheral lymphatic vasculature then results from centrifugal sprouting from the lymph sacs and remodeling of the LEC capillary plexus. Interestingly, the venous identity of lymphatic precursors is critical, because deletion of the gene encoding COUP-TFII in ECs results in arterialization of veins and inhibition of LEC specification of cardinal vein ECs.[27,78]

Although PROX1 is critical for formation of the lymphatic vasculature, the regulation of PROX1 expression in LECs remains elusive. The zinc finger transcription factor GATA2 binds a *Prox1* enhancer element, but it is not required for the onset of PROX1 expression or specification and early migration of LEC progenitors.[79] Yet, GATA2 does play an essential role in lymphovenous valve development and separation of the blood and lymphatic vasculatures.[79] Ablation of *Gata2* with Prox1-CreER[T2] confirms that GATA2 is pivotal for the initiation of lymphatic valve development and in adults for lymphatic vessel structure and transport.[79] Histone acetyltransferase 3 (HDAC3) regulates GATA2 expression epigenetically, and EC-specific *Hdac3* deletion mimics the phenotype of mice lacking *Gata2* in ECs.[79,80]

TUNICA MEDIA: SMOOTH MUSCLE AND EXTRACELLULAR MATRIX

Cellular and Extracellular Matrix Components

In large- and medium-sized vessels, radially outward from the EC layer is the tunica media consisting of VSMCs and ECM components including elastin and collagen. The dynamic contraction and relaxation of VSMCs allows for the tone of the blood vessel to be adjusted to the physiological demands of the relevant tissue and to maintain blood pressure and perfusion. Collagen provides strength to the vessel wall, and elastin is largely responsible for its elasticity such that upon receiving the cardiac output in systole, the arterial wall stretches to increase the lumen volume, and subsequently, in diastole, it recoils to help maintain blood pressure. The capillary wall is substantially thinner than that of larger vessels, thus facilitating the transfer of substances to and from the vascular compartment. Capillary mural cells consist of pericytes instead of VSMCs. Pericytes, VSMCs, and the ECM play critical roles in many vascular diseases; however, there are strikingly few studies of the development of these components in comparison with the vast number of investigations of the morphogenesis of EC networks and tubes.

Although differences exist between pericytes and VSMCs, these mural cell types are generally considered to exist along a continuum and lack firm distinctions.[81] Pericytes are imbedded in the basement membrane of capillary ECs and thus may be characterized as having an intimal location, whereas VSMCs are separated from the basement membrane in the media. VSMCs are oriented circumferentially around the vessel, whereas pericytes have an irregular orientation with elongated cytoplasmic processes contacting multiple ECs.[82,83]

VSMCs regulate vascular tone and blood flow distribution, whereas pericytes have diverse functions including intercellular communication, microvessel structure, phagocytosis, and perhaps vasoconstriction.[84] In the brain, pericytes play important roles in the formation and maintenance of the blood-brain barrier,[85–87] and their involvement in the regulation of blood flow has recently become controversial. Hall et al.[88] suggest that in response to neuronal activity, brain pericytes induce capillary dilation and increase blood flow, whereas a study by Hill et al.[89] indicates that cerebral blood flow is regulated predominantly by arteriole SMCs expressing α-smooth muscle actin (αSMA) but not by pericytes that express platelet-derived growth factor receptor

(PDGFR)-β, neuron glial 2 (NG2), and not αSMA. The controversy largely stems from a simple question: what is a pericyte?[90] However, the field continues to struggle to define this cell type, and molecular markers of pericytes and SMCs are overlapping. The commonly used markers of pericytes include PDGFR-β, NG2, CD13, desmin, and vimentin.[84] A study by Betsholtz's group using RNA sequencing identified a new set of genes to study in pericytes and validated pericyte-enriched expression of two genes of this set, *vitronectin* and *interferon-induced transmembrane protein1*.[91] VSMC markers include αSMA, transgelin (SM22α), calponin, and the more specific markers smooth muscle myosin heavy chain (SMMHC) and smoothelin.[1]

Vascular Smooth Muscle Cell Origins

The origins of VSMCs are diverse and differ among blood vessels and even within specific regions of individual blood vessels. Neural crest cells of the ectoderm give rise to SMCs of the cranial vessels, aorticopulmonary septum, and the proximal aorta from the root to the subclavian artery (Fig. 1.4).[2,92,93] The inner layers (on the luminal side) of the ascending aortic media derive from neural crest cells, and on the dorsal aspect of the ascending aorta, neural crest cells also contribute to SMCs in the outer layers of the media (on the adventitial side).[92] Second heart field cells give rise to aortic SMCs from the root to the innominate artery and in the ascending aorta are limited to the outer layers.[92,94]

SMCs of the descending aorta originate from the mesoderm.[2] Using HoxB6-Cre to mark cells derived from the LPM, Wasteson and colleagues suggest that these cells are the source of descending aortic ECs and that the ventral wall of the descending aorta is temporarily inhabited at E9.5 for approximately 1 day with early SMCs that derive from the LPM.[95] Subsequently, Meox1-Cre, which labels cells derived from both the presomitic paraxial mesoderm and the somites, marks SMCs that replace the LPM-derived aortic wall cells.[95] Thus, in the adult descending aorta, ECs and SMCs derive from distinct mesodermal populations, the LPM and the presomitic/somitic mesoderm, respectively. Importantly, a distinct study previously showed that aortic SMCs share a lineage with paraxial mesoderm-derived skeletal muscle cells.[96] Finally, Topouzis and Majesky suggest that the lineage of SMC populations has important functional implications.[97] In response to transforming growth factor (TGF)-β stimulation, ectodermally derived E14 chick-embryo aortic-arch SMCs increase DNA synthesis, whereas the growth of mesodermally derived abdominal aortic SMCs was inhibited.[97]

Coronary artery SMCs are critical players in atherosclerotic heart disease, and there have been significant investigations into their origin from the proepicardium/epicardium. The proepicardium is a transient tissue that forms on the pericardial surface of the septum transversum in the E9.5 mouse and, through a fascinating process, gives rise to epicardial cells that migrate as a mesothelial sheet over the myocardium. Signals emanating from the myocardial cells induce epithelial-to-mesenchymal transition in which some epicardial cells lose their cell-cell adhesion and invade the myocardium. Furthermore, lineage labeling has illustrated that the proepicardium and epicardium contribute to the coronary artery SMC lineage.[98,99] Recently, based on the results of lineage tracing and clonal analyses, it was suggested that developing coronary artery SMCs, at least partly, come from epicardial-derived NG2+ pericytes via a Notch3-dependent process.[100]

Related to these studies of the coronary artery, investigations of other organs suggest that the mesothelium could more generally be an important source of VSMCs. For instance, MSLN is a membrane glycoprotein expressed on the mesothelium, and a recent study found through lineage tracing with a Msln-Cre that the mesothelium contributes to SMCs of the trunk vasculature.[101] Previously, Wilm et al. showed

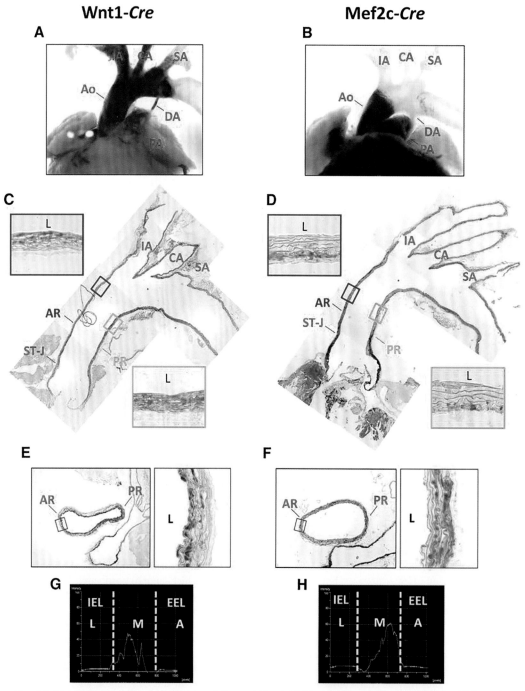

Fig. 1.4 Distribution of Neural Crest– and Second Heart Field–derived Cells in the Proximal Thoracic Aorta. Representative ventral views of β-galactosidase (β-gal) activity in proximal thoracic aortas from *Wnt1-Cre* (A) and *Mef2c-Cre* (B) mice in tissues acquired at 12 weeks of age, $n = 3$ to 4 for each group. Representative images of β-gal activity and eosin staining from sagittal sections of the aortic root and arch in *Wnt1-* (C) and *Mef2c-Cre* (D) male mice, $n = 3$ for each group. Magnified images were taken from the anterior *(blue box)* and posterior region *(green box)*. Cross-sections of mid-ascending aortas from *Wnt1-Cre* (E) and *Mef2c-Cre* (F) mice were stained with X-gal and eosin B, $n = 3$ for each group. Magnified images were taken from the anterior region *(blue box)*. Representative histograms measured β-gal activity from internal to external elastic lamina in the anterior region of ascending aortas from *Wnt1-Cre* (G) and *Mef2c-Cre* (H) mice, $n = 3$ for each group. Blue color is positive staining for distribution of Cre excision. Yellow dotted lines depict location of IEL and EEL. *A*, Adventitia; *Ao*, aorta; *AR*, anterior region; *CA*, common carotid artery; *DA*, ductus arteriosus; *EEL*, external elastin lamina; *IA*, innominate artery; *IEL*, internal elastin lamina; *L*, lumen; *LV*, left ventricle; *M*, media; *PA*, pulmonary artery; *PR*, posterior region; *SA*, subclavian artery; *ST-J*, sinotubular junction. (From Sawada H, Rateri DL, Moorleghen JJ, et al. Smooth muscle cells derived from second heart field and cardiac neural crest reside in spatially distinct domains in the media of the ascending aorta-brief report. *Arterioscler Thromb Vasc Biol* 2017;37:1722–1726.)

that expression of the Wt1 protein in the developing gut is limited to the serosal mesothelium, and a Wt1-Cre yeast artificial chromosome (YAC) transgene marked a lineage of cells that includes the SMCs of the major mesenteric blood vessels.[102]

The etiology of pulmonary artery SMCs is controversial. Using the Wt1-Cre YAC transgene and a panel of Cre reporters, the mesothelium of the lung was implicated as the source of approximately one-third of all pulmonary vascular cells expressing αSMA[103]; however, Morimoto et al. subsequently reported that embryos carrying the same Wt1-Cre YAC transgene and a ROSA26R-YFP Cre reporter have only rare YFP+ lung VSMCs.[104] Furthermore, using the Tie1-Cre, these authors suggested that most SMCs of the proximal pulmonary arteries arise from ECs.[104] Transdifferentiation of ECs into VSMCs has been raised in developmental and disease contexts.[105–108] For instance, embryonic stem cell–derived Flk1+ cells have the potential to differentiate into ECs or mural cells.[107] However, our results with the VE-cadherin-Cre[109] and mTomato/mGFP Cre reporter[110] indicated that ECs are not a significant source of the E18.5 pulmonary arterial SMCs, and additional experiments demonstrated that, instead, these cells largely derive from the local mesenchyme.[111] Studies by another group of *ROSA26R-tdTomato* mice also carrying *Gli-CreER^T2*, *Axin2-CreER^T2*, or *Acta2-CreER^T2*, induced with tamoxifen at E11.5 and analyzed 7 days later, suggest that GLI+ and AXIN2+ mesenchymal cells are a major, but not specific, pool of progenitors for lung vascular SMCs; however, SMA+ cells do not give rise to many distal vascular SMCs. Thus VSMCs in the lung predominantly derive from αSMA- lung mesenchyme that differentiate locally.

Smooth Muscle Cell Differentiation

A critical component of characterizing the morphogenesis of any tissue (e.g., vascular smooth muscle) is defining morphologic and molecular criteria which constitute the differentiated phenotype of specific cell types (e.g., VSMCs) that comprise the tissue. Early undifferentiated cells that are presumed to be destined to the VSMC fate have prominent endoplasmic reticulum and Golgi, a euchromatic nucleus and lack a distinctly filamentous cytoplasm.[112] In contrast, mature VSMCs have a heterochromatic nucleus, myofilaments, and decreased synthetic organelles.[112] In addition to these morphological changes, the differentiation of SMCs is marked by the expression of a number of contractile and cytoskeletal proteins. αSMA is the most abundant protein of SMCs, comprising 40% of the total protein in a differentiated SMC.[113] αSMA is an early marker of SMCs but is not specific, because it is expressed in skeletal muscle and a variety of other cell types, and is temporarily expressed in cardiac muscle during development.[113,114] The actin- and tropomyosin-binding protein SM22α is another early marker of SMCs and a more specific marker of adult SMCs; however, it also is expressed in the other muscle types during development.[114] The two isoforms of SMMHC are expressed slightly later during development than αSMA and SM22α, and in contrast to these other markers, SMMHC expression is ostensibly limited to the SMC lineage.[115] Smoothelin is another cytoskeletal protein that is also specific for SMCs but is not expressed until very late in the differentiation process when the cells are part of a contractile tissue.[116]

Studies of VSMCs in development or in mature blood vessels are challenging because these cells can assume a variety of phenotypes depending on their environment.[113] During the early stages of blood vessel development, many VSMCs rapidly proliferate, migrate substantial distances, and synthesize large amounts of ECM components. In contrast, more mature VSMCs are predominantly sedentary and nonproliferative and express contractile proteins but do not generate significant ECM. However, the distinctions between these synthetic and contractile states are not always firm. In contrast to cardiac and skeletal muscle, VSMCs in adults are not terminally differentiated, and thus, in

many vascular diseases, extracellular cues are implicated in inducing VSMCs to assume a dedifferentiated state through a process termed *phenotypic switching*.[117]

Tremendous efforts and advances have been made by numerous laboratories to elucidate the molecular mechanisms regulating phenotypic modulation, and the model that has emerged depends on combinatorial interactions of multiple factors that are either ubiquitously expressed or selective for smooth muscle (Fig. 1.5).[1] The most well-characterized underlying regulatory paradigm is the CArG-serum response factor (SRF)-dependent system. Expression of almost all smooth muscle contractile and cytoskeletal genes is modulated by the ubiquitous transcription factor SRF. SRF binds the 10-base-pair DNA consensus sequence $CC(A/T)_6GG$ known as the CArG box (i.e., C, AT rich, G box), which is found in the regulatory regions of virtually all smooth muscle genes. In fact, for most SMC genes, there are at least two CArG boxes. However, the CArG box sequence is also found within the 23-base-pair serum response enhancer element of early growth response genes. Because SRF is ubiquitous and the cis-regulatory CArG element is present in both growth and differentiation genes, a higher order of control is required to determine which of these disparate gene sets are expressed in a specific cell at a given time point.

Control of expression of contractile and cytoskeletal SMC genes is regulated through a competition for SRF between the transcriptional coactivator myocardin and ternary complex factors.[118] Myocardin is a master regulator of SMC differentiation, because ectopic expression of this factor in nonmuscle cells is sufficient to induce activation of the SMC differentiation gene program.[119] In addition, murine embryos null for *myocardin* lack VSMC differentiation and die at midgestation.[120] Many studies have focused on factors that counterbalance the effect of myocardin to promote dedifferentiation, including Kruppel-like factor 4 (KLF4),[121] E26 ETS-like transcription factor 1 (ELK-1),[118] and FOXO4.[122]

In addition, short and long noncoding RNA (lncRNA) genes modulate SMC phenotype.[123] Cordes et al. showed that expression of miR-143 and miR-145 is restricted to cardiac and SMCs and that these miRs target Klf4, Elk-1, and myocardin transcripts, inhibiting their expression.[124] The miR-143/145 gene cluster is a direct transcriptional target of SRF, myocardin, and NKX2-5, suggesting a positive feedback loop mechanism to maintain the differentiated SMC phenotype.[124,125] Beyond miR-143/145, additional miRNAs are implicated in the control of SMC differentiation state including miR-21,[126] miR-24,[127] miR-26a,[128] and miR-133a.[129] Emerging evidence points to the importance of lncRNAs, such as the SMC-specific MYOSLID,[130] as novel SMC regulators.[123] The expression of MYOSLID is transcriptionally regulated by SRF-myocardin and promotes SMC differentiation through a mechanism that may involve modulating the TGF-β pathway.[130]

Studies have emerged investigating the role of epigenetics in transcriptional regulation of SMC plasticity.[131,132] Epigenetics refers to mechanisms that regulate heritable changes in gene expression without altering DNA sequence but rather modifying DNA bases by methylation and hydroxymethylation, as well as posttranslational modifications of histones. Epigenetic regulation of chromatin structure of CArG-containing regions in SMC genes is critical for modulating SMC differentiation state. For instance, the histone modification H3K4me2 is enriched on SMC marker genes *Myh11*, *Acta2,* and *Tagln* in mature SMCs and progenitor cells committed to differentiate into SMCs.[1] Furthermore, the H3K4me2 mark persists through SMC phenotype modulation, and H3K4me2 at the *Myh11* locus is restricted to the SMC lineage.[131] This result is of major significance, because it has been used as a method for identifying whether SMC marker-cells in human tissues derive from cells that previously expressed SMC markers.[131,133] In addition to histone methylation, studies by Kathleen Martin and

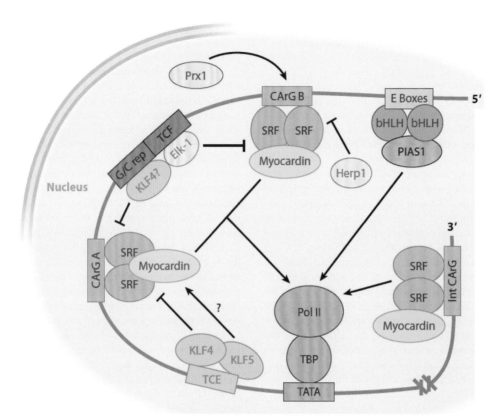

Fig. 1.5 Complex Interactions of Multiple Conserved *cis*-Regulatory Elements and Transcription Factors Govern Expression of Smooth Muscle–Enriched Genes. Myocardin promotes interactions of serum response factor *(SRF)* with CArG boxes within the promoters of SMC contractile and cytoskeletal genes to induce the recruitment of RNA polymerase II *(Pol II)* and drive expression of these genes. Additional factors support myocardin-SRF-CArG interactions and drive SMC gene expression, including paired-related homeobox gene 1 *(Prx1)* and complexes of the protein inhibitor of activated Stat1 *(PIAS1)* with basic helix-loop-helix *(bHLH)* factors at E-box cis-regulatory elements. In contrast, transcription factors such as Kruppel-like factors *(KLFs)*, E26 ETS-like transcription factor 1 *(Elk-1)*, and HES-related repressor protein 1 *(Herp1)* repress SMC gene expression, at least in part by disrupting myocardin-SRF-CArG interactions. Elk-1 binds to ternary complex factor *(TCF)* sites, whereas KLFs bind to TGFβ control elements *(TCEs)*. *TBP,* TATA binding protein. (Redrawn with permission from Alexander MR, Owens GK. Epigenetic control of smooth muscle cell differentiation and phenotypic switching in vascular development and disease. *Annu Rev Physiol.* 2012;74:13–40.)

colleagues[134] provide evidence that mature SMCs are enriched in ten-eleven translocation-2 (TET2), a member of a family of DNA demethylases that converts 5-methylcytosine to 5-hydroxymethylcytosine (5-hmc), resulting in DNA demethylation and gene activation. TET2 induces SMC differentiation and binds to CArG-rich regions of *Myocd* (encoding myocardin), *Srf*, and *Myh11*, and its product 5-hmC is enriched in these regions.[134]

Beyond dedifferentiating, VSMCs undergoing phenotypic switching can also acquire characteristics of other distinct cell types. In cultured SMCs, cholesterol loading induces downregulation of SMC markers and upregulation of macrophage markers.[135,136] Seminal in vivo fate mapping studies in the *Apoe*[(−/−)] atherosclerosis mouse model indicate that most smooth muscle–derived cells lose their classical SMC markers in plaques and many adopt phenotypic characteristics of other cell types, including macrophages and mesenchymal stem cells.[133,137]

Patterning of the Developing Vascular Smooth Muscle Cells Layers

Although a number of recent investigations describe the molecular mechanisms regulating SMC differentiation, there are relatively few studies of the patterning of the morphogenesis of SMC layers of a developing blood vessel.[112] Consequently, little is known about the

recruitment of SMCs and/or their precursors to the vascular wall, the investment of these cells around the nascent EC tube, and the pattern of differentiation of VSMC precursors within or in proximity to the vascular wall. Limited relevant studies have mostly focused on the histology and αSMA expression in the developing aortic wall. Early in development, the dorsal aortae exist as parallel tubes that subsequently fuse to generate the single descending aorta. The early EC tube is surrounded by loose undifferentiated mesenchymal cells, and as the aorta matures, the expression of αSMA proceeds in a cranial to caudal direction.[138,139] Within a cross-section of the descending aorta, the location of initial mesenchymal cell consolidation and αSMA expression depends on the cranial-caudal position: proximally these processes initially occur on the dorsal aspect of the aorta, whereas more distally they are first noted on the ventral side.[138,139] Studies published 45 years ago indicate that within the chick aortic media, the outer layers mature initially with condensation and elongation of early presumptive SMCs and accumulation of elastic tissue.[140,141] In contrast, in rodent or quail aortas, cells immediately adjacent to the EC layer are the first to consolidate and express SMC markers; subsequently, additional layers of SMCs are added.[138,139,142,143]

We conducted a meticulous investigation of murine pulmonary artery morphogenesis and found that the medial and adventitial wall of this vessel is constructed radially from inside out, by sequential induction and recruitment of successive layers.[111] The inner layer undergoes a series of morphological and molecular transitions that lasts approximately 3 days to build a relatively mature SMC layer. After this process commences in the first layer, the next layer initiates and completes a similar process. Finally, this developmental program arrests midway through the construction of the outer layer to generate a relatively "undifferentiated" adventitial cell layer.[111]

This inside-outside radial patterning is likely to involve an EC-derived signal and result from one or more potential mechanisms. For instance, in the morphogen gradient model,[144] an EC-derived signal diffuses through the media and adventitia and, depending on discrete concentration thresholds, induces responses in the cells of these compartments, such as changes in morphology, gene expression, and/or proliferation. Alternatively, in the relay mechanism,[145] a short-range or plasma membrane–bound EC signal induces adjacent cells, which, in turn, propagate the signal through either secreting a morphogen or inducing their neighbors and so on (i.e., "the bucket brigade model"). Such a bucket brigade mediated by Jagged1 on SMCs is implicated in regulating ductus arteriosus closure.[146] Finally, our results suggest a third mechanism, which we have termed "the conveyer belt model," in which some of the progeny of inner layer SMCs migrate radially outward to contribute to the next layer(s) of SMCs.[111]

A number of signaling pathways involving an EC-derived signal and mesenchymal receptors have been implicated in vascular wall morphogenesis.[147] The PDGF pathway is perhaps the most well-studied pathway in vascular mural cell development with a ligand that is expressed in ECs (PDGF-B) and receptors that are expressed in undifferentiated mesenchyme (PDGFR-α and -β) and pericytes (PDGFR-β). Mice null for *Pdgfb* or *Pdgfrb* have reduced SMC coverage of medium-sized arteries and reduced pericytes which results in microvascular hemorrhages and perinatal lethality.[148–151] In addition, when cocultured with ECs, undifferentiated embryonic mesenchymal 10T1/2 cells are induced to express SMC markers and elongate in a TGF-β–dependent manner.[152] Similar changes are also induced by directly treating 10T1/2 cells with TGF-β1.[152] Furthermore, the Notch pathway plays important roles in arterial SMC differentiation in vivo, and EC-derived Jagged1 is required for normal aortic and yolk sac vessel SMC differentiation.[153] In human adults, the receptor NOTCH3 is specifically expressed in arterial SMCs, and, at birth, blood vessels of *Notch3*-null mice and of *wild-type* mice are indistinguishable.[154,155] However, Notch3 is required for the postnatal maturation of the tunica media of small vessels in mice.[154] Furthermore, *NOTCH3* mutations in humans cause CADASIL (cerebral autosomal dominant arteriopathy with stroke and dementia) syndrome, characterized clinically by adult-onset recurrent subcortical ischemic strokes and vascular dementia, and pathologically by degeneration and eventual loss of VSMCs.[155,156] Finally, it is important to note that other signaling pathways, such as those mediated by angiopoietin-Tie and sphingosine-1-phosphate ligand-receptor pairs, do not involve an EC-derived ligand and/or mesenchymal receptors but play important roles in SMC development.[147]

Extracellular Matrix: Collagen and Elastic Fibers

In addition to maturation of the cellular constituents of the blood vessel wall, proper formation of the ECM is also critical for vascular function. Gene expression profiling of the developing mouse aorta demonstrates dynamic expression of most structural matrix proteins: an initial major increase of expression at E14 is often followed by a brief decrease at postnatal day 0 (P0), then a steady rise for approximately 2 weeks, and finally a decline to low levels at 2 to 3 months that persist into adulthood.[157,158] Fibrillar collagens, elastin, and most of the structural matrix proteins of the vascular wall follow this pattern. A similar pattern

for expression of structural matrix components has been documented in other animals and in humans.[159] SMCs are thought to secrete most of the elastin and collagens in the tunica media.[160]

The mechanical strength and viscoelastic properties of the aortic wall result from fibrillar collagens, elastic fibers, and associated proteins. In a healthy aorta, these molecules form a scaffolding allowing the aorta to withstand the pulsatile flow and high pressure of blood delivered by the heart. Collagen fibers have high tensile strength and bear most of the stressing forces at or above physiological blood pressures, shielding SMCs from excessive stress.[158,161] Seventeen different collagen types have been identified in the developing murine aortic wall with collagens I, III, IV, V, and VI having the highest expression.[158] Deletions and/or mutations in a number of collagens results in vascular phenotypes; for instance, *COLLAGEN3A1* mutations in humans are responsible for Ehlers-Danlos syndrome type IV, with vascular manifestations that include vessel fragility and large-vessel aneurysm and rupture.[158]

In contrast to collagen, elastin has low tensile strength, is distensible, and distributes stress throughout the wall, including onto the collagen fibers.[158] Elastin is the major protein of the arterial wall, composing up to 50% of the dry weight of the aorta.[162] VSMCs secrete tropoelastin monomers that undergo posttranslational modifications and cross-linking, and are organized into circumferential elastic lamellae in the tunica media.[160] These elastic lamellae alternate with rings of VSMCs to form lamellar units. $Eln^{(+/-)}$ mice have a normal life span despite being hypertensive and having a 50% reduction in elastin mRNA.[163,164] In comparison with *wild type*, the $Eln^{(+/-)}$ aorta has thinner elastic lamellae but a 35% increase in the number of lamellar units, which results in a similar tension per lamellar unit.[164,165] More dramatically, humans hemizygous for the *ELN* null mutant have a 2.5-fold increase in lamellar units and suffer an obstructive arterial disease, supravalvular aortic stenosis.[164] Similarly, at the end of gestation in the mouse, cells that are located subendothelium in $Eln^{(-/-)}$ arteries are hyperproliferative, resulting in increased number of αSMA+ cells and reduced luminal diameter, with lethality by approximately P4.5.[166] We recently reported that integrin β3 expression and activation are increased in the aortic media of $Eln^{(-/-)}$ mice.[167] Moreover, genetic or pharmacological inhibition of integrin β3 in elastin-null mice attenuates aortic SMC misalignment, hyperproliferation, and stenosis, suggesting inhibition of integrin β3–mediated signaling is a potential therapeutic strategy for supraventricular aortic stenosis patients (Fig. 1.6).[167]

Finally, *microfibrils* are fibrous structures that are intimately associated with elastic fibers surrounding the elastin core. Fibrillin1 is the major structural component of microfibrils, and its temporal pattern of expression during aortic development is similar to that of most structural proteins, such as elastin, except the peak expression of fibrillin1 occurs at P0.[157] In contrast, fibrillin2 expression is highest in the early embryonic period and then decreases linearly throughout maturation.[157] Mutations in the human *FBN1* gene result in Marfan syndrome, with vascular manifestations that include aortic root aneurysm and dissection.[168]

TUNICA ADVENTITIA

Components of the Adventitia

Owing to a paucity of studies, little is known about the development of the outer layer of blood vessels, which is referred to as the tunica adventitia or tunica externa. The tunica externa is composed of loose connective tissue (mostly collagen), and the cellular constituents include the fibroblast, which is the predominant cell type, as well as stem cell marker–positive cells and macrophages. Diffusion

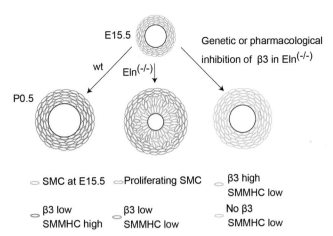

Fig. 1.6 The Effects of Integrin β3 Inhibition in Elastin-Null Mice. After E15.5, the pathology of the elastin-null aorta develops as characterized by subendothelial smooth muscle cells *(SMC)* that have increased integrin β3 levels and are misaligned (radially elongated). In addition, smooth muscle myosin heavy chain *(SMMHC)* expression is reduced, whereas SMC proliferation and radial migration are increased, resulting in hypermuscularization. Genetic or pharmacological inhibition of integrin β3 attenuates most of this pathobiology. (Redrawn with permission from Mazurek R, Dave JM, Chandran RR, et al. Vascular cells in blood vessel wall development and disease. *Adv Pharmacol.* 2017;78:323–350.)

of nutrients from the lumen to the adventitia and outer media is inadequate in larger vessels, and hence the adventitia of these vessels also includes small arteries, known as the vasa vasorum, which supply a capillary network extending through the adventitia and into the media. The adventitia of coronary vessels is thought to arise from the epicardium based on experiments with quail-chick transplants.[169] Quail epicardial cells grafted into the pericardial space of the E2 chick undergo epithelial-to-mesenchymal transition and contribute to both coronary vascular SMCs (consistent with the findings discussed previously in the section above on tunica media, VSMC origin) and coronary perivascular fibroblasts.[169] Our results suggest that adventitial cells of the pulmonary artery derive from PDGFR-β⁺ undifferentiated mesenchymal cells.[111]

Adventitial Cells Expressing Stem Cell Markers

More recently, a number of studies have investigated a population of adventitial cells expressing stem cell markers (e.g., SCA1, CD34). These investigations are largely a result of a paradigm shift: classically, the adventitia was considered a passive supportive tissue; however, adventitial fibroblast and progenitor cells are now implicated in playing important roles in neointimal formation during vascular disease.[170,171] A population of cells expressing CD34 but not expressing markers of other cell types including ECs (CD31) and leukocytes (CD45) reside in the adventitia of stromal vessels of human white adipose tissue and express mesenchymal stem cell markers.[172] When isolated, these cells give rise to clonogenic multipotent progenitor cells in culture, as do standard bone marrow–derived mesenchymal stem cells.[172] In human internal thoracic arteries, a niche for CD34⁺CD31⁻ cells has been identified at the interface between the media and adventitia of human internal thoracic arteries.[173]

SHH is expressed in this vascular "stem cell" niche of medium- and large-sized arteries of the perinatal mouse.[174] *Patched-1 (Ptc1)* and *Patched-2 (Ptc2)* are SHH target genes, and their gene products are SHH receptors. β-Galactosidase staining in SHH reporter mice, *Ptc1^lacZ* or *Ptc2^lacZ*, suggests that SHH signaling is active in the adventitia during the late embryonic period and early postnatal period.[174]

Cells expressing SCA1 are located in the adventitia of the mouse between the aortic and pulmonary trunks initially in the late embryonic stages and persisting into adulthood, and SHH signaling appears to be critical for this population of cells, because the number of adventitial SCA1⁺ cells is greatly diminished in *Shh* null mice.[174] In addition, in SCA1⁺ cells isolated from murine arteries, knockdown of the pluripotency factor KLF4 reduces SCA1 levels and conversely overexpression of KLF4 induces SCA1 expression.[175]

Interestingly, mature SMCs are apparently an important source of these adventitial stem cells. Fate mapping of adult SMCs in *Myh11-CreER^T2* mice also carrying the ROSA26R-YFP Cre reporter demonstrates that 8 weeks after tamoxifen induction, a subset of SMA⁻ cells expressing SCA1 or CD34 in the adventitia are YFP⁺.[175] This result suggests that some SMMHC⁺ cells dedifferentiate and migrate radially outward from the media to the adventitia.[175] In sum, the adventitia is apparently an important tissue in vascular development and disease; however, its role in these processes is critically understudied.

Macrophages

It is well accepted that macrophages reside in the adventitia; however, using fate mapping, the ontogeny of vascular wall macrophages was only recently revealed. Ensan et al. showed that arterial macrophages develop embryonically from early and late erythro-myeloid progenitors generated in the yolk sac.[176] In the early postnatal period, macrophage colonization of arteries occurs during a brief period of circulating monocyte recruitment, whereas in adulthood, arterial macrophages are replenished by local proliferation and not from circulating monocytes.[176] Similar to macrophages residing in the brain or kidney and to Ly-6C^low monocytes, arterial macrophage survival is promoted by interactions between the chemokine receptor CX3CR1 and its ligand CX3CL1.[176]

Given that macrophages are present in developing vessels, the question arises: what, if any, are the roles of macrophages in vascular morphogenesis? During development of the vasculature, macrophages engage in a number of heterotypic cell-cell interactions with other vascular cell types, including ECs, pericytes, and VSMCs. Macrophages direct neovessel pruning via phagocytosis during the maturation of microvessel networks. For example, in organogenesis of the testes, macrophages arise from primitive yolk sac–derived hematopoietic progenitors, and nearly all of them express CD206, a marker of the M2 macrophage state which is characteristic of angiogenic and tissue remodeling.[177] Macrophage depletion in this tissue results in disrupted vascular patterning due to inadequate remodeling.[177] Similar results were found in terms of the role of macrophages in pruning of the hyaloid vasculature of the developing eye.[178] Finally, macrophages have been shown to induce fusion of EC tip cells, linking distinct angiogenic sprouts.[179]

SUMMARY

Morphogenesis of the vascular system initiates shortly after gastrulation. The mesoderm gives rise to most vascular cells; however, the ectoderm contributes to SMCs of the aortic root, ascending aorta, and cranial vessels. The early vasculature develops through vasculogenesis in which mesodermal cells differentiate into angioblasts and then coalesce into blood vessels, and, in general, capillaries are generated thereafter predominantly through sprouting angiogenesis. Migratory tip and proliferative stalk ECs are crucial for sprouting angiogenesis. This early development of the tunica intima involves many molecular signaling pathways, including those mediated by VEGF and Notch, as well as metabolic processes. In addition to the blood vasculature, the lymphatic system is composed of lymphatic ECs, which derive from venous ECs. In large-caliber blood vessels, radially outward from ECs is the tunica media consisting of SMCs, elastin, and collagen. Among blood vessels and even within a single vessel (e.g., aorta), SMCs have diverse origins. The regulation of SMC gene expression is an active area of investigation and involves the CArG-SRF–dependent system, noncoding RNAs, and epigenetics. In capillaries, mural cells are pericytes, which are found embedded in the EC basement membrane. Finally, the outermost layer of blood vessels (i.e., the tunica adventitia) is composed of loose connective tissue, as well as fibroblasts, stem cell marker–positive cells, and macrophages.

REFERENCES

1. Alexander MR, Owens GK. Epigenetic control of smooth muscle cell differentiation and phenotypic switching in vascular development and disease. *Annu Rev Physiol.* 2012;74:13–40.
2. Majesky MW. Developmental basis of vascular smooth muscle diversity. *Arterioscler Thromb Vasc Biol.* 2007;27:1248–1258.
3. Pardanaud L, Yassine F, Dieterlen-Lievre F. Relationship between vasculogenesis, angiogenesis and haemopoiesis during avian ontogeny. *Development.* 1989;105:473–485.
4. Jin SW, Beis D, Mitchell T, et al. Cellular and molecular analyses of vascular tube and lumen formation in zebrafish. *Development.* 2005;132:5199–5520.
5. Vokes SA, Krieg PA. Endoderm is required for vascular endothelial tube formation, but not for angioblast specification. *Development.* 2002;129:775–785.
6. Dejana E, Hirschi KK, Simons M. The molecular basis of endothelial cell plasticity. *Nat Commun.* 2017;8:14361.
7. Marcelo KL, Goldie LC, Hirschi KK. Regulation of endothelial cell differentiation and specification. *Circ Res.* 2013;112:1272–1287.
8. Risau W, Flamme I. Vasculogenesis. *Annu Rev Cell Dev Biol.* 1995;11:73–91.
9. Byrd N, Becker S, Maye P, et al. Hedgehog is required for murine yolk sac angiogenesis. *Development.* 2002;129:361–372.
10. Dyer MA, Farrington SM, Mohn D, et al. Indian hedgehog activates hematopoiesis and vasculogenesis and can respecify prospective neurectodermal cell fate in the mouse embryo. *Development.* 2001;128:1717–1730.
11. Shalaby F, Rossant J, Yamaguchi TP, et al. Failure of blood-island formation and vasculogenesis in Flk-1-deficient mice. *Nature.* 1995;376:62–66.
12. Kataoka H, Hayashi M, Nakagawa R, et al. Etv2/ER71 induces vascular mesoderm from Flk1+PDGFRalpha+ primitive mesoderm. *Blood.* 2011;118:6975–6986.
13. Salanga MC, Meadows SM, Myers CT, Krieg PA. ETS family protein ETV2 is required for initiation of the endothelial lineage but not the hematopoietic lineage in the Xenopus embryo. *Dev Dyn.* 2010;239:1178–1187.
14. Risau W. Mechanisms of angiogenesis. *Nature.* 1997;386:671–674.
15. Adams RH, Wilkinson GA, Weiss C, et al. Roles of ephrinB ligands and EphB receptors in cardiovascular development: demarcation of arterial/venous domains, vascular morphogenesis, and sprouting angiogenesis. *Genes Dev.* 1999;13:295–306.
16. Gerety SS, Wang HU, Chen ZF, Anderson DJ. Symmetrical mutant phenotypes of the receptor EphB4 and its specific transmembrane ligand ephrin-B2 in cardiovascular development. *Mol Cell.* 1999;4:403–414.
17. Wang HU, Chen ZF, Anderson DJ. Molecular distinction and angiogenic interaction between embryonic arteries and veins revealed by ephrin-B2 and its receptor Eph-B4. *Cell.* 1998;93:741–753.
18. Chung AS, Ferrara N. Developmental and pathological angiogenesis. *Annu Rev Cell Dev Biol.* 2011;27:563–558.
19. Smithers L, Haddon C, Jiang YJ, Lewis J. Sequence and embryonic expression of deltaC in the zebrafish. *Mech Dev.* 2000;90:119–123.
20. Zhong TP, Childs S, Leu JP, Fishman MC. Gridlock signalling pathway fashions the first embryonic artery. *Nature.* 2001;414:216–220.
21. Zhong TP, Rosenberg M, Mohideen MA, et al. Gridlock, an HLH gene required for assembly of the aorta in zebrafish. *Science.* 2000;287:1820–1824.
22. Noden DM. Embryonic origins and assembly of blood vessels. *Am Rev Respir Dis.* 1989;140:1097–1103.
23. Lawson ND, Scheer N, Pham VN, et al. Notch signaling is required for arterial-venous differentiation during embryonic vascular development. *Development.* 2001;128:3675–3683.
24. Gu C, Rodriguez ER, Reimert DV, et al. Neuropilin-1 conveys semaphorin and VEGF signaling during neural and cardiovascular development. *Dev Cell.* 2003;5:45–57.
25. Lawson ND, Vogel AM, Weinstein BM. Sonic hedgehog and vascular endothelial growth factor act upstream of the Notch pathway during arterial endothelial differentiation. *Dev Cell.* 2002;3:127–136.
26. Herzog Y, Guttmann-Raviv N, Neufeld G. Segregation of arterial and venous markers in subpopulations of blood islands before vessel formation. *Dev Dyn.* 2005;232:1047–1055.
27. You LR, Lin FJ, Lee CT, et al. Suppression of Notch signalling by the COUP-TFII transcription factor regulates vein identity. *Nature.* 2005;435:98–104.
28. Red-Horse K, Ueno H, Weissman IL, Krasnow MA. Coronary arteries form by developmental reprogramming of venous cells. *Nature.* 2010;464:549–553.
29. Gerhardt H, Golding M, Fruttiger M, et al. VEGF guides angiogenic sprouting utilizing endothelial tip cell filopodia. *J Cell Biol.* 2003;161:1163–1177.
30. Blanco R, Gerhardt H. VEGF and Notch in tip and stalk cell selection. *Cold Spring Harb Perspect Med.* 2013;3:a006569.
31. Ausprunk DH, Folkman J. Migration and proliferation of endothelial cells in preformed and newly formed blood vessels during tumor angiogenesis. *Microvasc Res.* 1977;14:53–65.
32. Geudens I, Gerhardt H. Coordinating cell behaviour during blood vessel formation. *Development.* 2011;138:4569–4583.
33. Stone J, Itin A, Alon T, et al. Development of retinal vasculature is mediated by hypoxia-induced vascular endothelial growth factor (VEGF) expression by neuroglia. *J Neurosci.* 1995;15:4738–4747.
34. Hellström M, Phng LK, Hofmann JJ, et al. Dll4 signalling through Notch1 regulates formation of tip cells during angiogenesis. *Nature.* 2007;445:776–780.
35. Shutter JR, Scully S, Fan W, et al. Dll4, a novel Notch ligand expressed in arterial endothelium. *Genes Dev.* 2000;14:1313–1318.
36. Suchting S, Freitas C, le Noble F, et al. The Notch ligand Delta-like 4 negatively regulates endothelial tip cell formation and vessel branching. *Proc Natl Acad Sci U S A.* 2007;104:3225–3230.
37. Childs S, Chen JN, Garrity DM, Fishman MC. Patterning of angiogenesis in the zebrafish embryo. *Development.* 2002;129:973–982.
38. Siekmann AF, Lawson ND. Notch signalling limits angiogenic cell behaviour in developing zebrafish arteries. *Nature.* 2007;445:781–784.
39. Horowitz A, Simons M. Branching morphogenesis. *Circ Res.* 2008;103:784–795.
40. Affolter M, Caussinus E. Tracheal branching morphogenesis in Drosophila: new insights into cell behaviour and organ architecture. *Development.* 2008;135:2055–2064.
41. Cardoso WV, Lu J. Regulation of early lung morphogenesis: questions, facts and controversies. *Development.* 2006;133:1611–1624.
42. Metzger RJ, Klein OD, Martin GR, Krasnow MA. The branching programme of mouse lung development. *Nature.* 2008;453:745–750.
43. Min H, Danilenko DM, Scully SA, et al. Fgf-10 is required for both limb and lung development and exhibits striking functional similarity to Drosophila branchless. *Genes Dev.* 1998;12:3156–3161.
44. De Moerlooze L, Spencer-Dene B, Revest JM, et al. An important role for the IIIb isoform of fibroblast growth factor receptor 2 (FGFR2) in mesenchymal-epithelial signalling during mouse organogenesis. *Development.* 2000;127:483–492.
45. Costantini F, Kopan R. Patterning a complex organ: branching morphogenesis and nephron segmentation in kidney development. *Dev Cell.* 2010;18:698–712.
46. Dressler GR. Advances in early kidney specification, development and patterning. *Development.* 2009;136:3863–3874.
47. Skinner MA, Safford SD, Reeves JG, et al. Renal aplasia in humans is associated with RET mutations. *Am J Hum Genet.* 2008;82:344–351.

48. Simons M, Gordon E, Claesson-Welsh L. Mechanisms and regulation of endothelial VEGF receptor signalling. *Nat Rev Mol Cell Biol*. 2016;17: 611–625.

49. Carmeliet P, Ferreira V, Breier G, et al. Abnormal blood vessel development and lethality in embryos lacking a single VEGF allele. *Nature*. 1996;380:435–439.

50. Ferrara N, Carver-Moore K, Chen H, et al. Heterozygous embryonic lethality induced by targeted inactivation of the VEGF gene. *Nature*. 1996;380:439–442.

51. Breier G, Albrecht U, Sterrer S, Risau W. Expression of vascular endothelial growth factor during embryonic angiogenesis and endothelial cell differentiation. *Development*. 1992;114:521–532.

52. Fong GH, Rossant J, Gertsenstein M, Breitman ML. Role of the Flt-1 receptor tyrosine kinase in regulating the assembly of vascular endothelium. *Nature*. 1995;376:66–70.

53. Dumont DJ, Jussila L, Taipale J, et al. Cardiovascular failure in mouse embryos deficient in VEGF receptor-3. *Science*. 1998;282:946–949.

54. Coulon C, Georgiadou M, Roncal C, et al. From vessel sprouting to normalization: role of the prolyl hydroxylase domain protein/hypoxia-inducible factor oxygen-sensing machinery. *Arterioscler Thromb Vasc Biol*. 2010;30:2331–2336.

55. Olsson AK, Dimberg A, Kreuger J, Claesson-Welsh L. VEGF receptor signalling - in control of vascular function. *Nat Rev Mol Cell Biol*. 2006;7:359–371.

56. Yu P, Wilhelm K, Dubrac A, et al. FGF-dependent metabolic control of vascular development. *Nature*. 2017;545:224–228.

57. Downs KM. Florence Sabin and the mechanism of blood vessel lumenization during vasculogenesis. *Microcirculation*. 2003;10:5–25.

58. Folkman J, Haudenschild C. Angiogenesis by capillary endothelial cells in culture. *Trans Ophthalmol Soc U K*. 1980;100:346–353.

59. Davis GE, Bayless KJ. An integrin and Rho GTPase-dependent pinocytic vacuole mechanism controls capillary lumen formation in collagen and fibrin matrices. *Microcirculation*. 2003;10:27–44.

60. Bayless KJ, Davis GE. The Cdc42 and Rac1 GTPases are required for capillary lumen formation in three-dimensional extracellular matrices. *J Cell Sci*. 2002;115:1123–1136.

61. Kamei M, Saunders WB, Bayless KJ, et al. Endothelial tubes assemble from intracellular vacuoles in vivo. *Nature*. 2006;442:453–456.

62. Zeeb M, Strilic B, Lammert E. Resolving cell-cell junctions: lumen formation in blood vessels. *Curr Opin Cell Biol*. 2010;22:626–632.

63. Blum Y, Belting HG, Ellertsdottir E, et al. Complex cell rearrangements during intersegmental vessel sprouting and vessel fusion in the zebrafish embryo. *Dev Biol*. 2008;316:312–322.

64. Lubarsky B, Krasnow MA. Tube morphogenesis: making and shaping biological tubes. *Cell*. 2003;112:19–28.

65. Zovein AC, Luque A, Turlo KA, et al. Beta1 integrin establishes endothelial cell polarity and arteriolar lumen formation via a Par3-dependent mechanism. *Dev Cell*. 2010;18:39–51.

66. Carmeliet P, Lampugnani MG, Moons L, et al. Targeted deficiency or cytosolic truncation of the VE-cadherin gene in mice impairs VEGF-mediated endothelial survival and angiogenesis. *Cell*. 1999;98:147–157.

67. Strilić B, Kucera T, Eglinger J, et al. The molecular basis of vascular lumen formation in the developing mouse aorta. *Dev Cell*. 2009;17:505–515.

68. Li F, Sawada J, Komatsu M. R-Ras-Akt axis induces endothelial lumenogenesis and regulates the patency of regenerating vasculature. *Nat Commun*. 2017;8:1720.

69. Parker LH, Schmidt M, Jin SW, et al. The endothelial-cell-derived secreted factor Egfl7 regulates vascular tube formation. *Nature*. 2004;428:754–758.

70. De Bock K, Georgiadou M, Schoors S, et al. Role of PFKFB3-driven glycolysis in vessel sprouting. *Cell*. 2013;154:651–663.

71. Eelen G, de Zeeuw P, Simons M, Carmeliet P. Endothelial cell metabolism in normal and diseased vasculature. *Circ Res*. 2015;116:1231–1244.

72. Schoors S, Bruning U, Missiaen R, et al. Fatty acid carbon is essential for dNTP synthesis in endothelial cells. *Nature*. 2015;520:192–197.

73. Sabin FR. On the origin of the lymphatic system from the veins and the development of the lymph hearts and thoracic duct in the pig. *Am J Anat*. 1902;1:367–391.

74. Sabin FR. The lymphatic system in human embryos, with a consideration of the morphology of the system as a whole. *Am J Anat*. 1909;9:43–91.

75. Zheng W, Aspelund A, Alitalo K. Lymphangiogenic factors, mechanisms, and applications. *J Clin Invest*. 2014;124:878–887.

76. François M, Caprini A, Hosking B, et al. Sox18 induces development of the lymphatic vasculature in mice. *Nature*. 2008;456:643–647.

77. Irrthum A, Devriendt K, Chitayat D, et al. Mutations in the transcription factor gene SOX18 underlie recessive and dominant forms of hypotrichosis-lymphedema-telangiectasia. *Am J Hum Genet*. 2003;72:1470–1478.

78. Srinivasan RS, Dillard ME, Lagutin OV, et al. Lineage tracing demonstrates the venous origin of the mammalian lymphatic vasculature. *Genes Dev*. 2007;21:2422–2432.

79. Kazenwadel J, Betterman KL, Chong CE, et al. GATA2 is required for lymphatic vessel valve development and maintenance. *J Clin Invest*. 2015;125:2979–2994.

80. Janardhan HP, Milstone ZJ, Shin M, et al. Hdac3 regulates lymphovenous and lymphatic valve formation. *J Clin Invest*. 2017;127:4193–4206.

81. Armulik A, Genove G, Betsholtz C. Pericytes: developmental, physiological, and pathological perspectives, problems, and promises. *Dev Cell*. 2011;21:193–215.

82. Dore-Duffy P, Cleary K. Morphology and properties of pericytes. *Methods Mol Biol*. 2011;686:49–68.

83. Hartmann DA, Underly RG, Grant RI, et al. Pericyte structure and distribution in the cerebral cortex revealed by high-resolution imaging of transgenic mice. *Neurophotonics*. 2015;2:041402.

84. Trost A, Lange S, Schroedl F, et al. Brain and retinal pericytes: origin, function and role. *Front Cell Neurosci*. 2016;10:20.

85. Daneman R, Zhou L, Kebede AA, Barres BA. Pericytes are required for blood-brain barrier integrity during embryogenesis. *Nature*. 2010;468:562–566.

86. Armulik A, Genové G, Mäe M, et al. Pericytes regulate the blood-brain barrier. *Nature*. 2010;468:557–561.

87. Dave JM, Mirabella T, Weatherbee S, Greif DM. ALK5/TIMP3 axis in pericytes contributes to endothelial morphogenesis in the developing brain. *Dev Cell*. 2018;44:665–678. e6.

88. Hall CN, Reynell C, Gesslein B, et al. Capillary pericytes regulate cerebral blood flow in health and disease. *Nature*. 2014;508:55–60.

89. Hill RA, Tong L, Yuan P, et al. Regional blood flow in the normal and ischemic brain is controlled by arteriolar smooth muscle cell contractility and not by capillary pericytes. *Neuron*. 2015;87:95–110.

90. Attwell D, Mishra A, Hall CN, et al. What is a pericyte? *J Cereb Blood Flow Metab*. 2016;36:451–455.

91. He L, Vanlandewijck M, Raschperger E, et al. Analysis of the brain mural cell transcriptome. *Sci Rep*. 2016;6:35108.

92. Sawada H, Rateri DL, Moorleghen JJ, et al. Smooth muscle cells derived from second heart field and cardiac neural crest reside in spatially distinct domains in the media of the ascending aorta-brief report. *Arterioscler Thromb Vasc Biol*. 2017;37:1722–1726.

93. Jiang X, Rowitch DH, Soriano P, et al. Fate of the mammalian cardiac neural crest. *Development*. 2000;127:1607–1616.

94. Harmon AW, Nakano A. Nkx2-5 lineage tracing visualizes the distribution of second heart field-derived aortic smooth muscle. *Genesis*. 2013;51:862–869.

95. Wasteson P, Johansson BR, Jukkola T, et al. Developmental origin of smooth muscle cells in the descending aorta in mice. *Development*. 2008;135:1823–1832.

96. Esner M, Meilhac SM, Relaix F, et al. Smooth muscle of the dorsal aorta shares a common clonal origin with skeletal muscle of the myotome. *Development*. 2006;133:737–749.

97. Topouzis S, Majesky MW. Smooth muscle lineage diversity in the chick embryo. Two types of aortic smooth muscle cell differ in growth and receptor-mediated transcriptional responses to transforming growth factor-beta. *Dev Biol*. 1996;178:430–445.

98. Majesky MW. Development of coronary vessels. *Curr Top Dev Biol*. 2004;62:225–259.

99. Zhou B, Ma Q, Rajagopal S, et al. Epicardial progenitors contribute to the cardiomyocyte lineage in the developing heart. *Nature*. 2008;454:109–113.

100. Volz KS, Jacobs AH, Chen HI, et al. Pericytes are progenitors for coronary artery smooth muscle. *Elife*. 2015;4:e10036.

101. Rinkevich Y, Mori T, Sahoo D, et al. Identification and prospective isolation of a mesothelial precursor lineage giving rise to smooth muscle cells and fibroblasts for mammalian internal organs, and their vasculature. *Nat Cell Biol*. 2012;14:1251–1260.

102. Wilm B, Ipenberg A, Hastie ND, et al. The serosal mesothelium is a major source of smooth muscle cells of the gut vasculature. *Development*. 2005;132:5317–5328.

103. Que J, Wilm B, Hasegawa H, et al. Mesothelium contributes to vascular smooth muscle and mesenchyme during lung development. *Proc Natl Acad Sci U S A*. 2008;105:16626–16630.

104. Morimoto M, Liu Z, Cheng HT, et al. Canonical Notch signaling in the developing lung is required for determination of arterial smooth muscle cells and selection of Clara versus ciliated cell fate. *J Cell Sci*. 2010;123:213–224.

105. Arciniegas E, Frid MG, Douglas IS, Stenmark KR. Perspectives on endothelial-to-mesenchymal transition: potential contribution to vascular remodeling in chronic pulmonary hypertension. *Am J Physiol Lung Cell Mol Physiol*. 2007;293:L1–L8.

106. DeRuiter MC, Poelmann RE, VanMunsteren JC, et al. Embryonic endothelial cells transdifferentiate into mesenchymal cells expressing smooth muscle actins in vivo and in vitro. *Circ Res*. 1997;80:444–451.

107. Yamashita J, Itoh H, Hirashima M, et al. Flk1-positive cells derived from embryonic stem cells serve as vascular progenitors. *Nature*. 2000;408:92–96.

108. Chen PY, Qin L, Baeyens N, et al. Endothelial-to-mesenchymal transition drives atherosclerosis progression. *J Clin Invest*. 2015;125:4514–4528.

109. Alva JA, Zovein AC, Monvoisin A, et al. VE-Cadherin-Cre-recombinase transgenic mouse: a tool for lineage analysis and gene deletion in endothelial cells. *Dev Dyn*. 2006;235:759–767.

110. Muzumdar MD, Tasic B, Miyamichi K, et al. A global double-fluorescent Cre reporter mouse. *Genesis*. 2007;45:593–605.

111. Greif DM, Kumar M, Lighthouse JK, et al. Radial construction of an arterial wall. *Dev Cell*. 2012;23:482–493.

112. Hungerford JE, Little CD. Developmental biology of the vascular smooth muscle cell: building a multilayered vessel wall. *J Vasc Res*. 1999;36:2–27.

113. Owens GK, Kumar MS, Wamhoff BR. Molecular regulation of vascular smooth muscle cell differentiation in development and disease. *Physiol Rev*. 2004;84:767–801.

114. Li L, Miano JM, Cserjesi P, Olson EN. SM22 alpha, a marker of adult smooth muscle, is expressed in multiple myogenic lineages during embryogenesis. *Circ Res*. 1996;78:188–195.

115. Miano JM, Cserjesi P, Ligon KL, et al. Smooth muscle myosin heavy chain exclusively marks the smooth muscle lineage during mouse embryogenesis. *Circ Res*. 1994;75:803–812.

116. van der Loop FT, Schaart G, Timmer ED, et al. Smoothelin, a novel cytoskeletal protein specific for smooth muscle cells. *J Cell Biol*. 1996;134:401–411.

117. Gomez D, Owens GK. Smooth muscle cell phenotypic switching in atherosclerosis. *Cardiovasc Res*. 2012;95:156–164.

118. Wang Z, Wang DZ, Hockemeyer D, et al. Myocardin and ternary complex factors compete for SRF to control smooth muscle gene expression. *Nature*. 2004;428:185–189.

119. Wang Z, Wang DZ, Pipes GC, Olson EN. Myocardin is a master regulator of smooth muscle gene expression. *Proc Natl Acad Sci U S A*. 2003;100:7129–7134.

120. Li S, Wang DZ, Wang Z, et al. The serum response factor coactivator myocardin is required for vascular smooth muscle development. *Proc Natl Acad Sci U S A*. 2003;100:9366–9370.

121. Liu Y, Sinha S, McDonald OG, et al. Kruppel-like factor 4 abrogates myocardin-induced activation of smooth muscle gene expression. *J Biol Chem*. 2005;280:9719–9727.

122. Liu ZP, Wang Z, Yanagisawa H, Olson EN. Phenotypic modulation of smooth muscle cells through interaction of Foxo4 and myocardin. *Dev Cell*. 2005;9:261–270.

123. Miano JM, Long X. The short and long of noncoding sequences in the control of vascular cell phenotypes. *Cell Mol Life Sci*. 2015;72:3457–3488.

124. Cordes KR, Sheehy NT, White MP, et al. miR-145 and miR-143 regulate smooth muscle cell fate and plasticity. *Nature*. 2009;460:705–710.

125. Xin M, Small EM, Sutherland LB, et al. MicroRNAs miR-143 and miR-145 modulate cytoskeletal dynamics and responsiveness of smooth muscle cells to injury. *Genes Dev*. 2009;23:2166–2178.

126. Davis BN, Hilyard AC, Nguyen PH, et al. Smad proteins bind a conserved RNA sequence to promote microRNA maturation by Drosha. *Mol Cell*. 2010;39:373–384.

127. Chan MC, Hilyard AC, Wu C, et al. Molecular basis for antagonism between PDGF and the TGFbeta family of signalling pathways by control of miR-24 expression. *EMBO J*. 2010;29:559–573.

128. Leeper NJ, Raiesdana A, Kojima Y, et al. MicroRNA-26a is a novel regulator of vascular smooth muscle cell function. *J Cell Physiol*. 2011;226:1035–1043.

129. Torella D, Iaconetti C, Catalucci D, et al. MicroRNA-133 controls vascular smooth muscle cell phenotypic switch in vitro and vascular remodeling in vivo. *Circ Res*. 2011;109:880–893.

130. Zhao J, Zhang W, Lin M, et al. MYOSLID is a novel serum response factor-dependent long noncoding RNA that amplifies the vascular smooth muscle differentiation program. *Arterioscler Thromb Vasc Biol*. 2016;36:2088–2099.

131. Gomez D, Shankman LS, Nguyen AT, Owens GK. Detection of histone modifications at specific gene loci in single cells in histological sections. *Nat Methods*. 2013;10:171–177.

132. Liu R, Leslie KL, Martin KA. Epigenetic regulation of smooth muscle cell plasticity. *Biochim Biophys Acta*. 2015;1849:448–453.

133. Shankman LS, Gomez D, Cherepanova OA, et al. KLF4-dependent phenotypic modulation of smooth muscle cells has a key role in atherosclerotic plaque pathogenesis. *Nat Med*. 2015;21:628–637.

134. Liu R, Jin Y, Tang WH, et al. Ten-eleven translocation-2 (TET2) is a master regulator of smooth muscle cell plasticity. *Circulation*. 2013;128:2047–2057.

135. Rong JX, Shapiro M, Trogan E, Fisher EA. Transdifferentiation of mouse aortic smooth muscle cells to a macrophage-like state after cholesterol loading. *Proc Natl Acad Sci U S A*. 2003;100:13531–13536.

136. Vengrenyuk Y, Nishi H, Long X, et al. Cholesterol loading reprograms the microRNA-143/145-myocardin axis to convert aortic smooth muscle cells to a dysfunctional macrophage-like phenotype. *Arterioscler Thromb Vasc Biol*. 2015;35:535–546.

137. Feil S, Fehrenbacher B, Lukowski R, et al. Transdifferentiation of vascular smooth muscle cells to macrophage-like cells during atherogenesis. *Circ Res*. 2014;115:662–667.

138. de Ruiter MC, Poelmann RE, van Iperen L, Gittenberger-de Groot AC. The early development of the tunica media in the vascular system of rat embryos. *Anat Embryol (Berl)*. 1990;181:341–349.

139. Hungerford JE, Owens GK, Argraves WS, Little CD. Development of the aortic vessel wall as defined by vascular smooth muscle and extracellular matrix markers. *Dev Biol*. 1996;178:375–392.

140. el-Maghraby AA, Gardner DL. Development of connective-tissue components of small arteries in the chick embryo. *J Pathol*. 1972;108:281–291.

141. Kadar A, Gardner DL, Bush V. The relation between the fine structure of smooth-muscle cells and elastogenesis in the chick-embryo aorta. *J Pathol*. 1971;104:253–260.

142. Nakamura H. Electron microscopic study of the prenatal development of the thoracic aorta in the rat. *Am J Anat*. 1988;181:406–418.

143. Takahashi Y, Imanaka T, Takano T. Spatial and temporal pattern of smooth muscle cell differentiation during development of the vascular system in the mouse embryo. *Anat Embryol (Berl)*. 1996;194:515–526.

144. Turing AM. The chemical basis of morphogenesis. *Philosophical Transactions of the Royal Society of London Series B, Biological Sciences*. 1952;237:37–72.

145. Reilly KM, Melton DA. Short-range signaling by candidate morphogens of the TGF beta family and evidence for a relay mechanism of induction. *Cell*. 1996;86:743–754.

146. Feng X, Krebs LT, Gridley T. Patent ductus arteriosus in mice with smooth muscle-specific Jag1 deletion. *Development*. 2010;137:4191–4199.

147. Gaengel K, Genove G, Armulik A, Betsholtz C. Endothelial-mural cell signaling in vascular development and angiogenesis. *Arterioscler Thromb Vasc Biol*. 2009;29:630–638.

148. Hellstrom M, Kalen M, Lindahl P, et al. Role of PDGF-B and PDGFR-beta in recruitment of vascular smooth muscle cells and pericytes during embryonic blood vessel formation in the mouse. *Development*. 1999;126:3047–3055.

149. Leveen P, Pekny M, Gebre-Medhin S, et al. Mice deficient for PDGF B show renal, cardiovascular, and hematological abnormalities. *Genes Dev*. 1994;8:1875–1887.

150. Lindahl P, Johansson BR, Leveen P, Betsholtz C. Pericyte loss and microaneurysm formation in PDGF-B-deficient mice. *Science*. 1997;277:242–245.

151. Soriano P. Abnormal kidney development and hematological disorders in PDGF beta-receptor mutant mice. *Genes Dev*. 1994;8:1888–1896.

152. Hirschi KK, Rohovsky SA, D'Amore PA. PDGF, TGF-beta, and heterotypic cell-cell interactions mediate endothelial cell-induced recruitment of 10T1/2 cells and their differentiation to a smooth muscle fate. *J Cell Biol*. 1998;141:805–814.

153. High FA, Lu MM, Pear WS, et al. Endothelial expression of the Notch ligand Jagged1 is required for vascular smooth muscle development. *Proc Natl Acad Sci U S A*. 2008;105:1955–1959.

154. Domenga V, Fardoux P, Lacombe P, et al. Notch3 is required for arterial identity and maturation of vascular smooth muscle cells. *Genes Dev*. 2004;18:2730–2735.

155. Wang T, Baron M, Trump D. An overview of Notch3 function in vascular smooth muscle cells. *Prog Biophys Mol Biol*. 2008;96:499–509.

156. Joutel A, Corpechot C, Ducros A, et al. Notch3 mutations in CADASIL, a hereditary adult-onset condition causing stroke and dementia. *Nature*. 1996;383:707–710.

157. McLean SE, Mecham BH, Kelleher CM, et al. Extracellular matrix gene expression in the developing mouse aorta. *Adv Dev Biol*. 2005;15:81–128.

158. Kelleher CM, McLean SE, Mecham RP. Vascular extracellular matrix and aortic development. *Curr Top Dev Biol*. 2004;62:153–188.

159. Wagenseil JE, Mecham RP. Vascular extracellular matrix and arterial mechanics. *Physiol Rev*. 2009;89:957–989.

160. Xu J, Shi GP. Vascular wall extracellular matrix proteins and vascular diseases. *Biochim Biophys Acta*. 2014;1842:2106–2119.

161. Humphrey JD, Schwartz MA, Tellides G, Milewicz DM. Role of mechanotransduction in vascular biology: focus on thoracic aortic aneurysms and dissections. *Circ Res*. 2015;116:1448–1461.

162. Parks WC, Pierce RA, Lee KA, Mecham RP. Elastin. *Adv Mol Cell Biol*. 1993;6:133–181.

163. Faury G, Pezet M, Knutsen RH, et al. Developmental adaptation of the mouse cardiovascular system to elastin haploinsufficiency. *J Clin Invest*. 2003;112:1419–1428.

164. Li DY, Faury G, Taylor DG, et al. Novel arterial pathology in mice and humans hemizygous for elastin. *J Clin Invest*. 1998;102:1783–1787.

165. Wagenseil JE, Nerurkar NL, Knutsen RH, et al. Effects of elastin haploinsufficiency on the mechanical behavior of mouse arteries. *Am J Physiol Heart Circ Physiol*. 2005;289:H1209–H1217.

166. Li DY, Brooke B, Davis EC, et al. Elastin is an essential determinant of arterial morphogenesis. *Nature*. 1998;393:276–280.

167. Misra A, Sheikh AQ, Kumar A, et al. Integrin beta3 inhibition is a therapeutic strategy for supravalvular aortic stenosis. *J Exp Med*. 2016;213:451–463.

168. Ramirez F, Dietz HC. Marfan syndrome: from molecular pathogenesis to clinical treatment. *Curr Opin Genet Dev*. 2007;17:252–258.

169. Dettman RW, Denetclaw Jr W, Ordahl CP, Bristow J. Common epicardial origin of coronary vascular smooth muscle, perivascular fibroblasts, and intermyocardial fibroblasts in the avian heart. *Dev Biol*. 1998;193:169–181.

170. Hu Y, Zhang Z, Torsney E, et al. Abundant progenitor cells in the adventitia contribute to atherosclerosis of vein grafts in ApoE-deficient mice. *J Clin Invest*. 2004;113:1258–1265.

171. Majesky MW, Dong XR, Hoglund V, et al. The adventitia: a dynamic interface containing resident progenitor cells. *Arterioscler Thromb Vasc Biol*. 2011;31:1530–1539.

172. Corselli M, Chen CW, Sun B, et al. The tunica adventitia of human arteries and veins as a source of mesenchymal stem cells. *Stem Cells Dev*. 2012;21:1299–1308.

173. Zengin E, Chalajour F, Gehling UM, et al. Vascular wall resident progenitor cells: a source for postnatal vasculogenesis. *Development*. 2006;133:1543–1551.

174. Passman JN, Dong XR, Wu SP, et al. A sonic hedgehog signaling domain in the arterial adventitia supports resident Sca1+ smooth muscle progenitor cells. *Proc Natl Acad Sci U S A*. 2008;105:9349–9354.

175. Majesky MW, Horita H, Ostriker A, et al. Differentiated smooth muscle cells generate a subpopulation of resident vascular progenitor cells in the adventitia regulated by Klf4. *Circ Res*. 2017;120:296–311.

176. Ensan S, Li A, Besla R, et al. Self-renewing resident arterial macrophages arise from embryonic CX3CR1(+) precursors and circulating monocytes immediately after birth. *Nat Immunol*. 2016;17:159–168.

177. DeFalco T, Bhattacharya I, Williams AV, et al. Yolk-sac-derived macrophages regulate fetal testis vascularization and morphogenesis. *Proc Natl Acad Sci U S A*. 2014;111:E2384–E2393.

178. Lobov IB, Rao S, Carroll TJ, et al. WNT7b mediates macrophage-induced programmed cell death in patterning of the vasculature. *Nature*. 2005;437:417–421.

179. Fantin A, Vieira JM, Gestri G, et al. Tissue macrophages act as cellular chaperones for vascular anastomosis downstream of VEGF-mediated endothelial tip cell induction. *Blood*. 2010;116:829–840.

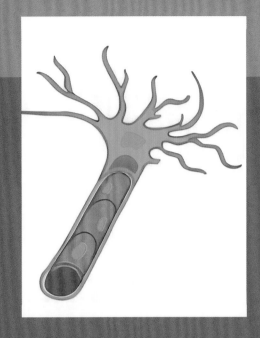

中文导读

第2章
血管内皮

　　本章讲述血管内皮的生理和功能：从内皮细胞的形态、结构到其功能。内皮细胞分布于全身的动脉、静脉和淋巴管内。内皮细胞的特殊解剖位置决定了其特殊的功能，如调节血栓和止血功能、调节免疫和炎症反应、调节血管渗透性及血管张力等。以上内皮细胞的功能都根据局部和系统的环境变化而发生改变，当然这一调节是极为复杂的。当内皮细胞无法对生理/病理的外部刺激做出适宜的调整时，将出现所谓的内皮细胞功能障碍，引起一系列的病理改变。利用生物化学和分子生物学评价方法对内皮细胞表型变化进行判断，在临床上将具有一定的价值。

舒　畅

The Endothelium

Jane A. Leopold

In 1839, the German physiologist Theodor Schwann became the first to describe a "thin, but distinctly perceptible membrane" that he observed as part of the capillary vessel wall that separated circulating blood from tissue.[1,2] The cellular monolayer that formed this membrane would later be named the *endothelium*; however, the term *endothelium* did not appear until 1865 when it was introduced by the Swiss anatomist Wilhelm His in his essay, "Die Häute und Höhlen des Körpers (The Membranes and Cavities of the Body)."[2,3] Owing to its anatomical location, the endothelium was believed initially to be a passive receptacle for circulating blood, cells, and macromolecules. It is now known that the endothelium is a dynamic cellular structure, and its biological and functional properties extend beyond that of a physical anatomical boundary. In its totality, the endothelium comprises approximately 10 trillion (10^{13}) cells with a surface area of $7\,m^2$, weighs 1.0 to 1.8 kg, and contributes 1.4% to total body mass.[4,5] Endothelium exists as a monolayer of cells that is present in all arteries, veins, capillaries, and the lymphatic system, and lies at the interface of the bloodstream or lymph and the vessel wall.

The paradigm shift in our understanding of the role of the endothelium in vascular function has occurred over the past half century and continues to evolve. As a cellular structure with its luminal surface in continuous contact with flowing blood, the endothelium serves as a thromboresistant, semipermeable barrier, and governs interactions with circulating inflammatory and immune cells. In response to pulsatile flow and pressure, the endothelium mechanotransduces these hemodynamic forces to synthesize and release vasoactive substances that regulate vascular tone as well as signals for compensatory vessel wall remodeling. This chapter will focus on the biology of the endothelium to provide insight into how perturbations of these homeostatic functions result in (mal)adaptive responses that determine vascular health or disease.

HOMEOSTATIC FUNCTIONS OF THE ENDOTHELIUM

The endothelium exhibits considerable regional heterogeneity that reflects its arterial or venous location in the vascular tree, as well as the specialized metabolic and functional demands of the underlying tissues.[4,6,7] Identity and heterogeneity of the arterial and venous endothelium is determined, in part, by a complex array of signaling pathways, including Notch, Wnt, and Sox, as well as by the stiffness of the regional extracellular matrix (ECM) and the distribution and density of F-actin-anchored focal adhesions.[8,9] Despite this heterogeneity, there are basal homeostatic properties that are common to all endothelial cell (EC) populations, although some of these functions may achieve greater importance in selected vascular beds (Box 2.1).[7]

Maintenance of a Thromboresistant Surface and Regulation of Hemostasis

The endothelium was first recognized as a cellular structure that compartmentalizes circulating blood.[5] As such, the endothelial luminal surface is exposed to cells and proteins in the bloodstream that possess prothrombotic and procoagulant activity and, when necessary, support hemostasis. Normal endothelium preserves blood fluidity by synthesizing and secreting factors that limit activation of the clotting cascade, inhibit platelet aggregation, and promote fibrinolysis.[10] These include the cell surface-associated anticoagulant factors thrombomodulin, protein C, tissue factor pathway inhibitor (TFPI), and heparan sulfate proteoglycans (HSPG) that act in concert to limit coagulation at the luminal surface of the endothelium.[10-12] For instance, thrombin-mediated activation of protein C is accelerated 10^4-fold by binding to thrombomodulin, Ca^{2+}, and the endothelial protein C receptor. Activated protein C (APC) engages circulating protein S, which is also synthesized and released by the endothelium, to inactivate factors Va and VIIIa proteolytically.[10,13] TFPI is a Kunitz-type protease inhibitor that binds to and inhibits factor VIIa; about 80% of TFPI is bound to the endothelium via a glycosylphosphatidylinositol anchor and forms a quaternary complex with tissue factor—factor VIIa to diminish its procoagulant activity.[14,15] Proteoglycan heparan sulfates (HSs) that are present in the EC glycocalyx attain anticoagulant properties by catalyzing the association of the circulating serine protease inhibitor antithrombin III to factors Xa, IXa, and thrombin.[10] Thus, these anticoagulant factors serve to limit activation and propagation of the clotting cascade at the endothelial luminal surface and thereby maintain vascular patency.

The endothelium also synthesizes and secretes tissue plasminogen activator (tPA) and the ecto-adenosine diphosphatase (ecto-ADPase) CD39 to promote fibrinolysis and inhibit platelet activation, respectively. tPA is produced and released into the bloodstream continuously, but unless tPA binds fibrin, it is cleared from the plasma within 15 minutes by the liver.[10] Fibrin binding accelerates tPA amidolytic activity by increasing the catalytic efficiency for plasminogen activation and plasmin generation. Platelet activation at the endothelial luminal surface is inhibited by the actions of the ectonucleotidase CD39/NTPDase1 that hydrolyzes adenosine diphosphate (ADP), prostacyclin (PGI_2), and nitric oxide (NO).[10,16,17] Together these agents maintain an environment on the endothelial surface that is profibrinolytic and antithrombotic.

By contrast, in the setting of an acute vascular injury or trauma, the endothelium initiates a rapid and measured hemostatic response through regulated synthesis and release of tissue factor and von Willebrand factor (vWF). Tissue factor is a multidomain transmembrane glycoprotein (GP) that forms a complex with circulating factor

VIIa to activate the coagulation cascade and generate thrombin.[18] Tissue factor is expressed by vascular smooth muscle cells (VSMCs) and fibroblasts and by ECs only after activation. Tissue factor acquires its biological activity by phosphatidylserine exposure, dedimerization, decreased exposure to TFPI, or posttranslational modification(s) including disulfide bond formation between Cys186 and Cys209.[19–21] This disulfide bond is important for tissue factor coagulation activity, and may be reduced by protein disulfide isomerase, which is located on the EC surface.

The endothelium also synthesizes and stores vWF, a large polymeric GP that is expressed rapidly in response to injury. Propeptides and multimers of vWF are packaged in Weibel-Palade bodies that are unique to the endothelium. Secretion of vWF from Weibel-Palade bodies is regulated by autophagy, which also plays a role in the processing and maturation of vWF.[22] Once released, vWF multimers form elongated strings that retain platelets at sites of endothelial injury. Weibel-Palade bodies also contain P-selectin, angiopoietin-2, osteoprotegerin, the tetraspanin CD63/Lamp3, as well as cytokines, which are believed to be present as a result of incidental packaging.[23] The stored pool of vWF may be mobilized quickly to the endothelial surface, where it binds to exposed collagen and participates in the formation of a primary platelet hemostatic plug. The endothelium modulates this response further by regulating vWF size, and thereby its activity, through the action of the EC product ADAMTS13 (a disintegrin and metalloproteinase with thrombospondin type I motif, number 13).[24] This protease cleaves released vWF at Tyr1605-Met1606 to generate smaller-sized polymers and to decrease the propensity for platelet thrombus formation.[24] Thus the endothelium uses geographical separation of factors that regulate its anti- and prothrombotic functions to maintain blood fluidity, yet allow for a hemostatic response to vascular injury.

Semipermeable Barrier and Transendothelial Transport Pathways

The endothelial monolayer serves as a size-selective semipermeable barrier that restricts the free bidirectional transit of water, macromolecules, and circulating or resident cells between the bloodstream and underlying vessel wall or tissues. Permeability function is determined in part by the architectural arrangement of the endothelial monolayer, as well as the activation of pathways that facilitate the transendothelial transport of fluids, molecules, and cells. This transport occurs via either transcellular pathways that involve vesicle formation, trafficking, and transcytosis, or by the loosening of interendothelial junctions and paracellular pathways (Fig. 2.1).[25] Molecules that traverse the endothelium by paracellular pathways are size restricted to a radius of 3 nm or less, whereas those of larger diameter may be actively transported across the cell in vesicles.[26] Although the diffusive flux of water occurs in ECs through aquaporin transmembrane water channels, the contribution of these channels to hydraulic conductivity and cellular permeability is limited.[27]

There is significant macrostructural heterogeneity of the endothelial monolayer that reflects the functional and metabolic requirements of the underlying tissue and has consequences for its permeability function. Endothelium may be arranged in either a continuous or discontinuous manner: continuous endothelium is either nonfenestrated or fenestrated.[4–6] Continuous nonfenestrated endothelium forms a highly exclusive barrier and is found in the arterial and venous blood vessels of the heart, lung, skin, connective tissue, muscle, retina, spinal cord, brain, and mesentery.[4–6] By contrast, continuous fenestrated endothelium is located in vessels that supply organs involved in filtration or with a high demand for transendothelial transport, including renal glomeruli, the ascending vasa recta and peritubular capillaries of the kidney, endocrine, and exocrine glands, intestinal villi, and the choroid plexus of the brain.[4–6] These ECs are characterized by fenestrae, or transcellular pores, with a diameter of 50 to 80 nm that, in the majority of cells, has a 5- to 6-mm nonmembranous diaphragm across the pore opening.[4–6,25] The distribution of these fenestrae may be polarized within the EC and allow for enhanced barrier size selectivity owing to the diaphragm.[4–6] Discontinuous endothelium is found in the bone marrow, spleen, and liver sinusoids. This type of endothelial monolayer is notable for its large-diameter fenestrae (100 to 200 nm) with absent diaphragms and gaps, and a poorly organized underlying basement membrane, which is permissive for transcellular flow of water and solutes as well as cellular trafficking.[4–6]

Transcellular and paracellular pathways are two distinct routes by which plasma proteins, solutes, and fluids traverse the endothelial monolayer. The transcellular pathway provides a receptor-mediated mechanism to transport albumin, lipids, and hormones across the endothelium.[25,28,29] The paracellular pathway is dependent upon the structural integrity of adherens, tight, and gap junctions and allows fluids and solutes to permeate between ECs but restricts the passage of large molecules.[28,29] Although these pathways were believed to function independently, it is now recognized that they are interrelated and together modulate permeability under basal conditions.

The transcellular transport of albumin and albumin-bound macromolecules is initiated by albumin binding to gp60, or albondin, a 60-kDa albumin-binding protein located in flask-shaped caveolae that reside at the cell surface.[30,31] These caveolae are cholesterol- and sphingolipid-rich structures that contain caveolin-1. Once activated, gp60 interacts with caveolin-1, followed by constriction of the caveolae neck and fission from the cell surface.[32,33] These actions lead to the formation of vesicles with a diameter of about 70 nm and vesicle transcytosis. Caveolae may contain as much as 15% to 20% of the cell volume, so they are capable of moving significant amounts of fluid across the cell through this mechanism.[32,33] Once vesicles have detached from the membrane, they undergo vectorial transit to the abluminal membrane, where they dock and fuse with the plasma membrane by interacting with vesicle-associated and membrane-associated target soluble N-ethylmaleimide-sensitive factor attachment receptors (SNAREs).[34] Once docked, the vesicles release their cargo to the interstitial space. Vesicles may traverse the cell as individual structures, or cluster to form channel-like structures with a diameter of 80 to 200 nm that span the cell.[4,6] Although transcellular vesicle trafficking is the predominant mechanism by which cells transport albumin, it is now appreciated that this pathway is not absolutely necessary for permeability function, owing to the compensatory capabilities of the paracellular pathway.

The junctions between ECs include the adherens, tight, and gap junctions; only the former two modulate permeability and comprise the paracellular pathway.[35] Adherens junctions are normally impermeant to albumin and other large molecules and are the major determinant of endothelial barrier function and permeability. The expression of tight

Transcellular   **Paracellular**

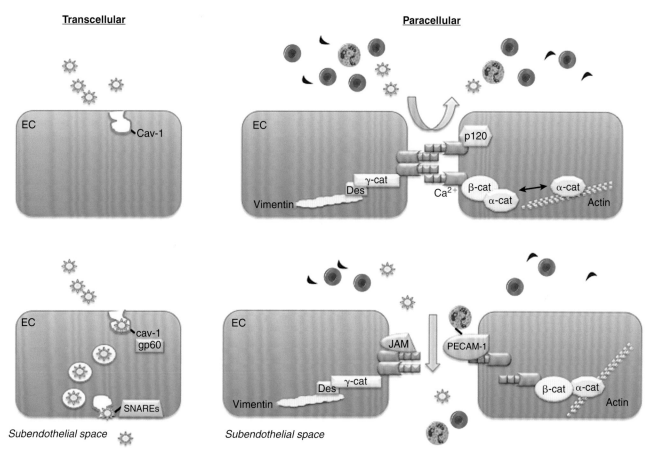

Fig. 2.1 Transendothelial Transport Mechanisms. The endothelium is a semipermeable membrane that facilitates transendothelial transport of solutes, macromolecules, and cells via a transcellular pathway *(left)* or a paracellular pathway *(right)*. The transcellular pathway allows for transit of albumin and other large molecules across the endothelium using caveolae as the transport mechanism. Once caveolin-1 *(cav-1)* interacts with gp60, caveolae separate from cell surface to form vesicles that undergo vectorial transit to the endoluminal surface. Here, the vesicles fuse with soluble *N*-ethylmaleimide-sensitive factor attachment receptors *(SNAREs)* and release their cargo to the subendothelial space. By contrast, the paracellular pathway relies on the integrity of adherens junctions between endothelial cells *(EC)*. Vascular endothelial (VE)-cadherin molecules from adjacent ECs form a barrier that is maintained by β-catenin *(β-cat)*, α-catenin *(α-cat)*, and γ-catenin *(γ-cat)*. Some mediators that increase permeability do so by promoting actin cytoskeletal rearrangement, leading to physical separation of the VE-cadherin molecules and passage of solutes and proteins. Platelet–endothelial cell adhesion molecule-1 *(PECAM-1)* and junctional adhesion molecules *(JAM)* present in the adherens junction also allow leukocytes to traffic through the adherens junction. (Modified from Komarova Y, Malik AB. Regulation of endothelial permeability via paracellular and transcellular transport pathways. *Annu Rev Physiol.* 2010;72:463–493.)

junctions, by contrast, is limited to the blood-brain or blood-retinal barriers where they restrict or prevent the passage of small molecules (<1 kDa) and some inorganic ions.[25] Gap junctions are composed of connexins that form a channel between adjacent cells to enhance cell-cell communication and facilitate the transit of water, small molecules, and ions.[25]

Adherens junctions are critical for maintaining endothelial barrier functional integrity and are composed of complexes of vascular endothelial (VE)-cadherin and catenins. VE-cadherin is a transmembrane GP with five extracellular repeats, a transmembrane segment, and a cytoplasmic tail. The external domains mediate the calcium-dependent hemophilic adhesion between VE-cadherin molecules expressed in adjacent cells.[28,29,36] The cytoplasmic tail interacts with β-catenin, plakoglobin (γ-catenin), and p120 catenin to control the organization of VE-cadherin and the actin cytoskeleton at adherens junctions. The actin binding proteins α-actinin, annexin 2, formin-1, and eplin may further stabilize this interaction. Other

proteins located in adherens junctions thought to provide stability include junctional adhesion molecules (JAMs) and platelet-EC adhesion molecule 1 (PECAM-1).[25]

Endothelial permeability may be increased or decreased through mechanisms that involve adherens junction remodeling or through interactions with the actin cytoskeleton.[28,29,37] These events may occur rapidly, be transient or sustained, and are reversible. Most commonly, mediators that increase endothelial permeability either destabilize adherens junctions through phosphorylation, and thereby internalization, of VE-cadherin or by RhoA activation and actin cytoskeletal rearrangement to physically pull apart VE-cadherin molecules and adherens junctions, resulting in intercellular gaps.[25] To counteract these effects, other mediators that attenuate permeability are present in the plasma or interstitial space. Fibroblast growth factor (FGF) stabilizes VE-cadherin by stabilizing VE-cadherin-gp120-catenin interaction. Sphingosine-1-phosphate and the protein tyrosine phosphatases (PTP) 1B, PTPμ, and PTPβ also stabilize adherens junctions.[38] This effect occurs through activation of Rac1/Rap1/Cdc42 signaling and reorganization of the actin cytoskeleton, recycling of VE-cadherin to the cell surface, and (re)assembly of adherens junctions. The cytokine angiopoietin-1 stabilizes adherens junctions by inhibiting endocytosis of VE-cadherin.[28,29,39,40] These actions are also mediated by calcium signaling, which regulates hyperpermeability of the endothelium via the transient receptor potential channel (TRPC) superfamily. The TRPC channels facilitate extracellular Ca^{2+} entry into ECs exposed to stimuli for edema and for angiogenesis.[38]

Endothelial tight junctions predominate in specialized vascular beds that require an impermeable barrier. These tight junctions are composed of the specific tight junction proteins occludin, claudins (3/5), and JAM-A.[25,39–41] Occludin and claudins are membrane proteins that contain four transmembrane and two extracellular loop domains. The extracellular loop domains of these proteins bind similar domains on neighboring cells to seal the intercellular cleft and to prevent permeability. Occludin, claudins, and JAM-A are also tethered to the actin cytoskeleton by α-catenin and zona occludens proteins (ZO-1, ZO-2).[38] The ZO proteins also function as guanylyl kinases or scaffolding proteins and use PDZ and Sc homology 3 (SH3)-binding domains to recruit other signaling molecules. Connections between tight junctions and the actin cytoskeleton are stabilized further via the actin cross-linking proteins spectrin or filamen, or by the accessory proteins cingulin and AF-6.[38,40] In this manner, the junctions remain stabilized and sealed to limit or prevent transendothelial transport of fluids and molecules.

Regulation of Vascular Tone

Since the early seminal studies of Furchgott and Zawadski, it has been increasingly recognized that the endothelium regulates vascular tone via endothelium-derived factors that maintain a balance between vasoconstriction and vasodilation (Fig. 2.2).[38,39,42,43] The endothelium produces both gaseous and peptide vasodilators, including NO, hydrogen sulfide, PGI_2, and endothelium-derived hyperpolarizing factor (EDHF). The effects of these substances on vascular tone are counterbalanced by vasoconstrictors that are either synthesized or processed by the endothelium, such as thromboxane A_2 (TxA_2), a product of arachidonic acid metabolism, and the peptides endothelin-1 (ET-1) and angiotensin II (Ang-II). The relative importance of these vasodilator or vasoconstrictor substances for maintaining vascular tone differs between vascular beds, with NO serving as the primary vasodilator in large conduit elastic vessels and non-NO mechanisms playing a greater role in the microcirculation.

NO is synthesized by three structurally similar NO synthase (NOS) isoenzymes: the constitutive enzyme identified in the endothelium (eNOS or NOS3) and neuronal cells (nNOS or NOS1) or the inducible enzyme (iNOS or NOS2) found in smooth muscle cells (SMCs), neutrophils, and macrophages following exposure to endotoxin or inflammatory cytokines.[44–46] NO is generated via a five-electron oxidation reaction of L-arginine to form L-citrulline and stoichiometric amounts of NO, and requires molecular oxygen and the reduced form of nicotinamide adenosine dinucleotide phosphate (NADPH) as co-substrates and flavin adenine dinucleotide, flavin mononucleotide,

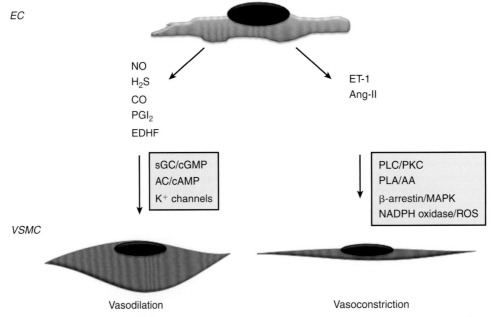

Fig. 2.2 Endothelium-derived Vasoactive Factors. Endothelium modulates vascular tone by synthesizing or participating in activation of vasoactive peptides that promote vascular smooth muscle cell *(VSMC)* vasodilation or relaxation. The vasodilator gases nitric oxide *(NO)* and carbon monoxide *(CO)* activate soluble guanylyl cyclase *(sGC)* to increase cyclic guanosine monophosphate *(cGMP)* levels, although NO has a far greater affinity for sGC than CO. Hydrogen sulfide *(H₂S)*, similar to endothelium-derived hyperpolarizing factor *(EDHF)* activates potassium channels. Prostacyclin *(PGI₂)* promotes vasodilation by activating adenylyl cyclase *(AC)* to increase cyclic adenosine monophosphate *(cAMP)* levels that influence calcium handling by sarcoplasmic reticulum calcium ATPase. Endothelium also synthesizes the vasoconstrictor peptide endothelin-1 *(ET-1)* and metabolizes angiotensin I *(Ang-I)* to angiotensin II *(Ang-II)*. These vasoconstrictor peptides activate phospholipase C *(PLC)* and protein kinase C *(PKC)* signaling, phospholipase A *(PLA)* and arachidonic acid *(AA)* metabolism, activate mitogen-activated protein kinase *(MAPK)* signaling through β-arrestin-cSrc signaling, or increase nicotinamide adenosine dinucleotide phosphate *(NADPH)* oxidase activity and reactive oxygen species *(ROS)* levels.

heme, and tetrahydrobiopterin as cofactors.[47–49] In the endothelium, eNOS expression is up-regulated by a diverse array of stimuli including transforming growth factor (TGF)-β1, lysophosphatidylcholine, hydrogen peroxide, tumor necrosis factor (TNF)-α, oxidized low-density lipoprotein (LDL) cholesterol, laminar shear stress, and hypoxia, and is subject to both posttranscriptional and posttranslational modifications that influence activity, including phosphorylation, acetylation, palmitoylation, and myristolation, as well as localization to caveolae.[49] Once generated, NO diffuses into SMCs and reacts with the heme iron of guanylyl cyclase to increase cyclic guanosine monophosphate (cGMP) levels and to promote vasodilation.[46] NO can also react with SH-containing molecules and proteins (e.g., peroxynitrite, N_2O_2) to generate S-nitrosothiols, a stable reservoir of bioavailable NO with recognized antiplatelet and vasodilator effects.[50–52] In the presence of oxygen, NO can be oxidized to nitrite and nitrate, which are stable end-products of NO metabolism; nitrite serves as a vasodilator, predominantly in the pulmonary and cerebral circulations.[52,53] In addition to vasodilator and antiplatelet effects, NO has other paracrine effects that include regulation of VSMC proliferation and migration, and leukocyte adhesion and activation.[17]

Hydrogen sulfide gas generated by the endothelium also possesses vasodilator properties. Hydrogen sulfide is membrane permeable and released as a byproduct of cysteine or homocysteine metabolism via the transulfuration/cystathionine-β-synthase and cystathionine-γ-lyase pathway or by the catabolism of cysteine via cysteine aminotransferase and 3-mercaptopyruvate sulfur transferase. Hydrogen sulfide-mediated vasodilation results from the activation of K_{ATP} and transient receptor membrane channel currents.[54–56]

PGI_2 is an eicosanoid generated by cyclooxygenase (COX) and arachidonic acid metabolism in the endothelium. It promotes vasodilation via adenylyl cyclase/cyclic adenosine monophosphate (cAMP) signal transduction pathways. PGI_2 also induces smooth muscle relaxation by reducing cytoplasmic Ca^{2+} availability; decreases VSMC proliferation through a cAMP-peroxisome proliferator-activated receptor (PPAR)-γ-mediated mechanism, and limits inflammation by decreasing interleukin (IL)-1 and IL-6.[57] Importantly, PGI_2 has significant antiplatelet effects and by decreasing TxA_2 levels, limits platelet aggregation. Because both COX-1 (constitutively expressed) and COX-2 (induced) contribute to basal PGI_2 production, selective pharmacological inhibition of either isoform may result in diminished PGI_2 levels, increased platelet aggregation, and impaired vasodilation.[58]

No single molecule has been identified as the vasodilator referred to as endothelium-derived hyperpolarizing factor (EDHF), and the effects attributed to EDHF likely represent the composite actions of several agents that share a common mechanism. EDHF is an important vasodilator in the microcirculation and acts by opening K^+ channels to allow for K^+ efflux, hyperpolarization, and vascular smooth muscle relaxation. Candidate EDHFs include the 11, 12-epoxyeicosatrienoic acids and hydrogen peroxide.[43,59–62]

To counterbalance the effects of endothelium-derived vasodilators, the endothelium also synthesizes the vasoconstrictor ET-1 and metabolizes Ang I to Ang II. ET-1, a 21-amino-acid peptide, is synthesized initially as inactive pre-proET-1 that is processed by endothelin-converting enzymes to its active form.[63,64] ET-1 binds to the G protein-coupled receptors (GPCRs) ET_A and ET_B: ECs express ET_B, whereas SMCs express both receptors. Although the activation of endothelial ET_B increases NO production, concomitant activation of SMC ET_A and ET_B results in prolonged and long-lasting vasoconstriction that predominates.[65]

There is no evidence that ET-1 is stored for immediate early release in the endothelium, indicating that acute stimuli such as hypoxia,

TGF-β, and shear stress that increase ET-1 production do so via a transcriptional mechanism; however, ET-1 and endothelin-converting enzyme are packaged in Weibel-Palade bodies.[66] Endothelium also expresses angiotensin-converting enzyme (ACE) and, as such, modulates processing of Ang-I to the vasoconstrictor peptide Ang-II.[67] Ang-II-stimulated activation of the Ang-I receptor results in vasoconstriction and SMC hypertrophy and proliferation, in part, by activating NADPH oxidase to increase reactive oxygen species (ROS) production.[68–70] Therefore vascular tone is determined by the balance of vasodilator and vasoconstrictor substances synthesized or processed by the endothelium in response to stimuli; each vasoactive mediator may attain individual importance in a different vascular bed.

Regulating Response to Inflammatory and Immune Stimuli

The endothelium monitors circulating blood for foreign pathogens, and participates in immunosurveillance by expressing Toll-like receptors (TLRs) 2, 3, and 4.[71–73] These TLRs identify pathogen-associated molecular patterns that are common to bacterial cell wall proteins or viral deoxyribonucleic acid (DNA) and ribonucleic acid (RNA) in the bloodstream. Once activated, TLRs elicit an inflammatory response through the activation of nuclear factor (NF)-κB and generation of chemokines that promote transendothelial migration of leukocytes, have chemoattractant and mitogenic effects, and increase endothelial oxidant stress and apoptosis.[71,72] The quiescent endothelium maintains its antiinflammatory phenotype through expression of cytokines with antiinflammatory properties and cytoprotective antioxidant enzymes that limit oxidant stress. The endothelium synthesizes TGF-β1, which inhibits synthesis of the proinflammatory cytokines monocyte chemotactic protein-1 (MCP-1) and IL-8; expression of the TNF-α receptor; NF-κB-mediated proinflammatory signaling; and leukocyte adherence to the luminal surface of the endothelium.[74,75] Endothelium also expresses a wide array of antioxidant enzymes, including catalase, the superoxide dismutases, glutathione peroxidase-1, peroxiredoxins, and glucose-6-phosphate dehydrogenase.[48] Through the actions of these antioxidant enzymes, ROS are reduced, and the redox environment remains stable. This homeostatic redox modulation also limits activation of ROS-stimulated transcription factors such as NF-κB, activator protein-1, specificity protein-1, and PPARs.[52] The inflammatory phenotype of the endothelium is also influenced by other circulating or paracrine factors that have antioxidant or antiinflammatory properties, such as high-density lipoprotein (HDL) cholesterol, IL-4, IL-10, IL-13, and IL-1 receptor antagonist.[76–78]

The endothelium is capable of mounting a rapid inflammatory response that involves the actions of chemoattractant cytokines, or chemokines, and their associated receptors to facilitate interactions between leukocytes and the endothelium. ECs express the chemokine receptors CXCR4, CCR2, and CCR8 on the luminal or abluminal surface of cells.[79] These receptors bind and transport chemokines to the opposite side of the cell to generate a chemoattractant gradient for inflammatory cell homing. HS, which is present in the endothelial glycocalyx, may serve as a chemokine presenter and is necessary for the action of some chemokines such as CXCL8, CCL2, CCL4, and CCL5.[80,81]

ECs also express the Duffy antigen receptor for chemokines (DARC) that participates in chemokine transcytosis across cells. DARC is a member of the silent chemokine receptor family that has high homology to GPCRs and can bind a broad spectrum of inflammatory CC and CXC chemokines, including MCP-1, IL-8, and CCL5 or Regulated upon Activation, Normal T-cell Expressed, and Secreted (RANTES), but does not activate G-protein signaling.[82–84] Exposure to chemokines, in turn, activates cellular signaling pathways that promote

EC-leukocyte interactions; however, homing of leukocytes to tissues is mediated directly by cell surface adhesion molecules.

Endothelium expresses selectins and immunoglobulin (Ig)-like cell surface adhesion molecules that regulate endothelial–leukocyte interactions. P-selectin and E-selectin are lectin-like transmembrane GPs. These selectins mediate leukocyte adhesion through Ca^{2+}-dependent binding of their N-terminal C-type lectin-like domain with a sialyl-Lewis X capping structure ligand present on leukocytes.[85-87] P-selectin is stored in Weibel-Palade bodies where it can be mobilized rapidly to the cell surface in response to thrombin, histamine, complement activation, ROS, and inflammatory cytokines. Cell surface expression of P-selectin is limited to minutes.[87] By contrast, E-selectin requires de novo protein synthesis for its expression. E-selectin is expressed on the cell surface, but it may also be found in its biologically active form in serum as a result of proteolytic cleavage from the cell surface.[86,87] These selectins bind the leukocyte ligands P-selectin glycoprotein ligand-1 (PSGL-1), E-selectin-ligand-1, and CD44, each of which appears to have a distinct function: PSGL-1 is implicated in the initial tethering of leukocytes to the endothelium, E-selectin-ligand-1 converts transient initial tethers to slower and more stable rolling, and CD44 controls the speed of rolling.[86-88]

The Ig-like cell surface adhesion molecules expressed by the endothelium are intercellular adhesion molecule (ICAM)-1, ICAM-2, vascular cell adhesion molecule (VCAM)-1, and PECAM-1. ICAM-1 is expressed at low levels in the endothelium, but its expression is upregulated several-fold by TNF-α or IL-1. ICAM-1 is active when it exists as a dimer and is able to bind macrophage adhesion ligand-1 or lymphocyte function-associated antigen-1[89] on leukocytes to facilitate transendothelial migration.[87,90] The clustering of ICAM-1 stimulates endothelial cytoskeletal rearrangements to form cuplike structures on the endothelial surface and remodel adherens junction complexes to enhance leukocyte transendothelial migration.[87,91] ICAM-2, by contrast, is constitutively expressed at high levels by the endothelium, but its expression is downregulated by inflammatory cytokines; however, ICAM-2 is believed to play a role in cytokine-stimulated migration of eosinophils and dendritic cells.[92,93] VCAM-1 is also up-regulated by inflammatory cytokines, binds to very late antigen-4 on leukocytes, and activates Rac-1 to increase NADPH oxidase activity and ROS production.[87] PECAM-1 is expressed abundantly in adherens junctions and is involved in homophilic interaction between endothelial and leukocyte PECAM-1. This interaction stimulates targeted trafficking of segments of EC membrane to surround a leukocyte in preparation for transendothelial migration and typically occurs within 1 or 2 μm of an intact endothelial junction.[87] Therefore the determination as to whether a leukocyte migrates paracellularly or transcellularly appears to be dependent upon the relative tightness of endothelial junctions.

Vascular Repair and Remodeling

The vessel wall undergoes little proliferation or remodeling under ambient conditions, with the exception of repair or remodeling associated with physiological processes such as wound healing or menses. When the endothelial monolayer sustains a biochemical or biomechanical injury resulting in EC death and denudation, loss of contact inhibition stimulates the normally quiescent adjacent ECs to proliferate. If the injury is limited, locally proliferating ECs will cover the injured site. However, if the area of injury is larger, circulating blood cells are recruited to aide proliferating resident ECs and reestablish vascular integrity.[94]

A subset of circulating blood cells that participate in vascular repair expresses cell surface proteins that were thought to be endothelial-specific and subsequently referred to as endothelial progenitor cells (EPCs). These cells were identified by the expression of CD31, lectin binding, and acetylated LDL uptake in culture; could be expanded in vitro to phenotypically resemble mature ECs; and when administered in vivo could promote vascular repair and regeneration at sites of ischemia. It is now recognized that these putative EPCs are likely not true progenitor cells for the endothelium, but represent a mixed population of cells that include proangiogenic hematopoietic cells (myeloid or monocyte lineage), circulating ECs that that are viable but nonproliferative, and endothelial colony-forming cells that are viable, proliferative, and emerge at day 14 when cultured in vitro.[94-96] This latter cell type is recognized as the repair effector in vascular injury and is defined as having an unequivocal EC phenotype, capacity to proliferate, and self-assembles into viable vascular networks. These endothelial colony-forming cells are distinguished by expression of CD31, vWF, CD146, VE-cadherin, and vascular endothelial growth factor receptor 2 (VEGFR2), and are negative for CD14 and CD45.[97] They reside in the bone marrow as well as in specific niches in postnatal organs and vessel wall. Within blood vessels, it is believed that they are located in niches in the subendothelial matrix or in the vasculogenic zone in the adventitia.[98]

Putative EPCs were initially thought to promote vascular repair by incorporating into and contributing structurally to the vessel wall, but more recent evidence supports a paracrine role. Once these cells are recruited to sites of injury, they secrete growth and angiogenic factors that promote and support endothelial proliferation. In fact, these cells are known to secrete high levels of vascular endothelial growth factor (VEGF), hepatocyte growth factor (HGF), granulocyte colony-stimulating factor, and granulocyte-macrophage colony-stimulating factor.[94,95] Other paracrine functions of putative EPCs include the release of exosomes that may transfer mediators directly to the endothelium.[99] These cells also provide transient residence as immediate placeholders at the site of endothelial injury and may reside there until proliferation of the endothelial monolayer is complete.[95]

Mechanotransduction of Hemodynamic Forces

The endothelium is subjected to the effects of hemodynamic forces such as hydrostatic pressure, cyclic stretch, and fluid shear stress, which occur as a consequence of blood pressure and pulsatile blood flow in the vasculature (Fig. 2.3). In the vascular tree, there is a gradient of pulsatile pressure that is proportional to vessel diameter, ranges from around 120 to 100 mm Hg in the aorta to about 0 to 30 mm Hg in the microcirculation, and modulates other hemodynamic forces.[92] ECs mechanotransduce these forces into cellular responses via ion channels, integrins, and GPCRs, as well as cytoskeletal deformations or displacements.[100,101]

Several key mechanotransducers expressed by the endothelium, such as the nonselective cationic ion channel PIEZO1 and the GPCR GPR68, respond to changes in shear stress by increasing intracellular calcium to stimulate flow-mediated vascular dilation and vascular remodeling.[102,103] The endothelial monolayer is exposed to variable levels of shear stress in the vascular tree that are inversely proportional to the radius of the vessel and range from 1 to 6 dyn/cm^2 in veins and from 10 to 70 dyn/cm^2 in arteries.[101] Physiological shear stress promotes a quiescent endothelial phenotype with cells that are aligned morphologically in the direction of flow, owing to the influence of laminar flow and shear on NO release. Increases in shear stress stimulate compensatory EC and SMC hypertrophy to expand the vessel and thereby return shear forces to basal levels. Conversely, a decrease in shear can narrow the lumen of the vessel in an endothelium-dependent manner.[101] Flow in tortuous vessels or at bifurcations is characterized by flow reversals, low flow velocities, and flow separation that cause shear stress gradients. Here, ECs acquire a polygonal shape with diminished cell and cytoskeletal alignment with flow.[5,76] This disturbed flow profile

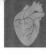

Atheroprotective

Atheroprone

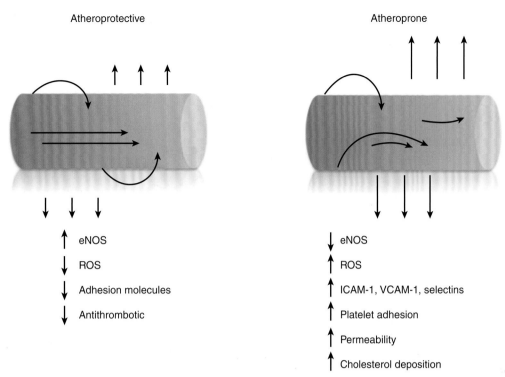

↑ eNOS

↓ ROS

↓ Adhesion molecules

↓ Antithrombotic

↓ eNOS

↑ ROS

↑ ICAM-1, VCAM-1, selectins

↑ Platelet adhesion

↑ Permeability

↑ Cholesterol deposition

Fig. 2.3 Effects of Hemodynamic Forces on Endothelial Functions. Endothelium is subjected to the effects of hemodynamic forces such as shear stress, cyclic strain, and pulsatile pressure. Under ambient conditions, these forces are generally atheroprotective and increase the expression of nitric oxide synthase *(eNOS)* to generate nitric oxide *(NO)*, decrease reactive oxygen species *(ROS)* and oxidant stress, decrease expression of proinflammatory adhesion molecules, and maintain an antithrombotic surface. When these forces are increased or perturbed, loss of laminar shear stress, increased cyclic strain, or increased pulse pressure leads to a decrease in eNOS expression, an increase in ROS levels, and the up-regulation of proinflammatory and prothrombotic mediators, which can lead to cholesterol oxidation and deposition to initiate atherosclerosis. *ICAM-1,* Intercellular adhesion molecule-1; *VCAM-1,* vascular cell adhesion molecule-1.

contributes to the development of endothelial dysfunction at these susceptible locations.[5,101] The association between endothelial dysfunction and perturbations in endothelial shear stress was confirmed in patients who underwent coronary artery endothelial function testing and computational fluid dynamics analysis of shear stress in the same vessel. The lowest levels of endothelial shear stress were detected in coronary artery segments with abnormal epicardial and microvascular endothelial function.[104]

Cyclic strain is circumferential deformation of the blood vessel wall associated with distension and relaxation with each cardiac cycle.[92] Under ambient conditions, cyclic strain averages roughly 2% at 1 Hz in the aorta, but may increase to over 30% when hypertension is present.[94,95] In the endothelial monolayer, individual cells are typically arranged so they are oriented perpendicular to the stretch axis. However, when strain levels are increased to pathophysiological levels, this orientation is lost, and stress fibers parallel the direction of stretch.[105,106] While physiologic levels of cyclic strain impart an antiproliferative effect on the endothelium via induction of CDKN1A,[107] elevated levels of cyclic strain increase endothelial matrix metalloproteinases (MMPs) and induce remodeling of the ECM as well as VE-cadherin and adherens junctions.[108]

In addition to physical forces imposed upon them, ECs are capable of generating traction stress and exerting force against the extracellular environment. These traction forces are mediated by stress fibers, actin–myosin interactions, and other proteins that anchor cells to focal adhesions. Traction forces are distributed heterogeneously within ECs with higher forces detected at cell-cell junctions; however, among neighboring ECs, junctional forces were asymmetrically dispersed.[109] These self-generated forces are important for cell shape stability, regulate endothelial permeability and connectivity by applying force to cell junctions, and promote endothelial network formation by creating tension-based guidance pathways by which ECs sense each other at a distance.[100,110–113]

ENDOTHELIAL HETEROGENEITY

Within the vascular tree, there is significant regional heterogeneity of the endothelium that occurs as a result of differences in developmental assignment, cellular structure, and surrounding environmental factors.[5,76,114] This heterogeneity is evidenced further by differences in endothelial protein expression of eNOS, HSP90, SOD1, SOD2, SOD3, and p67[phox] in different conduit arteries and between the conduit arteries and their corresponding veins. There are similar differences in transcriptional expression of eNOS, KLF2, and KLF4 between the endothelium in atheroresistant compared to atheroprone vessels prior to the development of disease.[115] This heterogeneity exists to support the specialized functions of the underlying vascular beds and tissues. As a result of these differences, the normal adult endothelium also exhibits functional heterogeneity in the homeostatic properties common to all ECs (Fig. 2.4). For instance, the endothelium functions as a semipermeable membrane that regulates transport of fluid, proteins, and macromolecules. Under basal conditions, this takes place primarily across capillaries, albeit at differing rates throughout the vascular beds with less permeability in nonfenestrated endothelium characterized

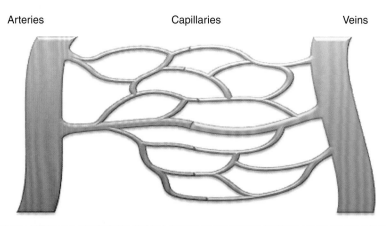

	Arteries	Capillaries	Veins
Hemostasis	TM tPA EPCR	TM TFPI	TM EPCR vWF
Inflammation	ICAM-1 VCAM-1	ICAM-1 VCAM-1	E-selectin P-selectin ICAM-1 VCAM-1
Permeability	+	+	+ +
Vascular tone	+ +	−	−

Fig. 2.4 Functional Heterogeneity of the Endothelium. The endothelium is adapted both structurally and functionally to serve the needs of the underlying vascular bed. Between the arterial, capillary, and venous systems, there are regional differences in the expression of anticoagulant and antithrombotic factors and inflammatory adhesion molecules. Permeability tends to be increased preferentially at postcapillary venules, whereas vascular tone is regulated by arterioles. *EPCR,* Endothelial protein C receptor; *ICAM-1,* intercellular adhesion molecule-1; *TFPI,* tissue factor plasminogen inactivator; *TM,* thrombomodulin; *tPA,* tissue plasminogen activator; *VCAM-1,* vascular cell adhesion molecule-1; *vWF,* von Willebrand factor.

by fewer caveolae and abundant tight junctions compared to vascular beds with fenestrated endothelium.[76] However, when stimulated with histamine, serotonin, bradykinin, or VEGF, the endothelium in post-capillary venules responds by increasing permeability either through the retraction of adherens junctions and the formation of interendothelial gaps, or via increased transendothelial transcytosis. This phenomenon is supported by increased expression of receptors for these agonists in the postcapillary venules.[5,76,116,117]

Transendothelial migration of leukocytes occurs at postcapillary venules in the skin, mesentery, and muscle, whereas in the lung and liver, this function takes place mostly at the level of the capillaries. In lymph nodes, this function occurs at the high endothelial venules.[118] Activated ECs that are largely restricted to postcapillary venules and express E-selectin mediate this function.[119] P-selectin, which is stored in Weibel-Palade bodies, is also preferentially expressed by endothelium in postcapillary venules, with levels of highest expression in the lung and mesentery.[120] By contrast, ICAM-1 and VCAM-1 may be expressed throughout the vasculature and respond rapidly to induction by lipopolysaccharide or cytokines. Although interactions between leukocytes and the endothelium occur typically in postcapillary venules, they can also occur in arterioles, capillaries, and large veins.[76]

The endothelium regulates hemostatic functions largely through expression of both anticoagulant and antiplatelet factors that are unevenly distributed throughout the vasculature. For instance, endothe-lium in the arterial system expresses thrombomodulin, tPA, and the endothelial protein C receptor; capillaries express thrombomodulin and TFPI; and thrombomodulin, the endothelial protein C receptor, and vWF are typically expressed in veins.[4,6,121] Owing to the differential expression of these factors across vascular beds, there are local differences in the endothelial regulation of blood fluidity and hemostasis commensurate with the endothelial phenotype. Endothelium also regulates vascular tone and does so at the level of the resistance arterioles through the release of site-specific vasodilator and vasoconstrictor molecules. The endothelium is the predominant source of NO generated by eNOS, and expression of eNOS is greater in the arterial than the venous system.[7] Thus, many of these functional heterogeneities allow the endothelium to respond to (patho)physiological stimuli and to adapt to a changing environment.

ENDOTHELIAL DYSFUNCTION AND VASCULAR DISEASE

Although the endothelium that resides at different locations within the vascular tree may be uniquely adapted to suit the local environment, there are circumstances where a prolonged or aberrant stimulus may lead to phenotype transition, endothelial dysfunction, and progress to frank vascular disease. When challenged with these (patho)physiological stimuli, the endothelium undergoes phenotype transition to an activated state. Activated ECs modulate their basal homeostatic functions to adapt to the aberrant stimuli and may display a broad spectrum of responses.

The endothelial monolayer can demonstrate increased permeability to plasma proteins and transendothelial migration of leukocytes, increased adhesion of inflammatory cells, and fluctuating imbalances in pro- and antithrombotic substances, vasodilators and vasoconstrictors, and growth factors. When these phenotypic changes are chronic and irreversible, they lead to maladaptive responses that result in permanent alterations in the structure and function of the endothelial monolayer; this phenomenon is known as endothelial dysfunction. Endothelial dysfunction is now understood to play an integral role in a number of vascular disease processes.

Thrombosis

Thrombus formation at sites of vascular injury is a physiological process localized to the endothelial surface. In contrast, intravascular thrombosis is a pathophysiological event that occurs at sites of vascular injury, and the response is augmented by concomitant endothelial dysfunction. These events may be associated with a chronic vascular injury process, such as atherosclerosis and plaque erosion, or with a more acute injury pattern that occurs with infection/autoimmune reactions, vascular compromise resulting from atherosclerotic encroachment on the vessel lumen, or percutaneous coronary intervention (PCI)-associated mechanical trauma to the endothelial monolayer. Emerging evidence also supports a role for immune-mediated thrombosis as a mechanism to protect the endothelium from circulating pathogens. The thrombus forms a physical barrier to prevent dissemination of pathogens to the endothelium and throughout the circulation, while individual platelets may engulf viruses to sequester them from the endothelium.[122] In conjunction with exposure to these pathophysiological stimuli, the activated endothelium is faced with loss of its anticoagulant cell surface-associated molecules, lower levels of antithrombotic NO, and expression of the prothrombotic factors tissue factor and vWF, as well as platelets that are recruited to the site of injury.[44,46,123–126] Thrombosis is augmented further by increases in endothelial ROS and oxidant stress, inhibition of tPA activity by plasminogen activator inhibitor-1 (PAI-1) generated by activated ECs, and alterations in shear stress and other mechanical forces as blood fluidity is diminished.[10,86,101]

Pulmonary Arterial Hypertension

Pulmonary arterial hypertension (PAH) is characterized by an angio-proliferative pulmonary vasculopathy localized to the precapillary pulmonary arterioles. This disorder occurs due to endothelial dysfunction, dysregulated apoptosis-resistant VSMC proliferation, inflammation, immune cell activation, and thrombosis that obliterates the vessel lumen to create plexiform lesions, which are pathognomonic for the disease.[127] This aberrant vascular remodeling results in a sustained increase in the mean pulmonary artery pressure ≥ 25 mm Hg and pulmonary vascular resistance greater than 3 Wood units, which ultimately leads to right ventricular hypertrophy, right ventricular failure, and death.[128] The observed increase in pulmonary vascular filling pressures is attributable to the remodeled pulmonary vasculature as well as to decreased bioavailable NO and PGI_2, increased endothelium-derived ROS generated by uncoupled eNOS and NADPH oxidase activation, and elevated levels of the TxA_2 and ET-1, which favor a state of persistent vasoconstriction.[129,130]

In heritable and idiopathic forms of PAH, downregulation of bone morphogenetic protein receptor type 2 (BMPR2) is associated with widespread loss of pulmonary artery EC viability and increased apoptosis causing the remaining ECs to hyperproliferate and contribute to neointima formation. This phenomenon has been attributed to impaired BRCA1-dependent DNA repair, Wnt signaling, and dimin-

ished apelin secretion.[131,132] Moreover, targeting endothelial apoptosis with the bone morphogenetic protein (BMP) ligand BMP9, which is a circulating vascular quiescence factor, reverses established PAH in preclinical models.[133] The pulmonary artery endothelium contributes to vascular remodeling through endothelial-to-mesenchymal transition (EndoMT) with myofibroblasts originating from ECs populating remodeled arteries in response to miR-21 and HIF-2α activation.[134] EndoMT myofibroblasts express both endothelial (CD31, CD34, VE-cadherin) and mesenchymal (αSMA, fibronectin 1) markers, as well as overexpress the transcription factors TWIST1, SNAIL, and SLUG.[135,136]

Metabolic reprogramming, reminiscent of the Warburg effect initially described for cancer cells, is characteristic of the pulmonary artery endothelium in PAH.[137] Pulmonary artery ECs demonstrate evidence of increased glycolytic flux, decreased oxidative phosphorylation, and upregulation of the pentose phosphate shunt, as well as enhanced glutaminolysis.[138] This metabolic switch under normoxic conditions underlies the PAH pulmonary artery EC pathophenotype.

Vasculitis

The primary systemic vasculitides differentially affect vessels based on size and, as such, are grouped accordingly. Takayasu arteritis is a large-vessel type that affects the aorta and its major branches, whereas granulomatosis with polyangiitis (formerly known as Wegener granulomatosis) affects mostly small vessels and occurs as a vasculitis that primarily affects the kidneys and lungs. Vasculitis affecting the coronary arteries and small vessels may also occur following cocaine exposure.[139–141] Although these vasculitides represent heterogeneous disease processes, they share the endothelium as the common target and propagator of an immuno-inflammatory reaction that occurs in the vessel wall. This immuno-inflammatory reaction may be so profound, as is seen in systemic lupus erythematosus (SLE), that antiendothelial antibodies are generated. These processes result in vascular immune-complex deposition, complement activation, and neutrophil-induced injury to the endothelial monolayer that results in EC activation, apoptosis, and in some areas, denudation.[142,143] Cocaine-induced vasculitis has been attributed to the levamisole component (used to dilute the cocaine), which causes an antineutrophil cytoplasmic antibody (ANCA)-associated vasculitis. This vasculitis is often proteinase 3 and myeloperoxidase positive. Other resident activated ECs synthesize and secrete cytokines, growth factors, and chemokines that include IL-1, IL-6, IL-8, and MCP-1.[123] Repeated injury to the endothelium from prolonged attack by immune and inflammatory cells can stimulate a prothrombotic and profibrotic response that ultimately leads to vessel occlusion and abnormal vascular remodeling.

Vascular Calcification

There is increasing preclinical evidence that the vascular endothelium contributes to the pathogenesis of vascular calcification, in part, by giving rise to osteoprogenitor cells, and lineage tracing studies have confirmed that some osteogenic cells in the vessel wall have an endothelial origin.[144] In addition, in the absence of calcification inhibitors, such as matrix Gla protein, EndoMT may occur via serine protease activation in the endothelium leading to a population of resident mesenchymal cells that calcify in the vessel wall.[145] Endothelial overexpression of tissue-non-specific alkaline phosphatase also promotes vascular calcification by stimulating the underlying VSMCs to acquire an osteoblast-like phenotype. The smooth muscle cells express key osteoblast transcription factors, such as Runx2, and calcification proteins, including osteocalcin and osteopontin, indicating that increased endothelial alkaline phosphatase activity is sufficient to induce vascular calcification.[146,147] Endothelial exposure to the procalcific mediator receptor activator of NF-κB ligand (RANKL) activates the noncanonical (NF-κB)/p52 signaling pathway and paracrine signaling to initiate vascular smooth muscle cell transition to an osteoblast-like phenotype.[148] The relationship between endothelial dysfunction and vascular calcification has been demonstrated in patients with chronic kidney disease: patients with vascular calcification had elevated levels of circulating endothelial microparticles as compared to those without evidence of vascular involvement.[149]

Atherosclerosis

Atherosclerosis is a progressive disease of blood vessels that is initiated by endothelial dysfunction and is now recognized as a chronic inflammatory and immune process. Atherosclerosis is characterized by the accumulation of lipid, thrombus, and inflammatory cells within the vessel wall.[52,150–152] This process may acutely occlude the vessel lumen, as occurs with plaque rupture and thrombosis, or result in a more chronic but stable process that eventually encroaches on the vessel lumen. In either event, atherosclerosis can lead to end-organ ischemia and ensuing infarction of the heart, brain, vital organs, or extremities. Early endothelial dysfunction associated with atherosclerosis is evidenced by the presence of a subendothelial accumulation of lipids and infiltration of monocyte-derived macrophages and other immune cells to form the fatty streak. Among the risk factors associated with the development of atherosclerosis, diabetes mellitus, tobacco use, hyperlipidemia, and hypertension are all known to induce endothelial dysfunction.[153] However, within the vasculature, the branch points and bifurcations tend to be the most atherosclerosis-prone segments, indicating that hemodynamic profiles and complex nonuniform flow is also of importance for endothelial dysfunction.[93,122] Once atherosclerosis is established, the endothelium continues to modify the progression of disease by recruiting inflammatory and immune cells and platelets; diminished NO production, enhanced permeability, and the production of prothrombotic species are believed to contribute to plaque progression.[52,150–152,154]

FUNCTIONAL ASSESSMENT OF THE ENDOTHELIUM

Nitric Oxide–mediated Vasodilation

Owing to the importance of endothelial function for vascular health, assessments of endothelial-dependent vasodilator responses, which reflect endothelial NO generation and NO bioavailability, have been advanced as predictors of adverse cardiovascular events. These studies are based on the principle that a healthy endothelium, when challenged with a physiological stress such as shear stress, or an endothelium-dependent vasodilator such as acetylcholine, will release NO, leading to a measurable vasodilatory response. In contrast, when the endothelium is dysfunctional or diseased, these stimuli will elicit a vasoconstrictor or significantly diminished vasodilator response. In humans, this phenomenon, which recapitulates the preclinical studies of Furchgott and Zawadski, was first demonstrated following the intracoronary administration of acetylcholine to patients with angiographically diseased or normal epicardial coronary arteries. Here, the patients with prevalent atherosclerosis demonstrated paradoxical vasoconstriction when infused with acetylcholine, but normal vasodilator responses when challenged with the NO donor nitroglycerin. Patients with normal vessels dilated appropriately to both agents.[155]

Subsequently, a close correlation between coronary artery vasodilation in response to acetylcholine and noninvasive measurements of flow-mediated dilation of the brachial artery was demonstrated. Imaging of the brachial artery with high-resolution vascular ultrasound to detect flow-mediated dilation or the use of strain-gauge forearm plethysmography to assess forearm blood flow in response to pharmacological stimuli that release NO are both accepted methodologies for evaluating endothelial function.[156–158] Analogous to flow-mediated dilation, low-flow-mediated constriction, which quantifies the decrease in artery diameter to restricted blood flow and altered shear stress in the conduit vessel, has been evaluated as a measure of endothelial function. Low-flow-mediated constriction is impaired in individuals with coronary artery disease (CAD) risk factors or established atherosclerosis. Low-flow-mediated constriction when combined with flow-mediated vasodilation provides additive information to improve the detection of CAD.[159] To date, these methods have been used to demonstrate impaired endothelium-dependent vascular reactivity in adults with risk factors for atherosclerosis in the absence of overt atherothrombotic cardiovascular disease; in children with diabetes mellitus, hypercholesterolemia, and congenital heart disease; and to demonstrate improved function in patients treated with 3-hydroxy-3-methylglutaryl-coenzyme A reductase inhibitors (statins) or ACE inhibitors.[160–164]

Measurement of peripheral arterial tonometry is a newer methodology to examine endothelial function. This device utilizes finger-mounted probes with an inflatable membrane that record a pulse wave in the presence and absence of flow-mediated dilation. This method has been shown to correlate well with endothelial dysfunction assessed by brachial artery flow-mediated dilation and to predict cardiovascular events.[165,166]

Newer techniques involving molecular imaging and gaseous microbubbles that are detectable by ultrasound are emerging as a methodology to evaluate endothelial function. This technique relies on the use of nanocarrier-encapsulated microbubbles, which may be tagged with antibodies such as P-selectin, to enhance targeting to the dysfunctional endothelium. Release of the microbubbles at the target destination provides the detectable signal.[167] Alternative strategies involve the infusion of a nanocarrier-encapsulated compound that reacts with a biomarker of interest, such as ROS, and generates a gas that is detected by ultrasound.[168]

Asymmetrical Dimethylarginine as a Biochemical Marker of Nitric Oxide Bioavailability

The endogenous competitive NOS inhibitor asymmetrical dimethylarginine (ADMA) has been suggested as a biomarker for decreased NO bioavailability and endothelial function. ADMA generated by the hydrolysis of methylated arginine residues is subject to intracellular degradation by dimethylarginine dimethylaminohydrolase (DDAH), but the activity of this enzyme is decreased significantly by oxidant stress.[169–172] This in turn leads to increases in plasma ADMA levels, a finding that has been demonstrated in patients with risk factors for atherosclerosis or established CAD.[173–176] With respect to endothelial function, a cross-sectional study of individuals enrolled in the Cardiovascular Risk in Young Finns Study confirmed a significant, albeit modest, inverse relationship between ADMA levels and endothelial function assessed by flow-mediated vasodilation.[177] Despite these findings, in a community-based sample, ADMA levels were not associated with cardiovascular disease incidence or all-cause mortality in diabetic patients.[178] Based on these observations, in certain populations, ADMA levels alone may not provide a full assessment of endothelial function; direct measurements of endothelial vasodilator capacity may be required.[179]

The Gut Microbiome and Trimethylamine N-Oxide

The gut metabolism of the dietary methylamines choline, L-carnitine, and phosphatidylcholine yields the proatherogenic species trimethylamine N-oxide (TMAO) via hepatic metabolism of its microbiome-derived precursor trimethylamine (TMA). Plasma levels of L-carnitine predict increased risk of cardiovascular disease and myocardial infarction, stroke, or death in individuals with high TMAO levels.[179] Elevated TMAO levels compared with levels in the lowest tertile were associated with a hazard ratio of 2.54 (95% CI: 1.96–3.28, $P < .01$) for increased risk of major adverse cardiovascular events and predicted risk of events after adjustment for traditional CAD risk factors.[180] Increased levels of TMAO also enhance platelet reactivity and thrombosis risk. Platelets directly exposed to TMAO have a multi-submaximal stimulus-dependent platelet activation through augmented calcium release.[181] In preclinical models, TMAO causes endothelial function by increasing ROS activation, proinflammatory cytokines, and decreasing eNOS expression that was associated with impaired endothelium-dependent relaxation.[182]

Endothelial Extracellular Matrix Vesicles

Endothelial ECM vesicles have been considered a surrogate biomarker for endothelial dysfunction.[183] ECs can release membrane vesicles with a diameter of approximately 0.1 to 1.0 μm that include microparticles, exosomes, and apoptotic bodies. These vesicles protect extracellular RNA from degradation, promote cellular communication, protect contents from phagocytosis, and remove molecular debris.[184] They are formed from plasma membrane blebbing and package endothelial proteins that include VE-cadherin, PECAM-1, ICAM-1, E-selectin, endoglin, VEGFR 2, S-endo, α_v integrin, and eNOS.[183,185] Although many of these proteins are expressed by microparticles derived from other cell types, the presence of VE-cadherin and E-selectin indicates EC origin. Endothelial microparticle formation is stimulated by TNF-α, ROS, inflammatory cytokines, lipopolysaccharides, thrombin, and low shear stress.[185] They have procoagulant properties as a result of exposed phosphatidylserines and tissue factor that is present in the microparticle, as well as proinflammatory properties. Endothelium-derived extracellular vesicles also transfer microRNAs to the recipient endothelium to regulate NF-κB signaling, inflammation, and EC activation.[184]

Techniques to measure circulating endothelial microparticles rely on differential centrifugation in platelet-free plasma and on the identification of cell-surface CD antigens.[183,185] Thus, they may not be as convenient a measure of endothelial function as currently available noninvasive imaging techniques. Nonetheless, circulating endothelial microparticles have been measured and found to be elevated in a number of patient populations with risk factors or diseases associated with endothelial dysfunction.[185] Increased levels of endothelial microparticles have been demonstrated and shown to correlate with flow-mediated dilation in individuals with end-stage renal disease, acute coronary syndromes (ACS), metabolic syndrome, diabetes, and systemic and pulmonary hypertension.[88,186–190]

CONCLUSIONS

The endothelium is a structurally and metabolically dynamic interface that resides between circulating blood elements, the vascular wall, and the underlying tissues served by these blood vessels. Owing to its unique anatomical location, the endothelium regulates thrombosis and hemostasis, immuno-inflammatory responses, vascular permeability, and vascular tone. These homeostatic functions are responsive to alterations in the local and systemic environments. Failure to adapt to (patho)physiological stimuli may activate aberrant compensatory mechanisms that alter the endothelial phenotype and promote endothelial dysfunction. As techniques to assess endothelial function advance, the clinical utility of this measure, coupled with biochemical and molecular assessments to define an endothelial phenotype profile, will provide a unique understanding of an individual's VE function and guide both prognosis and therapeutic interventions.

REFERENCES

1. Schwann T. *Microscopical Researches into the Accodance in the Structure and Growth of Animals and Plants.* London: Syndenham Society; 1847.
2. Hwa C, Aird WC. The history of the capillary wall: doctors, discoveries, and debates. *Am J Physiol Heart Circ Physiol.* 2007;293(5):H2667–H2679.
3. His W. *Die Häute und Höhlen des Körpers.* Basel: Schwighauser; 1865.
4. Aird WC. Phenotypic heterogeneity of the endothelium: I. Structure, function, and mechanisms. *Circ Res.* 2007;100(2):158–173.
5. Gimbrone M. Vascular endothelium: nature's blood container. In: Gimbrone M, ed. *Vascular Endothelium in Hemostasis and Thrombosis.* New York: Churchill Livingstone; 1986:1–13.
6. Aird WC. Phenotypic heterogeneity of the endothelium: II. Representative vascular beds. *Circ Res.* 2007;100(2):174–190.
7. dela Paz NG, D'Amore PA. Arterial versus venous endothelial cells. *Cell Tissue Res.* 2009;335(1):5–16.
8. Corada M, Morini MF, Dejana E. Signaling pathways in the specification of arteries and veins. *Arterioscler Thromb Vasc Biol.* 2014;34(11):2372–2377.
9. van Geemen D, Smeets MW, van Stalborch AM, et al. F-actin-anchored focal adhesions distinguish endothelial phenotypes of human arteries and veins. *Arterioscler Thromb Vasc Biol.* 2014;34(9):2059–2067.
10. van Hinsbergh VW. Endothelium-role in regulation of coagulation and inflammation. *Semin Immunopathol.* 2012;34(1):93–106.
11. Navarro S, Bonet E, Estelles A, et al. The endothelial cell protein C receptor: its role in thrombosis. *Thromb Res.* 2011;128(5):410–416.
12. Rezaie AR. Regulation of the protein C anticoagulant and antiinflammatory pathways. *Curr Med Chem.* 2010;17(19):2059–2069.
13. Conway EM. Thrombomodulin and its role in inflammation. *Semin Immunopathol.* 2012;34(1):107–125.
14. Kasthuri RS, Glover SL, Boles J, Mackman N. Tissue factor and tissue factor pathway inhibitor as key regulators of global hemostasis: measurement of their levels in coagulation assays. *Semin Thromb Hemost.* 2010;36(7):764–771.
15. Zhang J, Piro O, Lu L, Broze GJ Jr. Glycosyl phosphatidylinositol anchorage of tissue factor pathway inhibitor. *Circulation.* 2003;108(5):623–627.
16. Atkinson B, Dwyer K, Enjyoji K, Robson SC. Ecto-nucleotidases of the CD39/NTPDase family modulate platelet activation and thrombus formation: potential as therapeutic targets. *Blood Cells Mol Dis.* 2006;36(2):217–222.
17. Welch G, Loscalzo J. Nitric oxide and the cardiovascular system. *J Card Surg.* 1994;9(3):361–371.
18. Bazan JF. Structural design and molecular evolution of a cytokine receptor superfamily. *Proc Natl Acad Sci U S A.* 1990;87(18):6934–6938.
19. Jasuja R, Furie B, Furie BC. Endothelium-derived but not platelet-derived protein disulfide isomerase is required for thrombus formation in vivo. *Blood.* 2010;116(22):4665–4674.
20. Breitenstein A, Tanner FC, Luscher TF. Tissue factor and cardiovascular disease: quo vadis? *Circ J.* 2010;74(1):3–12.
21. Bach RR. Tissue factor encryption. *Arterioscler Thromb Vasc Biol.* 2006;26(3):456–461.
22. Torisu T, Torisu K, Lee IH, et al. Autophagy regulates endothelial cell processing, maturation and secretion of von Willebrand factor. *Nat Med.* 2013;19(10):1281–1287.
23. Valentijn KM, Sadler JE, Valentijn JA, et al. Functional architecture of Weibel-Palade bodies. *Blood.* 2011;117(19):5033–5043.
24. Lowenberg EC, Meijers JC, Levi M. Platelet-vessel wall interaction in health and disease. *Neth J Med.* 2010;68(6):242–251.
25. Komarova Y, Malik AB. Regulation of endothelial permeability via paracellular and transcellular transport pathways. *Annu Rev Physiol.* 2010;72:463–493.
26. Pappenheimer JR, Renkin EM, Borrero LM. Filtration, diffusion and molecular sieving through peripheral capillary membranes; a contribution to the pore theory of capillary permeability. *Am J Physiol.* 1951;167(1):13–46.
27. Fischbarg J. Fluid transport across leaky epithelia: central role of the tight junction and supporting role of aquaporins. *Physiol Rev.* 2010;90(4):1271–1290.
28. Dejana E, Orsenigo F, Molendini C, et al. Organization and signaling of endothelial cell-to-cell junctions in various regions of the blood and lymphatic vascular trees. *Cell Tissue Res.* 2009;335(1):17–25.

29. Dejana E, Tournier-Lasserve E, Weinstein BM. The control of vascular integrity by endothelial cell junctions: molecular basis and pathological implications. *Dev Cell.* 2009;16(2):209–221.

30. Tiruppathi C, Finnegan A, Malik AB. Isolation and characterization of a cell surface albumin-binding protein from vascular endothelial cells. *Proc Natl Acad Sci U S A.* 1996;93(1):250–254.

31. Tiruppathi C, Song W, Bergenfeldt M, et al. Gp60 activation mediates albumin transcytosis in endothelial cells by tyrosine kinase-dependent pathway. *J Biol Chem.* 1997;272(41):25968–25975.

32. Predescu D, Palade GE. Plasmalemmal vesicles represent the large pore system of continuous microvascular endothelium. *Am J Physiol.* 1993;265(2 Pt 2):H725–H733.

33. Predescu SA, Predescu DN, Palade GE. Endothelial transcytotic machinery involves supramolecular protein-lipid complexes. *Mol Biol Cell.* 2001;12(4):1019–1033.

34. Hu C, Ahmed M, Melia TJ, et al. Fusion of cells by flipped SNAREs. *Science.* 2003;300(5626):1745–1749.

35. Mehta D, Malik AB. Signaling mechanisms regulating endothelial permeability. *Physiol Rev.* 2006;86(1):279–367.

36. Weber C, Fraemohs L, Dejana E. The role of junctional adhesion molecules in vascular inflammation. *Nat Rev Immunol.* 2007;7(6):467–477.

37. Spindler V, Schlegel N, Waschke J. Role of GTPases in control of microvascular permeability. *Cardiovasc Res.* 2010;87(2):243–253.

38. Komarova YA, Kruse K, Mehta D, Malik AB. Protein interactions at endothelial junctions and signaling mechanisms regulating endothelial permeability. *Circ Res.* 2017;120(1):179–206.

39. Mochizuki N. Vascular integrity mediated by vascular endothelial cadherin and regulated by sphingosine 1-phosphate and angiopoietin-1. *Circ J.* 2009;73(12):2183–2191.

40. Curry FR, Adamson RH. Vascular permeability modulation at the cell, microvessel, or whole organ level: towards closing gaps in our knowledge. *Cardiovasc Res.* 2010;87(2):218–229.

41. Taddei A, Giampietro C, Conti A, et al. Endothelial adherens junctions control tight junctions by VE-cadherin-mediated upregulation of claudin-5. *Nat Cell Biol.* 2008;10(8):923–934.

42. Furchgott RF, Zawadzki JV. The obligatory role of endothelial cells in the relaxation of arterial smooth muscle by acetylcholine. *Nature.* 1980;288(5789):373–376.

43. Triggle CR, Ding H. The endothelium in compliance and resistance vessels. *Front Biosci (Schol Ed).* 2011;3:730–744.

44. Michel T, Vanhoutte PM. Cellular signaling and NO production. *Pflugers Arch.* 2010;459(6):807–816.

45. Searles CD, Miwa Y, Harrison DG, Ramasamy S. Posttranscriptional regulation of endothelial nitric oxide synthase during cell growth. *Circ Res.* 1999;85(7):588–595.

46. Walford G, Loscalzo J. Nitric oxide in vascular biology. *J Thromb Haemost.* 2003;1(10):2112–2118.

47. Bredt DS, Hwang PM, Glatt CE, et al. Cloned and expressed nitric oxide synthase structurally resembles cytochrome P-450 reductase. *Nature.* 1991;351(6329):714–718.

48. Bredt DS, Hwang PM, Snyder SH. Localization of nitric oxide synthase indicating a neural role for nitric oxide. *Nature.* 1990;347(6295):768–770.

49. Dudzinski DM, Michel T. Life history of eNOS: partners and pathways. *Cardiovasc Res.* 2007;75(2):247–260.

50. Handy DE, Loscalzo J. Nitric oxide and posttranslational modification of the vascular proteome: S-nitrosation of reactive thiols. *Arterioscler Thromb Vasc Biol.* 2006;26(6):1207–1214.

51. Upchurch GR, Welch GN, Loscalzo J. The vascular biology of S-nitrosothiols, nitrosated derivatives of thiols. *Vasc Med.* 1996;1(1):25–33.

52. Leopold JA, Loscalzo J. Oxidative risk for atherothrombotic cardiovascular disease. *Free Radic Biol Med.* 2009;47(12):1673–1706.

53. Stamler JS, Singel DJ, Loscalzo J. Biochemistry of nitric oxide and its redox-activated forms. *Science.* 1992;258(5090):1898–1902.

54. Bhatia M. Hydrogen sulfide as a vasodilator. *IUBMB Life.* 2005;57(9):603–606.

55. Wang R. Hydrogen sulfide: a new EDRF. *Kidney Int.* 2009;76(7):700–704.

56. Li L, Rose P, Moore PK. Hydrogen sulfide and cell signaling. *Annu Rev Pharmacol Toxicol.* 2011;51:169–187.

57. Parkington HC, Coleman HA, Tare M. Prostacyclin and endothelium-dependent hyperpolarization. *Pharmacol Res.* 2004;49(6):509–514.

58. Feletou M, Huang Y, Vanhoutte PM. Endothelium-mediated control of vascular tone: COX-1 and COX-2 products. *Br J Pharmacol.* 2011;164(3):894–912.

59. Matoba T, Shimokawa H, Nakashima M, et al. Hydrogen peroxide is an endothelium-derived hyperpolarizing factor in mice. *J Clin Invest.* 2000;106(12):1521–1530.

60. Edwards G, Dora KA, Gardener MJ, et al. K+ is an endothelium-derived hyperpolarizing factor in rat arteries. *Nature.* 1998;396(6708):269–272.

61. Campbell WB, Fleming I. Epoxyeicosatrienoic acids and endothelium-dependent responses. *Pflugers Arch.* 2010;459(6):881–895.

62. Shimokawa H. Hydrogen peroxide as an endothelium-derived hyperpolarizing factor. *Pflugers Arch.* 2010;459(6):915–922.

63. Kohan DE, Rossi NF, Inscho EW, Pollock DM. Regulation of blood pressure and salt homeostasis by endothelin. *Physiol Rev.* 2011;91(1):1–77.

64. Yanagisawa M, Kurihara H, Kimura S, et al. A novel potent vasoconstrictor peptide produced by vascular endothelial cells. *Nature.* 1988;332(6163):411–415.

65. Watts SW. Endothelin receptors: what's new and what do we need to know? *Am J Physiol Regul Integr Comp Physiol.* 2010;298(2):R254–R260.

66. Rondaij MG, Bierings R, Kragt A, et al. Dynamics and plasticity of Weibel-Palade bodies in endothelial cells. *Arterioscler Thromb Vasc Biol.* 2006;26(5):1002–1007.

67. Danser AH, Saris JJ, Schuijt MP, van Kats JP. Is there a local renin-angiotensin system in the heart? *Cardiovasc Res.* 1999;44(2):252–265.

68. Griendling KK, Minieri CA, Ollerenshaw JD, Alexander RW. Angiotensin II stimulates NADH and NADPH oxidase activity in cultured vascular smooth muscle cells. *Circ Res.* 1994;74(6):1141–1148.

69. Zafari AM, Ushio-Fukai M, Akers M, et al. Role of NADH/NADPH oxidase-derived H2O2 in angiotensin II-induced vascular hypertrophy. *Hypertension.* 1998;32(3):488–495.

70. Garrido AM, Griendling KK. NADPH oxidases and angiotensin II receptor signaling. *Mol Cell Endocrinol.* 2009;302(2):148–158.

71. Tobias PS. TLRs in disease. *Semin Immunopathol.* 2008;30(1):1–2.

72. Tobias PS, Curtiss LK. Toll-like receptors in atherosclerosis. *Biochem Soc Trans.* 2007;35(Pt 6):1453–1455.

73. Zimmer S, Steinmetz M, Asdonk T, et al. Activation of endothelial toll-like receptor 3 impairs endothelial function. *Circ Res.* 2011;108(11):1358–1366.

74. Feinberg MW, Jain MK. Role of transforming growth factor-beta1/Smads in regulating vascular inflammation and atherogenesis. *Panminerva Med.* 2005;47(3):169–186.

75. Kofler S, Nickel T, Weis M. Role of cytokines in cardiovascular diseases: a focus on endothelial responses to inflammation. *Clin Sci (Lond).* 2005;108(3):205–213.

76. Aird WC. Endothelial cell heterogeneity. *Cold Spring Harb Perspect Med.* 2012;2(1):a006429.

77. Haas MJ, Mooradian AD. Inflammation, high-density lipoprotein and cardiovascular dysfunction. *Curr Opin Infect Dis.* 2011;24(3):265–272.

78. de Vries JE. The role of IL-13 and its receptor in allergy and inflammatory responses. *J Allergy Clin Immunol.* 1998;102(2):165–169.

79. Speyer CL, Ward PA. Role of endothelial chemokines and their receptors during inflammation. *J Invest Surg.* 2011;24(1):18–27.

80. Lortat-Jacob H. The molecular basis and functional implications of chemokine interactions with heparan sulphate. *Curr Opin Struct Biol.* 2009;19(5):543–548.

81. Celie JW, Beelen RH, van den Born J. Heparan sulfate proteoglycans in extravasation: assisting leukocyte guidance. *Front Biosci.* 2009;14:4932–4949.

82. Peiper SC, Wang ZX, Neote K, et al. The Duffy antigen/receptor for chemokines (DARC) is expressed in endothelial cells of Duffy negative individuals who lack the erythrocyte receptor. *J Exp Med.* 1995;181(4):1311–1317.

83. Schnabel RB, Baumert J, Barbalic M, et al. Duffy antigen receptor for chemokines (Darc) polymorphism regulates circulating concentrations of monocyte chemoattractant protein-1 and other inflammatory mediators. *Blood.* 2010;115(26):5289–5299.

84. Horne K, Woolley IJ. Shedding light on DARC: the role of the Duffy antigen/receptor for chemokines in inflammation, infection and malignancy. *Inflamm Res.* 2009;58(8):431–435.

85. Huo Y, Xia L. P-selectin glycoprotein ligand-1 plays a crucial role in the selective recruitment of leukocytes into the atherosclerotic arterial wall. *Trends Cardiovasc Med.* 2009;19(4):140–145.

86. Langer HF, Chavakis T. Leukocyte-endothelial interactions in inflammation. *J Cell Mol Med.* 2009;13(7):1211–1220.

87. Muller WA. Mechanisms of leukocyte transendothelial migration. *Annu Rev Pathol.* 2010;6:323–344.

88. Amabile N, Guerin AP, Leroyer A, et al. Circulating endothelial microparticles are associated with vascular dysfunction in patients with end-stage renal failure. *J Am Soc Nephrol.* 2005;16(11):3381–3388.

89. Yang L, Froio RM, Sciuto TE, et al. ICAM-1 regulates neutrophil adhesion and transcellular migration of TNF-alpha-activated vascular endothelium under flow. *Blood.* 2005;106(2):584–592.

90. Miller J, Knorr R, Ferrone M, et al. Intercellular adhesion molecule-1 dimerization and its consequences for adhesion mediated by lymphocyte function associated-1. *J Exp Med.* 1995;182(5):1231–1241.

91. Shaw SK, Ma S, Kim MB, et al. Coordinated redistribution of leukocyte LFA-1 and endothelial cell ICAM-1 accompany neutrophil transmigration. *J Exp Med.* 2004;200(12):1571–1580.

92. Woodfin A, Voisin MB, Imhof BA, et al. Endothelial cell activation leads to neutrophil transmigration as supported by the sequential roles of ICAM-2, JAM-A, and PECAM-1. *Blood.* 2009;113(24):6246–6257.

93. Huang MT, Larbi KY, Scheiermann C, et al. ICAM-2 mediates neutrophil transmigration in vivo: evidence for stimulus specificity and a role in PECAM-1-independent transmigration. *Blood.* 2006;107(12):4721–4727.

94. Becher MU, Nickenig G, Werner N. Regeneration of the vascular compartment. *Herz.* 2010;35(5):342–351.

95. Richardson MR, Yoder MC. Endothelial progenitor cells: quo vadis? *J Mol Cell Cardiol.* 2011;50(2):266–272.

96. Torsney E, Xu Q. Resident vascular progenitor cells. *J Mol Cell Cardiol.* 2011;50(2):304–311.

97. Medina RJ, Barber CL, Sabatier F, et al. Endothelial progenitors: a consensus statement on nomenclature. *Stem Cells Transl Med.* 2017;6(5):1316–1320.

98. Watt SM, Athanassopoulos A, Harris AL, Tsaknakis G. Human endothelial stem/progenitor cells, angiogenic factors and vascular repair. *J R Soc Interface.* 2010;7(Suppl 6):S731–S751.

99. Li X, Chen C, Wei L, et al. Exosomes derived from endothelial progenitor cells attenuate vascular repair and accelerate reendothelialization by enhancing endothelial function. *Cytotherapy.* 2016;18(2):253–262.

100. Califano JP, Reinhart-King CA. Exogenous and endogenous force regulation of endothelial cell behavior. *J Biomech.* 2010;43(1):79–86.

101. Chiu JJ, Chien S. Effects of disturbed flow on vascular endothelium: pathophysiological basis and clinical perspectives. *Physiol Rev.* 2011;91(1):327–387.

102. Coste B, Mathur J, Schmidt M, et al. Piezo1 and Piezo2 are essential components of distinct mechanically activated cation channels. *Science.* 2010;330(6000):55–60.

103. Xu J, Mathur J, Vessieres E, et al. GPR68 senses flow and is essential for vascular physiology. *Cell.* 2018;173(3):762–775. e16.

104. Siasos G, Sara JD, Zaromytidou M, et al. Local low shear stress and endothelial dysfunction in patients with nonobstructive coronary atherosclerosis. *J Am Coll Cardiol.* 2018;71(19):2092–2102.

105. Lee T, Sumpio BE. Cell signalling in vascular cells exposed to cyclic strain: the emerging role of protein phosphatases. *Biotechnol Appl Biochem.* 2004;39(Pt 2):129–139.

106. Kaunas R, Nguyen P, Usami S, Chien S. Cooperative effects of Rho and mechanical stretch on stress fiber organization. *Proc Natl Acad Sci U S A.* 2005;102(44):15895–15900.

107. Peyton KJ, Liu XM, Durante W. Prolonged cyclic strain inhibits human endothelial cell growth. *Front Biosci (Elite Ed).* 2016;8:205–212.

108. Cummins PM, von Offenberg Sweeney N, Killeen MT, et al. Cyclic strain-mediated matrix metalloproteinase regulation within the vascular endothelium: a force to be reckoned with. *Am J Physiol Heart Circ Physiol.* 2007;292(1):H28–H42.

109. Valent ET, van Nieuw Amerongen GP, van Hinsbergh VW, Hordijk PL. Traction force dynamics predict gap formation in activated endothelium. *Exp Cell Res.* 2016;347(1):161–170.

110. Lu L, Feng Y, Hucker WJ, et al. Actin stress fiber pre-extension in human aortic endothelial cells. *Cell Motil Cytoskeleton.* 2008;65(4):281–294.

111. Lu L, Oswald SJ, Ngu H, Yin FC. Mechanical properties of actin stress fibers in living cells. *Biophys J.* 2008;95(12):6060–6071.

112. Kniazeva E, Putnam AJ. Endothelial cell traction and ECM density influence both capillary morphogenesis and maintenance in 3-D. *Am J Physiol Cell Physiol.* 2009;297(1):C179–C187.

113. Costa KD, Sim AJ, Yin FC. Non-Hertzian approach to analyzing mechanical properties of endothelial cells probed by atomic force microscopy. *J Biomech Eng.* 2006;128(2):176–184.

114. Atkins GB, Jain MK, Hamik A. Endothelial differentiation: molecular mechanisms of specification and heterogeneity. *Arterioscler Thromb Vasc Biol.* 2011;31(7):1476–1484.

115. Simmons GH, Padilla J, Laughlin MH. Heterogeneity of endothelial cell phenotype within and amongst conduit vessels of the swine vasculature. *Exp Physiol.* 2012;97(9):1074–1082.

116. Feng D, Nagy JA, Hipp J, et al. Reinterpretation of endothelial cell gaps induced by vasoactive mediators in guinea-pig, mouse and rat: many are transcellular pores. *J Physiol.* 1997;504(Pt 3):747–761.

117. McDonald DM, Thurston G, Baluk P. Endothelial gaps as sites for plasma leakage in inflammation. *Microcirculation.* 1999;6(1):7–22.

118. Miyasaka M, Tanaka T. Lymphocyte trafficking across high endothelial venules: dogmas and enigmas. *Nat Rev Immunol.* 2004;4(5):360–370.

119. Petzelbauer P, Bender JR, Wilson J, Pober JS. Heterogeneity of dermal microvascular endothelial cell antigen expression and cytokine responsiveness in situ and in cell culture. *J Immunol.* 1993;151(9):5062–5072.

120. McEver RP, Beckstead JH, Moore KL, et al. GMP-140, a platelet alpha-granule membrane protein, is also synthesized by vascular endothelial cells and is localized in Weibel-Palade bodies. *J Clin Invest.* 1989;84(1):92–99.

121. Laszik Z, Mitro A, Taylor Jr. FB, et al. Human protein C receptor is present primarily on endothelium of large blood vessels: implications for the control of the protein C pathway. *Circulation.* 1997;96(10):3633–3640.

122. Koupenova M, Kehrel BE, Corkrey HA, Freedman JE. Thrombosis and platelets: an update. *Eur Heart J.* 2017;38(11):785–791.

123. Levi M. The coagulant response in sepsis and inflammation. *Hamostaseologie.* 2010;30(1):10–12. 4-6.

124. Granger DN, Rodrigues SF, Yildirim A, Senchenkova EY. Microvascular responses to cardiovascular risk factors. *Microcirculation.* 2010;17(3):192–205.

125. Antoniades C, Bakogiannis C, Tousoulis D, et al. Platelet activation in atherogenesis associated with low-grade inflammation. *Inflamm Allergy Drug Targets.* 2010;9(5):334–345.

126. Freedman JE, Loscalzo J, Barnard MR, et al. Nitric oxide released from activated platelets inhibits platelet recruitment. *J Clin Invest.* 1997;100(2):350–356.

127. Leopold JA, Maron BA. Molecular mechanisms of pulmonary vascular remodeling in pulmonary arterial hypertension. *Int J Mol Sci.* 2016;17(5):E761.

128. Galie N, Humbert M, Vachiery JL, et al. 2015 ESC/ERS Guidelines for the diagnosis and treatment of pulmonary hypertension: The Joint Task Force for the Diagnosis and Treatment of Pulmonary Hypertension of the European Society of Cardiology (ESC) and the European Respiratory Society (ERS): endorsed by: Association for European Paediatric and Congenital Cardiology (AEPC), International Society for Heart and Lung Transplantation (ISHLT). *Eur Heart J.* 2016;37(1):67–119.

129. Ghouleh IA, Sahoo S, Meijles DN, et al. Endothelial Nox1 oxidase assembly in human pulmonary arterial hypertension; driver of Gremlin1-mediated proliferation. *Clin Sci (Lond).* 2017;131(15):2019–2035.

130. Lan NSH, Massam BD, Kulkarni SS, Lang CC. Pulmonary arterial hypertension: pathophysiology and treatment. *Diseases.* 2018;6(2):E38.

131. Li M, Vattulainen S, Aho J, et al. Loss of bone morphogenetic protein receptor 2 is associated with abnormal DNA repair in pulmonary arterial hypertension. *Am J Respir Cell Mol Biol.* 2014;50(6):1118–1128.

132. Diebold I, Hennigs JK, Miyagawa K, et al. BMPR2 preserves mitochondrial function and DNA during reoxygenation to promote endothelial cell survival and reverse pulmonary hypertension. *Cell Metab.* 2015;21(4):596–608.

133. Long L, Ormiston ML, Yang X, et al. Selective enhancement of endothelial BMPR-II with BMP9 reverses pulmonary arterial hypertension. *Nat Med.* 2015;21(7):777–785.

134. Ranchoux B, Harvey LD, Ayon RJ, et al. Endothelial dysfunction in pulmonary arterial hypertension: an evolving landscape (2017 Grover Conference Series). *Pulm Circ.* 2018;8(1):2045893217752912.

135. Ranchoux B, Antigny F, Rucker-Martin C, et al. Endothelial-to-mesenchymal transition in pulmonary hypertension. *Circulation.* 2015;131(11):1006–1018.

136. Cho JG, Lee A, Chang W, et al. Endothelial to mesenchymal transition represents a key link in the interaction between inflammation and endothelial dysfunction. *Front Immunol.* 2018;9:294.

137. Frump A, Prewitt A, de Caestecker MP. BMPR2 mutations and endothelial dysfunction in pulmonary arterial hypertension (2017 Grover Conference Series). *Pulm Circ.* 2018;8(2):2045894018765840.

138. Egnatchik RA, Brittain EL, Shah AT, et al. Dysfunctional BMPR2 signaling drives an abnormal endothelial requirement for glutamine in pulmonary arterial hypertension. *Pulm Circ.* 2017;7(1):186–199.

139. Berman M, Paran D, Elkayam O. Cocaine-induced vasculitis. *Rambam Maimonides Med J.* 2016;7(4).

140. Arnaud L, Haroche J, Mathian A, et al. Pathogenesis of Takayasu's arteritis: a 2011 update. *Autoimmun Rev.* 2011;11(1):61–67.

141. Jennette JC. Nomenclature and classification of vasculitis: lessons learned from granulomatosis with polyangiitis (Wegener's granulomatosis). *Clin Exp Immunol.* 2011;164(Suppl 1):7–10.

142. Duval A, Helley D, Capron L, et al. Endothelial dysfunction in systemic lupus patients with low disease activity: evaluation by quantification and characterization of circulating endothelial microparticles, role of anti-endothelial cell antibodies. *Rheumatology (Oxford).* 2010;49(6):1049–1055.

143. Savage CO. Vascular biology and vasculitis. *APMIS Suppl.* 2009;127:37–40.

144. Yao Y, Jumabay M, Ly A, et al. A role for the endothelium in vascular calcification. *Circ Res.* 2013;113(5):495–504.

145. Yao J, Guihard PJ, Blazquez-Medela AM, et al. Serine protease activation essential for endothelial-mesenchymal transition in vascular calcification. *Circ Res.* 2015;117(9):758–769.

146. Savinov AY, Salehi M, Yadav MC, et al. Transgenic overexpression of tissue-nonspecific alkaline phosphatase (TNAP) in vascular endothelium results in generalized arterial calcification. *J Am Heart Assoc.* 2015;4(12).

147. Romanelli F, Corbo A, Salehi M, et al. Overexpression of tissue-nonspecific alkaline phosphatase (TNAP) in endothelial cells accelerates coronary artery disease in a mouse model of familial hypercholesterolemia. *PLoS One.* 2017;12(10):e0186426.

148. Harper E, Rochfort KD, Forde H, et al. Activation of the non-canonical NF-kappaB/p52 pathway in vascular endothelial cells by RANKL elicits pro-calcific signalling in co-cultured smooth muscle cells. *Cell Signal.* 2018;47:142–150.

149. Soriano S, Carmona A, Trivino F, et al. Endothelial damage and vascular calcification in patients with chronic kidney disease. *Am J Physiol Renal Physiol.* 2014;307(11):F1302–F1311.

150. Libby P. Molecular and cellular mechanisms of the thrombotic complications of atherosclerosis. *J Lipid Res.* 2009;50(Suppl):S352–S357.

151. Libby P, Ridker PM, Hansson GK. Inflammation in atherosclerosis: from pathophysiology to practice. *J Am Coll Cardiol.* 2009;54(23):2129–2138.

152. Libby P, Ridker PM, Hansson GK. Progress and challenges in translating the biology of atherosclerosis. *Nature.* 2011;473(7347):317–325.

153. Reriani MK, Lerman LO, Lerman A. Endothelial function as a functional expression of cardiovascular risk factors. *Biomark Med.* 2010;4(3):351–360.

154. Borissoff JI, Spronk HM, ten Cate H. The hemostatic system as a modulator of atherosclerosis. *N Engl J Med.* 2011;364(18):1746–1760.

155. Ludmer PL, Selwyn AP, Shook TL, et al. Paradoxical vasoconstriction induced by acetylcholine in atherosclerotic coronary arteries. *N Engl J Med.* 1986;315(17):1046–1051.

156. Charakida M, Masi S, Luscher TF, et al. Assessment of atherosclerosis: the role of flow-mediated dilatation. *Eur Heart J.* 2010;31(23):2854–2861.

157. Corretti MC, Anderson TJ, Benjamin EJ, et al. Guidelines for the ultrasound assessment of endothelial-dependent flow-mediated vasodilation of the brachial artery: a report of the International Brachial Artery Reactivity Task Force. *J Am Coll Cardiol.* 2002;39(2):257–265.

158. Joyner MJ, Dietz NM, Shepherd JT. From Belfast to Mayo and beyond: the use and future of plethysmography to study blood flow in human limbs. *J Appl Physiol.* 2001;91(6):2431–2441.

159. Gori T, Muxel S, Damaske A, et al. Endothelial function assessment: flow-mediated dilation and constriction provide different and complementary information on the presence of coronary artery disease. *Eur Heart J.* 2012;33(3):363–371.

160. Jarvisalo MJ, Lehtimaki T, Raitakari OT. Determinants of arterial nitrate-mediated dilatation in children: role of oxidized low-density lipoprotein, endothelial function, and carotid intima-media thickness. *Circulation.* 2004;109(23):2885–2889.

161. Jarvisalo MJ, Raitakari M, Toikka JO, et al. Endothelial dysfunction and increased arterial intima-media thickness in children with type 1 diabetes. *Circulation.* 2004;109(14):1750–1755.

162. Pasquali SK, Marino BS, Powell DJ, et al. Following the arterial switch operation, obese children have risk factors for early cardiovascular disease. *Congenit Heart Dis.* 2010;5(1):16–24.

163. Wallace SM, Maki-Petaja KM, Cheriyan J, et al. Simvastatin prevents inflammation-induced aortic stiffening and endothelial dysfunction. *Br J Clin Pharmacol.* 2010;70(6):799–806.

164. Shahin Y, Khan JA, Samuel N, Chetter I. Angiotensin converting enzyme inhibitors effect on endothelial dysfunction: a meta-analysis of randomised controlled trials. *Atherosclerosis.* 2011;216(1):7–16.

165. Matsuzawa Y, Kwon TG, Lennon RJ, et al. Prognostic value of flow-mediated vasodilation in brachial artery and fingertip artery for cardiovascular events: a systematic review and meta-analysis. *J Am Heart Assoc.* 2015;4(11).

166. Lekakis J, Abraham P, Balbarini A, et al. Methods for evaluating endothelial function: a position statement from the European Society of Cardiology Working Group on Peripheral Circulation. *Eur J Cardiovasc Prev Rehabil.* 2011;18(6):775–789.

167. Daiber A, Steven S, Weber A, et al. Targeting vascular (endothelial) dysfunction. *Br J Pharmacol.* 2017;174(12):1591–1619.

168. Perng JK, Lee S, Kundu K, et al. Ultrasound imaging of oxidative stress in vivo with chemically-generated gas microbubbles. *Ann Biomed Eng.* 2012;40(9):2059–2068.

169. Cooke JP. Asymmetrical dimethylarginine: the Uber marker? *Circulation.* 2004;109(15):1813–1818.

170. Cooke JP, Ghebremariam YT. DDAH says NO to ADMA. *Arterioscler Thromb Vasc Biol.* 2011;31(7):1462–1464.

171. Ito A, Tsao PS, Adimoolam S, et al. Novel mechanism for endothelial dysfunction: dysregulation of dimethylarginine dimethylaminohydrolase. *Circulation.* 1999;99(24):3092–3095.

172. Teerlink T. ADMA metabolism and clearance. *Vasc Med.* 2005;10(Suppl 1):S73–S81.

173. Sibal L, Agarwal SC, Home PD, Boger RH. The role of asymmetric dimethylarginine (ADMA) in endothelial dysfunction and cardiovascular disease. *Curr Cardiol Rev.* 2011;6(2):82–90.

174. Abbasi F, Asagmi T, Cooke JP, et al. Plasma concentrations of asymmetric dimethylarginine are increased in patients with type 2 diabetes mellitus. *Am J Cardiol.* 2001;88(10):1201–1203.

175. Kielstein JT, Donnerstag F, Gasper S, et al. ADMA increases arterial stiffness and decreases cerebral blood flow in humans. *Stroke.* 2006;37(8):2024–2029.

176. Kielstein JT, Impraim B, Simmel S, et al. Cardiovascular effects of systemic nitric oxide synthase inhibition with asymmetrical dimethylarginine in humans. *Circulation.* 2004;109(2):172–177.

177. Juonala M, Viikari JS, Alfthan G, et al. Brachial artery flow-mediated dilation and asymmetrical dimethylarginine in the Cardiovascular Risk in Young Finns Study. *Circulation.* 2007;116(12):1367–1373.

178. Boger RH, Sullivan LM, Schwedhelm E, et al. Plasma asymmetric dimethylarginine and incidence of cardiovascular disease and death in the community. *Circulation.* 2009;119(12):1592–1600.

179. Koeth RA, Wang Z, Levison BS, et al. Intestinal microbiota metabolism of L-carnitine, a nutrient in red meat, promotes atherosclerosis. *Nat Med.* 2013;19(5):576–585.

180. Tang WH, Wang Z, Levison BS, et al. Intestinal microbial metabolism of phosphatidylcholine and cardiovascular risk. *N Engl J Med.* 2013;368(17):1575–1584.

181. Zhu W, Gregory JC, Org E, et al. Gut microbial metabolite TMAO enhances platelet hyperreactivity and thrombosis risk. *Cell.* 2016;165(1):111–124.

182. Li T, Chen Y, Gua C, Li X. Elevated circulating trimethylamine N-oxide levels contribute to endothelial dysfunction in aged rats through vascular inflammation and oxidative stress. *Front Physiol.* 2017;8:350.

183. Dignat-George F, Boulanger CM. The many faces of endothelial microparticles. *Arterioscler Thromb Vasc Biol.* 2010;31(1):27–33.

184. Hafiane A, Daskalopoulou SS. Extracellular vesicles characteristics and emerging roles in atherosclerotic cardiovascular disease. *Metabolism.* 2018;85:213–222.

185. Chironi GN, Boulanger CM, Simon A, et al. Endothelial microparticles in diseases. *Cell Tissue Res.* 2009;335(1):143–151.

186. Arteaga RB, Chirinos JA, Soriano AO, et al. Endothelial microparticles and platelet and leukocyte activation in patients with the metabolic syndrome. *Am J Cardiol.* 2006;98(1):70–74.

187. Bakouboula B, Morel O, Faure A, et al. Procoagulant membrane microparticles correlate with the severity of pulmonary arterial hypertension. *Am J Respir Crit Care Med.* 2008;177(5):536–543.

188. Mallat Z, Benamer H, Hugel B, et al. Elevated levels of shed membrane microparticles with procoagulant potential in the peripheral circulating blood of patients with acute coronary syndromes. *Circulation.* 2000;101(8):841–843.

189. Preston RA, Jy W, Jimenez JJ, et al. Effects of severe hypertension on endothelial and platelet microparticles. *Hypertension.* 2003;41(2):211–217.

190. Sabatier F, Darmon P, Hugel B, et al. Type 1 and type 2 diabetic patients display different patterns of cellular microparticles. *Diabetes.* 2002;51(9):2840–2845.

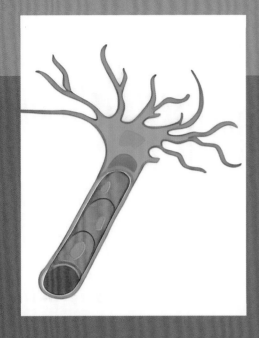

第3章
血管平滑肌

　　血管平滑肌细胞（vessel smooth muscle cells，VSMC）是血管的主要细胞成分之一，它对维持心血管系统的正常功能起着至关重要的作用。几十年来，随着对血管平滑肌细胞的生物物理学、细胞和分子机制研究的不断深入，人们发现血管平滑肌细胞不仅是维持正常心血管系统功能的关键，同时是介导心血管疾病和损伤反应的重要介质。本章重点介绍了血管平滑肌细胞生物学的重新评估；血管平滑肌细胞的起源、谱系、可塑性和基因表达调控的范式转变，以及以上几方面是如何将血管平滑肌细胞定位于正常和病理性血管功能的核心位置，如何将动脉粥样硬化是一种脂质功能障碍疾病的经典学说转变到一种包含炎症及其相关过程的炎症学说。本章讨论的核心是由不同的外源性和内源性因素产生的复杂信号网络，以及如何在不同转录和翻译后水平上调节和整合这些信号网络，从而介导各种不同表型的血管平滑肌细胞在正常生理或疾病、损伤病理中发挥不同的功能。最后，我们介绍了使用组学和成簇规律间隔短回文重复序列/CRISPR关联基因9（clustered regularly interspaced short palindromic repeats/CRISPR associated 9，CRISPRs/Cas 9）介导的基因组修饰等技术对血管细胞和心血管疾病进行的相关研究，这些具有前景的新技术能帮助我们更加全面和系统地了解心血管疾病。

薛　松

Vascular Smooth Muscle

Lula L. Hilenski and Kathy K. Griendling

The centrality of vascular smooth muscle cells (VSMCs) to normal functioning of the cardiovascular system has led to decades of intensive research into the physical, cellular, and molecular mechanisms regulating VSMC biology. VSMCs are the major cell type within the enclosed vascular continuum; they are primarily responsible for adaptations necessary for repeated cycles of contraction and relaxation resulting from cardiac-driven pulsatile blood flow. VSMCs maintain contractile tone by a highly organized architecture of contractile/cytoskeletal proteins and associated regulatory components within the cell cytoplasm and establish distensibility by the synthesis, secretion, and organization of extracellular matrix (ECM) components with elastic recoil and resilience properties.[2] The ability of VSMCs to adapt the expression of proteins involved in contraction and ECM synthesis, according to extrinsic and intrinsic cues during different developmental stages and in disease or response to injury, results from a phenomenon known as VSMC phenotypic modulation, or plasticity, and is a major feature distinguishing VSMCs from terminally differentiated cells.[3]

Just as VSMCs are central to normal physiology, they are also important mediators in cardiovascular disease (CVD) and response to injury. Data from recent clinical trials and advanced technologies have led to reappraisals of VSMC origin, plasticity, gene regulation, and contribution to CVD. Advances in developmental biology and genetic approaches have identified regions of the vascular tree with very distinct boundaries and distinct susceptibilities to CVD. These data suggest that intrinsic epigenetic marks, established early in development and maintained into adulthood, determine localized disease susceptibility and that environmental cues such as shear stress are not the only determinants of disease location.[4] Similar fate-mapping studies have shown that, in addition to the well-studied VSMC phenotypic switch from contractile to synthetic (de-differentiated) in atherosclerotic lesions and response to injury, resident VSMCs in the vascular wall can also transition to macrophage-like and osteoblast-like phenotypes, resulting in inflammation and calcification and leading to unstable atherosclerotic plaques.[5–7] The gene sequencing and "omics" revolution has identified multiple noncoding RNA regulatory molecules, including microRNAs (miRs) and long noncoding RNA (lncRNA), which impact the VSMC phenotype in CVD progression. As a result, current research is focusing on the roles of VSMCs in inflammation and inflammatory processes, calcification, and aging. Finally, there is an increasing appreciation for a more holistic view of the cross talk not only in the physical and chemical communication between vascular wall cells but also among the networks of signaling and molecular processes within cells, such as the redundancy among cellular processes relating to inflammation and aging.

This chapter highlights how these reappraisals of VSMC biology and shifting paradigms on VSMC origins, lineage, plasticity, and regulation of gene expression have positioned VSMCs at center stage in normal and pathological blood vessel function and how the canonical view of atherosclerosis as a disease of lipid dysfunction has been expanded to include inflammation and inflammation-related processes. The discussion centers on the complex webs of signaling networks generated by diverse extrinsic and intrinsic factors and how these networks are regulated and integrated at multiple transcriptional and posttranslational levels to mediate the diverse functions of multiple VSMC phenotypes in normal physiology and disease/injury pathology. Finally, studies of vascular cells and CVD using novel technologies, including omics and **C**lustered **R**egularly **I**nterspaced **S**hort **P**alindromic **R**epeats (CRISPRs)/Cas9-mediated genome modification, are discussed as promising tools for a more comprehensive understanding of CVD.[8]

ORIGINS OF VASCULAR SMOOTH MUSCLE CELLS DURING EMBRYONIC DEVELOPMENT

Initially in embryonic vasculature development, endothelial precursor cells form a common progenitor vessel, which then gives rise to the first artery (dorsal aorta) and vein (cardinal vein) by selective sprouting and subsequent arterial-venous cell segregation.[9] The distinct molecular identities of arteries and veins are regulated by complex interactions of several signaling pathways, including Sonic hedgehog (Shh), a member of the Hedgehog (Hh) family of secreted morphogens; secreted growth factors in the vascular endothelial growth factor family (VEGFs);[10] Notch receptors (Notch 1-4) and Notch ligands (Jagged1,2), and transmembrane proteins that can transduce cell-cell interactions into signals determining cell fates.[11] Interactions of these signals induce differential expression of VEGF receptors, ephrin ligands, and tyrosine kinase Eph receptors on the segregating arterial/venous cells, with ephrin B2 and EphB4 as markers expressed in arteries and veins, respectively.[9,10] Endothelial cells (ECs) within these primordial vascular networks, in response to VEGF signaling, recruit mural cells, including nascent VSMCs.[12]

Nascent VSMCs derive from at least eight independent embryonic origins, including the neural crest of the ectoderm, the lateral plate mesoderm, and the somites of the paraxial mesoderm.[13] These developmental regions are controlled by signaling through bone-morphogenetic protein (BMP), Wnt, and growth factors (fibroblast growth factor [FGF] and transforming growth factor β [TGF-β]) pathways. These embryonic origins are reflected in different anatomical locations within the adult. Ectodermal cardiac neural crest cells give rise to the large elastic arteries, such as the ascending and arch portions of the aorta, the ductus arteriosus, and the branches of the common carotid arteries; proepicardium mesothelial cells produce the coronary arteries; lateral plate mesodermal cells are origins for the abdominal aorta and small muscular arteries; paraxial mesoderm forms the descending aorta; secondary heart field cells form the base of the aorta and pulmonary trunk; and satellite-like mesoangioblasts give rise to the medial layers of arteries.[13]

There is increasing evidence that these lineage-diverse VSMCs exhibit morphologically and functionally distinct properties and respond differently to soluble factors in vitro and to morphogenetic cues in vivo, suggesting that the major determinants of VSMC responses to signals in vascular development and disease are principally lineage-dependent rather than environment-dependent.[14] For example, in vitro–derived VSMC subtypes produced from human pluripotent stem cells (hPSCs) that had initially been induced to form neuroectoderm, lateral plate mesoderm, or paraxial mesoderm showed that origin-specific VSMCs exhibited differential activation of matrix metalloproteinases (MMPs) 9 and tissue inhibitors of MMP (TIMPs) 1 in response to the inflammatory mediator IL-1β. Given that MMPs degrade ECM and induce VSMC migration in pathological remodeling in CVD, these results suggest that site-specific disease development could be due to hard-wired intrinsic differences in the VSMC's proteolytic ability and promigratory responses in disease settings.[15]

Genetic fate-mapping techniques and the use of a triple-transgenic mouse model have shown a new paradigm for the origins and fates of VSMCs. Roostalu et al.[16] used novel lineage tracking to follow the fate of immature VSMCs throughout the life of the animal. The earliest VSMCs formed in the mouse embryo dorsal aorta at E10.5 are uniquely identified by the coexpression of NG2 (neural/glial antigen 2) and CD146 (cell adhesion molecule and receptor for α4 chain of laminin). Aortic VSMCs exhibit a transient expression of CD146, whereas CD146 expression is retained into adulthood in smaller-caliber arteries such as mesenteric and superficial femoral arteries (SFAs). Using this mouse model——with fluorescence expression allowing for the identification of progenitor cells expressing two fluorescent colors and progeny expressing one fluorescent color——CD146/NG2 double-positive VSMCs, indicating immature cells, were found at arterial branch points and flow dividers in the adult. The authors speculate that if these "immature," double-labeled VSMCs at branch points are predisposed to clonal expansion and if equivalent cells exist in human arteries, this finding could support a monoclonal theory of VSMC accumulation in atherosclerotic plaque, as proposed by Benditt and Benditt in 1973.[17] Also expressed at these branching sites is YAP1 (yes-associated protein 1), a transcriptional regulator of CD146. YAP1 is involved in VSMC phenotypic switching and is downregulated in mature VSMCs. In additional studies using the same genetic tools, the authors examined the origin of intimal cells after different degrees of injury in adult mice. They found that after moderate injury to the SFA, most intimal cells came from double-labeled medial VSMCs. However, after severe injury, cells repopulating the injured site came from pluripotent Sca1+ progenitor cells in the adventitia.[18] These data indicate the presence of multiple subsets of immature VSMCs and progenitor cells with a division of labor in normal physiology and pathological remodeling after disease or injury.

The *Hox* genes, a family of conserved developmental control genes specifying positional identity at a given location, function as topographical ZIP codes for localization of VSMCs from different lineages to specific segments within the vascular tree during development, with implications for differential responses and different susceptibility to injury and inflammation in the adult. For example, VSMCs in the descending aorta (derived from paraxial mesoderm) versus atherogenic ascending thoracic and transverse aorta (AA) (derived from neural crest) express different levels of *HoxA9*, a repressor of NF-κB subunit p65; therefore, there are differences in responses in these arterial segments to the proinflammatory and proatherogenic tumor necrosis factor-α (TNF-α)–induced NF-κB activation. These anatomical differences are reflected in regional susceptibility to lesion development. Thus there are intrinsic phenotypic differences among VSMCs, defined by distinct differences in embryonic origin, that are maintained in the adult and determine responses

to inflammatory mediators (e.g., interplay between *HoxA9* and NF-κB), establishing atherosclerosis-resistant and atherosclerosis-susceptible regions in the vasculature independent of hemodynamic factors.[4,19] Therefore environmental cues such as shear stress are not the only important determinant of areas of disease progression.

VASCULAR SMOOTH MUSCLE CELL PHENOTYPIC MODULATION

Characterization of Vascular Smooth Muscle Cell Phenotypes

Given the multiple origins and distinct subpopulations of VSMCs, a compelling central question for understanding VSMC biology is how cells from these diverse embryonic origins, initially expressing lineage-specific pathways, differentiate to express the same marker genes specifically characteristic of VSMCs[14,20] and, additionally, how these same VSMCs, responding to both extrinsic and intrinsic cues, can alter expression of these genes and thus molecular pathways. VSMCs are one of the most plastic cells in the body,[21] but recent studies suggest that there is far more plasticity in these cells than previously acknowledged. Evidence suggests that not only can VSMCs transition to a synthetic phenotype during disease/response to injury, a transition supported by decades of research, but also that VSMCs can transition to macrophage-like cells——assuming macrophage-like characteristics such as phagocytosis, efferocytosis, and reverse cholesterol transport——and to an osteoblast-like phenotype with calcification function (Fig. 3.1). These phenotypic transitions are regulated by multiple different mechanisms: transcriptional, posttranscriptional, and epigenetic. Factors regulating the plasticity of VSMCs include master regulators of contractile genes, such as serum response factor (SRF) and myocardin; ligand-receptor interactions; additional cofactors and signaling pathways such as Kruppel-like factor 4 (KLF4), platelet-derived growth factor (PDGF)-BB, Notch pathway, and TGF-β; epigenetic factors controlling chromatin remodeling and thus the transcription of contractile genes; multiple miRs;[21] and lncRNAs.

Contractile Differentiated Vascular Smooth Muscle Cells

Contractile, or differentiated, VSMCs are characterized by a repertoire of contractile proteins, contractile-regulating proteins, contractile agonist receptors, and signaling proteins responsible for contraction and maintenance of vascular tone.[22-24] Of the VSMC "marker" proteins expressed in the contractile phenotype repertoire (see Fig. 3.1), the most discriminating markers are smooth muscle myosin heavy chain (SM-MHC) in conjunction with SM (smooth muscle) α-actin, smoothelin, SM-22α, h1-calponin, and h-caldesmon.[3] In addition to expression of these proteins associated with the contractile function, contractile VSMCs exhibit differential levels of ECM components (increased collagen types 1 and IV) and of matrix-modifying enzymes (decreased MMPs and increased TIMPs). Contractile VSMCs are further characterized by an elongated, spindle-shaped morphology in culture; a low proliferative rate; expression of α1β1, α7β1 integrins; and the dystrophin-glycoprotein complex (DGPC).[24,25]

Synthetic Dedifferentiated Vascular Smooth Muscle Cells

Synthetic, or dedifferentiated, VSMCs have decreased expression of SMC-related genes for contractile proteins, such as SM-MHC, with concomitantly increased osteopontin, l-caldesmon, nonmuscle myosin heavy chain B (NM-B MHC aka *MYH10*), vimentin, tropomyosin 4, and cellular-retinal binding-protein-1 *(CRBP1)*. "Positive" marker genes, such as *MYH10* or SM MHC embryonic (SMemb), expressed specifically in embryonic or phenotypically modified VSMCs, are

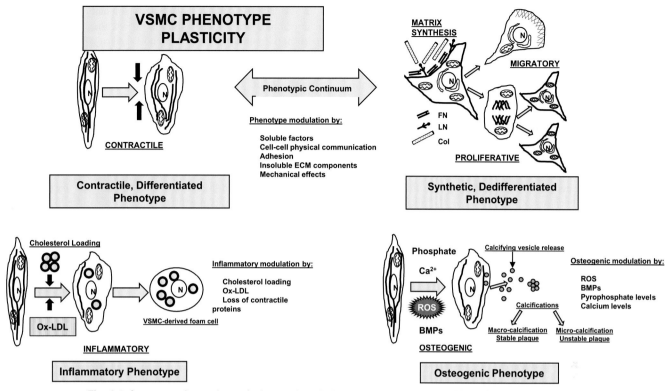

Fig. 3.1 Summary of vascular smooth muscle cell phenotype characteristics. *BMPs*, Bone morphogenetic proteins; *Col*, collagen; *FN*, fibronectin; *LN*, laminin; *N*, nucleus; *Ox-LDL*, oxidized LDL; *ROS*, reactive oxygen species; *VSMC*, vascular smooth muscle cell.

characteristic of dedifferentiated VSMCs in association with vascular injury.[3] Other characteristics of synthetic VSMCs include a decreased number of actin filaments, an increase in secretory vesicles, increased rates of proliferation and migration, extensive ECM synthesis/degradation capabilities, increased cell size and "hill and valley" morphology in culture, a high proliferative rate, and increased expression of α4β1 integrin.

Inflammatory/Macrophage-Like Vascular Smooth Muscle Cells

In addition to the phenotypic continuum between contractile and synthetic phenotypes, recent genetic inducible fate-mapping studies in ApoE[-/-] mice have shown that medial VSMCs can undergo clonal expansion in plaques, lose classic VSMC marker expression, and express the macrophage markers MAC-2 and CD68.[5] Quantitative assessments of these cells in plaques in murine models showed that 16% of CD68+ cells were derived from mature VSMCs and not from myeloid sources.[26] In further lineage tracing studies, Shankman et al.[18] showed that more than 80% of VSMCs in lesions were undetectable using conventional SM α-actin staining and undergo a phenotypic transition to a macrophage-like cell that expresses markers of macrophages. Importantly, VSMC-specific conditional knockout of KLF4 in ApoE[-/-] mice resulted in reduced plaque size and numbers of macrophage-like cells and increased fibrous cap thickness, providing further evidence that VSMC contributions to plaques have been underestimated and indicating an important role for VSMCs in foam cell formation and plaque progression. However, VSMC-derived macrophage-like cells, established by cholesterol loading and downregulation of the miR143/145 myocardin axis, exhibited a dysfunctional macrophage-like phenotype, suggesting that these cells are not "classical" macrophages.[27] In humans, a recent report stated that more than 40% of CD68-expressing cells in atherosclerosis of the human coronary artery were derived from resident VSMCs and not mono-

cytes.[6] These data are contrary to the paradigm that VSMCs, having undergone transition from a contractile to a synthetic/proliferative phenotype in the plaque, stabilize the plaque by secreting ECM components that contribute to protective fibrous cap formation. Instead these findings support a deleterious, proatherogenic role for VSMCs in plaque pathology.

A major environmental factor that contributes to the maintenance of the VSMC proinflammatory phenotype is the matrix milieu in which cells exist. In atherosclerotic plaques, VSMCs begin to secrete collagens I and III but they also, as a result of NF-κB activation, express the metalloproteinases MMP-1, MMP-3, and MMP-9, which degrade collagen fibrils to the monomeric form, thus promoting an inflammatory phenotype, as evidenced by an increase in the expression of vascular cell adhesion molecule-1 (VCAM-1).[28] A similar response is seen with regard to osteopontin, which is also increased in atherosclerosis.[29] The effects of these matrix proteins on VSMCs are mediated by binding to specific integrins, most likely α5β1 or αvβ3.[30] The nonintegrin matrix receptor CD44, which binds to hyaluronic acid in the matrix, has also been implicated in the transition to the proinflammatory phenotype, as shown by its ability to stimulate VCAM-1 expression.[31]

One of the primary stimuli for the development of the inflammatory phenotype is oxidized low-density lipoprotein (LDL), but ECs activated by disturbed flow also contribute to inflammatory changes in VSMC by secreting proinflammatory cytokines.[30] Oxidized LDL (oxLDL) and other cytokines like interleukin 1β (IL-1β) and TNF-α stimulate the VSMC expression of chemokines such as monocyte chemoattractant protein 1 (MCP-1), TNF-α, and chemokine (C-X-C motif) ligand 1 (CXCL1) as well as adhesion molecules such as VCAM-1, ICAM-1, and CCR-2, the receptors for MCP-1. Because many of these molecules activate NF-κB, with exposure to one often induces the expression of others, which results in the propagation of a positive feedback signaling mechanism to enhance the local inflammatory response. The end result is the recruitment and adhesion of T cells and monocytes to smooth muscle cells in the vessel wall.

Osteogenic Vascular Smooth Muscle Cells and Calcifying Extracellular Vesicles

Vascular calcification is a hallmark and one of the major risk factors for CVD.[32] One possible mechanism is the switch of VSMCs from a contractile to an osteoblastic phenotype. In the presence of proinflammatory mediators such as TNF-α and BMPs, procalcifying levels of phosphate, or oxidized forms of cholesterol, conditions endemic to plaque, VSMCs lose contractile markers and start to express bone-related genes, including BMPs, runt-related transcription factor 2 (Runx2), Msx, and osteocalcin.[7,32] Concomitant with this phenotypic switch are other cellular responses facilitating the calcification process. Responses on the cellular level include increased oxidation and stress on the endoplasmic reticulum (ER); the resultant stress repair processes, including DNA damage response signaling, in turn induce senescence and autophagy and inhibit matrix vesicle release.[7]

Osteogenic-like VSMCs deposit calcifying matrix vesicles (extracellular vesicles [EVs]), which serve as initial nucleation sites of calcium and phosphate mineralization.[33] These VSMC-derived calcifying EVs, originating in the endosomal pathway via multivesicular bodies (MVBs) that dock at the plasma membrane and release membrane-bounded exosomes, are enriched in alkaline phosphatase (ALP), annexins, MMP-2, and specific Rab GTPases implicated in vesicular trafficking. Matrix vesicles contain at least 79 proteins implicated in a wide range of functions including calcification, oxidant- and ER stress–related proteins, and matrix-modifying enzymes for both ECM biogenesis and degradation, contributing to disruption of the vessel wall.[7] In addition to proteins in matrix vesicles, there is selective loading of miRNAs, many of which target osteogenic marker genes in osteogenic differentiation.

Released EVs become entrapped within the ECM in the plaque, acting as multifoci for microcalcifications.[34] Contrary to the original paradigm that calcification stabilizes plaque, new evidence using computational modeling suggests that microcalcifications in the fibrous cap are plaque-destabilizing by serving as foci for high levels of local stress within the cap, making the cap prone to rupture, whereas large calcification areas stabilize plaque by reducing deformation of the fibrous cap during systole. Importantly, microcalcifications in the fibrous cap correlate with cardiovascular adverse events.[35] In fact, the calcium score is a better indicator of future acute events than the lipid scores.[36] Therefore the mechanisms for calcification, including the cell types involved, are of great interest owing to their considerable clinical impact, as there are no therapies for the treatment of cardiovascular calcification.

A recent genome-wide association study (GWAS) indicated an association of the *Sort1* gene with coronary artery calcification.[37] Sortilin, a multiligand sorting receptor with additional functions in lipid metabolism and inflammation, is a risk gene for hypercholesterolemia and myocardial infarction.[35] Of interest, sortilin is also a high-affinity receptor for PCSK9 (proprotein convertase subtilisin/kexin type 9), a potent regulator of LDL-C via its ability to shift LDLR traffic from recycling to degradation in the lysosome of hepatocytes, thus leading to excessive accumulation of LDL-C.[38] PCSK9 is constitutively expressed in cultured VSMCs and is found in VSMC regions in human atherosclerotic plaque.[39] In *Sort*[-/-] mice, vascular calcification was reduced by a single injection of a gain-of-function mutant PCSK9 adeno-associated virus vector into mice on a high-fat, high-cholesterol diet.[40]

In addition to a role for VSMC-derived EVs in calcification, VSMC-derived EVs loaded with Gla-containing coagulation factors have phosphatidylserine (PS) on their external surface, which can bind the vitamin K–dependent coagulation protein prothrombin (PT) and induce thrombogenesis, providing evidence for a dual role for VSMC-derived

EVs in calcification and coagulation.[41] Manipulation of exosome biogenesis/inhibition or cargo holds promise for either facilitating vascular repair or preventing excessive thrombosis and calcification.[42]

Upstream Mediators of Phenotypic Modulation
Growth-Inducing Factors

Soluble factors, including growth factors, hormones, and reactive oxygen species (ROS), serve as upstream mediators of the phenotypic switch from contractile to synthetic VSMCs, which results in large part from the coordinate activation/repression of VSMC marker genes important in the contractile response (Fig. 3.2).[3,24,43,44] Some of the most important growth-inducing factors include PDGF, epidermal growth factor (EGF), insulin-like growth factor (IGF), and basic fibroblast growth factor (bFGF). Growth factors bind to surface membrane receptor tyrosine kinases (RTKs), triggering sequential downstream signaling pathways mediated through the complex formation of activated RTKs with adaptor and signaling proteins Grb2/Shc/Sos, and activation of intracellular kinases, including phosphatidylinositol 3-kinase (PI3K), mitogen-activated protein kinases (MAPKs: extracellular signal regulated kinase, ERK1/2, p38MAPK, and c-jun NH$_2$-terminal kinase, JNK), Akt, MAPK activated protein kinases 2 (MAPKAPK2), and p70[S6] kinase

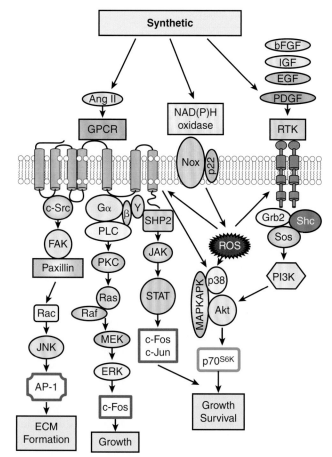

Fig. 3.2 Summary of multiple soluble extracellular factors, their receptors, their interacting signaling pathways, and various transcription factors responsible for expression of the synthetic/dedifferentiated vascular smooth muscle cell phenotype characterized by growth/survival pathways and extracellular matrix *(ECM)* formation. The details are outlined in the text. (Modified from Hilenski L, Griendling K, Alexander R. Angiotensin AT1 receptors. In: Re R, DiPette D, Schiffrin E, Sowers J, eds. *Molecular Mechanisms in Hypertension.* London: Taylor & Francis; 2006:25–40.)

($p70^{S6K}$). These signals not only transcriptionally mediate the switch to the synthetic phenotype but also serve to promote growth and survival. In addition, ROS such as hydrogen peroxide (H_2O_2), produced by activation of the nicotinamide adenine dinucleotide phosphate (NADPH) oxidase, a multimeric enzyme containing p22phox and other subunits depending upon the specific isoform, can act as second messengers for canonical G protein–coupled receptor (GPCR) and RTK pathways.[45]

Differentiation-Inducing Factors

In contrast to growth factor–stimulated proliferation, the cytokine TGF-β and members of the BMP subgroup of this family promote the differentiated contractile phenotype in VSMCs by inducing expression of the VSMC contractile genes SM α-actin (*ACTA2*) and calponin (*CNN1*) (Fig. 3.3). TGF-β binds to a tetrameric complex consisting of two type I and two type II receptors, resulting in the phosphorylation of Smads, transcription factors (TFs) named for *Caenorhabditis elegans* Sma and *Drosophila melanogaster* Mad (mothers against decapentaplegic).[46] Within the TGF-β signaling pathway itself, different Smads control expression of different markers. For example, Smad3 transactivates the SM22α (*TAGLN*; also known as transgelin) promoter, whereas Smad2 activates the *ACTA2* gene. Other soluble factors that inhibit proliferation and increase differentiation include heparin and retinoic acid.[47] Most smooth muscle differentiation markers share additional common

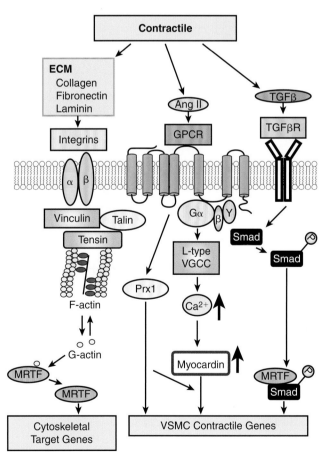

Fig. 3.3 Summary of soluble and insoluble extracellular factors, their receptors, their interacting signaling pathways, and transcription factors responsible for expression of the contractile/differentiated vascular smooth muscle cell *(VSMC)* phenotype. The details are outlined in the text. (Modified from Hilenski L, Griendling K, Alexander R. Angiotensin AT1 receptors. In: Re R, DiPette D, Schiffrin E, Sowers J, eds. *Molecular Mechanisms in Hypertension.* London: Taylor & Francis; 2006:25–40.)

transcriptional pathways, discussed in more detail further on. For example, both TGF-β–induced phosphorylated Smads and ECM-induced activation of integrins——mediated through focal adhesion components vinculin, talin, and tensin in concert with changes in cytoskeletal F/G actin dynamics——result in myocardin-related transcription factor (MRTF) induction of cytoskeletal/contractile genes (see Fig. 3.3).

Dual Factors

One factor with a potential dual role, depending on initial phenotype/developmental stage, is the octapeptide hormone angiotensin II (Ang II), the effector molecule of the renin-angiotensin II system.[48] Ang II can induce either contractile or synthetic phenotypes, with differential responses depending on cell context and locations within the artery (see Figs. 3.2 and 3.3). Ang II binding to its GPCR AT_1R activates VSMC marker gene expression indicative of the contractile phenotype through L-type voltage-gated Ca^{2+} channel–induced elevations in intracellular Ca^{2+} concentrations and subsequent increased myocardin transcription coactivator expression. This coactivator expression is dependent upon Prx1, a homeodomain protein that promotes SRF binding to conserved elements in VSMC marker gene promoters.[49] In addition, Ang II binding to AT_1R can induce signatures of the synthetic phenotype by activating multiple kinase and enzyme pathways that are interconnected in signaling networks (see Fig. 3.2). These include the (1) MAPKs; (2) RTKs, including ROS-sensitive transactivation of EGFR; (3) nonreceptor tyrosine kinases (c-Src/focal adhesion kinase [FAK]/paxillin/Rac/JNK/AP-1) and tyrosine phosphatase; (4) SHP2/Janus kinase and signal transducers and activators of transcription (JAK/STAT); and (5) GPCR classic signaling cascades (phospholipase C [PLC]/protein kinase C [PKC]/Ras/Raf/mitogen extracellular signal regulated kinase kinase (MEK)/ERK leading to stimulation of early growth response genes (*c-fos, c-jun*), survival pathways (e.g., Akt) and ECM formation (JNK/AP-1).

Notch Communication

In addition to its critical function in development, Notch signaling is also important in defining VSMC differentiation.[50,51] Downstream Notch effector gene activation results in the activation of "master regulators" of VSMC differentiation (myocardin, MRTFs, or SRF) or direct induction of contractile proteins SM-MHC and SM α-actin as well as the VSMC-specific differentiation marker SM22α.[11] The data regarding Notch signaling on VSMC differentiation, however, are conflicting, with some studies supporting a repressive effect, whereas others indicate a promoting effect on the expression of VSMC marker genes *MYH11* and *ACTA2*.[51] These discrepancies may be due to the antagonistic roles of Notch and the Notch effector Hairy-related transcription factor 1 (HRT1) on markers of VSMC differentiation.[52] HRT1 inhibits Notch/RBP-Jκ binding to the *ACTA2* promoter in a histone deacetylase-independent manner. The context-dependent roles of Notch and HRT1 on markers of VSMC differentiation may serve to fine tune VSMC phenotypic modulation during vascular development, injury, and disease.

There is considerable cross talk between Notch and other signaling pathways. Notch and TGF-β cooperatively induce a functional contractile, differentiated phenotype through parallel signaling axes,[53] whereas HRT factors block VSMC differentiation in both pathways. Other examples of cross talk among key signaling pathways for morphogenesis (Hh, Notch) and mitogenesis (VEGF-A, PDGF) include a Shh/VEGF-A/Notch signaling axis in VSMCs in the neointima to increase growth and survival[54] and Notch-induced upregulation of PDGF receptor β (PDGFR-β) to mediate growth and migration.[55]

Homotypic VSMC-VSMC Notch-mediated signaling pathways are also apparent in adult vascular pathologies and response to injury.[51] After injury, Notch receptors are increased along with elevated levels of HRT. Negative feedback between HRT and Notch may account for the adaptive response to injury in which initial Notch/HRT-induced suppression of the contractile phenotype is followed by arterial remodeling. As Notch/HRT signaling decreases, the contractile phenotype is reestablished.[53]

Transcriptional Regulation of Vascular Smooth Muscle Cell Diversity

The complex web of signaling pathways induced by these external signals——whether they are soluble, insoluble, structural, or mechanical——converge on a network of TFs that coordinately regulate gene expression and act as "masters switches" for growth and differentiation (Fig. 3.4).[56] Transcription of VSMC-specific differentiation or proliferative genes is regulated by cooperative interaction of TFs and their coregulators, including SRF,[57] myocardin and myocardin-related TFs (MRTF-A and –B),[58] Ets domain TFs known as ternary complex factors (TCFs),[59] zinc finger factors, GATA6[59] and PRISM (**PR** domain **I**n **S**mooth **M**uscle)/PRDM6,[60] and KLF.[61,62]

Serum Response Factor/Myocardin/CArG Axis

The discovery of the cell-restricted SRF transcriptional coactivator myocardin, which is expressed specifically in cardiac and VSMCs, resolved the paradoxical observations that SRF can regulate mutually exclusive gene expression programs for growth or differentiation.[59,63] In VSMCs, myocardin is a master regulator of marker gene expression and is sufficient for the smooth muscle–like contractile phenotype because conversion of cells to a VSMC-like phenotype involves transient ectopic expression of just one factor: myocardin.[64]

SRF, a widely expressed member of the MADS (MCM1, Agamous, Deficien, SRF) box of TFs, is a nodal point linking signaling pathways to differential gene expression related either to growth or differentiation, depending on which transcriptional partner is bound to SRF.[57] SRF self-dimerizes and binds with high affinity and specificity to a consensus DNA sequence CArG box found in the promoters of cyto-contractile genes.[63] More than half of the VSMC "marker" genes that define the VSMC molecular signature contain CArG boxes.[63] Included in these genes are three categories modulating actin filament dynamics: (1) structural (e.g., *ACTA2, TAGLN, CALD1, MYH11*); (2) effectors of actin turnover (e.g., *CFL1, GSN*); and (3) regulators of actin dynamics (four and a half LIM domains proteins [FHL1 and 2], MMP9, and myosin light chain kinase [MYCK]).[65]

To study the function of CArG boxes, precision-guided genome editing with CRISPR technology was used to edit the consensus intronic CArG box in the SMC-specific calponin (*Cnn1*) gene to drastically reduce calponin expression in the vessel wall without affecting other

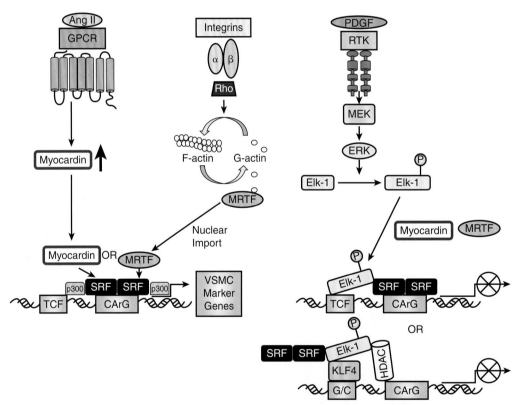

Fig. 3.4 A Model for the Opposing Roles of Transcription Factors, Their Coregulators, and Chromatin Remodeling Enzymes in the Control of Vascular Smooth Muscle Cell *(VSMC)* **Growth or Differentiation.** Differentiation-inducing extracellular cues——such as G protein–coupled receptor *(GPCR)* or integrin activation, which increase myocardin or modulate Rho-mediated actin dynamics, respectively——stimulate signaling pathways leading to the transcription factor serum response factor *(SRF)*. SRF binds to a CArG DNA sequence found in the promoters of many cytocontractile genes and interacts with myocardin/MRTF/p300 histone acetylase to promote the expression of VSMC marker genes. Growth factor signaling through the mitogen extracellular signal regulated kinase kinase *(MEK)*/extracellular signal–regulated kinase *(ERK)* pathway represses VSMC marker genes by phosphorylation of the ternary complex factor *(TCF)* Elk-1 and by increasing KLF4 expression. Phospho-Elk-1 inhibits SRF interaction with myocardin and KLF4, which binds to G/C-rich elements located in regulatory elements controlling expression of VSMC contractile genes, recruits histone deacetylase *(HDAC)*, and reduces SRF binding to CArG elements.

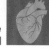

SMC-specific marker genes. Near elimination of calponin increased DNA synthesis, suggesting a role for calponin in VSMC quiescence.[66] These studies represent the first use of CRISPR-Cas9 technology for genome editing of a regulatory element in the control of an SRF target gene and show the importance of the CArG box for calponin-1 expression.[64]

SRF itself is a weak activator of CArG-dependent genes.[59] Potent SRF-dependent transcriptional activation is therefore dependent upon regulation at several levels: by interaction with different signal-regulated or tissue-specific regulatory SRF transcription cofactors/corepressors; by postranslational phosphorylation, acetylation, and sumoylation, modifications that affect these interactions; and by epigenetic alterations in chromatin structure in which myocardin serves as a scaffold for recruitment of chromatin-remodeling enzymes[67] that enable SRF and its cofactors to gain access to SRF target genes.[14] Myocardin association with histone acetyltransferases (HATs), including p300, enhances transcription of VSMC-restricted genes, whereas association with class II histone deacetylases (HDACs) suppresses myocardin-induced transcription of VSMC marker genes (see Fig. 3.4).[67]

SRF interacts with cofactors in two principal families: the TCF family of Ets-domain proteins (Elk, SAP-1, and Net)[68] that are activated by the MAPK pathway and lead to SRF binding to immediate early growth factor–inducible genes such as *c-fos*,[57] and the myocardin/MRTF-A/MRTF-B family[65] that promotes activation of VSMC-specific marker genes, most of which code for filamentous proteins that function in contractile activities or proteins that function in cell-matrix adhesions.[20] These alternative pathways provide the "plasticity" associated with VSMC phenotypic modulation, ranging from contractile functions to maintain vascular tone to synthetic or proliferative functions in response to vascular injury.[58]

Myocardin competes with Elk-1 for direct binding to SRF in VSMCs; thus, myocardin and Elk-1 can act as binary transcriptional switches that may regulate contractile versus synthetic VSMC phenotypes (see Fig. 3.4).[59] In addition, myocardin transduction leads to lower levels of the cell cycle–associated gene cyclin D1, resulting in repression of growth. Therefore myocardin is a nodal point for two features indicative of SMC differentiation: expression of the contractile apparatus and suppression of growth.[59]

Although myocardin functions exclusively as a transcriptional coactivator,[69] additional proteins function to regulate the transcriptional activity of myocardin. Positive regulators include myocyte-specific enhancer factor 2 (Mef2), TEA domain transcription factor 2 (Tead2), and forkhead transcription factor 4 (Foxo4), epigenetic markers such as ten-eleven translocation-2 (TET2) and TGF-β and Notch signaling pathways. Negative regulation of myocardin can occur by interaction of an upstream repressor region (URR) within the myocardin promoter (PrmM) with binding sites for KLF4 or PDGF-BB within the PrmM, mediating transcriptional repression of myocardin expression.[70]

In addition, miRNAs and lncRNAs regulate myocardin expression. The miR-143/145 cluster positively regulates myocardin expression by targeting inhibition of KLF4/5, itself an inhibitor of myocardin, regulating the phenotypic shift in VSMCs. miR-146a targets KLF4 to promote VSMC proliferation in vitro and neointimal hyperplasia in vivo.[71] Knockdown of the cytoplasmic lncRNAs *SENCR* (smooth muscle and endothelial cell–enriched migration/differentiation/associated long noncoding RNA) attenuates the expression of myocardin, decreases expression of VSMC contractile-associated genes, and increases expression of promigratory genes. Thus, *SENCR* seems to function in maintenance of the contractile, nonmotile phenotype.[72]

HRT-2 and GATA factors repress or enhance myocardin-induced transcriptional activity depending upon cell context.[59] In addition,

activation of Notch receptors by Jagged1 endogenous ligand induces translocation of Notch intracellular domain (ICD) to the nucleus, where it inhibits myocardin-induced SMC gene expression.[58] Ang II stimulation, as well as activation of L-type voltage-gated Ca^{2+} channels, activates SMC marker genes by inducing myocardin expression, and, in the case of Ang II, increasing SRF binding to CArG elements in the promoter regions of VSMC marker genes such as *ACTA2*.[49]

SRF transcriptional activity is also controlled by Rho-induced actin dynamics that facilitate the movement of MRTFs into or out of the nucleus (see Fig. 3.4).[58] In most cell types, MRTFs form a stable complex with monomeric G-actin and remain sequestered in the cytoplasm. MRTFs in VSMCs, however, are localized in the nucleus, where binding to SRF in the basal state promotes contractile gene expression and the differentiated phenotype. In response to growth factors or vascular injury, extracellular signals transduced through the Rho-actin pathway result in nuclear export of MRTF, downregulation of SRF/MRTF-induced VSMC contractile gene expression, and promotion of mitogen-induced ERK1/2 phosphorylation of TCFs, resulting in TCF displacement of MRTFs and SRF/TCF-mediated activation of growth responsive genes.[58] These differential pathways provide a switch in which SRF target genes are differentially regulated through growth factor–induced signaling for growth (active TCF, MRTF blocked) or Rho-actin signaling for differentiation (inactive TCF, MRTF active) (see Fig. 3.4).[59]

Myocardin has important roles beyond its role in activating transcription of VSMC-specific marker genes.[70] A recent study showed that myocardin is also a negative regulator of VSMC inflammation in CVD and after vessel injury.[73] Therefore, myocardin is a possible therapeutic target owing to its antiinflammatory properties. Furthermore, myocardin has been shown to suppress VSMC dedifferentiation and proliferation.[70] Myocardin inhibits VSMC proliferation by interaction with the NF-κB subunit p65 to suppress NF-κB activity independently of SRF.[70] Finally, myocardin has been shown to drive the formation of caveolae, or plasma membrane sphingolipid/cholesterol-rich domains, also in an SRF-independent manner, suggesting that myocardin has a role in lipid metabolism.[70] These antiinflammatory and lipid-regulatory roles of myocardin extend beyond its role in activating the transcription of VSMC-specific marker genes for a contractile phenotype.[70]

Hippo Kinase Pathway

The Hippo kinase pathway has been shown to modulate the myocardin/SRF pathway by inhibiting the phosphorylation of YAP, which, when phosphorylated, remains located in the cytosol and therefore cannot repress VSMC marker gene expression by interacting with myocardin and disrupting SRF binding. In rat carotid artery injury, YAP is induced in VSMCs in transition from contractile to synthetic phenotype; its expression promotes VSMC proliferation and migration. Deletion of YAP protects against neointimal formation after injury. Another kinase shown to regulate VSMC phenotypic switching by acting through MRTF-A is p38 MAPKα (*Mapk14*). Both the Hippo and the p38 MAPKα pathways are activated by extracellular cell-cell or cell-matrix contacts, which then modulate the cytoskeleton and cell adherence necessary for VSMC survival.[74]

Zinc Finger Proteins

GATA6, a zinc finger TF expressed in VSMCs, induces growth arrest by increasing expression of the general cyclin-dependent kinase inhibitor (CDKI) p21^{CIP1} and inhibiting S-phase entry.[59] PRISM is a smooth muscle–restricted member of zinc finger proteins belonging to the PRDM family and acts as a transcriptional repressor by interacting with class I HDACs and G9a histone methyltransferases (HMTs).

PRISM induces the proliferative phenotype while repressing differentiation regulators myocardin and GATA6.[60]

One of the most intensely studied zinc finger transcriptional regulators in VSMCs is the KLF subfamily, which bind to the TGF-β control element (TCE) in the regulatory sequences of target genes.[61,62,75] VSMCs express four KLFs (KLF4, KLF5, KLF13, and KLF15), each with individual biological functions implicated in regulating a range of processes in both growth and differentiation.[61] Individual KLFs may have opposing functions, depending upon temporal and developmental expression patterns and interactions with other factors. For example, KLF4 inhibits, whereas KLF5 and KLF13 induce, VSMC marker gene expression. Mechanisms that may account for these opposing functions of KLF factors include posttranslational modifications, interaction with specific cofactors, differential expression by growth factors, cytokines and differentiation state, or regulation by another KLF.[61]

KLF4 functions as both a VSMC growth repressor and as a repressor for VSMC differentiation, although the data on the effect of KLF4 on VSMC differentiation are conflicting (see Fig. 3.4).[62] As a growth repressor, KLF4 inhibits PDGF-BB–induced mitogenic signaling and induces expression of the negative cell cycle regulator p53 and its target gene p21^{CIP1}. As a differentiation repressor, KLF4 prevents SRF from binding to the TCE in the promoters of VSMC marker genes, suppresses expression of myocardin, inhibits myocardin-induced activation of SMC marker genes, reduces SRF binding to CArG elements in SMC contractile gene promoters,[62] and induces histone hypoacetylation at SMC CArG regions associated with gene silencing.[76] On the other hand, there is evidence that KLF4 promotes VSMC differentiation by directly activating VSMC marker gene transcription of SM22α and SM α-actin.[62] KLF4 thus functions as a bifunctional TF or "molecular switch" that can both activate and repress VSMC marker genes, depending upon regulation of KLF4.[62]

Even though the closely homologous KLF4 and KLF5 TFs share similar developmental and tissue pattern expression, they exert different, often opposing, effects on gene regulation and proliferation/differentiation.[62] Whereas KLF4 is associated with growth arrest, KLF5 exerts proproliferative effects, particularly in vascular remodeling in response to injury. KLF5 expression, which is abundant in fetal VSMCs but downregulated in the adult,[75] is induced after vascular injury by activation of immediate early response genes by Ang II and ROS.[77] KLF5 in turns mediates the reexpression of SMemb/NMHC-B, a marker for the dedifferentiated phenotype and activates other critical injury response genes involved in remodeling, such as PDGF-A/B, Egr-1, plasminogen activator inhibitor-1 (PAI-1), inducible NO synthase (iNOS) and VEGFR, implicating KLF5 as a key regulator for VSMC response to injury.[75] In additional injury responses, KLF5 increases cyclin D1 expression and inhibits the cyclin kinase inhibitor p21, thus leading to vascular remodeling by increased cell proliferation.[78] Similar to KLF4 regulation, KLF5 expression, and activity are regulated at multiple levels, including upstream Ras/MAPK, PKC, and TGF-β signaling pathways, downstream interactions with TFs——including retinoic acid receptor (RARα), NF-κB, and peroxisome proliferator-activated receptor gamma (PPARγ)——as well as posttranslational modifications that can positively or negatively regulate KLF activity.[75] In addition, KLF5 activity is regulated in the nucleus by chromatin-remodeling factors such as SET, a histone chaperone that inhibits the DNA-binding activity of KLF5[79]; p300, a coactivator/acetylase that coactivates KLF5 transcription; and HDAC1, which inhibits KLF5 binding to DNA.[61]

Two additional KLFs have been identified in VSMCs: KLF13 and KLF15.[61] After vascular injury, KLF13 is induced and activates the pro-

moter for the VSMC differentiation marker *TAGLN*, whereas KLF15 expression is downregulated, implicating KLF15 as a negative regulator of VSMC proliferation and a counterbalance to the growth promoting effects of KLF5 in vascular injury response.

RNA Regulation of Vascular Smooth Muscle Cell Diversity: Noncoding RNAs

The landscape for understanding protein-based regulation dramatically changed with the discovery of noncoding RNAs, previously referred to as "junk" DNA but now known to comprise 98% of the human genome.[80] These noncoding RNAs include the highly conserved miRs and the more recently described lncRNAs. These molecular rheostats are responsible for important regulatory control over the transcriptome or proteome in mediating VSMC phenotypic diversity.

microRNAs

Upstream signaling and downstream transcriptional pathways in VSMCs are intertwined with a multitude of miRs that act as "rheostats" and "switches" in regulating protein activity in development, function, and disease.[21,81,82] miRs are small noncoding RNAs, 20 to 25 nucleotides (nt) in length, that associate with an miRNA-induced silencing complex (miRISC) of regulatory proteins, including Argonaute family proteins, Argonaute interacting proteins of the GW182 family, eukaryotic initiation factors (eIFs), polyA-binding complexes, decapping enzymes/activators, and deadenylases to induce posttranscriptional silencing of their target genes.[83] These multiple components are assembled and interact in a multistep process with components of the translational machinery to inhibit translation initiation, to mark mRNAs for degradation through deadenylation, and to sequester targets into cytoplasmic P bodies.[84] Multiple mechanistic models for miRNA-induced gene silencing have been proposed that provide insight into the molecular mechanisms of translational inhibition, deadenylation, and mRNA decay, but questions remain concerning the kinetics and ordering of these translational events and whether these events are coupled or are independent.[83] A recent unifying model for miRNA-regulated gene repression is an attempt to reconcile the often conflicting existing data and proposes that recruitment of Argonaute and associated GW182 proteins to miRNA induces binding to the mRNA 5′m^7 cap, thus blocking translation initiation, potentially by mRNA deadenylation. Subsequent to miRNA-mediated deadenylation, mRNA is degraded through recruitment of decapping proteins.[85] In this model, inhibition of translation initiation is linked to subsequent rapid mRNA decay in a coupled process. Because miRs, which in general are negative regulators of gene expression, may be almost as important as TFs in controlling gene expression in the pathogenesis of human diseases,[86] insights into the functions of this class of noncoding RNAs are important in evaluating their potential use as therapeutic targets.[83]

Cardiovascular-specific, highly conserved miRNAs miR-143 and miR-145, the most abundant miRNAs in the vascular wall,[87] are key players in programming of VSMC fate from multipotent progenitors in embryonic development and in the reprogramming of VSMCs during phenotypic modulation in the adult (Fig. 3.5).[84,88] miR-143 and miR-145 have distinct sequences but are clustered together and transcribed as a bicistronic unit. Upstream in the genomic sequence of the miR143/145 is a conserved SRF-binding CArG box site, indicating control by SRF and myocardin.[88,89] These miRNAs cooperatively feed back to modulate the actions of SRF through targeting a network of TFs/coactivators/corepressors. This network includes miR-145-induced repression of KLF4, a positive regulator of proliferation and myocardin repressor; miR-143–induced repression of Elk-1,

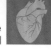

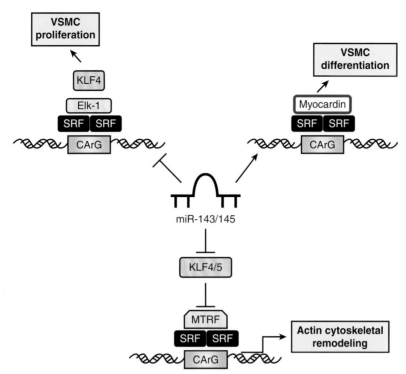

Fig. 3.5 A Model for the Regulation of Vascular Smooth Muscle Cell *(VSMC)* Phenotypes by the Cardiovascular-Specific microRNAs miR-143 and miR-145. These miRNAs act as signaling nodes to modulate serum response factor *(SRF)*-dependent transcription by regulating coactivators and corepressors to control VSMC proliferation or differentiation. miR-145 represses proliferation by repressing KLF4 and promotes differentiation by stimulating myocardin; miR-143 represses proliferation by repressing Elk-1. miR-143/145 also controls actin/cytoskeletal remodeling by repressing KLF4/5 and regulators of actin dynamics, including MTRF/SRF activity.

a myocardin competitor and positive regulator of proliferation; and, contrary to the usual inhibitory role of miRNA, miR-145–induced stimulation of myocardin, a positive regulator of differentiation. Thus miR-145 is necessary and sufficient for VSMC differentiation and the miR-143/miR-145 cluster acts as an integrated signaling node to promote differentiation while concurrently repressing proliferation.[88] Although mice with genetic deletions for miR-143/145 show no obvious abnormalities in early development, VSMCs in the adult exhibit both structural and phenotypic differences in injury- or stress-induced vascular remodeling. Ultrastructural analysis of arteries from miR-143/145 knockout mice shows reduced numbers of medial VSMCs with a contractile appearance and an increase in synthetic VSMCs.[90] These results suggest that miR-143 and miR-145 modulate cytoskeletal structure, actin dynamics, and modulation to a dedifferentiated phenotype (see Fig. 3.5).[89] Importantly, miR-143/145 knockout mice with increased synthetic VSMCs develop spontaneous neointimal lesions in the femoral artery in the absence of hyperlipidemia and inflammation, supporting a key role for phenotypically altered VSMCs in the pathogenesis of lesion formation.[90]

Whereas miR-143 and miR-145 play keys roles in the contractile phenotype of VSMCs and the response to injury,[91] miR-221 and miR-222 are modulators of VSMC proliferation, although largely by affecting growth-related signaling pathways rather than by controlling VSMC phenotype. miR-221 and miR-222, encoded by a gene cluster on the X chromosome, are upregulated in VSMCs in neointimal lesions and in proliferating cultured VSMCs stimulated by PDGF-BB.[92] Studies show that two CDKIs, p27^{KIP1} and p57^{KIP2}, have miR-221 and miR-222 binding sites and are gene targets for miR-221 and miR-222 in the rat carotid artery in vivo.[92] Thus miR-

221 and miR-222 are proproliferative because they repress two CDKIs, p27^{KIP1} and p57^{KIP2}. Furthermore, PDGF, via miR-221 induction, inhibits VSMC differentiation via c-kit–induced inhibition of myocardin.[93]

For a more comprehensive list of important miRs in VSMCs, see Table 3.1 and recent reviews.[64,94–96]

lncRNAs

High-throughput transcriptomics have identified over 100,000 genes for lncRNAs, indicating that lncRNAs outnumber both protein-coding and miR genes combined and are the majority transcript in the human genome. lncRNAs are noncoding RNAs more than 200 nt long transcribed by RNA polymerase. lncRNAs are generally expressed at low levels and are poorly conserved. In contrast to miRs, which usually act to downregulate mRNA and protein expression, lncRNAs have diverse functions and modulate gene expression at all levels: transcriptional, posttranscriptional, translational, and posttranslational via interaction with chromatin modifiers, RNA, RNA-binding proteins, and DNA.[97]

Subclasses of lncRNA are defined on the basis of genomic location relative to other gene loci: sense lncRNAs, antisense lncRNAs, bidirectional lncRNAs, intronic lncRNAs, and intergenic lncRNAs. lncRNAs can be also defined by localization within the cell: nuclear lncRNAs regulate gene transcription either in *cis* (local) or *trans* (distal) by acting as guides or scaffolds to localize chromatin remodeling factors on DNA loci; cytoplasmic lncRNAs can act as decoys for miRs or can affect mRNA stability and translation. In addition, lncRNAs in the cytoplasm can act to regulate nuclear translocation of TFs and signaling pathways by RNA-protein interactions. Although few vascular

TABLE 3.1   List of microRNAs in Vascular Smooth Muscle Cells

miR	Main Targets	Functions	Reference
Procontractile miRNAs (Differentiation)			
miR-10a	HDAC4	Regulates differentiation of VSMCs from embryonic stem cells	Huang et al.[261]
miR-21	*DOCK4, 5, 7*	Promotes contractility	Kang and Hata[262]
miR-143/145	KLF4, KLF5, myocardin, ELK-1, CamkIIδ, ACE, SSH2, SRGAP1/2, ADD3, MRTF-B	Phenotype switching	Boettger et al.[263] Cheng et al.[264] Cordes et al.[88] Xin et al.[89] Wang[265]
miR-143/145	miR-143 (PKC-ε and PDGF-Rα); miR-145 (fascin)	Regulates podosome formation and migration via downregulation of miR-143/145	Quintavalle et al.[266]
miR-143/145	KLF4, *ELK1*, CamkIIδ	miR-143/145 in exosomes from ECs transferred to VSMCs and prevents VSMC dedifferentiation (atheroprotective)	Hergenreider et al.[123]
miR-143/145		miR-143/145 mediates EC-VSMC-EC communication via tunneling nanotubes mediated by TGF-β	Climent et al.[128]
miR-143-3p		Modulates migration and apoptosis; miR-143 in PASMC-derived exosomes transferred to PAECs to induce migration	Deng et al.[125]
miR-145	KLF4	Restoration of contractile phenotype in metabolic syndrome	Hutcheson et al.[267]
miR-145	KLF4, myocardin	Promotes contractile phenotype	Lovren et al.[268]
Prosynthetic miRNAs (Proliferation, Migration)			
miR-1/33	KLF4, Sp-1	Proliferation	Chen et al.[269] Xie et al.[270] Torella et al.[271]
miR-9	PDGFR	Inhibits proliferation and migration	Ham et al.[272]
miR-15a	CDKN2B	Proliferation, decreases apoptosis	Gao et al.[273]
miR-21	*TPM1*, PDCD4, PPARα	Proliferation, migration, apoptosis	Lin et al.[274] Wang et al.[275] Davis et al.[276] Sarkar et al.[277]
miR-21	PTEN, Bcl-2	Promotes proliferation, decreases apoptosis	Ji et al.[278] Maegdefessel et al.[279]
miR-24	PDGFRB indirectly	Reduces migration and proliferation by myocardin-induced downregulation of PDGFRB	Talasila et al.[280]
miR-26	Contractile gene markers	Regulates VSMC contractile phenotype by exosome transfer of miR-26 from ECs to VSMCs	Lin et al.[124]
miR-26a	SMAD1, SMAD2	Promotes proliferation and migration, inhibits differentiation and apoptosis	Leeper et al.[281]
miR-29a	PDGFRB	Reduces migration and proliferation by myocardin-induced downregulation of PDGFRB	Talasila et al.[280]
miR-30c	PDGFRB	Inhibits PDGFRB expression and modulates proliferation and apoptosis	Xing et al.[282]
miR-31	CREG	Phenotypic modulation	Wang et al.[283]
miR-126 bound to Ago2 from ECs to VSMCs	FOXO3, Bcl2, IRS1	Modulates VSMC turnover	Zhou et al.[284]
miR-129	Wnt5a	Inhibits proliferation, induces apoptosis	Zhang et al.[285]
miR-132	LRRFIP1	Proliferation	Choe et al.[286]
miR-203	p63, Abl1	Inhibits proliferation by downregulating estradiol-induced Abl1 and p63	Zhao et al.[287]
miR-208	p21	Proliferation	Zhang et al.[288]
miR-221/222	p27, p57, c-kit	Promotes proliferation and migration, antiapoptosis	Liu et al.[92] Liu et al.[289] Davis et al.[93]
let-7d	*KRAS*	Proliferation	Yu et al.[290]

(Continued)

TABLE 3.1   List of microRNAs in Vascular Smooth Muscle Cells—cont'd

miR	Main Targets	Functions	Reference
let-7g	LOX-1	Proliferation and migration	Chen et al.[291]
Inflammation			
miR-24	CHI3L1	Inhibits vascular inflammation	Maegdefessel et al.[292]
miR-200 family	Zeb1	Upregulates proinflammatory COX-2 and MCP-1 in diabetic mice	Reddy et al.[293]
ECM Modifications			
miR-17 cluster	TIMP1, TIMP2	Downregulates ECM	Wu et al.[294]
miR-29	COL1A1, COL3A1, COL5A1, ELN, MMP2, MMP9	Downregulates ECM, regulates fibrosis	Boon et al.[295] Maegdefessel et al.[296]
miR-29	ELN	Elastin formation	Latronico et al.[297] Zhang et al.[298]
miR-29	ADAMTS-7	Promotes calcification by increasing ADAMTS-7 expression	Du et al.[299]
miR-29	COL1A, COL3A	Regulates ECM production	Ulrich et al.[300]
miR-29a	MMP2, MMP9	Downregulates ECM	Jones et al.[1]
miR-29b	ELN, MMP2	Upregulates ECM, promotes apoptosis	Merk et al.[301]
miR-133a	RUNX2	Osteogenic differentiation	Liao et al.[302]
miR-143	Versican mRNA	Attenuates ECM versican expression	Wang et al.[265]
miR-181a	OPN	Adhesion and osteopontin formation	Remus et al.[303]
miR-181b	TIMP3, ELN	Downregulates ECM	Di Gregoli et al.[304]
miR-195	COL1A1, COL1A2, COL3A1, ELN, MMP2, MMP9	Regulates ECM	Zampetaki et al.[305]
miR-516a	MTHFR, MMP2, TIMP1	Regulates ECM	Chan et al.[306]

ACE, Angiotensin-converting enzyme; *ADAMTS-7*, a disintegrin and metalloproteinase with thrombospondin motifs-7; *ADD3*, adducin-3; *Ago2*, Argonaute 2; *Bcl-2*, B-cell lymphoma 2; *CamkIIδ*, calcium/calmodulin kinase II-delta; *CDKN2B*, cyclin-dependent kinase inhibitor 2B; *CHI3L1*, chitinase 3-like 1; *COX-2*, cyclooxygenase-2; *CREG*, cellular repressor of E1A-stimulated genes; *DOCK*, dedicator of cytokinesis; *ECs*, endothelial cells; *ELK-1*, ETS oncogene family; *ELN*, elastin; *FOXO3*, forkhead box O3; *HDAC4*, histone deacetylase 4; *IRS1*, insulin receptor substrate 1; *KRAS*, Kirsten rat sarcoma virus oncogene; *KLF4*, Krupple-like factor 4; *LOX-1*, lectin-like oxidized LDL receptor-1; *LRRFIP1*, leucine-rich repeat (in Flightless 1) interacting protein-1; *MCP-1*, monocyte chemoattractant protein-1; *miR*, microRNAs; *MMP*, matrix metalloproteinases; *MRTF-B*, myocardin-related transcription factor B; *MTHFR*, ethylenetetrahydrofolate reductase; *PAEC*, pulmonary arterial endothelial cell; *PASMC*, pulmonary artery smooth muscle cell; *PDCD4*, programmed cell death protein-4; *PDGF-Rα*, PDGF receptor α; *PDGFRB*, PDGF receptor β; *PKC-ε*, protein kinase C epsilon; *PPARα*, peroxisome proliferator-activated receptor-α; *PTEN*, phosphatase and tensin homolog protein; *RUNX2*, runt-related transcription factor 2; *SMAD*, small mother against decapentaplegic; *Sp-1*, stimulating protein-1 (transcription factor); *SRGAP1/2*, Slit-Robo GTPase-activating protein 1/2; *SSH2*, Sling-shot 2 phosphatase; *TIMP*, tissue inhibitors of MMP; *TPM1*, tropomyosin-1; *VSMCs*, vascular smooth muscle cells.

lncRNAs have been identified and described, Table 3.2 contains a list of lncRNAs that have been found in VSMCs.[95,98–101]

Posttranslational Regulation of Vascular Smooth Muscle Cell Diversity: Epigenetics

The evolution of ideas about the regulation of gene expression started with the central dogma of molecular biology: the linear transfer of information of DNA to RNA to protein.[102] This classical paradigm underwent modification with the discovery of epigenetics, inherited changes in gene expression without alterations in the genomic sequence of DNA. Epigenetic mechanisms include methylation of DNA and histone modification of chromatin, which alters access to chromatin.

The "epigenetic landscape" controls gene expression by chemical modifications that mark regions of chromosomes either by methylation of promoter CpG sequences in the DNA itself or by covalent modification of histone proteins, which package DNA by the posttranslational addition of methyl, acetyl, phosphoryl, ubiquityl, or sumoyl groups, leading to the expression/repression of transcription.[103] In VSMCs, multiple levels of epigenetic controls exist for gene expression, leading to differentiation or dedifferentiation programs in healthy cells and for dysregulated gene expression in vascular disease. These epigenetic changes in VSMCs involve both DNA and histone methylation as well as histone acetylation/deacetylation. Methylation of histones, catalyzed by HMTs, results in a tight, stable epigenetic mark between methylated histones and chromatin that can be passed to daughter cells, thus providing "epigenetic memory," which defines cell lineage and identity by controlling SRF access to VSMC-specific marker genes.[103] Acetylation is controlled by HATs, which promote gene transcription by destabilizing chromatin structure to an "open," transcriptionally active conformation, and HDACs, which promote chromatin condensation to a "closed," transcriptionally silent conformation with restricted access to DNA. Histone acetylation/deacetylation thus serves to regulate transcription in a rapid and "on-off" manner in response to dynamic environmental changes and links the cell's genome with new extrinsic signals.[103] In VSMCs, SRF binding to CArG boxes in the promoters of SMC marker genes to promote the VSMC differentiated phenotype depends upon alterations of chromatin structure, including histone methylation and acetylation. In a model for the epigenetic regulation of VSMC phenotype,[104] SRF binding to CArG boxes in VSMC marker gene promoters is blocked by conditions, such as PDGF-BB exposure or vascular injury, which promote KLF4-induced myocardin suppression as well as KLF4-induced recruitment of HDACs, resulting in "closed" deacetylated chromatin and transcriptional repression of VSMC marker genes. Histone methylation, in contrast, is not affected

TABLE 3.2   List of Long Non-coding RNAs in Vascular Smooth Muscle Cells

lncRNA	Functions	References
ANRIL	Regulates cyclin dependent kinase inhibitors CDKN2A/B; promotes proliferation, increases adhesion and decreases apoptosis; resides on chromosome 9p21, the strongest genetic factor for coronary artery disease	Congrains et al.[307] Motterle et al.[308] Holdt et al.[309]
H19	Generates miR-675, inhibits tumor suppressor PTEN and promotes proliferation	Lv et al.[310]
HAS2_AS1	Regulates hyaluronan synthesis by altering *HAS2* gene chromatin structure and *HAS2* transcription; induces migration	Vigetti et al.[311]
HIF1A-AS1	Interacts with BRG1 to regulate proliferation and induce apoptosis	Wang et al.[312]
lincRNA-p21	Represses proliferation and induces apoptosis in atherosclerosis	Wu et al.[313]
lnc-Ang362	Ang II-regulated lnc-Ang362 modulates proliferation by targeting miR-221/222	Leung et al.[314]
lncRNA XR007793	Regulates cyclic strain-induced proliferation and migration	Yao et al.[315]
MYOSLID	Promotes differentiation and inhibits proliferation; first VSMC-selective and SRF/CArG-dependent lncRNA; amplifies differentiation through parallel pathways of TGF-β/SMAD and myocardin-related transcription factor A (MKL1)/SRF	Zhao et al.[316]
SENCR	Inhibits migration and stabilizes contractile phenotype	Bell et al.[72]
SMILR	Promotes proliferation by regulating proximal *HAS2* (hyaluronan synthase 2), an enzyme that synthesizes hyaluronic acid found in restenotic and atherosclerotic lesions	Ballantyne et al.[317]

Ang II, Angiotensin II; *ANRIL,* antisense ncRNA in the INK4 locus; *BRG1,* Brahma-related gene 1; *CArG,* CC(A+T-rich)₆GG; *CDKN2A/B,* cyclin-dependent kinase inhibitor A/B; *HAS2,* hyaluronan synthase 2; *HAS2-AS1,* hyaluronan synthase 2 antisense 1; *HIF1A-AS1,* HIF 1 alpha-antisense RNA 1; *lncRNA,* long non-coding RNA; *miR,* micro RNA; *MKL1,* myocardin-related transcription factor A; *MYOSLID,* MYOcardin-induced Smooth muscle LncRNA, Inducer of Differentiation; *PTEN,* phosphatase and tensin homolog; *SENCR,* Smooth muscle and Endothelial cell-enriched migration/differentiation-associated long Non-Coding RNA; *SMAD,* mothers against decapentaplegic homolog; *SMILR,* smooth muscle-induced lncRNA enhances replication; *SRF,* serum response factor; *TGF-β,* transforming growth factor-beta; *VSMC,* vascular smooth muscle cells.

by PDGF-BB and may serve as a permanent "memory" for VSMC identity during repression of SRF-dependent transcription and can, once repressive signals are terminated, reactivate the differentiation program by recruiting myocardin/SRF complexes or HATs to VSMC marker genes for reexpression. In the absence of KLF4 activation, SRF/myocardin can bind to HAT-induced acetylated "open" chromatin at CArG boxes for transcriptional activation of VSMC marker genes, thus promoting VSMC differentiation. In addition, myocardin induces acetylation of histones in the vicinity of SRF-binding promoters in VSMC marker genes by association with p300, a ubiquitous transcriptional coactivator with its own intrinsic HAT activity, leading to synergistic activation of VSMC marker gene expression. This promyogenic program is antagonized and repressed by myocardin binding to class II HDACs, which strongly inhibits expression of marker genes *ACTA2, TAGLN, MYCK, MYH11.* These opposing actions of HATs and HDACs on SRF/myocardin function to activate or repress, respectively, VSMC differentiation and serve to regulate transcription in a rapid and reversible manner in response to dynamic changes in the environment.[103]

Often, transcription mediators play roles in both classic signal transduction pathways and in epigenetic programming.[105] An example is the Smad proteins, which transmit TGF-β signals from the membrane to the nucleus to mediate gene transcription and VSMC differentiation. The balance between Smad-induced recruitment of corepressors or coactivators to TGF-β responsive genes is associated with activation of HDAC or HAT (p300), which then alters histone acetylation. TGF-β induces histone hyperacetylation at the VSMC marker gene SM22 promoter through recruitment of HATs, Smad3, SRF, and myocardin, demonstrating a role for HATs and HDACs in TGF-β activation of VSMC differentiation.[106]

A proposed example of metabolic memory stored in the histone code of VSMCs is found in the dysregulation of histone H3 methylation, an epigenetic mark usually associated with transcriptional repression, in type 2 diabetes.[107] In VSMCs derived from type 2 diabetic *db/db* mice, levels of H3K9me3 (H3 lysine-9 trimethylation), as well

as its HMT, are both reduced at the promoters of inflammatory genes. This loss of repressive histone marks, leading to increased inflammatory gene expression, is sustained in VSMCs from *db/db* mice cultured in vitro, suggesting persistence of metabolic memory. These results suggest that dysregulation in the histone code in VSMCs is a potential mechanism for increased and sustained inflammatory response in diabetic patients who continue to exhibit "metabolic memory" and vascular complications after glucose normalization.[108]

Recent data indicate that epigenetic mechanisms for DNA demethylation by the TET family of conserved dioxygenase enzymes is a powerful master regulator of VSMC phenotypic plasticity and development of vascular disease.[109] TET enzymes oxidize 5-methylcytosine (5mC) to 5-hydroxymethylcytosine (5hmC), which is subsequently converted to unmethylated cytosine via the DNA repair pathway and thymine-DNA glycosylase (TDG). DNA demethylation leads to gene activation. Of the three TET family isoforms (TET1–3), TET2 maintains hematopoietic stem cell (HSC) differentiation and is found to be mutated in myeloid malignancies, providing proliferative advantage.[110] In cultured coronary artery VSMCs, overexpression of TET2 induced differentiation-specific marker genes, including myocardin, *ACTA2, MYH11,* and *TAGLN,* whereas knockdown of TET2 resulted in increased expression of VSMC synthetic genes such as *KLF4,* indicating that TET2 activates VSMC-specific genes and represses dedifferentiation genes. Therefore TET2 is a master regulator of VSMC phenotype by regulating myocardin, SRF, and KLF4, thus activating VSMC-specific genes and repressing dedifferentiation genes.[111]

INFLUENCE OF CELL-CELL AND CELL-MATRIX INTERACTIONS

Communication among the various cell types within the vascular wall has undergone a paradigm shift, expanding from a model in which ECs responding to mechanical stimuli secrete diffusible paracrine factors to neighboring VSMCs to a model in which all layers in the vascular wall are interconnected and communicate via multiple mechanisms.[112] Many differential VSMC functions are influenced by cell-cell and cell-matrix adhesion receptors that are altered during phenotypic modulation and during response to injury or disease. Cell-cell adhesion receptors include cadherins and gap junction connexins, whereas cell-matrix interactions are dependent on combinations of integrins, syndecans, and α-dystroglycan.[22] Recently these intercellular mechanisms of communication among vascular wall cells have expanded to include physical connections in myoendothelial projections and long-range communication via exosomes and tunneling nanotubes (TNTs).

Cell-Cell Adhesion Molecules: Cadherins and Gap Junction Connexins

After investment of VSMCs to the EC layer of nascent vessels, vascular stabilization, also known as maturation,[113] is regulated by the sphingosine 1-phosphate (S1P) receptor S1P1, a GPCR on ECs. S1P1 activates the cell-cell adhesion molecule N-cadherin in ECs and induces formation of direct N-cadherin-based junctions between ECs and VSMCs required for vessel stabilization.[113] To maintain VSMC quiescence within the vascular wall, cadherin-mediated cell-cell adherens-type junctions between VSMCs inhibit VSMC proliferation, possibly by inhibiting the transcriptional activity of β-catenin, a component of the Wnt signaling pathway, which interacts with the ICD of cadherins.[114] Inhibition of β-catenin or stabilization of cadherin junctions in VSMCs may be useful in the treatment of vascular disease or injury.

Another type of direct intercellular junction between cells in the vasculature is the gap junction.[115] Gap junctions, formed by connexin proteins between ECs and VSMCs and between VSMCs, are intercellular channels that allow movement of metabolites, small signaling molecules and ions between cells.[115–117] Of the four connexin proteins expressed in VSMCs (Cx37, Cx40, Cx43, and Cx45), Cx45 is exclusively found in VSMCs, whereas Cx43 is the most prominent and is essential for the coordination of proliferation and migration.[115] Homotypic gap junctions between VSMCs coordinate changes in membrane potential and intracellular Ca^{2+}, while heterotypic contacts between ECs and VSMCs at the myoendothelial junction control vascular tone by EC-mediated VSMC hyperpolarization. Notably, the expression and/or activity of vascular connexins are altered in vascular disease such as hypertension, atherosclerosis, or restenosis[116] and in diabetes.[115]

Myoendothelial Projections

EC or VSMC protrusions less than 100 nm in diameter, known as myoendothelial junctions, extend through the internal elastic lamina and provide communications across basement membranes in both directions in the resistance vasculature.[118] Gap junction connexins have been shown within these projections, with Cx40 involved in EC to VSMC communication via endothelial-derived hyperpolarization-mediated vasodilation. Reverse signaling from VSMCs to ECs involves transmission of elevated calcium levels in phenylephrine-stimulated VSMCs to ECs, causing EC hyperpolarization and subsequent VSMC relaxation.[112] Thus myoendothelial junctions are signaling microdomains for regulation of calcium dynamics and membrane potential in control of blood flow.[119]

Exosomes

In addition to cell-cell junctions and the release of soluble messengers (hormones, cytokines, chemokines), ECs and VSMCs communicate by horizontal transfer and the delivery of bioactive molecules from cell to cell within secreted EVs, with significance not only for normal physiological function but also pathological vascular remodeling.[120]

As noted earlier, EVs are a heterogeneous collection of vesicles that vary in mode of formation and size.[121,122] Exosomes are 30- to 100-nm vesicles formed from intraluminal budding of MVBs. MVBs fuse with the plasma membrane and exosomes are released with the aid of Rab GTPases (Rab11/35, Rab27), tetraspanin, and the SNARE (soluble N-ethylmaleimide–sensitive attachment protein receptor) complex into the extracellular environment.[95] Exosomes can carry a wide variety of molecules——including proteins, DNAs, mRNAs, miRs, and lncRNAs——and can be taken up by neighboring or distant cells by fusion with the plasma membrane, receptor-mediated uptake, or endocytosis/micropinocytosis.[95]

In addition to a role for VSMC-derived EVs in pathological vascular calcification, as discussed earlier, exosome-mediated transfer has been documented from ECs to VSMCs and vice versa. Shear stress–activated ECs upregulate KLF2 and transfer the miR-143/145 cluster to VSMC via EC-derived exosomes, resulting in derepression of miR-143/145 target genes in VSMCs and promoting an atheroprotective contractile phenotypic state in vitro and in vivo.[123] Furthermore, human umbilical vein endothelial cells (HUVECs) regulate the smooth muscle cell phenotype through a miR-206/ARF6 (ADP-ribosylation factor 6)/NCS1 (sodium/calcium exchanger 1)/exosome axis.[124] HUVEC-derived exosomes decreased the expression of contractile phenotype markers SM α-actin, smoothelin, and calponin in VSMCs. These data suggest that miR-206 reduces HUVEC exosome production, thus maintaining the VSMC contractile phenotype.

Exosome transfer can also result in pathology. In a mouse model of pulmonary arterial hypertension (PAH), pulmonary arterial SMC-derived exosomes enriched in high levels of miR-143-3p were transferred from migrating pulmonary artery smooth muscle cells to pulmonary arterial endothelial cells (PAECs), inducing PAEC migration and angiogenesis. These results implicate exosomal transfer of functional miRNAs in the cross talk between vascular wall compartments in PAH development.[125] In addition, exosomes have been proposed as possible therapeutic "Trojan horses" for drug delivery or as biomarkers for disease.[42,126,127]

Tunneling Nanotubes

ECs and VSMCs can also communicate via TNTs. miR-143/145 transfer from VSMCs to ECs via TNTs has been shown using microscopy and fluorescent miR-143 and miR-145.[128] EC-VSMC cell-cell contact induces activation of miR-143/145 transcription in VSMCs and promotes transfer of miR-143/145 to ECs, where these miRs reduce angiogenesis potential in ECs, increasing vessel stability. In ex vivo experiments, TFG-β–induced miR-143 expression in VSMCs triggered the transfer of miR-143 from VSMCs to ECs via TNTs to inhibit target gene expression and induce cell proliferation and angiogenesis.[128]

Extracellular Matrix Components of Vascular Wall

VSMCs exist within an extracellular milieu of VSMC-secreted elastin and collagen fibers, conferring tensile strength and elasticity; proteoglycans (PGs; perlecan and hyaluronan) that allow for interfibrillar slippage, conferring viscosity; and adhesive glycoproteins (fibronectin [FN] and laminins) that bind PGs and collagen fibers. One of the most important functions of VSMCs is to secrete, organize, and maintain an elaborate ECM architecture, an "extended cytoskeleton," that varies according to the biomechanical stresses of the differing vascular beds. Large elastic arteries, such as the thoracic aorta, carotid, and renal arteries, are characterized by multiple concentric elastic lamellae that distribute cardiac-driven pulsatile stress evenly throughout the vessel wall. Smaller muscular arteries that experience less force, such as coronary, cerebral, and mesenteric arteries, contain only two elastic laminae. The elaboration of the ECM synthesized and organized by the VSMCs influences the same pathways that are regulated by growth/differentiation factors (see Fig. 3.3).[129] The changes acquired by VSMCs during acquisition of contractile properties are in turn maintained by the ECM in "dynamic reciprocity" between the matrix and gene expression. In addition to providing a structural, elastic scaffold for the extensible vessels, the ECM regulates gene expression through binding of matrix receptors on the cell surface and through acting as a reservoir for growth factors such as PDGF and FGF, which regulate cell function.[130]

Insoluble Extracellular Matrix Components

ECM components are classified as fiber-forming molecules (certain collagens and elastin); non–fiber-forming or interfibrillar molecules (PGs and glycoproteins); and matricellular proteins (thrombospondin-1 and -2, secreted protein acidic and rich in cysteine [SPARC/osteonectin], tenascin-C and osteopontin); which modulate cell-matrix interactions and tissue repair.[131] A list of ECM molecules and diseases resulting from ECM alterations can be found in a recent review.[131]

Basement Membrane

VSMCs in the intact vessel are surrounded by a basement membrane composed primarily of type IV collagen and laminin.[22] Laminins are basement membrane modular glycoproteins that interact with both cells and ECM to affect proliferation, migration, and differentiation.[129] Evidence from cultured VSMCs suggests that laminin induces the expression of contractile proteins and moderates the proliferative response to mitogens such as PDGF through a mechanism involving the laminin receptor $\alpha 7\beta 1$, which links the basement membrane to the VSMC contractile apparatus.[24]

Fibronectin, Collagens

FN is present in developing tissues prior to collagen and there is evidence that FN has an organizing role in ECM assembly as a "master orchestrator" for matrix assembly, organization, and stability.[132,133] FN binding to $\alpha 5\beta 1$ induces integrin-bound FN clustering, resulting in activation of actin polymerization, actin-myosin interactions, and signaling through kinase cascades. Thus FN modulates VSMCs toward the synthetic phenotype.[23]

Differential phenotypic modulation of VSMCs in response to different forms of collagen or to different isotypes of collagen illustrates the importance of cues from the physical and chemical ECM environment that regulate VSMC physiology in normal and disease states.[28] Cells cultured on fibrillar versus monomeric collagen type 1 exhibit very different gene expression profiles, responses to growth factors such as PDGF-BB, and migration properties.[23] Fibrillar collagen type 1 promotes the contractile phenotype, whereas monomeric collagen type 1, found in the degraded matrix of vascular lesions ("atherosclerotic matrix"), activates proliferation,[134] reduces contractile gene expression, and promotes a VSMC inflammatory phenotype with increased VCAM-1 expression.[28] VSMCs also exhibit different phenotypic profiles depending on contact with different collagen isotypes: collagen type IV, a component of the basement membrane surrounding VSMCs ("protective" matrix), promotes the expression of contractile proteins by regulating the SRF coactivator myocardin expression and mediating recruitment of SRF to CArG boxes in SM α-actin and SM MHC promoters.[28]

Elastins and Elastin-Associated Proteins

Elastic fibers are composed of tropoelastin, fibrillin-1, and fibrillin-2 and are assembled and deposited in a tightly regulated, hierarchical manner.[135,136] They not only provide unique elastomeric properties to the vessel wall but also influence phenotypes of VSMCs directly through adhesion and indirectly through TGF-β

signaling[135] to regulate migration, survival, and differentiation.[136] Elastin maintains the quiescent contractile phenotype of VSMCs by specifically regulating actin polymerization and organization via a signal transduction pathway involving Rho GTPases and their effector proteins.[137] Mechanical injury or inflammation that results in focal destruction of insoluble elastin into soluble elastin-derived peptides induces VSMC dedifferentiation and migration. Elastin-derived peptides can activate cyclins/cyclin-dependent kinases (CDKs), leading to cell cycle progression and proliferation found in neointimal formation.

Fibulins

Fibulins are elastic fiber–associated proteins.[136] VSMCs from fibulin-5 null mice exhibit enhanced proliferation and migration, indicating an inhibitory role for fibulin-5 in the VSMC response to mitogenic stimuli.[138] VSMC-specific deletion of the fibulin-4 gene results in the formation of large aneurysms exclusively in the ascending aorta and in the downregulation of SMC-specific contractile proteins and TFs for SMC differentiation. Thus fibulin-4 may serve a dual role in both elastic fiber formation and SMC differentiation and therefore may protect the aortic wall against aneurysm formation in vivo; it may also maintain an ECM environment for VSMC differentiation.

Glycosaminoglycans, Proteoglycans, and Matricellular Proteins

Glycosaminoglycans (GAGs) in the vascular ECM, including heparin and the related heparan sulfate, inhibit VSMC migration and proliferation. Heparin also induces the expression of contractile markers for maintenance of the differentiated phenotype.[24] Proteins bearing GAG chains, the PGs,[139] which include syndecan transmembrane heparan sulfate proteoglycans (HSPGs) and perlecan basement membrane HSPG, interact with FN in matrix assembly.[133] Different PGs can have opposing effects on VSMCs: the HSPG perlecan inhibits VSMC proliferation and intimal thickening by sequestering FGF-2,[23,140] whereas versican, a chondroitin sulfate proteoglycan, promotes VSMC proliferation.[141] Vasoactive agents acting through GPCRs, such as endothelin-1 and Ang II, stimulate the elongation of GAG chains on the proteoglycan core proteins.[142] These elongated GAG chains exhibit enhanced binding to LDL, providing a mechanism for atherogenic lipid retention in the vessel wall. Finally, matricellular proteins, such as thrombospondins, tenascins, and SPARC, are thought to be "antiadhesive proteins" with effects on VSMC migration and adhesion.[129] CCN (cysteine-rich protein, Cyr 61/CCN1) is a family of secreted matricellular proteins that mediate cellular responses to environmental stimuli through interaction with a variety of cell-surface proteins and adhesion receptors, including Notch receptors and integrins.[143] CCN1, which is upregulated in the VSMCs of injured arteries, stimulates VSMC proliferation through CCN1/α6β1 integrin interactions.[144] Knockdown of CCN1 in injury models suppresses neointimal hyperplasia. In contrast, CCN3 protein inhibits VSMC proliferation in a TGF-β–independent manner by increasing the CDKI p21 partly through Notch signaling, thus suppressing neointimal thickening.[145] These contrasting roles for proproliferative CCN1/α6β1 integrin signaling and antiproliferative CCN3/Notch signaling in VSMCs offer therapeutic strategies for reducing neointimal hyperplasia.[145]

Matrix Metalloproteinases and Tissue Inhibitors of Matrix Metalloproteinases

MMPs are zinc-containing enzymes that, along with extracellular proteases in the plasminogen activation system, induce remodeling of VSMC cell-matrix and cell-cell interactions[146-148] and release ECM-bound growth factors, cytokines and proteolyzed ECM fragments or "matrikines" with cytokine-like properties into the ECM. Members of the MMP family found in vascular tissues[149] include interstitial collagenases, basement membrane gelatinases, stromelysins, matrilysins, and membrane-type (MT) MMPs and metalloelastase. In the vascular wall, production of pro-MMP-2, MMP-14, and TIMP-1 and -2 is constitutive,[150] whereas other MMPs can be induced by inflammatory cytokines (IL-1 and -4 and TNF-α), hemodynamics, vessel injury, and ROS.[147] In addition, MMPs can act synergistically with growth factors such as PDGF and FGF-2.

MMP-induced remodeling of basement membrane components, laminin, polymerized type IV collagen, and HSPGs promotes a VSMC migratory phenotype. In addition, MMP cleavage and shedding of nonmatrix substrates, in particular adherens junction cadherins, act to remove physical constraints on cell movement.[147] Furthermore, ECM remodeling enables integrin signaling from the cell surface to focal adhesions, modulating cell cycle components cyclin D1 and p21/p27 CDK inhibitors.[150]

In vascular remodeling, MMP activities are tightly regulated at several levels: the transcriptional level, the activation of proforms, interaction with specific ECM components, and inhibition by TIMPs. The modulation of MMP activity is evident in VSMC migration and neointima formation after injury, plaque destabilization in atherosclerosis, aneurysm formation, hypertension, and coronary restenosis.[149] In atherosclerosis, MMPs have potential either to promote plaque instability, as in advanced plaques of hypercholesterolemia models, or to stabilize plaques by increasing VSMC migration/proliferation. Upregulation of MMPs in VSMCs may contribute to aneurysm formation.[24]

Cell-matrix Adhesion Molecules: Integrins and Syndecans

Integrins

Transmembrane integrin receptors are composed of combinations of α and β subunits, each combination with its own ligand-binding specificity and signaling properties. Integrins link the ECM with the actin cytoskeleton within VSMCs at focal adhesion attachment sites or adhesomes. In the adhesome are approximately 60 proteins involved in the transmission of external mechanical or internal contractile forces regulating focal adhesion dynamics and outside-in or inside-out signaling.[151,152]

The β1 subunit is the main β subunit in VSMCs in vivo and in vitro, whereas the major α integrin subunits expressed in VSMCs in vivo are α1, α3, and α5.[22] Integrin α1β1 is involved in collagen remodeling after injury, while integrin α5β1 binds to FN and effects FN polymerization.

Activation of different VSMC integrins results in expression of differential phenotypic programs. Beta-1 expression contributes to maintenance of the VSMC contractile phenotype, while integrins α2β1, α5β1, α7β1 and αvβ3 participate in SMC migration indicative of the synthetic phenotype.[22] Neointimal formation after vessel injury is reduced by blocking αvβ3, while apoptosis in the injured vessel is increased, potentially promoting plaque rupture. In addition, neointimal formation is prevented and the VSMC contractile phenotype is maintained by binding of α7β1 integrins to COMP (cartilage oligomeric matrix protein), a macromolecular ECM protein.[153]

Syndecans

Syndecans are members of a family of four transmembrane HSPGs consisting of a core protein covalently coupled with GAGs.[154,155] Syndecans function as coreceptors with growth factor or adhesion receptors and function to "tune" extracellular signal transfer across the cell surface to the cytoskeleton and cytoplasmic medi-

ators to effect activation of a variety of intracellular signaling cascades. All four syndecans are expressed in the artery and VSMC syndecans bind to ECM proteins, cell adhesion molecules, heparin-binding growth factors such as FGF and EGF, lipoproteins, lipoprotein lipases, and components of the blood-coagulation cascade.[22] Syndecan-1 inhibits VSMC growth in response to PDGF-BB and FGF2 after vascular injury,[140] whereas syndecan-4 has been implicated in thrombin-induced VSMC migration and proliferation by acting both as a mediator for bFGF signaling and as a cofactor for FGFR-1, suggesting that syndecan-4 is an early response gene after injury, whereas syndecan-1 is active during the proliferative and migratory phase.[155]

Mechanical Effects

Data on VSMC phenotypic modulation by the mechanical environment indicate that continuous cyclic mechanical strain acting directly on VSMCs increases collagen and FN synthesis, possibly by paracrine release of TGF-β1, resulting in increased ECM remodeling indicative of a VSMC synthetic phenotype.[23] In contrast, some studies have shown that mechanical strain can also stimulate the expression of contractile genes.[24] Although MAPK signaling pathways are induced following initiation of cyclic strain, the mechanisms for this induction are unclear. Activation of ion channels and tyrosine kinases and paracrine release of soluble mediators, such as Ang II, PDGF, and IGF, are postulated to play a role.[24] In addition, intra- and extracellular mechanical forces can stretch mechanosensitive molecules into different functional states, inducing biochemical signaling of varying quality and quantity, and inducing conformational changes regulating protein-protein interactions or enzymatically altering signaling molecules. Mechanotransduction can induce not only rapid changes in cellular mechanics but also long-term changes in gene expression.[156]

Mechanical signals play a role in stimulating cell cycle progression. Actin filament polymerization and organization induced by integrin ligation generate intracellular mechanical tensional forces that promote cell cycle progression.[157] In addition, "stiffness," or compliance of the ECM, can direct cellular functions through integrin-dependent signaling pathways involving FAK, the canonical mediator of integrin signaling, Rho family GTPase Rac, and cyclin D1.[158]

Central arterial stiffness is an independent risk factor for CVD and a predictor of future events.[159] VSMCs have a crucial role in controlling pathological arterial stiffness, as they both secrete mechanical load–bearing ECM components and also regulate actin/myosin-based contraction and mechanotransduction at cell-ECM interfaces.[160] (See Lacolley et al.[161] for review of VSMC molecules relevant to arterial stiffness.) Recently, intrinsic VSMC cellular properties in large arteries that modulate VSMC mechanical properties, in particular the SRF/myocardin/CArG pathway that governs genes encoding VSMC cytoskeletal/contractile proteins, have been shown to be important players in pathological aortic stiffening in hypertension and aging. These cell-based architectural changes are in addition to stiffness caused by changes in extracellular collagen content and wall thickness.[162] Inhibition of the SRF/myocardin/CArG pathway may therefore provide new therapeutic treatments for aortic wall stiffening and hypertension.

PHENOTYPE-SPECIFIC VASCULAR SMOOTH MUSCLE CELL FUNCTIONS

Contraction

The primary function of differentiated VSMC is to maintain vascular tone and blood pressure. This is an active process requiring significant energy expenditure, especially in resistance arterioles. A number of hormones and peptides regulate VSMC contraction, including catecholamines such as norepinephrine, Ang II, and endothelin-1. Contractions can be phasic, lasting only minutes, or tonic, depending on the stimulus.

In nearly all cases, stimulation of VSMC with contractile agents results in activation of a specific GPCR (Fig. 3.6). The immediate response is activation of PLC, which cleaves the membrane phospholipid phosphatidylinositol 4,5-bisphosphate (PIP_2) to release inositol 1,4,5-trisphosphate (IP_3) and diacylglycerol (DAG). IP_3, in turn, binds to its receptor (IP_3R, a ligand-gated Ca^{2+} channel) on the sarcoplasmic reticulum (SR), creating an open conformation and translocating Ca^{2+} to the cytoplasm. Simultaneously, receptor activation depolarizes the plasma membrane by altering the activity of pumps, such as the Na^+, K^+-ATPase, and channels, including Ca^{2+}-sensitive K^+ channels and TRP channels.[163] Membrane depolarization leads to activation of voltage-dependent L-type Ca^{2+} channels, calcium influx, and a more

sustained but less robust elevation of cytosolic calcium. Moreover, Ca^{2+} entry through these channels activates ryanodine receptors on the SR, further increasing Ca^{2+} release into the cytosol.

The increased cytoplasmic calcium binds to calmodulin (CaM) at a ratio of four calcium ions to one CaM molecule. CaM then undergoes a conformational change and binds to and activates MLCK, the enzyme responsible for phosphorylation of the 20-kDa regulatory myosin light chain (LC20) on serine 19. Activated LC20 facilitates actin-mediated myosin ATPase activity and cyclic interaction of myosin and actin,[164] leading to contraction. Contraction is maintained even when calcium drops, suggesting that LC20 becomes sensitized to calcium, likely by inhibition of myosin phosphatase (see further on).[165]

Because the increase in intracellular calcium caused by vasoconstrictors is largely responsible for activation of the contractile apparatus, essential mechanisms exist to limit Ca^{2+} entry and clear Ca^{2+} from the cytosol. Ryanodine receptors cluster to release calcium

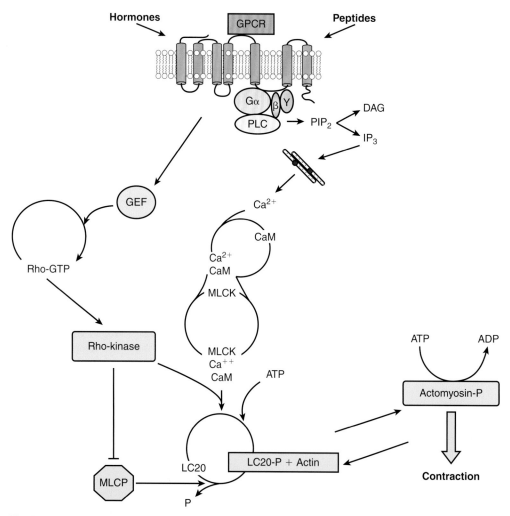

Fig. 3.6 A Model for the Contraction Cascade in Vascular Smooth Muscle Cells. Binding of contractile agonists to G protein–coupled receptor *(GPCR)* activates phospholipase C *(PLC)* and subsequent PLC-mediated hydrolysis of phosphtidylinositol 4,5-bisphosphate *(PIP₂)* to release inositol 1,4,5-trisphosphate *(IP₃)* and diacylglycerol *(DAG)*, leading to increased mobilization of Ca^{2+}. Ca^{2+} combines with calmodulin *(CaM)* and activates myosin light chain kinase *(MLCK)*–induced phosphorylation of myosin light chain *(MLC)*, which, together with actin, initiates contraction. In addition, guanine nucleotide exchange factor *(GEF)* activation of Rho leads to Rho kinase stimulation and inhibition of myosin light chain phosphatase *(MLCP)*, resulting in enhancement of contraction. (Modified from Griendling K, Harrison D, Alexander R. Biology of the vessel wall. In: Fuster V, Walsh R, Harrington R, eds. *Hurst's the Heart.* 13th ed. New York: McGraw-Hill; 2011:153–171. Courtesy Bernard Lassègue, PhD.)

sparks, which in turn stimulate Ca^{2+}-activated large-conductance K channels (BK channels) to cause hyperpolarization and limit L-type calcium channel activity.[166] Additionally, the sarcoplasmic reticulum Ca^{2+}-ATPase (SERCA) mediates Ca^{2+} reuptake into the SR, and serves to maximize Ca^{2+} extrusion from the cell because the newly taken up SR Ca^{2+} is released in a directed manner toward the plasma membrane, where a plasma membrane Ca^{2+}-ATPase extrudes Ca^{2+} from the cell. Importantly, SERCA is inhibited by CaM kinase II–mediated phosphorylation.[167]

Recently ROS and reactive nitrogen species (RNS) have emerged as effective modulators of contractile signaling.[168] Specifically, high levels of ROS oxidize SERCA, thereby inhibiting its activity. H_2O_2 applied externally increases IP_3 receptor–mediated release of Ca^{2+} into the cytosol, and calcium efflux from the SR is regulated in part by H_2O_2-induced reduction in IP_3Rs via proteasome degradation in VSMCs.[169] Activation of NADPH oxidases by contractile agonists sensitizes the IP_3 receptor to IP_3. Ryanodine receptors are also redox-sensitive. S-nitrosylation activates them, and exposure to endogenous levels of ROS and RNS can protect these receptors from inhibition by CaM at high concentrations of calcium. Both H_2O_2 and $O_2^{\bullet-}$ can stimulate Ca^{2+} entry via L- or T-type calcium channels (including TRP channels), but S-nitrosylation by NO is inhibitory. Thus, in general, ROS and RNS inhibit Ca^{2+} pumps and activate Ca^{2+} entry and release, resulting in an increase in intracellular Ca^{2+} concentration.

Myosin light chain phosphatase (MLCP) is also a vital regulator of vascular contraction. It is a multimeric enzyme composed of a regulatory myosin-binding subunit (MYPT1), a catalytic subunit (PP1c), and a 20-kDa protein (M20). The activity of MLCP is largely regulated by Rho kinase–mediated phosphorylation of MYPT1 on Thr695, either directly or via Rho-kinase activation of ZIP kinase.[165] MLCP activity can also be inhibited by CPI-17 (PKC-potentiated PP1 inhibitory protein of 17 kDa), which when phosphorylated by PKC, acts as a pseudosubstrate, binds to PP1c, and competes with LC20 for phosphorylation. Inhibition of MLCP activity enhances contraction, as mentioned, by inducing Ca^{2+} sensitization of the contractile apparatus.[170]

Rho kinase has thus emerged as an important part of the contraction cascade.[171] In addition to its role in enhancing contraction, as in response to Ang II, it is a major regulator of relaxation. Its activator, the low-molecular-weight GTPase RhoA, is a target of nitric oxide (NO), which by activating protein kinase G (PKG), inactivates Rho, thus indirectly inhibiting Rho kinase, increasing MLCP activity, and inhibiting contraction.

It is noteworthy that paracrine factors such as NO secreted by neighboring ECs represent the major mechanism of vasorelaxation. Shear stress forces and hormones such as acetylcholine or bradykinin stimulate ECs to secrete NO, which in turn initiates VSMC relaxation.[24,172,173] NO induces relaxation of smooth muscle potentially via a number of pathways, the most important of which depend on its ability to release cGMP. It can directly (via S-nitrosylation of cysteine residues) or indirectly (through PKG) activate BK channels,[174] thus causing membrane hyperpolarization and reducing influx through L-type Ca^{2+} channels. In addition, PKG phosphorylates IP_3 receptor–associated PKG-I substrate (IRAG), which inhibits Ca^{2+} release from IP_3 receptors. NO also increases Ca^{2+} uptake via S-glutathionylation of SERCA and decreases the Ca^{2+} sensitivity of contractile proteins. This pathway is perturbed in diabetic animal models, in which high levels of ROS derived from NADPH oxidase 4 irreversibly oxidize SERCA, rendering it insensitive to NO.[175] In addition to regulating Ca^{2+} levels, NO-mediated activation of PKG can phosphorylate PP1c and/or MYPT1 to block vasoconstrictor-mediated inhibition of MLCP.

Other relaxing factors secreted by ECs include H_2O_2, prostaglandins, and epoxyeicosatrienoic acids (EETs). In addition, perivascular adventitial adipocytes (PVAs) have also been shown to secrete factors that influence contractility.[176] These cytokines, collectively known as adipokines, are both vasoactive and pro- and antiinflammatory; they include cytokines TNF-α, IL-6, chemokines (IL-8 and MCP-1), and hormones (leptin, resistin, and adiponectin).[176,177]

Recent evidence has shown that cortical actin and actin contractile filaments form from different actin isoforms from separate gene products.[178] The α-smooth muscle actin is associated with the contractile apparatus, whereas β actin is associated with focal adhesions and cytoplasmic dense bodies that are actin filament insertion points for force transmission. Also, γ-nonmuscle actin is a major component of cortical actin networks. In response to stimulation, actin and actin networks are altered. Independent pathways activated by vasoconstrictors that regulate the actin cytoskeleton and promote F-actin formation include (1) p38MAPK through heat shock protein 27 (HSP27) and (2) cytosolic tyrosine kinase (Src and PYK2) through LIM protein paxillin and hydrogen peroxide inducible clone-5 (Hic-5). Cytosolic tyrosine kinases activated by vasoconstrictors in vascular tissue include Src, FAK, and PYK2, along with tyrosine phosphorylation of focal adhesion proteins paxillin, Hic-5, and p130 Crk–associated kinase (p130Cas). In differentiated VSMCs, Src and p130Cas relocalize between soluble and insoluble fractions after phenylephrine stimulation and focal adhesion proteins redistribute through an endocytic recycling pathway. Thus activation of cytosolic tyrosine kinases and phosphorylation of focal adhesion proteins result in remodeling of the actin cytoskeleton and focal adhesions. Importantly, this remodeling is essential to contractile response–independent myosin light chain phosphorylation. Focal adhesion sites are important for inside-out signaling (transducing internal contractile forces to the ECM) and outside-in signaling (transducing external forces such as mechanical stress/strain and ECM stiffness to the actin cytoskeleton in remodeling in response to vasoconstrictors, hypertension, and increased matrix stiffness).[179]

Proliferation

VSMC proliferation is important in early vascular development and in repair mechanisms in response to injury. However, excessive VSMC proliferation contributes to pathology not only in vascular proliferative diseases such as atherosclerosis but also, ironically, as a consequence of the intervention procedures used to treat these occlusive atherosclerotic diseases and their complications, including postangioplasty restenosis, vein bypass graft failure, and transplant failure.[180]

VSMC proliferation can be regulated by myriad soluble and insoluble factors that activate a variety of intracellular signaling pathways such as MAPK or Janus kinase/signal transducers, tyrosine phosphorylation, and mitogen-activated proteins.[181,182] Regardless of the initial proliferative stimulus, these signaling pathways ultimately converge onto the cell cycle (Fig. 3.7).[183] The four distinct phases of the cell cycle are (1) Gap 1 (G1) in which factors necessary for DNA replication are assembled; (2) DNA replication or S phase; (3) Gap 2 (G2) in preparation for mitosis; and (4) mitosis or M phase. Restriction points in the cell cycle exist at transitions between G1/S and G2/M. Progression through the cell cycle phases is regulated by CDKs and their regulatory cyclin subunits. Cyclins D/E and CDK2, 4, and 5 control G1, cyclin A and CDK2 control the S-phase along with the DNA polymerase cofactor proliferating cell nuclear antigen (PCNA), and cyclins A/B and CDK1 control the M phase. CDKIs such as $p27^{KIP1}$ and $p21^{CIP1}$ bind to and inhibit the activation of cyclin-CDK complexes (see Fig. 3.7). The activities of these enzymes depend on the phosphorylation status of CDKs, the levels of expression of cyclins, and the nuclear translocation of cyclin-CDK complexes. One regulatory protein is survivin, which competitively interacts with the CDK4/$p16^{INK4a}$ complex to form a CDK4/survivin complex, thus inducing CDK2/cyclin E activation

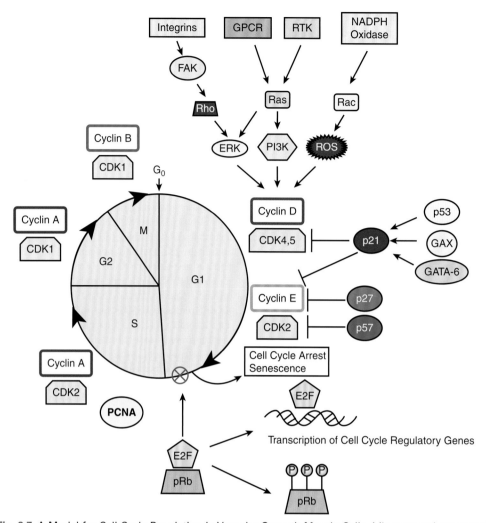

Fig. 3.7 A Model for Cell Cycle Regulation in Vascular Smooth Muscle Cells. Mitogens activate growth factor receptor tyrosine kinase *(RTK)*, G protein–coupled receptor *(GPCR)*, nicotinamide adenine dinucleotide phosphate *(NADPH)* oxidase, and integrins to stimulate extracellular signal–regulated kinase *(ERK)*, phosphatidylinositol 3-kinase *(PI3K)*, and Rho/Rac pathways, which converge onto cell cycle components, especially cyclin D, to regulate proliferation. Cyclin regulatory subunits and cyclin-dependent kinases *(CDKs)* catalytic subunits form holoenzymes, which are phase-specific for the four phases of the cell cycle: G1, DNA replication or S phase, G2 and mitosis or M phase. Endogenous cyclin-dependent kinase inhibitors *(CDKIs)*—— including p21, p27 and p57——inactivate cyclin/CDKs and therefore block cell cycle progression and proliferation. Other cell cycle regulators include the tumor suppressor p53 and the transcription factors GAX and GATA-6, which stimulate the CDKI p21^{CIP1} and induce cell cycle arrest. Cooperating with cyclin/CDKs is proliferating cell nuclear antigen *(PCNA)* for transition through G1 and S phases. Hyperphosphorylation of the retinoblastoma protein *(pRb)* releases elongation factor 2F *(E2F)*, allowing cell cycle progression through the G1 phase restriction point and the expression of genes required for DNA synthesis. Activation of p53 or Rb pathways results in cell cycle arrest and senescence.

and S phase entry and cell cycle progression.[184] TFs that transactivate CDKs and CDKIs also mediate cell cycle progression. p53, GAX, and GATA-6 induce p21^{CIP1} expression, leading to G1 phase arrest, whereas E2F TFs control the G1/S transition regulated by the retinoblastoma protein Rb, the product of the *rb* tumor suppressor gene. Rb exerts its negative regulation on the cell cycle by binding to E2F TFs, rendering them ineffective as TFs. When the Rb/E2F complex is phosphorylated by cyclin-dependent kinases in early G1, the complex is dissociated, leaving E2F available to activate genes required for S phase DNA synthesis.[183] It is worth noting that the HDAC inhibitor trichostatin A blocks proliferation by induction of the cell cycle inhibitor p21^{CIP1} and suppression of Rb protein phosphorylation, leading to subsequent cell cycle arrest at the G1/S phase.[184]

In addition to cell cycle regulatory proteins, telomerase activity is required for VSMC proliferation. Telomeres are noncoding DNA TTAGGG repeat sequences at the ends of chromosomes that cap and stabilize chromosomes against degradation, recombination, or fusion.[185] Associated with telomeric DNA are protein complexes, including telomerase, which synthesize new telomeric DNA in cells with high proliferative potential. Telomerase consists of an RNA component and two protein components, one of which is TERT (telomerase reverse transcriptase), the catalytic component and limiting factor for telomerase activation. When telomerase expression is low, telomere attrition with each mitotic cycle results in chromosome shortening and instability, replicative senescence, and growth arrest. In VSMCs, posttranslational phosphorylation of TERT is linked to telomerase activation,

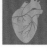

and levels of telomerase expression and activity correlate with proliferation.[185] Importantly, telomerase activation and telomere maintenance have been associated with excessive VSMC proliferation in both animal and human vascular injury and disease,[185] whereas disruption of telomerase activity reduces this proliferative response.

Growth of VSMC is initiated by exposure of the cells to proproliferative signals. Classical growth factors activate RTKs either directly or via GPCR-mediated transactivation.[183,184] Growth factors in VSMCs binding to RTKs include PDGF, bFGF, IGF1, TGF-β, and EGF, whereas mitogens that activate GPCRs include hormones such as Ang II,[43] endothelin, or oxidized LDL. Activation of these receptors stimulates sequential signaling cascades mediated by Ras, $p70^{S6K}$, Rac/NADPH/ROS, PI3K/Akt, MEK/ERK or MAPKK/p38MAPK, which induce cyclin D1 expression.[182] Src homology 2–containing protein tyrosine phosphatase 2 (SHP2), a member of the nonreceptor protein tyrosine phosphatase family, dephosphorylates tyrosine residues on target proteins in response to growth factors, hormones, and cytokines.[186] In VSMCs, SHP2 is a positive mediator of IGF-1- and LPA-induced MAPK signaling pathways, whereas SHP2 has negative effects on EGF- and Ang II–induced Akt signaling, implicating SHP2 in modulating cell cycle progression, growth, and migration.

An important integration point in growth factor signaling is mTOR (mammalian target of rapamycin), which regulates protein synthesis, cell cycle progression, and proliferation.[184] mTOR is a protein kinase that regulates translation initiation through effectors $p70^{S6K}$ and eIF4E, leading to the protein synthesis necessary for cell division. Rapamycin, an immunosuppressive macrolide antibiotic, inhibits mTOR downstream signaling cascades, with reductions in protein synthesis leading to cell cycle arrest.[183] In VSMCs, rapamycin inhibits the mTOR/$p70^{S6K}$ signaling axis and promotes a VSMC differentiated, contractile phenotype by regulating transcription of contractile proteins; it also induces expression of the antiproliferative CDKIs $p21^{CIP}$ and $p27^{KIP}$ to inhibit cell cycle progression.[184] The use of rapamycin (sirolimus)-coated coronary stents is highly effective in reducing the postangioplasty restenosis rate in interventional cardiology.[187]

Ion channels for Ca^{2+}, Mg^{2+}, and K^+ are also activated by growth factors and mediate proliferation. Transient increases in Ca^{2+} concentration, together with subsequent Ca^{2+} binding to its intracellular receptor CaM, are universally required for proliferation.[188] The mechanism for the Ca^{2+} sensitivity of this G1/S involves the Ca^{2+}-dependent binding of CaM to cyclin E and activation of CDK2 to promote G1/S transition and VSMC proliferation.[189,190] Elevated levels of Mg^{2+} increase expression of cyclin D1 and CDK4 and decrease activation of $p21^{CIP1}$ and $p27^{KIP1}$ through an ERK1/2-dependent, p38 MAP kinase–independent pathway.[191] Changes in VSMC K^+ channel expression profiles and activity are linked to cell cycle progression, implicating these ion channels as "internal timers" of VSMC cell division.[192] Growth factor–induced release of Ca^{2+} from intracellular Ca^{2+} storage organelles activates and upregulates intermediate-conductance Ca^{2+}-activated K^+ (IK_{Ca})-type K^+ channels, the predominant Ca^{2+}-sensitive K^+ channel in proliferating VSMCs.[193] In addition, voltage-gated K^+ channels $K_V1.3$[194] and $K_V3.4$[195] are upregulated in proliferating VSMCs. Blockade of these Ca^{2+} activated and voltage-gated K^+ channels inhibits proliferation and attenuates vascular disease/injury-induced remodeling in rodents.[196]

Signals from insoluble ECM-activated integrins and from soluble growth factor mitogens converge and jointly regulate upstream cytoplasmic signaling networks to mediate expression of cyclin D1 and cyclin E and associated CDK4/6 and CDK2 in the G1 phase, the part of the cell cycle most affected by extracellular stimuli.[197] In addition, joint RTK/integrin complex signaling networks impact G1 phase regulation by inhibiting $p21^{CIP1}$ and $p27^{KIP1}$, resulting in Rb phosphorylation and induction of E2F-dependent genes, with progression to autonomous stages of the cell cycle (S, G2, and M) that are independent of external stimuli.

As noted previously, Notch proteins are also important regulators of VSMC proliferation.[51] Notch4/HRT-induced repression of $p27^{KIP1}$ and Notch3/HRT1-induced repression of $p21^{CIP1}$, as well as upregulation of Akt signaling, an antiapoptosis pathway, result in promotion of VSMC proliferation. Furthermore, Notch1 is critical in mediating neointimal formation and remodeling after vascular injury.

PPARs, nuclear hormone receptors with regulatory roles in lipid and glucose metabolism, are beneficial in VSMCs by targeting genes for cell cycle progression, cellular senescence, and apoptosis to inhibit proliferation and neointimal formation in atherosclerosis and postangioplasty restenosis.[198] Activation of PPARα suppresses G1/S progression by inducing the expression of $p16^{INK4a}$ (a CDKI), thereby inhibiting phosphorylation of Rb.[199] This antiproliferative effect is mediated by repression of telomerase activity by inhibiting E2F binding sites in the TERT promoter.[198] Another PPAR isotype, PPARγ, also blocks G1/S cell cycle transition by preventing the degradation of $p27^{KIP1}$, resulting in inhibition of pRb phosphorylation and suppression of E2F-regulated genes responsible for DNA replication.[198] Similar to PPARα, PPARγ also inhibits telomerase activity in VSMCs by inhibition of early response gene Ets-1-dependent transactivation of the TERT promoter.[198] Thiazolidinediones (TZD), PPARγ agonists used clinically in the treatment of type 2 diabetes mellitus, decrease VSMC proliferation and prevent atherosclerosis in murine models of the disease.[198]

Cyclic adenosine 3′,5′-monophosphate (cAMP) and cyclic guanosine 3′,5′-monophosphate (cGMP) are second messengers in myriad signal transduction pathways.[200] In VSMCs, cAMP serves as an antagonist both to mitogenic signaling pathways, by inhibiting the MAPK kinase, PI3 kinase, and mTOR signaling axes, and to cell cycle progression by downregulating cyclins or upregulating CDKI $p27^{KIP1}$. An additional antiproliferative effect is due to downregulation of Skp2 (S-phase kinase-associated protein-2) mediated by inhibition of FAK phosphorylation and adhesion-dependent signaling. Skp2 is a ubiquitin ligase subunit that targets $p27^{KIP1}$ for proteasomal degradation, thus promoting VSMC proliferation.[201]

A more recently appreciated pathway that controls VSMC growth involves miRNAs. The potential involvement of these molecules was first noted in balloon-injured rat carotid arteries, where several miRNAs, including miR-21, are upregulated compared with control arteries.[202] Cell culture models show that miR-21 is a proproliferative and antiapoptotic regulator of VSMCs with target genes phosphatase and tensin homology deleted from chromosome 10 (PTEN), programmed cell death 4 (PDCD4), and B-cell lymphoma 2 (Bcl-2). miR-21 has opposite effects on PTEN and Bcl-2; overexpression downregulates PTEN and upregulates Bcl-2. PTEN modulates VSMCs through PI3K and Akt signaling pathways, while Bcl-2 mediates its downstream signaling through AP-1.

Finally, cell-cell junctions, as described above for cadherins and gap junction connexins, and cell-matrix contacts can greatly influence VSMC proliferation.[182] Normally, resident VSMCs, surrounded by and binding to polymerized collagen type 1 fibrils through α2β1 integrins, exhibit low proliferation indices, are arrested in the G1 phase of the cell cycle, and are refractory to mitogenic stimuli. In this quiescent state, levels of cell cycle regulatory proteins are modulated to inhibit the G1/S transition: cyclin E and CDK2 phosphorylation is inhibited, while CDKIs are upregulated and suppress cyclin E/CDK2 activity. Additionally, $p70^{S6K}$, a potent stimulator of mitogenesis and a regulator of $p27^{KIP1}$, is suppressed. In contrast, VSMCs on monomeric collagen matrices are responsive to growth factor signals which result in increased cyclin E–associated kinase activity and cell proliferation. These differential responses of VSMCs to structurally distinct forms of collagen type 1 are reflected in the differential regulation of cell cycle proteins and the differential response to mitogenic stimuli. Therefore perturbations or degradation of the collagen matrix, as found in sites of monomeric collagen in vascular lesions, result in altered VSMC proliferation, response to mitogens, and neointimal formation.[134]

Superoxide anion ($O_2^{\cdot-}$) is also increased in neointimal development and is necessary for VSMC proliferation. Manganese superoxide dismutase (SOD2) located in the mitochondria inhibits neointima formation in injured arteries, and inhibits Ang II–induced VSMC migration and proliferation by scavenging of $O_2^{\cdot-}$ and by suppressing PI3K/Akt signaling involved in Ang II–induced VSMC proliferation. Thus SOD2 is a negative regulator of injury-induced lesion formation by scavenging $O_2^{\cdot-}$.[203] Nox1 plays a role in VSMC proliferation in response to Ang II, PDGF, and thrombin, and its deficiency inhibits injury-induced neointimal formation.[204] Activation of Nox1 by NoxA1 increases neointimal formation via increased VSMC-induced $O_2^{\cdot-}$ and subsequent H_2O_2 formation.[205]

Migration

Smooth muscle migration is an essential element of wound repair, but unchecked migration and proliferation can contribute to neointimal thickening and the development of atherosclerotic plaques. A number of promigratory and antimigratory molecules regulate VSMC migration, including peptide growth factors, ECM components, and cytokines.[206] The extent of migration is also influenced by physical factors such as shear stress, stretch, and matrix stiffness. PDGF-BB, bFGF, and S1P are among the most potent promigratory stimuli in the vascular system. Intracellular signaling cascades initiated by these growth factors act in concert with those activated by integrin receptor interaction with matrix to mediate the migratory response. Matrix surrounding the migrating cell must be degraded by matrix metalloproteinases to allow a pathway into which the cell can protrude. Important promigratory matrix components include collagen I and IV, osteopontin, and laminin. Matrix interactions can also be antimigratory, as with the formation of stable focal adhesions, activation of tissue inhibitors of metalloproteinases, and heparin.

When a cell begins to migrate, a number of coordinated events must take place in a cyclic fashion (Fig. 3.8).[207] The signaling mechanisms that regulate migration have mostly been studied in fibroblasts,

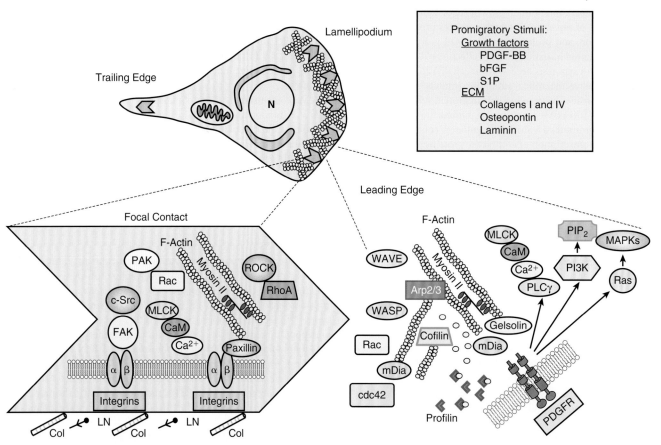

Fig. 3.8 Summary of Signaling and Effector Molecules Leading to Remodeling of the Actin Cytoskeleton at the Leading Edge and in Focal Contacts in Migrating Vascular Smooth Muscle Cells. In response to promigratory stimuli and the activation of multiple intracellular signaling pathways (details given in the text), cells extend lamellipodia and form new focal contacts, areas of dynamic actin turnover. Coordination of actin dynamics depends upon multiple actin-binding and associated proteins for actin filament nucleation and extension (actin-related protein (Arp2/3), WAVE, WASP, mDia, profilin) and actin filament depolymerization (cofilin) as well as filament capping and severing (gelsolin), remodeling events regulated by the small G proteins Rho, Rac and cdc42 and Rho-activated protein kinase (ROCK). Myosin II activation by Ca^{2+}/calmodulin (CaM)/myosin light chain kinase (MLCK) and p21-activated kinase (PAK) generates traction forces on the matrix to move the cell forward. In turn, matrix components exert traction forces by matrix/integrin binding-induced phosphorylation of focal contact components such as paxillin, focal adhesion kinase (FAK) and c-Src, which induce actomyosin motor protein interaction to move the cell forward.

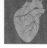

but recently many have been confirmed in VSMCs. Migration requires specialized signaling domains at the front and rear of the cell. When confronted with a migratory stimulus, the cell senses the gradient and established polarity. Plasma membrane in the form of lamellipodia is then extended in the direction of movement. This process is controlled by reorganization of the actin cytoskeleton just under the protruding membrane. New focal complexes are formed in the lamellipodia via cytoskeletal remodeling and integrin interaction with the matrix. The cell body begins to contract powered by engagement and phosphorylation of myosin II, and focal adhesions in the rear of the cell become detached, leading to retraction of the "tail" of the cell. Finally, adhesion receptors are recycled by endocytosis and vesicular transport. Successful migration is thus dependent on the proper temporal and spatial activation of many molecules, most of which are related to cytoskeletal elements.

Much is known or inferred about the signaling mechanisms activated by PDGF in migrating cells.[206] When PDGF-BB binds to PDGF receptors, receptor autophosphorylation creates binding sites for PLCγ, which mobilizes calcium; PI3K, which forms the membrane-targeting lipid PIP_2; and Ras, which activates MAPKs. Nucleation of new actin filaments at the leading edge is initiated by binding of nucleation promoting factors verprolin–homologous protein (WAVE) and Wiskott-Aldrich syndrome protein (WASP) to actin-related protein ARP2/3; phosphorylation of the actin binding coronin; and dissociation of actin capping proteins, many of which are regulated by PIP_2. Extension of new actin filaments is promoted by formins (mDia1 and mDia2), which act on the plus end of actin filaments in coordination with profilin. Regulation of mDia proteins is largely via conformational changes induced by the small G-proteins RhoA and cdc42. Profilin increases nucleotide exchange on G-actin monomers, thus enhancing actin polymerization.

Severing of existing actin filaments is a consequence of activation of gelsolin and cofilin, which limit the length of filaments and initiate turnover of existing filaments. Cofilin activity is regulated by cycling between phosphorylated (inactive) by LIM kinases 1 and 2, rendering cofilin unable to bind to F-actin, and nonphosphorylated (active) by protein phosphatase Slingshot (SSH) states.[208] Oxidation of cofilin by H_2O_2 at the leading edge in migrating cells inhibits cofilin-induced actin severing, increasing F-actin/G-actin ratios, enhancing F-actin stability, and promoting cell migration.[209,210]

The mechanism for H_2O_2-induced migration in VSMCs also involves H_2O_2 oxidation of cysteine residues in the α7 subunit of integrin α7β1 via binding of the integrin to laminin-111 in membrane protrusions, increasing migration.[211] PDGF induces VSMC migration via Nox-1 mediated, ROS-dependent activation of Src and Rac effectors (PAK1).[212] Thrombin stimulates VSMC migration and proliferation via Nox1-mediated transactivation of the EGFR.[208] In addition, Poldip2 (polymerase delta-interacting protein 2), a Nox4/p22phox interacting protein that regulates Nox4, modulates the Rho-dependent cytoskeleton and impacts cellular migration by mechanisms regulating actin cytoskeletal changes and focal adhesion turnover.[213]

Rac also regulates actin reorganization in the lamellipodium, perhaps by activation of p21-activated kinase (PAK)-mediated phosphorylation of actin-binding proteins. The result of these complicated coordinated events is protrusion of lamellipodia in the direction of the detected migratory stimulus (see Fig. 3.8). Once lamellipodial protrusion has occurred, it is necessary for the cell to create new contacts with the matrix and dissolve those no longer needed. These nascent focal contacts provide traction for eventual contraction of the cell body and propulsion of the cell forward.[206] Very little is known about focal adhesion composition in VSMCs, but signaling at focal adhesions is coordinated by integrin interaction with the matrix, integrin clustering, activation of a series of protein tyrosine kinases——including integrin-linked kinase (ILK), FAK, and Src——and interaction with the cortical F-actin cytoskeleton. Phosphorylation of focal adhesion components including FAK and paxillin occurs during VSMC migration, as does turnover of focal adhesion proteins by membrane-type metalloproteinases. Regulation of focal adhesion turnover is also intimately related to the microtubular network.

The final major event in cell migration is contraction of the cell body. Similar to contraction in differentiated cells, cell body contraction is initiated through calcium-mediated activation of MLCK and MLC phosphorylation following matrix interaction. RhoA and Rho kinase may also play a role, as pharmacological inhibition of Rho kinase blocks migration of VSMCs.[214] Current theory suggests that myosin II generates traction forces on the matrix, and the matrix in turn regulates myosin II activation.[206]

Much research remains to be done to fully elucidate the mechanisms underlying VSMC migration, but the potential for identifying new targets for prevention of restenosis and plaque formation is obvious (see Tang and Gerlach[215] for review on actin cytoskeleton, intermediate filaments, and microtubules on VSMC migration and Xu et al.[210] for a summary list of direct oxidation sites on actin, actin-binding proteins, and actin regulatory proteins as well as for components/pathways involved in redox regulation of the actin cytoskeleton in cell migration, contraction, and division).

INFLAMMATION AND INFLAMMATION-RELATED PROCESSES

The classical paradigm for the etiology of atherosclerosis, which focused on systemic cues such as blood pressure and impaired lipid metabolism, particularly increased LDL levels in the plasma, has recently expanded to include inflammation and inflammation-related processes. Clinical data from the CANTOS trial, which showed anti-inflammatory therapies reduced CVD without altering lipid profiles, demonstrate the need to look beyond LDL-C reduction and residual cholesterol risk for therapeutic intervention. The new paradigm for atherogenesis centers on inflammatory mediators[216] and the myriad intracellular processes that cross talk and link with the inflammatory response, particularly in VSMCs as these cells have key roles in pathological vascular remodeling.[217] These interrelated processes include oxidative and ER stress, mitochondrial damage and dysfunction, autophagy, apoptosis, and efferocytosis.

Oxidative Stress

ROS, including $O_2^{\cdot-}$, H_2O_2, and hydroxyl radicals, are generated as by-products of aerobic metabolism.[97] Under physiological conditions, ROS regulate signal transduction, gene expression, and proliferation. The shift in ROS levels from physiological to pathophysiological results in oxidative stress and leads to activation of VSMC proinflammatory genes via the stress-activated protein kinase p38MAPK and proinflammatory TFs such as NF-κB and STAT1/3. In addition, TNF-α–induced NF-κB signaling in VSMCs leads to increased expression of proinflammatory VCAM-1, MCP-1, fractalkine, and osteopontin. These responses are reduced in transgenic mice overexpressing VSMC-specific catalase, indicating that H_2O_2 produced in VSMCs regulates vascular inflammation. In addition, H_2O_2 induces expression of receptor activator of NF-κB ligand (RANKL) in VSMC, promoting macrophage infiltration. The combination of H_2O_2 produced from both activated VSMCs and the infiltrated monocytes/macrophages results in a vicious cycle of ROS and inflammation in the vasculature.[211]

The major sources of ROS in VSMCs are the mitochondrial respiratory enzymes and the NADPH oxidases (Noxs) family of transmembrane enzymes. Mitochondria generate the highly reactive, membrane-impermeable $O_2^{\cdot-}$, which is generally scavenged by SOD and converted to H_2O_2, a membrane-permeable signaling molecule.[210] The Nox enzymes in the vasculature consist of distinct isoforms and are differentially localized within the VSMC. Nox1, 2, 4, and 5 are the major Noxes in VSMC. Nox1, 2, and 4 require a second transmembrane subunit p22phox, while Nox5 is activated by calcium signaling. Nox1 produces $O_2^{\cdot-}$ and requires cytosolic p47phox, p67phox or NoxO1 and NoxA1, while Nox4 produces H_2O_2 and is constitutively active without requiring these cytosolic components.[210] Nox1, 2, and 4 in VSMC have all been implicated in multiple CVDs, including atherosclerosis, hypertension, and diabetic vasculopathy.

Inflammasomes

One of the primary stimuli for the development of inflammation is oxLDL which can activate inflammasomes. Inflammasomes are multiprotein complexes in the cytoplasm that "sense" danger signals, including pathogen-associated molecular patterns (PAMPs) and danger-associated molecular patterns (DAMPs).[218,219] The NLRP3 (nucleotide oligomerization domain-like receptor family, pyrin domain containing 3) inflammasome is the best-known and is implicated in atherogenesis. OxLDL-activated inflammasomes in turn activate caspase-1 and subsequent maturation of proinflammatory cytokines, such as IL-1β and IL-18, responsible for rapid lytic cell death or pyroptosis.[220] NLRP3 inflammasome activation mechanisms and atherogenesis mechanisms share similarities, including oxidative stress, ER stress, mitochondrial dysfunction, and lysosome rupture. In addition, the NLRP3 inflammasome contributes to atherosclerosis progression by affecting a sequence of cellular and molecular targets such as STAT, MAPK, JNK, the miR network, ROS, and protein kinase R (PRK).[218] In addition to its role in atherogenesis, the NLRP3 inflammasome is also involved in VSMC contractile protein degradation, leading to aortic aneurysm and dissection,[221] and in regulating VSMC phenotypic transformation and proliferation in hypertension.[222]

Endoplasmic Reticulum Stress and the Unfolded Protein Response Pathway

The ER is a membrane-like organelle responsible for protein translation, posttranscriptional modification of proteins, and maintenance of cellular Ca^{2+} homeostasis and lipid biosynthesis. The ER is responsive to stressors such as ROS, ischemia/reperfusion, disruption of Ca^{2+} homeostasis, and release of inflammatory cytokines and toxins which can cause misfolded/unfolded proteins to build up in the ER lumen.[223] ER stress is triggered by increased demand for protein secretion or an accumulation of misfolded/unfolded secretory proteins in the ER.[224]

ER stress is sensed by three resident sensors in the ER: (1) inositol requiring enzyme 1 (IRE-1α); (2) activating transcription factor-6 (ATF6); and (3) protein kinase RNA-like endoplasmic reticulum kinase (PERK). The TF CHOP (C/EBP homologous protein), which activates IL-1β signaling and mediates apoptosis and inflammation, can be activated by all three ER stress sensors.[223,225] ER stress leads to the unfolded protein response (UPR) which is activated to induce the expression of ER-localized chaperones to aid in the folding process or to upregulate genes for protein degradation in a conserved protein quality control mechanism.[226] ER stress in VSMCs has roles in (1) phenotypic switching, (2) trans/dedifferentiation, and (3) apoptosis, leading to atherosclerosis, hypertension, aneurysms, and vascular calcification.[217]

Activation of UPR sensors is triggered at different times during the progression of atherosclerosis.[227] In early lesions, the PERK pathway that reduces protein burden by blocking protein translation is activated

in VSMCs, playing a prosurvival role. Sustained ER stress in lesion progression leads to PERK pathway-induced death effector expression, with IRE1 activating apoptosis in VSMCs in advanced lesions. ER stress mechanisms are also implicated in autophagy and inflammation, illustrating tight integration and cross talk among these biological processes in the progression of CVD.[223]

The pathological progress of ER-stress–mediated atherosclerosis is similar to the development of abdominal aortic aneurysms (AAAs); both are complex diseases involving inflammation, ROS, degradative proteases, and apoptosis. A recent study in human AAA walls in ex vivo culture reported that statin (3-hydroxy-3-methyl-glutaryl-CoA reductase [HMG-CoA reductase]) therapy may have beneficial effects on AAA progression.[228] In a subsequent study using Ang II- or $CaCl_2$ mouse models of AAA, atorvastatin suppressed AAA development by reducing ER stress signaling proteins, ER stress–associated apoptosis, and the inflammatory response.[225]

Mitochondrial Dysfunction

Mitochondria are the "powerhouses" of the cell, generating ATP through oxidative phosphorylation. Importantly, mitochondria also produce potentially harmful reactive oxygen species (mtROS), which account for approximately 90% of total cellular ROS. mtROS products $O_2^{\cdot-}$ and H_2O_2 target phosphatases and other proteins via cysteine oxidation, inactivating phosphatase activity, and altering signaling cascades.[229]

Mitochondrial morphology is indicative of mitochondrial function: fusion of mitochondria results in elongated morphology maximizing ATP synthesis efficiency, whereas fission-generated mitochondrial fragments are transient and subject to autophagic degradation. PTEN-induced putative kinase-1 (PINK1) on healthy mitochondria is constitutively imported and degraded by protease presenilin–associated rhomboid-like (PARL) at the inner membrane. In dysfunctional mitochondria, import of PINK1 is inhibited and PINK1 accumulates at the outer membrane where its kinase activity recruits the lynchpin E3 ubiquitination ligase Parkin for mitophagy.[230] In a recent study, a subset of plaque VSMCs exhibited mitochondrial dysfunction with increased mtDNA damage, reduced oxidative phosphorylation, and PINK1 kinase expression as well as increased glycolytic activity.[231] These data suggest that PINK1 kinase may initiate a compensatory glycolytic switch in VSMCs in the context of mitochondrial dysfunction in atherosclerotic plaque.

In pulmonary hypertension, mitofusin 2 (Mfn2), a protein that mediates mitochondrial fusion, is decreased while mitochondrial fission proteins are increased. Furthermore, increased mitochondrial fission not only promotes VSMC proliferation in PAH but has also been reported to regulate arterial VSMC constriction, suggesting a mitochondrial fission-contraction coupling in VSMC and a novel mechanism for vasoconstriction in hypertension.[232]

Oxidative DNA damage and the DNA damage response (DDR) in both nuclear and mitochondrial DNA have been found in plaque VSMCs.[233] The DDR response attenuates the cell cycle, allowing DNA repair, or induces senescence or apoptosis if damage is severe. Although mtDNA damage and ROS are associated with atherosclerosis, whether oxidative stress-induced damage is a cause or consequence of atherosclerosis is controversial.[234] Targeting other parameters to increase mitochondrial health, such as enhancing mitochondrial fusion or mitophagy, may be important new therapies in the future.

Autophagy

Autophagy is a highly evolutionarily conserved and highly genetically regulated housekeeping process to promote cell survival by targeting damaged proteins and organelles to the lysosomal pathway for degradation, especially during nutrient/amino acid or energy deficiencies. Autophagy plays a key role in cell development and tissue remodeling and also protects against metabolic stress, ROS, and cytokines. However, in addition to enabling protective mechanisms, autophagy also functions in pathogenesis of vascular disease, especially when the autophagic process is impaired.[235-237]

The three types of autophagy include (1) macroautophagy, the most common and most studied form, in which large proteins and organelle components are sequestered into a double-membrane bounded autophagosome that fuses with acidic lysosome for degradation; (2) microautophagy, in which lysosome/late endosome membrane invaginates inward, engulfing cytosolic components for nonselective degradation and recycling of nutrients in starvation; and (3) chaperone-mediated autophagy, in which complexes of heat shock cognate (hsc70) and proteins bearing KFERQ-motifs are internalized into lysosomes via interaction with the lysosome-associate membrane protein (LAMP-2A).[238]

Autophagy is induced by growth factors, cytokines, and stress-sensing conditions (hypoxia, ROS, and ER stress). The best characterized signaling pathway in autophagosome biogenesis is the mTOR pathway, which is a negative regulator of autophagy.[236] The AMP-activated protein kinase (AMPK) is a positive regulator. Autophagy induction has differential consequences in VSMCs depending upon the stimulus. PDGF-BB–induced autophagy increases cell survival under oxidative stress conditions, whereas other growth factors, cytokines, and secreted signaling agents such as osteopontin, Shh, TNF-α, and Ang II promote cell death.[239] Many autophagic stimuli have a redox component. Reactive lipids, advanced glycation end products, and free radicals all regulate VSMC autophagy. VSMCs exposed to low levels of oxLDL showed increased LOX-1 (lectin-like oxidized low-density lipoprotein scavenger receptors-1) expression and increased autophagy, whereas increased oxLDL levels, with generation of large amounts of ROS and nonviable cells, could not be rectified by autophagy protection and induced apoptosis.[240] TNF-α stimulates autophagy and apoptosis, promoting cell death in VSMCs, whereas Ang II-induced autophagy in VSMC leads to cell death and has a role in initiation of vascular injury.[237] VSMCs treated with 7-ketocholesterol, an inducer of ER stress, accumulate ubiquitinated proteins, activating UPR leading to impaired autophagy and cell death.[241] In summary, autophagic flux in a VSMC can have protective or detrimental impacts on VSMC biology and can affect VSMC phenotypic switching.

Apoptosis and Efferocytosis

Apoptosis, or programmed cell death, is a tightly regulated process important in tissue homeostasis for clearance of aged and senescent cells, in remodeling events such as physiological remodeling after birth, and in response to flow dynamics, vessel injury, or disease.[242] Apoptosis is controlled by multiple signaling pathways that induce cell membrane shrinkage, membrane blebbing, nuclear and cytoplasmic condensation, and cellular fragmentation. Apoptotic cells and fragments are removed by programmed cell removal, or efferocytosis, from a Greek term meaning "to carry the dead to the grave," referring to the phagocytic removal of the dead cell "corpses."[243] There are multiple molecules implicated in cross talk between dying cells and potential phagocytes, including (1) chemoattractant "find me" ligands for recruitment of phagocytes to areas of cell death; (2) bridging molecules linking phagocytes and target cells; and (3) "eat me" cell surface ligands that engage and transactivate receptors on the phagocyte for engulfment and clearance.[243] Importantly, there are counterbalancing "don't eat me" ligands, such as the canonical signal CD47, on healthy cells; these ligands are downregulated in programmed cell death.

Apoptosis can be induced by both extrinsic and intrinsic mechanisms. Extrinsic apoptosis is triggered by binding of death receptors, TNFR1, Fas, and death receptor-4 and -5 to their cognate ligands: TNF (for TNFR1), Fas ligand (for Fas), and TNF-related apoptosis-inducing ligand (TRAIL) for DR4/5, with recruitment of death-inducing signaling complex (DISC), consisting of Fas-associated death domain and pro-caspase-8. DISC recruitment initiates caspase-3 activation resulting in apoptosis. In contrast to ligand-death receptor caspase activation in extrinsic apoptosis, intrinsic apoptosis requires intracellular signals for activation, including DNA damage induced-translocation of proapoptotic proteins Bax (BCL-2-associated X protein) and Bak (BCL-2 antagonist) to the outer membrane of mitochondria, resulting in loss of mitochondrial transmembrane potential, release of cytochrome *c* into the cytoplasm, caspase-9 and -3 activation, DNA fragmentation, membrane blebbing, and cell death.[244]

Clearance of cellular apoptotic bodies limits release of proinflammatory cytokines, such as TNF-α and IL-12, while increasing release of antiinflammatory cytokines, such as IL-10 and TGF-β, from phagocytes. VSMC apoptosis stimulates surrounding viable VSMCs to release mitogenic/chemoattractant factors, such as IL-6 and SDF-1 (stromal cell-derived factor-1), leading to the proliferation, migration, matrix synthesis, and recruitment of SMC progenitors to injured sites.[242] Apoptosing cells also release noninflammatory and "tolerate me" signals.[244]

Efficient phagocytosis of dying cells is normally swift. An important exception to swift efferocytosis occurs within the atherosclerotic plaque, where efferocytosis is reduced about 20-fold compared with other places in the body.[243] These deficiencies in clearance result in the accumulation of apoptotic cells and cellular debris, leading to expansion of the necrotic core and the acceleration of vascular inflammation. Loss of VSMCs through apoptosis promotes elastin fragmentation as well as increased GAGs and calcification, all features of vulnerable plaques.[242]

Because lineage-traced mice studies have shown that significant numbers of plaque macrophages are in fact of smooth muscle and not myeloid origin, there may be different mechanisms for efferocytosis for macrophages and VSMC-derived macrophage-like cells.[243] VSMCs, known to have efferocytic capabilities, are "nonprofessional" phagocytes, but their efferocytotic capabilities are impaired when they are exposed to oxidized lipids; thus VSMC-derived foam cells would be inefficient efferocytes in the oxidized conditions in plaque.

As indicated in this section, inflammation and related processes interact and share common pathways and mechanisms not only with each other but also with pathways leading to proproliferative phenotypes. Autophagy shares pathways with other cellular mechanisms: (1) autophagy-protein-6 (ATG6 or Beclin1) signaling functions in both autophagy and apoptosis; (2) autophagy gene product Atg7 modulates p53 activity for regulation of the cell cycle; and (3) autophagy proteins AMBRA1 and Beclin1 regulate c-Myc and have roles in cross talk between autophagy and proliferation.[237] Cell death and inflammation are coupled through inflammasomes, which regulate cytokine release in inflammation. Apoptosis and autophagy share complementary pathways. Furthermore, apoptosis is regulated by ER stress and the UPR.

SENESCENCE AND AGING

Aging is the dominant risk factor for CVD and atherosclerotic lesion formation.[245] Over 400 years ago, Thomas Syndenham commented that "a man is as old as his arteries."[236] Aging VSMCs in particular are important contributors to vascular aging, with extrinsic factors, such as environmental changes, leading to vascular deterioration or disease, and intrinsic factors, such DNA/mitochondrial damage and defects in proteostasis or nutrient sensing, contributing to vascular aging. Aging and senescence are interrelated and share similar pathways.[229]

Senescence

Cellular senescence is the progressive decline of normal cell function but it paradoxically serves as a protective mechanism in response to excessive stresses, including mitochondrial dysfunction, DNA damage, and increased ROS. Senescence induces permanent cell-cycle arrest in the G1 phase, thus preventing the transmission of damage to progeny cells. Multiple stresses——including DNA-damaging radiation or chemicals, mitochondrial dysfunction, and oxidant stress——can invoke two types of senescence programs: stress-induced premature senescence (SIPS) and replicative senescence associated with accelerated telomere uncapping or shortening.[246] Senescence stimulatory pathways converge onto two effector pathways: the p53 and p16[ink4a]-Rb pathway. p53 is normally targeted to proteasome-mediated degradation by MDM2 (mouse double minute2). Mitogenic stress or DNA damage suppresses MDM2 activity, resulting in p53-mediated activation of the CDKI p21 and cell cycle arrest.[247] Atherogenic stimuli such as Ang II initially stimulate proliferation, followed by mitogen-induced SIPs or replicative senescence via telomere uncapping. Inflammatory cytokine/chemokine release by senescent VSMCs results in ECM degradation. The decreased cellularity and increased inflammation contribute to plaque instability.[248]

In the second pathway, stress or damage activates Rb, which then binds to and inhibits E2F, a TF required for the G1 phase/S phase transition to cell cycle progression (see Fig. 3.7). These two senescence pathways exhibit cross talk at the level of p53 and can overlap death pathways. Senescent cells release degradative proteases, growth factors, and inflammatory cytokines, which affect neighboring cells.

Senescent VSMCs in aged and atherosclerotic vessels express the senescent marker senescent associated-β-galactosidase (SA-β-Gal) and exhibit other senescence features such as decreased proliferation, decreased cyclin expression, and increased expression of cell cycle inhibitors p21 and p16[ink4a]. Senescent human VSMCs actively secrete IL-1α and develop an IL-1α–driven senescence-associated secretory phenotype (SASP), releasing high levels of multiple inflammatory cytokines including IL-6 and chemokines including IL-8. Thus, VSMCs actively promote chemotaxis of mononuclear cells via MCP-1 secretion, release MMP-9, upregulate inflammasome components, and prime ECs and VSMCs for a proadhesive and proinflammatory state, leading to chronic inflammation and matrix degradation in lesions. Although senescent VSMCs exist in small numbers in the plaque, the SASP response is persistent and is not dependent on external stimulation. In addition, IL-1α secreted into the environment can act on responsive ECs and VSMCs, which produce even more proinflammatory cytokines and chemokines, amplifying inflammation.

In VSMCs, DNA damage caused by ROS, such as $O_2^{\cdot-}$, H_2O_2, and hydroxyl radicals, incites rapid (within days) SIPS. There are increased levels of ROS in all diseased layers of an atherosclerotic lesion, particularly in the plaque itself,[246] and senescent VSMCs have been identified in injured arteries and in the intima of atherosclerotic plaques.[248] Senescent VSMCs are also implicated in vascular calcification. They exhibit enhanced expression of osteoblastic genes such as ALP, type 1 collagen, and RUNX-2, while the expression of matrix Gla protein (MGP), an anticalcification factor, is downregulated.[249]

The therapeutic removal of senescent cells using "senolytics" was recently demonstrated in an LDL-null mice model. Atherosclerotic plaques from these animals showed markers of senescence, including SA-β-Gal and SASPs, in ECs, VSMCs, and macrophages identified by transmission electron microscopy ultrastructure.[250] When the investigators then used transgenic mice containing reporter and/or suicide genes to kill cells with p16[ink4a] promoter activity, all three senescent cell types were eliminated, and removal of these cells reduced plaque formation and progression. Therefore, removal of p16[ink4a+]/SA-β-Gal+ senescent cells or use of the senolytic drug ABT263, an inhibitor of antiapoptotic proteins Bcl-2 and Bcl-xL, may be useful for age-associated diseases such as atherosclerosis.[251]

Aging

As organisms age chronologically, they experience a time-dependent functional decline with the accumulation of cellular damage.[252] There are multiple "hallmarks of aging" common across all tissues and extensive interconnectedness among these aging hallmarks (see recent reviews of common denominators of aging in cells/tissues[252] and in VSMCs in particular[229,253]). Extrinsic systemic or environmental factors mediating vascular aging include disease and alterations in vascular cell communication. Hallmarks of aging due to intrinsic factors include evidence of senescence, proinflammatory secretory phenotype, epigenetic changes, DNA damage (including telomere attrition), mitochondrial dysfunction producing oxidative stress, defects in protein homeostasis, defective nutrient sensing, loss of nuclear organization, and exhaustion of progenitor cells.[253] Some of these mechanisms were discussed earlier.

In diseases such as atherosclerosis and hypertension, normally contractile VSMCs modulate to express a secretory or inflammatory phenotype characteristic of arterial aging, with increased proliferation, migration, oxidative stress, inflammation, senescence, and apoptosis in the plaque environment or in the remodeled vascular wall. Arterial stiffness in central arteries, one of the important factors in vascular aging, is due to increased collagen-to-elastin ratios, and enhanced collagen cross-linking and calcification.[161] In addition, EC-VSMC communication via paracrine signaling or myoendothelial junctions is defective in age-related vascular dysfunction and disease.[229]

DNA Damage

DNA damage in aged VSMCs in human atherosclerosis includes strand breaks, chromosome damage, telomere shortening, and the oxidation of guanosine.[253] The DNA damage response includes recruitment of the histone 2A protein X (H2AX), which is then phosphorylated by kinases such as ataxia telangiectasia–mutated (ATM) protein and ATM-Rad3-related (ATR) in the PI3K pathway. Another marker of DNA damage is the phosphorylated form of γ-H2AX. ATM and ATR also activate p53, the main regulator of DNA damage response. p53 acts via multiple mechanisms such as cell cycle arrest and apoptosis by inducing expression of pro- and antiapoptotic genes.[229] VSMCs in plaques show increased ATM and γ-H2AX levels.

Telomere Attrition

Telomeres serve as protective caps against degradation, recombination, and fusion. Telomere length is regulated through telomerase and the protein complex Shelterin. Telomere loss leads to DNA damage response with subsequent cellular senescence, apoptosis, or inflammation. Factors reducing telomere length include genetics, cell division, inflammation, hypertension, and cholesterol levels. Short telomere length and reduced telomerase expression are evident in aged and atherosclerotic VSMCs.[229]

Defective Nutrient Sensing

Protective pathways for nutrient deficiencies include the glucose-sensing IGF-1/Akt and insulin signaling, the most conserved aging-controlling pathways. Other nutrient-sensing systems include

5′-AMPK, which senses low-energy conditions by detecting high AMP levels, mTOR for sensing high amino acid concentrations, and the sirtuin HDACs, which sense low-energy states by detecting high NAD+ levels. The effectors of these pathways include forkhead box protein O (FOXO) proteins, mTOR and PPAR-γ coactivator-1α (PGC1α), the master regulator of metabolism, which mediates mitochondriogenesis and increased antioxidant defenses.[252]

In atherosclerosis, downregulation of IGF1 receptor and subsequent reduction in Akt signaling result in activation of FOXO proteins leading to increased features of vulnerable plaques.[253] Knockout of PGC1α leads to increased oxidative stress and mitochondrial abnormalities, and reductions in telomerase activity and levels of sirtuin1 and the antioxidant catalase. These changes lead to increased VSMC senescence, which promotes the progression of atherosclerosis and inhibits plaque repair.[254]

Mitochondrial Dysfunction

Mitochondrial aging effects are due to (1) defective antioxidant mechanisms, with aging mice exhibiting reduced levels of SOD1, SOD2, glutathione peroxidase (Gpx3, Gpx4), catalase, and glutathione S-transferase Mu 1; (2) defective mitochondrial biogenesis/dynamics; and (3) mtDNA damage. Aging and disease alter mitochondrial dynamics, characterized by biogenesis, fusion, and fission. Aged VSMCs have reduced expression of biogenesis markers such as mitochondrial transcription factor A (TFAM) and PGC-1α.

Defects in Protein Homeostasis

There are multiple quality-control mechanisms to preserve proteostasis by ensuring that biogenesis, folding, trafficking, and degradation of proteins all occur in a coordinated manner, thus preventing accumulation of damaged components and renewal of intracellular proteins. Aging impairs chaperone-mediated protein folding and stability, and also results in a decline in the autophagy-lysosomal and ubiquitin-proteasome systems.[252] Defects in protein storage, misfolding or secretion can lead to ER stress and the UPR discussed earlier, as well as oxidative stress signaling through Nox4 and Nox2 pathways, which are important ROS sources during the UPR.[255] UPR is activated in VSMCs in atherosclerosis and can lead to VSMC death within the plaque, resulting in decreased collagen production and consequent thinning of the protective fibrous cap.[224]

Loss of Nuclear Organization

Lamins, intermediate filaments inside the nuclear envelope, not only provide structure for the nucleus but also function in chromatin organization, transcription, and DNA replication and repair. Functional lamin protein requires posttranslational modifications including farnesylation and methylation; in aging VSMCs, permanently farnesylated pre-lamin A accumulations cause DNA damage and mitotic defects. Interestingly, mutations in the *LMNA* gene, associated with the genetic disease Hutchinson-Gilford progeria syndrome (HGPS), cause an aging-like phenotype in VSMCs, which exhibit decreased telomere length, DNA damage, and premature senescence. HGPS patients have premature atherosclerosis and die of stroke or myocardial infarction.[229]

Exhaustion of Stem/Progenitor Cells

Aging is accompanied by decline in the regenerative potential of tissue and the attrition of functional stem/progenitor cells.[252] Some VSMCs in plaque have been proposed to derive from HSCs or endothelial progenitor cells (EPCs) that migrate into the vascular wall. Dysfunctional EPCs and HSCs are seen in aged and atherosclerotic mouse models.[253] Furthermore, there may be a multipotent vascular stem cell niche

giving rise to VSMCs[256] that could become exhausted by multiple divisions or damage.[257]

CONCLUSIONS

The protean nature of VSMCs is fundamental not only to their contractile and synthetic functions within the normal vessel wall during development and maturation but also to vascular remodeling in response to injury and disease. As outlined in this chapter, advances in technology have led to reassessments of "classical" dogmas in VSMC biology and caused paradigm shifts in multiple areas. These shifts have resulted from (1) developmental and genetic studies showing that——in addition to environmental cues such as shear stress on the EC——the embryonic origins of VSMCs determine disease location; (2) from lineage tracing in transgenic animal models suggesting that foam cells in the atherosclerotic neointima are derived in part from resident transdifferentiated VSMCs in the vascular wall and not exclusively by invasion of circulating bone marrow–derived monocytes; (3) from the omics revolution, such as transcriptomics, which demonstrated the existence and importance of regulatory noncoding RNAs, including miRNAs and, more recently, lncRNAs, that impact mechanisms of VSMC biology at every level; (4) from clinical trials that shifted emphasis from hyperlipidemia to inflammation in the etiology of atherosclerosis, thus focusing attention on the myriad interrelationships, cross talk, and redundancy among inflammation and inflammation-stimulated processes in VSMCs; (5) from high resolution microcomputed tomography (CT) clinical data and finite element modeling of stress mechanics showing the importance of plaque microcalcification in predicting future adverse CVD events, thus focusing interest on VSMC-derived calcifying exosomes; (6) and from whole-exome sequencing that showed association between somatic mutation–driven clonal hematopoiesis and increased coronary artery disease.

As some paradigms were overturned, earlier ones were brought back into favor, as in the Benditt and Benditt monoclonal origin theory of atherosclerosis that VSMC-derived cells in lesions came from only a few medial VSMCs,[17] a theory recently supported by data showing that SMCs in plaque or after injury are produced by mono- or oligoclonal expansion.[258–260] Integration of these areas will require a holistic and an increasingly multidisciplinary approach, combining data from basic scientists, clinicians, chemists, biomechanical engineers, and computer scientists. Future challenges include the question of how to translate this new understanding into clinically effective pharmacological interventions for the treatment of CVD. Future scientists have a rich resource of data from multiple disciplines and increasingly sophisticated tools to study the "biological symphony"[64] of interactions among vascular cells and to generate new hypotheses regarding the contribution of VSMC plasticity to physiology and disease.

REFERENCES

1. Jones JA, Stroud RE, O'Quinn EC, et al. Selective microRNA suppression in human thoracic aneurysms: relationship of miR-29a to aortic size and proteolytic induction. *Circ Cardiovasc Genet*. 2011;4:605–613.
2. Wagenseil JE, Mecham RP. Vascular extracellular matrix and arterial mechanics. *Physiol Rev*. 2009;89:957–989.
3. Owens GK, Kumar MS, Wamhoff BR. Molecular regulation of vascular smooth muscle cell differentiation in development and disease. *Physiol Rev*. 2004;84:767–801.
4. Trigueros-Motos L, Gonzalez-Granado JM, Cheung C, et al. Embryological-origin-dependent differences in homeobox expression in

adult aorta: role in regional phenotypic variability and regulation of NF-kappaB activity. *Arterioscler Thromb Vasc Biol.* 2013;33:1248–1256.

5. Feil S, Fehrenbacher B, Lukowski R, et al. Transdifferentiation of vascular smooth muscle cells to macrophage-like cells during atherogenesis. *Circ Res.* 2014;115:662–667.

6. Allahverdian S, Chehroudi AC, McManus BM, et al. Contribution of intimal smooth muscle cells to cholesterol accumulation and macrophage-like cells in human atherosclerosis. *Circulation.* 2014;129:1551–1559.

7. Leopold JA. Vascular calcification: mechanisms of vascular smooth muscle cell calcification. *Trends Cardiovasc Med.* 2015;25:267–274.

8. Cheng X, Waghulde H, Mell B, et al. Positional cloning of quantitative trait nucleotides for blood pressure and cardiac QT-interval by targeted CRISPR/Cas9 editing of a novel long non-coding RNA. *PLoS Genet.* 2017;13:e1006961.

9. Herbert SP, Huisken J, Kim TN, et al. Arterial-venous segregation by selective cell sprouting: an alternative mode of blood vessel formation. *Science.* 2009;326:294–298.

10. Swift MR, Weinstein BM. Arterial-venous specification during development. *Circ Res.* 2009;104:576–588.

11. Anderson LM, Gibbons GH. Notch: a mastermind of vascular morphogenesis. *J Clin Invest.* 2007;117:299–302.

12. Jain RK. Molecular regulation of vessel maturation. *Nat Med.* 2003;9:685–693.

13. Shen EM, McCloskey KE. Development of mural cells: from in vivo understanding to in vitro recapitulation. *Stem Cells Dev.* 2017;26:1020–1041.

14. Majesky MW. Developmental basis of vascular smooth muscle diversity. *Arterioscler Thromb Vasc Biol.* 2007;27:1248–1258.

15. Cheung C, Bernardo AS, Trotter MW, et al. Generation of human vascular smooth muscle subtypes provides insight into embryological origin-dependent disease susceptibility. *Nat Biotechnol.* 2012;30:165–173.

16. Roostalu U, Aldeiri B, Albertini A, et al. Distinct cellular mechanisms underlie smooth muscle turnover in vascular development and repair. *Circ Res.* 2018;122:267–281.

17. Benditt EP, Benditt JM. Evidence for a monoclonal origin of human atherosclerotic plaques. *Proc Natl Acad Sci U S A.* 1973;70:1753–1756.

18. Shankman LS, Gomez D, Cherepanova OA, et al. KLF4-dependent phenotypic modulation of smooth muscle cells has a key role in atherosclerotic plaque pathogenesis. *Nat Med.* 2015;21:628–637.

19. Bentzon JF, Majesky MW. Lineage tracking of origin and fate of smooth muscle cells in atherosclerosis. *Cardiovasc Res.* 2018;114:492–500.

20. Larsson E, McLean SE, Mecham RP, et al. Do two mutually exclusive gene modules define the phenotypic diversity of mammalian smooth muscle? *Mol Genet Genomics.* 2008;280:127–137.

21. Maegdefessel L, Rayner KJ, Leeper NJ. MicroRNA regulation of vascular smooth muscle function and phenotype: early career committee contribution. *Arterioscler Thromb Vasc Biol.* 2015;35:2–6.

22. Moiseeva EP. Adhesion receptors of vascular smooth muscle cells and their functions. *Cardiovasc Res.* 2001;52:372–386.

23. Rensen SS, Doevendans PA, van Eys GJ. Regulation and characteristics of vascular smooth muscle cell phenotypic diversity. *Neth Heart J.* 2007;15:100–108.

24. Beamish JA, He P, Kottke-Marchant K, et al. Molecular regulation of contractile smooth muscle cell phenotype: implications for vascular tissue engineering. *Tissue Eng Part B Rev.* 2010;16:467–491.

25. Rzucidlo EM. Signaling pathways regulating vascular smooth muscle cell differentiation. *Vascular.* 2009;17(Suppl 1):S15–S20.

26. Albarran-Juarez J, Kaur H, Grimm M, et al. Lineage tracing of cells involved in atherosclerosis. *Atherosclerosis.* 2016;251:445–453.

27. Vengrenyuk Y, Nishi H, Long X, et al. Cholesterol loading reprograms the microRNA-143/145-myocardin axis to convert aortic smooth muscle cells to a dysfunctional macrophage-like phenotype. *Arterioscler Thromb Vasc Biol.* 2015;35:535–546.

28. Orr AW, Lee MY, Lemmon JA, et al. Molecular mechanisms of collagen isotype-specific modulation of smooth muscle cell phenotype. *Arterioscler Thromb Vasc Biol.* 2009;29:225–231.

29. Yin BL, Hao H, Wang YY, et al. Downregulating osteopontin reduces angiotensin II-induced inflammatory activation in vascular smooth muscle cells. *Inflamm Res.* 2009;58:67–73.

30. Orr AW, Hastings NE, Blackman BR, et al. Complex regulation and function of the inflammatory smooth muscle cell phenotype in atherosclerosis. *J Vasc Res.* 2010;47:168–180.

31. Cuff CA, Kothapalli D, Azonobi I, et al. The adhesion receptor CD44 promotes atherosclerosis by mediating inflammatory cell recruitment and vascular cell activation. *J Clin Invest.* 2001;108:1031–1040.

32. Bardeesi ASA, Gao J, Zhang K, et al. A novel role of cellular interactions in vascular calcification. *J Transl Med.* 2017;15:95.

33. Kapustin AN, Chatrou ML, Drozdov I, et al. Vascular smooth muscle cell calcification is mediated by regulated exosome secretion. *Circ Res.* 2015;116:1312–1323.

34. Krohn JB, Hutcheson JD, Martinez-Martinez E, et al. Extracellular vesicles in cardiovascular calcification: expanding current paradigms. *J Physiol.* 2016;594:2895–2903.

35. Goettsch C, Hutcheson JD, Aikawa M, et al. Sortilin mediates vascular calcification via its recruitment into extracellular vesicles. *J Clin Invest.* 2016;126:1323–1336.

36. Ruiz JL, Weinbaum S, Aikawa E, et al. Zooming in on the genesis of atherosclerotic plaque microcalcifications. *J Physiol.* 2016;594:2915–2927.

37. O'Donnell CJ, Kavousi M, Smith AV, et al. Genome-wide association study for coronary artery calcification with follow-up in myocardial infarction. *Circulation.* 2011;124:2855–2864.

38. Glerup S, Schulz R, Laufs U, et al. Physiological and therapeutic regulation of PCSK9 activity in cardiovascular disease. *Basic Res Cardiol.* 2017;112:32.

39. Ferri N, Marchiano S, Tibolla G, et al. PCSK9 knock-out mice are protected from neointimal formation in response to perivascular carotid collar placement. *Atherosclerosis.* 2016;253:214–224.

40. Goettsch C, Hutcheson JD, Hagita S, et al. A single injection of gain-of-function mutant PCSK9 adeno-associated virus vector induces cardiovascular calcification in mice with no genetic modification. *Atherosclerosis.* 2016;251:109–118.

41. Kapustin AN, Schoppet M, Schurgers LJ, et al. Prothrombin loading of vascular smooth muscle cell-derived exosomes regulates coagulation and calcification. *Arterioscler Thromb Vasc Biol.* 2017;37:e22–e32.

42. Kapustin AN, Shanahan CM. Emerging roles for vascular smooth muscle cell exosomes in calcification and coagulation. *J Physiol.* 2016;594:2905–2914.

43. Berk BC. Vascular smooth muscle growth: autocrine growth mechanisms. *Physiol Rev.* 2001;81:999–1030.

44. Griendling K, Harrison D, Alexander R. Biology of the vessel wall. In: Fuster V, Walsh R, O'Rourke R, Poole-Wilson P, eds. *Hurst's the heart.* 12th ed. New York: McGraw Hill;2008:135–154.

45. Garrido AM, Griendling KK. NADPH oxidases and angiotensin II receptor signaling. *Mol Cell Endocrinol.* 2009;302:148–158.

46. Pardali E, Goumans M-J, ten Dijke P. Signaling by members of the TGF-b family in vascular morphogenesis and disease. *Trends Cell Biol.* 2010;20:556–567.

47. Hao H, Gabbiani G, Bochaton-Piallat M-L. Arterial smooth muscle cell heterogeneity: implications for atherosclerosis and restenosis development. *Arterioscler Thromb Vasc Biol.* 2003;23:1510–1520.

48. Mehta PK, Griendling KK. Angiotensin II cell signaling: physiological and pathological effects in the cardiovascular system. *Am J Physiol Cell Physiol.* 2007;292:C82–C97.

49. Yoshida T, Owens GK. Molecular determinants of vascular smooth muscle cell diversity. *Circ Res.* 2005;96:280–291.

50. High FA, Zhang M, Proweller A, et al. An essential role for Notch in neural crest during cardiovascular development and smooth muscle differentiation. *J Clin Invest.* 2007;117:353–363.

51. Gridley T. Notch signaling in the vasculature. *Curr Top Dev Biol.* 2010;92:277–309.

52. Tang Y, Urs S, Liaw L. Hairy-related transcription factors inhibit Notch-induced smooth muscle a-actin expression by interfering with Notch intracellular domain/CBF-1 complex interaction with the CBF-1-binding site. *Circ Res.* 2008;102:661–668.

53. Tang Y, Urs S, Boucher J, et al. Notch and transforming growth factor-beta (TGFb) signaling pathways cooperatively regulate vascular smooth muscle cell differentiation. *J Biol Chem.* 2010;285:17556–17563.

54. Morrow D, Cullen JP, Liu W, et al. Sonic Hedgehog induces Notch target gene expression in vascular smooth muscle cells via VEGF-A. *Arterioscler Thromb Vasc Biol.* 2009;29:1112–1118.

55. Jin S, Hansson EM, Tikka S, et al. Notch signaling regulates platelet-derived growth factor receptor-b expression in vascular smooth muscle cells. *Circ Res.* 2008;102:1483–1491.

56. Wang D-Z, Olson EN. Control of smooth muscle development by the myocardin family of transcriptional coactivators. *Curr Opin Genet Dev.* 2004;14:558–566.

57. Miano JM, Long X, Fujiwara K. Serum response factor: master regulator of the actin cytoskeleton and contractile apparatus. *Am J Physiol Cell Physiol.* 2007;292:C70–C81.

58. Parmacek MS. Myocardin-related transcription factors: critical coactivators regulating cardiovascular development and adaptation. *Circ Res.* 2007;100:633–644.

59. Pipes GC, Creemers EE, Olson EN. The myocardin family of transcriptional coactivators: versatile regulators of cell growth, migration, and myogenesis. *Genes Dev.* 2006;20:1545–1556.

60. Davis CA, Haberland M, Arnold MA, et al. PRISM/PRDM6, a transcriptional repressor that promotes the proliferative gene program in smooth muscle cells. *Mol Cell Biol.* 2006;26:2626–2636.

61. Haldar SM, Ibrahim OA, Jain MK. Kruppel-like factors (KLFs) in muscle biology. *J Mol Cell Cardiol.* 2007;43:1–10.

62. Zheng B, Han M, Wen JK. Role of Krüppel-like factor 4 in phenotypic switching and proliferation of vascular smooth muscle cells. *IUBMB Life.* 2010;62:132–139.

63. Miano JM. Deck of CArGs. *Circ Res.* 2008;103:13–15.

64. Miano JM, Long X. The short and long of noncoding sequences in the control of vascular cell phenotypes. *Cell Mol Life Sci.* 2015;72:3457–3488.

65. Olson EN, Nordheim A. Linking actin dynamics and gene transcription to drive cellular motile functions. *Nat Rev Mol Cell Biol.* 2010;11:353–365.

66. Han Y, Slivano OJ, Christie CK, et al. CRISPR-Cas9 genome editing of a single regulatory element nearly abolishes target gene expression in mice—brief report. *Arterioscler Thromb Vasc Biol.* 2015;35:312–315.

67. Liu N, Olson EN. Coactivator control of cardiovascular growth and remodeling. *Curr Opin Cell Biol.* 2006;18:715–722.

68. Posern G, Treisman R. Actin' together: serum response factor, its cofactors and the link to signal transduction. *Trends Cell Biol.* 2006;16:588–596.

69. Parmacek MS. Myocardin: dominant driver of the smooth muscle cell contractile phenotype. *Arterioscler Thromb Vasc Biol.* 2008;28:1416–1417.

70. Xia XD, Zhou Z, Yu XH, et al. Myocardin: a novel player in atherosclerosis. *Atherosclerosis.* 2017;257:266–278.

71. Sun SG, Zheng B, Han M, et al. miR-146a and Kruppel-like factor 4 form a feedback loop to participate in vascular smooth muscle cell proliferation. *EMBO Rep.* 2011;12:56–62.

72. Bell RD, Long X, Lin M, et al. Identification and initial functional characterization of a human vascular cell-enriched long noncoding RNA. *Arterioscler Thromb Vasc Biol.* 2014;34:1249–1259.

73. Ackers-Johnson M, Talasila A, Sage AP, et al. Myocardin regulates vascular smooth muscle cell inflammatory activation and disease. *Arterioscler Thromb Vasc Biol.* 2015;35:817–828.

74. Wall VZ, Bornfeldt KE. Arterial smooth muscle. *Arterioscler Thromb Vasc Biol.* 2014;34:2175–2179.

75. Dong J-T, Chen C. Essential role of KLF5 transcription factor in cell proliferation and differentiation and its implications for human diseases. *Cell Mol Life Sci.* 2009;66:2691–2706.

76. Kawai-Kowase K, Owens GK. Multiple repressor pathways contribute to phenotypic switching of vascular smooth muscle cells. *Am J Physiol Cell Physiol.* 2007;292:C59–C69.

77. Liu Y, J-k Wen, Dong L-h, et al. Kruppel-like factor (KLF) 5 mediates cyclin D1 expression and cell proliferation via interaction with c-Jun in Ang II-induced VSMCs. *Acta Pharmacol Sin.* 2009;31:10–18.

78. Suzuki T, Sawaki D, Aizawa K, et al. Kruppel-like factor 5 shows proliferation-specific roles in vascular remodeling, direct stimulation of cell growth, and inhibition of apoptosis. *J Biol Chem.* 2009;284:9549–9557.

79. Nagai R, Suzuki T, Aizawa K, et al. Significance of the transcription factor KLF5 in cardiovascular remodeling. *J Thromb Haemostasis.* 2005;3:1569–1576.

80. Mazurek R, Dave JM, Chandran RR, et al. Vascular cells in blood vessel wall development and disease. *Adv Pharmacol.* 2017;78:323–350.

81. Laffont B, Rayner KJ. MicroRNAs in the pathobiology and therapy of atherosclerosis. *Can J Cardiol.* 2017;33:313–324.

82. Barwari T, Joshi A, Mayr M. MicroRNAs in cardiovascular disease. *J Am Coll Cardiol.* 2016;68:2577–2584.

83. Eulalio A, Huntzinger E, Izaurralde E. Getting to the root of miRNA-mediated gene silencing. *Cell.* 2008;132:9–14.

84. Liu N, Olson EN. MicroRNA regulatory networks in cardiovascular development. *Dev Cell.* 2010;18:510–525.

85. Djuranovic S, Nahvi A, Green R. A parsimonious model for gene regulation by miRNAs. *Science.* 2011;331:550–553.

86. Bartel DP. MicroRNAs: target recognition and regulatory functions. *Cell.* 2009;136:215–233.

87. Cheng Y, Liu X, Yang J, et al. MicroRNA-145, a novel smooth muscle cell phenotypic marker and modulator, controls vascular neointimal lesion formation. *Circ Res.* 2009;105:158–166.

88. Cordes KR, Sheehy NT, White MP, et al. miR-145 and miR-143 regulate smooth muscle cell fate and plasticity. *Nature.* 2009;460:705–710.

89. Xin M, Small EM, Sutherland LB, et al. MicroRNAs miR-143 and miR-145 modulate cytoskeletal dynamics and responsiveness of smooth muscle cells to injury. *Genes Dev.* 2009;23:2166–2178.

90. Boettger T, Beetz N, Kostin S, et al. Acquisition of the contractile phenotype by murine arterial smooth muscle cells depends on the Mir143/145 gene cluster. *J Clin Invest.* 2009;119:2634–2647.

91. Song Z, Li G. Role of specific microRNAs in regulation of vascular smooth muscle cell differentiation and the response to injury. *J Cardiovasc Transl Res.* 2010;3:246–250.

92. Liu X, Cheng Y, Zhang S, et al. A necessary role of miR-221 and miR-222 in vascular smooth muscle cell proliferation and neointimal hyperplasia. *Circ Res.* 2009;104:476–487.

93. Davis BN, Hilyard AC, Nguyen PH, et al. Induction of microRNA-221 by platelet-derived growth factor signaling is critical for modulation of vascular smooth muscle phenotype. *J Biol Chem.* 2009;284:3728–3738.

94. Santulli G. microRNAs distinctively regulate vascular smooth muscle and endothelial cells: functional implications in angiogenesis, atherosclerosis, and in-stent restenosis. *Adv Exp Med Biol.* 2015;887:53–77.

95. Deng L, Bradshaw AC, Baker AH. Role of noncoding RNA in vascular remodelling. *Curr Opin Lipidol.* 2016;27:439–448.

96. Li Y, Maegdefessel L. Non-coding RNA contribution to thoracic and abdominal aortic aneurysm disease development and progression. *Front Physiol.* 2017;8:429.

97. Kim C, Kang D, Lee EK, et al. Long noncoding RNAs and RNA-binding proteins in oxidative stress, cellular senescence, and age-related diseases. *Oxid Med Cell Longev.* 2017;2017:2062384.

98. Leung A, Stapleton K, Natarajan R. Functional long non-coding RNAs in vascular smooth muscle cells. *Curr Top Microbiol Immunol.* 2016;394:127–141.

99. Liu Y, Zheng L, Wang Q, et al. Emerging roles and mechanisms of long noncoding RNAs in atherosclerosis. *Int J Cardiol.* 2017;228:570–582.

100. Gomes CPC, Spencer H, Ford KL, et al. The function and therapeutic potential of long non-coding RNAs in cardiovascular development and disease. *Mol Ther Nucleic Acids.* 2017;8:494–507.

101. Simion V, Haemmig S. Feinberg MW. LncRNAs in vascular biology and disease. *Vascul Pharmacol.* 2018.

102. Elia L, Quintavalle M. Epigenetics and vascular diseases: influence of non-coding RNAs and their clinical implications. *Front Cardiovasc Med.* 2017;4:26.

103. McDonald OG, Owens GK. Programming smooth muscle plasticity with chromatin dynamics. *Circ Res.* 2007;100:1428–1441.

104. McDonald OG, Wamhoff BR, Hoofnagle MH, et al. Control of SRF binding to CArG box chromatin regulates smooth muscle gene expression in vivo. *J Clin Invest.* 2006;116:36–48.

105. Mohammad HP, Baylin SB. Linking cell signaling and the epigenetic machinery. *Nat Biotech.* 2010;28:1033–1038.

106. Qiu P, Ritchie RP, Gong XQ, et al. Dynamic changes in chromatin acetylation and the expression of histone acetyltransferases and histone deacetylases

regulate the SM22a transcription in response to Smad3-mediated TGFb1 signaling. *Biochem Biophys Res Commun.* 2006;348:351–358.

107. Villeneuve LM, Reddy MA, Lanting LL, et al. Epigenetic histone H3 lysine 9 methylation in metabolic memory and inflammatory phenotype of vascular smooth muscle cells in diabetes. *Proc Natl Acad Sci U S A.* 2008;105:9047–9052.

108. Ceriello A, Ihnat MA, Thorpe JE. The "metabolic memory": is more than just tight glucose control necessary to prevent diabetic complications? *J Clin Endocrinol Metab.* 2009;94:410–415.

109. Liu R, Jin Y, Tang WH, et al. Ten-eleven translocation-2 (TET2) is a master regulator of smooth muscle cell plasticity. *Circulation.* 2013;128:2047–2057.

110. Jaiswal S, Natarajan P, Silver AJ, et al. Clonal hematopoiesis and risk of atherosclerotic cardiovascular disease. *N Engl J Med.* 2017;377:111–121.

111. Liu R, Bauer AJ, Martin KA. A new editor of smooth muscle phenotype. *Circ Res.* 2016;119:401–403.

112. Freed JK, Gutterman DD. Communication is key: mechanisms of intercellular signaling in vasodilation. *J Cardiovasc Pharmacol.* 2017;69:264–272.

113. Paik JH, Skoura A, Chae SS, et al. Sphingosine 1-phosphate receptor regulation of N-cadherin mediates vascular stabilization. *Genes Dev.* 2004;18:2392–2403.

114. George SJ, Dwivedi A. MMPs, cadherins, and cell proliferation. *Trends Cardiovasc Med.* 2004;14:100–105.

115. Figueroa XF, Duling BR. Gap junctions in the control of vascular function. *Antioxid Redox Signal.* 2009;11:251–266.

116. Brisset AC, Isakson BE, Kwak BR. Connexins in vascular physiology and pathology. *Antioxid Redox Signal.* 2009;11:267–282.

117. Johnstone S, Isakson B, Locke D. Biological and biophysical properties of vascular connexin channels. *Int Rev Cell Mol Biol.* 2009;278:69–118.

118. Straub AC, Zeigler AC, Isakson BE. The myoendothelial junction: connections that deliver the message. *Physiology (Bethesda).* 2014;29:242–249.

119. Lilly B. We have contact: endothelial cell-smooth muscle cell interactions. *Physiology (Bethesda).* 2014;29:234–241.

120. Chen X, Liang H, Zhang J, et al. Secreted microRNAs: a new form of intercellular communication. *Trends Cell Biol.* 2012;22:125–132.

121. Cocucci E, Racchetti G, Meldolesi J. Shedding microvesicles: artefacts no more. *Trends Cell Biol.* 2009;19:43–51.

122. Osteikoetxea X, Nemeth A, Sodar BW, et al. Extracellular vesicles in cardiovascular disease: are they Jedi or Sith? *J Physiol.* 2016;594:2881–2894.

123. Hergenreider E, Heydt S, Treguer K, et al. Atheroprotective communication between endothelial cells and smooth muscle cells through miRNAs. *Nat Cell Biol.* 2012;14:249–256.

124. Lin X, He Y, Hou X, et al. Endothelial cells can regulate smooth muscle cells in contractile phenotype through the miR-206/ARF6&NCX1/exosome axis. *PLoS One.* 2016;11:e0152959.

125. Deng L, Blanco FJ, Stevens H, et al. MicroRNA-143 activation regulates smooth muscle and endothelial cell crosstalk in pulmonary arterial hypertension. *Circ Res.* 2015;117:870–883.

126. Emanueli C, Shearn AI, Angelini GD, et al. Exosomes and exosomal miRNAs in cardiovascular protection and repair. *Vascul Pharmacol.* 2015;71:24–30.

127. Barile L, Vassalli G. Exosomes: therapy delivery tools and biomarkers of diseases. *Pharmacol Ther.* 2017;174:63–78.

128. Climent M, Quintavalle M, Miragoli M, et al. TGFbeta triggers miR-143/145 transfer from smooth muscle cells to endothelial cells, thereby modulating vessel stabilization. *Circ Res.* 2015;116:1753–1764.

129. Kelleher CM, McLean SE, Mecham RP. Vascular extracellular matrix and aortic development. *Curr Top Dev Biol.* 2004;62:153–188.

130. Hynes RO. The extracellular matrix: not just pretty fibrils. *Science.* 2009;326:1216–1219.

131. Järveläinen H, Sainio A, Koulu M, et al. Extracellular matrix molecules: potential targets in pharmacotherapy. *Pharmacol Rev.* 2009;61:198–223.

132. Mao Y, Schwarzbauer JE. Fibronectin fibrillogenesis, a cell-mediated matrix assembly process. *Matrix Biol.* 2005;24:389–399.

133. Singh P, Carraher C, Schwarzbauer JE. Assembly of fibronectin extracellular matrix. *Annu Rev Cell Dev Biol.* 2010;26:397–419.

134. Koyama H, Raines EW, Bornfeldt KE, et al. Fibrillar collagen inhibits arterial smooth muscle proliferation through regulation of Cdk2 inhibitors. *Cell.* 1996;87:1069–1078.

135. Kielty CM, Sherratt MJ, Shuttleworth CA. Elastic fibres. *J Cell Sci.* 2002;115:2817–2828.

136. Kielty CM. Elastic fibres in health and disease. *Expert Rev Mol Med.* 2006;8:1–23.

137. Karnik SK, Brooke BS, Bayes-Genis A, et al. A critical role for elastin signaling in vascular morphogenesis and disease. *Development.* 2003;130:411–423.

138. Yanagisawa H, Davis EC. Unraveling the mechanism of elastic fiber assembly: the roles of short fibulins. *Int J Biochem Cell Biol.* 2010;42:1084–1093.

139. Couchman JR. Transmembrane signaling proteoglycans. *Annu Rev Cell Dev Biol.* 2010;26:89–114.

140. Fukai N, Kenagy RD, Chen L, et al. Syndecan-1: an inhibitor of arterial smooth muscle cell growth and intimal hyperplasia. *Arterioscler Thromb Vasc Biol.* 2009;29:1356–1362.

141. Wight TN. Arterial remodeling in vascular disease: a key role for hyaluronan and versican. *Front Biosci.* 2008;13:4933–4937.

142. Ballinger ML, Ivey ME, Osman N, et al. Endothelin-1 activates ETA receptors on human vascular smooth muscle cells to yield proteoglycans with increased binding to LDL. *Atherosclerosis.* 2009;205:451–457.

143. Chen C-C, Lau LF. Functions and mechanisms of action of CCN matricellular proteins. *Int J Biochem Cell Biol.* 2009;41:771–783.

144. Matsumae H, Yoshida Y, Ono K, et al. CCN1 knockdown suppresses neointimal hyperplasia in a rat artery balloon injury model. *Arterioscler Thromb Vasc Biol.* 2008;28:1077–1083.

145. Shimoyama T, Hiraoka S, Takemoto M, et al. CCN3 inhibits neointimal hyperplasia through modulation of smooth muscle cell growth and migration. *Arterioscler Thromb Vasc Biol.* 2010;30:675–682.

146. Newby AC. Dual role of matrix metalloproteinases (matrixins) in intimal thickening and atherosclerotic plaque rupture. *Physiol Rev.* 2005;85:1–31.

147. Newby AC. Matrix metalloproteinases regulate migration, proliferation, and death of vascular smooth muscle cells by degrading matrix and non-matrix substrates. *Cardiovasc Res.* 2006;69:614–624.

148. Nagase H, Visse R, Murphy G. Structure and function of matrix metalloproteinases and TIMPs. *Cardiovasc Res.* 2006;69:562–573.

149. Raffetto JD, Khalil RA. Matrix metalloproteinases and their inhibitors in vascular remodeling and vascular disease. *Biochem Pharmacol.* 2008;75:346–359.

150. Newby AC. Metalloproteinases and vulnerable atherosclerotic plaques. *Trends Cardiovasc Med.* 2007;17:253–258.

151. Winograd-Katz SE, Fassler R, Geiger B, et al. The integrin adhesome: from genes and proteins to human disease. *Nat Rev Mol Cell Biol.* 2014;15:273–288.

152. Horton ER, Humphries JD, James J, et al. The integrin adhesome network at a glance. *J Cell Sci.* 2016;129:4159–4163.

153. Wang L, Zheng J, Du Y, et al. Cartilage oligomeric matrix protein maintains the contractile phenotype of vascular smooth muscle cells by interacting with a7b1 integrin. *Circ Res.* 2010;106:514–525.

154. Tkachenko E, Rhodes JM, Simons M. Syndecans: new kids on the signaling block. *Circ Res.* 2005;96:488–500.

155. Alexopoulou AN, Multhaupt HAB, Couchman JR. Syndecans in wound healing, inflammation and vascular biology. *Int J Biochem Cell Biol.* 2007;39:505–528.

156. Sun Z, Guo SS, Fassler R. Integrin-mediated mechanotransduction. *J Cell Biol.* 2016;215:445–456.

157. Assoian RK, Klein EA. Growth control by intracellular tension and extracellular stiffness. *Trends Cell Biol.* 2008;18:347–352.

158. Klein EA, Yin L, Kothapalli D, et al. Cell-cycle control by physiological matrix elasticity and in vivo tissue stiffening. *Curr Biol.* 2009;19:1511–1518.

159. Ben-Shlomo Y, Spears M, Boustred C, et al. Aortic pulse wave velocity improves cardiovascular event prediction: an individual participant meta-analysis of prospective observational data from 17,635 subjects. *J Am Coll Cardiol.* 2014;63:636–646.

160. Lyle AN, Raaz U. Killing me unsoftly: causes and mechanisms of arterial stiffness. *Arterioscler Thromb Vasc Biol.* 2017;37:e1–e11.

161. Lacolley P, Regnault V, Segers P, et al. Vascular smooth muscle cells and arterial stiffening: relevance in development, aging, and disease. *Physiol Rev*. 2017;97:1555–1617.

162. Zhou N, Lee JJ, Stoll S, et al. Inhibition of SRF/myocardin reduces aortic stiffness by targeting vascular smooth muscle cell stiffening in hypertension. *Cardiovasc Res*. 2017;113:171–182.

163. Watanabe H, Murakami M, Ohba T, et al. TRP channel and cardiovascular disease. *Pharmacol Ther*. 2008;118:337–351.

164. Akata T. Cellular and molecular mechanisms regulating vascular tone. Part 1: basic mechanisms controlling cytosolic Ca2+ concentration and the Ca2+-dependent regulation of vascular tone. *J Anesth*. 2007;21:220–231.

165. Kim HR, Appel S, Vetterkind S, et al. Smooth muscle signalling pathways in health and disease. *J Cell Mol Med*. 2008;12:2165–2180.

166. Essin K, Gollasch M. Role of ryanodine receptor subtypes in initiation and formation of calcium sparks in arterial smooth muscle: comparison with striated muscle. *J Biomed Biotechnol*. 2009;2009:135249.

167. Sathish V, Thompson MA, Bailey JP, et al. Effect of proinflammatory cytokines on regulation of sarcoplasmic reticulum Ca2+ reuptake in human airway smooth muscle. *Am J Physiol Lung Cell Mol Physiol*. 2009;297:L26–L34.

168. Trebak M, Ginnan R, Singer HA, et al. Interplay between calcium and reactive oxygen/nitrogen species: an essential paradigm for vascular smooth muscle signaling. *Antioxid Redox Signal*. 2010;12:657–674.

169. Martin-Garrido A, Boyano-Adanez MC, Alique M, et al. Hydrogen peroxide down-regulates inositol 1,4,5-trisphosphate receptor content through proteasome activation. *Free Radic Biol Med*. 2009;47:1362–1370.

170. Berk B. Vascular smooth muscle. In: Creager M, Dzau V, Loscalzo J, eds. *Vascular medicine: a companion to Braunwald's heart disease*. Philadelphia: Saunders; 2006:17–30.

171. Hilgers RHP, Webb RC. Molecular aspects of arterial smooth muscle contraction: focus on Rho. *Exp Biol Med*. 2005;230:829–835.

172. Masaki T. Historical review: endothelin. *Trends Pharmacol Sci*. 2004;25:219–224.

173. Tsutsui M, Shimokawa H, Otsuji Y, et al. Pathophysiological relevance of NO signaling in the cardiovascular system: novel insight from mice lacking all NO synthases. *Pharmacol Ther*. 2010;128:499–508.

174. Gao Y, Yang Y, Guan Q, et al. IL-1beta modulate the Ca(2+)-activated big-conductance K channels (BK) via reactive oxygen species in cultured rat aorta smooth muscle cells. *Mol Cell Biochem*. 2010;338:59–68.

175. Tong X, Hou X, Jourd'heuil D, et al. Upregulation of Nox4 by TGFb1 oxidizes SERCA and inhibits NO in arterial smooth muscle of the prediabetic Zucker rat. *Circ Res*. 2010;107:975–983.

176. Rajsheker S, Manka D, Blomkalns AL, et al. Crosstalk between perivascular adipose tissue and blood vessels. *Curr Opin Pharmacol*. 2010;10:191–196.

177. Zhang H, Cui J, Zhang C. Emerging role of adipokines as mediators in atherosclerosis. *World J Cardiol*. 2010;2:370–376.

178. Yamin R, Morgan KG. Deciphering actin cytoskeletal function in the contractile vascular smooth muscle cell. *J Physiol*. 2012;590:4145–4154.

179. Ohanian J, Pieri M, Ohanian V. Non-receptor tyrosine kinases and the actin cytoskeleton in contractile vascular smooth muscle. *J Physiol*. 2015;593:3807–3814.

180. Fuster JJ, Fernandez P, Gonzalez-Navarro H, et al. Control of cell proliferation in atherosclerosis: insights from animal models and human studies. *Cardiovasc Res*. 2010;86:254–264.

181. Griendling KK, Ushio-Fukai M, Lassegue B, et al. Angiotensin II signaling in vascular smooth muscle: new concepts. *Hypertension*. 1997;29:366–370.

182. Schwartz MA, Assoian RK. Integrins and cell proliferation: regulation of cyclin-dependent kinases via cytoplasmic signaling pathways. *J Cell Sci*. 2001;114:2553–2560.

183. Dzau VJ, Braun-Dullaeus RC, Sedding DG. Vascular proliferation and atherosclerosis: new perspectives and therapeutic strategies. *Nat Med*. 2002;8:1249–1256.

184. Marsboom G, Archer SL. Pathways of proliferation: new targets to inhibit the growth of vascular smooth muscle cells. *Circ Res*. 2008;103:1047–1049.

185. Fuster JJ, Andres V. Telomere biology and cardiovascular disease. *Circ Res*. 2006;99:1167–1180.

186. Kandadi MR, Stratton MS, Ren J. The role of Src homology 2 containing protein tyrosine phosphatase 2 in vascular smooth muscle cell migration and proliferation. *Acta Pharmacol Sin*. 2010;31:1277–1283.

187. Abizaid A. Sirolimus-eluting coronary stents: a review. *Vasc Health Risk Manag*. 2007;3:191–201.

188. Kahl CR, Means AR. Regulation of cell cycle progression by calcium/calmodulin-dependent pathways. *Endocr Rev*. 2003;24:719–736.

189. Koledova VV, Khalil RA. Ca2+, calmodulin, and cyclins in vascular smooth muscle cell cycle. *Circ Res*. 2006;98:1240–1243.

190. Choi J, Husain M. Calmodulin-mediated cell cycle regulation: new mechanisms for old observations. *Cell Cycle*. 2006;5:2183–2186.

191. Touyz RM, Yao G. Modulation of vascular smooth muscle cell growth by magnesium—role of mitogen—activated protein kinases. *J Cell Physiol*. 2003;197:326–335.

192. Burg ED, Remillard CV, Yuan JXJ. Potassium channels in the regulation of pulmonary artery smooth muscle cell proliferation and apoptosis: pharmacotherapeutic implications. *Br J Pharmacol*. 2008;153:S99–S111.

193. Neylon CB. Potassium channels and vascular proliferation. *Vasc Pharmacol*. 2002;38:35–41.

194. Cidad P, Moreno-Dominguez A, Novensa L, et al. Characterization of ion channels involved in the proliferative response of femoral artery smooth muscle cells. *Arterioscler Thromb Vasc Biol*. 2010;30:1203–1211.

195. Miguel-Velado E, Perez-Carretero FD, Colinas O, et al. Cell cycle-dependent expression of Kv3.4 channels modulates proliferation of human uterine artery smooth muscle cells. *Cardiovasc Res*. 2010;86: 383–391.

196. Jackson WF. KV1.3: a new therapeutic target to control vascular smooth muscle cell proliferation. *Arterioscler Thromb Vasc Biol*. 2010;30:1073–1074.

197. Assoian RK, Schwartz MA. Coordinate signaling by integrins and receptor tyrosine kinases in the regulation of G1 phase cell-cycle progression. *Curr Opin Genet Dev*. 2001;11:48–53.

198. Gizard F, Bruemmer D. Transcriptional control of vascular smooth muscle cell proliferation by peroxisome proliferator-activated receptor-gamma: therapeutic implications for cardiovascular diseases. *PPAR Res*. 2008;2008:429123.

199. Gizard F, Amant C, Barbier O, et al. PPAR A inhibits vascular smooth muscle cell proliferation underlying intimal hyperplasia by inducing the tumor suppressor p16INK4a. *J Clin Invest*. 2005;115:3228–3238.

200. Koyama H, Bornfeldt KE, Fukumoto S, et al. Molecular pathways of cyclic nucleotide-induced inhibition of arterial smooth muscle cell proliferation. *J Cell Physiol*. 2001;186:1–10.

201. Wu Y-J, Sala-Newby GB, Shu K-T, et al. S-phase kinase-associated protein-2 (Skp2) promotes vascular smooth muscle cell proliferation and neointima formation in vivo. *J Vasc Surg*. 2009;50:1135–1142.

202. Cheng Y, Zhang C. MicroRNA-21 in cardiovascular disease. *J Cardiovas Trans Res*. 2010;3:251–255.

203. Wang JN, Shi N, Chen SY. Manganese superoxide dismutase inhibits neointima formation through attenuation of migration and proliferation of vascular smooth muscle cells. *Free Radic Biol Med*. 2012;52:173–181.

204. Lee MY, San Martin A, Mehta PK, et al. Mechanisms of vascular smooth muscle NADPH oxidase 1 (Nox1) contribution to injury-induced neointimal formation. *Arterioscler Thromb Vasc Biol*. 2009;29:480–487.

205. Niu XL, Madamanchi NR, Vendrov AE, et al. Nox activator 1: a potential target for modulation of vascular reactive oxygen species in atherosclerotic arteries. *Circulation*. 2010;121:549–559.

206. Gerthoffer WT. Mechanisms of vascular smooth muscle cell migration. *Circ Res*. 2007;100:607–621.

207. San Martín A, Griendling KK. Redox control of vascular smooth muscle migration. *Antioxid Redox Signal*. 2010;12:625–640.

208. Burtenshaw D, Hakimjavadi R, Redmond EM, et al. Nox, reactive oxygen species and regulation of vascular cell fate. *Antioxidants (Basel)*. 2017;6.

209. Cameron JM, Gabrielsen M, Chim YH, et al. Polarized cell motility induces hydrogen peroxide to inhibit cofilin via cysteine oxidation. *Curr Biol*. 2015;25:1520–1525.

210. Xu Q, Huff LP, Fujii M, et al. Redox regulation of the actin cytoskeleton and its role in the vascular system. *Free Radic Biol Med*. 2017;109:84–107.

211. Byon CH, Heath JM, Chen Y. Redox signaling in cardiovascular pathophysiology: a focus on hydrogen peroxide and vascular smooth muscle cells. *Redox Biol.* 2016;9:244–253.

212. Weber DS, Taniyama Y, Rocic P, et al. Phosphoinositide-dependent kinase 1 and p21-activated protein kinase mediate reactive oxygen species-dependent regulation of platelet-derived growth factor-induced smooth muscle cell migration. *Circ Res.* 2004;94:1219–1226.

213. Lyle AN, Deshpande NN, Taniyama Y, et al. Poldip2, a novel regulator of Nox4 and cytoskeletal integrity in vascular smooth muscle cells. *Circ Res.* 2009;105:249–259.

214. Seasholtz TM, Majumdar M, Kaplan DD, et al. Rho and Rho kinase mediate thrombin-stimulated vascular smooth muscle cell DNA synthesis and migration. *Circ Res.* 1999;84:1186–1193.

215. Tang DD, Gerlach BD. The roles and regulation of the actin cytoskeleton, intermediate filaments and microtubules in smooth muscle cell migration. *Respir Res.* 2017;18:54.

216. Ridker PM. How common is residual inflammatory risk? *Circ Res.* 2017;120:617–619.

217. Furmanik M, Shanahan CM. Endoplasmic reticulum stress in arterial smooth muscle cells: a novel regulator of vascular disease. *Curr Cardiol Rev.* 2017;13:94–105.

218. Hoseini Z, Sepahvand F, Rashidi B, et al. NLRP3 inflammasome: its regulation and involvement in atherosclerosis. *J Cell Physiol.* 2018;233:2116–2132.

219. Malik A, Kanneganti TD. Inflammasome activation and assembly at a glance. *J Cell Sci.* 2017;130:3955–3963.

220. Sagulenko V, Thygesen SJ, Sester DP, et al. AIM2 and NLRP3 inflammasomes activate both apoptotic and pyroptotic death pathways via ASC. *Cell Death Differ.* 2013;20:1149–1160.

221. Wu D, Ren P, Zheng Y, et al. NLRP3 (nucleotide oligomerization domain-like receptor family, pyrin domain containing 3)-caspase-1 inflammasome degrades contractile proteins: implications for aortic biomechanical dysfunction and aneurysm and dissection formation. *Arterioscler Thromb Vasc Biol.* 2017;37:694–706.

222. Sun HJ, Ren XS, Xiong XQ, et al. NLRP3 inflammasome activation contributes to VSMC phenotypic transformation and proliferation in hypertension. *Cell Death Dis.* 2017;8:e3074.

223. Zhang C, Syed TW, Liu R, et al. Role of endoplasmic reticulum stress, autophagy, and inflammation in cardiovascular disease. *Front Cardiovasc Med.* 2017;4:29.

224. Scull CM, Tabas I. Mechanisms of ER stress-induced apoptosis in atherosclerosis. *Arterioscler Thromb Vasc Biol.* 2011;31:2792–2797.

225. Li Y, Lu G, Sun D, et al. Inhibition of endoplasmic reticulum stress signaling pathway: a new mechanism of statins to suppress the development of abdominal aortic aneurysm. *PLoS One.* 2017;12: e0174821.

226. Lindholm D, Korhonen L, Eriksson O, et al. Recent insights into the role of unfolded protein response in ER stress in health and disease. *Front Cell Dev Biol.* 2017;5:48.

227. Zhou AX, Tabas I. The UPR in atherosclerosis. *Semin Immunopathol.* 2013;35:321–332.

228. Yoshimura K, Nagasawa A, Kudo J, et al. Inhibitory effect of statins on inflammation-related pathways in human abdominal aortic aneurysm tissue. *Int J Mol Sci.* 2015;16:11213–11228.

229. Mistriotis P, Andreadis ST. Vascular aging: molecular mechanisms and potential treatments for vascular rejuvenation. *Ageing Res Rev.* 2017;37:94–116.

230. Durcan TM, Fon EA. The three 'P's of mitophagy: PARKIN, PINK1, and post-translational modifications. *Genes Dev.* 2015;29:989–999.

231. Docherty CK, Carswell A, Friel E, et al. Impaired mitochondrial respiration in human carotid plaque atherosclerosis: a potential role for Pink1 in vascular smooth muscle cell energetics. *Atherosclerosis.* 2018;268:1–11.

232. Liu MY, Jin J, Li SL, et al. Mitochondrial fission of smooth muscle cells is involved in artery constriction. *Hypertension.* 2016;68:1245–1254.

233. Gray K, Kumar S, Figg N, et al. Effects of DNA damage in smooth muscle cells in atherosclerosis. *Circ Res.* 2015;116:816–826.

234. Davidson SM, Yellon DM. Mitochondrial DNA damage, oxidative stress, and atherosclerosis: where there is smoke there is not always fire. *Circulation.* 2013;128:681–683.

235. Ryter SW, Bhatia D, Choi ME. Autophagy: a lysosome-dependent process with implications in cellular redox homeostasis and human disease. *Antioxid Redox Signal.* 2019;30:138–159.

236. Nussenzweig SC, Verma S, Finkel T. The role of autophagy in vascular biology. *Circ Res.* 2015;116:480–488.

237. Tai S, Hu XQ, Peng DQ, et al. The roles of autophagy in vascular smooth muscle cells. *Int J Cardiol.* 2016;211:1–6.

238. Yan Y, Finkel T. Autophagy as a regulator of cardiovascular redox homeostasis. *Free Radic Biol Med.* 2017;109:108–113.

239. Salabei JK, Hill BG. Autophagic regulation of smooth muscle cell biology. *Redox Biol.* 2015;4:97–103.

240. Ding Z, Wang X, Schnackenberg L, et al. Regulation of autophagy and apoptosis in response to ox-LDL in vascular smooth muscle cells, and the modulatory effects of the microRNA hsa-let-7 g. *Int J Cardiol.* 2013;168:1378–1385.

241. Brophy ML, Dong Y, Wu H, et al. Eating the dead to keep atherosclerosis at bay. *Front Cardiovasc Med.* 2017;4:2.

242. Bennett M, Yu H, Clarke M. Signalling from dead cells drives inflammation and vessel remodelling. *Vascul Pharmacol.* 2012;56:187–192.

243. Kojima Y, Weissman IL, Leeper NJ. The role of efferocytosis in atherosclerosis. *Circulation.* 2017;135:476–489.

244. Kavurma MM, Rayner KJ, Karunakaran D. The walking dead: macrophage inflammation and death in atherosclerosis. *Curr Opin Lipidol.* 2017;28:91–98.

245. Head T, Daunert S, Goldschmidt-Clermont PJ. The aging risk and atherosclerosis: a fresh look at arterial homeostasis. *Front Genet.* 2017;8:216.

246. Gorenne I, Kavurma M, Scott S, et al. Vascular smooth muscle cell senescence in atherosclerosis. *Cardiovasc Res.* 2006;72:9–17.

247. Vicencio JM, Galluzzi L, Tajeddine N, et al. Senescence, apoptosis or autophagy? When a damaged cell must decide its path—a mini-review. *Gerontology.* 2008;54:92–99.

248. Minamino T, Miyauchi H, Yoshida T, et al. Vascular cell senescence and vascular aging. *J Mol Cell Cardiol.* 2004;36:175–183.

249. Burton DG, Matsubara H, Ikeda K. Pathophysiology of vascular calcification: pivotal role of cellular senescence in vascular smooth muscle cells. *Exp Gerontol.* 2010;45:819–824.

250. Childs BG, Baker DJ, Wijshake T, et al. Senescent intimal foam cells are deleterious at all stages of atherosclerosis. *Science.* 2016;354:472–477.

251. Bennett MR, Clarke MC. Basic research: killing the old: cell senescence in atherosclerosis. *Nat Rev Cardiol.* 2016;14:8–9.

252. Lopez-Otin C, Blasco MA, Partridge L, et al. The hallmarks of aging. *Cell.* 2013;153:1194–1217.

253. Uryga AK, Bennett MR. Ageing induced vascular smooth muscle cell senescence in atherosclerosis. *J Physiol.* 2016;594:2115–2124.

254. Xiong S, Patrushev N, Forouzandeh F, et al. PGC-1alpha modulates telomere function and DNA damage in protecting against aging-related chronic diseases. *Cell Rep.* 2015;12:1391–1399.

255. Laurindo FR, Araujo TL, Abrahao TB. Nox NADPH oxidases and the endoplasmic reticulum. *Antioxid Redox Signal.* 2014;20:2755–2775.

256. Tang Z, Wang A, Yuan F, et al. Differentiation of multipotent vascular stem cells contributes to vascular diseases. *Nat Commun.* 2012;3:875.

257. Psaltis PJ, Simari RD. Vascular wall progenitor cells in health and disease. *Circ Res.* 2015;116:1392–1412.

258. Chappell J, Harman JL, Narasimhan VM, et al. Extensive proliferation of a subset of differentiated, yet plastic, medial vascular smooth muscle cells contributes to neointimal formation in mouse injury and atherosclerosis models. *Circ Res.* 2016;119:1313–1323.

259. Gomez D, Owens GK. Reconciling smooth muscle cell oligoclonality and proliferative capacity in experimental atherosclerosis. *Circ Res.* 2016;119:1262–1264.

260. Jacobsen K, Lund MB, Shim J, et al. Diverse cellular architecture of atherosclerotic plaque derives from clonal expansion of a few medial SMCs. *JCI Insight.* 2017;2.

261. Huang H, Xie C, Sun X, et al. miR-10a contributes to retinoid acid-induced smooth muscle cell differentiation. *J Biol Chem.* 2010;285: 9383–9389.

262. Kang H, Hata A. MicroRNA regulation of smooth muscle gene expression and phenotype. *Curr Opin Hematol.* 2012;19:224–231.

263. Boettger T, Beetz N, Kostin S, et al. Acquisition of the contractile phenotype by murine arterial smooth muscle cells depends on the Mir143/145 gene cluster. *J Clin Invest*. 2009;119:2634–2647.

264. Cheng Y, Liu X, Yang J, et al. MicroRNA-145, a novel smooth muscle cell phenotypic marker and modulator, controls vascular neointimal lesion formation. *Circ Res*. 2009;105:158–166.

265. Wang X, Hu G, Zhou J. Repression of versican expression by microRNA-143. *J Biol Chem*. 2010;285:23241–23250.

266. Quintavalle M, Elia L, Condorelli G, et al. MicroRNA control of podosome formation in vascular smooth muscle cells in vivo and in vitro. *J Cell Biol*. 2010;189:13–22.

267. Hutcheson R, Terry R, Chaplin J, et al. MicroRNA-145 restores contractile vascular smooth muscle phenotype and coronary collateral growth in the metabolic syndrome. *Arterioscler Thromb Vasc Biol*. 2013;33:727–736.

268. Lovren F, Pan Y, Quan A, et al. MicroRNA-145 targeted therapy reduces atherosclerosis. *Circulation*. 2012;126:S81–S90.

269. Chen J, Yin H, Jiang Y, et al. Induction of microRNA-1 by myocardin in smooth muscle cells inhibits cell proliferation. *Arterioscler Thromb Vasc Biol*. 2011;31:368–375.

270. Xie C, Huang H, Sun X, et al. MicroRNA-1 regulates smooth muscle cell differentiation by repressing Kruppel-like factor 4. *Stem Cells Dev*. 2011;20:205–210.

271. Torella D, Iaconetti C, Catalucci D, et al. MicroRNA-133 controls vascular smooth muscle cell phenotypic switch in vitro and vascular remodeling in vivo. *Circ Res*. 2011;109:880–893.

272. Ham O, Lee SY, Song BW, et al. Small molecule-mediated induction of miR-9 suppressed vascular smooth muscle cell proliferation and neointima formation after balloon injury. *Oncotarget*. 2017;8:93360–93372.

273. Gao P, Si J, Yang B, et al. Upregulation of microRNA-15a contributes to pathogenesis of abdominal aortic aneurysm (AAA) by modulating the expression of cyclin-dependent kinase inhibitor 2B (CDKN2B). *Med Sci Monit*. 2017;23:881–888.

274. Lin Y, Liu X, Cheng Y, et al. Involvement of microRNAs in hydrogen peroxide-mediated gene regulation and cellular injury response in vascular smooth muscle cells. *J Biol Chem*. 2009;284:7903–7913.

275. Wang M, Li W, Chang GQ, et al. MicroRNA-21 regulates vascular smooth muscle cell function via targeting tropomyosin 1 in arteriosclerosis obliterans of lower extremities. *Arterioscler Thromb Vasc Biol*. 2011;31:2044–2053.

276. Davis BN, Hilyard AC, Lagna G, et al. SMAD proteins control DROSHA-mediated microRNA maturation. *Nature*. 2008;454:56–61.

277. Sarkar J, Gou D, Turaka P, et al. MicroRNA-21 plays a role in hypoxia-mediated pulmonary artery smooth muscle cell proliferation and migration. *Am J Physiol Lung Cell Mol Physiol*. 2010;299:L861–L871.

278. Ji R, Cheng Y, Yue J, et al. MicroRNA expression signature and antisense-mediated depletion reveal an essential role of MicroRNA in vascular neointimal lesion formation. *Circ Res*. 2007;100:1579–1588.

279. Maegdefessel L, Azuma J, Toh R, et al. MicroRNA-21 blocks abdominal aortic aneurysm development and nicotine-augmented expansion. *Sci Transl Med*. 2012;4:122ra22.

280. Talasila A, Yu H, Ackers-Johnson M, et al. Myocardin regulates vascular response to injury through miR-24/-29a and platelet-derived growth factor receptor-beta. *Arterioscler Thromb Vasc Biol*. 2013;33:2355–2365.

281. Leeper NJ, Raiesdana A, Kojima Y, et al. MicroRNA-26a is a novel regulator of vascular smooth muscle cell function. *J Cell Physiol*. 2011;226:1035–1043.

282. Xing Y, Zheng X, Li G, et al. MicroRNA-30c contributes to the development of hypoxia pulmonary hypertension by inhibiting platelet-derived growth factor receptor beta expression. *Int J Biochem Cell Biol*. 2015;64:155–166.

283. Wang J, Yan CH, Li Y, et al. MicroRNA-31 controls phenotypic modulation of human vascular smooth muscle cells by regulating its target gene cellular repressor of E1A-stimulated genes. *Exp Cell Res*. 2013;319:1165–1175.

284. Zhou J, Li YS, Nguyen P, et al. Regulation of vascular smooth muscle cell turnover by endothelial cell-secreted microRNA-126: role of shear stress. *Circ Res*. 2013;113:40–51.

285. Zhang Y, Liu Z, Zhou M, et al. MicroRNA-129-5p inhibits vascular smooth muscle cell proliferation by targeting Wnt5a. *Exp Ther Med*. 2016;12:2651–2656.

286. Choe N, Kwon JS, Kim JR, et al. The microRNA miR-132 targets Lrrfip1 to block vascular smooth muscle cell proliferation and neointimal hyperplasia. *Atherosclerosis*. 2013;229:348–355.

287. Zhao J, Imbrie GA, Baur WE, et al. Estrogen receptor-mediated regulation of microRNA inhibits proliferation of vascular smooth muscle cells. *Arterioscler Thromb Vasc Biol*. 2013;33:257–265.

288. Zhang Y, Wang Y, Wang X, et al. Insulin promotes vascular smooth muscle cell proliferation via microRNA-208-mediated downregulation of p21. *J Hypertens*. 2011;29:1560–1568.

289. Liu X, Cheng Y, Yang J, et al. Cell-specific effects of miR-221/222 in vessels: molecular mechanism and therapeutic application. *J Mol Cell Cardiol*. 2012;52:245–255.

290. Yu ML, Wang JF, Wang GK, et al. Vascular smooth muscle cell proliferation is influenced by let-7d microRNA and its interaction with KRAS. *Circ J*. 2011;75:703–709.

291. Chen KC, Hsieh IC, Hsi E, et al. Negative feedback regulation between microRNA let-7g and the oxLDL receptor LOX-1. *J Cell Sci*. 2011;124:4115–4124.

292. Maegdefessel L, Spin JM, Raaz U, et al. miR-24 limits aortic vascular inflammation and murine abdominal aneurysm development. *Nat Commun*. 2014;5:5214.

293. Reddy MA, Jin W, Villeneuve L, et al. Pro-inflammatory role of microrna-200 in vascular smooth muscle cells from diabetic mice. *Arterioscler Thromb Vasc Biol*. 2012;32:721–729.

294. Wu J, Song HF, Li SH, et al. Progressive aortic dilation is regulated by miR-17-associated miRNAs. *J Am Coll Cardiol*. 2016;67:2965–2977.

295. Boon RA, Seeger T, Heydt S, et al. MicroRNA-29 in aortic dilation: implications for aneurysm formation. *Circ Res*. 2011;109:1115–1119.

296. Maegdefessel L, Azuma J, Toh R, et al. Inhibition of microRNA-29b reduces murine abdominal aortic aneurysm development. *J Clin Invest*. 2012;122:497–506.

297. Latronico MV, Catalucci D, Condorelli G. Emerging role of microRNAs in cardiovascular biology. *Circ Res*. 2007;101:1225–1236.

298. Zhang P, Huang A, Ferruzzi J, et al. Inhibition of microRNA-29 enhances elastin levels in cells haploinsufficient for elastin and in bioengineered vessels—brief report. *Arterioscler Thromb Vasc Biol*. 2012;32:756–759.

299. Du Y, Gao C, Liu Z, et al. Upregulation of a disintegrin and metalloproteinase with thrombospondin motifs-7 by miR-29 repression mediates vascular smooth muscle cell calcification. *Arterioscler Thromb Vasc Biol*. 2012;32:2580–2588.

300. Ulrich V, Rotllan N, Araldi E, et al. Chronic miR-29 antagonism promotes favorable plaque remodeling in atherosclerotic mice. *EMBO Mol Med*. 2016;8:643–653.

301. Merk DR, Chin JT, Dake BA, et al. miR-29b participates in early aneurysm development in Marfan syndrome. *Circ Res*. 2012;110:312–324.

302. Liao XB, Zhang ZY, Yuan K, et al. MiR-133a modulates osteogenic differentiation of vascular smooth muscle cells. *Endocrinology*. 2013;154:3344–3352.

303. Remus EW, Lyle AN, Weiss D, et al. miR181a protects against angiotensin II-induced osteopontin expression in vascular smooth muscle cells. *Atherosclerosis*. 2013;228:168–174.

304. Di Gregoli K, Mohamad Anuar NN, Bianco R, et al. MicroRNA-181b controls atherosclerosis and aneurysms through regulation of TIMP-3 and elastin. *Circ Res*. 2017;120:49–65.

305. Zampetaki A, Attia R, Mayr U, et al. Role of miR-195 in aortic aneurysmal disease. *Circ Res*. 2014;115:857–866.

306. Chan CYT, Cheuk BLY, Cheng SWK. Abdominal aortic aneurysm-associated microRNA-516a-5p regulates expressions of methylenetetrahydrofolate reductase, matrix metalloproteinase-2, and tissue inhibitor of matrix metalloproteinase-1 in human abdominal aortic vascular smooth muscle cells. *Ann Vasc Surg*. 2017;42:263–273.

307. Congrains A, Kamide K, Oguro R, et al. Genetic variants at the 9p21 locus contribute to atherosclerosis through modulation of ANRIL and CDKN2A/B. *Atherosclerosis*. 2012;220:449–455.

308. Motterle A, Pu X, Wood H, et al. Functional analyses of coronary artery disease associated variation on chromosome 9p21 in vascular smooth muscle cells. *Hum Mol Genet.* 2012;21:4021–4029.

309. Holdt LM, Hoffmann S, Sass K, et al. Alu elements in ANRIL non-coding RNA at chromosome 9p21 modulate atherogenic cell functions through trans-regulation of gene networks. *PLoS Genet.* 2013;9:e1003588.

310. Lv J, Wang L, Zhang J, et al. Long noncoding RNA H19-derived miR-675 aggravates restenosis by targeting PTEN. *Biochem Biophys Res Commun.* 2018;497:1154–1161.

311. Vigetti D, Deleonibus S, Moretto P, et al. Natural antisense transcript for hyaluronan synthase 2 (HAS2-AS1) induces transcription of HAS2 via protein O-GlcNAcylation. *J Biol Chem.* 2014;289:28816–28826.

312. Wang S, Zhang X, Yuan Y, et al. BRG1 expression is increased in thoracic aortic aneurysms and regulates proliferation and apoptosis of vascular smooth muscle cells through the long non-coding RNA HIF1A-AS1 in vitro. *Eur J Cardiothorac Surg.* 2015;47:439–446.

313. Wu G, Cai J, Han Y, et al. LincRNA-p21 regulates neointima formation, vascular smooth muscle cell proliferation, apoptosis, and atherosclerosis by enhancing p53 activity. *Circulation.* 2014;130:1452–1465.

314. Leung A, Trac C, Jin W, et al. Novel long noncoding RNAs are regulated by angiotensin II in vascular smooth muscle cells. *Circ Res.* 2013;113:266–278.

315. Yao QP, Xie ZW, Wang KX, et al. Profiles of long noncoding RNAs in hypertensive rats: long noncoding RNA XR007793 regulates cyclic strain-induced proliferation and migration of vascular smooth muscle cells. *J Hypertens.* 2017;35:1195–1203.

316. Zhao J, Zhang W, Lin M, et al. MYOSLID is a novel serum response factor-dependent long noncoding RNA that amplifies the vascular smooth muscle differentiation program. *Arterioscler Thromb Vasc Biol.* 2016;36:2088–2099.

317. Ballantyne MD, Pinel K, Dakin R, et al. Smooth muscle enriched long noncoding RNA (SMILR) regulates cell proliferation. *Circulation.* 2016;133:2050–2065.

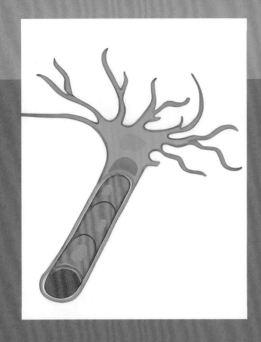

中文导读

第4章
正常血管止血机制

　　止血是限制血液从受损血管中流出的过程，是一种对血管损伤的反应，止血过程主要包括局部血管收缩、血小板血栓形成和血液凝固。血管对病变的反应具备迅速性、高度调节性和局部性。血液凝固对于防止失血和启动伤口修复过程都是必不可少的。如果这一过程失衡，可能会导致异常出血或非生理性血栓形成，进而导致疾病的发生。例如，在动脉粥样硬化斑块区域形成异常血栓会显著提高心血管疾病的发病率和死亡率。本章将侧重于正常的止血机制，重点强调：①血小板和受损的血管内皮细胞在受损部位形成血小板血栓的过程（一期止血）；②凝血因子在受损的内皮细胞和血小板表面被激活，通过凝血级联系统形成纤维蛋白凝块，稳定血小板血栓的过程（二期止血）；③纤维蛋白溶解系统清除纤维蛋白，溶解血小板血栓，并恢复内皮正常结构和正常血流的过程（三期止血）。同时还强调了这些途径的调节方式，并基于此了解这些过程中的异常导致血栓和出血性疾病的具体机制。

薛　松

Normal Mechanisms of Vascular Hemostasis

Elisabeth M. Battinelli and Joseph Loscalzo

Hemostasis occurs in response to vessel injury. The clot is essential both for the prevention of blood loss and the initiation of the wound repair process. When there is a lesion present in the blood vessel, the response is rapid, highly regulated, and localized. If the process is not balanced, abnormal bleeding or nonphysiological thrombosis, can result. In cardiovascular disease, the formation of abnormal thrombus at the area of an atherosclerotic plaque results in significant morbidity and mortality. This chapter will focus on normal mechanisms of hemostasis with specific attention to the role of the platelet in the process, as well as the coagulation cascade, and fibrinolytic mechanisms, as a basis for understanding how abnormalities in these processes can lead to thrombotic and hemorrhagic disorders.

ENDOTHELIAL FUNCTION AND PLATELET ACTIVATION

Platelets are anucleate cells that are produced by megakaryocytes in the bone marrow. Once they have traversed from the bone marrow to the general circulation, their lifespan is approximately 10 days. They function mainly to limit hemorrhage after trauma resulting in vascular injury. Normally in the vasculature, platelets are in a resting state and only become activated after exposure to a stimulus leads to a shape change and a release reaction that causes the platelets to export many of its biologically important proteins. Some of the agonists that can initiate this response include thromboxane A_2, adenosine diphosphate (ADP), thrombin, and serotonin. In areas of vascular injury, platelets are attracted to the impaired site by collagen through binding with von Willebrand factor via the glycoprotein Ib/V/IX (GPIb/V/IX) complex. This initial binding results in platelet activation with a subsequent feedback mechanism in which ADP, thrombin, and thromboxane A_2 further activate the platelets and recruit additional platelets to the area. The complex firmly binds the platelet to the area of injury so that there is no disruption by the high shear forces of turbulent blood flow that occur with vessel disruption. This amplification of the response is essential to form a hemostatic plug, and represents the first stage in the hemostatic process. When von Willebrand factor is not present, hemostatic abnormalities result with deficiencies leading to von Willebrand disease, which can be associated with severe bleeding. Hemostasis issues also arise when the platelet receptor complex GPIb/V/IX is mutated, resulting in the inability for von Willebrand to bind, a disorder termed Bernard-Soulier syndrome.[1,2]

Additional platelet aggregation occurs through the activation of G-protein–coupled receptors with the final pathway relying on the glycoprotein IIb/IIIa complex, which is the main receptor for platelet aggregation and adhesion.[3,4] Fibrinogen tethers glycoprotein IIb/IIIa complexes on different platelets stabilizing the clot. The integral role of this receptor is manifest in Glanzmann thrombasthenia, a disorder in which fibrinogen binding is impaired leading to mucocutaneous bleeding episodes that occur spontaneously.[5]

Recently, the role of the platelet has been expanded to include a subset of platelets termed procoagulant platelets. The main characteristic of this subtype of platelets is the presence of phosphatidylserine (PS) on the plasma membrane presenting a surface for binding of tenase and the prothrombinase complexes, thereby upregulating coagulation.[6] These platelets have been characterized as ballooning platelets or as containing the mitochondrial permeability transition pore. This subgroup of platelets is dependent on collagen as the main agonist that regulates their phenotype making them ideal to accelerate hemostasis at the site of vessel injury.[7]

The vascular endothelium is essential to this hemostatic process as this is the cellular site at which the regulation and initiation of coagulation begins. Endothelial cells modulate vascular tone, generate mediators of inflammation, and provide a resistant surface that allows for platelets to experience laminar flow with minimal shear. The endothelial cells regulate hemostasis through the release of a number of inhibitors of platelets and of inflammation. The vascular endothelium is essential for regulating uncontrolled platelet activity through mechanisms of inhibition including the arachidonic acid-prostacyclin pathway, the L-arginine-nitric oxide pathway, and the endothelial ectoadenosine diphosphatase (ecto-ADPase) pathways (Table 4.1).[8]

Nitric oxide (NO) is produced constitutively by endothelial cells via an endothelial isoform of nitric oxide synthase (eNOS) in a process that is dependent on the conversion of L-arginine to L-citrulline. Vascular tone is regulated by NO as it controls smooth muscle cell contraction. It also inhibits platelets directly, thereby blocking platelet aggregation through the stimulation of guanylyl cyclase and cyclic guanosine-monophosphate (cGMP) formation and the inhibition of platelet phosphoinositol-3-kinase (PI-3 kinase). NO functions by decreasing the intracellular Ca^{2+} level through cGMP, which inhibits the conformational change in glycoprotein IIb/IIIa suppressing fibrinogen's ability to bind to the receptor, thereby attenuating platelet aggregation.[9]

Prostacyclin, which is synthesized in the endothelial cells from arachidonic acid through cyclooxygenase-1 or -2 (COX-1 and COX-2)-dependent pathways, inhibits platelet function through increasing cyclic adenosine-monophosphate (cAMP). This is essential for aspirin's ability to diminish platelet function through the acetylation of platelet COX-1 at serine 529.

The last pathway important in modulation of the vascular endothelium's interaction with platelets is the endothelial ecto-ADPase pathway, which impairs ADP-mediated platelet activation. By hydrolyzing ADP, this enzyme inhibits the critical state of platelet recruitment to a growing aggregate, thereby limiting thrombus formation. Once the platelet aggregate has been stabilized by fibrin with red cells to the vessel wall, the next stage of hemostasis involves activation of the highly regulated coagulation cascade (Fig. 4.1).

TABLE 4.1   Factors Involved in Fibrinolysis

Prohemostatic	Antihemostatic
Circulating	
α₂-Antiplasmin	Antithrombin III
Thrombin	Protein C
Thrombin-activatable fibrinolysis inhibitor (TAFI)	Protein S
	Tissue factor pathway inhibitor (TFPI)
Endothelium-Derived	
Plasminogen activator inhibitor-1 (PAI-1)	Ecto-ADPase/CD39
Tissue factor (TF)	Heparan sulfate
von Willebrand factor (vWF)	Nitric oxide (NO)
	Prostacyclin (PGI₂)
	Thrombomodulin
	Tissue plasminogen activator (tPA)
	Urokinase plasminogen activator (uPA)

THE COAGULATION CASCADE LEADING TO FIBRIN FORMATION

Disruption in the endothelium not only recruits platelets for plug formation, but also stimulates the activation of the coagulation cascade, which is essential for secondary clot formation through fibrin generation. The coagulation cascade is a dynamic, integrated process in which each step is dependent on another step for activation of pro-enzymes or zymogens to their active forms through proteolytic cleavage. This process is dependent upon calcium and the phospholipid bilayer allowing inactive clotting factors to be converted to active enzymes through serine protease activity. These coagulation proteins function in a step-by-step fashion in order to activate downstream members of the cascade leading to production of the penultimate clotting factor, thrombin. Thrombin is versatile, playing a role in many of the essential stages of hemostasis. Not only is it important for platelet activation, but it is also necessary for the cross-linking of fibrin. Recently, there have been attempts to limit thrombus formation by directly inhibiting thrombin activity through anticoagulants such as ximelagatran and the oral medication, dabigatran, which is now available for clinical use.[10]

The clotting cascade is divided into two main pathways: intrinsic and extrinsic.

The extrinsic pathway begins through the establishment of a complex between tissue factor found on the cell surface or on microparticles and factor VIIa. This complex leads to activation of factor X to Xa, which can then further the response by looping back and converting factor VII to VIIa in a feedback mechanism. When factor Xa is present, it binds to factor Va on the membrane surface and again generates prothrombinase, which converts prothrombin to thrombin and then generates fibrin as detailed above. The activity of factor Xa is accelerated by the presence of factor Va through calcium and the formation of a noncovalent association between the gamma-carboxyglutamate residues of factor Xa and the phospholipid surface of activated platelets.[11] The extrinsic pathway is measured by the prothrombin time, which is determined by adding an extrinsic substance, such as tissue factor or thromboplastin.[12]

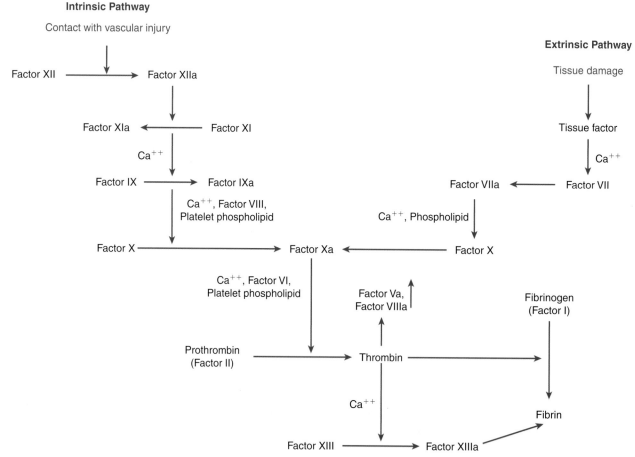

Fig. 4.1 Coagulation Cascade.

The extrinsic pathway, which is dependent on tissue factor, appears to be the main pathway responsible for hemostasis with the intrinsic pathway playing a supporting role. Tissue factor is a membrane-bound glycoprotein that is constitutively expressed by smooth muscle cells and fibroblasts, but it is selectively expressed by endothelial cells when there is vessel wall injury. The "encrypted," activated form of factor VIIa is made functional through a conformational change that occurs at cysteines 186 and 209 leading to disulfide bond formation upon vessel wall injury. Protein disulfide isomerase, glutathione, and NO all may have a role in these allosteric changes; however, recent studies have questioned the importance of "de-encryption" in this process.[13–16] Tissue factor functions through activation of factors X and IX after interactions with factor VII as a complex. Factor VII, although at low levels in an active state (factor VIIa) in the circulation, only becomes biologically important after it is bound to tissue factor in complex with factors X and IX. This complex formation is essential for the activation of thrombin.[11]

The role of tissue factor has recently been expanded. It circulates in the blood in association with microvesicles that are derived from cellular membranes, which are produced from lipid rafts on monocytes and macrophages.[17] These tissue factor-bearing microvesicles can directly initiate coagulation cascade on activated platelets in a process that may be important for understanding the hypercoagulable state.[18,19]

Once thrombin is activated in the tissue factor X-IX-VIIa complex, it initiates further activation within the coagulation cascade. In addition to activating platelets and factor V, it also activates factor VIII, which exists in the circulation in association with von Willebrand factor. Activated factor VIII (factor VIIIa) works in a feedback loop with factor IXa to activate further factor X to Xa and therefore yield more thrombin to accelerate its own activation. Factors VIII and IX are essential in coagulation as is evident in patients who suffer deficiencies of these factors leading to hemophilia A and B, respectively. These disorders lead to severe bleeding through the loss of activation of factor X leading to decreased thrombin formation. Another deficiency that is seen occurs when factor XI is mutated, resulting in a disorder associated with delayed bleeding in the postoperative setting. The importance of this coagulation cascade is highlighted by the severity of this disorder, which suggests that the feedback mechanism by which thrombin activates factor XI with subsequent activation of IX and then further generation of thrombin is an essential stage of amplification necessary for hemostasis.

The extrinsic pathway as described above joins up with the intrinsic pathway through factor X to form the common pathway. The intrinsic pathway is initiated by contact and results in the activation of factor IXa, which then goes on to activate factor X as described above. It is generally accepted that the intrinsic pathway is of less importance in coagulation than the tissue factor–mediated extrinsic pathway, although it plays an essential role in inflammation and fibrinolysis. The intrinsic pathway is based on the exposure of blood to a negatively charged surface, and is classically initiated by the activation of factor XIIa by kallikrein, which is facilitated by kininogen. Kallikrein is generated from prekallikrein through proteolytic cleavage by activated factor XII in a reaction that is dependent on the presence of high-molecular-weight kininogen (HMWK). When kallikrein has been generated, it also functions to cleave HMWK to bradykinin, which functions as an inflammatory mediator to potentiate vasodilating and vascular permeability, thereby expanding the role of factor XIIa to inflammation, and regulating vascular tone and fibrinolysis.[20] Activated factor XII catalyzes the conversion of factor XI to the active enzyme form factor XIa. When calcium is present, factor Xa next functions to convert IX to IXa, which then binds to VIIIa on membrane surfaces converting X to its active form, factor Xa. Factor Xa then binds to factor Va on the membrane surface to generate prothrombinase, which converts prothrombin to thrombin. As thrombin is formed, two small prothrombin fragments, termed molecules F1 and F2, are released and can be used as markers of thrombin formation in the serum.[21] The intrinsic pathway is monitored through the activated partial thromboplastin time (aPTT), which relies on foreign substances, such as glass or silicates, to activate factor XII to initiate the pathway. Deficiencies in the earliest states of the intrinsic pathway when prekallikrein, HMWK, and factor XII are involved are not associated with any bleeding tendencies; therefore they do not lead to a bleeding diathesis even though there is an elevation in the PTT. Mutations in factor XII have been reported in a group of patients with hereditary angioedema, although there does not appear to be a bleeding diathesis with this disorder. Some initial studies have suggested that factor XII polymorphisms may be associated with an increased propensity for thrombosis, but this has not been validated.[22,23]

The importance of the intrinsic pathway has recently been debated. Previously it was thought that its role is mainly to augment the role of the primary, extrinsic pathway. However, recent evidence suggests that the intrinsic and extrinsic pathways are activated simultaneously, and that there are more activators than initially thought.[24] These include collagen, linear phosphate polymers, and neutrophil extracellular traps (NETs).[25–27]

It has been established that polyphosphates can directly activate factor XII, thereby leading to activation of the intrinsic pathway. The polyphosphates that are most likely to be at the site of vascular injury are present on the platelet surface, further involving the platelet in coagulation.[28]

Recently, the role of polyphosphates in hemostasis has been highlighted. Polyphosphates are released from dense granules in platelets upon platelet activation, and function as a driver of coagulation. Not only do they stimulate the intrinsic pathway through factor XII, but also they have other effects, including augmentation of factor V and factor XI activation as well as the inhibition of tissue factor pathway inhibitor (TFPI), to enhance fibrin formation.[29]

Another important regulator of the intrinsic pathway is NETs. NETs are released by neutrophils in a manner dependent on cell death, termed NETosis. They consist of nucleic acids with histones on their surface, which physically trap bacteria and fungi for destruction. However, these histones can also directly activate platelets, further augmenting coagulation. In addition, NETs have taken center stage in the extrinsic pathway. Also, they have been demonstrated to impact fibrinolysis through the inactivation of TFPI.[30]

The two pathways merge into the common pathway. When factor Xa generates thrombin, the intrinsic and extrinsic pathways have merged into the common pathway. Thrombin is essential for fibrinogen to generate fibrin, which is released through proteolytic cleavage.[31] The fibrin molecules that are generated have polymerization sites exposed making it easier for fibrin to cross-link noncovalently. This cross-linking enables platelets to be entrapped in a meshwork of fibrin strands to form the secondary clot through the action of factor XIII that is activated by thrombin.[32] In the process of cross-linking, there is also an inherent mechanism of auto-regulation with the binding sites necessary to initiate fibrinolysis being blocked so the clot does not self-destruct.

This process of platelet activation and upregulation of the coagulation cascade occurs in a swift and efficient manner in order to prevent excessive bleeding. However, it can lead to thrombosis if left unchecked. Therefore other mechanisms are in place whose main role is to modulate coagulation activities to avoid such complications. These mechanisms involve mechanical means, such as dilution of coagulation factors in blood, and also removal of factors after activation through the reticulo-endothelial system, as well as antithrombotic pathways, which are separate from the coagulation cascade. Patients with deficiencies in these natural antithrombotic mechanisms often present with thrombosis. These pathways include antithrombin, proteins C and S, and TFPI.

Antithrombin is a serine protease inhibitor that binds specifically to factors IXa, Xa, and thrombin, thereby rendering them inactive. Antithrombin has two main binding sites that maintain its functionality, including the reactive center at Arg 3930Ser394 and the heparin binding site at the aminoterminal end of the molecule. Binding of both endogenous and exogenous heparins at this site causes a conformational change in antithrombin that enables it to inactivate its targets at an accelerated rate. The glycosaminoglycan heparan sulfate that is present on the surface of endothelial cells mediates antithrombin's ability to increase its activity and functions as the physiological equivalent to heparin.[33] The deficiency of antithrombin is associated with a genetic propensity to venous thromboembolic disease, as discussed in Chapter 8.[34]

Activated protein C (APC) and protein S are also important mechanisms for the prevention of excessive clotting. During the clotting process, thrombin binds to thrombomodulin, which is also present on the endothelial cell surface. It then undergoes a conformational change leading to the activation of protein C.[35] APC complexes with protein S and proteolytically cleaves factors Va and VIIIa, resulting in their inactivation and decreasing the generation of factors Xa and thrombin. The cleavage of factor Va occurs at Arg 506, Arg 306, and Arg 679 by APC in a sequential manner such that the cleavage at Arg 506 exposes the other cleavage sites through a conformational change. Mutation of the arginine located at position 506 to glutamine leads to factor V Leiden, which is associated with a hypercoagulable state.

Another important natural anticoagulant is the TFPI, which acts as a multivalent protease inhibitor to inactivate both factor Xa and IXa. TFPI is also present within endothelial cells with the majority remaining localized to the endothelial surface with very little circulating in the plasma. However, the concentration in plasma is increased in the presence of heparin, which modulates its release from the endothelial surface.

Although TFPI has been viewed as the main inhibitor of coagulation through the inhibition of TF/factor VIIa, it has recently been demonstrated that TFPI can inhibit prothrombinase assembly directly through its association with factor V.[36] In this new capacity, factor V mediates TFPI inhibition of prothrombinase in conjunction with protein S. These results demonstrate a new means of regulating TFPI functionality to limit hemostasis.

FIBRINOLYSIS

The importance of fibrinolysis lies in its removing blood clots and maintaining hemostasis without excessive clotting. The mechanism of serine protease activity is preserved in the fibrinolytic system and accounts for the mechanism of action of many of its components (Fig. 4.2). The main factor responsible for fibrinolysis is plasmin. The process begins when plasminogen in its inactive form is converted to the active enzyme, plasmin, which functions to convert fibrin to soluble fibrin degradation products (FDPs). Two molecules that mimic this function include tissue plasminogen activator (tPA) and urokinase plasminogen activator (uPA). The motif that is responsible for its action is the kringle domain, which resides in the aminoterminal end. Kringles are 80 amino acids in length and have a unique folded-sheet structure that results from disulfide linkages, which yields a homotypic binding site specific for plasminogen, fibrinogen, and fibrin. There

is homology between the kringles contained in all three of these molecules.

These kringle domains are essential for providing a mechanism for binding many components of the developing thrombus, including fibrinogen and fibrin. The kringle domains shared by tPA and plasminogen allow fibrinogen and fibrin to bind and therefore to be incorporated into the developing clot. Plasminogen is converted to plasmin through the proteolytic cleavage achieved by tPA and uPA at the Arg 560 and Val561 sites.[37] The plasmin that is generated can then bind to a number of proteins involved in the process of fibrinolysis.[38] Relevant properties include its high affinity for fibrin, its ability to cleave Glu-plasminogen to Lys-plasminogen, its ability to activate factor XII, and its ability to inactivate factors V and VIII in the coagulation cascade. Plasmin cleaves the fibrin molecule into differentially sized degradation or split products (FDP), the smallest of which is D-dimer, which is used as a marker of venous thromboembolism and disseminated intravascular coagulopathy (DIC).

The plasminogen pathway is complex and tightly regulated.[39] The main proteins involved in its modulation are plasminogen activator inhibitor 1 (PAI-1) and PAI-2. The activators and inhibitors of plasminogen regulate fibrinolysis upon release from the endothelial cells. These activators of the fibrinolytic process are under the control of plasminogen activator inhibitors, which complex with tPA and uPA to inactivate them and therefore block plasmin generation.

tPA is more important than uPA for normal hemostasis as is evident by how endothelial cells upregulate production of this protein when injured. tPA is stimulated by a variety of substances, including thrombin, serotonin, bradykinin, cytokines, and epinephrine. This binding affords tPA some protection from degradation, and enables it to survive for longer than its expected half-life of 4 minutes. The role of tPA in hemostasis is of such significance that recombinant tPA (alteplase) and its derivatives that incorporate the kringle domains, including reteplase and tenecteplase, are used as thrombolytic agents in patients with acute thrombotic events, including myocardial infarction and thrombotic stroke.[39,40]

The other essential plasminogen activator in this process is uPA, which exists in a high-molecular-weight (HMW) form and a low-molecular-weight (LMW) form, both of which have the ability to activate plasminogen through cleavage at Arg560-Val561. Urokinase is present in high concentration in the urine. While tPA is mainly important for intravascular fibrinolysis, urokinase has more of a role in the extravascular compartment. However, unlike tPA, uPA does not bind to fibrin and therefore is not involved in activation of plasminogen incorporated into clots through fibrin binding.[41] uPA is derived from urokinase, which consists of a single chain precursor molecule termed scuPA, which is hydrolyzed by plasmin or kallikrein to the two-chain active uPA, which is biologically active.[42] In plasma, scuPA does not activate plasminogen; however, in the presence of fibrin it is actually the scuPA that induces clot lysis. Interestingly, the role of urokinase has been expanded to include the support of invasion and metastasis in malignancy.[43,44] uPA has been shown to play a role in extracellular matrix degradation, allowing for the migration and invasion of metastatic cells. There is now a growing interest in developing targeted therapy that blocks this pathway as a means of controlling metastasis.

Streptokinase does not participate in normal hemostasis, but is used as a therapeutic agent for acute thrombosis. It is isolated from beta-hemolytic streptococci, and since it is not an enzyme, it must combine with plasminogen to form an active molecule, which then has the ability to cleave plasminogen to plasmin.[45] However, its use as a therapeutic agent is limited because, as a foreign substance, it is often recognized by the immune system and antistreptokinase antibodies are generated.

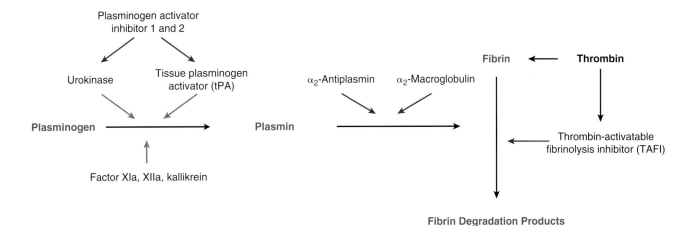

Fig. 4.2 Pathway of Fibrinolysis. Inhibition is signified by red arrows, and stimulation is signified by green arrows.

There are multiple endogenous proteins that can rapidly inhibit the fibrinolytic response. These include PAI-1, alpha-2 anti-plasmin, α1 antitrypsin, and C1 inhibitor. Most of these inhibitors act through serine protease inhibition (serpin) and therefore affect many aspects of coagulation. The most important of these inhibitors is PAI-1, which is expressed by endothelial cells or platelets after exposure to thrombin; inflammatory mediators such as tumor necrosis factor-α; and growth factors, lipids, insulin, angiotensin II, and endotoxin.[46] Recently, the role of PAI-1 as an inhibitor of tissue factor has been postulated to regulate hemostasis in inflammatory conditions, such as sepsis or acute lung injury.[47] It has been shown that platelets release PAI-1 as a mechanism of preventing premature clot dissolution. Patients who are deficient in PAI-1 have a bleeding diathesis with trauma or surgery. In addition, PAI-1 appears to accelerate the aging process by as yet unclear mechanisms.[45,48]

Another important mechanism for the regulation of fibrinolysis is thrombin-activatable fibrinolysis inhibitor (TAFI), which is not a member of the serpin family. It is known for its ability to cleave the carboxyterminal lysine in fibrin, impairing plasminogen binding.[49] The activation of TAFI is dependent upon the thrombin-thrombomodulin complex, which can expedite the inhibitory process in a similar manner to thrombin.[50] This process has recently been shown to be inhibited by platelet factor 4, which is secreted by activated platelets.[51] If the feedback mechanisms of thrombin generation through factors V, VIII, and XI is impaired, leading to diminution of the thrombin-thrombomodulin complex and therefore decreased activation of TAFI, clinical consequences can occur. It has been suggested that in chronic liver disease where coagulation factors are decreased, the low amounts of TAFI may account for the low-grade fibrinolysis which is observed.[52] The opposite can also occur, as is seen in patients with the G20210A prothrombin gene mutation in which thrombin generation is increased, leading to increased activation of TAFI and an increased thrombotic propensity through the inhibition of fibrinolysis.[53]

Recently, it has been shown that there is yet another important mechanism by which to regulate the fibrinolytic process via matrix metalloproteinases (MMPs). MMPs (including MMP-3, 7, 9, and 12) are found in the endothelial cells and have the ability to cleave uPA and plasminogen. The importance of MMPs in downregulating cellular fibrinolysis still remains to be elucidated, although it is clear that they function through reducing the availability of plasminogen. MMP-3 and 7 also have the ability to degrade fibrinogen and cross-linked fibrin, and MMP-11 can degrade fibrinogen and not fibrin. MMPs also

can modulate the activity of many of the inhibitors of fibrinolysis, including alpha 2 antiplasmin and PAI-1.[54,55]

SUMMARY

In this chapter, we have described the intricate pathways involved in coagulation and fibrinolysis with specific emphasis on the regulation of hemostasis. Future endeavors focused on understanding the complex nature of these processes and how they relate to human disease processes, including inflammation, malignancy, and arterial and venous thrombotic events, will provide additional targeted therapies to modulate hemostasis and thrombosis.

REFERENCES

1. Kunishima S, Kamiya T, Saito H. Genetic abnormalities of Bernard-Soulier syndrome. *Int J Hematol.* 2002;76(4):319–327.
2. Sadler JE. Von Willebrand disease type 1: a diagnosis in search of a disease. *Blood.* 2003;101(6):2089–2093.
3. Offermanns S. Activation of platelet function through G protein-coupled receptors. *Circ Res.* 2006;99(12):1293–1304.
4. Kulkarni S, Dopheide SM, Yap CL, et al. A revised model of platelet aggregation. *J Clin Invest.* 2000;105(6):783–791.
5. Bellucci S, Caen J. Molecular basis of Glanzmann's Thrombasthenia and current strategies in treatment. *Blood Rev.* 2002;16(3):193–202.
6. Agbani EO, Poole AW. Procoagulant platelets: generation, function, and therapeutic targeting in thrombosis. *Blood.* 2017;130(20):2171–2179.
7. Agbani EO, van den Bosch MT, Brown E, et al. Coordinated membrane ballooning and procoagulant spreading in human platelets. *Circulation.* 2015;132(15):1414–1424.
8. Davi G, Patrono C. Platelet activation and atherothrombosis. *N Engl J Med.* 2007;357(24):2482–2494.
9. Moncada S. Adventures in vascular biology: a tale of two mediators. *Philos Trans R Soc Lond B Biol Sci.* 2006;361(1469):735–759.
10. Mehta RS. Novel oral anticoagulants. Part II: direct thrombin inhibitors. *Expert Rev Hematol.* 2010;3(3):351–361.
11. Mann KG, Butenas S, Brummel K. The dynamics of thrombin formation. *Arterioscler Thromb Vasc Biol.* 2003;23(1):17–25.
12. Bajaj SP, Joist JH. New insights into how blood clots: implications for the use of APTT and PT as coagulation screening tests and in monitoring of anticoagulant therapy. *Semin Thromb Hemost.* 1999;25(4):407–418.
13. Mandal SK, Pendurthi UR, Rao LV. Cellular localization and trafficking of tissue factor. *Blood.* 2006;107(12):4746–4753.
14. Chen VM, Ahamed J, Versteeg HH, et al. Evidence for activation of tissue factor by an allosteric disulfide bond. *Biochemistry.* 2006;45(39):12020–12028.

15. Kothari H, Nayak RC, Rao LV, Pendurthi UR. Cystine 186-cystine 209 disulfide bond is not essential for the procoagulant activity of tissue factor or for its de-encryption. *Blood*. 2010;115(21):4273–4283.

16. Bach RR, Monroe D. What is wrong with the allosteric disulfide bond hypothesis? *Arterioscler Thromb Vasc Biol*. 2009;29(12):1997–1998.

17. Bogdanov VY, Balasubramanian V, Hathcock J, et al. Alternatively spliced human tissue factor: a circulating, soluble, thrombogenic protein. *Nat Med*. 2003;9(4):458–462.

18. Del Conde I, Shrimpton CN, Thiagarajan P, Lopez JA. Tissue-factor-bearing microvesicles arise from lipid rafts and fuse with activated platelets to initiate coagulation. *Blood*. 2005;106(5):1604–1611.

19. Panes O, Matus V, Saez CG, et al. Human platelets synthesize and express functional tissue factor. *Blood*. 2007;109(12):5242–5250.

20. Skidgel RA, Alhenc-Gelas F, Campbell WB. Prologue: kinins and related systems. New life for old discoveries. *Am J Physiol Heart Circ Physiol*. 2003;284(6):H1886–H1891.

21. Horan JT, Francis CW. Fibrin degradation products, fibrin monomer and soluble fibrin in disseminated intravascular coagulation. *Semin Thromb Hemost*. 2001;27(6):657–666.

22. Cochery-Nouvellon E, Mercier E, Lissalde-Lavigne G, et al. Homozygosity for the C46T polymorphism of the F12 gene is a risk factor for venous thrombosis during the first pregnancy. *J Thromb Haemost*. 2007;5(4):700–707.

23. Reuner KH, Jenetzky E, Aleu A, et al. Factor XII C46T gene polymorphism and the risk of cerebral venous thrombosis. *Neurology*. 2008;70(2):129–132.

24. Versteeg HH, Heemskerk JW, Levi M, Reitsma PH. New fundamentals in hemostasis. *Physiol Rev*. 2013;93(1):327–358.

25. Renne T, Gailani D. Role of factor XII in hemostasis and thrombosis: clinical implications. *Expert Rev Cardiovasc Ther*. 2007;5(4):733–741.

26. van der Meijden PE, Munnix IC, Auger JM, et al. Dual role of collagen in factor XII-dependent thrombus formation. *Blood*. 2009;114(4):881–890.

27. von Bruhl ML, Stark K, Steinhart A, et al. Monocytes, neutrophils, and platelets cooperate to initiate and propagate venous thrombosis in mice in vivo. *J Exp Med*. 2012;209(4):819–835.

28. Muller F, Mutch NJ, Schenk WA, et al. Platelet polyphosphates are proinflammatory and procoagulant mediators in vivo. *Cell*. 2009;139(6):1143–1156.

29. Morrissey JH, Choi SH, Smith SA. Polyphosphate: an ancient molecule that links platelets, coagulation, and inflammation. *Blood*. 2012;119(25):5972–5979.

30. Geddings JE, Mackman N. New players in haemostasis and thrombosis. *Thromb Haemost*. 2014;111(4):570–574.

31. Mosesson MW, Siebenlist KR, Meh DA. The structure and biological features of fibrinogen and fibrin. *Ann N Y Acad Sci*. 2001;936:11–30.

32. Ariens RA, Lai TS, Weisel JW, et al. Role of factor XIII in fibrin clot formation and effects of genetic polymorphisms. *Blood*. 2002;100(3):743–754.

33. Weitz JI. Heparan sulfate: antithrombotic or not? *J Clin Invest*. 2003;111(7):952–954.

34. Patnaik MM, Moll S. Inherited antithrombin deficiency: a review. *Haemophilia*. 2008;14(6):1229–1239.

35. Esmon CT. The protein C pathway. *Chest*. 2003;124(3 Suppl):26S–32S.

36. Santamaria S, Reglinska-Matveyev N, Gierula M, et al. Factor V has an anticoagulant cofactor activity that targets the early phase of coagulation. *J Biol Chem*. 2017;292(22):9335–9344.

37. Miles LA, Castellino FJ, Gong Y. Critical role for conversion of glu-plasminogen to Lys-plasminogen for optimal stimulation of plasminogen activation on cell surfaces. *Trends Cardiovasc Med*. 2003;13(1):21–30.

38. Kolev K, Machovich R. Molecular and cellular modulation of fibrinolysis. *Thromb Haemost*. 2003;89(4):610–621.

39. Cassella CR, Jagoda A. Ischemic stroke: advances in diagnosis and management. *Emerg Med Clin North Am*. 2017;35(4):911–930.

40. Kunadian V, Gibson CM. Thrombolytics and myocardial infarction. *Cardiovasc Ther*. 2012;30:e81–e88.

41. Rijken DC, Sakharov DV. Basic principles in thrombolysis: regulatory role of plasminogen. *Thromb Res*. 2001;103(Suppl 1):S41–S49.

42. Colman RW. Role of the light chain of high molecular weight kininogen in adhesion, cell-associated proteolysis and angiogenesis. *Biol Chem*. 2001;382(1):65–70.

43. Mekkawy AH, Morris DL, Pourgholami MH. Urokinase plasminogen activator system as a potential target for cancer therapy. *Future Oncol*. 2009;5(9):1487–1499.

44. Hildenbrand R, Allgayer H, Marx A, Stroebel P. Modulators of the urokinase-type plasminogen activation system for cancer. *Expert Opin Investig Drugs*. 2010;19(5):641–652.

45. Bell WR. Present-day thrombolytic therapy: therapeutic agents—pharmacokinetics and pharmacodynamics. *Rev Cardiovasc Med*. 2002;3(Suppl 2):S34–S44.

46. Kohler HP, Grant PJ. Plasminogen-activator inhibitor type 1 and coronary artery disease. *N Engl J Med*. 2000;342(24):1792–1801.

47. Sen P, Komissarov AA, Florova G, et al. Plasminogen activator inhibitor-1 inhibits factor VIIa bound to tissue factor. *J Thromb Haemost*. 2010;9:531–539.

48. Khan SS, Shah SJ, Klyachko E, et al. A null mutation in SERPINE1 protects against biological aging in humans. *Sci Adv*. 2017;3(11): eaao1617.

49. Zhao L, Buckman B, Seto M, et al. Mutations in the substrate binding site of thrombin-activatable fibrinolysis inhibitor (TAFI) alter its substrate specificity. *J Biol Chem*. 2003;278(34):32359–32366.

50. Mosnier LO, Meijers JC, Bouma BN. Regulation of fibrinolysis in plasma by TAFI and protein C is dependent on the concentration of thrombomodulin. *Thromb Haemost*. 2001;85(1):5–11.

51. Mosnier LO. Platelet factor 4 inhibits thrombomodulin-dependent activation of thrombin-activatable fibrinolysis inhibitor (TAFI) by thrombin. *J Biol Chem*. 2010;286:502–510.

52. Van Thiel DH, George M, Fareed J. Low levels of thrombin activatable fibrinolysis inhibitor (TAFI) in patients with chronic liver disease. *Thromb Haemost*. 2001;85(4):667–670.

53. Colucci M, Binetti BM, Tripodi A, et al. Hyperprothrombinemia associated with prothrombin G20210A mutation inhibits plasma fibrinolysis through a TAFI-mediated mechanism. *Blood*. 2004;103(6):2157–2161.

54. Lijnen HR, Van Hoef B, Collen D. Inactivation of the serpin alpha(2)-antiplasmin by stromelysin-1. *Biochim Biophys Acta*. 2001;1547(2): 206–213.

55. Lijnen HR, Arza B, Van Hoef B, et al. Inactivation of plasminogen activator inhibitor-1 by specific proteolysis with stromelysin-1 (MMP-3). *J Biol Chem*. 2000;275(48):37645–37650.

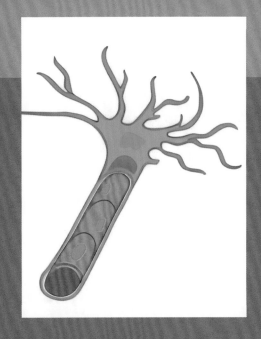

第5章
血管药理学

　　大多数治疗血管系统疾病的药物是通过增强内源性保护介质的释放，或抑制病理介质的异常活动产生药理作用。这类药物对血管组织的选择性越高，其对机体的不良反应越低。而直接调节血管内皮细胞（vascular endothelial cell，VEC）和血管平滑肌细胞（vascular smooth muscle cell，VSMC）的功能是实现高选择性的重要途径。其中作用于血管内皮细胞受体或血管平滑肌细胞受体的激动剂或拮抗剂类药物居多。从疾病发生角度来看，血管内皮细胞受损是导致血管舒缩障碍、血栓及炎症的重要诱因。首先，血管内皮细胞可释放一氧化氮（NO）和前列腺素（PG）等内源介质干预血管平滑肌细胞的相应信号以调控其舒缩功能；但在血管内皮细胞受损时，该功能受限进而导致血压失衡。此外，血管内皮细胞受损时细胞间的紧密连接被打破，各种损伤因素如低密度脂蛋白（low density lipoprotein，LDL）及单核细胞进入平滑肌层，可影响血管平滑肌细胞的功能，加速动脉粥样硬化的进程。同时，血管内皮细胞在正常情况下抑制血小板活化，而在受到外源性损伤时激活血小板，发挥生理性止血作用，但其在长期受到内源性损伤或慢性炎症时也会激活血小板并抑制纤溶系统引发血栓栓塞性疾病，在此过程中，环氧合酶（COX）系统活化是血管内皮细胞传递的重要内源性信号。因此，从药物治疗的角度来看，直接调控血管平滑肌细胞舒缩功能是对血压异常最为直接的治疗。去甲肾上腺素（norepinephrine，NE）类药物可激动血管平滑肌细胞上的 α 受体引起血管收缩，升高血压，而酚妥拉明等药物通过阻断α受体扩张血管，下调血压。从另一方面来看，离子通道阻断剂、G蛋白受体拮抗剂等通过调控血管平滑肌细胞内的钙离子含量影响其舒缩功能，也可发挥治疗作用。由于血管平滑肌细胞的收缩也受血管内皮细胞释放的介质影响，故而拟一氧化氮及前列腺素类药物能够模拟血管内皮细胞功能，从而干预血管平滑肌细胞的舒缩。血管紧张素转化酶抑制剂类药物则主要通过抑制机体肾素-血管紧张素-醛固酮系统从整体调节血管内皮细胞及血管平滑肌细胞的细胞连接与舒缩功能，实现血管重构，在多种心血管疾病中都显现出疗效。最后，诸如阿司匹林、氯吡格雷等药物主要通过抑制血管内皮细胞的环氧合酶系统来抑制血小板的激活，从而实现对血栓栓塞性疾病的治疗。

薛　松

Vascular Pharmacology

Nicholas A. Flavahan

Therapeutic intervention is optimized when we understand the normal physiological signaling processes that are disrupted by a disease process, the abnormal molecular and cellular mechanisms driving disease pathogenesis, and the pharmacological profile of the intervention. Indeed, the majority of vascular drugs act as replacement therapy to augment endogenous protective signaling processes or as reversal therapy to block or reduce the abnormal activity of pathological mediators or signaling processes. This chapter discusses current and potential future therapies within the context of these processes.

THE PHARMACOLOGICAL FRAMEWORK OF DRUG ACTION

Pharmacology provides a guiding scientific framework to help define optimal approaches to correcting abnormal or perturbed systems. It encompasses the area of pharmacokinetics, which characterizes how our bodies interact with and process drugs, including their absorption, distribution, metabolism, and elimination; and the area of pharmacodynamics, which characterizes the mechanism of action of drugs and how they interact with our bodies to modify cellular and organ function. This chapter focuses mainly on pharmacodynamics and the mechanisms of action of drugs.

The action of most drugs involves their chemical interaction with macromolecular species that regulate cellular activity within important regulatory systems. Indeed, drug receptors generally serve as receptors or signaling intermediates for endogenous mediators. Exogenous drugs and endogenous stimuli that bind to and cause activation of receptor-dependent signaling are termed agonists. Their activity is determined by agonist-dependent and tissue-dependent characteristics. Agonist-dependent activity at receptors is determined by two main drug characteristics: the affinity of the drug for the receptor, which defines the concentration range over which the agonist effectively engages the receptor, and the intrinsic efficacy of the agonist, which defines how well the agonist activates the receptor after it has bound to the site (Fig. 5.1). A key aspect of receptor systems is their remarkable ability, via activation of ion channels and/or serial activation of enzyme systems, to amplify signaling systems. This enables initial discrete agonist-receptor molecular interactions to cause profound alterations in cellular and organ function. High-efficacy agonists are very effective at activating receptors and can generate a maximal response of the system while occupying only a fraction of the receptors. As a result, they are also described as "full" agonists, and the fraction of receptors not required for the maximal response are described as spare receptors or the receptor reserve (see Fig. 5.1). In contrast, low-efficacy agonists are less effective at activating the receptors and must engage and activate a greater proportion of receptors to generate a functional response equivalent to that of the higher-efficacy agonists. Low-efficacy agonists will therefore have fewer spare receptors or a smaller receptor reserve as compared with

higher-efficacy agonists. When receptor systems are limited (or agonist efficacy is sufficiently low), low-efficacy agonists will not generate the full maximal response in the system; under these conditions, they are also described as "partial" agonists (see Fig. 5.1). Receptor systems can become limited as a result of decreased receptor expression or from the reduced efficiency of downstream signaling events, which could reflect reduced expression of signaling mediators or concurrent activation of opposing mechanisms (functional antagonism). Because of their ability to occupy receptors coupled with a reduced ability to activate them, low-efficacy or partial agonists can actually block the activity of higher-efficacy agonists. Indeed, if the receptor system is severely limited or the intrinsic efficacy of the partial agonists is sufficiently low, they may not generate an agonist response and would act like pure antagonists to block the response to higher-efficacy agonists. This variable activity is observed with the low-efficacy α-adrenergic agonist clonidine, which is approved by the US Food and Drug Administration (FDA) for the treatment of hypertension. It activates α2-adrenergic receptors (α2-adrenoceptors, α2-ARs) in the central nervous system to reduce sympathetic outflow, which is thought to be the major mechanism for its hypotensive activity (see the section titled "Therapeutic Intervention and the Autonomic Vascular Innervation"). In the vascular system, clonidine can activate α1- and α2-ARs to cause vasoconstriction, but in the presence of high-efficacy agonists such as the physiological agonists norepinephrine and epinephrine, clonidine has the opposite effect and causes vasodilatation. It is unclear whether this contributes to its antihypertensive activity.

Pure receptor antagonists have significant affinity for receptors but no intrinsic efficacy and are therefore unable to provide activation. Competitive antagonists bind reversibly to the receptor and inhibit the ability of the agonist to bind and cause receptor activation. Increasing the concentration of the agonist will compete away the antagonist and regain functional activity, resulting in a parallel rightward shift in the concentration-response curve with no change in the maximal response (see Fig. 5.1). The magnitude of the rightward shift of the curve depends on the concentration of the antagonist and its affinity for the receptor. Indeed, the affinity of the antagonist for the receptors can be determined based on the magnitude of the shift (see Fig. 5.1). If the antagonist binds irreversibly or pseudo-irreversibly (i.e., slow dissociation), it will function in a similar manner to a reduced number of receptors, with rightward shifts in the concentration-effect curve (no change in the maximal response) until the receptor reserve is lost, after which it will cause downward shifts in the curve with progressive depression of the maximal response (see Fig. 5.1). This type of action is described as noncompetitive antagonism. Phenoxybenzamine, which is FDA-approved for the treatment of pheochromocytoma, is an irreversible noncompetitive antagonist at α-ARs (see section titled "Therapeutic Intervention and the Autonomic Vascular Innervation").

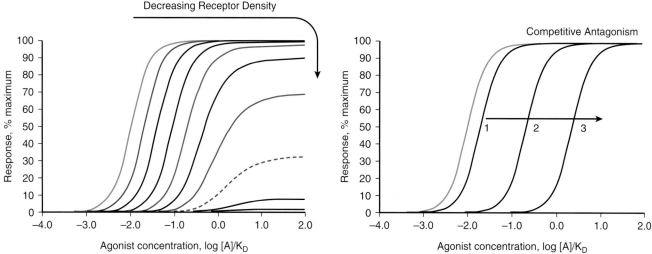

Fig. 5.1 The Interaction of Agonists and Antagonists With Drug Receptors (modeled as previously described[111]). In the upper panel, agonist concentration-response curves were generated by 50% stepwise reductions in the density of receptors. Agonist concentration [A] is expressed relative to K_D, the dissociation constant of the agonist for the receptors, to provide insight into the receptor-response coupling. For example, at −2, the agonist will be bound to approximately 1% of the receptors, whereas at 0 (i.e., [A] = K_D), the agonist will be bound to 50% of the receptors. Therefore the control curve *(green curve)* represents an effector system with a large receptor reserve. Stepwise reductions in receptor density cause rightward shifts in the agonist concentration-response curve, with no change in the maximal response until the receptor reserve has been depleted *(blue curve)*. At that point, decreases in receptor density cause downward shifts in the concentration-response curves with stepwise reductions in the maximal response. A similar progression in concentration-response curves could be produced by analyzing a series of agonists with the same affinity (or K_D) for the receptors and same receptor density, but with stepwise reductions in agonist intrinsic efficacy. For example, the green curve would represent a full agonist with high intrinsic efficacy, whereas the red curve would represent a partial agonist with the same affinity but much lower intrinsic efficacy. The lower panel presents the impact of increasing concentrations of a competitive antagonist on the concentration-response curve to a high-efficacy agonist *(green curve)*. The antagonist would have a similar impact on a lower-efficacy agonist, assuming that the agents all act in a simple manner with a single population of receptors. Under these conditions, the antagonist will cause parallel rightward shifts in the agonist's concentration-effect curve. The magnitude of the rightward shift (calculated as the agonist concentration ratio [CR]) is determined by the affinity of the antagonist for the receptor: CR-1 = [B]/K_B, where [B] is the concentration of the antagonist and K_B is the dissociation constant of the antagonist for the receptors. K_B can be calculated using a single concentration of the antagonist, but it is most often analyzed using an Arunlakshana and Schild plot, where log (CR-1) is plotted against log [B] for a series of agonist concentrations.[112,113] The resulting plot should have a slope of 1 and an x-intercept, when y = 0, equal to the log K_B. When [B] equals the K_B, the antagonist will cause a twofold shift in the agonist concentration-response curve (curve 1); with each additional 10-fold increase in antagonist concentration, there should be a further ~11-fold shift in the agonist concentration–effect curve (curves 2 and 3). This relationship, and the slope of the Arunlakshana and Schild plot can be adversely affected when the agonist but not the antagonist interacts with multiple receptor subtypes or when the agonist saturates a disposition mechanism.[112,113] Interestingly, the impact of a competitive antagonist is analogous to a decrease in the affinity of the agonist for the receptor (or an increase in K_D), whereas the effect of a noncompetitive antagonist is analogous to a reduction in the intrinsic efficacy of the agonist or of receptor density. For example, in the upper panel, if the green and red concentration-response curves represent two distinct agonists with the same affinity but different intrinsic efficacies at the same receptor system, then the same concentration of a noncompetitive antagonist (or reduction in receptor density) would cause a parallel shift in the concentration-response curve to the high efficacy agonist *(pink curve)* and a downward shift in the curve to the low-efficacy agonist *(dashed pink curve)*.

Some receptors can display spontaneous activity or be activated in an agonist-independent manner. For example, in addition to being activated by angiotensin II (ANGII), AT1 receptors (AT1Rs) are thought to function as mechanoreceptors and to be activated by mechanical stretch independently of ANGII.[1] Because no agonist is bound to the receptor, this type of activity cannot be reversed by simple receptor antagonists. However, some antagonists actually function as inverse agonists: they have negative intrinsic efficacy and cause the receptors to have reduced activity. Inverse agonists therefore have the ability to inhibit receptor activation by agonists and agonist-independent mechanisms. Regarding the example of AT1Rs, both losartan and valsartan are FDA-approved as selective AT1R antagonists to treat hypertension (see section titled

"Therapeutic Intervention and the Vascular Media"); however, unlike losartan, valsartan can function as an inverse agonist at AT1Rs and therefore block the ANGII-dependent and independent activity of AT1Rs.[1]

Drug selectivity is a relative, not an absolute quality. In general, as the concentration of a drug is increased, it will interact with additional receptor sites, resulting in distinct concentration-effect curves for its multiple effects. The concentration difference between these concentration-response curves provides a measure of drug selectivity. Although the additional activity could contribute to the therapeutic activity of the drug, it often reflects an unwanted or problematic activity; the selectivity of the compound therefore also provides a measure of its therapeutic index.

Receptors are generally regulated by a negative feedback signaling system whereby sustained activation causes downregulation or desensitization of the receptor system, whereas sustained absence of activation can result in receptor sensitization or increased reactivity to a stimulus. These processes can complicate treatment strategies, causing a diminution in effectiveness of agonist-based therapeutics or rebound activity following cessation or interruption of antagonist-based approaches. For example, treatment of pulmonary arterial hypertension (PAH) with the prostacyclin IP receptor agonist eproprostenil requires continual dose escalation to maintain clinical efficacy (see section titled "Therapeutic Intervention and the Endothelium").[2,3] Alterations in the clinical efficacy of drugs can also reflect adaptive changes in pharmacokinetics, including absorption and disposition mechanisms or changes in pharmacodynamics processes resulting, for example, from an ongoing disease process.

The nature of therapeutic intervention is evolving. Emerging therapeutics include biologics such as genetically engineered enzymes, humanized antibodies, and RNA-silencing approaches. Gene therapy approaches using viral vectors to correct genetic mutations are now being approved in the United States and Europe. However, pharmacological concepts can still provide a guiding framework to optimize traditional and novel approaches for correcting abnormal or perturbed systems.

THERAPEUTIC INTERVENTION AND THE ENDOTHELIUM

Normal endothelial function is crucial for maintaining cardiovascular and organismal health. Endothelial cells are important regulators of blood vessel constriction, thrombosis, inflammation, permeability, and vascular remodeling.[4] Under physiological conditions, the endothelium exerts a powerful protective influence to inhibit these processes and maintain vascular stability and homeostasis; however, during the development of vascular disease, the endothelium becomes "dysfunctional," promoting these same processes and contributing to pathological changes in vascular function and structure.[4] Not surprisingly, endothelial-dependent mechanisms are targeted by numerous therapeutics to treat vascular diseases.

Vasoconstriction and Vasodilatation

Under normal conditions, endothelial cells generate two prominent vasodilator mediators, prostacyclin (prostaglandin I_2, or PGI_2) and nitric oxide (NO) (Fig. 5.2). Although endothelial cells can release another vasodilator, endothelium-derived hyperpolarizing factor (EDHF), it has not yet been implicated or utilized in vascular therapies and is not discussed further here. PGI_2 production is dependent on the enzyme cyclooxygenase (COX), whereas endothelium-derived NO is produced by endothelial NO synthase (eNOS). Basal production of these mediators can be rapidly increased following endothelial activation by numerous stimuli that may be present in the vessel wall and bloodstream, including norepinephrine, thrombin, and bradykinin. Endothelial cells are also mechanosensitive and are regulated by the shear stress exerted by the bloodstream itself, including increased production of PGI_2 and NO (see Fig. 5.2). Such flow-mediated dilatation (FMD) has become an important noninvasive mechanism to assess endothelial function and vascular health. Under physiological conditions, endothelial FMD enables dilatation in small arterioles, for example, in response to cellular metabolism, to be conducted upstream to more proximal arterioles and arteries, facilitating targeted increases in blood flow and preventing tissue ischemia.[5,6]

The COX enzyme converts arachidonic acid to an unstable intermediate PGH_2, which is then converted via specific synthase enzymes to numerous prostanoids, including PGI_2 generated by endothelial PGI_2 synthase (see also the section titled "COX Inhibitors and the Human Vascular System"). A key step in this process is the availability of arachidonic acid, which is released from membrane phospholipids by phospholipase A_2. eNOS comprises an N-terminal oxygenase domain that binds heme, zinc, tetrahydrobiopterin (BH_4), calmodulin and the substrate L-arginine, and a C-terminal reductase domain that binds flavin mononucleotide (FMN), flavin adenine dinucleotide (FAD), and nicotinamide adenine dinucleotide phosphate (NADPH). Normal enzyme activity requires the formation of homodimers that enables the transfer of electrons from the reductase domain of one eNOS monomer to the oxygenase domain of the other monomer, culminating in the oxidation of L-arginine and NO formation.[7,8] Owing to their very short half-lives, NO and PGI_2 act locally and are not circulating mediators. PGI_2 activates IP receptors, which are plasma membrane receptors predominantly coupled to the G_S-protein, resulting in activation of adenylyl cyclase and increased production of cyclic adenosine monophosphate (AMP). NO diffuses through plasma membranes and activates the cytosolic enzyme soluble guanylyl cyclase and increases production of cyclic guanosine monophosphate (GMP). In vascular smooth muscle cells (VSMCs), cyclic AMP and cyclic GMP activate protein kinase A (PKA) and protein kinase G (PKG), respectively, to initiate vasodilation (see Fig. 5.2) (see also the section titled "Therapeutic Intervention and the Vascular Media"). These agents have important additional effects on endothelial, VSMCs, and circulating cells to regulate thrombosis/hemostasis, vascular remodeling, and inflammation.

The activity of NO and PGI_2 is reduced during the development of vascular diseases, resulting in diminished endothelial-mediated dilatation and an increased propensity for vasoconstriction (see Fig. 5.2). Indeed, the presence of endothelial dilator dysfunction is predictive of future cardiovascular events, and the assessment of endothelial function may help direct vascular therapy to improve cardiovascular outcomes.[9] Reduced activity of these mediators can reflect alterations in the ability of endothelial cells to be activated or reflect specific changes in enzyme/mediator dynamics such as, for PGI_2, inactivation of PGI_2 synthase by the pathological oxidant $OONO^-$ and/or expression of alternate synthases, and for NO, inactivation by superoxide radical.[10] Indeed, decreased levels of cofactor BH_4 or substrate arginine causes uncoupling of enzyme function resulting in the generation of superoxide rather than NO.[7,8] eNOS uncoupling is thought to contribute to endothelial dysfunction in numerous vascular disorders including atherosclerosis, diabetes, hypertension and aging. In the setting of endothelial dysfunction, there is not only a decrease in the activity of protective vasodilator mediators but also increased production of the potent vasoconstrictor endothelin-1 (ET-1). ET-1 is formed from precursor peptides by proteolytic processing. PreproET-1 mRNA is translated, stripped of its signal sequence, and further cleaved by a furin-like peptidase to generate BigET-1.[11] Further processing to biologically active ETs is achieved by endothelin-converting enzyme (ECE). BigET-1 and to a lesser extent mature ET-1 are stored in granules within the endothelium. Following stimulation by endothelial secretagogues, for example, thrombin, these peptides are released by exocytosis, resulting in an explosive generation of ET-1 and blood vessel constriction.[11] Endothelium-derived NO is an important functional inhibitor of ET-1, reducing its expression and blocking its exocytotic release and generation. Not surprisingly, there is a minimal role for ET-1 in the normal endothelial regulation of contractility in mature arteries. Indeed, the diminution in NO activity occurring during endothelial dysfunction is likely an important contributor to the increased prominence of ET-1.[11] ET-1 activates two receptor subtypes: the ET_A receptor, which is

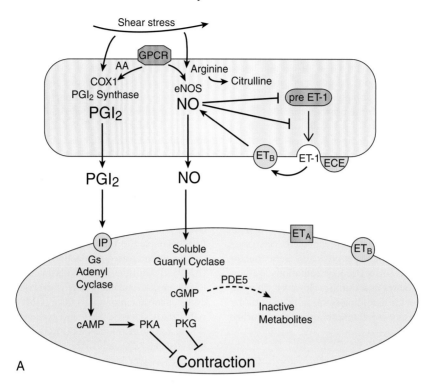

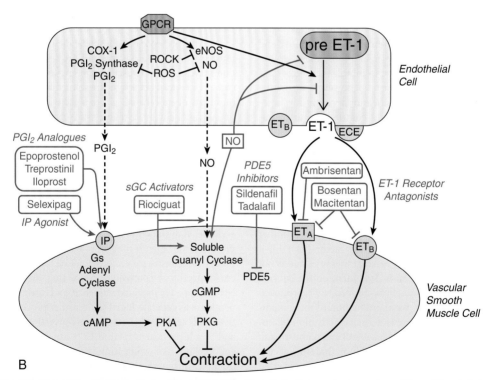

Fig. 5.2 Regulation of vasomotor function by the vascular endothelium under normal conditions (A) and during endothelial dilator dysfunction (B) and current therapeutic interventions that mimic or modulate endothelial activity, particularly with regard to those approved for the treatment of pulmonary arterial hypertension. *AA*, Arachidonic acid; *pre ET-1*, precursor ET-1 peptide (BigET-1).

expressed on smooth muscle cells and mediates constriction, and the ET_B receptor, which also can be present on VSMCs to mediate constriction but is prominently expressed on endothelial cells and mediates increased production of PGI_2 and NO (see Fig. 5.2).

Therapeutic intervention to correct endothelial dilator dysfunction is best exemplified by current approaches to treat PAH (see Fig. 5.2). Indeed, first-line therapeutic intervention for PAH is directed toward augmenting or replacing the reduced signaling activity of the endogenous protective mediators NO or PGI_2 and reducing the heightened activity of ET-1.[12–14] PAH results from a progressive increase in pulmonary vascular resistance and is defined as an elevated mean pulmonary arterial pressure ($\geq$25 mm Hg) and increased pulmonary arterial resistance, but with normal pulmonary venous pressure (pulmonary wedge pressure $\leq$15 mm Hg).[12–14] The disease is predominantly of idiopathic (or unknown) origin but is also associated with other disease processes including scleroderma and ingestion of certain drugs or toxins (e.g., toxic rapeseed oil, fenfluramine).[12,13] The condition results in right heart failure, which is the major cause of morbidity and mortality. PAH is associated with endothelial dysfunction including reduced activity of NO and PGI_2 and increased expression and circulating levels of ET-1.[12,13] Before this targeted endothelial mechanistic approach to treatment, the median survival was 2.8 years. This has been dramatically extended to over 7 years, although PAH still represents a devastating disease process.[12,15]

Intravenous synthetic PGI_2 (epoprostenol) was the first targeted therapy approved for PAH. Epoprostenol improves symptoms, exercise capacity, and hemodynamics and is the only treatment shown to reduce mortality in severe PAH.[12,13,16] It is still considered the cornerstone of therapy for PAH, particularly in advanced stages of the disease.[12] As with endogenous PGI_2, epoprostenol has a very short half-life (~3 min) and requires the use of a drug delivery pump system for continuous intravenous infusion.[12,13] Side effects are consistent with vasodilator therapy and include headaches, flushing, dizziness, and systemic hypotension; potential adverse events are also associated with the delivery system.[12,13] Two other structural analogues of PGI_2 are FDA-approved for treating PAH.[14] Treprostinil has a longer half-life than epoprostenol and is available for continuous intravenous infusion as well as subcutaneous, inhalation, and oral delivery, whereas iloprost is available in an inhaled formulation.[12–14] These analogues have favorable effects on exercise capacity, hemodynamics, symptoms, and clinical events, and the vasodilator side effects are similar to those of epoprostenol.[12–14] Selexipag belongs to a distinct class of PGI_2-related, FDA-approved treatment options in PAH. It is a selective IP receptor agonist that is structurally distinct from PGI_2 and has shown favorable clinical efficacy in PAH.[12–14] The active metabolite of selexipag, ACT-333697, has lower intrinsic efficacy at IP receptors compared with iloprost or trepinostil.[2] This reduced intrinsic efficacy results in reduced desensitization and reduced internalization of IP receptors compared with the higher-efficacy agonists.[2] It is unclear how this difference in pharmacodynamics might affect clinical efficacy in PAH.[2]

Cyclic GMP, the predominant signaling mediator of NO activity, is degraded by a family of phosphodiesterase (PDE) enzymes whose expression varies in a cell- and tissue-specific manner. Inhibition of relevant PDE enzymes will augment the basal and stimulated levels of cyclic GMP and therefore amplify the activity of endothelium-derived NO. Pulmonary VSMCs have a high level of expression of the PDE5 subtype.[12,13] Two orally active selective inhibitors of the PDE5 enzyme, sildenafil and tadalafil, are FDA-approved for the treatment of PAH.[12–14] Tadalafil differs structurally from sildenafil and has a longer half-life. PDE5 inhibition has shown favorable results in improving exercise capacity, symptoms, and hemodynamics and in decreasing

time to clinical worsening.[12,13] Side effects are mild to moderate and mainly related to vasodilation (headache, flushing, and epistaxis).[12,13] The therapeutic activity of PDE5 inhibitors will be dependent on the catalytic activity of PDE5 and the basal and NO-stimulated activity of soluble guanylyl cyclase. Endothelial dysfunction is generally associated with reduced bioactivity of endothelium-derived NO. If NO activity is severely limited, it would be expected to negatively affect the clinical efficacy of these agents. In contrast, a new class of agent that directly activates soluble guanylyl cyclase has recently been approved for use in PAH.[12–14] The first-in-class agent, riociguat, not only directly stimulates soluble guanylyl cyclase independently of NO but also amplifies NO activity by sensitizing soluble guanylyl cyclase to endogenous NO.[12] It has shown favorable effects in improving exercise capacity, symptoms, and hemodynamics and decreasing time to clinical worsening.[12,13]

Three ET-1 competitive receptor antagonists are currently FDA-approved for treating PAH. Bosentan, macitentan, and ambrisentan are all orally effective.[12–14] Two of them, bosentan and macitentan, do not discriminate between ET_A and ET_B receptors and inhibit both receptor subtypes. In contrast, ambrisentan is selective for ET_A receptors, displaying an approximate 200-fold increased affinity when compared with ET_B receptors. Clinical trials have demonstrated beneficial effects of all three agents in PAH, and data from monotherapy trials do not indicate a difference in clinical efficacy.[12,13]

Inhaled NO gas is FDA-approved to treat persistent pulmonary hypertension of the newborn, a rare subtype of PAH, and acute hypoxemic respiratory failure.[13] Inhaled NO causes preferential vasodilatation in better-ventilated lung regions rather than poorly inflated areas, resulting in improved ventilation/perfusion matching and increased PaO_2 levels. Because of its mode of delivery and extremely short half-life (2 to 6 seconds), inhaled NO is a selective pulmonary vasodilator that can lower pulmonary artery pressure without altering systemic blood pressure. Although inhaled NO is not approved for use in adult PAH, it is used in this patient group to acutely test sensitivity to vasodilator therapy and to treat acute pulmonary hypertensive crises.

Although it might be assumed that these endothelial-related therapies target vasoconstriction in PAH, they are likely acting through multiple mechanisms. The pathogenesis of PAH involves both functional and structural changes in the pulmonary arterial system. In addition to vasoconstriction, there is hypertrophy and proliferation of VSMCs, with increased muscularization and pulmonary arterial thickening, deposition of extracellular matrix proteins, and increased thrombotic activity, which conspire to increase vascular stiffness and precipitate luminal narrowing or occlusion (see also the section titled "Therapeutic Intervention and the Vascular Media").[12–14] Chronic treatment with intravenous epoprostenol has beneficial hemodynamic and clinical effects in PAH even in individuals who lack significant pulmonary arterial vasodilatation to acute administration of the drug.[3,16,17] The conclusion is that the long-term beneficial effects of epoprostenol may be only partially related to its vasodilator properties and may reflect alternate actions on disease pathogenesis.[16] Indeed, current guidelines suggest that selected PAH patients should undergo acute vasodilator testing (e.g., inhaled NO or intravenous epoprostenol) to identify the small subgroup of responders (defined as a $\geq$10 mm Hg decrease in pulmonary artery pressure to achieve an absolute level $\leq$40 mm Hg) who might benefit from long-term calcium channel blocker therapy.[13,15] Only about 10% of idiopathic PAH patients will meet this criterion.[13] In addition to acutely controlling vascular contractility, PGI_2, NO, cyclic GMP, and ET-1 have important regulatory effects on hemostasis/thrombosis, inflammation, and vascular wall remodeling that likely contribute to the therapeutic effects of drugs targeting these mediators.

Current approaches emphasize combination therapy to treat PAH even as an initial approach to treatment.[12,13] This is an attractive approach based on the disparate and potentially synergistic mechanisms utilized by these drugs (see Fig. 5.2).[13] Indeed, current data suggest that patients may benefit from triple combination therapy comprising intravenous PGI_2 analogues, PDE5 inhibition, and ET-1 receptor blockade.[13,14]

The endothelium-related therapeutic approaches to treat PAH are also being used in other vascular pathological processes. Intravenous PGI_2 analogues (iloprost, epoprostenol), PDE5 inhibitors (sildenafil, tadalafil, vardenafil), ET receptor antagonists (bosentan) and topical NO-based therapy (topical nitroglycerin) are currently used to treat cutaneous vasospastic episodes and prevent ischemic injury in scleroderma.[5,18] Scleroderma is associated with a cold-induced cutaneous vasospastic disorder (secondary Raynaud phenomenon) and disruption of endothelial dilator function, which limits FMD, resulting in digital ulceration and necrosis.[5,18]

Penile erection, which reflects vasodilatation of the venous corpus cavernosum system and results in the organ's engorgement with blood, is mediated by increased activity of NO and relaxation of cavernosal VSMCs.[19] Cavernosal endothelial cells can produce and liberate NO in response to endothelial agonists and to physical stimuli.[20] However, the predominant source of NO responsible for penile erection is not endothelium-derived but is neuronal NOS (nNOS) located in parasympathetic nonadrenergic noncholinergic nerve fibers innervating the blood vessel wall.[21] In contrast, the sympathetic adrenergic nervous system, acting through norepinephrine and α-ARs, constricts cavernosal smooth muscle and is responsible for maintaining a flaccid penis and the induction of detumescence following erection. Erectile dysfunction can result from psychologic, hormonal, and vascular etiologies, including reduced NO signaling—for example, as a result of increased oxidant activity. Indeed, erectile dysfunction is strongly associated with cardiovascular arterial disease.[19] As with pulmonary smooth muscle cells, cavernosal VSMCs have a high expression of PDE5, responsible for the degradation of cyclic GMP and diminution in NO activity. PDE5 inhibitors—including sildenafil, vardenafil, tadalafil, and avanafil—are approved for use in treating erectile dysfunction and have demonstrated beneficial effects in patients with varying etiologies of sexual dysfunction.[19] As mentioned earlier, their activity is dependent on NO-stimulated activity of soluble guanylyl cyclase, and their use still requires sexual stimulation to create arousal and raise the available levels of NO.[19] Additional vasodilator therapies are being investigated for use in erectile dysfunction, including inhibition of Rho-associated coiled-coil protein kinase or Rho-kinase (ROCK) (see the section titled "Therapeutic Intervention and the Vascular Media") and direct activation of soluble guanylyl cyclase.[19]

Nitrovasodilators, which generate NO, have been employed for over 150 years to alleviate the chest pain associated with myocardial ischemia.[22] Their activity is reviewed in the section titled "Therapeutic Intervention and the Vascular Media."

Hemostasis, Thrombosis, and Fibrinolysis

Normally the endothelium actively inhibits hemostasis/thrombosis and promotes fibrinolysis by producing and regulating numerous mediators (Fig. 5.3). It also passively inhibits hemostasis/thrombosis by separating blood from the procoagulant environment of the subendothelium. Indeed, after endothelial injury, hemostasis proceeds in three overlapping phases.[23,24]—initiation, amplification, and propagation:

- *Initiation*, when subendothelial tissue factor (TF) and activated plasma factor VII (TF/FVIIa) generate trace amounts of thrombin.

- *Amplification*, when platelets are activated by thrombin, by adhesive interactions with the injured vessel, and by platelet-derived mediators (including adenosine diphosphate [ADP], serotonin, and thromboxane A_2 [TXA_2]), resulting in their aggregation, release of granule contents, production of procoagulant mediators, increased avidity of adhesion receptors, and reorientation of membrane lipids to expose negatively charged phosphatidylserine. This surface enables positively charged, vitamin K-dependent factors including FIX and FX to assemble the terminal coagulation complexes on the platelet surface.

- *Propagation*, when the tenase (FVIIIa:FIXa) and prothrombinase complexes (FVa:FXa) are assembled on the activated platelet surface. The tenase complex activates FX, whereas the prothrombinase complex generates the burst of thrombin necessary to cleave soluble fibrinogen into insoluble fibrin and formation of the clot.[23,24]

Both endothelium-derived NO and PGI_2 have important antithrombotic activity, acting in a synergistic manner to inhibit platelet activity, inhibit platelet adhesion to the endothelium, and stimulate platelet disaggregation (see Fig. 5.3). Importantly, mediators generated during thrombosis—including thrombin, ADP, and serotonin—activate the endothelium to increase the release of NO and PGI_2. NO is also the most important physiological inhibitor of the exocytosis of Weibel Palade bodies (WPBs), which are endothelial granules containing a highly prothrombotic form of von Willebrand factor (VWF) (ultra-large VWF [ULVWF]) and P-selectin.[11] It is unclear whether antiplatelet and antithrombotic activity contributes to the clinical efficacy of PGI_2 and NO-related therapies (e.g., epoprostenol, riociguat).

There are three major anticoagulant pathways: activated protein C (APC), tissue factor pathway inhibitor (TFPI), and antithrombin. Each pathway is intimately dependent on the endothelium (Fig. 5.4; also see Fig. 5.3).[23] Endothelial cells express thrombomodulin, which binds and inhibits the procoagulant activity of thrombin. Moreover, the thrombin-thrombomodulin complex activates protein C, causing an approximately 1000-fold increase in its rate of activation. Endothelial cells also express the endothelial protein C receptor (EPCR), which binds protein C and increases the ability of thrombin-thrombomodulin to activate the protein by another 10-fold. APC inhibits the clotting process by degrading FVa and FVIIIa, key cofactors in the prothrombinase and tenase complexes. Antithrombin is a circulating irreversible inhibitor of several proteinases of the coagulation process, including thrombin, FXa, and FIXa. However, antithrombin circulates in a repressed reactivity state with reduced activity against these mediators.[25] This repression is reversed following the interaction of antithrombin with heparan sulfate, expressed on the endothelial surface.[25] Heparan sulfate is a glycosaminoglycan that forms the bulk of the endothelial glycocalyx, a luminal mesh that covers the endothelial surface.[25,26] The high-affinity interaction of antithrombin with a small pentasaccharide sequence on heparan sulfate causes a conformational change in the proteinase inhibitor and specifically enhances its activity against FXa and FIXa.[25] Engagement of antithrombin with longer polysaccharide chains of heparan sulfate provides the bridging mechanism that is required for the proteinase inhibitor to block thrombin while also increasing its inhibitory activity against FXa and FIXa.[25] The fourth major anticoagulant mediator, TFPI, is produced predominantly by the endothelium and inhibits FXa and TF/FVIIa activity (see Figs. 5.3 and 5.4).[23]

Endothelial cells play a crucial role in fibrinolysis by producing and releasing tissue plasminogen activator (tPA), which converts plasminogen to plasmin, resulting in the degradation of fibrin and dissolution of clot (see Figs. 5.3 and 5.4).

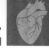

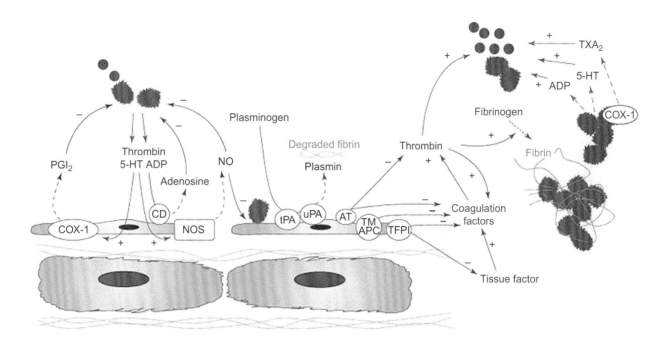

Fig. 5.3 **Regulation of Thrombosis in the Human Vascular System.** Under normal conditions, endothelial cells have a key role in preventing thrombosis by inhibiting platelet activity and the coagulation cascade and by stimulating thrombus dissolution (fibrinolysis). Following vascular and endothelial injury, this protection is lost and the prothrombotic properties of the subendothelium are revealed, including the activation of platelets and the coagulation cascade, culminating in the generation of thrombin and fibrin. Antithrombotic processes are shown in blue; prothrombotic processes are shown in red. *CD*, CD39, and CD72; *TM-APC*, thrombomodulin-thrombin activation of protein C; *uPA*, urokinase plasminogen activator; *5-HT*, 5-hydroxytryptamine. (From Flavahan NA. Balancing prostanoid activity in the human vascular system. *Trends Pharmacol Sci.* 2007;2:106–110.)

Healthy Venous Endothelium

Fig. 5.4 See legend on next page.

Continued

Venous Thrombosis

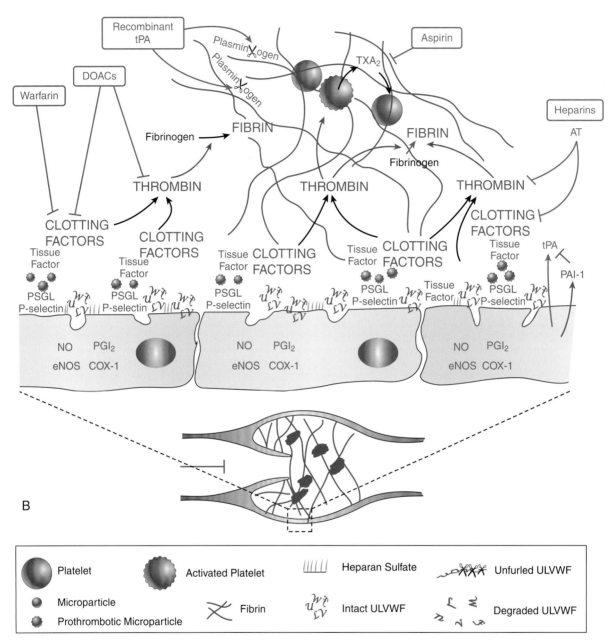

Fig. 5.4 Regulation of Thrombosis in the Venous System. Potential mechanisms contributing to venous thrombosis and currently approved therapies to combat the disease process. Healthy venous endothelium (A) contributes to the antithrombotic process in a similar manner to arterial endothelium. However, disruption of blood flow, for example, stasis, and inflammatory activation of the endothelium can diminish this antithrombotic activity and promote prothrombotic activity (B). In addition, increased levels of prothrombotic microparticles expressing tissue factor can interact with this prothrombotic endothelium and accelerate the thrombotic process. *AT,* Antithrombin; *TF,* tissue factor; *ThrM:Thr,* thrombomodulin:thrombin.

Atherothrombosis and Venous Thromboembolism

Arterial thrombosis occurs predominantly within the context of atherothrombosis and the structural deterioration of atherosclerotic lesions (see the section titled "Atherosclerosis and Intimal Lesion Development").[23,27] Atherosclerosis and its clinical sequelae—including coronary heart disease (CHD), ischemic stroke, and peripheral vascular disease—represent the leading cause of death and morbidity in the Western world. The principal mechanism contributing to acute coronary syndromes (ACSs)—such as unstable angina,

myocardial infarction, and sudden cardiac death—is rupture of the atherosclerotic plaque, which exposes the bloodstream to large quantities of TF, precipitating arterial thrombosis and blood vessel occlusion.[23] Thrombotic ACS events can also result from superficial erosion of the endothelium, which may reflect endothelial apoptosis.[23,27]

Non-ST–segment elevation myocardial infarction and unstable angina, which together are defined as NSTE-ACS, represent the leading causes of morbidity and mortality from cardiovascular disease worldwide.[28] The cornerstone of therapy for NSTE-ACS is dual therapy with antiplatelet agents.[28] This approach targets two key platelet-derived mediators involved in platelet activation, TXA_2 and ADP. Low doses of aspirin (ranging from 81 to 325 mg/day) are recommended for all NSTE-ACS patients to inhibit the platelet COX-1 enzyme and platelet generation of TXA_2, whereas $P2Y_{12}$ receptor antagonists (e.g., clopidogrel, ticagrelor) are included to inhibit ADP activity.[28] Because of the rapid inactivation of aspirin in the presystemic circulation and because of its assumed preferential activity at the COX-1 enzyme in platelets, it is often considered that these low doses of aspirin do not influence endothelial COX and therefore do not inhibit the antiplatelet activity of endothelium-derived PGI_2 (see the section titled "COX Inhibitors and the Human Vascular System"). Although the $P2Y_{12}$ receptor is expressed on other cell types, including promoting the inflammatory activity of leukocytes and macrophages, distinct purinergic receptors mediate the ADP-induced activation of endothelial cells, suggesting that these agents would preserve the antiplatelet activity resulting from ADP-mediated endothelial production of PGI_2 and NO.[29,30]

Venous thromboembolism (VTE) is observed clinically as deep-vein thrombosis (DVT) and pulmonary embolism, and is the third most common cause of cardiovascular death after CHD and stroke.[31] Mechanisms contributing to VTE are usually considered within a modern interpretation of the historic Virchow triad, namely endothelial dysfunction, blood flow abnormalities (chiefly stasis), and procoagulant changes in blood constituents.[31] In contrast to atherothrombosis, thrombus formation in human veins is rarely associated with vessel injury and forms on a largely intact endothelium.[31] Furthermore, although platelets make up the core of arterial thrombi and are the closest component to the blood vessel wall, in venous thrombi, fibrin appears to be the substance attaching the thrombus to the vessel wall with platelets attaching to the fibrin downstream. Venous thrombosis is initiated predominantly at venous valves, where blood flow can be sluggish under normal conditions.[31] If blood flow is halted, then this fragile environment can experience a dramatic reduction in oxygen tension. Although venous and valvular endothelial cells express anticoagulant proteins and mediators, hypoxia or inflammation can lead to the downregulation of these protective factors and cause upregulation of procoagulant activity (see Fig. 5.4). For example, during inflammatory stimulation, endothelial expression of anticoagulant mediators—including NO, thrombomodulin, EPCR, TFPI, and heparan sulfate—is decreased, whereas endothelial expression of prothrombotic mediators—including PAI-1, TF, and FV—is increased.[23,26,31] Moreover, the phosphatidylserine-rich anionic surface necessary for clot formation can result from hypoxia-induced reorientation of endothelial membrane lipids or fusion of the endothelium with circulating microparticles. These are small (<1 μm) phospholipid vesicles generated by leukocytes, platelets, and endothelial cells.[32] A subpopulation of microparticles, which is increased in individuals at risk for developing VTE, contains high levels of TF and a phosphatidylserine-rich surface.[31,32] Fusion of these microparticles with venous endothelium can occur subsequent to their interaction with endothelial P-selectin via P-selectin glycoprotein ligand 1 (PSGL-1) expressed by microparticles. Endothelial cells do not normally express P-selectin on their surface, but hypoxia, thrombotic, and inflammatory mediators cause exocytosis of WPBs, which will be amplified by reduced activity of endothelium-derived NO, enabling the translocation of P-selectin to the endothelial cell surface and release of ULVWF onto the luminal surface.[11] P-selectin would then be available to capture PSGL-1–expressing microparticles and focus the crucial components of the coagulation system. ULVWF is normally unfurled by blood flow, enabling it to be degraded by an endothelial surface protease ADAMTS13. However, during stasis, this activity would be diminished preserving the hyperreactive activity of ULVWF

on the venous endothelium (see Fig. 5.4). Analysis of veins from patients dying of VTE has revealed consistent presence of VWF in venous thrombi, whereas P-selectin is considered a potential biomarker for individuals at risk of VTE, and inhibition of VWF or P-selectin inhibits VTE in preclinical models of the disease.

Unlike atherothrombosis, treatment strategies in venous thrombosis are targeted toward inhibiting prothrombotic mediators. The initial traditional treatment of VTE has been concurrent treatment with heparan/heparin-based anticoagulants and vitamin K antagonists, in particular warfarin, with termination of the heparin-based treatment after a few days once the vitamin K antagonism has become effective.[31,33] Warfarin inhibits the vitamin K–dependent production of coagulation factors including FIX and FX. Heparin, a product of mast cells, shares considerable structural similarity in its polysaccharide chains to endothelial heparan sulfate and acts in a similar manner to amplify the inhibitory effect of antithrombin against thrombin, FXa, and FIXa (see Fig. 5.4). Heparin-based approaches include intravenous unfractionated heparin (UFH), subcutaneous low-molecular-weight heparins (LMWHs), or subcutaneous fondaparinux. UFH is a heterogeneous mixture of heparin polysaccharide chains derived from animal intestines, and only approximately 30% of the molecular species bind to antithrombin.[31,34] As with endothelial heparan sulfate, the amplification of antithrombin activity against thrombin requires longer polysaccharide chains compared with its activity against FXa and FIXa. The polysaccharide chains in UFH are of sufficient length to support antithrombin-mediated inhibition of thrombin and FXa, resulting in relatively equal inhibitory activity against these mediators. LMWHs are generated by the depolymerization of UFH, resulting in a smaller and variable molecular size, which translates into higher activity against FXa compared with thrombin.[34] Fondaparinux is a synthetic drug based on the small pentasaccharide sequence of heparin/heparan sulfate, which enables it to support antithrombin-mediated inhibition of FXa but not to block thrombin.[31,34]

Current guidelines recommend the use of direct oral anticoagulants (DOACs), which directly inhibit the enzymatic activity of factor Xa or thrombin, rather than vitamin K antagonists in patients without cancer.[33] Clinical trials have demonstrated that DOACs are noninferior to vitamin K antagonists in preventing recurrent VTE and are associated with less major bleeding.[31,33] DOACs include the direct thrombin inhibitor dabigatran and the FXa inhibitors rivaroxaban, apixaban, and edoxaban.[31,33] In patients with cancer, current guidelines recommend long-term use of LMWH, based on clinical trials observing improvement in outcomes compared with vitamin K inhibitors.[33] Aspirin is reported to have beneficial effects in VTE, suggesting that platelets are important contributors to this disease process (see Fig. 5.4)[31]; however, aspirin is inferior to anticoagulants, with DOACs reducing the risk of VTE recurrence by at least 80%, whereas aspirin showed only a 32% risk reduction. Current guidelines recommend aspirin as an available option in individuals with unprovoked VTE who are stopping anticoagulant therapy, but it is not recommended as an alternative to anticoagulant therapy.[33]

Anticoagulants including heparin analogues (e.g., the LMWH enoxaparin) and direct thrombin inhibitors (e.g., bivalirudin) are recommended as additional therapy for NSTE-ACS patients undergoing invasive procedures.[28] Some patients, including those with NSTE-ACS at high risk for VTE, may benefit from long-term triple therapy, combining dual antiplatelet therapy with anticoagulant treatments.[28] In addition to standard warfarin treatment, emerging options for triple therapy anticoagulation include PDE-3 inhibitors, FXa inhibitors, thrombin receptor antagonists, and direct thrombin inhibitors, although this aggressive approach is associated with an increased risk of bleeding.[28,35]

Thrombolytic therapy (using recombinant tissue-type plasminogen activators, e.g., alteplase) converts endogenous plasminogen to plasmin, which then degrades fibrin in clots (see Fig. 5.4).[31] Thrombolytic treatment is indicated for patients with severe pulmonary embolism; it is administered systemically or by catheter infusion directly into the thrombus.[31,33] Local catheter-directed thrombolysis is occasionally used for the treatment of extensive DVT.[31,33] Thrombolytic therapy is also utilized to counter arterial thrombotic events, including ischemic stroke and myocardial infarction.[36]

Cyclooxygenase Inhibitors and the Human Vascular System

Two COX enzyme subtypes, COX-1 and COX-2, are expressed in human cells. The COX enzyme in mature platelets that is responsible for TXA_2 production is the COX-1 subtype. The nature of the enzyme in endothelial cells that is responsible for PGI_2 production is the surprising subject of debate.[10,37,38] The COX-2 subtype is generally an inducible form and is the major source of prostanoids contributing to inflammatory responses. Indeed, inhibition of COX-2 mediates the antipyretic, analgesic, and antiinflammatory actions of nonsteroidal antiinflammatory drugs (NSAIDs) such as ibuprofen or naproxen. The original NSAIDs inhibit both COX-1 and COX-2, although there is variation in their relative selectivity. In contrast, aspirin is a preferential inhibitor of COX-1. This explains why low doses of aspirin (from as low as 75 mg/day) have protective cardiovascular activity by blocking platelet COX-1, but much higher doses are needed for NSAID-like activity mediated by COX-2 inhibition (up to 4 g/day). In each case, the inhibitory effect of aspirin is irreversible. Because COX-1 inhibition in gastric epithelial cells was thought to be responsible for the gastric adverse events associated with NSAID use, a distinct class of NSAIDs with high selectivity for COX-2 was developed.[10,37,38] These selective COX-2 inhibitors, described as COXIBs, including rofecoxib and celecoxib, did reduce gastric toxicity while retaining the therapeutic efficacy of NSAIDs. However, there was concern that COXIBs might increase the risk for adverse cardiovascular events, which resulted in a reduction in their use and the withdrawal of rofecoxib from the market.[10,37,38] The proposal that endothelial PGI_2 is dependent on COX-2 activity has been promoted to support an increased cardiovascular risk associated with COXIBs compared with traditional NSAIDs.[37] Within that context, arterial thrombosis is considered to be dependent on a balance between the COX-1–dependent generation of TXA_2 in platelets and the COX-2–dependent generation of PGI_2 in the endothelium.[37] Accordingly, low-dose aspirin would be cardioprotective because it selectively inhibits COX-1 in platelets, eliminating prothrombotic TXA_2 while preserving COX-2–mediated endothelial production of antithrombotic PGI_2. In contrast, COXIBs, by selectively inhibiting COX-2–dependent production of endothelial PGI_2, would tip the balance in favor of TXA_2 and precipitate vasoconstriction, platelet activation, and atherothrombosis.[37] This "imbalance theory" is based on incorrect assumptions, ignores compelling evidence to the contrary, and is invalid.[10,38]

Overwhelming evidence confirms that the endothelial COX enzyme responsible for PGI_2 production in the human vascular system is the COX-1 enzyme.[10,38] However, numerous reports propose that endothelial PGI_2 is derived from COX-2.[37] This proposal is based on the analysis of basal urinary levels of 2,3-dinor-6-keto $PGF1\alpha$ (PGI-M) in healthy volunteers.[10] PGI-M is a PGI_2 metabolite derived from 6-keto $PGF1\alpha$, the more immediate hydration byproduct of PGI_2. In healthy volunteers, the basal urinary levels of PGI-M are unaffected or minimally affected by low doses of aspirin (<160 mg/day), which preferentially inhibit COX-1, but are markedly reduced (up to 80%) by selective COX-2 inhibition with COXIBs.[10] Therefore the basal generation of urinary PGI-M in healthy human volunteers is dependent on COX-2.

However, the cellular source of human urinary PGI-M has never been identified. PGI_2 synthase is widely expressed in human nonvascular cells, and COX systems have considerable capacity to generate prostaglandins.[10] Therefore generation of PGI_2 from nonendothelial sources could easily dominate the basal urinary excretion of this PGI_2 metabolite. Although this COX-2–dependent basal urinary excretion of PGI-M was not significantly affected by low-dose aspirin,[39,40] infusion of the endothelial agonist bradykinin to human volunteers caused a six-fold increase in PGI-M that was abolished by a very low dose of aspirin (75 mg/day).[10,41] Therefore, in healthy human volunteers, although the basal level of urinary PGI-M is dependent on COX-2 and is derived from an unknown cellular source, the increase in PGI_2 (and urinary PGI-M) resulting from endothelial cell stimulation is entirely dependent on COX-1.

Sensitive molecular, biochemical, and immunochemical analyses of human arteries and veins have consistently demonstrated that native endothelial cells express high levels of COX-1 but do not express COX-2.[10] However, if cells and arteries are placed into the stressful conditions of cell culture, then they begin to express COX-2.[10] One exception is the kidney, where multiple cell types naturally express COX-2, which likely explains why basal levels of urinary 6-keto $PGF1\alpha$ (and perhaps of PGI-M) are thought to be derived from renal COX-2 systems.[10] Unlike urinary 6-keto $PGF1\alpha$, circulating levels of 6-keto $PGF1\alpha$ were not affected by selective inhibition of COX-2 but were abolished by very low doses of aspirin (35–75 mg/day). Likewise, selective COX-1 inhibition by prior ingestion of low-dose aspirin inhibited the subsequent vascular and endothelial production of PGI_2 from human arteries and veins.[10] Aspirin is rapidly degraded in the bloodstream, and this pharmacokinetic profile was thought to favor inhibition of platelet COX-1 by repetitive administration of low doses of the drug.[10,37] The ability of low doses of aspirin to inhibit vascular production of PGI_2 is additional compelling evidence that it is derived from COX-1.

Therefore analysis of the human vascular system provides convincing evidence that the endothelial production of PGI_2 is dependent predominantly, if not exclusively, on the COX-1 enzyme.[10] This appears to be valid in normal healthy blood vessels as well as during the development of vascular disease, which can be associated with decreased endothelial production of PGI_2, likely reflecting inactivation of PGI_2 synthase by reactive oxygen species (ROS).[10]

Atherosclerosis and the Development of Intimal Lesions

Atherosclerotic lesions develop preferentially at sites of disturbed blood flow (branches, curvatures) where normal laminar shear stress is distorted by flow separation and directional changes.[4,42,43] Although exposure of endothelial cells to sustained normal shear stress is antiinflammatory and atheroprotective, disturbed atheroprone shear stress increases the transcriptional activity of nuclear factor kappa B (NF-κB), a master regulator of the atherosclerotic process, and increases the expression of inflammatory and thrombotic mediators (Fig. 5.5).[4] Regions prone to atherosclerosis also display increased endothelial permeability to macromolecules, including low-density lipoprotein (LDL), and the subendothelial deposition and modification of LDL is an important early amplification step in the atherosclerotic process.[4,42,43] These modified lipids further increase inflammatory activity, reducing the activity of protective mediators such as NO and amplifying NF-κB activation.[4] These key changes in endothelial function including increased permeability and inflammatory activity likely reflect the disruptive effects of atheroprone shear stress and modified LDL on endothelial adherens junctions and VE-cadherin–dependent signaling (see Fig. 5.5 and the section titled "Endothelial and Vascular Stabilization").[4] Expression of inflammatory mediators such as vascular cell adhesion molecule-1 (VCAM-1), monocyte chemoattractant protein-1 (MCP-1), and macrophage colony-stimulating factor (MCSF) increase monocyte recruitment and stimulate their survival and differentiation to macrophages (see Fig. 5.5).[4,42,43] These cells attempt to clear the modified LDL particles but become engorged with lipids and die, releasing their lipid content into the developing lesion. The evolving lesion reflects interactions between endothelial, immune, and inflammatory cells, with continual remodeling of the atheroma resulting in the formation of a lipid-rich necrotic core, which is capped by a fibrous layer of VSMCs and extracellular matrix that provides stability to the plaque.[4,42,43] Although they may remain relatively stable, plaques can develop into chronic active inflammatory lesions with accumulation and activation of macrophages and T cells, which can remodel and weaken the stabilizing fibrous cap, precipitating thrombosis and luminal occlusion (see the section titled "Atherothrombosis and Venous Thromboembolism").[4,42,43]

VSMCs expressing endothelial and smooth muscle (mesenchymal) proteins are present in human atherosclerotic lesions, suggesting that they are derived from the endothelium rather than from the arterial media (see Fig. 5.5).[4,44] During endothelial-to-mesenchymal transition (EndoMT), endothelial cells can change their phenotype to that of mesenchymal cells. Indeed, atheroprone shear stress or modified LDL stimulates EndoMT, whereas normal laminar shear stress increases resistance to EndoMT.[4] Because EndoMT cells contribute to vascular and tissue fibrosis, EndoMT-derived mesenchymal cells might be expected to expand and stabilize the protective fibrous cap.[4,5] However, there is an inverse relationship between the number of EndoMT-derived cells and cap thickness, and an increased number of EndoMT-derived cells are present in ruptured versus nonruptured plaques.[44] The lineage and activity of VSMCs in atherosclerotic plaques is complex: although some VSMC populations contribute to plaque stability, cholesterol accumulation can transform VSMCs into macrophage-like cells and foam cells

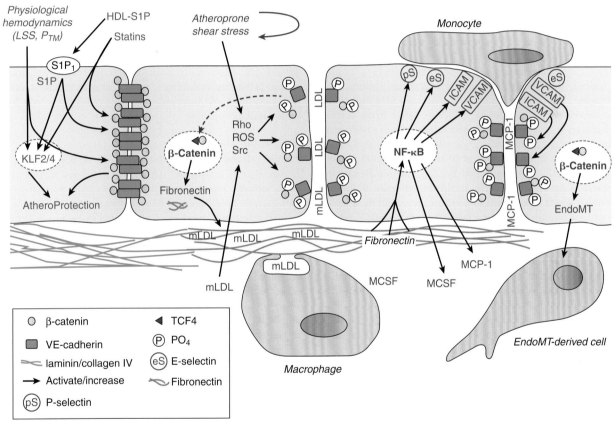

Fig. 5.5 The Potential Importance of Adherens Junction Disruption in the Atherosclerotic Process. Arterial regions prone to atherosclerosis are sites of increased endothelial proliferation and increased endothelial permeability to low-density lipoprotein *(LDL)*, effects consistent with reduced junctional clustering of vascular endothelial *(VE)*-cadherin. Indeed, atherosclerosis-prone shear stress, modified LDL, or inflammatory mediators (including interaction with monocytes) all cause disruption of endothelial adherens junctions. In contrast, normal laminar shear stress (and exposure to high-density lipoprotein *[HDL]*) protects the integrity of the junctions. Disruption of adherens junctions and VE-cadherin–dependent signaling increases endothelial permeability and contributes to proinflammatory activity of the endothelium. This appears to be mediated at least in part by the increased transcriptional activity of β-catenin, which increases the deposition of subendothelial fibronectin and activation of nuclear factor kappa B *(NF-κB)*, the master regulator of the atherosclerotic process. Transcriptional activity of β-catenin is also a key mediator of endothelial-to-mesenchymal transition *(EndoMT)*, which is thought to contribute to destabilization of the atherosclerotic plaque. Therefore the status of endothelial adherens junctions likely plays a key role in the initiation, progression and clinical expression of the atherosclerotic process. *KLF,* Kruppel-like factor; *LSS,* laminar shear stress; *mLDL,* modified LDL; *MCSF,* macrophage colony-stimulating factor; *MCP-1,* monocyte chemoattractant protein-1; *PTM,* transmural pressure; *S1P,* sphingosine 1-phosphate; *S1P1,* SIP receptor. (Redrawn and modified from Flavahan NA. In development—a new paradigm for understanding vascular disease. *J Cardiovasc Pharmacol.* 2017;69:248–263.)

that contribute to plaque development.[45,46] EndoMT-derived cells may therefore have an increased propensity to develop a macrophage-like phenotype and contribute to destabilization of the plaque. Preventing the phenotypic switching of VSMCs to macrophage-like cells or inhibiting the EndoMT process may be beneficial in preventing plaque destabilization (see Fig. 5.5) (see also the section titled "Endothelial and Vascular Stabilization").[4,46]

Owing to their efficacy in reducing morbidity and mortality associated with atherosclerosis, HMG-CoA reductase inhibitors, termed statins, are among the most widely prescribed classes of cardiovascular drugs.[42,47] Their primary mechanism of action is to inhibit cholesterol biosynthesis, thereby increasing the expression of hepatic LDL clearance receptors and reducing circulating LDL levels.[42,47] However, the HMG-CoA reductase pathway also plays a fundamental role in cell signaling by generating isoprenoid intermediates involved in the lipid modification and activity of the small GTP-binding proteins (G proteins) Rho, Ras, and Rac.[47] Statins inhibit the activity of these G proteins in numerous cell types, and these pleiotropic effects of statins can produce vascular protective effects that are independent of LDL lowering.[47] Indeed, statins have direct protective effects on endothelial cells that appear to be mediated predominantly by the inhibition of RhoA/ROCK signaling, a key signaling pathway promoting multiple aspects of endothelial dysfunction (see Figs. 5.2 and 5.5).[4,47] Indeed, with regard to reversing endothelial dysfunction, statins increase eNOS expression, eNOS activity, and NO production; they also decrease ET-1 expression, reduce oxidative stress, inhibit apoptosis, increase progenitor cell mobilization, reduce endothelial permeability, reduce prothrombotic activity, enhance fibrinolytic activity, and reduce the production of inflammatory cytokines and mediators.[4,47,48] Statins can also inhibit EndoMT.[4] These pleiotropic effects of statins represent a powerful stabilizing influence on the endothelium that would be expected to dramatically inhibit the atherosclerotic process (see also the section titled "Endothelial and Vascular Stabilization").

Although the idea is appealing, it is currently unclear whether these pleiotropic effects of statins are activated during clinical therapy or contribute to their clinical efficacy.[47] Clinical studies have shown that inflammatory biomarkers predict the risk of initial and recurrent major cardiovascular events (myocardial infarction, stroke, and cardiovascular death).[42,49] C-reactive protein (CRP), produced by the liver in response to systemic inflammatory mediators, is an independent biomarker of cardiovascular disease.[42] In addition to their effects on lipids, statins have been shown to reduce the level of CRP.[42] Clinical evidence indicates that statins can stabilize vulnerable plaque; this is associated with a decrease in inflammatory biomarkers, suggesting that in addition to LDL lowering, the pleiotropic effects of statins may be involved.[42,43,47] Currently available statins are lovastatin, simvastatin, pravastatin, fluvastatin, atorvastatin, rosuvastatin, and pitavastatin.[47] They are competitive and reversible inhibitors of HMG-CoA reductase but vary in their elimination half-lives, potency, and lipophilicity.[47]

Although statins are highly effective at lowering LDL cholesterol levels and preventing cardiovascular disease events, there is still a clear need for additional therapies.[42,49a] Indeed, nonstatin approaches are indicated only as adjunctive therapy for patients who are unable to reach their lipid goals despite optimal statin therapy.[47] Ezetimibe, which reduces cholesterol absorption in the small intestine and may increase hepatic LDL clearance, lowers LDL levels by 15% to 25%.[42,47] A new class of lipid-lowering agents, the proprotein convertase subtilisin–kexin type 9 (PCSK9) inhibitors, has the potential to achieve a 50% to 65% decrease in LDL cholesterol levels.[42,43,47] PCSK9 promotes degradation of the hepatic LDL clearance receptor.[42,43] PCSK9 inhibitors therefore increase the LDL receptor–mediated hepatic uptake of LDL, a mechanism shared by statins.[43,47] However, they do not inhibit the HMG-CoA reductase pathway and therefore do not have similar pleiotropic effects to statins. For example, despite their potent LDL-lowering effects, PCSK9 inhibitors, unlike statins, do not reduce serum markers of inflammation such as CRP, interleukins (ILs), or tumor necrosis factor-α (TNF-α).[47] Two fully human monoclonal antibodies against PCSK9 (evolocumab, alirocumab) are approved for clinical use.[49b] Placebo-controlled randomized clinical trials have demonstrated that an aggressive approach to lowering LDL cholesterol levels by combining statin therapy with ezetimibe or a PCSK9 inhibitor can significantly reduce the risk of major adverse cardiovascular events compared to statin use alone.[49a,49c–49e] Current clinical guidelines recommend a combined therapeutic approach (statin plus ezetimibe, with or without a PCSK9 inhibitor) in certain patient groups, including individuals at very high risk for atherosclerotic events and whose LDL cholesterol remains ≥70 mg/dL despite maximally tolerated statin use.[49a]

Because of the importance of inflammatory mechanisms in the pathogenesis of atherosclerosis, there is increased awareness of the potential for antiinflammatory approaches in treatment for the disease.[42,49] These approaches include mAbs against IL-6 (e.g., tocilizumab), TNF-α (e.g., infliximab), IL-1β (e.g., canakinumab), and MCP-1 (e.g., MLN-1202). Some of these approaches are already providing promising preliminary results in atherosclerotic disease.[42,49] These agents would be expected to have protective effects to reverse endothelial dysfunction.

Angiogenesis

Because cell and tissue function is dependent on adequate vascular perfusion, normal growth and development requires parallel expansion of the vascular system.[50,51] Healthy tissues can be adequately supplied with oxygen by diffusion only over distances up to 150 μ, requiring cells to maintain a close association with a vascular network and vascular capillaries.[51] Normal cellular expansion beyond this vascular perfusion zone will result in hypoxia, which is the primary stimulus for the necessary expansion of the microvasculature (angiogenesis).[50] Angiogenesis is regulated by a complex interplay between numerous interconnected signaling systems that cause destabilization of the existing microvasculature, enabling invasion and proliferation of "tip" and "stalk" endothelial cells through the extracellular matrix, fusion of neighboring endothelial branches, lumen formation and perfusion of the nascent vessel, followed by stabilization and maturation of the blood vessel.[50] A key regulator of the process is vascular endothelial growth factor (VEGF), which is released by multiple cells types following activation of the hypoxic transcription factor HIF-1α (hypoxia inducible factor). VEGF stimulates angiogenesis following activation of the endothelial VEGFR-2 receptor subtype.[50] Not surprisingly, the angiogenic process can be disrupted by disease processes and is the target of existing and developing therapies to amplify or to inhibit microvascular expansion.[50]

Therapeutic angiogenesis to counter pathological tissue ischemia, such as in peripheral artery disease, has been pursued for decades.[52] However, despite numerous clinical trials targeting a variety of angiogenic mediators and mechanisms including VEGF, the results have been disappointing and no approved therapeutic interventions are currently available.[52]

Folkman originally proposed the groundbreaking hypothesis that the growth of tumors was dependent on angiogenesis and that antiangiogenic therapy would be an effective treatment for human cancers.[51,53] Angiogenesis is now considered to be an essential component of malignant growth and a "hallmark of cancer."[54] However, tumor angiogenesis can be a highly abnormal process resulting in heterogeneous, tortuous, and chaotic channels, with an uneven vessel lumen.[50] In addition to abnormal or absent endothelial cells, the stabilizing pericytes are also abnormal or absent, culminating in highly leaky vessels.[50] Such unstable vessels are thought to contribute to metastases and to increased interstitial fluid pressure resulting in heterogeneous blood flow, which can disrupt delivery of therapeutic agents.[50] Although future antiangiogenic therapy will likely take advantage of specific abnormal traits of tumor angiogenesis, current therapy is targeted to mediators involved in normal angiogenesis.[50] FDA-approved antiangiogenic drugs for treating solid tumors are targeted predominantly to VEGF-dependent signaling.[55] Bevacizumab is a recombinant humanized monoclonal antibody that targets circulating VEGF, aflibercept is a recombinant molecule comprising VEGFR-binding domains to sequester VEGF, and ramucirumab is a humanized monoclonal antibody that targets and blocks endothelial VEGFR-2 receptors.[55] A number of protein kinase inhibitors that target the activity of VEGFR receptors have also been approved as antiangiogenic treatment, including sorafenib, sunitinib, axitinib, and cabozantinib.[55] These agents have variable selectivities for the VEGFR-2 receptor, with some agents effectively blocking other mechanisms involved in angiogenesis (including platelet-derived growth factor receptors) and in lymphangiogenesis (e.g., VEGFR-3 receptors).[55] A major problem with current therapies is that the tumors become refractory to VEGF blockade, resulting in treatment failure.[50,55] A number of mechanisms have been proposed to account for this, including activation of alternate angiogenesis pathways.[50,55] The inhibition of endothelial VEGFR-2–receptor activity by these different approaches results in a similar spectrum of adverse effects, including hypertension, cardiac toxicity, and thromboembolic events.[55]

Endothelial and Vascular Stabilization

Normal endothelial activity is of vital importance to vascular and organismal health, and the destabilization of endothelial structure and function is a common precipitating event in the pathogenesis of vascular disease.[4] Although numerous therapeutic interventions can mimic aspects of endothelial function, no current approaches are specifically targeted toward reversing the diseased endothelial phenotype and re-establishing endothelial stability.

The maintenance of the normal protective endothelial phenotype is an active rather than a passive process.[4] The protective features of the arterial endothelium appear to become fully engaged during the initial postnatal period and to be mediated by increased clustering of VE-cadherin and the formation of adherens junctions.[4] VE-cadherin clustering stimulates the assembly of a macromolecular complex that regulates endothelial cell signaling, function, morphology, and phenotypic identity (Fig. 5.6).[4,56] This includes increasing eNOS and NO activity, promoting endothelial barrier function (decreased permeability), inhibiting apoptosis, and inhibiting inflammatory activation such as inhibiting leukocyte extravasation and the expression of inflammatory mediators (see Fig. 5.5).[4,56] Inflammatory mediators cause the transient interruption of VE-cadherin clustering, enabling increased endothelial inflammatory activity, increased permeability, and inflammatory cell extravasation. However, chronic disruption of VE-cadherin–dependent signaling precipitates endothelial and vascular destabilization and promotes the development of vascular disease.[4,56] Indeed, the degradation and loss of VE-cadherin from adherens junctions is responsible for the endothelial dilator dysfunction associated with aging and likely contributes to the prominent endothelial frailty of the aging vasculature, a key aspect of vascular aging.[4,56,57] In addition to the loss of protective activity, VE-cadherin degradation and junctional disruption can result in nuclear translocation of its binding partner β-catenin, a transcription factor that stimulates the expression of numerous pathological and inflammatory mediators including the renin angiotensin system (angiotensinogen, renin, angiotensin-converting enzyme [ACE], AT1 receptors), ET-1, TNF-α, IL-6, and fibronectin

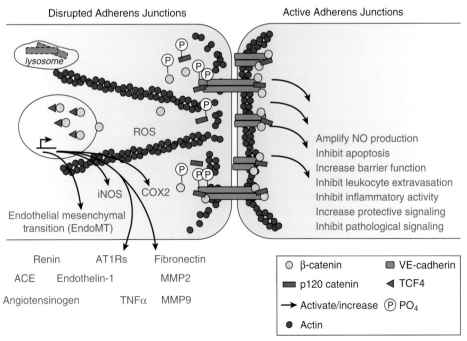

Fig. 5.6 Regulatory impact of endothelial adherens junctions, with protective activity of normal active junctions *(right)* and the potential pathological effects of disrupted junctions *(left)*. The red font mediators and processes reflect effects that can be induced by the disruption of adherens junctions. (Redrawn and modified from Flavahan NA. In development—a new paradigm for understanding vascular disease. *J Cardiovasc Pharmacol.* 2017;69:248–263.)

(see Figs. 5.5 and 5.6).[4] Disruption of endothelial adherens junctions and β-catenin transcriptional activity are essential components of EndoMT. Indeed, disruption of VE-cadherin–dependent activity likely contributes to the initiation, progression, and destabilization of atherosclerotic lesions (see Fig. 5.5).[4]

Numerous endogenous protective factors, including sphingosine-1-phosphate, associated with high-density lipoprotein (HDL) and angiopoietin-1, amplify VE-cadherin clustering at adherens junctions (see Fig. 5.5).[4] Not surprisingly, vascular disease is associated with alternate signaling mediators that diminish the activity of these protective factors and may be responsible for junctional disruption.[4] Targeted approaches to increasing VE-cadherin clustering at adherens junctions not only decrease inflammatory activity and frailty of endothelial cells but also reduce β-catenin transcriptional activity and stabilize endothelial function and phenotype.[4] This type of therapeutic approach is associated with organ protection and reduced mortality in preclinical inflammatory models. Therapeutic amplification of VE-cadherin–dependent signaling and endothelial adherens junctions would likely be a powerful mechanism to reverse endothelial dysfunction, restore protective endothelial activity and vascular stability, and inhibit the initiation and progression of vascular disease.[4]

THERAPEUTIC INTERVENTION AND THE AUTONOMIC VASCULAR INNERVATION

The normal regulation of blood flow requires integration of the metabolic requirements of individual organs and tissues with the overall needs of the entire organism.[6] The complex central regulation of the cardiovascular system is achieved in large part though the sympathetic nervous system.[6,58] The central nervous system receives numerous inputs regarding sensory, emotional, environmental, and hemodynamic challenges and directs acute vascular responses by altering sympathetic activity.[6,58] Sympathetic nerves innervate and provide a powerful vasoconstrictor influence in most vascular beds, with their activity increasing in arterioles (the vascular faucets)[6] compared with more proximal arteries.[6,58] Notable exceptions are the cerebral system, where the sympathetic system minimally affects blood flow, and the coronary circulation, where sympathetic activation can initiate vasodilatation. Sympathetic nerves are widely distributed in the venous system, where they play an important role to increase venous return and support an increase in cardiac output and blood pressure. In the arterial system, sympathetic nerves are restricted to the adventitia, requiring sympathetic neurotransmitters to diffuse through the blood vessel wall and regulate vascular cell function. In contrast, in the venous system, the sympathetic nerves penetrate the medial layer to provide a more direct delivery of neurotransmitters to VSMCs, which may contribute to heightened responsiveness of the venous system.[6,59] The predominant autonomic control of the vasculature is achieved through the sympathetic system, and only a small subset of blood vessels receive a prominent parasympathetic innervation—for example, the pulmonary vasculature. In an upright human, the sympathetic nervous system exerts significant vasoconstrictor activity to numerous tissues and organs, including the splanchnic, renal, skeletal muscle, and cutaneous circulations.[6,59]

Arterial baroreceptors located in the carotid sinus and aortic arch continually sense blood pressure through the resulting mechanical stretch of the arterial wall.[6,58] Elevated sensory afferent activity resulting from increased blood pressure is processed in the central nervous system to cause a reflex decrease in efferent sympathetic activity.[6,58,60] Likewise, a fall in blood pressure will result in increased sympathetic activity. Although originally considered to be important only for the acute control of blood pressure, it is now believed that the reflex can contribute to long-term blood pressure regulation.[58,59] Other reflexes contribute to regulation of sympathetic outflow, including peripheral and central chemoreceptors, which respond to changes in the partial pressures of oxygen and carbon dioxide in arterial blood.[58,60] For example, hypoxia increases sympathetic outflow and is thought to contribute to the chronic sympathoexcitation and hypertension occurring in obstructive sleep apnea.[58,59]

The primary neurotransmitter released by vascular sympathetic nerves is norepinephrine, which activates α1- and α2-ARs expressed on VSMCs to initiate vasoconstriction (Fig. 5.7).[5,6] There is generally minimal activation of vasodilator β-ARs by nerve-released norepinephrine except, for example, in the coronary circulation. VSMCs in the peripheral circulation are predominantly of the β2-AR subtype and are activated preferentially by circulating epinephrine, released by the adrenal medulla.[58] Sympathetic nerves also release secondary constrictor neurotransmitters including adenosine triphosphate (ATP) and neuropeptide Y, which can cause vasoconstriction directly or indirectly by amplifying the response to norepinephrine.[6,58] Following its release from sympathetic nerves, norepinephrine is recaptured by sympathetic nerve varicosities via the norepinephrine transporter (NET) and is then either metabolized by cytoplasmic monoamine oxidase (MAO) or taken into storage vesicles via the vesicular monoamine transporter (VMAT) (see Fig. 5.7).

α1-Adrenoceptors are expressed by the VSMCs of most blood vessels regardless of their innervation density. In contrast, functional constrictor α2-ARs have a unique distribution in the human vasculature.[5,6] VSMC α2-ARs are generally not functional in large proximal arteries, and their activity increases in distal arterioles. This reflects variable expression of VSMC α2-ARs resulting from differential transcriptional activation of α2-AR genes. In most vascular beds, the activity of α2-ARs in distal arteries and arterioles still remains relatively weak compared with α1-ARs, whereas in some systems, notably the cutaneous circulation, α2-AR constrictor activity is greatly increased. This reflects the physiological role of α2-ARs in vascular thermoregulation.[5,6] In contrast to their selective distribution in the arterial circulation, α2-ARs are widely expressed and functional within the venous system.[5,6] α2-ARs are also expressed on nerve fibers, including sympathetic nerves, where their activation inhibits the release of neurotransmitters. With vascular sympathetic nerves, this contributes to negative feedback regulation, with prejunctional α2-AR activation causing inhibition of norepinephrine release and vasodilatation (see Fig. 5.7).[6] α2-ARs are also expressed by endothelial cells, with their stimulation increasing production of NO and PGI₂.[61]

In addition to its direct effects to cause arterial and venous constriction in most vascular beds and to stimulate the heart, increasing cardiac output, the sympathetic nervous system has important regulatory effects on the kidneys to increase blood pressure. Increased renal sympathetic nerve activity can elevate blood pressure by three independent mechanisms: (1) increasing renin secretion from the juxtaglomerular apparatus through activation of β1-ARs, (2) increasing sodium reabsorption in the proximal tubules through activation of epithelial α1-ARs, and (3) increasing renal vascular resistance through activation of VSMC α1-ARs.[58,60]

Therapies Causing Adrenergic or Sympathetic Activation

Over 100 years ago, a pioneer of adrenergic pharmacology, Sir Henry Dale, introduced the term *sympathomimetic* to describe a "range of compounds" that "simulate the effects of sympathetic nerves" without regard to the "precise mechanism of the action."[62] The term is still widely used to describe agents that stimulate any component of sympathetic neuroeffector mechanisms, including indirect agents that release sympathetic neurotransmitters and agents that directly activate

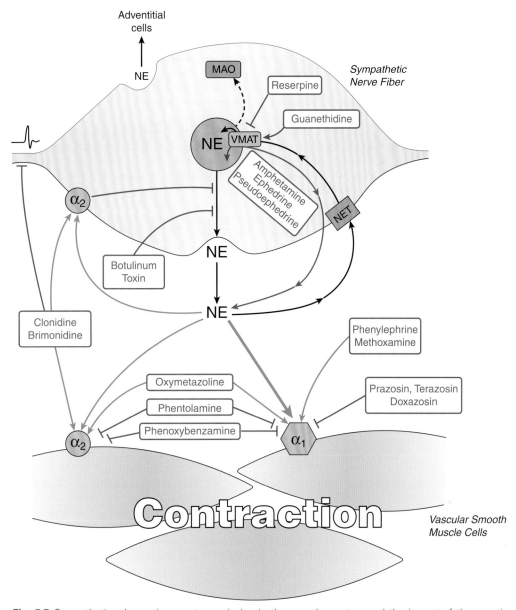

Fig. 5.7 Sympathetic adrenergic neurotransmission in the vascular system and the impact of therapeutic drugs, as well as drugs of abuse, on the different components of neurotransmission. *NE,* Norepinephrine; α1, α1-ARs; α2, α2-ARs.

adrenoceptors. Although including such a broad spectrum of activity is consistent with Dale's original concept of sympathomimetics, it creates problems for the continued use of the term. For example, although α2-AR agonists are defined as sympathomimetics, they actually inhibit rather than mimic sympathetic nerve activity. Thus the term is no longer viable and is not used here.

A number of drugs stimulate sympathetic mechanisms and initiate vascular effects but are not designed or approved for this activity. Agents such as amphetamine and tyramine act on sympathetic nerves to cause norepinephrine release. Their mechanism of action is distinct from the exocytotic release of storage vesicles stimulated by neuronal impulses. They are instead substrates for NET and VMAT, resulting in the rapid release of norepinephrine from storage vesicles into the cytoplasm, followed by the reverse transport of norepinephrine into the extracellular compartment. Because cytoplasmic norepinephrine can be degraded by MAO, the concomitant use of antidepressant MAO

inhibitors can amplify indirect activity—for example, precipitating increased blood pressure during ingestion of tyramine-rich foods. In contrast to these agents, cocaine inhibits NET and so prevents the reuptake of norepinephrine and prolongs its activity. Consistent with these effects on sympathetic nerves, adverse cardiovascular effects dominate the toxicity profile of cocaine and amphetamine abuse.

Activation of sympathetic mechanisms and α-ARs are used by therapeutics to treat a number of vascular conditions (see Fig. 5.7).

Nasal Decongestion

FDA-approved nasal decongestants, phenylephrine and d-pseudoephedrine (a stereoisomer of ephedrine), are vasoconstrictors that decrease airflow resistance by reducing the volume of the nasal mucosa. Inflammation will contribute to arteriolar dilation, increased blood flow, and edema formation as well as dilation of venous capacitance vessels in the nasal mucosa. The venous system is a high-volume system that contains most of the blood volume,[6] and the nasal mucosal veins have erectile characteristics.[63] Indeed, therapeutic decongestion most likely reflects venoconstriction in the nasal mucosa. Phenylephrine is considered a selective α1-AR agonist; at slightly higher concentrations, however, it can also activate α2-AR and β-ARs.[64] In contrast, the predominant mechanism of action of d-pseudoephedrine is as an indirect agonist to cause the release of norepinephrine from sympathetic nerves (see Fig. 5.7).[65] Neither phenylephrine nor d-pseudoephedrine can be considered selective nasal vasoconstrictors; their systemic administration could therefore result in blood flow restriction to other vascular beds and contribute to an increase in blood pressure. Phenylephrine is extensively metabolized in the intestinal wall and liver, contributing to a low bioavailability and diminished vasoconstrictor potential.[66] Special care is therefore required in individuals with diminished MAO activity, including those concurrently receiving MAO inhibitors.[66] Pseudoephedrine can cross the blood-brain barrier and has the potential for central stimulant activity.[66] Pseudoephedrine but not phenylephrine is on the current list of banned substances released by the World Anti-Doping Agency.

Consistent with their increased activity in cutaneous and venous systems, α2-ARs have considerable activity in blood vessels of the nasal mucosa, where their activity can predominate over α1-ARs in regulating blood flow and the constriction of mucosal collecting veins.[63] Indeed, activation of α2-ARs may be the preferred choice for causing nasal vasoconstriction and nasal decongestion.[63] Although the nasal decongestant activity of the widely used phenylpropanolamine likely reflected its agonist activity at α2-AR, it was withdrawn in 2000 because of concerns that it might increase the risk of hemorrhagic stroke.[63]

Blood Pressure Reduction

Although the α2-AR agonist clonidine was originally developed as a nasal decongestant, its ability to lower blood pressure led to its approval as an antihypertensive agent in 1974.[67] It is a lipid-soluble compound that traverses the blood-brain barrier and acts on α2-ARs in the central nervous system to reduce sympathetic outflow. Although generally described as a selective α2-AR agonist, clonidine has poor selectivity at α1-ARs and α2-ARs and is a low-efficacy agonist of these receptor systems. Indeed, when administered during venoconstriction with norepinephrine, clonidine causes direct vasodilatation. Although clonidine administration has the potential to cause vasoconstriction through partial agonism at α1-ARs and α2-ARs, its antagonism of sympathetic activity normally prevails and direct vasoconstriction is observed only following interruption of sympathetic activity. It is unclear whether activation of α2-ARs on peripheral sympathetic nerves or partial agonism/antagonism of α1-ARs contributes to clonidine's antihypertensive effects. Other centrally acting α2-AR agonists have been developed for the treatment of hypertension, including guanfacine. These drugs share a significant class effect to cause sedation, which is also mediated by activation of centrally located α2-ARs. Although they are still approved as antihypertensive agents, these drugs are now reserved only for a "last-line" approach.[68] The unwanted side effect of sedation has led to the development of centrally acting selective α2-AR agonists such as dexmedetomidine for sedation and light anesthesia.

Cutaneous Vasoconstriction

Rosacea is a chronic inflammatory skin disease that causes facial erythema and flushing.[69] Approved treatments for the condition include two α-AR agonists: brimonidine (or UK 14,304), which is a highly selective and high-efficacy α2-AR agonist, and oxymetazoline, which is a nonselective and low-efficacy agonist at α1 and α2-ARs.[69] By causing cutaneous vasoconstriction, the topical application of these agents

to the face is effective in reducing the facial erythema in rosacea (see Fig. 5.7). Based on increased α2-AR activity in cutaneous blood vessels and differences in intrinsic efficacy between these compounds, brimonidine would be expected to have a more powerful vasoconstrictor potential. However, both treatments should be used with caution to prevent excessive vasoconstriction and ischemic injury, which could worsen the condition.

Blood Pressure Support

Numerous sympathetic agonists are used to raise or support blood pressure during intensive care conditions, including perioperative care, hemorrhage, reactions to medications, and shock. They include intravenous delivery of the physiological agonists (norepinephrine, epinephrine), selective α1-AR agonists (e.g., phenylephrine and methoxamine), and indirect-acting agonists that stimulate the release of norepinephrine (e.g., l-ephedrine) (see Fig. 5.7). Likewise, droxidopa, which is converted into norepinephrine, and midodrine, which is converted to the selective α1-AR agonist desglymidodrine, are available for the treatment of orthostatic hypotension.

A key challenge in providing blood pressure support in the intensive care setting has been defining an appropriate blood pressure target. A recent innovative approach has been to assess cerebral autoregulation and provide an individualized approach to blood pressure management. Autoregulation is mediated by pressure or stretch-induced constriction of arteriolar VSMCs.[6] Arterioles, the vascular faucets, are embedded within an organ making them ideally suited to provide local control of blood flow—for example, to vasodilator metabolites as a result of cellular activity.[6] If blood pressure is maintained within the autoregulatory zone, then the control of blood flow can be achieved predominantly by local mechanisms, ensuring that perfusion is matched to metabolic activity. When blood pressure is below the autoregulatory zone, perfusion may not be adequate, whereas above the zone, the downstream transmission of high pressure could injure the microcirculation. Clinical studies have confirmed that there is wide interindividual variation in the autoregulation zone and that a standardized approach to blood pressure management causes a significant percentage of patients to be outside their zone.[70] Failure to maintain blood pressure within the autoregulatory zone during cardiac surgery was found to be independently associated with poorer outcomes, including major morbidity or operative mortality, acute kidney injury, and postoperative delirium.[70]

Local Anesthetics

Adrenergic agonists, predominantly epinephrine and oxymetazoline, are included in local anesthetic injections to cause local vasoconstriction, which decreases removal of the anesthetic and so prolongs its activity. Likewise, the nonselective α1-AR and α2-AR antagonist phentolamine is FDA-approved to reverse local anesthesia by blocking the vasoconstriction.

Therapies Causing Inhibition of Sympathetic Activity

Increased sympathetic activity has been reported in numerous cardiovascular disease processes and is regarded as an independent predictor of outcomes and mortality.[58,59,71] Sympathetic overdrive is thought to contribute to the development and maintenance of hypertension and is present in the early stages of the disease, particularly in young patients and in the stable hypertensive state of middle-aged and elderly individuals.[58,59,71] The sympathetic nervous system is also thought to contribute to the development and progression of organ damage in hypertension, including cardiac and renal injury and arterial remodeling.[71,72] The increase in sympathetic activity is not uniform in hypertension, with a disproportionate increase in sympathetic

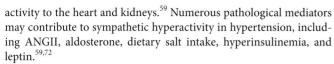

activity to the heart and kidneys.[59] Numerous pathological mediators may contribute to sympathetic hyperactivity in hypertension, including ANGII, aldosterone, dietary salt intake, hyperinsulinemia, and leptin.[59,72]

The first therapeutic approach to hypertension, from the 1930s to 1950s, was surgical sympathectomy, which comprised cutting sections of the spinal sympathetic chain and severing as many vasopressor nerves as possible to remove their vasoconstrictor activity.[59,71] The approach successfully lowered blood pressure and reduced mortality in patients with severe hypertension. However, as might be expected, it was associated with profound side effects, including postural and postprandial hypotension and syncope as well as procedural mortality.[59,71]

The surgical approach ended with the discovery and introduction of ganglion-blocking drugs such as hexamethonium in the 1950s, which represented the first line of therapeutics to inhibit the sympathetic nervous system in hypertension. Although they achieved similar clinical efficacy as surgical sympathectomy, they also retained similar significant side effects, although without the surgical risk.[71] Over the next two decades, increased understanding of sympathetic adrenergic pharmacology fueled a revolution in antihypertensive therapies, from sympathetic neuronal blockers such as reserpine and guanethidine, centrally acting α2-AR agonists such as clonidine, β-AR antagonists including propranolol, and α1-AR antagonists such as prazosin (see Fig. 5.7).[71] Indeed, these antiadrenergic drugs, coupled with diuretics and direct-acting vasodilators such as hydralazine, were the preferred antihypertensive therapy for 30 years until the introduction of ACE inhibitors and AT1R antagonists.[71] ACE inhibitors and AT1R antagonists were at least as effective as antiadrenergic agents, and they were substantially better tolerated (see the section titled "Therapeutic Intervention and the Renin Angiotensin System").[71] Since the 1990s, they have come to occupy the top rung of hypertension treatment in international guidelines, with antiadrenergic drugs drifting toward the bottom.[67,68,71]

Reserpine was one of the earliest drugs used for treating hypertension, gaining FDA approval in 1955, and there is still support for its continued use.[67,73] Reserpine inhibits the VMAT-mediated transport of dopamine and norepinephrine into vesicular storage vesicles in sympathetic nerve fibers. In contrast to tyramine or amphetamine, reserpine causes a much slower depletion of the adrenergic transmitter from the vesicles, where it is metabolized by MAO (see Fig. 5.7).[67] Recovery of sympathetic nerve function requires the formation of new storage vesicles, which can take days to weeks after the cessation of drug treatment.[67] Reserpine's antihypertensive effect resulted from its inhibitory effects on peripheral nerves, reducing cardiac output and peripheral resistance with minimal postural hypotension, but its major side effects of sedation and depression reflected its effects on the central nervous system.[67] Reserpine was a highly effective antihypertensive drug and, when combined with a diuretic and vasodilator, was associated with reduced mortality and morbidity, including a reduced incidence of stroke.[67] As with reserpine, guanethidine was initially approved by the FDA in 1960 and was only recently discontinued from the US market.[67] Guanethidine is a false neurotransmitter and is taken up by storage vesicles in sympathetic nerve fibers, where it displaces the natural transmitter norepinephrine (see Fig. 5.7). During subsequent nerve stimulation, guanethidine, which lacks activity at adrenoceptors, is released instead of norepinephrine, producing a block of sympathetic neurotransmission.[67] Its use was traditionally reserved for hypertensive patients who were refractory to other treatments. Although its therapeutic effects were similar to those of reserpine, it did not cross the blood-brain barrier and therefore was without central effects.[67]

Prazosin was the first selective α1-AR antagonist to be approved for the treatment of hypertension, with a selectivity of at least 1000-fold for α1-ARs compared with α2-ARs (see Fig. 5.7). Subsequent α1-AR antagonists included doxazosin and terazosin.[68] By blocking α1-ARs in arterioles, prazosin, doxazosin, and terazosin decrease peripheral resistance. Their use is associated with marked hypotension and syncope during initial dosing and with orthostatic hypotension, especially in older adults.[68] Because of these side effects, they are no longer recommended as primary agents in the treatment of hypertension, but they should be considered as second-line agents in patients with concomitant benign prostatic hyperplasia (BPH).[68] In contrast to the changing role of α1-AR antagonists in the treatment of hypertension, α-AR antagonists are still the first-line agents of choice for the perioperative control of blood pressure in pheochromocytomas or paragangliomas.[74] Pheochromocytomas are neuroendocrine tumors of the adrenal medulla; when they occur outside of the medulla, they are referred to as paragangliomas. The tumors produce and store excessive amounts of norepinephrine and epinephrine, which, when released, especially during surgical removal, can produce life-threatening cardiovascular complications.[74] The most commonly used agent, which has not changed in over 50 years, is the irreversible noncompetitive and nonselective α-AR antagonist phenoxybenzamine (see Fig. 5.7). This drug reduces perioperative hypertensive crises and contributes to improved surgical outcomes, although, as expected, it is associated with orthostatic hypotension, reflex tachycardia, syncope, and nasal congestion.[74]

β-AR antagonists were a popular first-line approach to treat hypertension until the 1990s, when ANGII inhibitors and calcium channel blockers (CCBs) became more frequently used.[71,75] They are no longer recommended as first-line therapy and are generally to be used only as add-on therapy—for example, with an ACE inhibitor or AT1R antagonist.[68,75,76] Approved β-blockers are highly heterogeneous with regard to their pharmacological and pharmacokinetic profiles, including β-AR subtype selectivity, intrinsic efficacy, supplemental antihypertensive mechanisms (e.g., β-1-AR antagonism), and lipid solubility.[75,77] Mechanisms contributing to the antihypertensive effects of β-blockers are still debated, but the primary mechanism is considered to be a reduction in cardiac output resulting from antagonism of cardiac β-ARs.[75,77] However, their long-term use is associated with a decrease in peripheral vascular resistance.[75,77] The so-called third-generation β-blockers can cause vasodilatation and reduce peripheral vascular resistance through unique mechanisms: nebivolol increases endothelial NO activity, which appears to reflect activation of endothelial β3-ARs and inhibition of oxidant stress, whereas carvedilol is an α1-AR antagonist.[75,78] Individual β-blockers may also contribute to reduced peripheral vascular resistance through partial agonism at VSMC β-ARs (e.g., celiprolol), by inhibiting renin release from the juxtaglomerular apparatus through β1-AR antagonism, by reducing central sympathetic outflow, and by antagonizing prejunctional β-ARs on sympathetic nerve fibers that act to increase the stimulated release of norepinephrine.[75,77,78]

The downgrading of β-blocker therapy reflected clinical trial data indicating that β-blockers were inferior to other agents for reducing stroke, cardiovascular mortality, and all-cause mortality despite similar reductions in blood pressure.[75] Specifically, the second-generation β-blocker atenolol did not demonstrate benefit compared with placebo; and when compared with other active treatments, atenolol was associated with an increased risk of all-cause mortality, cardiovascular mortality, and stroke.[75] One of the issues raised with β-blockers such as atenolol is their inability to reduce central arterial pressure as effectively as brachial blood pressure (see the section titled "Therapeutic Intervention and the Vascular Media").[75,77,78] Blood pressure measured in the periphery at the brachial artery is the standard approach and is an established predictor of cardiovascular morbidity and mortality. However, central arterial pressure, which reflects the summation of afferent and efferent pressure waves, is also an independent predictor of cardiovascular events and may be a better predictor of certain aspects of cardiovascular morbidity and mortality than peripheral brachial pressure.[75,78] Although it is as effective as other agents in lowering brachial blood pressure, atenolol does not reduce central arterial pressure indices to the same extent as other antihypertensive drugs.[75,78] Importantly, this lack of clinical efficacy with atenolol does not appear to extend to vasodilator β-blockers such as nebivolol, which is highly effective at decreasing peripheral and central arterial pressures.[75,77,78] Continuing studies with newer-generation β-blockers will likely stimulate a reassessment and reassignment of their status in treating hypertension.

Despite major advances in the pharmacological treatment of hypertension, there is still a substantial group of patients whose blood pressure cannot be adequately controlled.[60,71] In a stunning reversal of history, one of the most promising approaches to treating drug-resistant hypertension has been the catheter-based denervation of renal sympathetic nerves.[58–60,71] In hypertension, sympathetic neural outflow is activated to numerous organs, including the heart and skeletal muscle, but it is the hyperactivity of the renal sympathetic system that is thought to play a central role in the pathogenesis of hypertension.[59,60,71] Furthermore, among patients with hypertension, renal sympathetic activation is at its highest level in drug-resistant hypertension.[71] As described earlier, renal sympathetic nerves can drive increased blood pressure through their multiple effects on the tubular processing of sodium, on renin secretion, and on renal vascular resistance.[59,71] Moreover, Harrison has proposed that an initial increase in sympathetic activity, such as a prehypertensive state, causes oxidative protein modification, creating neoantigens that are processed and presented by dendritic cells, leading to T-cell activation. Activated T cells then infiltrate the kidney and arterial adventitia, producing cytokines that promote renal sodium and water retention, vasoconstriction and arterial remodeling, and culminate in overt hypertension.[60,72] Indeed, in this experimental model of hypertension, renal denervation blunted the renal accumulation of T cells and the resulting hypertension.[60]

Renal sympathetic nerves enter the kidneys via the outer adventitia of the renal arteries, within reach of radiofrequency energy delivered by an intraluminal catheter.[60,71] This catheter-based approach to cause renal sympathetic denervation demonstrated consistent antihypertensive efficacy in early clinical trials, with office systolic blood pressure falling on average by 20 to 30 mm Hg.[60,71] Moreover, the effect was durable, persisting for 3 years after a single procedure.[60,71] In confirming sympathetic denervation, the procedure caused a 47% reduction in renal spillover of norepinephrine, which was less than expected but apparently sufficient for clinical efficacy.[60,71] Subsequent expansion in a larger clinical analysis of the approach was associated with reduced clinical efficacy and has resulted in an unsure future for the technique. However, the expansion was also associated with inconsistency in the approach, a failure to confirm sympathetic denervation, and a realization that the technique must be more thoroughly optimized.[60,71] Although the original success of the denervation procedure is consistent with a key role for renal sympathetic nerves in maintaining hypertension, disruption of afferent sensory fibers may also have contributed to the antihypertensive effect. Activation of afferent renal nerves, which respond to mechanosensitive (e.g., to increases in urine flow), chemosensitive (e.g., PGE$_2$), or nociceptive (e.g., noxious renal) stimuli, can result in a reflex increase in sympathetic activity to other organs, resulting in increased peripheral vascular resistance and increased blood pressure.[60,71] Also, chronic inflammation in the kidneys

and infiltration of immune and inflammatory cells may activate afferent fibers to drive sympathetic-mediated hypertension.[60]

A similar evolution in treatment strategies to inhibit sympathetic activity is evident in therapeutic approaches to treating primary and secondary Raynaud phenomenon,[5,18,79] which reflects exaggerated sympathetic-mediated vasoconstriction of the cutaneous vascular system in response to cold exposure.[5,18,79] The condition causes characteristic color changes in the affected extremities, with an initial pallor followed by a blue phase, which is interpreted as ischemia or cyanosis, and a final red or rubor phase, which is ascribed to ischemic hyperemia. However, all the color changes can be explained by temporal differences in constrictor activity of the sympathetic nervous system on arteries, arteriovenous anastomoses, and the venous system.[5,79] Primary Raynaud phenomenon is uncomfortable but ultimately benign, whereas secondary Raynaud phenomenon (e.g., in scleroderma) is associated with pathological remodeling of the vasculature and extravascular compartments, resulting in substantial tissue pathology and injury.[5,18,79] As with hypertension, treatment strategies explored cervical sympathectomy, reserpine and guanethidine, and the use of selective and nonselective α-AR antagonists.[79,80] The treatment approach to Raynaud phenomenon is particularly challenging because of the key role played by VSMC α2-ARs, which are uniquely sensitive to cold temperatures.[5,79,81] Systemic administration of α2-ARs antagonists increases sympathetic outflow and amplifies peripheral sympathetic neurotransmission, thus counteracting the desired effect.[5] An interesting recent development has been exploration of the potentially beneficial effects of botulinum toxin in Raynaud phenomenon and scleroderma.[5,18,79] The toxin inhibits macromolecular SNARE complexes involved in the fusion of storage vesicles with the plasma membrane, thereby preventing their exocytosis and blocking neurotransmission.[5,79] Although botulinum toxin A preferentially inhibits cholinergic neurotransmission, which likely reflects increased numbers of toxin receptors on these nerves, at higher doses it also inhibits sympathetic neurotransmission.[5] The potential of this modern version of reserpine in Raynaud phenomenon and other vascular disorders remains to be confirmed. Its activity profile will be determined by optimizing the dose and delivery of the toxin so as to increase its effects on sympathetic nerves while reducing its impact on other nerve fibers, including parasympathetic nerves, peptidergic nerves, and skeletal muscle motoneurons.[5]

Adventitial Vascular Biology

The adventitial perivascular compartment is the most diverse and complex component of the blood vessel wall.[82,83] In addition to sympathetic nerve fibers, the vascular adventitia can contain numerous interacting cell types including fibroblasts, inflammatory and immune cells (macrophages, dendritic cells, T cells, B cells, mast cells), perivascular adipose tissue (PVAT), a distinct microvascular network (vasa vasorum), lymphatic vessels, and vascular progenitor cells.[82,83] These diverse adventitial cells can be the source of protective as well as pathological vascular mediators. Indeed, inflammatory and fibrotic activity originating in the adventitial compartment can contribute to pathological functional and structural changes throughout the vascular wall, including the media and intima.[82,83] For example, the activation of adventitial fibroblasts may contribute to adventitial fibrosis and arterial stiffening, including during hypertension, as well as to remodeling of the media and intima.[82,83] Increased inflammatory activity of the adventitia and PVAT in response to exogenous and endogenous stress signals can lead to the generation of pathological mediators—including cytokines, ROS, and a local renin angiotensin system—that can contribute to endothelial dysfunction and pathological changes in vascular function and structure.[82,83] Furthermore, expansion of a dysfunctional vasa vasorum during the progression of atherosclerotic lesions can ultimately lead to structural destabilization of the plaque and plaque rupture.[83] An intriguing aspect of adventitial biology is the presence of sympathetic nerve fibers, placing them in an ideal location to regulate the activity of these diverse cell types that express adrenoceptors and receptors for other sympathetic neurotransmitters.[6,72,83] Indeed, sympathetic-dependent activation of immune/inflammatory cells, including in the arterial adventitia, may contribute to end-organ injury in hypertension, including arterial remodeling and endothelial dysfunction.[72] Existing vascular and antiinflammatory therapies undoubtedly modulate adventitial cell biology. With increased understanding of the regulatory role of this vascular compartment, future therapies may be designed to specifically target the adventitial compartment or adventitial mechanisms.[82]

THERAPEUTIC INTERVENTION AND THE VASCULAR MEDIA

VSMCs are ultimately responsible for acutely regulating blood vessel diameter and vascular resistance, and are important contributors to the regulation of arterial structure and vascular remodeling.

Mechanisms of Vasoconstriction

The main mechanism for VSMC contraction and blood vessel constriction is increased phosphorylation of myosin light chains (MLCs), which enables actin-myosin interaction, cross-bridge cycling, and contraction.[84] The process is initiated by an increase in cytosolic free calcium that, following its binding to calmodulin (CaM), causes activation of MLC kinase (MLCK), increased MLC phosphorylation, and VSMC contraction (Fig. 5.8).[84] Vasoconstrictor agonists initiate VSMC contraction by triggering an increase in cytosolic free calcium through

the opening of plasma membrane calcium channels, which enables influx of extracellular calcium, as well as the release of calcium from intracellular stores.[84] Vasoconstrictor agonists can also increase the sensitivity of the myofilament contractile process to calcium.[84]

Calcium influx into VSMCs can be mediated by a number of distinct plasma membrane ion channels, including voltage-dependent calcium channels (VDCCs), the transient receptor potential (TRP) family of channels, store-operated channels, and stretch-activated calcium channels (see Fig. 5.8).[84] VDCCs, which are activated by membrane depolarization, comprise two distinct channels and currents. L-type calcium channels are activated by relatively large depolarizations, provide a long-lasting calcium current, and are inactivated relatively slowly. In contrast, T-type calcium channels are activated by smaller depolarizations and inactivate more rapidly.[84] Although vasoconstrictor agonists (e.g., activation of α1-ARs by norepinephrine, ET_A receptors by ET-1, AT1Rs by ANGII, or TP receptors by TXA_2) can stimulate calcium influx by depolarizing VSMCs and activating VDCC, they can also activate a distinct set of plasma membrane calcium channels. Originally described as receptor-operated channels, these channels are now known to be part of the TRP family of ion channels.[84,85] The human TRP channels comprise a family of 27 cation channels with diverse ion selectivity and regulatory properties.[84,85] Multiple TRP channels are expressed in VSMCs, although the level of expression and activity can vary depending on blood vessel location. The canonical subfamily of TRP channels, termed TRPC channels, are activated by vasoconstrictor agonists and also by depletion of internal calcium stores (i.e., store operated calcium channels).[84,85] TRP channels simultaneously allow the influx of sodium and calcium ions, thereby triggering cell membrane depolarization and increasing cytosolic free calcium directly as well as indirectly through the activation of VDCCs.[84,85]

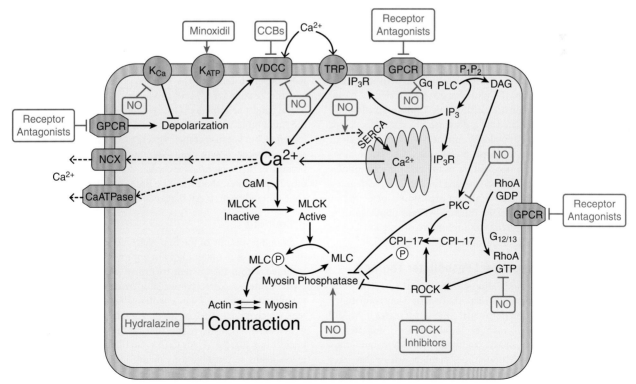

Fig. 5.8 The regulation of vascular smooth muscle cell contraction and the currently approved therapeutic agents targeted to those regulatory components. *CaATPase,* Calcium ATPase pump; K_{Ca} and K_{ATP}, calcium-sensitive and ATP-sensitive potassium channels, respectively; *NCX,* sodium-calcium exchanger.

The main intracellular calcium storage site involved in regulating VSMC contraction is the sarcoplasmic reticulum (SR), an intracellular system of tubules or flattened cisternae that can occupy up to 7.5% of the cellular volume.[84] The SR compartment is larger in the VSMCs of proximal arteries compared with arterioles. The release of calcium from the SR can be induced by vasoconstrictor receptor stimulation and by calcium itself, which is termed calcium-induced calcium release.[84] Caffeine initiates the contraction of VSMCs by directly stimulating calcium release from the SR.

Vasoconstrictor G protein–coupled receptors (GPCRs)—including $\alpha 1$-ARs, ET_A receptors, AT1Rs, and TP receptors—are coupled to the Gq protein, which activates membrane-associated phospholipase C (PLC), leading to the hydrolysis of plasma membrane phosphatidylinositol 4,5-bisphosphate (PIP_2) to inositol 1,4,5-trisphosphate (IP_3) and diacylglycerol (DAG) (see Fig. 5.8).[84,86] IP_3 binds to IP_3 receptors located on the SR, resulting in opening of calcium release channels and the release of stored calcium, and to IP_3 receptors associated with plasma membrane TRP channels, leading to opening of the channels and the influx of extracellular calcium.[84,85] In contrast to IP_3, DAG is lipophilic and remains in the plasma membrane, where it activates protein kinase C (PKC), a family of serine/threonine kinases comprising 10 isoforms.[84] PKC contributes to VSMC contraction by increasing influx of extracellular calcium, doing so by inhibiting the activity of plasma membrane potassium channels, leading to membrane depolarization (see Fig. 5.8).[84] PKC also increases the sensitivity of the myofilament contractile process to calcium, enabling maintained VSMC contraction with lower levels of cytosolic free calcium.[84,86] PKC phosphorylates and activates PKC-potentiated phosphatase inhibitor protein-17 (CPI-17), which then inhibits MLC phosphatase, resulting in the increased phosphorylation of MLCs and augmented VSMC contraction (see Fig. 5.8). PKC also inhibits MLC phosphatase directly via phosphorylation of its myosin phosphatase target subunit 1 (MYPT1).[84,86]

Activation of vasoconstrictor agonist receptors can also increase the calcium sensitivity of the contractile process by coupling to the G12/G13 family of heterotrimeric G proteins. G12/G13 activate the small G protein RhoA, which subsequently stimulates the Ser/Thr kinase, ROCK.[84,86] ROCKs can amplify contraction directly by phosphorylating MLCs, and they can also increase the calcium sensitivity of VSMC contraction by phosphorylating MYPT-1 and by phosphorylating and activating CPI-17, which lead to inhibition of MLC phosphatase (see Fig. 5.8).[84,86]

On cessation of the vasoconstrictor stimulus, VSMC relaxation and blood vessel dilation is mediated by a decrease in cytosolic calcium levels resulting from calcium uptake by intracellular stores and from extrusion of calcium across the plasma membrane.[84] The fall in cytosolic calcium levels results in dissociation of the calcium-calmodulin complex and deactivation of MLCK, enabling the MLCs to be dephosphorylated by MLC phosphatase.[84] Calcium extrusion is mediated by two plasma membrane proteins, the calcium-ATPase pump and the sodium-calcium exchanger, whereas the recapture of calcium by the SR is mediated by SERCA, the SR calcium ATPase (see Fig. 5.8).[84]

Mechanisms Underlying Direct Vasodilator Therapy

Endothelial dysfunction and diminution in the activity of endothelium-derived vasodilator mediators is clearly a key contributor to augmented vasoconstriction in vascular disease. Increases in VSMC calcium levels and increased vascular activity of PKC and ROCK also contribute to increased VSMC contractile activity in numerous disease processes including hypertension, cerebral vasospasm, and coronary artery disease.[84,86] However, it is also apparent that these vascular mechanisms are closely linked. For example, PKC reduces NO-mediated vasodilation by inhibiting soluble guanylyl cyclase and increasing production of ROS, and ROCK inhibits the expression and

activation of eNOS.[84] Likewise, NO can inhibit PKC and ROCK activity (see Fig. 5.8).

Direct vasodilators are used in numerous vascular disorders including systemic and pulmonary hypertension, cerebral and peripheral vasospasm, and coronary artery disease (see Fig. 5.8).

Calcium Channel Blockers

CCBs are divided into two groups: dihydropyridines, which includes nifedipine, amlodipine, felodipine, israpidine, nicardipine, and nisoldipine; and nondihydropyridines, which comprise verapamil (a benzothiazepine) and diltiazem (a phenylalkylamine).[77,84] CCBs selectively inhibit L-type VDCCs, thereby inhibiting depolarization-induced influx of calcium and the component of VSMC contraction mediated by this mechanism.[77,84] Their clinical efficacy does not involve inhibition of other major pathways for calcium influx, including TRP, T-type voltage-dependent channels, or other contractile pathways initiated by vasoconstrictor agonists or stimuli (see Fig. 5.8).[77,84]

The dihydropyridines are considered to have vascular selectivity, preferentially inhibiting L-type calcium channels in vascular compared with cardiac muscle, whereas verapamil and diltiazem are more effective in blocking L-type channels in cardiac compared with vascular muscle.[77] This difference in selectivity is thought to reflect differences in the activation kinetics of the channels in vascular compared with cardiac muscle.[77] CCBs acutely decrease peripheral vascular resistance and blood pressure.[77] Although tachycardia is observed after dihydropyridine CCBs as a result of baroreflex activation, it is minimal or absent after verapamil and diltiazem because of their direct negative chronotropic effects.[77] Likewise, verapamil and diltiazem are negative inotropic agents, whereas dihydropyridines have minimal effects because any direct effect is compensated by afterload reduction and a baroreflex-mediated inotropic effect. The tachycardia associated with the dihydropyridine CCBs is reduced after more chronic administration because of resetting of the baroreceptor reflex.[68,77]

Because they have a well-documented effect on cardiovascular end points and total mortality, CCBs remain among the preferred drugs for the treatment of systemic hypertension, both as monotherapy and with other antihypertensive agents.[68,77] CCBs are also used in the treatment of coronary vasospasm, in some patients with pulmonary hypertension (see the section titled "Therapeutic Intervention and the Endothelium") and to alleviate the cold-induced vasospasm of Raynaud phenomenon (see section "Therapeutic Intervention and the Autonomic Vascular Innervation").[13,18,27,84] CCBs are generally well tolerated, but because of their generalized vasodilator activity, their use can be associated with headache, flushing, and edema.[77] Importantly, because of their potential for cardiac depression, CCBs, especially nondihydropyridines, should not be used in patients with heart failure or concomitantly with β-AR blockers.[68,77]

Hydralazine

Although it was one of the first pharmacological approaches for treating hypertension, obtaining FDA approval in 1953, hydralazine is still included within the current treatment guidelines for the disease.[67,68] Hydralazine is a direct vasodilator of resistance arterioles, reducing peripheral vascular resistance with negligible effects on the venous system, which reduces the risk for postural hypotension.[67] Despite its longevity, the mechanisms responsible for the vasodilator response remain unclear (see Fig. 5.8). Hydralazine can directly relax VSMCs, inhibiting mechanisms responsible for calcium influx and calcium release, and may also amplify endothelium-dependent vasodilator mechanisms.[67] The decrease in blood pressure evoked by hydralazine results in compensatory stimulation of the sympathetic nervous system and the renin-angiotensin-aldosterone system. As a result, side effects include

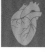

tachycardia and fluid retention as well as effects associated with generalized vasodilatation such as headache and flushing.[67,77] Because of these side effects, its use as an antihypertensive has diminished considerably; it is now recommended only as a secondary agent to treat drug-resistant hypertension and must be combined with a diuretic and β-AR blocker to counter the increase in sympathetic activity.[67,68,77]

Nitric Oxide, Nitrovasodilators, and Cyclic Guanosine Monophosphate

Endothelium-derived NO is a powerful vasodilator with multiple mechanisms of action (see Fig. 5.8). Its main signaling pathway in VSMCs is activation of soluble guanylyl cyclase, resulting in increased production of cyclic GMP and activation of the cyclic GMP-specific serine/threonine kinase PKG.[7,84,86] Activated PKG regulates multiple calcium regulatory systems to decrease intracellular calcium levels and reduce the activity of MLCK. PKG phosphorylates and activates the large-conductance Ca^{2+}-sensitive potassium channels, causing VSMC hyperpolarization and decreasing the open probability of VDCC.[84,86] PKG inhibits TRPC channels, further reducing calcium influx, and also increases calcium uptake into the SR by phosphorylating phospholamban, a key regulator of SERCA activity.[7,85] In addition to reducing intracellular calcium levels and indirectly inhibiting MLCK activity, activated PKG reduces the calcium sensitivity of the contractile process by phosphorylating and increasing MLC phosphatase activity. PKG also inhibits the ability of the vasoconstrictor agonist receptor system to increase the calcium sensitivity of contraction by inhibiting RhoA/ROCK signaling via the phosphorylation of RhoA.[86] Likewise, PKG directly inhibits the coupling of vasoconstrictor receptors through the Gq protein, thereby reducing the ability of receptor systems to activate PLC and generate the IP_3 and DAG signaling mediators.[86] This inhibitory effect is mediated by PKG-dependent activation of RGS2, a GTPase activating protein (GAP), which accelerates the hydrolysis of GTP by Gqα, resulting in inactivation of the Gq protein.[86] In addition to this impressive vasodilator activity mediated through PKG, NO can also contribute to VSMC relaxation via S-nitrosylation reactions, resulting in inhibition of PKC, RhoA, and L-type calcium channels.[7,84]

As discussed in the section titled "Therapeutic Intervention and the Endothelium," NO-dependent vasodilator mechanisms can be activated, amplified, and/or mimicked by therapies such as inhaled NO, PDE5 inhibitors, and direct activators of soluble guanylyl cyclase. NO-induced vasodilatation also mediates the therapeutic activity of the organic nitrates (e.g., nitroglycerin, isosorbide dinitrate, isosorbide mononitrate) and sodium nitroprusside. Sodium nitroprusside readily releases NO within the circulation, whereas the organic nitrates require extensive cellular processing to generate NO.[22] Their biotransformation is initiated in the mitochondria via aldehyde dehydrogenase (ALDH-2).[22] The clinical efficacy of organic nitrates is mediated through vasodilation of capacitance veins and proximal arteries. NO-dependent venous dilation reduces ventricular preload, whereas NO-mediated dilatation of large and medium-sized arteries decreases afterload, resulting in reduced left ventricular wall tension and decreased myocardial oxygen demand.[22] Nitrates can also dilate stenotic portions of epicardial coronary arteries and improve coronary collateral blood flow by decreasing collateral resistance.[22] Nitroglycerin is the most frequently used treatment for acute episodes of angina; it is usually administered as a sublingual tablet but also as a sublingual spray. Oral formulations of organic nitrates, including isosorbide dinitrate and isosorbide mononitrate, have also been shown to increase exercise tolerance and improve chronic stable angina.[22] Intravenous nitroglycerin and sodium nitroprusside can be used to treat patients experiencing hypertensive emergencies.[22]

Tolerance is a common result of chronic nitrate use; the underlying mechanisms have not been clearly defined but may reflect desensitization of soluble guanylyl cyclase, increased production of ROS, a compensatory increase in vasoconstrictor activity, or reduced biotransformation.[22] The major side effects of nitrate therapy are consistent with vasodilator therapy and include headache, flushing, lightheadedness, and postural hypotension. An additional rare side effect with sodium nitroprusside relates to the presence of five cyanide groups within its molecular structure and the generation of cyanide toxicity.[22]

Rho Kinase Inhibition

Fasudil is an isoquinoline derivative that inhibits ROCK kinase by competing with ATP for the active site.[84] Although fasudil is available in Japan for the treatment of cerebral vasospasm associated with subarachnoid hemorrhage, it is not currently available in the United States. After its oral administration, fasudil is metabolized to a more selective ROCK inhibitor hydroxyfasudil.[84] Indeed, although fasudil inhibits ROCK and PKA with similar potency, hydroxyfasudil is 15-fold more selective for ROCK than for PKA.[84] There is considerable interest in the role of ROCK in vascular disease pathogenesis and the potential for ROCK inhibition in treating numerous vascular diseases, including pulmonary and systemic hypertension, erectile dysfunction, Raynaud phenomenon, and coronary artery disease. Indeed, fasudil reduces the rate of coronary spasm episodes in patients with vasospastic angina.[27] As described in the section titled "Therapeutic Intervention and the Endothelium," RhoA/ROCK signaling mediates multiple aspects of endothelial dysfunction, including reducing eNOS and NO activities. Therefore the vascular benefits of ROCK inhibition could reflect actions in multiple cell types. As also detailed in the section titled "Therapeutic Intervention and the Endothelium," statins exert pleiotropic effects independent of LDL lowering that are mediated predominantly by inhibition of RhoA/ROCK signaling. There could therefore be some overlap in the protective vascular effects of statins and ROCK inhibitors.

Potassium Channel Agonists

Potassium channel openers hyperpolarize VSMCs and produce vasodilation by diminishing the open probability of VDCCs (see Fig. 5.8).[86] Currently only one potassium channel opener, minoxidil, is FDA-approved for use in hypertension. Minoxidil opens ATP-sensitive potassium channels, permitting potassium efflux and hyperpolarization, and resulting in VSMC relaxation.[67,77,86] It acts predominantly on the arterial side of the circulation, reducing peripheral vascular resistance and blood pressure.[67,77] As with hydralazine, minoxidil is associated with reflex activation of the sympathetic nervous system and renin-angiotensin-aldosterone systems, resulting in an increased heart rate, myocardial contractility, and fluid retention.[67,77] Fluid retention may also reflect direct effects of minoxidil on renal tubules by increasing tubular sodium retention.[67] Minoxidil use is also associated with excess hair growth, and minoxidil cream is specifically marketed for this "side effect." Because of the severity of its adverse effects, minoxidil is now reserved for the treatment of severe hypertension in patients who respond poorly to other medications; it should be used in combination with a diuretic and β-AR blocker to counter the compensatory increase in sympathetic activity.[68,77]

Prostaglandin I2 and Prostaglandin I2 Analogues

As indicated in the section titled "Therapeutic Intervention and the Endothelium," PGI_2 and its analogues relax VSMCs by activating IP receptors, which are coupled predominantly through the G_S protein leading to activation of adenylyl cyclase and increased production of cyclic AMP. Cyclic AMP can act through two major signaling pathways: activation of the cyclic AMP–specific serine/threonine kinase PKA and activation of exchange proteins directly activated by cyclic AMP (EPAC), which are guanine exchange factors (GEFs) that activate the small G proteins Rap1 and Rap2.[84,86,87] Mechanisms contributing to PGI$_2$ or cyclic AMP–dependent relaxation of VSMCs have not been studied as extensively as those relating to NO. However, these mechanisms are thought to be similar to those initiated by PKG and include inhibition of RhoA/ROCK signaling, increased activity of MLC phosphatase, and activation of calcium-sensitive potassium channels, leading to a decrease in calcium influx.[84,86,87] In addition, IP receptor activation can also activate endothelium-dependent dilator mechanisms.

The Renin Angiotensin System, Vasoconstriction, and Vascular Remodeling

The renin-angiotensin system is a complex signaling cascade that acts through multiple mechanisms to regulate blood pressure and the vascular system, including volume homoeostasis, vascular cell function, and vascular structure.[88,89] Although it is an important physiological regulatory system, increased activity of renin angiotensin systems plays a critical role in driving the pathogenesis of numerous cardiovascular diseases.[88,89]

Renin Angiotensin Systems

The traditional system involves the synthesis and release of renin from the juxtaglomerular apparatus of the renal afferent arterioles, which cleaves circulating hepatic angiotensinogen to form the decapeptide ANGI.[88,89] The ACE enzyme, which is located predominantly on en-dothelial cells, hydrolyzes inactive ANGI to the biologically active octa-peptide ANGII (Fig. 5.9). In addition to generating active ANGII, ACE also metabolizes and inactivates the vasodilator bradykinin. Most of the recognized effects of ANGII are mediated by activation of AT1Rs, including VSMC contraction, aldosterone secretion from the adrenal cortex, renal tubular sodium reabsorption, and activation of the sympathetic nervous system.[88,89] Likewise, the prominent pathological roles of ANGII are to disrupt endothelial cell function, including reduced NO activity and increased ROS and inflammatory activity, and to increase VSMC fibrotic and inflammatory activity, all of which contribute to vascular dysfunction and remodeling, are mediated by AT1Rs (see Fig. 5.9). AT1Rs initiate multiple signaling cascades to mediate these diverse effects.[88,89] Although ANGII also activates AT2Rs, these receptors are developmentally regulated and generally have low expression in adult tissues. AT2R activation may counter the effects of AT1R activation and promote vasodilatation, natriuresis, antiinflammatory and antifibrotic activity, and inhibition of cell growth (see Fig. 5.9).[88–90]

This traditional view of the renin angiotensin system has expanded to include new enzymes and new active ANG peptides (see Fig. 5.9).[88,89] An important development has been the recent discovery of ACE-2, a homologue of ACE that metabolizes ANGI and ANGII to generate the novel peptides ANG-(1-9) and ANG-(1-7), respectively.[88,89] ANG-(1-9) can be further metabolized to ANG-(1-7) by ACE. ACE-2 is considered to be part of a counterregulatory system to the classic RAS pathway. By utilizing ANGI and ANGII as substrates, ACE-2 will directly inhibit ANGII activity. Furthermore, ANG-(1-7) activates Mas receptors to counter the biological effects of ANGII (see Fig. 5.9). For example, in endothelial cells, Mas activation by ANG-(1-7) increases NO production and reduces the generation of ROS (see Fig. 5.9).[88] The

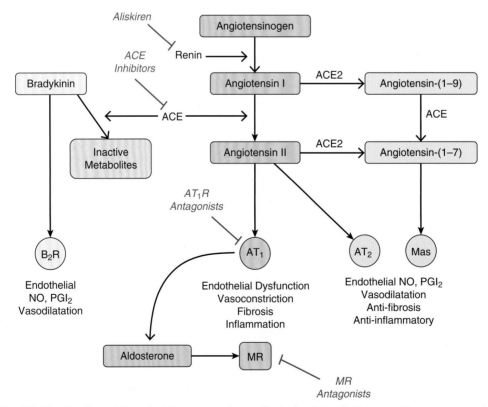

Fig. 5.9 The Classic and Proposed Counterregulatory Renin Angiotensin Systems. The systems can be expanded further to include additional potentially biologically active mediators and enzymes. (Redrawn and modified from Nguyen Dinh Cat A, Touyz RM. A new look at the renin-angiotensin system—focusing on the vascular system. *Peptides*. 2011;32:2141–2150; and Briet M, Schiffrin EL. Vascular actions of aldosterone. *J Vasc Res*. 2013;50:89–99.)

traditional concept of a circulating systemic renin angiotensin system has also expanded to include fully compartmentalized systems that are expressed and active within individual tissues and organs, including potentially at intracellular sites.[88,89] Local intact renin angiotensin systems have been reported in numerous organs and tissues including the vasculature, adipose tissue, heart, kidney, and brain. Increased expression and activity of local renin angiotensin systems is thought to contribute to the progression of vascular disease, including atherosclerosis and hypertension.[88,89] For example, in hypertension, increased expression of the vascular angiotensin system is thought to contribute to vascular dysfunction and remodeling, the brain angiotensin system to pathological activation of the sympathetic nervous system, and the cardiac angiotensin system to pathological remodeling.[4,91,92]

Arterial Wall Remodeling

Age is the most important determinant of cardiovascular health.[93] For example, the prevalence of hypertension increases exponentially with aging: 11.6% among those 20 to 39 years of age, 37.3% among those 40 to 59 years of age, and 67.2% among those 60 years of age and older.[94] Similarly, rates of atherosclerosis increase markedly in old versus young individuals.[95,96] Normal aging is associated with structural and functional deterioration of the arterial system, causing a lower threshold for cardiovascular diseases as well as their increased severity and poorer prognosis.[95,97] A key aspect of vascular aging is increased inflammatory and fibrotic activity, causing central arterial remodeling and increased arterial stiffness.

Central elastic arteries normally contribute to optimal organ perfusion by stabilizing the pulsatile pressure and flow from the heart.[98] These elastic arteries expand during systole to store a significant portion of the heart's stroke volume, which is then released during diastole to support continuous organ blood flow. This is facilitated by a partial reflection of the pulse wave, which returns during diastole to augment central diastolic pressure.[98] However, in the aging vasculature, central arterial remodeling reduces their compliance and increases pulse wave velocity. As a result, the reflected wave returns during systole, causing summation of the incident and reflected waves and augmentation of the central pulse and systolic pressures. This disruption of central arterial dynamics is a significant predictor of cardiovascular complications including myocardial infarction, stroke, and cardiovascular death.[97,98]

Arterial compliance is determined by the relative content of distensible wall components (e.g., elastin) and less distensible, stiffer elements (e.g., collagens, fibronectin). Aging central arteries have prominent intimal fibrous lesions characterized by invasion and expansion of VSMCs, increased deposition of poorly distensible proteins (collagens, fibronectin), and by degradation of the highly distensible elastin fibers.[96] The stiffness of aging arteries is further amplified by increased fragility and reduced compliance of aging elastin fibers, and by increased cross-linking and resilience of collagen and fibronectin matrices.[96] Importantly, this aging-associated arterial remodeling and stiffening is mediated by increased expression and activity of a local intravascular renin-angiotensin system, with increased expression of renin, ACE, AT1Rs and ANGII, and activation of ANGII signaling cascades.[95,99,100] These mediators are colocalized within the endothelium and intimal VSMCs of the developing lesion.[95,99] ANGII-dependent increases in fibrotic (e.g., TGFβ), inflammatory (e.g., MCP-1, TNF-α), and proteolytic activity (e.g., MMP2, MMP9) by endothelial and intimal VSMCs drive the remodeling process by sustaining inflammatory stress and by promoting the secretory and invasive phenotype of intimal VSMCs, culminating in the deposition of collagens and fibronectin and elastin degradation.[95,99] The intimal VSMCs are immature synthetic cells, with reduced expression of mature contractile marker proteins (e.g., SM2) and increased expression of immature VSMC

marker proteins (e.g., NMHC-B).[95,99] In contrast to expanding intimal VSMCs, the content of mature contractile VSMCs within the arterial media actually decreases in aging arteries.[95,96] Synthetic immature VSMCs have increased capacity to synthesize collagens and fibronectin, whereas mature SMCs have an increased ability to generate elastin.[101] The increased activity of inflammatory and fibrotic mediators in aged arteries or VSMCs is reduced by blocking local ANGII activity. Likewise, chronic ANGII inhibition using ACE or AT1R inhibitors markedly inhibits the inflammatory activity and progression of central arterial remodeling.[95]

Endothelial dysfunction is thought to contribute importantly to the age-associated remodeling and increase in central arterial stiffness.[95,96,102] Normal endothelial cell activity helps maintain a quiescent vascular phenotype, inhibiting inflammatory activity and arterial remodeling.[4] Indeed, PGI_2 and NO inhibit whereas ET-1 amplifies VSMC proliferation.[13] Likewise, activation of PKG, the cyclic GMP-specific kinase involved in NO signaling, promotes the phenotypic maturation of immature synthetic VSMCs to mature contractile cells.[103] Furthermore, the increased cross-linking and resilience of collagen and fibronectin matrices, which contributes to arterial stiffening, is mediated in part by tissue transglutaminase (TG2).[102,104] TG2 is normally inhibited by endothelium-derived NO, but endothelial dysfunction and reduced activity of NO causes increased TG2 activity and increased cross-linking activity.[102,104] Therefore endothelial dysfunction would be expected to amplify arterial remodeling and arterial stiffness by increasing the inflammatory and fibrotic activity of intimal VSMCs. Importantly, endothelial dysfunction in aging arteries appears to be mediated by the same local renin angiotensin system that directly promotes the pathological activity of intimal VSMCs.[100]

The increased inflammatory and fibrotic activity of aging arteries, which results in pathological changes in arterial structure and compliance, is likely to provide a "fertile soil" for vascular diseases to flourish.[96,97,99] This would certainly be consistent with the fundamental role of aging in the development of vascular disease. Cross-sectional studies have demonstrated a strong association between arterial stiffness and hypertension, which was generally assumed to reflect hypertensive end-organ injury to the arterial wall.[97,98] However, longitudinal studies suggest that central arterial stiffening, rather than being the consequence of hypertension, actually contributes to the development of hypertension.[98,105,106] The role of ANGII-dependent signaling in central arterial stiffening and in other mechanisms contributing to hypertension—including volume regulation, vasoconstriction, endothelial dysfunction, and activation of the sympathetic nervous system—explains why therapies targeted to ANGII signaling dominates the hierarchy of treatment options for the disease process.[68]

Therapeutic Intervention and the Renin Angiotensin System

ACE inhibitors first became available in the 1980s with the introduction of captopril to treat hypertension, which was quickly followed by additional ACE inhibitors including enalapril, perindopril, lisinopril, ramipril, quinapril, benazepril, cilazapril, trandolapril, fosinopril, moexipril, imidapril, and zofenopril.[77] AT1R antagonists became available much later, with the introduction of losartan for the treatment of hypertension in the late 1990s, followed by additional antagonists including candesartan, eprosartan, irbesartan, valsartan, telmisartan, and olmesartan.[77] AT1R antagonists were developed to address some perceived deficiencies regarding ACE inhibitors, including the potential for non–ACE dependent generation of ANGII and class-specific side effects associated with ACE inhibition.[77] ACE inhibition reduces the degradation of bradykinin and other peptides such as substance P, resulting in a common side effect of cough and the rarer side effect of angioedema (see Fig. 5.9).[77,91] These effects are much less common with AT1R antagonists. Otherwise, the ACE inhibitors and AT1R antagonists are generally well-tolerated therapeutics.[77]

The hemodynamic effects of ACE inhibitors and AT1R antagonists are similar, with vasodilatation of arterioles, reduction in peripheral vascular resistance, and a decrease in blood pressure.[77] Because of the multiple mechanisms employed by the renin angiotensin systems in the pathogenesis of hypertension, the therapeutic actions of ACE inhibitors and AT1R antagonists are also myriad, including blood pressure–dependent and independent protective effects on tissue and organ function.[77,91]

Within the vascular system, treatment with ACE inhibitors or AT1R antagonists improves endothelial function in hypertensive patients, which is thought to reflect blood pressure–dependent and independent effects, including reduced ANGII-mediated oxidative stress and increased NO activity.[77,107] Consistent with the key role of the ANGII system in arterial stiffening, ACE inhibitors or AT1R antagonists are highly effective at reducing central arterial stiffness, which is thought to reflect a long-term reduction in arterial wall fibrosis.[77] This is associated with a slower propagation of pressure waves along the aorta, a reduction in adverse pressure wave summation, and a fall in central systolic and pulse pressures.[77] These beneficial effects of ANGII inhibition are independent of changes observed in brachial blood pressure.[77] Indeed, when different classes of antihypertensive agents producing similar reductions in brachial artery blood pressure are compared, ACE inhibitors or AT1R antagonists are more effective at reducing central arterial stiffening.[77,107]

Hypertension is associated with target-organ damage, which contributes to the progression of cardiovascular diseases including heart failure, ischemic heart disease, cerebrovascular disease, and renal failure.[107] In the treatment of hypertension, there is increased awareness of addressing these comorbidities.[91] Drugs such as inhibitors of the renin angiotensin system that not only lower blood pressure but are also organ-protective have added benefit in this approach.[77,107] Indeed, ACE inhibitors and AT1R antagonists are widely used to treat heart failure and ischemic heart disease and have beneficial effects on cardiac and renal function in hypertensive patients, which reflect decreases in blood pressure and direct protective effects.[77,91]

There is an ongoing debate as to potential differences in clinical efficacy between ACE inhibitors and AT1R antagonists—for example, with regard to reducing the risk of CHD.[91,107] There are theoretical advantages and disadvantages to these agents (see Fig. 5.9). For example, unlike ACE inhibitors, AT1Rs can inhibit ANGII generated by ACE-independent pathways (e.g., chymase) and would preserve the potential protective counterregulatory systems of AT2Rs and the ACE2/ANG-(1-7)/Mas.[91] However, unlike AT1R antagonists, ACE protects bradykinin, which is an endothelial agonist and may have protective vasodilator activity.[91,107]

The only direct renin inhibitor currently available for treating hypertensive patients is aliskiren, a highly potent and selective inhibitor of human renin.[77] Aliskiren is effective at reducing blood pressure but has not been demonstrated to have beneficial effects on major cardiovascular events in patients with hypertension or coronary artery disease.[107,108] In contrast to ACE inhibitors and AT1R antagonists, aliskiren is to considered a secondary agent for therapy and should not be used in combination with other ANGII inhibitors.[68]

Aldosterone and the activation of mineralocorticoid receptors (MRs) are thought to contribute to vascular dysfunction resulting from increased activity of the renin angiotensin system. MRs are expressed in endothelial and VSMCs, with their activation contributing to endothelial dysfunction, increased inflammatory activity, and vascular remodeling (see Fig. 5.9).[102,109,110] Indeed, MR expression is increased in aging central arteries and appears to contribute to the proinflammatory and profibrotic activity of intimal VSMCs and the increase in arterial stiffening.[95] Likewise, as with inhibition of ANGII activity, MR antagonism can decrease central arterial stiffening independently of changes in blood pressure.[77] Furthermore, MR antagonists have also been shown to be an effective therapeutic addition in drug-resistant hypertension.[90] Two steroidal compounds, spironolactone and eplerenone, are currently approved for antagonism of MRs. However, both drugs present significant disadvantages that limit their clinical use.[108] Spironolactone is a nonselective MR antagonist that activates progesterone receptors and inhibits androgen receptors. Interestingly, this pharmacological profile is similar to that of natural progesterone. Spironolactone use is associated with adverse sexual effects, including impotence and gynecomastia.[68,108] Eplerenone is a spironolactone derivative that was designed to have enhanced selectivity at MRs by reducing activity at progesterone and androgen receptors. Its use is associated with a very low occurrence of sexual side effects. However, both drugs are associated with hyperkalemia, especially in patients with renal dysfunction.[109] Although listed as secondary agents for treating hypertension, they are the preferred agents in primary aldosteronism and resistant hypertension.[68]

The expanded network of renin angiotensin systems and ANG-dependent signaling present numerous opportunities for therapeutic intervention in cardiovascular and other disease processes, including activators of the ACE-2/ANG-(1-7)/Mas system and of AT2Rs (see Fig. 5.9).[90,108] Although this is an active area of investigation, no drugs are currently approved to specifically target these additional processes.[108]

REFERENCES

1. Zhao Y, Flavahan S, Leung SW, et al. Elevated pressure causes endothelial dysfunction in mouse carotid arteries by increasing local angiotensin signaling. *Am J Physiol Heart Circ Physiol.* 2015;308:H358–H363.
2. Gatfield J, Menyhart K, Wanner D, et al. Selexipag active metabolite ACT-333679 displays strong anticontractile and antiremodeling effects but low beta-arrestin recruitment and desensitization potential. *J Pharmacol Exp Ther.* 2017;362:186–199.
3. Shapiro SM, Oudiz RJ, Cao T, et al. Primary pulmonary hypertension: improved long-term effects and survival with continuous intravenous epoprostenol infusion. *J Am Coll Cardiol.* 1997;30:343–349.
4. Flavahan NA. In development - a new paradigm for understanding vascular disease. *J Cardiovasc Pharmacol.* 2017;69:248–263.
5. Flavahan NA. A vascular mechanistic approach to understanding Raynaud phenomenon. *Nat Rev Rheumatol.* 2015;11:146–158.
6. Flavahan NA. Thermoregulation: the normal structure and function of the cutaneous vascular system. In: Wigley F, Herrick A, Flavahan NA, eds. *Raynaud's Phenomenon: A Guide to Pathogenesis and Treatment.* New York: Springer; 2015:37–55.
7. Farah C, Michel LYM, Balligand JL. Nitric oxide signalling in cardiovascular health and disease. *Nat Rev Cardiol.* 2018;15:292–316.
8. Qian J, Fulton D. Post-translational regulation of endothelial nitric oxide synthase in vascular endothelium. *Front Physiol.* 2013;4:347.
9. Matsuzawa Y, Kwon TG, Lennon RJ, et al. Prognostic value of flow-mediated vasodilation in brachial artery and fingertip artery for cardiovascular events: a systematic review and meta-analysis. *J Am Heart Assoc.* 2015;4.
10. Flavahan NA. Balancing prostanoid activity in the human vascular system. *Trends Pharmacol Sci.* 2007;28:106–110.
11. Goel A, Su B, Flavahan S, et al. Increased endothelial exocytosis and generation of endothelin-1 contributes to constriction of aged arteries. *Circ Res.* 2010;107:242–251.
12. Lau EMT, Giannoulatou E, Celermajer DS, et al. Epidemiology and treatment of pulmonary arterial hypertension. *Nat Rev Cardiol.* 2017;14:603–614.
13. Galie N, Humbert M, Vachiery JL, et al. 2015 ESC/ERS Guidelines for the diagnosis and treatment of pulmonary hypertension: The Joint Task

Force for the Diagnosis and Treatment of Pulmonary Hypertension of the European Society of Cardiology (ESC) and the European Respiratory Society (ERS): endorsed by: Association for European Paediatric and Congenital Cardiology (AEPC), International Society for Heart and Lung Transplantation (ISHLT). *Eur Respir J.* 2015;46:903–975.

14. Barnett CF, Alvarez P, Park MH. Pulmonary arterial hypertension: diagnosis and treatment. *Cardiol Clin.* 2016;34:375–389.

15. Lyle MA, Davis JP, Brozovich FV. Regulation of pulmonary vascular smooth muscle contractility in pulmonary arterial hypertension: implications for therapy. *Front Physiol.* 2017;8:614.

16. Barst RJ, Rubin LJ, Long WA, et al. A comparison of continuous intravenous epoprostenol (prostacyclin) with conventional therapy for primary pulmonary hypertension. *N Engl J Med.* 1996;334:296–301.

17. Barst RJ, Rubin LJ, McGoon MD, et al. Survival in primary pulmonary hypertension with long-term continuous intravenous prostacyclin. *Ann Int Med.* 1994;121:409–415.

18. Wigley FM, Flavahan NA. Raynaud's phenomenon. *N Engl J Med.* 2016;375:556–565.

19. Yafi FA, Jenkins L, Albersen M, et al. Erectile dysfunction. *Nat Rev Dis Primers.* 2016;2:16003.

20. Toda N, Ayajiki K, Okamura T. Nitric oxide and penile erectile function. *Pharmacol Ther.* 2005;106:233–266.

21. Forstermann U, Sessa WC. Nitric oxide synthases: regulation and function. *Eur Heart J.* 2012;33:829–837.

22. Divakaran S, Loscalzo J. The role of nitroglycerin and other nitrogen oxides in cardiovascular therapeutics. *J Am Coll Cardiol.* 2017;70:2393–2410.

23. De Caterina R, Husted S, Wallentin L, et al. General mechanisms of coagulation and targets of anticoagulants (Section I). Position Paper of the ESC Working Group on Thrombosis–Task Force on Anticoagulants in Heart Disease. *Thromb Haemost.* 2013;109:569–579.

24. Hoffman M, Monroe 3rd DM. A cell-based model of hemostasis. *Thromb Haemost.* 2001;85:958–965.

25. Olson ST, Richard B, Izaguirre G, et al. Molecular mechanisms of antithrombin-heparin regulation of blood clotting proteinases. A paradigm for understanding proteinase regulation by serpin family protein proteinase inhibitors. *Biochimie.* 2010;92:1587–1596.

26. Ushiyama A, Kataoka H, Iijima T. Glycocalyx and its involvement in clinical pathophysiologies. *J Intensive Care.* 2016;4:59.

27. Crea F, Libby P. Acute coronary syndromes: the way forward from mechanisms to precision treatment. *Circulation.* 2017;136:1155–1166.

28. Rodriguez F, Mahaffey KW. Management of patients with NSTE-ACS: a comparison of the recent AHA/ACC and ESC guidelines. *J Am Coll Cardiol.* 2016;68:313–321.

29. Cattaneo M. P2Y12 receptors: structure and function. *J Thromb Haemost.* 2015;13(Suppl 1):S10–S16.

30. Burnstock G. Purinergic signaling in the cardiovascular system. *Circ Res.* 2017;120:207–228.

31. Wolberg AS, Rosendaal FR, Weitz JI, et al. Venous thrombosis. *Nat Rev Dis Primers.* 2015;1:15006.

32. van Es N, Bleker S, Sturk A, et al. Clinical significance of tissue factor-exposing microparticles in arterial and venous thrombosis. *Semin Thromb Hemost.* 2015;41:718–727.

33. Piran S, Schulman S. Management of venous thromboembolism: an update. *Thromb J.* 2016;14:23.

34. Laux V, Perzborn E, Heitmeier S, et al. Direct inhibitors of coagulation proteins - the end of the heparin and low-molecular-weight heparin era for anticoagulant therapy? *Thromb Haemost.* 2009;102:892–899.

35. Spinthakis N, Farag M, Rocca B, et al. More, more, more: reducing thrombosis in acute coronary syndromes beyond dual antiplatelet therapy-current data and future directions. *J Am Heart Assoc.* 2018;7(3).

36. Klegerman ME. Translational initiatives in thrombolytic therapy. *Front Med.* 2017;11:1–19.

37. Grosser T, Yu Y, Fitzgerald GA. Emotion recollected in tranquility: lessons learned from the COX-2 saga. *Annu Rev Med.* 2010;61:17–33.

38. Kirkby NS, Lundberg MH, Harrington LS, et al. Cyclooxygenase-1, not cyclooxygenase-2, is responsible for physiological production of prostacyclin in the cardiovascular system. *Proc Natl Acad Sci U S A.* 2012;109:17597–17602.

39. Braden GA, Knapp HR, FitzGerald GA. Suppression of eicosanoid biosynthesis during coronary angioplasty by fish oil and aspirin. *Circulation.* 1991;84:679–685.

40. FitzGerald GA, Oates JA, Hawiger J, et al. Endogenous biosynthesis of prostacyclin and thromboxane and platelet function during chronic administration of aspirin in man. *J Clin Invest.* 1983;71:676–688.

41. Clarke RJ, Mayo G, Price P, et al. Suppression of thromboxane A2 but not of systemic prostacyclin by controlled-release aspirin. *N Engl J Med.* 1991;325:1137–1141.

42. Bertrand MJ, Tardif JC. Inflammation and beyond: new directions and emerging drugs for treating atherosclerosis. *Expert Opin Emerg Drugs.* 2017;22:1–26.

43. Bom MJ, van der Heijden DJ, Kedhi E, et al. Early detection and treatment of the vulnerable coronary plaque: can we prevent acute coronary syndromes? *Circ Cardiovasc Imaging.* 2017;10.

44. Evrard SM, Lecce L, Michelis KC, et al. Endothelial to mesenchymal transition is common in atherosclerotic lesions and is associated with plaque instability. *Nat Commun.* 2016;7:11853.

45. Lacolley P, Regnault V, Segers P, et al. Vascular smooth muscle cells and arterial stiffening: relevance in development, aging, and disease. *Physiol Rev.* 2017;97:1555–1617.

46. Bennett MR, Sinha S, Owens GK. Vascular smooth muscle cells in atherosclerosis. *Circ Res.* 2016;118:692–702.

47. Oesterle A, Laufs U, Liao JK. Pleiotropic effects of statins on the cardiovascular system. *Circ Res.* 2017;120:229–243.

48. Zhou Q, Liao JK. Pleiotropic effects of statins. Basic research and clinical perspectives. *Circ J.* 2010;74:818–826.

49. Libby P. Interleukin-1 beta as a target for atherosclerosis therapy: biological basis of CANTOS and beyond. *J Am Coll Cardiol.* 2017;70:2278–2289.

49a. Grundy SM, Stone NJ, Bailey AL, et al. AHA/ACC/AACVPR/AAPA/ABC/ACPM/ADA/AGS/APhA/ASPC/NLA/PCNA Guideline on the Management of Blood Cholesterol: A Report of the American College of Cardiology/American Heart Association Task Force on Clinical Practice Guidelines. *J Am Coll Cardiol.* 2018. [Epub ahead of print].

49b. Sabatine MS. PCSK9 inhibitors: clinical evidence and implementation. *Nat Rev Cardiol.* 2018. [Epub ahead of print].

49c. Sabatine MS, Giugliano RP, Keech AC, et al. Evolocumab and clinical outcomes in patients with cardiovascular disease. *N Engl J Med.* 2017;376:1713–1722.

49d. Schwartz GG, Steg PG, Szarek M, et al. Alirocumab and cardiovascular outcomes after acute coronary syndrome. *N Engl J Med.* 2018. [Epub ahead of print].

49e. Cannon CP, Blazing MA, Giugliano RP, et al. Ezetimibe added to statin therapy after acute coronary syndromes. *N Engl J Med.* 2015;372:2387–2397.

50. Carmeliet P, Jain RK. Molecular mechanisms and clinical applications of angiogenesis. *Nature.* 2011;473:298–307.

51. Folkman J. The vascularization of tumors. *Sci Am.* 1976;234:58–64.

52. Iyer SR, Annex BH. Therapeutic angiogenesis for peripheral artery disease: lessons learned in translational science. *JACC Basic Transl Sci.* 2017;2:503–512.

53. Folkman J. Tumor angiogenesis: therapeutic implications. *N Engl J Med.* 1971;285:1182–1186.

54. Hanahan D, Weinberg RA. The hallmarks of cancer. *Cell.* 2000;100:57–70.

55. Gougis P, Wassermann J, Spano JP, et al. Clinical pharmacology of anti-angiogenic drugs in oncology. *Crit Rev Oncol Hematol.* 2017;119:75–93.

56. Chang F, Flavahan S, Flavahan NA. Impaired activity of adherens junctions contributes to endothelial dilator dysfunction in ageing rat arteries. *J Physiol.* 2017;595:5143–5158.

57. Chang F, Flavahan S, Flavahan NA. Superoxide inhibition restores endothelium-dependent dilatation in aging arteries by enhancing impaired adherens junctions. *Am J Physiol Heart Circ Physiol.* 2018;314:H805–H811.

58. Charkoudian N, Wallin BG. Sympathetic neural activity to the cardiovascular system: integrator of systemic physiology and interindividual characteristics. *Compr Physiol.* 2014;4:825–850.

59. Malpas SC. Sympathetic nervous system overactivity and its role in the development of cardiovascular disease. *Physiol Rev.* 2010;90:513–557.

60. Osborn JW, Foss JD. Renal nerves and long-term control of arterial pressure. *Compr Physiol.* 2017;7:263–320.

61. Flavahan NA, Shimokawa H, Vanhoutte PM. Pertussis toxin inhibits endothelium-dependent relaxations to certain agonists in porcine coronary arteries. *J Physiol (Lond).* 1989;408:549–560.

62. Barger G, Dale HH. Chemical structure and sympathomimetic action of amines. *J Physiol.* 1910;41:19–59.

63. Flavahan NA. Phenylpropanolamine constricts mouse and human blood vessels by preferentially activating alpha2-adrenoceptors. *J Pharmacol Exp Ther.* 2005;313:432–439.

64. Crassous PA, Flavahan S, Flavahan NA. Acute dilation to alpha(2)-adrenoceptor antagonists uncovers dual constriction and dilation mediated by arterial alpha(2)-adrenoceptors. *Br J Pharmacol.* 2009;158:1344–1355.

65. Kobayashi S, Endou M, Sakuraya F, et al. The sympathomimetic actions of l-ephedrine and d-pseudoephedrine: direct receptor activation or norepinephrine release? *Anesth Analg.* 2003;97:1239–1245.

66. Kanfer I, Dowse R, Vuma V. Pharmacokinetics of oral decongestants. *Pharmacotherapy.* 1993;13:116S–128S. discussion 143S-146S.

67. Slim HB, Black HR, Thompson PD. Older blood pressure medications-do they still have a place? *Am J Cardiol.* 2011;108:308–316.

68. Whelton PK, Carey RM, Aronow WS, et al. ACC/AHA/AAPA/ABC/ACPM/AGS/APhA/ASH/ASPC/NMA/PCNA Guideline for the prevention, detection, evaluation, and management of high blood pressure in adults: a report of the American College of Cardiology/American Heart Association Task Force on Clinical Practice Guidelines. *J Am Coll Cardiol.* 2018;71:e127–e248.

69. van Zuuren EJ Rosacea. *N Engl J Med.* 2017;377:1754–1764.

70. Ono M, Brady K, Easley RB, et al. Duration and magnitude of blood pressure below cerebral autoregulation threshold during cardiopulmonary bypass is associated with major morbidity and operative mortality. *J Thorac Cardiovasc Surg.* 2014;147:483–489.

71. Grassi G, Mark A, Esler M. The sympathetic nervous system alterations in human hypertension. *Circ Res.* 2015;116:976–990.

72. Harrison DG. The immune system in hypertension. *Trans Am Clin Climatol Assoc.* 2014;125:138–140. discussion 138–140.

73. Barzilay J, Grimm R, Cushman W, et al. Getting to goal blood pressure: why reserpine deserves a second look. *J Clin Hypertens (Greenwich).* 2007;9:591–594.

74. Naranjo J, Dodd S, Martin YN. Perioperative management of pheochromocytoma. *J Cardiothorac Vasc Anesth.* 2017;31:1427–1439.

75. Ripley TL, Saseen JJ. Beta-blockers: a review of their pharmacological and physiological diversity in hypertension. *Ann Pharmacother.* 2014;48:723–733.

76. Aronow WS, Frishman WH. Contemporary drug treatment of hypertension: focus on recent guidelines. *Drugs.* 2018;78(5):567–576.

77. Laurent S. Antihypertensive drugs. *Pharmacol Res.* 2017;124:116–125.

78. Giles TD, Cockcroft JR, Pitt B, et al. Rationale for nebivolol/valsartan combination for hypertension: review of preclinical and clinical data. *J Hypertens.* 2017;35:1758–1767.

79. Flavahan NA. Pathophysiological regulation of the cutaneous vascular system in Raynaud's phenomenon. In: Wigley F, Herrick A, Flavahan NA, eds. *Raynaud's Phenomenon: A Guide to Pathogenesis and Treatment.* New York: Springer; 2015:57–79.

80. Fava A, Boin F. Historical perspective of Raynaud's phenomenon. In: Wigley F, Herrick A, Flavahan NA, eds. *Raynaud's Phenomenon: A Guide to Pathogenesis and Treatment.* New York: Springer; 2015:1–11.

81. Chotani MA, Flavahan NA. Intracellular alpha(2C)-adrenoceptors: storage depot, stunted development or signaling domain? *Biochim Biophysica Acta.* 2011;1813:1495–1503.

82. Majesky MW. Adventitia and perivascular cells. *Arterioscler Thromb Vasc Biol.* 2015;35:e31–e35.

83. Stenmark KR, Yeager ME, El Kasmi KC, et al. The adventitia: essential regulator of vascular wall structure and function. *Annu Rev Physiol.* 2013;75:23–47.

84. Liu Z, Khalil RA. Evolving mechanisms of vascular smooth muscle contraction highlight key targets in vascular disease. *Biochem Pharmacol.* 2018;153:91–122.

85. Alonso-Carbajo L, Kecskes M, Jacobs G, et al. Muscling in on TRP channels in vascular smooth muscle cells and cardiomyocytes. *Cell Calcium.* 2017;66:48–61.

86. Brozovich FV, Nicholson CJ, Degen CV, et al. Mechanisms of vascular smooth muscle contraction and the basis for pharmacologic treatment of smooth muscle disorders. *Pharmacol Rev.* 2016;68:476–532.

87. Roberts OL, Kamishima T, Barrett-Jolley R, et al. Exchange protein activated by cAMP (Epac) induces vascular relaxation by activating Ca2+-sensitive K+ channels in rat mesenteric artery. *J Physiol.* 2013;591:5107–5123.

88. Nguyen Dinh Cat A, Touyz RM. A new look at the renin-angiotensin system—focusing on the vascular system. *Peptides.* 2011;32:2141–2150.

89. van Thiel BS, van der Pluijm I, te Riet L, et al. The renin-angiotensin system and its involvement in vascular disease. *Eur J Pharmacol.* 2015;763:3–14.

90. Te Riet L, van Esch JH, Roks AJ, et al. Hypertension: renin-angiotensin-aldosterone system alterations. *Circ Res.* 2015;116:960–975.

91. Borghi C, Force ST, Rossi F, et al. Role of the renin-angiotensin-aldosterone system and its pharmacological inhibitors in cardiovascular diseases: complex and critical issues. *High Blood Press Cardiovasc Prev.* 2015;22:429–444.

92. Young CN, Davisson RL. Angiotensin-II, the brain, and hypertension: an update. *Hypertension.* 2015;66:920–926.

93. North BJ, Sinclair DA. The intersection between aging and cardiovascular disease. *Circ Res.* 2012;110:1097–1108.

94. Benjamin EJ, Virani SS, Callaway CW, et al. Heart disease and stroke statistics-2018 update: a report from the American Heart Association. *Circulation.* 2018;137:e67–e492.

95. Wang M, Jiang L, Monticone RE, et al. Proinflammation: the key to arterial aging. *Trends Endocrinol Metab.* 2014;25:72–79.

96. Wang JC, Bennett M. Aging and atherosclerosis: mechanisms, functional consequences, and potential therapeutics for cellular senescence. *Circ Res.* 2012;111:245–259.

97. Barton M, Husmann M, Meyer MR. Accelerated vascular aging as a paradigm for hypertensive vascular disease: prevention and therapy. *Can J Cardiol.* 2016;32:680–686. e4.

98. Kaess BM, Rong J, Larson MG, et al. Aortic stiffness, blood pressure progression, and incident hypertension. *JAMA.* 2012;308:875–881.

99. Wang M, Monticone RE, Lakatta EG. Arterial aging: a journey into subclinical arterial disease. *Curr Opin Nephrol Hypertens.* 2010;19:201–207.

100. Flavahan S, Chang F, Flavahan NA. Local renin-angiotensin system mediates endothelial dilator dysfunction in aging arteries. *Am J Physiol Heart Circ Physiol.* 2016;311:H849–H854.

101. Wanjare M, Kuo F, Gerecht S. Derivation and maturation of synthetic and contractile vascular smooth muscle cells from human pluripotent stem cells. *Cardiovasc Res.* 2013;97:321–330.

102. Aroor AR, Demarco VG, Jia G, et al. The role of tissue renin-angiotensin-aldosterone system in the development of endothelial dysfunction and arterial stiffness. *Front Endocrinol (Lausanne).* 2013;4:161.

103. Lincoln TM, Wu X, Sellak H, et al. Regulation of vascular smooth muscle cell phenotype by cyclic GMP and cyclic GMP-dependent protein kinase. *Front Biosci.* 2006;11:356–367.

104. Santhanam L, Tuday EC, Webb AK, et al. Decreased S-nitrosylation of tissue transglutaminase contributes to age-related increases in vascular stiffness. *Circ Res.* 2010;107:117–125.

105. Mukherjee D. Atherogenic vascular stiffness and hypertension: cause or effect? *JAMA.* 2012;308:919–920.

106. Koivistoinen T, Lyytikainen LP, Aatola H, et al. Pulse wave velocity predicts the progression of blood pressure and development of hypertension in young adults. *Hypertension.* 2018;71:451–456.

107. Cameron AC, Lang NN, Touyz RM. Drug treatment of hypertension: focus on vascular health. *Drugs.* 2016;76:1529–1550.

108. Tamargo M, Tamargo J. Future drug discovery in renin-angiotensin-aldosterone system intervention. *Expert Opin Drug Discov.* 2017;12:827–848.

109. Briet M, Schiffrin EL. Vascular actions of aldosterone. *J Vasc Res*. 2013;50:89–99.

110. Brown NJ. Contribution of aldosterone to cardiovascular and renal inflammation and fibrosis. *Nat Rev Nephrol*. 2013;9:459–469.

111. Flavahan NA, Vanhoutte PM. Alpha-1 and alpha-2 adrenoceptor: response coupling in canine saphenous and femoral veins. *J Pharmacol Exp Ther*. 1986;238:131–138.

112. Flavahan NA, Rimele TJ, Cooke JP, et al. Characterization of postjunctional alpha-1 and alpha-2 adrenoceptors activated by exogenous or nerve-released norepinephrine in the canine saphenous vein. *J Pharmacol Exp Ther*. 1984;230:699–705.

113. Flavahan NA, Hales MA, Aleskowitch TD, et al. Alpha1L-adrenoceptors in canine pulmonary artery. *J Cardiovasc Pharmacol*. 1998;32:308–316.

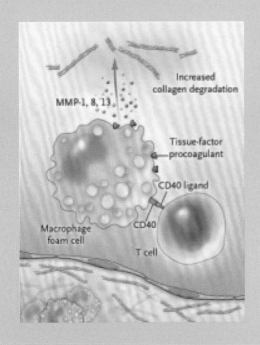

Pathobiology of
Blood Vessels

血管病理生理学

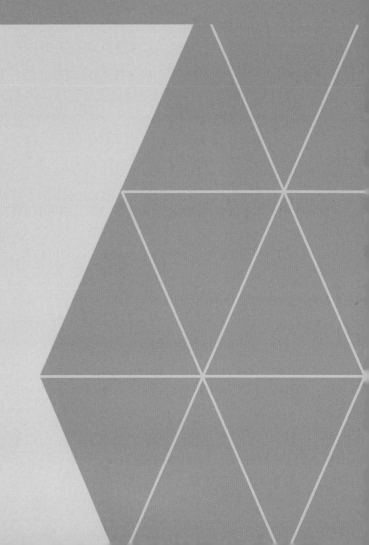

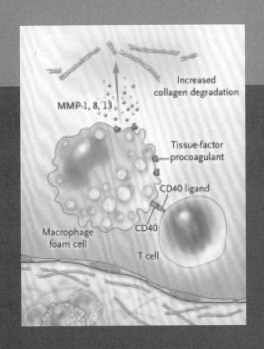

第6章
动脉粥样硬化的病理生理学

　　动脉粥样硬化的概念和病理生理学知识在快速更新发展。传统观念认为动脉粥样硬化是一种胆固醇累积性疾病，但目前我们认识到它是一种由多种危险因素参与的，与血管细胞、血细胞及脂蛋白相互作用的全身性疾病。除外冠状动脉粥样硬化，外周血管、脑血管粥样硬化也需关注。细胞相互作用使白细胞黏附并进入血管内膜，促进炎症介质释放、主动脉平滑肌细胞迁移和增殖、细胞外基质沉积和钙化等，形成纤维化斑块，晚期可导致动脉狭窄和并发症。一方面，动脉粥样硬化是局灶性的，它常始于血流紊乱、低剪切应力的血管分叉部位，引起管腔狭窄和明显血流受限；另一方面，它又是弥漫性的，因血管内超声发现非狭窄血管存在早期动脉粥样硬化迹象。通常，急性动脉血栓不发生于最狭窄的动脉段，因此，斑块病变大小与血管狭窄程度是不同的概念。4种斑块破坏机制（纤维帽破裂、浅表侵蚀、斑块中新生血管破裂出血及钙化结节侵蚀）可形成动脉粥样硬化血栓性并发症。总之，动脉粥样硬化是一种全身性疾病，尽管药物干预可有效改变斑块的生物学特性，取得较好的临床成效，但我们仍面临生活方式改变的挑战，仍需寻求更深入的科学理解和创新治疗来进一步减少动脉粥样硬化相关的并发症，降低死亡率。

陈良万

Pathobiology of Atherosclerosis

Peter Libby

Knowledge of the pathobiology of atherosclerosis has continued to evolve at a rapid pace. Previously regarded as a mainly segmental disease, we now increasingly appreciate the condition's diffuse nature. The traditional clinical focus on atherosclerosis has emphasized coronary artery disease. The attention of physicians in general and of cardiovascular specialists in particular now embraces other arterial beds, including the peripheral and cerebrovascular arterial circulations.[1]

Formerly considered an inevitable and relentlessly progressive degenerative process, we now recognize that, quite to the contrary, atherogenesis progresses at varied paces. Increasing clinical and experimental evidence indicates that atheromatous plaques can evolve in vastly different fashions. Atheromas behave much more dynamically than traditionally conceived from both structural and biologic points of view. Plaques not only progress but may also regress and/or alter their qualitative characteristics in ways that decisively influence their clinical behavior.[2]

Concepts of the pathobiology of atherosclerosis have likewise undergone perpetual revision. During much of the 20th century, most considered atherosclerosis a cholesterol storage disease. Recognition of the key role of interactions of vascular cells, blood cells including leukocytes and platelets, and lipoproteins challenged this model later in the 20th century.[3] Current thinking further broadens this schema, incorporating an appreciation of the global metabolic status of individuals and extending far beyond traditional risk factors as triggers to the atherogenic process.

This chapter delineates the concepts of the widespread and diffuse distributions of atherosclerosis and its clinical manifestations; it also describes current progress in elucidating its fundamental biology.

RISK FACTORS FOR ATHEROSCLEROSIS: TRADITIONAL, EMERGING, AND ON THE RISE

Traditional Risk Factors for Atherosclerosis

Cholesterol

Experimental data have repeatedly shown a link between plasma cholesterol levels and the formation of atheromas. Pioneering work performed in Russia in the early 20th century showed that consumption by rabbits of a cholesterol-rich diet caused the formation of arterial lesions that shared features with human atheromas.[4] By mid-century, application of the ultracentrifuge to the analysis of plasma proteins led to the recognition that various classes of lipoproteins

transported cholesterol and other lipids through the aqueous medium of the blood. Multiple epidemiologic studies verified a link between one cholesterol-rich lipoprotein particle in particular, low-density lipoprotein (LDL), and risk for coronary heart disease (CHD).[5] The characterization of familial hypercholesterolemia as a genetic disease provided further evidence linking LDL cholesterol levels with CHD. Heterozygotes for this condition had a markedly elevated risk for atherosclerotic disease. Individuals homozygous for familial hypercholesterolemia commonly develop CHD within the first decade of life.

The elucidation of the LDL-receptor pathway and findings that mutations in the LDL receptor cause familial hypercholesterolemia provided proof positive of LDL's role in atherogenesis.[5,6] Yet the cholesterol hypothesis of atherogenesis still encountered skepticism. Many critics—some lay people and some respected professionals—questioned aspects of the theory, pointing out that dietary cholesterol levels did not always correlate with cholesterolemia. The lack of proof that either dietary or drug intervention could modify outcomes dogged proponents of the cholesterol hypothesis of atherogenesis.[7]

Ultimately, controlled clinical trials that lowered LDL by interventions including partial intestinal bypass, bile acid–binding resins, and statin drugs showed reductions in coronary events and vindicated the cholesterol hypothesis. In appropriately powered trials conducted with sufficiently potent agents, lipid lowering also reduced overall mortality.[8,9] Yet the very success of these interventions suggested that there must be more to atherogenesis than cholesterol, because a majority of events still occurred despite increasingly aggressive control of LDL cholesterol levels. The identification of proprotein convertase subtilisin/kexin type 9 (*PCSK9*) as the gene involved in autosomal dominant hypercholesterolemia has furnished new insight in this regard. Reduced function of this enzyme raises cellular LDL receptor numbers and hence augments LDL clearance, leading to lower plasma LDL levels. Individuals with reduced function variants of *PCSK9* who experience lifelong lower exposure to LDL show protection from atherosclerotic events even in the presence of other cardiovascular risk factors. These observations strengthen the case for the involvement of LDL in atherogenesis and for the aggressive management of LDL in practice.[10,11]

Of course aspects of the lipoprotein profile other than LDL can influence atherogenesis (see later).[12] Yet as atherosclerotic events commonly occur in individuals with average levels of the major lipoprotein classes, a full understanding of atherogenesis requires consideration of factors other than blood lipids.

Systemic arterial hypertension

The relationship between arterial blood pressure and mortality emerged early from actuarial studies. Insurance underwriters had a major financial stake in mortality prediction. A simple measurement of blood pressure with a cuff sphygmomanometer powerfully predicted longevity. Data emerging from the Framingham Study and other observational cohorts verified a relationship between systemic arterial pressure and CHD events.[13] Concordant observations from experimental animals and epidemiologic studies bolstered the link between hypertension and atherosclerosis.

As in the case of high cholesterol, clinical evidence that the pharmacologic reduction of blood pressure could reduce CHD events proved fairly elusive. Early intervention studies readily showed decreases in stroke and congestive heart failure endpoints following the administration of antihypertensive drugs. Studies indicating clear-cut reductions in CHD events with antihypertensive treatment have accumulated much more recently.[14]

Mechanistically, antihypertensive drug therapy likely benefits atherosclerosis and its complications principally by lowering blood pressure, although some have posited other beneficial actions of various antihypertensive agents. A large randomized clinical trial, the Antihypertensive and Lipid-Lowering Treatment to Prevent Heart Attack Trial (ALLHAT), showed no advantage over a 5-year period over a thiazide diuretic of an angiotensin receptor blocker, a calcium channel antagonist, or a β-adrenergic blocking agent.[15,16] Recent studies affirm the benefits of antihypertensive therapy in reducing the risk of atherosclerosis.[17]

Clinical observations provide strong additional support for the concept that hypertension itself can promote atherogenesis. Atherosclerosis of the pulmonary arteries seldom occurs in individuals with normal pulmonary artery pressures, but even in relatively young patients with pulmonary hypertension, pulmonary artery atheromas occur quite commonly. This "experiment of nature" supports the direct proatherogenic effect of hypertension in humans.

Cigarette smoking

Tobacco abuse, and cigarette smoking in particular, accentuates the risk of cardiovascular events.[18] In the context of noncoronary artery disease, cigarette smoking appears particularly important. The rapid return toward baseline rates of cardiovascular events after smoking cessation suggests that tobacco use alters the risk of thrombosis as much or more than it may accentuate atherogenesis per se. Classic studies in nonhuman primates have shown little effect of 2 to 3 years of cigarette smoke inhalation on experimental atherosclerosis in the presence of moderate hyperlipidemia.

Smoking has many adverse systemic effects, including eliciting the chronic inflammatory response implicated in atherothrombosis.[19] Cigarette smoking seems to contribute particularly to the formation of abdominal aortic aneurysms. The mechanistic link between cigarette smoking and arterial aneurysm formation may resemble that invoked in the pathogenesis of smoking-related emphysema. Studies in genetically altered mice that inhale tobacco smoke have delineated a role for elastolytic enzymes such as matrix metalloproteinase (MMP)-12 in the destruction of lung extracellular matrix. Smoke-induced inflammation appears to release tumor necrosis factor-α (TNF-α) from macrophages, which can elevate the activity of elastolytic enzymes and promote pulmonary emphysema.[20] A similar mechanism might well promote the destruction of elastic laminae in the tunica media of the abdominal aorta, which characterizes aneurysm formation.

Age

Multiple observational studies have identified age as a potent risk factor for atherosclerotic events. Indeed, age contributes substantially to risk calculation in most algorithms. Demographic trends portend a marked expansion in the elderly population, particularly women, in coming years. Although age-adjusted rates of cardiovascular disease may appear stable or even be declining in men, the actual burden of disease in the elderly will increase because of their sheer number. In view of the expanding elderly population, evidence supporting the mutability of atherosclerosis assumes even greater importance (see later). Recent studies have established that somatic mutations in bone marrow stem cells give rise to clones of leukocytes that accumulate with age and confer substantial cardiovascular risk. This new field of clonal hematopoiesis should provide new insights and links between age and atherosclerosis.[21,22]

Sex

Male sex contributes to heightened cardiovascular risk in numerous observational studies. The mechanisms for this increased burden of disease may reflect male-related proatherogenic factors and/or lack of protection conferred by female sex. As cardiovascular risk increases after menopause in women, many previously attributed the vascular protection enjoyed by premenopausal women to estrogen. But estrogen therapy in women (in recent large-scale clinical trials) and in men (in the older Coronary Drug Project study) seems to confer hazard rather than benefit in the circumstances studied.[23] Thus estrogen, certainly in combination with progesterone, does not provide a panacea for protection against cardiovascular events, although the timing of intervention may influence outcomes.[24,25]

High-density lipoprotein and triglyceride-rich lipoproteins

High-density lipoprotein (HDL) indubitably relates inversely to cardiovascular risk; however, current genetic data suggest that HDL does not protect against atherosclerotic risk.[26] Moreover, numerous attempts to raise HDL pharmacologically have failed to improve outcomes. Although various functional properties of HDL are still considered possibly beneficial, there is currently no actionable information regarding the therapeutic modification of HDL.[27] Indeed, low HDL concentrations associated with increased cardiovascular risk probably reflect the inverse relationship between HDL and triglycerides (Fig. 6.1). In contrast to HDL, current genetic evidence strongly supports a causal role for triglyceride-rich lipoproteins in atherosclerotic risk.[28,29]

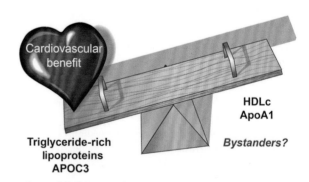

Fig. 6.1 The High-Density Lipoprotein/Triglyceride Seesaw. High-density lipoprotein and triglycerides tend to vary inversely. Traditional thought has focused on the benefits of raising high-density lipoprotein and high-density lipoprotein as a protective factor for atherosclerosis. Triglycerides have received less attention as a causal risk factor, as adjustment for high-density lipoprotein attenuates its association with risk. The new clinical and genetic data described in this commentary indicate that triglycerides and specifically the apolipoprotein constituent of many triglyceride-rich lipoproteins, apolipoprotein C3, may actually lie in the causal pathway for atherosclerosis, as well as lipoprotein lipase itself and its inhibitors ANGPTL 3 and 4. Thus, contrary to common belief, current data suggest that we should focus more on triglyceride-rich lipoproteins as a target for cardiovascular risk reduction. (Modified from Libby P. Triglycerides on the rise: should we swap seats on the seesaw? *Eur Heart J.* 2015;36:774–776.)

Emerging Risk Factors for Atherosclerosis

Homocysteine

Homocysteine, a product of amino acid metabolism, may contribute to atherothrombosis.[30] Individuals with monogenic defects that lead to elevated homocysteine levels (e.g., homocystinuria, commonly due to deficiency in cystathionine β-synthase) have a thrombotic diathesis. Yet recent genetic studies do not substantiate a causal role for modest alterations in atherosclerotic outcomes.[31] Reliable clinical tests for hyperhomocysteinemia exist. Although clearly associated with elevated thrombotic risk in patients with homocystinuria, elevated levels of homocysteine in unselected populations predict cardiovascular risk only weakly (Fig. 6.2). Moreover, randomized trials using vitamin treatments to lower homocysteine levels have not documented improvements in cardiovascular outcomes.[32] The enrichment of cereals and flour with folate in the United States has shifted dietary intake and should lower blood homocysteine levels in the American population.

Lipoprotein(a)

Lipoprotein(a) (Lp[a]; commonly pronounced "L P little a") consists of an LDL particle with apolipoprotein a (apo a)—covalently attached to the apo B, the major apolipoprotein of LDL particles.[33] Apo a should not be confused with apolipoprotein A—the family that includes apolipoprotein AI, the principal apolipoprotein of HDL. Lp(a) has considerable heterogeneity, which is determined genetically and related to the number of repeats of a structural motif known as a "kringle" in the apo a moiety of the special lipoprotein particle. The structural resemblance of apo a to plasminogen suggests that Lp(a) may inhibit fibrinolysis. Lp(a) levels in the general population have high skew. Many individuals lie in the lower range of distribution, with fewer in the higher levels of Lp(a). Black Americans have a higher frequency of elevated Lp(a). Those with Lp(a) levels substantially above normal appear to have increased cardiovascular risk, yet we currently have no evidence-based therapy, although promising avenues are being explored.[34,35] Genetic studies suggest a causal role of Lp(a) in contributing to cardiovascular events and aortic stenosis (see Fig. 6.2).[35–37]

Fibrinogen

Fibrinogen, the substrate of thrombin, provides the major meshwork of arterial thrombi. Levels of fibrinogen increase in inflammatory states as part of the acute-phase response. A consistent body of observational evidence links elevated levels of fibrinogen with cardiovascular risk.[38,39] Standardization of assays for fibrinogen has proved difficult. Moreover, diurnal variation in plasma fibrinogen levels weakens the potential of fibrinogen as a biomarker of cardiovascular risk despite its obvious biological plausibility as a major participant in thrombosis. Fibrin deposition in plaques, first hypothesized by von Rokitansky in the mid-19th century, provides evidence of fibrinogen's involvement in atherogenesis.[40]

Infection

The possibility that infectious agents or responses to infection may contribute to atherogenesis or precipitate atherosclerotic events has periodically captured the fancy of students of atherosclerosis. Many infectious agents could contribute to aspects of atherogenesis by direct cytopathic effect or through mediators they release or elicit as part of a host defense. The hemodynamic stresses of acute infection, accentuated thrombotic risk, or impaired fibrinolysis due to acute-phase reactants such as fibrinogen or plasminogen activator inhibitor-1 (PAI-1) might transiently heighten the risk for thrombotic complications of atherosclerosis.[41,42] Some seroepidemiologic studies have suggested links between exposure to viral and bacterial pathogens and various measures of atherosclerosis or risk of atherosclerotic events. Prospective studies properly controlled for confounding factors have shown weak if any correlation of antibody titers against various microbial or viral pathogens and cardiovascular events. Trials of various antibiotic regimens in patients with coronary artery disease have not shown reductions in recurrent events.[43,43a]

Inflammation and Atherosclerosis

The recognition that inflammation provides a unifying theme for many of the pathophysiologic alterations that occur during atherogenesis has provoked both interest and controversy. A subsequent section of this chapter discusses in detail the links between inflammatory processes/risk factors/atherogenesis and the complications of atherosclerosis. The emergence of C-reactive protein (CRP) as a validated marker of prospective cardiovascular risk has spawned countless studies proposing other inflammatory markers as potential predictors of atherosclerotic risk.[44] Although some markers of inflammation, such as fibrinogen and PAI-1, have defined roles as mediators and as markers, CRP serves as a risk marker rather than as an effector.

Genetic Predisposition

The example of familial hypercholesterolemia, recounted earlier, illustrates irrefutably the link between gene mutation and atherosclerosis. The accelerated development of molecular genetic technology and increasing ease of identifying and cataloging genetic polymorphisms have facilitated the search for genetic variants that predispose toward atherosclerosis or its complications.[26] Monogenic conditions, such as familial hypercholesterolemia, do not appear to explain the majority of the burden or risk of atherosclerotic disease. The quest for genetic polymorphisms that predispose to atherosclerosis has yielded many potential candidates. Genome-wide association studies have identified reproducible regions of the genome associated with increased cardiovascular risk.[45–49] Some of the genes at locations so identified have well-established functions in pathogenic pathways for atherosclerosis.[50] Rare variant approaches have recently identified the NOS3 and GUCY1A3 genes, both involved in vascular nitric oxide signaling, as associated with atherosclerotic risk.[51] Other sites emerging from genome-wide association studies have unknown functions and have not previously been associated with cardiovascular disease. Notably, the chromosome 9p21 region concordantly associates with cardiovascular events in several independent large population studies. Genetic markers of atherosclerotic risk have proven useful in providing new understanding of disease mechanisms and may identify new avenues for intervention and for risk stratification.[52–54]

Risk Factors on the Rise

We are witnessing a transition in the pattern of atherosclerotic risk factors in the United States and indeed worldwide.[55] Certain traditional atherosclerotic risk factors are on the wane. For example, rates of smoking in the United States are declining, particularly in men.[56] Dissemination of effective antihypertensive therapies has provided a means of reducing the degree or prevalence of this traditional atherosclerotic risk factor. Although many patients do not achieve the currently established targets for blood pressure, effective therapies have become much more widely implemented in recent decades.

We have made striking progress in combating high levels of LDL, a major traditional risk factor for atherosclerosis, as discussed earlier. In particular, the introduction of statins and accumulating evidence of their effectiveness as preventive therapies, combined with their relative ease of use and tolerability, should foster a secular trend toward lower LDL levels in the higher-risk segments of our population.[57,58]

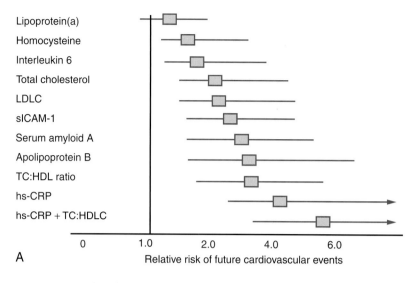

A
Relative risk of future cardiovascular events

Novel risk factors as predictors of peripheral arterial disease

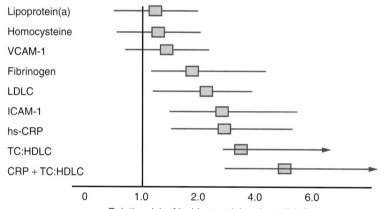

B
Relative risk of incident peripheral arterial disease
(Adjusted for age, smoking, DM, HTN, family history, exercise level, and BMI)

C-reactive protein concentration and risk of cardiovascular events: 2010
Direct comparison of hsCRP, SBP, total cholesterol, and non-HDLC

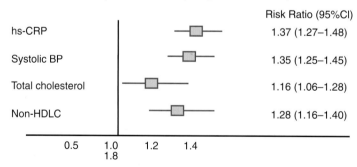

Risk ratio (95%CI) per 1-SD higher usual values

Adjusted for age, sex, smoking, diabetes, BMI, BP, triglycerides, alcohol, lipid levels, and hsCRP

C

Fig. 6.2 See legend on opposite page.

Although we justly derive considerable satisfaction from these pharmacologic inroads into the traditional profile of cardiovascular risk, we are losing ground rapidly in other respects. The astounding increase in obesity in the US population in the last decade alone represents a change in body habitus of substantial proportion that, on an evolutionary time scale, has occurred in an instant.[59,60] Short of major disasters or famines, this kind of rapid shift in body habitus may have no precedent in the history of our species. From the perspective of cardiovascular risk, the metabolic alterations that accompany this increased girth of our population should sound an alarm. Current data point to a significant increase in the prevalence of the components of the clustered risk factors often referred to as the "metabolic syndrome."

Although individuals with the metabolic syndrome cluster commonly have dyslipidemia, their levels of LDL cholesterol may be average or even below average. This finding may provide false reassurance to physicians and patients alike. Although LDL cholesterol levels in such patients may not be especially elevated, the quality of the lipoprotein particles may prove particularly atherogenic. LDL particles in those with high levels of triglycerides and low levels of HDL tend to be small and dense. Such small dense LDL particles appear to bind to proteoglycans in the arterial intima with more avidity. Their retention in the intima may facilitate their oxidative modification. Thus small dense LDL particles may have particularly atherogenic properties. Prolonged retention and increased entry may promote lipoprotein accumulation in the artery wall.[61]

Hyperglycemia

Hyperglycemia may contribute independently to the pathogenesis of atherosclerosis. In the presence of higher levels of glucose, the nonenzymatic glycation and other types of oxidative posttranslational modification of various macromolecules increases. The accumulation of glycated macromolecules ultimately leads to the formation of complex condensates known as advanced glycation end products (AGEs), which may trigger inflammatory and oxidative responses implicated in atherogenesis.[62] A cell surface receptor for AGEs known as RAGE may transduce proinflammatory signals when occupied by AGE-modified ligands.[63] This and other mechanisms link hyperglycemia and insulin resistance to aspects of host defenses considered essential for the atherogenic process. Although strict glycemic control does not necessarily improve cardiovascular outcomes, certain antidiabetic medications can lower cardiovascular risk.[64,65]

Interactions of Risk Factors With Cells in the Artery Wall and With Leukocytes During Atherogenesis

We increasingly understand atherosclerosis as a process that involves cellular interactions with risk factors such as high levels of LDL. This contemporary view contrasts with previous notions that the artery wall passively accumulates cholesterol. This cross talk among cells of varying types during atherogenesis involves more than just the intrinsic cells of the artery wall, the endothelium, and vascular smooth muscle cells (see Chapters 2 and 3).[3,66] Indeed, the mononuclear phagocyte also contributes importantly to atherogenesis.[67] The normal endothelium resists prolonged contact with leukocytes, including blood monocytes, the precursors of the tissue macrophages that accumulate in atheromas. A mechanism involving the expression of particular leukocyte adhesion molecules on the endothelial surface likely mediates the recruitment of blood monocytes to sites of formation of the earliest atherosclerotic lesions. The heterogeneity of monocytes and the macrophages to which they give rise has generated considerable recent interest. A particularly proinflammatory subset of monocytes accumulates in the blood of hypercholestrolemic mice.[68–70] Macrophages exhibiting atherogenic functions also appear to accumulate in atherosclerotic lesions, and therapeutic interventions may modulate these functions.

Adhesion molecules considered important in this process include members of the selectin superfamily, such as P-selectin.[71,72] Leukocytes passing through the arterial circulation can bind to patches of endothelial cells expressing P-selectin, which mediates a rolling or saltatory slowing of the leukocytes. The more permanent adhesion of the tethered white cell depends on the expression of another category of leukocyte adhesion molecule expressed on the endothelial surface at sites prone to lesion formation—members of the IgG superfamily, including vascular cell adhesion molecule-1 (VCAM-1). Both P-selectin and VCAM-1, among other adhesion molecules, show increased expression in regions of human atherosclerotic plaques and on the macrovascular endothelium overlying nascent atherosclerotic plaques in experimental animals. Whereas other leukocyte adhesion molecules certainly participate in this capture of blood leukocytes, considerable evidence from genetically altered mice supports the essential involvement of P-selectin and VCAM-1 in lesion formation.

Once firmly bound to the endothelial surface, white blood cells must receive chemoattractant stimuli to penetrate into the intima.[73,74] Among such signals, monocyte chemoattractant protein-1 (MCP-1, CCL2) may be particularly important. Again, experiments in genetically altered mice support the involvement of MCP-1/CCL2 in the formation of experimental atherosclerotic lesions. Other chemokines, such as the cell surface–associated molecule fractalkine, may also contribute to this process. In addition to mononuclear phagocytes, T lymphocytes accumulate in human atherosclerotic plaques, where they may play important regulatory roles. Adhesion molecules such as intracellular adhesion molecule-1 (ICAM-1), overexpressed by endothelial cells overlying atheromas, may participate with VCAM-1 in the adhesion of T lymphocytes. In addition, a trio of chemokines induced by the T-cell

Fig. 6.2 The Predictive Power of Some Established and Emerging Risk Markers for Coronary and Peripheral Atherosclerosis. Relative risk for overall cardiovascular events (A) and the incidence of peripheral artery disease (B) from the Women's Health Study and the Physicians' Health Study, respectively. The whisker plots show the point estimates and confidence intervals (CI) for various emerging and established risk factors for atherosclerotic complications. The rank, order, and magnitude of risk of peripheral artery disease in the Women's Health Study and of cardiovascular events in the Physicians' Health Study due to these established and emerging risk factors resemble those reported earlier (not shown). (C) Direct comparison of C-reactive protein measured by high-sensitivity assay (hsCRP), systolic blood pressure (SBP), total cholesterol, and non–high density lipoprotein cholesterol (HDLC), adjusted for age, sex, smoking, diabetes mellitus (DM), body mass index (BMI), blood pressure (BP), triglycerides, alcohol, lipid levels, and hsCRP. Comparisons use data from 91,990 participants (5373 coronary heart disease events) from 31 studies. HTN, Hypertension; LDLC, low-density lipoprotein cholesterol; SD, standard deviation; sICAM-1, soluble intercellular adhesion molecule-1; TC:HDL ratio, total cholesterol:high-density lipoprotein ratio; TC:HDLC, total cholesterol:high-density lipoprotein cholesterol; VCAM-1, soluble vascular cell adhesion molecule. ([A] From Ridker PM. Clinical application of C-reactive protein for cardiovascular disease detection and prevention. Circulation. 2003;107:363–369. [B] Data from Ridker PM, Stampfer MJ, Rifai N. Novel risk factors for systemic atherosclerosis: a comparison of C-reactive protein, fibrinogen, homocysteine, lipoprotein(a), and standard cholesterol screening as predictors of peripheral artery disease. JAMA. 2001;285:2481–2485. [C] Modified from The Emerging Risk Factors Collaboration, Kaptoge S, Di Angelantonio E, et al. C-reactive protein concentration and risk of coronary heart disease, stroke, and mortality: an individual participant meta-analysis. Lancet. 2010;375:132–140.)

activator interferon gamma may promote the chemoattraction of adherent T cells into the arterial intima. Mast cells, long recognized in the leukocyte population of the arterial adventitia, also localize within the intimal lesions of atherosclerosis. Although vastly outnumbered by macrophages, mast cells may also contribute to lesion formation or complication. The chemokine exotaxin may participate in the recruitment of mast cells to the arterial intima.

Once present in the arterial intima, these various classes of leukocytes undergo diverse activation reactions that may potentiate atherogenesis. For example, monocytes mature into macrophages in the atherosclerotic plaque, where they overexpress a series of scavenger receptors that can capture modified lipoproteins; these then accumulate in the atherosclerotic intima.[75] Because their levels do not decrease as cells accumulate cholesterol, these scavenger receptors permit the formation of foam cells, a hallmark of the atheromatous plaque. Macrophages within the atherosclerotic intima proliferate and become a rich source of mediators, including reactive oxygen species and proinflammatory cytokines, that may contribute to the progression of atherosclerosis.[76]

The T cells in the atherosclerotic plaque also appear to modulate aspects of atherogenesis.[77-79] Gamma interferon, a strong activating stimulus for macrophages produced by activated type 1 helper T (Th1) cells, localizes in plaques. Indicators of the action of gamma interferon, such as induction of the class II major histocompatibility antigen molecules, provide evidence for the biologic activity of gamma interferon in atherosclerotic plaques.

Once recruited to the intima, white blood cells can perpetuate, amplify, or mitigate the ongoing inflammatory response that led to their recruitment.[78,80] The function of the "professional phagocytes" adds to the proinflammatory mediators elaborated by the intrinsic vascular wall cells, and perpetuates and amplifies the local inflammatory response. T-lymphocyte subsets may also quell inflammation. Th2 cells that produce interleukin-10 (IL-10), a putative antiatherosclerotic cytokine, also localize in plaques. Regulatory T cells (T$_{reg}$) produce transforming growth factor β (TGF-β), another antiinflammatory and fibrogenic mediator that may modulate plaque biology. The role in atherogenesis of another T-cell subset, Th17, remains unsettled. Dendritic cells, specialized in surveying the environment and presenting antigens to T cells, arrive early in the arterial intima of mice subjected to hyperlipidemia. The nature of the antigenic stimulus to T-cell activation remains speculative, although animal experiments have suggested some candidates.

Progression of Atherosclerosis

The recruitment of blood leukocytes and their activation in the arterial intima sets the stage for the progression of atherosclerosis. The proinflammatory mediators produced by these various cell types lead to the elaboration of factors that can stimulate the migration of smooth muscle cells from the tunica media into the intima. The normal human tunica intima contains resident smooth muscle cells. Growth factors produced locally by activated leukocytes provide a paracrine stimulus to the proliferation of smooth muscle cells.[81] Activated smooth muscle cells also appear capable of producing growth factors that can stimulate their own proliferation or that of their neighbors, an autocrine pathway of proliferation. Some evidence supports the ability of smooth muscle cells to undergo metaplasia to form macrophage-like foam cells.[82] Smooth muscle cells also die in atheromas. Depletion of smooth muscle cells may influence the biology of plaques by disturbing the repair and maintenance of the fibrous cap.

Other mediators present in atheromatous plaques, such as TGF-β, can augment the production of macromolecules of the extracellular matrix, including interstitial collagen. Thus "maturing" atherosclerotic lesions assume fibrous as well as fatty characteristics. Ultimately the established atherosclerotic plaque develops a central lipid core encapsulated in a fibrous extracellular matrix. In particular, the fibrous cap—the layer of connective tissue overlying the lipid core and separating it from the lumen of the artery—forms during this phase of lesion progression.

Calcification, another characteristic of the advancing atherosclerotic plaque, also involves tightly regulated biological functions.[83,84] The expression of certain calcium-binding proteins within the plaque may sequester calcium hydroxyapatite. Such deposits, far from fixed, can undergo resorption as well as deposition. Inflammatory pathways participate in the regulation of mineralization of atheromas.[85] Reminiscent of bone metabolism, activated macrophages within the plaque appear to function as osteoclasts. Indeed, mice deficient in macrophage colony-stimulating factor, the macrophage activator, show increased accumulation of calcified deposits.[86] This observation supports the dynamic nature of the calcium accretion in the plaque. Microparticles or vesicles may form the nidus of calcium mineral accretions in cardiovascular structures as well as plaques.[87,88]

The atheroma eventually develops a central region filled with lipid, inflammatory cells, and cellular debris. Macrophage death, including apoptotic (programmed) death, contributes to the formation of this lipid-rich core.[89,90] Indeed, classical pathologists often referred to this region of the plaque as the "necrotic core" of atheroma. Defective clearance of apoptotic cells, a process called "efferocytosis," may contribute to the formation of the plaque's lipid core.[91]

Thus, during the progression of atherosclerotic plaques, migration and proliferation of smooth muscle cells, accumulation of extracellular matrix, and calcification lead to the transition from the fatty streak, dominated by the lipid-laden macrophages known as foam cells, to the fibrocalcific plaque, which can produce arterial stenoses and other complications. Although this phase of lesion progression in humans may begin in youth, it often continues for many decades. Notably, atherosclerotic plaques often produce no symptoms during this generally prolonged phase of lesion evolution. Although traditionally viewed as a disease of middle and later life, the seeds of atherosclerosis are sown much earlier. This recognition highlights the importance of the early and aggressive reduction of risk factors, which is best accomplished by lifestyle modification rather than pharmacological intervention during the formative phase of the disease process.[92,93]

THE DIVERSITY OF ATHEROSCLEROSIS

Heterogeneity of Atherosclerosis Lesions

Although in the past we have focused on atherosclerosis of the coronary arteries, we now recognize increasingly that atherosclerosis reaches beyond the coronary bed.[1] For example, atherosclerosis underlies many ischemic strokes. Although peripheral artery disease jeopardizes limb more than life, the limitation of exercise capacity and the considerable burden of nonhealing ulcers and other complications render this manifestation of atherosclerosis important from both medical and economic points of view (see Chapter 17). In addition, atherosclerotic involvement of the renal arteries contributes to end-stage renal disease and refractory hypertension in many instances (see Chapter 22).

From a pathophysiologic perspective, atherosclerosis in different distributions of the arterial tree overlap considerably. Although the fundamental cellular and molecular events that underlie atherosclerosis in various arterial trees seem similar, certain complications appear distinct. For example, ectasia and eventual aneurysm formation affect the atherosclerotic abdominal aorta more commonly than do stenosis and thrombosis leading to total aortic occlusion. In addition, the aorta, and particularly the proximal portions of its trunk, appears especially important as a source for atheroemboli that may cause cerebral or renal infarctions.[94] Atherosclerosis of the extracranial vessels that perfuse the brain often leads to stenosis, but ulceration of carotid plaques with embolization of atheromatous material commonly causes transient ischemic attacks or monocular blindness.[95]

Some of the regional variations in the expressions of atherosclerosis may depend on embryologic factors. Endothelial cells in different regions of the arterial tree can display considerable heterogeneity, as determined by a variety of markers.[96] Developmental biologists have long recognized that smooth muscle cells found in various segments of the arterial tree may have distinct embryologic origins. For example, smooth muscle cells in the ascending aorta and other arteries of the upper body derive from neural crest cells rather than mesenchyme.[81] Thus smooth muscle cells can arise even from different germ layers in the lower body and neurectoderm in certain upper body arteries. The developmental biology of arteriogenesis and the determination of smooth muscle and endothelial cell lineages constitute a frontier of contemporary vascular biology research.

Atherosclerosis: A Focal or Diffuse Disease?

We classically understand atherosclerosis as a segmental process. Much of our traditional diagnostic armamentarium and treatment modalities aim to identify stenoses and restore flow by revascularization. Nonetheless, we recognize increasingly the diffuse nature of atherosclerosis. Classic comparison of histopathological examination with angiograms showed that the arteriogram vastly underestimates the involvement of coronary arteries by atherosclerosis. More recently, the application of intravascular ultrasound has renewed our appreciation of the diffuse nature of coronary atherosclerosis. Arterial stenoses often cause ischemia and bring the patient to the attention of clinicians. Various noninvasive modalities can disclose ischemia. Contrast angiography readily localizes the focal stenoses that most often cause demand ischemia. Yet cross-sectional images obtained by intravascular ultrasound reveal that segments of arteries that appear absolutely normal by angiography may nonetheless harbor a substantial burden of atherosclerotic disease.[97]

The process of arterial remodeling during atherogenesis explains this apparent paradox. During much of its life history, an atherosclerotic plaque grows in an outward, or abluminal, direction. Thus the plaque can grow silently without producing stenosis. Morphometric studies in nonhuman primates by Clarkson and colleagues first called attention to this compensatory enlargement of arteries, which preserves the lumen during atherogenesis.[98] Oft-cited studies by Glagov and colleagues established the relevance of this process to human coronary atherosclerosis.[99] Remodeling also occurs in atherosclerotic peripheral arteries.[100] Expansive arterial remodeling can influence the clinical manifestations of atheromas, with those with increased compensatory enlargement more prone to cause clinical events.[101] Luminal encroachment usually occurs relatively late in the life history of an atheromatous plaque.

Well-performed and systematic histopathologic studies have shown that atherosclerotic disease begins early in life. In the Pathobiological Determinants of Atherosclerosis in Youth (PDAY) study, the aortas and coronary arteries of Americans 34 years of age or younger who died of noncardiac causes revealed consistent involvement of the dorsal surface of the abdominal aorta by both fatty and raised arterial plaques.[102] The coronary arteries, including the proximal portion of the left anterior descending coronary artery, also disclosed involvement, even in this young population. The Bogalusa Heart Study also showed a correlation between risk factors during life and the degree of atherosclerotic involvement at autopsy.[103] These systematic observations agree

with reports of a substantial burden of coronary arterial atherosclerosis in young American male casualties during the Korean and Vietnam wars.[104] Indeed, maternal hypercholesterolemia associates with the formation of fatty streaks in fetuses.[105]

These various data indicate that atherosclerosis affects arteries far more diffusely than we believed only a few years ago. The process begins much earlier in life than is generally acknowledged. Indeed, intravascular ultrasound studies have shown that 1 in 6 American teenagers has significant atherosclerotic involvement of the coronary arteries.[106] These findings have considerable importance for understanding the pathophysiology of the clinical manifestations of atherosclerosis. They also have important implications for the management of this disease (see later).

Shear Stress and Atheroprotection: Why Atherosclerosis Begins Where It Does

The foregoing section emphasizes the diffuse nature of atherosclerosis in adults. Yet both in humans and experimental animals, atherosclerosis begins in certain stereotyped locales. The predilection of atherosclerosis for branch points and flow dividers appears quite consistent across species.

Why do these sites have a predisposition to early atherogenesis? Decades of sophisticated biomechanical analysis have established that atheromas tend to form at sites of disturbed blood flow, particularly areas of low shear stress.[72,107,108] Endothelial cells can sense shear stress through a variety of mechanotransduction mechanisms (Fig. 6.3).[109,110] In areas of laminar shear stress in vivo and in vitro, endothelial cells align their long axes parallel to the direction of flow. At branch points and dividers in the arterial tree, the well-ordered cobblestone array of the endothelial monolayer changes—cells appear more polygonally and irregularly shaped. Areas of low shear stress show heightened endothelial cell turnover, increased permeability, and prolonged retention of lipoprotein particles in the subendothelial regions of the intima. Such data, accumulated over many decades, provide answers to the question of what goes awry at sites of lesion predilection.

A distinct and complementary hypothesis can also explain the focality of atherosclerosis initiation. Transcriptional profiling provides a "snapshot" of the expression of a large number of genes in a single experiment. The pattern of genes expressed by endothelial cells subjected to controlled physiologic levels of laminar shear stress in vitro differs strikingly from that of resting endothelial cells in vitro. A number of genes differentially expressed by endothelial cells experiencing laminar shear stress appear to have "atheroprotective" functions. A number of putative atheroprotective genes rise selectively under conditions of physiologic laminar shear stress. These findings suggest that regions of undisturbed, laminar shear stress enjoy tonic endogenous antioxidant, vasodilatory, and antiinflammatory properties conferred by the function of these putative "atheroprotective" genes.[72] The transcription factor Krüppel-like factor 2 (KLF-2) has emerged as an integrator of shear stress and altered endothelial functions implicated in "atheroprotection."[111]

At regions of disturbed flow—for example, near branch points and flow dividers—expression of these endogenous atheroprotective genes should decline. Indeed, regions predisposed to early lesion formation show activation of nuclear factor kappa B (NF-κB), the master regulator of inflammatory gene expression.[112] Because nitric oxide can antagonize the activation of NF-κB, the absence of laminar flow in these regions may explain, at least in part, the tendency of nascent atheromas to form at such sites.[113]

Thus atherosclerosis is both a focal and diffuse disease. It begins focally for reasons we understand in increasing detail. The stenoses that cause flow-limiting lesions tend to localize in similar regions.

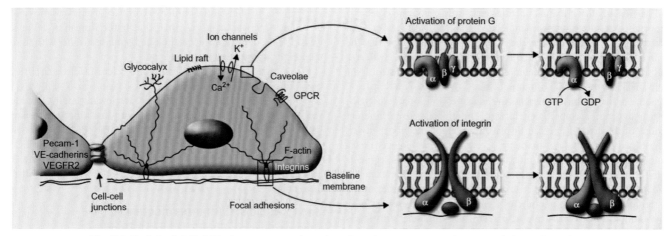

Fig. 6.3 Endothelial Cell Mechanosensors. Location of mechanosensors such as cytoskeleton, integrins, cell-cell junctions, caveolae, lipid rafts, cell surface glycocalyx, G protein–coupled receptors *(GPCR)*, and ion channels. While mechanosensors in the apical region (luminal) are activated directly by shear stress (such as G proteins), the cytoskeleton (represented by actin fibers, F-actin) is responsible for transmitting forces to the mechanosensors at the basal region of endothelial cells (such as integrins). The activation of G protein occurs due to local changes in plasma membrane fluidity; therefore it is directly due to shear stress and independent from an agonist, causing hydrolysis of guanosine triphosphate *(GTP)* into guanosine diphosphate *(GDP)*. Shear stress changes the structure of mechanosensitive integrins from inactive to active, possibly due to transmission of the mechanical force to the cytoskeleton. In their active conformation, integrins have higher affinity for cognate proteins in the extracellular matrix. *VE,* Vascular endothelial; *VEGFR2,* vascular endothelial growth factor receptor 2. (From Fernandes DC, Araujo TLS, Laurindo FRM, Tanaka LY. Hemodynamic forces in the endothelium: from mechanotransduction to implications on development of atherosclerosis. In: da Luz PL, Libby P, Chagas ACP, Laurindo FRM, eds. *Endothelium and Cardiovascular Diseases: Vascular Biology and Clinical Syndromes.* Cambridge, MA: Elsevier; 2018.)

Much of our diagnostic and therapeutic activity in contemporary cardiology and vascular medicine has traditionally focused on these stenoses. Advances in both arterial biology and clinical science heighten our appreciation of the diffuse distribution of atherosclerosis and the systemic nature of the risk factors that promote its development. These considerations help to clarify how optimum medical management with systemic therapies can confer benefits on par with those derived from revascularization procedures in many patients.

The Pathophysiology of the Thrombotic Complications of Atherosclerosis

As noted, flow-limiting stenoses have driven much of the diagnostic and therapeutic activity in clinical atherosclerosis for many decades. Patients with flow-limiting lesions often experience symptoms due to ischemia—such as angina pectoris in the coronary circulation and intermittent claudication in peripheral artery disease. We can readily diagnose ischemia by various noninvasive modalities. We can localize stenoses through invasive and noninvasive angiographic techniques. The percutaneous and surgical approaches can effectively relieve ischemia due to focal stenoses but do not address lesions that do not limit flow. In many cases acute thrombosis does not occur in the most tightly narrowed segments of an artery.

A common confusion surrounds the distinction between lesion size and degree of stenosis. Based on our traditional angiographically centered view of atherosclerosis, many assume that lesions that cause high-grade stenoses are larger than those that cause less obstruction. This fallacy fails to consider the importance of outward remodeling or compensatory enlargement. The outward growth of most atherosclerotic plaques before they begin to encroach on the lumen protects the lumen from obstruction and conceals the growing lesion from visualization by angiography until the later stages of its evolution. Thus low-grade

stenoses do not equate with smaller plaques. Indeed, larger and eccentrically remodeled plaques may cause acute coronary syndromes more frequently than smaller plaques that do not exhibit compensatory enlargement and/or produce greater degrees of stenosis.[114]

Concordant evidence from several avenues of investigation suggests that a physical disruption of the atherosclerotic plaque commonly precipitates arterial thromboses.[115,116] Four mechanisms of plaque disruption may cause thrombosis or rapid plaque expansion (Fig. 6.4).[117] A through-and-through fracture of the plaque's fibrous cap causes most fatal coronary thromboses (see Fig. 6.4). Our group hypothesized a model of the pathophysiology of this common mechanism of atherosclerotic plaque disruption, focusing on the metabolism of interstitial collagen. This extracellular matrix macromolecule accounts for much of the biomechanical strength of the plaque's fibrous cap. Further hypothesizing that inflammation regulates the metabolism of interstitial forms of collagen and might regulate the stability of an atherosclerotic plaque (Fig. 6.5), we found that certain proinflammatory cytokines expressed in the atherosclerotic plaque can inhibit the ability of the smooth muscle cell to synthesize the new collagen required to repair and maintain the integrity of the plaque's fibrous cap. The signature Th1 cytokine gamma interferon can inhibit the expression of interstitial collagen genes in human vascular smooth muscle cells.[118]

The interstitial collagen triple helix resists breakdown by most proteinases. We described the overexpression of proteolytic enzymes specialized in the catabolism of collagen in the atherosclerotic plaque and further demonstrated that inflammatory mediators found in the atheroma can enhance the expression of these collagenolytic enzymes, members of the MMP family. Cells in human atheromas overexpress all three members of the human interstitial collagenase family (MMP-1, MMP-13, and MMP-8). We have furnished evidence that collagen breakdown occurs in situ in human atherosclerotic plaques.[115] These findings indicate that the interstitial collagenase MMPs exist in their

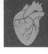

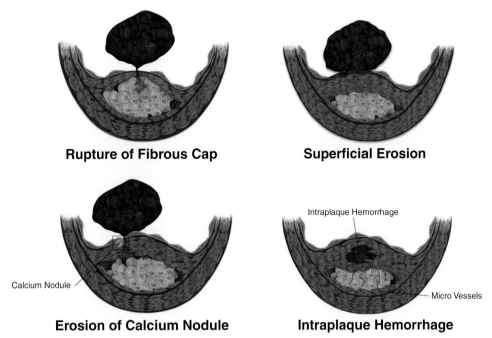

Rupture of Fibrous Cap

Superficial Erosion

Calcium Nodule

Erosion of Calcium Nodule

Intraplaque Hemorrhage

Micro Vessels

Intraplaque Hemorrhage

Fig. 6.4 Mechanisms of Plaque Disruption. Rupture of the fibrous cap *(upper left)* causes two-thirds to three-fourths of fatal coronary thrombosis. Superficial erosion *(upper right)* occurs in one-fifth to one-fourth of all cases of fatal coronary thrombosis. Certain populations, such as diabetic individuals and women, appear more susceptible to superficial erosion as a mechanism of plaque disruption and thrombosis. Erosion of a calcium nodule may also cause plaque disruption and thrombosis *(lower left)*. In addition, the friable microvessels in the base of the atherosclerotic plaque may rupture and cause intraplaque hemorrhage *(lower right)*. The consequent local generation of thrombin may stimulate smooth muscle proliferation, migration, and collagen synthesis, promoting fibrosis and plaque expansion on a subacute basis. Severe intraplaque hemorrhage can also cause sudden lesion expansion by a mass effect acutely. (From Libby P, Theroux P. Pathophysiology of coronary artery disease. *Circulation.* 2005;111:3481–3488.)

active forms rather than their precursor zymogen forms. Furthermore, the demonstration of collagenolysis in situ indicates that these collagenases overwhelm their endogenous inhibitors, including the tissue inhibitors of MMPs (TIMPs). A preponderance of proteinases over their inhibitors prevails in the atherosclerotic plaque.

Colocalization of proteinases with inflammatory cells and regulation of their expression by products of inflammatory cells strongly implicate disordered collagen metabolism as a key mechanism for atherosclerotic plaque destabilization. Experiments using genetically altered mice have demonstrated the importance of collagen catabolism due to MMP collagenases in the regulation of the steady-state level of this extracellular matrix macromolecule in experimental atheromas using both loss-of-function and gain-of-function strategies.[115] The finding that inflammatory mediators elicit overexpression of MMP collagenases from macrophages supports the view that inflammation promotes the thrombotic complications of atherosclerosis. This mechanistic insight aids the understanding of how biomarkers of inflammation can help predict such events.

Superficial erosion of the endothelial monolayer constitutes an important cause of a minority of coronary thromboses. The morphology, cellular content, and biochemical features of plaques complicated by erosion differ distinctly from those that have undergone rupture of the fibrous cap (see Figs. 6.4 and 6.6).[116,119,120] Eroded plaques have abundant extracellular matrix and many smooth muscle cells but little lipid and few macrophages, whereas plaques that rupture tend to have thin fibrous caps, large lipid accumulations, and abundant macrophages but a relative paucity of smooth muscle cells in the regions of fracture.

Women, the elderly, and patients with diabetes may have a higher frequency of superficial erosion as a cause of fatal throm-

bosis than do younger male hypercholesterolemic individuals. Various molecular and cellular mechanisms may underlie superficial erosion.[121] Excessive proteolysis of the extracellular matrix macromolecules that make up the subendothelial basement membrane may predispose toward endothelial desquamation and superficial erosion. Apoptosis of endothelial cells may also promote superficial erosion. Various proinflammatory stimuli can sensitize endothelial cells to apoptosis, some through engagement of the innate immune receptor Toll-like receptor 2 (TLR2).[122,123] In addition, hypochlorous acid, a product of myeloperoxidase—an enzyme found in leukocytes in atherosclerotic plaques—can provoke endothelial cell apoptosis.[124] Local generation of tissue factor from dying endothelial cells may also contribute to thrombosis at sites of superficial erosion.

Atherosclerotic plaques often harbor rich plexi of microvessels. The neovascularization of plaques provides an additional portal for trafficking of leukocytes, which may promote the inflammatory process. Neovessels in the plaque, like those in the diabetic retina, may be friable and fragile. Intraplaque hemorrhage due to the disruption of microvessels may cause sudden plaque expansion (see Fig. 6.4). Local generation of thrombin and other mediators associated with coagulation in situ may promote lesion growth. For example, platelet-derived growth factor (PDGF), TGF-β, and platelet factor 4 (PF4), released by platelets at sites of microvascular hemorrhage and intramural thrombosis may hasten local fibrosis. Thrombin can stimulate smooth muscle cell migration, division, and collagen synthesis. Thus microvascular disruption, though not provoking an occlusive thrombus, may promote lesion evolution nonetheless.

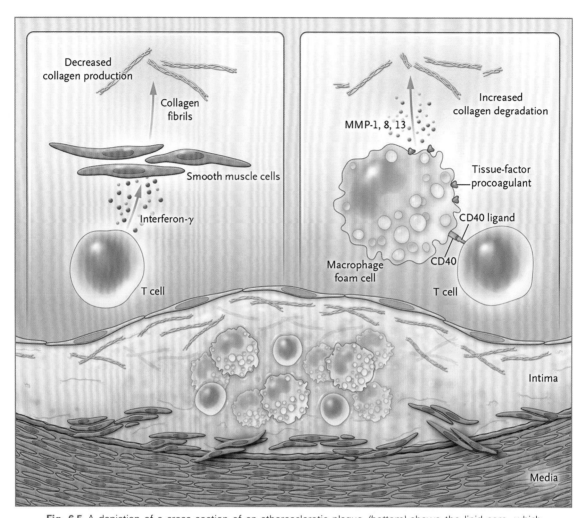

Fig. 6.5 A depiction of a cross section of an atherosclerotic plaque *(bottom)* shows the lipid core, which contains macrophage foam cells *(yellow)* and T cells *(blue)*. The intima and media also contain arterial smooth muscle cells *(red)*, which produce arterial collagen (depicted as triple helical coiled structures). Activated T cells (of the type-1 helper T-cell subtype) secrete cytokine interferon-γ, which inhibits the production of new interstitial collagen that can repair and maintain the plaque's protective fibrous cap *(upper left)*. The T cells can also activate the macrophages in the intimal lesion by expressing CD40 ligand (CD154), which engages its cognate receptor (CD40) on the phagocyte. This inflammatory signaling causes overproduction of interstitial collagenases (matrix metalloproteinases *[MMP]* 1, 8, and 13), which effect the initial rate-limiting step in collagen breakdown *(top right)*. CD40 ligation also causes macrophages to elaborate tissue-factor procoagulant. Thus inflammatory signaling puts the collagen in the plaque's fibrous cap in double jeopardy—decreased synthesis and increased breakdown—weakening the cap and making it susceptible to rupture. Inflammatory activation also augments the production of tissue factor, which triggers thrombus formation over disrupted plaque. These mechanisms illustrate inflammation in the plaque can precipitate the thrombotic complications of atherosclerosis, including acute coronary syndromes (From Libby P. Mechanisms of acute coronary syndromes and their implications for therapy. *N Engl J Med.* 2013;369:2004–2013.)

Erosion through the intima of a calcified nodule represents another less common form of atherosclerotic plaque disruption associated with thrombosis (see Fig. 6.4). The active metabolism of calcium hydroxyapatite, with its accretion and removal as described earlier, can contribute to calcium accumulation in regions of atherosclerotic plaques. The tendency of atheromas to accumulate calcium has given rise to clinical testing. Increasing evidence supports the contention that the amount of coronary artery calcification correlates with the burden of atherosclerotic disease. Moreover, considerable data suggest a correlation between calcium score and risk of future cardiovascular events. Yet neither calcium scoring nor any other imaging modality (such as computed tomographic coronary angiography) has garnered evidence that it can direct therapy that improves outcome in atherosclerosis.

Indeed, statin treatment increases coronary calcification but decreases events.[125,126] Thus there is no rational basis for serially performing coronary artery calcium scoring in individuals on statins.

The Mutability of the Atherosclerotic Plaque

The classic concept of atherosclerosis assumed a steady, relentless, and continuous progression of the disease. But serial angiographic studies suggest that stenoses evolve in a discontinuous fashion, with periods of relative quiescence punctuated by spurts in growth. Our current understanding of plaque pathobiology suggests a plausible mechanism to explain this angiographically discontinuous evolution of arterial stenoses. Careful study of the coronary arteries of individuals who succumb to noncardiac death and of coronary arteries perfusion-fixed in the

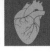

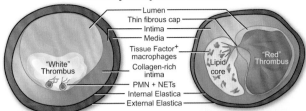

Coronary Artery Cross Sections

Lumen
Thin fibrous cap
Intima
Media
Tissue Factor⁺ macrophages
Collagen-rich intima
PMN + NETs
Internal Elastica
External Elastica

"White" Thrombus

Lipid core

"Red" Thrombus

Thrombosis due to Erosion	Thrombosis due to Rupture
Fibrous cap thick & intact	Thin fibrous cap with fissure
"White" platelet-rich thrombus	"Red" fibrin-rich thrombus
Collagen trigger	Tissue Factor trigger
Smooth muscle cells prominent	Macrophages prominent
Often sessile, non-occlusive Thrombus	Often occlusive thrombus
Usually less remodelled outward	Usually expansively remodelled
Neutrophil extracellular traps (NETs) involved	Less NET involvement?
More frequent in non-STEMI?	More frequently cause STEMI?

Fig. 6.6 Distinct mechanisms may trigger coronary thrombosis due to superficial erosion versus fibrous cap rupture. This diagram depicts cross sections of coronary arteries. On the left, thrombosis due to erosion shows a sessile, "white" thrombus superimposed on an extracellular matrix–rich lesion with little or no expansive remodeling. Endothelial cell sloughing or death can expose plaque collagen, which can initiate such platelet-rich thrombi. Recruited polymorphonuclear leukocytes (PMN) can contribute to a second wave of thrombus amplification and propagation due to their elaboration of neutrophil extracellular traps (NETs). Further, erosion may associate more frequently with non–ST-segment elevation myocardial infarction (non-STEMI) than with STEMI.[5] The right side of this illustration depicts thrombosis due to rupture, which typically results from a lesion with a fissured thin fibrous cap. Such thrombi tend to slant toward a "red" fibrin-rich clot. Tissue factor derived from the abundant macrophages probably triggers thrombosis in plaque rupture. In thrombosis due to plaque rupture, the underlying lesions may more often exhibit expansive remodeling and the thrombi may more often occlude the vessel and provoke a STEMI versus a non-STEMI. (From Libby P. Superficial erosion and the precision management of acute coronary syndromes: not one-size-fits-all. *Eur Heart J.* 2017;38:801–803.)

operating room from hearts of transplantation recipients with ischemic cardiomyopathy as well as observations of cholesterol-fed nonhuman primates all indicate that areas of plaque disruption or superficial erosion with nonocclusive mural thrombus formation occur frequently. The picture that arises from an amalgamation of these human and experimental observations indicates that most plaque disruptions with thrombosis in situ do not proceed to a total occlusion and indeed usually pass unnoticed by the patient or physician (Fig. 6.7). For various reasons, plaque disruptions with mural thrombosis may not proceed to a disastrous occlusive thrombosis in all events. In many patients, the endogenous fibrinolytic mechanisms or antithrombotic effects of dietary or pharmacologic intervention may prevent thrombi from propagating. Larger arteries such as the aorta have sufficient flow to prevent mural thrombi from progressing to total occlusion in most instances. Indeed, although inspection of the aortas of many patients with atherosclerosis discloses many ulcerated lesions with mural thrombi, aortic occlusion due to thrombosis fortunately occurs relatively rarely (Fig. 6.8).

The failure of most mural thrombi to progress to total occlusion does not imply that such events have a benign course. Although subclinical at the time that they occur, the mural thrombi elicit a local "wound healing" response that tends to promote plaque progression. Indeed, one of the types of "crisis" in the history of a plaque that can lead to its sudden evolution, as disclosed by serial angiographic studies, likely reflects such a scenario (see Fig. 6.7). A localized plaque disrup-

tion with mural thrombus can engender a healing response induced by platelet products released at short range, such as TGF-β, a potent stimulus to collagen gene expression by smooth muscle cells. PDGF, also released during platelet aggregation, stimulates smooth muscle cell migration. Thrombin locally generated at sites of thrombosis can stimulate smooth muscle cell proliferation, migration, and collagen gene expression. All of these molecular and cellular mechanisms conspire to promote a cycle of smooth muscle cell migration, proliferation, and local collagen synthesis. Quite plausibly, this scenario leads to evolution from a lipid-rich plaque with abundant inflammatory cells to a more fibrous lesion, rich in connective tissue, often with a paucity of inflammatory cells due to their death or departure, accretion of calcium deposits, and a relative lack of lipid accumulation. Careful study of atheromas obtained at autopsy shows signs of healed plaque disruption in some fibrous lesions (Fig. 6.9).[127,128]

The biologic scenario just described depicts a more dynamic life history of the atherosclerotic plaque than that heretofore recognized (see Fig. 6.7). The heterogeneity of human atherosclerotic plaques, a concept now gaining considerable currency, highlights the importance of the qualitative characteristics of a lesion, not just its size. Whereas previous concepts emphasized the structure of atherosclerotic plaques, contemporary thinking accords a greater contribution to the biologic characteristics of the plaque.

"Stable" Versus "Vulnerable" Plaques

This recognition of the heterogeneity of atherosclerotic plaques has fostered the adoption of a dichotomous view of atheromas—"stable" versus "vulnerable" plaques. The notion of the vulnerable plaque has engendered considerable interest from pathologists and practitioners alike. Current cardiologic parlance uses the term "vulnerable plaque" to designate a lesion characterized by a thin fibrous cap, a large lipid core, and a surfeit of inflammatory cells. Use of this term and its opposite, the "stable plaque," extends findings largely obtained at postmortem examination of humans who succumbed to acute myocardial infarction. Although the dichotomization of plaques into vulnerable and stable provides a useful shorthand, we should exercise care in extrapolating morphologic findings uncritically to foretell clinical complications.[129]

This pigeon-holing of plaques has engendered considerable effort to develop methods for identifying vulnerable or high-risk lesions, but such a view of atherosclerosis oversimplifies a disease of staggering complexity. For example, considerable evidence suggests that a given arterial tree has not one but many vulnerable plaques. Angioscopic and intravascular ultrasonographic study of coronary arteries as well as interpretation of angiographic observations support the multiplicity of disrupted plaques in patients with acute coronary syndromes.[130,131]

Inflammation may provide a mechanistic link between "instability" of coronary and carotid plaques in the same individuals. As previously mentioned, the aorta in an atherosclerotic individual often shows multiple ulcerated lesions, often within millimeters of fatty streaks, raised fibrous lesions, and resorbing, healing thrombi (see Fig. 6.7). Thus the quest to identify a single vulnerable plaque underestimates the complexity of the clinical challenge. Our broader view of the risk of atherosclerotic complications seeks the "vulnerable patient" and targets intervention more widely than to a single vulnerable plaque.[132]

How could one approach such a vulnerable patient? Experimental and clinical considerations provide grounds for considerable optimism in this regard. Atherosclerosis exhibits considerable mutability; lipid lowering and other manipulations can alter features of plaques paramount to the clinical expression of the disease. Preclinical studies have shown that lipid lowering by diet or by treatment with statins can alter features

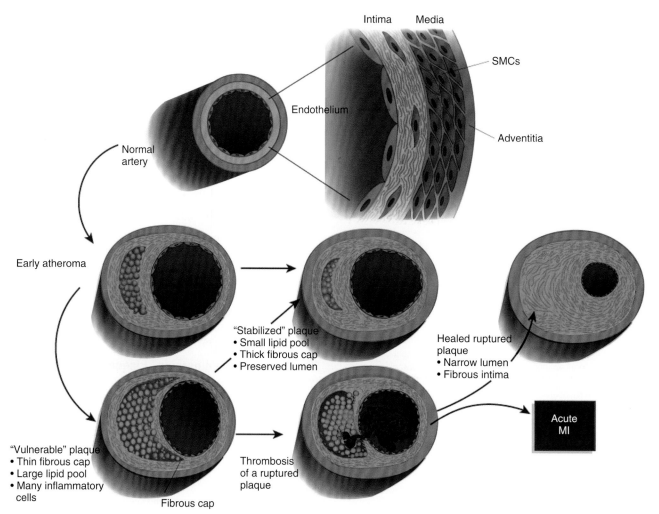

Fig. 6.7 Schematic of the Life History of an Atheroma. The normal human coronary artery has a typical trilaminar structure. The endothelial cells in contact with the blood in the arterial lumen rest on a basement membrane. The intimal layer in adult humans generally contains a small amount of smooth muscle cells *(SMCs)* scattered within the intimal extracellular matrix. The internal elastic lamina forms the barrier between the tunica intima and the underlying tunica media. The media consists of multiple layers of SMCs, much more tightly packed than in the diffusely thickened intima and embedded in a matrix rich in elastin as well as collagen. In early atherogenesis, recruitment of inflammatory cells and the accumulation of lipids lead to the formation of a lipid-rich core, as the artery enlarges in an outward, abluminal direction to accommodate the expansion of the intima. If inflammatory conditions prevail and risk factors such as dyslipidemia persist, the lipid core can grow and proteinases secreted by the activated leukocytes can degrade extracellular matrix, whereas proinflammatory cytokines such as interferon-gamma can limit the synthesis of new collagen. These changes can thin the fibrous cap and render it friable and susceptible to rupture. When the plaque ruptures, blood coming in contact with the tissue factor in the plaque coagulates; platelets activated by thrombin generated from the coagulation cascade as well as by contact with collagen in the intimal compartment instigate thrombus formation. If the thrombus occludes the vessel persistently, an acute myocardial infarction *(MI)* can result. The thrombus may eventually resorb due to endogenous or therapeutic thrombolysis, but a wound-healing response triggered by thrombin generated during blood coagulation can stimulate smooth muscle proliferation. Platelet-derived growth factor released from activated platelets stimulates SMC migration. Transforming growth factor β, also released from activated platelets, stimulates interstitial collagen production. This increased migration, proliferation, and extracellular matrix synthesis by SMCs thickens the fibrous cap and causes further expansion of the intima, often in an inward direction, constricting the lumen. Such stenotic lesions, produced by the luminal encroachment of the fibrosed plaque, may restrict flow, particularly in situations of increased cardiac demand, leading to ischemia and commonly provoking symptoms such as angina pectoris. Such advanced stenotic plaques, being more fibrous, may prove less susceptible to rupture and renewed thrombosis. Lipid lowering can reduce lipid content and calm the intimal inflammatory response, yielding a more stable plaque with a thick fibrous cap and a preserved lumen *(center).* (From Libby P. Inflammation in atherosclerosis. *Nature.* 2002;420:868–874.)

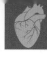

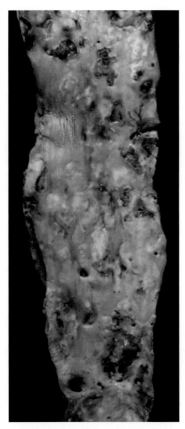

Fig. 6.8 Widespread Atheromatous Involvement of the Abdominal Aorta in a Patient With Atherosclerosis. Note the variety of atheromas at different stages of evolution within a few centimeters of one another. There are ulcerated plaques, raised lesions, and fatty streaks among other types of lesions demonstrated in this example.

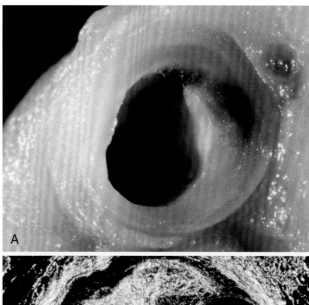

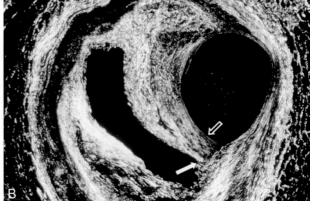

Fig. 6.9 Hemorrhage, Thrombosis, and Plaque Healing as a Mechanism of Atheroma Progression. (A) Photograph of a coronary artery with a plaque rupture that has led to an intraplaque hematoma without an occlusive thrombus. As explained in the text, thrombin and platelet products such as platelet-derived growth factor and transforming growth factor β, elaborated locally at the site of microthrombosis and hematoma formation, can stimulate fibrosis. (B) This Sirius red–stained preparation of a cross section of a coronary artery shows an area of plaque rupture (*solid arrow*) that healed, causing further accretion of a layer of collagen (*open arrow*) and luminal encroachment. This example illustrates the "archaeology" of the atherosclerotic plaque: distant plaque rupture, followed by healing and fibrosis, with progression of the lesion to stenosis. Note that the arterial lumen at the time of the original plaque rupture would not have shown a critical narrowing. (Courtesy the late Prof. Michael J. Davies.)

of plaques associated with vulnerability in humans, such as proteinase activity or collagen content.[115] Studies in atherosclerosis-prone mice have demonstrated that interruption of inflammatory signaling pathways or manipulation of TGF-β can alter features of plaques associated with their propensity to rupture and provoke thrombosis. In addition to structural changes relating to the collagen content of plaques that may determine their biomechanical integrity, interventions such as lipid lowering can reduce the expression of tissue factor, hence lowering the thrombogenic potential of the atherosclerotic plaque.[115]

Clinical studies also support the mutability of atherosclerosis, abundantly demonstrated in animals by the experiments described earlier. Aggressive lipid-lowering therapy with a statin can arrest or even reverse the accumulation of atherosclerotic plaque, as determined by serial ultrasonographic study.[2,133–135] These preclinical and clinical observations inspire considerable optimism regarding our ability to manipulate atherosclerotic plaques to benefit patient outcomes. The disease appears much more mutable than has generally been appreciated in the past.

ATHEROSCLEROSIS: A SYSTEMIC DISEASE

Our traditional medical focus on atherosclerosis as a segmental disease caused by cholesterol accumulation has undergone an accelerated revision. We increasingly understand the global nature of factors that encompass the entire metabolic state of the patient, not just the serum cholesterol level. As the spectrum of risk factors in our population shifts, our attention must likewise broaden to encompass not just hypercholesterolemia but also the dyslipidemia associated with the components of the metabolic syndrome and diabetes. As elevated LDL

cholesterol and smoking recede as risk factors in our society, we must acknowledge the increasing contribution of obesity, insulin resistance, and triglyceride-rich lipoproteins.

We also recognize increasingly the importance of atherosclerosis beyond the coronary arteries. Our purview should now embrace the entire arterial tree with all of its beds. We must strive to fill the knowledge gaps about regional differences in human atherosclerosis as well as to clarify differences in the biology and clinical manifestations of atherosclerosis associated with the shifting pattern of risk factors.

Our comprehension of the pathophysiology of atherosclerosis has undergone a revolution in recent decades. Emerging data and deeper understanding of this process will continue to change our concepts of this disease in the future. We should take immense satisfaction in the therapeutic inroads furnished by contemporary pharmacologic tools. The reduction in CHD and cerebrovascular events accruing from such treatments as statins and angiotensin converting enzyme inhibitors has changed medicine irrevocably, and provides striking benefits to patients. The advent of PCSK9 inhibitors constitutes a victory of rapid translation of fundamental science to effective therapies.[10] The therapeutic advances that have emerged from the application of progress in basic science have proved effective in randomized clinical trials furnishing cardiovascular medicine with an enviable and unparalleled database for the practice of evidence-based medicine.

Yet, despite the victory of clinical science, much remains undone. The majority of cardiovascular events still occur despite optimal therapy that addresses multiple facets of our current understanding of the pathophysiology of this disease. Our challenge for the future is clear. We must strive to turn the tide on the alarming trends toward increased cardiovascular risk due to obesity and physical inactivity. We must not relent in our quest to advance the scientific understanding of atherogenesis and the translation to innovative therapies that address the residual and ever-growing burden of disease.

Many of the current landmark studies in the cardiovascular arena have focused on death and acute coronary syndromes as "major adverse coronary events." These end points offer relative ease of study, adjudication, and quantification. Although the mortality of patients with peripheral artery disease often comes from coronary artery disease, we must not lose sight of the enormous impediment to their quality of life due to intermittent claudication and the loss of ability to communicate and live independently due to cerebrovascular disease. In addition to the human costs of these manifestations of noncoronary atherosclerosis, our society shoulders a substantial economic burden due to the ravages of peripheral artery and cerebrovascular disease. We must pursue these issues with the same fervor we have accorded to the exploration of coronary artery disease. This goal will become even more important as elder segments of our population continue to increase in numbers. The powerful tools available to investigators today provide grounds for optimism. Further inroads against the residual morbidity and mortality from atherosclerosis will emerge from future application of basic science to alter the biology of this disease, regarded not so long ago as an inevitable companion of the aging process.

REFERENCES

1. Gallino A, Aboyans V, Diehm C, et al. Non-coronary atherosclerosis. *Eur Heart J.* 2014;35:1112–1119.
2. Libby P. How does lipid lowering prevent coronary events? New insights from human imaging trials. *Eur Heart J.* 2015;36:472–474.
3. Libby P, Hansson GK. Inflammation and immunity in diseases of the arterial tree: players and layers. *Circ Res.* 2015;116:307–311.
4. Anitschkow N, Chalatow S. On experimental cholesterin steatosis and its significance in the origin of some pathological processes, 1913. *Arteriosclerosis.* 1983;3:178–182.
5. Goldstein JL, Brown MS. A century of cholesterol and coronaries: from plaques to genes to statins. *Cell.* 2015;161:161–172.
6. Goldstein JL, Brown MS. The LDL receptor. *Arterioscler Thromb Vasc Biol.* 2009;29:431–438.
7. Steinberg D. *The Cholesterol Wars: The Skeptics vs. the Preponderance of Evidence.* 1 ed. San Diego: Academic Press; 2007.
8. Collins R, Reith C, Emberson J, et al. Interpretation of the evidence for the efficacy and safety of statin therapy. *Lancet.* 2016;388:2532–2561.
9. Pedersen TR. The success story of LDL cholesterol lowering. *Circ Res.* 2016;118:721–731.
10. Sabatine MS, Giugliano RP, Keech AC, et al. Evolocumab and clinical outcomes in patients with cardiovascular disease. *N Engl J Med.* 2017;376:1713–1722.
11. Ference BA, Ginsberg HN, Graham I, et al. Low-density lipoproteins cause atherosclerotic cardiovascular disease. 1. Evidence from genetic, epidemiologic, and clinical studies. A consensus statement from the European Atherosclerosis Society Consensus Panel. *Eur Heart J.* 2017;38:2459–2472.
12. Di Angelantonio E, Sarwar N, Perry P, et al. Major lipids, apolipoproteins, and risk of vascular disease. *JAMA.* 2009;302:1993–2000.
13. Lloyd-Jones DM, Evans JC, Levy D. Hypertension in adults across the age spectrum: current outcomes and control in the community. *JAMA.* 2005;294:466–472.
14. Blood Pressure Lowering Treatment Trialists' Collaboration. Blood pressure-lowering treatment based on cardiovascular risk: a meta-analysis of individual patient data. *Lancet.* 2014;384:591–598.
15. ALLHAT. Officers and Coordinators for the ALLHAT Collaborative Research Group. The Antihypertensive and Lipid-Lowering Treatment to Prevent Heart Attack Trial. Major outcomes in high-risk hypertensive patients randomized to angiotensin-converting enzyme inhibitor or calcium channel blocker vs diuretic: The Antihypertensive and Lipid-Lowering Treatment to Prevent Heart Attack Trial (ALLHAT). *JAMA.* 2002;288:2981–2997.
16. Onuigbo MA. ALLHAT findings revisited in the context of subsequent analyses, other trials, and meta-analyses. *Arch Intern Med.* 2009;169:1810. author reply 1810-1811.
17. Yusuf S, Lonn E. The SPRINT and the HOPE-3 trial in the context of other blood pressure-lowering trials. *JAMA Cardiol.* 2016;1:857–858.
18. National Center for Chronic Disease Prevention and Health Promotion (US). *Office on Smoking and Health. The health consequences of smoking—50 years of progress: a report of the Surgeon General.* Atlanta: Centers for Disease Control and Prevention; 2014.
19. Yanbaeva DG, Dentener MA, Creutzberg EC, et al. Systemic effects of smoking. *Chest.* 2007;131:1557–1566.
20. Churg A, Wang RD, Tai H, et al. Macrophage metalloelastase mediates acute cigarette smoke-induced inflammation via tumor necrosis factor-alpha release. *Am J Respir Crit Care Med.* 2003;167:1083–1089.
21. Jaiswal S, Fontanillas P, Flannick J, et al. Age-related clonal hematopoiesis associated with adverse outcomes. *N Engl J Med.* 2014;371:2488–2498.
22. Jaiswal S, Natarajan P, Silver AJ, et al. Clonal hematopoiesis and risk of atherosclerotic cardiovascular disease. *N Engl J Med.* 2017;377:111–121.
23. Bhupathiraju SN, Grodstein F, Stampfer MJ, et al. Exogenous hormone use: oral contraceptives, postmenopausal hormone therapy, and health outcomes in the Nurses' Health Study. *Am J Public Health.* 2016;106:1631–1637.
24. Marjoribanks J, Farquhar C, Roberts H, et al. Long-term hormone therapy for perimenopausal and postmenopausal women. *Cochrane Database Syst Rev.* 2017;1: CD004143.
25. Bassuk SS, Manson JE. The timing hypothesis: do coronary risks of menopausal hormone therapy vary by age or time since menopause onset? *Metabolism.* 2016;65:794–803.
26. Khera AV, Kathiresan S. Genetics of coronary artery disease: discovery, biology and clinical translation. *Nat Rev Genet.* 2017;8:331–334.
27. Siddiqi HK, Kiss D, Rader D. HDL-cholesterol and cardiovascular disease: rethinking our approach. *Curr Opin Cardiol.* 2015;30:536–542.
28. Libby P. Triglycerides on the rise: should we swap seats on the seesaw? *Eur Heart J.* 2015;36:774–776.
29. Musunuru K, Kathiresan S. Surprises from genetic analyses of lipid risk factors for atherosclerosis. *Circ Res.* 2016;118:579–585.
30. Handy DE, Loscalzo J. Homocysteine and atherothrombosis: diagnosis and treatment. *Curr Atheroscler Rep.* 2003;5:276–283.
31. van Meurs JB, Pare G, Schwartz SM, et al. Common genetic loci influencing plasma homocysteine concentrations and their effect on risk of coronary artery disease. *Am J Clin Nutr.* 2013;98:668–676.
32. Clarke R, Halsey J, Lewington S, et al. Effects of lowering homocysteine levels with B vitamins on cardiovascular disease, cancer, and cause-specific mortality: meta-analysis of 8 randomized trials involving 37 485 individuals. *Arch Intern Med.* 2010;170:1622–1631.
33. Marcovina SM, Albers JJ. Lipoprotein (a) measurements for clinical application. *J Lipid Res.* 2016;57:526–537.
34. Libby P. Lipoprotein (a) - a frustrating final frontier in lipid management? *JACC: Basic Transl Sci.* 2016;1:428–431.
35. Tsimikas S, Fazio S, Ferdinand KC, et al. NHLBI Working Group recommendations to reduce lipoprotein(a)-mediated risk of cardiovascular disease and aortic stenosis. *J Am Coll Cardiol.* 2018;71:177–192.
36. Tsimikas S, Hall JL. Lipoprotein(a) as a potential causal genetic risk factor of cardiovascular disease: a rationale for increased efforts to understand its pathophysiology and develop targeted therapies. *J Am Coll Cardiol.* 2012;60:716–721.

37. Thanassoulis G, Campbell CY, Owens DS, et al. Genetic associations with valvular calcification and aortic stenosis. *N Engl J Med*. 2013;368:503–512.

38. Danesh J, Lewington S, Thompson SG, et al. Plasma fibrinogen level and the risk of major cardiovascular diseases and nonvascular mortality: an individual participant meta-analysis. *JAMA*. 2005;294:1799–1809.

39. Mora S, Rifai N, Buring JE, Ridker PM. Additive value of immunoassay-measured fibrinogen and high-sensitivity C-reactive protein levels for predicting incident cardiovascular events. *Circulation*. 2006;114:381–387.

40. Bini A, Kudryk BJ. Fibrinogen in human atherosclerosis. *Ann N Y Acad Sci*. 1995;748:461–471. Discussion 471-463.

41. Corrales-Medina VF, Madjid M, Musher DM. Role of acute infection in triggering acute coronary syndromes. *Lancet Infect Dis*. 2010;10:83–92.

42. Kwong JC, Schwartz KL, Campitelli MA, et al. Acute myocardial infarction after laboratory-confirmed influenza infection. *N Engl J Med*. 2018;378:345–353.

43. Andraws R, Berger JS, Brown DL. Effects of antibiotic therapy on outcomes of patients with coronary artery disease: a meta-analysis of randomized controlled trials. *JAMA*. 2005;293:2641–2647.

43a. Libby P, Loscalzo J, Ridker PM, et al. Inflammation, immunity, and infection in atherothrombosis: JACC review topic of the week. *J Am Coll Cardiol*. 2018;72:2071–2081.

44. Ridker PM. A test in context: high-sensitivity c-reactive protein. *J Am Coll Cardiol*. 2016;67:712–723.

45. Samani NJ, Erdmann J, Hall AS, et al. Genomewide association analysis of coronary artery disease. *N Engl J Med*. 2007;357:443–453.

46. Schunkert H, Gotz A, Braund P, et al. Repeated replication and a prospective meta-analysis of the association between chromosome 9p21.3 and coronary artery disease. *Circulation*. 2008;117:1675–1684.

47. Kathiresan S, Melander O, Guiducci C, et al. Six new loci associated with blood low-density lipoprotein cholesterol, high-density lipoprotein cholesterol or triglycerides in humans. *Nat Genet*. 2008;40:189–197.

48. Palomaki GE, Melillo S, Bradley LA. Association between 9p21 genomic markers and heart disease: a meta-analysis. *JAMA*. 2010;303:648–656.

49. Teslovich TM, Musunuru K, Smith AV, et al. Biological, clinical and population relevance of 95 loci for blood lipids. *Nature*. 2010;466:707–713.

50. Nurnberg ST, Zhang H, Hand NJ, et al. From loci to biology: functional genomics of genome-wide association for coronary disease. *Circ Res*. 2016;118:586–606.

51. Emdin CA, Khera AV, Klarin D, et al. Phenotypic consequences of a genetic predispostion to enhanced nitric oxide signaling. *Circulation*. 2018;137:222–232.

52. Paynter NP, Ridker PM, Chasman DI. Are genetic tests for atherosclerosis ready for routine clinical use? *Circ Res*. 2016;118:607–619.

53. McPherson R, Tybjaerg-Hansen A. Genetics of coronary artery disease. *Circ Res*. 2016;118:564–578.

54. Emdin CA, Khera AV, Natarajan P, et al. Evaluation of the pooled cohort equations for prediction of cardiovascular risk in a contemporary prospective cohort. *Am J Cardiol*. 2017;119:881–885.

55. Gaziano JM. Fifth phase of the epidemiologic transition: the age of obesity and inactivity. *JAMA*. 2010;303:275–276.

56. Jamal A, Homa DM, O'Connor E, et al. Current cigarette smoking among adults - United States, 2005-2014. *MMWR Morb Mortal Wkly Rep*. 2015;64:1233–1240.

57. Schreiner PJ, Jacobs Jr. DR, Wong ND, Kiefe CI. Twenty-five year secular trends in lipids and modifiable risk factors in a population-based biracial cohort: the Coronary Artery Risk Development in Young Adults (CARDIA) study, 1985-2011. *J Am Heart Assoc*. 2016;5(7); pii: e003864.

58. Hopstock LA, Bonaa KH, Eggen AE, et al. Longitudinal and secular trends in total cholesterol levels and impact of lipid-lowering drug use among Norwegian women and men born in 1905-1977 in the population-based Tromso Study 1979-2016. *BMJ Open*. 2017;7: e015001.

59. Flegal KM, Kruszon-Moran D, Carroll MD, et al. Trends in obesity among adults in the United States, 2005 to 2014. *JAMA*. 2016;315:2284–2291.

60. Ogden CL, Carroll MD, Lawman HG, et al. Trends in obesity prevalence among children and adolescents in the United States, 1988-1994 through 2013-2014. *JAMA*. 2016;315:2292–2299.

61. Tabas I, Williams KJ, Boren J. Subendothelial lipoprotein retention as the initiating process in atherosclerosis: update and therapeutic implications. *Circulation*. 2007;116:1832–1844.

62. Giacco F, Brownlee M. Oxidative stress and diabetic complications. *Circ Res*. 2010;107:1058–1070.

63. Yan SF, Ramasamy R, Schmidt AM. The RAGE axis: a fundamental mechanism signaling danger to the vulnerable vasculature. *Circ Res*. 2010;106:842–853.

64. Lupsa BC, Inzucchi SE. Diabetes medications and cardiovascular disease: at long last progress. *Curr Opin Endocrinol Diabetes Obes*. 2018;25:87–93.

65. Cefalu WT, Kaul S, Gerstein HC, et al. Cardiovascular outcomes trials in type 2 diabetes: where do we go from here? Reflections from a Diabetes Care editors' expert forum. *Diabetes Care*. 2018;41:14–31.

66. Tabas I, Garcia-Cardena G, Owens GK. Recent insights into the cellular biology of atherosclerosis. *J Cell Biol*. 2015;209:13–22.

67. Moore KJ, Tabas I. Macrophages in the pathogenesis of atherosclerosis. *Cell*. 2011;145:341–355.

68. Tabas I, Bornfeldt KE. Macrophage phenotype and function in different stages of atherosclerosis. *Circ Res*. 2016;118:653–667.

69. Swirski FK, Nahrendorf M, Libby P. Mechanisms of myeloid cell modulation of atherosclerosis. *Microbiol Spectr*. 2016;4. doi: 10.1128/microbiolspec.MCHD-0026.2015.

70. Buscher K, Marcovecchio P, Hedrick CC, Ley K. Patrolling mechanics of non-classical monocytes in vascular inflammation. *Front Cardiovasc Med*. 2017;4:80.

71. Gerhardt T, Ley K. Monocyte trafficking across the vessel wall. *Cardiovasc Res*. 2015;107:321–330.

72. Gimbrone MA, García-Cardeña G. Endothelial cell dysfunction and the pathobiology of atherosclerosis. *Circ Res*. 2016;118:620–636.

73. Soehnlein O, Drechsler M, Doring Y, et al. Distinct functions of chemokine receptor axes in the atherogenic mobilization and recruitment of classical monocytes. *EMBO Mol Med*. 2013;5:471–481.

74. Zernecke A, Weber C. Chemokines in atherosclerosis: proceedings resumed. *Arterioscler Thromb Vasc Biol*. 2014;34:742–750.

75. Canton J, Neculai D, Grinstein S. Scavenger receptors in homeostasis and immunity. *Nat Rev Immunol*. 2013;13:621–634.

76. Mallat Z. Macrophages. *Arterioscler Thromb Vasc Biol*. 2017;37:e92–e98.

77. Ketelhuth DFJ, Hansson GK. Adaptive response of T and B cells in atherosclerosis. *Circ Res*. 2016;118:668–678.

78. Nus M, Mallat Z. Immune-mediated mechanisms of atherosclerosis and implications for the clinic. *Expert Rev Clin Immunol*. 2016;12:1217–1237.

79. Libby P, Hansson GK. Taming immune and inflammatory responses to treat atherosclerosis. *J Am Coll Cardiol*. 2018;71:173–176.

80. Libby P, Nahrendorf M, Swirski FK. Leukocytes link local and systemic inflammation in ischemic cardiovascular disease. *J Am Coll Cardiol*. 2016;67:1091–1103.

81. Bennett MR, Sinha S, Owens GK. Vascular smooth muscle cells in atherosclerosis. *Circ Res*. 2016;118:692–702.

82. Nguyen AT, Gomez D, Bell RD, et al. Smooth muscle cell plasticity: fact or fiction? *Circ Res*. 2013;112:17–22.

83. Ruiz JL, Weinbaum S, Aikawa E, Hutcheson JD. Zooming in on the genesis of atherosclerotic plaque microcalcifications. *J Physiol*. 2016;594:2915–2927.

84. Aikawa E, Libby P. A rock and a hard place: chiseling away at the multiple mechanisms of aortic stenosis. *Circulation*. 2017;135:1951–1955.

85. Hjortnaes J, Butcher J, Figueiredo JL, et al. Arterial and aortic valve calcification inversely correlates with osteoporotic bone remodelling: a role for inflammation. *Eur Heart J*. 2010;31:1975–1984.

86. Rajavashisth T, Qiao JH, Tripathi S, et al. Heterozygous osteopetrotic (op) mutation reduces atherosclerosis in LDL receptor–deficient mice. *J Clin Invest*. 1998;101:2702–2710.

87. New SE, Goettsch C, Aikawa M, et al. Macrophage-derived matrix vesicles: an alternative novel mechanism for microcalcification in atherosclerotic plaques. *Circ Res*. 2013;113:72–77.

88. Kapustin AN, Chatrou ML, Drozdov I, et al. Vascular smooth muscle cell calcification is mediated by regulated exosome secretion. *Circ Res*. 2015;116:1312–1323.

89. Geng YJ, Libby P. Progression of atheroma: a struggle between death and procreation. *Arterioscler Thromb Vasc Biol*. 2002;22:1370–1380.

90. Gautier EL, Huby T, Witztum JL, et al. Macrophage apoptosis exerts divergent effects on atherogenesis as a function of lesion stage. *Circulation*. 2009;119:1795–1804.

91. Yurdagul A, Doran AC, Cai B, et al. Mechanisms and consequences of defective efferocytosis in atherosclerosis. *Front Cardiovasc Med*. 2018;4:86.

92. Khera AV, Emdin CA, Drake I, et al. Genetic risk, adherence to a healthy lifestyle, and coronary disease. *N Engl J Med*. 2016;375:2349–2358.

93. Ference BA, Majeed F, Penumetcha R, et al. Effect of naturally random allocation to lower low-density lipoprotein cholesterol on the risk of coronary heart disease mediated by polymorphisms in NPC1L1, HMGCR, or both: a 2 x 2 factorial Mendelian randomization study. *J Am Coll Cardiol*. 2015;65:1552–1561.

94. Russo C, Jin Z, Rundek T, et al. Atherosclerotic disease of the proximal aorta and the risk of vascular events in a population-based cohort: the Aortic Plaques and Risk of Ischemic Stroke (APRIS) study. *Stroke*. 2009;40:2313–2318.

95. Takaya N, Yuan C, Chu B, et al. Association between carotid plaque characteristics and subsequent ischemic cerebrovascular events: a prospective assessment with MRI–initial results. *Stroke*. 2006;37: 818–823.

96. Aird WC. Mechanisms of endothelial cell heterogeneity in health and disease. *Circ Res*. 2006;98:159–162.

97. Lavoie AJ, Bayturan O, Uno K, et al. Plaque progression in coronary arteries with minimal luminal obstruction in intravascular ultrasound atherosclerosis trials. *Am J Cardiol*. 2010;105:1679–1683.

98. Clarkson TB, Prichard RW, Morgan TM, et al. Remodeling of coronary arteries in human and nonhuman primates. *JAMA*. 1994;271:289–294.

99. Glagov S, Weisenberg E, Zarins C, et al. Compensatory enlargement of human atherosclerotic coronary arteries. *N Engl J Med*. 1987;316: 371–375.

100. Vink A, Schoneveld AH, Borst C, Pasterkamp G. The contribution of plaque and arterial remodeling to de novo atherosclerotic luminal narrowing in the femoral artery. *J Vasc Surg*. 2002;36:1194–1198.

101. Schoenhagen P, Sipahi I. Arterial remodelling: an independent pathophysiological component of atherosclerotic disease progression and regression. Insights from serial pharmacological intervention trials. *Eur Heart J*. 2007;28:2299–2300.

102. McGill Jr. HC, McMahan CA, Herderick EE, et al. Effects of coronary heart disease risk factors on atherosclerosis of selected regions of the aorta and right coronary artery. PDAY Research Group. Pathobiological Determinants of Atherosclerosis in Youth. *Arterioscler Thromb Vasc Biol*. 2000;20:836–845.

103. Li S, Chen W, Srinivasan SR, et al. Childhood cardiovascular risk factors and carotid vascular changes in adulthood: the Bogalusa Heart Study. *JAMA*. 2003;290:2271–2276.

104. Virmani R, Robinowitz M, Geer JC, et al. Coronary artery atherosclerosis revisited in Korean war combat casualties. *Arch Pathol Lab Med*. 1987;111:972–976.

105. Palinski W. Maternal-fetal cholesterol transport in the placenta: good, bad, and target for modulation. *Circ Res*. 2009;104:569–571.

106. Tuzcu EM, Kapadia SR, Tutar E, et al. High prevalence of coronary atherosclerosis in asymptomatic teenagers and young adults: evidence from intravascular ultrasound. *Circulation*. 2001;103:2705–2710.

107. Gimbrone Jr. MA, Garcia-Cardena G. Vascular endothelium, hemodynamics, and the pathobiology of atherosclerosis. *Cardiovasc Pathol*. 2013;22:9–15.

108. Gitsioudis G, Chatzizisis YS, Wolf P, et al. Combined non-invasive assessment of endothelial shear stress and molecular imaging of inflammation for the prediction of inflamed plaque in hyperlipidaemic rabbit aortas. *Eur Heart J Cardiovasc Imaging*. 2017;18:19–30.

109. Baeyens N, Schwartz MA. Biomechanics of vascular mechanosensation and remodeling. *Mol Biol Cell*. 2016;27:7–11.

110. Fernandes DC, Araujo TLS, Laurindo FRM, Tanaka LY. Hemodynamic forces in the endothelium: from mechanotransduction to implications on development of atherosclerosis. In: da Luz PL, Libby P, Chagas ACP, Laurindo FRM, eds. *Endothelium and Cardiovascular Disease: Vascular Biology and Clinical Syndromes*. Cambridge, MA: Elsevier; 2018.

111. Jain MK, Sangwung P, Hamik A. Regulation of an inflammatory disease: Kruppel-like factors and atherosclerosis. *Arterioscler Thromb Vasc Biol*. 2014;34:499–508.

112. Hajra L, Evans AI, Chen M, et al. The NF-kappa B signal transduction pathway in aortic endothelial cells is primed for activation in regions predisposed to atherosclerotic lesion formation. *Proc Natl Acad Sci U S A*. 2000;97:9052–9057.

113. Peng HB, Libby P, Liao JK. Induction and stabilization of I kappa B alpha by nitric oxide mediates inhibition of NF-kappa B. *J Biol Chem*. 1995;270:14214–14219.

114. Schoenhagen P, Ziada KM, Kapadia SR, et al. Extent and direction of arterial remodeling in stable versus unstable coronary syndromes : an intravascular ultrasound study. *Circulation*. 2000;101:598–603.

115. Libby P. Mechanisms of acute coronary syndromes and their implications for therapy. *N Engl J Med*. 2013;369:2004–2013.

116. Bentzon JF, Otsuka F, Virmani R, Falk E. Mechanisms of plaque formation and rupture. *Circ Res*. 2014;114:1852–1866.

117. Crea F, Libby P. Acute coronary syndromes. *Circulation*. 2017;136:1155–1166.

118. Amento EP, Ehsani N, Palmer H, Libby P. Cytokines and growth factors positively and negatively regulate intersitial collagen gene expression in human vascular smooth muscle cells. *Arterioscler Thromb Vasc Biol*. 1991;11:1223–1230.

119. Bentzon JF, Falk E. Plaque erosion - new insights from the road less travelled. *Circ Res*. 2017;121:8–10.

120. Partida RA, Libby P, Crea F, Jang IK. Plaque erosion: a new in vivo diagnosis and a potential major shift in the management of patients with acute coronary syndromes. *Eur Heart J*. 2018;39:2070–2076.

121. Quillard T, Franck G, Mawson T, et al. Mechanisms of erosion of atherosclerotic plaques. *Curr Opin Lipidol*. 2017;28:434–441.

122. Quillard T, Araujo HA, Franck G, et al. TLR2 and neutrophils potentiate endothelial stress, apoptosis and detachment: implications for superficial erosion. *Eur Heart J*. 2015;36:1394–1404.

123. Franck G, Mawson T, Sausen G, et al. Flow perturbation mediates neutrophil recruitment and potentiates endothelial injury via tlr2 in mice - implications for superficial erosion. *Circ Res*. 2017;121:31.

124. Sugiyama S, Kugiyama K, Aikawa M, et al. Hypochlorous acid, a macrophage product, induces endothelial apoptosis and tissue factor expression: involvement of myeloperoxidase-mediated oxidant in plaque erosion and thrombogenesis. *Arterioscler Thromb Vasc Biol*. 2004;24:1309–1314.

125. Henein M, Granasen G, Wiklund U, et al. High dose and long-term statin therapy accelerate coronary artery calcification. *Int J Cardiol*. 2015;184:581–586.

126. Puri R, Nicholls SJ, Shao M, et al. Impact of statins on serial coronary calcification during atheroma progression and regression. *J Am Coll Cardiol*. 2015;65:1273–1282.

127. Mann J, Davies MJ. Mechanisms of progression in native coronary artery disease: role of healed plaque disruption. *Heart*. 1999;82:265–268.

128. Burke AP, Kolodgie FD, Farb A, et al. Healed plaque ruptures and sudden coronary death: evidence that subclinical rupture has a role in plaque progression. *Circulation*. 2001;103:934–940.

129. Finn AV, Nakano M, Narula J, et al. Concept of vulnerable/unstable plaque. *Arterioscler Thromb Vasc Biol*. 2010;30:1282–1292.

130. Bavendiek U, Zirlik A, LaClair S, et al. Atherogenesis in mice does not require CD40 ligand from bone marrow-derived cells. *Arterioscler Thromb Vasc Biol*. 2005;25:1244–1249.

131. Sugiyama T, Yamamoto E, Bryniarski K, et al. Nonculprit plaque characteristics in patients with acute coronary syndrome caused by plaque erosion vs plaque rupture: a 3-vessel optical coherence tomography study. *JAMA Cardiol*. 2018;3:207–214.

132. Arbab-Zadeh A, Fuster V. The myth of the "vulnerable plaque": transitioning from a focus on individual lesions to atherosclerotic disease burden for coronary artery disease risk assessment. *J Am Coll Cardiol*. 2015;65:846–855.

133. Nissen SE, Nicholls SJ, Sipahi I, et al. Effect of very high-intensity statin therapy on regression of coronary atherosclerosis: the ASTEROID trial. *JAMA*. 2006;295:1556–1565.

134. Puri R, Libby P, Nissen SE, et al. Long-term effects of maximally intensive statin therapy on changes in coronary atheroma composition: insights from SATURN. *Eur Heart J Cardiovasc Imaging*. 2014;15:380–388.

135. Raber L, Taniwaki M, Zaugg S, et al. Effect of high-intensity statin therapy on atherosclerosis in non-infarct-related coronary arteries (IBIS-4): a serial intravascular ultrasonography study. *Eur Heart J*. 2015;36:490–500.

中文导读

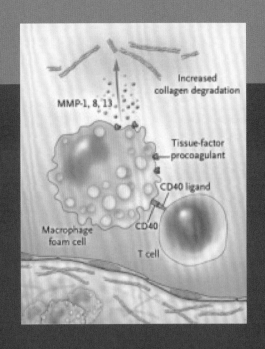

第7章
主动脉瘤的病理生理学

    主动脉瘤根据动脉瘤发生部位分为胸主动脉瘤和腹主动脉瘤。不同的主动脉疾病累及其特定的主动脉节段，这可能与不同主动脉部位的胚胎起源不同，导致不同主动脉节段弹性纤维蛋白分布存在差异有关。主动脉瘤存在共同的病理机制，即由细胞外基质蛋白水解、主动脉平滑肌细胞失调（表型转化：由相对静止的收缩型转变为具有促炎特征的增殖、迁移、分泌型）、炎症和氧化应激（多因素促进蛋白水解酶增加）及生物力学应激改变等相互作用的复杂过程。主动脉瘤也与单基因或多基因遗传缺陷、表观遗传学改变（DNA甲基化、组蛋白修饰）及MicroRNAs改变等相关。目前主动脉瘤尚无有效的临床治疗措施，但基于其多病因性和复杂性特点，针对其常见的病理机制进行治疗或同时干扰其多个机制靶点，未来或许可以获得主动脉瘤的突破性治疗。

陈良万

Pathobiology of Aortic Aneurysms

Uwe Raaz, Joshua M. Spin, Lars Maegdefessel, and Philip S. Tsao

Aortic aneurysms (AAs) can develop in either the thoracic or the abdominal aorta, termed thoracic aortic aneurysm (TAA) (Fig. 7.1) or abdominal aortic aneurysm (AAA) (Fig. 7.2), respectively. AAs are further subclassified according to their specific location in the thoracic (ascending aorta, aortic arch, descending aorta) or abdominal (suprarenal or infrarenal) aortic segments (Fig. 7.3). Although this classification may appear purely descriptive at first glance, it is important to note that TAA and AAA generally represent quite distinct diseases with heterogeneous etiology.

AAs due to genetic disorders with single-gene mutations, as seen in syndromic connective tissue disorders (e.g., Marfan syndrome or Loeys-Dietz syndrome), primarily affect the ascending aorta, and, less often, the descending and abdominal segments.[1] In addition, less common aortopathies, including inflammatory vasculitides (e.g., Takayasu arteritis, giant cell arteritis) and chronic infections such as tertiary syphilis, typically affect thoracic segments.[2] In contrast, age-related, degenerative (sporadic) AAs primarily occur in the descending aorta and are most frequently observed in the form of infrarenal AAAs. These have historically been considered as a manifestation of atherosclerosis but—as increasing epidemiological and pathomechanistic evidence suggests—may, in fact, represent a distinct disease.[3]

The differential susceptibility of specific aortic segments to different etiological factors may partly be explained by embryological, as well as structural, aspects. Embryologically, the aorta is composed of cells originating from the neural crest, mesenchyme, and splanchnic mesoderm (see Fig. 7.3). Primitive arteries are surrounded by smooth muscle cells (SMCs) of mesodermal origin; however, during later development, the primitive SMCs of the ascending thoracic aorta are replaced in part by SMCs that migrate from the neural crest.[4] These neural crest-derived SMCs exhibit distinctive biology compared with mesodermal SMCs, particularly regarding their response to stimulation with cytokines/growth factors, such as transforming growth factor-β (TGFβ).[5] Moreover, neural crest–derived SMCs lead to adaptive remodeling of the thoracic aorta, producing more elastic lamellae during development and growth. Structurally, this results in significantly higher elastin content of the thoracic aorta compared with the abdominal segment, leading to greater mechanical distensibility and buffering cyclical mechanical stress from pulsatile cardiac action (aortic *Windkessel* function).[6,7] In contrast, the lower elastin content of the abdominal aorta may render this segment particularly susceptible to age-related stiffening and degenerative aneurysm formation (see Biomechanical Stress). Despite the variety of etiologies and triggers underlying human AA, and the noted spatial tendencies, AAs to a variable extent exhibit common pathobiological and mechanistic features, including degradation of the medial extracellular matrix (ECM proteolysis), smooth muscle phenotypic switching, and apoptosis, as well as inflammation and oxidative stress (Fig. 7.4).

DEGRADATION OF THE MEDIAL EXTRACELLULAR MATRIX

Remodeling and destruction of elastin and collagen fibers, the two major mechanical load-bearing components of the aortic ECM, are a hallmark of AA disease. Medial elastin and interstitial collagen (types I and III) determine much of the structural integrity and stability of arteries.[8] The mechanistic importance of ECM breakdown, and elastin fragmentation in particular, for AA pathogenesis has been made apparent in a variety of animal models where local treatment of previously intact aortic segments with elastolytic agents (such as porcine pancreatic elastase or calcium chloride) results in subsequent aneurysm development.[9,10]

One critical mechanism leading to increased ECM proteolysis is an imbalance between matrix-degrading matrix metalloproteinases (MMPs) and their endogenous antagonists, the tissue inhibitors of metalloproteinases (TIMPs). MMPs are divided into subclasses based upon substrate specificity and include gelatinases, elastases, and collagenases.[11] Members of the gelatinase subclass (MMP-2 and MMP-9) degrade denatured fibrillar collagen (gelatin), elastin, and native collagen types IV, V, and VII, along with other ECM components, and are thought to be of particular importance in AA. MMP-2 (gelatinase A) is constitutively expressed by SMCs. MMP-9 (gelatinase B) can be produced by macrophages, fibroblasts, or SMCs with a secretory phenotype. MMP-2 and MMP-9 have been extensively studied in both TAA and AAA. Expression and activity of MMP-2 and MMP-9 are increased in human AAA,[12–14] and gene knockout of these enzymes abolishes experimental AAA formation.[15,16] Similarly, MMP-9 levels are increased in human TAA,[17] and MMP-9 knockdown is protective in preclinical TAA models.[18] (The significance of MMP-2 in TAA pathogenesis is less clear.) Regarding the role of TIMPs, there is no consistent evidence that TIMP levels are altered in aneurysmal compared with healthy aortic tissue. As such, TIMP dysregulation alone may not serve as a causative factor for AA; however, a multitude of animal studies indicate that manipulation of TIMP activity clearly affects AA progression,[19,20] suggesting that altered MMP/TIMP balance influences aneurysmal disease. Notably, therapeutic strategies that focus on MMP inhibition (e.g., the use of doxycycline or roxithromycin for MMP-9 inhibition) have not thus far translated into attenuated AAA growth in humans.[21] The expression of serine proteases (such as tissue-type plasminogen activator [t-PA], urokinase-type plasminogen activator [u-PA], and plasmin) that may activate MMPs, as well as cysteine proteases that exhibit potent elastolytic activity (e.g., cathepsins S and K), is also increased in AA.[22]

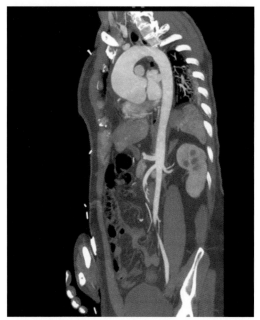

Fig. 7.1 Computed Tomographic Angiogram of Aortic Root/Ascending Aortic Aneurysm in Marfan Syndrome. Maximum diameter is 5.6 cm (normal ≤4 cm). (Courtesy Johannes T. Kowallick, MD, Diagnostic and Interventional Radiology, Georg-August-University Göttingen, Germany.)

SMOOTH MUSCLE DYSREGULATION

A common thread that links the pathobiology of nearly all arterial diseases is the progressive dysfunction of mural SMCs. During AA formation, aortic SMCs manifest phenotypic switching away from

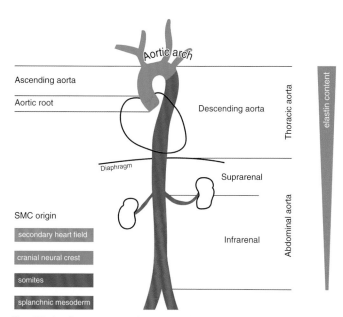

Fig. 7.3 Aortic anatomy and segmental heterogeneity of aortic smooth muscle cell *(SMC)* embryology and aortic elastin content. (Illustration by K. Mattern.)

their relatively quiescent contractile form and toward a proliferative, migratory, and secretory phenotype with proinflammatory characteristics.[23] Later in AA development, SMC dropout due to apoptosis predominates, which leads to mural weakening, progressive expansion, and ultimately dissection or rupture.[24] Degradation of the mural ECM framework surrounding aortic SMCs breaks cell-matrix contacts, triggering phenotypic switching. In addition,

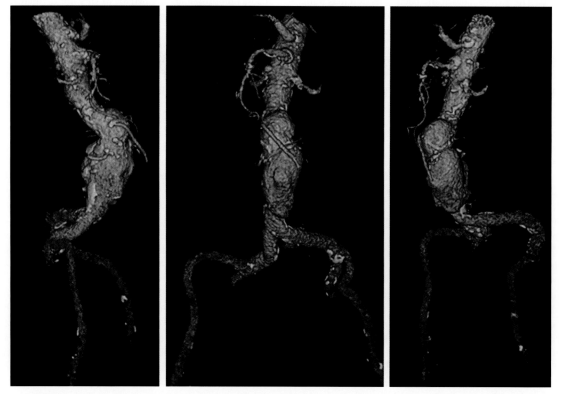

Fig. 7.2 Computed tomographic angiogram 3D reconstruction of an infrarenal abdominal aortic aneurysm. (Courtesy Johannes T. Kowallick, MD, Diagnostic and Interventional Radiology, Georg-August-University Göttingen, Germany.)

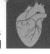

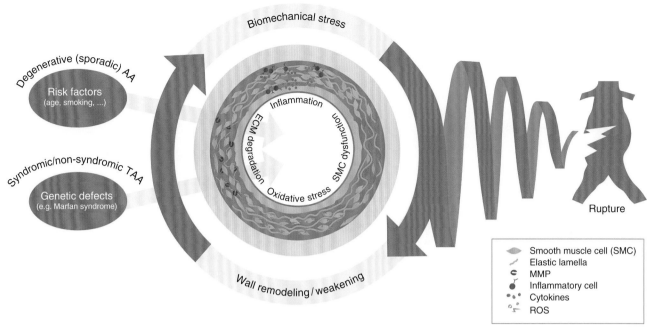

Fig. 7.4 Synopsis of Aortic Aneurysm Pathobiology. Aortic aneurysm *(AA)* formation/progression is driven by a vicious cycle of increasing biomechanical stress (due to AA stiffening and dilatation) and aneurysmal wall remodeling/weakening, eventually resulting in potentially fatal dissection or rupture. AA wall remodeling features extensive degradation of the extracellular matrix *(ECM)*, inflammation, smooth muscle cell *(SMC)* dysregulation, and apoptosis, as well as oxidative stress. AA formation may be initiated/promoted by aging-related degenerative matrix remodeling and other risk factors such as smoking (degenerative AA; AAA in particular), as well as genetic abnormalities in connective tissue homeostasis (syndromic and nonsyndromic TAA). (Illustration by K. Mattern.)

the local inflammatory milieu found in AA encourages SMC dedifferentiation.

Genetically, aneurysmal aortopathies (typically in thoracic aortic segments) may occur as a consequence of heritable, single-gene smooth muscle cell protein mutations leading to abnormal function or signaling, or premature breakdown. These include both structural elements of the SMC contractile apparatus (e.g., smooth muscle alpha-actin [ACTA2], or smooth muscle myosin heavy chain [MYH11]), as well as signaling molecules that regulate SMC tone (e.g., myosin light chain kinase [MYLK], or type I cyclic guanosine monophosphate [cG-MP]-dependent protein kinase [PRKG1]).[25]

As noted previously, a key element of AA formation involves TGFβ signaling. SMC responses to TGFβ can vary depending on growth factor subtype and embryological SMC origin. The role of TGFβ in AA formation is somewhat controversial, because decreased canonical signaling is thought to drive TAA formation, whereas, at the same time, the disease has been attributed to TGFβ hyperactivity. Inactivating mutations in TGFβ receptors and in TGFβ subtypes lead to several syndromic conditions featuring AA. Recent work has suggested that in heritable disease, the underlying aortic wall structure develops improperly, and it is the SMC response to hemodynamic load that leads to aneurysm formation, with TGFβ overactivity acting as a secondary, ineffective corrective response.[25]

INFLAMMATION AND OXIDATIVE STRESS

AAA disease involves chronic transmural infiltration of inflammatory cells, such as polymorphonuclear neutrophils, T cells, B cells, macrophages, mast cells, and natural killer cells. Moreover, an inflammatory component can be identified in TAAs of various etiologies (e.g., Marfan syndrome, familial, and sporadic) during medial degeneration, composed primarily of T cells and macrophages.[26] These infiltrating

cells secrete a cascade of inflammatory mediators, including cytokines, chemokines, and reactive oxygen species (ROS), some of which may induce proteolytic enzymes (e.g., MMPs).

In contrast to stenotic atherosclerosis, which is commonly associated with the T helper cell type 1 (Th1) response and associated cytokines (such as interferon [IFN]-γ, IL-2, and tumor necrosis factor), human AAA inflammation is characterized by the predominance of Th2 cytokine expression (IL-4, IL-5, IL-6, IL-10) and a relative paucity of Th1 cytokines, especially IFN-γ.[27] Murine studies have indicated that skewing the Th1/Th2 balance toward Th2 (with augmented IL-4/IL-6 and attenuated IFN-γ signaling) may promote proteolysis and AAA development.[28]

ROS also contribute to the pathogenesis of AA.[29] AA segments have been shown to feature both increased levels of ROS (along with ROS-producing enzymes), as well as reduced amounts of antioxidants (including ascorbic acid, superoxide dismutase, and glutathione peroxidase). In addition, ROS-scavenging interventions reduce AA progression in animal models.[30,31]

Inflammation and ROS generation may be triggered or augmented by various mechanisms during AA development. For instance, AA formation is associated with increased biomechanical stress, which has been shown to induce ROS signaling, expression of proinflammatory adhesion molecules (e.g., ICAM, VCAM, E-selectin), inflammatory cytokine release (e.g., IL-6), and vascular monocyte adhesion.[29,32,33] Furthermore, the elastin fragmentation that accompanies AA development leads to exposure of tropoelastin and elastin-derived peptides (EDPs) that may mediate neutrophil and monocyte/macrophage chemotaxis, as well as proinflammatory macrophage M1 polarization, partly through an interaction with a cell surface receptor known as the 67-kDa elastin-binding protein (EBP).[34] Interventions blocking EDP signaling have reduced experimental AA progression.[35]

In AAA, it is common to find layered intraluminal thrombus (ILT), which is thought to form a barrier to the diffusion of oxygen and nutrients from the aortic lumen into the vascular wall. This phenomenon is particularly critical in the infrarenal abdominal aorta, which lacks the nutritive intramural vasa vasorum found in more proximal aortic segments. The relatively hypoxic environment may induce subsequent neovascularization and inflammation.[36] Moreover, the ILT forms a reservoir for platelets and inflammatory cells, contributing to the production of proteolytic enzymes and cytokines that may further degrade the aortic wall.[37]

BIOMECHANICAL STRESS

Biomechanical stress is a critical driver of AA pathogenesis (see Fig. 7.4). Clinically, there is a close correlation between AA diameter and rupture risk, which, in the case of AAA, increases steeply at a diameter greater than 5 to 5.5 cm. Laplace's law is commonly used to explain this phenomenon, dictating that increasing diameter of a pressurized vessel directly translates into increased wall stress, which, in turn, increases rupture risk. Although clinically useful, most AAs do not follow "Laplacian" ideal symmetrical geometry to justify an assessment of wall stress and rupture risk solely on the basis of diameter. As such, more complex biomechanical modeling that also includes a patient's individual complex AA geometry (e.g., assessment by computed tomography angiography or magnetic resonance angiography) has been shown to improve AA wall stress assessment and subsequent rupture risk prediction.[38-40]

One endogenous protective mechanism to lower AA wall stress may be the generation of ILT found in most AAA, as described previously, which may act to shield the aneurysmal wall from aortic pressure.[38,39] In fact, computational analyses reveal that the presence of ILT lowers peak aortic wall stress by up to 38%.[41] By contrast, as detailed previously, the ILT may also pathogenically contribute to AA growth. Larger AAA thrombus has been associated with higher aneurysm growth rate, despite lower wall stress.[42]

Biomechanical factors may also help to explain the particular susceptibility of the (infrarenal) abdominal aorta to AAA formation. Aortic aging is generally associated with fragmentation of medial elastic lamella resulting in increasing aortic stiffness[43]; however, because of embryologic differences, the low elastin content of the infrarenal abdominal aorta (compared with more proximal regions) renders this segment most susceptible to age-related stiffening (see Fig. 7.3). Accordingly, aging results in heterogeneous aortic stiffness and resultant stiffness gradients along the abdominal aorta.[44-46] Mechanistically, stiffness gradients may locally enhance aortic wall stress and drive early AA formation.[46] The dramatic elastin breakdown that accompanies AA formation also increases mechanical stiffness, aggravating gradients with respect to the adjacent nonaneurysmal aorta. From a therapeutic aspect, interventional reduction of aortic stiffness gradients (by increasing the mechanical stiffness of the AA-adjacent aorta) was able to reduce aortic inflammation and ECM remodeling and limit AA growth in a murine model.[46] Interestingly, diabetes mellitus—a protective factor for AAA disease—generally increases aortic stiffness.[47] As such, diabetes mellitus may reduce aortic stiffness gradients, thereby blunting AAA growth.

In addition, perturbations in blood flow at the iliac bifurcation may induce detrimental oscillatory wall shear stress (at the expense of physiological laminar shear stress), thereby facilitating proximal AA formation. In this regard, experimental augmentation of physiological laminar shear stress (via creation of a femoral arteriovenous fistula) reduced AAA growth in an animal model.[31]

On a gross scale, the effects of biomechanical stress may be related to straightforward physical damage to the aortic tissue, leading to AA growth and rupture. However, these mechanical stimuli may also elicit subtler biological responses through a variety of signaling mechanisms in various vascular cell types. Mechanical stress can induce ROS generation (e.g., via activation of NADPH oxidases), proinflammatory cytokines, chemokines, and adhesion molecules (e.g., through increased NF-κB signaling), and MMP expression, thereby regulating a variety of mechanisms critical to AA progression.[29]

RISK FACTORS AND GENETICS OF AORTIC ANEURYSMS

A number of genetic defects that lead to abnormalities in connective tissue homeostasis can predispose to AA formation (Table 7.1).[48] In fact, approximately 5% of all TAAs have a genetic basis.

Syndromic TAAs (e.g., Marfan syndrome, Loeys-Dietz syndrome, subtypes of Ehlers-Danlos syndrome, or aneurysm-osteoarthritis syndrome) are associated with specific extra-aortic abnormalities and signs, with single-gene mutations leading to defects in connective tissue homeostasis (see Fig. 7.4). Marfan and vascular Ehlers-Danlos syndrome patients have mutations leading to abnormal ECM proteins (fibrillin-1 [FBN1] and type III collagen [COL3A1], respectively). In Loeys-Dietz syndrome (with mutations in *TGFBR1-* or *TGFBR2* gene) or aneurysm-osteoarthritis syndrome (with mutations in the *SMAD3* gene), ECM perturbations are thought to be the consequence of altered TGFβ signaling.

In the case of nonsyndromic TAA, including various types of familial thoracic aortic aneurysm and dissection (FTAAD), the pathology appears to be more restricted to the thoracic aorta. Several of these conditions have been associated with specific single-gene mutations, whereas others, such as the TAAs that often accompany bicuspid aortic valve, are thought to be multifactorial.[25,49]

In contrast to the aforementioned monogenetic disorders, the pathogenesis of degenerative (sporadic) aneurysms that represent the majority of AAs (including AAAs) are associated with a variety of risk factors.[3,50] Traditional AAA risk factors include advanced age, male sex, and Caucasian race, with smoking as the most significant modifiable risk factor. Interestingly, and in contrast to obstructive atherosclerosis, diabetes mellitus seems to be a negative risk factor (protective) for AAA disease, suggesting pathomechanistic differences between atherosclerosis and AAA.[3,50] Of note, a positive family history increases AAA risk twofold to fivefold with variable polygenic inheritance patterns. In this context, genome-wide association studies have been able to identify associations between a broad panel of gene variants and AAA formation[51]; however, their individual pathomechanistic significance is unknown to date.

EPIGENETICS/MICRORNAS IN AORTIC ANEURYSMS

A recent appreciation has developed for the crucial role played by epigenetic factors in disease regulation. These include microRNAs, which are short, single-stranded RNAs with the ability to affect posttranscriptional gene expression. microRNAs, unlike other forms of noncoding RNAs, are typically conserved across species. Dysregulation of several key microRNAs and their targets have been identified within diseased human AA tissue, as well as in experimental models of AA development and progression.[52]

Several microRNAs are strongly deregulated with aortic dilation including miR-21, a crucial regulator of smooth muscle proliferation and survival; miR-29b, an inducer of collagen gene regulation and matrix reconstruction; miR-205, which controls matrix remodeling and

TABLE 7.1 Genes Associated with Syndromic and Nonsyndromic Thoracic Aneurysm and Dissection

Gene	Location	Protein	Associated Disease/Syndrome	Syndromic TAAD	Nonsyndromic FTAAD	Inheritance	OMIM No. (Phenotype)
ACTA2	10q23.31	Smooth muscle α-actin	AAT6, multisystemic smooth muscle dysfunction, MYMY5	+	+	AD	611788 613834 614042
BGN	Xq28	Biglycan	Meester-Loeys syndrome	+	-	X-linked	300989
COL1A2	7q21.3	Collagen 1 α2 chain	Ehlers-Danlos syndrome, arthrochalasia type (VIIb) and cardiac valvular type	+	-	AD, AR	130060 225320
COL3A1	2q23.2	Collagen 3 α1 chain	Ehlers-Danlos syndrome, vascular type (IV)	+	-	AD	130050
COL5A1	9q34.3	Collagen 5 α1 chain	Ehlers-Danlos syndrome, classic type (I)	+	-	AD	130000
COL5A2	2q23.2	Collagen 5 α2 chain	Ehlers-Danlos syndrome, classic type (II)	+	-	AD	130000
EFEMP2	11q13.1	Fibulin-4	Cutis laxa, AR type Ib	+	-	AR	614437
ELN	7q11.23	Elastin	Cutis laxa, AD	+	-	AD	123700
EMILIN1	2p23.3	Elastin microfibril interfacer 1	Unidentified CTD	+	-	AD	Unassigned
FBN1	15q21.1	Fibrillin-1	Marfan syndrome	+	+	AD	154700
FBN2	5q23.3	Fibrillin-2	Contractural arachnodactyly	+	-	AD	121050
FLNA	Xq28	Filamin A	Periventricular Heterotopia	+	-	XLD	300049
FOXE3	1p33	Forkhead box 3	AAT11	-	+	AD	617349
LOX	5q23.1	Lysyl oxidase	AAT10	-	+	AD	617168
MAT2A	2p11.2	Methionine adenosyltransferase II alpha	FTAA	-	+	AD	Unassigned
MFAP5	12p13.31	Microfibril-associated glycoprotein 2	AAT9	-	+	AD	616166
MYH11	16p13.11	Smooth muscle myosin heavy chain	AAT4	-	+	AD	132900
MYLK	3q21.1	Myosin light chain kinase	AAT7	-	+	AD	613780
NOTCH1	9q34.3	NOTCH1	AOVD1	-	+	AD	109730
PRKG1	10q11.2-q21.1	Type 1 cGMP-dependent protein kinase	AAT8	-	+	AD	615436
SKI	1p36.33-p36.32	Sloan Kettering proto-oncoprotein	Shprintzen-Goldberg syndrome	+	-	AD	182212
SLC2A10	20q13.12	Glucose transporter 10	Arterial tortuosity syndrome	+	-	AR	208050
SMAD2	18q21.1	SMAD2	Unidentified CTD with arterial aneurysms/dissections	+	-	AD	Unassigned
SMAD3	15q22.33	SMAD3	Loeys-Dietz syndrome type 3	+	+	AD	613795
SMAD4	18q21.2	SMAD4	JP/HHT syndrome	+	-	AD	175050
TGFB2	1q41	TGFβ2	Loeys-Dietz syndrome type 4	+	+	AD	614816
TGFB3	14q24.3	TGFβ3	Loeys-Dietz syndrome type 5	+	-	AD	615582
TGFBR1	9q22.33	TGFβ receptor type 1	Loeys-Dietz syndrome type 1, AAT5	+	+	AD	609192
TGFBR2	3p24.1	TGFβ receptor type 2	Loeys-Dietz syndrome type 2, AAT3	+	+	AD	610168

A "+" symbol in the syndromic TAAD column indicates that the gene is causative of syndromic TAAD (same for the nonsyndromic TAAD column). A "-" symbol in the syndromic TAAD column indicates that the gene is not known to cause syndromic TAAD (same for the nonsyndromic TAAD column).

AAT, Aortic aneurysm, familial thoracic; AD, autosomal dominant; AOVD, aortic valve disease; AR, autosomal recessive; cGMP, cyclic guanosine monophosphate; CTD, connective tissue disease; FTAA, familial thoracic aortic aneurysm; FTAAD, familial thoracic aortic aneurysm and dissection; HHT, hereditary hemorrhagic telangiectasia; JP, juvenile polyposis; MYMY, moyamoya disease; OMIM, Online Mendelian Inheritance in Man; TAAD, thoracic aortic aneurysm and dissection; TGF, transforming growth factor; TGFBR, TGFβ receptor; XLD, X-linked dominant.
From Brownstein AJ, Ziganshin BA, Elefteriades JA. Genetic disorders of the vasculature. In: Vasan RS, Sawyer DB. eds. *Encyclopedia of Cardiovascular Research and Medicine.* Philadelphia: Elsevier; 2018:327–367.

protease activity; and miR-24, which is involved in aortic inflammation and macrophage activity.[52] Evidence suggests that all the previously mentioned microRNAs are involved in human AA disease, and all have shown mechanistic contribution to aneurysm progression in experimental models.

Recent studies have begun to explore other noncoding RNA species, including circular RNAs and long noncoding RNAs. These two RNA subclasses appear particularly interesting as some of them display tissue and cell-type specificity. For AA, noncoding RNAs with specific expression patterns in smooth muscle cells could offer novel therapeutic strategies for limiting AA progression and rupture rates.

Inhibition of microRNAs, as well as other RNA subclasses, is possible through the utilization of nucleotide sequence–specific inhibition with antisense oligonucleotides (ASOs). In particular, ASOs using a locked nucleic acid (LNA) formulation are a powerful class of potential therapeutic agents on the threshold of entering daily clinical routine.

Other epigenetic factors involved in AA include acquired, as well as inherited, modifications to the genome affecting gene expression without altering the DNA sequence. Abnormal DNA methylation or imprinting is believed to lead to numerous human diseases and syndromes, including Silver-Russell, Angelman, and Prader-Willi syndromes, as well as autism, schizophrenia, and cancer.[53] Many of these epigenetic modifications appear mainly related to environmental factors and are thus quite volatile, and a few might be capable of being passed on to future generations.[54] Apart from the aforementioned noncoding RNAs, histone modifications, as well as DNA methylation, appear as the most common forms of epigenetic regulation, directly interacting with nucleotide sequences and gene expression patterns. DNA methylation, in particular, occurs naturally as a consequence of vascular aging and cell differentiation, and appears to be involved in AA expansion and ultimately dissection and rupture.[55]

A key modifiable risk factor that leads to both widespread epigenetic changes and disease progression in aneurysm patients is smoking. It has been established that prenatal cigarette smoke exposure, as well as current smoking, can distinctly affect DNA methylation status.[56] Changes in DNA methylation for genes associated with aneurysmal disease can be observed in promoters of the protease-activated receptor-4 (PAR4 or F2RL3) and 15-lipoxygenase (ALOX15) genes.[55]

CONCLUSION

AA formation is driven by a complex interplay between ECM proteolysis, SMC dysregulation, inflammation, and oxidative stress. Unfortunately, our extensive knowledge of those processes has not yet translated into effective medical therapies. However, therapeutic strategies that sufficiently address the multifactorial and complex nature of AA disease, for example, by targeting common pathomechanistic triggers (e.g., mechanical stress and mechanosignaling) or through simultaneous interference with various disease pathways (e.g., microRNA-based interventions), may overcome this unmet need in the future.

REFERENCES

1. Verstraeten A, Luyckx I, Loeys B. Aetiology and management of hereditary aortopathy. *Nat Rev Cardiol.* 2017;14:197–208.
2. Tavora F, Burke A. Review of isolated ascending aortitis: differential diagnosis, including syphilitic, Takayasu's and giant cell aortitis. *Pathology.* 2006;38:302–308.
3. Blanchard JF, Armenian HK, Friesen PP. Risk factors for abdominal aortic aneurysm: results of a case-control study. *Am J Epidemiol.* 2000;151:575–583.
4. Majesky MW. Developmental basis of vascular smooth muscle diversity. *Arterioscler Thromb Vasc Biol.* 2007;27:1248–1258.
5. Gadson Jr PF, Dalton ML, Patterson E, et al. Differential response of mesoderm- and neural crest-derived smooth muscle to TGF-beta1: regulation of c-myb and alpha1 (I) procollagen genes. *Ex Cell Res.* 1997;230:169–180.
6. Wolinsky H, Glagov S. Comparison of abdominal and thoracic aortic medial structure in mammals. Deviation of man from the usual pattern. *Circ Res.* 1969;25:677–686.
7. Halloran B, Davis V, McManus B, et al. Localization of aortic disease is associated with intrinsic differences in aortic structure. *J Surg Res.* 1995;59:17–22.
8. Wagenseil J, Mecham R. Vascular extracellular matrix and arterial mechanics. *Physiol Rev.* 2009;89:957–989.
9. Azuma J, Asagami T, Dalman R, Tsao PS. Creation of murine experimental abdominal aortic aneurysms with elastase. *J Vis Exp.* 2009;29 pii: 1280.
10. Wang Y, Krishna S, Golledge J. The calcium chloride-induced rodent model of abdominal aortic aneurysm. *Atherosclerosis.* 2013;226:29–39.
11. Visse R, Nagase H. Matrix metalloproteinases and tissue inhibitors of metalloproteinases: structure, function, and biochemistry. *Circ Res.* 2003;92:827–839.
12. Freestone T, Turner R, Coady A, et al. Inflammation and matrix metalloproteinases in the enlarging abdominal aortic aneurysm. *Arterioscler Thromb Vasc Biol.* 1995;15:1145–1151.
13. Thompson R, Holmes D, Mertens R, et al. Production and localization of 92-kilodalton gelatinase in abdominal aortic aneurysms. An elastolytic metalloproteinase expressed by aneurysm-infiltrating macrophages. *J Clin Invest.* 1995;96:318–326.
14. Davis V, Persidskaia R, Baca-Regen L, et al. Matrix metalloproteinase-2 production and its binding to the matrix are increased in abdominal aortic aneurysms. *Arterioscler Thromb Vasc Biol.* 1998;18:1625–1633.
15. Pyo R, Lee J, Shipley J, et al. Targeted gene disruption of matrix metalloproteinase-9 (gelatinase B) suppresses development of experimental abdominal aortic aneurysms. *J Clin Invest.* 2000;105:1641–1649.
16. Longo G, Xiong W, Greiner T, et al. Matrix metalloproteinases 2 and 9 work in concert to produce aortic aneurysms. *J Clin Invest.* 2002;110:625–632.
17. Schmoker JD, McPartland KJ, Fellinger EK, et al. Matrix metalloproteinase and tissue inhibitor expression in atherosclerotic and nonatherosclerotic thoracic aortic aneurysms. *J Thorac Cardiovasc Surg.* 2007;133:155–161.
18. Ikonomidis JS, Barbour JR, Amani Z, et al. Effects of deletion of the matrix metalloproteinase 9 gene on development of murine thoracic aortic aneurysms. *Circulation.* 2005;112:I242–I248.
19. Silence J, Collen D, Lijnen HR. Reduced atherosclerotic plaque but enhanced aneurysm formation in mice with inactivation of the tissue inhibitor of metalloproteinase-1 (TIMP-1) gene. *Circ Res.* 2002;90:897–903.
20. Allaire E, Forough R, Clowes M, et al. Local overexpression of TIMP-1 prevents aortic aneurysm degeneration and rupture in a rat model. *J Clin Invest.* 1998;102:1413–1420.
21. Erbel R, Aboyans V, Boileau C, et al. 2014 ESC Guidelines on the diagnosis and treatment of aortic diseases: document covering acute and chronic aortic diseases of the thoracic and abdominal aorta of the adult. The Task Force for the Diagnosis and Treatment of Aortic Diseases of the European Society of Cardiology (ESC). *Eur Heart J.* 2014;35:2873–2926.
22. Ailawadi G, Eliason JL, Upchurch GR. Current concepts in the pathogenesis of abdominal aortic aneurysm. *J Vasc Surg.* 2003;38:584–588.
23. Ailawadi G, Moehle CW, Pei H, et al. Smooth muscle phenotypic modulation is an early event in aortic aneurysms. *J Thorac Cardiovasc Surg.* 2009;138:1392–1399.
24. Thompson RW, Liao S, Curci JA. Vascular smooth muscle cell apoptosis in abdominal aortic aneurysms. *Coron Artery Dis.* 1997;8:623–631.
25. Milewicz DM, Prakash SK, Ramirez F. Therapeutics targeting drivers of thoracic aortic aneurysms and acute aortic dissections: insights from predisposing genes and mouse models. *Annu Rev Med.* 2017;68:51–67.
26. He R, Guo DC, Sun W, et al. Characterization of the inflammatory cells in ascending thoracic aortic aneurysms in patients with Marfan syndrome, familial thoracic aortic aneurysms, and sporadic aneurysms. *J Thorac Cardiovasc Surg.* 2008;136:922-9, 929 e1.

27. Shimizu K, Mitchell RN, Libby P. Inflammation and cellular immune responses in abdominal aortic aneurysms. *Arterioscler Thromb Vasc Biol.* 2006;26:987–994.

28. Shimizu K, Shichiri M, Libby P, et al. Th2-predominant inflammation and blockade of IFN-gamma signaling induce aneurysms in allografted aortas. *J Clin Invest.* 2004;114:300–308.

29. Raaz U, Toh R, Maegdefessel L, et al. Hemodynamic regulation of reactive oxygen species: implications for vascular diseases. *Antioxid Redox Signal.* 2014;20:914–928.

30. Gavrila D, Li W, McCormick M, et al. Vitamin E inhibits abdominal aortic aneurysm formation in angiotensin II-infused apolipoprotein E-deficient mice. *Arterioscler Thromb Vasc Biol.* 2005;25:1671–1677.

31. Nakahashi T, Hoshina K, Tsao P, et al. Flow loading induces macrophage antioxidative gene expression in experimental aneurysms. *Arterioscler Thromb Vasc Biol.* 2002;22:2017–2022.

32. Zampetaki A, Zhang Z, Hu Y, Xu Q. Biomechanical stress induces IL-6 expression in smooth muscle cells via Ras/Rac1-p38 MAPK-NF-kappaB signaling pathways. *Am J Physiol Heart Circ Physiol.* 2005;288:H2946–H2954.

33. Riou S, Mees B, Esposito B, et al. High pressure promotes monocyte adhesion to the vascular wall. *Circ Res.* 2007;100:1226–1233.

34. Duca L, Blaise S, Romier B, et al. Matrix ageing and vascular impacts: focus on elastin fragmentation. *Cardiovasc Res.* 2016;110:298–308.

35. Guo G, Munoz-Garcia B, Ott CE, et al. Antagonism of GxxPG fragments ameliorates manifestations of aortic disease in Marfan syndrome mice. *Hum Mol Genet.* 2013;22:433–443.

36. Vorp DA, Lee PC, Wang DH, et al. Association of intraluminal thrombus in abdominal aortic aneurysm with local hypoxia and wall weakening. *J Vasc Surg.* 2001;34:291–299.

37. Fontaine V, Jacob MP, Houard X, et al. Involvement of the mural thrombus as a site of protease release and activation in human aortic aneurysms. *Am J Pathol.* 2002;161:1701–1710.

38. Humphrey J, Holzapfel G. Mechanics, mechanobiology, and modeling of human abdominal aorta and aneurysms. *J Biomech.* 2012;45:805–814.

39. Vorp D. Biomechanics of abdominal aortic aneurysm. *J Biomech.* 2007;40:1887–1902.

40. Fillinger MF, Marra SP, Raghavan ML, Kennedy FE. Prediction of rupture risk in abdominal aortic aneurysm during observation: wall stress versus diameter. *J Vasc Surg.* 2003;37:724–732.

41. Wang DH, Makaroun MS, Webster MW, Vorp DA. Effect of intraluminal thrombus on wall stress in patient-specific models of abdominal aortic aneurysm. *J Vasc Surg.* 2002;36:598–604.

42. Speelman L, Schurink GW, Bosboom EM, et al. The mechanical role of thrombus on the growth rate of an abdominal aortic aneurysm. *J Vasc Surg.* 2010;51:19–26.

43. O'Rourke M, Hashimoto J. Mechanical factors in arterial aging: a clinical perspective. *J Am Coll Cardiol.* 2007;50:1–13.

44. Hickson S, Butlin M, Graves M, et al. The relationship of age with regional aortic stiffness and diameter. *JACC Cardiovasc Imaging.* 2010;3:1247–1255.

45. Zhang J, Zhao X, Vatner DE, et al. Extracellular matrix disarray as a mechanism for greater abdominal versus thoracic aortic stiffness with aging in primates. *Arterioscler Thromb Vasc Biol.* 2016;36:700–706.

46. Raaz U, Zollner AM, Schellinger IN, et al. Segmental aortic stiffening contributes to experimental abdominal aortic aneurysm development. *Circulation.* 2015;131:1783–1795.

47. Raaz U, Schellinger IN, Chernogubova E, et al. Transcription factor Runx2 promotes aortic fibrosis and stiffness in type 2 diabetes mellitus. *Circ Res.* 2015;117:513–524.

48. Brownstein AJ, Ziganshin BA, Elefteriades JA. Genetic disorders of the vasculature. In: Vasan RS, Sawyer DB, eds. *Encyclopedia of Cardiovascular Research and Medicine.* Philadelphia: Elsevier; 2018:327–367.

49. Losenno KL, Goodman RL, Chu MW. Bicuspid aortic valve disease and ascending aortic aneurysms: gaps in knowledge. *Cardiol Res Pract.* 2012; article ID; https://doi.org.10.1155/2012/145202.

50. Lederle FA, Johnson GR, Wilson SE, et al. Prevalence and associations of abdominal aortic aneurysm detected through screening. Aneurysm Detection and Management (ADAM) Veterans Affairs Cooperative Study Group. *Ann Intern Med.* 1997;126:441–449.

51. Tromp G, Kuivaniemi H, Hinterseher I, Carey DJ. Novel genetic mechanisms for aortic aneurysms. *Curr Atheroscler Rep.* 2010;12:259–266.

52. Li Y, Maegdefessel L. Non-coding RNA contribution to thoracic and abdominal aortic aneurysm disease development and progression. *Front Physiol.* 2017;8:429.

53. Wilkins JF, Ubeda F. Diseases associated with genomic imprinting. *Prog Mol Biol Transl Sci.* 2011;101:401–445.

54. Skinner MK, Manikkam M, Guerrero-Bosagna C. Epigenetic transgenerational actions of endocrine disruptors. *Reprod Toxicol.* 2011;31:337–343.

55. Kim HW, Stansfield BK. Genetic and epigenetic regulation of aortic aneurysms. *Biomed Res Int.* 2017;2017:7268521.

56. Lee KW, Pausova Z. Cigarette smoking and DNA methylation. *Front Genet.* 2013;4:132.

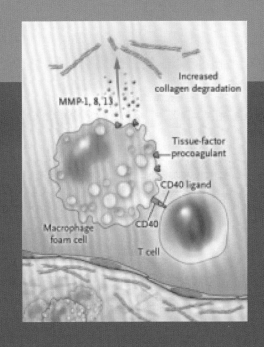

第8章
血栓形成的病理生理学

　　血栓形成和血栓栓塞是造成人类死亡的重要原因之一。血管壁、血液成分及血液流体力学的改变引发血栓形成。血栓形成可发生于心脏、动脉及静脉系统。静脉血栓所导致的血栓栓塞事件（VTE）每年可造成10万～20万人死亡，其发生主要是由于血液成分及血液流变学的改变等。血液成分的改变常见于凝血因子Ⅴ基因*Leiden*突变、凝血酶原*20210A*突变等。血液流变学的改变常见于术后卧床、长途航空期间的制动等。抗磷脂抗体综合征是临床常见的增加凝血及血栓栓塞事件风险的后天因素。肝素、维生素K拮抗剂（华法林）及新型口服抗凝剂（new oral anticoagulant，NOACs）等多种药物可用于静脉血栓形成的治疗。动脉血栓形成常见于动脉粥样硬化斑块破裂等所导致的血小板募集、激活。动脉血栓形成与血小板、纤维蛋白原及其相关基因的先天缺陷有关，也与吸烟、糖尿病、高血压、高脂血症等风险因素有关。因此，动脉血栓治疗以抗血小板为主。本章将主要阐述动静脉血栓形成的病理生理学机制、发病风险因素及治疗处理原则，同时对炎症与血栓形成之间的关系也进行了概述。

辛世杰

Pathobiology of Thrombosis

Elisabeth M. Battinelli, Jane A. Leopold, and Joseph Loscalzo

OVERVIEW OF THROMBOSIS

Abnormal hemostasis leads to thrombus formation. Thrombosis in either the arterial or the venous system is a leading cause of significant morbidity and mortality. When thrombosis occurs in the arterial system, myocardial infarction and stroke may occur, whereas thrombosis in the venous system results in venous thromboembolic disease. Thrombosis and thrombotic-related events are among the most common causes of mortality in the Western world. It is estimated that 695,000 people had new thrombotic events within the coronary circulation in 2017 in the United States and that more than 325,000 people had recurrent events; an additional 165,000 silent myocardial infarctions are estimated to occur annually. Stroke also accounts for significant morbidity, with 795,000 people per year suffering from a thrombotic event within the cerebral circulation. There are 300,000 to 600,000 new cases of venous thromboembolism each year, approximately 30% of which result in death in the first 30 days after diagnosis, the majority of deaths being sudden in the setting of a pulmonary embolism. In fact, thromboembolism is the cause of one in four deaths worldwide, and, although mortality rates have declined, the cases worldwide continue to increase.[1] This is largely due to the fact that the population is aging, because the majority of events occur in the elderly.[2]

The pathogenesis of thrombosis was elucidated as early as 1856 when Virchow first described its major determinants, including abnormalities in the vessel wall, platelets, and coagulation proteins as essential for establishing a thrombus. The composition of arterial thrombi is distinct from that of thrombi that form in the venous circulation: arterial thrombi are composed mainly of platelets and occur in areas of vascular wall injury; by contrast, venous thrombi are rich in fibrin and dependent on a hypercoagulable response associated with individual coagulation factor abnormalities or mechanical issues related to blood flow limitation. Under normal circumstances, the endothelial lining is not a thrombotic surface with endothelial cells constantly interacting with other cell types, including platelets to directly inhibit thrombus formation through the release of antithrombotic factors, such as thrombomodulin, tissue factor pathway inhibitor system, plasmin, and antithrombin systems. At the same time, platelet aggregation is inhibited through prostacyclins and nitric oxide (NO), which are released from platelets directly. However, when the endothelial surface becomes damaged, release of many procoagulant proteins, especially tissue factor, and activation of platelets result in uncontrolled hemostasis at the site of vascular injury.[3] As the thrombus begins to form, it recruits additional platelets to the area, leading to further platelet activation. Initially tethering of platelets is dependent on exposure of glycoprotein Ib-V-IX in damaged collagen, which binds to von Willebrand factor, resulting in adhesion of platelets to the area of injury. Further recruitment of platelets is mediated through activation of the glycoprotein IIb/IIIa (GPIIb/IIIa) platelet receptor, which undergoes a conformational change leading to increased affinity for fibrinogen. These events culminate with further platelet activation, which results in the release of many essential components for thrombus formation, including adenosine diphosphate (ADP), serotonin, and thromboxane A_2 (TXA_2). Exposure of vascular collagen also leads to activation of the normal mechanisms of hemostasis, including the coagulation cascade, through exposure of tissue factor leading to "hemostasis in the wrong place." The coagulation regulatory system is outlined in Fig. 8.1 and is discussed in Chapter 4. Briefly, both the tissue factor–mediated pathway (extrinsic) and the contact-mediated pathway (intrinsic) rely on activation of inactive enzyme precursors of serine proteases, which then lead to activation of another downstream protein within the cascade. The ultimate step (factor XIII activation) results in cross-linking of fibrin to stabilize a platelet plug and evolving thrombus. The tissue factor–initiated pathway is essential for thrombus formation. When tissue factor is released during cellular injury, factor VII is activated and complexes. This complex next activates factor X and factor XI. Activation of factor X is essential for conversion of prothrombin (factor II) to thrombin through the prothrombinase complex assembled on activated platelets. This cascade of coagulation proteins is essential for hemostasis but also can have deleterious effects when it occurs in an unregulated fashion, leading to unwanted thrombotic complications.

Walton and colleagues have established that erythrocytes also play a significant role in thrombus formation.[4] The authors demonstrated that erythrocytes can affect thrombus formation by increasing platelet deposition at the site of injury. This finding was especially notable in cases where the hematocrit was elevated, demonstrating that elevations in hematocrit can have a negative impact on overall thrombus risk.

PLATELETS, THROMBOSIS, AND VASCULAR DISEASE

Venous Thrombosis

It is estimated that 100,000 to 200,000 deaths occur yearly because of a venous thromboembolic event (VTE). These events occur mainly in the vasculature at the area of the vessel sinus where stasis can lead to a hypercoagulable microenvironment. The hemostatic process is activated when tissue factor is exposed at the site of vascular injury, leading to initiation of the coagulation cascade with subsequent formation of thrombin and conversion of fibrinogen to fibrin. This process evolves at the same time that platelets are actively being recruited to the area of injury through collagen exposure, leading to platelet and fibrin thrombus formation. There are a number of physiological anticoagulants that

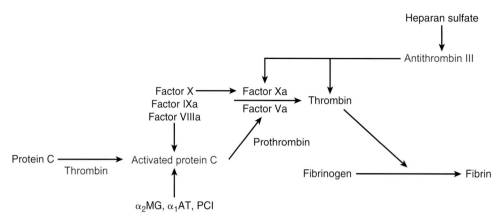

Fig. 8.1 **Physiological Regulation of Blood Coagulation.** $\alpha_1 AT$, α_1-antitrypsin; $\alpha_2 MG$, α_2-macroglobin; *PCI*, protein C inhibitor.

are also present and modulate this response, including antithrombin, tissue factor pathway inhibitor, and activated protein C and its cofactor protein S. Defects in these hemostatic proteins can lead to disorders that elevate the risk of thrombus formation.

The risk factors for venous thromboembolism are associated with venous stasis or acquired and congenital hypercoagulable states and include obesity, smoking, malignancy, pregnancy, hormone therapy, and recent trauma or surgery. Immobilization resulting from prolonged hospitalization following surgical intervention and during long-distance air-travel also contributes to the risk of VTE. Genetic risk factors that are associated with increased risk of VTE include mutations in factor V (Leiden) and prothrombin 20210, as well as mutations leading to deficiencies in antithrombin, protein C, and protein S. Approximately 5% of the Caucasian population has at least one mutation for factor V Leiden, and 15% to 20% of patients who present with a VTE carry the mutation.[5–8] Approximately 2% of the population carry the prothrombin gene mutation, but it may be present in approximately 5% to 15% of persons with VTE.[9] The population frequencies of mutations in other coagulation factor genes, such as protein C, are estimated to be 1 in 500 individuals. Antithrombin III deficiency has a frequency of 1 in 300 in the general population and 3% to 5% among those with thrombotic events. Previously it was thought that genetic mutations in the genes important for methylene tetrahydrofolate reductase and hyperhomocysteinemia increased the risk of VTEs; however, recently this association has been shown to be less likely.[10] One of the acquired risk factors known to be important in both venous and arterial thrombosis is the acquisition of antiphospholipid antibodies, which represent a family of antibodies against phospholipids, such as cardiolipins, and phospholipid binding proteins, such as beta 2 glycoprotein I. The mechanisms responsible for thrombosis are still based on speculation but may include inhibition of protein C, antithrombin, and annexin A5 expression; binding and activation of platelets; enhanced endothelial cells tissue factor expression; activation of the complement cascade; and impaired assembly of fibrinolytic proteins on the endothelial cell surface owing to antibody-mediated impairment of annexin A2 availability for tissue plasminogen activator and plasminogen binding to the endothelium.[11,12] The criteria for the diagnosis of the associated disorder, antiphospholipid syndrome, include the presence of both clinical events and laboratory evidence for the presence of antiphospholipid antibodies.[13]

Because it is clear that other genes could also be responsible for increased risk of VTE, a number of studies have been performed using genome-wide association studies (GWAS) to identify new genetic loci.[14,15] Recently, Germain and colleagues published the results of a meta-analysis of 12 GWAS compiling more than 7500 cases of VTE.[16]

The results identified a number of new potential loci for genetics-associated VTE, including some genes which were previously not understood to be associated with thrombosis, thereby setting the stage for a new understanding of the pathobiology and the risk of VTE. Although it is clear that there are strong genetic links that increase the risk of VTE, the utility of uncovering these genetic predispositions often does not affect clinical therapeutic strategies, making discovery of these underlying genetic disorders less appealing. In fact, the overuse of these screening tests in patients with provoked events is greatly discouraged by the Choosing Wise Campaign of the American Society of Hematology, as well as the British Committee.[17] Most physicians currently do not pursue a hypercoagulable work-up in those individuals who present with a provoked VTE. However, these work-ups are still used in those with spontaneous events, as well is individuals whose family members would benefit from the knowledge of an increased propensity for thrombosis.

New Drugs for Treating Venous Thrombosis

Recently, a number of new drugs have been approved for the treatment of VTEs. In the past the main stays of treatment included mainly heparin products and the vitamin K antagonist warfarin. Owing to issues with frequent blood testing to maintain therapeutic ranges, food and drug interactions, and fluctuations in drug levels, new oral agents were developed which provided a steady state of drug delivery without concerns for drug interactions and no need for frequent monitoring. These drugs target factor Xa and thrombin in the coagulation cascade and are termed direct oral anticoagulants (DOACs). These drugs have been especially effective in providing a therapeutic option for long-term therapy for prevention of venous thrombosis recurrence in unprovoked clots. These DOACs include a direct thrombin inhibitor, dabigatran etexilate, as well as three factor Xa inhibitors, rivaroxaban, apixiban, and edoxaban. All these drugs have a rapid onset of action, hepatic metabolism, and renal clearance. Studies using these DOACs in comparison with therapeutic warfarin demonstrated noninferiority for the treatment of an acute deep vein thrombosis or pulmonary embolism. Although there was no difference in efficacy for treatment, the bleeding profile of the DOACs was better than that of warfarin, with lower risk of significant bleeding. Briefly, RECOVER I and II, which included more than 5000 patients, were randomized double-blinded control trials comparing the use of dabigatran to warfarin for VTE.[46] The pooled analysis of these two trials demonstrated similar rates of recurrent VTE but fewer episodes of clinically relevant bleeding. Similarly the factor Xa inhibitors demonstrated noninferiority in terms of VTE, with less significant bleeding. At this time, it is unclear if there is one

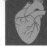

DOAC that offers improved VTE prevention in comparison with the others. Recently, studies have demonstrated the efficacy of this novel anticoagulant in patients with malignancy, which often leads to a hypercoagulable state, making this patient population more vulnerable to thrombosis. Edoxaban was demonstrated to be noninferior to the standard of care (low-molecular-weight heparin) with respect to risk of recurrent venous thromboembolism or major bleeding.[46a] However, there are differences that make some more well utilized than others. Dabigatran and apixaban are taken twice daily, whereas edoxaban and rivaroxaban are once-daily medications. Both dabigatran and edoxaban require bridging therapy with a parenteral anticoagulant during the first 5 to 10 days prior to primary therapy, whereas apixaban and rivaroxaban can be used as initial therapy. Perhaps the greatest difference at the time of writing this chapter is that dabigatran is the only agent with a known reversal agent (idarucizumab). Of note, the utility of all these drugs in patients with obesity, cancer, hepatic cirrhosis, antiphospholipid syndrome, and other special clinical circumstances has yet to be established, making these drugs less likely to be used in those situations.

Arterial Thrombosis

Arterial thrombosis, which accounts for myocardial infarction and thrombotic cerebrovascular events, initiates from damage to the vessel wall, leading to a cascade of platelet-mediated cellular interactions. Endothelial injury resulting from plaque rupture with exposure of subendothelial collagen and von Willebrand factor is the core event leading to arterial thrombosis. Platelet activation through direct interaction with exposed collagen or thrombin generated by tissue factor leads to thrombus formation. Important in this process are platelet factors that are released with activation, including ADP, serotonin, and TXA_2. The recruitment of additional platelets leads to thrombus growth as platelets aggregate through bridges formed from the binding of fibrinogen to the platelet receptor, GPIIb/IIIa. The recruitment and activation of platelets are modulated by a tightly regulated process that involves factors released from the platelet, as well as the endothelium, including prostacyclin, NO, and ecto-AD(T)Pase. Prostacyclin, which is generated from arachidonic acid by the endothelium, works through cAMP to inhibit platelet function. NO, through stimulation of the soluble guanylyl cyclase to produce cyclic GMP (cGMP), directly inhibits platelet activation and prevents thrombosis. cGMP signaling cascades lead to a decrease in fibrinogen binding to GPIIb/IIIa and inhibits the phospholipase A_2 and C pathways. A primary mechanism of arterial thrombosis is rupture of atherosclerotic plaques precipitating platelet-rich aggregates. Arterial thrombosis can have catastrophic consequences when it occurs in the coronary or carotid artery circulation. Factors that can exacerbate these types of thrombotic events include smoking, diabetes, hypertension, and hyperlipidemia. Thrombosis generally occurs when there is a disruption in the hemostatic balance, which results when procoagulant and anticoagulant molecules are at disequilibrium. Endothelial damage shifts this balance toward a greater procoagulant propensity, leading to exposure of collagen and tissue factor. The collagen that is now exposed can activate platelets in the blood flowing through the vessel, and, concomitantly, thrombin is generated as the coagulation cascade is initiated in the presence of tissue factor. Genetic modifications of proteins important in coagulation can alter this process, leading to a greater likelihood of forming thrombi in the arterial system (Box 8.1). These mutations affect platelet function, thereby leading to increased propensity to aggregation. Polymorphisms in the eNOS gene, which is essential for NO production by endothelial cells, have been described. The 894-G/T polymorphism I exon 7 results in a glutamate-to-aspartate change at position 298. This polymorphism is associated with decreased levels of nitrogen oxides leading to increased risk of hypertension, myocardial infarction, and stroke in

---

BOX 8.1 Genetic Polymorphisms and Arterial Thrombosis

Polymorphism

Coagulation Factors
Fibrinogen beta chain 455 G/A
Fibrinogen beta-chain 854 G/A
Fibrinogen beta-chain Bcl1
Fibrinogen alpha chain Thr312 Ala
FVII Arg353Gln
FVII HVR4
FVII 401G/T
FV Leiden
Prothrombin 20210G/A
FXIII Val34Leu

Platelet Receptors
GPIIIa Leu33Pro
GPIb alpha VNTR
GPIb alpha Thr145Met
GPIa/IIa alpha$_2$ 807C/T
GPIa/IIa alpha$_2$ 1648A/G

Fibrinolytic System
PAI-1 675 4G/5G
PAI-1 (CA)$_n$
PAI-1 HindIII
t-PA Alu insertion/deletion
t-PA 7351C/T
TAFI ala147Thr
TAFI 1542C/G

Vascular Factors
eNOS Glu298Asp
Guanylyl cyclase-1 rs7692387
Glutathione peroxidase-3 h2 promoter haplotype

---

patients who are homozygous for the abnormality.[18,19] A risk variant (rs7692387) in the α3-subunit of the soluble guanylyl cyclase-1 gene (*GUCY1A3*) decreases gene expression in whole blood, reduces platelet inhibition by NO (donors), and accounts for the increase in coronary heart disease risk associated with chromosomal $4_q32.1$ locus.[20,21] A unique polymorphism in the promoter of the glutathione peroxidase-3 gene has been associated with thrombotic strokes in children. Genome-wide associations have identified other loci associated with cardiovascular thrombotic disease.[22]

Increased levels of fibrinogen have been associated with an increased risk of myocardial infarction, ischemic stroke, and peripheral artery disease.[23] Age, elevated lipids, and smoking increase the risk associated with fibrinogen. Beta chain variants, such as Arg448Lys, BclI, -148C/T, -455G/A, and -854G/A, with the -455G/A polymorphism are present in 10% to 20% of the population and are associated with a significant rise in fibrinogen levels.[24] However, studies have not been consistent, and the association between this polymorphism and risk of arterial thrombosis is not established.[25] Another site of potential polymorphisms in the fibrinogen gene is the Thr312Ala substitution in the alpha-chain. When this polymorphism is present, the fibrin stranding is thicker and there is increased cross-linking that may predispose to an increased thrombotic risk.[26] Other potential associations between arterial thrombosis and increased risk include hyperhomocysteinemia, elevated C-reactive protein, factor VII polymorphisms, increased plasminogen activator inhibitor-1 (PAI-1), and platelet hyperreactivity. Wald and colleagues performed a meta-analysis of 72 prospective cohort studies focusing on a mutation in the methylenetetrahydrofolate reductase (MTHFR) C677T gene and the occurrence of various thrombotic events, including stroke and cardiovascular disease, and found a weak association between the mutation and the risk of arterial events.[27] Other factors including CRP, factor VII, and PAI-1 have shown even less promising results.[24]

Drugs That Modulate Arterial Thrombosis

Because arterial thrombi are mainly composed of platelets and platelet activation is key to their formation, manipulation of platelet function is central to prevent arterial thrombosis. The most commonly used drugs that affect platelet function include aspirin, thienopyridines (clopidogrel and ticlopidine), dipyridamole, and GPIIb/IIIa antagonists. Aspirin's mechanism of action is to irreversibly inhibit acetylation at serine-529 in the active site of platelet cyclooxygenase (COX)-1. In this manner, the COX-1 enzyme is unable to interact with arachidonic acid, and therefore the generation of prostaglandin H_2 and TXA_2 is inhibited. TXA_2 plays an essential role in regulation of platelet activation and aggregation upon stimulation with platelet agonists, including collagen, thrombin, and ADP. When TXA_2 binds to its receptor, phospholipase C is activated and intracellular calcium increases, leading to amplification of platelet aggregation and feedback-dependent release of more ADP and TXA_2. Aspirin functions by producing a dose-dependent inhibition of COX, which prevents the aforementioned feedback loop leading to platelet aggregation. The use of aspirin to prevent arterial thrombosis was first definitively established in the ISIS-2 trial, in which aspirin was shown to reduce the mortality rate associated with a myocardial infarction. Other studies showed that aspirin resulted in a 25% relative risk reduction from all vascular-associated events, including myocardial infarction and stroke, and the benefit occurred with treatment with low-dose aspirin.[28] Although the half-life of aspirin is only 20 minutes and inhibitory effects of aspirin on COX occur as quickly as 5 minutes after administration, the irreversible inhibition of COX ensures that its effects are preserved for the lifespan of the platelet (7 to 10 days) such that COX activity does not return to normal levels until a new generation of platelets is produced. Interestingly, aspirin's inhibitory properties appear to be most effective when exposed to weak platelet agonists, such as TXA_2 and ADP, whereas exposure to stronger agonists, such as thrombin, leaves platelet function (as measured by aggregation) intact. For this reason, many of the essential functions of platelets, such as platelet adhesion to von Willebrand factor or activation by thrombin, are not inhibited by aspirin. Aspirin resistance may explain some of the clinical failure that is seen with its use. There have recently been two meta-analyses regarding aspirin resistance showing that laboratory evidence of irresponsiveness to aspirin may be associated with a high risk of recurrent thrombotic cardiovascular events.[29,30] Another important modulator of platelet function is ADP, which acts as a weak platelet agonist through two different platelet membrane receptors, P2Y1 and P2Y12.[31] When ADP stimulates the P2Y1 receptor, the platelet undergoes a shape change and Ca^{2+} is mobilized through activation of phospholipase C to initiate platelet aggregation in a reversible manner. The P2Y12 receptor is essential for secretion and stabilization of platelet aggregation by lowering cyclic AMP levels. There are two available thienopyridine derivatives that act as inhibitors of ADP-induced platelet aggregation: ticlopidine and clopidogrel. Clopidogrel is metabolized by cytochrome P450 into an active metabolite, which irreversibly blocks the P2Y12 receptor. Clopidogrel reduces recurrent thrombotic events in patients with cardiovascular disease.[32–34] The CAPRIE trial found that clopidogrel is more effective than aspirin in reducing the risk of cardiovascular

events in patients with recent myocardial infarction, recent ischemic stroke, and established peripheral artery disease. Ticlopidine is metabolized by cytochrome P450 to an active metabolite which functions to block the PGY12 receptor. Although it functions in a similar manner to clopidogrel, it is associated with a higher degree of neutropenia and thrombotic thrombocytopenic purpura and therefore is not used as readily as clopidogrel.[35,36] A new class of antiplatelet agents targeting the PAR-1 thrombin receptor have recently been developed as a novel platelet therapeutic agent; their use, however, has been limited due to questions of safety and efficacy, and new pharmacological approaches are in development.[36a] Other antiplatelet drugs in the same general class include ticagrelor, cangrelor, and elinogrel, all of which reversibly inhibit the P2Y12 receptor.[37]

Another class of drugs in the armamentarium of antithrombotic agents is that which specifically target the GPIIb/IIIa receptor to prevent the binding of fibrinogen essential for platelet aggregation. This approach blocks platelet aggregation independent of the platelet agonist, because GPIIb/IIIa activation is a final common pathway for almost all platelet agonists. The GPIIb/IIIa receptor is the most abundant receptor on platelets and is also found on the surface of megakaryocytes. Under normal circumstances, this glycoprotein receptor is inactive, but when the platelets become activated, a signal transduction cascade is initiated, which leads to a conformational change and activation of the receptor allowing it to bind to fibrinogen or, if high-shear conditions are in place, von Willebrand factor. Binding is mediated by the ARg-Gly-Asp (RGD) and the Lys-Gly-Asp (KGD) sequences in both macromolecules. Drugs that inhibit GPIIb/IIIa include abciximab, eptifibatide, and tirofiban. Abciximab is derived from a murine monoclonal antibody and was one of the first GPIIb/IIIa receptor antagonists to be developed. It functions as a high-affinity antibody to inhibit platelet function through binding to the GPIIb/IIIa receptor, thereby blocking fibrinogen from interacting with its binding site. Abciximab also binds to integrins in the vitronectin receptor, as well as MAC1 and CD11b-CD18, although the clinical significance of these interactions is not understood. Eptifibatide is a cyclic heptapeptide that binds to GPIIb/IIIa through the KGD motif. Tirofiban is a tyrosine derivative that functions as an RGD mimetic. These drugs work on the final common pathway of platelet aggregation to inhibit binding to fibrinogen in a similar manner to abciximab. These actions are thought to be regulated by inhibition of thrombin generation via tissue factor and a decrease in microparticle formation. Multiple clinical trials have shown that inhibition of GPIIb/IIIa is effective in preventing recurrent thrombotic events. The use of these drugs leads to a 35% decrease in acute ischemic events and a 26% decrease in recurrent events within the 6 months. The long-term use of these drugs was shown to be efficacious in the Evaluation of PTCA to Improve Long-Term Outcome by c7E3 GPIIb/IIIa Receptor Blockade (EPILOG) trial with a reduction in the incidence of death. Other trials have supported the use of GPIIb/IIIa blockade in management of acute coronary syndromes.[38,39] However, their use has been reserved for high-risk circumstances such as percutaneous coronary intervention in acute coronary syndromes, due to the recent finding of the long-term benefits of ADP receptor antagonists.[40] Oral GPIIb/IIIa inhibitors have not been shown to limit cardiovascular events to date,[41] which may be due to persistent conformational changes in the GPIIb/IIIa receptor after the antagonist dissociates from it. In this case the receptor remains active and increases binding to fibrinogen and von Willebrand factor, leading to a paradoxical thrombotic effect. Novel GPIIb/IIIa antagonists that do cause such conformational changes are under development. In one study, RUC-1, which is a novel compound discovered through high-throughput screening, induced partial exposure of the binding site yet still led to decreased platelet aggregation without the enhanced fibrinogen

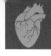

binding. RUC-1 may represent a prototype molecule for these types of derivative drugs.[42]

Other antiplatelet agents that may inhibit thrombus formation yet preserve hemostasis so that bleeding complications do not result are under investigation. One potential new therapeutic target is the glycoprotein GPIb-V-IX complex (GPIb). Initial studies of patients who have Bernard-Soulier syndrome identified a deficiency of the GPIb complex. The GPIb complex is important for building a platelet bridge through von Willebrand factor at areas of damage to the endothelium. Drugs under development act as antagonists for the GPIb–von Willebrand factor interaction, including specific monoclonal antibodies, GPIb complex antagonists isolated from snake venoms,[43,44] and the Fab fragment of 6B4, which is a murine monoclonal antibody that targets human GPIb and prevents binding to vWF. Nonhuman primate studies have suggested that thrombus formation can be attenuated using these drugs.[45]

INFLAMMATION AND THROMBOSIS

Recent evidence has clearly established a role for inflammation in the atherothrombotic process. Patients with acute coronary syndromes have increased interactions between platelets and leukocytes forming detectable aggregates. The process of inflammation involves a variety of cell types, including leukocytes, endothelial cells, and platelets. The endothelium is activated and multiple cell adhesion molecules are released, including P-selectin, which essentially has two important roles in inflammation: recruitment of proinflammatory cells and establishing signaling cascades leading to increased expression of CD11b/CD18 (MAC-1).[47] Platelets are instrumental in the inflammatory aspects of atherosclerosis. Thrombin activation of platelets leads to release of many procoagulant molecules and release of inflammatory molecules, including platelet factor 4 (PF4), PDGF, and RANTES, which is regulated upon normal T cell activation. In addition, platelets that have been activated in the presence of thrombin secrete CD40 ligand (CD40L). This chemoattractant is key to the recruitment of endothelial cells, smooth muscle cells, and macrophages. CD40L also recruits a variety of proinflammatory cytokines, such as IL-1, IL-6, and IL-8, and increases expression of the adhesion molecules ICAM-1, VCAM-1, and P-selectin.[48] CD40L is also important for the release of matrix metalloproteinases (MMPs), which are needed for plaque progression, neovascularization, and plaque rupture. The CD40L also initiates release of tissue factor, which then interacts with other cells to create a thrombogenic microenvironment. T lymphocytes orchestrate an inflammatory cascade that begins by binding to VCAM-1 through signaling regulated by interferon-γ–inducible chemokine ligands (CXCLs), protein-10, and chemoattractant (I-TAC). Through this binding, a number of inflammatory cytokines are released, including the CD40L; CD154, which leads to metalloproteinase generation; and tissue factor expression, which initiates the coagulation cascade. Mice that are lacking the CD40L have less atherothrombosis. Patients with acute coronary syndromes have elevated levels of CD40L, and plasma levels of CD40L predict the risk of future cardiovascular events.[49–51] Elevated soluble CD40L levels can be decreased by treatment with abciximab.[52]

The role of inflammation in the thrombotic response is supported by many clinical studies that have shown an association between bacterial infections and increased risk of myocardial infarction or stroke and by recent complex molecular network analysis[53]; however, further studies are needed to prove this association.[54,55] One possible mechanism is through the Toll-like receptors (TLRs), which are present in platelets. Platelet activation through stimulation of TLR2 activates signaling mechanisms responsible for both thrombotic and inflammatory responses. These effects underlie the mechanism by which bacteria induce a proinflammatory cascade in platelets, suggesting that bacteria can directly activate platelet-dependent thrombotic responses.[56] Recently, this process was further refined by demonstrating that TLR2 stimulation leads to platelet activation through PI3-Kinase, which is known to be important in platelet activation-associated shape change, calcium release, and granular content secretion.[57] A link between thrombosis and inflammation has emerged, implicating neutrophil extracellular traps (NETs) in inflammatory disease. NETs are chromatin fibers that are released from neutrophils at the time of clearance.[58] Increased NETs have been observed in a variety of inflammatory states, including autoimmune disease, cardiovascular disease, cancer, and VTE. Their role in atherosclerosis has recently been attributed to their release of reactive oxygen species. A review of the evidence suggests that the link between both arterial and VTEs may indeed be the inflammatory state and its associated "NETosis." In summary, as our understanding of hemostasis and thrombosis continues to evolve, so does the development of novel agents directed toward treating thromboembolic diseases. This development continues to be driven by scientific discovery, the growing number of patients, and the increasing indications for antithrombotics. Targets for antiplatelet drugs continue to be defined, leading to novel therapies and the development of additional agents in existing successful classes.

REFERENCES

1. Benjamin EJ, Blaha MJ, Chiuve SE, et al. American Heart Association Statistics Committee and Stroke Statistics Subcommittee. Heart and stroke statistics: 2017 update. A report from the American Heart Association. *Circulation.* 2017;135:e146–e603.
2. Weitz JI, Eikelboom JW. Advances in thrombosis and hemostasis: an introduction to the compendium. *Circ Res.* 2016;118(9):1337–1339.
3. Alfirevic Z, Alfirevic I. Hypercoagulable state, pathophysiology, classification and epidemiology. *Clin Chem Lab Med.* 2010;48 Suppl 1:S15-26.
4. Walton BL, Lehmann M, Skorczewski T, et al. Elevated hematocrit enhances platelet accumulation following vascular injury. *Blood.* 2017;129(18):2537–2546.
5. Prandoni P. Acquired risk factors for venous thromboembolism in medical patients. *Hematology Am Soc Hematol Educ Program.* 2005;458–461.
6. Rosendaal FR. Venous thrombosis: the role of genes, environment, and behavior. *Hematology Am Soc Hematol Educ Program.* 2005;2005:1–12.
7. Cushman M. Inherited risk factors for venous thrombosis. *Hematology Am Soc Hematol Educ Program.* 2005;2005:452–457.
8. Vossen CY, Conard J, Fontcuberta J, et al. Risk of a first venous thrombotic event in carriers of a familial thrombophilic defect. The European Prospective Cohort on Thrombophilia (EPCOT). *J Thromb Haemost.* 2005;3(3):459–464.
9. Kottke-Marchant K. Genetic polymorphisms associated with venous and arterial thrombosis: an overview. *Arch Pathol Lab Med.* 2002;126(3):295–304.
10. Ray JG. Hyperhomocysteinemia: no longer a consideration in the management of venous thromboembolism. *Curr Opin Pulm Med.* 2008;14(5):369–373.
11. Luo M, Hajjar KM. Annexin A2 system in human biology: cell surface and beyond. *Semin Thromb Hemost.* 2013;39:338–346.
12. Lim W. Antiphospholipid antibody syndrome. *Hematology Am Soc Hematol Educ Program.* 2009;2009:233–239.
13. Cohen D, Berger SP, Steup-Beekman GM, et al. Diagnosis and management of the antiphospholipid syndrome. *BMJ.* 2010;340:c2541.
14. Tang W, Teichert M, Chasman DI, et al. A genome-wide association study for venous thromboembolism: the extended cohorts for heart and aging research in genomic epidemiology (CHARGE) consortium. *Genet Epidemiol.* 2013;37(5):512–521.
15. Germain M, Saut N, Oudot-Mellakh T, et al. Caution in interpreting results from imputation analysis when linkage disequilibrium extends over a large distance: a case study on venous thrombosis. *PloS One.* 2012;7(6):e38538.

147 ⋘

16. Germain M, Chasman DI, de Haan H, et al. Meta-analysis of 65,734 individuals identifies TSPAN15 and SLC44A2 as two susceptibility loci for venous thromboembolism. *Am J Hum Genet.* 2015;96(4):532–542.

17. Connors JM. Thrombophilia testing and venous thrombosis. *N Engl J Med.* 2017;377(12):1177–1187.

18. Elbaz A, Poirier O, Moulin T, et al. Association between the Glu298Asp polymorphism in the endothelial constitutive nitric oxide synthase gene and brain infarction. *The GENIC Investigators Stroke.* 2000;31(7):1634–1639.

19. Hingorani AD, Liang CF, Fatibene J, et al. A common variant of the endothelial nitric oxide synthase (Glu298-->Asp) is a major risk factor for coronary artery disease in the UK. *Circulation.* 1999;100(14):1515–1520.

20. Kessler T, Wobst J, Wolf B, et al. Functional characterization of the GUCY1A3 coronary artery disease risk locus. *Circulation.* 2017;136(5):476–489.

21. Loscalzo J. Nitric oxide signaling and atherothrombosis risk redux. Evidence from experiments of nature and implications for therapy. *Circulation.* 2018;137:233–236.

22. Malarstig A, Hamsten A. Genetics of atherothrombosis and thrombophilia. *Curr Atheroscler Rep..* 2010;12(3):159–166.

23. Scarabin PY, Arveiler D, Amouyel P, et al. Plasma fibrinogen explains much of the difference in risk of coronary heart disease between France and Northern Ireland. The PRIME study. *Atherosclerosis.* 2003;166(1):103–109.

24. Voetsch B, Loscalzo J. Genetic determinants of arterial thrombosis. *Arterioscler Thromb Vasc Biol.* 2004;24(2):216–229.

25. Endler G, Mannhalter C. Polymorphisms in coagulation factor genes and their impact on arterial and venous thrombosis. *Clin Chim Acta.* 2003;330(1-2):31–55.

26. Standeven KF, Grant PJ, Carter AM, et al. Functional analysis of the fibrinogen Aalpha Thr312Ala polymorphism: effects on fibrin structure and function. *Circulation.* 2003;107(18):2326–2330.

27. Wald DS, Law M, Morris JK. Homocysteine and cardiovascular disease: evidence on causality from a meta-analysis. *BMJ.* 2002;325(7374):1202.

28. Jneid H, Bhatt DL. Advances in antiplatelet therapy. *Expert Opin Emerg Drugs.* 2003;8(2):349–363.

29. Snoep JD, Hovens MM, Eikenboom JC, et al. Association of laboratory-defined aspirin resistance with a higher risk of recurrent cardiovascular events: a systematic review and meta-analysis. *Arch Intern Med.* 2007;167(15):1593–1599.

30. Krasopoulos G, Brister SJ, Beattie WS, Buchanan MR. Aspirin "resistance" and risk of cardiovascular morbidity: systematic review and meta-analysis. *BMJ.* 2008;336(7637):195–198.

31. Daniel JL, Dangelmaier C, Jin J, et al. Role of intracellular signaling events in ADP-induced platelet aggregation. *Thromb Haemost.* 1999;82(4):1322–1326.

32. Yusuf S, Zhao F, Mehta SR, et al. Effects of clopidogrel in addition to aspirin in patients with acute coronary syndromes without ST-segment elevation. *N Engl J Med.* 2001;345(7):494–502.

33. Mehta SR, Yusuf S, Peters RJ, et al. Effects of pretreatment with clopidogrel and aspirin followed by long-term therapy in patients undergoing percutaneous coronary intervention: the PCI-CURE study. *Lancet.* 2001;358(9281):527–533.

34. Steinhubl SR, Berger PB, Mann 3rd JT, et al. Early and sustained dual oral antiplatelet therapy following percutaneous coronary intervention: a randomized controlled trial. *JAMA.* 2002;288(19):2411–2420.

35. Michelson AD. P2Y12 antagonism: promises and challenges. *Arterioscler Thromb Vasc Biol.* 2008;28(3):s33–s38.

36. Bertrand ME, Rupprecht HJ, Urban P, Gershlick AH. Double-blind study of the safety of clopidogrel with and without a loading dose in combination with aspirin compared with ticlopidine in combination with aspirin after coronary stenting: the clopidogrel aspirin stent international cooperative study (CLASSICS). *Circulation.* 2000;102(6):624–629.

36a. Flaumenhaft R, De Ceunynck K. Targeting PAR1: now what? *Trends Pharmacol Sci.* 2017;38(8):701–716.

37. Michelson AD. Antiplatelet therapies for the treatment of cardiovascular disease. *Nat Rev Drug Discov..* 2010;9(2):154–169.

38. van 't Hof AW, Valgimigli M. Defining the role of platelet glycoprotein receptor inhibitors in STEMI: focus on tirofiban. *Drugs.* 2009;69(1):85–100.

39. Tamhane UU, Gurm HS. GP IIb/IIIa inhibitors during primary percutaneous coronary intervention for STEMI: new trial and registry data. *Curr Cardiol Rep.* 2008;10(5):424–430.

40. Mukherjee D, Roffi M. Glycoprotein IIb/IIIa receptor inhibitors in 2008: do they still have a role? *J Interv Cardiol.* 2008;21(2):118–121.

41. Chew DP, Bhatt DL, Sapp S, Topol EJ. Increased mortality with oral platelet glycoprotein IIb/IIIa antagonists: a meta-analysis of phase III multicenter randomized trials. *Circulation.* 2001;103(2):201–206.

42. Blue R, Murcia M, Karan C, et al. Application of high-throughput screening to identify a novel alphaIIb-specific small- molecule inhibitor of alphaIIbbeta3-mediated platelet interaction with fibrinogen. *Blood.* 2008;111(3):1248–1256.

43. Chang MC, Lin HK, Peng HC, Huang TF. Antithrombotic effect of crotalin, a platelet membrane glycoprotein Ib antagonist from venom of Crotalus atrox. *Blood.* 1998;91(5):1582–1589.

44. Yeh CH, Chang MC, Peng HC, Huang TF. Pharmacological characterization and antithrombotic effect of agkistin, a platelet glycoprotein Ib antagonist. *Br J Pharmacol.* 2001;132(4):843–850.

45. Fontayne A, Meiring M, Lamprecht S, et al. The humanized anti-glycoprotein Ib monoclonal antibody h6B4-Fab is a potent and safe antithrombotic in a high shear arterial thrombosis model in baboons. *Thromb Haemost.* 2008;100(4):670–677.

46. Rosovsky R, Merli G. Anticoagulation in pulmonary embolism: update in the age of direct oral anticoagulants. *Tech Vasc Interv Radiol.* 2017;20(3):141–151.

46a. Raskob GE, van Es N, Verhamme P, et al. Edoxaban for the treatment of cancer-associated venous thromboembolism. *N Engl J Med.* 2018;378(7):615–624.

47. Neumann FJ, Zohlnhofer D, Fakhoury L, et al. Effect of glycoprotein IIb/IIIa receptor blockade on platelet-leukocyte interaction and surface expression of the leukocyte integrin Mac-1 in acute myocardial infarction. *J Am Coll Cardiol.* 1999;34(5):1420–1426.

48. Schonbeck U, Libby P. The CD40/CD154 receptor/ligand dyad. *Cell Mol Life Sci.* 2001;58(1):4–43.

49. Aukrust P, Muller F, Ueland T, et al. Enhanced levels of soluble and membrane-bound CD40 ligand in patients with unstable angina. Possible reflection of T lymphocyte and platelet involvement in the pathogenesis of acute coronary syndromes. *Circulation.* 1999;100(6):614–620.

50. Schonbeck U, Varo N, Libby P, et al. Soluble CD40L and cardiovascular risk in women. *Circulation.* 2001;104(19):2266–2268.

51. Varo N, de Lemos JA, Libby P, et al. Soluble CD40L: risk prediction after acute coronary syndromes. *Circulation.* 2003;108(9):1049–1052.

52. Freedman JE. CD40 ligand—assessing risk instead of damage? *N Engl J Med.* 2003;348(12):1163–1165.

53. Ghiassian D, Menche J, Chasman DI, et al. Endophenotype network models: common core of complex diseases. *Sci Rep.* 2016;6:27414.

54. Fagoonee S, De Angelis C, Elia C, et al. Potential link between Helicobacter pylori and ischemic heart disease: does the bacterium elicit thrombosis? *Minerva Med.* 2010;101(2):121–125.

55. Stassen FR, Vainas T, Bruggeman CA. Infection and atherosclerosis. An alternative view on an outdated hypothesis. *Pharmacol Rep.* 2008;60(1):85–92.

56. Balogh S, Kiss I, Csaszar A. Toll-like receptors: link between "danger" ligands and plaque instability. *Curr Drug Targets.* 2009;10(6):513–518.

57. Rex S, Beaulieu LM, Perlman DH, et al. Immune versus thrombotic stimulation of platelets differentially regulates signalling pathways, intracellular protein-protein interactions, and alpha-granule release. *Thromb Haemost.* 2009;102(1):97–110.

58. Mozzini C, Garbin U, Fratta Pasini AM, Cominacini L. An exploratory look at NETosis in atherosclerosis. *Intern Emerg Med.* 2017;12(1):13–22.

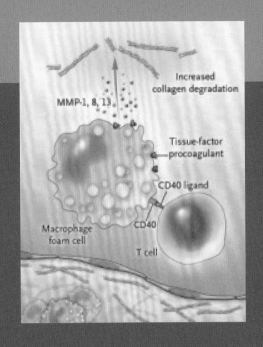

第9章
心血管系统纤维化的
病理生理学和评估

　　纤维化是指疏松细胞外基质（extracellular matrix，ECM）的重组和成纤维细胞的增殖导致的结缔组织增厚。当创伤发生，实质细胞无法恢复正常结构完整性时，作为一种代偿机制，促纤维化信号通路就会上调。细胞外基质蛋白，如胶原蛋白、弹性蛋白等在纤维化部位沉积，同时激活的金属蛋白酶降解细胞外基质蛋白以促进组织重塑和瘢痕形成。纤维化的结果部分取决于所涉及的组织亚型。纤维化在生理上是机体应对创伤的适应性反应。然而，纤维化又是许多心血管疾病的致病因素，包括特发性肺动脉高压（pulmonary arterial hypertension，PAH）、动脉硬化、肥厚性心肌病等。病理性纤维化是完全有害的，而胶原蛋白的数量常被认为是判断纤维化致病性的标准，但并不是唯一独立衡量标准。了解血管纤维化的差别需要了解其病理生理学，因为仅仅根据其分布进行分类是不科学的，需要同时考虑胶原的生物学功能。同样，把纤维化归结为单一原因引起也是不对的，因为这样无法证实细胞外基质和胶原沉积参与到心血管组织损伤的重要机制。对调节纤维化的分子机制的了解是心血管纤维化潜在治疗新靶点研发的重要一步。本章节将阐述胶原蛋白的合成与代谢调节，以及心血管病理性纤维化的发生机制及检测手段。

辛世杰

Pathobiology and Assessment of Cardiovascular Fibrosis

Evan L. Brittain and Bradley A. Maron

Fibrosis refers to the reorganization of loose extracellular matrix (ECM) and proliferation of fibroblasts that causes connective tissue thickening.[1] Upregulation of profibrotic signaling pathways occurs in response to tissue destruction as a compensatory mechanism when parenchymal cells are unable to restore the normal structural integrity of affected organs. Recruitment of ECM proteins such as collagens, elastin, fibrillin, adhesive glycoproteins, integrins, and other secreted matricellular proteins is counterbalanced by activation of metalloproteinase enzymes that degrade ECM proteins to promote tissue remodeling and scar.

The functional consequences of fibrosis are diverse and hinge, in part, on the involved tissue subtype. For example, activation of preprogrammed mechanisms in response to dermal injury results in a highly coordinated series of molecular and histological events that causes the formation of a discrete collagen plug. In this scenario, fibrosis is physiological by generating an adaptive response to trauma that regulates hemostasis and decreases the probability of infection. By contrast, fibrosis is a pathogenic finding in numerous cardiovascular diseases, including idiopathic pulmonary arterial hypertension (PAH),[2] atherosclerosis,[3] systemic sclerosis,[4] fibromuscular dysplasia,[5] and hypertrophic cardiomyopathy,[6] among many other examples. Pathogenic fibrosis is solely detrimental and therefore contradistinctive to maladaptive fibrosis, which may have favorable and unfavorable consequences. For example, replacement fibrosis following myocardial infarction maintains the structural integrity of the myocardium but also serves as a nidus for unstable reentry tachyarrhythmia and progression to heart failure.[7]

Collagen quantity is often regarded as the standard for characterizing the pathogenicity of fibrosis. However, collagen content is an insufficient metric in isolation, as increased collagen is critical to physiological fibrosis, detrimental in pathogenic fibrosis, and of ambiguous relevance to benign tumors of fibroblast proliferation, such as keloid,[8] and normal aging (Fig. 9.1). Understanding the nuances of vascular fibrosis requires appreciation for its pathobiology, because classifying fibrosis based only on its distribution without regard to collagen biofunctionality is an incomplete paradigm. Similarly, as will be discussed in greater detail, traditional paradigms that ascribe global fibrosis to activation of a single master switch, particularly via transforming growth factor (TGF)-β signaling,[9] may also fail to capture a wide range of important mechanisms that regulate ECM and collagen deposition related to end-organ injury in cardiovascular tissue. In turn, a contemporary understanding of the molecular mechanisms that regulate fibrosis is an important step toward potentially identifying novel treatment targets for fibrotic cardiovascular diseases.

OVERVIEW OF COLLAGEN

The ECM is composed of water, proteins, glycosaminoglycans, and minerals but is acellular.[10] Collagen is the principal structural protein of the ECM and accounts for approximately one-third of the total protein mass in mammals.[11] There is disagreement on the optimal criteria for defining collagen: although all 28 isoform members of the collagen family are glycoproteins containing a triple helix, not all profibrotic triple helix proteins are identified as collagen, such as adiponectin.[12,13] The stereometric conformation of collagen is a three parallel polypeptide motif: a polyproline II–type helical coil wrapped tightly forming a right-handed triple helix (Fig. 9.2). (2S)-proline and 2S,4R-4-hydroxyproline account for 28% and 38% of collagen amino acids, respectively[14]; every third residue is glycine, which by virtue of its smaller size and polarity, allows for tight packing of each strand that ultimately is the basis for the tensile strength of collagen (e.g., Gly-Xaa-Yaa). Thus the most common triplet sequence is glycine-proline-hydroxyproline (predicted denaturation enthalpy $\Delta G° = -1.8$ kcal/mol),[15,16] resulting in a helical pitch of 7/2 (20.0 Å axial repeat).[17]

In general, unique collagen isoforms are identified with respect to their corresponding encoding gene (designated by a Roman numeral). Each of three polypeptide α-chains (662 to 3152 amino acids)[13] is labeled by an Arabic numeral that indicates unique structural properties. Thus the *Col2A1* gene encodes collagen II, which has three identical α-chains (homotrimer), designated as $(\alpha 1[II])_3$. By contrast, the *Col1A* gene encodes the heterotrimer collagen I, which may have either two α1-chains and one α2-chain $(\alpha1[I]_2, \alpha2[I])$, or, alternatively, three α1-chains $(\alpha1[I])_3$ (Table 9.1).

COLLAGEN STRUCTURE, PROPERTIES, AND RELEVANCE TO HUMAN BIOLOGY

Proline is derived from the amino acid L-glutamate and synthesized by cyclization of glutamate-5-semialdehyde into its biosynthetic precursor 1-pyrroline-5-carbyoxylic acid. Owing to its secondary amino group, proline may exist in the *cis* or *trans* conformation. However, the beneficial effect of proline on thermodynamic stability of collagen requires isomerization from the *cis* to *trans* orientation. Posttranslational modification of proline residues by prolyl 4-hydroxylase results in hydroxylation of its γ-carbon to form hydroxyproline, which provides a thermodynamic and mechanical advantage of this modification when in the Yaa position.[18]

Fibrillar collagen refers to collagen subtypes that generate striated fibrils; specifically, type I-III, V, XI, XXIV, and XXVII. In human biology, fibrillar collagens constitute the majority of ECM. The tensile strength of an individual collagen fibril is high, ranging from 0.2 to 0.86 GPa,[19] which suits its functionality as a tissue scaffold and anchor for matrix metalloproteinases (MMPs). The *C*-propeptides are enzymes that coordinate selection, alignment, and organization of α-chains, which is required for formation and elongation of the triple helix to generate procollagen in the endoplasmic reticulum. Next, the procollagen is transported in a coat protein II complex to the

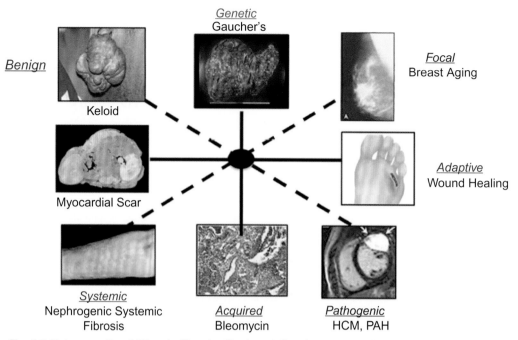

Genetic
Gaucher's

Benign
Keloid

Focal
Breast Aging

Myocardial Scar

Adaptive
Wound Healing

Systemic
Nephrogenic Systemic
Fibrosis

Acquired
Bleomycin

Pathogenic
HCM, PAH

Fig. 9.1 Heterogeneity of Fibrosis. The classification of fibrosis must consider collagen distribution and biofunctionality. Fibrosis contributing to cardiovascular disease is generally maladaptive or pathogenic. In maladaptive fibrosis, collagen deposition occurs in response to necrosis, such as following myocardial infarction or other injury, and increases the probability of adverse cardiovascular events through, for example, malignant arrhythmias. In pathogenic fibrosis, increased collagen characterizes a circumspect disease, such a myocardial fibrosis in hypertrophic cardiomyopathy *(HCM)* or pulmonary vascular fibrosis in pulmonary arterial hypertension *(PAH)*.

endoplasmic reticulum-Golgi apparatus,[10] where it may be modified further by *N*- and *C*-proteinases to form fibrils.[20] Ultimately, procollagen is transported from the Golgi apparatus to the extracellular space via a range of processes, including bulk flow, microtubule docking, and cell membrane fission.[21] Stabilization of collagen fibrils is modulated by lysyl oxidase, which occurs via the formation of highly reactive aldehydes from lysine and subsequent interaction between reactive aldehyde pairs causing mechanical cross-links. The fundamental hallmarks of the fibrosis phenotype are increased cellular stiffness and impaired tissue compliance.

REGULATION OF COLLAGEN SYNTHESIS

A wide range of perturbations to the vascular environment is associated with upregulation of collagen synthesis, ECM remodeling, and histopathological fibrosis. For example, vascular inflammation and thrombotic remodeling promote synthesis, release, and recruitment of growth factors, angiogenic simulators, and vasoactive cytokines. If unopposed or sustained, injury to the endothelial basement membrane occurs and results in the initiation of a larger cascade characterized by increased vascular permeability, platelet degranulation, and clot formation. Ultimately, activation of fibroblasts, myofibroblasts, macrophages, and endothelial or epithelial cell phenotype switching to profibrotic cells of mesenchymal origin (e.g., endothelial-mesenchymal transition) ensues and results in increased collagen protein synthesis.[22]

Profibrotic signaling has been studied largely through activation of the TGF-β superfamily of cytokines. This includes various TGF-β isoforms, bone morphogenetic proteins, and growth and differentiation factors.[23] Overactivation of canonical TGF-β signal transduction is complex and regulated by a wide spectrum of processes implicated in cardiovascular disease, including increased oxidant stress, necrosis, neurohumoral signaling (e.g., renin-angiotensin-aldosterone axis), and local hypoxia that stimulate TGF-β ligand binding to serine/threonine kinase type I or type II receptors (TGF-β-R1/2, respectively). Stimulation of the TGF-β-R1/2 complex results in phosphorylation of TGF-β-R2 by TGF-β-R1, which is required for downstream activation of various SMAD targets, particularly SMADs 3-5. Counteractivation of inhibitory SMADs, particularly SMADs 6 and 7, offsets nuclear accumulation of SMAD-DNA binding in the cell nucleus, preventing transcription of profibrotic genes, including connective tissue growth factor (CTGF). Under pathogenic circumstances, tonic upregulation of this pathway promotes excessive fibrillar collagen synthesis and deposition. In the case of heart failure, for example, increased circulating levels of angiotensin II (Ang II) activate TGF-βR1–dependent collagen synthesis in vascular smooth muscle cells (VSMCs) and left ventricular cardiomyocytes through a mechanism involving Erk1/2 signaling. Alternatively, Ang II also induces SMAD2 association with the CTGF promoter in VSMCs in vivo, supporting converging lines of evidence suggesting TGF-β–independent pathways also regulate vascular fibrosis.[24]

Similarly, aldosterone promotes fibrosis, in part, by modulating the redox potential of vascular cells. Activation of NADPH oxidase activity by aldosterone has been shown to increase reactive oxygen species (ROS) generation in macrophages, systemic vascular endothelial cells, pulmonary artery endothelial cells (PAECs), and cardiomyocytes.[25–27] Cultured proximal tubular cells treated with pathophysiologically relevant levels of aldosterone demonstrate increased mitochondrial ROS accumulation that induces epithelial-mesenchymal transition via ERK1/2 and p66Shc phosphorylation. Conversely, inhibition of the antioxidant enzyme glucose-6-phosphodehydrogenase (G6PD) by aldosterone perturbs the redox balance of vascular endothelial cells and results in diminished nitric oxide bioavailability and endothelial dysfunction.[28] Aldosterone-induced

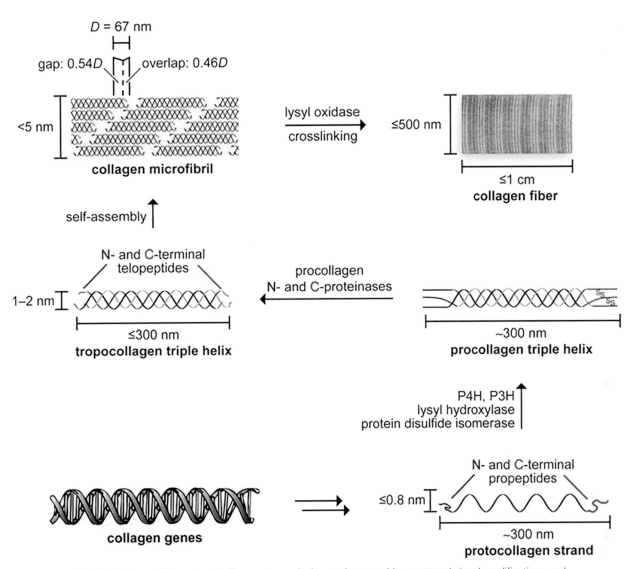

Fig. 9.2 Collagen Biosynthesis. Size and complexity are increased by posttranslational modifications and self-assembly. Oxidation of lysine side chains leads to the spontaneous formation of hydroxylysyl pyridinoline and lysylpyridinoline cross-links. (From Shoulders MD, Raines RT. Collagen structure and stability. *Annu Rev Biochem.* 2009;78:929–958.)

oxidant stress, in turn, is associated with increased expression of plasminogen activator inhibitor (PAI)-1, CTGF, and galectin-3. These proinflammatory mediators regulate crosstalk with TGF-βR-1–dependent signaling, providing a molecular basis for overlap between inflammatory and fibrotic pathophenotypes commonly observed in cardiovascular diseases associated with increased aldosterone.

Importantly, the angiotensin type 1 (AT-1) receptor and mineralocorticoid receptor (MR) are important in mediating the genomic and profibrotic effects of Ang II and aldosterone, respectively. Thus these are bona fide treatment targets by which to prevent or attenuate cardiovascular fibrosis. For example, in experimental PAH, nonselective and selective MR antagonism with spironolactone and eplerenone, respectively, prevents or reverses vascular fibrosis of distal pulmonary arterioles (Fig. 9.3).[27] However, there are alternative stimuli that may directly or indirectly result in AT-1/MR-signal transduction, which are important potential treatment targets for cardiovascular fibrosis. The vasoactive peptide endothelin-1 (ET-1), for example, is increased in heart failure, systemic hypertension, and pulmonary vascular disease and is a potent stimulator of aldosterone synthesis in the zona glomerulosa of the adrenal gland and in pulmonary endothelium.[29] In addition to its vasoconstrictor effects, ET-1 stimulates fibroblast activation, which is linked to cardiac fibrosis, and ET-1–CTGF signaling is reported in VSMCs via endothelin type-A receptor signaling.[30]

Upregulation of noncanonical TGF-β signaling targets TRAF4, TRAF6, TAK1, MAPKs, ERK, NF-κB, PI3K-Akt, and JNK.[23] These intermediaries are promiscuous and implicated in a wide range of adverse signaling cascades. However, several of these pathways have been studied in association with microRNA (miR) regulation of vascular fibrosis, particularly via miR130/301,[31] miR-29a,[32] and miR-181 a/b[33] that target YAP/TAZ, collagen and elastin, and p27, respectively. A list of some profibrotic miRs and their putative targets are provided in Table 9.2.[34] The mechanisms by which these and other miRs regulate fibrosis are diverse but, importantly, include paracrine signaling. In particular, cardiac fibroblasts exert a range of transcellular communication capabilities through miR signaling involving exosomes, apoptotic bodies, and microvesicles, which are important for propagation of fibrotic remodeling beyond the site of initial cardiovascular injury.

TABLE 9.1 Individual α-Chains, Molecular Species, and Supramolecular Assemblies of Selected Collagen Types of Relevance to Human Disease

Collagen Type	α-Chains	Molecular Species
Collagen I	α1(I), α2(I)	(α1[I])₂, α2(I)
Collagen II	α1(II)	(α1[I])₃
Collagen III	α1(III)	(α1[III])₃
Collagen IV	α1(IV), α2(IV), α3(IV), α4(IV), α5(IV), α6(IV)	(α1[IV])₂, α2(IV) α3(IV), α4(IV), α5(IV) (α5[IV])₂, α6(IV)
Collagen V	α1(V), α 2(V), α 3(V), α 4(V)	(α1[V])₂, α2(V) (α1[V])₃ (α1[V])₂, α4(V) α1(XI), α1(V), α3(XI)
Collagen VI	α1(VI), α2(VI), α3(VI), α4(VI), α5(VI)c, α6(V)	
Collagen VII	α1(VII)	(α1[VII])₃
Collagen VIII	α1(VIII)	(α1[VIII])₂, α2(VIII) α1(VIII), (α2[VIII])₂ (α 1[VIII])₃ (α2[VIII])₃
Collagen IX	α1(IX), α2(IX), α3(IX)	(α1[IX], α2[X], α3[X])
Collagen X	α1(X)	(α1[X])₃
Collagen XI	α1(XI), α2(XI), α3(XI)	α1(XI), α2(XI), α3(XI) α1(XI), α1(V), α3(XI)
Collagen XII	α1(XII)	(α1[XII])₃
Collagen XIII	α1(XIII)	(α1[XIII])₃
Collagen XIV	α1(XIV)	(α [XIV])₃
Collagen XV	α1(XV)	(α1[XV])₃
Collagen XVI	α1(XVI)	(α1[XVI])₃
Collagen XVII	α1(XVII)	(α [XVII])₃
Collagen XVIII	α1(XVIII)	(α1[XVIII])₃
Collagen XIX	α1(XIX)	(α1[XIX])₃
Collagen XX	α1(XX)	(α1[XX])₃

Modified from Ricard-Blum S. The collagen family. *Cold Spring Harb Perspect Biol.* 2011;3(1):a004978.

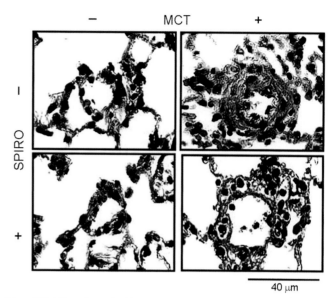

Fig. 9.3 Mineralocorticoid receptor inhibition prevents vascular fibrosis in experimental pulmonary arterial hypertension in vivo. The preventative effect of aldosterone receptor antagonism with spironolactone *(SPIRO)* was assessed using the monocrotaline *(MCT)* experimental model of pulmonary arterial hypertension (PAH). Gomori trichrome stain performed on paraffin-embedded lung sections demonstrates that SPIRO significantly decreased perivascular collagen deposition in pulmonary arterioles measuring compared with MCT-PAH rats. (From Maron BA, Zhang YY, White K, et al. Aldosterone inactivates the endothelin-B receptor via a cysteinyl thiol redox switch to decrease pulmonary endothelial nitric oxide levels and modulate pulmonary arterial hypertension. *Circulation.* 2012;126:963–974.)

REGULATION OF COLLAGEN METABOLISM

The MMP family consists of zinc-dependent endopeptidases that exert collagenolytic activity by virtue of site-specific hydrolysis. For collagen I, for example, MMP-2 and the two membrane-type MMP, MT-1-MMPs, target the Pro-Gln-Gly[775] ~Ile[776]-Ala-Gly for cleavage.[35] The final common pathways for degradation via hydrolysis involve proteolysis or urokinase plasminogen activator receptor–associated protein/Endo180–mediated endocytosis.[36] In addition to the interaction between MMP and MT-MMP proteins with collagen, alternative pathways relevant to cardiovascular fibrosis for collagen catabolism have been reported, including α2β1 integrin–dependent phagocytosis in the lysosome. The initiation of collagen degradation generally involves mechanical strain on the fibrils, which facilitates their physical dissociation and breakdown. Although fibronectin, other α2β1-targeting proteins, and the tetraspanins CD63 and CD151 have been implicated in the initiation of collagen degradation,[37,38] the factors that prompt these critical steps relevant to vascular fibrosis in cardiovascular diseases are not well characterized.

FIBROSIS IN CLINICAL CARDIOVASCULAR DISEASE

Myocardial Fibrosis: Background

The ECM provides strength and structure to the myocardium and permits signal transduction among surrounding cells. Executing these functions is a dynamic process that involves continuous collagen deposition and breakdown. Cardiac fibroblasts secrete procollagen chains that organize into fibrils and undergo posttranslational cross-linking, which maintains tissue strength. Type I collagen comprises the majority of the ECM in the myocardium and provides strength, whereas type III collagen provides (recoil) elasticity. Pathological fibrosis arises when there is aberrant healing or response to injury in which collagen deposition exceeds clearance. Overall, myocardial fibrosis results in increased tissue stiffness, decreased cardiac compliance, and, ultimately, impaired contractility with increased susceptibility to malignant arrhythmias and sudden cardiac death.

Two characteristic patterns of fibrosis occur in the myocardium: replacement fibrosis and interstitial fibrosis. Replacement fibrosis occurs in response to injury in which myocytes die and are "replaced" by fibrotic scar. The most common example of replacement fibrosis occurs as a result of myocardial infarction and is observed in the blood flow distribution of the involved coronary artery. Additional myocardial diseases in which replacement fibrosis is observed include hypertrophic cardiomyopathy and dilated cardiomyopathy, which exhibit stereotypical fibrosis patterns (Fig. 9.4).

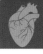

TABLE 9.2 MicroRNAs Involved in Cardiac Fibrosis

miRNA	Target	Mode of Action
miR-1	Fibulin-1	Delivery during left ventricular pressure overload attenuates fibrosis
miR-21	Protein sprouty homologue 1, protein sprouty homologue 2, PTEN	Inhibits fibroblast apoptosis and increases fibroblast growth factor 2 secretion; leads to endothelial dedifferentiation
miR-26a	Collagen α-1(1) chain, connective tissue growth factor	Regulates nuclear factor κB and fibrosis development
miR-29	Collagens, elastin, other matrix genes	Targets extracellular matrix genes
miR-34	Vascular endothelial growth factor, neurogenic locus notch homologue protein 1, vinculin, PPP1R10	Involved in cardiomyocyte aging; inhibits miR-34 and limits cardiac fibrosis
miR-101	c-fos	Overexpression rescues pressure overload–induced fibrosis
miR-122	Transforming growth factor-β1	Reciprocally regulated in patients with aortic stenosis
miR-132	Ras/Rap GTPase-activating protein SynGAP; methyl-CpG-binding domain protein 2	Saphenous vein–derived pericyte progenitor cells mediate antifibrotic signaling in the infarcted heart
miR-133/miR-30	Connective tissue growth factor	Involved in fibrosis development through connective tissue growth factor targeting
miR-133a	Collagen α-1(1) chain	Transgenic overexpression in cardiomyocytes prevents fibrosis development during pressure overload and diabetic cardiomyopathy
miR-155	Unknown	A macrophage-derived miRNA involved in cardiac inflammation and fibrosis
miR-199b	Dual-specificity tyrosine-(Y)-phosphorylation regulated kinase 1A	Inhibition prevents cardiac fibrosis under left ventricular pressure overload
miR-208	Myosin-6, myosin-7	Inhibition leads to reduced fibrosis development under cardiac stress
miR-214	Sodium/calcium exchanger 1	Inhibition leads to excessive cardiac fibrosis development after myocardial infarction

miR, MicroRNA; *PTEN*, phosphatidylinositol 3,4,5-triphosphate 3-phosphatase.
From Thum T. Noncoding RNAs and myocardial fibrosis. *Nat Rev Cardiol.* 2014;11(11):655–663.

Interstitial fibrosis arises from excess collagen deposition by activated myocardial fibroblasts, known as myofibroblasts. The composition of interstitial fibrosis is disproportionately type I collagen, which increases collagen crosslinking leading to myocardial stiffness. The underlying triggers for fibroblast activation and the factors that contribute to individual variation in the development of interstitial fibrosis are unknown.

Processes implicated in interstitial fibrosis include inflammation, immune response, infection, and metabolic diseases, among others. Specific mediators of fibroblast activation, among many others, include TGF-β, tumor necrosis factor-α, CTGF, proteolytic enzymes, angiogenic factors, and miRNAs. The relative contributions of these molecular mediators and specific diseases in which they exert their effects are incompletely understood. Nonetheless, these factors represent potential targets to prevent or reverse myocardial fibrosis by virtue of their involvement in fibroblast activation. Interstitial fibrosis increases with age and is observed in patients with systemic hypertension, heart failure with preserved ejection fraction, and systemic sclerosis. Importantly, interstitial fibrosis is reversible and thus an important target for intervention to improve cardiovascular outcomes.

Methods of Detection

The "gold standard" for detection of myocardial fibrosis is endomyocardial biopsy. Biopsy is typically performed on the interventricular septal surface of the right ventricle because of increased thrombosis and systemic embolism risk when performed in the left ventricle. The extent of fibrosis is assessed by Masson trichrome and picrosirius red staining, among other collagen stains. The percentage of myocardium occupied by collagen and the relative abundance of types I and III collagen can be determined using modern semiquantitative immunohistochemistry methods.[39] Despite the clear advantage of direct tissue studies, biopsy is limited in clinical practice to situations in which definitive diagnosis of myocardial disease will alter clinical management. Major limitations of endomyocardial biopsy include the invasive nature of the procedure, with limited access to left ventricular tissue, and sampling error, in which patchy areas of fibrosis may be missed.

Cardiac magnetic resonance (CMR) has revolutionized the clinical approach to assessing myocardial fibrosis. Myocardial fibrosis on CMR is identified by two different techniques, which parallel the two types of fibrosis. Replacement fibrosis is detected by late gadolinium enhancement (LGE), whereas interstitial fibrosis is detected by T1 mapping and related techniques. Both methods require administration of gadolinium-based contrast, which is cleared more slowly in tissues with expanded extracellular space and reduced capillary density (e.g., after myocardial infarction). Pixel intensity on CMR is related to the magnetic properties of hydrogen nuclei in the tissue of interest. Myocardial gadolinium accumulation shortens the longitudinal relaxation time, which increases signal intensity and can be quantified.

LGE is identified based on signal contrast with neighboring myocardium to identify focal areas of scar. LGE appears in stereotypical patterns based on the etiology of myocardial disease. CMR LGE is clinically useful because it provides incremental prognostic prediction over clinical and biochemical variables in myocardial diseases that involve fibrosis. Moreover, LGE extent after myocardial infarction (i.e., subendocardial vs. transmural) predicts functional recovery of the involved myocardial segment after revascularization. An important limitation of LGE imaging is that there is no consensus on which signaling threshold discriminates normal and abnormal myocardium. Most studies have favored high signaling thresholds (e.g., six standard deviations above normal), resulting in high specificity but low sensitivity, which may misclassify abnormal areas of myocardium.

T1 mapping allows identification of interstitial fibrosis that cannot be seen with the "naked eye." T1 time reflects the longitudinal relaxation time of hydrogen nuclei (expressed in milliseconds) and is an inherent property of the myocardium. Precontrast or "native" T1 time is longer in areas of interstitial fibrosis, whereas postcontrast T1 is decreased in fibrotic areas. Diffuse fibrosis can also be expressed as a

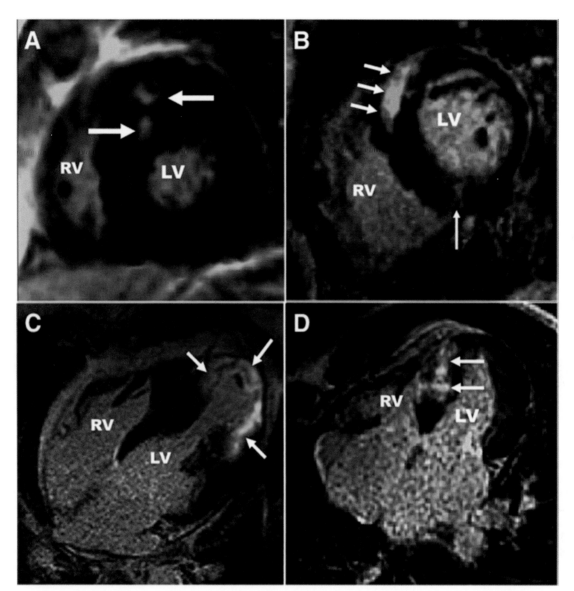

Fig. 9.4 Heterogeneity of Cardiac Fibrosis in Hypertrophic Cardiomyopathy. Contrast-enhanced cardiovascular magnetic resonance images in four patients with hypertrophic cardiomyopathy. (A) Basal left ventricular *(LV)* short-axis image shows focal areas of late gadolinium enhancement (LGE) are confined to the midmyocardial anterior wall *(arrows)*. (B) Mid-LV short-axis image from a 61-year-old woman with substantial LGE (23% of LV mass) involving the basal anterior septum and contiguous anterolateral free wall *(thick arrows)*, as well as focally at the intersection of right ventricular *(RV)* free wall and posterior septum *(thin arrow)*. (C) A four-chamber long-axis image from mildly symptomatic 54-year-old man without conventional sudden cardiac death risk factors and normal ejection fraction (60%) but with transmural LGE involving the distal posterior septum, apex, and lateral free wall *(arrows)* encompassing 36% of the LV mass. (D) A four-chamber long-axis image from 29-year-old man with extensive LGE involving large portions of the ventricular septum *(arrows)* encompassing 32% of the overall LV mass. (From Chan RH, Maron BJ, Oliviotto I, et al. Prognostic value of quantitative contrast-enhanced cardiovascular magnetic resonance for the evaluation of sudden death risk in patients with hypertrophic cardiomyopathy. *Circulation.* 2014;130:484–495.)

ratio of pre/post T1 values to calculate the extracellular volume (ECV), which represents the volume of fibrosis.[40] Measuring ECV overcomes technical limitations related to "windowing" and timing between contrast and T1 measurement because T1 time is highly dynamic. T1 time and ECV become abnormal before circulating markers of myocardial fibrosis emerge, which may allow detection of subclinical myocardial disease. ECV and T1 mapping are particularly powerful because interstitial fibrosis is modifiable, positioning CMR as a valuable tool for clinical studies assessing longitudinal changes or response to therapy.

MYOCARDIAL FIBROSIS IN SPECIFIC CARDIOVASCULAR CONDITIONS

Ischemic Heart Disease

Myocardial infarction assessment was the initial application of LGE to cardiovascular disease. Early studies in experimental models demonstrated strong agreement between the distribution of the coronary vessel in the infarct model and the distribution of LGE. The intensity of

LGE also correlated with the biochemical severity of the infarct. After myocardial infarction, LGE appears in the subendocardium and extends to the epicardium in the setting of transmural infarction, mirroring the loss of blood flow after coronary occlusion. The extent and transmural thickness of LGE are independently associated with risk of subsequent heart failure, ventricular arrhythmia, and death.[40] In subjects without a prior history of myocardial infarction, identification of occult LGE is strongly associated with an increased risk of adverse cardiovascular events.[41] CMR LGE is also clinically useful in predicting recovery of infarcted segments after revascularization. Segments with greater than 50% LGE thickness have only an 8% chance of improved contractility after revascularization.[42] In addition to providing information on prognosis and response to therapy, CMR offers gold-standard measurements of cardiac structure and function.

Nonischemic Cardiomyopathy

CMR LGE allows accurate discrimination of nonischemic and ischemic cardiomyopathies. A nonischemic etiology is suggested by either absence of LGE in the setting of systolic dysfunction and normal coronary arteries on angiography or a midwall distribution of LGE.[43] Midwall myocardial fibrosis on CMR is independently associated with all-cause mortality and sudden cardiac death, and provides prognostic information that is incremental to left ventricular ejection fraction.[44] The clinical use of T1 mapping to quantify interstitial fibrosis is likely to increase as a tool to detect subclinical myocardial fibrosis in populations at risk of developing overt cardiomyopathy. For example, increased myocardial ECV has been identified in lamin A/C mutation carriers with normal LV size and function and no LGE, suggesting subclinical disease.

Hypertrophic Cardiomyopathy

LGE in hypertrophic cardiomyopathy may be observed in several patterns, including at the septal right ventricular insertion sites, in the midwall, or as patchy fibrosis in the hypertrophied segments. Proposed mechanisms of LGE in hypertrophic cardiomyopathy include fibrosis due to microvascular ischemic injury in hypertrophied segments and expanded ECM in areas of myocyte disarray. Similar to other conditions, fibrosis in hypertrophic cardiomyopathy is associated with increased risk of malignant arrhythmias and sudden cardiac death,[45] including in subjects without other high-risk features.[46] A linear relationship exists between LGE by percent of left ventricular mass and the risk of sudden cardiac death, without a clear threshold at which risk plateaus. In a study of 1293 subjects with hypertrophic cardiomyopathy and greater than 3 years of follow-up, the presence of any LGE improved the net reclassification index when added to conventional risk factors for sudden cardiac death.[6]

Myocarditis

LGE in myocarditis typically involves the subepicardium or midwall. The mechanism of LGE in the acute phase of myocarditis is necrosis, whereas persistence of LGE is likely the result of progression to replacement fibrosis.

Amyloidosis

LGE is highly specific for the diagnosis of amyloidosis, although endomyocardial biopsy remains the reference standard. The characteristic pattern of LGE in light chain amyloidosis is a global subendocardial distribution, which may also involve the atria and right ventricle. LGE in amyloid is believed to represent expansion of the extracellular space from amyloid deposition. Some evidence exists from necropsy studies that LGE distribution mirrors areas of myocardial fibrosis from perivascular amyloid deposition. Unlike most other conditions involving myocardial fibrosis, there is no evidence that LGE in patients with amyloidosis is associated with prognosis.

Atrial Myopathy in Atrial Fibrillation

Fibrosis of the myocardium may also involve the atria and contribute to the risk of persistent atrial fibrillation and thromboembolic stroke. Fibrotic atrial cardiomyopathy results from fibroblast activation by atrial injury and stretch from atrial fibrillation risk factors (e.g., hypertension, ischemia, etc.).[47] Collagen deposition further impairs electrical conduction, worsening atrial distension and triggering a cycle in which "atrial fibrillation begets atrial fibrillation." Atrial LGE on CMR correlates well with fibrosis on histopathological samples and is associated with both an increased risk of stroke and atrial fibrillation recurrence after ablation. The risk of stroke appears to persist after restoration of sinus rhythm in patients with atrial fibrosis, suggesting that fibrotic substrate may contribute directly to the risk of thrombosis. Preventing atrial fibrosis has thus emerged as an additional therapeutic target to reduce stroke risk.

Endomyocardial Fibrosis

Endomyocardial fibrosis most commonly affects young adults in low-income tropical areas. It is characterized by an acute febrile illness, myocardial inflammation, and eosinophilic infiltration leading to subendocardial myocardial fibrosis.[48] Subendocardial fibrosis can be seen on echocardiography or LGE CMR and is often complicated by mural thrombi on the endocardial surface. In the chronic phase, endomyocardial fibrosis typically involves the apices of both ventricles and manifests clinically as a restrictive cardiomyopathy with congestion, edema, and ascites.

Myocardial fibrosis is also observed in genetic cardiomyopathies (arrhythmogenic right ventricular cardiomyopathy), autoimmune conditions (systemic sclerosis, Churg-Strauss syndrome), and infectious diseases (Lyme disease, Chagas disease).

BIOMARKERS OF MYOCARDIAL FIBROSIS

Numerous circulating markers involved in ECM formation and degradation correlate with outcomes in patients with cardiovascular disease.[49] A major limitation of translating these markers to clinical use is lack of specificity to the myocardium. Moreover, levels of some markers are affected by the function of other organs (e.g., galactin-3 is influenced by liver and renal disease). Lack of specificity limits the diagnostic potential of these potential biomarkers of fibrosis. Only two serum peptides consistently correlate with myocardial fibrosis on histological specimens: propeptides of collagen type I (PCIP) and propeptides of collagen type III (PIIICP). Both markers correlate well with the fibrosis fraction on histology, are higher in patients with known heart disease, and decline in response to heart failure therapies. Other candidate fibrosis markers, such as MMPs, miRs, galactin-3, and soluble ST2, do not correlate with myocardial fibrosis, have not been directly compared, or produced conflicting results. Emerging biomarkers, such as ST2 and galactin-3, maintain value as prognostic markers in heart failure, but lack of validation with myocardial fibrosis limits their use in mechanistic studies.[50]

TARGETING MYOCARDIAL FIBROSIS

Expansion of the ECM leading to myocardial fibrosis is an important target for intervention because it represents a common pathological pathway in many cardiovascular diseases, directly impairs myocardial function, and is strongly associated with clinical outcomes. Replacement or "scar" fibrosis is thought to be irreversible, whereas interstitial fibrosis is modifiable. Evidence of ECM regression has been shown in biopsy samples in early clinical trials of angiotensin-converting enzyme inhibitors, angiotensin receptor blockers, and MR. Although absolute reductions in collagen were modest, regression correlated with improved cardiac function, providing important proof of principle.

Active areas of investigation in early-phase clinical trials to prevent or reduce interstitial fibrosis include modulating TGF-β activity, nonsteroidal MR antagonism, reduction of collagen cross-linking (lysyl oxidase-like 2), blocking miR-21 activity, and thromboxane receptor antagonism.[51] Serelaxin, a recombinant relaxin receptor agonist, was initially approved by the US Food and Drug Administration as a breakthrough therapy on the basis of efficacy in early studies but failed to meet the primary end point in a phase III trial, halting further clinical investigations targeting myocardial fibrosis.

VASCULAR FIBROSIS IN SYSTEMIC HYPERTENSION

Maintenance of vascular ECM function is a dynamic process involving production and breakdown of its major components, collagen and elastin. As in the myocardium, vascular ECM is primarily composed of collagen types I and III. The relative abundance of these collagen types determines the vascular biomechanical properties, arterial stiffness, and hemodynamics. Imbalance of collagen and elastin in a proinflammatory milieu leads to vascular fibrosis. ECM turnover is regulated by MMPs and tissue inhibitors of metalloproteinases (TIMPs). In particular, MMP2/MMP9 activation by TGF-β1/SMAD leads to fibroblast activation and vascular wall injury.[52] Inhibiting MMPs reduces vascular fibrosis in experimental models, further supporting a pathological role of MMP activation. Aging, the most common risk factor for hypertension, also increases MMP activation by proinflammatory cytokines and interleukins. Fibrosis in small vessels contributes to endothelial dysfunction, increased vascular tone, and reduced tissue perfusion. The latter can lead to replacement of parenchymal tissue with fibrosis, ultimately resulting in organ damage. Fibrosis in large vessels leads to hemodynamic changes such as systemic arterial hypertension.

The clinical consequence of macrovascular fibrosis is increased arterial stiffness. Stiffening is caused by dysregulated collagen deposition and elastin degeneration, medial calcification, and cross-linking of collagen by advanced glycation end products. Arterial stiffening and vascular fibrosis precede the development of overt clinical hypertension.[53] When present, hypertension leads to alterations in all layers of the vasculature, from endothelial dysfunction and increased vascular smooth muscle growth and tone to ECM remodeling in the adventitia. Therefore hypertension is both a cause and a consequence of increased arterial stiffening.

Vasoactive peptides and hormones that contribute to hypertension are profibrotic. The renal-angiotensin-aldosterone system plays an important role in changes in vascular tone and structure. Ang II binding to AT-1 increases production of ECM proteins, and antagonism of Ang II reduces vascular fibrosis in experimental models. The mechanism of Ang II–induced fibrosis is incompletely understood, but evidence suggests its effects are exerted through activation of TGF-β1, p38 MAPK, and galactin-3. Aldosterone, signaling through the MR, increases collagen type I synthesis and promotes medial hypertrophy. Aldosterone antagonism improves vascular remodeling in mice overexpressing Ang II and reduces vascular stiffness and myocardial fibrosis in humans with hypertension.[54,55] Antagonism of ET_A and ET_B receptors reduce ET-1-induced MMP activity and decrease collagen type I gene expression, resulting in regression of renal vascular fibrosis.

In clinical studies, arterial stiffness is used as a surrogate for fibrosis. Stiffness is most commonly quantified using the pulse wave amplitude and velocity (PWV), a measurement of the rate at which a pressure wave moves along a conduit vessel. PWV is calculated as the distance traveled divided by time, most often measured using Doppler ultrasound or magnetic resonance imaging. Higher PWV is associated with longitudinal risk of hypertension, and pulse wave amplitude is associated with increased risk of cardiovascular events.[53] These observations suggest that vascular stiffness may be an intermediate phenotype (endophenotype) and a target for intervention to prevent hypertension and other vascular outcomes. Indeed, ACE inhibitors, angiotensin receptor blockers, and aldosterone antagonists have all been shown to reduce arterial stiffness in patients with established hypertension. The salutary effects of antagonizing the angiotensin system in patients with Marfan syndrome appear to be explained in part by reductions in arterial stiffness.[56] In addition to fibrosis of the vasculature itself, hypertension is associated with increased myocardial fibrosis. Myocardial fibrosis has been demonstrated on biopsy studies and CMR T1 mapping which show increased interstitial fibrosis in hypertensive subjects and translates to worse left ventricular diastolic function.

VASCULAR FIBROSIS IN PULMONARY ARTERIAL HYPERTENSION

Vascular effacement of distal pulmonary arterioles is a cornerstone feature of the PAH vasculopathy. Increased collagen III expression is observed in PAECs, pulmonary artery smooth muscle cells (PASMCs), and adventitial fibroblasts isolated from PAH patients. Increased collagen bioactivity, in turn, underpins pathological changes to pulmonary arterial compliance and is an important cause of elevated pulmonary vascular resistance and pulmonary artery pressure in PAH.

The molecular basis of PAH is heterogeneous and a feature that is also observed when considering disease-associated factors regulating vascular collagen. Germline mutation causing loss of function in the gene encoding BMPR2 is the most common genetic risk factor for PAH, in part, through its effect on fibrotic remodeling via endothelial-mesenchymal transition.[57] Dysregulated BMPR2-signal transduction is also implicated in overactivation of the TGF-β axis; however, this pathway is linked to variable patterns of vascular fibrosis in PAH. One mechanism by which BMPR-2–TGF-β may cause fibrosis involves overactivation of SMAD3 directly by virtue of the BMPR2 mutation or through increased susceptibility to SMAD3 activation under environmental conditions commonly associated with PAH, such as local hypoxia in the pulmonary vasculature.[58] Several genes encoding collagens are predicted targets of SMAD3 or have been shown previously to regulate SMAD3-dependent collagen expression, providing the basis for a complete pathway between BMPR2 and fibrosis.

Elevated circulating plasma levels of the angiostatic peptide endostatin (ES) are observed in patients with idiopathic PAH, which has potential relevance to fibrosis since the gene coding for ES is COL18α1.[59] Indeed, ES[60] and other collagen-associated processing enzymes have been proposed as biomarkers in PAH patients. For example, it was recently shown that PIIINP levels correlate inversely with measurements of clinical status in PAH, such as functional class and 6-minute walk distance.[61]

More recently, the Cas protein NEDD9, long established as a critical regulator of cell growth and metastasis in some solid tumors, emerged from network analyses as a key profibrotic mediator in PAH. Oxidation of a functionally essential NEDD9 cysteinyl thiol at position 18 was associated with impaired SMAD3-dependent degradation of NEDD9. In turn, increased NEDD9 bioavailability upregulated binding of the transcription factor Nkx2-5 to the Col3A1 gene resulting in increased Col3A1 mRNA and protein levels in PAECs, and NEDD9-dependent fibrotic remodeling of PAECs and PASMCs.[62]

Despite the importance of vascular fibrosis in PAH, fibrosis-specific treatment targets are lacking. The tyrosine kinase inhibitor imatinib inhibits fibrosis in other cardiovascular diseases, presumably by preventing activation of the TGF-β effector molecule, c-Abl. For this reason, and anecdotal reports suggesting clinical benefit by imatinib for end-stage PAH patients, this inhibitor was the focus of a randomized clinical trial in PAH. However, the findings from that study were mixed, and any signal toward clinical benefit in selected patients was offset by increased intracranial hemorrhage in the study population.[63] Aldosterone, angiotensin, and other neurohumoral intermediaries are promising drug targets for abrogating vascular fibrosis in PAH, have been shown to activate TGF-β–CTGF signaling in pulmonary vascular cells, but remain the focus of experimental investigations and ongoing clinical research.

CONCLUSIONS

The pathobiology of vascular fibrosis is complex, which corresponds to the diversity of collagen biofunctionality observed across the spectrum of cardiovascular diseases. The synthesis and regulation of collagen fibrils is a highly coordinated biochemical event that may be stimulated by a wide range of insults commonly observed in cardiovascular diseases, such as necrosis, inflammation, thrombosis, hypoxia, and pathophysiological levels of profibrotic hormones. Cardiovascular fibrosis plays a crucial role in the pathology and clinical risk in many diseases; however, fibrosis-specific drug therapies generally remain lacking. Greater emphasis on the disease-specific mechanisms underlying fibrosis, rather than targeting master switch molecules alone, may provide much needed insight for the development of effective therapeutics to decrease or prevent fibrosis in affected patients.

REFERENCES

1. Cotran RS, Kumar V, Collins T, eds. *Robbins Pathological Basis of Disease.* 6th ed. Philadelphia: WB Saunders; 1999.
2. Maron BA, Oldham WM, Chan SY, et al. Upregulation of steroidogenic acute regulatory protein by hypoxia stimulates aldosterone synthesis in pulmonary artery endothelial cells to promote vascular fibrosis. *Circulation.* 2014;130:168–179.
3. Stone GW, Maehara A, Lansky AJ, et al. A prospective natural-history study of coronary atherosclerosis. *N Engl J Med.* 2011;364:226–235.
4. Denton CP, Khanna D. Systemic sclerosis. *Lancet.* 2017;390:1685–1699.
5. Shivapour DM, Erwin P, Kim ESH. Epidemiology of fibromuscular dysplasia: a review of the literature. *Vasc Med.* 2016;21:376–381.
6. Chan RH, Maron BJ, Olivotto I, et al. Prognostic value of quantitative contrast-enhanced cardiovascular magnetic resonance for the evaluation of sudden death risk in patients with hypertrophic cardiomyopathy. *Circulation.* 2014;130:484–495.
7. Soejima K, Stevenson WG, Maisel WH, et al. Electrically unexcitable scar mapping based on pacing threshold for identification of the reentry circuit isthmus: feasibility for guiding ventricular tachycardia ablation. *Circulation.* 2002;106:1678–1683.
8. Hu ZC, Shi F, Liu P, et al. TIEG1 represses Smad7-mediated activation of TGF-β1/Smad signaling in keloid pathogenesis. *J Invest Dermatol.* 2017;137:1051–1059.
9. Kang JH, Jung MY, Yin X, et al. Cell-penetrating peptides selectively targeting Smad3 inhibit profibrotic TGF-β signaling. *J Clin Invest.* 2017;127:2541–2554.
10. Unlu G, Levic DS, Melville DB, et al. Trafficking mechanisms of extracellular matrix macromolecules: insights from vertebrate development and human disease. *Int J Biochem Cell Biol.* 2014;47:57–67.
11. Ricard-Blum S. The collagen family. *Cold Spring Harb Perspect Biol.* 2011;3: a004978.
12. Guo C, Ricchiuti V, Lian BQ, et al. Mineralocorticoid receptor blockade reverses obesity-related changes in expression of adiponectin, peroxisome proliferator-activated receptor-gamma, and proinflammatory adipokines. *Circulation.* 2008;117:2253–2261.
13. Ricard-Blum S, Dublet B, van der Rest M. *Unconventional Collagens: Types VI, VII, VIII, IX, X, XII, XIV, XVI and XIX.* New York: Oxford University Press; 2000.
14. Shoulders MD, Raines RT. Collagen structure and stability. *Ann Rev Biochem.* 2009;78:929–958.
15. Ramshaw JAM, Shah NK, Brodsky B. Gly-X-Y tripeptide frequencies in collagen: a context for host-guest triple-helical peptides. *J Struct Biol.* 1998;122:86–91.
16. Boryskina OP, Bolbukh TV, Semenov MA, et al. Energies of peptide-peptide and peptide-water hydrogen bonds in collagen: evidences from infrared spectroscopy, quartzpiezo gravimetry, and differential scanning calorimetry. *J Mol Struct.* 2007;827:1–10.
17. Cowan PM, McGavin S, North ACT. The polypeptide chain configuration of collagen. *Nature.* 1955;176:1062–1064.
18. Berg RA, Prockop DJ. The thermal transition of a non-hydroxylated form of collagen. Evidence for a role of hydroxyproline in stabilizing the triple-helix of collagen. *Biochem Biophys Res Comm.* 1973;52:115–120.
19. Yang L, van der Werf KO, Feijen J. Mechanical properties of native and cross-linked type I collagen fibrils. *Biophys J.* 2008;94:2204–2211.
20. Exposito J-Y, Valcourt U, Cluzel C, et al. The fibrillar collagen family. *Int J Mol Sci.* 2010;11:407–426.
21. Polishchuk EV, Di Pentima A, Luini A, et al. Mechanism of constitutive export from the Golgi: bulk flow via the formation, protrusion, and en bloc cleavage of large trans-Golgi network tubular domains. *Mol Biol Cell.* 2003;14:4470–4485.
22. Wynn TA. Common and unique mechanisms regulate fibrosis in various fibroproliferative diseases. *J Clin Invest.* 2007;117:524–529.
23. Akhurst RJ, Hata K. Targeting TGFβ signaling pathway in disease. *Nat Rev Drug Discov.* 2012;11:790–811.
24. Rodriguez-Vita J, Sanchez-Lopez E, Esteban V, et al. Angiotensin II activates the Smad pathway in vascular smooth muscle cells by a transforming growth factor-beta-independent mechanism. *Circulation.* 2005;111:2509–2517.
25. Brown NJ. Contribution of aldosterone to cardiovascular and renal inflammation and fibrosis. *Nat Rev Nephrol.* 2013;9:459–469.
26. Sun Y, Zhang J, Lu L, et al. Aldosterone-induced inflammation in the rat heart: role of oxidative stress. *Am J Pathol.* 2002;161:1773–1781.
27. Maron BA, Zhang YY, White K, et al. Aldosterone inactivates the endothelin-B receptor via a cysteinyl thiol redox switch to decrease pulmonary endothelial nitric oxide levels and modulation pulmonary arterial hypertension. *Circulation.* 2012;126:963–974.
28. Leopold JA, Dam A, Maron BA, et al. Aldosterone impairs vascular reactivity by decreasing glucose-6-phosphate dehydrogenase activity. *Nat Med.* 2007;13:189–197.
29. Maron BA, Leopold JA. Aldosterone receptor antagonists: effective but often forgotten. *Circulation.* 2010;121:934–939.
30. Rodriquez-Vita J, Ruiz-Ortega M, Ruperez M, et al. Endothelin-via ETA receptor and independently of transforming growth factor-beta, increases the connective tissue growth factor in vascular smooth muscle cells. *Circ Res.* 2005;97:125–134.
31. Bertero T, Cottrill KA, Annis S, et al. A YAP/TAZ-miR-130/301 molecular circuit exerts systems-level control of fibrosis in a network of human diseases and physiologic conditions. *Sci Rep.* 2015;5:18277.
32. Wang Y, Li M, Xu L, et al. Expression of Bcl-2 and microRNA in cardiac tissue of patients with dilated cardiomyopathy. *Mol Med Rep.* 2017;15:359–365.
33. Wang B, Li W, Guo K, et al. miR-181b promotes hepatic stellate cells proliferation by targeting p27 and is elevated in the serum of cirrhosis patients. *Biochem Biophys Res Commun.* 2012;421:4–8.
34. Thum T. Noncoding RNAs and myocardial fibrosis. *Nat Rev Cardiol.* 2014;11:655–663.
35. Hotary K, Allen E, Penturieri A, et al. Regulation of cell invasion and morphogenesis in a three-dimensional type I collagen matrix by membrane-type matrix metalloproteinases 1, 2, and 3. *J Cell Biol.* 2000;149:1309–1323.

36. Rosenblum G, Van den Steen PE, Cohen SR, et al. Direct visualization of protease action on collagen triple helical structure. *PLoS One.* 2010;5: e11043.

37. Murphy G, Nagase H. Localizing matrix metalloproteinase activities in the pericellular environment. *FEBS J.* 2011;278:2–15.

38. Fields GB. Interstitial collagen catabolism. *J Biol Chem.* 2013;288: 8785–8793.

39. Lopez B, Ravassa S, Gonzalez A, et al. Myocardial collagen cross-linking is associated with heart failure hospitalization in patients with hypertensive heart failure. *J Am Coll Cardiol.* 2016;67:251–260.

40. Mewton N, Liu CY, Croisille P, et al. Assessment of myocardial fibrosis with cardiovascular magnetic resonance. *J Am Coll Cardiol.* 2011;57:891–903.

41. Kwong RY, Chan AK, Brown KA, et al. Impact of unrecognized myocardial scar detected by cardiac magnetic resonance imaging on event-free survival in patients presenting with signs or symptoms of coronary artery disease. *Circulation.* 2006;113:2733–2743.

42. Kim RJ, Wu E, Rafael A, et al. The use of contrast-enhanced magnetic resonance imaging to identify reversible myocardial dysfunction. *N Engl J Med.* 2000;343:1445–1453.

43. Japp AG, Gulati A, Cook SA, et al. The diagnosis and evaluation of dilated cardiomyopathy. *J Am Coll Cardiol.* 2016;67:2996–3010.

44. Gulati A, Jabbour A, Ismail TF, et al. Association of fibrosis with mortality and sudden cardiac death in patients with nonischemic dilated cardiomyopathy. *JAMA.* 2013;309:896–908.

45. Adabag AS, Maron BJ, Appelbaum E, et al. Occurrence and frequency of arrhythmias in hypertrophic cardiomyopathy in relation to delayed enhancement on cardiovascular magnetic resonance. *J Am Coll Cardiol.* 2008;51:1369–1374.

46. Briasoulis A, Mallikethi-Reddy S, Palla M, et al. Myocardial fibrosis on cardiac magnetic resonance and cardiac outcomes in hypertrophic cardiomyopathy: a meta-analysis. *Heart.* 2015;101:1406–1411.

47. Hirsh BJ, Copeland-Halperin RS, Halperin JL. Fibrotic atrial cardiomyopathy, atrial fibrillation, and thromboembolism: mechanistic links and clinical inferences. *J Am Coll Cardiol.* 2015;65:2239–2251.

48. Grimaldi A, Mocumbi AO, Freers J, et al. Tropical endomyocardial fibrosis: natural history, challenges, and perspectives. *Circulation.* 2016;133:2503–2515.

49. Lopez B, Gonzalez A, Ravassa S, et al. Circulating biomarkers of myocardial fibrosis: the need for a reappraisal. *J Am Coll Cardiol.* 2015;65:2449–2456.

50. Bayes-Genis A, de Antonio M, Vila J, et al. Head-to-head comparison of 2 myocardial fibrosis biomarkers for long-term heart failure risk stratification: ST2 versus galectin-3. *J Am Coll Cardiol.* 2014;63: 158–166.

51. Schelbert EB, Fonarow GC, Bonow RO, et al. Therapeutic targets in heart failure: refocusing on the myocardial interstitium. *J Am Coll Cardiol.* 2014;63:2188–2198.

52. Harvey A, Montezano AC, Lopes RA, et al. Vascular fibrosis in aging and hypertension: molecular mechanisms and clinical implications. *Can J Cardiol.* 2016;32:659–668.

53. Kaess BM, Rong J, Larson MG, et al. Aortic stiffness, blood pressure progression, and incident hypertension. *JAMA.* 2012;308:875–881.

54. Sakurabayashi-Kitade S, Aoka Y, Nagashima H, et al. Aldosterone blockade by spironolactone improves the hypertensive vascular hypertrophy and remodeling in angiotensin II overproducing transgenic mice. *Atherosclerosis.* 2009;206:54–60.

55. Savoia C, Touyz RM, Amiri F, et al. Selective mineralocorticoid receptor blocker eplerenone reduces resistance artery stiffness in hypertensive patients. *Hypertension.* 2008;51:432–439.

56. Bhatt AB, Buck JS, Zuflacht JP, et al. Distinct effects of losartan and atenolol on vascular stiffness in Marfan syndrome. *Vasc Med.* 2015;20:317–325.

57. Ranchoux B, Antigny F, Rucker-Martin C, et al. Endothelial-to-mesenchymal transition in pulmonary hypertension. *Circulation.* 2015;131:1006–1018.

58. Upton D, Davies RJ, Tamara T, et al. Transforming growth factor-β_1 represses bone morphogenetic protein-mediated Smad signaling in pulmonary artery smooth muscle cells via Smad3. *Am J Respir Cell Mol Biol.* 2013;49:1135–1145.

59. Hoffmann J, Marsh LM, Pieper M, et al. Compartment specific expression of collagens and their processing enzymes in intrapulmonary arteries of IPAH patients. *Am J Physiol Lung Cell Mol.* 2015;308:L1002–L1013.

60. Damico R, Kolb TM, Valera L, et al. Serum endostatin is a genetically determined predictor of survival in pulmonary arterial hypertension. *Am J Respir Crit Care Med.* 2015;191:208–218.

61. Safdar Z, Tamez E, Chan W, et al. Circulating collagen biomarkers as indicators of disease severity in pulmonary arterial hypertension. *JACC Heart Fail.* 2014;2:412–421.

62. Samokhin AO, Maron BA, Alba GA, et al. Genetic ablation or molecular inhibition of NEDD9 prevents vascular fibrosis and pulmonary arterial hypertension in vivo. *Circulation.* 2017;136:A16762. Abstract.

63. Hoeper MM, Barst RJ, Bourge RC, et al. Imatinib mesylate as an add-on therapy for pulmonary arterial hypertension: results of the randomized IMPRES study. *Circulation.* 2013;127:1128–1138.

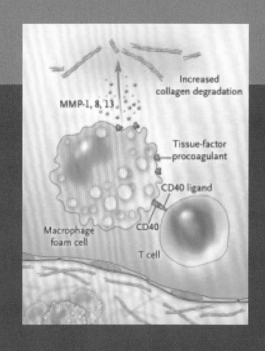

第10章
血管炎的病理生理学

　　血管炎是以血管或血管周围炎症破坏为特征的一组疾病。血管炎可累及一个或多个器官，一种或多种组织类型。主动脉及其主要分支动脉的血管炎可导致动脉狭窄及动脉瘤等病变，而发生于小血管的血管炎可导致皮肤、肺部及肾等多种组织及器官病变。激素联合免疫抑制剂是处理血管炎的常规药物治疗手段。托珠单抗、利妥昔单抗等靶向生物制剂的开发与应用具有广泛的临床前景。同时，多学科联合对于血管炎及其并发症的诊治尤为重要。血管炎的罕见性和动物模型的缺乏导致我们对其病理及分子机制认识尚不明确。在目前的研究知识背景下，发生于不同层级血管的血管炎在机制上有所不同。本章将主要阐述不同血管炎发病的病理及免疫学机制。

辛世杰

Pathobiology of Vasculitis

Paul A. Monach

The term "vasculitis" encompasses diseases that share the feature of inflammatory destruction of blood vessels but otherwise include diverse clinical phenotypes and pathophysiologies. The rarity of the vasculitides and the paucity of animal models means that their pathophysiologies are not as well understood as in many other inflammatory diseases. However, a combination of genetic, epidemiologic, and laboratory-based studies has provided insight into ways that the vasculitides resemble or differ from each other, and, in a few cases, serology has provided breakthroughs into disease mechanisms leading to changes in strategies for treatment.

Some of the localizing symptoms and objective findings of vasculitis are directly attributable to inflammation, but most are attributable to tissue ischemia or infarction. The sizes of the involved vessels, density of vessel involvement, structure of vascular beds, and pace of disease all play important roles in determining the severity of tissue injury. For example, patchy destruction of capillaries and venules in the upper part of the dermis in a single episode of vasculitis will yield discrete purpuric lesions that heal without scarring. Repeated episodes, confluent purpura, and involvement of vessels in the deeper dermis are more likely to produce hyperpigmentation and atrophy. Dense involvement of the microvasculature or destruction of small arteries is more likely to produce ulceration. Whether there is scarring or not, skin heals well and integrity is usually restored. In contrast, ischemia within a peripheral nerve sheath causes local edema that magnifies damage, and functioning nerve tissue is often not restored along the path of an infarcted nerve. Destruction of capillaries in the lung will cause bleeding but will heal without scarring. Destruction of glomerular capillaries will often cause permanent failure of the filtering unit. Stenosis of large arteries where there is limited anastomosis, such as the heart or brain, can be devastating, whereas scalp necrosis is extremely rare even when both temporal arteries are occluded or removed by biopsy. In the extremities, narrowing of large arteries occurs slowly unless there is superimposed thrombosis, for which reason critical limb ischemia is rare.

At the microscopic level, fundamentally different processes appear to cause vasculitis in the microvasculature and in large arteries, with less clarity about the mechanism(s) of injury in small arteries. This chapter will focus on how diverse underlying causes proceed through a more limited number of mechanisms to produce a narrow range of pathologies. The clinical syndromes that include these pathologies are diverse in their epidemiology, spectrum of organ involvement, and course of disease. Classification criteria are undergoing revision through an international effort. The diseases recognized in the current classification schemes are summarized in Chapter 39. The diseases that affect arteries large enough to come to the attention of specialists in vascular medicine are described in detail in Chapters 39–43.

LARGE-VESSEL VASCULITIS

In vasculitis affecting the aorta and its primary branches ("large-vessel vasculitis" [LVV]), the artery wall can be considered the site of an immune-mediated process, either directed against an undefined set of autoantigens or local deposition of undefined infectious agents or potentially against antigens derived from them (Fig. 10.1). In contrast to atherosclerosis, in which the fundamental lesion is in the intima, inflammation in LVV occurs in the media with or without involvement of the adventitia; inflammation limited to the adventitia is referred to as "periaortitis" or "periarteritis." In all forms of LVV, leukocytes are known or presumed to exit the circulation via the vasa vasorum in the manner of a regulated inflammatory reaction to injury or infection, rather than via the endovasculature of the large artery. Even in cases in which bacterial infection of the aorta may have occurred via the endothelium, the intima has usually already been damaged by atherosclerosis, and it is not clear how the resulting transmural inflammation developed.

Four patterns of aortitis have been defined and have been associated with particular diseases (Fig. 10.2)[1]; it is reasonable to propose that LVV involving the primary and secondary branches of the aorta would show a similar pattern. The granulomatous/giant cell pattern is the most common and is characteristic of the two quintessential forms of LVV: giant cell arteritis (GCA) and Takayasu arteritis. Although noninfectious aortitis is often seen in isolation, the pathology is often granulomatous, and the demographics of the patients affected also suggest that this condition is a variant of GCA in many cases.[1] GCA is the only form of LVV in which large numbers of tissue samples have been available outside the aorta, and the pathology of temporal arteritis is similarly granulomatous and focused on the media. Although the pathology of GCA and Takayasu is similar, there are some differences in the location and appearance of granulomatous disease, more differences in the arteries most commonly affected, and striking differences in epidemiology, including genetics (see Chapters 39 and 40).

The other causes of granulomatous aortitis/arteritis are rare complications of several infectious and noninfectious diseases that have little in common in their pathophysiologies otherwise, with the reasons for occasional localization to the aorta or other large arteries are unknown. The suppurative form, not surprisingly, is associated only with conventional gram-positive and gram-negative bacterial infections.

Whether by coincidence or not, aortitis with a mixed inflammatory appearance is associated with diseases in which aortitis and/or LVV is relatively common (5% to 10%): Behçet disease, relapsing polychondritis, and Cogan syndrome. It may be notable that Behçet disease has a strong "autoinflammatory" component to it. Analogous to the pathergy reaction that produces inflammation in the skin after minor sharp trauma, inflammation in large arteries and veins has been described anecdotally as occurring after vascular interventions in patients with

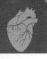

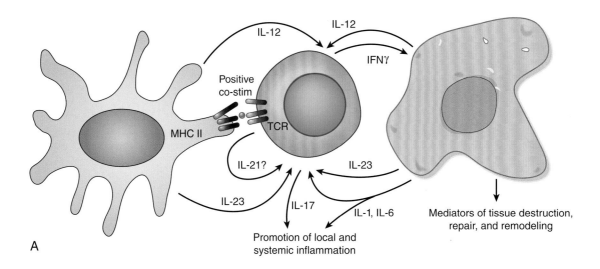

A

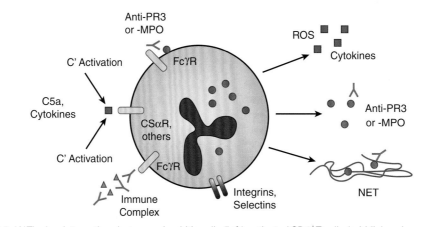

B

Fig. 10.1 (A) The key interactions between dendritic cells *(left),* activated CD4⁺ T cells *(middle),* and macrophages *(right)* in the artery wall in giant cell arteritis. The balance of costimulatory and coinhibitory molecules turns to favor activation rather than inhibition (positive costimulation) when antigenic peptides bound to MHC class II molecules on antigen-presenting cells (APCs) are recognized by T cell receptors *(TCR).*[25] IL-12 made by APCs favors development of Th1 T cells secreting IFN-γ. IL-23, IL-1β, IL-6, and IL-21 favor development of Th17 cells secreting IL-17, GM-CSF, and other proinflammatory cytokines. Macrophages, including giant cells, are a major source of enzymes and growth factors leading to tissue damage, repair, and remodeling. (B) Mechanisms of activation of neutrophils by immune complexes or ANCAs in small-vessel vasculitis. In both cases, Fc receptors, the receptor for C5a (C5aR), and likely other chemotactic factors and cytokines are involved, as are adhesion molecules. The exact order of activation through these receptors is unknown and may vary. Immune complexes may bind first to circulating cells, or the endothelium, or subendothelial tissues. ANCAs may bind to proteinase-3 or myeloperoxidase on the surface of neutrophils, the endothelium, in solution, and/or attached to neutrophil extracellular traps *(NETs).* Neutrophil effector functions that could damage tissues and perpetuate inflammation include release of granule enzymes, cytokines and other mediators, reactive oxygen species *(ROS),* and NETs. Not shown in (A) and (B) is the initial development of antigen-specific T cells and APCs, which are presumed to occur in lymphoid organs. *ANCAs,* Antineutrophil cytoplasmic antibodies; *MPO,* myeloperoxidase.

Behçet disease who have vascular involvement.[2] Nothing similar has been described in other causes of LVV, but few data are available, including a dearth of tissue.

The lymphoplasmacytic pattern of aortitis also includes diseases with no clear pathophysiologic relationship to each other. Of these, immunoglobulin G4–related disease (IgG4-RD) involves the aorta and large arteries in multiple ways. It appears to be a major cause of periaortitis, including retroperitoneal fibrosis, and it can involve the aorta and the surrounding tissue simultaneously.[3] Identification of IgG4-RD in many cases limited to the artery wall, however, indicates

that the inflammation does not always represent extension from surrounding tissues.

In all forms of noninfectious LVV, it is thought that T cells recognizing local autoantigens or extrinsic antigens are central to the pathobiology and, via local activation of innate immune cells, lead to tissue damage (see Fig. 10.1).[4] In GCA, T cells secreting either interferon-γ (Th1) or interleukin-17 (Th17) are prominent, and in an experimental model of human temporal arteries transplanted into immune-deficient mice, the Th17, but not Th1, cells are eliminated by treatment with glucocorticoids.[5]

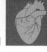

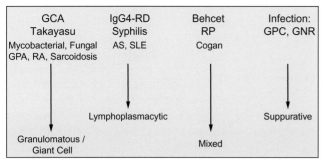

Fig. 10.2 Pathologic Patterns of Aortitis and Their Association With Different Underlying Diseases. Although all of the diseases listed other than giant cell arteritis *(GCA)* are considered rare, those in the smaller font are probably less common than the diseases in the larger font in the same columns. *AS*, Ankylosing spondylitis; *GNR*, gram-negative rods; *GPA*, granulomatosis with polyangiitis (Wegener); *GPC*, gram-positive cocci; *IgG4-RD*, IgG4-related disease; *RA*, rheumatoid arthritis; *RP*, relapsing polychondritis; *SLE*, systemic lupus erythematosus. (Data from Stone JR, Bruneval P, Angelini A, et al. Consensus statement on surgical pathology of the aorta from the Society for Cardiovascular Pathology and the Association for European Cardiovascular Pathology: I. Inflammatory diseases. *Cardiovasc Pathol.* 2015;24:267–278.)

Whether the presence of an elastic lamina, present only in relatively large arteries, is essential for any of the forms of LVV is unknown. Initial implication of different microbes in temporal arteries has not been borne out in subsequent studies. Although autoantibodies have been described in LVV, they typically are found in a minority of patients and disappear quickly after treatment. If they contribute to pathology, it is thought to be a secondary process. IgG4-RD is the form of LVV in which a search for antibody targets seems most likely to be fruitful, in light of the remarkable presence of IgG4-secreting plasma cells in the tissue. The leading hypothesis is that IgG4 itself is not the cause of tissue changes, but rather a side effect of a T cell process that induces both local plasma cell maturation and fibrosis.[3]

Although epidemiologic differences are striking, the objective genetic contributions to risk of GCA, Takayasu arteritis, and Behçet disease are modest, and they have not been determined for LVV seen rarely in other settings. In GCA, most of the risk is attributable to alleles in the HLA class II region, typical of autoimmune diseases known to be associated with one or more specific target antigens. Association of disease with HLA class II indicates that antigen-specific CD4+ T cells play a key role at some point in pathogenesis but does not give insight as to whether autoantibodies, cell-mediated immunity and inflammation, or both are important in initiation or evolution of disease. In contrast, by far the most important risk alleles in Takayasu arteritis and Behçet disease are in the HLA class I region. At first glance, this finding would appear to implicate CD8+ T cells, but there is no other reason to suspect CD8+ cells as being critical, which is also true of the quintessential HLA–class I–associated disease, ankylosing spondylitis. Because ankylosing spondylitis and Behçet disease both have features also found in autoinflammatory diseases and weak evidence for antigen-specific immunity, the finding of a class I association in Takayasu arteritis invites speculation that this disease progresses to an inflammatory lesion resembling GCA via a different basic mechanism rather than merely activation of a different type of T cell.

Intimal hyperplasia is an important feature of GCA and does not require inflammation extending into the intima but rather indicates a response to mediators produced by inflammation in the media. This inflammation also produces a fibrotic response. In the aorta, severe, permanent damage, whatever the underlying disease, often causes aneurysmal dilatation. In the primary and secondary branches, the result

in GCA and Takayasu arteritis is usually stenosis. In Behçet disease, aneurysm and pseudoaneurysm formation appear to be more common; more data are needed to assess the long-term consequences of LVV beyond the aorta in IgG4-RD.

SMALL-VESSEL VASCULITIS

In the great majority of cases of small-vessel vasculitides, the initial injury is damage to the endothelium of capillaries, venules, and arterioles by neutrophils (see Fig. 10.1). Activation of neutrophils in the vessel wall and adjacent tissue produces necrosis. Many of the neutrophils die in a manner that produces fragments of condensed nuclear material (karyorrhexis), and loss of vessel integrity leads to extravasation of red blood cells. The focal necrosis is called "fibrinoid" because of its color on routine staining; fibrin is only one of many proteins present. These features comprise "leukocytoclastic vasculitis" (LCV) and are a common end point of many underlying processes. These processes can be grouped as being secondary to antineutrophil cytoplasmic antibodies (ANCAs) or to deposition of immune complexes (see Fig. 10.1).

The ANCAs that are clearly associated with vasculitis are directed against proteinase-3 (PR3) or myeloperoxidase (MPO). Three clinical syndromes have been associated with ANCAs: granulomatosis with polyangiitis (GPA, Wegener), microscopic polyangiitis (MPA), and eosinophilic granulomatosis with polyangiitis (EGPA, Churg-Strauss). GPA is strongly but not exclusively associated with PR3-ANCAs and always features extravascular, necrotizing granulomatous inflammation in addition to necrotizing vasculitis. MPA is more strongly associated with MPO-ANCAs. EGPA is characterized by eosinophilic inflammation; only 40% of patients have MPO-ANCAs, and this subset has more features of vasculitis than does the ANCA-negative subset.

Although both PR3 and MPO are predominantly intracellular and stored in the granules of neutrophils, they are also translocated to the external surface of the plasma membrane. PR3 is found on the surface of normal neutrophils and is increased after neutrophil activation, whereas MPO is found on the surface only after activation.[6] PR3 and MPO are also released from neutrophils, either in the process of degranulation or as components of neutrophil extracellular traps (NETs).[6] Thus deposits of NETs could serve as targets of ANCAs in small vessels; however, notably, the lesions of ANCA-associated vasculitis are "pauci-immune," meaning that there is little deposition of immunoglobulin or complement. Both MPO-ANCA and PR3-ANCA can activate neutrophils in vitro.[6,7] Most convincingly with regard to pathobiology, MPO-ANCA, raised by immunization of MPO-deficient mice, can cause neutrophil-dependent pauci-immune glomerulonephritis when transferred into normal mice (Fig. 10.3).[6,8,9] Although few immune deposits are seen, the process is still dependent on activation of complement to generate C5a that activates the C5aR on neutrophils.[6,10] In addition to NETs serving as an intravascular deposit of the target antigen, it has been proposed that NETs may contribute to breaking of tolerance and production of specific autoantibodies in a susceptible host.[11] Although CD4+ T cells must play an important role in the pathogenesis of any disease that features high-affinity IgG antibodies, there is strong evidence for additional roles of T-cell subsets in established GPA, which can only be summarized briefly as "complex."[12]

The genes discovered thus far as conferring risk of ANCA-associated vasculitis segregate by the target antigen: PR3 or MPO.[13] The strongest risk is conferred by different alleles in the HLA class II region, but the additional genes associated with PR3-ANCAs encode proteins related to PR3: SERPINA1 (α-1-antitrypsin) and PRTN3 (proteinase-3 itself). However, overall genetic risk is modest, considering that the risk alleles are mostly common, and the diseases affect

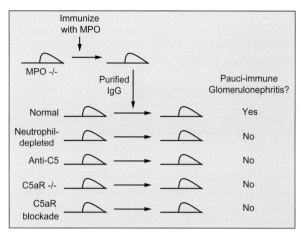

Fig. 10.3 Induction of Pauci-immune Glomerulonephritis (GN) by Autoantibodies to Myeloperoxidase (MPO) in Mice. High-titer antibodies to MPO were raised by immunizing genetically MPO-deficient (MPO -/-) mice with purified MPO antibodies. IgG purified from these mice causes GN when transferred into normal mice. Recipient mice depleted of neutrophils, or treated with antibodies to C5, or genetically deficient in the receptor for C5a (C5aR -/-), or treated with a small-molecule inhibitor of C5aR, do not develop GN. (Data from Xiao H, Heeringa P, Hu P, et al. Antineutrophil cytoplasmic autoantibodies specific for myeloperoxidase cause glomerulonephritis and vasculitis in mice. *J Clin Invest.* 2002;110:955–963; Xiao H, Heeringa P, Liu Z, et al. The role of neutrophils in the induction of glomerulonephritis by anti-myeloperoxidase antibodies. *Am J Pathol.* 2005;167:39–45; Xiao H, Dairaghi DJ, Powers JP, et al. C5a receptor [CD88] blockade protects against MPO-ANCA GN. *J Am Soc Nephrol.* 2014;25:225–231.)

approximately 1 in 10,000 persons. Several drugs—most convincingly, propothiouracil, hydralazine, and minocycline, but likely others—can lead to production not only of MPO-ANCAs but also severe vasculitis and glomerulonephritis.[14] Exposure to silica and chronic carriage of staphylococcus in the upper airway confer modest increases in risk of GPA associated with PR3-ANCAs, but the majority of cases of ANCA-associated vasculitis are idiopathic.[15]

The vasculitides mediated by immune complex deposition include cryoglobulinemic vasculitis, IgA vasculitis (Henoch-Schönlein purpura), and, presumably, most forms of vasculitis caused by reactions to medications, following infection, associated with systemic autoimmune diseases, or (less commonly) associated with malignancy. The skin is by far the most commonly involved organ system, often in isolation, but vasculitis can be found isolated to almost any organ system, and the syndromes of cryoglobulinemic vasculitis and IgA vasculitis typically involve organ systems in addition to the skin. The common involvement of the kidney in IgA vasculitis is not surprising in light of isolated IgA nephropathy being a common condition; however, the common involvement of the gastrointestinal tract remains unexplained.

The Arthus reaction is an animal model of immune-complex disease discovered more than a century ago. The model involves either the local injection of antigen and systemic delivery ("passive" Arthus reaction), de novo induction of antibodies, or the local injection of antibody and systemic delivery of antigen ("reverse passive" Arthus reaction). LCV is a feature of the Arthus reaction, but deliberate local deposition of antigen or antibody via a mechanism that causes mechanical injury calls into question its alignment with immune complex–mediated vasculitis in humans. However, "serum sickness," in which both antigen and antibody circulate, proves that immune complexes derived from the circulation cause LCV. In mice, the cutaneous reverse passive Arthus reaction is dependent on C5a and its receptor, Fc receptors for

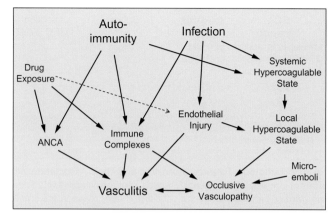

Fig. 10.4 Pathways to Small-Vessel Vasculitis and Occlusive Vasculopathy. Larger fonts and thicker arrows denote the more common pathways. *ANCAs,* Antineutrophil cytoplasmic antibodies.

IgG, P-selectin and P-selectin glycoprotein ligand-1 (PSGL-1), and the chemokine CX3CL1 and its receptor.[16,17]

Cryoglobulinemic vasculitis comes in three forms, which are worth discussing in light of the most common mimics of small vessel vasculitis, considered together as "occlusive vasculopathies." Type I cryoglobulinemia consists of high concentrations of self-aggregating monoclonal immunoglobulins derived from malignant or premalignant B cell clones. Physical blockage of the microvasculature in cold-exposed areas is thought to be part of this condition in many patients, whereas vasculitis is not always present. In contrast, types II and III cryoglobulinemia involve immune complexes, with (type II) or without (type III) a monoclonal anti-IgG component, that precipitate in the cold in the laboratory. The clinical syndromes are more reliably those of immune complex vasculitis, with more glomerulonephritis, less relationship to cold exposure, and thus less of the acrocyanosis and ulceration that are characteristic of type I cryoglobulinemia.[18,19]

The primary occlusive vasculopathies involve hypercoagulable states initiated in the microvasculature, often in association with antiphospholipid antibodies. In a finding likely analogous to some cases of type I cryoglobulinemia, thrombotic vasculopathy may sometimes be accompanied by vasculitis but usually is not. Damage to the microvascular endothelium by direct infection (such as rickettsia) or by a systemic state of infection (such as bacteremia and sepsis) also produces a local thrombotic state, and, ultimately, completely occluded vessels probably involve thrombosis to some degree, regardless of the original insult. Thus it is appropriate to conceive of small-vessel vasculitis and its main mimics as having some overlapping mechanisms as depicted in Fig. 10.4.

MEDIUM-VESSEL VASCULITIS

The mechanisms of injury to medium-sized vessels are less clear. The term polyarteritis nodosa (PAN), although encompassing a more limited spectrum of conditions than it did originally, may still be a wastebasket term, because it includes any form of vasculitis affecting only arteries ranging in size from the secondary branches of the aorta to the smallest vessels that still have a smooth muscle layer. Biopsies show diverse findings, ranging from necrotizing, neutrophilic lesions to an infiltrate composed of mononuclear cells, sometimes without evidence of necrosis. Whether the mononuclear pathology represents a completely different process or is merely the transition from a focal, necrotizing neutrophilic process to a "chronic" infiltrate that can spread longitudinally in the vessel wall[20]—known to happen within a few days—is

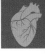

controversial and challenging to answer definitively. For example, authors of a recent series on arteritis limited to the skin argued that a proposed entity called "lymphocytic arteritis" could not be distinguished from PAN,[21] in line with what a leading vascular pathologist has concluded about PAN more generally.[20]

Even if one considers PAN to be initiated invariably by a neutrophilic process originating at the endothelium of the artery lumen, the underlying causes are unclear.[22] PAN secondary to chronic infection with hepatitis B virus (HBV)—historically up to 30% of cases but now fewer than 5% except in endemic areas—suggests that such a syndrome could be mediated by immune complexes. Involvement of small arteries in some patients with cryoglobulinemia or with vasculitis secondary to systemic rheumatic diseases also supports a possible role for immune complexes, although the microvasculature is almost always also involved in those diseases, and more extensively than larger vessels. Similarly, many patients with ANCA-associated vasculitis have involvement of small arteries but only in addition to the microvasculature. The great majority of patients who fall under the current definition of PAN test negative for ANCA and show no staining for immune complexes on biopsies.[20]

Although the pathologies of PAN and Kawasaki disease are regarded as distinct,[20] a recent pathologic study of Kawasaki arteritis suggests that mononuclear arteritis of medium-sized vessels need not be preceded by a neutrophilic phase.[23] Two main types of active inflammation were described: a necrotizing, neutrophilic type originating at the endothelium and extending outward, and a nonnecrotizing, mononuclear arteritis originating with extravasation from the vasa vasorum and extending inward. The neutrophilic inflammation, which was proposed to be a response to viral infection in the artery wall, produced a type of damage that was not seen in samples with the mononuclear type of inflammation. A study of idiopathic PAN in sheep similarly concluded that lesions featuring fibrinoid necrosis might be distinct from a more common mononuclear inflammatory lesion, without evidence of immune complex deposition in either case.[24]

Although Kawasaki disease is a unique syndrome (see Chapter 43), and an epidemic disease in a small number of animals deserves skepticism about its applicability to human PAN, it is fair to conclude that these studies demonstrate the plausibility of reconciling the controversy surrounding the pathobiology, and even the essential pathology, of PAN. Small and medium-sized arteries can be damaged in more than one way. There is no evidence that a large proportion of cases of non-HBV–associated PAN are attributable to one pathogen or one autoimmune response, but a key study to make such assessment—a genetics study to seek HLA linkage, for example—has not been performed.

SUMMARY

The mechanisms of vasculitis differ radically comparing the microvasculature to large arteries (see Fig. 10.1). Although the biology of endothelial cells differs substantially in vessels of different sizes and in vessels of the same size in different organs, the way vasculitis expresses itself may start with dynamic vascular physiology. Owing to differences in flow rate and the likelihood of cells or circulating proteins encountering the endothelium, activation of neutrophils at the vessel wall is prominent only in the microvasculature, co-opting mechanisms that evolved to fight infection in the surrounding tissues. It appears that deposition of immune complexes or binding of autoantibodies to neutrophils accounts for the great majority of cases of dysregulated neutrophil activation that destroys vessels at the sites where the leukocytes would normally exit in response to infection or injury: venules, capillaries, and to a lesser extent, arterioles. At the other end of the spectrum, the largest arteries might be thought of as the "target organ" of a

cellular immune process directed against either intrinsic autoantigens or foreign antigens, with exit of predominantly mononuclear cells via the vasa vasorum. Although the mechanisms of inflammatory destruction of small arteries are less clear, it is reasonable to propose that the larger the vessel, the more likely that its inflammation will be initiated via the vasa vasorum, and the smaller the vessel, the more likely that its inflammation will be initiated by damage to the endothelium by neutrophils.

REFERENCES

1. Stone JR, Bruneval P, Angelini A, et al. Consensus statement on surgical pathology of the aorta from the Society for Cardiovascular Pathology and the Association for European Cardiovascular Pathology: I. Inflammatory diseases. *Cardiovasc Pathol.* 2015;24:267–278.
2. Kim SW, Lee DY, Kim MD, et al. Outcomes of endovascular treatment for aortic pseudoaneurysm in Behcet's disease. *J Vasc Surg.* 2014;59:608–614.
3. Kamisawa T, Zen Y, Pillai S, Stone JH. IgG4-related disease. *Lancet.* 2015;385:1460–1471.
4. Weyand CM, Goronzy JJ. Immune mechanisms in medium and large-vessel vasculitis. *Nat Rev Rheumatol.* 2013;9:731–740.
5. Deng J, Younge BR, Olshen RA, et al. Th17 and Th1 T-cell responses in giant cell arteritis. *Circulation.* 2010;121:906–915.
6. Xiao H, Hu P, Falk RJ, Jennette JC. Overview of the pathogenesis of ANCA-associated vasculitis. *Kidney Dis.* 2016;1:205–215.
7. Falk RJ, Terrell RS, Charles LA, Jennette JC. Anti-neutrophil cytoplasmic autoantibodies induce neutrophils to degranulate and produce oxygen radicals in vitro. *Proc Natl Acad Sci U S A.* 1990;87:4115–4119.
8. Xiao H, Heeringa P, Hu P, et al. Antineutrophil cytoplasmic autoantibodies specific for myeloperoxidase cause glomerulonephritis and vasculitis in mice. *J Clin Invest.* 2002;110:955–963.
9. Xiao H, Heeringa P, Liu Z, et al. The role of neutrophils in the induction of glomerulonephritis by anti-myeloperoxidase antibodies. *Am J Pathol.* 2005;167:39–45.
10. Xiao H, Dairaghi DJ, Powers JP, et al. C5a receptor (CD88) blockade protects against MPO-ANCA GN. *J Am Soc Nephrol.* 2014;25:225–231.
11. Kessenbrock K, Krumbholz M, Schonermarck U, et al. Netting neutrophils in autoimmune small-vessel vasculitis. *Nat Med.* 2009;15:623–625.
12. Abdulahad WH, Lamprecht P, Kallenberg CG. T-helper cells as new players in ANCA-associated vasculitides. *Arthritis Res Ther.* 2011;13:236.
13. Lyons PA, Rayner TF, Trivedi S, et al. Genetically distinct subsets within ANCA-associated vasculitis. *N Engl J Med.* 2012;367:214–223.
14. Choi HK, Merkel PA, Walker AM, Niles JL. Drug-associated antineutrophil cytoplasmic antibody-positive vasculitis: prevalence among patients with high titers of antimyeloperoxidase antibodies. *Arthritis Rheum.* 2000;43:405–413.
15. Mahr AD, Neogi T, Merkel PA. Epidemiology of Wegener's granulomatosis: lessons from descriptive studies and analyses of genetic and environmental risk determinants. *Clin Exp Rheumatol.* 2006;24:S82–S91.
16. Morimura S, Sugaya M, Sato S. Interaction between CX3CL1 and CX3CR1 regulates vasculitis induced by immune complex deposition. *Am J Pathol.* 2013;182:1640–1647.
17. Yanaba K, Komura K, Horikawa M, et al. P-selectin glycoprotein ligand-1 is required for the development of cutaneous vasculitis induced by immune complex deposition. *J Leukoc Biol.* 2004;76:374–382.
18. Ramos-Casals M, Stone JH, Cid MC, Bosch X. The cryoglobulinaemias. *Lancet.* 2012;379:348–360.
19. Terrier B, Karras A, Kahn JE, et al. The spectrum of type I cryoglobulinemia vasculitis: new insights based on 64 cases. *Medicine (Baltimore).* 2013;92:61–68.
20. Jennette JC. Implications for pathogenesis of patterns of injury in small- and medium-sized-vessel vasculitis. *Cleve Clin J Med.* 2002;69(Suppl 2):SII33–SII38.
21. Buffiere-Morgado A, Battistella M, Vignon-Pennamen MD, et al. Relationship between cutaneous polyarteritis nodosa (cPAN) and macular lymphocytic arteritis (MLA): blinded histologic assessment of 35 cPAN cases. *J Am Acad Dermatol.* 2015;73:1013–1020.

22. Hernandez-Rodriguez J, Alba MA, Prieto-Gonzalez S, Cid MC. Diagnosis and classification of polyarteritis nodosa. *J Autoimmun.* 2014;48-49:84–89.

23. Orenstein JM, Shulman ST, Fox LM, et al. Three linked vasculopathic processes characterize Kawasaki disease: a light and transmission electron microscopic study. *PLoS One.* 2012;7:e38998.

24. Ferreras MC, Benavides J, Fuertes M, et al. Pathological features of systemic necrotizing vasculitis (polyarteritis nodosa) in sheep. *J Comp Pathol.* 2013;149:74–81.

25. Watanabe R, Zhang H, Berry G, et al. Immune checkpoint dysfunction in large and medium vessel vasculitis. *Am J Physiol Heart Circ Physiol.* 2017;312:H1052–H1059.

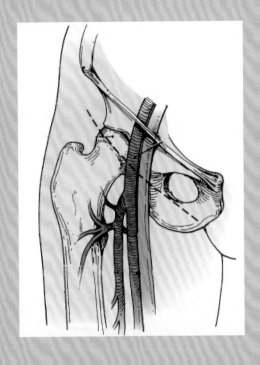

Principles of Vascular
Examination

血管检查相关原则

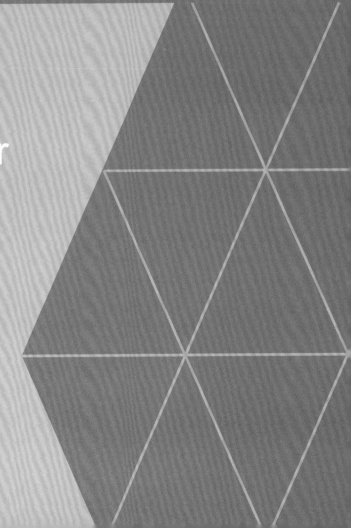

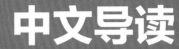

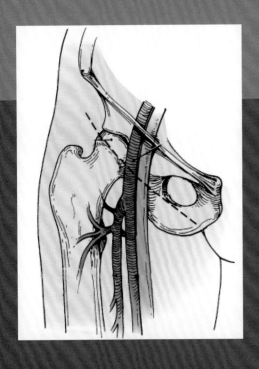

第11章
病史采集与体格检查

　　血管疾病与单一脏器损伤不同，动脉、静脉与淋巴脉管遍布于全身，其损伤和病变可发生于身体的任何部位，所以对于患有血管疾病的患者，充分且全面的评估尤为重要。本章节将介绍血管疾病患者初始评估的核心组成部分：病史采集与体格检查。临床中合理应用这些方法及特殊检查操作可辅助特定的血管检查，从而进行血管疾病的诊断。本章节病史采集部分将根据动脉疾病、静脉疾病及淋巴管疾病分别进行讲述，而体格检查部分将按照上肢、下肢及腹部等不同部位进行概述。关于特定血管疾病的病史、常见主诉及体格检查的具体特点，将在各个血管疾病的相关章节中进行更深入的讲解。

郑月宏

The History and Physical Examination

Joshua A. Beckman and Mark A. Creager

The ubiquitous nature of arteries, veins, and lymphatic vessels allows for any region of the body to develop vascular disease. This chapter describes the vascular medical history and physical examination—the core components of evaluating patients with vascular diseases. Application of these methods and tailored use of special examination maneuvers facilitate the diagnosis of vascular disease, especially when used in conjunction with vascular tests described elsewhere in this section. This chapter will review the cardinal complaints of patients with vascular disease, and then the physical findings associated with common arterial, venous, and lymphatic diseases. More specific features of the vascular history and examination are discussed in the relevant chapters of each vascular disease.

VASCULAR HISTORY

The medical history is the foundation of the physician-patient interaction, guiding the physical examination, testing, and treatment decisions. A comprehensive medical history can identify the diagnosis the vast majority of the time, but an inadequate one can result in excess testing and inappropriate therapy.

Arterial Disease

Symptoms of arterial disease typically arise as a result of either arterial stenoses or occlusions, although aneurysms also may cause symptoms. The important historical features of arterial disease in selected regional circulations are reviewed first.

Peripheral Artery Disease

In addition to carotid and coronary artery disease (CAD), peripheral artery disease (PAD) is one of the most common clinical manifestations of atherosclerosis. Approximately 50% of patients with PAD have symptoms, described in the following discussion as typical or atypical, and the remainder are asymptomatic. The importance of making the diagnosis of PAD, even in the absence of symptoms, derives from the prognostic information implicit with its diagnosis (see Chapter 16). Notably, patients with PAD often have coexisting coronary and cerebrovascular atherosclerosis and are twofold to fourfold more likely than patients without PAD to die of cardiovascular disease.[1] The risk of adverse cardiovascular events is increased in patients with PAD, even among asymptomatic patients. The presence of limb symptoms further increases the risk of adverse cardiovascular and limb outcomes.

Therefore the history of patients with PAD should seek to determine whether the patient has known risk factors for atherosclerosis and whether or not there are concomitant clinical manifestations of atherosclerosis. The historian should elicit information regarding dyslipidemia, diabetes mellitus, hypertension, family history of premature atherosclerosis, and cigarette smoking. Historical evidence of CAD, including prior myocardial infarction (MI), symptoms of angina, or prior coronary revascularization procedures and history of stroke or symptoms of cerebrovascular ischemia, including hemiparesis, hemiparesthesia, aphasia, or amaurosis fugax, should be sought and documented.

Intermittent claudication. A cardinal symptom of PAD is intermittent claudication (see Chapter 18). Claudication occurs when limb skeletal muscle ischemia is produced with effort because increased muscle energy requirements are not served by sufficient augmentation in blood supply. Symptoms develop *intermittently* with activity; the blood flow limitation imposed by peripheral artery stenosis typically does not compromise muscular function at rest. Claudication is variably described as aching, heaviness, burning, fatigue, cramping, and/or tightness in the affected limb. Symptoms occur with reproducible amounts of exercise: for example, one block of walking, one flight of stairs, or 5 minutes on a bicycle. Discomfort may develop in any muscular portion of the leg—buttocks, hip, thigh, calf, or foot. Areas of the limb to develop discomfort are related to the arterial segments with stenoses. Iliac artery disease typically produces hip or buttock claudication, whereas femoral artery disease causes thigh or calf claudication. Arm claudication is unusual but may occur in patients with innominate, subclavian, axillary, or brachial artery stenosis. Cessation of activity relieves the exercising muscle's demand-supply mismatch and enables restoration of oxidative metabolism. Therefore patients typically report that discontinuation of activity relieves the discomfort after several minutes.

Atypical symptoms also occur and may include reduction of leg discomfort despite continued effort, gait disturbance, and slower walking speed.[2] Atypical claudication may be more common than traditional symptoms because of the high frequency of other conditions present in this older age group: spinal stenosis, venous insufficiency, and degenerative joint disease. Patients with intermittent claudication often slow their walking speed by a third to regulate muscle use and prolong walking distance. Thus, when a physician solicits the history of walking impairment, patients may report no change in distance walked before symptoms occur, despite a progressive decline in functional ability.

Several questionnaires for PAD have been devised and validated. These provide a standard to accompany the interview when querying patients about symptoms of PAD.[3] The Rose questionnaire was the initial PAD-related questionnaire, but limited diagnostic sensitivity minimized its utility. The San Diego questionnaire is a modified version of the Rose questionnaire and a more reliable instrument to assess intermittent claudication (see Chapter 18). The disease-specific Walking Impairment Questionnaire has been validated and can be used to assess walking difficulty in patients with PAD. It has four subscales: severity of pain with walking, distance, speed, and stair climbing.[4]

Critical limb ischemia. Critical limb ischemia (CLI) occurs when limb blood flow is inadequate to meet the metabolic demands of the tissues at rest.[5] This may result in persistent pain, especially in the acral portions of the leg (toes, ball of the foot, heel). Additional foot symptoms include sensitivity to cold, joint stiffness, and hypesthesia. As a consequence of the effects of gravity on perfusion pressure, patients may report worsening of pain with leg elevation, or even when lying in bed, and reduction in pain with limb dependency (e.g., when the feet hang over the bed onto the floor). CLI may cause tissue breakdown (ulceration) or gangrene.

Acute limb ischemia. Acute limb ischemia is most often due to embolism or in situ thrombosis (see Chapter 44).[6] Other causes include arterial dissection or trauma. The presentation of acute arterial occlusion ranges from asymptomatic loss of a pulse, to worsened claudication, to sudden onset of severe pain at rest. Symptoms may develop suddenly over several hours, or over several days. Acute ischemic symptoms are more likely to occur when no or few collateral vessels are present, rather than when there is a well-developed collateral network. Acute arterial occlusion may cause symptoms in any portion of the leg distal to the obstruction. The five Ps—pain, pallor, poikilothermia, paresthesias, and paralysis—characterize the historical features and findings of patients with acute limb ischemia. Severity of symptoms does not discriminate among etiologies.

Atheroembolism. Atheroembolism is embolization of atherosclerotic debris that compromises distal arteries (see Chapter 45). Atheroemboli vary in composition, from larger fibroplatelet particles that occlude small arteries to cholesterol emboli, nanometers in size, that occlude arterioles. Causes of atheroemboli include catheterization and cardiovascular surgery, but approximately half of such events occur without a known precipitant.[7]

Symptoms reflect occlusion of the small distal vessels in the limb, and patients will commonly present with calf, foot, or toe pain and areas of violaceous discoloration or cyanosis in the toes *(blue toe syndrome).* Symptoms develop hours to days after the event; ulcerations may develop and are slow to resolve. Symptoms may be unilateral or bilateral, depending upon the origin of emboli proximal to or beyond the aortic bifurcation. If atheroemboli arise proximal to the renal arteries, renal insufficiency is a potential sequela.

Other peripheral artery diseases. Uncommon diseases of the peripheral arteries should be considered in patients with claudication or evidence of ischemia but whose age is less than that typically affected by atherosclerosis or in those with atypical symptoms. These diseases include thromboangiitis obliterans (TAO) (see Chapter 42), Takayasu arteritis (see Chapter 40), and giant cell arteritis (GCA; see Chapter 40), and vascular compression syndromes, such as those affecting the thoracic outlet, iliac artery, and popliteal artery (see Chapter 63).

Takayasu arteritis is a large-vessel vasculitis that generally occurs between the ages of 20 and 40 years.[8] Women are more likely to develop the disease than are men. Constitutional and vascular symptoms occur (e.g., fevers, weight loss, fatigue, arthralgias, myalgias) and may be present months to years without overt evidence of vascular disease.

Approximately 50% of patients complain of muscle or joint pains, and headache has been reported in up to 40%. More than 50% of patients will have a diminished pulse or claudication of an upper extremity. Approximately 30% of patients will report neck pain and have a tender carotid artery (i.e., *carotidynia*). Lightheadedness is also common and may be secondary to vertebral artery involvement.

Patients with *GCA* are typically older than 50 years of age.[9] GCA predominantly affects the branches of the thoracic aorta and the intracranial arteries. Some 50% of patients have constitutional symptoms related to inflammation, and 50% have coexisting polymyalgia rheumatica. The most common complaint is headache that typically affects the occipital or temporal region; it occurs in more than 60% of patients with GCA. In patients with headache, scalp tenderness may be present. Partial or complete vision loss develops in 20% of patients, and approximately 50% of these individuals report *amaurosis fugax* (i.e., transient episodes that involve one eye and last 10 minutes or less). Patients may present with upper limb claudication, and 40% report jaw claudication. Tongue claudication and swallowing difficulties are less common.

TAO (Buerger disease) is a small- to medium-vessel vasculitis that affects the distal vessels of the arms or legs and usually occurs before 40 years of age in cigarette smokers.[10] It affects more men than women. The classic triad of TAO is claudication, Raynaud phenomenon, and superficial thrombophlebitis. Claudication of the hands or feet may progress to ulceration of the fingers or toes.

Neurovascular compression syndromes. Claudication in the upper extremities raises the possibility of *thoracic outlet syndrome* (see Chapter 63).[11] Compression of the axillary or subclavian artery by a cervical rib, abnormal insertion of the scalene anticus muscle, or apposition of the clavicle and first rib may result in arterial compression during head turning, arm use above or behind the head, or arm extension. Weakness, burning, aching, or fatigue in the arms can result. Examples of triggers include wall painting, hair washing, and housecleaning.

Popliteal artery entrapment should be considered in a young person with leg claudication but preserved pulses at rest.[12,13] Anatomical variants in the course of the popliteal artery may result in its compression by the gastrocnemius muscle during exercise and can cause symptoms of claudication.

Vasospastic and Related Diseases

Raynaud phenomenon is the most common vasospastic disorder encountered in clinical practice (see Chapter 46).[12,13] Patients typically report that the digits become pale or cyanotic during cold exposure. Fingers are most commonly affected, but the toes develop symptoms in 40% of affected individuals. Less commonly involved areas include the tongue, nose, and ear lobes. Patients may experience paresthesias or pain in the digits if ischemia persists. With rewarming and release of vasospasm, digital rubor due to reactive hyperemia may develop. A pulsating or flushed feeling may accompany the hyperemic phase. All color phases are not required for diagnosis. Indeed, with an appropriate history, the diagnosis can be made with only one color change.

There are two categories of Raynaud phenomenon: primary and secondary. Differentiating between the two is important because of the information it provides about cause and prognosis. *Primary Raynaud disease* is benign, typically affects fingers (and toes) symmetrically, and recovery is predictable with rewarming. Some 70% to 80% of patients with primary Raynaud disease are women. In patients with *secondary Raynaud phenomenon*, pallor may occur in only one or several digits. In severe cases, cyanosis is unremitting and tissue loss may occur.

Raynaud phenomenon that has its onset after age 45 years should prompt an investigation for an underlying cause. The history should include questions to elicit evidence of disease or conditions that cause secondary Raynaud phenomenon, including connective tissue disorders, arterial occlusive disease, trauma (vibration, hypothenar hand injury), neurovascular compression syndromes, blood dyscrasias, and drug use.

Acrocyanosis is a vascular disorder characterized by bluish discoloration of the hands and feet exacerbated by cold exposure (see Chapter 47). Unlike Raynaud phenomenon, the discoloration is not confined to the digits, and pallor does not occur. However, warming can ameliorate cyanosis and restore normal skin color. Acrocyanosis typically occurs in persons aged 20 to 45 years, and women are affected more often than men.

Pernio is a vascular inflammatory disorder in which skin lesions and swelling occur in fingers and toes, particularly in cold moist climates (see Chapter 49). Other exposed portions of the body may be affected. The typical lesions described by the patient are pruritic and painful blisters or superficial ulcers.

The *complex regional pain syndromes*, reflex sympathetic dystrophy (RSD), and causalgia are associated with limb symptoms, often following a relatively minor injury. Hand or foot pain is a frequent complaint. This may be associated with hyperpathia, hyperesthesias, coolness, cyanosis, hyperhidrosis, and swelling. Symptoms are typically out of proportion to severity of the initial injury. Patients may observe brittle nails that develop ridges and report muscle, skin, and subcutaneous tissue wasting and limited joint mobility in the affected limb.

Renal Artery Disease

No symptoms specific to renal artery stenosis are elicited by history. Unlike other end organs, symptoms of chronic renal ischemia are not localized to the kidney but reflect systemic pathophysiological alterations that result from activation of the renin-angiotensin system and disturbances of salt and water balance. Historical clues that raise suspicion of renal artery stenosis include onset of hypertension younger than age 30 or older than age 55, malignant hypertension, hypertension refractory to three concurrently prescribed antihypertensive medications, azotemia subsequent to administration of an angiotensin-converting enzyme (ACE) inhibitor or angiotensin receptor blocker, unexplained azotemia, recurrent congestive heart failure, and episodic pulmonary edema (see Chapter 23). Renal artery stenosis should be considered in patients with these clinical clues, particularly if they have evidence of atherosclerosis in other regional circulations (e.g., CAD, PAD, aortic disease).

Mesenteric Artery Disease

Most patients with atherosclerosis of the celiac, superior mesenteric, or inferior mesenteric arteries are asymptomatic unless two or all three of these arteries are occluded. Symptoms of chronic mesenteric ischemia include postprandial epigastric or midabdominal pain that may radiate to the back (see Chapter 26). Onset of abdominal discomfort is 15 to 30 minutes after eating, and symptoms may persist for several hours. Patients tend to avoid food to prevent these symptoms, and weight loss ensues.

Carotid Artery Disease

The majority of patients with significant stenoses of the common or internal carotid arteries are asymptomatic (see Chapter 29).[14] When they do occur, symptoms may be temporary (minutes to hours) or fixed, indicating a transient ischemic attack (TIA) or stroke, respectively. Symptoms of carotid artery disease reflect compromise of the neural territory subtended by its principal intracranial branch, the middle cerebral artery, and include contralateral hemiparesis, hemiparesthesia, and aphasia. Ipsilateral amaurosis fugax or blindness may also occur because the ophthalmic artery is supplied by the internal carotid artery.

The prevalence of carotid artery disease is increased in patients with CAD or PAD, both of which increase the risk of stroke by twofold to fourfold.

Venous and Lymphatic Systems

A history soliciting evidence of venous and lymphatic diseases is required when patients complain of leg pain or swelling, or express concerns regarding leg ulcers, varicose veins, or localized inflammation on a limb. In patients presenting with leg edema, the history should seek to determine whether the swelling is secondary to venous or lymphatic diseases, trauma, or arthritis, or whether it is associated with a systemic condition such as congestive heart failure, cirrhosis, nephrotic syndrome, renal insufficiency, or endocrinopathy (e.g., hypothyroidism, Cushing syndrome).

Deep Vein Thrombosis

Patients with thrombosis of a deep vein of a limb may present with swelling or discomfort or no symptoms at all (see Chapter 51). Symptoms are usually but not always unilateral. Historical queries should seek potential causes of deep vein thrombosis (DVT) when it is suspected. Information regarding recent trauma, surgery, hospitalization, prolonged period of immobility, cancer, thrombophilic disorder, or family history of venous thrombosis should be acquired. An uncommon cause of left leg DVT is May-Thurner syndrome, in which the left iliac vein is compressed by the right iliac artery. In patients with arm symptoms, questions should seek evidence of indwelling catheters or cancer because these are the most common causes of upper extremity DVT. In addition, a history of repetitive arm motion should be sought when considering the possibility of Paget-Schroetter syndrome, in which compression of the axillosubclavian vein by muscular, tendinous, or bony components of the thoracic outlet may cause thrombosis. Thrombosis or extrinsic compression of the superior vena cava may cause symptoms of superior vena cava syndrome, which include headache, face and neck fullness and flushing, and bilateral arm swelling.

Superficial Thrombophlebitis

Thrombosis of a superficial vein is a local phenomenon that presents with pain and tenderness over the affected vein. Predisposing factors sought by history include intravenous catheters, varicose veins, injury, and malignancy. It is important to consider the possibility of malignancy, especially pancreatic, lung, and ovarian cancers in patients with recurrent or migratory superficial thrombophlebitis (i.e., Trousseau syndrome). Uncommon disorders associated with superficial thrombophlebitis include TAO and Behçet syndrome.

Chronic Venous Insufficiency

Venous insufficiency should be considered in patients who present with chronic unilateral or bilateral leg swelling. Causes of venous insufficiency include deep venous obstruction and deep venous valvular incompetence (also see Chapter 54). Approximately 30% of patients with DVT will ultimately develop chronic venous insufficiency.[15] Valvular incompetence may be a consequence of recanalized venous thrombus or a primary valvular abnormality. Queries should address the duration of leg swelling, knowledge of prior DVT, presence of focal hyperpigmentation, pain, pruritus, or ulcers. Symptoms may include a heavy, dull, or "bursting" sensation of the edematous leg. Patients may report that discomfort in the affected leg increases with dependency

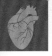

and improves with leg elevation. Some individuals with severe leg swelling note that calf discomfort worsens with walking, a symptom termed *venous claudication.*

Varicose Veins

Most patients with varicose veins do not have specific symptoms but present to a physician's office with cosmetic concerns. Symptoms of varicose veins include leg discomfort or aching, particularly with prolonged standing. These symptoms are most likely to occur along long segments of the greater and lesser saphenous veins and their tributaries. Burning or pruritus may develop, particularly if complicated by accompanying skin ulceration.

Lymphedema

Lymphedema should be considered in patients who present with limb swelling (see Chapter 57).[16] This condition may affect the arms or legs and is usually unilateral, although it can be bilateral. Lymphedema should be suspected if limb swelling occurs early in life, particularly during childhood or adolescence. Congenital lymphedema typically appears at birth or shortly thereafter. Lymphedema praecox often presents around puberty but can occur any time before age 35. Lymphedema tarda generally occurs after age 35. Lymphedema is also associated with genetic disorders such as Turner and Noonan syndromes. It is important to elicit history of conditions that may predispose a patient to lymphedema, including recurrent skin infection, lymphangitis, filariasis, trauma, malignancy of the lymphatic system, and radiation or surgical resection of lymph nodes and lymphatic vessels as adjunctive therapy for cancer.

Lymphangitis

Patients with lymphangitis may report an erythematous patch or linear streak that affects the limb and tends to propagate proximally over time. The erythematous area may be painful and tender. These patients usually present with systemic signs of infection, including fever and shaking chills. History might determine whether lesions induced by trauma or infection may have served as a portal of entry.

VASCULAR EXAMINATION

As in any comprehensive physical examination, vital signs (blood pressure, heart rate, respiratory rate) should be assessed and recorded. Blood pressure should be measured in both arms and preferably in supine, seated, and upright positions. Overall appearance of the patient should be noted.

The vascular examination includes inspection, palpation, and auscultation of vascular structures in many areas of the body. A systematic approach ensures a complete evaluation, so the examination described in this chapter will cover principal anatomical regions that are particularly relevant to the peripheral vasculature. The heart, lungs, and neurological and musculoskeletal systems should be examined, but details of these examinations are beyond the scope of this chapter.

Limbs

The limbs should be inspected carefully, assessing their appearance, symmetry, color, and evidence of edema or muscle wasting.

Pulse Examination

The pulse examination of the arms and legs is a critical part of the vascular examination. Asymmetry, decreased intensity, or absence of pulses provide clinical evidence of PAD and indicate the location of stenotic lesions. Some examiners describe pulses as absent, diminished, or normal, or use a numerical scale (e.g., from 0 [absent] to 2+).

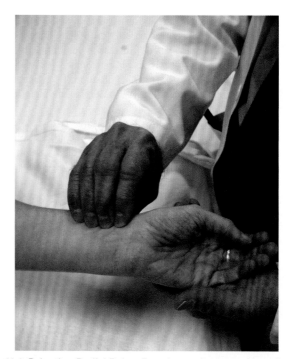

Fig. 11.1 Palpating Radial Pulse. Examiner, using two or three fingers, lightly palpates the superficial radial pulse over stylus of radius near base of thumb.

Bounding pulses may be evidence of aortic valve insufficiency, and dilated expansive pulses a sign of ectasia or aneurysm.

Pulses of the arms—brachial, radial, and ulnar pulses—should be palpated using two or three fingertips. The brachial pulse is superficial and in the medial third of the antecubital fossa. The radial pulse, also superficial, can be found over the stylus of the radius near the base of the thumb (Fig. 11.1). The ulnar pulse is palpated on the volar aspect of the wrist, over the head of the ulnar bone. Wrist support by the examiner improves pulse detection by decreasing overlying muscle tension.

Pulse examination of the leg (femoral, popliteal, posterior tibial, and dorsalis pedis pulses) should be undertaken with the patient supine. The femoral pulse is located deep, below the inguinal ligament, approximately midway between the symphysis pubis and iliac spine. Obesity may obscure local landmarks. Lateral rotation of the leg, pannus retraction, and two hands may be required for adequate palpation. On occasion, the increase in flow velocity caused by a stenosis may create a thrill in the common or superficial femoral artery that is appreciated by palpation of the femoral pulse or by a bruit that can be heard with auscultation.

Palpation of the popliteal pulse can be difficult. The leg should be straight yet relaxed to decrease overlying muscle stiffness. The popliteal pulse should be palpated with three fingers from each hand while the thumbs are applying moderate opposing force to the top of the knee, indenting the surface of the skin by approximately 1 cm (Fig. 11.2). The popliteal pulse typically can be found at the junction of the medial and lateral thirds of the fossa. In contrast to superficial pulses like the radial or dorsalis pedis pulse, the popliteal pulse is diffuse and deep. Widened popliteal pulses may be indicative of popliteal artery aneurysm.

The posterior tibial pulse can be found slightly below and behind the medial malleolus. Counterpressure with the thumb and passive dorsiflexion of the foot may increase the likelihood of palpation (Fig. 11.3). The posterior tibial pulse should be present. Its absence is diagnostic for lower extremity artery PAD. In contrast, the dorsalis pedis pulse, which can be appreciated just lateral to the extensor

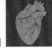

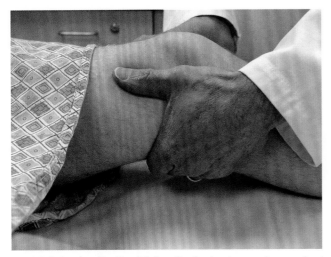

Fig. 11.2 Palpating Popliteal Pulse. Popliteal pulse requires moderate pressure for its appreciation. Examiner uses both thumbs for moderate opposing force while placing digits two, three, and four in lateral third of popliteal fossa. Patient's leg should be relaxed while examiner induces mild flexion. A widened popliteal artery pulse may indicate presence of aneurysm.

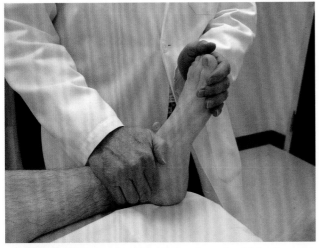

Fig. 11.3 Palpating Posterior Tibial Pulse. Posterior tibial pulse resides slightly below and behind medial malleolus. It should be approached from the lateral aspect, with digits applied to lower curvature of malleolus. Passive foot dorsiflexion may enhance appreciation of pulse.

tendon on the dorsum of the foot, normally may be absent in 2% to 12% of persons. An abnormal pulse examination is indicative of PAD. Confirmation of PAD is made by measuring the ankle-brachial index (ABI) (see Chapters 12 and 18). A reduction in the ankle systolic pressure to ≤90% of brachial artery systolic pressure (i.e., an ABI ≤0.90, is diagnostic of PAD).

Allen Test

The radial and ulnar arteries supply blood flow to the hand. Within the hand, these arteries form the superficial and deep palmar arches, enabling blood supply to the digits from either vessel; 5% to 10% of the population has a congenitally incomplete arch. Disease states associated with interruption of the palmar arch include connective tissue diseases like the CREST variant (calcinosis, Raynaud phenomenon, esophageal dysmotility, sclerodactyly, telangiectasia) of scleroderma, vasculitides such as TAO, and thromboemboli. The Allen test can

differentiate between a complete and incomplete palmar arch. The examiner occludes both the radial and ulnar pulses (Fig. 11.4), and the patient then opens and closes the fist several times, creating palmar pallor. Upon release of one pulse, normal skin color should return within seconds. The other artery is then tested and observed similarly. Persistent pallor is indicative of an incomplete palmar arch or occluded artery distal to the remaining pulse occluded by the examiner.

Nearly three-quarters of all patients with TAO will have a positive Allen test, and 50% will report Raynaud phenomenon. Digital ischemia in these patients is more likely to progress and cause persistent cyanosis and lead to digital ulcers. Patients with TAO also may develop migratory superficial thrombophlebitis, which appears as painful, tender, red nodules.

Thoracic Outlet Maneuvers

Thoracic outlet syndrome results from compression of the neurovascular bundle as it leaves the thoracic cavity (see Chapter 63).[11] Each component of the bundle may be affected, including the brachial plexus, subclavian/axillary artery, and subclavian/axillary vein.

Thoracic outlet maneuvers seek to elicit positional interruption of arterial flow. During the examination, the physician holds the radial pulse in one hand and maneuvers the arm with the other. The subclavian artery is auscultated in the supraclavicular fossa. An abnormal thoracic outlet maneuver is characterized by development of a subclavian bruit followed by loss of the radial pulse. Several thoracic outlet maneuvers have been described, and each may be relevant to compression at different sites in the thoracic outlet. Each side is examined in sequence. The *Adson maneuver* assesses the segment of the subclavian artery in the scalene triangle. The patient rotates his/her head toward the symptomatic side, extends the neck (i.e., looking up and over the shoulder), and simultaneously performs an exaggerated inspiration. The *costoclavicular maneuver* assesses the segment of the subclavian artery coursing between the clavicle and first rib. The patient thrusts the shoulders back and inferiorly. The *hyperabduction maneuver* evaluates the subclavian artery as it courses near the insertion of the pectoralis major muscle. The patient is seated, and the head is looking forward. The arm is abducted 180 degrees to a position along the side of the head. Abduction of the arm to 90 degrees may be combined with external rotation in evaluating symptoms suggestive of thoracic outlet syndrome (Fig. 11.5). This maneuver is often used to assess subclavian venous or arterial compression during ultrasonography or angiography.

For patients in whom clinical suspicion for thoracic outlet syndrome is present, sensitivity and specificity for these provocative tests are 72% and 53%, respectively.[17] However, routine application of these maneuvers is not warranted, because up to 50% of the population may have a positive finding.[18]

Limb Ischemia

Skin color and temperature can provide information about severity of limb arterial perfusion. The feet, hands, fingers, and toes should be examined for temperature and skin color and the nails for evidence of fragility and pitting. Limb temperature can best be appreciated using the back of the examiner's hand. Temperature changes of adjacent segments on the ipsilateral limb and comparisons with the contralateral limb can be made. Presence of foot pallor while the leg is horizontal is indicative of poor perfusion and may be a sign of ischemia. Foot pallor may be precipitated in patients with PAD (who do not have CLI) by elevating the patient's leg to 60 degrees for 1 minute. Repetitive dorsiflexion and plantar flexion of the foot may also precipitate pallor on the sole of the foot when PAD is present. To qualitatively assess collateral blood flow, the leg is then lowered as the patient moves to the

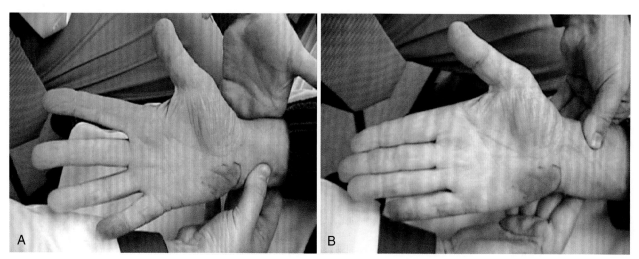

Fig. 11.4 Allen Test. The Allen test determines presence or absence of a complete palmar arch. Both radial and ulnar pulses are occluded while patient opens and closes hand to create palmar pallor. Once pallor is evident, examiner releases one pulse. In this example, patient presented with persistent fifth digit and hypothenar cyanosis. (A) Release of radial artery pulse results in expected hyperemia and palmar erythema. (B) In contrast, release of ulnar artery pulse does not result in palmar erythema, indicating proximal occlusion in ulnar segment of palmar arch. This test is considered a positive Allen test.

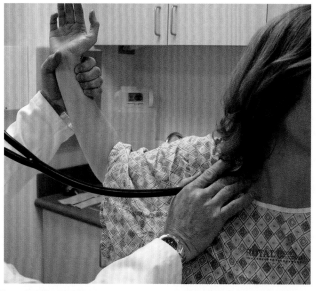

Fig. 11.5 Elevated arm stress test may be used to evaluate subclavian artery as it courses near insertion of pectoralis major muscle. Patient initially sits looking forward while arms are abducted 90 degrees, elbows are abducted 90 degrees, and patient repeatedly makes a clenched fist. During maneuver, radial pulse should be palpated while subclavian artery is auscultated. Loss of pulse or development of subclavian artery bruit is a positive study.

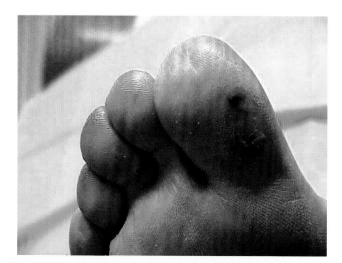

Fig. 11.6 Digital Ulceration. Pernio is associated with persistent sensation of cold, with pain in the toes. Painful blue nodules are noted in association with a discrete ulcer.

Ulcers

Ischemia arising from arterial occlusive disease or emboli may cause formation of ischemic ulcers (see Chapter 61).[19] They tend to be small, annular, pale, and desiccated (Fig. 11.6) and are usually located in distal areas of the limbs (e.g., toes, heels, fingertips). Ischemic ulcers vary in size but may be as small as 3 mm in diameter. Arterial ischemic ulcers are tender. Neurotrophic ulcers that develop in patients with diabetes typically occur at sites of trauma, such as areas of callus formation, bony prominence, or parts of the foot exposed to mild chronic trauma caused by ill-fitting shoes. Ischemic ulcers also develop in diabetic patients with PAD and may have features of neuropathic ulcers. Without proper treatment, ulceration may progress to tissue necrosis and gangrene. *Gangrene* can be characterized as an area of dead tissue that blackens, mummifies, and sloughs.

seated position. This is done to elicit rubor, indicative of arteriolar and venular dilation, indicative of reactive hyperemia, and to determine pedal vein refill time. The time to development of dependent rubor is indicative of the severity of PAD. Severe PAD and poor collateral blood flow may prolong reactive hyperemia by more than 30 seconds. Normally, pedal venous refill occurs in less than 15 seconds. Moderate PAD subserved by collateral vessels is suspected if venous refill is 30 to 45 seconds; severe disease with poor collateral development is likely when venous filling time is longer than 1 minute.

Digital Vasospasm

It is unusual for patients with Raynaud phenomenon to present to the physician's office during an attack in which the fingers are blanched. Moreover, it is difficult to precipitate digital ischemia in these patients, even with local cold exposure, such as placing the hands in ice water. Digital ischemia may be apparent in patients with fixed obstructive lesions of the digital arteries. Persistent digital ischemia may occur in patients with connective tissue disorders such as scleroderma or systemic lupus erythematosus, atheroemboli, TAO, or atherosclerosis. The fingers and toes are cool and appear cyanotic or pale. Fissures, pits, ulcerations, or necrosis or gangrene may be evident on the ischemic digits (see Fig. 11.6).

Livedo Reticularis

Livedo reticularis can be described as a lacelike or netlike pattern in the skin (Fig. 11.7). The "laces" may vary in color from red to blue and surround a central area of clearing. Cold exposure exacerbates the changes in hue. Both primary and secondary forms may occur and may be complicated by ulceration. The primary benign form is more common in women. The secondary forms are usually associated with vasculitis, atheroemboli, hyperviscosity syndromes, endocrine abnormalities, and infections. In the secondary forms of livedo reticularis, lesions may be more diffuse and ominous. Purpuric lesions and cutaneous nodules that progress to ulceration in response to cold may develop.

Edema

The limbs should be evaluated for edema. The most common location is in the legs, adjacent to the malleoli and over the tibia. With deep digital palpation, development of a divot or finger impression is indicative of pitting edema. Edema can be graded in each leg or arm as absent, mild, moderate, or severe, or on a numerical scale of 4, with 0 being the absence of edema. Unilateral edema may be evidence of DVT, chronic venous insufficiency, or lymphedema.

The most common physical findings of DVT include unilateral leg swelling, warmth, and erythema. The affected vein may be tender. A common femoral vein cord is detected by palpating along its course just below the inguinal ligament vein, and a femoral vein cord would be appreciated along the anteromedial aspect of the thigh. In the absence of obvious edema, a subtle clue may be unilateral absence of contours of the thigh, calf, or ankle. Muscular groups subtended by the thrombosed vein may be edematous due to poor venous drainage, conferring a boggy feeling to the affected calf or thigh muscles. Inflammation associated with a thrombosis may make the leg feel warm.

Homans sign is nonspecific and misses the diagnosis as commonly as it makes it. In John Homans' essay on lower extremity venous thrombosis, he states, "The clinical signs of a deep thrombosis of the muscles of the calf are entirely lacking when the individual lies or even reclines in bed. It is possible there may be a little discomfort upon forced dorsiflexion of the foot (tightening of the posterior muscles) but it is not yet clear whether or not this is a sign upon which to depend."[20]

Presence of thrombus just below the skin makes the diagnosis of superficial thrombophlebitis relatively easy. The patient may present with local venous engorgement, a palpable cord, warmth, erythema, or tenderness.

Chronic Venous Insufficiency

With chronic venous insufficiency, the physical examination may demonstrate fibrosis, tenderness, excoriation, and skin induration from hyperkeratosis, cellulitis, and ulceration (Fig. 11.8).[21] Chronic venous edema may impart hemosiderin deposition in the skin and confer a brawny appearance, typically in the pretibial calf. The severity of chronic venous disease may be classified using the CEAP (clinical signs, etiology, anatomy, pathophysiology) classification (Table 11.1).[22]

In contrast to arterial ulcers, which are circumscribed and pallid, venous ulcers are large with irregular borders, erythematous, and moist, giving the skin a shiny appearance (see Chapter 61). They are usually located near the medial or lateral malleolus. Venous ulcers may be painless, but many are associated with pain.

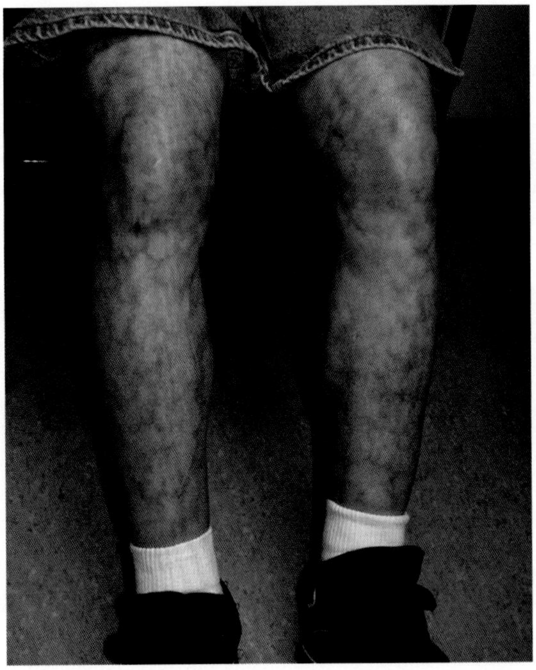

Fig. 11.7 Livedo Reticularis. Note lacelike pattern of superficial skin vessels surrounding a clear area.

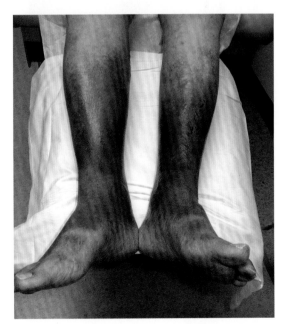

Fig. 11.8 Skin Changes of Chronic Venous Insufficiency. Chronic venous insufficiency and edema result in deposition of hemosiderin, causing darkening and toughening of skin and giving calf a brawny appearance. Note small superficial venous ulcers midcalf above shin.

TABLE 11.1   CEAP Clinical Classification

Class	Clinical Signs
0	No visible or palpable signs of venous disease
1	Telangiectasis or reticular veins
2	Varicose veins
3	Edema
4	Skin changes ascribed to venous disease
4a	pigmentation, venous eczema
4b	lipodermatosclerosis, atrophie blanche
5	Skin changes as defined above, with healed ulceration
6	Skin changes as defined above, with active ulceration

CEAP, Clinical signs, etiology, anatomy, pathophysiology.

Varicose Veins

Varicose veins are dilated, serpentine, superficial veins. If they cluster, they may feel and appear like a bunch of grapes (Fig. 11.9). Varicose veins should be inspected and palpated. Areas of erythema, tenderness, or induration may identify superficial thrombophlebitis. Varicose veins are most prominent with leg dependence (e.g., with standing). Once filled, the veins may be balloted, and a fluid wave may be detected. Venous telangiectasias, also known as *spider veins*, are commonly confused with varicose veins. Spider veins are typically small, cutaneous veins in a caput medusa pattern.

Superficial venous varicosities may be primary or result from DVT or insufficiency. An examiner can distinguish between superficial venous insufficiency and deep venous insufficiency at the bedside using the *Brodie-Trendelenburg test*. With the patient lying supine, the leg is elevated to 45 degrees and a tourniquet applied after the veins have drained. The patient then stands. The veins below the tourniquet should fill slowly. If venous refill distal to the site of tourniquet

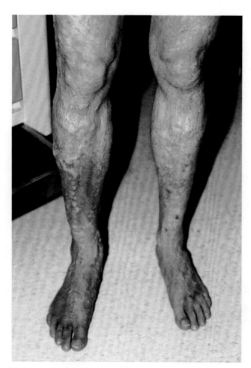

Fig. 11.9 Varicose Veins. Severe bilateral varicose veins with extension into both feet.

application occurs in less than 30 seconds, this is evidence of an incompetent deep and perforator system. Slower refills suggest a competent deep and perforator system. The varicose veins are examined upon tourniquet release. Superficial venous insufficiency will be confirmed with rapid retrograde superficial venous filling.

The *Perthes test* can differentiate between deep venous insufficiency and a deep venous obstruction as the cause of varicose veins. The patient is asked to stand, and once the superficial veins are engorged, a tourniquet is applied around the midthigh. The patient then walks for 5 minutes. If the varicose veins collapse below the level of the tourniquet, the perforator veins are presumed competent and the deep veins patent. If the superficial veins remain engorged, either the superficial and/or communicating veins are incompetent. If the varicose veins increase in prominence, and walking causes leg pain, the deep veins are occluded.

Lymphedema

During the initial stages of lymphedema, leg swelling will be similar to venous insufficiency: soft and pitting. Extension of edema into the foot to the origin of the toes may help to differentiate lymphedema from venous edema (Fig. 11.10). In addition, the inability to pinch dorsal skin at the base of the second toe, the *Stemmer sign*, also may differentiate early lymphedema from venous edema. Subsequently, the limb becomes wooden as progressive deposition of protein-rich fluid causes induration and fibrosis of affected tissues. Lymphedema increases production of subcutaneous and adipose tissue, thickening the skin. Advanced disease may be identified when the leg feels wooden, edema is no longer pitting, and the limb is enlarged; the skin may appear verrucous at the toes. Palpation for lymphadenopathy should be performed when considering secondary causes of lymphedema.

Lymphangitis

Lymphangitis can usually be visualized as a red streak that extends proximally from an inciting lesion. If left untreated, the entire limb may become edematous, erythematous, and warm, without evidence of venous congestion or impairment of arterial flow. Commonly, the regional lymph nodes are indurated.

Neck Examination

The neck is inspected for any areas of swelling or asymmetry. Jugular venous pressure is assessed to investigate the possibility of a volume-overloaded state or congestive heart failure. Patients typically are placed at 45 degrees and the height of jugular venous pressure estimated. If necessary, the angle of head elevation should be adjusted to see the top of the jugular venous column.

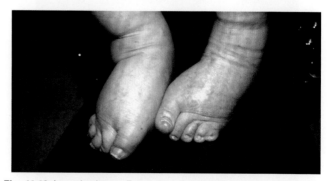

Fig. 11.10 Lymphedema. Extension of edema into foot to level of toe is a useful physical sign to differentiate between venous edema and lymphedema. Foot swelling ending abruptly at toes is called squared toe sign.

The carotid arteries are palpated between the trachea and the sternocleidomastoid muscles. In older patients especially, the carotid body may be sensitive, and carotid pulses may induce bradycardia and hypotension. Pulses should be symmetrical with a rapid upstroke. Pulse asymmetry may indicate a proximal carotid or brachiocephalic stenosis. Parvus and tardus pulses (decreased amplitude and a delayed slow upstroke) may indicate aortic valve stenosis or proximal occlusive disease. Stenosis of the carotid bifurcation or internal carotid artery usually does not affect carotid pulse contour or amplitude. Occasionally, severe stenosis will create a thrill that can be appreciated by palpation.

The carotid pulses are auscultated to elicit evidence of bruits. Bruits are caused by blood flow turbulence as a result of arterial stenosis, extrinsic compression, aneurysmal dilation, or arteriovenous connection. The bell of the stethoscope is recommended to appreciate low-frequency bruits and eliminate any adventitious sounds heard through the diaphragm. The entire cervical portion of each carotid artery should be auscultated, including the segment near the angle of the jaw where the carotid bifurcation is often located (Fig. 11.11). The sensitivity and specificity of a carotid bruit for the presence of stenosis ranges from 50% to 79% and 61% to 91%, respectively.[23,24] Auscultation of the subclavian arteries for bruits is performed in the supraclavicular fossa and between the lateral aspect of the clavicle and pectoralis muscle. Although the proximal location of a bruit defines the area of turbulent flow, a bruit may be appreciated for an additional several centimeters. The pitch of bruits increases with worsening severity. Continuation of the bruit into diastole is another marker of severity and implies advanced stenosis. Paradoxically, severe stenosis causing subtotal arterial occlusion may not evoke an audible bruit.

Abdominal Vascular Examination

Vascular examination of the abdomen is performed as the patient lies supine on the examining table, with legs outstretched. From this position, the abdominal wall should be relaxed and not rigid. Prior to palpation, the abdomen should be inspected. Engorged superficial veins in the abdomen indicate the possibility of inferior vena cava obstruction. After inspection, all four quadrants are auscultated with the stethoscope. The presence of bruits is indicative of aortic or branch vessel occlusive disease. Bruits may arise as a result of mesenteric, renal, or aortic disease. Following auscultation, the abdomen is palpated for masses and to detect an aortic aneurysm. Deepest palpation can generally be obtained by gradually increasing pressure in the midline

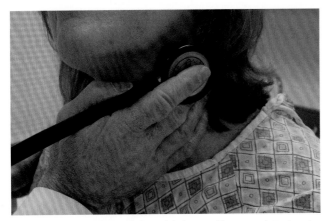

Fig. 11.11 Auscultation of Carotid Artery. To appreciate low-tone bruits, examiner should use stethoscope bell and apply mild to moderate pressure. Entire length of artery should be examined, with particular attention paid to region just below jaw, at approximation of carotid artery bifurcation.

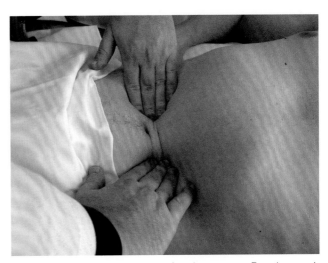

Fig. 11.12 Abdominal Palpation for Aneurysm. Examiner, using progressively increasing force, palpates until aorta can be defined between both sets of fingers. Examiner should appreciate lateral pulsation with every heart beat. Aneurysm sizing is performed by estimating distance between closest fingers of each hand.

using both hands (Fig. 11.12). In asthenic patients, the aorta can be palpated. In subjects with a waist size greater than 40 inches, the likelihood of palpating an aneurysm is quite limited.

Presence of an aneurysm can be determined when there is a distinct and expansive pulsatile configuration to the aorta. An aneurysm should be sized by determining the lateral borders with both hands and the space estimated with a measuring tape. Tenderness during the abdominal vascular examination is unusual and may suggest aneurysmal expansion, an inflammatory aneurysm, or a contained rupture. Nonaortic pathology, including appendicitis, cholecystitis, diverticulitis, and peritonitis, are more common causes of tenderness.

REFERENCES

1. Fowkes FG, Murray GD, Butcher I, et al. Ankle brachial index combined with Framingham Risk Score to predict cardiovascular events and mortality: a meta-analysis. *JAMA*. 2008;300:197–208.
2. McDermott MM. Lower extremity manifestations of peripheral artery disease: the pathophysiologic and functional implications of leg ischemia. *Circ Res*. 2015;116:1540–1550.
3. Schorr EN, Treat-Jacobson D. Methods of symptom evaluation and their impact on peripheral artery disease (PAD) symptom prevalence: a review. *Vasc Med*. 2013;18:95–111.
4. Nead KT, Zhou M, Diaz Caceres R, et al. Walking Impairment Questionnaire improves mortality risk prediction models in a high-risk cohort independent of peripheral arterial disease status. *Circ Cardiovasc Qual Outcomes*. 2013;6:255–261.
5. Teraa M, Conte MS, Moll FL, Verhaar MC. Critical limb ischemia: current trends and future directions. *J Am Heart Assoc*. 2016;5: e002938.
6. Creager MA, Kaufman JA, Conte MS. Clinical practice. Acute limb ischemia. *N Engl J Med*. 2012;366:2198–2206.
7. Kronzon I, Saric M. Cholesterol embolization syndrome. *Circulation*. 2010;122:631–641.
8. Kim ESH, Beckman J. Takayasu arteritis: challenges in diagnosis and management. *Heart*. 2018;104:558–565.
9. Hoffman GS. Giant cell arteritis. *Ann Intern Med*. 2016;165:ITC65–ITC80.
10. Piazza G, Creager MA. Thromboangiitis obliterans. *Circulation*. 2010;121:1858–1861.
11. Hussain MA, Aljabri B, Al-Omran M. Vascular thoracic outlet syndrome. *Semin Thorac Cardiovasc Surg*. 2016;28:151–157.

12. Hameed M, Coupland A, Davies AH. Popliteal artery entrapment syndrome: an approach to diagnosis and management. *Br J Sports Med.* 2018;52:1073–1074.

13. Wigley FM, Flavahan NA. Raynaud's phenomenon. *N Engl J Med.* 2016;375:556–565.

14. Beckman JA. Management of asymptomatic internal carotid artery stenosis. *JAMA.* 2013;310:1612–1618.

15. Bergan JJ, Schmid-Schonbein GW, Smith PD, et al. Chronic venous disease. *N Engl J Med.* 2006;355:488–498.

16. Rockson SG. Lymphedema. *Vasc Med.* 2016;21:77–813.

17. Gillard J, Perez-Cousin M, Hachulla E, et al. Diagnosing thoracic outlet syndrome: contribution of provocative tests, ultrasonography, electrophysiology, and helical computed tomography in 48 patients. *Joint Bone Spine.* 2001;68:416–424.

18. Nord KM, Kapoor P, Fisher J, et al. False positive rate of thoracic outlet syndrome diagnostic maneuvers. *Electromyogr Clin Neurophysiol.* 2008;48:67–74.

19. Armstrong DG, Boulton AJM, Bus SA. Diabetic foot ulcers and their recurrence. *N Engl J Med.* 2017;376:2367–2375.

20. Homans J. Venous thrombosis in the lower limbs: its relation to pulmonary embolism. *Am J Surg.* 1937;38:316–326.

21. Eberhardt RT, Raffetto JD. Chronic venous insufficiency. *Circulation.* 2014;130:333–346.

22. Eklöf B, Rutherford RB, Bergan JJ, et al. Revision of the CEAP classification for chronicvenous disorders: consensus statement. *J Vasc Surg.* 2004;40:1248–1252.

23. Magyar MT, Nam EM, Csiba L, et al. Carotid artery auscultation—anachronism or useful screening procedure? *Neurol Res.* 2002;24:705–708.

24. Ratchford EV, Jin Z, Di Tullio MR, et al. Carotid bruit for detection of hemodynamically significant carotid stenosis: the Northern Manhattan Study. *Neurol Res.* 2009;31:748–752.

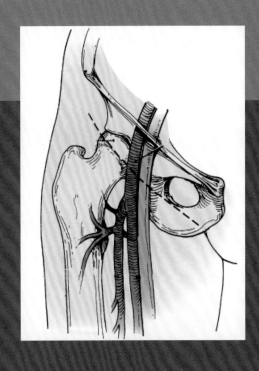

中文导读

第12章
血管相关实验室检查

　　在当下血管医学实践中，有许多费用相对低廉但实用的血管实验室检查技术，这些技术被广泛应用于血管功能检查及多种血管疾病的检测。临床上常用的血管检查技术包括血管生理功能测试与多普勒超声检查。本章将主要介绍血管生理功能测试的基本原理和应用，包括节段压力测量、脉冲体积记录（PVR）、连续波多普勒及体积描记法。这些生理功能测试通过使用袖带、多普勒仪器和体积描记设备即可完成。多普勒超声检查通过将灰度和多普勒成像与光谱及彩色多普勒结合，可用于大多数部位的血管检查。超声机由硬件和软件两部分组成：软件用于分析及成像；硬件，即超声探头则用于体表探测及信息采集。不同部位的多普勒超声检查需要使用不同规格的超声探头，如颈部和四肢血管超声需要5～12 MHz探头，腹部血管超声应配备2.25～3.5 MHz探头。目前临床上已有6～15 MHz的探头可供选择。根据目标血管选用适宜的探头能够获取更清晰、准确的超声检查结果。

郑月宏

Vascular Laboratory Testing

Marie Gerhard-Herman and Mark A. Creager

Vascular laboratory technology offers many cost-effective applications in the practice of vascular medicine. Vascular testing includes both physiological testing and duplex ultrasonography. Physiological testing includes segmental pressure measurements, pulse volume recordings (PVRs), continuous wave (CW) Doppler, and plethysmography. These tests use sphygmomanometric cuffs, Doppler instruments, and plethysmographic recording devices. Duplex ultrasonography combines gray-scale and Doppler imaging with spectral and color Doppler and is used for the majority of vascular laboratory tests. An ultrasound machine should be equipped with vascular software and two transducers/probes, at least 5- to 12-MHz transducers for the neck and extremities and 2.25- to 3.5-MHz transducers for the abdomen. There are currently many options available, such as 6- to 15-MHz transducers.

LIMB PRESSURE MEASUREMENT AND PULSE VOLUME RECORDINGS

Limb segmental systolic blood pressure measurements and PVRs are used to confirm a clinical diagnosis of peripheral artery disease (PAD) and further define the level and extent of the obstruction.[1] Segmental pressures are typically measured in conjunction with segmental limb plethysmography (PVRs). These techniques are used predominantly in the lower extremities but are also applicable to the arms. Both procedures are performed using sphygmomanometric cuffs that are appropriately sized to the diameter of the limb segment under study. The patient rests in the supine position for at least 10 minutes prior to measuring limb pressures. Commercially available machines with automatic cuff inflation are able to digitally store the pressures and waveforms. A CW Doppler instrument with a 4- to 8-MHz transducer frequency is used to detect the arterial flow signal. The cuff is quickly inflated to a suprasystolic pressure and then slowly deflated until a flow signal occurs. The cuff pressure at which the flow signal is detected is the systolic pressure in the arterial segment beneath the cuff. For example, if the cuff is on the high thigh and the sensor is over the posterior tibial artery at the ankle, the measured pressure is reflective of the proximal superficial and deep femoral arteries beneath the cuff, as well as any collateral arteries, and not only the posterior tibial artery. The Doppler flow signal from an artery at the ankle is typically used for all limb measurements. It is more accurate, although less convenient, to place the Doppler transducer probe close to the cuff being inflated.

Sphygmomanometric cuffs are positioned on each arm above the antecubital fossa, on the upper portion of each thigh (high thigh), on the lower portions of the thighs above the patella (low thigh), on the calves below the tibial tubercle, and on the ankles above the malleoli. Typically, foot pressures are measured by insonating the posterior tibial and anterior tibial arteries at the ankle level. Both arm pressures at the brachial artery are determined. A difference of greater than 20 mm Hg between the arm pressures indicates the presence of stenosis on the side of the lower pressure. Pressure measurements are made at the high thigh, low thigh, calf, and ankle levels with a tibial or dorsalis pedis signal selected as the flow indicator. There is a second method which uses one long contoured thigh cuff rather than two separate thigh cuffs. The lower extremity pressure evaluation should begin at the ankle level and proceed proximally. Patients who are found to have a normal pressure measurement at rest may require a treadmill exercise test to detect PAD. If disease distal to the ankle is suspected, pedal or digital artery obstruction can be evaluated with cuffs sized appropriately for the toes.

Segmental Doppler Pressure Interpretation

Segmental limb pressures are compared with the highest arm pressure. The ankle pressures are used to calculate the ankle-brachial indices (ABIs) for each extremity. This is accomplished by dividing each of the ankle pressures by the higher of the brachial artery pressures.[2] A normal ABI is between 1.0 and 1.4, whereas an ABI >0.9 to 1.0 is borderline abnormal. Studies that evaluated the ABI in healthy subjects and patients with PAD confirmed by arteriography found that an ABI of ≤0.9 was diagnostic of PAD with 79% to 95% specificity and 96% to 100% sensitivity. Pressures are compared between levels. A 20 mm Hg or greater reduction in pressures from one level to the next is considered significant and indicates stenosis between those two levels. In healthy subjects, the high thigh pressure determined by cuff typically exceeds the brachial artery pressure by approximately 30 mm Hg. A thigh/brachial index >1 is interpreted as normal, and an index ≤1 indicates stenosis proximal to the thigh (Fig. 12.1). When the high thigh pressures are low compared with the arm pressure, the site of obstruction could be in the aorta or in the ipsilateral iliac artery, common femoral artery, or proximal superficial femoral artery (see Fig. 12.1). If only one high thigh pressure is less than the brachial pressure, then an ipsilateral iliofemoral artery stenosis is inferred.

In the presence of severe vascular calcification, systolic pressures cannot be determined because the vessels are noncompressible. An index ≥1.4 suggests vascular calcification artifact and makes interpretation of the pressure measurement unreliable. The presence or absence of a significant pressure gradient cannot be determined in the presence of vascular calcification artifact. In this setting the toe-brachial index (TBI) is a useful measurement. The TBI is the ratio of the systolic pressure in the toe to the brachial artery systolic pressure. This should be performed in a warm room, because cold-induced vasoconstriction may lower the digital pressure.[3] To perform the procedure, a cuff is placed on a toe. Typically, the great toe is used. The pulse waveform is obtained by photoplethysmography or Doppler. The cuff is inflated to suprasystolic pressure and then deflated. Systolic pressure is determined as the pressure at which the waveform reappears. A normal value for TBI is 0.70, and a value less than 0.70 indicates the presence of PAD.

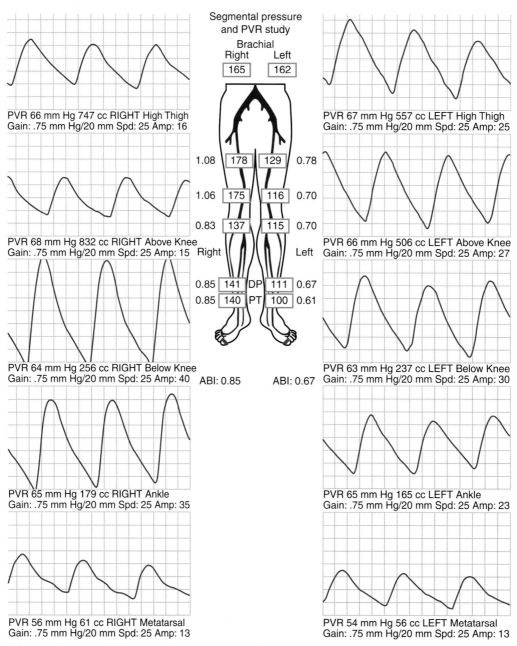

Fig. 12.1 Segmental Pressure Measurements and Pulse Volume Recording. Pressure at each level is shown within the box. The right leg has a pressure drop between the low thigh and calf, consistent with superficial femoral/popliteal artery stenosis. The left leg has a pressure drop at the level of the high thigh relative to the brachial artery and right high thigh, consistent with iliofemoral artery stenosis.

Pulse Volume Recording Interpretation

The same cuffs used to measure segmental pressures may be attached to a plethysmographic instrument and used to record the change in volume of a limb segment with each pulse, designated the pulse volume. The pulse volume waveform evaluation allows assessment of arterial flow in regions of calcified vessels because the test does not rely on cuff occlusion of the calcified artery. Each cuff is inflated in sequence to a predetermined reference pressure, up to 65 mm Hg. The change in volume in the limb segment causes a corresponding change in pressure in the cuff throughout the cardiac cycle. Interpretation of the PVR requires calibration of the amount of air in the cuff.

A pulse volume waveform is recorded for each limb segment. PVR analysis is based on evaluation of waveform shape, signal, and amplitude (Fig. 12.2). The configuration of the normal pulse volume waveform resembles the arterial pressure waveform and is composed of a sharp systolic upstroke followed by a downstroke that contains a prominent dicrotic notch.[4] A hemodynamically significant stenosis manifests as a change in the PVR contour with broadening of the wave toward a tardus parvus waveform. Both the slope and amplitude decrease when there is more severe disease. Severity of PAD can be defined by the slope of the upstroke and the amplitude of the pulse volume (see Fig. 12.2).

Pulse waveforms can also be obtained using photoplethysmography, recording reflected infrared light. In photoplethysmography, the signal is proportional to the quantity of red blood cells in the cutaneous circulation; it does not measure volume changes. Waveform shape is

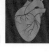

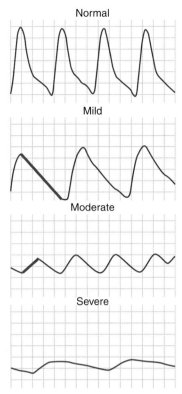

Fig. 12.2 Pulse Volume Recording. The normal waveform has a sharp upstroke, dicrotic notch, and a period of diastasis. The mildly abnormal waveform has a delay in the upstroke and a straightened downslope *(blue line)*. The moderately abnormal waveform has a delay in upstroke *(blue line)*, flat systolic peak, and diminished amplitude. The severely abnormal waveform has a flat systolic peak and very diminished amplitude.

assessed in a similar fashion in pulse volume and photoplethysmography recordings. Low photoplethysmographic waveforms in the toes identify increased risk of amputation, in addition to the toe pressure.

Exercise Testing for Peripheral Artery Disease

Exercise testing is an adjunctive physiologic test to evaluate PAD. It is useful to assess functional capacity and determine the distance patients with claudication are able to walk.[5] Moreover, it can be used to clarify whether leg symptoms are related to PAD. This is relevant in patients with symptoms that are atypical for claudication and in those who have a history of intermittent claudication, yet normal ABIs at rest. There is also a role for TBI and transcutaneous tissue oxygen pressure in the evaluation of PAD.[6] Relative contraindications to treadmill exercise testing for PAD include rest pain in the leg, shortness of breath with minimal exertion, or unstable angina. The test cannot be performed if the patient cannot walk on a treadmill.

Patients are instructed to fast for 12 hours prior to walking on the treadmill. The constant load treadmill test is performed at a speed of 2 miles per hour and an incline of 12%. Graded exercise protocols increase the grade and/or speed in 2- to 3-minute stages. The Gardner protocol is the most commonly used graded protocol to evaluate walking exercise capacity. It begins at a speed of 2 mph and an incline of 0% and the grade increases by 2% progressively every 2 minutes, allowing for a wider range of responses to be measured. It is often used to determine clinical trial end points, such as change in walking time in response to therapy. Other graded exercise protocols, such as the Bruce protocol, are not commonly used because the rapid rate of speed and incline limits the assessment of exercise capacity in claudicants.

The treadmill exercise test is terminated when the patient cannot continue due to leg claudication or chest pain or is limited by other symptoms such as shortness of breath or fatigue. The patient then immediately lies down on the stretcher. The ankle pressures are obtained starting with the symptomatic leg, followed by the highest brachial pressure. The pressures are repeated approximately every 1 to 2 minutes until they return to baseline. Data recorded from the exercise test should include ankle pressures, length of time the patient could walk, time required for the pressures to return to baseline, nature and location of the patient's symptoms, and reason for discontinuing the test. A decrease in ABI to <0.90 or decrease in ABI of more than 20% immediately following exercise is diagnostic for PAD. The time before ankle pressure returns to normal is increased in more severe disease (e.g., from 2 minutes in mild disease to 10 minutes in more severe disease).

TRANSCUTANEOUS OXIMETRY

By exploiting the variations in color absorbance of oxygenated and deoxygenated hemoglobin, transcutaneous oximetry can determine the state of blood oxygenation.[7] Oximeters use two light frequencies, red at 600 to 750 nm and infrared at 800 to 1050 nm, to differentiate oxygenated and deoxygenated hemoglobin. Deoxygenated blood absorbs more red light, whereas oxygenated blood absorbs more infrared light. Oximeters typically use both an emitter and receiver. Red and infrared light is emitted and passes through a relatively translucent structure, such as the finger or earlobe. A photodetector determines the ratio of red and infrared light received to derive blood oxygenation. When measured continuously, oxygenation peaks with each heartbeat as fresh, oxygenated blood arrives in the zone of measurement. The normal values for oxygen tension are from 50 to 75 mm Hg. One probe is placed on the chest as a control to ensure that the oxygen tension is from 50 to 75 mm Hg. A second probe is placed on the limb in the area of interest. Measurements are obtained from the probe, which is sequentially positioned from proximal to distal segments of the limb. The normal limb TcO_2 should approximate that of the chest. Transcutaneous oximetry is most often used to determine the level of amputation. A value of >20 mm Hg can predict healing at the site with 80% accuracy. This measurement is not affected by arterial calcification.

PHYSICAL PRINCIPLES OF ULTRASONOGRAPHY

Ultrasound Image Creation

An ultrasound transducer, or probe, emits sound waves in discrete bundles or pulses into the tissue of interest. On encountering a tissue, a portion of the waves are reflected to the transducer. The fraction of returning waves depends on the density and size of the tissue examined. The depth of tissue is determined by the time required for pulse emission and return. Thus, by integrating the number of returning pulses and the time required for return, a B-mode, or gray-scale, image may be created. The time for wave reflection decreases with higher ultrasound probe frequencies. Transducer probes with higher frequencies image superficial tissues better than probes with lower frequencies but lose depth imaging because of attenuation of the returning emitted pulses.

Improvements in technology have permitted a widening of the bandwidth of vascular transducers and can improve gray-scale imaging using harmonics of the fundamental frequency. A harmonic represents a whole number multiple of the emitted frequency. Because the tissue compresses and expands in response to the application of ultrasound, the fundamental wave may become distorted, impairing image quality. However, the distortion also creates harmonics of the original frequency that can be detected by the transducer. By detecting only the fundamental frequency and its harmonics, artifact (e.g., speckle and reverberation) may be reduced to create a clearer image.

Detection of Blood Flow

Normal blood flow is laminar in a straight segment of an artery. If thought of as a telescopic series of flow rings, blood moves forward most rapidly in the middle ring and velocity decreases in the outer rings as blood comes closer to the vessel wall. The cardiac cycle, defined by its pulsatile nature of flow, causes a continual variation in blood flow velocity, highest with systole and lowest with diastole. The concentric or laminar flow of blood may be disturbed at a normal branching point or with abnormal vessel contours, such as those caused by atherosclerotic plaque. Disturbed or turbulent flow causes a much greater loss of pressure than does laminar flow.

Determination of flow velocity is a mainstay of vascular ultrasonography.[8] Abnormalities in the vessel wall cause changes in flow velocity and permit the detection and assessment of stenotic regions within the vessel. Flow in a normal vessel is proportional to the difference of pressure between the proximal and distal end of the vessel. The prime determinant or limitation of flow is the radius of the vessel because volume of blood flow is determined by the fourth power of the radius. For example, a 50% reduction in vessel radius causes a greater than 90% reduction in blood flow. Thus blood flow represents an example of Poiseuille's law, which determines flow of a viscous fluid through a tube. Specifically,

$$Q = \frac{\pi \times \Delta P \times r^4}{8 \eta L}$$

where Q denotes the volume of flow; ΔP is pressure at inflow minus the pressure at outflow; r is the radius; η is the viscosity; and L is tube length. Because blood viscosity, blood vessel length, and pressure remain relatively stable, the most important determinant of blood flow is vessel lumen size.

Vascular ultrasonography can depict flow velocity by taking advantage of Doppler shift frequencies. The frequency will shift, either positively or negatively, depending on the direction of blood flow. The variables, which determine the size of the shift, include the speed of sound, the speed of the moving object, and the angle between the transmitted beam and the moving object. Christoph Doppler described this relationship using the following equation:

$$F_d = \left(2F_t \bullet V \bullet \cos\theta\right) \div c$$

where F_d is the Doppler frequency shift; F_t is the Doppler frequency transmitted from the probe; V is the velocity of flow; cos is the cosine, θ is the angle between the beam and direction of the moving object, and c is the velocity of sound.

Artifact

Although a highly reliable imaging modality, ultrasound does suffer from occasional image artifact.[9] Dense objects, such as vessel wall calcium deposits, permit few sound waves to penetrate, resulting in acoustic shadowing and diminishing imaging of deeper tissues. Tissue imaging enhancement may be noted on the far side of echo-free or liquid-filled zones. Tissue interfaces may generate multiple sound wave reflections, causing "additions" to the tissue termed reverberation artifact. Refraction of the sound pulse may cause improper placement of a structure of an image and shadowing at the edge of a large structure. Highly reflective surfaces may create mirror images because the reflecting tissue alters the timing of the returning sound wave. The mirror image should be equidistant from the reflecting surface or tissue.

Gray-Scale (B-Mode) Imaging

Ultrasound images are generated using a pulse echo system. The position of the tissue interface is determined by the time between pulse generation and returning echo. Each returning echo is displayed as a gray dot on a video screen using a brightness mode (B mode), in which the brightness of the dot depends on the strength of the reflected wave. A two-dimensional (2D) image is created by sequentially transmitting waves in multiple directions within a single plane and combining the reflected echoes into a single display. The image can be refreshed rapidly, permitting real-time display of the gray-scale image. The surface of interest should be perpendicular to the ultrasound beam to obtain the brightest echo with B-mode imaging. This is readily achieved in vascular imaging because the neck, extremity, and visceral vessels generally lie parallel to the surface of the transducer. Higher-frequency probes are used to image vessels close to the surface, and lower-frequency probes are used to image deeper vessels. Details of the vessel wall can be seen more clearly with the use of harmonics. The wide bandwidth of transducers allows analysis of returning harmonics (whole number multiples) of the fundamental frequency. The use of ultrasound contrast agents also allows for accurate imaging of the lumen wall interface; however, these agents are not yet approved for vascular imaging.

Spectral Doppler Waveform Analysis

Velocity recordings are obtained with an angle of 60 degrees between the Doppler insonation beam and the flow.[8] In ultrasound practice, the optimal angle of measurement between the beam and blood flow is 60 degrees. Although maximal shift is detected at 0 degrees, this angle cannot be reliably obtained in vascular imaging because the vessels are parallel to the surface of the body. Insonation angles below and above 60 degrees influence the measurement, such that small reductions in the insonation angle may alter velocity by 10%, whereas small increases in insonation angle may change flow velocity by 25% (Fig. 12.3). Thus the sample volume cursor is placed parallel to the inner wall, and a Doppler angle from 30 to 60 degrees between the wall and the insonation beam (or flow jet) is used. A normal peripheral artery Doppler waveform consists of a narrow, sharply defined tracing.[10] This indicates that all blood cells are moving at an equivalent speed at any time in the cardiac cycle. Waveforms are also characterized as high resistance due to limited flow during diastole (e.g., normal peripheral arterial Doppler velocity waveform), or low resistance with continuous flow

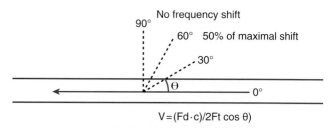

Fig. 12.3 The Doppler angle is the angle between the insonation beam and the sample cursor aligned with flow. The dashed lines represent different insonation beams. The solid arrow represents the direction of flow and the position of the Doppler sample cursor. The velocity is determined using the Doppler equation, with the cosine (cos) in the denominator. The cos 0 degrees = 1, cos 30 degrees = 0.86, cos 60 degrees = 0.5, and cos 90 degrees = 0. c, Velocity of sound; F_d, Doppler frequency shift; F_t, transmitted Doppler frequency; V, velocity.

during diastole as when downstream resistance arterioles are widely dilated or there is contiguity with low-resistance circuits (e.g., normal internal carotid artery [ICA] velocity waveform) (Fig. 12.4). The normal high-resistance waveform is typically triphasic. The first component is caused by initial high-velocity forward flow during ventricular systole. A range of normal peak systolic velocity (PSV) measurements have been defined for each arterial segment, as described later in this chapter.

The second phase of the waveform consists of early diastolic flow reversal, as the left ventricular pressure falls below the aortic pressure prior to aortic valve closure.[11] The final or third component is a small amount of forward flow when there is elastic recoil of vessel walls. Flow is typically not uniform or laminar at bifurcations and sites of stenosis; at these sites, flow becomes turbulent. For these locations, the spectral Doppler waveform reflects the fact that blood cells move with varying velocities. Instead of a narrow, well-defined tracing (see Fig. 12.4), spectral broadening becomes evident (Fig. 12.5), with partial or complete filling-in of the area under the spectral waveform. This third, or late, diastolic component is usually absent in atherosclerotic vessels that have lost compliance or elasticity.

Color Doppler

Color Doppler is the phase or frequency shift information that is contained in the returning echoes and processed in real time to form a velocity map over the entire imaging field.[12] Doppler frequency-shift

data are available for every point imaged. This information is then superimposed on the gray-scale image to provide a composite real-time display of both anatomy and flow. When motion is detected, it is assigned a color, typically red or blue, determined by whether the frequency shift is toward or away from the probe. Color assignment is arbitrary and can be altered by the user, but most choose to assign red to arteries and blue to veins. With increasing Doppler frequency shifts, the hue and intensity of the color display change, with a progressive desaturation of the color and a shift toward white at the highest detectable velocities. The pulse repetition frequency (velocity) scale determines the degree of color saturation and filling of the vessel lumen. The pulse repetition frequency (radio frequency pulses per second from the probe) is adjusted so that in a normal vessel, laminar flow appears as a homogeneous color. The color appearance changes throughout the cardiac cycle. Increasing flow velocity and turbulence in the region of a stenosis results in the production of a high-velocity jet and an abrupt change in the color-flow pattern (Fig. 12.6). Color aliasing occurs at the site of stenosis when the flow velocity exceeds the Nyquist limit (i.e., when the Doppler frequency shift exceeds one half the pulse repetition frequency). Aliasing (see Fig. 12.6) causes the color display to appear as if there is an abrupt reversal in the direction of the flow (wraparound). This suggests a high-velocity flow jet, requiring confirmation by pulsed-wave Doppler analysis. Color persistence is a continuous flow signal that is the color of the forward direction only, in contrast to the alternating color in normal arteries. There is loss of early diastolic flow reversal. Color persistence corresponds to the monophasic spectral Doppler waveform and is indicative of severe stenosis. Poststenotic regions display mosaic patterns indicating turbulent flow. A color bruit in the surrounding soft tissue also indicates flow disturbance. This color artifact is associated with turbulence and occurs with flow disturbances associated with high-velocity jets. The color bruit is particularly useful in locating postcatheterization arteriovenous fistulae.

Assessment of Arterial Stenosis

Characteristic duplex ultrasound features of a stenosis include elevated systolic velocity, elevated end-diastolic velocity (EDV), color aliasing, color bruit, spectral broadening of the Doppler waveform, poststenotic flow, and poststenotic turbulence.[13] An auditory "thump" occurs in the presence of total arterial occlusion. Doppler velocity measurements are the main tools used to evaluate stenosis severity. When flow rate is constant, a decrease in vessel cross-sectional area is balanced by an increase in velocity.

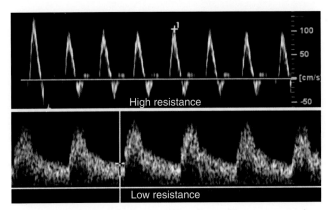

Fig. 12.4 High and Low Resistance Waveforms. These two waveforms are distinguished by the absence (high resistance) and a presence (low resistance) of flow during diastole.

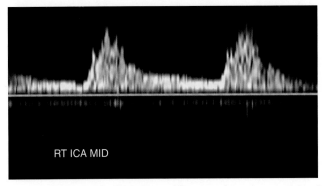

Fig. 12.5 Poststenotic Waveform. The waveform has a delay in upstroke, diminished amplitude, and marked turbulence. *RT ICA MID,* Midportion of the right internal carotid artery.

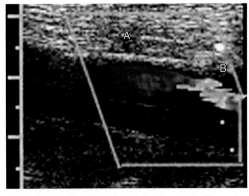

Fig. 12.6 Aliasing at the Site of Arterial Stenosis. There is an abrupt change from low-velocity laminar flow *(A)* to high-velocity flow with aliasing *(B)* as the velocity exceeds the Nyquist limits. An echolucent (dark) plaque is evident at the site of stenosis within the superficial femoral artery stent.

As blood flow turbulence increases, spectral broadening of the Doppler waveform becomes a clear indicator of turbulent flow seen in the poststenotic region. The poststenotic waveform is dampened with a delayed upstroke (see Fig. 12.5). If no poststenotic turbulence can be identified, inappropriate angle alignment or a tortuous vessel should be suspected. Power (or amplitude) Doppler is a complementary imaging technique that displays the total strength or amplitude of the returning Doppler signal. In comparison with conventional color flow imaging, color-flow sensitivity is increased by a factor of 3 to 5 times with power Doppler. This enhanced dynamic range can depict very slow flow in the area of a subtotal occlusion that may not be detected by conventional color-flow Doppler. Contrast agents can also help to differentiate between occlusion and high-grade stenosis in carotid and renal arteries and especially in cases where multiple renal arteries are present.

CAROTID DUPLEX ULTRASOUND

The standard carotid duplex examination includes assessment of the carotid arteries, as well as the vertebral, subclavian, and brachiocephalic arteries. Indications for this test include a bruit, transient ischemic attack, amaurosis fugax, stroke, and surveillance after revascularization.[14] The examination begins with a gray-scale survey of the extracranial carotid arteries in transverse and longitudinal views. The operator images the region from the clavicle to the angle of the jaw, in both the anterolateral and posterolateral views. The common carotid artery (CCA) is typically medial to the internal jugular vein, and the bifurcation is often located near the cricoid cartilage. The ICA is usually posterolateral, with a diameter at its origin greater than that of the anteromedially located external carotid artery (ECA).

Carotid artery stenosis can be focal, and flow patterns can normalize within a short distance. Therefore the pulse wave sample volume should be methodically advanced along the length of the vessel; color Doppler may be used for guidance in delineating areas of abnormal flow requiring change in the position of the sample volume (Figs. 12.7 and 12.8). Representative velocity measurements should be recorded from the proximal, mid-, and distal CCA. The CCA spectral waveform is a combination of the ECA and ICA waveforms, with greater diastolic flow than the ECA but less than that of the ICA. Atherosclerosis, when present, is usually most evident at the ICA origin, whereas fibromuscular dysplasia may be more evident distally. Using spectral Doppler, the sample volume is advanced throughout the entire ICA. At a minimum, PSV and EDV from the proximal, mid-, and distal ICA segments should be recorded. The vertebral artery is then located posterior to the carotid artery. The vertebral artery and vein lie between the spinous processes. The vertebral artery is followed as far cephalad as possible, sampling the spectral Doppler in the accessible portions of the vertebral artery.

Distinguishing the internal and ECA is critical to the examination (Fig. 12.9; see Fig. 12.7). The ECA is usually smaller and more anteromedial and has less diastolic flow than the ICA. The ECA will also have branches in the cervical region, whereas the ICA will not. A direct comparison of the waveforms from the two vessels is critical. A velocity waveform obtained from the proximal vessel or the site of maximal velocity should be obtained while intermittently tapping on the preauricular branch of the temporal artery. The intermittent tapping is reflected clearly in the diastolic portion of the ECA waveform but not in the ICA waveform (see Fig. 12.9).

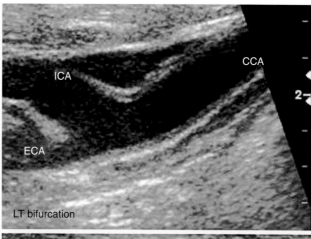

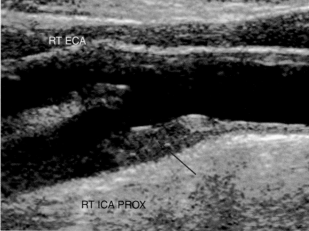

Fig. 12.7 Gray Scale of Right and Left Carotid Bifurcation. The internal carotid artery *(ICA)* in each is slightly wider at the origin than the external carotid artery *(ECA)*. The red arrow indicates plaque in the proximal right ICA. A branch is evident arising from the left ECA. In the absence of identified branches, waveforms are necessary to distinguish the ICA from the ECA. *CCA,* common carotid artery.

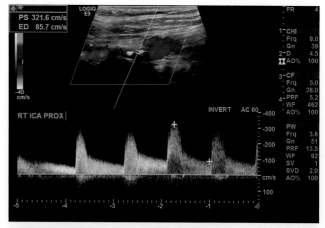

Fig. 12.8 Color Doppler of the Internal Carotid Artery *(ICA)*. Color Doppler is added to the gray-scale picture of the right ICA seen in Fig. 12.7. Color aliasing identifies an area of high velocity adjacent to the plaque. This guides the placement of the spectral Doppler sample volume, identified by the parallel white lines.

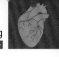

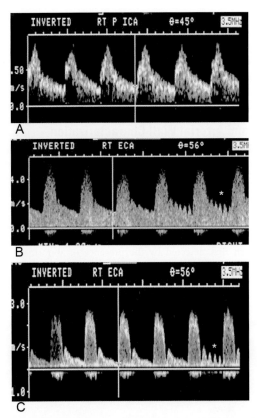

Fig. 12.9 Spectral Waveforms of the Internal and External Carotid Arteries (*ICA* and *ECA*) During Intermittent Tapping of the Ipsilateral Temporal Artery. (A) Has no clear "tapping" pattern and is therefore likely ICA. (B) Has high-peak systolic velocity *(PSV)* of 400 cm/s. Tapping *(asterisk)* clearly identified in the diastolic component of the waveform identifies the artery as the ECA and indicates that the high PSV represents ECA stenosis. (C) The typical ECA waveform is high resistance with low-peak systolic velocity and obvious tapping pattern of the temporal artery during diastole.

The interpretation of the spectral waveforms is based on parameters such as PSV, EDV, shape, and the extent of spectral broadening (Fig. 12.10). Delay in the systolic upstroke of the wave should be seen just beyond a high-grade stenosis. There are a number of criteria for ICA stenosis that have been proposed, each having their own strengths and weaknesses (Table 12.1). PSV criteria for ICA stenosis have identified a cut point of 230 cm/s as the threshold for detecting greater than 70% stenosis and 125 cm/s as the cut point for identifying greater than 50% stenosis. Criteria that include EDV use a cut point of greater than 140 cm/s to identify greater than 80% stenosis. The ratio of the peak ICA systolic velocity to the mid-CCA velocity may be particularly useful in determining the presence or stenosis in the hemodynamic setting of low cardiac output or critical aortic stenosis. At a minimum, the velocity criteria must distinguish less than 50% stenosis, 50% to 69% stenosis, and greater than 70% stenosis.[15] Selection of criteria for use in an individual laboratory requires review of the published parameters and selection of those that are appropriate to the laboratory practice. Individual vascular laboratories must validate the results of their own criteria for stenosis against a suitable standard, such as arteriography.

Waveform analysis depends on evaluation of acceleration, diastolic flow, direction of flow, and comparison to the contralateral vessel. If the ICA is totally occluded, there will be absent or severely

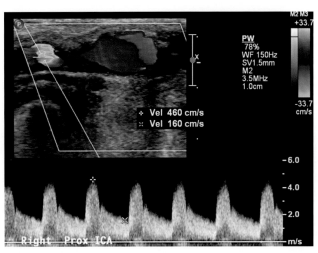

Fig. 12.10 Internal Carotid Artery Stenosis. The pulsed wave sample volume is placed at the site of aliasing. There is marked spectral broadening. The waveform resembles that in Fig. 12.9C.

TABLE 12.1 Criteria for Internal Carotid Artery Stenosis

Stenosis	ICA PSV	Lumen Plaque	ICA/CCA PSV	ICA EDV
0	<125	0	<2	<40
1–49	<125	+	<2	<40
50–69	>125	+	2–4	40–100
>70	>230	+	>4	>100
Subtotal	VAR.	+++	VAR.	>0
Total	0	+++	0	0

This table summarizes multiple criteria—including peak-systolic velocity alone, peak systolic and end-diastolic velocities, and ICA/CCA ratio. *CCA*, Common carotid artery; *EDV*, end-diastolic velocity; *ICA*, internal carotid artery; *PSV*, peak systolic velocity; *VAR.*, variable.
From Grant EG, Benson CB, Moneta GL, et al. Carotid artery stenosis: grayscale and Doppler ultrasound diagnosis—Society of Radiologists in Ultrasound consensus conference. *Ultrasound Q.* 2003;19:190–198.

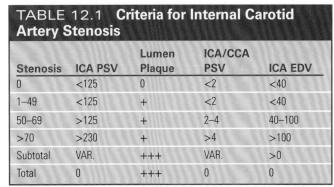

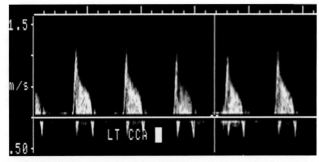

Fig. 12.11 Absent diastolic flow in the common carotid artery *(CCA)* suggesting the presence of total occlusion of the ipsilateral internal carotid artery.

diminished diastolic flow in the ipsilateral CCA (Fig. 12.11). A delay in the upstroke suggests more proximal stenosis. For example, severe stenosis of the brachiocephalic artery will result in dampened right CCA waveforms. A step-up in systolic velocity in the cervical portion of the CCA indicates stenosis, with doubling indicating at least 50% stenosis and tripling indicating at least 75% stenosis.

Waveform evaluation is particularly valuable in the vertebral artery because the segments within the bone cannot be directly evaluated with ultrasound. Specific velocity criteria have not been developed for vertebral artery stenosis. Velocities greater than 125 cm/s and dampened waveforms are two indicators of vertebral artery stenosis. Absent flow in the vertebral artery is confirmed when flow is detected in the vertebral vein but not in the vertebral artery. Retrograde flow in the vertebral artery indicates subclavian steal (i.e., the subclavian circulation is stealing from the cerebral circulation).[16] Reverse flow is confirmed by comparing the direction of vertebral artery flow with that of the carotid artery (Fig. 12.12). Reverse flow typically will have a diminished diastolic component because flow is into the high resistance bed of the subclavian artery (Fig. 12.13). If flow is cephalad but notching is evident in the systolic portion of the wave, subclavian steal can be elicited by reexamining flow after arm exercise or following deflation of a blood pressure cuff that had been inflated to suprasystolic pressures on the ipsilateral arm. These maneuvers will increase demand in the subclavian bed, and vertebral flow will completely reverse in the setting of subclavian stenosis proximal to the vertebral

origin. The vast majority of these patients with subclavian stenosis are asymptomatic.

The subclavian artery is evaluated as close to the origin as possible. The probe is placed longitudinally above the clavicle and angled to obtain a scanning plane below the clavicle. Color Doppler surveillance is used to detect nonlaminar flow. The Doppler spectrum is obtained throughout the vessel. A doubling of the PSV is consistent with ≥50% stenosis.

Plaque and Arterial Wall Characterization

Gray-scale imaging is used to evaluate carotid plaque and arterial wall characteristics. Atherosclerotic plaque is evident on ultrasound examination as material that thickens the media and intima, and protrudes into the arterial lumen. Plaque surface and echo characteristics can be determined and described. Ulceration refers to an excavation within the plaque containing flow. Echolucent plaque is characterized as plaque that is less echogenic than the surrounding muscle (Fig. 12.14) and is often first detected by the presence of abnormal color flow (Fig. 12.15). The volume of plaque is appreciated best in the transverse view and with 3D reconstruction.

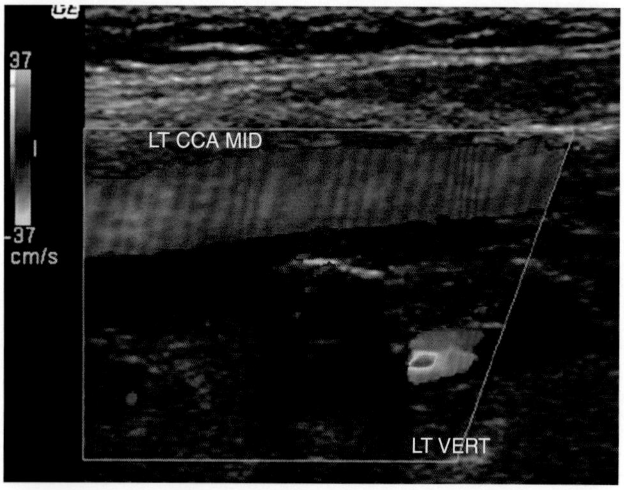

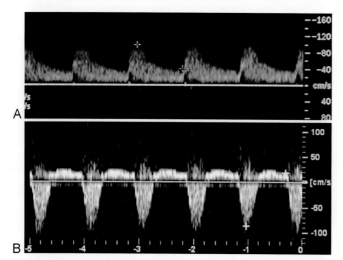

Fig. 12.12 Color Doppler of the common carotid artery (CCA) and vertebral arteries demonstrating flow in two different directions, antegrade carotid artery flow and retrograde vertebral artery flow.

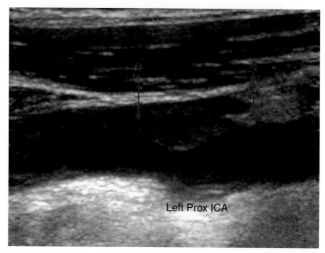

Fig. 12.14 Gray-Scale Image of Atherosclerotic Plaque. Echolucent plaque is indicated (arrow B) adjacent to more echobright plaque (arrow A) in the gray-scale image of this internal carotid artery.

Fig. 12.13 Spectral waveform of normal, antegrade vertebral flow (A) with low resistance waveform and (B) reversed, retrograde vertebral flow with high resistance waveform.

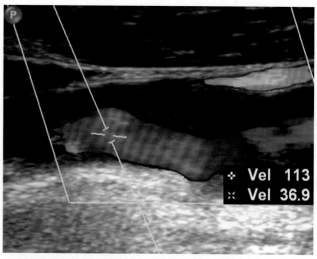

Fig. 12.15 Duplex Imaging of Atherosclerotic Plaque. Echolucent plaque is now clearly evident with the addition of color Doppler.

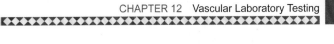

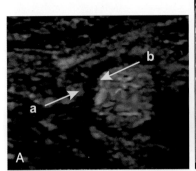
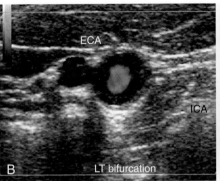
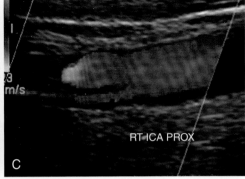

Fig. 12.16 Arterial Wall Characteristics. (A) Contrast is used to identify the lumen wall interface. Wall thickening is evident between the intima lumen interface *(a)* and the media adventitia interface *(b)*. (B) Power Doppler is used to identify the lumen wall interface. The thickened echolucent wall suggests the presence of arteritis. (C) Dissection of the internal carotid artery *(ICA)* with flow evident in both the true and false lumen. *ECA,* External carotid artery.

Another potential technique to characterize the arterial wall is contrast-enhanced ultrasound to detect ulceration, dissection, and inflammation.[17] Contrast can be used to define the wall-lumen interface (Fig. 12.16A). The plaque thickness can be severely overestimated or underestimated in the longitudinal image and is best evaluated in transverse images. Ultrasound can also evaluate findings such as edema (see Fig. 12.16B) and dissection of the carotid wall (see Fig. 12.16C). Circumferential arterial wall edema creating a "halo" appearance indicates the presence of arteritis.[18] Dissection can originate in the ICA (see Fig. 12.16C) or extend from the arch into the CCA. Flow can be present in both the true and false lumen. The flap may be apparent on gray-scale imaging but generally requires color or contrast for elucidation. A flutter is occasionally identified in the down-slope of the waveform on the affected side. Evaluation should identify both the proximal and distal extent of dissection, flow velocities in the true lumen, and flow to the end organ.

Carotid Intimal Medial Thickness

Carotid ultrasonography has traditionally been used to evaluate the presence of obstructive atherosclerosis in the setting of symptomatic cerebrovascular disease or asymptomatic carotid bruit. More recently, carotid ultrasonography has been performed in epidemiological studies to detect nonobstructive plaque and intimal-medial thickness (IMT).[19] IMT refers to the distance from the intima lumen interface to the media adventitia border. Protocols have measured ICA, CCA, ICA plus CCA, and carotid bulb IMT. The yield and reproducibility appear to be greatest for the far wall CCA IMT measurement. IMT measurement is most commonly made from longitudinal images with the assistance of semiautomated edge detection software (Fig. 12.17). There is variability in this measurement from systole to diastole and by age and gender. A single threshold value for abnormal IMT has not been determined. Ideally, threshold values derived from large population-based studies should be used in the evaluation of IMT. Both plaque and IMT correlate with cardiovascular morbidity and mortality. Indeed, the presence of carotid plaque resulting in 50% stenosis is included in the Adult Treatment Panel III guidelines as a coronary heart disease equivalent.

ABDOMINAL AORTA EVALUATION

Abdominal ultrasound is used to diagnose and follow abdominal aortic aneurysms (AAAs). The US Preventive Services Task Force recommendation is screening in all men 65 to 75 years who have ever smoked and selectively to those in this age group who have never

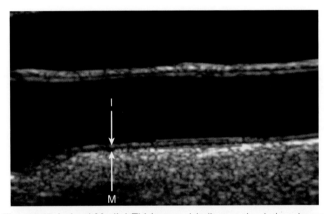

Fig. 12.17 Intimal-Medial Thickness. *I* indicates the intima lumen border and *M* indicates the media adventitia border. The distance between the intima lumen border and the media adventitia border is determined using an automated edge detection program that averages the thickness of wall over the region identified by the purple lines laid over these borders.

smoked.[20] There should also be targeted AAA family screening for female and male relatives of all AAA patients.[21]

An ultrasound machine with a low-frequency transducer (e.g., 2.5 MHz) is used to determine the aneurysm size, shape, location (infrarenal or suprarenal), and distance from other arterial segments. The patient is required to fast prior to the study because bowel gas will obscure imaging. Aortic ultrasound scanning begins with the patient supine and the transducer placed in a subxiphoid position. The aorta is located slightly left of midline. The abdominal aorta from the diaphragm to the bifurcation is evaluated using three sonographic views: the sagittal plane (A-P diameter), transverse plane (A-P diameter and transverse diameters), and coronal plane (longitudinal and transverse diameters). Diameter is measured from outer wall to outer wall. If overlying bowel gas obstructs the aorta from view, patients are instructed to lie in the decubitus position and the aorta is visualized via the coronal plane through either flank.[22] As the transducer is moved caudally, the celiac trunk will be evident branching into the common hepatic and splenic arteries (Fig. 12.18). The superior mesenteric artery (SMA) originates approximately 1 cm distal to the celiac trunk (Fig. 12.19). Next, the right renal artery may be seen emerging from the aorta and traveling under the inferior vena cava. The left renal vein then crosses over the aorta, and the left renal artery will be seen posterior to the

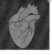

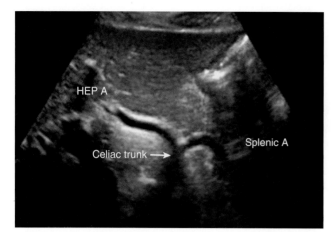

Fig. 12.18 Transverse Gray-Scale Image of the Splenic and Hepatic Arteries Arising From the Celiac Trunk. The celiac trunk is the first branch from the abdominal aorta.

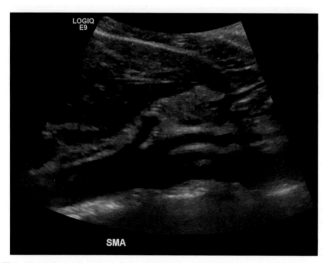

Fig. 12.19 Longitudinal Gray-Scale Image of the Aorta. The superior mesenteric artery (SMA) is the second branch of the abdominal aorta and is seen running parallel to the aorta just after the celiac artery in this longitudinal image of the abdominal aorta.

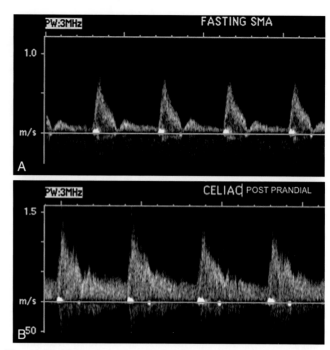

Fig. 12.20 (A) Fasting spectral waveform in the superior mesenteric artery (SMA). (B) Postprandial spectral waveform in the celiac trunk.

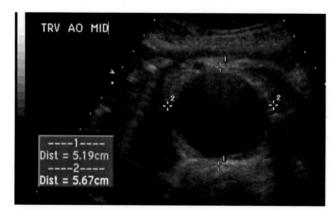

Fig. 12.21 Gray-Scale Image From an Abdominal Aortic Aneurysm Screening Examination. This transverse image of the abdominal aorta has a maximum diameter of >5.6 cm, indicating aneurysm.

vein. The inferior mesenteric artery is the final branch arising from the aorta before it bifurcates into the iliac vessels. Spectral Doppler evaluation of the celiac and mesenteric vessels will demonstrate low-resistance waveforms following a meal and high-resistance waveforms in the normal, fasting patient (Fig. 12.20). In contrast, evaluation of the normal renal arteries always demonstrates low-resistance waveforms.

An AAA is defined as an aortic diameter of at least 1.5 times the adjacent normal segment or a distal aorta diameter of greater than 3.0 cm (Fig. 12.21). Normal abdominal aortic diameters range from 1.4 to 3.0 cm. The shape of the AAA is described as saccular, fusiform, or cylindrical. Most AAAs are fusiform in shape, located below the renal arteries, and involve one or both of the iliac arteries. Atherosclerotic plaque, mural thrombus, and dissection can be detected in the wall of the aneurysm.

Ultrasound evaluation is also performed after endograft repair of an AAA.[23] Flow within the graft is evaluated with longitudinal and transverse imaging. Endoleak is diagnosed when there is flow outside the graft but within the aneurysm. Dissection, pseudoaneurysm, and thrombus within the graft are other potential complications that can be detected using ultrasound evaluation.

RENAL ARTERY DUPLEX ULTRASONOGRAPHY

Atherosclerotic renal artery stenosis is recognized as a cause of hypertension and may contribute to decline in renal function (see Chapter 22). Duplex ultrasound of the renal arteries includes spectral Doppler evaluations of the aorta, the renal arteries and renal parenchyma, and B-mode determination of kidney size (also see Chapter 23). Abdominal obesity and bowel gas are barriers to adequate renal artery duplex examination.[24]

A longitudinal view of the aorta is obtained with the patient in the supine position. The origins of the celiac artery and SMA are seen on the anterior aspect of the aorta cephalad to the renal arteries. The PSV in the aorta is then recorded using a 60-degree Doppler angle. The probe is turned transverse to localize the renal arteries. The Doppler cursor is "walked" from the aorta into the ostium of the renal artery (Fig. 12.22). The right renal artery is generally seen most easily. It is followed from the origin to the hilum of the kidney. The left lateral decubitus position can also be used for examination of the right renal artery. The left renal artery is best evaluated in the right lateral

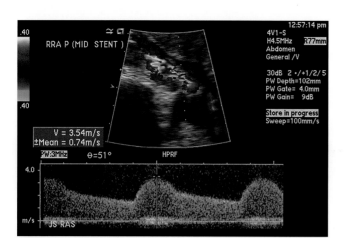

Fig. 12.22 Duplex Ultrasound Image of the Right Renal Artery *(RRA)* **in Which a Stent Had Been Inserted.** Turbulent flow is evident within the stent, suggesting the possibility of restenosis. Spectral Doppler at this site identifies stenosis with high peak systolic and end diastolic velocities. Spectral bruit of high-grade stenosis is seen in the baseline at peak systole. The renal vein *(blue)* runs parallel to the artery.

decubitus position using a posterolateral transducer position. Ideally, the renal arteries are evaluated from two views to ensure that stenosis is not missed. Kidney length is measured from pole to pole with the patient in the decubitus position.

Color and spectral Doppler are obtained throughout the course of each renal artery. A low-velocity range and a low wall filter setting are used in the spectral Doppler evaluations of the segmental renal arteries and the hilar flow. The renal artery normally has a low resistance waveform. A ≥60% renal artery stenosis is characterized by a renal-to-aortic PSV ratio of >3.5, combined with a PSV within the stenosis of >200 cm/s. Elevated EDV of ≥150 cm/s suggests ≥80% stenosis (see Fig. 12.22). The same criteria are used in native and stented renal arteries.[25] There is high-grade stenosis therefore in the renal artery seen in Fig. 12.22. Low systolic flow, poststenotic turbulence, and a color mosaic appearance indicate subtotal occlusion of the renal artery. Low parenchymal Doppler velocities support the diagnosis of an occluded renal artery in those cases where no flow can be detected in the renal artery. In addition, the ipsilateral kidney is often small, <9 cm in length. The overall sensitivity of duplex ultrasonography for renal artery stenosis is 98% and specificity is 98% compared with arteriography.

Evaluation of the renal arteries may also reveal aneurysms and pseudoaneurysms. A 50% increase in more distal arterial diameter is diagnostic for aneurysm, typically fusiform. A "sac" of extra-arterial flow may represent aneurysm or pseudoaneurysm. A pseudoaneurysm is present if there is "to and fro" flow in the neck connecting the extravascular blood and the artery.

Measurement of the resistive index (RI) is used to evaluate renal parenchymal disease. Spectral Doppler waveforms are obtained from at least three regions of each kidney. The RI is calculated using the formula, $RI = [1 - (V_{min} \div V_{max})] \times 100$, where V_{min} denotes EDV and V_{max} denotes PSV. In severe renal artery stenosis, where there is significant renal parenchymal disease, the EDV is often low. An RI >0.80 suggests significant parenchymal renal disease and may have implications regarding the outcome of therapy. Similarly, the PSV and EDV can be used to monitor renal transplants.

PERIPHERAL ARTERIAL ULTRASONOGRAPHY

Ultrasound of the lower extremities is used in the diagnosis of PAD in the setting of claudication, limb pain, or ulcers. It is also indicated

following lower extremity revascularization and in planning therapy for known PAD.[26] The goal of the examination is to elucidate the location and severity of limb arterial stenoses.[1,27] The study is tailored to individual requirements and can be limited to a given arterial segment or extended to evaluate both lower extremities in their entirety or to evaluate the upper extremity.

Color Doppler is used initially to detect normal or abnormal flow states throughout the arterial segments or bypass grafts being evaluated. Laminar flow is visible in the absence of disease (Fig. 12.23A), whereas turbulence and aliasing are present at the sites of disease. When an abnormal flow pattern is detected by color Doppler, pulsed (spectral) Doppler sampling is used to characterize the degree of stenosis (see Fig. 12.23B). The pulse Doppler signal is acquired throughout the arterial segments. PSV determination and waveform analyses are the primary parameters used to quantify and localize disease. PSV measurements are obtained at the level of the lesion and from vascular segments proximal and distal to the lesion. Aneurysmal dilation is another etiology for abnormal color flow. The velocities will decrease as the diameter doubles at the site of the aneurysm. The iliac, superficial femoral, and popliteal arteries are all sites of aneurysm (Fig. 12.24).

Peripheral arterial stenosis is categorized by pulsed wave Doppler examination as percentage reduction of luminal diameter that is mild (0% to 19%), moderate (20% to 49%), or severe (50% and greater).[28,29]

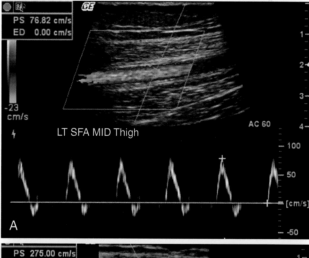
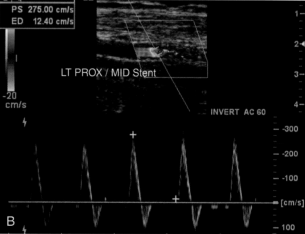

Fig. 12.23 Duplex Ultrasound of a Superficial Femoral Artery *(SFA)* **Stent.** (A) Laminar flow is evident in the longitudinal image of the proximal portion of the stent. (B) Color aliasing and elevated velocity are present at the site of stenosis within the mid-distal portion of the SFA stent.

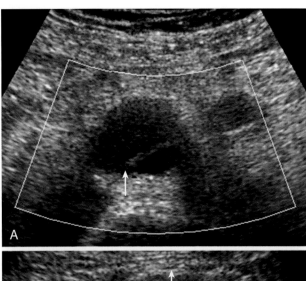

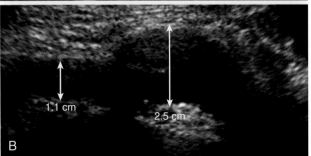

Fig. 12.24 (A) Transverse gray-scale image of right common iliac artery aneurysm with dissection. The arrow indicates the dissection flap. (B) Longitudinal gray-scale image of the right common iliac artery aneurysm. Aneurysm is defined by a 1.5 or greater increase in arterial diameter compared with the proximal segment. Thrombus develops in these aneurysms and can result in occlusion or distal embolization.

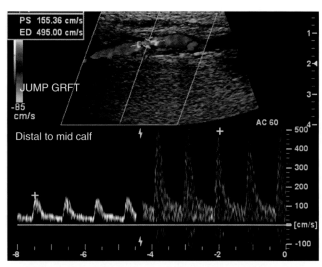

Fig. 12.25 Duplex Ultrasound of Peripheral Bypass Graft. The proximal velocity is 155 cm/s and increases to 495 cm/s at the site of stenosis. Aliasing of the Doppler is also evident at the site of stenosis.

With mild stenosis, there is some spectral broadening and a slight increase in PSV. With moderate stenosis, there is increased spectral broadening and a rise in PSV that is less than double that of the proximally sampled segment. Pulsed Doppler interrogation at the level of a severe stenosis reveals marked spectral broadening and a monophasic waveform. The waveform loses its normal diastolic reverse flow component and flow is forward throughout the cardiac cycle. In addition, the PSV is more than double the velocity measured in the proximal segment (Fig. 12.25). An occlusion is present when flow is absent within an arterial segment. If there are no collateral vessels, high-resistance waveforms are present in the artery proximal to the occlusion. Antegrade diastolic flow is present in the proximal artery if there are collateral vessels. The reconstituted distal artery will have the characteristic poststenotic, tardus et parvus waveform. This Doppler waveform is particularly important to recognize because it signifies a proximal high-grade lesion.

Duplex ultrasound examination is accurate for diagnosing PAD. The comparison of duplex ultrasound evaluation with arteriography to detect significant stenoses in patients with symptomatic aortoiliac and femoropopliteal disease reveals a high sensitivity (82%) and specificity (92%) for identifying significant stenoses. Ratios of PSV between the stenosis and the proximal artery are preferred over the absolute PSV measurements for the classification of peripheral arterial stenosis because there is a wide range of absolute PSV measurements obtained in normal and abnormal patients. There is a stronger correlation between PSV ratio and degree of stenosis than between absolute PSV and degree of stenosis. PSV ratios of 2 and 7 correspond to stenoses

≥50% and ≥90%, respectively. There are conflicting data regarding the precision of the duplex ultrasound examination in the determination of stenosis severity when serial stenoses are present.

Extremity Arterial Ultrasound Following Revascularization

Ultrasound evaluation following endovascular procedures is performed to detect recurrence of stenoses at sites of intervention. The concept is similar to that for graft surveillance (i.e., early detection of lesions assists in identifying the need for reintervention to maintain arterial patency).[26] Duplex ultrasonography is performed following the intervention prior to discharge; 1, 3, and 6 months postintervention; then yearly. The color Doppler and pulsed wave Doppler evaluations focus on the vessel proximal to the site of intervention, at the site of intervention, and distal to the site of intervention. Waveform analysis is used to categorize stenosis in a manner like that used in native vessels. A doubling of PSV is consistent with hemodynamically significant stenosis (see Figs. 12.23B and 12.25). Increases in velocity measurements and change in waveform shape from triphasic to monophasic on serial examinations suggest developing stenosis and warrant close interval follow-up and consideration for revision.

Graft surveillance is extremely useful in efforts to preserve the patency of peripheral arterial bypass grafts.[30] Graft failure in the first month is usually caused by technical factors. Between 1 month and 2 years postoperatively, it is often due to intimal hyperplasia. Graft failure after 2 years is likely the result of progression of atherosclerotic disease.[31] The 5-year primary patency rate for an infrainguinal vein bypass graft ranges from 60% to 85%. Surgical revision of these stenoses identified with ultrasound surveillance improves the 5-year patency rate to 82% to 93%. By contrast, segmental pressure measurements have not proved useful to predict bypass graft thrombosis. To detect graft abnormalities before frank graft failure, standard graft surveillance protocols recommend duplex ultrasound evaluation at 1, 3, and 6 months during the first postoperative year and 12 months thereafter. The location and type of graft are identified before performing the ultrasound examination. Scanning techniques in the supine patient are similar to native arterial examinations. Color Doppler is used initially to scan the entire graft. The color pulse repetition frequency is adjusted so focal stenoses or arteriovenous fistulae appear as regions of aliasing, persistence, or bruit color flash artifact. Based on color Doppler findings, pulsed Doppler interrogation is used to determine the PSV. Sampling is done routinely at the proximal native artery, proximal anastomosis, throughout the graft, distal anastomosis, distal native vessel, and throughout sites of flow disturbance. These measurements are used also for serial comparison during subsequent examinations.

Pulsed Doppler is used to determine PSV ratios within the graft similar to its use in the native arterial examination (see Fig. 12.25). A segment distal (rather than proximal) to the lesion may be chosen for the ratio when there is a diameter mismatch in the graft or there are tandem lesions proximal to the flow disturbance. Doubling of the velocity ratio indicates a significant graft stenosis (>50% diameter reduction) with a sensitivity of 95% and specificity of 100%. Vein graft lesions also have been classified using PSV: (1) a minimal stenosis (<20%) has PSV ratio up to 1.4 with a PSV of less than 125 cm/s; (2) a moderate stenosis (20% to 50%) has a PSV ratio of 1.5 to 2.4 with a PSV up to 180 cm/s; (3) a severe stenosis (50% to 75%) has a PSV ratio of 2.5 to 4 with a PSV of more than 180 cm/s; and (4) a high-grade stenosis (>75%) has a PSV ratio greater than 4 with a PSV greater than 300 cm/s. Intervention is recommended for lesions categorized as severe or high grade.[32] Detection of low-flow velocities within the graft with pulsed Doppler suggests either proximal or distal stenosis. Low velocity flow can also be caused by large graft diameter or poor arterial inflow. Nonetheless, velocities within a functioning graft that are less

than 45 cm/s indicate that subsequent graft failure is likely to occur. Other worrisome findings are a significant decrease or increase in PSV on serial examination.

PSEUDOANEURYSM

A pseudoaneurysm is a contained arterial rupture. A hole through all layers of the arterial wall results in extravasation of blood which is then enclosed by the surrounding soft tissues. Any patient who has undergone an arterial puncture for arteriography and experiences sudden pain at the access site, or is found to have pulsatile mass or a bruit on auscultation over the access site, should be evaluated for the presence of pseudoaneurysm.[33]

Ultrasound evaluation is performed in the region of the puncture. Spectral waveforms are obtained in the native artery proximal and distal to the site of puncture and in the femoral vein proximal and distal to the site of puncture. Color Doppler evaluation should focus on detecting an extravascular collection of flowing blood, most commonly anterior to the native artery (Fig. 12.26A and B). Posterior extravasation is less common. The neck is the connection between the native artery and the pseudoaneurysm sac. The neck is identified by a to and fro pattern of the Doppler waveform that is pathognomonic for pseudoaneurysm (see Fig. 12.26C). This waveform results from systolic flow out of the native artery into the contained rupture,

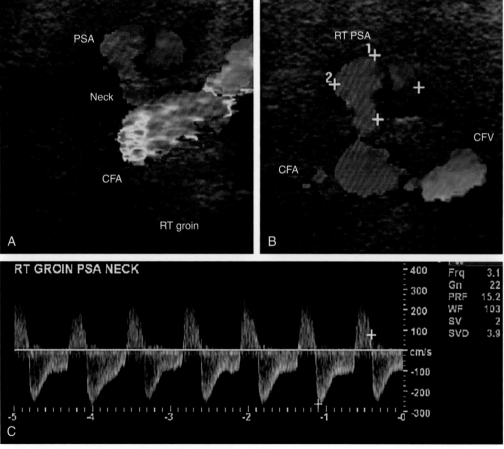

Fig. 12.26 Duplex Ultrasound Evaluation of a Pseudoaneurysm *(PSA)*. The "yin-yang" appearance of the PSA cavity is evident in the longitudinal (A) and transverse (B) images. Although the artery is longer in the longitudinal image, the contained rupture sac of the PSA retains its saccular shape. (C) Pulsed Doppler placed in the neck of the pseudoaneurysm demonstrates the pathognomonic "to-and-fro" pattern of bidirectional flow into and out of the contained rupture. *CFA,* Common femoral artery; *CFV,* common femoral vein.

and diastolic flow back into the native artery. In addition to the to and fro signal in the neck, the segment of native artery proximal to the origin of the pseudoaneurysm may have a lower resistance waveform when compared with that found in the artery distal to the pseudoaneurysm.

There are several options for treatment of pseudoaneurysms, including observation, surgical repair, manual compression, ultrasound-guided compression, or thrombin injection.[34] Ultrasound-guided compression is performed with visualization of the pseudoaneurysm neck while compressing until flow is absent in the neck. Pressure is applied for 20 minutes and may need to be maintained for much longer before thrombosis of the pseudoaneurysm sac is achieved. Reported success rate of compression varies from 60% to 80%. Ultrasound-guided thrombin injection is best suited for those pseudoaneurysms with a long, narrow neck. Thrombin injection is contraindicated in those with allergy to bovine thrombin, in those with overlying skin infections, in the presence of ipsilateral arteriovenous fistula, and in those with active limb ischemia. The injection is performed under sterile conditions, using a syringe equipped with a three-way stopcock. The needle is placed into the sac while drawing back gently on the syringe. The tip of the needle is seen in the cavity, and blood return is noted. The stopcock is then switched to a position open to the thrombin, and 0.1 to 0.2 mL of thrombin are injected. The duplex ultrasound examination should include final pictures documenting thrombosis of the pseudoaneurysm, and a patent artery of origin. Complications of thrombin injection include limb ischemia if thrombin enters the native artery and causes a thrombus to form, and anaphylaxis.

ARTERIOVENOUS FISTULAE

Arteriovenous fistulae occur secondary to trauma, including catheterization, or are created intentionally for dialysis. The duplex ultrasound findings include turbulent and pulsatile venous flow.[35] The turbulence may result in a color "bruit" adjacent to the vein, caused by vibration of the surrounding soft tissue. Arterial flow proximal to the fistula will have a low resistance pattern, rather than the typical high resistance peripheral waveform (Fig. 12.27). The arterial flow distal to the fistula

will have a high resistance waveform. The venous flow pattern at the connection will resemble an arterial waveform. The actual arteriovenous connection may be too small to be seen in postcatheterization arteriovenous fistulae.

Evaluation of dialysis fistulae uses specific criteria for the Doppler spectra obtained from arterial inflow and venous outflow. PSV is recorded throughout the native system and the graft. The arterial limb should demonstrate high velocities and continuous forward flow with a low-resistance waveform. The venous limb is expected to have slightly lower velocities. The normal PSV at the anastomosis is 300 cm/s. The normal outflow vein has a PSV greater than 180 cm/s and appears distended. PSV less than 150 cm/s at the anastomosis indicates a fistula in jeopardy of failure. The fistula may result in arterial steal from the distal circulation. If this is suspected, the direction of distal flow should be evaluated before and after compression of the arteriovenous fistula.

VENOUS DUPLEX ULTRASOUND

Duplex examination of the extremity veins enables accurate noninvasive evaluation for deep vein thrombosis (DVT).[36,37] Normal veins have thin walls and an echo-free lumen. The vein lumen can be obliterated (compressed) with a small amount of extrinsic pressure (Fig. 12.28). However, the walls do not coapt when the lumen contains thrombus, even when enough pressure is applied to distort the shape of an adjacent artery. Vein compressibility is best tested in an image plane transverse to the vein axis. Veins are characterized by anatomical location as deep or superficial and as proximal or distal. The major veins of the thigh and arm are larger in diameter than the corresponding arteries. Extremity veins have valves, which permit only cephalad flow, and these increase in number from proximal to distal. Valve sinuses are widened areas of the lumen that accommodate the valve cusps.

Doppler evaluation of flow in normal veins has four important characteristics (1) respirophasic variation; (2) augmentation with distal compression; (3) unidirectional flow toward the heart; and (4) and abrogation of flow in the lower extremities by the Valsalva maneuver. Complete analysis of venous spectral waveforms requires comparison of the waveforms from both right and left limbs. The presence of a flattened, unvarying waveform (loss of respirophasic variation in flow) on one side compared with the other suggests the presence of more proximal obstruction of venous return proximal to the site of the Doppler interrogation.

Neck and Upper Extremity Venous Duplex Ultrasound

Neck and upper extremity duplex evaluation includes assessments of the internal jugular, subclavian, axillary, brachial, cephalic, and basilic veins.[38] The innominate veins and the superior vena cava cannot be

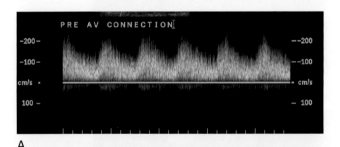
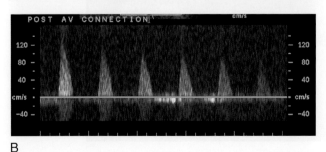

Fig. 12.27 Spectral Doppler evaluation of a peripheral artery proximal (A) and distal (B) to an arteriovenous connection. The low resistance pattern in A occurs because the artery is flowing into the high-capacitance venous bed.

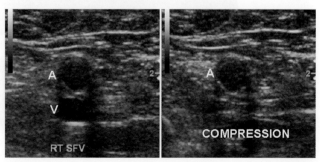

Fig. 12.28 Transverse Gray-Scale Imaging of the Superficial Femoral Artery *(A)* and Vein *(V) (Left)*. With gentle compression *(right)* the artery is unchanged and the vein is obliterated.

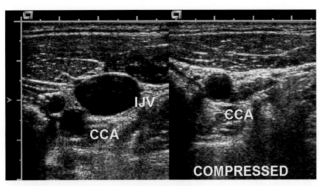

Fig. 12.29 Transverse gray-scale imaging of the internal jugular vein *(IJV)* and common carotid artery *(CCA)* without compression *(Left)* and with gentle compression *(Right)* obliterating the lumen of the vein.

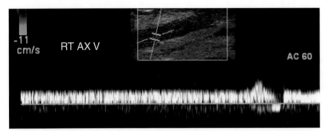

Fig. 12.30 Spectral Doppler Evaluation of the Axillary Vein Demonstrating Loss of Phasic Variation in Flow with Respiration. This finding suggests more proximal venous obstruction. The transient increase in flow on the right results from compression of the forearm (augmenting venous return).

evaluated with duplex ultrasound because of their location within the bony thorax. The examination begins with evaluation of the internal jugular (Fig. 12.29) and subclavian veins. The subclavian vein can be imaged from a supraclavicular or subclavicular approach. The arm is extended in a comfortable position for the evaluation of the axillary vein, paired brachial veins, basilic vein (medial), and cephalic vein (lateral). The examination includes color and spectral Doppler evaluation of flow in all of these veins. Loss of respirophasic variation in the waveform in the subclavian or axillary veins suggests the presence of more proximal venous obstruction (due to thrombosis or extrinsic compression) (Fig. 12.30). The subclavian vein cannot be compressed where it lies directly below the clavicle, and venous thrombosis is suspected when flow is absent or echogenic material is seen within the lumen.

Loss of compressibility is the pathognomonic feature of venous thrombosis. As the thrombus progresses from acute to chronic, there is increased echogenicity of the thrombus and decreased diameter of the vein. Elastography is being evaluated as a means of determining thrombus age.[39] Over time, collateral veins may develop and recanalization may occur in the thrombosed vessel. In the upper arm, both superficial and deep venous systems have a significant role in venous drainage. The majority of upper extremity DVTs are secondary to indwelling venous catheters, pacemaker leads or hypercoagulability. Upper extremity DVT is a disorder that is rarely idiopathic but is more often attributed to effort thrombosis (Paget-Schroetter syndrome) related to thoracic outlet obstruction or occurs in the setting of malignancy (see Chapter 51).[40] An unusual etiology of noncompressible veins is intravascular tumor. This is suspected when the echogenic material within the lumen appears to extend through the vessel wall and may contain arterial flow signals.

Lower Extremity Venous Duplex Ultrasound

The venous ultrasound examination to evaluate the presence or absence of leg DVT begins at the inguinal ligament with identification of the common femoral vein and extends to the calf.[41] The proximal deep veins evaluated include the common femoral, femoral (previously known as superficial femoral), and popliteal veins. The deep calf veins include posterior tibial, peroneal, gastrocnemius (sural), and soleal veins. Special attention is given to the saphenofemoral and saphenopopliteal junctions because thrombus in the superficial veins of these regions deserve more aggressive treatment than thrombus limited to other parts of the superficial venous system. The examination includes color and spectral Doppler evaluation of flow in all these veins (Fig. 12.31). Loss of respirophasic variation in the waveform of the common femoral vein would suggest obstruction proximal to the site of Doppler interrogation is preventing venous return. Augmentation of flow with calf compression is not prevented by proximal venous obstruction. Proximal obstruction may be caused by extrinsic compression or venous thrombosis.

B-mode transverse images are used to determine compressibility along the entire course of the veins examined (see Video 12.1 on ExpertConsult.com). Normally, the vein walls fully coapt with gentle pressure. Lack of compressibility, which occurs because of a thrombosis in the vein, is the most reliable finding for determining venous thrombosis. With acute thrombosis, there is low echogenicity of the intraluminal thrombus and the vein is dilated. As the thrombus ages, it becomes more echogenic and less central within the lumen. The vein

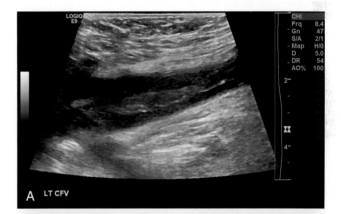

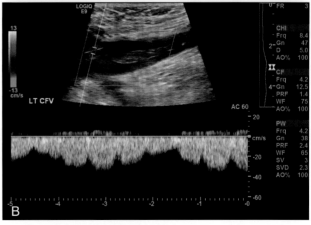

Fig. 12.31 Ultrasound Evaluation of the Femoral Vein Thrombosis. (A) Gray-scale imaging with echogenic material seen within the lumen of the common femoral vein. (B) Color Doppler in the femoral vein shows a flow void within the lumen. Spectral Doppler demonstrates flow with respirophasic variation. (See also Video 12.1 on ExpertConsult.com.)

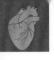
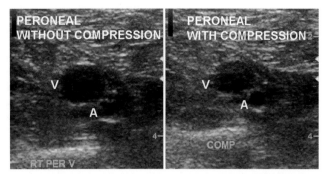

Fig. 12.32 Transverse Gray-scale Imaging of the Peroneal (Deep) Veins of the Calf. The vein *(V)* appears dilated in the noncompression image on the left. The vein lumen is not obliterated by gentle compression, indicating the presence of calf-vein thrombosis. *A,* Artery.

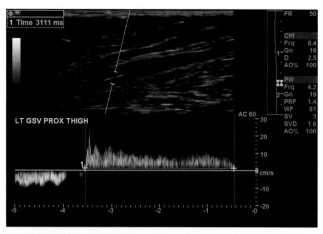

Fig. 12.33 Spectral Doppler of Venous Insufficiency. The greater saphenous vein *(GSV)* is imaged. The spectral Doppler demonstrates prolonged retrograde flow at this site following an augmentation maneuver.

diameter decreases as the thrombus retracts. Recanalization occurs and flow can be detected by pulsed or color Doppler. The thrombus often appears eccentric and adjacent to the vein wall. When image quality is poor because of significant soft tissue edema, it is not possible to exclude the presence of small, nonocclusive thrombi. Sensitivity for the detection of common femoral vein thrombosis is 91% and for both the femoral and popliteal veins is 94%.

Duplex ultrasound is accurate for the diagnosis of deep calf vein thrombosis in symptomatic patients, as long as the calf veins can be seen clearly (Fig. 12.32). Sensitivity of compression ultrasound for deep calf vein thrombosis is 94% and specificity is 100% when compared with angiography. The small calf veins cannot be visualized well in all patients. However, the specificity and positive predictive value are high even when those individuals with poor calf vein images are included in the evaluation. Thus the diagnosis of DVT is made when calf veins are seen and cannot be compressed.

Lower extremity venous ultrasound testing is often ordered when a patient is undergoing evaluation for pulmonary embolism. This test will provide information about the presence or absence of venous thrombosis but will not determine whether or not someone has had a pulmonary embolism.[36] The increase in point-of-care ultrasound has contributed to the ultrasound evaluation for DVT taking place at only two or three points in the lower extremity is also being evaluated.[42] Although accuracy can be reported as high as 90%, there are clear limitations imposed by the ultrasound training of the provider.

Duplex Ultrasound Evaluation of Venous Insufficiency

The use of duplex ultrasound has been extended to detect reflux or obstruction and determine the anatomical extent of venous disease in patients with chronic venous insufficiency.[43] This development has been facilitated by the use of color Doppler imaging to provide instant determination of the direction of blood flow. A 4- to 7-MHz linear array transducer is used. The saphenofemoral junction is examined first with the patient standing and then in the supine, reverse Trendelenburg position. Compressibility is determined in transverse views of the veins. A longitudinal view of the saphenofemoral junction is then obtained.

One of two maneuvers can be used to elicit reflux. The first is the Valsalva maneuver. Intra-abdominal pressure increases as the patient bears down, and venous outflow from the legs decreases. The venous return from the legs increases with release of the maneuver. The second is thigh cuff inflation and deflation. Venous return is stopped with inflation of a cuff, typically to a level approximating arterial diastolic pressure. There is a transient increase in venous return that accompanies cuff deflation. Color flow is evaluated before and after one of these

two maneuvers to elicit reflux. Baseline antegrade flow is displayed by blue color Doppler. Red color after the maneuver indicates retrograde flow. Reflux is present if red color persists for >0.5 seconds after either maneuver. Spectral Doppler can also be used to evaluate reflux. The Doppler cursor is placed midstream with an angle of 60 degrees with respect to the wall. Reverse flow >0.5 seconds in duration is consistent with reflux (Fig. 12.33). Ideally, the remainder of the examination is performed with the patient standing with the weight on the leg that is not being examined.[44]

The extent of reflux can be determined by repeating this assessment throughout the deep and superficial veins of the leg. For evaluation of the small saphenous and popliteal veins, the patient sits on the edge of the examination table with his/her foot resting on a stool. The probe is placed over the popliteal fossa. The gastrocnemius veins can be seen between the popliteal vein (which is deep) and small saphenous vein (which is superficial). Compressibility and reflux following a Valsalva maneuver are determined in these veins. The posterior tibial and peroneal veins are assessed for reflux using the posteromedial and anterolateral views.

Perforating veins are vessels connecting superficial and deep veins. Incompetent perforating veins are identified by sliding the transducer up and down dilated superficial varicose veins. Color Doppler is then used while distal compression of the superficial vein is performed. The presence of different colors during compression and release indicates that the direction of venous flow changes with compression and relief. This finding is diagnostic of reflux in the perforator veins.

PLETHYSMOGRAPHIC EVALUATION OF VENOUS REFLUX

Duplex ultrasound identifies reflux in individual veins, and plethysmographic methods evaluate the volume of venous reflux in the limb.[45] Air or strain gauge plethysmography is a simple screening test that has the potential to provide a complete analysis of venous hemodynamics (also see Chapter 54). The air chamber is filled with air to 6 mm Hg and connected to a pressure transducer and recorder. Changes in the volume of the leg as a result of emptying or filling veins produce changes in the pressure of the air chamber. Recordings are made with the patient supine, and the leg elevated at a 45-degree angle. The patient then stands with the leg flexed slightly and bearing weight on the nonstudy leg. Venous filling time and venous volume are determined. The time until the volume plateaus after the raised limb is dropped is the venous filling time. Venous volumes of 80 to 150 mL are normal. The venous filling index (VFI) correlates best with the clinical severity of reflux.

$$VFI = 0.90 \left(\text{venous volume} \right) \div 0.9 \left(\text{venous filling time} \right)$$

Values <2 mL/s indicate the absence of significant reflux, whereas values >10 mL/s indicate high risks of edema, skin changes, and ulceration.

Postexercise plethysmography can be used to evaluate the ejecting capacity of the calf muscle pump. Venous volume is measured at rest and again post exercise. The rest volume minus the postexercise volume equals the ejected volume. The ejection fraction is the ejected volume/rest volume × 100. Calf ejection fractions <40% indicate patients most likely to benefit from deep vein reconstruction.

VASCULAR LABORATORY ACCREDITATION

Laboratory accreditation is obtained through organizations such as the Intersocietal Accreditation Commission for Vascular Testing (www.intersocietal.org) and the American College of Radiology (www.acr.org). The accreditation process reviews the educational credentials of the interpreting physicians and sonographers, as well as laboratory procedures. It provides excellent standards for setting up examination protocols and quality assurance programs.

REFERENCES

1. Gerhard-Herman MD, Gornik HL, Barrett C, et al. 2016 AHA/ACC guideline on the management of patients with lower extremity peripheral artery disease: executive summary: a report of the American College of Cardiology/American Heart Association Task Force on Clinical Practice Guidelines. *J Am Coll Cardiol.* 2017;69(11):1465–1508.
2. Aboyans V, Criqui MH, Abraham P, et al. Measurement and interpretation of the Ankle-Brachial Index: a scientific statement from the American Heart Association. *Circulation.* 2012;126(24):2890–2909.
3. Ahmed O, Hanley M, Bennett SJ, et al. ACR Appropriateness Criteria® vascular claudication—assessment for revascularization. *J Am Coll Radiol.* 2017;14(5):372–4379.
4. Gerhard-Herman M, Gardin JM, Jaff M, et al. Guidelines for noninvasive vascular laboratory testing: a report from the American Society of Echocardiography and the Society for Vascular Medicine and Biology. *Vasc Med.* 2006;11(3):183–200.
5. Aboyans V, Ricco JB, Bartelink MEL, et al. 2017 ESC guidelines on the diagnosis and treatment of peripheral arterial diseases, in collaboration with the European Society for Vascular Surgery (ESVS). *Eur J Vasc Endovasc Surg.* 2017;55(3):305–308.
6. Kovacs D, Csiszar B, Biro K, et al. Toe-brachial index and exercise test can improve the exploration of peripheral artery disease. *Atherosclerosis.* 2018;269:151–158.
7. Young DA, Blake DF, Brown LH. Transcutaneous oximetry measurement: normal values for the upper limb. *Diving Hyperb Med.* 2012;42(3):208–213.
8. Kremkau FW. Principles of spectral Doppler. *J Vasc Ultrasound.* 2011;35(4):15.
9. Abreu I, Roriz D, Barros M, et al. B-mode ultrasound artifacts. *Eur Soc Radiol.* 2015;1–48.
10. Wood MM, Romine LE, Lee YK, et al. Spectral doppler signature waveforms in ultrasonography: a review of normal and abnormal waveforms. *Ultrasound Q.* 2010;26(2):83–99.
11. Beulen BW, Bijnens N, Koutsouridis GG, et al. Toward noninvasive blood pressure assessment in arteries by using ultrasound. *Ultrasound Med Biol.* 2011;37(5):788–797.
12. Grant EG. Vascular ultrasound. *Ultrasound Clin.* 2006;1(6).
13. Ascher E, Salles-Cunha SX, Marks N, Hingorani A. Lower extremity arterial mapping: duplex ultrasound as an alternative to arteriography prior to femoral and popliteal reconstruction. *Noninvasive Peripheral Arterial Diagnosis.* 2010;89–98.
14. Mohler III ER, Gornik HL, Gerhard-Herman M, et al. ACCF/ACR/AIUM/ASE/ASN/ICAVL/SCAI/SCCT/SIR/SVM/SVS 2012 Appropriate use criteria for peripheral vascular ultrasound and physiological testing part I: arterial ultrasound and physiological testing. *J Am Coll Cardiol.* 2012;60(3):649–655.
15. Grant EG, Benson CB, Moneta GL, et al. Carotid artery stenosis: grayscale and Doppler ultrasound diagnosis—Society of Radiologists in Ultrasound Consensus Conference. *Ultrasound Q.* 2003;19(4):190–198.
16. Ginat DT, Bhatt S, Sidhu R, Dogra V. Carotid and vertebral artery Doppler ultrasound waveforms. *Ultrasound Q.* 2011;27(2):81–85.
17. Mehta KS, Lee JJ, Taha AA, et al. Vascular applications of contrast-enhanced ultrasound imaging. *J Vasc Surg.* 2017;66(1):266–274.
18. Germanò G, Monti S, Ponte C, et al. The role of ultrasound in the diagnosis and follow-up of large-vessel vasculitis: an update. *Clin Exp Rheumatol.* 2017;35(1):194–198.
19. Polak JF, Pencina MJ, O'Leary DH, D'Agostino RB. Common carotid artery intima-media thickness progression as a predictor of stroke in multi-ethnic study of atherosclerosis. *Stroke.* 2011;42(11):3017–3021.
20. LeFevre ML. Screening for abdominal aortic aneurysm: U.S. Preventive Services Task Force recommendation statement. *Ann Intern Med.* 2014;161(4):281–290.
21. van de Luijtgaarden KM, Rouwet EV, Hoeks SE, et al. Risk of abdominal aortic aneurysm (AAA) among male and female relatives of AAA patients. *Vasc Med.* 2017;22(2):112–118.
22. Beales L, Wolstenhulme S, Evans JA, et al. Reproducibility of ultrasound measurement of the abdominal aorta. *Br J Surg.* 2011;98(11):1517–1525.
23. Cao P, De Rango P, Verzini F, Parlani G. Endoleak after endovascular aortic repair: classification, diagnosis and management following endovascular thoracic and abdominal aortic repair. *J Cardiovasc Surg (Torino).* 2010;51(1):53–69.
24. Hedayati N, Del Pizzo DJ, Harris SE, et al. Predictors of diagnostic success with renal artery duplex ultrasonography. *Ann Vasc Surg.* 2011;25(4):515–519.
25. Fleming SH, Davis RP, Craven TE, et al. Accuracy of duplex sonography scans after renal artery stenting. *J Vasc Surg.* 2010;52(4):953–957.
26. Mohler III ER, Gornik HL, Gerhard-Herman M, et al. ACCF/ACR/AIUM/ASE/ASN/ICAVL/SCAI/SCCT/SIR/SVM/SVS 2012 appropriate use criteria for peripheral vascular ultrasound and physiological testing part I: arterial ultrasound and physiological testing. *J Vasc Surg.* 2012;56(1):17–51.
27. Shrikhande GV, Graham AR, Aparajita R, et al. Determining criteria for predicting stenosis with ultrasound duplex after endovascular intervention in infrainguinal lesions. *Ann Vasc Surg.* 2011;25(4):454–460.
28. Gerhard-Herman M, Roman MJ, Naqvi TZ, et al. Guidelines for noninvasive vascular laboratory testing: a report from the American Society of Echocardiography and the Society for Vascular Medicine and Biology. *Vasc Med.* 2006;11(3):183–200.
29. Tendera M, Aboyans V, Bartelink M-L, et al. ESC Guidelines on the diagnosis and treatment of peripheral artery diseases. *Eur Heart J.* 2011;32(22):2851–2906.
30. Tinder CN, Bandyk DF. Detection of imminent vein graft occlusion: what is the optimal surveillance program? *Semin Vasc Surg.* 2009;22(4):252–260.
31. Slim H, Tiwari A, Ritter JC, Rashid H. Outcome of infra-inguinal bypass grafts using vein conduit with less than 3 millimeters diameter in critical leg ischemia. *J Vasc Surg.* 2011;53(2):421–425.
32. Franz R, Jump M, Spalding MC, Jenkins J. Accuracy of duplex ultrasonography in estimation of severity of peripheral vascular disease. *Int J Angiol.* 2013;22(3):155–158.
33. Lenartova M, Tak T. Iatrogenic pseudoaneurysm of femoral artery: case report and literature review. *Clin Med Res.* 2003;1(3):243–247.
34. Kapoor BS, Haddad HL, Saddekni S, Lockhart ME. Diagnosis and management of pseudoaneurysms: an update. *Curr Probl Diagn Radiol.* 2009;38(4):170–188.
35. Venkatanarasimha N, Freeman S. Ultrasound features of arteriovenous fistula. *Am J Roentgenol.* 2010;194(6):W540.

36. Bounameaux H, Perrier A, Righini M. Diagnosis of venous thromboembolism: an update. *Vasc Med.* 2010;15(5):399–406.

37. Lin EP, Bhatt S, Dogra VS. Lower extremity venous Doppler. *Ultrasound Clin.* 2008;3(1):147–158.

38. Pozniak MA. Upper extremity venous Doppler. *Ultrasound Clin.* 2011;6(4):435–444.

39. Hoang P, Wallace A, Sugi M, et al. Elastography techniques in the evaluation of deep vein thrombosis. *Cardiovasc Diagn Ther.* 2017;7(Suppl 3):S238–S245.

40. Alexander KM, Vaduganathan M, Qamar A, Gerhard-Herman MD. Grim messenger: Virchow's node presenting with Virchow's triad. *Am J Med.* 2016;129(9):948–951.

41. Elliott CG, Lovelace TD, Brown LM, Adams D. Diagnosis: imaging techniques. *Clin Chest Med.* 2010;31(4):641–657.

42. Pedraza García J, Valle Alonso J, Ceballos García P, et al. Comparison of the accuracy of emergency department-performed point-of-care-ultrasound (POCUS) in the diagnosis of lower-extremity deep vein thrombosis. *J Emerg Med.* 2018;54(5):656–664.

43. Eberhardt RT, Raffetto JD. Chronic venous insufficiency. *Circulation.* 2014;130(4):333–346.

44. Coleman DM, Campbell DN, Shuster KA, et al. Implications of the expanded venous reflux study. *J Vasc Ultrasound.* 2013;37(1):26–29.

45. Rosfors S, Blomgren L. Venous occlusion plethysmography in patients with post-thrombotic venous claudication. *J Vasc Surg.* 2013;58(3):722–726.

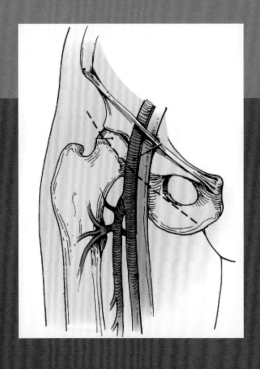

中文导读

第13章
磁共振血管成像

　　MRI是一种很有价值的成像工具，磁共振血管成像（MR angiography，MRA）则是利用血液流动的MRI特点对血管和血流信号特征进行显示的一种无创造影技术，在血管成像中被广泛应用，包括周围动脉造影和肾动脉造影。其中，钆对比增强（CE）磁共振血管成像可以用相对短的采集时间获得高空间分辨率图像，现已广泛应用于临床。磁共振血管成像作为一种无创、无电离辐射的血管造影技术，在临床上广受青睐，但并非适用于所有血管疾病。各种血管成像技术优缺点对比见表13.1，这可为临床医师在选择最佳成像技术以评估特定患者时提供非常重要的参考。本章将介绍MRI和磁共振血管成像技术的基本原理，重点介绍从胸部血管到外周肢体血管使用MRI技术的适应证。

常光其

Magnetic Resonance Imaging

Amy West Pollak and Christopher M. Kramer

Magnetic resonance imaging (MRI) is a valuable vascular imaging tool and is a modality of choice for many indications, including peripheral and renal arteriography.[1-3] Gadolinium-based contrast-enhanced magnetic resonance angiography (CE-MRA) yields high-quality spatial resolution images with relatively short acquisition times. An overview of the relative advantages and disadvantages compared with other imaging technologies are outlined in Table 13.1, which is important for the clinician to consider when faced with choosing the best imaging technology to evaluate a particular patient. This chapter will cover the basic principles of MRI and magnetic resonance angiography (MRA) techniques and then focus on vascular indications for MRI from the thorax to the peripheral extremity vessels.

BASIC PRINCIPLES

MRI detects the magnetic moment created by hydrogen protons in the human body. MRI of blood vessels relies upon the intrinsic magnetic properties of blood flow and the surrounding static tissue to produce tissue contrast. Because any moving electric charge produces a magnetic field, spinning protons produce small magnetic fields or "spins." When a patient is placed in the MRI scanner, which is essentially the bore of a large magnet, hydrogen protons align with the externally applied static magnetic field (B_0) to create a net magnetization vector. On a quantum level, most protons will distribute randomly, either with or against the scanner's B_0. However, a slight excess of spins aligns with the field, causing net tissue magnetization. The time required for this alignment is denoted by the longitudinal relaxation time, T1. T1 variations between tissues is used to provide contrast.

Spinning protons wobble or "precess" about the axis of B_0. The frequency of the wobble is proportional to the strength of B_0. If a radiofrequency (RF) pulse is applied at the resonance frequency of the wobble, protons can absorb energy and jump to a higher energy state. This RF pulse deflects the protons, creating a new net magnetization vector distinct from the major axis of the applied magnetic field. The net magnetization vector tips from the longitudinal to the transverse plane (transverse magnetization). After the RF pulse tips the spinning protons out of alignment with the main magnetic field, new protons begin to align with the main magnetic field at a rate determined by the T1 relaxation time.

Energy is given off as the spins move from high to low energy states. The absorbed RF energy is retransmitted at the resonance frequency and can be detected with RF antennas or "coils" placed around the patient. These signals are compiled and, after mathematical transformation, become the MR images. Proton excitation with an externally applied RF field is repeated at short intervals to obtain signals. This MR parameter is referred to as *repetition time* (TR). Throughout the dephasing process, the MR signal decays. This loss of phase is termed *T2 relaxation time* or *transverse relaxation*. T2, like T1, is unique among tissues and is used for image contrast.

In addition to the intrinsic T2 of tissue, inhomogeneity of B_0 results in rapid loss of transverse magnetization. The relaxation time that reflects the sum of these random defects with tissue T2 is called *T2**. To obtain an MRI signal, these spins must be brought back in phase and produce a signal or echo. The time at which it happens is referred to as *echo time* (TE). In gradient echo (GRE) imaging, the echo is obtained by gradient reversal rather than by RF pulse. Because this includes effects from tissue homogeneity, TE-dependent signal loss reflects T2*. Recently, balanced steady-state free precession (SSFP) sequences have been developed that are insensitive to magnet field inhomogeneities and reflective of actual tissue T2.

Longitudinal and transverse magnetizations occur simultaneously but are two different processes that reflect properties of various tissues in the body. Because T1 measures signal recovery, tissues with short T1 are bright, whereas tissues with long T1 are dark. Fat has a very short T1. In contrast, T2 is a measure of signal loss. Therefore tissues with short T2 are dark, and those with long T2 are bright. Simple fluids, such as cerebrospinal fluid and urine, have long T2. To differentiate between the tissues based on these relaxation times, MR images can be designed to be T1-weighted (W), T2-W, or proton-density W.

Magnetic resonance echoes are digitized and stored in "k-space" composed of either two axes (for two-dimensional [2D] imaging) or three axes (for three-dimensional [3D] imaging). K-space represents frequency data and is related to image space by Fourier transformation. An important feature of k-space is that tissue contrast is determined by the center of k-space (central phase encoding lines), whereas the periphery of the k-space encodes the image detail. The order in which k-space lines are collected can be varied, strongly influencing tissue contrast. For example, in CE-MRA, the central contrast-defining portion of k-space may be acquired early in the scan (centric acquisition) during peak intra-arterial contrast concentration to maximize arterial contrast.

MAGNETIC RESONANCE ANGIOGRAPHY TECHNIQUES

MRA imaging relies on selective imaging of moving blood where the signals from within the blood vessels are maximized, in contrast to the signals from the adjacent stationary tissues which are suppressed. There are both noncontrast MRA, as well as contrast-enhanced MRA techniques (Table 13.2), with intrinsic advantages and limitations of each approach. For a given MRA, reformatting algorithms are used to create a set of images which are similar to those from conventional x-ray angiography (Table 13.3).

MRA methods can depict blood as either black or white (Fig. 13.1A). For those "black-blood" methods that use standard spin echo (SE) sequences, the excitation RF pulse is applied at 90 degrees and followed by a refocusing pulse at 180 degrees. If the imaging slice cuts across a vessel, then depending on the flow velocity and time interval between the pulses,

TABLE 13.1 Advantages and Disadvantage of Vascular Imaging Methods

Method	Advantages	Disadvantages
MR	No ionizing radiation	Image acquisition requires technical expertise during imaging
CE-MRA	High signal from gadolinium-based agents Less nephrotoxic than comparable iodine-based imaging (CTA)	Nephrogenic systemic fibrosis can occur rarely in patients with severe renal insufficiency
Noncontrast MRA	Eliminates gadolinium toxicity concern	Longer acquisition times compared to CE-MRA protocol Increased risk of artifacts when compared to CE-MRA
CTA	Rapid, high signal, high-quality image acquisition Less technical expertise required compared to MR	Ionizing radiation Nephrotoxicity of iodine
DSA	Intervention can be performed at time of diagnosis Highest spatial resolution	Invasive Nephrotoxicity of iodine Projectional data may be inferior to volumetric acquisitions (CT, MR) that can be viewed in any plane
Ultrasonography	No ionizing radiation Inexpensive Flow information obtained Portable	Good for superficial imaging Limited by artifacts from bone, air, and sonographic interfaces Lower CNR, SNR compared to CT and MRI Operator-dependent

CE, Contrast-enhanced; *CNR*, contrast-to-noise ratio; *CT*, computed tomography; *DSA*, digital subtraction angiography; *MR*, magnetic resonance; *MRA*, magnetic resonance angiography; *MRI*, magnetic resonance imaging; *SNR*, signal-to-noise ratio.
Modified from Mathew RC, Kramer CM. Recent advances in magnetic resonance imaging for peripheral artery disease. *Vasc Med.* 2018;23:143–152.

TABLE 13.2 Types of Clinically Available MRA Sequences

Technique	Advantages	Limitations
Noncontrast MRA Options		
Time-of-flight MRA	High spatial resolution	Long imaging times, sensitive to patient motion and turbulent flow lead to artifacts
Phase-contrast MRA	Allows for flow quantification at the same time	Difficult imaging with both slow and turbulent flow
3D half-Fourier spin echo	High spatial resolution Requires gated imaging	If gating difficulties due to arrhythmia or low electrocardiographic voltage, then artifacts
Balanced SSFP MRA	High signal-to-noise ratio Requires gated imaging	Long imaging time
Quiescent-interval single shot MRA	Excellent image quality Shorter acquisition time and less sensitive to patient motion	In-plane vessels can have reduced image quality
Contrast-enhanced MRA	Excellent image quality	Caution related to gadolinium contrast in severe renal disease (GFR <30 mL/min). Imaging improved with moving table technique to follow the contrast peripherally.

3D, Three dimensional; *GFR*, glomerular filtration rate; *MRA*, magnetic resonance angiography; *SSFP*, steady-state free precession.

TABLE 13.3 Types of Postprocessing Techniques

Technique	Description
MPR	Cross-sectional images can be evaluated in planes different from acquisition plane
MIP projection	Production of full- or partial-volume images along any desired axis
Volume rendering	Manipulation of MRI slices to produce full volumetric images; structures optimized for viewing after applying intensity thresholds and removal of unwanted adjacent structures

MIP, Maximum-intensity projection; *MPR*, multiplanar reconstruction; *MRI*, magnetic resonance imaging.

the blood volume originally excited by the first pulse may not "see" the second pulse. This results in a black-appearing signal void in the vessel lumen. This technique allows detailed examination of arterial wall morphology. Fast spin echo (FSE) sequences produce images more rapidly. The double inversion recovery (DIR) FSE uses two consecutive inversion pulses: the first nulls or blackens the blood everywhere in the coil, and the second restores magnetization in the image slice. This produces the most reliable black blood images, which aids in evaluation of wall thickness, dissection flaps, and the presence of mural thrombus or inflammation.

"Bright blood" MRA techniques use GRE sequences and are generally divided into those measuring signal amplitude (time-of-flight [TOF]) and those based on phase effects (phase-contrast [PC]). In each GRE sequence, a single RF pulse is applied in short time intervals, which eliminates the signal loss due to flow void. TOF-MRA techniques depend on the flow of unsaturated protons in blood from outside the field of view (FOV) into the stationary tissue within an imaging plane that is already saturated by exposure to repeated RF pulses, which results in

"saturated" stationary protons that cannot contribute significant signal to the image. However, the "unsaturated" protons in blood flowing into the imaging plane give a maximal signal because they have not experienced the RF pulses. The unsaturated flowing blood appears bright compared with background static tissue (see Fig. 13.1B). The time required for blood to flow through an image slice and the resulting effect on the signal is known as TOF. If blood vessels have slow moving flow due to stenotic lesions, this can result in saturation of signals within the blood vessels due to the repeated RF excitation in the acquisition plane during the slow transit of blood. This can result in artifacts within vessels with slow flow due to stenotic lesions or occlusions.

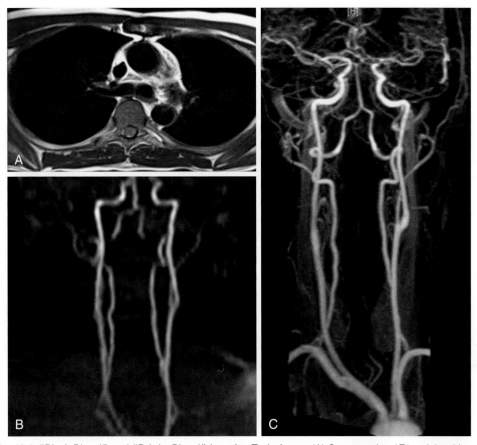

Fig. 13.1 "Black-Blood" and "Bright-Blood" Imaging Techniques. (A) Cross-sectional T1-weighted image of ascending and descending aorta; lumen appears black. (B) Time-of-flight (TOF) image of carotid-vertebral system. (C) Maximum-intensity projection reconstruction of arterial phase of contrast-enhanced magnetic resonance angiography images in same patient shows normal carotid-vertebral arteries at higher spatial resolution than corresponding TOF acquisition.

TOF techniques can be obtained in 2D or 3D. The 2D TOF imaging takes sequentially acquired, overlapping thin slices to form an image. Because of this, the patient needs to breath-hold during image acquisition to minimize motion artifact. Spatial misregistration may occur if patients cannot hold their breath at the same level each time. Therefore one or two slices are typically acquired per breath-hold. 2D TOF has good sensitivity for identifying vessels with slow flow because blood must move only 3 to 5 mm per slice. 3D TOF consists of GRE acquisition of an imaging plane to which blood is flowing. The advantage of this technique is higher signal-to-noise ratio (SNR) and improved resolution. A successful TOF image requires the section to be thin enough to allow for sufficient inflow between RF pulse repetitions but thick enough to ensure adequate SNR and anatomical coverage. Cardiac gating can be used to minimize artifacts at the expense of increased imaging time.

Although TOF uses differences in signal amplitude to differentiate between stationary and flowing spins, the PC technique observes the phase shifts of signals to determine the speed of blood flow. Strength and orientation of the applied magnetic field are varied to encode different phase shifts for flowing protons relative to stationary protons. The faster the spins are moving, the greater their phase shift, and protons of flowing blood can be distinguished from stationary protons. The phase shifts result in contrast between moving and stationary tissues and form the basis for PC imaging. By acquiring a pair of images at the same location with different sensitivities to flow and then subtracting the images to cancel out the background signal, the remaining signal is due to flowing blood. Phase shift is proportional to velocity, so

that blood flow can be quantified. PC acquisitions may be acquired in two or three dimensions.

Visualization of the arterial system with PC and TOF has limitations of long acquisition times that cannot be completed in one breath-hold, thus increasing the risk of motion artifact. Overestimating the degree of stenosis is often due to signal loss in the areas of complex flow, or "intravoxel dephasing." Undergrading may be due to inadequate spatial resolution.

Newer noncontrast techniques have been developed in the past decade and are still being evaluated in clinical studies. These include 3D half-Fourier FSE, balanced SSFP (b-SSFP), and quiescent-interval single shot (QISS) MRA techniques. 3D FSE uses the contrast difference between fast-moving arterial blood and slow-moving venous blood to create contrast and requires electrocardiographic (ECG) gating, which can be a limitation. b-SSFP MRA takes advantage of the differences in T2/T1-W imaging ratios between the blood and surrounding tissue to create an angiographic image and requires ECG gating. The QISS MRA is a type of b-SSFP imaging wherein the stationary tissues and venous signal are suppressed and then magnetized blood flow is imaged during diastole as it enters the imaging plane. However, the most commonly used MRA technique remains CE-MRA.

Contrast-Enhanced Magnetic Resonance Angiography

The introduction of CE-MRA has revolutionized MRA. This technique overcomes many of the limitations of traditional bright blood modalities: respiratory motion artifacts, poor SNR, and flow- and saturation-related artifacts (Fig. 13.2). Gadolinium increases the signal intensity of blood on contrast-enhanced 3D T1-W GRE images. With the use of gadolinium, blood contrast is not flow dependent, instead it is determined by the concentration of contrast agent (such as gadolinium) within the arterial tree during image acquisition. This technique acquires large-volume data sets in coronal or sagittal orientation within a single breath-hold during the first pass of the contrast material. The most commonly used contrast agent, gadolinium, is a heavy metal which is inert when bound to a chelator. Intravenous (IV) administration of gadolinium chelates dramatically shortens the T1 or longitudinal relaxation time of blood, thus reducing the effects of spin saturation. Moreover, the very short TE reduces spin dephasing to allow for accurate evaluation of vascular stenoses.

Contrast-enhanced MRA is much faster than TOF-MRA. The current CE-MRA allows imaging within a single breath-hold that minimizes motion artifacts through the use of high-performance gradient systems with ultra-short TR and TE. Digital subtraction, spoiling, and fat saturation techniques suppress background signal and enhance the contrast signal from within the vessels (see Fig. 13.1C). The subtracted data sets can then be postprocessed to generate 3D projectional images. Although CE-MRA provides a road map of the vessels similar to a conventional angiogram, it is important to still use axial images through the vessels to determine the true lumen diameter and presence of thrombus.

The goal of CE-MRA is to image the vessel of interest when the gadolinium concentration is highest in that vessel, which requires attention to the timing of the gadolinium bolus. Imaging during the arterial

phase of gadolinium infusion takes advantage of higher arterial SNR and significantly reduces adjacent venous enhancement. Image acquisition too late after the gadolinium reaches the vessel of interest results in venous and tissue enhancement which contaminates the arterial signal. This can be challenging for CE-MRA of the extremities, because the images are obtained in multiple segments. Contrast transit time from the point of injection through the arterial system can be affected by low cardiac output, valvular regurgitation, large abdominal aneurysms, and flow-limiting stenoses. Correct timing of the contrast bolus can be achieved by one of three means: (1) using an empirical estimation of transit time for a given arterial location, (2) giving a test bolus in the anatomical field of interest, or (3) using automated triggering wherein a pulse sequence is designed to sense the arrival of contrast in the desired vessel and automatically trigger image acquisition. It is important to remember that anatomical regions which require higher spatial resolution, such as the lower extremities, will need larger doses of contrast for longer acquisition times.

CE-MRA is limited by venous and soft-tissue enhancement. Contrast media not only passes into venous structures, dependent on the arteriovenous transit time of the tissue, but also rapidly leaks out of the vascular compartment, resulting in tissue enhancement. Newer "blood pool" agents are retained within blood vessels and selectively enhance the blood pool on T1-weighted MR images. The "blood pool" agents have one of the following characteristics: (1) gadolinium compounds that bind to albumin, (2) are large enough to stay within the vascular space, or (3) are very-small iron particles. Another agent, gadobenate, has a high T1 relaxation time because of its capacity for weak and transient interaction with serum albumin. It provides a higher and longer-lasting vascular signal enhancement in the abdominal aorta compared with gadolinium, which does not interact with proteins and has been studied in lower extremity peripheral artery disease (PAD).[4]

A limitation to gadolinium-based contrast is the potential for nephrogenic systemic fibrosis (NSF) in patients who have chronic renal insufficiency with a glomerular filtration rate (GFR) less than 30 mg/mL.[5] NSF primarily involves the skin with a scleroderma-like effect; however, it is a systemic process can also affect the muscle, joints, or internal organs, such as the lungs, liver, and heart, in patients with renal failure who are exposed to gadolinium. NSF occurs in patients with severe renal disease who are exposed to high doses of gadolinium agents or in patients who receive multiple standard doses of contrast agents in a short period of time. The reported prevalence of NSF among patients with GFR less than 30 mL/min is 3% to 5%.[6] Therefore MR protocols should caution against administration of gadolinium in cases of GFR <30 mg/mL. For patients with mild-moderate renal impairment, the goal is to minimize contrast volume.

Metal objects, such as stents or surgical clips, lead to susceptibility artifacts in MRA. Cavagna et al. evaluated CE-MRA of seven stent types in the aortic, iliac, and popliteal artery positions.[7] Of the available stent materials, those made from nitinol, tantalum, or polytetrafluoroethylene (PTFE) caused less artifact with CE-MRA. Overall, there were only a few stent types that allowed for adequate visualization of the intrastent lumen.

Approach to Imaging Analysis

Magnetic resonance data can be viewed as standard source images in the plane they were acquired, or image postprocessing allows reformatting in any desired plane to improve vessel evaluation with MR angiography (see Table 13.3, Fig. 13.3). One advantage of MR versus digital subtraction angiography (DSA) is that the latter may require multiple injections to assess arterial origins. The details of image interpretation are beyond the scope of this review, but source image data, multiplanar

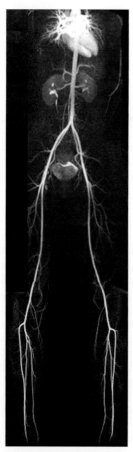

Fig. 13.2 Contrast-enhanced magnetic resonance angiography in a patient without obstructive atherosclerotic disease with images obtained from the chest through to the ankle.

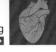

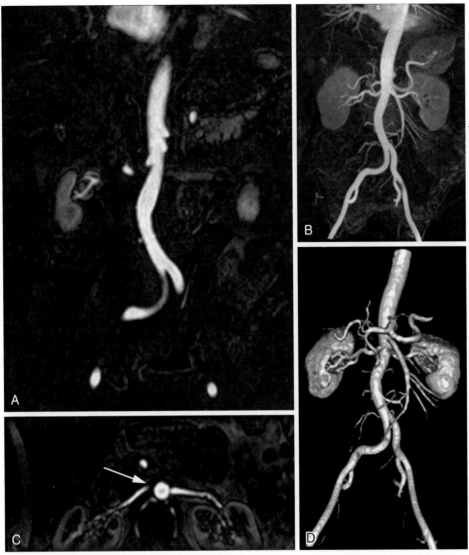

Fig. 13.3 Postprocessing Techniques; Contrast-Enhanced Magnetic Resonance Angiography of Abdominal Aorta and Branches. (A) Coronal thin-section image of abdominal aorta. Summation of these images, projected with maximum intensity, is used for (B) coronal maximum-intensity projection that includes normal renal and mesenteric arteries. (C) Axial multiplanar reconstruction image at level of left renal ostium does not include entire extent of both renal arteries, giving false impression of a proximal right renal artery occlusion *(arrow)*. (D) Three-dimensional volume-rendered image shows entire course of abdominal aorta and its branches.

reconstruction (MPR), maximum-intensity projection (MIP), and volume rendering (VR) are used. Source images are the initial acquisitions and should be used for detailed analysis and to confirm findings from the reformatted images. Interpretation often begins with a vascular survey using MPR and MIP data sets. MPRs are very useful in volumetric acquisitions because the desired imaging plane can be prescribed to enhance vascular separations. Subtracted MIPs are routinely created from CE-MRA. The noncontrast (mask) images are subtracted from the enhanced images, and resulting high SNR data sets undergo projection of maximum intensity. By performing the projections of all angles around the z-axis of the patient, the data sets can be viewed *in cine*. These projections are referred to as *rotating MIPs*.

Clinical Applications

Extracranial Carotid and Vertebral Arteries

The extracranial carotid arteries and the vertebral arteries can be affected by atherosclerosis, dissection, and inflammatory diseases such

as giant cell arteritis. CE-MRA is considered the standard for MRI-based evaluation of these vessels given that one can image the entirety of their course with good SNR and relative insensitivity to artifacts from turbulence (Fig. 13.4). TOF imaging for the extracranial carotid and vertebral arteries is limited by turbulent flow near the carotid bifurcation which can overestimate the burden of atherosclerosis at this site. PC sequences offer flow quantification which can aid in the assessment of stenotic lesion severity.

Accuracy of CE-MRA for carotid artery stenosis is excellent. In a meta-analysis of 41 studies, the sensitivity is 94% and specificity is 93% for severe (70% to 99%) carotid artery stenosis.[8] Despite advancements in TOF imaging at 3T, there remains an increased sensitivity to artifacts, which could overestimate the degree of stenosis; therefore CE-MRA is favored for carotid artery evaluation.[9] In patients with severe renal failure, TOF MRA may be considered as an option to evaluate the degree of carotid artery stenosis if ultrasound is indeterminate. Alternatively, 3D fast black-blood MR carotid artery imaging

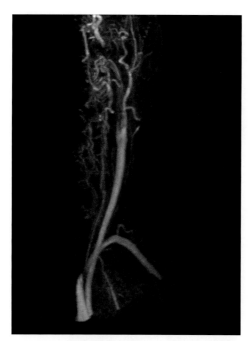

Fig. 13.4 Carotid Artery Disease. Left internal carotid artery dissection resulted in a thrombotic occlusion of proximal vessel. Internal carotid artery reconstitutes more distally.

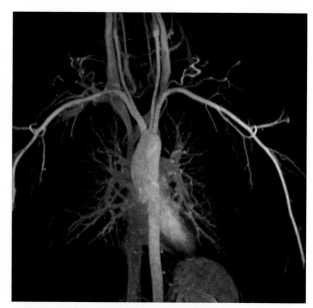

Fig. 13.5 Normal Thoracic Aorta. Maximum-intensity projection image shows normal thoracic aorta, and origin and course of supra-aortic vessels.

performed well compared with DSA, with a high sensitivity (91.7%) and specificity (96.5%) for the detection of severe carotid artery stenosis.[10] Compared with computed tomography angiography (CTA) for carotid artery stenosis, CE-MRA is not limited by the presence of arterial wall calcifications.

High-resolution MRI (HR-MRI) for vessel wall imaging typically includes T1/T2-W imaging, proton-density imaging, or contrast-enhanced T1-W imaging with FSE sequencers or black-blood techniques.[11] The HR-MR vessel imaging can aid in determining the presence of vulnerable carotid artery plaque, which has contrast enhancement and is associated with acute ischemic stroke, as well as detecting inflammatory diseases such as vasculitis.[12] It is important to remember that cerebrovascular events can occur in the setting of mild-moderate carotid artery stenosis and, in these settings, atherosclerotic plaque composition evaluation by HR-MRI can provide insight into the presence of a vulnerable plaque.[13]

Carotid and vertebral artery dissection flaps can be visualized with either CE-MRA or CTA; however, CTA is preferred if a patient requires a rapid exam such as with a hemodynamically unstable patient. CE-MRA has the advantage for stable patients of not being associated with ionizing radiation or exposure to iodinated contrast so that serial exams can be compared with minimal risk using MRI. With MRI, dissections of the cervical arteries can show evidence of intramural hematoma with cross-sectional images. The appearance varies based on timing of imaging from the onset of the dissection due to the hemoglobin breakdown within the hematoma.[14] TOF imaging does not completely suppress stationary tissues; therefore it can show subacute intramural hematoma.

Thoracic Aorta and Branches

The thoracic aorta can be evaluated with a single breath-hold 3D CE-MRA (Fig. 13.5), usually with electrocardiographic monitoring so that there is minimal pulsation artifact. The main thoracic aorta indications for MRA include aneurysm, dissection, congenital vascular anomalies, and thoracic outlet obstruction.

Thoracic aortic aneurysm. The location, size, shape, and associated vessel involvement of thoracic aortic aneurysms can be easily determined by CE-MRI. Measurements of the maximal aortic aneurysmal size need to be done on source images (including noncontrast) where there is clear delineation of the vessel wall rather than on MIP reformatted images where the 3D outline of the lumen is shown.[15] CE-MRA allows for visualization of associated mural thrombus. SSFP cine imaging of the aortic valve aids in the determination of whether the ascending aortic aneurysm is related to a congenital bicuspid valve. For patients who cannot receive gadolinium, native SSFP 3D MRA provides the same final diagnosis for thoracic aortic aneurysm size and extent as compared with CE-MRA.[16]

Thoracic aortic dissection. Patients who present with symptoms or signs of acute thoracic aortic dissection typically are evaluated with CTA due to the rapid exam and easier time monitoring acutely ill patients compared with the MR scanner (see Chapter 32). For the most part, MRI is used to evaluate patients with a more subacute presentation or in the follow-up of patients managed conservatively for a type B dissection. A comprehensive MRI exam of the thoracic aorta is associated with a nearly 100% sensitivity for the detection of an aortic dissection and intramural hematoma (Fig. 13.6).[17] The MR examination includes SE black-blood sequences which can show an aortic intimal flap. GRE sequences can differentiate slow flow versus thrombus in the false lumen. CE-MRA of the thoracic aorta is performed rapidly and without ECG gating. The complete thoracic aorta MR examination visualizes true and false lumens, location and extent of the dissection, and the involvement of any aortic branch vessels or pericardial effusion.

Aortic coarctation and pseudocoarctation. Aortic coarctation is a common congenital defect, with a focal narrowing of the thoracic aorta near the ductus arteriosus, most commonly post ductal when diagnosed in adults (Fig. 13.7). The combination of cardiac MRI and CE-MRA are used for a comprehensive evaluation of aortic coarctation[18] and any associated congenital heart diseases (such as a bicuspid aortic valve). ECG-gated black-blood DIR T1-W images provide detail about the coarctation segment. MRA with or without contrast will illustrate the location of the stenosis, associated tortuosity of the aorta, and any collateral vessels. PC images across the stenotic lesion can measure the peak pressure gradient to aid in the decision for intervention. The use

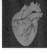

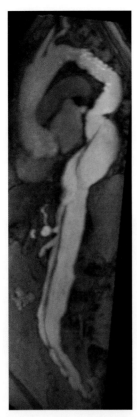

Fig. 13.6 Aortic Dissection. Contrast-enhanced magnetic resonance angiography in a patient with a Stanford type B dissection with an intimal flap and flow shown in both the true and false lumen in the descending aorta.

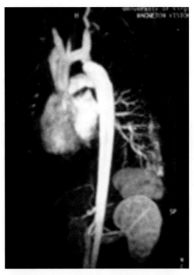

Fig. 13.7 Aortic Coarctation. Contrast-enhanced magnetic resonance angiography in a pediatric patient with an aortic coarctation shown just below the left subclavian artery. Prominent intercostal collaterals are also seen.

of time-resolved velocity-encoded 3D PC MRI (4D flow MRI) to measure the degree of stenosis across the coarctation correlates well with invasive measurements from the catheterization lab.[19] Collateral flow assessment with MR velocity mapping can accurately evaluate the hemodynamic significance of a coarctation.[20] A comprehensive MR study of the thoracic aorta has excellent diagnostic ability for coarctation, with sensitivity of 95% and specificity of 82%.[21] Follow-up MR studies are used after a coarctation repair or angioplasty to evaluate for long-term complications of stenosis or aneurysm formation.[18]

MRA also can distinguish between coarctation and pseudocoarctation. Pseudocoarctation rarely occurs in the descending thoracic aorta, wherein there is an elongated redundant thoracic aorta with buckling distal to the origin of the left subclavian artery. The key differentiator is that there is no stenotic gradient across the area of buckling.

Thoracic outlet syndrome. Thoracic outlet syndrome (TOS) can result in symptoms from compression of the brachial plexus (neurogenic TOS), subclavian vein (venous TOS) or the subclavian artery (arterial TOS) as this neurovascular bundle exits the thoracic outlet (see Chapter 63). Arterial TOS is the most rare, accounting for less than 3% of cases. Venous TOS is often associated with repetitive upper arm exercises and associated deep vein thrombosis. Because the anatomy of the thoracic outlet is dynamic, it is important to image for arterial or venous TOS with abduction of the arms (Fig. 13.8). MRI is considered the preferred cross-sectional imaging modality for evaluation of arterial or venous TOS.[22] Because the MRI for thoracic obstruction includes MRA, it is important to have the patient's IV on the side opposite to their symptoms to prevent any artifact from the concentrated

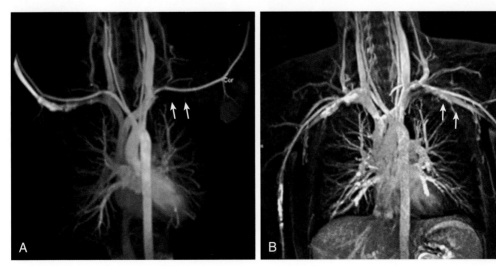

Fig. 13.8 Thoracic Outlet Syndrome. (A) Severe compression of left subclavian vein with arms up *(arrows)*. (B) Left subclavian vein becomes widely patent *(arrows)* with arms down; no evidence of thrombosis.

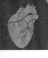
gadolinium bolus. A series of images are performed with the arms adducted and then abducted to show any positional narrowing of the axillary and subclavian vessels. If a "blood pool" contrast agent such as gadofosveset trisodium is used, then a single injection can be used for both arm positions; however, if an extracellular gadolinium contrast agent is used, then the dose needs to be divided for the two arm positions.

Pulmonary Vessels

RF ablation for atrial fibrillation uses preprocedure noninvasive angiographic mapping of the pulmonary veins to determine the number, location, and size of the pulmonary veins for planning of the ablation procedure (Fig. 13.9).[23] Multidetector computed tomography (CT) is considered the "gold standard" for preprocedure assessment of the pulmonary veins and also allows for evaluation of left atrial appendage thrombus using delayed postcontrast images. The overall spatial resolution and quality of the 3D reconstructions are better with CT than with MRA. Certain institutions may have greater levels of success with preatrial fibrillation pulmonary vein studies with cardiac MRI and CE-MRA and therefore preferentially use this modality.[24] Postprocedural evaluation of pulmonary vein stenosis with MRA has the advantage of avoiding radiation or iodinated contrast for serial studies. Pulmonary MRA could be performed in patients with suspected pulmonary embolism only if they are prohibited from

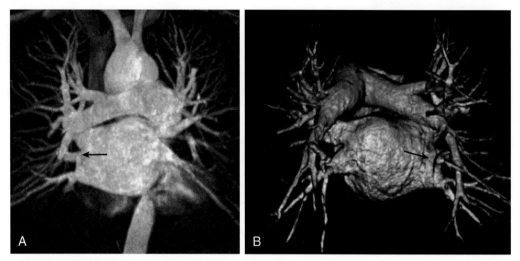

Fig. 13.9 Pulmonary Veins. (A) Coronal maximum-intensity projection image. (B) Posterior aspect of three-dimensional volume-rendered image shows pulmonary arteries, left atrium and pulmonary veins, and separate opening of right middle lobe vein to left atrium *(arrow)*.

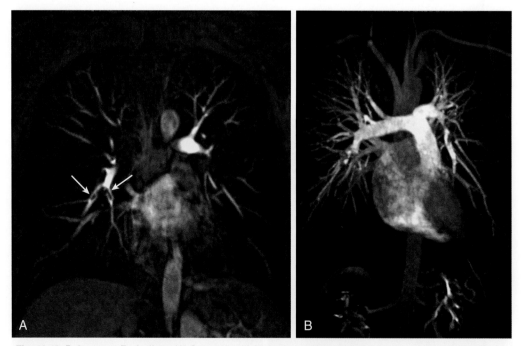

Fig. 13.10 Pulmonary Embolism. (A) Coronal multiplanar reconstructed image shows embolic filling defects in right lower lobe pulmonary artery branches *(arrows)*. (B) Coronal maximum-intensity projection image shows whole branching pattern of pulmonary arteries but hides details. Embolic filling defects in right lower lobe pulmonary artery cannot be seen clearly.

receiving iodinated contrast given that multidetector CTA is the current gold standard noninvasive study for the detection of pulmonary embolism (Fig. 13.10).

Upper Extremity Peripheral Arteries

Although most brachiocephalic and subclavian artery disease is due to atherosclerosis (Fig. 13.11), large vessel vasculitis (such as Takayasu arteritis [Fig. 13.12] or giant cell arteritis [Fig. 13.13]) or fibromuscular dysplasia can lead to stenotic lesions in these vessels. CE-MRA is helpful to evaluate for the presence of arterial stenosis, as well as inflammation.[25] Vessel wall edema and thickening can occur even before luminal narrowing. Black-blood imaging evaluates the arterial wall morphology, and postgadolinium imaging demonstrates any mural enhancement as a sign of inflammation. MRA of the upper extremities is limited by a brief acquisition window of only a few seconds between maximal arterial enhancement and the beginning of venous contamination. Blood pressure cuff inflation proximal to the imaged area can extend imaging time and enhance image quality.

Lower Extremity Peripheral Arteries

The overwhelming majority of lower extremity arterial disease is due to atherosclerosis; however, nonatherosclerotic diseases can result in reduced blood flow to the legs such as: peripheral artery aneurysms, popliteal artery entrapment (Fig. 13.14), cystic adventitial disease, thromboangiitis obliterans (TAO), vasculitis (Fig. 13.15), giant cell and Takayasu arteritis, and (rarely) fibromuscular dysplasia. Popliteal artery entrapment uncommonly occurs due to an anomalous relationship between the popliteal artery and the medial head of the gastrocnemius muscle. MRI defines the anatomical relationships, and MRA can show evidence of vascular compromise during provocative plantar flexion and

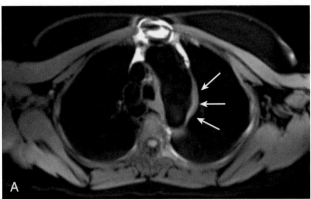
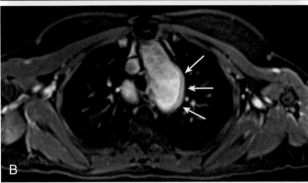

Fig. 13.12 Takayasu Arteritis. Axial precontrast (A) and postcontrast (B) T1-weighted images show aneurysmatic dilation, thickening, and contrast enhancement of aortic arch, consistent with aortitis (arrows) in patient with Takayasu arteritis.

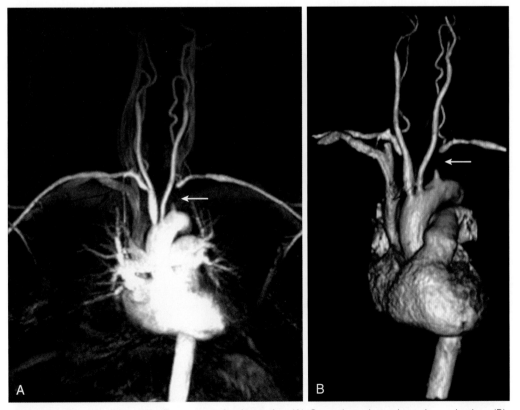

Fig. 13.11 Thoracic Magnetic Resonance Angiography. (A) Coronal maximum-intensity projection. (B) Three-dimensional volume-rendered image shows proximal left subclavian artery occlusion (arrows) causing subclavian steal syndrome.

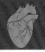

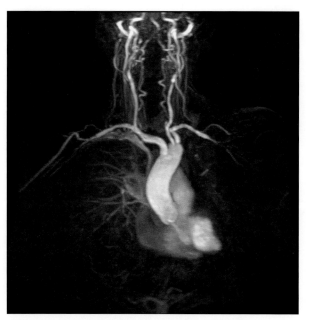

Fig. 13.13 Giant Cell Arteritis. Both subclavian arteries have smooth, tapered stenoses in mid- to distal segments.

at rest.[25] Cystic adventitial disease occurs when a mucin-containing cyst in the popliteal artery wall impairs arterial flow and causes claudication. The presence of water in the cyst gives a bright appearance on T2-weighted images, and MRA reveals popliteal artery stenosis.[26]

MRI of the lower extremities for evaluation of atherosclerotic PAD begins at the distal abdominal aorta and extends through the level of the ankle (Fig. 13.16). A routine MRA of the abdominal

aorta with peripheral run-off protocol uses 3D CE-MRA to evaluate the peripheral arteries. After a patient is diagnosed with symptomatic PAD, usually based on the results of an ankle-brachial index, noninvasive angiography with either MRI or CT is often done to evaluate the location and degree of stenosis for consideration of revascularization (Fig. 13.17) (see Chapter 18). One of the challenges in lower extremity CE-MRA is optimizing the gadolinium contrast bolus so that adequate vessel opacification is achieved in the abdomen through the feet with rapid imaging that follows the contrast media distally. As the imaging approaches the distal lower extremities, gadolinium can enter the venous system and cause venous opacification or "contamination" of the arterial images. The MRA can be done with a continuous moving table which allows the patient examination table to move in tandem with the contrast bolus as it progresses distally.[27]

To have adequate visualization of the peripheral arteries to assess for obstructive atherosclerotic lesions, a peripheral MRA requires high spatial resolution to visualize the distal arteries. Given the length of arteries evaluated, a relatively fast scan is required so that the risk of venous enhancement is minimized. Venous contamination of the peripheral arterial MRA can be particularly problematic in diabetic patients due to the presence of distal vessel atherosclerotic disease. The use of calf compression during CE-MRA at 3.0 T significantly reduced the venous opacification in the leg and foot for diabetic patients which resulted in improved accuracy.[28]

The diagnostic performance of CE-MRA for identification of significant peripheral arterial stenosis is excellent. A meta-analysis of 32 studies from 1998 to 2009 found a pooled sensitivity of 94.7% and specificity of 95.6% for CE-MRA to diagnose segmental steno-occlusive lesions in peripheral arteries.[29] Similarly, when compared against CTA and ultrasound, CE-MRA had excellent diagnostic

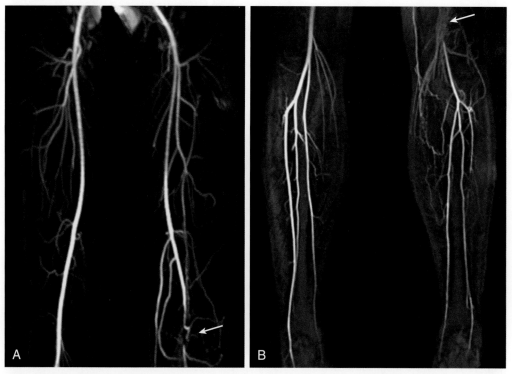

Fig. 13.14 Popliteal Artery Entrapment. (A) and (B) Arterial-phase maximum-intensity projection images of leg show left popliteal artery entrapment *(arrows)*.

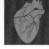

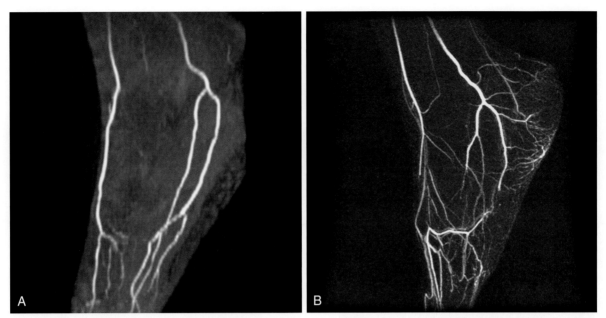

Fig. 13.15 Pedal Arteries. (A) Time-of-flight image of normal pedal arteries. (B) Contrast-enhanced magnetic resonance angiography maximum intensity projection reconstruction of pedal arteries in patient with cryoglobulinemia and small-vessel vasculitis. Arteries of pedal arch are occluded. Moderate venous enhancement is present.

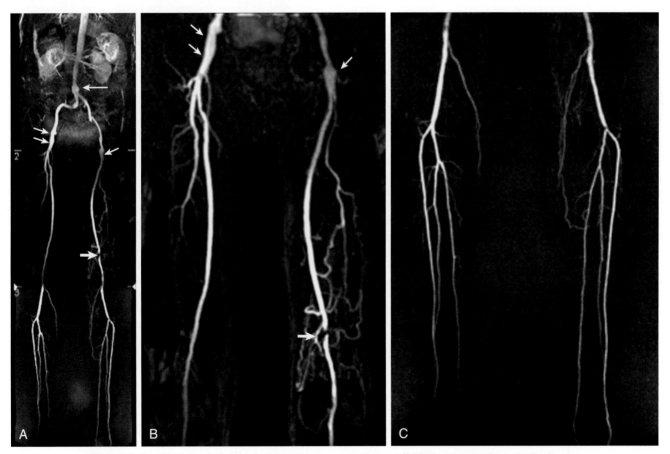

Fig. 13.16 (A to C) Abdominal aorta and bilateral lower-extremity run-off. Maximum-intensity projection images show fusiform ectasia of infrarenal abdominal aorta *(long arrow)*, mild ectasia of right distal external iliac artery and left proximal common femoral artery *(short arrows)*, short-segment moderate to severe stenosis in left popliteal artery *(thick arrow)*, and collateral vascularization. Normal three-vessel run-off is seen in each calf.

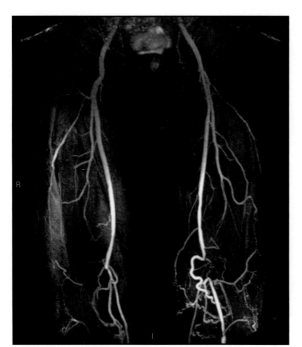

Fig. 13.17 Superficial Femoral Artery Atherosclerosis. Contrast-enhanced magnetic resonance angiography in a patient with peripheral artery disease demonstrating bilateral occluded superficial femoral arteries, although the left is reconstituted by a collateral.

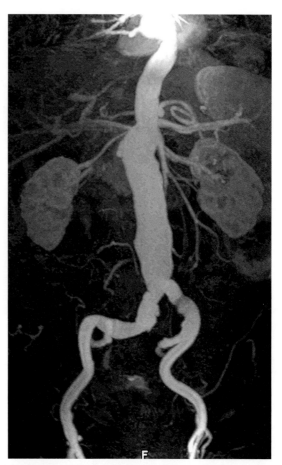

Fig. 13.18 Abdominal Aortic Aneurysm. Contrast-enhanced magnetic resonance angiography in a patient with an infrarenal abdominal aortic aneurysm.

ability for the detection of PAD with stenosis greater than 50%.[30] Traditionally CE-MRA has been performed at 1.5 Tesla, although the diagnostic accuracy is similar at 3 Tesla with improved contrast-to-noise ratio for the same contrast dose.[30] Current techniques for MRA also include noncontrast studies, as discussed previously (see Table 13.2).[3]

There are novel MRI techniques to evaluate lower extremity PAD, which are used primarily in the research setting, with some limited clinical use depending upon the center.[3,31] These techniques measure blood flow in the calf muscles and include arterial spin labeling, blood oxygen level–dependent MRI, and first pass gadolinium-enhanced perfusion.

In addition to the initial evaluation of PAD for planning a revascularization, MRA can be done to follow patients post intervention for graft patency.[32] However, the presence of metallic surgical clips causes a susceptibility artifact which can obscure evaluation of the graft or native vessels. The evaluation of patients after peripheral arterial stent traditionally was limited with MRI. However, the use of a blood pool agent, such as gadofosveset trisodium for CE-MRA, has excellent sensitivity and specificity (>95%) for the detection of superficial femoral artery stenosis.[33]

Abdominal Aorta Imaging

MRI is well suited to image the abdominal aorta. CE-MRA permits high contrast between the aorta, its branching vessels, and surrounding organs. After contrast injection, both an arterial and a delayed phase are acquired. The delayed images can be helpful in cases of slow flow in large aneurysms or with a false lumen where the initial acquisition does not have sufficient contrast enhancement. In addition, black-blood images are available to aid in the measurement of the aorta lumen, diameter, and overall assessment of the aorta wall.

Abdominal aorta aneurysm. Abdominal aortic aneurysm (AAA) can be evaluated by either CTA or MRA (see Chapter 36). The American College of Radiology guidelines for evaluation of a pulsatile aortic mass advocate for contrast-enhanced MRA as an alternative to CTA (Fig. 13.18).[34] The use of blood pool contrast agents allows for longer imaging time with MRI with improved image quality and resolution.[35] A typical MRI protocol for AAA includes axial T1-W GRE images and CE-MRA with arterial and late phase imaging, as well as time-resolved MRA with flow analysis to further evaluate the flow in the aneurysm sac.

With regard to planning endovascular repair of AAA, CT is the preferred imaging modality due to the visualization of aortic calcifications. However, CE-MRA is an alternative. Postaortic stent graft imaging can be done with MRA to determine patency of the aortic lumen, positioning of the device and the presence of an endoleak.[36] Stents made from nitinol have minimal artifact with MRI; however, stainless steel and cobalt-chromium-nickel alloy stents both can have significant artifact due to being ferromagnetic.[37] The use of superparamagnetic iron oxide–enhanced dynamic MRI may be an alternative to a gadolinium-based MRA for patients with renal failure and suspected endoleak.[38]

Abdominal aorta dissection. The evaluation for abdominal aortic dissection with MRI uses essentially the same sequences as the protocol outlined previously for AAA. With suspected dissection, the use of the rapid black-blood images over the entire abdominal aorta shows delineation between the true lumen and vessel wall. CE-MRA then allows for differentiation between the true and false lumen. In the setting of suspected acute abdominal aortic dissection, CTA is typically performed due to the rapid image acquisition and timely diagnosis of an emergent condition.

Mesenteric Arteries

MRA along with flow measurements using PC MRI can evaluate the origins of the mesenteric vessels in patients with suspected chronic mesenteric ischemia (Fig. 13.19) (see Chapter 26).[39] The accuracy for diagnosis of chronic mesenteric ischemia with MRI is more limited because the stenosis occurs farther from the arterial ostium. Given clinical concern for acute mesenteric ischemia, a CT is done typically to enable rapid imaging in acutely ill patients. For stable patients or suspected chronic mesenteric ischemia, MRI is a viable alternative to CT. In addition to atherosclerosis affecting the mesenteric arteries, dissection, vasculitis, or median arcuate ligament syndrome can all affect arterial flow to the abdominal organs.

Renal Arteries

The two primary causes of renal artery stenosis (RAS), atherosclerosis and fibromuscular dysplasia, can both be evaluated with contrast-enhanced MRA (see Chapter 23). With atherosclerotic RAS, MRI has the distinct advantage over CT because the presence of calcium does not obscure accurate classification of stenosis with MR. Meta-analysis including 25 studies for the use of MRA for the evaluation of suspected RAS found that gadolinium-enhanced MRA has a higher sensitivity (97%) and specificity (93%) than noncontrast MRA (94% sensitivity and 85% specificity).[40] With fibromuscular dysplasia, CE-MRA has excellent sensitivity (97%) for the diagnosis of FMD based on the "string

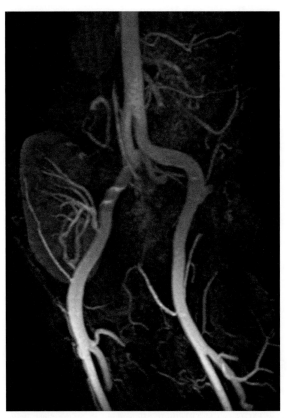

Fig. 13.20 Renal Artery Anastomosis of a Transplanted Kidney. Oblique coronal maximum-intensity projection contrast-enhanced magnetic resonance angiography reconstruction shows patency of renal artery anastomosis of transplanted kidney.

of beads" appearance, and a specificity of 93%.[41] However, the sensitivity for detecting a >50% RAS due to FMD is limited with CE-MRA (68%).[41] An additional indication for renal artery MRA is in the renal transplant population to evaluate anastomoses (Fig. 13.20).

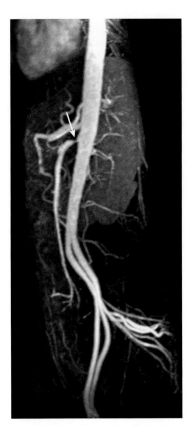

Fig. 13.19 Mesenteric Artery Stenosis. Sagittal maximum-intensity projection contrast-enhanced magnetic resonance angiography shows severe stenosis of superior mesenteric artery *(arrow)*.

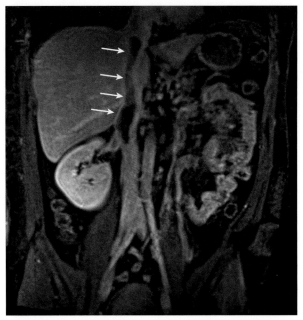

Fig. 13.21 Abdominal Magnetic Resonance Venography. Coronal maximum-intensity projection image; large hypointense filling defect due to thrombosis seen in inferior vena cava lumen *(arrows)*.

Magnetic Resonance Venography

Magnetic resonance venography (MRV) protocols often use contrast-enhanced imaging within similar rapid 3D sequences that are used for MRA followed by subtraction data sets to produce venograms by limiting arterial signal.[42] The noncontrast, gradient-recalled echo venogram has a lower accuracy for detection of deep venous thrombosis than does CE-MRV, particularly when performed with gadofosveset, a blood-pool agent.[43] With regard to the detection of thrombus using MRI, thrombus has a high T1 signal due to the presence of methemoglobin. For the lower extremities, ultrasound remains the diagnostic modality of choice to evaluate for deep venous thrombosis. CE-MRV with gadolinium of the pelvic and lower extremity veins showed similar image quality compared with conventional venogram for postthrombotic changes and suitability prior to bypass surgery.[44] MRV can evaluate the central thoracic veins, abdominal/pelvic veins (Fig. 13.21), and the renal vein.

ACKNOWLEDGMENT

Drs. Pollak and Kramer acknowledge the prior contributions of Dr. Cihan Duran, Dr. Piotr S. Sobieszczyk, and Dr. Frank J. Rybicki to the sections on principles of MRI and image analysis.

REFERENCES

1. Ho VB, Corse WR. MR angiography of the abdominal aorta and peripheral vessels. Radiol Clin North Am. 2003;41:115–144.
2. Vogt FM, Goyen M, Debatin JF. MR angiography of the chest. Radiol Clin North Am. 2003;41:29–41.
3. Mathew RC, Kramer CM. Recent advances in magnetic resonance imaging for peripheral artery disease. Vasc Med. 2018;23:143–152.
4. Thurnher S, Miller S, Schneider G, et al. Diagnostic performance of gadobenate dimeglumine enhanced MR angiography of the iliofemoral and calf arteries: a large-scale multicenter trial. AJR Am J Roentgenol. 2007;189:1223–1237.
5. Cowper SE, Robin HS, Steinberg SM, et al. Scleromyxoedema-like cutaneous diseases in renal-dialysis patients. Lancet. 2000;356:1000–1001.
6. Sadowski EA, Bennett LK, Chan MR, et al. Nephrogenic systemic fibrosis: risk factors and incidence estimation. Radiology. 2007;243:148–157.
7. Cavagna E, Berletti R, Schiavon F. In vivo evaluation of intravascular stents at three-dimensional MR angiography. Eur Radiol. 2001;11:2531–2535.
8. Wardlaw JM, Chappell FM, Best JJ, et al. Non-invasive imaging compared with intra-arterial angiography in the diagnosis of symptomatic carotid stenosis: a meta-analysis. Lancet. 2006;367:1503–1512.
9. Weber J, Veith P, Jung B, et al. MR angiography at 3 Tesla to assess proximal internal carotid artery stenoses: contrast-enhanced or 3D time-of-flight MR angiography? Clin Neuroradiol. 2015;25:41–48.
10. Zhao H, Wang J, Liu X, et al. Assessment of carotid artery atherosclerotic disease by using three-dimensional fast black-blood MR imaging: comparison with DSA. Radiology. 2015;274:508–516.
11. Choi YJ, Jung SC, Lee DH. Vessel wall imaging of the intracranial and cervical carotid arteries. J Stroke. 2015;17:238–255.
12. Dieleman N, van der Kolk AG, Zwanenburg JJ, et al. Imaging intracranial vessel wall pathology with magnetic resonance imaging: current prospects and future directions. Circulation. 2014;130:192–201.
13. Saam T, Cai J, Ma L, et al. Comparison of symptomatic and asymptomatic atherosclerotic carotid plaque features with in vivo MR imaging. Radiology. 2006;240:464–472.
14. Marteau V, Gerber S, et al. Craniocervical arterial dissection: spectrum of imaging findings and differential diagnosis. Radiographics. 2008;28:1711–1728.
15. Sakamoto I, Sueyoshi E, Uetani M. MR imaging of the aorta. Radiol Clin North Am. 2007;45:485–497. viii.
16. von Knobelsdorff-Brenkenhoff F, Gruettner H, Trauzeddel RF, et al. Comparison of native high-resolution 3D and contrast-enhanced MR angiography for assessing the thoracic aorta. Eur Heart J Cardiovasc Imaging. 2014;15:651–658.
17. Moore AG, Eagle KA, Bruckman D, et al. Choice of computed tomography, transesophageal echocardiography, magnetic resonance imaging, and aortography in acute aortic dissection: International Registry of Acute Aortic Dissection (IRAD). Am J Cardiol. 2002;89:1235–1238.
18. Karaosmanoglu AD, Khawaja RD, Onur MR, Kalra MK. CT and MRI of aortic coarctation: pre- and postsurgical findings. AJR Am J Roentgenol. 2015;204:W224–W233.
19. Goubergrits L, Riesenkampff E, Yevtushenko P, et al. MRI-based computational fluid dynamics for diagnosis and treatment prediction: clinical validation study in patients with coarctation of aorta. J Magn Reson Imaging. 2015;41:909–916.
20. Holmqvist C, Stahlberg F, Hanseus K, et al. Collateral flow in coarctation of the aorta with magnetic resonance velocity mapping: correlation to morphological imaging of collateral vessels. J Magn Reson Imaging. 2002;15:39–46.
21. Nielsen JC, Powell AJ, Gauvreau K, et al. Magnetic resonance imaging predictors of coarctation severity. Circulation. 2005;111:622–628.
22. Raptis CA, Sridhar S, Thompson RW, et al. Imaging of the patient with thoracic outlet syndrome. Radiographics. 2016;36:984–1000.
23. Ohana M, Bakouboula B, Labani A, et al. Imaging before and after catheter ablation of atrial fibrillation. Diagn Interv Imaging. 2015;96:1113–1123.
24. Groarke JD, Waller AH, Vita TS, et al. Feasibility study of electrocardiographic and respiratory gated, gadolinium enhanced magnetic resonance angiography of pulmonary veins and the impact of heart rate and rhythm on study quality. J Cardiovasc Magn Reson. 2014;16:43.
25. Cosottini M, Zampa V, Petruzzi P, et al. Contrast-enhanced three-dimensional MR angiography in the assessment of subclavian artery diseases. Eur Radiol. 2000;10:1737–1744.
26. Elias DA, White LM, Rubenstein JD, et al. Clinical evaluation and MR imaging features of popliteal artery entrapment and cystic adventitial disease. AJR Am J Roentgenol. 2003;180:627–632.
27. Koziel K, Attenberger UI, Lederle K, et al. Peripheral MRA with continuous table movement: imaging speed and robustness compared to a conventional stepping table technique. Eur J Radiol. 2011;80:537–542.
28. Li J, Zhao JG, Li MH. Lower limb vascular disease in diabetic patients: a study with calf compression contrast-enhanced magnetic resonance angiography at 3.0 Tesla. Acad Radiol. 2011;18:755–763.
29. Menke J, Larsen J. Meta-analysis: accuracy of contrast-enhanced magnetic resonance angiography for assessing steno-occlusions in peripheral arterial disease. Ann Intern Med. 2010;153:325–334.
30. Collins R, Cranny G, Burch J, et al. A systematic review of duplex ultrasound, magnetic resonance angiography and computed tomography angiography for the diagnosis and assessment of symptomatic, lower limb peripheral arterial disease. Health Technol Assess. 2007;11:iii–iv, xi–xiii, 1–184.
31. van den Bosch HC, Westenberg JJ, Caris R, et al. Peripheral arterial occlusive disease: 3.0-T versus 1.5-T MR angiography compared with digital subtraction angiography. Radiology. 2013;266:337–346.
32. Meissner OA, Verrel F, Tato F, et al. Magnetic resonance angiography in the follow-up of distal lower-extremity bypass surgery: comparison with duplex ultrasound and digital subtraction angiography. J Vasc Interv Radiol. 2004;15:1269–1277.
33. Plank CM, Wolf F, Langenberger H, et al. Improved detection of in-stent restenosis by blood pool agent-enhanced, high-resolution, steady-state magnetic resonance angiography. Eur Radiol. 2011;21:2158–2165.
34. Reis SP, Majdalany BS, AbuRahma AF, et al. ACR Appropriateness Criteria® pulsatile abdominal mass suspected abdominal aortic aneurysm. J Am Coll Radiol. 2017;14:S258–S265.
35. Wolf F, Plank C, Beitzke D, et al. Prospective evaluation of high-resolution MRI using gadofosveset for stent-graft planning: comparison with CT angiography in 30 patients. AJR Am J Roentgenol. 2011;197:1251–1257.
36. Pitton MB, Schweitzer H, Herber S, et al. MRI versus helical CT for endoleak detection after endovascular aneurysm repair. AJR Am J Roentgenol. 2005;185:1275–1281.

37. Shah A, Stavropoulos SW. Imaging surveillance following endovascular aneurysm repair. *Semin Intervent Radiol*. 2009;26:10–16.

38. Ichihashi S, Marugami N, Tanaka T, et al. Preliminary experience with superparamagnetic iron oxide-enhanced dynamic magnetic resonance imaging and comparison with contrast-enhanced computed tomography in endoleak detection after endovascular aneurysm repair. *J Vasc Surg*. 2013;58:66–72.

39. Shih MC, Hagspiel KD. CTA and MRA in mesenteric ischemia: part 1. Role in diagnosis and differential diagnosis. *AJR Am J Roentgenol*. 2007;188:452–461.

40. Tan KT, van Beek EJ, Brown PW, et al. Magnetic resonance angiography for the diagnosis of renal artery stenosis: a meta-analysis. *Clin Radiol*. 2002;57:617–624.

41. Willoteaux S, Faivre-Pierret M, Moranne O, et al. Fibromuscular dysplasia of the main renal arteries: comparison of contrast-enhanced MR angiography with digital subtraction angiography. *Radiology*. 2006;241:922–929.

42. Lebowitz JA, Rofsky NM, Krinsky GA, et al. Gadolinium-enhanced body MR venography with subtraction technique. *AJR Am J Roentgenol*. 1997;169:755–758.

43. Huang SY, Kim CY, Miller MJ, et al. Abdominopelvic and lower extremity deep venous thrombosis: evaluation with contrast-enhanced MR venography with a blood-pool agent. *AJR Am J Roentgenol*. 2013;201:208–214.

44. Ruehm SG, Wiesner W, Debatin JF. Pelvic and lower extremity veins: contrast-enhanced three-dimensional MR venography with a dedicated vascular coil-initial experience. *Radiology*. 2000;215:421–427.

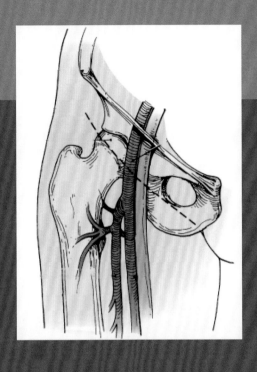

第14章
CT血管成像

　　多排螺旋CT容积数据采集促进了CT血管造影（CT angiography，CTA）的发展，而CT血管造影作为一种诊断工具使血管疾病的诊断发生了极大的变革。1998年4排螺旋CT面世后，单次造影剂注射和数据采集即可完成充分的周围血管成像。直至16排CT的出现，实现了解剖学意义上的容积数据采集，空间分辨率达到了亚毫米级各向同性，可常规完成周围血管CT成像，清楚显示直径<1 mm的小血管。2004年64排CT机的出现带来了新的重大进步，不同厂家引入了2种不同的扫描仪理念。通用电气、飞利浦、东芝公司追求容积理念，目标是利用更宽的探测器在单次旋转中进行更大的覆盖。西门子公司追求分辨率理念，利用相同的探测器结合双倍z轴采样，目的是增加z轴方向分辨率和减少螺旋伪影。采用这种方法，图像的数量增加而探测器的宽度不变，从而避免了锥束伪影和图像噪声。不仅在冠状动脉成像方面优势明显，在血管成像上亦优势突出，包括动脉期成像和血管疾病诊断（如夹层和动静脉畸形）。此外，双能CT和能谱CT为进一步的组织显影提供了额外的可能性。本章主要论述多排螺旋CT的基本原理及其在血管疾病方面的应用，同时涉及图像阅读的方法，图像显示、分析、定量等常规后处理方法。CT血管造影的优缺点，包括辐射剂量的问题也会一并讲解。

常光其

Computed Tomographic Angiography

Rahul B. Thomas, Armando Ugo Cavallo, and Sanjay Rajagopalan

Volumetric data acquisition with multidetector computed tomography (MDCT) has enabled the development of computed tomographic angiography (CTA), a diagnostic modality that has revolutionized the diagnosis of vascular disorders. Adequate imaging of the peripheral vascular system during a single acquisition and a single injection of contrast medium became feasible with the introduction of a 4-slice computed tomography (CT) system with a 0.5 second gantry rotation (thinnest collimation 4 × 2.5 mm) in 1998.[1] The introduction of 8-slice CT in 2000 enabled shorter scan times, but did not yet provide improved longitudinal resolution (thinnest collimation 8 × 1.25 mm). The introduction of 16-slice CT made it possible to routinely acquire substantial anatomic volumes with isotropic submillimeter spatial resolution.[2] CT angiographic scans of the peripheral vasculature could now routinely be acquired with 16 × 0.625 mm or 16 × 0.75 mm collimation which provided the level of resolution required to investigate small vessel involvement (<1 mm). Sixty-four–slice CT-systems introduced in 2004 were the next major advance, when two different scanner concepts were introduced by the different vendors. The "volume concept" pursued by General Electric, Philips, and Toshiba aimed at a further increase in volume coverage. Wider detector panels allowed larger coverage in a single rotation. This concept has been pursued with systems, capable of covering 16 cm volume with 256 rows.

The "resolution concept" uses the same physical detector rows in combination with double z-sampling, a refined z-sampling technique enabled by a periodic motion of the focal spot in the z-direction, to simultaneously acquire overlapping slices with the goal of pitch-independent increase of longitudinal resolution and reduction of spiral artifacts. With this approach the number of slices doubles, but the total width of the detector panel does not change thus obviating cone beam artifact and image noise.[3] Although clearly advantageous in coronary imaging, these have provided advantages for vascular imaging including arterial phase imaging and diagnosis of vascular disorders such as dissection and arteriovenous malformations. Furthermore, dual energy CT and spectral CT have added additional possibilities for further tissue characterization.

This chapter discusses the basic principles of MDCT and provides an overview of its application in vascular diseases. Image interpretation methods have also evolved with routine postprocessing methods for image display, analysis, and quantitation. These methods will be discussed as well as the strengths and weaknesses of CTA, including radiation dose concerns.

FUNDAMENTALS OF COMPUTED TOMOGRAPHY IMAGING

Major Components of a Computed Tomography Scanner

The major components of a CT scanner are an x-ray tube and generator, a collimator, and photon detectors. These components are mounted on a rotating gantry which produces the x-rays necessary for imaging. The predetector collimator helps shape the beams that emanate from the x-ray tube in order to cut out unnecessary radiation. The detectors consist of multiple rows of detector elements (>900 elements per row in the current scanners), which receive x-ray photons that have traversed through the patient, with the postdetector collimators preventing backscatter which degrades image quality. The newer scanners have as many as 320 detector rows and the width of each detector ("detector collimation") has decreased from 2.5 mm in 4-slice systems to 0.5 mm. The most important benefit of increasing the detector rows is the increased coverage per gantry rotation (a 320-row detector CT with a detector width of 0.5 mm will have 160 mm z-axis coverage). The submillimeter detector width improves spatial resolution in the z-axis while increased coverage shortens the scan time. Each detector element contains radiation-sensitive solid state material (such as cadmium tungstate, gadolinium oxide or gadolinium oxysulfide), which converts the absorbed x-rays into visible light.[4] The light is then detected by a silicone photodiode, amplified, and converted into a digital signal. The gantry rotation time determines the temporal resolution of the images with older scanners having a rotation time of 0.75 second while the more contemporary scanners have a rotation time of 0.33 second.[2] The temporal resolution of a single-source scanner, one x-ray generator mounted on the gantry, is slightly higher than half the time it takes for the gantry to rotate 360 degrees. Thus a 0.33 second gantry rotation will effectively provide a temporal resolution of 0.17 second. With a dual-source scanner, two x-ray generators mounted on the gantry, the temporal resolution will improve by a factor of 2.

Computed Tomography Attenuation Data for Image Reconstruction

CT measures the local x-ray attenuation coefficients of the tissue volume elements, or voxels, in an axial slice of the patient's anatomy. The attenuation coefficients are then translated into gray-scale values (CT value) of the corresponding picture elements (pixels) in the displayed two-dimensional image of the slice. The numerical CT value is normalized to the attenuation properties of water and is reported as "Hounsfield units" (HU). Pixel values are stored as integers, in the range–1024 HU to 3071 HU, corresponding to 4096 different gray-scale values. By convention water = 0 HU, air = −1000 HU, and is independent of the x-ray spectrum. The CT values of human tissue, however, depend on the x-ray spectrum. In general, lung and fat have negative CT values, muscle has a positive HU and bone has rather large CT values up to 2000 HU. Administration of iodine contrast agent increases the CT value with contrast-filled vessels typically having CT values in the range 200 HU to 600 HU. In most cases contrast-filled vessels can be easily differentiated from the surrounding tissue, which does not exceed a CT value of 100 HU with the exception of bone. This easy, threshold-based differentiation is the basis for CTA and related image postprocessing techniques. The gantry rotates around the patient collecting attenuation data from different angles. The attenuation coefficient also varies depending on the energy of the photons (measured in keV). The measured intensity of photons at the CT detector is related to the photon flux (number of photons) coming through the x-ray tube and that detected at the detector elements. Consequently, as the attenuation of the tissue increases, the fraction of photons that are detected at the detector element decreases. Photon energy (keV) and photon flux (milliamperes [mA]) are variables that are set by the user. Increasing tube current (mA) will improve image quality at the expense of increasing radiation dose. Certain manufacturers have introduced an "effective" mAs concept for spiral/helical scanning, which incorporates the amount of time the tube current is being generated. Tube voltage (kV) determines the energy of the x-ray beam or the hardness of the x-ray. A higher kV results in a smaller fraction of the x-ray beam being absorbed (reduced attenuation) but will result in improvements in contrast.

Scanning Modes

The two scanning modes used in CT are the axial mode and the spiral/helical mode. The major differences between these modes include (1) differences in table movement during image acquisition, (2) differences in assignment of data to each channel, and (3) need for interpolation for data reconstruction. Each mode has its benefits; however, the mode used for vascular CTA is the spiral/helical mode. For coronary CTA, there has been a shift toward using the axial mode due to its benefit in significantly reducing radiation exposure.

Spiral/Helical

During spiral scanning, there is continuous table movement while x-rays are generated the entire time; however, the tube current can be made to fluctuate. Since the table is moving during the acquisition, the detector channels are not dedicated to a slice position of the patient and hence it receives data from multiple contiguous slices of the patient. An interpolation algorithm is necessary to reconstruct "virtual" axial slices with some loss in image quality. Spiral imaging is fast and can provide infinite reconstruction of data, however at the cost of higher radiation.

Beam Pitch

Pitch is an expression of the relationship between the table distance moved per gantry rotation and the coverage of the scanner. Pitch = (table feed per gantry rotation [mm]/coverage [mm]). If the pitch is 1 then there would be no gaps between the data set; however, if the pitch is greater than 1, gaps would be present, and if the pitch is less than 1 there would be overlap in the data acquisition. The pitch for electrocardiographic (ECG) gated cardiac scanning is typically 0.2–0.3, whereas for vascular CT the pitch ranges between 0.5–1.2.

General Acquisition Parameters

The selection of the specific acquisition parameters of imaging depends on the employed scanner model, the patient's body habitus, and the clinical question. The two main adjustable parameters are the tube voltage and current. The voltage is typically set at 120 kV although 100 kV provides acceptable images with significantly reduced radiation and can be employed in most individuals for vascular imaging who are not obese. Tube current is usually 200–300 mA and again can be adjusted upward if the patient is very large. Breath-holding is required for chest and abdomen CTA acquisitions in order to reduce motion artifact. In MDCT spiral scans, the volume coverage speed (v, cm/s) can be estimated by the following formula:

$$v = \frac{M s_{coll} p}{t_{rot}}$$

where M = number of simultaneous acquired slices, s_{coll} = collimated slice-width, p = pitch, and t_{rot} = gantry rotation time. Although current

generation scanners offer improved spatial resolution, their increased coverage and rotation speeds pose the risk of "out-running" the bolus of contrast in CTA applications. Accordingly, adjustments in both the pitch and the gantry rotation speed must be made to achieve a table translation speed of no more than 30–32 mm/s for CTA applications. In a 64-slice scanner, this usually is achieved by a reduction in t_{rot} to 0.5 second and a decrease in pitch to ≤0.8.

Electrocardiogram Gating

ECG gating is a method of gating imaging events to portions in the cardiac cycle where motion may be minimal, namely diastole. ECG gating is indispensable for coronary imaging and vascular structures that are prone to cardiac motion artifact such as the ascending aorta. The two most common ECG gating methods are retrospective and prospective gating. With traditional spiral scanning the ECG gating is performed retrospectively where the data and ECG information are acquired and subsequent reconstructions can be performed at various time points in the R-R interval.[5] Compared to prospective ECG gating, which is the method used for axial scanning, the scan is triggered at the R wave and image acquisition occurs at a fixed point in the cardiac cycle. However with recent advances in CT imaging, it is also now possible to perform a prospective ECG triggered helical scan using high pitch with extremely low radiation exposure.[6] These have been referred to as "flash" scans and are gaining significant popularity for coronary imaging.

Contrast Administration

All angiographic x-ray contrast remains in the extracellular space and rapidly distributes between the intravascular and extravascular spaces immediately after intravenous administration.[7] It is the process during the early phase of rapid contrast distribution and redistribution that determines the vascular enhancement. Vascular enhancement differs significantly from parenchymal (soft tissue) enhancement characteristics. The two key components that determine arterial enhancement are the amount of contrast per unit time (mL/s) and the duration of administration (seconds). The resulting product of the two is the volume of contrast (flow rate × duration). For example, 100 mL of contrast media given at 5 mL/s will require 20 seconds to deliver. The relationship between flow rate, volume of contrast, and duration of administration is the most important concept to understanding injection protocols for vascular imaging.

Currently, low- or iso-osmolar nonionic contrast agents are the most commonly used for CTA. It is imperative to assess renal function prior to administration of contrast so decisions can be made in regard to prophylactic measures, type of contrast used, and whether the study should be cancelled. The contrast is given intravenously using a power injector. Since contrast arrival time to the region of interest may vary, appropriate timing needs to be determined by using a test bolus or automated bolus tracking technique.[8] The less commonly used technique of using a test bolus is performed by giving a small dose of contrast material and determining the time it takes for the region of interest to opacify. More commonly, a triggered or automated bolus tracking technique is used where a region of interest is drawn on the aorta closest to the area of interest. A repetitive low-dose acquisition is acquired 5 to 10 seconds after contrast administration until an HU threshold is achieved (typically 110 HU). The actual CTA will be acquired once this threshold is obtained. The typical volume of contrast used is 100–120 mL with an iodine concentration between 320–370 mg/mL administered at a rate of 4 mL/s followed by a saline flush.

Contrast Considerations

Although MDCT angiography uses substantially lower contrast volumes compared with prior generations of CT, the inherent nephrotoxicity of contrast media must be considered, especially in individuals with preexisting renal dysfunction (e.g., diabetes mellitus, chronic kidney disease). For these individuals, except in emergency situations, creatinine clearance should be determined before scheduling the patient. An allergy to iodinated contrast material is a major contraindication for performing contrast CT studies. However, based on the severity of previous contrast reactions, an assessment may be made whether the study can be safely performed after premedication with oral steroids and antihistamines. Fasting is not mandatory except for patients with previous contrast-induced gastrointestinal reactions.

Image Reconstruction at the Scanner Console

There are various image reconstruction filters offered by each manufacturer. Filters are referred to as "sharp" or "soft" filters. Sharper reconstruction filters will provide more details but also more noise and are best for assessment of stents and areas of calcification. Softer reconstruction filters provide less image detail but less noise as well. Soft to medium filters are usually used for most CTA applications. Image reconstruction can also be performed at different cardiac phases of cardiac gated acquisitions. It may be important in assessment of coronary anatomy in cases of thoracic aortic dissection and thoracic aortic aneurysms.[9] This is most important for cardiac CTA where coronary anatomy may need to be assessed at different phases to ensure accurate delineation of coronary stenosis. When ECG gated thoracic aortic imaging is performed, various phases can be reconstructed to assess the aorta.

Slice width and slice increment used for image reconstruction at the scanner console depends on the anatomy being assessed and scanner capabilities. Reconstruction thickness for vascular imaging can be performed at the same width (thin) or several times the detector width (thick) to reduce noise. Thinner slices are associated with higher image noise compared to thicker slices and take longer time to review. A slice increment of approximately 50% of the slice thickness is typically used.

Image Postprocessing

Similar to vascular magnetic resonance angiography (MRA) (see Chapter 13), multiple postprocessing techniques can be used in vascular CTA to assess the hundreds to thousands of images that are generated. Usually two data sets are reconstructed including "thick" and "thin" sets. The thick set (5.0 mm) is used for general assessment, whereas the thin set (0.5–0.75 mm) is better suited for detailed evaluation. Image formats used for evaluation include (1) multiplanar reformats (MPR), (2) maximal intensity projections (MIP), (3) curved planer reformats (CPR), (4) volume rendering (VR), and (5) shaded surface display (SSD). (See Chapter 13 for a description of these techniques.) For CTA, the evaluation of the data set begins with review of the axial images to assess gross anatomy and scan quality. A MIP format is used to view the vascular structure of interest in the traditional projections as well as in oblique orientations. A major caveat is the presence of calcium when viewing MIP images, as it can overestimate the severity of stenosis. For detailed evaluation, especially when calcium and/or stents are present, the raw MPR images need to be reviewed. Curved planar reconstruction is a unique technique that makes it possible to follow the course of any single vessel and displays it in a nontraditional plane where the entire vessel can be seen in a single image. 3D-VR images can also be reviewed to get a general appreciation of the anatomic variations if necessary. Each of these reconstruction methods has its pitfalls and it is important to develop a systematic process to identify and evaluate an abnormality.

RADIATION EXPOSURE AND RADIATION DOSE REDUCTION

Radiation exposure of the patient by CT and the resulting potential radiation hazard has gained considerable attention both in the public and in the scientific literature.[10-13] Radiation exposure is defined as the total charge of ions produced in a unit of dry air by a given amount of x-ray or γ-ray radiation. In the International System of Units (SI), exposure is measured in terms of Coulombs (C)/kg or amperes (A) seconds/kg. Exposure is also commonly measured in units of roentgens, where 1 roentgen (R) equals 2.58×10^{-4} C/kg. Absorbed dose is the energy imparted to a volume of matter by ionizing radiation, divided by the mass of the matter. The SI unit of absorbed dose is the gray (Gy), where 1 Gy equals 1 J/kg. The traditional unit is the rad, short for radiation absorbed dose, which equals 1 cGy or 10^{-2} Gy. While absorbed dose is a useful concept, the biological effect of a given absorbed dose varies depending on the type and quality of radiation emitted. A dimensionless radiation-weighting factor is used to normalize for this effect, where the weighting factor ranges from 1 for photons (including x-rays and γ rays) and electrons to 20 for α particles. A special SI unit to represent the equivalent dose, the Sievert (Sv), was adopted to avoid confusion with absorbed dose. One Sv equals 1 J/kg. The traditional unit for equivalent dose is the rem, short for roentgen equivalent man. One rem equals 1 cSv, that is 10^{-2} Sv. Equivalent dose multiplied by the tissue-weighting factor is often termed weighted equivalent dose, properly measured in Sv or rem. The sum of the weighted equivalent dose over all organs or tissues in an individual is termed the effective dose (E).

Computed Tomography Specific Dosimetry

In addition to the nomenclature for radiation dosimetry described above, a particular set of terms has been developed for CT.[14,15] The dose profile (D[z]) for a CT scanner is a mathematical description of the dose as a function of position on the z axis (perpendicular to the tomographic plane). The CT dose index (CTDI), measured in units of Gy, is the area under the radiation dose profile for a single rotation and fixed table position along the axial direction of the scanner, divided by the total nominal scan width or beam collimation. CTDI is difficult to measure and therefore not commonly reported. Instead, the CTDI 100 is measured. CTDI 100 represents the integrated radiation exposure from acquiring a single scan over a length of 100 mm. To estimate the average radiation dose to a cross-section of a patient's body, a weighted CTDI ($CTDI_w$) is calculated. This is determined by the equation:

$$CTDI_w = \frac{2}{3} CTDI_{100} \text{ at periphery} + \frac{1}{3} CTDI_{100} \text{ at center}$$

$CTDI_w$, given in mGy, is always measured in an axial scan mode and depends on scanner geometry, slice collimation, and beam prefiltration as well as x-ray tube voltage, tube current (mA), and gantry rotation time (t_{rot}). The product of mA and t_{rot} is the mAs-value of the scan. To obtain a parameter characteristic for the scanner used, it is helpful to eliminate the mAs-dependence and to introduce a *normalized* $(CTDI_w)_n$ given in mGy per mAs:

$$CTDI_w = mA \times t_{rot} \times (CTDI_w)_n = mAs \times (CTDI_w)_n$$

The important CT-specific dosimetry term is the *volume weighted CTDI*, or $CTDI_{vol}$. This quantity represents the average radiation dose over the volume scanned in a helical or sequential sequence. It is determined from the $CTDI_w$ by the equation:

$$CTDI_{vol} = CTDI_w / \text{pitch} = CTDI_w \cdot$$
$$\text{total nominal scan width} / \text{distance between scans.}$$

$CTDI_{vol}$ is used to determine the *dose-length product (DLP)*, measured in units of mGy · cm. *DLP* reflects the integrated radiation dose for a complete CT examination, and is calculated by:

$$DLP = CTDI_{vol} \cdot \text{length irradiated.}$$

Many CT scanner consoles report the $CTDI_{vol}$ and DLP for a study. DLP can be related to E by the formula:

$$E = E_{DLP} \times DLP$$

where E_{DLP}, measured in units of mSv/(mGy · cm), is a body region-specific conversion factor. The most commonly used E_{DLP} values are reported in the 2004 CT Quality Criteria.[16] These E_{DLP} values are determined using Monte Carlo methods, averaged for multiple scanners.

Dose Reduction Techniques

There are several ways to lower the dose delivered to a patient.[15,17] These methods can be used either in isolation or combined to lower the exposure exponentially. Reducing tube current will lead to a direct reduction in the radiation dose to a patient. However, a conscious decision needs to be made on whether the trade off on radiation reduction outweighs image quality. This becomes very important in obese patients where the reduction in tube current may result in rather poor images. The contrast to noise ratio increases with decreasing x-ray tube voltage.[6] As a consequence, to obtain the adequate contrast to noise ratio, the dose to the patient may be reduced by lowering the kV setting. There is nearly a 50% reduction in the radiation exposure when using 80 kV instead of 120 kV when performing CTA. A recent study recommends 100 kV as the standard mode for aortoiliac CTA and reports dose savings of 30% without loss of diagnostic information.[18]

ECG-controlled dose modulation is a method that is employed during continuous imaging with retrospective studies. Typically, the output is kept at its nominal value during a user-defined phase (in general the mid- to end-diastolic phase) while during the rest of the cardiac cycle, the tube output is reduced to 20% of its nominal value to allow for image reconstruction throughout the entire cardiac cycle. Using this technique, dose reduction of 30% to 50% has been demonstrated in clinical studies.[19–23]

Anatomical tube current modulation is a technique adapted to the patient geometry during each rotation of the gantry. The tube output is modulated on the basis of the tissue attenuation characteristics of the localizer scan or determined online by evaluating the signal of a detector row. By employing such a technique, dose can be reduced by 15% to 35% without degrading image quality depending on the body region.[24] A more sophisticated variation of anatomic tube current modulation varies the tube output according to the patient geometry in the longitudinal direction in order to maintain adequate dose when moving to different body regions, for instance from thorax to abdomen (automatic exposure control). Automatic adaptation of the tube current to patient size prevents both over- and under-irradiation, considerably simplifies the clinical workflow for the technician, and eliminates the need to look up tables of patient weight and size for adjusting the mAs settings.

EMERGING TECHNOLOGIES IN COMPUTED TOMOGRAPHY

Dual Energy Computed Tomography

Within the last few years, certain technological advancements have occurred including dual energy and spectral CT. Standard CT contains a polychromatic range of x-ray photon energies. Lower level photons exhibit the photoelectric effect while higher energy levels produce the Compton effect. The photoelectric process predominates when lower energy photons interact with materials of high atomic number and Compton scattering predominates at higher photon energies with materials of lower atomic numbers.[25]

Spectral CT or dual energy CT takes advantage of different x-ray photon energy levels to highlight differences in tissue properties.[26] Several photon energies can be used, but typically a low and high energy profile are utilized to highlight differences in tissue attenuation (80 kVp vs. 140 kVp and hence "dual energy"). Siemens provides a dual source-detection scanner that operates at two different energy levels. General Electric provides a single source detector that switches between high and low tube potentials, while Phillips provides a single x-ray source that operates at a constant polychromatic range and that uses a double layer of detectors to produce both low and high energy images.

Spectral Computed Tomography

Spectral detector CT (IQon, Philips Healthcare) can provide numerous new applications for vascular imaging. Virtual monoenergetic images can illustrate different tissue attenuation properties depending on the photon energy selected. Low monoenergetic images improve the appearance of vasculature by increasing the attenuation of iodinated contrast.[27] In fact, CT numbers of iodine are 70% higher in 80 kVp images compared to those acquired at 140 kVp.[28] Higher monoenergetic images lead to less beam hardening artifact, which aid in the examination of bone and calcium within various structures. Iodine maps can be created between known material pairs, usually iodine and water, and this allows for a new way to illustrate tissue composition beyond just attenuation values. In fact, effective atomic number images based on the properties of the tissue in relation to the high and low spectrum can be generated. These maps are constructed from pixels that equal the effective atomic number of the tissue (the z value) and can be displayed as gray or color scale images. Finally, such technology allows for the ability to create virtual noncontrast images by removing the iodine from the contrast study, thereby obviating the need for a noncontrast preliminary scan.[27]

Spectral CT can allow for improved vascular enhancement at lower contrast loads without compromising image quality. Such technology would aid elderly or chronic kidney disease patients in terms of reducing their risk for contrast induced nephropathy. Such a technology may prove useful for preprocedural planning of complex vascular procedures where patient demographics may indicate high or prohibitive risk.[29] In CT pulmonary embolism (PE) studies, iodine or effective atomic maps may be able to display smaller perfusion defects to improve the sensitivities.

Given the advantage of lower contrast use, the technology has been pursued in examinations for peripheral artery disease. Images using normal contrast volume compared to those on a spectral CT scanner with lower contrast volume revealed less attenuation and improved signal-to-noise ratio and contrast-to-noise ratio. The reconstructions at 65 keV yielded the best results and the radiation dose between the cohorts was not statistically different.[30] Furthermore, for peripheral stents, reconstructions at 72 keV with 50% adaptive iterative reconstructions for common iliac, external iliac, and superficial femoral artery stents when compared to conventional CTA protocols adds information without any significant increase in radiation.[31] This added information comes without any significant increase in radiation.[32] Information such as the different monochromatic energies, iodine maps, effective atomic number maps, and virtual noncontrast images are reconstructed from the scanner's standard polychromatic range. Hence such technology will allow to decrease phases of a multiphase scan and perhaps save suboptimal scans without the need for repeating.[26]

ARTIFACTS AND PITFALLS OF COMPUTED TOMOGRAPHIC ANGIOGRAPHY

There are several artifacts that can been seen with CT imaging. Artifacts include those that are patient related, procedure related, or reconstruction related. Three of the most common artifacts include motion artifact, beam hardening, and partial volume effects. Motion artifacts occur due to body motion during scanning or inability to hold breath. Beam hardening artifacts occur due to the passage of photons through structures such as pacemaker leads, metal clips, or calcium, resulting in lower energy photons being filtered out. As a consequence, dark areas are created next to these structures, which can affect assessment of lumen patency. Partial volume effects occur when parts of the voxel of a structure are affected by other structures with different attenuation properties. This results in averaging of the CT values for that voxel. As a consequence the image appears distorted. The most frequent artifact that affects interpretation of the CTA is deviation from vascular segments affected by moderate-to-severe calcification or occupied by a stent. The selection of the adequate windowing set (~1500 window width) may reduce the unavoidable blooming effect caused by structures with high signal attenuation. Cross-sectional MPR images of the vessel of interest are helpful in visualizing, at least in part, the underlying lumen in the presence of intense calcification or a stent. Other interpretation pitfalls such as pseudo-stenoses or pseudo-occlusions may potentially be generated by inadequate image postprocessing (e.g., partial or total vessel removal during MIP image editing and inaccurate centerline definition in CPR images).

CLINICAL APPLICATIONS OF COMPUTED TOMOGRAPHIC ANGIOGRAPHY IN VASCULAR DISEASE

Computed Tomographic Angiography of the Neurovascular Circulation

Technical Considerations

CTA is comparable to digital subtraction angiography (DSA) for the measurement of residual carotid artery stenosis and is the preferred method of assessment at many institutions.[33-35] To perform CTA of the head and neck arteries, the patient is placed in the supine position with the arms along the sides of the body. The topogram is used to assist planning of the imaging volume, which should start from the aortic arch and end at the level of the circle of Willis. A submillimeter detector collimation is required for images with the greatest spatial resolution in the z axis. A test bolus or bolus tracking algorithm can be used to determine the start of the scan. The pitch can range from 0.5 to 1.0 depending on the vendor and the number of detector rows. Breath-holding and cessation of swallowing are critical to eliminate motion artifacts. Reconstruction is performed with smooth reconstruction kernels using a slice thickness between 0.6 and 1.0 mm, and a 50% to 80% reconstruction increment is typically used for the assessment of the carotid circulation.

Attention to the appropriate window settings will have significant impact on measured variances in luminal contrast density. Differences in the measured residual lumen and beam-hardening from calcified plaque will overestimate the degree of stenosis. To avoid this problem a simple formula may be used to calculate the optimal window settings for the assessment of carotid stenosis with CTA.[36] The window width used is the product of the intraluminal HU × 2.07, and the window level is the product of the intraluminal HU × 0.72. The degree of stenosis should be reported in terms of percent stenosis or residual luminal area. Percent stenosis is defined as the ratio of the maximal luminal narrowing to the normal internal carotid artery distal to the bulb as was described in the North American Symptomatic Carotid Endarterectomy Trial (NASCET).[37] However, the segment of normal internal carotid artery measurement can range from 5 to 8 mm, which will affect the calculated degree of stenosis. This can be averted by using the residual luminal diameter instead of the percent stenosis,[38-42] or using a simple visual estimation of the degree of stenosis rather than using a caliper-based method.[43] The current standard is using the percent stenosis measurement based on NASCET; however, there are papers describing the use of residual lumen diameter, where 1.5 mm

is used as the cutoff for hemodynamically significant stenosis, which correlates with an ultrasound peak systolic velocity of >250 cm/s and a NASCET measurement of >70% stenosis.[44]

If the clinical question is whether there is a total or subtotal internal carotid occlusion, an immediate delayed acquisition through the neck is helpful in the detection of slow opacification through a residual lumen. It is important to be aware that sometimes, the ascending pharyngeal artery may mimic a subtotally occluded internal carotid artery. This is easily differentiated by the fact that the ascending pharyngeal artery does not reach the skull base, whereas the internal carotid artery will. Accurate distinction is critically important, as a subtotally stenosed internal carotid artery may be amenable to revascularization.[45-47]

Clinical Application

Atherosclerotic and Nonatherosclerotic Disease

Technical advances in CTA have allowed unprecedented imaging for a number of neurovascular applications, including the evaluation for carotid artery stenosis, acute ischemic and hemorrhagic stroke, intracranial vascular anomalies, or craniocervical trauma. By far the most common indication for CTA of the extracranial circulation is for suspected carotid artery stenosis due to atherosclerosis (Fig. 14.1). CTA is also part of the comprehensive evaluation of the patient with an acute stroke where nonenhanced brain CT, vascular angiography, and perfusion imaging can be acquired during the comprehensive CT examination. Nonatherosclerotic diseases such as fibromuscular dysplasia (FMD), aneurysms or pseudoaneurysms, or dissections also can be imaged with high spatial resolution (Fig. 14.2). Additionally, CTA has a unique role in the follow-up after carotid artery stenting procedures (see Fig. 14.1) instead of using MRA, which typically has significant susceptibility artifacts.

Performance of Computed Tomographic Angiography in the Diagnosis of Carotid Disease

MDCT has shown a 100% correlation with invasive angiography for the location of significant stenosis.[33,48] The interobserver agreement in evaluating total versus subtotal occlusion, stenosis length, retrograde internal carotid artery flow, and the location of the stenotic site is 1.0, 0.94, 0.86, and 0.89 respectively.[33,48] Additionally MDCT is helpful in identifying the underlying etiology such as dissection, atherosclerosis, or thrombosis. Berg et al. studied 35 consecutive, symptomatic patients with cerebrovascular disorders such as minor stroke, transient ischemic attack, amaurosis fugax, and dizziness, and performed MDCT angiography.[33] The main focus of the study was the comparison of MDCT to conventional x-ray DSA and rotational DSA as reference standards. In this study, the degree of stenosis was slightly underestimated with CTA, with mean differences (± standard deviation) per observer of 6.9% ± 17.6% and 10.7% ± 16.1% for cross-sectional and 2.8% ± 19.2% and 9.1% ± 16.8% for oblique sagittal MPRs compared with x-ray and rotational angiography, respectively. CTA was somewhat inaccurate for measuring the absolute minimal diameter of subtotally occluded carotid arteries. For symptomatic lesions, interactive CTA interpretation combined with MPR measurements of lesions with a visual estimate of ≥50% diameter narrowing had a sensitivity of 95% and specificity of 93% for the detection of carotid stenosis compared with DSA. Certain imaging characteristics of the carotid arteries on CTA can illustrate further downstream events. In a recent meta-analysis, soft plaque, plaque ulceration, and increased common carotid artery wall thickness was associated with ipsilateral cerebrovascular ischemia, while calcified plaques had a negative association with downstream events.[49]

Carotid arteries CTA is also a valid tool in the follow-up of patients with carotid atherosclerosis to estimate plaque progression and assess

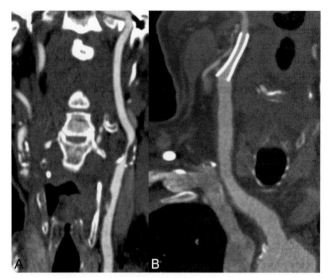

Fig. 14.1 Carotid Artery Atherosclerosis. Curved planar reformation from the left carotid artery shows significant stenosis and noncalcified plaque with minor calcifications at the bifurcation, and hemodynamically insignificant but ulcerated plaque at the common carotid artery (A), and a widely patent right carotid artery stent (B). (Modified from Berg M, Kangasniemi M, Manninen H, Vanninen RL. CT angiography of the extracranial and intracranial circulation with imaging protocols. In: Mukherjee D, Rajagopalan S, eds. CT and MR Angiography of the Peripheral Circulation. Boca Raton, FL: CRC Press; 2007:67.)

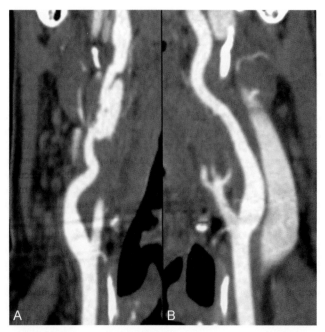

Fig. 14.2 Carotid Artery Pseudoaneurysm. Curved planar reformation of the right carotid artery shows a large pseudoaneurysm (A) of the right internal carotid with normal-appearing left common and internal carotid artery (B).

ischemic cerebrovascular events risk. Moreover, this technique allows a good definition of plaque surface and eventual ulceration, enabling assessment of plaque vulnerability.[50,51]

Although MDCT angiography is a very effective noninvasive means of assessing the cervicocranial circulation, there are multiple limitations that may occasionally limit its usefulness. CTA does not include flow dynamics. Calcification in segments can obscure the lumen

due to blooming artifact and lead to overestimation of stenosis severity. Surgical clips also can preclude accurate assessment. The radiation dose of neurovascular CTA is between 1.7 mSv and 3.0 mSv depending on the imaged volume, the type of scanner, and the use of radiation reduction algorithms. There may be overlapping veins that prevent detection of small cerebral artery aneurysms.

Computed Tomographic Angiography of the Thorax

Computed Tomographic Angiography of the Pulmonary Artery: Technical Consideration and Clinical Applications

PE is the third most common cause of cardiovascular death in the United States, following ischemic heart disease and stroke, with an estimated annual incidence of 300,000 to 600,000 cases per year.[52] Even though there is a high prevalence of PE, it continues to be under diagnosed, with only 43 to 53 patients per 100,000 being accurately identified.[53]

CT of the pulmonary arteries (CTPA) is the current diagnostic test of choice for the assessment of pulmonary thromboembolic disease (see Chapter 51). In the PIOPED-II study, CTPA was principally performed on 4-slice CT with a slice thickness of 1–1.25 mm.[54] In this study, the overall positive predictive value in diagnosing PE was 86% (97% for proximal, 68% for segmental, and 25% for subsegmental thrombus), and the negative predictive value was 95%.[54] The value of CTPA varied with the clinical pretest probability of PE; in patients with high or intermediate clinical probability, the positive predictive value for PE was 96%. However, in the face of low clinical pretest likelihood, 42% of patients had a false-positive CTPA result. Therefore a positive CTPA that was discordant with clinical data had little diagnostic value at least on the basis of this study. There are randomized controlled studies using later generation CT scanners that have addressed the issue of their superiority over 4-slice systems used in PIOPED-II.[55–57] The expectation is that thinner detectors and larger detector assemblies would allow rapid imaging of the pulmonary artery and branches in a few seconds avoiding motion artifact.

To perform a CTPA, the patient is placed supine with the hands above the head. Following the topogram, the field of view is prescribed to include the adrenals to the lung apices. The goal is to acquire the study with the thinnest slice collimation with a single short breath hold in full-suspended respiration. The voltage, current, and pitch will vary depending on vendor and patient characteristics. There are two main methods for image acquisition: timing bolus and bolus tracking techniques. In the timing bolus technique, a region of interest is placed in the pulmonary trunk and repeated scans are acquired at the same level repeatedly. A time density curve is obtained allowing for calculation of the scan delay. The alternate approach is using an automated bolus tracking technique, where a region of interest is placed over the pulmonary trunk and the image acquisition initiates once a specified attenuation threshold is achieved. The pulmonary arteries are imaged with the first pass of intravenous contrast, while the pelvis and lower extremity veins are can be imaged later with a scan delay of 2.5 to 3.5 minutes. There are multiple artifacts that can limit the detection of true pulmonary emboli and hence careful scrutiny of the acquired images with active scrolling in and out of each main, lobar, segmental, and subsegmental artery is necessary, to avoid overcalling or missing pulmonary emboli. Similarly CT venography of the proximal lower extremities is difficult to interpret and suffers from several technical limitations, such as flow artifacts from suboptimal timing of contrast, arterial inflow contamination, streak artifacts from orthopedic hardware, arterial calcification, or dense contrast within the bladder.

The CTPA findings of acute PE can be divided into arterial findings and ancillary findings. Intraluminal filling defects may partially

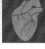

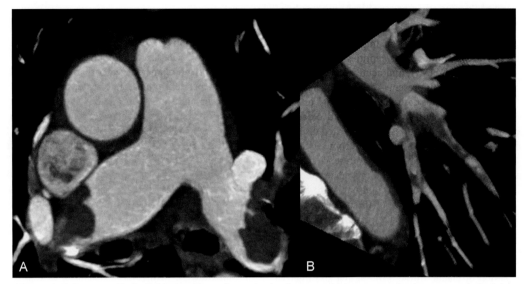

Fig. 14.3 Pulmonary Emboli. Maximal intensity projection images with large central pulmonary emboli of the left and right main pulmonary artery (PA) (A) and subsegmental emboli involving the branches of the left PA (B).

or completely occlude a pulmonary artery and typically cause significant dilation of the vessel. Acute emboli typically appear as adherent intravascular filling defects that form acute angles to the vessel wall, whereas chronic thrombi have the appearance of mural adherent thrombi contiguous with the vessel wall. Acute pulmonary emboli which straddle the bifurcation of the left and right pulmonary arteries are referred to as "saddle emboli" (Fig. 14.3). Lung infarcts, atelectasis, and oligemia of the affected territory are common lung parenchymal findings with a PE. CTPA examinations should have optimized window settings, where the window width is equal to the mean attenuation of the pulmonary artery plus 2 standard deviations, and the window level should be half this value. Active scrolling in and out each main, lobar, segmental, and subsegmental artery avoids confusion with veins or mucous-filled bronchi. MPR and MIP of the pulmonary arteries can be used to improve reader confidence for subtle or questionable findings; however improved diagnostic accuracy has not been proven.[58,59] An important fact to keep in mind while interpreting a CTPA study is that most pulmonary emboli are larger than 1 to 2 mm. Therefore, filling defects seen on only a 1.25 mm image are more likely to be an artifact rather than true emboli. Pulmonary emboli typically originate from the pelvic and lower extremity deep venous anatomy. Less commonly, the source of emboli will be from the thorax, such as the superior vena cava or brachiocephalic veins likely as a complication from indwelling catheters.

Computed Tomographic Venography Findings of Acute Deep Venous Thrombosis

The usual findings of a pelvic or proximal lower extremity deep venous thrombosis is a partial or complete intravenous filling defect. There is commonly associated generalized leg and perivenous edema seen on the acquired images.[60]

Computed Tomography of the Pulmonary Arteries Predictors of Patient Outcome

There are many CTPA findings that give powerful prognostic information. These include the presence of right ventricular dilatation, interventricular septal flattening suggesting significant right ventricular pressure overload, and reflux of contrast into the inferior vena cava all of which may result from a massive acute PE. The short axis diameter ratio of the right to left ventricles of 1 to 1.5 or greater is an indicator for severe right ventricular strain and carries a poor prognosis.[61] A right to left ventricular diameter ratio of >0.9 in a 4-chamber view is associated with increased 30-day mortality, cardiopulmonary resuscitation, ventilator support, and the use of vasopressors.[62]

Other clinical applications of CTPA include assessment of pulmonary artery aneurysms and pseudoaneurysms, congenital anomalies such as pulmonary artery atresia, palliative shunts, arteriovenous malformations, and pre-procedure planning for percutaneous pulmonary valve replacement or stenting of branch pulmonary artery stenosis.

Computed Tomographic Angiography of the Thoracic Aorta

Technical considerations. The development of 16-slice multidetector CTA and beyond has granted the ability to acquire nearly isotropic submillimeter images within seconds. The standard protocol for acute aortic pathology should include pre-contrast CT to assess whether intramural hematoma (IMH) is present or if there is blood, which is high density, within the pericardium, pleural space, or mediastinum, indicating aortic rupture. Pre-contrast CT is performed with a low dose technique using 1.5 mm collimation, to reduce the total radiation dose.[63,64] While the scan range of the pre-contrast CT should be restricted to an area from the lung apex to the upper abdomen, the contrast-enhanced CT portion should cover from the thoracic inlet to the femoral head.[65] A bolus tracking method using an HU of 100 with a scan delay of 5 to 7 seconds followed by a saline chaser to minimize venous contamination is the ideal method to obtain contrast-enhanced CTA images.[64] Adequate opacification of the entire aorta is achieved by administering the contrast material at least as long as the scan time plus the delay time. For example, if the scan time and scan delay time are 15 and 5 seconds, respectively, a 20-second injection of contrast material followed by a 50-mL saline chaser would be sufficient. With 64-slice MDCT and beyond, it is possible to scan the entire aorta with submillimeter collimation (collimation, 0.625 mm; slice thickness, 0.625 mm; reconstruction interval, 0.3 mm) within a single breath-hold, thus making high-resolution 3-dimensional displays possible. Cardiac motion may simulate an intimal flap resembling aortic root dissection, which can be eliminated with the use of an ECG-gated acquisition.[66,67]

Clinical Application of Computed Tomographic Angiography of Thoracic Aorta

Acute aortic syndromes. CTA plays an important role in the assessment of acute aortic syndromes. These entities comprise penetrating aortic ulcerations (PAU), IMH, and acute aortic dissection (AAD) (see Chapter 32). Dissection presents with severe chest and/or back pain with sudden onset that is described as "ripping" or "tearing." This is typically associated with hypertension and older age. However, there are other strong associations with inherited disorders of collagen including Marfan and Ehlers Danlos syndrome. MDCT is the imaging modality of choice for evaluating the presence of AAD. The major advantage of MDCT is its ability to visualize the entire aorta and the branch vessels and its rapid through-put. With MDCT, it is important to discern potential artifacts that are caused by motion of the aortic root and which may simulate an intimal flap. With ECG-gating, motion artifact can be eliminated. This may be important in cases when also assessing coronary patency and left ventricular wall motion.

PAU is the protrusion of plaque through the intima and internal elastic membrane of the aorta. PAU can be seen when the lumen is filled with contrast. It appears as a focal contrast outpouching that may enhance the aortic wall. The most common site of PAU is the middle or lower descending thoracic aorta.[68] PAU needs to be differentiated from a nonpenetrating atheromatous ulcer, where the ulceration is confined within the intima layer. The location of intimal calcification can be helpful in this situation.[69] Atheromatous ulcers overlie the aortic contour and calcified intima, whereas PAU extends beyond this margin.[63,69,70] However, differentiating a calcified mural thrombus, IMH, and PAU can be quite challenging.[71] The natural history of PAU can vary depending on the location.[72–74] The attenuation of the aortic wall

on pre-contrast images can help distinguish acute IMH or PAU with some mural hemorrhage from chronic IMH. Typically, acute IMH has high attenuation (50 to 70 HU), in contrast to lower attenuation with chronic IMH. The size of a PAU has influence on its natural history.[75] PAU depth and diameter greater than 10 mm and 20 mm respectively were independent predictors of extension of IMH or dissection and rupture in one study.[76] In another study, however, no predictors of adverse outcomes were acknowledged except for overt rupture upon presentation.[77] The interval change in diameter on follow up CT may be more important than the size of the PAU on the initial CT exam to determine treatment options or patient prognosis.[68]

The pathogenesis of IMH is not well understood, however hypertension is the major predisposing factor. The two pathophysiologic mechanisms of IMH are spontaneous bleeding into the media from the vasa vasorum and intimal tear with complete thrombosis of the false lumen. More recent studies suggest that most IMH result from an entry tear similar to aortic dissection.[71,78,79] The identification of an intimal tear is often underappreciated on pre-operative CT, but is seen intraoperatively.[71] An IMH is visualized as a crescent or ring shaped region of the aortic wall with characteristic high attenuation.[63,80] In the International Registry of Aortic Dissection (IRAD), the location of the IMH was associated with adverse outcome.[81] A Korean study, however, contradicted the findings of IRAD.[82] A new ulceration on follow-up CT and the progression of IMH to a thickness greater than 11 mm is associated with progression to overt aortic dissection.[83,84]

AAD is easily detected by MDCT and is a first line imaging study for evaluating patients (Fig. 14.4).[70] The Stanford classification is based on the extent of the intimal flap, where type A dissection involves the ascending aorta and type B only involves the descending aorta.[85] Important aspects of the evaluation of AAD include location

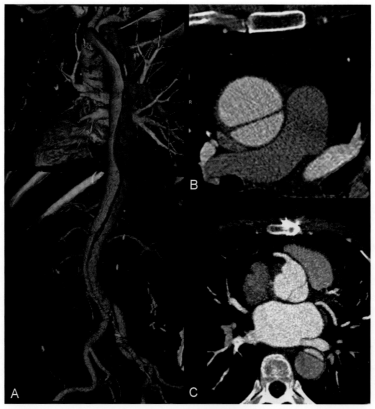

Fig. 14.4 Aortic Dissection. Three-dimension computed tomographic angiography volume-rendered image showing an extensive aortic dissection (A) and maximal intensity projection images in the axial projection depicting ascending (B) and descending (C) dissection propagation.

and extent, site of entry/exit, side branch involvement, presence of aortic rupture, patency of false lumen and associated complications. An inward displacement of intimal calcification can be a sign of aortic dissection on pre-contrast MDCT. Identifying the location of the entry tear is extremely important as this may affect endovascular treatment options. Likewise, reentry tears can be visualized in the descending and abdominal aorta, or iliac arteries.[86] The differentiation between the true and false lumen is extremely important because of the major side branches originating from the false lumen may be occluded after stent graft placement.[70] The dissection flap may directly extend into or obstruct the ostium of an affected side branch vessel. A simple method to differentiate true from false lumen is to identify the communication with uninvolved aortic segment. The larger lumen is typically the false lumen because the pressure in the false lumen is higher than that of the true lumen.[63,70,80] Typically the true lumen has greater opacification with contrast from the higher velocity of blood through the lumen compared to the false lumen.[63,70] The false lumen may also show a beak sign which is the acute angle between the intimal flap and outer false lumen on axial images.[63,70,80] Intraluminal thrombus is much more commonly seen within the false lumen due to the slower flow of blood. Less commonly seen is strands from incompletely torn connective tissue of the aortic media that is also known as the cobweb sign.[87]

Thoracic aortic aneurysms. A true aortic aneurysm is a dilation of the aorta greater than 50% comprising the intima, media, and adventitial layers (see Chapter 36). The aortic root and ascending aorta are affected in nearly 60% of patients with a thoracic aneurysm, the aortic arch in 10%, the descending thoracic aorta in 40%, and the thoracoabdominal aorta in 10% of cases.[88] MDCT can determine the extent, location, and size of the aneurysm. The diameter of the aneurysm should be measured in the true aortic short axis. MDCT also can detect complications such as rupture, infection, and fistulas.

Congenital anomalies of the thoracic aorta. CTA can be used for the assessment of congenital anomalies such as aortic coarctation and anomalous origin of the head and neck vessels. MRA, however, is more useful in this circumstance as it provides additional hemodynamic data that is not possible with CTA. CT has a unique role in assessing the relationship of vascular structures such as main pulmonary artery, ascending aorta, and mammary arteries to the sternum.

Aortitis. CTA also can be used for the assessment of inflammatory diseases that involve the aorta and its proximal branches including giant cell arteritis and Takayasu arteritis. A recent meta-analysis showed that the sensitivity and specificity of CT angiography for the diagnosis of Takayasu arteritis were >90%.[89] Wall thickness can be easily assessed and arterial phase wall enhancement has been at times used as a marker of ongoing inflammatory disease activity.

Computed Tomographic Angiography of the Abdominal Aorta

Technical Considerations

CTA has an important role in abdominal aortic imaging due to its ability to assess intrinsic vessel pathology and branches such as the renal and mesenteric arteries with a high degree of accuracy. The protocols for image acquisition vary significantly based on the clinical question and the CT scanner used for imaging. The patient is placed in the supine position, with imaging collimation placed at the lowest possible setting by the scanner. The scanning volume can range from the upper edge of the 12th rib superiorly to the femoral heads or the iliac crest inferiorly. Scanning is performed in the cranio-caudal direction without cardiac gating. Breath-holding will improve image quality especially of the upper abdominal vessels and is recommended whenever possible. A noncontrast study may be performed using larger collimation to assess for hemorrhage or aortic hematoma. This is followed by a contrast study with triggering at the diaphragmatic or supraceliac aorta. A post contrast study may be performed to evaluate venous anatomy, renal perfusion, or slow bleeding. Images can be reconstructed using a softer filter at submillimeter slice thickness with 50% slice increments.

Clinical Applications

Abdominal Aortic Dissection

The most common cause for dissection of the abdominal aorta and iliac arteries is propagation of a thoracoabdominal aortic dissection. Focal dissection of the abdominal aorta is rare, occurring in only 1.3% of all aortic dissections.[90] A focal dissection is usually associated with hypertension, smoking, diabetes, previous aneurysm surgery, and hyperlipidemia.[91] CTA, in addition to assessing the vasculature, also can provide information on soft tissue structures including complications such as hemorrhage. A noncontrast study may illustrate acute hemorrhage or IMH within an aortic dissection plane and may reveal complications. In addition, a pre-contrast study in conjunction with a post-contrast study, may allow for comparison of subtle changes in thrombus opacification, suggesting a slow bleed. An additional delayed acquisition 1 to 2 minutes post contrast, can help identify slow hemorrhage and venous abnormalities.

Abdominal Aortic Aneurysm

An abdominal aortic aneurysm (AAA) is defined by a greater than 50% enlargement of the abdominal aorta compared to a normal aortic segment, and a less than 50% dilation of the aorta is referred to as ectasia (see Chapter 36).[92,93] Although ultrasound is the preferred screening modality for AAA, CTA is often required to assess the extent and complications of an AAA and to plan treatment.[92] Regardless of the indication for a CTA exam, true short and long axis measurements of the aneurysm need to be reported. The distance between the lower, most renal artery to the superior border of the aneurysm, referred to as the (neck), provides a standardized description of its location. CTA can assess the shape and angulation of the neck, measure the maximal diameter of the AAA, and provide a thorough assessment of the iliac and femoral arteries. These determinations are important especially when consideration is being made for endovascular aneurysm repair (EVAR) (Fig. 14.5). CTA can visualize mural thrombus and calcification within the aneurysm, which have important implications for EVAR (Fig. 14.6) (see Chapter 38). Identifying the number and location of the renal arteries, the presence of a retroaortic left renal vein and assessment of the mesenteric and hypogastric arteries also are important for operative planning.

Surveillance following EVAR: CTA is the modality of choice for the surveillance of patients who have undergone EVAR as it assesses potential complications including endoleaks. A post-stent graft examination consists of pre-contrast, dynamic first circulation imaging, and immediate delayed post-contrast imaging. The pre-contrast study allows identification of calcification so that it is not confused with endoleak. The immediate delayed post-contrast study may identify a slow leaking endoleak which may be missed on the dynamic first circulation study.[94] CTA is used to measure the maximum external dimensions of the aneurysm sac, the lumen of the aortic stent graft along with its two limbs, the distance between the proximal margin of the stent graft and the inferior margin of the most inferior renal artery, and the lower margin of the stent graft and the iliac artery bifurcation of each side.

Endoleaks cause increased pressure within the aneurysm sac and thereby increase the potential for continued aneurysm growth and rupture. A type I endoleak is either a proximal or distal attachment site endoleak, and is usually discovered during implantation. Delayed type I endoleak may be related to changes in tortuosity of the aorta

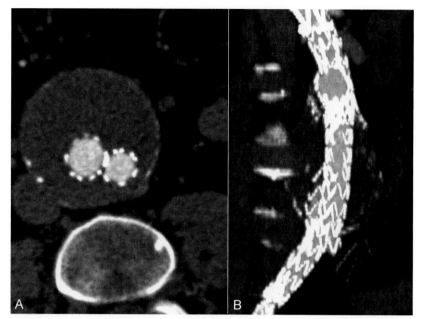

Fig. 14.5 Aortoiliac Composite Stent Graft. Multiplanar projection reformation images depicting the usual appearance of an aortoiliac stent graft in the axial (A) and sagittal oblique views (B).

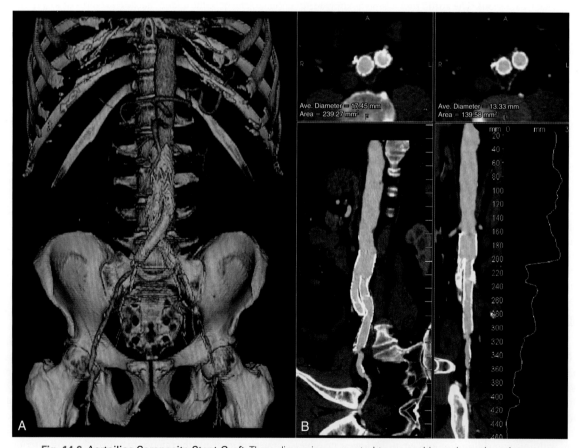

Fig. 14.6 Aortoiliac Composite Stent Graft. Three-dimension computed tomographic angiography volume-rendered image (A) and curved planar reformation (B) showing an aortoiliac stent graft.

secondary to aneurysm reshaping, and should be suspected on CT when acute hemorrhage or contrast pooling is found in the aneurysm sac adjacent to the device attachment site.[95] Type II endoleak, the most common form of endoleak, is caused by continued blood flow into the aneurysm sac through a small arterial branch that is excluded by the stent graft. This type of endoleak resolves spontaneously in most instances and is seen as a small area of contrast opacification within the aneurysm. It is often located at a distance from the graft.[96] Type III endoleak is caused by mechanical disruption of the material of an endograft or by separation of an iliac extender from the main graft. This type of endoleak is considered "high pressure" and carries a high risk for rupture. It appears as a large central collection of contrast, distant from the landing zone of the graft.[97] A type IV endoleak is due to graft porosity, which is often detected near the time of implantation, prior to the endothelialization of the graft conduit. This type of endoleak is self-healing and resolves with cessation of anticoagulation. A type V endoleak is result of endotension from arterial pressurization within the aneurysm sac, and is without an identifiable cause. This is a diagnosis of exclusion after CTA and invasive angiography fail to identify an alternative type of endoleak.[95]

Vasculitis

In the abdomen, CTA also has a role in assessing vascular wall and branch vessel changes associated with large and medium vessel vasculitis, such as Takayasu arteritis and polyarteritis nodosa respectively. There are four subtypes of Takayasu arteritis (see Chapter 40); type I is confined to the aortic arch and branches, type 2 involves the descending thoracic and abdominal aorta, type 3 includes type 1 and 2 components, and type 4 combines type 1, 2, and 3 with pulmonary artery involvement. In patients in the acute stage of vasculitis, CTA findings include thickening and enhancement of the vessel wall. In the chronic form of the disease, there may be arterial stenosis, occlusion, or aneurysm formation.[98]

Renal Artery Disease

The superb isotropic spatial resolution ($0.5 \times 0.5 \times 0.5$ mm) from CTA enables assessment of the renal arteries that is unsurpassed by other imaging modalities. There is approximately 6 seconds between initial renal arterial and venous opacification because of the rapid transit time within the kidney.[99] This requires acquiring images with a very high temporal resolution to decrease the degree of venous contamination. Common applications for CTA of the renal arteries include renal artery stenosis either from atherosclerosis or FMD, acute renal artery occlusion, and renal artery aneurysms (see Chapter 23). Atherosclerotic renal artery disease manifests as a stenosis occurring at the vessel origin or proximal segment (typically within 2 cm of the ostium).[100] FMD often involves the mid to distal renal artery and appears as multiple sequential stenoses ("string of pearls"), and possibly renal artery aneurysm.[101] Acute renal artery occlusion may rapidly lead to renal infarction.[100] The CTA appearance includes occlusion of a renal artery, with or without an intimal flap, the former indicting propagation of dissection. Renal

artery infarction is manifest by wedge-shaped or global perfusion abnormalities. Renal artery aneurysms are rare and are most commonly detected incidentally (Fig. 14.7). The most common cause of renal artery aneurysms is associated with atherosclerosis, but may also be related to FMD, connective tissue disease, mycotic infection, or vasculitis (such as Behçet syndrome and polyarteritis nodosa).[100,102] CTA also has a role in the surveillance of patients after renal artery stenting. The biggest limitation of CTA use is the fact that a large proportion of patients with renal artery disease also have advanced renal dysfunction, hence precluding a contrast-enhanced CTA study.

Mesenteric Artery Disease

CTA is useful in the assessment of mesenteric artery disease, including mesenteric artery aneurysms, dissection, and vasculitis and FMD (Fig. 14.8) (see Chapter 26). Mesenteric artery aneurysms involve

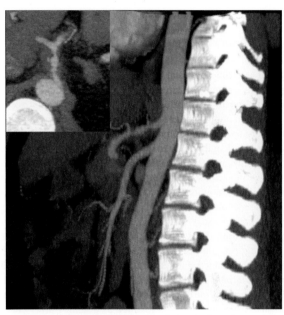

Fig. 14.8 Fibromuscular Dysplasia of the Celiac Artery. Maximal intensity projection images showing proximal fibromuscular dysplasia of the celiac artery in the lateral oblique and axial (inset, upper left) orientations.

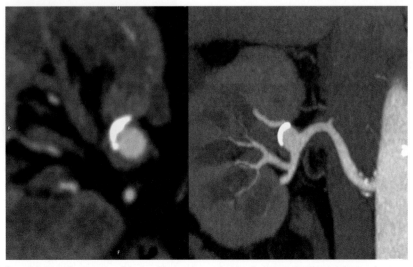

Fig. 14.7 Renal Artery Aneurysm. Maximal intensity projection images of a distal right renal artery aneurysm with peripheral calcification.

the splenic (60%), hepatic (20%), superior mesenteric (5.5%), celiac (4%), pancreatic (2%), and gastroduodenal arteries (1.5%).[103,104] Traditionally, these types of aneurysms were diagnosed by invasive angiography. With the increased speed and resolution of CTA, these aneurysms are increasingly detected noninvasively. Usually, celiac artery and superior mesenteric artery dissections result from propagation of aortic dissection. On CTA, the dissection flap may be visualized in the proximal vessel and may cause complete occlusion. Rarely, spontaneous dissections may occur of the SMA. These have a relatively high mortality rate.[105,106] Stenosis of the celiac axis may be caused by a fibrous band that unites the crura on both sides of the aortic hiatus. This is termed median arcuate ligament syndrome (see Chapter 63). Typically the ligament crosses superior to the origin of the celiac axis, but in some people there is a variant in which it crosses inferiorly and can cause compression of the proximal portion of the celiac axis.[107] This diagnosis is suggested by CTA when there is focal narrowing with a "hook-like" appearance in the proximal celiac axis.

Peripheral Artery Diseases

Technical considerations. Contemporary MDCT scanners are capable of assessing the distal vessels in lower extremities. In order to image vessels <1 mm in diameter, as is the case in pedal vessels, submillimeter detector collimation is necessary. Patients are placed in a supine position on the scanner table in a feet-first orientation. The typical field-of-view should extend from the diaphragm to the toes, with an average scan length of 110 to 130 cm. The scanning protocol begins with a scout image of the entire field of view followed by a test bolus or bolus triggering acquisition. Breath-holding may be necessary for the more proximal abdominal station, but not for the distal stations. This is followed by a contrast-enhanced angiographic acquisition during the arterial contrast phase. With newer scanners, care must be taken to set the gantry rotation times and pitch appropriately to avoid the risk of "out running" the contrast bolus. A second late acquisition of the calf vessels can be obtained in the event of inadequate pedal opacification during the arterial phase. For most CTA applications, 100 to 140 mL of contrast (with an iodine concentration between 350 and 370 mg/mL) is administered at a rate of 4 mL/s followed by a saline flush.[108] Recently a fixed time strategy has been recommended to image peripheral artery disease (PAD) (Table 14.1).[109] In this strategy, the pitch is varied to accomplish a fixed scan time of 40 seconds in all patients. A biphasic injection protocol is used to provide sustained opacification of the arterial system. This approach standardizes PAD imaging protocols and

consistently enables good quality scans. Images are reconstructed using a smooth kernel into one data set of thicker slices at 5.0 mm slice thickness for general assessment, and another data set of thinner slices of 0.6 to 0.75 mm, incorporating a 25% to 50% overlap. When stenosis is present, the determination of severity is typically by visual estimation rather than a computer-based technique. The combination of MIP, CPR, and axial plane imaging will allow the experienced reader to discern mild (0% to 50%), moderate (50% to 70%), and severe (>70%) stenosis.[110,111]

Clinical Application

Atherosclerotic peripheral artery disease. The major indication for CTA in the evaluation of PAD is in the diagnosis and preinterventional evaluation of symptomatic patients (Fig. 14.9) (see Chapter 18). Findings from CTA can assist the decision to use open surgical or endovascular therapy for revascularization.[112] CTA is less useful in patients with tibioperoneal atherosclerotic disease, since these patients are typically diabetic and have heavily calcified vessels that may preclude accurate assessment of the degree of stenosis. A meta-analysis of CTA in PAD including mostly 4-slice systems reported a pooled sensitivity and specificity for detecting a stenosis of greater than 50% per segment of 92% (95% confidence interval [CI] of 89% to 95%) and 93% (95% CI of 91% to 95%), respectively.[113] The diagnostic performance of CTA in the infrapopliteal tract is lower, but not significantly different from that in the aortoiliac and femoropopliteal levels.[113–115] At least

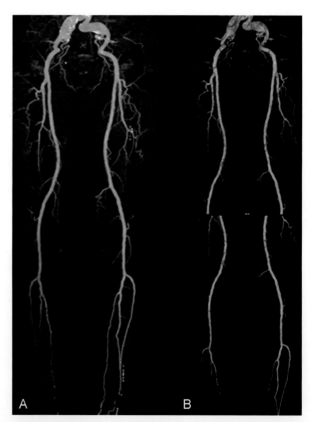

Fig. 14.9 Abdominal Computed Tomographic Angiography With Runoff. Maximal intensity projection (A) and three-dimensional computed tomography angiography volume-rendered (B) images showing bilateral common iliac aneurysms with distal runoff disease of the right lower extremity. (Modified from Cohen EI, Doshi A, Lookstein R. CT angiography of the lower extremity circulation with protocols. In: Mukherjee D, Rajagopalan S, eds. *CT and MR Angiography of the Peripheral Circulation.* Boca Raton, FL: CRC Press; 2007:140.)

TABLE 14.1 **Biphasic Injection Protocol for Peripheral Artery Disease Imaging**	
Contrast agent	**Low-osmolar nonionic 350–370 mg/mL**
Scan time	Fixed at 40 s
Injection duration	35 s
Pitch	Variable and adjusted to scan time of 40 s
Delay	Bolus trigger to occur on reaching threshold of 150–200 HU
Weight-based biphasic injection rate	<55 kg: 20 mL (4 mL/s) + 96 mL (3.2 mL/s) 56–65 kg: 23 mL (4.5 mL/s) + 108 mL (3.6 mL/s) 66–85 kg: 25 mL (5.0 mL/s) + 120 mL (4.0 mL/s) 86–95 kg: 28 mL (5.5 mL/s) + 132 mL (4.4 mL/s) >95 kg: 30 mL (6.0 mL/s) + 144 mL (4.8 mL/s)

HU, Hounsfield units.

one study has compared the comparative effectiveness of various imaging approaches in PAD. The outcome measures included the clinical utility, functional patient outcomes, quality of life, and diagnostic and therapeutic costs related to the initial imaging test during 6 months of follow-up. Higher confidence and less additional imaging were found for MRA and CTA, compared with duplex sonography, and at lower costs.[116] Further development with 256 detector scanners and curved 3D multipath reconstructions have allowed for improved examination of peripheral disease when compared to DSA.[117,118] CTA showed higher sensitivity and specificity in the assessment of stenosis for aortic and lower limb occlusive disease. As mentioned before, the assessment of infrapopliteal lesions was worse (sensitivity 91.6%, accuracy 73.3%, and positive predictive value 78.5%), and more so in significantly calcified vessels. However, the 256-slice CTA can provide a fast and reliable imaging of most of the peripheral vascular tree with DSA only for certain segments.[117]

Peripheral artery aneurysm. Approximately 10% of patients with abdominal aortic aneurysms have femoral and/or popliteal artery aneurysms (Fig. 14.10). The definition of a popliteal artery aneurysm is when the arterial diameter is greater than 7 mm, and a femoral artery aneurysm is when the diameter is greater than 10 mm.[119,120] CTA is very helpful in diagnosing concomitant aneurysms and also allows the distinction of popliteal artery aneurysm from Baker cyst or cystic adventitial disease. In the case of femoral artery aneurysm, CTA is appropriate to define the presence of iliac and native femoral vessel disease and to plan revascularization strategies.[121]

Vasculitis. The most common type of arteritis affecting the lower extremity is thromboangiitis obliterans (Buerger disease) (see Chapter 42). Thromboangiitis obliterans disease typically affects the small-to-medium–sized arteries of the extremities and primarily affects young male smokers. The distal nature of the disease may favor the use of CTA over MRA in light of the submillimeter resolution of the technique, which permits imaging of femoropopliteal occlusive disease extending into the tibioperoneal circuit. The angiographic appearance is one of abrupt vessel occlusion or focal high-grade concentric stenoses associated with extensive collateral circulation resulting in a "corkscrew appearance." Takayasu arteritis mostly involves the thoracic aorta and brachiocephalic vessels with less frequent involvement of the abdominal aorta and visceral branches.[122]

Other forms of arteritis may affect the peripheral circulation; however, this is uncommon. These include giant cell arteritis, polyarteritis nodosa, Behçet disease, and Kawasaki disease. The pattern and type of vessels involved as seen on CTA are useful in distinguishing these entities.

Endovascular stent evaluation. CTA may be used for evaluation of in-stent restenosis particularly in proximal vessels, such as the iliac and femoral arteries (see Chapter 20). This may require reconstruction with alternate kernels and adjustment of window levels. There is only limited data comparing CT to other modalities for the evaluation of peripheral stents.[123]

CTA is used to evaluate patients who have aortoiliac, aortofemoral, or axillofemoral bypass grafts (see Chapter 21).[124] Surveillance of

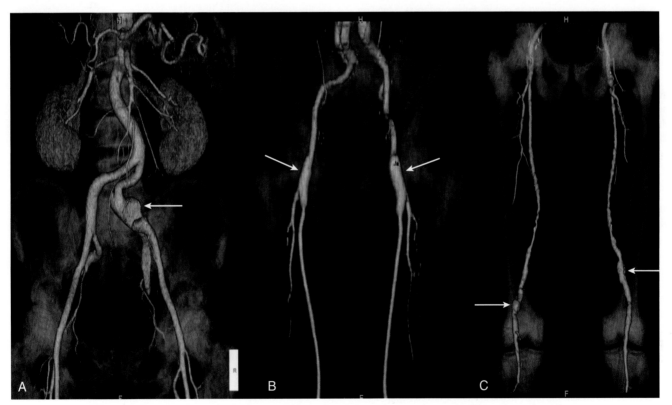

Fig. 14.10 Peripheral Arterial Aneurysms. Three-dimensional computed tomographic angiography volume-rendered images showing a focal aneurysmal dilatation of the distal portion of the left common iliac artery (*arrow,* A); aneurysms of the common femoral arteries bilaterally (*arrows,* B), extending to the origins of the superficial femoral arteries; and focal aneurysmal dilatation of the bilateral popliteal arteries (*arrows,* C). (Modified from Cohen E, Doshi A, Lookstein R. CT angiography of the lower extremity circulation with protocols. In: Mukherjee D, Rajagopalan S, eds. *CT and MR Angiography of the Peripheral Circulation.* Boca Raton, FL: CRC Press; 2007:140.)

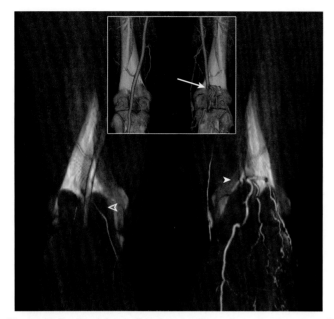

Fig. 14.11 Popliteal Artery Entrapment. Three-dimensional computed tomographic angiography volume-rendered image (posteroanterior view) of a young patient with right calf pain on exertion. The medial head of the right gastrocnemius muscle demonstrates an abnormal origin lateral to the popliteal artery *(closed arrowhead).* Inset image shows complete occlusion of the right popliteal artery *(arrow)* with multiple superficial collateral arteries originating just proximal to this level. The normal origin of the medial head of the left gastrocnemius medial to the popliteal artery *(open arrowhead)* is shown for comparison. (Modified from Cohen E, Doshi A, Lookstein R. CT angiography of the lower extremity circulation with protocols. In: Mukherjee D, Rajagopalan S, eds. *CT and MR Angiography of the Peripheral Circulation.* Boca Raton, FL: CRC Press; 2007:143.)

grafts is important and is primarily performed by duplex ultrasound evaluation. Recent studies, however, suggest that CTA may be superior to duplex ultrasound evaluation.[125] Attention must be paid to the cumulative radiation dose and the use of contrast agents. Assessment of the graft should include careful evaluation of the proximal anastomotic area to exclude stenosis or aneurysm, the body of the graft, and the touch-down site of the graft.

Other Indications

A variety of other conditions represent less common indications for the use of a peripheral CTA. These include persistent sciatic artery, popliteal entrapment, and cystic medial adventitial disease (Fig. 14.11). Arteriovenous malformations and fistulas may be well delineated by acquiring images during the arterial and venous phase. CTA imaging may be used to characterize congenital vascular anomalies.

REFERENCES

1. Ligon BL. Biography: history of developments in imaging techniques: Egas Moniz and angiography. *Semin Pediatr Infect Dis.* 2003;14:173–181.
2. Fleischmann D. Present and future trends in multiple detector-row CT applications: CT angiography. *Eur Radiol.* 2002;12(Suppl 2):S11–S15.
3. Li B, Toth TL, Hsieh J, Tang X. Simulation and analysis of image quality impacts from single source, ultra-wide coverage CT scanner. *J Xray Sci Technol.* 2012;20:395–404.
4. Kalender WA. Technical foundations of spiral CT. *Semin Ultrasound CT MR.* 1994;15:81–89.
5. Kalender WA, Seissler W, Klotz E, Vock P. Spiral volumetric CT with single-breath-hold technique, continuous transport, and continuous scanner rotation. *Radiology.* 1990;176:181–183.
6. Petersilka M, Bruder H, Krauss B, et al. Technical principles of dual source CT. *Eur J Radiol.* 2008;68:362–368.
7. Dawson P, Blomley MJ. Contrast media as extracellular fluid space markers: adaptation of the central volume theorem. *Br J Radiol.* 1996;69:717–722.
8. van Hoe L, Marchal G, Baert AL, et al. Determination of scan delay time in spiral CT-angiography: utility of a test bolus injection. *J Comput Assist Tomogr.* 1995;19:216–220.
9. Leschka S, Wildermuth S, Boehm T, et al. Noninvasive coronary angiography with 64-section CT: effect of average heart rate and heart rate variability on image quality. *Radiology.* 2006;241:378–385.
10. Einstein AJ, Henzlova MJ, Rajagopalan S. Estimating risk of cancer associated with radiation exposure from 64-slice computed tomography coronary angiography. *JAMA.* 2007;298:317–323.
11. Fazel R, Krumholz HM, Wang Y, et al. Exposure to low-dose ionizing radiation from medical imaging procedures. *N Engl J Med.* 2009;361:849–857.
12. Ron E. Cancer risks from medical radiation. *Health Phys.* 2003;85:47–59.
13. Einstein AJ, Moser KW, Thompson RC, et al. Radiation dose to patients from cardiac diagnostic imaging. *Circulation.* 2007;116:1290–1305.
14. Martin CJ. The application of effective dose to medical exposures. *Radiat Prot Dosimetry.* 2008;128:1–4.
15. Martin CJ. Radiation dosimetry for diagnostic medical exposures. *Radiat Prot Dosimetry.* 2008;128:389–412.
16. Bongartz G, Golding SJ, Jurik AG, et al. *European guidelines for multislice computed tomography.* http://biophysicssite.com/html/msct_quality_criteria_2004.html; 2004. Accessed April 19, 2018.
17. Blankstein R, Shah A, Pale R, et al. Radiation dose and image quality of prospective triggering with dual-source cardiac computed tomography. *Am J Cardiol.* 2009;103:1168–1173.
18. Wintersperger B, Jakobs T, Herzog P, et al. Aorto-iliac multidetector-row CT angiography with low kV settings: improved vessel enhancement and simultaneous reduction of radiation dose. *Eur Radiol.* 2005;15:334–341.
19. Lee EJ, Lee SK, Agid R, et al. Comparison of image quality and radiation dose between fixed tube current and combined automatic tube current modulation in craniocervical CT angiography. *AJNR Am J Neuroradiol.* 2009;30:1754–1759.
20. Arnoldi E, Johnson TR, Rist C, et al. Adequate image quality with reduced radiation dose in prospectively triggered coronary CTA compared with retrospective techniques. *Eur Radiol.* 2009;19:2147–2155.
21. Hurwitz LM, Yoshizumi TT, Goodman PC, et al. Radiation dose savings for adult pulmonary embolus 64-MDCT using bismuth breast shields, lower peak kilovoltage, and automatic tube current modulation. *AJR Am J Roentgenol.* 2009;192:244–253.
22. Hausleiter J, Meyer T, Hadamitzky M, et al. Radiation dose estimates from cardiac multislice computed tomography in daily practice: impact of different scanning protocols on effective dose estimates. *Circulation.* 2006;113:1305–1310.
23. Raff GL, Chinnaiyan KM, Share DA, et al. Radiation dose from cardiac computed tomography before and after implementation of radiation dose-reduction techniques. *JAMA.* 2009;301:2340–2348.
24. Meeson S, Alvey CM, Golding SJ. The in vivo relationship between cross-sectional area and CT dose index in abdominal multidetector CT with automatic exposure control. *J Radiol Prot.* 2010;30:139–147.
25. Bushberg JT. The AAPM/RSNA physics tutorial for residents. X-ray interactions. *Radiographics.* 1998;18(2):457–468.
26. Johnson TR. Dual-energy CT: general principles. *AJR Am J Roentgenol.* 2012;199(5 Suppl):S3–S8.
27. Rajiah P, Abbara S, Halliburton SS. Spectral detector CT for cardiovascular applications. *Diagn Interv Radiol.* 2017;23:187–193.
28. Vlahos I, Chung R, Nair A, Morgan R. Dual-energy CT: vascular applications. *AJR Am J Roentgenol.* 2012;199(5 Suppl):S87–S97.
29. Dubourg B, Caudron J, Lestrat JP, et al. Single-source dual-energy CT angiography with reduced iodine load in patients referred for

aortoiliofemoral evaluation before transcatheter aortic valve implantation: impact on image quality and radiation dose. *Eur Radiol.* 2014;24:2659–2668.

30. Almutairi A, Sun Z, Poovathumkadavi A, Assar T. Dual energy CT angiography of peripheral arterial disease: feasibility of using lower contrast medium volume. *PLoS One.* 2015;10: e0139275.

31. Almutairi A, Al Safran Z, AlZaabi SA, Sun Z. Dual energy CT angiography in peripheral arterial stents: optimal scanning protocols with regard to image quality and radiation dose. *Quant Imaging Med Surg.* 2017;7:520–531.

32. Lu GM, Zhao Y, Zhang LJ, Schoepf UJ. Dual-energy CT of the lung. *AJR Am J Roentgenol.* 2012;199(5 Suppl):S40–S53.

33. Berg M, Zhang Z, Ikonen A, et al. Multi-detector row CT angiography in the assessment of carotid artery disease in symptomatic patients: comparison with rotational angiography and digital subtraction angiography. *AJNR Am J Neuroradiol.* 2005;26:1022–1034.

34. Josephson SA, Bryant SO, Mak HK, et al. Evaluation of carotid stenosis using CT angiography in the initial evaluation of stroke and TIA. *Neurology.* 2004;63:457–460.

35. Zhang Z, Berg MH, Ikonen AE, et al. Carotid artery stenosis: reproducibility of automated 3D CT angiography analysis method. *Eur Radiol.* 2004;14:665–672.

36. Saba L, Mallarin G. Window settings for the study of calcified carotid plaques with multidetector CT angiography. *AJNR Am J Neuroradiol.* 2009;30:1445–1450.

37. Fisher M, Martin A, Cosgrove M, Norris JW. The NASCET-ACAS plaque project. North American Symptomatic Carotid Endarterectomy Trial. Asymptomatic Carotid Atherosclerosis Study. *Stroke.* 1993;24(12 Suppl):I24–I25. discussion I31-I32.

38. Zhang Z, Berg M, Ikonen A, et al. Carotid stenosis degree in CT angiography: assessment based on luminal area versus luminal diameter measurements. *Eur Radiol.* 2005;15:2359–2365.

39. Bartlett ES, Walters TD, Symons SP, Fox AJ. Quantification of carotid stenosis on CT angiography. *AJNR Am J Neuroradiol.* 2006;27:13–19.

40. Bartlett ES, Walters TD, Symons SP, Fox AJ. Carotid stenosis index revisited with direct CT angiography measurement of carotid arteries to quantify carotid stenosis. *Stroke.* 2007;38:286–291.

41. Bartlett ES, Symons SP, Fox AJ. Correlation of carotid stenosis diameter and cross-sectional areas with CT angiography. *AJNR Am J Neuroradiol.* 2006;27:638–642.

42. Bartlett ES, Walters TD, Symons SP, et al. Classification of carotid stenosis by millimeter CT angiography measures: effects of prevalence and gender. *AJNR Am J Neuroradiol.* 2008;29:1677–1683.

43. Waaijer A, Weber M, van Leeuwen MS, et al. Grading of carotid artery stenosis with multidetector-row CT angiography: visual estimation or caliper measurements? *Eur Radiol.* 2009;19:2809–2818.

44. Suwanwela N, Can U, Furie KL, et al. Carotid Doppler ultrasound criteria for internal carotid artery stenosis based on residual lumen diameter calculated from en bloc carotid endarterectomy specimens. *Stroke.* 1996;27:1965–1969.

45. Lev MH, Romero JM, Goodman DN, et al. Total occlusion versus hairline residual lumen of the internal carotid arteries: accuracy of single section helical CT angiography. *AJNR Am J Neuroradiol.* 2003;24:1123–1129.

46. Chen CJ, Lee TH, Hsuy HL, et al. Multi-slice CT angiography in diagnosing total versus near occlusions of the internal carotid artery: comparison with catheter angiography. *Stroke.* 2004;35:83–85.

47. Bartlett ES, Walters TD, Symons SP, Fox AJ. Diagnosing carotid stenosis near-occlusion by using CT angiography. *AJNR Am J Neuroradiol.* 2006;27:632–637.

48. Delgado Almandoz JE, Romero JM, Pomerantz SR, Lev MH. Computed tomography angiography of the carotid and cerebral circulation. *Radiol Clin North Am.* 2010;48:265–281.

49. Baradaran H, Al-Dasuqi K, Knight-Greenfield A, et al. Association between carotid plaque features on CTA and cerebrovascular ischemia: a systematic review and meta-analysis. *AJNR Am J Neuroradiol.* 2017;38:2321–2326.

50. van Gils MJ, Vukadinovic D, van Dijk AC, et al. Carotid atherosclerotic plaque progression and change in plaque composition over time: a 5-year follow-up study using serial CT angiography. *AJNR Am J Neuroradiol.* 2012;33:1267–1273.

51. Rafailidis V, Chryssogonidis I, Tegos T, et al. Imaging of the ulcerated carotid atherosclerotic plaque: a review of the literature. *Insights Imaging.* 2017;8:213–225.

52. Albrecht MH, Bickford MW, Nance Jr. JW, et al. State-of-the-art pulmonary CT angiography for acute pulmonary embolism. *AJR Am J Roentgenol.* 2017;208:495–504.

53. Stein PD, Beemath A, Olson RE. Trends in the incidence of pulmonary embolism and deep venous thrombosis in hospitalized patients. *Am J Cardiol.* 2005;95:1525–1526.

54. Stein PD, Fowler SE, Goodman LR, et al. Multidetector computed tomography for acute pulmonary embolism. *N Engl J Med.* 2006;354:2317–2327.

55. Coche E, Verschuren F, Keyeux A, et al. Diagnosis of acute pulmonary embolism in outpatients: comparison of thin-collimation multi-detector row spiral CT and planar ventilation-perfusion scintigraphy. *Radiology.* 2003;229:757–765.

56. Qanadli SD, Hajjam ME, Mesurolle B, et al. Pulmonary embolism detection: prospective evaluation of dual-section helical CT versus selective pulmonary arteriography in 157 patients. *Radiology.* 2000;217:447–455.

57. Winer-Muram HT, Rydberg J, Johnson MS, et al. Suspected acute pulmonary embolism: evaluation with multi-detector row CT versus digital subtraction pulmonary arteriography. *Radiology.* 2004;233: 806–815.

58. Brader P, Schoellnast H, Deutschmann HA, et al. Acute pulmonary embolism: comparison of standard axial MDCT with paddlewheel technique. *Eur J Radiol.* 2008;66:31–36.

59. Chiang EE, Boiselle PM, Raptopoulos V, et al. Detection of pulmonary embolism: comparison of paddlewheel and coronal CT reformations— initial experience. *Radiology.* 2003;228:577–582.

60. Coche EE, Hamoir XL, Hammer FD, et al. Using dual-detector helical CT angiography to detect deep venous thrombosis in patients with suspicion of pulmonary embolism: diagnostic value and additional findings. *AJR Am J Roentgenol.* 2001;176:1035–1039.

61. Sista AK, Kuo WT, Schiebler M, Madoff DC. Stratification, imaging, and management of acute massive and submassive pulmonary embolism. *Radiology.* 2017;284:5–24.

62. Quiroz R, Kucher N, Schoepf UJ, et al. Right ventricular enlargement on chest computed tomography: prognostic role in acute pulmonary embolism. *Circulation.* 2004;109:2401–2404.

63. Bhalla S, West OC. CT of nontraumatic thoracic aortic emergencies. *Semin Ultrasound CT MR.* 2005;26:281–304.

64. Salvolini L, Renda P, Fiore D, et al. Acute aortic syndromes: role of multi-detector row CT. *Eur J Radiol.* 2008;65:350–358.

65. Batra P, Bigoni B, Manning J, et al. Pitfalls in the diagnosis of thoracic aortic dissection at CT angiography. *Radiographics.* 2000;20: 309–320.

66. Manghat NE, Morgan-Hughes GJ, Roobottom CA. Multi-detector row computed tomography: imaging in acute aortic syndrome. *Clin Radiol.* 2005;60:1256–1267.

67. Roos JE, Willmann JK, Weishaupt D, et al. Thoracic aorta: motion artifact reduction with retrospective and prospective electrocardiography-assisted multi-detector row CT. *Radiology.* 2002;222:271–277.

68. Hayashi H, Matsuoka Y, Sakamoto I, et al. Penetrating atherosclerotic ulcer of the aorta: imaging features and disease concept. *Radiographics.* 2000;20:995–1005.

69. Macura KJ, Corl FM, Fishman EK, Bluemke DA. Pathogenesis in acute aortic syndromes: aortic dissection, intramural hematoma, and penetrating atherosclerotic aortic ulcer. *AJR Am J Roentgenol.* 2003;181:309–316.

70. Chiles C, Carr JJ. Vascular diseases of the thorax: evaluation with multidetector CT. *Radiol Clin North Am.* 2005;43:543–569. viii.

71. Park KH, Lim C, Choi JH, et al. Prevalence of aortic intimal defect in surgically treated acute type A intramural hematoma. *Ann Thorac Surg.* 2008;86:1494–1500.

72. Quint LE, Williams DM, Francis IR, et al. Ulcerlike lesions of the aorta: imaging features and natural history. *Radiology*. 2001;218: 719–723.

73. Harris JA, Bis KG, Glover JL, et al. Penetrating atherosclerotic ulcers of the aorta. *J Vasc Surg*. 1994;19:90–98. discussion 98-99.

74. Maddu KK, Shuaib W, Telleria J, et al. Nontraumatic acute aortic emergencies: part 1, acute aortic syndrome. *AJR Am J Roentgenol*. 2014;202:656–665.

75. Jeudy J, Waite S, White CS. Nontraumatic thoracic emergencies. *Radiol Clin North Am*. 2006;44:273–293. ix.

76. Ganaha F, Miller DC, Sugimoto K, et al. Prognosis of aortic intramural hematoma with and without penetrating atherosclerotic ulcer: a clinical and radiological analysis. *Circulation*. 2002;106:342–348.

77. Cho KR, Stanson AW, Potter DD, et al. Penetrating atherosclerotic ulcer of the descending thoracic aorta and arch. *J Thorac Cardiovasc Surg*. 2004;127:1393–1399. discussion 1399-1401.

78. Beauchesne LM, Veinot JP, Brais MP, et al. Acute aortic intimal tear without a mobile flap mimicking an intramural hematoma. *J Am Soc Echocardiogr*. 2003;16:285–288.

79. Mussa FF, Horton JD, Moridzadeh R, et al. Acute aortic dissection and intramural hematoma. *JAMA*. 2016;316:754–763.

80. Castañer E, Andreu M, Gallardo X, et al. CT in nontraumatic acute thoracic aortic disease: typical and atypical features and complications. *Radiographics*. 2003;23. Spec No:S93-S110.

81. Hagan PG, Nienaber CA, Isselbacher EM, et al. The International Registry of Acute Aortic Dissection (IRAD): new insights into an old disease. *JAMA*. 2000;283:897–903.

82. Song JK, Kim HS, Song JM, et al. Outcomes of medically treated patients with aortic intramural hematoma. *Am J Med*. 2002;113:181–187.

83. Sueyoshi E, Matsuoka Y, Imada T, et al. New development of an ulcerlike projection in aortic intramural hematoma: CT evaluation. *Radiology*. 2002;224:536–541.

84. Song MO, Kim KJ, Chung SI, et al. Distribution of human group a rotavirus VP7 and VP4 types circulating in Seoul, Korea between 1998 and 2000. *J Med Virol*. 2003;70:324–328.

85. Nienaber CA, Clough RE. Management of acute aortic dissection. *Lancet*. 2015;385:800–811.

86. Manghat NE, Walsh M, Roobottom CA, Williams MP. Can the 'vortex sign' be used as an imaging indicator of the false lumen in acute aortic dissection? *Clin Radiol*. 2005;60:1037–1038.

87. McMahon MA, Squirrell CA. Multidetector CT of aortic dissection: a pictorial review. *Radiographics*. 2010;30:445–460.

88. Isselbacher EM. Thoracic and abdominal aortic aneurysms. *Circulation*. 2005;111:816–828.

89. Barra L, Kanji T, Malette J, et al. Imaging modalities for the diagnosis and disease activity assessment of Takayasu's arteritis: a systematic review and meta-analysis. *Autoimmun Rev*. 2018;17:175–187.

90. Trimarchi S, Tsai T, Eagle KA, et al. Acute abdominal aortic dissection: insight from the International Registry of Acute Aortic Dissection (IRAD). *J Vasc Surg*. 2007;46:913–919.

91. Jonker FH, Schlosser FJ, Moll FL, Muhs BE. Dissection of the abdominal aorta. Current evidence and implications for treatment strategies: a review and meta-analysis of 92 patients. *J Endovasc Ther*. 2009;16:71–80.

92. Pande RL, Beckman JA. Abdominal aortic aneurysm: populations at risk and how to screen. *J Vasc Interv Radiol*. 2008;19:S2–S8.

93. Annambhotla S, Bourgeois S, Wang X, et al. Recent advances in molecular mechanisms of abdominal aortic aneurysm formation. *World J Surg*. 2008;32:976–986.

94. Rozenblit AM, Patlas M, Rosenbaum AT, et al. Detection of endoleaks after endovascular repair of abdominal aortic aneurysm: value of unenhanced and delayed helical CT acquisitions. *Radiology*. 2003;227:426–433.

95. Bashir MR, Ferral H, Jacobs C, et al. Endoleaks after endovascular abdominal aortic aneurysm repair: management strategies according to CT findings. *AJR Am J Roentgenol*. 2009;192:W178–W186.

96. Tolia AJ, Landis R, Lamparello P, et al. Type II endoleaks after endovascular repair of abdominal aortic aneurysms: natural history. *Radiology*. 2005;235:683–686.

97. Görich J, Rilinger N, Sokiranski R, et al. Leakages after endovascular repair of aortic aneurysms: classification based on findings at CT, angiography, and radiography. *Radiology*. 1999;213:767–772.

98. Gotway MB, Araoz PA, Macedo TA, et al. Imaging findings in Takayasu's arteritis. *AJR Am J Roentgenol*. 2005;184:1945–1950.

99. Foley WD. Special focus session: multidetector CT: abdominal visceral imaging. *Radiographics*. 2002;22:701–719.

100. Kawashima A, Sandler CM, Ernst RD, et al. CT evaluation of renovascular disease. *Radiographics*. 2000;20:1321–1340.

101. Beregi JP, Louvegny S, Gautier C, et al. Fibromuscular dysplasia of the renal arteries: comparison of helical CT angiography and arteriography. *AJR Am J Roentgenol*. 1999;172:27–34.

102. Sabharwal R, Vladica P, Law WP, et al. Multidetector spiral CT renal angiography in the diagnosis of giant renal artery aneurysms. *Abdom Imaging*. 2006;31:374–378.

103. Chiesa R, Astore D, Guzzo G, et al. Visceral artery aneurysms. *Ann Vasc Surg*. 2005;19:42–48.

104. Dohan A, Dautry R, Guerrache Y, et al. Three-dimensional MDCT angiography of splanchnic arteries: pearls and pitfalls. *Diagn Interv Imaging*. 2015;96:187–200.

105. Barmeir E, Halachmi S, Croitoru S, Torem S. CT angiography diagnosis of spontaneous dissection of the superior mesenteric artery. *AJR Am J Roentgenol*. 1998;171:1429–1430.

106. Dong Z, Fu W, Chen B, et al. Treatment of symptomatic isolated dissection of superior mesenteric artery. *J Vasc Surg*. 2013;57:69S–76S.

107. Loukas M, Pinyard J, Vaid S, et al. Clinical anatomy of celiac artery compression syndrome: a review. *Clin Anat*. 2007;20:612–617.

108. Cohen EI, Doshi A, Lookstein RA. CT angiography of the lower extremity circulation with protocols. In: Mukherjee D, Rajagopalan S, eds. *CT and MR Angiography of the Peripheral Circulation. Practical Approach with Clinical Protocols*: Boca Raton, FL: CRC Press; 2007:133–146.

109. Fleischmann D. CT angiography: injection and acquisition technique. *Radiol Clin North Am*. 2010;48:237–247. vii.

110. Catalano C, Fraioli F, Laghi A, et al. Infrarenal aortic and lower-extremity arterial disease: diagnostic performance of multi-detector row CT angiography. *Radiology*. 2004;231:555–563.

111. Schernthaner R, Stadler A, Lomoschitz F, et al. Multidetector CT angiography in the assessment of peripheral arterial occlusive disease: accuracy in detecting the severity, number, and length of stenoses. *Eur Radiol*. 2008;18:665–671.

112. Norgren L, Hiatt WR, Dormandy JA, et al. Inter-Society Consensus for the Management of Peripheral Arterial Disease (TASC II). *Eur J Vasc Endovasc Surg*. 2007;33(Suppl 1):S1–S75.

113. Heijenbrok-Kal MH, Kock MC, Hunink MG. Lower extremity arterial disease: multidetector CT angiography meta-analysis. *Radiology*. 2007;245:433–439.

114. Schernthaner R, Fleischmann D, Lomoschitz, et al. Effect of MDCT angiographic findings on the management of intermittent claudication. *AJR Am J Roentgenol*. 2007;189:1215–1222.

115. Dellegrottaglie S, Sanz J, Macaluso F, et al. Technology insight: magnetic resonance angiography for the evaluation of patients with peripheral artery disease. *Nat Clin Pract Cardiovasc Med*. 2007;4:677–687.

116. Ouwendijk R, de Vries M, Stijnen T, et al. Multicenter randomized controlled trial of the costs and effects of noninvasive diagnostic imaging in patients with peripheral arterial disease: the DIPAD trial. *AJR Am J Roentgenol*. 2008;190:1349–1357.

117. Mishra A, Jain N, Bhagwat A. CT angiography of peripheral arterial disease by 256-slice scanner: accuracy, advantages and disadvantages compared to digital subtraction angiography. *Vasc Endovasc Surg*. 2017;51:247–254.

118. Schreiner MM, Platzgummer H, Unterhumer S, et al. Multipath curved planar reformations of peripheral CT angiography: diagnostic accuracy and time efficiency. *Cardiovasc Intervent Radiol*. 2018;41:718–725.

119. Jarraya M, Simmons S, Farber A, et al. Uncommon diseases of the popliteal artery: a pictorial review. *Insights Imaging*. 2016;7:679–688.

120. Diwan A, Sarkar R, Stanley JC, et al. Incidence of femoral and popliteal artery aneurysms in patients with abdominal aortic aneurysms. *J Vasc Surg*. 2000;31:863–869.

121. Lopera JE, Trimmer CK, Josephs SG, et al. Multidetector CT angiography of infrainguinal arterial bypass. *Radiographics*. 2008;28:529–548. discussion 549.

122. Chung JW, Kim HC, Choi YH, et al. Patterns of aortic involvement in Takayasu arteritis and its clinical implications: evaluation with spiral computed tomography angiography. *J Vasc Surg*. 2007;45:906–914.

123. Li XM, Li YH, Tian JM, et al. Evaluation of peripheral artery stent with 64-slice multi-detector row CT angiography: prospective comparison with digital subtraction angiography. *Eur J Radiol*. 2010;75:98–103.

124. Foley WD, Stonely T. CT angiography of the lower extremities. *Radiol Clin North Am*. 2010;48:367–396. ix.

125. Willmann JK, Mayer D, Banyai M, et al. Evaluation of peripheral arterial bypass grafts with multi-detector row CT angiography: comparison with duplex US and digital subtraction angiography. *Radiology*. 2003;229:465–474.

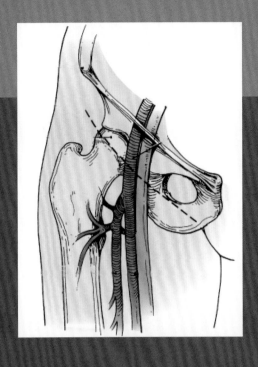

中文导读

第15章
基于导管的周围血管造影术

导管法介入血管对比造影术是诊断外周动脉疾病（peripheral artery disease，PAD）的金标准，其准确度高于其他所有方法。血管造影是通过导管注入造影剂，由于X线无法穿透造影剂，可通过成像系统显示造影剂在血管中的流动情况，提供血管的"路径图"，其不仅能显示目标血管的病变，还能评价血管节段中的流入和流出节段，为临床医师提供更为全面的血管情况，从而协助其做出治疗决策。进行血管造影时，患者的安全是重中之重，医师的血管解剖结构知识和对正常生理变异的了解是保证周围血管造影和干预治疗安全进行的关键。本章将介绍导管法介入血管对比造影术的基本原理及其在全身各处血管造影方面的应用，以及其在血管疾病诊疗方面的适应证，同时会论述该技术在应用过程中可能会发生的一些并发症，旨在为临床医师选择使用该项技术时提供参考。

常光其

Catheter-Based Peripheral Angiography

Christopher J. White

Catheter-based invasive contrast angiography is the standard method for diagnosing peripheral artery disease (PAD), and against which all other methods are compared for accuracy. Angiography provides the "road map" on which therapeutic decisions are based. Knowledge of the vascular anatomy and its normal variations is a core element in the skill set required to safely perform peripheral vascular angiography and interventions.

IMAGING EQUIPMENT

There are many radiographic equipment vendors and many different room layout schemes suitable for performing peripheral vascular angiography. However, if both cardiac and noncardiac types of peripheral vascular angiography are to be performed in the same room, equipment options become much more limited. One angiographic suite designed to perform both coronary and peripheral vascular angiography is a *dual-plane system* (Fig. 15.1). A dual-plane system economically provides a layout with two independent C-arm image intensifiers operated by a single x-ray generator and one computer. A dual-plane system is not synonymous with a biplane system, which is the simultaneous operation of an anteroposterior (AP) and lateral (LAT) image acquisition system. In a dual-plane system, the cardiac C-arm is a three-mode, 8- or 9- inch flat-panel image intensifier, and the noncardiac C-arm should be as large as possible, usually a 15- or 16-inch flat-panel image intensifier. For peripheral vascular imaging, particularly bilateral lower-extremity runoff angiography, an image intensifier smaller than 15 inches may not be able to include both legs in the same field. The noncardiac C-arm should be capable of head-to-toe digital imaging.

The ability to angulate (rotational as well as cranial and caudal) the image intensifier is necessary to resolve bifurcation lesions and optimally image aorto-ostial branch lesions. Of the many imaging options available, those most often used include digital subtraction angiography (DSA), roadmapping, and a stepping table for lower-extremity (digital subtraction) runoff angiography.

RADIOGRAPHIC CONTRAST

Ionic low-osmolar or nonionic iodinated radiographic contrast is preferred for angiography of the peripheral vessels to avoid patient discomfort. Low-osmolar contrast agents produce fewer side effects (e.g., nausea, vomiting, local pain) and offer better patient tolerability. In addition, low-osmolar agents deliver a lesser osmotic load and thereby a lower intravascular volume, which may be important in patients with impaired left ventricular or renal function. DSA is often preferred because nonvascular structures are removed from the image and less contrast is required. Frequently, it is possible to dilute radiographic contrast 1:1 with saline and still preserve image quality with DSA.

Alternatives to iodine-based radiographic contrast include carbon dioxide (CO_2) and gadolinium (gadopentetate dimeglumine).[1,2]

To minimize the risk of distal embolization and stroke, it is recommended that CO_2 not be used for angiograms above the diaphragm. Gadolinium, traditionally used with magnetic resonance angiography, is relatively nontoxic in patients with adequate renal function at a recommended dose not exceeding 0.4 mmol/kg, but provides suboptimal image quality.

IMAGING TECHNIQUE

Many of the technical aspects of diagnostic cardiac imaging also apply to performing angiography of the aorta and peripheral vasculature. The basic principle of vascular angiography is not only to visualize the target lesion but also to demonstrate the inflow and outflow vascular segments. Inflow anatomy constitutes the vascular segment preceding the target lesion, and outflow constitutes the vascular segment immediately distal to the target vessel and includes the runoff bed. For example, the inflow segment for the common iliac artery (CIA) is the infrarenal aorta, and the outflow segment is the external iliac and femoral vessels. The runoff bed would be the tibioperoneal vessels.

When performing selective arterial imaging, it is important for patients' safety that a coronary manifold with pressure measurement be used to monitor hemodynamic status and ensure that damping of the catheter has not occurred prior to injecting contrast. The use of pressure monitoring during selective angiography can prevent a myriad of complications, including the creation of dissections and air injection.

Angiography may be performed using a "bolus chase" cineangiographic method or with a digital subtraction stepping mode. The bolus chase technique involves injecting a bolus of contrast at the inflow of the territory, then "panning" or manually moving the image intensifier or table to follow the bolus of contrast through the target lesion and into the run-off segment. The bolus chase technique does not allow for subtraction to occur. In digital subtraction stepping mode, the patient lies motionless on the angiographic table. A "mask" of the segments to be imaged is taken, and then contrast is injected. The table moves in steps to image the contrast-filled vessels, from which the mask is then subtracted, leaving only the contrast-filled vascular structures.

OBTAINING VASCULAR ACCESS

Vascular access for noncardiac diagnostic angiography is most commonly achieved at the common femoral artery (CFA), with alternative upper-extremity sites at the radial, brachial, or axillary artery. For diagnostic, nonselective lower extremity run-off angiography, 4F catheters inserted into the radial artery and positioned in the infrarenal aorta is becoming more common. The most common complications of angiographic procedures occur at vascular access sites.

A thorough understanding of the relationship of the CFA to anatomical landmarks is necessary to ensure safe CFA puncture (Fig. 15.2). The femoral artery and vein lie below the inguinal ligament, which is

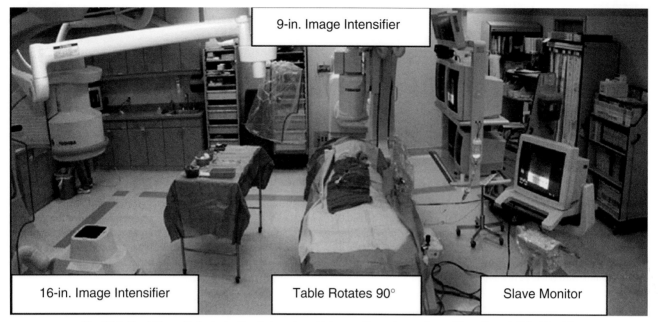

9-in. Image Intensifier

16-in. Image Intensifier   Table Rotates 90°   Slave Monitor

Fig. 15.1 Dual-Plane Catheterization Laboratory. Note two C-arm image intensifiers (9- and 16-inch), with catheterization table able to rotate 90 degrees.

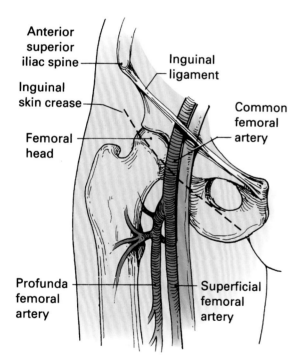

Anterior superior iliac spine

Inguinal skin crease

Femoral head

Profunda femoral artery

Inguinal ligament

Common femoral artery

Superficial femoral artery

Fig. 15.2 Schematic of common femoral artery anatomical landmarks.

a band of dense fibrous tissue connecting the anterior superior iliac spine to the pubic tubercle. The inguinal skin crease, which is variable in location, is shown as a dotted line in the figure. Current recommendations are to use either fluoroscopic guidance or ultrasound guidance to image the femoral head to guide CFA puncture.[3,4]

The most important anatomic landmark for femoral arterial access is the head of the femur. In a morphological study using computed tomography (CT) images, there was not a single case in which a puncture would have passed cranial to the inguinal ligament or caudal to the femoral artery bifurcation if the CFA were entered at the level of the center of the femoral head.[5] Caudal to the femoral head, the CFA is

encased in the femoral sheath and bifurcates into the superficial femoral artery (SFA) medially and the deep femoral artery (DFA) laterally. With these anatomical observations in mind, the importance of osseous support and entry of the needle into the CFA at the center of the femoral head is obvious.

Anatomical landmarks are initially identified by palpation of the anterior superior iliac spine and pubic tubercle to locate the inguinal ligament; the position of the femoral head is confirmed fluoroscopically. Depending on the amount of subcutaneous fat, a skin incision should be made 1 to 2 cm caudal to the level of the center of the femoral head. The needle is directed in an oblique direction while palpating the CFA over the center of the femoral head. Once the CFA has been entered and brisk blood flow returns through the needle, a soft guidewire is advanced into the iliac artery, and a vascular sheath is inserted to secure vascular access.

For ultrasound-guided CFA access, after sterile draping, the ultrasound probe is used to visualize the femoral bifurcation with a transverse view. With the bifurcation kept in focus, the view is switched to longitudinal, and the femoral bifurcation and femoral head are identified, giving a clear view of the CFA. Keeping the bifurcation at the inferior edge of the screen also aids in avoiding a high puncture. A nick in the skin is made with a No. 11 blade, and the subcutaneous tissue is spread to create a track for the arterial sheath. A micropuncture needle is then inserted under ultrasound guidance, with care taken to see the entire length of the needle as well as the length of the CFA filling the ultrasound screen with the long view. If fluoroscopy demonstrates a puncture above the femoral head, the needle is removed and reinserted lower.[6]

Complications of CFA puncture are most commonly related to arterial entry that is either too high or too low. When the puncture is too high, a retroperitoneal hemorrhage may occur. The presence of loose connective tissue in the retroperitoneal space can lead to large hematomas that can result in life-threatening hemorrhage. Lack of osseous support and the presence of a tense inguinal ligament at the arterial puncture site make manual compression difficult. Low punctures may be complicated by formation of arteriovenous fistulas (AVFs), false aneurysms, and hematomas.

Abdominal Aortography and Lower-extremity Runoff

For abdominal aortography, vascular access with a 4 F to 6 F catheter is obtained in the CFA, although brachial or radial access may also be used. The angiographic catheter (e.g., pigtail, tennis racquet, omni flush) is positioned in the abdominal aorta such that the tip of the catheter reaches the level of the last rib. A power injector is used to deliver 20 to 30 mL of contrast at 15 mL/s for digital subtraction (Fig. 15.3). Either biplane angiography may be obtained or, if needed, two separate angiograms with single-plane systems. Three visceral (mesenteric) arterial branches, the celiac trunk, superior mesenteric artery (SMA), and inferior mesenteric artery (IMA), arise from the anterior surface of the abdominal aorta (Fig. 15.4). The renal arteries originate from the lateral aspect of the abdominal aorta at the level of L1 to L2. The AP projection allows visualization of the aorta, renal arteries, and iliac artery bifurcation, whereas the LAT view demonstrates the origin of the celiac trunk and mesenteric arteries. Commonly in the AP view, the proximal portion of the SMA obscures the origin of the right renal artery. When this occurs, selective angiography of the renal artery may be required to visualize the origin of this vessel.

Generally, a nonselective abdominal aortogram is obtained before selective renal angiography, using a large format (9- to 16-inch) image intensifier with digital subtraction imaging. The nonselective aortogram demonstrates the level at which the renal arteries arise, the presence of any accessory renal arteries and their location, the severity and location of aortoiliac pathology, and the presence of significant renal artery stenosis. To optimize viewing of the renal arteries, the angiographic catheter should be placed below the origin of the SMA, and the image intensifier should be positioned such that the superior, inferior, and lateral borders of both kidneys are visualized. The ostia of the renal arteries are often better seen with slight rotation of the image intensifier, usually into left anterior oblique (LAO) position.

Selective Renal Angiography

Selective renal angiography is indicated to identify suspected renovascular disease. Selective renal artery engagement allows the measurement of pressure gradients, particularly if ostial lesions are suspected. When measuring pressure gradients across lesions, it is important to

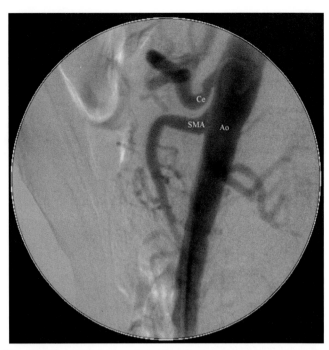

Fig. 15.4 Femoral Access. Lateral aortogram. Aorta *(Ao)*, with celiac trunk *(Ce)* and superior mesenteric artery *(SMA)* arising from anterior aortic surface.

use the smallest catheter possible (i.e., ≤4 F) to avoid creating an artificial gradient. The 0.014-inch pressure wire is the optimal method of pressure gradient measurement. Usually, selective renal angiography is performed with 4 F to 6 F diagnostic catheters (Fig. 15.5) and a 9-inch image intensifier. Selective renal angiography is performed using hand injections with shallow oblique angulations to optimize visualization of the renal ostia (Figs. 15.6 and 15.7). Caudal or cranial angulation (15 to 20 degrees) may occasionally be necessary for better visualization of some ostial lesions. An optimal image will reveal the ostial portion of the renal artery and distal branches at the cortex of the kidney.

Selective Mesenteric Angiography

As is the case for the renal arteries, nonselective aortography (AP and LAT) generally precedes selective angiography of the mesenteric arteries. Once the origin of the mesenteric vessel has been identified,

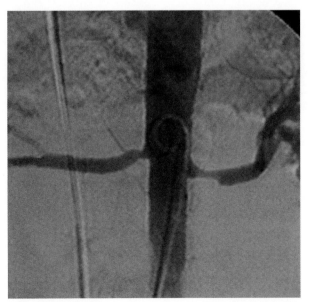

Fig. 15.3 Femoral Access. Pigtail catheter contrast injection of 20 mL/s for 30 mL (5 degrees left anterior oblique) using a digital subtraction angiography technique. Note bilateral renal artery stenosis.

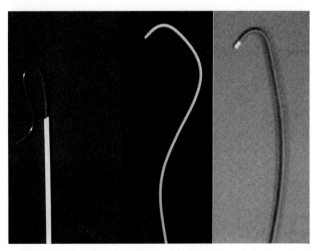

Fig. 15.5 Selective Renal Angiographic Catheters. *Left,* Sos; *Middle,* Cobra; *Right,* Internal mammary artery catheter.

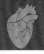

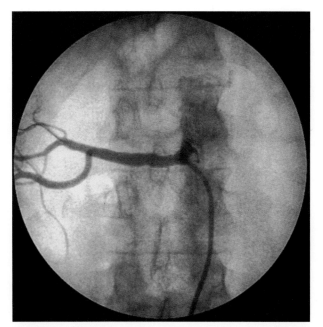

Fig. 15.6 Femoral Access. Internal mammary artery catheter selectively engaged in right renal artery.

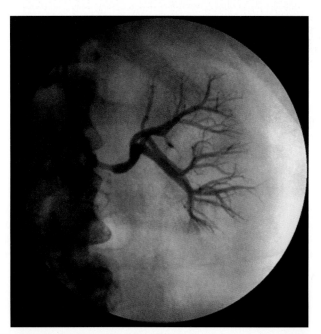

Fig. 15.7 Upper-Extremity Access. Selective left renal artery engagement with multipurpose catheter.

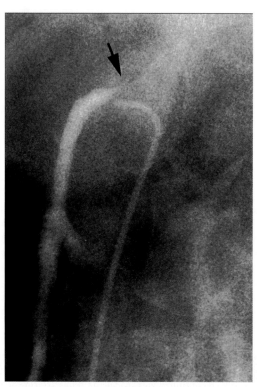

Fig. 15.8 Selective superior mesenteric angiography in lateral projection, with internal mammary artery catheter. Note ostial stenosis *(arrow)*.

measurement of the pressure gradient. Selective angiographic images in multiple views are obtained with hand injections of contrast.

Aortoiliac and Lower-extremity Angiography

The abdominal aorta bifurcates into the CIA, which bifurcates into the internal iliac arteries (IIA) and external iliac arteries (EIA; Fig. 15.9). The IIA is often referred to as the *hypogastric artery* because this vessel

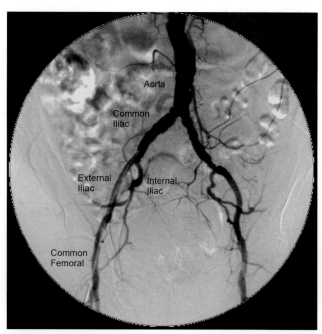

Fig. 15.9 Aortoiliac Angiography. Pigtail catheter contrast injection of 20 mL/s for a total of 30 mL.

selective angiography may be carried out in the LAT and oblique views using 4 F to 6 F catheters (Fig. 15.8). The celiac trunk, SMA, and IMA arteries arise from the anterior surface of the aorta. There are usually collaterals between the mesenteric vessels, and it is uncommon for stenosis or occlusion of a single branch to cause clinical symptoms.

The mesenteric arteries often arise at an inferior (caudal) angle from the abdominal aorta, for which a shepherd's crook catheter via femoral artery access is helpful for selective engagement. Alternatively, upper-extremity vascular access allows the mesenteric arteries to be engaged with a multipurpose-shaped catheter. Analogous to the renal arteries, selective engagement of the mesenteric arteries also allows

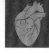

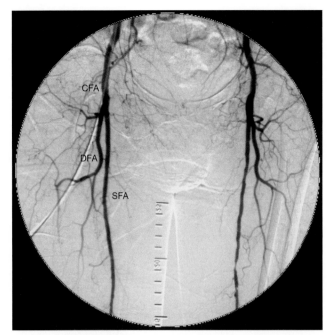

Fig. 15.10 Common femoral arteries *(CFA)* branching into deep femoral artery *(DFA)* and superficial femoral artery *(SFA).*

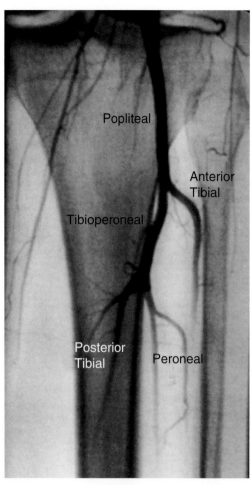

Fig. 15.11 Left popliteal artery bifurcates into anterior tibial (lateral) and tibioperoneal trunk, which then divides into posterior tibial (medial) and peroneal arteries.

commonly provides collateral circulation to the viscera. The EIA emerges from the pelvis just posterior to the inguinal ligament. At the level of the inguinal ligament, two small branches originate from the EIA: the inferior epigastric artery, which follows a medial direction, and the deep iliac circumflex artery, which takes a LAT and superior direction.

On crossing the inguinal ligament, the EIA becomes the CFA, which lies over the femoral head. When it reaches the lower third of the femoral head, the CFA divides into the SFA and profunda femoris, or DFA. The DFA runs posterolaterally along the femur. The SFA continues down the anteromedial thigh, and in its distal portion dives deeper to enter the Hunter (adductor) canal and emerges as the popliteal artery (Fig. 15.10).

Below the knee, the popliteal artery bifurcates into the anterior tibial (AT) artery and tibioperoneal trunk (TPT). The AT artery runs laterally and anterior to the tibia toward the foot and continues onto the foot as the dorsalis pedis (DP) artery. The TPT bifurcates into the posterior tibial (PT) and peroneal arteries (Fig. 15.11). The PT artery courses posteriorly and medially in the calf, whereas the peroneal artery runs near the fibula between the AT and PT arteries. On the dorsum of the foot, the DP artery has lateral and medial tarsal branches. After the PT artery passes behind the medial malleus, it divides into medial and lateral plantar arteries. The lateral plantar and distal DP arteries join to form the plantar arch.

Vascular access for diagnostic aortoiliac and lower-extremity angiography is obtained in the CFA, preferentially in the least symptomatic extremity, although upper-extremity access (axillary, brachial, or radial) also may be used. A 4 F to 6 F pigtail catheter is positioned above the aortic bifurcation. The preferred technique is to use DSA with a stepping table and a large (15- or 16-inch) format image intensifier so that both legs are imaged together. A single bolus of contrast is injected from the catheter at the aortic bifurcation at 8 to 12 mL/s for 8 to 10 seconds, and sequential images are obtained from the aorta to the feet.

Selective angiograms performed in angulated views of a particular artery or arterial segments are useful when clarification of a potential stenosis is needed. One option is to place a diagnostic catheter at different levels in the iliac, femoral, or popliteal artery for a more detailed examination of a particular arterial segment. If access has been obtained in the CFA and the arterial segment in question is located in the

contralateral extremity, a 4 F internal mammary catheter is positioned at the level of the aortic bifurcation, with the tip of the catheter selectively engaged in the contralateral CIA (Fig. 15.12). An angled guidewire is advanced to the CFA, and the diagnostic catheter is advanced over the guidewire to the area of interest.

Several angiographic views are important to mention because they help clarify anatomical detail. In the AP view, there is often overlapping of the origin of the external and IIA, and ostial stenoses in either or both vessels may be missed. The contralateral oblique view (20 degrees) with 20 degrees of caudal angulation is very useful to separate these vessels (Fig. 15.13).

Overlap at the origin of the SFA and DFA arteries commonly occurs in the AP projection and can be improved with a 20 to 30 degrees LAT oblique view.[7] Another common source of artifact may occur when the tibial arteries overlie the relatively radiodense bony periosteum of the tibia or fibula. In that case, slight angulation will move the artery in question off the bony density to allow better visualization.

Aortic Arch and Brachiocephalic Vessels

The aortic arch includes portions of the ascending, transverse, and descending aorta (Fig. 15.14). The thoracic aorta gives rise to the brachiocephalic trunk in the proximal portion of the arch, the left common carotid artery in the mid-portion, and the left subclavian artery in the distal portion. In 10% to 20% of cases, the left common carotid artery originates from the brachiocephalic trunk, an anatomical variation known as a *bovine arch* (Fig. 15.15). Other common variations include

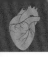

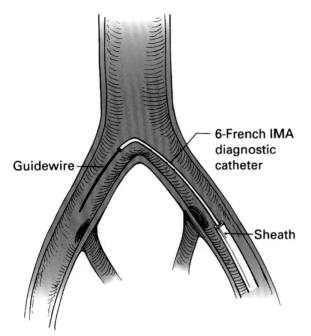

Fig. 15.12 Drawing illustrating contralateral iliac access for selective angiography. *IMA*, Internal mammary artery.

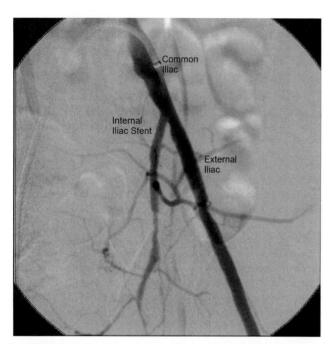

Fig. 15.13 Selective left common iliac angiography (20 degrees left anterior oblique and 20 degrees caudal view) demonstrating origin of internal iliac artery (ostial stent present) and external iliac artery.

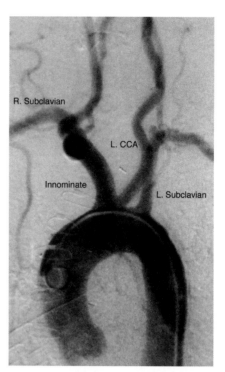

Fig. 15.14 Aortic Arch and Brachiocephalic Vessels. Digital subtraction angiogram injection of 15 mL/s of contrast material for 3 seconds, with image obtained at 30 degrees left anterior oblique. *L.CCA*, Left common carotid artery.

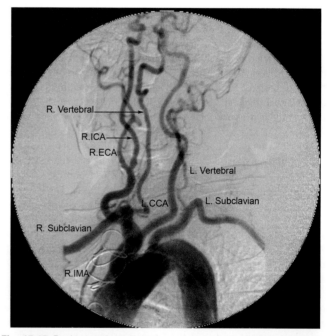

Fig. 15.15 Bovine aortic arch angiogram injection of 15 mL of contrast per second for 3 seconds (total 45 mL contrast) at 45 degrees left anterior oblique. *L.CCA*, Left common carotid artery; *R.ECA*, right external carotid artery; *R.ICA*, right internal carotid artery; *R.IMA*, right internal mammary artery.

the left vertebral artery originating directly from the aortic arch, between the left common carotid artery and left subclavian artery, and the right subclavian artery originating from the aortic arch distal to the origin of the left subclavian artery.

Thoracic aortography is commonly performed to diagnose pathological entities, such as stenoses of the origin of the great vessels, aneurysms, aortic dissection, coarctation of the aorta, patent ductus arteriosus, and vascular rings, and to evaluate vascular injuries caused by blunt or penetrating chest trauma.[8] Vascular access is most often obtained at the CFA, although the brachial or radial approaches are

also useful. A pigtail catheter is advanced into the ascending aorta and positioned proximal to the brachiocephalic trunk. Using a power injector, radiographic contrast material is injected at 15 to 20 mL/s for a total of 2 to 3 seconds. The LAO projection (30 to 60 degrees) separates the ascending from the descending aorta and allows good visualization of the origin of the great vessels (see Fig. 15.14).

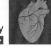

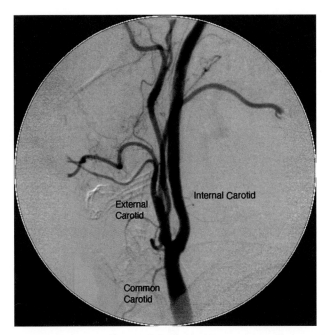

Fig. 15.16 Common Carotid Bifurcation. External carotid artery is marked by presence of branch vessels.

The brachiocephalic trunk, left common carotid artery, and subclavian arteries originate from the transverse thoracic aorta. The brachiocephalic trunk or innominate artery divides into the right common carotid artery and the right subclavian artery. The common carotid arteries run lateral to the vertebral bodies and bifurcate into the external and the internal carotid arteries at about the level of the fourth cervical vertebra (Fig. 15.16). In its extracranial portion, the internal carotid artery has no branches. On entering the skull, the internal carotid artery makes a sharp turn at the carotid siphon and thereafter divides into the middle cerebral arteries (MCA) and anterior cerebral arteries (ACA), from which the anterior communicating artery forms the anterior portion of the circle of Willis (Fig. 15.17).

Carotid Angiography

Selective carotid angiography is usually performed after obtaining an aortic arch aortogram in the LAO view, which allows the operator to visualize the origin of the brachiocephalic trunk and left common carotid artery. Using that same LAO angle, the brachiocephalic trunk is engaged with a diagnostic catheter (Fig. 15.18).

Once the origin of the common carotid artery has been engaged with a guidewire, the catheter is advanced into the common carotid artery over the wire. Care must be taken to clear the catheters and manifold of air and debris before injecting into the carotid artery. Carotid angiograms are obtained in the AP, oblique, and LAT views.

Because of the dense bony structure of the skull, it is preferable to use digital subtraction techniques for diagnostic images of the intracranial vascular anatomy. A 12-inch or larger image intensifier is optimal for intracranial angiography. It is important to emphasize using DSA for the intracranial portion of the internal carotid artery and its branches in the AP and LAT views. This enables assessment of the circle of Willis and demonstrates the presence of any collateral circulation.

Subclavian Angiography

Important branches of the subclavian artery include the vertebral (superior) and internal mammary (inferior) arteries (Fig. 15.19). The vertebral artery, the first and usually largest branch of the subclavian artery, arises from the superior and posterior surface of the subclavian. The AP view will disclose stenosis in the proximal subclavian artery (the left subclavian artery is affected three to four times as frequently as the right subclavian artery). In patients with a tortuous proximal left subclavian artery, a steep right anterior oblique (RAO) view with caudal angulation may help elucidate a proximal stenosis. If the proximal portion of the right subclavian artery is suspected of having a lesion, the AP view may not show the stenosis because of overlap with the origin of the right common carotid artery. A steep RAO caudal view (40 to 60 degrees RAO and 15 to 20 degrees caudal) will usually separate the ostia of these two vessels (Fig. 15.20).

Vertebral Angiography

The vertebral arteries are identified on the aortic arch aortogram. Often, a nonselective injection of contrast in the subclavian artery near the origin of the vertebral artery is performed to view ostial lesions. Cranial angulation (30 to 40 degrees) with shallow oblique views (RAO or LAO), may be necessary to view the origin (see Fig. 15.19). Nonselective angiography is preferred to avoid trauma when engaging the ostium of the vertebral artery with an angled catheter (Judkins right

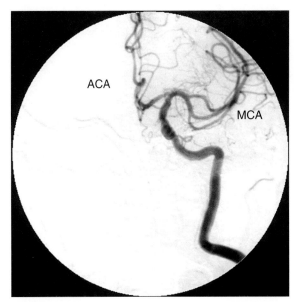

Fig. 15.17 Intracranial Carotid Arteries (Anteroposterior View). Internal carotid artery branches into middle cerebral artery *(MCA)* and anterior cerebral artery *(ACA)*.

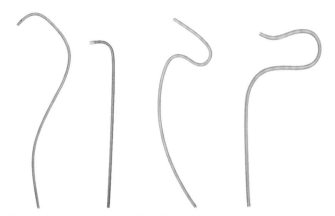

Fig. 15.18 Commonly used brachiocephalic and carotid angiographic catheters.

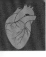

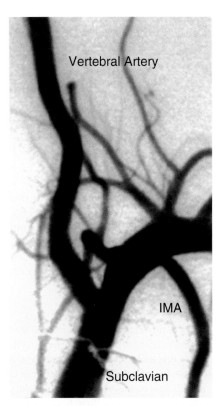

Fig. 15.19 Left subclavian angiogram showing vertebral artery arising superiorly and internal mammary artery *(IMA)* arising inferiorly.

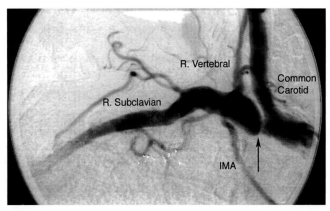

Fig. 15.20 Proximal right subclavian stenosis *(arrow)*, seen best at 40 degrees right anterior oblique and 20 degrees of caudal angulation. *IMA,* Interior mammary artery.

coronary, Berenstein, Cobra, or internal mammary artery catheter). Typically, the catheter is placed very near the ostium, and hand injections of contrast are made to visualize the vertebral artery.

The vertebral artery runs cranially through the foramina of the transverse processes of the cervical vertebrae to the base of the skull (Fig. 15.21). After penetrating the foramen of the atlas, it enters the cranial cavity through the foramen magnum. The first branch of the vertebral artery, located in its V4 segment, is the posterior inferior cerebellar artery (PICA). The vertebral artery joins with the contralateral vertebral artery to form the basilar artery (Fig. 15.22).

Nonselective angiography is performed with hand injections, using a coronary manifold with pressure monitoring, analogous to selective coronary angiography. AP and LAT views of the extracranial and intracranial course of the vertebral and basilar arteries should

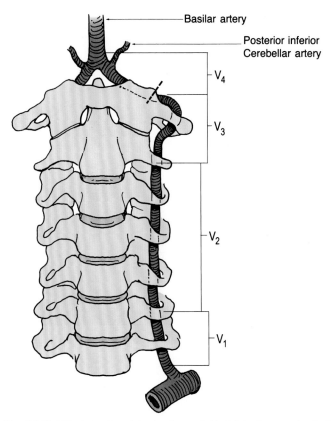

Fig. 15.21 Drawing of vertebral artery, divided into four anatomical segments that course through cervical spine foramina.

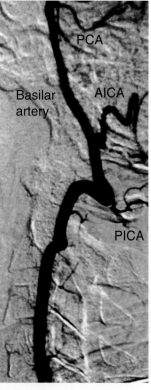

Fig. 15.22 Proximal vertebral artery segment visualized with subclavian angiography. *AICA,* Anterior inferior cerebellar artery; *PCA,* posterior cerebral artery; *PICA,* posterior inferior cerebellar artery.

be performed with a DSA technique. Similar to views of the anterior cerebral circulation, it is important to determine the contribution of the posterior circulation to the circle of Willis.

COMPLICATIONS OF PERIPHERAL VASCULAR ANGIOGRAPHY

Complications of peripheral vascular angiography may lead to significant morbidity or even mortality. Complications may be thought of in three categories: (1) access site related, (2) systemic, or (3) catheter induced. The best strategy to minimize complications is to anticipate and avoid them.

Access Site–related Complications

Vascular access site–related complications include hematoma formation, retroperitoneal hemorrhage, pseudoaneurysm formation, AVF creation, and infection. Access site bleeding is the most frequent complication following femoral arterial access.[9] It is important to note that femoral closure devices shorten time to ambulation and add cost without reducing complications.[10] The management of access site bleeding depends on the severity and hemodynamic consequences of bleeding. In general, access site bleeding is usually controlled by manual compression and reversal of anticoagulation. If bleeding continues despite these steps, more aggressive therapies—including percutaneous intervention or surgical therapy—should be considered.

Signs and symptoms of retroperitoneal bleeding include hypotension, abdominal distention or fullness, and pain. Diagnosis of retroperitoneal bleeding may be confirmed by CT or abdominal/pelvic ultrasound. If retroperitoneal bleeding is suspected, anticoagulation should be reversed and discontinued. Volume resuscitation with crystalloid solutions and/or blood products should be administered if volume depletion is clinically evident. If bleeding causes hemodynamic embarrassment (hypotension), emergency angiography from the contralateral femoral artery access site should be performed to identify the bleeding site. Once the bleeding site has been identified, tamponade of bleeding with balloon occlusion will stabilize the patient. If prolonged balloon inflation is not effective in stopping blood loss, consideration may be given to placing a covered stent to seal the leak. Open surgical repair may also be an option to consider.[11]

A pseudoaneurysm occurs when a hematoma communicates with the arterial lumen. Low arterial punctures (SFA or profunda femoris artery entry) are associated with pseudoaneurysm formation. Other risk factors include female sex, age older than 70 years, diabetes mellitus, and obesity. Patients with pseudoaneurysms often present with pain at the access site several days following the intervention. On physical examination, a pulsatile hematoma may be present with a systolic bruit. The diagnosis of a femoral pseudoaneurysm is confirmed with color-assisted duplex ultrasonography. The management of a femoral pseudoaneurysm depends on its size, the severity of symptoms, and the need for continued anticoagulation. A small pseudoaneurysm (<2 cm) may be observed and often will resolve spontaneously. Larger pseudoaneurysms may be treated with ultrasound-guided compression, percutaneous off-label thrombin injection, endovascular coil insertion, or covered stents.[11] Surgical repair of pseudoaneurysms is reserved for failure of less invasive approaches.

An AVF complicates vascular access when the needle punctures the femoral artery and nearby vein, creating a fistulous communication when the sheath is removed. The risk of creating an AVF is increased by either a high or low femoral puncture, multiple puncture attempts, or prolonged clotting times. Fistulae may not be clinically evident for several days following the procedure. An AVF is characterized by a continuous to-and-fro murmur over the access site. In some cases, there may be a swollen and tender extremity due to venous dilation, and in severe circumstances, arterial insufficiency (steal syndrome) may occur. Diagnosis of an AVF can be confirmed by color flow Doppler ultrasound.

Most AVFs following femoral access are small, not hemodynamically significant, and close spontaneously. Symptomatic AVFs require closure to prevent increased shunting and distal swelling and tenderness.[11] Surgical repair, traditional therapy for the closure of catheterization-related AVFs when necessary, has been replaced by percutaneous methods in most circumstances. Surgical correction is reserved for those patients who fail a less invasive approach.

Vascular access closure devices are designed to facilitate hemostasis, reduce time to ambulation, and decrease length of hospital stay. All devices currently approved by the US Food and Drug Administration (FDA) have shown favorable results. However, these devices are prone to specific complications and have not been demonstrated to reduce access site complications.[10]

Systemic Complications

Systemic complications relate to allergic and anaphylactic reactions, as well as nephrotoxicity caused by iodinated contrast agents. Allergic or anaphylactic reactions occur in fewer than 3% of cases, and fewer than 1% require hospitalization.

Nonoliguric creatinine elevation, which peaks within 2 to 3 days and returns to baseline by 7 days, is the usual clinical scenario of contrast-induced nephrotoxicity. Patients at risk for contrast-induced nephropathy are those with baseline chronic renal insufficiency, diabetes mellitus, multiple myeloma, and those who are receiving other nephrotoxic drugs (e.g., aminoglycosides). All patients in general, but those at risk to develop contrast-induced nephropathy in particular, should be well hydrated before and after the procedure, and the amount of contrast volume should be minimized.

Diuretics do not protect against contrast-induced nephrotoxicity. Hydration with half-normal saline for 12 hours before and after the procedure provides better protection against creatinine rise than the combination of hydration and diuretics. Two prospective trials have demonstrated that mannitol does not reduce contrast nephropathy.

The POSEIDON trial is the first randomized trial to directly compare different normal saline fluid administration protocols and to use the left ventricular end-diastolic pressure, a measure of intravascular volume status.[12] Left ventricular end-diastolic pressure-guided intravenous fluid administration significantly reduced the rates of contrast-induced acute kidney injury and major adverse clinical events.

Catheter Related Complications

Catheters may disrupt atherosclerotic plaque and cause atheroemboli (also see Chapter 45). When catheters are manipulated in the aorta or brachiocephalic vessels during a thoracic aortogram, stroke is a rare but potentially devastating complication. Patients who develop a neurological complication should have an immediate neurological assessment, and angiography of the culprit vessel should be obtained. If an embolic stroke has occurred, one option is to perform catheter-directed thrombolysis and/or thrombectomy.[13] In the presence of intracerebral hemorrhage, anticoagulants and antiplatelet agents should be discontinued or reversed.

Atheroembolism is another cause of renal insufficiency following angiography. Unlike contrast-induced nephropathy, renal dysfunction after atheroembolization usually develops slowly (weeks to months) and some of these patients progress to renal failure. Diagnosis is confirmed by tissue examination (biopsy), and treatment is supportive. Systemic manifestations of atheroembolism include livedo reticularis, abdominal or foot pain, and purple toes associated with systemic eosinophilia (blue toe syndrome).

REFERENCES

1. Saleh L, Juneman E, Movahed MR. The use of gadolinium in patients with contrast allergy or renal failure requiring coronary angiography, coronary intervention, or vascular procedure. *Catheter Cardiovasc Interv.* 2011;78:747–754.

2. Dogan M, Un H, Aparci M, et al. Carbon dioxide angiography. *Angiology.* 2016;67:973.

3. Sobolev M, Slovut DP, Lee Chang A, et al. Ultrasound-guided catheterization of the femoral artery: a systematic review and meta-analysis of randomized controlled trials. *J Invasive Cardiol.* 2015;27:318–323.

4. Lee MS, Applegate B, Rao SV, et al. Minimizing femoral artery access complications during percutaneous coronary intervention: a comprehensive review. *Catheter Cardiovasc Interv.* 2014;84:62–69.

5. Abu-Fadel MS, Sparling JM, Zacharias SJ, et al. Fluoroscopy vs. traditional guided femoral arterial access and the use of closure devices: a randomized controlled trial. *Catheter Cardiovasc Interv.* 2009;74:533–539.

6. Lo RC, Fokkema MTM, Curran T, et al. Routine use of ultrasound-guided access reduces access site-related complications after lower extremity percutaneous revascularization. *J Vasc Surg.* 2015;61:405–412.

7. Samal AK, White CJ. Percutaneous management of access site complications. *Catheter Cardiovasc Interv.* 2002;57:12.

8. Waigand J, Uhlich F, Gross C, et al. Percutaneous treatment of pseudoaneurysms and atriovenous fistulas after invasive vascular procedures. *Catheter Cardiovasc Interv.* 1999;47:157.

9. Jolly SS, Amlani S, Hamon M, et al. Radial versus femoral access for coronary angiography or intervention and the impact on major bleeding and ischemic events: a systematic review and meta-analysis of randomized trials. *Am Heart J.* 2009;157(1):132–140.

10. Patel MR, Jneid H, Derdeyn CP, et al. Arteriotomy closure devices for cardiovascular procedures: a scientific statement from the American Heart Association. *Circulation.* 2010;122:1882–1893.

11. Tsetis D. Endovascular treatment of complications of femoral arterial access. *Cardiovasc Intervent Radiol.* 2010;33:457–468.

12. Brar SS, Aharonian V, Mansukhani P, et al. Haemodynamic-guided fluid administration for the prevention of contrast-induced acute kidney injury: the POSEIDON randomised controlled trial. *Lancet.* 2014;383:1814–1823.

13. Evans MRB, White P, Cowley P, et al. Revolution in acute ischaemic stroke care: a practical guide to mechanical thrombectomy. *Pract Neurol.* 2017;17:252–265.

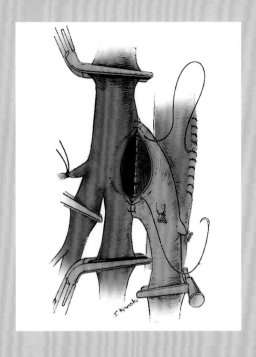

PART IV

第四部分

Peripheral Artery
Disease

外周动脉疾病

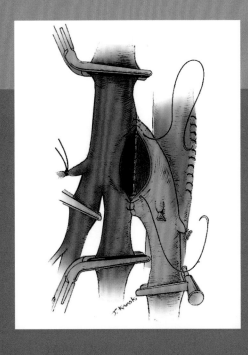

第16章
外周动脉疾病流行病学

外周动脉疾病（peripheral artery disease，PAD）的发病率很高，最近估计，美国患有外周动脉疾病的总人数超过800万，全球超过2亿。外周动脉疾病的发生率与年龄、性别、人种、收入状况有明显的相关性，与该病发生发展相关的危险因素有吸烟、糖尿病、代谢综合征、高血压、高脂血症、肥胖、酗酒、高同型半胱氨酸血症、慢性肾疾病、遗传因素等。在该病的诊断上，除了依据典型的临床表现外，踝肱比（ankle-brachial index，ABI）也是用于诊断和评估该病严重程度的客观指标，具有较好的敏感度和特异度。该病的自然病理过程并不系统地遵循从无症状进展到间歇性跛行，进而出现静息痛、坏疽的过程，部分患者可以从无症状很快进展为严重肢体缺血状态。在临床外周动脉疾病患者中，有40%～60%的患者同时合并有冠心病和脑血管狭窄性疾病，已有研究发现外周动脉疾病与冠心病和脑血管狭窄性疾病存在显著的相关性。外周动脉疾病是其他动脉硬化性疾病的独立危险因素，明显增加动脉硬化性疾病的致残率和致死率，极大增加了患者和社会的经济负担。

谷涌泉

The Epidemiology of Peripheral Artery Disease

Victor Aboyans and Michael H. Criqui

Peripheral artery disease (PAD) is one of several terms referring to a partial or complete obstruction of one or more arteries that supply blood to the limbs. Although the term PAD is sometimes inclusive of all peripheral arteries and/or any etiology, in this chapter PAD refers to atherosclerotic occlusive disease of lower extremity arteries. Other terms used for this condition in the literature are "peripheral vascular disease (PVD)" and "lower extremity arterial disease (LEAD)."

While the first studies on PAD epidemiology focused on symptomatic disease only, the development of investigative methods applicable in large cohorts enabled the identification of asymptomatic PAD. Indeed, symptomatic PAD is preceded by a long asymptomatic period, and several studies showed that even at the initial stage of the disease, patients affected by asymptomatic PAD are already at higher risk of cardiovascular (CVD) events. Consequently, more recent studies have used objective investigation methods, and typically included both symptomatic and asymptomatic forms of the disease. This has led to better estimates of PAD prevalence and incidence. Recent estimates place the total number of persons with PAD at more than 8 million in the United States and 200 million worldwide.[1,2]

SYMPTOMS AND MEASURES OF PERIPHERAL ARTERY DISEASE IN EPIDEMIOLOGY

Insufficient blood supply to the legs can cause pain and dysfunction. This type of pain is generally known as intermittent claudication (IC), characterized as leg muscle pain occurring when walking and relieved at rest, which is indicative of exercise-induced ischemic pain.

A number of questionnaires have been developed to uniformly identify IC and distinguish it from other causes of leg pain. The first was the Rose questionnaire, also referred to as the World Health Organization questionnaire. However, this questionnaire presents a low sensitivity, ranging from 9% to 68% in different studies.[1] Two other questionnaires attempted to improve the diagnostic performances;[1] The Edinburgh Claudication Questionnaire is a modification of the Rose questionnaire, with 47% to 91% sensitivity and 95% to 99% specificity in different studies. The San Diego Claudication Questionnaire is another modified version of the Rose questionnaire that additionally captures information on the laterality of symptoms (Table 16.1).

Although considered as typical, it should be emphasized that classical IC is not the sole clinical pattern related to PAD. Besides rest pain, occurring at a more evolved stage of the disease, several patterns of atypical pain can be related to PAD. For example, in the PAD Awareness, Risk, and Treatment: New Resources for Survival (PARTNERS) program, more than half of the PAD patients reported symptoms, but few reported classic Rose claudication.[3] The definitional distinctions used to separate IC from other types of leg pain make the former more specific to arterial disease, but less sensitive to other types of pain that may in some cases be related to PAD.

Two attempts have been made to qualify different patterns of non-typical pain, both using the San Diego Claudication Questionnaire (Table 16.2). In one report, five categories of symptoms have been proposed: no pain, pain on exertion and rest, noncalf pain, atypical calf pain, and classic claudication (see Table 16.2).[4] There is a respectively increasing prevalence of PAD in these five groups. In another study, McDermott et al.[5] proposed a sixth category, splitting the "no pain" group according to whether people walk enough to experience exertional pain (see Table 16.2). They also divided atypical leg pain according to whether the subject stops or carries on with this pain. The authors not only found different mean ankle-brachial index (ABI) values in different categories, but also found several concomitant disorders (i.e., neurological and articular), which can make symptoms of ischemic muscle cramp less typical. More recently, the concept of "masked PAD" has been proposed to cover all situations where patients do not complain of pain despite the presence of PAD: this encompasses patients unable to walk, or other conditions limiting walking distance before the occurrence of ischemia and pain (e.g., general conditions such as heart failure, or local conditions such as joint/muscular diseases), or when pain sensitivity is altered, especially in the elderly and/or conditions responsible for neuropathy (e.g., diabetes).[6] These cases of "masked PAD" should be conceptually distinct from truly asymptomatic PAD, but further studies are necessary to better delineate this subgroup. Masked PAD can explain why a patient can suddenly present with a severe form of PAD without any complaint beforehand.

More severe clinical forms of PAD include leg pain at rest, trophic lesions, or both. In this situation the vitality of the limb is threatened due to severe arterial insufficiency and the risk of limb loss in the absence of medical care is high. Consequently, this clinical pattern has been defined as critical limb ischemia (CLI), grouping typical chronic ischemic rest pain and ischemic skin lesions, either ulcers or gangrene.[6] This situation is more recently defined in the European Society of Cardiology PAD Guidelines as critical limb threatening ischemia (CLTI) because of the high risk of limb loss, not only because of severe ischemia, but also wounds and infection which can be present in the most severe cases.[6]

Ankle-Brachial Index

Because PAD often has a long silent course before symptoms, and given the variety of clinical signs ranging from atypical pain to severe trophic lesions, an objective method to define the disease is warranted.

TABLE 16.1   The San Diego Claudication Questionnaire (Interviewer Administered Version)

		Right	Left
1. Do you get pain or discomfort in either leg or either buttock on walking? (If no, stop)	No	1	1
	Yes	2	2
2. Does this pain ever begin when you are standing still or sitting?	No	1	1
	Yes	2	2
3. In what part of the leg or buttock do you feel it?	No	1	1
a. Pain includes calf/calves	Yes	2	2
b. Pain includes thigh/thighs	No	1	1
	Yes	2	2
c. Pain includes buttock/buttocks	No	1	1
	Yes	2	2
4. Do you get it when you walk uphill or hurry?	No	1	1
	Yes	2	2
	Never walks uphill/hurries	3	3
5. Do you get it when you walk at an ordinary pace on the level?	No	1	1
	Yes	2	2
6. Does the pain ever disappear while you are walking?	No	1	1
	Yes	2	2
7. What do you do if you get it when you are walking?	Stop or slow down	1	1
	Continue on	2	2
8. What happens to it if you stand still? (if unchanged, stop)	Lessened or relieved	1	1
	Unchanged	2	2
9. How soon?	10 min or less	1	1
	More than 10 min	2	2

1. No Pain—Q1 = 1
2. Pain at rest—Q1 = 2 and Q2 = 2
3. Noncalf—Q1 = 2 and Q2 = 1 and Q3a = 1 and Q3b = 2 or Q3c = 2
4. Non-Rose calf—Q1 = 2 and Q2 = 1 and Q3a = 2, and not Rose
5. Rose—Q1 = 2 and Q2 = 1 and Q3a = 2 and Q4 = 2 or 3 (and if Q4 = 3, then Q5 = 2), and Q6 = 1 and Q7 = 1 and Q8 = 1 and Q9 = 1
Modified from Criqui MH, Aboyans V. Epidemiology of peripheral artery disease. *Circ Res.* 2015;116(9):1509–1526.

The ABI is the ratio of the systolic blood pressure at the ankle to that in the arm. Although there is no clear-cut threshold to confirm or exclude the presence of PAD, an ABI ≤0.90 is commonly used in both clinical practice and epidemiologic research to define PAD,[7] although an ABI between 0.90 and 1.00 should be considered as borderline requiring further investigation. It is estimated that one out of four subjects with an ABI in the 0.90 to 1.00 range actually have PAD.[7] In a large German primary care cohort, compared to the reference group with an ABI ≥1.1, mortality rates were increased for ABI values within the 0.9 to 1.1 interval.[8] The ABI has been shown to have good receiver operating curve characteristics as a test for PAD.

The major advantage of ABI-defined PAD is that it covers both symptomatic and asymptomatic PAD. In the Rotterdam study, 99.4% of subjects with ABI ≥0.90 did not have IC; but only 6.3% of subjects with ABI <0.90 had claudication.[9] In another study in elderly women in the United States, these percentages were 93.3% and 18.3%, respectively.[10] In another study, even in limbs with ABI ≤0.50, considered as severe PAD, any exertional pain was not present in 17% of limbs.[11] This supports the concept of "masked PAD" presented above.[6]

In the general population, it is estimated that for every prevalent case of typical IC, two to five asymptomatic cases are generally found with the use of ABI.[1] Based on this, PAD defined by ABI is much more common than when defined by claudication in the general population, and large numbers of patients with PAD but without IC have a low (<0.90) ABI.

To validate the ABI, early studies compared the ABI measurement to angiography, considered as the "gold standard" for the visualization of atherosclerosis in the legs, and reported sensitivity and specificity

in the 97% to 100% range.[1] These studies involved comparisons of patients with angiographically-confirmed PAD with young, healthy individuals assumed not to have PAD. The reported diagnostic performances are therefore based on the ability of the ABI to discriminate between extremes of disease and health. Also using angiography as the gold standard, another study assessed the verification bias, related to the fact that only highly suspect cases are referred to angiography. Even after correcting the diagnostic performance results by the estimation of this selection bias, they found an area under the ROC curve at 0.95 when using ABI to detect >50% stenosis at angiography.[1,7] In that study, the corrected sensitivity and specificity of an ABI <0.91 was estimated at 79% and 96%, respectively.[7] This lower sensitivity can be explained in part by some PAD patients with stiff peripheral arteries and false normal ABIs.[7] Another explanation can be that normal values are different between sexes and among different ethnic groups (see below).[1,7] More recently, taking color-duplex ultrasound as a reference, a study comparing the ABI ability to diagnose PAD showed lower accuracy in diabetic than nondiabetic patients.[12]

The ABI has been demonstrated to have a strong association with CVD risk factors and disease outcomes. In a meta-analysis[13] of 16 cohort studies including over 48,000 individuals, the mortality risk by ABI had a reverse J-shaped distribution with a normal (low risk) ABI of 1.11 to 1.40. The 10-year mortality in men and women with an ABI <0.90 was 18.7% and 12.6%, respectively, with a significant risk-excess as compared to counterparts with normal (1.10 to 1.40) ABI.[13] In a clinical study, patients with ABI <0.90 who did not have exertional leg pain were shown to have poorer lower extremity functioning, even

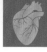

TABLE 16.2 Different Classifications of Typical/Atypical Pain in Peripheral Artery Disease Based on the San Diego Claudication Questionnaire

	CRIQUI ET AL.		MCDERMOTT ET AL.	
	Pain Category	Definition	Pain Category	Definition
Asymptomatic	No pain	No pain in either leg or buttock on walking.	No exertional pain/active	No pain in either leg or buttock on walking. Subject walking >6 blocks.
			No exertional pain/inactive	No pain in either leg or buttock on walking. Subject not walking >6 blocks.
Atypical pain	Pain on exertion/rest	Pain in either leg or buttock on walking, can sometimes begin when standing still or sitting.	Pain on exertion/rest	Pain in either leg or buttock on walking, can sometimes begin when standing still or sitting.
	Noncalf pain	Pain not in calf region but in thighs or buttocks, only when walking.	Atypical exertional leg pain/stop	Noncalf pain, starting only when walking, the subject stops walking.
	Atypical calf pain	Pain in calf region, starting only when walking, but different from classic claudication pain.	Atypical exertional leg pain/carry on	Pain starting only when walking, the subject carries on walking.
Typical "Rose" pain	Classic claudication	Pain in calf region, starting only when walking, does not disappear during walk, causing subject to halt or slow down. Pain is lessened or relieved within 10 min if walking halted.	Intermittent claudication	Pain in calf region, starting only when walking, does not disappear during walk, causing subject to halt or slow down. Pain is lessened or relieved within 10 min if walking halted.

after adjustment for traditional risk factors and comorbidities.[14] The ABI correlates with the ability to exercise as measured on an accelerometer, and an ABI <0.6 is related to the development of walking impairment.[15] The ABI also has been shown to have high intra- and inter-rater reliability.[7] Thus, even aside from its association with claudication, the ABI is considered a powerful marker for functional outcomes, risk factors, and associated CVD diseases.

However, the ABI has several limitations for PAD diagnosis. Occlusive disease located in arteries distal to the site of pressure measurement is not detected by the ABI. PAD affecting pedal arteries can be detected by the measurement of toe-brachial index (TBI), which is particularly relevant in diabetic patients who often present with more distal disease. It is suggested that ABI might also be related to the subject's height, with taller patients having slightly higher ABIs; however, this is not a consistent finding in all studies.[1] Similarly, it has been noted in several studies that the ABI in the left foot is slightly lower on average than the ABI in the right foot. It is unlikely that these differences are related to real differences in the presence of PAD.

Arterial calcification (e.g., those occurring with medial calcinosis or intimal calcification) can make the arteries of the ankle stiff and less compressible, and lead to artificially high values of the ABI. This is particularly common in patients with diabetes or chronic kidney disease (CKD).[1,7] Patients with ABI values >1.50 are often excluded in epidemiologic analyses.[1] In two large population-based studies in the United States, the proportion of patients with such elevated values was approximately 0.5%.[16,17] Some investigators use the more conservative cutpoint of 1.3. New evidence suggests 1.40 may be a good compromise and is considered as the threshold to qualify as high ABI.[7] In one study, in more than 80% of cases with an ABI >1.40, concomitant occlusive disease could be identified when using other diagnostic methods.[18] This can explain the similar rates of IC and the association with subclinical disease in other vascular beds found in patients in this elevated ABI range, compared to an ABI <0.90.

INCIDENCE AND PREVALENCE OF PERIPHERAL ARTERY DISEASE

The current prevalence of PAD worldwide is estimated at approximately 200 million people.[2] In the United States, pooling and adjusting the data of seven US population studies provided an estimate of approximately 6.8 million people aged ≥40 years affected by this condition in the year 2000,

corresponding to 5.8% of that population.[19] This estimation includes both people with an abnormal (<0.90) ABI and those with normal ABI values after lower limb revascularization. A recent meta-analysis also estimated the prevalence of PAD in the United States. In men, this prevalence ranged from 6.5% at age of 60 to 69 to 11.6% in those at age of 70 to 79, and 29.4% in those over the age of 80 years. A similar age-related rise in PAD prevalence was found in women, with a corresponding prevalence rate of 5.3%, 11.5%, and 24.7%, respectively.[19] Given the larger number of women surviving to older age, the burden of PAD (defined as the total number of individuals with prevalent PAD in the population) is significantly greater in women than in men. This is particularly true in low- and middle-income countries.[2]

More recently, several studies shed light on PAD epidemiology in the populations of non-Western countries. In a population cohort of 4055 Chinese men and women aged >60 years, the prevalence of PAD (ABI <0.90) was 2.9% and 2.8%, respectively.[20] In one Japanese community study, the prevalence of ABI <0.90 was very low at 1.4% after the age of 40.[21] In another population-based cohort of 1871 individuals above 65 years of age in two countries in Central Africa, the prevalence was considerably higher, nearing 15%.[22]

Data suggesting that PAD is more common in the black population are compelling in studies from both the United States and Africa.[1,22–24] Several large cohort studies have reported that blacks are more likely to have PAD than whites.[1,24,25] The prevalence of PAD in the >40 years old population in 2000 were estimated at 5.5%, 8.8%, 2.8%, 2.6%, and 6.1% in non-Hispanic whites, African-Americans, Hispanics, Asians, and Native-Americans, respectively. The higher prevalence of PAD in African-Americans is consistent in all large American epidemiological studies.[1,24,25]

Differences in PAD incidence and prevalence in different ethnic groups could be related to non-genetic factors, for example social and nutritional factors, and these issues are only partially controlled when comparing different ethnic groups in the same country. However, a study performed in a subset of the Multi-Ethnic Study on Atherosclerosis (MESA) population free of PAD and without any of the four traditional risk factors of PAD (smoking, hypertension, diabetes, and dyslipidemia), found that even after adjustments for a full range of anthropometric, biological, and social variables, black subjects had a lower normal ABI, about 0.02 less than non-Hispanic whites.[26] This small difference affects the prevalence of low ABI, overestimating the PAD prevalence by about +10% in this ethnic group. Nonetheless, even taking this into account, there is still a higher prevalence of PAD in blacks compared to whites. Similar findings have been found in another cohort of siblings of subjects with premature atherosclerosis.[27] Interestingly, hospital-based studies suggest that the anatomic distribution of disease may differ in blacks, with a higher percentage of distal disease in black subjects, even after adjustment for diabetes and other CVD risk factors.[1]

There is also evidence that Asians and Hispanics have a lower prevalence of PAD than whites.[25] A study of Native Americans suggested PAD prevalence comparable to that in non-Hispanic whites.[28] The explanation for these differences among races may in part reflect differences in traditional risk factors and socio-economic status.

Fig. 16.1 shows prevalence estimates of ABI-based PAD in population studies by age in women and men, in high- and low/middle-income

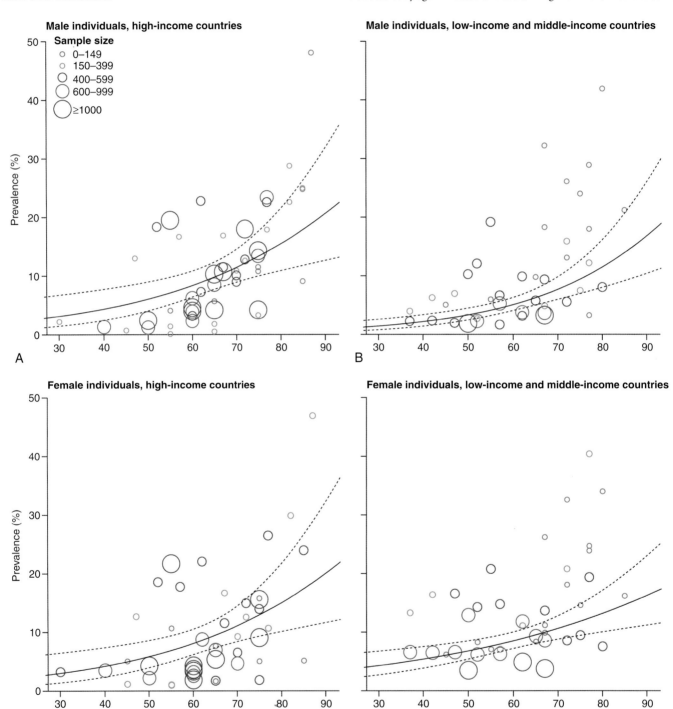

Fig. 16.1 Prevalence of Peripheral Artery Disease by Age in Men and Women in High-Income Countries and Low-Income or Middle-Income Countries According to the Global Burden Disease 2010 Study. The size and color of circles equivalent to the sample size of the population from which the datapoint was derived. Note that at younger (<40 years) and older (>80 years) ages, regression lines are based on projection only or very few datapoints. (Reprinted with permission from Elsevier. Fowkes FG, Rudan D, Rudan I, et al. Comparison of global estimates of prevalence and risk factors for peripheral artery disease in 2000 and 2010: a systematic review and analysis. *Lancet.* 2013;38:1329–1340.)

countries in 2010.[2] The figure shows a curvilinear relationship of prevalence with age in both genders. In younger populations, PAD is a newer problem for certain geographic regions, notably in the western Pacific and Southeast Asia.[2]

Estimates of PAD incidence are reported somewhat less frequently in the literature, with more data for claudication incidence than for ABI. Fig. 16.2 presents the incidence of IC according to age in available studies. Data from the Framingham study show IC in men rising from <0.4 per 1000 per year in men aged 35 to 45 years to over 6 per 1000 per year in men aged 65 years and older.[1] Incidence among women ranged from 40% to 60% lower by age, although estimates in men and women were similar by age 65 to 74. In a group of Israeli men, the incidence of claudication ranged from 6.3 per 1000 per year at ages 40 to 49 to 10.5 per 1000 at age 60 and greater.[29] In a study of 4570 men from Quebec, claudication incidence rose from 0.7 per 1000 per year at ages 35 to 44, to 3 per 1000 per year at ages 45 to 54; 7 per 1000 per year at ages 55 to 63; and 9 per 1000 at age 65 and greater.[30] In the Speedwell study, which followed English men aged 45 to 63 years for 10 years, claudication incidence per 1000 per year ranged from 3.1 in the youngest to 4.9 in the oldest age group based on age at baseline exam.[31] A higher incidence of 15.5 per 1000 per year was reported among men and women aged 55 to 74 in the Edinburgh Artery Study; however, this study did not apply strict Rose criteria for probable claudication.[32]

There are very few ABI-based studies of PAD incidence, given the time and resources required to periodically retest study subjects for incident disease. In male participants of the Limburg Study, the annual incidence of developing PAD based on an ABI <0.95 was 1.7 per 1000 at ages 40 to 54; 1.5 per 1000 at ages 55 to 64; and 17.8 per 1000 at ages ≥65.[33] The annual incidence in women was higher: 5.9, 9.1, and 22.9 per 1000 for the same age groups. More recently, in a Spanish cohort of 5434 PAD-free subjects aged 35 to 79 years recruited between 2003 and 2006 and followed on average for >5 years, the cumulative incidence of PAD (based on ABI <0.90 or clinical events) was estimated at 548 and 234 cases per 100,000 person-years in men and women, respectively.[34]

Data on temporal changes in PAD incidence and prevalence are very scarce. In the Reykjavik study, Ingolfsson and colleagues concluded that IC rates among Icelandic men dropped significantly between 1968

and 1986.[35] Among 50-year-old men, the estimate of claudication rates dropped from 1.7 per 1000 per year in 1970 to 0.6 per 1000 per year in 1984, while in 70-year-olds, this rate dropped from 6.0 to 2.0 per 1000 per year.[35] The authors attributed this to decreased smoking and cholesterol levels. In the Framingham study, a decrease of incident IC was reported, from 282 per 100,000 person-years during the 1950 to 1959 period to 225 per 100,000 person-years during the 1990 to 1999 period.[36] More recently, a population-based study in the United Kingdom showed a significant drop in incident cases of symptomatic PAD from 38.6 per 10,000 person-years (men: 51.0; women: 28.7) in 2000 to 17.3 (men: 23.1; women: 12.4) in 2014.[14] Similarly, the prevalence dropped during the same period from 3.4% (men: 4.5%; women: 2.5%) in 2000 to 2.4% (men: 3.1%; women: 1.7%) in 2014.[37]

Sex differences in the incidence and prevalence of PAD are less clear than those of other CVD diseases. Claudication incidence and prevalence have usually been found to be higher in men than women. For example, in the Framingham study, the annual claudication incidence for all ages combined was 7.1 per 1000 in men versus 3.6 per 1000 in women, for a male/female ratio of 1.97.[38] In the Framingham Offspring Study, claudication prevalence was 1.9% in men versus 0.8% in women (ratio = 2.38), while in the Rotterdam study it was 2.2% in men versus 1.2% in women (ratio = 1.83).[9]

The case for an excess of disease among males is even weaker for PAD diagnosed based on ABI. When using the usual 0.90 ABI threshold to define ABI, the male/female ratio in population studies varies from 0.71 to 1.68.[1] This is true even in those studies finding clear male excess with respect to claudication. For example, in the Framingham Offspring Study, the male/female PAD prevalence ratio based on ABI <0.90 was of 1.18.[38] In the CVD Health Study, an ABI <0.9 was somewhat more prevalent in men than women (13.8% vs. 11.4%, ratio = 1.21), but the association of disease with sex was not significant after adjusting for age and CVD status.[16] In the Atherosclerosis Risk in Communities (ARIC) study, this male/female ratio was similar in whites and blacks, at 0.71.[39] Interestingly, this sex ratio became inverted when using lower ABI thresholds, suggesting more frequent cases of severe PAD among men.[39] However, this also can be explained by potential different normal ABI values in both sexes. It has been suggested

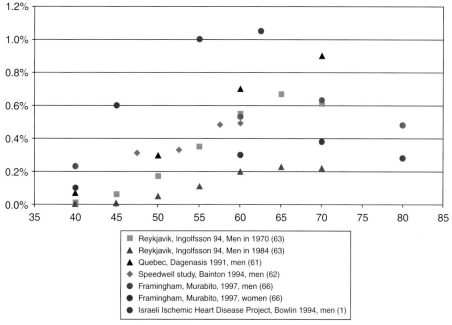

Fig. 16.2 Incidence of intermittent claudication by age in population-based studies.

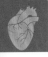

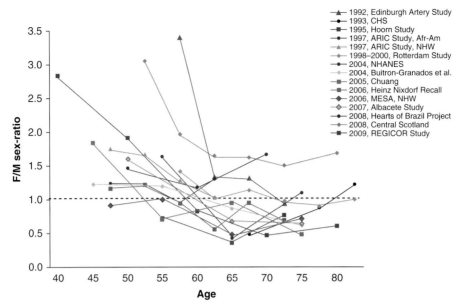

Fig. 16.3 Sex-ratio according to main epidemiological studies using ABI <0.90 to define peripheral artery disease.

that women have multiple risk factors–adjusted lower normal ABI values than men by 0.02.[26] Consequently the same threshold for both sexes would lead to PAD prevalence overestimation in women, which corresponded to a 36% increase in prevalence of PAD in women participating in the MESA study.[26] Also, the gender-ratio varies according to age groups, with an unexpectedly higher female-to-male ratio at younger ages, suggesting that young women may have lower normal values of ABI, leading to an overestimation of PAD rates at younger ages. The female-to-male ratio declines with age (Fig. 16.3) suggesting some false positive PAD diagnoses in women in younger age groups.

Data on the prevalence of CLTI are scarcer. In a 2013 meta-analysis, the prevalence of CLTI from six studies (a total of 82,923) was 0.74% (95% confidence interval [CI], 0.26 to 1.46), with marked heterogeneity among studies (ranging from 0.11% to 1.59%).[40] The contemporary retrospective analysis of the MarketScan database provides the best estimate of CLTI incidence and prevalence in the United States, with a large cohort of approximately 12 million individuals, and well-defined cases by an expert committee.[41] The study reported a prevalence of CLTI estimated at 1.33% among individuals >40 years of age with an annual incidence of CLTI at 0.35%, which equates to almost 3500 new cases per million individuals per year.[41] All patients with CLTI represented 11.08% (95% CI, 11.03% to 11.13%) of total cases of incident clinical PAD.

PERIPHERAL ARTERY DISEASE RISK FACTORS

The epidemiologic assessment of PAD and its associated risk factors is dependent on several methodological issues. First, as aforementioned, the definition of disease has evolved over time, with earlier studies focusing more on claudication, defined by Rose and other criteria, and later studies using an ABI <0.90 to define this condition. Second, the strongest epidemiological evidence for a causal relationship between disease and putative risk factors comes from studies of incident disease, while the greatest majority of the available epidemiological studies on PAD are cross-sectional. While such studies are informative, the reported associations are more subject to bias than prospective studies. Caution should therefore be exercised in reviewing the results of such cross-sectional studies, particularly where reverse causation is plausible. For example, low physical activity might cause claudication, but claudication might just as plausibly cause

low physical activity. Third, the strength of association between some risk factors and PAD may be underestimated, due to competitive outcomes (e.g., smokers may die because of coronary death prior to the diagnosis of PAD). Fourth, since the risk factors for PAD are themselves interrelated in various ways, adjustments for multiple potential risk factors in a single statistical model are necessary, in order to estimate accurately the independent contribution of any single risk factor. The following discussion of risk factors focuses on the results from five large epidemiologic studies referred to as index studies (Table 16.3).[16,38,42–44] These studies each had over 3000 subjects drawn from the general population, and included both genders. These studies are similar enough in their selection and manner of measuring risk factors, and in their statistical analyses, to allow reasonable comparisons for most of the common risk factors. Table 16.3 also includes 12 other large studies.[29,30,33,35,45–49] Although the discussion draws on data from many other studies, data are presented from these five index studies across all the conventional CVD risk factors to provide some consistency and comparability for the reader.

Another important source of information regarding the association between CVD risk factors and PAD comes from the Global Burden of Disease study[2] compiling evidence through epidemiological studies performed until 2010 worldwide (Fig. 16.4).

Smoking

Smoking is the single most important risk factor for PAD in virtually all studies (see Fig. 16.4 and Table 16.4). For current smoking, this attributable risk was estimated at 18% to 26% when PAD was defined by the ABI.[10,43] Using a clinical definition of PAD, the Health Professionals Follow-up Study estimated the attributable risk up to 44%.[49] Studies vary as to their measurement of smoking, often combining a categorical assessment of smoking status (current, past, or never) with some measure of current or historical volume of smoking; these multiple approaches to measurement make comparisons difficult (see Table 16.4). All of the large, population-based studies that were reviewed found a significant, independent association between PAD and smoking (see Table 16.4).

In several studies, an increasing risk of IC and PAD was found with a greater number of cigarettes smoked, and smoking cessation was systematically followed by a consistent decrease of PAD occurrence or progression. Smoking cessation was followed by a rapid decline in the

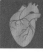

TABLE 16.3   Major Epidemiological Studies on PAD

Study Name	First Author, Year[a]	No. of Subjects	Country	Population	Study Design	PAD Definition
Index Studies						
Cardiovascular Health Study[16]	Newman, 1993	5084	USA	Ages 65+	Cross-sectional	ABI <0.90
Framingham Study[42]	Murabito, 1997	5209	USA		Cross-sectional	IC
Rotterdam Study[43]	Meijer, 2000	6450	Netherlands		Cross-sectional	ABI <0.90
Framingham Offspring Study[38]	Murabito, 2002	3313	USA		Longitudinal	ABI <0.90
Multi-ethnic Study of Atherosclerosis[44]	Allison, 2006	6653	USA		Cross-sectional	ABI <0.90
Other Large Studies						
Honolulu Heart Program[45]	Curb, 1996	3450	USA	Japanese American men	Cross-sectional and longitudinal	ABI <0.90
Edinburgh Artery Study[46]	Fowkes, 1992	1592	Scotland		Cross-sectional	ABI and reactive hyperemia
Limburg PAOD Study[33]	Hooi, 2001	2327	Netherlands		Longitudinal	ABI <0.95
Israeli Ischemic Heart Disease[29]	Bowlin, 1994	10,059	Israel	Middle-aged men	Longitudinal	IC projected
Reykjavik Study[35]	Ingolfsson, 1994	9141	Iceland	Men only	Longitudinal	IC
Quebec Cardiovascular Study[30]	Dagenais, 1991	4570	Canada	Men only	Longitudinal	IC
Physicians' Health Study[47]	Ridker, 2001	14,916	USA	Male physicians	Nested case-control	IC or PAD surgery
San Diego Population Study[48]	Criqui, 2005	2343	USA	Multiethnic	Cross-sectional	ABI ≤0.90, abnormal waveform, PAD revascularization
Health Professionals Follow-Up Study[49]	Joosten, 2012	51,529	USA	Male health professionals	Longitudinal	Clinical PAD[b]

[a] Where multiple papers were published, this refers to the paper most frequently referenced herein.
[b] Includes: limb amputation or revascularization, angiography with vascular obstruction ≥50%, ABI ≤0.90, or physician-diagnosed PAD.
ABI, Ankle-brachial index; *IC*, intermittent claudication; *PAD*, peripheral artery disease.
Modified from Criqui MH, Aboyans V. Epidemiology of peripheral artery disease. *Circ Res*. 2015;116(9):1509–1526.

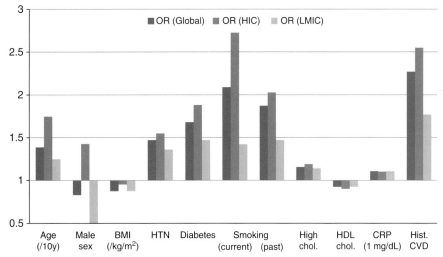

Fig. 16.4 Association of risk factors with prevalent peripheral artery disease. *BMI*, Body mass index; *CRP*, C-reactive protein; *CVD*, cardiovascular disease; *HDL*, high-density lipoprotein; *HIC*, high income countries; *HTN*, hypertension; *LMIC*, low/middle income countries; *OR*, odds ratio. (Data from Fowkes FG, Rudan D, Rudan I, et al. Comparison of global estimates of prevalence and risk factors for peripheral artery disease in 2000 and 2010: a systematic review and analysis. *Lancet*. 2013;382:1329–1340.)

TABLE 16.4 Association Between Smoking and Peripheral Artery Disease in Index Studies

Study	Variable	OR	95% CI Low	95% CI High
Framingham study	Current packs/day	1.96	1.69	2.25
Framingham offspring study	Current smoker (vs. former or never)	2.00	1.10	3.40
	Pack-years of smoking	1.03	1.02	1.03
Cardiovascular health study	Current smoker (vs. former or never)	2.55	1.76	3.68
	Pack-years of smoking	1.01	1.01	1.02
Rotterdam study	Current smoker (vs. never)	2.69	1.67	4.33
	Former smoker (vs. never)	1.15	0.75	1.78
Multi-ethnic study of atherosclerosis	Current smoker (vs. never)	3.42	2.48	4.73

CI, Confidence interval; OR, odds ratio.
From Criqui MH, Aboyans V. Epidemiology of peripheral artery disease. *Circ Res*. 2015;116(9):1509–1526.

incidence of IC. In the Health Professionals Follow-up Study, smoking was associated with increased risk of incident clinical PAD even after 20 years of smoking cessation, although this association was substantially diminished beyond 10 years after quitting smoking cigarettes.[49] In claudicants, smoking cessation has been shown to improve various functional and physiologic measures related to PAD, as well as increasing survival.[1] However, because symptomatic PAD patients have long been advised to quit smoking, it is possible that observational comparisons of patients who quit smoking with those who do not are confounded by differences in compliance with other medical advice between the two groups. Nevertheless, substantial bias is unlikely given the large effect size for cigarette smoking.

Due to the remarkable decline of smoking in general population following smoking ban legislation in several Western countries, the relative influence of smoking on incident PAD is changing. In a 50-year trend of IC in the Framingham Study, the proportion of smokers in incident cases dropped from 42% in the 1950s to 16% during the 1990s.[36]

Diabetes and Metabolic Syndrome

Diabetes is strongly associated with elevated risk of PAD (see Fig. 16.4). Intermittent claudication was more frequently observed in cases of diabetes in the Framingham, Quebec, Speedwell and Israeli civil servants studies, whereas this association was not found in the Reykjavik Study.[29–31,42] In the Edinburgh study, the association between diabetes and IC was not significant, whereas a significant inverse relationship was found with the ABI.[46]

Four of the five index studies found diabetes, dichotomized based on different criteria, to be associated with PAD after multivariable adjustment, with odds ratios (ORs) ranging from 1.89 to 4.05.[9,16,42,44] However, the Framingham Offspring Study found such an association on an age- and sex-adjusted basis, but not in multivariable models.[38] Despite its strong association with PAD but because of its lower prevalence in the population compared to other traditional risk factors, the population attributable fraction of type-2 diabetes for incident PAD was estimated at 14% in a longitudinal study on US professionals.[49]

Some inconsistencies may be related to the definition of PAD using the ABI, as this index may be falsely normal or even elevated because of concomitant vascular calcification—a condition mostly encountered in long-lasting diabetes and/or with renal failure, leading to stiffened arteries and overestimated ankle arteries pressures.[7]

Severe and/or longstanding diabetes appears to be more strongly related to PAD. In the Hoorn study, it was shown that known diabetes was associated with PAD in multivariable analysis, while newly diagnosed diabetes was only of borderline significance, and impaired glucose tolerance was not associated with PAD.[50] In that study, after excluding

patients with known diabetes, none of the common glycemic indices that were tested were significantly associated with PAD as determined by ABI, although significant associations were observed when the PAD criteria were broadened to include patients with additional criteria. Studies conducted in patients with diabetes have shown that the duration of diabetes and the use of insulin are associated with PAD.[1]

Outcomes of PAD in diabetic patients have been shown to be worse. In one study, diabetic patients with PAD were five times more likely to have an amputation than other patients with PAD, and had over three times the odds of mortality.[51] There is also some evidence to support a somewhat different anatomic distribution of disease, with greater involvement of the profunda femoris, crural, and infragenicular arteries in diabetic patients.[52]

Due to the epidemic of diabetes in Western countries, the proportion of diabetes-related PAD may increase dramatically. In the Framingham study, the proportion of incident cases with diabetes increased from 5% in the 1950s to 11% in the 1990s.[36]

Diabetes is often part of the metabolic syndrome. The recent analysis of the MESA and Cardiovascular Heart Study (CHS) longitudinal cohort studies evidenced the significant association between metabolic syndrome and incident PAD.[53,54]

Hypertension and Blood Pressure

The association of hypertension with PAD has been demonstrated in most studies in which blood pressure was studied. All five of the index studies reported a significant association between hypertension as a categorical variable and PAD. The lowest reported OR was 1.32 as reported in the Rotterdam Study; this is somewhat lower relative to the others, as it was based on a model that included both a categorical hypertension variable and an adjustment for systolic blood pressure level, which was also significant.[43] Other than this, ORs for hypertension ranged from 1.50 to 2.20.[1]

Most other large, population-based studies have also found a significant, independent association of hypertension or systolic blood pressures with PAD.[a] Where both systolic and diastolic pressures were considered, systolic pressure was usually found to be associated with PAD, whereas diastolic pressure was not significantly associated.[16,43]

Although the relative risks associated with hypertension are modest in some studies, its high prevalence, particularly among older patients, makes it a significant contributor to the total burden of PAD in the population. For example, in one large study from the Netherlands, the OR for hypertension was 1.32, but its attributable fraction (a measure of the proportion of PAD in the population attributable to hypertension) was

[a]References 30, 31, 33, 46, 48, 49.

17.0%.[43] In the Framingham Study, 30% of the risk of IC in the population was attributable to blood pressure in excess of 160/100 mm Hg.[42] Even higher population risk attributable to hypertension, 41%, was recently reported in the Health Professionals Follow-up Study (HPFS).[49] In these three latter studies, hypertension was second only to current smoking as the most contributive risk factor for PAD in the population.

Lipids

The challenge of defining the roles of the various lipid fractions in PAD lies in identifying the strongest independent risk factors from among multiple correlated measures. Results from the major population studies are presented in Table 16.5.

Total cholesterol was examined as a potential risk factor in four of the index studies, and it was significantly associated with PAD in multivariable analysis in three;[16,43,55] in the remaining study, total cholesterol was significant in a univariate analysis but dropped out of multivariable models in which other lipid measures were considered.[38] In other studies, total cholesterol has usually been found to be associated with PAD with occasional null findings in multivariable analyses in which other lipid measures are considered.[1] According to the HPFS, the population attributable fraction for PAD related to hypercholesterolemia is 17%.[49] High-density lipoprotein cholesterol (HDL-C) has been shown to be protective against PAD in most studies where it was evaluated, usually in models that also considered total cholesterol. HDL-C was included among the potential risk factors in three of the five index studies and the total cholesterol/HDL-C ratio in the fourth, and it was significantly associated with PAD in multivariable analysis in all four. In two studies, both HDL-C and total cholesterol were significant in multivariable analysis, whereas in one study, HDL-C (but not total cholesterol) was significant. Other studies have also shown a protective effect of HDL-C.[1] In a large cohort of Israeli men, non–HDL-C (total cholesterol minus HDL-C) was significantly associated with incident IC; neither total cholesterol nor HDL-C were significantly associated with disease in models that included non–HDL-C.[29] In a comparison of incident cases of IC with healthy controls in the Physician's Health Follow-up Study, the ratio of total cholesterol/HDL-C was the lipid measure most strongly associated with disease, with patients in the highest quartile having 3.9× the IC risk of patients in the lowest quartile, while screening for other lipid fractions was judged to have little clinical usefulness beyond the measurement of this ratio.[47]

Previous case-control studies showed a consistent relationship between hypertriglyceridemia and PAD. However, using multivariable modeling, the Edinburgh Artery Study challenged these findings.[46] Among the index studies, only two included triglycerides among the potential risk factors evaluated. In both cases, triglycerides were significant in univariate analysis but dropped out of multivariable models based on stepwise logistic regression.[16,38] Other studies have shown triglycerides to be significantly and independently associated with PAD in multivariable analysis.[31,56] There is also some evidence suggesting that elevated triglycerides may have a role in disease progression or more severe PAD.[46]

In summary, although total cholesterol, HDL-C, and triglycerides all seem to be associated with PAD on a univariate basis, in multivariable analysis, triglycerides frequently drop out as an independent risk factor. It is unclear whether total cholesterol is the strongest independent risk factor for PAD; in one comparison of patients with PAD with healthy controls, it was found that mean total cholesterol did not differ significantly, whereas triglycerides, very low-density lipoprotein (LDL) cholesterol, LDL cholesterol, HDL-C, and the total-cholesterol/HDL-cholesterol ratio all did.[57] Total cholesterol and HDL-C seem to provide distinct information, and they lend themselves to summarization in a single ratio.

A growing amount of evidence suggests that the plasma levels of lipoprotein (a) (Lp[a]) are a determining risk factor for PAD. This has been observed in cases of PAD occurring at a young age, in diabetic patients, as well as a case control study.[58] Lp(a) was found as an independent factor of PAD progression. The InChianti study, which enrolled 1002 Italian individuals aged 60 to 92 years, studied the prevalence of PAD as well as its incidence over 6 years of follow-up, and found that participants in the highest quartile of the Lp(a) distribution ($\geq$32.9 mg/dL) were more likely to have prevalent PAD compared to those in the lowest quartile (OR = 1.83, 95% CI 1.01 to 3.33), but the study did not find a significant association between high Lp(a) levels and incident PAD.[59]

Lipoprotein-associated phospholipase A2 (Lp-PLA$_2$) is an enzyme highly expressed by macrophages in atherosclerotic lesions and is responsible for the hydrolysis of oxidized phospholipids on LDL particles. Recently, the analysis of several cohort studies assessed the association of Lp-PLA$_2$ with incident PAD. Two studies[60,61] showed a significant association of Lp-PLA$_2$ activity with incident PAD, while the MESA has not found such an association.[62]

TABLE 16.5   Association Between Dyslipidemia and Peripheral Artery Disease in Index Studies

Study	Variable	OR	95% CI	
			Low	High
Framingham Study[a]	Total cholesterol (10 mg/dL)	1.05	1.02	1.07
Framingham Offspring Study[b]	HDL cholesterol (5 mg/dL)	0.90	0.80	1.00
Cardiovascular Health Study[c]	Total cholesterol (10 mg/dL)	1.10	1.06	1.14
	HDL cholesterol (5 mg/dL)	0.95	0.90	1.00
Rotterdam Study[d]	Total cholesterol (10 mg/dL)	1.05	1.01	1.08
	HDL cholesterol (5 mg/dL)	0.93	0.87	1.00
Multi-ethnic Study of Atherosclerosis[e]	Dyslipidemia (yes/no)	1.58	1.22	2.05

[a] Only total cholesterol was tested.
[b] Hypercholesterolemia ($\geq$240 mg/dL or medication) and triglycerides dropped out of stepwise logistic regression model.
[c] Triglycerides dropped out of stepwise logistic regression model.
[d] Triglycerides not tested.
[e] Total/HDL cholesterol ratio >5.0 or lipid medication use.
CI, Confidence interval; HDL, high-density lipoprotein; OR, odds ratio.

Obesity

Among the conditions known as being harmful for the CVD system, obesity presents the most conflicting results regarding its association to PAD. To date, the preponderance of evidence fails to support a consistent, independent positive association between obesity and PAD. In a study of 10,059 Israeli men, for every increase of body mass index (BMI) per $5 kg/m^2$, the risk of occurrence of intermittent claudication was independently increased by 24%.[29] Three of the index studies and many other large, population-based studies have failed to find a significant association between obesity and PAD or claudication after multivariable adjustment. There have also been many studies, including the other two index studies, in which higher relative weight or BMI was actually shown to be protective against PAD. In the Framingham Study, claudication was significantly inversely related to relative weight in men in multivariable analysis and seemed to have a U-shaped nonlinear relationship with relative weight in women.[63] The CHS found higher BMI to be significantly protective against PAD after multivariable adjustment in a large sample of Medicare beneficiaries.[16] BMI was significantly protective against PAD (defined based on a combination of ABI, Doppler flow curves, and history of surgery) in the Hoorn Study.[50] Similarly, the odds of PAD among subjects in the highest quintile of BMI compared with the lowest quintile were found to be significantly reduced in a cross-sectional analysis of elderly Japanese American men in Honolulu.[45] Subjects with higher BMI also were shown to be at significantly lower risk of PAD in a study of Taiwanese subjects with diabetes mellitus.[62] Finally, the multiethnic San Diego Population Study (SDPS) reported a significant inverse association of BMI and PAD.[48] Obesity has been implicated in the causes of other risk factors for PAD, such as hypertension, type II diabetes mellitus, and dyslipidemia. Adjusting for factors that are on the causal pathway between a risk factor and disease is known to attenuate the observed strength of that risk factor. Therefore, estimates of risks related to obesity in multivariable models are estimates of the risk of obesity that artificially ignore most of the mechanisms by which obesity might reasonably cause PAD. In a few cases, unadjusted models or models adjusted only for age and sex show a significant association with PAD, although obesity was not significant or protective after multivariable adjustment.[38,46,64] However, in other studies, obesity was found to be either protective or not significant even in unadjusted models or models adjusted only for age and sex.[16,31,43,45,63] Thus the failure to find more cases of a positive association between PAD and obesity is not simply an artifact of adjusting for factors on the causal pathway in multivariable modeling. Unaccounted for in the multivariable analyses just cited is possible residual confounding by cigarette smoking, which is strongly associated with both PAD and lower BMI. In addition, chronic illness in older patients, including PAD, may lead to weight loss, allowing for a spurious inverse correlation between obesity and PAD. In cross-sectional analysis of the CHS cohort, each $5 kg/m^2$ increase in BMI was inversely associated with PAD (PR [prevalence ratio], 0.92).[65] However, among people in good health who had never smoked, the direction of association was opposite (PR = 1.20). Similar results were observed between BMI calculated using weight at the age of 50 years and PAD prevalence (prevalence ratio, 1.30), and between BMI at baseline and incident PAD events occurring during follow-up (hazard ratio [HR], 1.32), among never smokers in good health. Thus, the reported inverse associations between BMI and PAD may be artifactual. As in coronary artery disease epidemiology, there is some evidence to suggest that central adiposity may be more closely related to an increased risk of PAD. Vogt et al. found that, after adjustment for BMI, higher waist/hip ratio was associated with significantly higher risk of PAD.[10] In a group of patients with diabetes mellitus, it was shown that waist/hip ratio, but not BMI or body fat percentage, was associated with PAD.[62]

Alcohol Consumption

Evidence for a protective effect of light to moderate alcohol consumption is less consistent for PAD. In the Rotterdam Study, moderate alcohol consumption was found protective in women but not in men, whereas the opposite—a protective effect of alcohol—was seen in men but not women in the Edinburgh Artery Study; this association disappeared after adjustment for social class.[66] The most protective effect of moderate alcohol for PAD was found in the Strong Heart Study, which is exclusively focused on Native Americans Indians.[28] Conversely, in the Honolulu study, alcohol intake was found to increase rather than decrease the risk of incident PAD in Japanese American men.[45] Data from the Physician's Health Study suggest that a protective effect related to moderate alcohol consumption may exist.[67] In that study, there was no univariate association between alcohol and claudication incidence but further adjustment for cigarette smoking actually revealed a significant protective association, reflecting the positive correlation of alcohol consumption with smoking, a strong risk factor for PAD. Based on this, it seems possible that incomplete adjustment for smoking in other studies might allow residual confounding that would obscure any protective effect of alcohol despite multivariate adjustment.

Homocysteine

The association of homocysteine with PAD has been debated because of conflicting results, but a meta-analysis of 14 studies showed that homocysteine was significantly elevated (pooled mean difference, +4.31 $\mu mol/L$) in patients with PAD compared with controls.[68] Two nested case-control studies within the Nurses Health Study and the HPFS cohorts found homocysteine levels positively associated, and dietary folate intake inversely associated, with the risk of PAD in men but not in women.[69]

Inflammatory Markers

Fibrinogen and C-reactive protein are two inflammatory markers that have been shown to be associated with PAD in several studies. In an analysis from the Physician's Health Study, each was found to be significantly associated with IC in multivariable models, with ORs for the upper versus lower population quartiles of 2.2 for fibrinogen and 2.8 for C-reactive protein.[47] In studies using ABI, fibrinogen was significantly associated with PAD in multivariable analysis in six studies.[b] Only Carbayo et al.[72] reported a negative result, but converse with other studies, their fibrinogen variable in the model was categorical (> vs. $\leq$400 mg/dL). Beyond a marker of inflammation, fibrinogen is a major determinant of blood viscosity. Hence, the relationship between PAD and fibrinogen also can be due to rheological factors affecting distal limb perfusion. Other studies have also reported significant and independent associations of PAD with C-reactive protein.[27]

Chronic Kidney Disease

In patients at end-stage renal disease, the prevalence of PAD (ABI <0.90) is extremely high, estimated at 38% in a single-center study, to which should be added 14% of cases with noncompressible ankle arteries.[73] CKD and PAD share several common risk factors, especially age, hypertension, and diabetes. Nevertheless, in the Cardiovascular Health Study, creatinine levels were independently associated with prevalent PAD, after adjusting for usual risk factors.[16] In the NHANES, CKD defined as glomerular filtration rate <60 mL/mn/$1.73 m^2$ was an independent factor associated for PAD (OR = 2.17, 95% CI 1.10–4.30).[74]

---

[b]References 9, 28, 43, 45, 70, 71.

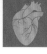

Among the 14,280 middle-aged men enrolled in the ARIC study and followed for a mean period of 13 years, CKD was shown to be significantly associated with incident PAD defined by an ABI <0.90, with an HR at 1.56 in a multivariable model including usual risk factors.[75] In a more recent analysis of the same cohort, renal failure was independently associated with future PAD risk, using new makers of CKD, particularly cystatin C and β-2-microglobulin.[76] The well-known association of CKD with vascular calcification likely results in many falsely high ABIs, which will artifactually attenuate the CKD-PAD association.

Genetic Factors

Genetic factors appear to have a role in PAD, but data are limited. Wassel et al. reported that in the SDPS, a family history of PAD was independently and strongly associated with PAD prevalence and severity.[77] This indicates a role for genetic factors or other shared environmental factors, or both, contributing to PAD. Similarly, in the Framingham Study, a family history of IC significantly predicted incident IC.[78] In a study of fraternal and identical twins, Carmelli and colleagues estimated that 48% of the variability in ABI could be explained by additive genetic effects.[79] It also has been shown that familial hypercholesterolemia, a genetic disorder, is related to a higher prevalence of PAD.[80]

A meta-analysis of 21 genome-wide association studies (GWAS) in 41,692 persons evaluated both categorical PAD (ABI ≤0.90) and the continuous distribution of ABI as outcomes.[81] One genome-wide significant association on chromosome 9p21, rs10757269, was identified for ABI. Two candidate genes for PAD and 1 SNP for coronary artery disease were associated with ABI, DAB21P (rs13290547), CYBA (rs3794624), and rs1122608 (LDLR). No significant associations were found for categorical PAD. Using a categorical PAD definition, including revascularization, Kullo et al. reported that in a GWAS the SNP rs653178 in the ATXN2-SH2B3 locus was significantly associated with PAD.[82] However, Wassel et al. reported from the candidate gene association resource (CARe) consortium no strong genetic associations for either categorical PAD or the continuous measure of ABI.[83] Further studies regarding this topic are ongoing.

Other Risk Factors

A variety of other potential risk factors for PAD have been examined: In several studies, various measures of oral health have been shown to be independently associated with PAD.[84,85] During a follow-up of 1110 male veterans during 25 years, men with periodontal disease had a 2.3 times higher risk of incidence of PAD versus men without periodontal disease.[85] Similar findings were noted in the Health Professionals' Follow-up Study, with an excess risk for incident PAD in cases of periodontal disease or tooth loss (OR = 1.40, $P < .05$), independent of age and traditional CVD risk factors.[84] These findings are possibly explained by common inflammatory pathways. Psychosocial factors were found to be associated with PAD in one large cohort in Scotland, while in a large study of Israeli men, anxiety, job-related stress and manner of coping with job-related conflicts were all significantly related to incident claudication even after adjustment for traditional risk factors.[29] In the MESA study, a low level of education and income were both associated with PAD.[44]

There is a growing amount of evidence for an association between osteoporosis and atherosclerosis, and this association is also found with PAD.[1] In the study of osteoporotic fractures, cross-sectional and prospective data have shown that among elderly women the mineral density measured in several bones was positively correlated with the ABI, and the annual ABI decrease was positively correlated with bone loss rates.[1,87-90] In the Rotterdam Study,[88] the risk of PAD (ABI <0.90) was increased in women (but not in men) who had a low femoral neck bone mineral density (BMD), whereas no association

was found between PAD and lumbar spine BMD. Similarly, in an Italian cross-sectional study[89] when BMD was assessed at the femoral neck, ABI levels were lower in postmenopausal women with osteoporosis compared to osteoporosis-free counterparts, and this association remained significant even after multivariate analysis controlling PAD and osteoporosis risk factors. This study also did not find any relationship between lumbar spine BMD and PAD. In MESA, there was an association between lower lumbar vertebral BMD and lower ABI in men.[87] In the postmenopausal women study, ABI was also correlated with BMD assessed in the wrist, excluding the hypothesis of a direct role of obstructed arteries impeding the bone cells nutrient supply.[90] Several studies generated other hypotheses regarding mechanisms, such as the calcium transfer from bones to the atherosclerotic plaque, as well as potential roles for estrogen deficiency, a direct role of LDL oxidative products inhibiting osteoblastic differentiation, secondary hypoparathyroidism, vitamin D excess and vitamin K deficiency, and the inflammatory process favoring the osteoclastic activity.

Other possible risk factors for which some supporting data exist include antiphospholipid antibodies, hypothyroidism, sedentary lifestyle, and pollution.[1] Regarding the last of these, higher lead and cadmium blood levels were associated with increased risk of prevalent PAD.[91] Long-term air pollution exposure has been shown to have an effect on the development of atherosclerotic diseases, including PAD. In Germany, pollution (in particular, from road traffic) was associated with a reduced ABI in exposed individuals.[91]

Possible protective effects have been reported for antioxidants, high dietary intake of vitamin E, fibers, and vegetable lipids as well as hormone replacement therapy.[1] However, the Women's Health Initiative's randomized, clinical trial of combined estrogen/progestin therapy showed no beneficial effect on incident PAD.[92]

INTERACTION AND RISK FACTOR COMPARISONS

Some research has been conducted into potential variations in the significance and strength of the various risk factors as they are estimated in different subgroups and for different PAD-related outcomes. Differences in the relative strength and significance of risk factors in men and women have been examined in several studies. Many of these studies have concluded that risk factors do not differ substantially in men and women.[1]

Regarding potential interactions between ethnicity and CVD risk factors, the SDPS showed no evidence that a greater sensitivity of blacks to traditional CVD risk factors explained ethnic differences in PAD.[48]

Peripheral Artery Disease Risk Scores

PAD risk scoring systems have been proposed, including a scoring system involving novel biomarkers not routinely measured, but none has yet gained acceptance. Of note, the General Framingham score is used to predict a composite outcome of coronary heart disease, stroke, IC, or congestive heart failure.[93] Analyses of prediction of the individual outcome components showed that an IC-specific model and prediction of IC with the general score showed high concordance.

PROGRESSION OF PERIPHERAL ARTERY DISEASE

The natural history of PAD can be estimated through studies performed years ago, prior to the advent of revascularization techniques and medications that improve the local and general prognosis. A classical study included a cohort of 520 patients with the diagnosis of "arteriosclerosis obliterans" based only on symptoms and clinical examination and was managed between 1939 and 1948 at the Mayo

Clinic.[94] Two-thirds presented with IC, while the others presented with pain at rest and/or trophic lesions. The survival rates of these patients at 5 and 10 years were approximately 75% and 50%, respectively. Among deceased patients, 75% were related to CVD causes. Amputation was required in 8.9% of cases (almost 15% of the survivors) during the 5 years follow-up, but this occurred in only 3% of patients who initially had an IC. Importantly, 11.3% of patients who continued smoking experienced an amputation, but none who abstained from smoking had an amputation. In a Finnish series of PAD patients (three-quarters with IC, one-quarter with more progressed disease) followed for approximately 10 years, half of the patients died.[1] Among the survivors, one-quarter clinically improved, one-half were clinically stable, and one-quarter experienced clinical worsening. In a population >65 years of age with IC, the 5-year clinical progression can be summarized as: symptoms deteriorated in 25% of patients, with claudication worsening in almost 15% of cases, while 5% to 10% progressed to CLI with approximately 5% requiring amputation.[95] In a study defining disease progression by the occurrence of rest pain or gangrene, PAD progressed in 2.5% of patients annually, with a progression rate approximately three times greater in the first year following diagnosis than in subsequent years.[96] Nowadays, the limb prognosis of patients with symptomatic PAD has not substantially improved, though direct comparisons are difficult since the access to healthcare for PAD probably differs in different periods and different countries, and the patterns of risk factors—especially the prevalence of diabetic patients—has changed, and the overall survival improved. In the SMART study conducted in the Netherlands in this century, during a mean follow-up of 5.5 years of patients with clinical PAD, 7.6% experienced amputation.[97] However, these results are related to cases referred to vascular centers, and it is well known that almost one-half of patients with clinical symptoms, probably those at a less severe stage, are not referred for specialized management. In two large epidemiological studies, only 1.6% and 1.8% of patients who developed claudication came to amputation.[63,98] In the Edinburgh Artery Study, 8.2% of patients with claudication at baseline underwent vascular surgery or amputation.[32] However, it should be emphasized that the clinical progression of PAD does not systematically follow the asymptomatic—exercise pain—rest pain—trophic lesions scheme. A patient can directly switch from asymptomatic PAD to chronic limb ischemia, especially the elderly and in the presence of diabetes, when subjects might have walking limitations for other reasons masking exertional pain, and a minor trauma can have delayed healing and quickly turn the limb's clinical state into CLI. This is the concept of "masked PAD" presented earlier in this chapter. In one of the largest series of CLI, about 15% of cases did not have prior intermittent claudication.[99] This proportion was even higher (37%) in another smaller series.[100]

Little is known about the early natural history of PAD, particularly the progression of the disease during the asymptomatic period, and the transition from asymptomatic to early symptomatic disease. In the Edinburgh Artery Study, the 5-year occurrence of IC was estimated at 3.2% in those who initially had no PAD (normal ABI and reactive hyperemia test), while the occurrence of IC was 9.3% among those who initially had asymptomatic PAD.[32] In a recent meta-analysis of available studies between 1990 and 2015, it was estimated that over 5 years, 7% of patients with asymptomatic PAD progress to clinical PAD, mostly intermittent claudication.[101]

The average annual change in ABI has been estimated as −0.01 and −0.02 in various groups.[102,103] However, these figures may be somewhat misleading, because average change in ABI is subject to considerable variability and is biased by arterial stiffening. A more meaningful approach may be to look at the percentage of the population achieving some categorically defined measure of change. Nicoloff and colleagues found that in 5 years, 37% of patients experienced a significant (≥0.15) worsening of ABI, while 22% of patients experienced clinical progression of PAD based on a change in symptoms or a need for surgical intervention.[104] Among 415 English smokers with PAD referred for a surgical opinion, about half experienced a significant (≥0.14) drop in ABI over the following 48 months.[105] Bird and colleagues defined a ranked series of six categories of PAD based on ABI and other tests in a study of patients referred to a vascular laboratory. In this study, 30.2% of limbs progressed to a more serious category of PAD over an average follow-up time of 4.6 years, but 22.8% of limbs regressed to a less severe category during the same period.[103]

Two studies addressed the epidemiology of PAD progression based on the ABI change.[106–108] Over approximately 5 years, the ABI change was at −0.06 in a clinical cohort[108] and −0.03 in a general population cohort.[106] In the clinical cohort composed of subjects with and without PAD having visited a vascular laboratory, active smoking, the total cholesterol/HDL-C ratio, Lp(a), and C-reactive protein were significant markers of substantial ABI decrease.[108] Interestingly, in this study, diabetes was not associated with ABI decline, but was the sole significant risk factor for small-vessels disease progression, defined by a substantial TBI drop without any noticeable ABI change. Markers of inflammation were also found as independent and significant factors associated with ABI decline in the Edinburgh Artery Study, with fibrinogen and interleukin-6 as the most significant factors.[107]

In the CVD Health Study, cystatin C, a marker of renal function, was positively correlated with the rates of further interventions (revascularization/amputation) in patients with PAD.[109]

Additionally, it has been shown that patients with a more progressive PAD were at a higher risk of CV death.[110] In this instance, the progression of PAD in longitudinal studies might be underestimated due to selective mortality in patients with greater progression.

CO-PREVALENCE OF PERIPHERAL ARTERY DISEASE AND OTHER ATHEROSCLEROTIC DISEASE

Given the common risk factors for PAD and other CVD and cerebrovascular disease, it is not surprising that patients with PAD are more likely to have these other disorders concomitantly, and vice versa. In patients with clinical PAD, 40% to 60% also have clinical CAD.[1,3] In a seminal report of a series of 1000 PAD patients undergoing revascularization surgery, systematic coronary angiography revealed that 90% them had angiographically significant lesions.[111] In two smaller but more recent series using coronary CT-scans, one-third of patients with PAD had significant coronary obstructive lesions.[112,113] In the CVD Health Study, the prevalence of a history of myocardial infarction (MI) was 2.5 times as high in subjects with PAD (based on ABI <0.9) versus those without; for angina, congestive heart failure, stroke, and transient ischemic attack, the prevalence was 1.9, 3.3, 3.1, and 2.3 times as high, respectively.[114] Similarly, the prevalence of PAD was 2.1 times higher in patients with a history of MI versus those without. The corresponding ratios for angina, congestive heart failure, stroke, and transient ischemic attack were 1.7, 2.6, 2.4, and 2.1, respectively.[24] Other cross-sectional studies have found similar correlation.[115–118] Subjects with PAD have also been shown to have an elevated prevalence of carotid artery stenosis with a prevalence of >30% carotid stenosis estimated between 51% and 72% of cases.[119,120] A modest but significant correlation between the two diseases' severity has been demonstrated. Fig. 16.5 summarizes the rates of concomitant arterial diseases in other main territories in patients with PAD.[6]

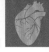

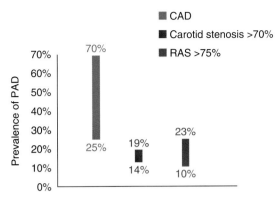

Fig. 16.5 Association of peripheral artery disease *(PAD)* with other arterial diseases. *CAD,* Coronary artery disease; *RAS,* renal artery stenosis. (Data from Aboyans V, Ricco JB, Bartelink MEL, et al. 2017 ESC guidelines on the diagnosis and treatment of peripheral arterial diseases, in collaboration with the European Society for Vascular Surgery [ESVS]: Document covering atherosclerotic disease of extracranial carotid and vertebral, mesenteric, renal, upper and lower extremity arteries. *Eur Heart J.* 2018;39:763–816.)

PERIPHERAL ARTERY DISEASE AS A PREDICTOR OF MORTALITY AND MORBIDITY

Patients with PAD, even when asymptomatic, are at increased risk of incident morbidity and mortality from other types of atherosclerotic disease, even after adjustment for known common risk factors. Although PAD is unlikely to directly cause these other diseases, the presence of PAD serves as a marker for underlying atherosclerotic processes or susceptibilities affecting other vascular beds. These prospective relationships are clinically important, to the extent that the PAD has prognostic value independent of other known risk factors.

Table 16.6 provides a summary of studies of the association of PAD with various mortality and morbidity outcomes. The table is limited to studies using a noninvasive measure of PAD (usually ABI at various cut-points). In addition, included studies used logistic or proportional hazard regression models, with multivariable adjustment for conventional CVD risk factors. Results are shown with multivariable adjustments and after the exclusion of subjects with baseline CVD disease where such exclusion was attempted.

TABLE 16.6   Association of PAD with Various Mortality and Morbidity Outcomes

Study	PAD Definition	Hazard Ratio	95% CI Lower	95% CI Upper	Model Specifications
Total Mortality					
Criqui, 1992	Large-vessel PAD	3.1	1.8	5.3	Adjusted for conventional risk factors; excludes subjects with baseline angina, MI, stroke (multiple criteria)
Newman, 1993	ABI <0.9	3.4	1.6	7.1	Adjusted for conventional risk factors; excludes subjects with baseline cardiovascular disease
Vogt, 1993	ABI <0.9	3.1	1.5	6.7	Adjusted for conventional risk factors; excludes subjects with baseline cardiovascular disease
Ogren, 1993	ABI <0.90	2.3	1.4	3.8	Adjusted for conventional risk factors
Kornitzer, 1995	ABI <0.9	2.1	0.90	4.8	Adjusted for conventional risk factors other than blood pressure; excludes baseline CHD
Jager, 1999	ABI <0.9	1.5	0.8	2.8	Adjusted for conventional risk factors
Newman, 1999	ABI <0.9	1.6	1.2	2.1	Adjusted for conventional risk factors; excludes subjects with baseline cardiovascular disease
Hooi, 2002	ABI <0.7 (vs. >0.95)	2.1	1.6	2.8	Adjusted for conventional risk factors
Murabito, 2003	ABI <0.9	1.4	0.9	2.1	Adjusted for conventional risk factors
Lee, 2004	ABI ≤0.9	1.1	0.9	1.4	Adjusted for conventional risk factors
Resnick, 2004	ABI ≤0.9	1.7	1.3	2.1	Adjusted for conventional risk factors
Cardiovascular Disease Mortality					
Criqui, 1992	Large-vessel PAD	6.3	2.6	15.0	Adjusted for conventional risk factors; excludes subjects with baseline angina, MI, stroke (multiple criteria)
Vogt, 1993	ABI <0.9	4.5	1.5	6.7	Adjusted for conventional risk factors; excludes subjects with baseline cardiovascular disease
Kornitzer, 1995	ABI <0.9	3.3	1.0	10.6	Adjusted for conventional risk factors other than blood pressure; excludes baseline CHD

TABLE 16.6   Association of PAD with Various Mortality and Morbidity Outcomes—cont'd

Study	PAD Definition	Hazard Ratio	95% CI		Model Specifications
			Lower	Upper	
Jager, 1999	ABI <0.9	2.4	0.9	6.1	Adjusted for conventional risk factors
Newman, 1999	ABI <0.9	2.1	1.2	3.4	Adjusted for conventional risk factors; excludes subjects with baseline cardiovascular disease
Hooi, 2002	ABI <0.7 (vs. >0.95)	2.3	1.7	3.1	Adjusted for conventional risk factors
Lee, 2004	ABI ≤0.9	1.3	0.9	1.8	Adjusted for conventional risk factors
Resnick, 2004	ABI ≤0.9	2.5	1.7	3.6	Adjusted for conventional risk factors
Coronary Heart Disease Mortality					
Criqui, 1992	Large-vessel PAD	4.3	1.4	12.8	Adjusted for conventional risk factors; excludes subjects with baseline angina, MI, stroke (multiple criteria)
Kornitzer, 1995	ABI <0.9	3.6	1.1	11.8	Adjusted for conventional risk factors other than blood pressure; excludes baseline CHD
Cardiovascular Morbidity					
Newman, 1993	ABI <0.9	2.1	1.1	4.1	Adjusted for conventional risk factors
Hooi, 2002	ABI <0.7 (vs. >0.95)	1.7	1.3	2.4	Adjusted for conventional risk factors
Myocardial Infarction					
Newman, 1999	ABI <0.9	1.4	0.9	2.2	Adjusted for conventional risk factors; excludes subjects with baseline cardiovascular disease
Stroke					
Newman, 1999	ABI <0.9	1.1	0.7	1.7	Adjusted for conventional risk factors; excludes subjects with baseline cardiovascular disease
All Coronary Heart Disease Morbidity and Mortality					
Ogren, 1993	ABI ≤0.9	2.3	1.2	4.3	Adjusted for conventional risk factors
Newman, 1999	ABI <0.9	1.4	0.9	2.2	Adjusted for conventional risk factors; excludes subjects with baseline cardiovascular disease
Abbott, 2000	ABI <0.8 (vs. >1.0)	2.7	1.6	4.5	Adjusted for conventional risk factors
Lee, 2004	ABI ≤0.90	1.1	0.8	1.5	Adjusted for conventional risk factors
Van der Meer, 2004	ABI <0.90	1.1	0.8	1.5	Adjusted for conventional risk factors
Criqui, 2010	ABI <1.0	1.8	1.3	2.7	Adjusted for conventional risk factors; excludes subjects with baseline cardiovascular disease
	ABI >1.4	2.2	1.1	4.2	
All Stroke Morbidity and Mortality					
Newman, 1999	ABI <0.9	1.1	0.7	1.7	Adjusted for conventional risk factors; excludes subjects with baseline cardiovascular disease
Abbott, 2000	ABI <0.9	2.0	1.1	3.5	Adjusted for conventional risk factors
Tsai, 2001	ABI <0.9	1.4	0.7	2.6	Adjusted for conventional risk factors
Hollander, 2003	ABI <1.01 (vs. >1.17)	1.3	0.9	1.9	Adjusted for conventional risk factors
Murabito, 2003	ABI <0.9	2.0	1.1	3.7	Adjusted for conventional risk factors
Lee, 2004	ABI ≤0.90	1.1	0.7	1.7	Adjusted for conventional risk factors
Criqui, 2010	ABI <1.0	1.6	0.9	3.0	Adjusted for conventional risk factors; excludes subjects with baseline cardiovascular disease
	ABI >1.4	2.7	0.9	7.6	

ABI, Ankle-brachial index; *CHD*, coronary heart disease; *CI,* confidence interval; *MI,* myocardial infarction; *PAD*, peripheral artery disease.
Modified from Criqui MH, Aboyans V. Epidemiology of peripheral artery disease. *Circ Res.* 2015;116(9):1509–1526.

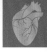

Elevated mortality rates among subjects with IC were reported in the 1970s and 1980s in the Framingham cohort, although this excess risk was markedly attenuated when subjects with baseline cerebrovascular and coronary heart disease were excluded.[1] Similarly, a Finnish study failed to find an association between IC and total or CVD mortality in men after adjustment for CVD risk factors and baseline CVD.[1] In a large and methodologically rigorous study, data from the 18,403 men in the Whitehall cohort were used to show that after adjusting for CVD risk factors, IC was a significant predictor of CVD mortality, even after excluding subjects with baseline disease.[121]

The development of the ABI and other noninvasive measures of PAD permitted further investigation of the association of PAD and CVD. In 1985, it was first demonstrated that a combination of noninvasive measures, including ABI, were prospectively related to all-cause mortality, even after adjustment for CVD risk factors and exclusion of subjects with baseline CVD.[122] Relative risks in this study were in the range of 4 to 5; a later re-analysis of the same cohort with additional mortality follow-up demonstrated elevated relative risks for CVD disease and coronary heart disease in particular, with no significant increase in noncardiovascular death.[123]

In the 1990s, a number of other prospective studies confirmed that ABI was related to CVD disease, based on either mortality or combined mortality and morbidity. This was found to be true in a variety of populations: vascular laboratory patients, elderly patients with hypertension, elderly women, an employment-based cohort from Belgium, the Edinburgh Artery Study cohort, and the CHS cohort.[16,32,124–126] Most of these studies controlled for various known CVD disease risk factors and the presence of CVD disease at baseline. The relative risks reported ranged from approximately 2 to 5. Many of these studies also found PAD to be significantly associated with incident coronary heart disease in particular, although the CHS failed to find such associations for either total MI or angina.[1,16]

The data regarding the association of PAD with cerebrovascular disease are less conclusive. A 1991 study showed a strong association between multiple noninvasive measures of PAD and cerebrovascular disease morbidity and mortality, with risk ratios of 3.3 for men and 9.0 for women after multivariable adjustment.[127] Data from the Edinburgh Artery Study also showed such an association based on ABI, although after multivariable adjustment, the association persisted for nonfatal but not fatal stroke.[32] However, data from the CHS failed to show a relationship between low ABI and incident stroke.[16] The ARIC Study showed a significant association between ABI as a continuous variable and ischemic stroke after multivariable adjustment, but failed to show such an association when ABI was categorized based on a 0.80 cut-point.[128]

A meta-analysis of 16 population-based cohort studies evaluated the association of ABI with subsequent coronary events, CVD mortality, and total mortality.[13] An ABI of <0.90 was associated with approximately twice the 10-year event rates in each of these three categories. In addition, these results held across the full range of Framingham Risk Score categories. The ABI was also evaluated as a continuous variable. As shown in Fig. 16.6, there was a graded association of increasing risk with decreasing ABIs below 1.00, with an HR of 4 for ABIs <0.60. Risk was essentially flat for ABIs in the normal range, 1.00 to 1.40.

Population studies suggest a high ABI, >1.40, is also associated with elevated risk of CVD. In the meta-analysis of 16 population studies, ABIs >1.40 were associated with a modest but significant increase in total mortality, with an HR of approximately 1.3.[13] Such high ABIs are caused by stiff, often calcified ankle arteries, which may mask underlying PAD.[7] Recently, the MESA reported that both "low" (<1.00) and "high" (>1.40) ABI were associated with an increased risk of incident CVD events, even after adjustment for traditional and novel risk factors.[1] Interestingly, high ABI showed a stronger association for stroke than low ABI. Also, this was the first report to show that the ABI predicted events independent of other measures of extant atherosclerosis; specifically, coronary artery calcium, carotid intimal-medial thickness, and major electrocardiogram abnormalities. Evidence is contradictory as to whether the increased risk in persons with a high ABI is restricted to those with underlying PAD. A vascular lab study from France in persons with diabetes reported that increased risk of mortality for an ABI ≥1.40 was restricted to persons with underlying PAD.[129] In contrast, a report from the Mayo clinic vascular lab showed an independent risk for a high ABI, which was further increased in the presence of underlying PAD.[130] Further studies on this question are needed.

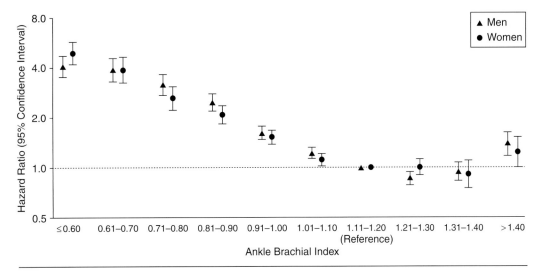

Hazard ratios are not adjusted for age or cardiovascular risk factors.

Fig. 16.6 Association of peripheral artery disease and mortality, according to the ankle brachial index collaboration meta-analysis. (From Ankle Brachial Index Collaboration, Fowkes FG, Murray GD, et al. Ankle brachial index combined with Framingham Risk Score to predict cardiovascular events and mortality: a meta-analysis. *JAMA.* 2008;300:197–208.)

Recent evidence also indicates that, independent of baseline ABI, a more rapid deterioration in ABI carries a worse prognosis. Decreases in ABI of more than 0.15 are significantly associated with an increased risk of all-cause mortality (risk ratio 2.4) and CVD mortality (risk ratio 2.8) at 3 years, independent of baseline ABI and potential confounding variables.[110]

Through walking impairment and amputation, PAD is associated with significant disability worldwide. Data from Global Burden Disease projects in 1990 and 2010 show that along with mortality, disability associated with PAD has significantly increased; this increase in burden is even greater among women than among men.[131] In 2010, the disability-adjusted life years (DALYs) were the highest in Australasia, Western Europe, and North America, but the overall relative change in median DALYs was larger in developing nations than in developed nations.

REFERENCES

1. Criqui MH, Aboyans V. Epidemiology of peripheral artery disease. *Circ Res.* 2015;116(9):1509–1526.
2. Fowkes FG, Rudan D, Rudan I, et al. Comparison of global estimates of prevalence and risk factors for peripheral artery disease in 2000 and 2010: a systematic review and analysis. *Lancet.* 2013;382(9901):1329–1340.
3. Hirsch AT, Criqui MH, Treat-Jacobson D, et al. Peripheral arterial disease detection, awareness and treatment in primary care. *JAMA.* 2001;286(11):1317–1324.
4. Criqui MH, Denenberg JO, Bird CE, et al. The correlation between symptoms and non-invasive test results in patients referred for peripheral arterial disease testing. *Vasc Med.* 1996;4(1):65–71.
5. McDermott MM, Greenland P, Liu K, et al. Leg symptoms in peripheral arterial disease. Associated clinical characteristics and functional impairment. *JAMA.* 2001;286(13):1599–1606.
6. Aboyans V, Ricco JB, Bartelink MEL, et al. 2017 ESC guidelines on the diagnosis and treatment of peripheral arterial diseases, in collaboration with the European Society for Vascular Surgery (ESVS): document covering atherosclerotic disease of extracranial carotid and vertebral, mesenteric, renal, upper and lower extremity arteries. *Eur Heart J.* 2018;39(9):763–816.
7. Aboyans V, Criqui MH, Abraham P, et al. Measurement and interpretation of the ankle-brachial index: a scientific statement from the American Heart Association. *Circulation.* 2012;126(24):2890–2909.
8. Diehm C, Lange S, Darius H, et al. Association of low ankle brachial index with high mortality in primary care. *Eur Heart J.* 2006;27(14):1743–1749.
9. Meijer WT, Hoes AW, Rutgers D, et al. Peripheral arterial disease in the elderly: the Rotterdam Study. *Arterioscler Thromb Vasc Biol.* 1998;18(2):185–192.
10. Vogt MT, Cauley JA, Newman AB, et al. Decreased ankle/arm blood pressure index and mortality in elderly women. *JAMA.* 1993;270(4):465–469.
11. Wang JC, Criqui MH, Denenberg JO, et al. Exertional leg pain in patients with and without peripheral arterial disease. *Circulation.* 2005;112(22):3501–3508.
12. Tehan PE, Barwick AL, Sebastian M, Chuter VH. Diagnostic accuracy of the postexercise ankle-brachial index for detecting peripheral artery disease in suspected claudicants with and without diabetes. *Vasc Med.* 2018;23(2):116–125.
13. Fowkes FG, Murray GD, Butcher I, et al. Ankle brachial index combined with Framingham Risk Score to predict cardiovascular events and mortality: a meta-analysis. *JAMA.* 2008;300(2):197–208.
14. McDermott MM, Fried L, Simonsick E, et al. Asymptomatic peripheral arterial disease is independently associated with impaired lower extremity functioning: the women's health and aging study. *Circulation.* 2000;101(9):1007–1012.
15. McDermott MM, Criqui MH, Liu K, et al. Lower ankle/brachial index, as calculated by averaging the dorsalis pedis and posterior tibial arterial

16. pressures, and association with leg functioning in peripheral arterial disease. *J Vasc Surg.* 2000;32(6):1164–1171.
16. Newman AB, Siscovick DS, Manolio TA, et al. Ankle-arm index as a marker of atherosclerosis in the Cardiovascular Health Study. Cardiovascular Heart Study (CHS) Collaborative Research Group. *Circulation.* 1993;88(3):837–845.
17. McDermott MM, Liu K, Criqui MH, et al. Ankle-brachial index and subclinical cardiac and carotid disease. The Multi-Ethnic Study of Atherosclerosis. *Am J Epidemiol.* 2005;162(1):33–41.
18. Aboyans V, Ho E, Denenberg JO, et al. The association between elevated ankle systolic pressures and peripheral occlusive arterial disease in diabetic and nondiabetic subjects. *J Vasc Surg.* 2008;48(5):1197–1203.
19. Allison MA, Ho E, Denenberg JO, et al. Ethnic-specific prevalence of peripheral arterial disease in the United States. *Am J Prev Med.* 2007;32(4):328–333.
20. Sheng CS, Li Y, Huang QF, et al. Pulse waves in the lower extremities as a diagnostic tool of peripheral arterial disease and predictor of mortality in elderly Chinese. *Hypertension.* 2016;67(3):527–534.
21. Kojima I, Ninomiya T, Hata J, et al. A low ankle brachial index is associated with an increased risk of cardiovascular disease: the Hisayama study. *J Atheroscler Thromb.* 2014;21(9):966–973.
22. Desormais I, Aboyans V, Guerchet M, et al. Prevalence of peripheral artery disease in the elderly population in urban and rural areas of Central Africa: the EPIDEMCA study. *Eur J Prev Cardiol.* 2015;22(11):1462–1472.
23. Guerchet M, Aboyans V, Mbelesso P, et al. Epidemiology of peripheral artery disease in elder general population of two cities of Central Africa: Bangui and Brazzaville. *Eur J Vasc Endovasc Surg.* 2012;44(2):164–169.
24. Criqui MH, McClelland RL, McDermott MM, et al. The ankle-brachial index and incident cardiovascular events in the MESA (Multi-Ethnic Study of Atherosclerosis). *J Am Coll Cardiol.* 2010;56(18):1506–1512.
25. Forbang NI, Hughes-Austin JM, Allison MA, Criqui MH. Peripheral artery disease and non-coronary atherosclerosis in Hispanics: another paradox? *Prog Cardiovasc Dis.* 2014;57(3):237–243.
26. Aboyans V, Criqui MH, McClelland RL, et al. Intrinsic contribution of gender and ethnicity to normal ankle-brachial index values: The Multi-Ethnic Study of Atherosclerosis (MESA). *J Vasc Surg.* 2007;45(2):319–327.
27. Danyi P, Yanel LR, Moy TF, et al. Ankle-brachial index is lower in asymptomatic African Americans independent of risk factors and body mass index in families at high risk of premature coronary disease. *Circulation.* 2007;115.
28. Fabsitz RR, Sidawy AN, Go O, et al. Prevalence of peripheral arterial disease and associated risk factors in American Indians: the Strong Heart Study. *Am J Epidemiol.* 1999;149(4):330–338.
29. Bowlin SJ, Medalie JH, Flocke SA, et al. Epidemiology of intermittent claudication in middle-aged men. *Am J Epidemiol.* 1994;140(5):418–430.
30. Dagenais GR, Maurice S, Robitaille NM, et al. Intermittent claudication in Quebec men from 1974-1986: the Quebec Cardiovascular Study. *Clin Invest Med.* 1991;14(2):93–100.
31. Bainton D, Sweetnam P, Baker I, et al. Peripheral vascular disease: consequence for survival and association with risk factors in the Speedwell prospective heart disease study. *Br Heart J.* 1994;72(2):128–132.
32. Leng GC, Lee AJ, Fowkes FG, et al. Incidence, natural history and cardiovascular events in symptomatic and asymptomatic peripheral arterial disease in the general population. *Int J Epidemiol.* 1996;25(6):1172–1181.
33. Hooi JD, Kester AD, Stoffers HE, et al. Incidence of and risk factors for asymptomatic peripheral arterial occlusive disease: a longitudinal study. *Am J Epidemiol.* 2001;153(7):666–672.
34. Velescu A, Clara A, Peñafiel J, et al. Peripheral arterial disease incidence and associated risk factors in a Mediterranean population-based cohort. The REGICOR Study. *Eur J Vasc Endovasc Surg.* 2016;51(5):696–705.
35. Ingolfsson IO, Sigurdsson G, Sigvaldason H, et al. A marked decline in the prevalence and incidence of intermittent claudication in Icelandic men 1968-1986: a strong relationship to smoking and serum cholesterol—the Reykjavik Study. *J Clin Epidemiol.* 1994;47(11):1237–1243.
36. Murabito JM, Evans JC, D'Agostino B, et al. Temporal trends in the incidence of intermittent claudication from 1950 to 1999. *Am J Epidemiol.* 2005;162(5):430–437.

37. Cea-Soriano L, Fowkes FGR, Johansson S, et al. Time trends in peripheral artery disease incidence, prevalence and secondary preventive therapy: a cohort study in The Health Improvement Network in the UK. *BMJ Open.* 2018;8(1):e018184.

38. Murabito JM, Evans JC, Nieto K, et al. Prevalence and clinical correlates of peripheral arterial disease in the Framingham Offspring Study. *Am Heart J.* 2002;143(6):961–965.

39. Zheng ZJ, Rosamond WD, Chambless LE, et al. Lower extremity arterial disease assessed by ankle-brachial index in a middle-ages population of African Americans and Whites. *Am J Prev Med.* 2005;29(5S1):42–49.

40. Biancari F. Meta-analysis of the prevalence, incidence and natural history of critical limb ischemia. *J Cardiovasc Surg (Torino).* 2013;54(6):663–669.

41. Nehler MR, Duval S, Diao L, et al. Epidemiology of peripheral arterial disease and critical limb ischemia in an insured national population. *J Vasc Surg.* 2014;60(3):686–695.

42. Murabito JM, D'Agostino RB, Silbershatz H, et al. Intermittent claudication. A risk profile from The Framingham Heart Study. *Circulation.* 1997;96(1):44–49.

43. Meijer WT, Grobbee DE, Hunink MG, et al. Determinants of peripheral arterial disease in the elderly: the Rotterdam study. *Arch Intern Med.* 2000;160(19):2934–2938.

44. Allison MA, Criqui MH, McClelland RL, et al. The effect of novel cardiovascular risk factors on the ethnic-specific odds for peripheral arterial disease in the Multi-Ethnic Study of Atherosclerosis (MESA). *J Am Coll Cardiol.* 2006;48(6):1190–1197.

45. Curb JD, Masaki K, Rodriguez BL, et al. Peripheral artery disease and cardiovascular risk factors in the elderly. The Honolulu Heart Program. *Arterioscler Thromb Vasc Biol.* 1996;16(12):1495–1500.

46. Fowkes FG, Housley E, Riemersma RA, et al. Smoking, lipids, glucose intolerance, and blood pressure as risk factors for peripheral atherosclerosis compared with ischemic heart disease in the Edinburgh Artery Study. *Am J Epidemiol.* 1992;135(4):331–340.

47. Ridker PM, Stampfer MJ, Rifai N. Novel risk factors for systemic atherosclerosis: a comparison of C-reactive protein, fibrinogen, homocysteine, lipoprotein(a), and standard cholesterol screening as predictors of peripheral arterial disease. *JAMA.* 2001;285(19):2481–2485.

48. Criqui MH, Vargas V, Denenberg JO, et al. Ethnicity and peripheral arterial disease. The San Diego Population Study. *Circulation.* 2005;112(17):2703–2707.

49. Joosten MM, Pai JK, Bertoia ML, et al. Associations between conventional cardiovascular risk factors and risk of peripheral artery disease in men. *JAMA.* 2012;308(16):1660–1667.

50. Beks PJ, Mackaay AJ, de Neeling JN, et al. Peripheral arterial disease in relation to glycaemic level in an elderly Caucasian population: the Hoorn study. *Diabetologia.* 1995;38(1):86–96.

51. Jude EB, Oyibo SO, Chalmers N, et al. Peripheral arterial disease in diabetic and nondiabetic patients: a comparison of severity and outcome. *Diabetes Care.* 2001;24(8):1433–1437.

52. Haltmayer M, Mueller T, Horvath W, et al. Impact of atherosclerotic risk factors on the anatomical distribution of peripheral arterial disease. *Int Angiol.* 2001;20(3):200–207.

53. Vidula H, Liu K, Criqui MH, et al. Metabolic syndrome and incident peripheral artery disease—the Multi-Ethnic Study of Atherosclerosis. *Atherosclerosis.* 2015;243(1):198–203.

54. Garg PK, Biggs ML, Carnethon M, et al. Metabolic syndrome and risk of incident peripheral artery disease: the cardiovascular health study. *Hypertension.* 2014;63(2):413–419.

55. Fowkes FG, Housley E, Cawood EH, et al. Edinburgh Artery Study: prevalence of asymptomatic and symptomatic peripheral arterial disease in the general population. *Int J Epidemiol.* 1991;20(2):384–392.

56. Katsilambros NL, Tsapogas PC, Arvanitis MP, et al. Risk factors for lower extremity arterial disease in non-insulin-dependent diabetic persons. *Diabet Med.* 1996;13(3):243–246.

57. Mowat BF, Skinner ER, Wilson HM, et al. Alterations in plasma lipids, lipoproteins and high density lipoprotein subfractions in peripheral arterial disease. *Atherosclerosis.* 1997;131(2):161–166.

58. Valentine RJ, Grayburn PA, Vega DL, et al. Lp(a) lipoprotein is an independent discriminating risk factor for premature peripheral atherosclerosis among white men. *Arch Intern Med.* 1994;154(7):801–806.

59. Volpato S, Vigna GB, McDermott MM, et al. Lipoprotein(a), inflammation, and peripheral arterial disease in a community-based sample of older men and women (the InCHIANTI study). *Am J Cardiol.* 2010;105(12):1825–1830.

60. Garg PK, Norby FL, Polfus LM, et al. Lipoprotein-associated phospholipase A(2) and risk of incident peripheral arterial disease: findings from The Atherosclerosis Risk in Communities study (ARIC). *Atherosclerosis.* 2018;268(1):12–18.

61. Garg PK, Arnold AM, Hinckley Stukovsky KD, et al. Lipoprotein-associated phospholipase A2 and incident peripheral arterial disease in older adults: the Cardiovascular Health Study. *Arterioscler Thromb Vasc Biol.* 2016;36(4):750–756.

62. Tseng CH. Prevalence and risk factors of peripheral arterial obstructive disease in Taiwanese type 2 diabetic patients. *Angiology.* 2003;54(3):331–338.

63. Kannel WB, McGee DL. Update on some epidemiologic features of intermittent claudication: the Framingham study. *J Am Geriatr Soc.* 1985;33(1):13–18.

64. Ness J, Aronow WS, Ahn C. Risk factors for symptomatic peripheral arterial disease in older persons in an academic hospital-based geriatrics practice. *J Am Geriatr Soc.* 2000;48(3):312–314.

65. Ix JH, Biggs ML, Kizer JR, et al. Association of body mass index with peripheral arterial disease in older adults: the Cardiovascular Health Study. *Am J Epidemiol.* 2011;174(9):1036–1043.

66. Jepson RG, Fowkes FG, Donnan PT, et al. Alcohol intake as a risk factor for peripheral arterial disease in the general population in the Edinburgh Artery Study. *Eur J Epidemiol.* 1995;11(1):9–14.

67. Camargo Jr CA, Stampfer MJ, Glynn RJ, et al. Prospective study of moderate alcohol consumption and risk of peripheral arterial disease in US male physicians. *Circulation.* 1997;95(3):577–580.

68. Khandanpour N, Loke YK, Meyer FJ, et al. Homocysteine and peripheral arterial disease: systematic review and meta-analysis. *Eur J Vasc Endovasc Surg.* 2009;38(3):316–322.

69. Bertoia ML, Pai JK, Cooke JP, et al. Plasma homocysteine, dietary B vitamins, betaine, and choline and risk of peripheral artery disease. *Atherosclerosis.* 2014;235(1):94–101.

70. Wildman RP, Muntner P, Chen J, et al. Relation of inflammation to peripheral arterial disease in the National Health and Nutrition Examination Survey, 1999-2002. *Am J Cardiol.* 2005;96(11):1579–1583.

71. Lowe GD, Fowkes FG, Dawes J, et al. Blood viscosity, fibrinogen, and activation of coagulation and leukocytes in peripheral arterial disease and the normal population in the Edinburgh Artery Study. *Circulation.* 1993;87(6):1915–1920.

72. Carbayo JA, Divison JA, Escribano J, et al. Using ankle-brachial index to detect peripheral arterial disease: prevalence and associated risk factors in a random population sample. *Nutr Metab Cardiovasc Dis.* 2007;17(1):41–49.

73. Fishbane S, Youn S, Kowalski EJ, et al. Ankle-arm blood pressure index as a marker for atherosclerotic vascular diseases in hemodialysis patients. *Am J Kidney Dis.* 1995;25(1):34–39.

74. Selvin E, Erlinger TP. Prevalence of and risk factors for peripheral arterial disease in the United States: results from the National Health and Nutrition Examination Survey, 1999–2000. *Circulation.* 2004;110(6):738–743.

75. Wattanakit K, Folsom AR, Selvin E, et al. Kidney function and risk of peripheral arterial disease: results from the Atherosclerosis Risk in Communities (ARIC) Study. *J Am Soc Nephrol.* 2007;18(2):629–636.

76. Yang C, Kwak L, Ballew SH, et al. Kidney function, bone-mineral metabolism markers, and future risk of peripheral artery disease. *Atherosclerosis.* 2017;267(12):167–174.

77. Wassel CL, Loomba R, Ix JH, et al. Family history of peripheral artery disease is associated with prevalence and severity of peripheral artery disease: the San Diego population study. *J Am Coll Cardiol.* 2011;58(13):1386–1392.

78. Prushik SG, Farber A, Gona P, et al. Parental intermittent claudication as risk factor for claudication in adults. *Am J Cardiol.* 2012;109(5):736–741.

79. Carmelli D, Fabsitz RR, Swan GE, et al. Contribution of genetic and environmental influences to ankle-brachial blood pressure index in the

NHLBI Twin Study. National Heart, Lung, and Blood Institute. *Am J Epidemiol*. 2000;151(5):452–458.

80. Kroon AA, Ajubi N, van Asten WN, Stalenhoef AF. The prevalence of peripheral vascular disease in familial hypercholesterolaemia. *J Intern Med*. 1995;238(5):451–459.

81. Murabito JM, White CC, Kavousi M, et al. Association between chromosome 9p21 variants and the ankle-brachial index identified by a meta-analysis of 21 genome-wide association studies. *Circ Cardiovasc Genet*. 2012;5(1):100–112.

82. Kullo IJ, Shameer K, Jouni H, et al. The ATXN2-SH2B3 locus is associated with peripheral arterial disease: an electronic medical record-based genome-wide association study. *Front Genet*. 2014;5:166.

83. Wassel CL, Lamina C, Nambi V, et al. Genetic determinants of the ankle-brachial index: a meta-analysis of a cardiovascular candidate gene 50K SNP panel in the candidate gene association resource (CARe) consortium. *Atherosclerosis*. 2012;222(1):138–147.

84. Hung HC, Willett W, Merchant A, et al. Oral health and peripheral arterial disease. *Circulation*. 2003;107(8):1152–1157.

85. Mendez MV, Scott T, LaMote W, et al. An association between periodontal disease and peripheral vascular disease. *Am J Surg*. 1998;176(2):153–157.

86. Deleted in review.

87. Hyder JA, Allison MA, Barrett-Connor E, et al. Bone mineral density and atherosclerosis: the Multi-Ethnic Study of Atherosclerosis. *Abdominal Aortic Calcium Study Atherosclerosis*. 2010;209(1):283–289.

88. van der Klift M, Pols HA, Hak AE, et al. Bone mineral density and the risk of peripheral arterial disease: the Rotterdam Study. *Calcif Tissue Int*. 2002;70(6):443–449.

89. Mangiafico RA, Russo E, Riccobene S, et al. Increased prevalence of peripheral arterial disease in osteoporotic postmenopausal women. *J Bone Miner Metab*. 2006;24(2):125–131.

90. Vogt MT, Cauley JA, Kuller LH, et al. Bone mineral density and blood flow to the lower extremities: the study of osteoporotic fractures. *J Bone Miner Res*. 1997;12(2):283–289.

91. Fowkes FG, Aboyans V, Fowkes FJ, et al. Peripheral artery disease: epidemiology and global perspectives. *Nat Rev Cardiol*. 2017;14(3):156–170.

92. Hsia J, Criqui MH, Rodabough R, et al. Estrogen plus progestin and the risk of peripheral arterial disease: the Women's Health Initiative. *Circulation*. 2004;109(5):620–626.

93. D'Agostino Sr RB, Vasan RS, Pencina MJ, et al. General cardiovascular risk profile for use in primary care: the Framingham Heart Study. *Circulation*. 2008;117(6):743–753.

94. Juergens JE, Parker NW, Hines EA. Arteriosclerosis obliterans: review of 520 cases with special reference to pathogenic and prognostic factors. *Circulation*. 1960;21:188–195.

95. Meru AV, Mittra S, Thyagarajan B, et al. Intermittent claudication: an overview. *Atherosclerosis*. 2006;187(2):231–237.

96. Jelnes R, Gaardsting O, Hougaard Jensen K, et al. Fate in intermittent claudication: outcome and risk factors. *Br Med J (Clin Res Ed)*. 1986;293(6555):1137–1140.

97. Goessens BMB, van der Graaf Y, Olijhoek JK, et al. The course of vascular risk factors and the occurrence of vascular events in patients with symptomatic peripheral arterial disease. *J Vasc Surg*. 2007;45(1):47–54.

98. Widmer LK, Biland L, DaSilva A. Risk profile and occlusive peripheral arterial disease (OPAD). In: *Proceedings of 13th International Congress of Angiology*. Athens; 1985.

99. Bertele V, Roncaglioni MC, Pangrazzi J, et al. Clinical outcome and its predictors in 1560 patients with critical leg ischemia. *Eur J Vasc Endovasc Surg*. 1999;18(5):401–410.

100. Mätzke S, Lepäntalo M. Claudication does not always precede critical leg ischemia. *Vasc Med*. 2001;6(2):77–80.

101. Sigvant B, Lundin F, Wahlberg E. The risk of disease progression in peripheral arterial disease is higher than expected: a meta-analysis of mortality and disease progression in peripheral arterial disease. *Eur J Vasc Endovasc Surg*. 2016;51(3):395–403.

102. Fowkes FG, Lowe GD, Housley E, et al. Cross-linked fibrin degradation products, progression of peripheral arterial disease, and risk of coronary heart disease. *Lancet*. 1993;342(8863):84–86.

103. Bird CE, Criqui MH, Fronek A, et al. Quantitative and qualitative progression of peripheral arterial disease by non-invasive testing. *Vasc Med*. 1999;4(1):15–21.

104. Nicoloff AD, Taylor Jr LM, Sexton GJ, et al. Relationship between site of initial symptoms and subsequent progression of disease in a prospective study of atherosclerosis progression in patients receiving long-term treatment for symptomatic peripheral arterial disease. *J Vasc Surg*. 2002;35(1):38–46.

105. Smith I, Franks PJ, Greenhalgh RM, et al. The influence of smoking cessation and hypertriglyceridaemia on the progression of peripheral arterial disease and the onset of critical ischaemia. *Eur J Vasc Endovasc Surg*. 1996;11(4):402–408.

106. Smith FB, Lee AJ, Price JF, et al. Changes in ankle brachial index in symptomatic and asymptomatic subjects in the general population. *J Vasc Surg*. 2003;38(6):1323–1330.

107. Tzoulaki I, Murray GD, Lee AJ, et al. C-reactive protein, interleukin-6, and soluble adhesion molecules as predictors of progressive peripheral atherosclerosis in the general population. Edinburgh artery study. *Circulation*. 2005;112(7):976–983.

108. Aboyans V, Criqui MH, Denenberg JO, et al. Risk factors for progression of peripheral arterial disease in large and small vessels. *Circulation*. 2006;113(22):2623–2629.

109. O'Hare AM, Newman AB, Katz R, et al. Cystatin C and incident peripheral arterial disease events in the elderly. Results from the Cardiovascular Health Study. *Arch Intern Med*. 2005;165(22):2666–2670.

110. Criqui MH, Ninomiya JK, Wingard DL, et al. Progression of peripheral arterial disease predicts cardiovascular disease morbidity and mortality. *J Am Coll Cardiol*. 2008;52(21):1736–1742.

111. Hertzer NR, Beven EG, Young JR, et al. Coronary artery disease in peripheral vascular patients. Classification of 1000 coronary angiograms and results of surgical management. *Ann Surg*. 1984;199(2):223–233.

112. Khandelwal A, Kondo T, Amanuma M, et al. Single injection protocol for coronary and lower extremity CT angiographies in patients suspected for peripheral arterial disease. *Medicine (Baltimore)*. 2016;95(46):e5410.

113. Miszalski-Jamka T, Lichołai S, Karwat K, et al. Computed tomography characteristics of coronary artery atherosclerosis in subjects with lower extremity peripheral artery disease and no cardiac symptoms. *Pol Arch Med Wewn*. 2013;123(12):657–663.

114. Newman AB, Shemanski L, Manolio TA, et al. Ankle-arm index as a predictor of cardiovascular disease and mortality in the Cardiovascular Health Study. The Cardiovascular Health Study Group. *Arterioscler Thromb Vasc Biol*. 1999;19(3):538–545.

115. Zheng ZJ, Sharrett AR, Chambless LE, et al. Associations of ankle-brachial index with clinical coronary heart disease, stroke and preclinical carotid and popliteal atherosclerosis: the Atherosclerosis Risk in Communities (ARIC) Study. *Atherosclerosis*. 1997;131(1):115–125.

116. Kröger K, Stang A, Kondratieva J, et al. Prevalence of peripheral arterial disease—results of the Heinz Nixdorf recall study. *Eur J Epidemiol*. 2006;21(4):279–285.

117. Ness J, Aronow WS. Prevalence of coexistence of coronary artery disease, ischemic stroke, and peripheral arterial disease in older persons, mean age 80 years, in an academic hospital-based geriatrics practice. *J Am Geriatr Soc*. 1999;47(10):1255–1256.

118. Criqui MH, Denenberg JO, Langer RD, et al. The epidemiology of peripheral arterial disease: importance of identifying the population at risk. *Vasc Med*. 1997;2(3):221–226.

119. Alexandrova NA, Gibson WC, Norris JW, et al. Carotid artery stenosis in peripheral vascular disease. *J Vasc Surg*. 1996;23(4):645–649.

120. Pilcher JM, Danaher J, Khaw KT. The prevalence of asymptomatic carotid artery disease in patients with peripheral vascular disease. *Clin Radiol*. 2000;55(1):56–61.

121. Smith GD, Shipley MJ, Rose G. Intermittent claudication, heart disease risk factors, and mortality. The Whitehall Study. *Circulation*. 1990;82(6):1925–1931.

122. Criqui MH, Coughlin SS, Fronek A. Noninvasively diagnosed peripheral arterial disease as a predictor of mortality: results from a prospective study. *Circulation*. 1985;72(4):768–773.

123. Criqui MH, Langer RD, Fronek A, et al. Mortality over a period of 10 years in patients with peripheral arterial disease. *N Engl J Med*. 1992;326(6):381–386.

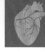

124. Kornitzer M, Dramaix M, Sobolski J, et al. Ankle/arm pressure index in asymptomatic middle-aged males: an independent predictor of ten-year coronary heart disease mortality. *Angiology*. 1995;46(3):211–219.

125. McDermott MM, Feinglass J, Slavensky R, et al. The ankle-brachial index as a predictor of survival in patients with peripheral vascular disease. *J Gen Intern Med*. 1994;9(8):445–449.

126. Newman AB, Sutton-Tyrrell K, Vogt MT, et al. Morbidity and mortality in hypertensive adults with a low ankle/arm blood pressure index. *JAMA*. 1993;270(4):487–489.

127. Criqui MH, Langer RD, Fronek A, Feigelson HS. Coronary disease and stroke in patients with large-vessel peripheral arterial disease. *Drugs*. 1991;42(Suppl 5):16–21.

128. Tsai AW, Folsom AR, Rosamond WD, et al. Ankle-brachial index and 7-year ischemic stroke incidence: the ARIC study. *Stroke*. 2001;32(8):1721–1724.

129. Aboyans V, Lacroix P, Tran MH, et al. The prognosis of diabetic patients with high ankle-brachial index depends on the coexistence of occlusive peripheral artery disease. *J Vasc Surg*. 2011;53(4):984–991.

130. Arain FA, Ye Z, Bailey KR, et al. Survival in patients with poorly compressible leg arteries. *J Am Coll Cardiol*. 2012;59(4):400–407.

131. Sampson UK, Fowkes FG, McDermott MM, et al. Global and regional burden of death and disability from peripheral artery disease: 21 world regions, 1990 to 2010. *Glob Heart*. 2014;9(1):145–158.

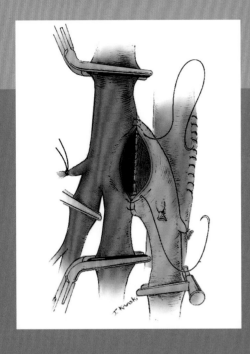

中文导读

第17章
外周动脉疾病的病理生理学

　　外周动脉疾病正在对全世界人民的心血管健康产生相当大且不断增长的影响。外周动脉疾病是下肢系统性动脉粥样硬化的表现，会明显增加心脑血管事件的发生风险，如心肌梗死和中风。动脉粥样硬化病变导致的动脉阻塞是导致外周动脉疾病发生的决定性因素。外周动脉疾病患者肢体缺血会引起腿部疼痛，限制行走能力，并可能发展为截肢。该病进展为严重肢体缺血后，截肢率和致死率会出现明显的升高。一方面，动脉狭窄会改变下肢的动脉血流动力学，增大远端动脉压力梯度，降低外周动脉灌注压，同时狭窄动脉内一氧化氮的生物利用度降低会干扰正常运动引起的血流量增加，血管内皮功能障碍引起人体对血管收缩物质（包括儿茶酚胺和血栓素）反应增强，加之动脉狭窄患者血液黏度的升高会进一步降低远端动脉的灌注。另一方面，炎症和氧化应激也会引起血管内皮损伤及血管内皮功能障碍，进而加重动脉狭窄引起的肢体缺血，此外，肢体缺血引起的骨骼肌功能障碍和细胞线粒体功能障碍也是引起患者行走障碍的重要因素之一。总之，外周动脉疾病患者腿部疼痛和导致组织坏死的机制是多因素的，包括全身炎症、内皮功能障碍、血管生成受损和微循环流量减少及骨骼肌功能障碍等，需要进一步的深入研究。

谷涌泉

Pathophysiology of Peripheral Artery Disease

Naomi M. Hamburg and Mark A. Creager

Peripheral artery disease (PAD) has a considerable and growing impact on cardiovascular health worldwide.[1,2] PAD represents systemic atherosclerosis in the lower extremities that elevates the risk for cardiovascular events including myocardial infarction and stroke (see Chapter 16).[3] Patients with PAD experience limb manifestations that lead to substantial suffering. Limb ischemia induces leg pain, limits walking ability, and may progress to amputation (see Chapter 18).[4] Arterial obstruction from atherosclerotic lesions is a defining event of PAD. See Chapter 6 for discussion of the pathobiology of atherosclerosis. The focus of the current chapter is to review the mechanistic pathways that produce limb symptoms in PAD, including functional limitations, intermittent claudication, critical chronic limb ischemia (CLI), and acute limb ischemia (ALI). A thorough understanding of the pathophysiology of the clinical manifestations of PAD is critical to both patient management and the creation of novel therapeutic approaches. An overview of the pathophysiological mechanisms that contribute to limb symptoms is included in Fig. 17.1.

CLINICAL EXPRESSIONS OF PERIPHERAL ARTERY DISEASE

Disability attributable to PAD is rising worldwide, with the greatest increases observed in women, and in low- and middle-income countries.[2] The pathophysiology of PAD begins with obstruction to flow in the leg arteries by atherosclerotic plaques. Typically, PAD is a chronic ischemic disease that impairs limb function; although recent clinical studies demonstrate the high incidence of ALI in clinically established PAD, it is indicative of thrombosis superimposed on atherosclerotic plaque or in bypass grafts.[5–7] PAD is readily detectable by measuring the ankle-brachial index (ABI), comparing ankle and arm systolic blood pressures (see Chapter 12). The diagnosis of obstructive PAD is made with an ABI ≤0.90.[8]

Functional Limitation and Cardiovascular Risk

Patients with PAD develop limb symptoms that impair walking ability.[9] The classic clinical manifestation of PAD is intermittent claudication, characterized by leg discomfort with activity that resolves with rest (see Chapter 18). The term *claudication* is derived from the Latin word *claudicato*, meaning "to limp," which is typical of the gait pattern of the patient who experiences limb ischemia when walking. Patients describe leg cramping, heaviness, or fatigue in the muscles of the buttock, thigh, or calf, which comes on exclusively with exercise, escalates with increasing activity, and diminishes rapidly with rest. This sequence of exercise-induced progression and complete relief with rest are important clinical differentiators of claudication from other lower-extremity musculoskeletal conditions.[10] The pain is not positional or precipitated by standing alone. Typical intermittent claudication is present in only

10% to 20% of patients with PAD defined by ABI. A much larger group of PAD patients experience atypical leg symptoms, leading to reduced walking capacity. Impaired functional ability is present in PAD patients regardless of symptom category, and asymptomatic patients with PAD are at risk for progressive functional impairment.[4] Compared to healthy individuals of the same age, patients with claudication have a marked reduction in peak treadmill performance.[11] There are multiple contributing factors driving exercise limitations in PAD, including self-restriction of activity to minimize leg pain.

Functional limitations in patients with PAD leads to poor clinical outcomes. Several studies demonstrate that these patients have reduced quality of life related to leg pain and activity restriction.[12] Reduced walking ability measured by questionnaires or direct assessment is associated with higher cardiovascular events, limb events, and mortality.[13,14] Longitudinal declines in exercise performance predict mortality risk in PAD, and lower physical function predicts decline in ABI.[13,15] Thus, a key therapeutic goal in PAD is preservation and restoration of walking ability.

In addition to limb manifestations, patients with PAD have high rates of cardiovascular events (see Chapter 16). In clinical registries, more than half of PAD patients have coexistence of clinical coronary artery disease and/or cerebrovascular disease.[16] PAD predicts a high risk for cardiovascular events regardless of symptom status.[17] Patients with polyvascular disease, in which atherosclerosis is manifest in multiple territories, have particularly poor outcomes. Thus treatment to reduce atherosclerotic risk is a key component of PAD treatment (see Chapter 19).

Chronic and Acute Limb Threatening Ischemia

CLI is critically severe arterial insufficiency leading to inadequate tissue perfusion at rest. CLI is defined by rest pain in the leg for more than 2 weeks and/or the presence of nonhealing wounds or gangrene in the presence of arterial obstructive disease. ALI is the rapid onset of severe ischemia of less than 2 weeks' duration and the classic clinical signs of pallor, pulselessness, coolness (poikilothermia), paresthesia, and paralysis (see Chapter 44). A key outcome in symptomatic PAD is the occurrence of major adverse limb events (MALE) defined as amputation, CLI, or ALI. In the overall adult US population, the annual incidence of CLI is estimated at 0.2% to 0.4% in an analysis of recent administrative datasets, with a prevalence of 0.23% to 1.33%.[18–20] In analyses based on insurance claims data, out of the total number of patients diagnosed with PAD, 11% had prevalent CLI.[20] Patients with CLI have poor limb-related outcomes, including 35% to 67% amputation rates, and mortality rates as high as 40%, particularly in patients with tissue loss.[21] CLI patients typically have arterial obstructions in multiple segments, which usually involve the infrainguinal and tibial vessels. The arterial stenoses and occlusions reduce limb perfusion,

Healthy Artery

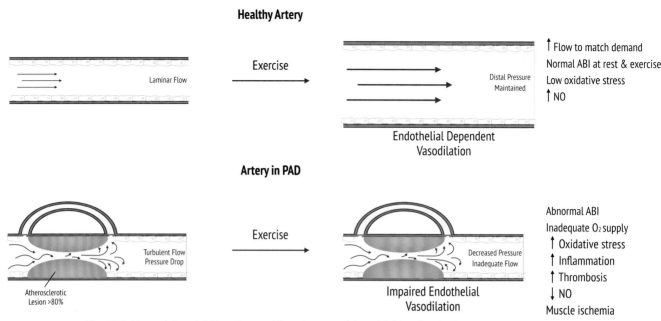

Fig. 17.1 Normal Arterial Function and Impairment of Arterial Function in Peripheral Artery Disease. In healthy arteries *(top)*, flow is laminar. Endothelial function is intact, permitting vasodilation in response to increased blood flow and muscle oxygen demand, including that associated with exercise. Blood flow and oxygen delivery match muscle metabolic demand at rest and with exercise. The absence of ischemia keeps oxidative stress low. In contrast, in peripheral artery disease *(bottom)*, arterial stenosis results in turbulent flow. Increased resistance associated with stenosis and loss of kinetic energy results in a pressure drop across the stenosis that is only partially compensated by collateral vessel formation. Endothelial function is impaired, leading to lack of exercise-induced vasodilation and increased oxidative stress. These changes limit blood flow response to exercise, resulting in inadequate oxygen delivery to meet skeletal muscle demand. Oxidative stress perpetuates muscle damage and impairs muscle metabolism. *ABI*, Ankle-brachial index; *NO*, nitric oxide; *PAD*, peripheral artery disease.

and limit oxygen and nutrient supply to an extent that produces resting ischemia and progresses to tissue compromise. ALI occurs when there is an abrupt reduction in limb blood flow related to thrombosis or embolism. The overall incidence of ALI is low, approximating 1.5 cases per 10,000 person-years.[22] In clinical trials, the annual rate of ALI is 1.3% in established PAD patients, with higher rates in patients with prior peripheral revascularization and in patients who continue to smoke.[6] Rates of amputation and recurrent limb events remain high following ALI. Revascularization for limb preservation is crucial in both ALI and CLI.

HEMODYNAMICS IN PERIPHERAL ARTERY DISEASE

Arterial Flow and Oxygen Delivery to Skeletal Muscle

Muscle oxygen consumption involves oxygen delivery (mediated by pulmonary oxygen uptake, oxygen content of hemoglobin, and blood flow) and oxygen extraction by the skeletal muscle. In healthy people, both at rest and during exercise, muscle oxygen consumption is determined primarily by maximal oxygen delivery. Muscle oxidative capacity, the amount of oxygen converted to energy by mitochondria, remains tightly coupled with maximal exercise capacity and increases with exercise training. Blood flow to skeletal muscle also increases with exercise and with exercise training.[23]

Determinants of Limb Blood Flow

At any given systemic blood pressure, the major determinant of blood flow in regional circulations is the peripheral resistance of the vascular

bed supplied by major conduit vessels. This basic relation can be expressed as:

$$\text{Blood flow} = \text{Pressure} \div \text{Vascular Resistance}$$

Delivery of blood flow is matched to demand by adjustments in the arteriolar vascular resistance through vasoconstriction or vasodilation. In the healthy blood vessels without obstruction, exercise is a major stimulus for vasodilation, causing a decrease in peripheral resistance, which, when combined with an increase in arterial pressure, results in a large increase in limb arterial flow to supply sufficient oxygen to accommodate exercising muscular oxygen consumption.[24] Normal arteries have the capacity to support large volumetric increases in blood flow without a significant drop in pressure across the large and medium conduit vessels (Fig. 17.1).

Alterations in Limb Hemodynamics in Peripheral Artery Disease

Altered limb perfusion in PAD is due to atherosclerotic stenosis in limb arteries resulting in fixed-resistance elements. Obstructive arterial lesions create drops in pressure and flow that are additive. Major factors that determine the pressure drop across an arterial stenosis include the magnitude of blood flow and the resistance caused by the narrowing. The resistance across an individual stenosis is defined by the length, the internal radius, and the blood viscosity as described by the Poiseuille equation:

$$\text{Pressure drop across stenosis} = \frac{\text{Blood flow}\left[8L_{\eta}\right]}{\pi r^4}$$

where L is the length of the stenosis, r is the internal radius of the artery, and η is blood viscosity.

As shown by the equation, the radius or cross-sectional area of the stenosis is the primary factor in determining the drop in pressure across a stenosis. A reduction by 50% in the vessel diameter results in a 16-fold increase in resistance and, consequently, a fall in pressure. As a stenosis worsens, perfusion pressure and the maximal achieved blood flow decreases dramatically. The length of the stenosis also contributes to the dissipation of energy that occurs as blood flow traverses a stenosis. Whereas the length of an individual stenosis may have only a modest impact on the pressure gradient, the hemodynamic effect of two equivalent lesions in series is double that of a single lesion. Thus, individual noncritical stenosis may become hemodynamically significant when combined in the same limb. A patient with mild claudication may have single vessel stenosis, but a patient with more advanced claudication could have occlusive disease at multiple sites, such as the iliac, femoral, and tibial arteries. Patients with CLI often have diffuse disease affecting multiple arterial segments and levels. These lesions in series create more hemodynamic compromise threatening limb viability. Adequate flow at rest requires sufficient tissue perfusion to provide nutrient delivery to the foot to prevent skin breakdown and to promote wound healing. Tibial artery disease is quite common in CLI and is predictive of a higher risk of ischemic ulceration and amputation.[25,26] Progression of the disease from intermittent claudication to chronic CLI is modulated by many factors, including the severity and number of stenotic or occlusive lesions, and the availability of collateral vessels to maintain adequate blood flow.[27] Chronically reduced blood flow induces compensatory vasodilation producing the characteristic dependent rubor observed in patients with CLI; however, the hypoperfusion leads to resistance vessel remodeling with impaired myogenic regulation and peripheral edema, which contributes to skin ischemia and ulcer formation.[28]

Critical Degree of Arterial Stenosis

The term *critical arterial stenosis* is defined as the degree of luminal narrowing that causes a decrease in distal blood flow. The concept integrates the relation of a stenotic narrowing and the resultant limitation in volumetric flow distal to the stenosis. At rest, stenosis of 50% may only produce a mild pressure gradient and a minimal, or no, decrease in distal flow at rest. With more severe stenosis, the pressure gradient is greater and distal flow decreases.

When blood flow across a stenosis increases, as occurs with exercise, a pressure gradient will occur. Indeed, during exercise, blood flow to the limb may increase more than 10-fold. Thus, a pressure drop across an arterial stenosis may limit distal perfusion pressure augmentation during exercise, even with a stenosis of only 50%. The magnification of pressure drop across fixed lesions with exercise is relevant not only for the manifestation of claudication but also in the diagnosis of PAD. In patients with claudication symptoms, the pedal pulse examination and ABI may be normal at rest but abnormal with activity. The exercise ABI has greater sensitivity to detect PAD than the ABI at rest. Further, an abnormal exercise ABI has greater prognostic value for future limb events compared to the resting ABI alone.[29–32]

Blood Flow Response to Exercise in Peripheral Artery Disease

In most patients with PAD, blood flow at rest is sufficient to meet the relatively low metabolic needs of skeletal muscle. At the onset of leg exercise, patients with PAD have an initial rise in leg blood flow and a delayed rise in leg oxygen consumption. Further increases in muscle oxidative work are supported by increases in oxygen extraction.[23]

As exercise intensity increases, blood flow reaches a plateau because of the limitation imposed by fixed arterial obstructions. The plateau reflects dissipation of energy across arterial stenoses. Moreover, the severity of arterial disease correlates inversely with the maximal increase in flow. With continuous exercise, leg oxygen demand increases and there is a mismatch between supply and demand in patients, leading to the symptom of claudication. With cessation of exercise, the hyperemic phase (duration of increased flow over resting levels) is prolonged in patients with PAD relative to healthy controls.

Functional Limitation and Anatomic Stenosis in Peripheral Artery Disease

The extent of arterial obstruction in PAD is not the only determinant of symptoms and prognosis. In some studies of patients with PAD, there is a modest association of ABI and functional status; other studies have not observed any relation between ABI and walking ability.[24] Similarly, calf blood flow at rest has modest or no association with functional capacity. When measured by magnetic resonance imaging (MRI), resting calf blood flow is modestly associated with walking distance; however, calf blood flow measured at rest by plethysmography is not predictive of treadmill walking time.[33] Overall plaque burden measured by MRI predicts mobility loss in patients with PAD.[34] Hyperemic blood flow measured by plethysmography also does not predict exercise capacity in patients with PAD.[35] However, microvascular blood flow to skeletal muscle, when assessed by contrast-enhanced ultrasound, is associated with time to claudication in patients with PAD.[36] Overall, the available evidence indicates that arterial lesion severity and perfusion pressure or flow do not fully govern symptom status in PAD.

CONTRIBUTORS TO LIMB SYMPTOMS IN PERIPHERAL ARTERY DISEASE: BEYOND ARTERIAL STENOSIS

A classic demand-supply mismatch model (as discussed above) attributes intermittent claudication to insufficient augmentation of skeletal muscle blood flow during exercise due to arterial stenosis. Additional disease processes co-exist with atherosclerosis that interfere with walking ability and promote tissue loss. Current evidence supporting the role of vascular dysfunction, altered hemorheology, impaired angiogenesis, impaired skeletal muscle metabolic function, and systemic inflammation—as characteristic to limb symptoms—is discussed in this section (Fig. 17.2).

Endothelial Dysfunction in Peripheral Artery Disease

Vascular dysfunction exacerbates fixed arterial obstruction in PAD by limiting dynamic increases in blood flow to exercising muscle.[37] Endothelium-derived nitric oxide is central to the physiological regulation of arteriolar tone. Nitric oxide and prostaglandins are major autocrine and paracrine mediators of local vascular resistance during exercise in healthy individuals. In addition, nitric oxide promotes vascular health by inhibiting platelet aggregation, limiting smooth muscle proliferation, reducing inflammation, and augmenting angiogenesis. Reduced nitric oxide bioavailability in leg arteries of patients with PAD interferes with the normal exercise-induced increases in blood flow. Endothelial dysfunction in atherosclerotic arteries is also manifested as enhanced production and reaction to vasoconstrictor substances, including catecholamines and thromboxane.[38]

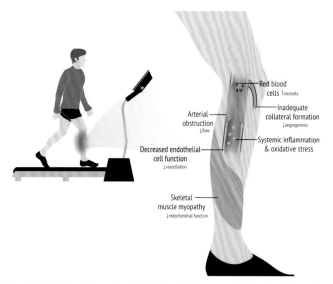

Fig. 17.2 Mechanisms Contributing to Abnormal Exercise Capacity in Peripheral Artery Disease. Arterial stenosis leads to a pressure drop and an inability to increase flow relative to demand. Collateral formation attempts to compensate for arterial obstruction, but impaired angiogenesis limits efficacy. Endothelial dysfunction limits the vasodilator response to exercise. Systemic inflammation and oxidative stress damage the endothelium and skeletal muscle. Skeletal muscle myopathy from oxidant damage leads to atrophy, and mitochondrial dysfunction limits skeletal muscle metabolism.

Measures of endothelium-dependent vasodilation are lower in conduit arteries and resistance vessels of patients with PAD.[39] Endothelial dysfunction in the femoral artery is associated with lesion severity.[40] Impairment of vascular function is associated with functional limitation and reduced physical activity in daily life.[41–43] Endothelial dysfunction predicts the risk of cardiovascular events in patients with PAD.[44–46] Revascularization and supervised exercise training improve endothelial function in PAD.[47] Limb amputation in CLI is associated with improved markers of endothelial function, suggesting local generation of oxidative stress from an ischemic limb.[48]

Arterial stiffening accentuates small vessel damage and may contribute to vascular events.[49] Patients with PAD have higher central and peripheral arterial stiffness that predicts cardiovascular events.[50,51] Higher arterial stiffness is observed in association with impaired walking distance in patients with PAD, suggesting that structural changes in central arteries may relate to functional limitations.[52,53]

Hemorheology in Peripheral Artery Disease

PAD is associated with altered hemorheology (flow properties of blood and its cellular components). PAD patients have higher blood viscosity than age-matched controls. Increased viscosity leads to altered flow as described by the Poiseuille equation. Patients with PAD have increased blood concentrations of fibrinogen, von Willebrand factor, and plasminogen activator inhibitor, as well as increased fibrin turnover.[54] These circulating factors may affect blood flow characteristics, though an association with exercise performance has not been shown. Red cell flexibility is reduced in patients with intermittent claudication, and thus the passage of erythrocytes through capillaries might be compromised by microcirculatory vessel plugging. In patients with CLI, erythrocyte fluidity and erythrocyte volume fraction are reduced.[23,55]

Inadequate Angiogenesis and Altered Microcirulatory Flow in Peripheral Artery Disease

Insufficient angiogenesis and inadequate collateral formation may amplify limb ischemia. The angiogenic response to ischemia is complex and involves the elaboration of many factors that regulate vascular growth, including vascular endothelial growth factor (VEGF), fibroblast growth factor, hepatocyte growth factor, and hypoxia-inducible factor 1-alpha, as well as cellular regeneration from bone-marrow–derived cells and endothelial progenitor cells targeted to ischemic territories to promote vessel growth.[56]

Several microRNAs (miRNAs) are altered in PAD in the circulation including miRNAs known to be relevant to inflammation and cell adhesion.[57,58] In animal models with limb ischemia, there is lower microRNA93 expression, and treatment with antagonists to selected microRNAs improves hindlimb recovery.[59–61] Increased expression of an inhibitory isoform of VEGF is present in PAD patients and contributes to impaired hindlimb recovery in animal models.[62]

Therapeutic approaches that stimulate angiogenesis restore functional status in animal models of PAD. In patients with PAD, insufficient growth of collateral vessels and impaired angiogenesis may contribute to limb ischemia. In skeletal muscle biopsies, patients with PAD had reduced capillary density, which are associated with lower peak walking time.[36] Reduced exercise blood flow in the muscle microvasculature is related to a greater degree of claudication symptoms and lower 6-minute walking time.[63] Insufficient formation of collateral vessels may be a mediator of the association of both diabetes and chronic renal disease with progression to CLI.[26] In addition, microthrombosis reflecting both endothelial injury and hemostasis contributes to the development of tissue loss in CLI.[28]

Inflammatory Activation in Peripheral Artery Disease

In patients with claudication, markers of systemic inflammation, including interleukin-8 (IL-8), soluble intracellular adhesion molecule-1 (sICAM-1), soluble vascular cell adhesion molecule-1 (sVCAM-1), and thrombomodulin are increased. The acute inflammatory response to skeletal muscle ischemia may exacerbate symptoms and alter muscle metabolism. Systemic inflammation is associated with altered muscle structure, including lower calf muscle area and higher fat content.[64] Inflammation also drives endothelial dysfunction by increasing oxidative stress and reducing nitric oxide bioactivity.

Circulating markers of vascular inflammation also relate to reduced walking capacity in PAD.[65,66] Expression levels of tumor necrosis factor alpha (TNF-α) in peripheral monocytes are associated with lower walking time in patients with claudication.[67] Higher expression of the pro-inflammatory, anti-angiogenic mediator, Wnt5a, in circulating leukocytes is associated with lower ABI.[62] Higher levels of C-reactive protein, IL-6, sICAM-1, and sVCAM-1 are present in PAD patients and relate to lower physical activity in daily life.[68] C-reactive protein levels predict the degree of functional decline over time in PAD patients,[65] and there are reduced levels of resolvin D2, an anti-inflammatory regulator of tissue repair. Increased resolvin D2 augments vessel growth and reduces inflammation in PAD models.[69]

Oxidative Injury in Peripheral Artery Disease

In animal models, ischemia and ischemia-reperfusion are associated with oxidative stress, and are mediated by higher reactive oxygen species generation.[70] Patients with claudication do not deliver sufficient oxygen to exercising muscle and have a prolonged hyperemic oxygen-rich phase during recovery from exercise.[23] Muscle ischemia during exercise is associated with an increase in oxidant stress measured by malondialdehyde levels.[71] Production of oxygen-derived free radicals may be a unifying mechanism of skeletal muscle and endothelial injury in PAD. Oxidative injury may, in turn, promote chronic changes in muscle structure and metabolism leading to loss of function in PAD, which cannot be explained simply by a reduction in blood flow. Mitochondrial damage and subsequent oxidant production may be particularly relevant in PAD. Mitochondria are a source of reactive oxygen species and are particularly sensitive to oxidative damage.[72] Mitochondrial DNA damage is greater in atherosclerosis, and specific acquired mutations are present in PAD.[73] As discussed below, altered mitochondrial energetics induced by oxidant injury also contribute to skeletal muscle dysfunction in PAD. Strategies to treat PAD with antioxidant therapies have been tried without success; however, approaches with targeted antioxidant therapies that reduce mitochondrial oxidative stress and promote bioenergetics may have greater potential to improve symptoms.

ALTERED SKELETAL MUSCLE STRUCTURE AND FUNCTION IN PERIPHERAL ARTERY DISEASE

Changes in Muscle Structure in Peripheral Artery Disease

Patients with PAD develop a skeletal muscle myopathy that may contribute to walking impairment. In patients with claudication, myofiber damage relates to shorter walking distance and decreased muscle strength.[74,75] In a 2-year prospective study, calf muscle fat content predicted functional decline.[76,77] Gait abnormalities include slowed walking speed with decreased step length and cadence. The gait abnormalities may reflect muscle weakness, denervation, and adaptations to minimize pain.

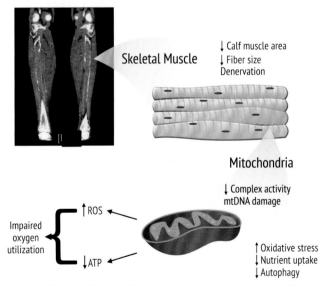

Fig. 17.3 Skeletal Muscle Myopathy in Peripheral Artery Disease. Oxidative damage and inflammation produced by repeated ischemic episodes lead to reduced calf muscle size and smaller myofibers with altered fiber type. Nutrient delivery to the skeletal muscle is reduced. Mitochondrial function is impaired with decreased complex activity, reduced autophagy, DNA damage leading to decreased energy production, and increased reactive oxygen species *(ROS)* generation. *ATP,* Adenosine triphosphate.

Lower extremity skeletal muscle shows evidence of damage at multiple levels in PAD, as shown in Fig. 17.3. Decreased calf muscle area and fiber type changes are associated with lower walking time.[78] Recurrent ischemic bouts, disuse due to exercise limitation, and chronic inflammation each contribute to histological and gross structural changes in skeletal muscle in PAD. Calf muscle area measured on computed tomography scan is smaller in patients with PAD, and is characterized by lower density and higher fat content.[76] Muscle biopsy studies show oxidative damage that worsens with the advancing degree of ischemia and preferentially affects type II fast-twitch fibers.[79,80] Fiber type distribution varies across patients with PAD, but overall larger muscle fiber size is associated with greater walking performance.[81] Oxidative stress markers including 4-hydroxy-2-nonenol adducts are associated with muscle fiber degeneration.[79] Patients with claudication also demonstrate extensive peripheral denervation, with evidence of poor nerve conduction in patients with severe PAD. Impaired peripheral nerve function is associated with self-reported walking function in PAD.[82]

Changes in Muscle Metabolism in Peripheral Artery Disease

Both muscle oxygen saturation and phosphocreatine levels are normal at rest in patients with PAD. However, at the onset of exercise there is a marked delay in systemic oxygen uptake, which parallels a slowed response in skeletal muscle oxygen uptake. In patients with PAD, phosphocreatine is used preferentially for energy creation at similar exercise work load.[83–85]

Patients with PAD have changes in oxidative metabolism that are intrinsic to skeletal muscle. A potential site of impairment of oxidative metabolism in PAD is the mitochondria. In the muscle tissue, mitochondrial mass is paradoxically higher with more severe PAD; however, the activity of several mitochondrial complexes, including complex I and complex III, is lower, leading to decreased adenosine triphosphate generation and increased reactive oxygen species production.[86,87] Impaired mitochondrial bioenergetics and oxidative stress underlies restricted oxygen utilization and lowers nitric oxide bioavailability.[88] The increased mitochondrial content may represent a compensatory mechanism aimed at improving oxygen extraction under ischemic conditions, and overcoming abnormalities in mitochondrial oxidative capacity. Overall, mitochondrial metabolism is lower, as indicated by higher circulating levels of oxidative phosphorylation intermediates, including acylcarnitines, and by lower phosphocreatine recovery on magnetic resonance spectroscopy.[33] Systemic metabolic disturbances also contribute to altered muscle function by reducing nutrient delivery. In patients with intermittent claudication, skeletal muscle glucose uptake is lower, reflecting calf muscle insulin resistance.[89]

Mitochondrial dysfunction contributes to functional status and symptoms in PAD. Reduced mitochondrial respiration assessed by magnetic resonance phosphocreatine recovery is associated with lower treadmill walking time.[33] Interestingly, the accumulation of desmin, a cytoskeletal protein, occurs in the skeletal muscle of PAD patients, and is associated with lower mitochondrial function and reduced walking ability.[88] Damaged mitochondria produce more reactive oxygen species, and the mitochondria are cleared by the cellular clearance process, autophagy. Skeletal muscle biopsies show evidence of inadequate mitochondrial autophagy—the process for clearing damaged organelles—and this may contribute to impaired mitochondrial oxidative capacity.[81] Inadequate autophagy is associated with walking time.[81] Unfortunately, treatment with resveratrol, a polyphenol that improves mitochondrial function in experimental models, did not improve walking performance in a clinical trial in patients with PAD.[90]

SUMMARY

Patients with PAD suffer from reduced walking ability, accelerated functional decline, atypical leg pain, intermittent claudication, and in severe cases critical limb ischemia. Arterial atherosclerotic lesions that obstruct large artery flow characterize PAD. With exercise there is a drop in pressure across severe obstructive stenosis, resulting in reduced blood flow and oxygen delivery to the leg muscle inciting ischemic symptoms. Arterial hemodynamics and altered large vessel blood flow do not fully account for exercise limitations. The mechanisms that generate leg pain and lead to tissue loss in patients with PAD are multifactorial and include systemic inflammation, endothelial dysfunction, impaired angiogenesis with reduced microcirculatory flow, and skeletal muscle dysfunction.

REFERENCES

1. Sampson UK, Fowkes FG, McDermott MM, et al. Global and regional burden of death and disability from peripheral artery disease: 21 world regions, 1990 to 2010. *Glob Heart.* 2014;9:145–158. e21.
2. Fowkes FG, Rudan D, Rudan I, et al. Comparison of global estimates of prevalence and risk factors for peripheral artery disease in 2000 and 2010: a systematic review and analysis. *Lancet.* 2013;382:1329–1340.
3. Creager MA. The crisis of vascular disease and the journey to vascular health: presidential address at the American Heart Association 2015 Scientific Sessions. *Circulation.* 2016;133:2593–2598.
4. McDermott MM. Lower extremity manifestations of peripheral artery disease: the pathophysiologic and functional implications of leg ischemia. *Circ Res.* 2015;116:1540–1550.
5. Bonaca MP, Bhatt DL, Storey RF, et al. Ticagrelor for prevention of ischemic events after myocardial infarction in patients with peripheral artery disease. *J Am Coll Cardiol.* 2016;67:2719–2728.
6. Bonaca MP, Gutierrez JA, Creager MA, et al. Acute limb ischemia and outcomes with vorapaxar in patients with peripheral artery disease: results from the trial to assess the effects of vorapaxar in preventing heart attack and stroke in patients with atherosclerosis-thrombolysis in myocardial infarction 50 (TRA2 degrees P-TIMI 50). *Circulation.* 2016;133:997–1005.
7. Anand SS, Caron F, Eikelboom JW, et al. Major adverse limb events and mortality in patients with peripheral artery disease: the COMPASS trial. *J Am Coll Cardiol.* 2018;71:2306–2315.
8. Aboyans V, Criqui MH, Abraham P, et al. Measurement and interpretation of the ankle-brachial index: a scientific statement from the American Heart Association. *Circulation.* 2012;126:2890–2909.
9. McDermott MM, Liu K, Ferrucci L, et al. Decline in functional performance predicts later increased mobility loss and mortality in peripheral arterial disease. *J Am Coll Cardiol.* 2011;57:962–970.
10. Gerhard-Herman MD, Gornik HL, Barrett C, et al. 2016 AHA/ACC guideline on the management of patients with lower extremity peripheral artery disease: a report of the American College of Cardiology/American Heart Association Task Force on Clinical Practice Guidelines. *Circulation.* 2017;135(12):e726–e779.
11. McDermott MM, Guralnik JM, Tian L, et al. Associations of borderline and low normal ankle-brachial index values with functional decline at 5-year follow-up: the WALCS (Walking and Leg Circulation Study). *J Am Coll Cardiol.* 2009;53:1056–1062.
12. Ramirez JL, Drudi LM, Grenon SM. Review of biologic and behavioral risk factors linking depression and peripheral artery disease. *Vasc Med.* 2018;23:478–488.
13. Nead KT, Zhou M, Diaz Caceres R, et al. Walking impairment questionnaire improves mortality risk prediction models in a high-risk cohort independent of peripheral arterial disease status. *Circ Cardiovasc Qual Outcomes.* 2013;6:255–261.
14. McDermott MM, Guralnik JM, Ferrucci L, et al. Community walking speed, sedentary or lying down time, and mortality in peripheral artery disease. *Vasc Med.* 2016;21:120–129.
15. Delaney JA, Jensky NE, Criqui MH, et al. The association between physical activity and both incident coronary artery calcification and ankle brachial index progression: the multi-ethnic study of atherosclerosis. *Atherosclerosis.* 2013;230:278–283.
16. Bhatt DL, Eagle KA, Ohman EM, et al. Comparative determinants of 4-year cardiovascular event rates in stable outpatients at risk of or with atherothrombosis. *JAMA.* 2010;304:1350–1357.
17. Diehm C, Allenberg JR, Pittrow D, et al. Mortality and vascular morbidity in older adults with asymptomatic versus symptomatic peripheral artery disease. *Circulation.* 2009;120:2053–2061.
18. Willey J, Mentias A, Vaughan-Sarrazin M, et al. Epidemiology of lower extremity peripheral artery disease in veterans. *J Vasc Surg.* 2018;68:527–535. e5.
19. Reinecke H, Unrath M, Freisinger E, et al. Peripheral arterial disease and critical limb ischaemia: still poor outcomes and lack of guideline adherence. *Eur Heart J.* 2015;36:932–938.
20. Nehler MR, Duval S, Diao L, et al. Epidemiology of peripheral arterial disease and critical limb ischemia in an insured national population. *J Vasc Surg.* 2014;60:686–695. e2.
21. Agarwal S, Sud K, Shishehbor MH. Nationwide trends of hospital admission and outcomes among critical limb ischemia patients: from 2003-2011. *J Am Coll Cardiol.* 2016;67:1901–1913.
22. Baril DT, Ghosh K, Rosen AB. Trends in the incidence, treatment, and outcomes of acute lower extremity ischemia in the United States Medicare population. *J Vasc Surg.* 2014;60:669–677. e2.
23. Hiatt WR, Armstrong EJ, Larson CJ, Brass EP. Pathogenesis of the limb manifestations and exercise limitations in peripheral artery disease. *Circ Res.* 2015;116:1527–1539.
24. Hamburg NM, Creager MA. Pathophysiology of intermittent claudication in peripheral artery disease. *Circ J.* 2017;81(3):281–289.
25. Shishehbor MH, White CJ, Gray BH, et al. Critical limb ischemia: an expert statement. *J Am Coll Cardiol.* 2016;68:2002–2015.
26. Farber A, Eberhardt RT. The current state of critical limb ischemia: a systematic review. *JAMA Surg.* 2016;151:1070–1077.
27. Breton-Romero R, Hamburg NM. Every PACE counts: learning about blood cells and blood flow in peripheral artery disease. *Circulation.* 2017;135:1429–1431.
28. Coats P, Wadsworth R. Marriage of resistance and conduit arteries breeds critical limb ischemia. *Am J Physiol Heart Circ Physiol.* 2005;288:H1044–H1050.
29. Hammad TA, Strefling JA, Zellers PR, et al. The effect of post-exercise ankle-brachial index on lower extremity revascularization. *JACC Cardiovasc Interv.* 2015;8:1238–1244.
30. Diehm C, Darius H, Pittrow D, et al. Prognostic value of a low post-exercise ankle-brachial index as assessed by primary care physicians. *Atherosclerosis.* 2011;214:364–372.
31. Sheikh MA, Bhatt DL, Li J, et al. Usefulness of postexercise ankle-brachial index to predict all-cause mortality. *Am J Cardiol.* 2011;107:778–782.
32. Drachman DE, Beckman JA. The exercise ankle-brachial index: a leap forward in noninvasive diagnosis and prognosis. *JACC Cardiovasc Interv.* 2015;8:1245–1247.
33. Anderson JD, Epstein FH, Meyer CH, et al. Multifactorial determinants of functional capacity in peripheral arterial disease: uncoupling of calf muscle perfusion and metabolism. *J Am Coll Cardiol.* 2009;54:628–635.
34. McDermott MM, Carroll T, Carr J, et al. Femoral artery plaque characteristics, lower extremity collaterals, and mobility loss in peripheral artery disease. *Vasc Med.* 2017;22:473–481.
35. Szuba A, Oka RK, Harada R, Cooke JP. Limb hemodynamics are not predictive of functional capacity in patients with PAD. *Vasc Med.* 2006;11:155–163.
36. Robbins JL, Jones WS, Duscha BD, et al. Relationship between leg muscle capillary density and peak hyperemic blood flow with endurance capacity in peripheral artery disease. *J Appl Physiol.* 2011;111:81–86.
37. Vita JA, Hamburg NM. Does endothelial dysfunction contribute to the clinical status of patients with peripheral arterial disease? *Can J Cardiol.* 2010;26(Suppl A):45A–50A.
38. Flammer AJ, Anderson T, Celermajer DS, et al. The assessment of endothelial function: from research into clinical practice. *Circulation.* 2012;126:753–767.

39. Kiani S, Aasen JG, Holbrook M, et al. Peripheral artery disease is associated with severe impairment of vascular function. *Vasc Med.* 2013;18:72–78.

40. Heinen Y, Stegemann E, Sansone R, et al. Local association between endothelial dysfunction and intimal hyperplasia: relevance in peripheral artery disease. *J Am Heart Assoc.* 2015;4. pii: e001472.

41. Payvandi L, Dyer A, McPherson D, et al. Physical activity during daily life and brachial artery flow-mediated dilation in peripheral arterial disease. *Vasc Med.* 2009;14:193–201.

42. Grenon SM, Chong K, Alley H, et al. Walking disability in patients with peripheral artery disease is associated with arterial endothelial function. *J Vasc Surg.* 2014;59:1025–1034.

43. Silva Rde C, Wolosker N, Yugar-Toledo JC, Consolim-Colombo FM. Vascular reactivity is impaired and associated with walking ability in patients with intermittent claudication. *Angiology.* 2015;66:680–686.

44. Gokce N, Keaney Jr. JF, Hunter LM, et al. Predictive value of non-invasively-determined endothelial dysfunction for long-term cardiovascular events in patients with peripheral vascular disease. *J Am Coll Cardiol.* 2003;41:1769–1775.

45. Huang AL, Silver AE, Shvenke E, et al. Predictive value of reactive hyperemia for cardiovascular events in patients with peripheral arterial disease undergoing vascular surgery. *Arterioscler Thromb Vasc Biol.* 2007;27:2113–2119.

46. van Mil A, Pouwels S, Wilbrink J, et al. Carotid artery reactivity predicts events in peripheral arterial disease patients. *Ann Surg.* 2017 [Epub ahead of print].

47. Mika P, Konik A, Januszek R, et al. Comparison of two treadmill training programs on walking ability and endothelial function in intermittent claudication. *Int J Cardiol.* 2013;168:838–842.

48. Newton DJ, Khan F, Kennedy G, Belch JJ. Improvement in systemic endothelial condition following amputation in patients with critical limb ischemia. *Int Angiol.* 2008;27:408–412.

49. Cooper LL, Palmisano JN, Benjamin EJ, et al. Microvascular function contributes to the relation between aortic stiffness and cardiovascular events: the Framingham Heart Study. *Circ Cardiovasc Imaging.* 2016;9. pii: e004979.

50. Husmann M, Jacomella V, Thalhammer C, Amann-Vesti BR. Markers of arterial stiffness in peripheral arterial disease. *Vasa.* 2015;44:341–348.

51. Kals J, Lieberg J, Kampus P, et al. Prognostic impact of arterial stiffness in patients with symptomatic peripheral arterial disease. *Eur J Vasc Endovasc Surg.* 2014;48:308–315.

52. Amoh-Tonto CA, Malik AR, Kondragunta V, et al. Brachial-ankle pulse wave velocity is associated with walking distance in patients referred for peripheral arterial disease evaluation. *Atherosclerosis.* 2009;206:173–178.

53. Brewer LC, Chai HS, Bailey KR, Kullo IJ. Measures of arterial stiffness and wave reflection are associated with walking distance in patients with peripheral arterial disease. *Atherosclerosis.* 2007;191:384–390.

54. Lowe GD, Fowkes FG, Dawes J, et al. Blood viscosity, fibrinogen, and activation of coagulation and leukocytes in peripheral arterial disease and the normal population in the Edinburgh Artery Study. *Circulation.* 1993;87:1915–1920.

55. Holmberg A, Sandhagen B, Bergqvist D. Hemorheologic variables in critical limb ischemia before and after infrainguinal reconstruction. *J Vasc Surg.* 2000;31:691–695.

56. Cooke JP, Losordo DW. Modulating the vascular response to limb ischemia: angiogenic and cell therapies. *Circ Res.* 2015;116:1561–1578.

57. Stather PW, Sylvius N, Wild JB, et al. Differential microRNA expression profiles in peripheral arterial disease. *Circ Cardiovasc Genet.* 2013;6:490–497.

58. Hamburg NM, Leeper NJ. Therapeutic potential of modulating microRNA in peripheral artery disease. *Curr Vasc Pharmacol.* 2015;13:316–323.

59. Hazarika S, Farber CR, Dokun AO, et al. MicroRNA-93 controls perfusion recovery after hindlimb ischemia by modulating expression of multiple genes in the cell cycle pathway. *Circulation.* 2013;127:1818–1828.

60. Grundmann S, Hans FP, Kinniry S, et al. MicroRNA-100 regulates neovascularization by suppression of mammalian target of rapamycin in endothelial and vascular smooth muscle cells. *Circulation.* 2011;123:999–1009.

61. Bonauer A, Carmona G, Iwasaki M, et al. MicroRNA-92a controls angiogenesis and functional recovery of ischemic tissues in mice. *Science.* 2009;324:1710–1713.

62. Kikuchi R, Nakamura K, MacLauchlan S, et al. An antiangiogenic isoform of VEGF-A contributes to impaired vascularization in peripheral artery disease. *Nat Med.* 2014;20:1464–1471.

63. Lindner JR, Womack L, Barrett EJ, et al. Limb stress-rest perfusion imaging with contrast ultrasound for the assessment of peripheral arterial disease severity. *JACC Cardiovasc Imaging.* 2008;1:343–350.

64. McDermott MM, Ferrucci L, Guralnik JM, et al. Elevated levels of inflammation, d-dimer, and homocysteine are associated with adverse calf muscle characteristics and reduced calf strength in peripheral arterial disease. *J Am Coll Cardiol.* 2007;50:897–905.

65. McDermott MM, Ferrucci L, Liu K, et al. D-dimer and inflammatory markers as predictors of functional decline in men and women with and without peripheral arterial disease. *J Am Geriatr Soc.* 2005;53:1688–1696.

66. McDermott MM, Liu K, Ferrucci L, et al. Circulating blood markers and functional impairment in peripheral arterial disease. *J Am Geriatr Soc.* 2008;56:1504–1510.

67. Pande RL, Brown J, Buck S, et al. Association of monocyte tumor necrosis factor alpha expression and serum inflammatory biomarkers with walking impairment in peripheral artery disease. *J Vasc Surg.* 2015;61:155–161.

68. Craft LL, Guralnik JM, Ferrucci L, et al. Physical activity during daily life and circulating biomarker levels in patients with peripheral arterial disease. *Am J Cardiol.* 2008;102:1263–1268.

69. Zhang MJ, Sansbury BE, Hellmann J, et al. Resolvin D2 enhances postischemic revascularization while resolving inflammation. *Circulation.* 2016;134:666–680.

70. Paradis S, Charles AL, Meyer A, et al. Chronology of mitochondrial and cellular events during skeletal muscle ischemia-reperfusion. *Am J Physiol Cell Physiol.* 2016;310:C968–C982.

71. Ciuffetti G, Mercuri M, Mannarino E, et al. Free radical production in peripheral vascular disease. A risk for critical ischaemia? *Int Angiol.* 1991;10:81–87.

72. Kluge MA, Fetterman JL, Vita JA. Mitochondria and endothelial function. *Circ Res.* 2013;112:1171–1188.

73. Fetterman JL, Holbrook M, Westbrook DG, et al. Mitochondrial DNA damage and vascular function in patients with diabetes mellitus and atherosclerotic cardiovascular disease. *Cardiovasc Diabetol.* 2016;15:53.

74. Brass EP, Hiatt WR, Green S. Skeletal muscle metabolic changes in peripheral arterial disease contribute to exercise intolerance: a point-counterpoint discussion. *Vasc Med.* 2004;9:293–301.

75. Koutakis P, Myers SA, Cluff K, et al. Abnormal myofiber morphology and limb dysfunction in claudication. *J Surg Res.* 2015;196:172–179.

76. McDermott MM, Hoff F, Ferrucci L, et al. Lower extremity ischemia, calf skeletal muscle characteristics, and functional impairment in peripheral arterial disease. *J Am Geriatr Soc.* 2007;55:400–406.

77. McDermott MM, Ferrucci L, Guralnik J, et al. Pathophysiological changes in calf muscle predict mobility loss at 2-year follow-up in men and women with peripheral arterial disease. *Circulation.* 2009;120:1048–1055.

78. Askew CD, Green S, Walker PJ, et al. Skeletal muscle phenotype is associated with exercise tolerance in patients with peripheral arterial disease. *J Vasc Surg.* 2005;41:802–807.

79. Weiss DJ, Casale GP, Koutakis P, et al. Oxidative damage and myofiber degeneration in the gastrocnemius of patients with peripheral arterial disease. *J Transl Med.* 2013;11:230.

80. Koutakis P, Weiss DJ, Miserlis D, et al. Oxidative damage in the gastrocnemius of patients with peripheral artery disease is myofiber type selective. *Redox Biol.* 2014;2:921–928.

81. White SH, McDermott MM, Sufit RL, et al. Walking performance is positively correlated to calf muscle fiber size in peripheral artery disease subjects, but fibers show aberrant mitophagy: an observational study. *J Transl Med.* 2016;14:284.

82. Evans NS, Liu K, Criqui MH, et al. Associations of calf skeletal muscle characteristics and peripheral nerve function with self-perceived physical functioning and walking ability in persons with peripheral artery disease. *Vasc Med.* 2011;16:3–11.

83. Bauer TA, Brass EP, Barstow TJ, Hiatt WR. Skeletal muscle StO2 kinetics are slowed during low work rate calf exercise in peripheral arterial disease. *Eur J Appl Physiol.* 2007;100:143–151.

84. Bauer TA, Brass EP, Hiatt WR. Impaired muscle oxygen use at onset of exercise in peripheral arterial disease. *J Vasc Surg.* 2004;40:488–493.

85. Kemp GJ, Roberts N, Bimson WE, et al. Mitochondrial function and oxygen supply in normal and in chronically ischemic muscle: a combined 31P magnetic resonance spectroscopy and near infrared spectroscopy study in vivo. *J Vasc Surg.* 2001;34:1103–1110.

86. Makris KI, Nella AA, Zhu Z, et al. Mitochondriopathy of peripheral arterial disease. *Vascular.* 2007;15:336–343.

87. Pipinos II, Judge AR, Zhu Z, et al. Mitochondrial defects and oxidative damage in patients with peripheral arterial disease. *Free Radic Biol Med.* 2006;41:262–269.

88. Koutakis P, Miserlis D, Myers SA, et al. Abnormal accumulation of desmin in gastrocnemius myofibers of patients with peripheral artery disease: associations with altered myofiber morphology and density, mitochondrial dysfunction and impaired limb function. *J Histochem Cytochem.* 2015;63:256–269.

89. Pande RL, Park MA, Perlstein TS, et al. Impaired skeletal muscle glucose uptake by [18F]fluorodeoxyglucose-positron emission tomography in patients with peripheral artery disease and intermittent claudication. *Arterioscler Thromb Vasc Biol.* 2011;31:190–196.

90. McDermott MM, Leeuwenburgh C, Guralnik JM, et al. Effect of resveratrol on walking performance in older people with peripheral artery disease: the RESTORE randomized clinical trial. *JAMA Cardiol.* 2017;2:902–907.

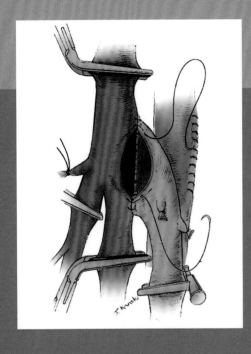

中文导读

第18章
外周动脉疾病的临床评估

　　外周动脉疾病是动脉粥样硬化疾病最不常见的表现之一。许多心血管医师并不常规进行外周动脉疾病的临床评估，对于老年患者、冠状动脉或脑动脉粥样硬化患者及有动脉粥样硬化危险因素（如糖尿病、吸烟、肾功能衰竭）的患者，应当给予充分的重视，特别是上述人群，需要进行踝肱比的筛查，因为相当一部分患者是无症状的外周动脉疾病患者，而对于表现为间歇性跛行和下肢静息痛等典型外周动脉疾病表现的患者，需要将其与腘动脉陷迫综合征、纤维肌发育不良、静脉功能不全、血栓闭塞性脉管炎及非血管性下肢疼痛相鉴别。对于该病的鉴别需要综合患者的临床体征、踝肱比、下肢动脉彩色多普勒超声、CT血管造影、磁共振血管成像和血管造影等检查。

谷涌泉

Peripheral Artery Disease: Clinical Evaluation

Joshua A. Beckman and Mark A. Creager

The least often recognized of the commonly occurring manifestations of atherosclerosis is peripheral artery disease (PAD). Epidemiological studies suggest that approximately 7.1 million people in the United States have PAD.[1] Among 7458 participants aged 40 years and older from the 1999 to 2004 National Health and Nutrition Examination Survey (NHANES), the prevalence of PAD was 5.9%.[2] Despite its relative frequency, predictable patient population, and prognostic implications for life and limb, many cardiovascular physicians do not undertake clinical evaluation of PAD. This chapter will focus on the history, physical examination, and diagnostic tests important to the management of limb atherosclerosis.

PATIENT HISTORY

The diagnosis of PAD begins with clinical suspicion in the typical patient population. This includes avid questioning and seeking to elicit historical evidence of limb and systemic atherosclerosis. Clinical suspicion should be heightened in older persons, in those with coronary or cerebral atherosclerosis, and in patients with atherosclerotic risk factors, such as diabetes or tobacco use, as well as renal failure (see Chapter 16). PAD is uncommon before the age of 40 years. In the German Epidemiological Trial on Ankle Brachial Index (getABI) of 6990 unselected patients aged 65 years or older, the prevalence of PAD in men and women was 20% and 17%, respectively.[3] In the PAD Awareness, Risk, and Treatment: New Resources for Survival (PARTNERS) program, a study of 6979 patients in 350 primary care practices across the United States, ankle-brachial index (ABI) screening was performed in subjects older than age 70, or older than age 50 if they were smokers or had diabetes.[4] In this primary care population, 29% of those screened with an ABI met the criteria for PAD. In the recent Danish Viborg Vascular (VIVA) trial of men aged 65 to 75 years, PAD was diagnosed in 11% of the men who attended a screening examination.[5]

Despite the relative frequency of disease, the diagnosis of PAD is not often considered because the majority of patients with PAD are asymptomatic. In the PARTNERS program, only 11% of PAD patients had classic symptoms.[6] Similar data have been reported in other large cross-sectional studies (see Chapter 16). Even in high-risk subgroups with a higher population frequency of PAD, the diagnosis may be missed because PAD is often asymptomatic. The decision to look for PAD in the outpatient should be predicated on the pretest probability of finding it. Application of the PARTNERS criteria, for example, demonstrated the importance of risk factors in enriching the population with PAD to make ABI screening worthwhile. Thus the presence of risk factors for atherosclerosis should lower the threshold for routine screening.

Symptoms of Peripheral Artery Disease

The most commonly ascribed symptom that develops as a result of PAD is intermittent claudication. The word *claudication* derives from the Latin word *claudicato*, which was used to describe the limp gait of a lame horse. As defined in the Rose questionnaire,[7] claudication is the development of an ischemic muscular pain on exertion. The pain can be characterized as aching, burning, heaviness, feeling leaden, tightness, or cramping. Pain should originate in a muscular bed, such as the calf, thigh, hip, or buttock, and not localize to a joint. The area of the worst blood flow limitation usually subtends the site of muscular discomfort. For example, patients who develop hip or buttock discomfort with walking most likely have distal aorta or iliac artery occlusive disease, whereas patients with calf claudication likely have superficial femoral or popliteal arterial stenoses or occlusions. The reduction of muscular work upon activity cessation rebalances the available blood supply with muscle demand and quickly resolves the pain.

Both time of activity to pain onset and time to pain resolution should be consistent and predictable. The distance walked to the onset of leg discomfort is called the *initial claudication distance*, and the maximal distance the patient can walk without stopping because of leg discomfort is called the *absolute claudication distance*. Several classification schemes are used to categorize the severity of claudication, including the Fontaine (Table 18.1) and Rutherford classifications (Table 18.2).[8] When the interview is complete, the physician should have insight into the nature of discomfort, how long it has been present, the typical duration of exercise required to cause the discomfort, and the amount of rest necessary to relieve the symptoms.

Classic symptoms of claudication occur in a minority of patients with PAD, including those with functional limitations. The application of questionnaires for claudication, such as the World Health Organization (WHO)/Rose questionnaire or the Walking Impairment Questionnaire,[9] may underestimate PAD prevalence by 50%. Data from McDermott et al. indicate that complaints other than claudication are common.[6] They evaluated functional tolerance across a range of symptoms in cross-sectional analyses of patients with and without PAD.[10] PAD patients demonstrated several types of leg discomfort, including leg pain at rest and with walking, pain with walking alone requiring cessation of activity, and pain patients could "walk through." This variety of presentations would be missed with questioning only for classic symptoms. Moreover, the type of discomfort predicted function. Patients with pain at rest and with walking had worse functional capacity than those whose pain occurred with walking and stopped with walking cessation, and those who were able to "walk through" the pain. Quality of leg pain, whether it is atypical or classic, does not predict severity of reduction in limb perfusion pressure as measured by the ABI.[6]

TABLE 18.1   Fontaine Classification

Stage	Description
I	Asymptomatic, ABI <0.9
II	Intermittent claudication
III	Daily rest pain
IV	Focal tissue necrosis

ABI, Ankle-brachial index.

TABLE 18.2   Rutherford Classification

Grade	Category	Description
0	0	Asymptomatic
I	1	Mild claudication
I	2	Moderate claudication
I	3	Severe claudication
II	4	Ischemic rest pain
III	5	Minor tissue loss
IV	6	Major tissue loss

The presence of intermittent claudication has important prognostic implications regarding functional capacity and mortality. Three quarters of patients with intermittent claudication will have stable symptoms over the next 10 years; approximately 25% will progress to more disabling claudication or critical limb ischemia (CLI) requiring revascularization or culminating in amputation. Moreover, they will suffer a mortality more than twice that of the general population, approximating 15% to 30% at 5 years.[8]

Differential Diagnosis of Claudication

Once exercise-related discomfort has been established, several alternate vascular and nonvascular diagnoses should be considered (Box 18.1). Vascular disorders include popliteal artery entrapment (see Chapter 63), compartment syndrome, fibromuscular dysplasia (FMD), venous insufficiency (see Chapter 54), and vasculitis (see Chapters 39 through 42). Popliteal artery entrapment typically occurs in very active persons or athletes. Because of an abnormal origin of the medial (or less commonly, lateral) head of the gastrocnemius muscle, the popliteal artery may be compressed with walking and yield symptoms of claudication. Endofibrosis of the external iliac artery (EIA), a rare occurrence in highly trained cyclists and other endurance athletes, may cause claudication.

FMD is a noninflammatory arterial occlusive disease that most commonly affects the renal and carotid arteries but may involve other arterial beds (see Chapter 58).[11] Any of the arteries in the lower extremities may be affected, but the iliac arteries are the most common. Fibroplasias may involve the intimal, medial, or adventitial layer of the artery. The most common histological type is medial fibroplasia, which is the most frequent cause of the "string of beads" appearance of FMD on angiography, depicting areas of stenosis and dilatation. FMD has a predilection for the nonbranching points of vessels. The etiology of FMD remains unknown.

Increased calf muscle size with exercise may inhibit venous outflow, cause exertional compartment syndrome—in which tissue pressure is increased and microvascular flow is impeded—and bring about complaints of calf pain or tightness with exertion. Symptoms improve with leg elevation after exercise cessation. Venous claudication may occur as a result of iliofemoral thrombosis with poor collateral vein formation. When venous outflow is impaired, the increase in arterial inflow with exercise increases venous pressure markedly and causes a severe tightness or bursting sensation in the limb. Patients may report improvement in symptoms with leg elevation following exercise cessation. These patients frequently have leg edema. Vasculitides such as Takayasu arteritis, giant-cell arteritis (GCA), and thromboangiitis obliterans (TAO) are infrequent causes of claudication.

Nonvascular causes of exertional leg pain include lumbar radiculopathy, hip and knee arthritis, and myositis. Perhaps the most common nonvascular diagnosis is lumbar radiculopathy causing nerve-based pain. Patients may complain of leg pain or paresthesias as a result of compression of the lumbar nerve roots from disk herniation or degenerative osteophytes. The paresthesias or pain tend to affect the posterior aspect of the leg and occur with specific positions, such as standing, or develop at the beginning of ambulation. These symptoms may improve with continued walking or when leaning forward because pressure on the nerve roots is reduced.

Osteoarthritis of the hip or knee may cause pain associated with walking. The pain may be confused with intermittent claudication because it typically occurs with exercise. However, the discomfort is usually referable to a joint such as the hip or knee. It can be distinguished from claudication in that the level of activity required to precipitate symptoms varies and does not resolve rapidly with activity cessation.

BOX 18.1   Nonatherosclerotic Causes of Exertional Leg Pain

Nonatherosclerotic arterial disease
Atheroembolism
Vasculitis
Extravascular compression
Popliteal artery entrapment
Adventitial cysts
Fibromuscular dysplasia
Endofibrosis of the internal iliac artery
Venous claudication
Compartment syndrome
Lumbar radiculopathy
Spinal stenosis
Hip/knee arthritis
Myositis

CRITICAL LIMB ISCHEMIA

CLI is the most debilitating manifestation of PAD (Fig. 18.1). The TransAtlantic Inter-Society Consensus (TASC) Working Group estimates that the incidence of CLI is between 300 and 1000 persons per million per year.[12] Across the globe, the incidence of amputation varies from 7.4 to 41.3 per 100,000 person-years in subjects without diabetes and 78 to 704 per 100,000 person-years in patients with diabetes.[13] The prevalence of CLI was 1.2% and affected more women than men in a population study of 8000 persons between 60 and 90 years of age.[14]

Diabetes and smoking increase the risk of developing CLI. Diabetes is the cause of most nontraumatic lower-extremity amputations in the United States. Diabetes increases the risk of amputation nearly fourfold, even with similar levels of blood flow limitation as in nondiabetic patients.[15] Cigarette smoking also increases the risk that PAD will progress to CLI. In a study of 343 consecutive patients with intermittent claudication, 16% of those who continued to smoke developed CLI, compared to none in those who were able to stop smoking.[16] CLI occurs

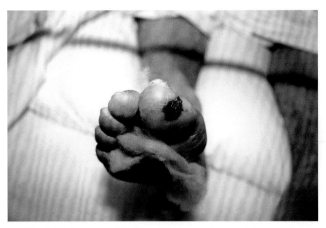

Fig. 18.1 A nonhealing first-digit ulcer with overlying eschar.

Arterial Occlusive Disease
Atherosclerosis
Atheroemboli
Acute arterial occlusion
    in situ thrombosis
    Emboli

Vasculitis
Thromboangiitis obliterans
Scleroderma
Systemic lupus erythematosus
Mixed connective tissue disease
Cryoglobulinemia

Vasospasm
Raynaud pheomenon
Acrocyanosis

Ulcers
Neuropathy
Venous insufficiency
Trauma

Pain
Neuropathy

Arthritis
Gout
Rheumatoid arthritis

Other
Fasciitis
Trauma

as a consequence of tissue ischemia at rest, and it manifests as foot pain, nonhealing ulceration, or tissue gangrene. The pain is often severe, unremitting, and localized to the acral portion of the foot or toes, notably at the site of ulceration or gangrene. Blood flow limitation is so severe that the gravitational effects of leg position may affect symptoms. Patients commonly report that leg elevation worsens pain. This is typically worse at night when the patient is in bed and the leg, now at heart level, no longer benefits from the dependent position. Placing the foot on the floor beside the bed is a common action used by patients to reduce pain. The inability to use the leg and chronically placing the leg in a dependent position may cause peripheral edema, a finding occasionally mistaken for venous disease in these patients. With severe ischemia, any skin perturbation, including bedclothes or blankets, may cause pain; in ischemic neuropathy, this causes a lancinating pain in the foot. Other symptoms of CLI include hypesthesia, cold intolerance, muscular weakness, and joint stiffness of the affected limb. The severity of CLI is categorized in both the Fontaine and Rutherford classification schemes (see Tables 18.1 and 18.2).

Differential Diagnosis of Critical Limb Ischemia

The differential diagnosis of CLI includes vascular and nonvascular diseases (Box 18.2). Atheroembolism, or *blue toe syndrome*, occurs when components of large-vessel atherosclerotic plaque embolize to distal vessels (Fig. 18.2) (see Chapter 45). The embolized material is composed of fibroplatelet debris and cholesterol crystals. A common cause of atheroembolism is iatrogenic disruption of the vessel, whether from catheterization or surgery. Several features may help in differentiating atheroembolism from traditional CLI. Patients typically have pulses palpable down to the ankle, because the emboli require a patent pathway to distal portions of the extremities. Other clinical clues include new renal insufficiency and blood eosinophilia. On examination, the patient will have areas of cyanosis or violaceous discoloration of the toes or portions of the feet and areas of livedo reticularis.

Acute limb ischemia may occur from thrombosis in situ or from thromboemboli of large fibroplatelet accumulations that originate in the heart or large arteries and occlude conduit arteries (see Chapter 44). These patients have an accelerated course and may present with the "five Ps" of acute ischemia: pain, pallor, poikilothermia, paresthesia, and paralysis. Other causes of limb ischemia include vasospasm, TAO, other vasculitides, and connective tissue disorders (see Chapters 40–42, and 46). Other causes of ulcers include neuropathy, venous disease, and trauma (see Chapter 61).

Nonvascular causes of foot pain include neuropathy, arthritides such as gout, fasciitis, and trauma (see Box 18.1).

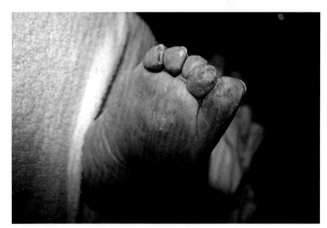

Fig. 18.2 Atheroembolism After Catheterization. Note areas of cyanosis and surrounding livedo reticularis. This patient had a palpable dorsalis pedis pulse.

PHYSICAL EXAMINATION

A comprehensive physical examination that includes the general appearance of the patient, integument, heart, lungs, abdomen, and limbs should be performed during the initial patient encounter to elucidate evidence of systemic disease and to provide insight into cause and

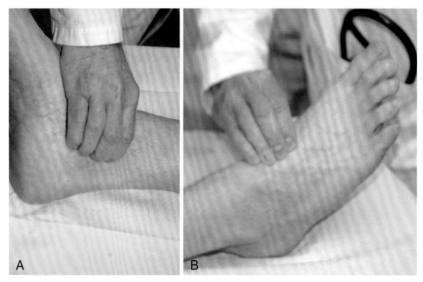

Fig. 18.3 Palpation of Pedal Pulses. (A) Palpation of posterior tibial (PT) pulse. Examiner should place his/her fingers in the curve below the malleolus with light pressure and reposition as needed. Application of passive foot dorsiflexion occasionally makes PT palpation easier. (B) Dorsalis pedis pulse is typically appreciated within 1 cm of the dorsum, most prominent near navicular bone.

manifestation of the patient's vascular disease. The entire vascular system should be examined. Blood pressure is measured in each arm. A blood pressure difference of 10 mm Hg or more may be indicative of innominate, subclavian, axillary, or brachial artery stenosis. The carotid, brachial, radial, ulnar, femoral, popliteal, dorsalis pedis, and posterior tibial pulses should be palpated in every patient (Fig. 18.3). Several pulse-descriptive schemes have been promulgated. One is to grade the pulses as 0 (absent), 1 (diminished), and 2 (normal). A very prominent or forceful pulse may occur in patients with aortic regurgitation or high cardiac output states. The absence of any pulse in the lower extremity, except in the dorsalis pedis, increases the likelihood of PAD.[17] The dorsalis pedis pulse is not palpable in approximately 8% of healthy patients.[18] The absence of a peripheral pulse may indicate a significant stenosis between the present and the absent pulse. Occasionally, pulses may be palpable below the level of a significant stenosis. This most commonly occurs in the setting of iliac artery disease when there may be sufficient collateral vessels to maintain perfusion to distal arteries.

The abdominal aorta also should be palpated to elicit evidence of an aortic aneurysm if permitted by body habitus. A widened pulse in the abdomen or over a peripheral artery (e.g., the popliteal artery) may be indicative of an aneurysm. Once palpated, the abdomen and several peripheral vessels also should be auscultated. Palpation of an expansile or pulsatile periumbilical mass is indicative of an abdominal aortic aneurysm. Proper auscultation of normal vessels with a stethoscope should reveal no sound. Bruits should be sought over the carotid and subclavian arteries, in the abdomen, in the lower back, and over the femoral arteries. Presence of a bruit, indicative of turbulent blood flow, typically occurs as a result of arterial stenosis, but may indicate extrinsic compression or arteriovenous malformation. Vessels with no flow, resulting from complete occlusion, do not convey bruits.

A skin examination should be performed, looking for alterations in temperature, edema, signs of active or healed lesions, or signs of chronic ischemia—including thin shiny skin, thickened yellow nails, and loss of hair. Foot or toe cyanosis or pallor may be a forerunner of ulceration. Inspection of the skin may reveal trophic signs of chronic ischemia, including sympathetic denervation (impaired hair growth or impaired sweating) and sensorimotor neuropathy (lack of vibratory sense). CLI may cause muscle and subcutaneous tissue atrophy, hair loss, petechiae,

and thin or encrusted skin. In CLI, the toes and foot are cool and pallor may be present when the foot is in the neutral (or horizontal) position.

Changes in skin appearance with elevation and dependency may provide a gauge for PAD severity. The leg should be elevated to 45 to 60 degrees for 1 minute. If pallor develops quickly (within 10 to 15 seconds), severe PAD is likely. After 1 minute, the patient sits up and the leg is placed in a dependent position. The time to pedal vein refill should be recorded. Ischemic-induced arteriolar and venular dilation may lead to development of a violaceous appearance of the foot with dependency, called *dependent rubor* (Fig. 18.4). Normal refill occurs rapidly, typically within 10 to 15 seconds. Prolongation of venous filling or the development of numbness beyond 1 minute suggests severe PAD.

Arterial fissures most commonly develop in the heel, toes, in the web space between the toes, or in segments subjected to pressure (the ball of the foot). Arterial ulcers are circumscribed, tender, and prone to infection. The base of the ulcer is usually pale. The ulcers, in contrast to venous ulcers, are dry; however, the devitalized tissue is prone to infection, which may generate a purulent exudate. The ulcer may be covered by an eschar. In CLI, gangrene most commonly occurs in the digits, but may occur on the ball of the foot or heel. In the absence of infection, gangrene tends to be dry, and the skin is mummified.

Two classification schemes are used to categorize the clinical assessment of patients with PAD: the Fontaine Stage Classification of PAD and the Rutherford Categorical Classification of PAD. In the system described by Fontaine, the severity of PAD is classified into 1 of 4 stages ranging from asymptomatic in stage 1, intermittent claudication in stage 2, daily rest pain in stage 3, and focal tissue necrosis in stage 4 (see Table 18.1). The Rutherford system employs seven categories, dividing the severity of claudication into three categories (mild, moderate, and severe) and CLI into three categories (rest pain, minor tissue loss, and major tissue loss) (see Table 18.2).

DIAGNOSTIC TESTING

Office-Based Ankle-Brachial Index

Measurement of the ABI is a simple method employed to corroborate the historical and physical findings of PAD. The ABI is the ratio of the

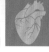

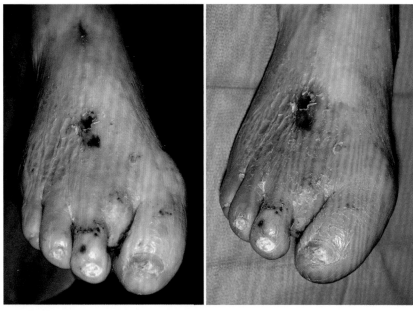

Fig. 18.4 Dependent Rubor. This patient with severe peripheral artery disease (note previously amputated second digit) develops a ruborous appearance of the forefoot with dependent positioning as a result of arteriolar and venular dilation.

systolic blood pressure at the ankle and brachial artery. The latter is an estimate of central aortic pressure. Brachial artery systolic blood pressure is measured in both arms and ankles using a handheld 5- or 10-MHz Doppler ultrasound device and sphygmomanometric cuff. The cuffs are placed on each arm above the antecubital fossa and above each ankle. The cuffs are sequentially inflated above systolic pressure and then are slowly depressurized. The Doppler probe, placed over the brachial artery and the dorsalis pedis and posterior tibial arteries, monitors the pressure (Fig. 18.5). As the cuff is slowly deflated, reappearance of a Doppler signal indicates the systolic pressure at the level of the cuff.

Brachial artery pressures must be measured in both arms because atherosclerosis may occur in subclavian and axillary arteries. The higher of the two brachial systolic blood pressures is used for reference in the ABI calculation. Hence, the ABI is the systolic pressure at each ankle divided by the higher pressure of the two brachial artery pressures; an ABI may be generated for each leg. When assessing foot perfusion, the ABI uses the highest of the pedal pressures in each leg.[19] Both pedal pressures (dorsalis pedis and posterior tibial artery) are considered when seeking evidence of atherosclerosis.

Normal systolic pressure at the ankle should be at least the same as in the arm, yielding an ABI of 1.0 or greater. As a result of reflected arterial

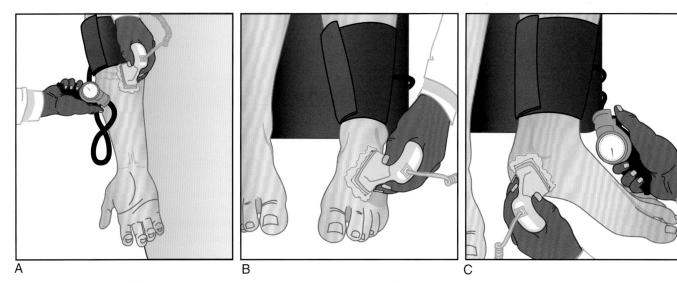

A   B   C

Fig. 18.5 Measurement of the Ankle-Brachial Index (ABI). Brachial artery systolic blood pressure is determined in both arms and both ankles using a handheld 5- or 10-MHz Doppler ultrasound and sphygmomanometric cuff. Because atherosclerosis may occur in subclavian and axillary arteries, brachial artery pressures must be measured in both arms (A). The higher of the two brachial systolic blood pressures is used as the reference pressure in ABI calculation. In each ankle, pressure should be measured at the dorsalis pedis pulse (B) and the posterior tibial pulse (C). ABI is the quotient of the highest systolic pressure at each ankle divided by the highest pressure of the two brachial artery pressures.

pressure waves, healthy persons tend to have an ABI ranging from 1.0 to 1.4. Recognizing an intrinsic (up to 10%) variability of blood pressure when measured sequentially, since ankle pressures are not measured simultaneously, an abnormal ABI consistent with the diagnosis of PAD is categorized as 0.9 or less, whereas an ABI above 0.9 to 1.0 is borderline abnormal.[8] The ABI is a reliable determinant of PAD, with a sensitivity for ABI 0.9 or less ranging from 79% to 95% with a specificity of 96% to 100%.[19] An ABI of 0.4 or less is extremely abnormal and typically present in patients with CLI. Arterial calcification may introduce a false elevation in ABI, typically >1.4, as a result of noncompressible vessels at the ankle. Arterial calcification occurs more commonly in patients with diabetes or end-stage renal disease, and in the elderly.[20]

The ABI provides prognostic information because it is a gauge of the burden of systemic atherosclerosis. In the ABI Collaboration, the incidence of adverse events rose as the ABI dropped below 1.0, even in the absence of symptoms.[17] The lower the ABI, the greater the cardiovascular morbidity and mortality. An ABI of 0.8 or less is associated with twice the age-adjusted 10-year mortality, and an ABI of 0.4 or less is associated with a fourfold increase in mortality.[17] Measuring the ABI provides an assessment of both PAD and cardiovascular risk.

There are limitations to ABI measurement. The correlation between ABI, functional capacity, and symptoms is weak. Resting ABI is occasionally normal in patients with PAD; this may occur in patients with aortoiliac stenoses and a well-collateralized arterial system that maintains perfusion pressure. In patients with a normal ABI but a strong suspicion of significant PAD, office-based exercise testing may be performed. Exercise accentuates arterial gradients by increasing the turbulence across the flow-limiting lesion and decreasing muscular arteriolar resistance to significantly attenuate lower-extremity perfusion pressure. In fact, arterial pressure at the ankle may reach zero in patients who develop claudication and recover more than 10 minutes after exercise cessation. In the office, stair climbing or active pedal plantar flexion may be used to elicit symptoms and to document a decrease in ankle pressure (and ABI) to confirm the diagnosis of intermittent claudication.

Noninvasive Laboratory Testing for Peripheral Artery Disease

For patients in whom revascularization is considered, such as those with CLI or disabling claudication, the location and severity of disease should be evaluated by additional noninvasive testing. There are two general formats of noninvasive testing to discern the location and severity of PAD: physiological testing and anatomical imaging.

Physiological testing

Physiological or functional testing most commonly occurs in a noninvasive vascular laboratory (see Chapter 12). The measurement of limb segmental systolic pressures employs methods similar to ABI measurement (Fig. 18.6). Sphygmomanometric cuffs are placed on the proximal thigh, distal thigh, calf, and ankle. The cuffs are inflated sequentially to suprasystolic pressure and then deflated to determine systolic pressure at each site. A Doppler probe is placed on the posterior tibial or dorsalis pedis artery. Arterial stenosis or occlusion will decrease the perfusion pressure. Arterial pressure gradients of more than 20 mm Hg between thigh cuffs and 10 mm Hg between cuffs below the knee indicate the presence of a stenosis. As with the ABI, the most common source of error for the test is vascular calcification. In the setting of vascular calcification, a toe brachial index may be obtained. Pressures in the toe may be measured with strain gauge photoplethysmography. Pressure is measured in the toes and a ratio of toe pressure to brachial artery pressure is generated; a value of 0.7 or less is consistent with PAD.

Pulse volume recordings (PVRs), or segmental pneumatic plethysmography, determines the relative change in limb volume with each

pulse and can be obtained along with segmental pressure measurements. The pulse-volume waveform represents the product of pulse pressure and vascular wall compliance. In a healthy person, the pulse-volume waveform is similar to a normal arterial pressure waveform and includes rapid upstroke, dicrotic notch, and downstroke (see Fig. 18.6). The waveform changes when it is recorded distal to a significant stenosis as perfusion pressure falls. Initially, there is a loss of the dicrotic notch. As the stenosis worsens, the waveform upstroke (anacrotic slope) is delayed, the amplitude is less, and the downstroke (catacrotic slope) is slower. The combined use of segmental pressure measurements and PVRs improves the accuracy of identifying significant stenosis.

Treadmill testing. As described earlier, eliciting symptoms through exercise may permit the diagnosis of PAD, despite a normal or near-normal ABI.[21] When a vessel has a significant stenosis, increasing flow through the lesion decreases energy delivered beyond the area of stenosis. Treadmill exercise increases blood flow through a stenosed vessel and can increase sensitivity of the ABI. In the vascular laboratory, a diagnosis of intermittent claudication and a quantification of exercise tolerance may be obtained through treadmill exercise testing. Many treadmill protocols exist to test walking ability, but each one falls into one of two types: constant or graded exercise. In constant exercise protocols (e.g., Carter protocol), a specific speed (1.5 to 2.0 mph) and treadmill grade (0% to 12%) is chosen, whereas in the graded exercise protocols (e.g., Hiatt or Gardner protocol), speed and/or treadmill grade may increase. In both protocols, the brachial and ankle pressures are determined pretest at rest, patients exercise until they are unable to continue, and brachial and ankle pressures are redetermined within 1 minute of exercise cessation.[22] Patients with PAD as a cause of exercise limitation will have an attenuated rise in ankle pressure compared to brachial artery pressure or, more commonly, a fall in ankle pressure, thus lowering the ABI. The fall in ankle pressure is directly related to severity of arterial occlusive disease. Analogously, length of recovery is also directly related to disease severity. Two parameters are recorded in addition to the ABI: the time claudication begins (initial claudication time), and the time until exhaustion or cessation (absolute claudication time). Variability of walking distance is greater in the constant exercise protocols than the graded protocols, making the latter more commonly used.

Anatomical Imaging of the Peripheral Circulation

Defining arterial anatomy is not typically necessary to make the diagnosis of PAD but is required for patients who will be undergoing revascularization. The following is a discussion of the major methods used to image peripheral arteries.

Duplex ultrasonography. Duplex ultrasonography of the lower extremities is performed in most vascular laboratories (see Chapter 12). The combination of bright (B)-mode ultrasound, color Doppler imaging, and pulsed-Doppler velocity analysis can accurately identify the location and severity of atherosclerotic lesions in the legs. Normally, flow through each arterial segment should be laminar, with a uniform homogeneous color appearance. Blood flow becomes turbulent and velocity increases at sites of stenosis, creating areas of color discordance. Pulsed Doppler measurements in the area of stenosis demonstrate increased flow velocity and spectral broadening.

Applying the concepts of the Poiseuille law regarding movement of incompressible viscous fluids through a tube, the ratio of peak systolic velocity in the area of a stenosis is compared with the normal area of artery proximal to the stenosis. A ratio of 2 or greater is consistent with stenosis of 50% or more (Fig. 18.7). In one meta-analysis of seven studies, the sensitivity and specificity of duplex ultrasound to detect 50% or greater stenosis or occlusion were 88% and 96%, respectively, and to detect complete occlusion were 90% and 99%, respectively.[23] In another

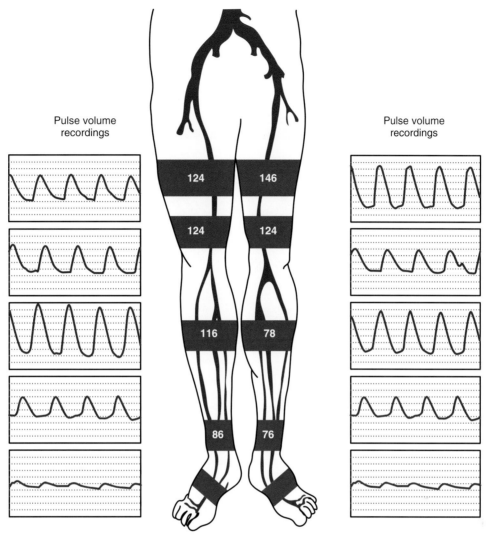

Fig. 18.6 Segmental Pressure Measurements. Sequential Doppler pressures are measured by placing sphygmomanometric cuffs on the proximal thigh, distal thigh, calf, and ankle. Cuffs are inflated above systolic pressure and then slowly depressurized. Simultaneously, a Doppler probe placed over the dorsalis pedis or posterior tibial artery monitors pressure. As the cuff is slowly deflated, the reappearance of Doppler signal indicates systolic pressure at the level of the cuff. Arterial stenosis or occlusion will decrease perfusion pressure. Arterial pressure gradients between cuffs indicate the presence of a stenosis. In this example, arterial pressures (mm Hg) are noted in the location of each sphygmomanometric cuff. The patient has evidence of a systolic gradient between both upper thigh cuffs, which is suggestive of right iliac and/or common femoral arterial occlusive disease, and a gradient between right calf and ankle, which is suggestive of arterial occlusive disease in the infrapopliteal arteries. A significant gradient between the left lower thigh cuff and the calf cuff is indicative of distal superficial femoral artery and/or popliteal artery occlusive disease.

meta-analysis of 14 studies, the sensitivity and specificity of duplex ultrasound with and without color-guided Doppler analysis to detect 50% or greater stenosis or occlusion was 93% and 95%, respectively.[24] Duplex ultrasonography is less accurate at the site of calcified plaque because of the acoustic shadowing caused by the dense calcium. Serial stenoses are more difficult to diagnose because ultrasound diagnosis relies on comparing peak arterial velocities between adjacent segments, and there are altered hemodynamics between sequential stenoses. Single-center studies have found that ultrasound may be used alone in planning both percutaneous and surgical peripheral revascularization.

Duplex ultrasonography is also used in the postoperative surveillance of infrainguinal arterial bypass grafts. Routine ultrasound surveillance may be part of a strategy to identify graft stenosis and prompt repair before graft occlusion occurs. Some studies reported that duplex ultrasound is useful to predict vein graft failure.[25,26] However, a recent meta-analysis

of 15 studies found that duplex ultrasound surveillance was not associated with a significant change in primary, secondary, or assisted primary patency or mortality when compared with ABI and clinical examination.[27] There are limited data for ultrasound surveillance of prosthetic bypass grafts, though studies have found that abnormal velocity predicts graft failure.[28] Duplex ultrasound after angioplasty or stenting is useful to detect restenosis and to plan repeat revascularization, but it is not known whether routine surveillance affects outcomes.[29]

Magnetic resonance angiography. Magnetic resonance angiography (MRA) is an accurate imaging modality to diagnose PAD, visualize peripheral arteries, and to determine the location of stenoses (see Chapter 13). Techniques used to image the arterial tree include black blood, phase contrast, time of flight (TOF), and contrast-enhanced MRA.[30] The application of two magnetic pulses to suppress the signal in the vessel lumen yields a dark appearance of flowing blood, with the

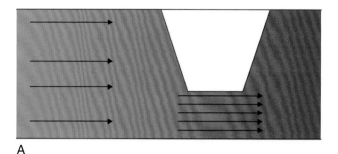

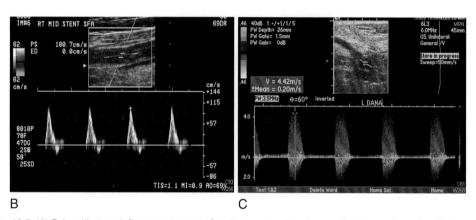

Fig. 18.7 (A) Poiseuille law defines movement of an incompressible viscous fluid through a tube. Fluid entry into tube must equal its exit; thus, the ratio of peak-systolic velocity in the area of stenosis is proportional to the segment of normal vessel proximal to stenosis. When the ratio is >2, stenosis of more than 50% is diagnosed. Sensitivity and specificity of duplex ultrasound evaluation in the determination of stenoses of 50% or greater range from 90% to 95%. Normal arterial flow velocity is approximately 100 cm/s. (B) Doppler ultrasound is passed through a recently placed superficial femoral artery *(SFA)* stent, demonstrating normal flow velocity. This is indicative of a patent stent without evidence of restenosis. (C) Doppler ultrasound is passed through distal anastomosis of a femoral–popliteal bypass graft, demonstrating a flow velocity of 4.4 m/s. This is consistent with >75% stenosis. Velocity in proximal normal segment is 1.3 m/s (not shown).

vessel wall remaining white. Selective removal of blood from the image causes the lumen to appear black, and the technique is therefore called *black blood.* When the phase shift of moving electrons spins in, flowing blood is compared with surrounding stable tissue, blood volume and velocity can be measured to permit the assessment of blood flow. The application of electrocardiographic gating while interrogating the flow-related enhancement of spins into a partially saturated area provides a TOF angiogram. Limitations of a flow-based TOF MRA include lengthy acquisition types, turbulence, nonlinear vascular structures, and retrograde flow.[30]

Most MRAs are performed using contrast, most commonly gadolinium. Contrast-enhanced MRA provides a high-resolution angiogram, and is useful as a noninvasive imaging test to define lower-extremity vascular anatomy. In a meta-analysis comparing contrast-enhanced MRA with TOF MRA, the contrast-enhanced study had a much greater diagnostic accuracy.[31] The use of contrast has improved scan quality and efficiency, and has enhanced vessel visualization and identification, especially in distal vessels (Fig. 18.8). MRA can identify the presence of stenoses and reveal distal vessels suitable for bypass, which is not demonstrated by contrast angiography. In a meta-analysis of 32 studies of contrast-enhanced MRA and intraarterial digital subtraction angiography (DSA), the pooled sensitivity of MRA was 95%, and specificity was 96%.[32]

One potential limitation is a tendency for MRA to overestimate lesion severity. Similar benefits and limitations exist in the imaging of bypass grafts. MRA has a sensitivity as high as 91% for the identification of arterial bypass graft stenoses, but overestimates lesion severity in up to 30% of stenoses.[32] A sound strategy may involve the use of MRA initially because of the noninvasive nature of the test and its superior identification of bypass vessels, reserving DSA for cases requiring greater definition. Technological advancement is rapid in MRA, including three-dimensional (3D) MRA, and is likely to improve the detection and assessment of PAD.

Computed tomographic angiography. Computed tomography angiography (CTA) has recently undergone rapid improvements in technology and imaging, allowing its entry into peripheral vascular imaging (see Chapter 14). Much of this advance results from the development of multidetector-row CT scanners and improved resolution of arteries. Availability of higher resolution to scanners is particularly relevant for smaller and more distal arteries.

In meta-analyses of studies mostly using multidetector CT scanners, pooled sensitivity and specificity for detecting stenoses of 50% or greater in leg arteries were 91% to 92% and 91% to 93%, respectively.[23,33] Newer CT scanners should have even greater accuracy.

CTA is commonly presented using a maximal intensity projection (MIP) or with a volume rendering technique (Fig. 18.9). The MIP algorithm displays only the pixel with the highest intensity along a ray perpendicular to the plane of projection. This algorithm creates a 2D projectional image similar in appearance to MRA or contrast angiography. Volume rendering applies shades of gray to pixels of varying density. Fourier transfer functions allow modification of the relative contribution of various pixel values. Volume rendering considers pixels that are only partially filled with contrast material. Arterial calcification limits imaging with both CT techniques. Optimal techniques used for postprocessing are being developed. As resolution

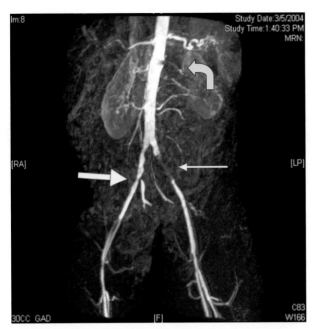

Fig. 18.8 Gadolinium-Enhanced Magnetic Resonance Angiogram (MRA). This MRA was performed in a patient with Takayasu arteritis. Several findings are notable. The patient has an occluded left upper renal artery *(curved arrow)*, and the right internal iliac artery has severe stenosis *(thick arrow)*. At the thin arrow is an area of dropout due to image interference by a previously placed stent.

improves, CTA may become a regular instrument in the diagnostic armamentarium because of its rapid study time (typically <1 minute) or because of the 75% reduction in ionizing radiation compared with angiography.

Contrast angiography. Contrast angiography is the most venerable and widely available method for imaging arterial anatomy (see Chapter 15). Angiography commonly serves as the standard for determining the sensitivity and specificity of newer techniques and is an excellent method to clarify arterial anatomical queries (Fig. 18.10). Technical improvements in equipment, including smaller catheters, image resolution, and digital subtraction, have enhanced the capability of angiography. Digital subtraction eliminates bony and soft-tissue shadows from the angiographic image, enhancing angiographic detail. Despite wide acceptance of angiography as a reliable method for defining arterial anatomy, its invasive nature, requirement for contrast, nephrotoxicity, risk of atheroembolism, and risk of pseudoaneurysms or arteriovenous fistula (AVF) continue to foster the development of alternative angiographic methods.

SUMMARY

An algorithm for evaluating the patient with PAD is depicted in Fig. 18.11. The diagnosis and evaluation of PAD is required in patients predisposed to develop PAD because of age or the presence of atherosclerotic risk factors, and in patients whose history or examination are suggestive of PAD. An office evaluation should include measurement of the ABI. An exercise test with measurement of the ABI after exercise is appropriate if resting ABI is normal, yet clinical suspicion remains high. Patients with noncompressible ankle vessels should be referred to a vascular laboratory for additional testing, including segmental pressure measurements, pulse-volume recordings, and/or duplex ultrasonography. Symptomatic patients, particularly those with CLI, should undergo anatomical imaging with CT, MRA, or conventional contrast angiography prior to revascularization.

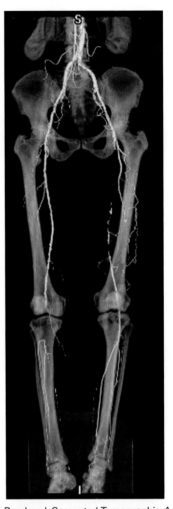

Fig. 18.9 Volume-Rendered Computed Tomographic Angiogram of the Lower Extremities. Note the left superficial femoral artery occlusion and collateral formation depicted by this study. (Image courtesy Dr. Joseph Schoepf.)

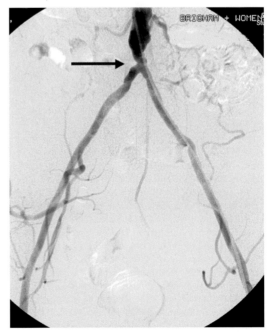

Fig. 18.10 Contrast abdominal angiogram demonstrating significant aortic stenosis just proximal to bifurcation into iliac arteries *(arrow)*.

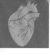

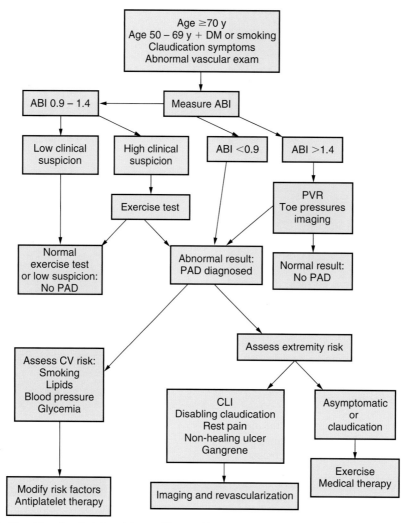

Fig. 18.11 Algorithm for Peripheral Artery Disease Evaluation. History, physical examination, and ankle-brachial index *(ABI)* make the diagnosis of peripheral artery disease *(PAD)* in the majority of cases. Treadmill exercise testing is performed in conjunction with the measurement of ABI performed prior to and immediately following exercise. Segmental pressure measurements, pulse volume recordings *(PVR)*, toe pressures, and arterial duplex ultrasound imaging are noninvasive vascular tests used to consider and assess severity of PAD. Anatomical imaging by duplex ultrasonography, computed tomography angiography, magnetic resonance angiography, or conventional contrast angiography is used to assess symptomatic patients who require revascularization. Patients with PAD require risk factor assessment and treatment. The physician should more aggressively inquire about leg symptoms and inspect the patient's feet for evidence of critical limb ischemia *(CLI)*. *CV,* Cardiovascular; *DM,* diabetes mellitus.

REFERENCES

1. Benjamin EJ, Virani SS, Callaway CW, et al. Heart disease and stroke statistics—2018 update: a report from the American Heart Association. *Circulation.* 2018;137(12):e67-e492.
2. Pande RL, Perlstein TS, Beckman JA, Creager MA. Secondary prevention and mortality in peripheral artery disease: National Health and Nutrition Examination Study, 1999 to 2004. *Circulation.* 2011;124:17–23.
3. Diehm C, Schuster A, Allenberg JR, et al. High prevalence of peripheral arterial disease and co-morbidity in 6880 primary care patients: cross-sectional study. *Atherosclerosis.* 2004;172:95–105.
4. Hirsch AT, Criqui MH, Treat-Jacobson D, et al. Peripheral arterial disease detection, awareness, and treatment in primary care. *JAMA.* 2001;286:1317–1324.
5. Grondal N, Sogaard R, Lindholt JS. Baseline prevalence of abdominal aortic aneurysm, peripheral arterial disease and hypertension in men aged 65-74 years from a population screening study (VIVA trial). *Br J Surg.* 2015;102:902–906.
6. McDermott MM. Lower extremity manifestations of peripheral artery disease: the pathophysiologic and functional implications of leg ischemia. *Circ Res.* 2015;116:1540–1550.
7. Rose GA. The diagnosis of ischaemic heart pain and intermittent claudication infield surveys. *Bull World Health Organ.* 1962;27: 645–658.
8. Gerhard-Herman MD, Gornik HL, Barrett C, et al. 2016 AHA/ACC guideline on the management of patients with lower extremity peripheral artery disease: a report of the American College of Cardiology/American Heart Association Task Force on Clinical Practice Guidelines. *Circulation.* 2017;135:e726–e779.
9. Regensteiner JG, Steiner JF, Panzer RJ, Hiatt WR. Evaluation of walking impairment by questionnaire in patients with peripheral arterial disease. *J Vasc Med Biol.* 1990;2:142–152.
10. McDermott MM, Ferrucci L, Guralnik JM, et al. The ankle-brachial index is associated with the magnitude of impaired walking endurance among men and women with peripheral arterial disease. *Vasc Med.* 2010;15:251–257.

11. Olin JW, Froehlich J, Gu X, et al. The United States Registry for Fibromuscular Dysplasia: results in the first 447 patients. *Circulation*. 2012;125:3182–3190.

12. Norgren L, Hiatt WR, Dormandy JA, et al. Inter-Society Consensus for the Management of Peripheral Arterial Disease (TASC II). *J Vasc Surg*. 2007;45:S5–67. Suppl S.

13. Epidemiology of lower extremity amputation in centres in Europe, North America and East Asia. The Global Lower Extremity Amputation Study Group. *Br J Surg*. 2000;87:328–337.

14. Sigvant B, Wiberg-Hedman K, Bergqvist D, et al. A population-based study of peripheral arterial disease prevalence with special focus on critical limb ischemia and sex differences. *J Vasc Surg*. 2007;45:1185–1189.

15. Jude EB, Oyibo SO, Chalmers N, Boulton AJ. Peripheral arterial disease in diabetic and nondiabetic patients: a comparison of severity and outcome. *Diabetes Care*. 2001;24:1433–1437.

16. Jonason T, Bergstrom R. Cessation of smoking in patients with intermittent claudication. Effects on the risk of peripheral vascular complications, myocardial infarction and mortality. *Acta Med Scand*. 1987;221:253–260.

17. Fowkes FG, Murray GD, Butcher I, et al. Ankle brachial index combined with Framingham Risk Score to predict cardiovascular events and mortality: a meta-analysis. *JAMA*. 2008;300:197–208.

18. Khan NA, Rahim SA, Anand SS, et al. Does the clinical examination predict lower extremity peripheral arterial disease? *JAMA*. 2006;295:536–546.

19. Aboyans V, Criqui MH, Abraham P, et al. Measurement and interpretation of the ankle-brachial index: a scientific statement from the American Heart Association. *Circulation*. 2012;126:2890–2909.

20. Rocha-Singh KJ, Zeller T, Jaff MR. Peripheral arterial calcification: prevalence, mechanism, detection, and clinical implications. *Catheter Cardiovasc Interv*. 2014;83:E212–E220.

21. Hiatt WR, Rogers RK, Brass EP. The treadmill is a better functional test than the 6-minute walk test in therapeutic trials of patients with peripheral artery disease. *Circulation*. 2014;130:69–78.

22. Hiatt WR, Hirsch AT, Regensteiner JG, et al. Clinical trials for claudication. Assessment of exercise performance, functional status, and clinical end points. Vascular Clinical Trialists. *Circulation*. 1995;92:614–621.

23. Collins R, Burch J, Cranny G, et al. Duplex ultrasonography, magnetic resonance angiography, and computed tomography angiography for diagnosis and assessment of symptomatic, lower limb peripheral arterial disease: systematic review. *BMJ*. 2007;334:1257–1261.

24. de Vries SO, Hunink MG, Polak JF. Summary receiver operating characteristic curves as a technique for meta-analysis of the diagnostic performance of duplex ultrasonography in peripheral arterial disease. *Acad Radiol*. 1996;3:361–369.

25. Gibson KD, Caps MT, Gillen D, et al. Identification of factors predictive of lower extremity vein graft thrombosis. *J Vasc Surg*. 2001;33:24–31.

26. Rehfuss J, Scali S, He Y, et al. The correlation between computed tomography and duplex evaluation of autogenous vein bypass grafts and their relationship to failure. *J Vasc Surg*. 2015;62:1546–1554.

27. Dabrh AMA, Mohammed K, Wigdan Farah W, et al. Systematic review and meta-analysis of duplex ultrasound surveillance for infrainguinal vein bypass grafts. *J Vasc Surg*. 2017;66:1885–1891.

28. Brumberg RS, Back MR, Armstrong PA, et al. The relative importance of graft surveillance and warfarin therapy in infrainguinal prosthetic bypass failure. *J Vasc Surg*. 2007;46:1160–1166.

29. Sobieszczyk P, Eisenhauer A. Management of patients after endovascular interventions for peripheral artery disease. *Circulation*. 2013;128:749–757.

30. Pollak AW, Norton PT, Kramer CM. Multimodality imaging of lower extremity peripheral arterial disease: current role and future directions. *Circ Cardiovasc Imaging*. 2012;5:797–807.

31. Nelemans PJ, Leiner T, de Vet HC, et al. Peripheral arterial disease: meta-analysis of the diagnostic performance of MR angiography. *Radiology*. 2000;217:105–114.

32. Menke J, Larsen J. Meta-analysis: accuracy of contrast-enhanced magnetic resonance angiography for assessing steno-occlusions in peripheral arterial disease. *Ann Intern Med*. 2010;153:325–334.

33. Heijenbrok-Kal MH, Kock MC, Hunink MG. Lower extremity arterial disease: multidetector CT angiography meta-analysis. *Radiology*. 2007;245:433–439.

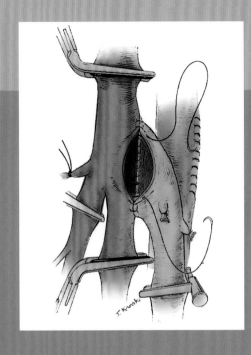

中文导读

第19章
外周动脉疾病的内科治疗

外周动脉疾病患者内科治疗目的如下。

防止心脑血管和肢体的不良事件，主要包括：①戒烟：需给患者切实的戒烟建议和措施安排；②血压控制：最新的指南要求控制目标值<130/80 mmHg，血管紧张素转化酶抑制剂和血管紧张素受体阻断剂（ARBs）是外周动脉疾病患者控制血压的一线药物；③降糖：降糖是外周动脉疾病患者内科治疗的核心，二甲双胍是口服降糖的一线药物，钠-葡萄糖协同转运蛋白2（SGLT2）抑制剂和胰高糖素样肽1（GLP-1）拮抗剂等新型降糖药物则具有降糖和减少微血管并发症的双重功效；④抗感染治疗：现有应用卡那单抗进行抗感染治疗的研究证据尚不充分；⑤降脂：降脂治疗的重点是尽可能多地降低低密度脂蛋白，可使用他汀、Ezetimibe或PCSK9抑制剂；⑥抗栓治疗：采用单抗血小板治疗还是更高强度的联合用药方案取决于对外周动脉疾病、心脑血管事件的获益及出血风险的评估。

改善外周动脉疾病症状与肢体功能，包括：①锻炼疗法：有监督的行走锻炼是间歇性跛行患者的初始治疗手段；②药物治疗：他汀类药物应用于所有外周动脉疾病患者，西洛他唑也是指南推荐的治疗间歇性跛行的药物；③其他疗法：包括血管扩张剂、代谢类药物、细胞疗法和血管生长因子等仍在研究中。

包俊敏

Medical Treatment of Peripheral Artery Disease

Marc P. Bonaca and Mark A. Creager

Medical treatment of patients with peripheral artery disease (PAD) is targeted at preventing adverse cardiovascular and limb outcomes and improving limb function. Atherothrombotic complications such as myocardial infarction (MI), ischemic stroke, and cardiovascular death are referred to as major adverse cardiovascular events (MACE), with risk related to the systemic nature of atherosclerosis (see Chapter 16). In addition, patients with PAD are at risk of major adverse limb events (MALE), including acute limb ischemia (ALI), chronic critical limb ischemia (CLI), and ischemic amputation (Fig. 19.1).[1,2]

Although all patients with PAD are at heightened risk of both MACE and MALE, there is growing appreciation of the heterogeneity of risk within the broad population of patients with PAD.[3-5] Risk is related to the presence of concomitant symptomatic disease in other vascular beds (polyvascular disease), especially coronary artery disease (CAD), and also to the severity of disease in the limbs.[5-8] The risk of MACE in patients with PAD is 60% to 80% greater than that in patients with history of MI or stroke without symptomatic PAD; however, the greatest risk is in those who have both symptomatic PAD and symptomatic CAD exceeding that of symptomatic PAD or CAD alone (Fig. 19.2).[6,9,10] The risk of MALE is highest in those with prior peripheral revascularization, followed by those with symptomatic PAD but no history of peripheral revascularization, and with relatively low risk in those without symptoms but with an ankle-brachial index (ABI) less than 0.9 (Table 19.1 and Fig. 19.3).[3,11-14] The therapeutic approach to patients with PAD therefore depends on the severity of symptoms and manifestation of disease in the lower extremities, the presence of concomitant symptomatic disease in other vascular territories, and the presence of comorbid disease such as diabetes. Preventive measures such as diet, smoking cessation, blood pressure control, and lipid optimization apply to all patients (Fig. 19.4). Targeted therapies such as those for glucose lowering apply only to those with specific risk factors such as diabetes. The intensity of antithrombotic therapy must be balanced against the associated risk of bleeding, when considered for those with the highest risk of MACE (e.g., those with polyvascular disease) or MALE (e.g., those with prior peripheral revascularization). Similarly, although intensive low-density lipoprotein cholesterol (LDL-C) lowering may have the same relative benefits for all patients with PAD, expensive therapies with limited availability may first be considered in those patients at the highest absolute risk, who are likely to derive the greatest absolute risk reductions.

This chapter reviews the evidence to support medical treatments to reduce the risk of MACE and MALE in patients with PAD, and the physical and medical therapies used to improve functional capacity in patients with intermittent claudication. Investigational therapies are briefly discussed. Catheter-based revascularization for PAD is reviewed in Chapter 20, and surgical revascularization for PAD is reviewed in Chapter 21. Multisocietal consensus guidelines for management of the patient with PAD are available and helpful for guiding clinical practice.[2,4]

INTERVENTIONS TO REDUCE CARDIOVASCULAR RISK AND ADVERSE LIMB EVENTS

Prevention guidelines recommend lifestyle modification, such as a heart-healthy diet, regular exercise habits, and maintenance of a healthy weight.[15,16] Specific diet recommendations include Mediterranean diets and the DASH (Dietary Approaches to Stop Hypertension) diet.[15] PAD guidelines advocate for interdisciplinary care, including nutritionists/dieticians.[2] Lifestyle modifications should be recommended for all patients with PAD regardless of the severity of disease or comorbidities. These interventions have little risk and low cost and have the potential to reduce risk of MACE, improve limb function, and improve quality of life.

Smoking Cessation

Tobacco smoking is associated strongly with the development and progression of PAD, and the risk of PAD among smokers is as high as threefold that of nonsmokers (see Chapter 16). Smoking cessation is a critical component of risk factor modification for patients with PAD.[2]

Smoking cessation has salutary effects on claudication symptoms, exercise physiology, and limb-related outcomes in patients with symptomatic PAD.[1,2,17] Patients with intermittent claudication who quit smoking have longer pain-free walking times and maximal walking times compared with patients who continue to smoke. Smoking cessation is also associated with improved clinical outcomes in patients with PAD. Continued smoking in patients with claudication is associated with higher rates of CLI, need for peripheral revascularization, and MACE. Similarly, in patients undergoing bypass surgery, continued smoking is associated with lower patency rates both for venous and prosthetic grafts. Ongoing smoking is also associated with development of MI and a trend toward decreased overall survival at 10 years of follow-up. In the Spanish Factores de Riesgo y ENfermedad Arterial (FRENA) Registry, patients with vascular disease (467 of the 1182 smokers had PAD) who stopped smoking had lower mortality over a mean of 14 months follow-up.[18]

Despite the multiple benefits of smoking cessation in patients with PAD, it is an extremely difficult goal to accomplish and initial success rates are low. The efficacy of physician advice in achieving smoking cessation is less than 5%.[2] The effectiveness of smoking cessation interventions in patients with PAD was evaluated in a randomized trial of 124 patients with PAD who were currently smoking.[19] Patients randomized to a PAD-specific tailored counseling program had higher rates of abstinence at 6 months compared with those receiving minimal

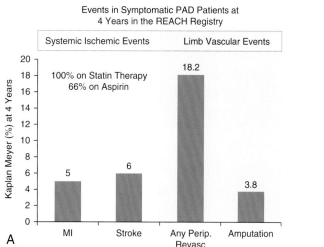

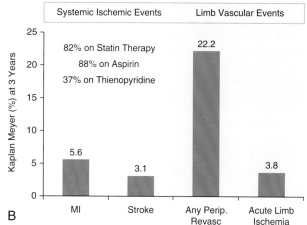

Fig. 19.1 Outcomes in patients with symptomatic peripheral artery disease at 4 years in the REACH registry (A) and the TRA2P-TIMI 50 trial (B). (From Bonaca MP, Creager MA. Pharmacological treatment and current management of peripheral artery disease. *Circ Res.* 2015;116:1579–1598.)

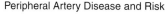

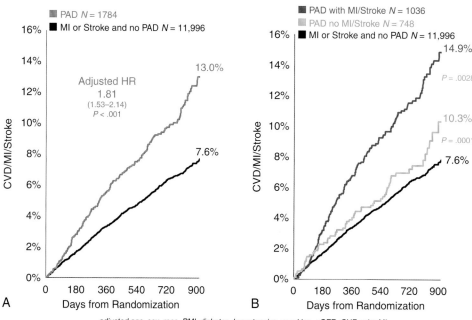

Fig. 19.2 Outcomes in patients with symptomatic peripheral artery disease *(PAD)* randomized to placebo in the FOURIER trial and followed for 2.5 years. All patients with PAD are shown in orange (A) and then stratified by PAD only *(yellow)* or PAD with prior myocardial infarction *(MI)* and/or prior stroke *(red,* B). *BMI,* Body mass index; *CABG/PCI,* coronary artery bypass grafting/percutaneous coronary intervention; *CHF,* congestive heart failure; *CVD,* cardiovascular death; *eGFR,* estimated glomerular filtration rate; *HR,* hazard ratio; *TIA,* transient ischemic attack. (Data from Bonaca MP, Nault P, Giugliano RP, et al. Low-density lipoprotein cholesterol lowering with evolocumab and outcomes in patients with peripheral artery disease: insights from the FOURIER trial [Further Cardiovascular Outcomes Research with PCSK9 Inhibition in Subjects with Elevated Risk]. *Circulation.* 2018;137:338–350.)

intervention (21.3% vs. 6.8%). Although the intervention was successful, almost 80% were no longer abstinent at 6 months, underscoring the need for more effective interventions.

Smoking cessation programs are more successful when coupled with pharmacologic therapy, including both nicotine and nonnicotine agents. The antidepressant bupropion has been demonstrated to

improve tobacco abstinence rates at 12 months relative to placebo when used alone or in combination with the nicotine patch.[2] Varenicline, a partial agonist of the nicotinic acetylcholine receptor (nAchR) α4β, improves tobacco abstinence rates among subjects with or without cardiovascular disease, including patients with PAD.[20] Among those with cardiovascular disease, varenicline is associated with a threefold

TABLE 19.1	Independent Predictors of Acute Limb Ischemia in Peripheral Artery Disease Trials[12–14]		
	TRA2P-TIMI 50	PEGASUS-TIMI 54 PAD	EUCLID
Prior peripheral revascularization	HR 3.60 (2.10–6.18) $P < .001$	HR 3.76 (2.26–6.25) $P < .001$	HR 4.23 (2.86–6.25) $P < .001$
ABI ≤0.50	HR 2.86 (1.81–4.51)		
ABI ≥1.30	HR 2.71 (1.09–6.72)		
Current smoking	HR 2.17 (1.01–4.67) $P = .046$		

ABI, Ankle-brachial index; *HR,* hazard ratio.

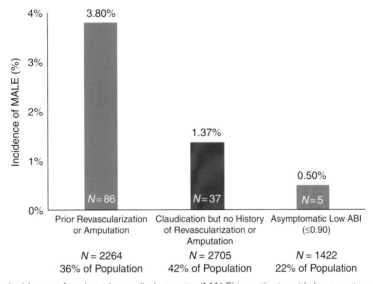

Fig. 19.3 The incidence of major adverse limb events *(MALE)* in patients with lower extremity peripheral artery disease randomized in the COMPASS trial and stratified by peripheral artery disease history. *ABI,* Ankle-brachial index. (From Bonaca MP, Creager MA. Antithrombotic therapy and major adverse limb events in peripheral artery disease: a step forward. *J Am Coll Cardiol.* 2018;71:2316–2318.)

likelihood of abstinence at 1-year follow-up compared with placebo, although the absolute abstinence rate is only approximately 20%. Side effects of varenicline include sleep abnormalities, nausea, and flatulence. Both varenicline and bupropion are associated with an increased risk of neuropsychiatric side effects. Package labeling for both agents includes a black box warning recommending observation for changes in behavior or mood or development of suicidal ideation while receiving these agents for smoking cessation treatment.

Recommendations

Smoking cessation advice and encouragement of cessation efforts should be key components of each office visit. Although time intensive, achievement of smoking cessation is one of the most powerful interventions to reduce risk in patients with PAD. Evaluation using the "5 A" algorithm (Ask, Advise, Assess, Assist, and Arrange) may be useful.[21] For patients motivated to quit smoking, treatment with nicotine replacement therapy, bupropion, or varenicline should be considered. These efforts may be incorporated into a formal smoking cessation program that includes longitudinal counseling on an individual basis or in a small group.

Blood Pressure Lowering

Optimizing blood pressure reduces cardiovascular risk, including stroke, MI, and congestive heart failure. A number of therapies are effective at reducing blood pressure, and large randomized trials have demonstrated the benefits of pharmacotherapy on outcomes, including mortality.[22] The SPRINT trial demonstrated greater risk reduction with more intensive blood pressure lowering.[23] The current American Heart Association/American College of Cardiology (AHA/ACC) blood pressure–lowering guidelines recommend treating patients with established cardiovascular disease, including patients with PAD, to a target of <130/80 mm Hg.[22] There are few studies of blood pressure lowering in patients with PAD and which focus either on specific drugs or optimal targets.[2] No specific antihypertensive agent or class has been shown to improve limb vascular outcomes or symptoms of claudication, nor is convincing evidence for harm, specifically with β-blocker therapy. The Appropriate Blood Pressure Control in Diabetes (ABCD) study enrolled 950 patients, with 53 having symptomatic PAD. Patients were randomized to treatment with enalapril or nisoldipine (intensive treatment) or placebo (moderate control) and followed for 5 years.[1] Although the number of events was modest, there appeared to be a

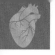

| Asymptomatic Low ABI Without Symptomatic Vascular Disease | Symptomatic PAD or Asymptomatic Low ABI With Concomitant Symptomatic Vascular Disease |

Prevention of Progression to Symptomatic Disease

Reduction of MACE Risk
- Risk high in patients with symptomatic PAD
- Risk highest in patients with polyvascular disease, particularly concomitant coronary disease

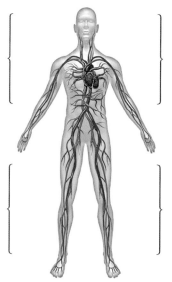

Prevention of Progression to Symptomatic Disease

Reduction in MALE Risk
- Risk highest in patients with prior peripheral revascularization

Functional Improvement
- Symptoms most evident in patients with typical claudication
- Most patients with low ABI have some degree of functional impairment

Fig. 19.4 Markers of risk and goals of prevention in patients with peripheral artery disease *(PAD)* diagnosed by ankle-brachial index *(ABI)* and symptoms. *MACE,* Major adverse cardiovascular events; *MALE,* major adverse limb events.

significant reduction in risk reduction in MACE in those with PAD who received intensive treatment (achieving a mean of 128/75 mm Hg).[24] Benefits appeared to be greater in patients with more severe disease as measured by ABI. These observations were further supported by the International Verapamil-SR/Trandolapril study.[25] In a post hoc subgroup analysis of patients with PAD, treatment to a target <130/80 mm Hg reduced the risk of MACE. Although a J-shaped relationship was seen overall, this was not seen in the PAD subgroup.[25]

There are few trials comparing classes of agents for blood pressure lowering in patients with PAD. Several studies evaluating the benefits of angiotensin-converting enzyme inhibitors (ACEIs) and angiotensin receptor blockers (ARBs) have reported consistent benefits in subgroups of patients with PAD. The Heart Outcomes Prevention Evaluation (HOPE) trial randomized patients with vascular disease or diabetes to ramipril 10 mg daily or placebo and followed them for 5 years.[26] The trial showed a 22% reduction in MACE with ramipril with consistent benefits for components of the MACE end point. The HOPE trial included 4051 patients with PAD (44% of the overall trial), and benefits in this subgroup were similar to those observed in the overall trial. Of note is that the reductions in adverse outcomes were observed even though there was only a modest blood pressure–lowering effect overall (5 mm Hg at 1 month, 3 mm Hg at study completion).[26] Similar benefits were observed in the EUROPA trial, which randomized 12,218 patients to the ACEI, perindopril, or placebo and observed a 20% reduction in MACE with consistent benefits in the subgroup of patients with PAD.[27] These observations were extended to ARBs in the ON TARGET trial, which randomized more than 25,000 patients to telmisartan, ramipril, or the combination of both.[28] Overall, telmisartan and ramipril showed similar efficacy with consistent findings in the approximately 3000 patients with PAD, supporting the use of ACEI or ARB therapy in this population.[24]

The use of β-blockade may be indicated in patients with PAD in the comorbid setting of atrial fibrillation or CAD or as an additional class of drugs when multiagent therapy is needed for blood pressure lowering. Although there have been theoretic concerns about risk in patients with PAD stemming from reductions in cardiac output or resulting unopposed α-agonism potentially leading to adverse limb outcomes, these risks have not been observed in studies or meta-analyses; however, the number of patients included in these studies is small, and there are no large prospective trials of β-blockade in PAD patients evaluating limb outcomes.[2,29,30] One study evaluated 177 patients with Fontaine stage II claudication who were randomized to nebivolol or hydrochlorothiazide for 24 weeks. Both therapies appeared to be well tolerated with no difference in adverse effects between agents.[31]

Recommendations

Blood pressure control is an important component of cardiovascular risk reduction in all patients, including those with PAD. Recent AHA/ACC guidelines recommend treating to a target of <130/80 mm Hg. It is reasonable to measure blood pressure in both upper extremities to exclude the possibility of occult subclavian stenosis leading to inaccurate blood pressure assessment in one of the arms. Although limited data exist comparing specific agents, the benefits of ACEI and ARB therapy have been shown, and these agents should be considered first line antihypertensive therapy in patients with PAD. In patients with another indication for β-blocker therapy, it can be safely used without an excess in limb risk.

Glucose-Lowering Therapies in Patients with Diabetes

Robust observational datasets show a clear association between diabetes mellitus and PAD, with associated risks of PAD 2 to 4 times that of patients without diabetes (see Chapter 16). Diabetes mellitus is associated with heightened risk of microvascular, as well as macrovascular complications.[32] Elevated glucose is associated with lower patency rates after peripheral vascular intervention and higher risk of amputation.[33] Independent risk factors for amputation include poor vision, neuropathy, and ABI ≤0.5, suggesting both microvascular and macrovascular etiologies to limb loss in this complex population.[34] Tissue loss in the setting of chronic CLI may have a particularly complex pathobiology, with significant contributions of ischemia, microvascular disease, and infection.[35] Therapies to lower glucose have shown consistent benefit for reduction of microvascular complications but mixed effects on macrovascular outcomes. For the latter, the specific mechanism of the therapy may be more important than the effect of the therapy on glucose levels.

Treating to Lower Glycemic Targets

The Action to Control Cardiovascular Risk in Diabetes (ACCORD) trial investigated whether more intensive glucose-lowering control to achieve a lower glycated hemoglobin would reduce outcomes in patients with cardiovascular disease (35% with PAD) or risk factors. Patients in the intensive therapy arm achieved a glycated hemoglobin of 6.4% versus 7.5% in those randomized to standard therapy and at 3.5 years had higher rates of cardiovascular and all-cause mortality.[2,36] The ADVANCE trial similarly showed no benefit among patients randomized to achieve a lower glycated hemoglobin target (6.5% vs. 7.3%) at 5 years of follow-up but did not show an excess in mortality. A third trial of more intensive glucose lowering in veterans, with a median follow-up of 5.6 years, also showed no benefit.[37]

The Look AHEAD trial investigated whether intensive lifestyle intervention targeted at lowering glucose would be beneficial.[38] Of the 5145 patients randomized, 714 had established cardiovascular disease. At 10 years the intensive intervention led to weight loss, improved fitness, and lower glycated hemoglobin; however, these benefits did not translate into lower rates of MACE. There was statistical heterogeneity with a trend toward benefit in those without established cardiovascular disease and a trend toward harm in those with cardiovascular disease.[38]

Although data for the macrovascular benefits of glucose lowering are mixed, there are some data to suggest that benefits may emerge only over longer periods of time than that included in most clinical trial observation periods. For example, the United Kingdom Prospective Diabetes Study (UKPDS) randomized patients with newly diagnosed type II diabetes mellitus to either dietary restriction only or intensive medical therapy (with sulfonylurea, insulin, or metformin). At 5 years of follow-up, there were reductions in microvascular complications with intensive medical therapy relative to diet; however, there was no benefit for MACE. At 10 years a benefit for MACE became evident with a 15% relative risk reduction for MI and a 6% relative risk reduction in mortality.[1,39] Taken together these studies suggest that macrovascular benefits attributable to glucose lowering may be present over long periods of time, largely in patients without evident cardiovascular disease.

Class Specific Glucose-Lowering Therapies

Several trials have investigated the effects of class glucose-lowering agents both for safety and efficacy in high-risk populations. Two large trials have evaluated dipeptidyl peptidase 4 (DPP-4) inhibitors in patients with diabetes at high risk for cardiovascular events. Neither agent (saxagliptin or alogliptin) reduced MACE risk over relatively short follow-up, but both had some microvascular benefits in the setting of modest glucose lowering and appeared safe.[40,41] The Prospective Pioglitazone Clinical Trial in Macrovascular Events (PROactive) trial randomized patients to the peroxisome proliferator–activated receptor gamma (PPAR-γ) agonist, pioglitazone, or placebo. Patients with established vascular disease, including 1043 with symptomatic PAD, were included. Over a mean follow-up of 34.5 months, there was no benefit for a broad macrovascular composite of MACE, revascularization, or amputation; however, there was a reduction in the key secondary end point of MACE, which included MI, stroke, and cardiovascular death.[42] These data suggest that PPAR-γ may be a target that reduces cardiovascular risk in patients with diabetes and vascular disease.

Three agents targeting the sodium glucose cotransporter 2 (SGLT2) are currently available. Two have completed large outcomes trials, and a third trial of a third in this class is in progress. This class of drugs reduces plasma glucose by inducing glucosuria, with associated reductions in body weight and blood pressure and increased risk of urinary tract infections. The EMPA-REG trial enrolled approximately 7000 patients with diabetes mellitus and stable cardiovascular disease and randomized them to empagliflozin or matching placebo. The trial was designed to evaluate cardiovascular safety and was not powered for superiority; nonetheless, at the conclusion, empagliflozin significantly reduced the MACE composite of cardiovascular death, MI, or stroke by 14%.[43] In addition to significant reductions in mortality and ischemic events, there was a reduction in hospitalizations for heart failure.[43] Benefits observed were robust, leading to regulatory approval for cardiovascular risk reduction in patients with diabetes and vascular disease; however, the mechanism of benefit has not been clearly defined and is out of proportion to what would be expected based on glucose or blood pressure lowering alone. In addition to the macrovascular benefits, there were also improvements in renal outcomes.[44]

The outcomes in EMPA-REG were evaluated in the subgroup of approximately 1400 patients with PAD at baseline. A consistent benefit was observed for MACE, with a significant 43% reduction in cardiovascular mortality and 38% reduction in all-cause mortality. There was no differential in the safety profile of empaglifozin among patients with PAD, including no increased risk of lower extremity amputation.[45,46]

The CANVAS program evaluated the safety and efficacy of the SGLT2 inhibitor canagliflozin in a population of patients with either established cardiovascular disease or risk factors.[47] Consistent with EMPA-REG, canagliflozin reduced MACE overall; however, the results were most notable in patients with established cardiovascular disease. CANVAS also showed similar benefits for the composite of cardiovascular death and heart failure, with consistent risk reductions in those with and without established cardiovascular disease.[47] Observational analyses have also supported a class effect for cardiovascular benefit.[48] The results of CANVAS confirmed the benefits observed in EMPA-REG and reinforced the notion that SGLT2 inhibition is an important mechanism for risk reduction in patients with diabetes. However, there was an approximately twofold excess in the risk of lower extremity amputation with canagliflozin compared with placebo.[47,49] The risk was consistent for major and minor amputations in patients with or without PAD, but with the greatest absolute excess in patients with PAD, and particularly those with prior amputation. These findings, which also have been seen in observational analyses, led to a black box warning by the US Food and Drug Administration (FDA) for amputation.[35,49,50]

A third SGLT2 inhibitor, dapagliflozin, is available for treating patients with diabetes. A large outcomes trial, DECLARE-TIMI 58, is currently evaluating the efficacy and safety of dapagliflozin in high-risk patients with established cardiovascular disease or risk factors.[51,52] The study is powered for ischemic efficacy and will include well-characterized limb outcomes. Results are anticipated in late 2018.[52]

Another target specific class of diabetes therapy are the glucagon-like peptide-1 (GLP-1) agonists. These, delivered parenterally by injection, induce weight loss and lower glucose levels. In two large outcomes trials, GLP-1 agonists have shown significant reductions in ischemic risk, largely in patients with established cardiovascular disease.[53,54] GLP-1 agonists appear to have primary benefit in ischemic risk reduction, but there have been no signals for limb benefits or adverse limb events.

Recommendations

Diabetes mellitus is a risk factor for PAD and a common comorbid condition. Patients with diabetes and PAD are at high risk of MACE, microvascular complications, and complex limb events that are highly morbid. Glucose lowering remains a core aspect of medical management, with the primary goal of reducing microvascular complications with targets as outlined by professional society guidelines, with metformin being first line oral therapy.[2] SGLT2 inhibitors reduce MACE; however, signals for amputation raise concerns for canagliflozin, particularly in PAD patients; this is not the case for empagliflozin. The mechanisms of benefit and harm with this class of glucose-lowering drugs are unclear. The GLP-1 agonists reduce ischemic risk. Because the benefits of SGLT2 inhibitors and GLP-1 agonists appear independent of their glucose-lowering effects, they should be considered in appropriate patients for macrovascular risk reduction. In patients on insulin or secretagogue therapy, addition of drugs from other classes may necessitate reductions in the intensity of therapy to avoid hypoglycemia.

Antiinflammatory Therapy

A growing body of evidence supports a causal role for inflammation in the pathogenesis of atherothrombosis. The recently completed Cardiovascular Risk Reduction Study (Reduction in Recurrent Major CV Disease Events) (CANTOS) trial evaluated the efficacy and safety of antiinflammatory therapy in patients with vascular disease. CANTOS randomized approximately 10,000 patients with prior MI and a high sensitivity C-reactive protein greater than 2 mg/dL to canakinumab, a monoclonal antibody targeting interleukin-1β (IL-1β) or placebo, and followed them for 48 months. Treatment with canakinumab reduced the risk of MACE by 17%, with broader benefits for reducing cancer deaths. However, there was an increased risk of fatal infections. MACE and MALE outcomes in the subgroup with PAD have not been reported. The CANTOS trial establishes the importance of inflammatory risk in atherothrombosis and the potential benefit of targeting IL-1β. Additional studies will be necessary to define the role of antiinflammatory therapies in patients with PAD.

Recommendations

Currently there is no established role for antiinflammatory therapy with canakinumab in patients with PAD. Future trials of therapies targeting inflammation are needed to establish the role of these therapies in patients with vascular disease.

Lipid-Lowering Therapy

Dyslipidemia is associated with adverse cardiovascular risk in epidemiologic studies. LDL-C has shown the strongest association and is considered a true risk factor for adverse outcomes. Therapies to reduce LDL-C have shown benefit particularly in patients with established vascular disease. Although high-density lipoprotein cholesterol (HDL-C) and triglycerides have also been associated with outcomes, therapies to modify these factors have not shown robust benefits for risk reduction. The body of data supporting the use of LDL-C–lowering therapies and targets for LDL-C are largely derived from large datasets evaluating broad populations with established vascular disease. Several of these studies include large PAD subgroups showing consistency of benefit.

Lowering Low-Density Lipoprotein Cholesterol for Reducing Major Adverse Cardiovascular Events

The Scandinavian Simvastatin Survival Study (4S) randomized patients with CAD and high cholesterol to an HMG-CoA reductase inhibitor, simvastatin, or placebo.[55] The use of simvastatin resulted in a survival benefit. In addition to broad benefits for MACE and mortality, a secondary analysis described reductions in claudication. The Heart Protection Study (HPS) randomized 20,536 patients with stable vascular disease to simvastatin or placebo, including a large subgroup of patients with PAD.[56] Overall, simvastatin reduced major vascular events by 24%, including an 18% reduction in all-cause mortality, with consistent benefits in patients with PAD.[1,2] This benefit extended to patients with PAD and no history of MI or other evident coronary heart disease.

Whether the benefits observed with statin therapy in patients with vascular disease are specific to statins per se or driven by LDL-C lowering remained unknown until the Examining Outcomes in Subjects With Acute Coronary Syndrome: Vytorin (Ezetimibe/Simvastatin) vs. Simvastatin (IMPROVE-IT) trial demonstrated benefit with addition of nonstatin therapy, ezetimibe, which inhibits cholesterol absorption from the intestine.[57] IMPROVE-IT randomized approximately 18,000 patients with acute coronary syndrome (ACS), including approximately 1000 with PAD, to ezetimibe or placebo. All patients received a high- or moderate-intensity statin, with a median LDL-C in the placebo group of 69.5 mg/dL and a reduction of approximately 14 mg/dL in the intervention arm to a median LDL-C of 53.7 mg/dL.[57] This reduction translated into an approximately 6% relative risk reduction (2% absolute risk reduction) in the primary MACE composite at 7 years of follow-up. Risk in patients with ACS and concomitant PAD was higher than in those with ACS and without PAD, and translated into greater absolute risk reductions.[7]

Recently, inhibitors of proprotein convertase subtilisin kexin type 9 (PCSK9), a protein which chaperones the LDL receptor on the liver to its destruction, thereby reducing update and increasing LDL-C levels, have been studied in clinical trials.[58–60] Two inhibitors to PCSK9, alirocumab and evolocumab, have shown benefit in large cardiovascular outcomes trials, with the latter showing benefits in a dedicated PAD subgroup.[58,60]

The Further Cardiovascular Outcomes Research With PCSK9 Inhibition in Subjects With Elevated Risk (FOURIER) trial studied evolocumab versus placebo on a background of statin therapy in a broad population of patients with stable atherosclerotic vascular disease, including 3642 with symptomatic lower extremity PAD.[58] Overall patients had approximately 60% reduction in LDL-C, from 92 mg/dL to 30 mg/dL, and a 15% reduction in MACE over a relatively short follow-up with a median of 2.2 years.[58] Subsequent analysis demonstrated that the benefits were present regardless of baseline LDL-C.[61] There were no adverse effects observed with evolocumab beyond injection site reactions and no adverse neurocognitive outcomes, even in those patients achieving single digit LDL-C.[58] The Evaluation of Cardiovascular Outcomes After an Acute Coronary Syndrome During Treatment With Alirocumab (ODYSSEY Outcomes) trial studied patients with ACS showed a similar LDL-C reduction, and the magnitude of benefit was consistent with that seen in FOURIER; and there was an associated reduction in mortality.

A prespecified subgroup analysis from FOURIER evaluated the MACE and MALE efficacy and safety of evolocumab in the 3642 patients with lower extremity symptomatic PAD. Patients with PAD were higher risk than those with coronary disease or cerebrovascular disease without PAD. The efficacy of evolocumab was consistent in patients with PAD, but by nature of their higher risk, there was a more robust 3.5% absolute risk reduction and more favorable number needed to treat (NNT) of 29. As was seen in the HPS with statins, the benefit was present also in those with PAD and no prior MI or stroke, with an absolute risk reduction (ARR) of 4.8% and NNT of 21. MALE were reduced by 42%, and when combined in patients with PAD and no prior MI

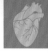

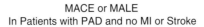

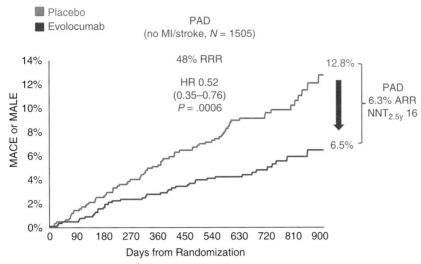

Fig. 19.5 The incidence of the composite of major adverse cardiovascular events *(MACE)* or major adverse limb events *(MALE)* in patients with peripheral artery disease *(PAD)* randomized to placebo *(blue)* or evolocumab *(red)* in the FOURIER trial. Relative risk reduction *(RRR)*, absolute risk reduction *(ARR)*, and hazard ratio *(HR)* are shown. *NNT*, Number needed to treat. (Reproduced with permission from Bonaca MP, Nault P, Giugliano RP, et al. Low-density lipoprotein cholesterol lowering with evolocumab and outcomes in patients with peripheral artery disease: insights from the FOURIER Trial [Further Cardiovascular Outcomes Research with PCSK9 Inhibition in Subjects with Elevated Risk]. *Circulation.* 2018;137:338–350.)

or stroke, there was an ARR and NNT for the composite of MACE or MALE of 6.3% at 2.5 years and 16, respectively (Fig. 19.5).

Other Lipid Targets and Outcomes

Epidemiologic studies observe an association between HDL-C and reduced cardiovascular risk. Strategies to increase HDL include the addition of niacin, as well as the use of cholesterol ester transfer protein (CETP) inhibitors. In the AIM-HIGH trial, the addition of niacin to patients with low HDL-C receiving statins was not beneficial in spite of raising HDL and lowering triglycerides.[62] The CETP inhibitor anacetrapib reduced risk in patients with vascular disease when added to statin therapy; however, the magnitude of benefit was attributable to the degree of LDL-C lowering and not to the 138% increase in HDL-C. This agent will not be commercialized and is not available for patients. The use of fibrates in selected populations has not shown convincing benefit when added to statin therapy. Bezafibrate did not reduce MACE.[17] The Fenofibrate Intervention and Event Lowering in Diabetes (FIELD) study was a randomized study of fenofibrate or placebo in patients with diabetes. Fenofibrate similarly did not reduce the composite of MACE but did decrease secondary end points such as nonfatal MI and coronary and peripheral revascularization.[17]

Lowering Low-Density Lipoprotein Cholesterol for Reducing Major Adverse Limb Events

Overall there are few studies that evaluated the effects of lipid lowering on limb vascular events. 4S reported a reduction in claudication with simvastatin,[55] and in HPS there was a 16% reduction in peripheral vascular events with simvastatin compared with placebo in patients with PAD, driven largely by a 20% relative risk reduction in noncoronary revascularizations.[56] Effects on this outcome were independent of baseline LDL-C.

In the REACH Registry, of 5861 patients with symptomatic PAD, 62.2% were using statin therapy at baseline. After adjustment for differences, statin therapy was associated with an 18% reduction in the composite of worsening claudication or CLI, as well as a 17% reduction in peripheral revascularization procedures. In addition, there was an as-

sociated 56% reduction in amputation. Although the comparison was nonrandomized, the analyses were adjusted for potential confounders and were consistent through a series of sensitivity analyses.[63] Analyses from other large registries have observed an association between amputation rates and statin therapy; however, intensity of statin therapy or achieved LDL-C was not reported.[63–65] Observational studies in patients with CLI treated with statins have shown mixed results for the limb outcomes, with some showing neutral findings and others showing improved outcomes.[66–68]

Broader benefits of LDL-C lowering on limb outcomes have recently been shown in the PAD subgroup from the FOURIER trial.[6] A composite of MALE included ALI, major amputation, and urgent revascularization for ischemia. Lowering LDL-C with evolocumab reduced MALE by 42% in the overall population, with consistent benefits for all components of the MALE composite end point. In patients with PAD, evolocumab reduced the risk of MALE at 2.5 years by 57%, with an ARR of 1.3%.[6] Reduction in elective or total peripheral revascularization procedures was not observed; however, exposure was relatively short at 2.2 years, whereas outcomes in the HPS were after approximately twice that duration of exposure.

An analysis from FOURIER explored the benefit in MALE reduction by achieved LDL-C. Similar to that seen for MACE, there was ongoing benefit of LDL-C reduction extending to levels below 10 mg/dL (Fig. 19.6). These data along with those from 4S, HPS, and observational studies support the notion that LDL-C lowering reduces the risk of adverse limb vascular outcomes.

It is unknown whether HDL raising or fibrates impact limb outcomes. A single study has reported a 36% reduction in amputations with fenofibrate relative to placebo over 5 years in patients with diabetes and PAD, possibly through non–LDL-C–mediated mechanisms.[69] These observations require confirmation in prospective studies.

Lipid-Lowering Therapy Recommendations

Emerging data demonstrate that intensively lowering LDL-C improves outcomes in patients with PAD, with robust absolute risk

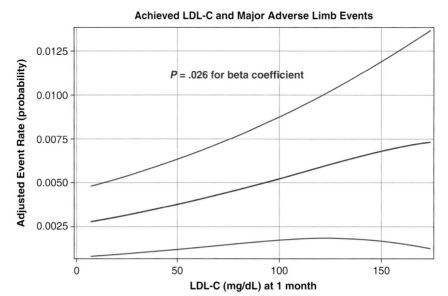

Fig. 19.6 The probability of major adverse limb event in patients randomized in the FOURIER trial by achieved low-density lipoprotein cholesterol *(LDL-C)* at month 1 in the FOURIER trial. Analyses adjusted for significant (*P* < .05) predictors of LDL-C at 1 month after randomization including age, body mass index, LDL-C at baseline, male sex, race, randomized in North America, current smoker, and high-intensity statin. (From Bonaca MP, Nault P, Giugliano RP, et al. Low-density lipoprotein cholesterol lowering with evolocumab and outcomes in patients with peripheral artery disease: insights from the FOURIER Trial [Further Cardiovascular Outcomes Research with PCSK9 Inhibition in Subjects with Elevated Risk]. *Circulation.* 2018;137:338–350.)

reductions. This, coupled with the excellent safety profile of LDL-C–lowering therapies, supports the notion to lower LDL-C as much as possible in patients with PAD with statins, ezetimibe, and PCSK9 inhibitors.

Antithrombotic Therapy

The rationale for antithrombotic therapy in patients with clinical manifestations of atherosclerosis is based on observations that acute cardiovascular events often are atherothrombotic in origin, with underlying lipid-rich plaque and inflammation leading to plaque rupture and then activation of platelets and the coagulation cascade. The acute thrombotic occlusion of the arterial blood supply then leads to downstream tissue injury, including spontaneous MI, ischemic stroke, and potentially ALI. In spite of this pathobiologic basis, outcome data for antithrombotic therapies in PAD show complex and inconsistent results, in part due to the populations studied, comorbid vascular disease, and differences in outcome definitions and antithrombotic drugs administered.

Antiplatelet Monotherapy

The Antithrombotic Trialists' (ATT) Collaboration meta-analyses have evaluated the use of antiplatelet therapy in patients across a spectrum of risk,[70,71] including more than 9000 patients with symptomatic PAD, defined as claudication or prior revascularization. Overall, there was a 23% reduction in MACE with antiplatelet therapy, which included aspirin at various doses, and other agents such as thienopyridines, dipyridamole, and picotamide (a thromboxane inhibitor).[70,71] There was an associated 60% excess in major extracranial (mostly gastrointestinal) bleeding. Taken broadly, the ATT meta-analysis provides evidence that antiplatelet therapy reduces ischemic risk in patients with symptomatic PAD, and it is most often translated as evidence for aspirin monotherapy. It should be noted that these meta-analyses did not include patients who were asymptomatic, and subsequent meta-analyses that have included broader populations of patients with PAD have not shown clear benefit of aspirin.[72]

Several studies have shown no benefit for aspirin, specifically in patients with abnormal ABI and no other evident vascular disease. The Prevention of Progression of Arterial Disease with Diabetes (POPADAD) trial randomized patients with diabetes and an ABI <0.99 to aspirin 100 mg daily or placebo. Patients were followed for a median of approximately 7 years.[73] Overall there was no benefit for MACE, or amputation for ischemia. The Aspirin for Prevention of Cardiovascular Events in a General Population Screened for a Low Ankle-Brachial Index (AAA) trial evaluated evidently healthy patients with an ABI ≤0.95.[74] A total of 3350 patients were randomized to aspirin 100 mg daily or placebo and followed for a mean of 8.2 years. Event rates were low, and only 357 primary end points (CV death, MI, stroke, or revascularization) occurred. There was no benefit of aspirin for MACE or MALE; however, there was a 71% excess in bleeding. A subsequent meta-analysis evaluated the efficacy of aspirin versus placebo in 5269 patients broadly defined as having PAD.[72] Overall the number of events was low and there were fewer with aspirin (125 vs. 144), with a nonsignificant 25% reduction in MACE.

Several studies have evaluated $P2Y_{12}$ inhibition as a target for MACE reduction in patients with PAD. The Swedish Ticlopidine Multicenter Study (STIMS) randomized 687 patients with intermittent claudication to the first-generation $P2Y_{12}$ inhibitor ticlopidine or placebo and followed them for a median of 5.6 years.[75] In patients treated with ticlopidine, there was a 30% reduction in mortality, as well as a 51% reduction in the need for vascular surgery.[76]

A second-generation thienopyridine, clopidogrel, was subsequently studied in the Clopidogrel versus Aspirin in Patients at Risk of Ischaemic Events (CAPRIE) trial.[77] More than 19,000 patients with stable vascular disease, including 6452 with symptomatic PAD (ABI ≤0.85 with a history of claudication or prior revascularization or amputation for ischemia), were randomized to clopidogrel 75 mg daily or aspirin 325 mg daily. The primary results were that clopidogrel was superior to aspirin, although the relative risk reduction was modest at 8.7%. There was statistical heterogeneity based on baseline disease state, with the most robust benefit in those randomized with PAD showing a 23.8% relative risk reduction. Safety of aspirin and clopidogrel were comparable, with numerically but not statistically significant lower rates of gastrointestinal bleeding and intracranial hemorrhage with clopidogrel.

The third-generation P2Y$_{12}$ inhibitor ticagrelor was compared as monotherapy to clopidogrel in A Study Comparing Cardiovascular Effects of Ticagrelor and Clopidogrel in Patients with Peripheral Artery Disease (EUCLID).[78] EUCLID enrolled only patients with symptomatic PAD (ABI < 0.80 or prior peripheral revascularization), and concomitant CAD was present in approximately 29% of patients. A total of 13,885 patients were randomized and followed for 30 months. MACE was similar with both treatments (10.8% with ticagrelor, 10.6% with clopidogrel), with no evidence for superiority with ticagrelor compared with clopidogrel. Results were similar for components of the primary end point, with the exception of ischemic stroke, which was lower with ticagrelor. Results were consistent across subgroups, but there was statistical heterogeneity when evaluating patients with prior coronary revascularization (patients with polyvascular disease), where MACE was lower with ticagrelor than with clopidogrel. Patients with prior peripheral revascularization were at approximately fourfold risk of MALE relative to those without, driving the greatest risk of limb outcomes.[14] There was no reduction in MALE with ticagrelor compared with clopidogrel in patients with or without prior peripheral revascularization. Safety was similar between treatment arms.

Overall, these data demonstrate that antiplatelet therapy reduces MACE risk in patients with symptomatic PAD. Aspirin is likely efficacious in patients with symptomatic PAD, as it is in patients with other manifestations of atherosclerosis, although efficacy based on clinical trials is not as well established as it is in other clinical manifestations of atherosclerosis. P2Y$_{12}$ inhibition may be more effective than aspirin with similar safety. Patients with marginally abnormal ABI but no other evidence of vascular disease are characterized by low risk of MACE and little if any benefit of antiplatelet monotherapy.

More Intensive Antithrombotic Therapies

Various combinations of antithrombotic agents have been evaluated in patients with PAD, either in dedicated populations or as subgroups of broader trials. The Clopidogrel for High Atherothrombotic Risk and Ischemic Stabilization, Management and Avoidance (CHARISMA) trial randomized 15,603 patients with vascular disease or risk factors to dual antiplatelet therapy (DAPT), consisting of the combination of low-dose aspirin plus clopidogrel versus aspirin alone.[79] Overall there was a 7% relative risk reduction in MACE with DAPT versus aspirin alone, which was not statistically significant. A post hoc subgroup evaluation of a population similar to that in the CAPRIE trial showed a significant 17% reduction in MACE, with the most robust signal in patients with prior MI. A specific analysis of the 2383 patients with symptomatic PAD was performed, which showed no significant reduction in MACE but lower rates of MI and hospitalization for ischemic events.[80] There was no reported effect on MALE. DAPT increased bleeding compared with aspirin alone, with statistically significant excesses in minor and moderate bleeding and a trend for more severe bleeding.

The benefits of DAPT with aspirin and clopidogrel were evaluated also in the CASPAR trial of patients with PAD undergoing lower extremity bypass surgery.[81] A total of 851 patients were randomized to DAPT versus aspirin alone and followed for a maximum of 24 months. The primary end point was a broad composite, including graft occlusion, revascularization, amputation, or death from any cause. There was no benefit of DAPT in this trial. Post hoc subgroup analyses of this overall negative trial suggested that DAPT reduced the risk of prosthetic graft occlusions. A similar trial, called CAMPER, designed to

evaluate the same regimen after endovascular revascularization, failed to enroll enough patients and was halted.

A growing appreciation for the role of thrombin-mediated platelet activation led to the evaluation of agents to either inhibit thrombin's actions or thrombin generation (see anticoagulants later). There are four known protease-activated receptors (PARs), with PAR-1 and PAR-4 expressed on human platelets, and with PAR-1 as the predominant receptor leading to platelet activation. The PAR-1 receptor antagonist vorapaxar has been evaluated in a series of clinical studies leading to its approval by the FDA for patients with prior MI or PAD. The pivotal study for this indication was the Trial to Assess the Effects of Vorapaxar in Preventing Heart Attack and Stroke in Patients With Atherosclerosis (TRA 2°P–TIMI 50).[82] This trial enrolled a broad population including patients with prior MI, symptomatic PAD (ABI ≤0.85 with history of claudication or prior peripheral revascularization for ischemia) or prior stroke, and randomized them to vorapaxar or placebo. A broad range of background therapy was allowed, including aspirin, P2Y$_{12}$ inhibitors, or the combination of both. A total of 26,449 patients were randomized and hierarchically assigned to a disease group (if MI or stroke within 12 months, then they were assigned to the MI or stroke groups even if PAD was present). Vorapaxar significantly reduced the risk or MACE by 13%. There was an excess in moderate or severe bleeding with vorapaxar, most notably in patients with stroke, who suffered an excess of intracranial bleeding. In patients with prior MI or PAD and no history of stroke or transient ischemic attack, there was a significant 17% reduction in MACE with no heterogeneity in those who qualified with MI or PAD.[83]

In the PAD population of this trial, including those with abnormal ABI (≤0.90) and symptomatic PAD, there was a significant 15% reduction in MACE and 30% reduction in MALE. One of the most notable effects of vorapaxar was a robust 42% reduction in ALI (Fig. 19.7; see Chapter 44).[12,84,85] This benefit was present regardless of the cause of ALI but particularly in reduction of graft thrombosis. Patients with prior lower extremity revascularization were at an approximately fourfold risk of ALI relative to patients with claudication but no history of revascularization. In addition to the reduction in ALI, there were significant reductions in urgent peripheral revascularization and elective revascularization. Treatment with vorapaxar was associated with an increased risk of major bleeding. Overall, a net clinical outcome defined as the composite of MACE, MALE, fatal bleeding, or symptomatic bleeding into a critical organ was 18% lower with vorapaxar relative to placebo, with an absolute risk reduction of approximately 3% at 3 years.[83]

Anticoagulant Therapy with a Vitamin K Antagonist

The Warfarin Antiplatelet Vascular Evaluation (WAVE) trial is the largest randomized study to test warfarin added to aspirin versus aspirin alone in patients with PAD.[86] A total of 2161 patients were randomized. Overall there was no benefit for MACE or MALE with the combination of warfarin and aspirin compared with aspirin alone, but there was greater than threefold excess in the risk of life-threatening bleeding.

Warfarin has also been studied for lower extremity bypass graft patency. In the Dutch Bypass Oral Anticoagulants or Aspirin (BOA) Study Group trial, 2690 patients with PAD undergoing infrainguinal bypass grafting were randomized to warfarin or aspirin. There was no benefit for ischemic outcomes, including graft occlusion and MACE. There was a 3.48-fold excess in hemorrhagic stroke and a twofold excess in hemorrhage overall. A post hoc exploratory analysis suggested a benefit for vein grafts, but these findings have not been confirmed.

Taken together, available data do not support the use of vitamin K antagonist therapy for patients with PAD for either MACE or MALE reduction, and demonstrate unacceptable rates of bleeding with greater than threefold excesses in life-threatening bleeding and hemorrhagic stroke.

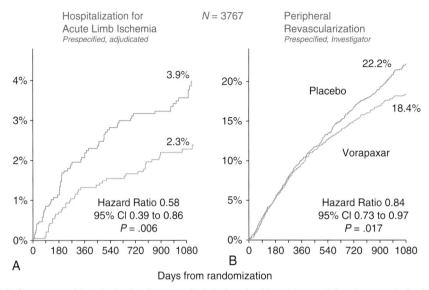

Fig. 19.7 Outcomes of hospitalization for acute limb ischemia (A) and any peripheral revascularization (B) in patients with symptomatic peripheral artery disease randomized in the TRA2P-TIMI 50 trial and stratified by allocation to vorapaxar *(green)* or placebo *(blue)*. *CI,* Confidence interval. (Redrawn from Bonaca MP, Scirica BM, Creager MA, et al. Vorapaxar in patients with peripheral artery disease: results from TRA2{degrees} P-TIMI 50. *Circulation.* 2013;127:1522–1529, 1529e1–6.)

Adding a Factor Xa Inhibitor to Aspirin

The ATLAS-TIMI 46 and ATLAS-TIMI 51 studies evaluated low doses of rivaroxaban, a factor Xa inhibitor, added to DAPT in patients with coronary disease. The most efficacious and safest dose was 2.5 mg twice daily.[87,88] Added to DAPT (aspirin and clopidogrel), rivaroxaban 2.5 mg twice daily reduced MACE and all-cause mortality. There was an excess in TIMI major bleeding and intracranial hemorrhage with rivaroxaban.

These observations were carried forward into the Rivaroxaban for the Prevention of Major Cardiovascular Events in Coronary or Peripheral Artery Disease (COMPASS) trial, which evaluated rivaroxaban for long-term prevention in stable patients with coronary disease or PAD, in this trial broadly defined as disease outside the coronary circulation.[89,90] Patients enrolled were enriched for risk with either revascularizations in two vascular territories, two additional risk factors, or advanced age. Of the overall cohort of 27,396 patients, 90% had coronary disease. Patients randomized were allocated to one of three strata: low-dose aspirin monotherapy, low-dose aspirin monotherapy plus rivaroxaban 2.5 mg twice daily, or rivaroxaban 5 mg twice daily as monotherapy. After a mean follow-up of 23 months, the trial was prematurely terminated for overwhelming efficacy in the rivaroxaban plus aspirin group relative to the control group of aspirin monotherapy.

Treatment with rivaroxaban 2.5 mg twice daily and aspirin relative to aspirin alone reduced the primary end point of MACE, with a significant reduction in CV death. All-cause mortality was numerically lower with low-dose rivaroxaban plus aspirin but did not meet the prespecified *P* value and was not statistically significant. Efficacy came at the cost of a 70% increase in major bleeding. Rates of fatal bleeding and intracranial hemorrhage were low overall but not statistically significantly increased with rivaroxaban.

Patients randomized into the COMPASS PAD cohort included 1919 patients with coronary disease plus carotid disease, 1422 patients with coronary disease and asymptomatic ABI <0.90, and 4129 with symptomatic lower extremity PAD. Approximately 70% had concomitant CAD or prior stroke, and approximately 84% were on lipid-lowering therapy. In the PAD cohort, low-dose rivaroxaban plus aspirin reduced MACE by 28%, with a nonsignificant trend for lower CV death that was consistent with the overall trial. All-cause mortality was not reduced (Fig. 19.8). In the PAD patients in COMPASS, low-dose rivaroxaban plus aspirin compared with aspirin alone reduced MALE, defined as ALI, revascularization for ischemia within 30 days, or ischemic amputation, by 46%. Rates of major ischemic amputation were low (5 of 2492 patients with rivaroxaban plus aspirin and 17 of 2504 patients on aspirin alone) but were significantly reduced by 70% with rivaroxaban plus aspirin. The safety of rivaroxaban in patients with PAD was like that in the overall trial, with an excess in major bleeding but no significant excess in major bleeding or intracranial hemorrhage. There was a net benefit demonstrated for low-dose rivaroxaban plus aspirin compared with aspirin alone in the overall trial population and in the PAD subset when counting fatal bleeding or intracranial hemorrhage. A subsequent analysis of limb outcomes showed consistent reductions in MALE in patients with lower extremity PAD only.[3,11] Of note, most events occurred in patients with prior peripheral revascularization, with few events occurring in those with asymptomatic low ABI.

The results of COMPASS trial suggest that the combination of low-dose rivaroxaban plus aspirin may be an important therapeutic option for patients with PAD. The clearest benefit for MACE was in patients with polyvascular disease (CAD + PAD), and the benefit for MALE reduction was particularly notable in patients with symptomatic PAD who had prior peripheral revascularization. Rivaroxaban 2.5 mg twice daily added to aspirin is approved by the FDA for use in patients with PAD for MACE reduction.

More Intensive Antithrombotic Therapy in Patients with Polyvascular Disease

Patients with PAD and concomitant CAD (particularly prior MI) are at approximately 60% greater risk for MACE beyond patients with CAD only, even after adjusting for other risk factors. The risk associated with polyvascular disease has been demonstrated in registries and in at least three clinical trial cohorts.

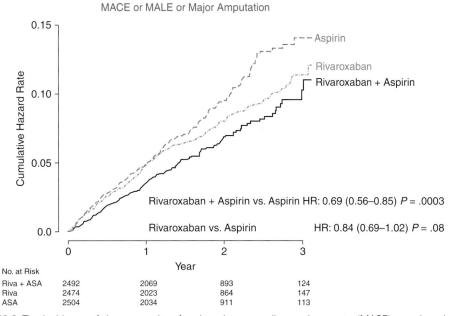

Fig. 19.8 The incidence of the composite of major adverse cardiovascular events *(MACE)* or major adverse limb events *(MALE)* in patients with peripheral artery disease randomized to aspirin *(ASA)* monotherapy *(red)*, rivaroxaban 5 mg twice daily monotherapy *(blue)*, or aspirin and rivaroxaban 2.5 mg twice daily *(black)* in the COMPASS trial. Hazard ratios *(HRs)* for each comparison are shown. (Modified from Anand SS, Bosch J, Eikelboom JW, et al. Rivaroxaban with or without aspirin in patients with stable peripheral or carotid artery disease: an international, randomised, double-blind, placebo-controlled trial. *Lancet.* 2018;391:20–26.)

The Prevention of Cardiovascular Events (Death From Heart or Vascular Disease, Heart Attack, or Stroke) in Patients With Prior Heart Attack Using Ticagrelor Compared to Placebo on a Background of Aspirin (PEGASUS-TIMI 54) trial randomized stable patients with prior MI to aspirin monotherapy or aspirin combined with ticagrelor 60 mg twice daily or ticagrelor 90 mg twice daily. Overall, ticagrelor reduced the risk of MACE by 15%, with an associated approximately twofold excess in major bleeding. The ticagrelor 60-mg dose was better tolerated and is approved for long-term use in patients with prior MI.[13,91] A subgroup analysis of approximately 1000 patients with concomitant symptomatic PAD found higher risk overall relative to those without PAD, with an event rate of 19% at 3 years. There was a substantial reduction in MACE (ARR 5.2%, NNT 20) in patients with prior MI and concomitant PAD, which translated into significant 53% reduction in CV death and 48% reduction in all-cause mortality, with an excess in bleeding as was observed in the overall trial (Fig. 19.9). In addition to benefits in MACE and mortality, ticagrelor reduced MALE by 35%, with the greatest absolute risk reduction in patients with symptomatic PAD. As has been observed in the TRA2P-TIMI-50, EUCLID, and COMPASS trials, patients with prior lower extremity revascularization were at the highest risk of MALE, with an approximately fourfold excess after adjustment for other risk factors.

The results of PEGASUS-TIMI 54 were supported by observations from the PRODIGY trial, which looked at longer versus shorter durations of DAPT with aspirin and clopidogrel after coronary stenting. Overall there was no difference between strategies for the outcome of MACE; however, there was statistical heterogeneity by PAD at baseline, demonstrating a reduction in MACE with extended DAPT versus shorter DAPT in the patients with CAD and PAD, and particularly those with prior ACS and PAD.[92] In this subgroup there was a 54% reduction in MACE and a significant 55% reduction in all-cause mortality. Prolonged DAPT increased bleeding compared with shorter DAPT. Limb outcomes were not ascertained or reported in PRODIGY.

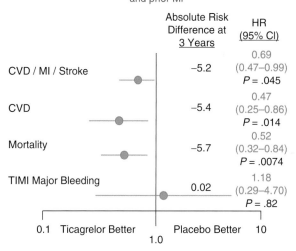

Fig. 19.9 Outcomes in patients with symptomatic peripheral artery disease *(PAD)* randomized in the PEGASUS-TIMI 54 trial randomized to ticagrelor 60 mg twice daily added to low-dose aspirin *(ASA)* versus aspirin alone. Cardiovascular death *(CVD)*, myocardial infarction *(MI)*, stroke, and major adverse limb events *(MALE)* are shown. *CI,* Confidence interval; *HR,* hazard ratio; *TIMI,* Thrombolysis in Myocardial Infarction. (Modified from Bonaca MP, Bhatt DL, Storey RF, et al. Ticagrelor for prevention of ischemic events after myocardial infarction in patients with peripheral artery disease. *J Am Coll Cardiol.* 2016;67:2719–2728.)

When considering COMPASS PAD, which was largely enriched for polyvascular disease, along with PEGASUS-TIMI 54 PAD and PRODIGY PAD, greater MACE reductions are seen with more potent antithrombotic strategies. The totality of the data suggests that a more potent regimen should be considered for these patients unless bleeding risk is prohibitive.

Antithrombotic Therapy Recommendations

Patients with atherosclerotic vascular disease, including PAD, benefit from antithrombotic therapy with a reduction of MACE, although at the risk of increased bleeding. Antiplatelet monotherapy with either as-

superior. More intensive antithrombotic strategies further reduce the risk of MACE but at the cost of increased bleeding, with the clearest benefit in patients with PAD and concomitant coronary disease, particularly prior ACS. More intensive regimens also reduce MALE, with the greatest absolute benefits in patient with prior peripheral revascularization. Current guidelines assign a class I recommendation to antiplatelet monotherapy in symptomatic PAD, with dual antiplatelet or other more intensive regimens receiving lesser levels of recommendation, indicating that clinicians should tailor therapy based on ischemic and bleeding risk.[2,4] An algorithm for considering the intensity of antithrombotic therapy is provided in Fig. 19.10 and Table 19.2.

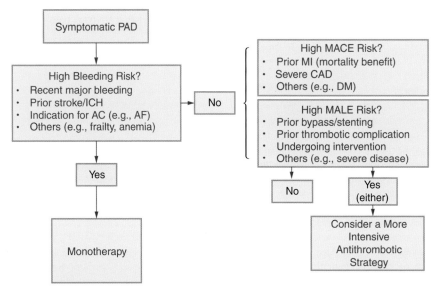

Fig. 19.10 A framework for optimizing antithrombotic therapy in patients with peripheral artery disease *(PAD). AC,* Anticoagulation; *AF,* atrial fibrillation; *CAD,* coronary artery disease; *DM,* diabetes mellitus; *ICH,* intracranial hemorrhage; *MACE,* major adverse cardiovascular events; *MALE,* major adverse limb events; *MI,* myocardial infarction.

TABLE 19.2   Risk Stratification and Considerations for Antithrombotic Therapy in Patients with PAD

Antithrombotic Regimens Studied in PAD	PATIENT RISK PROFILES IN PAD			
	Low Risk for MACE and MALE	High Risk for MALE and Low Risk for MACE	High Risk for MACE and Low Risk for MALE	High Risk for MACE and MALE
Monotherapy with aspirin or P2Y$_{12}$ inhibitor *(n.b. clopidogrel monotherapy FDA approved for PAD)*	Standard	Consider if high bleeding risk	Consider if high bleeding risk	Consider if high bleeding risk
Aspirin and P2Y$_{12}$ inhibitor *(n.b. DAPT with ticagrelor FDA approved for prior MI)*			Consider in PAD patients with high MACE risk (e.g., prior MI)	Consider in PAD patients with high MACE risk (e.g., prior MI) with benefit for MALE reduction
Aspirin or clopidogrel + vorapaxar *(n.b. vorapaxar FDA approved in PAD added to aspirin or clopidogrel)*		Consider if at low bleeding risk	Consider if at low bleeding risk	Consider if at low bleeding risk
Aspirin + rivaroxaban 2.5 mg twice daily		Consider if at low bleeding risk if approved in PAD	Consider if at low bleeding risk if approved in PAD	Consider if at low bleeding risk if approved in PAD

DAPT, dual antiplatelet therapy; *FDA,* US Food and Drug Administration; *MACE,* major adverse cardiovascular events; *MALE,* major adverse limb events; *MI,* myocardial infarction; *PAD,* peripheral artery disease.

pirin or P2Y$_{12}$ inhibition is recommended, although the latter is likely

INTERVENTIONS TO IMPROVE SYMPTOMS AND FUNCTION

Exercise Therapy

The most effective, safest, and most rigorously studied therapy to improve function and reduce symptoms is exercise therapy. Although underutilized in the United States, recent changes in coverage determinations are expected to increase availability. Several complementary mechanisms likely account for this benefit (Fig. 19.11).[93] Although claudication is associated with reduced perfusion, the association between ABI and walking distance is variable.[93] Imaging measures of perfusion such as magnetic resonance imaging (MRI) show modest associations between perfusion and functional capacity. Therefore functional limitations in PAD are more complex than simply obstruction of the large arteries (see Chapters 13 and 17).[93] Although reduced perfusion from luminal narrowing contributes to functional limitation, contributions by structural and metabolic changes at the level skeletal muscle are also important.[93] Changes to skeletal muscle include reductions in mass and density, and efficiency of cellular energetics and metabolism. Mitochondrial dysfunction may also contribute to functional limitations, both by disordered energetics and by proinflammatory changes leading to cellular damage.[93]

Exercise training may provide benefit through several mechanisms, including promotion of growth factors and collateral development, increased endothelial nitric oxide synthase (eNOS) activity and enhanced endothelium-dependent vasodilitation.[93] In addition, exercise improves skeletal muscle efficiency through improvements in metabolic and mitochondrial function (see Fig. 19.11).[93,94] Improved endothelial function and reduced blood cell viscosity may improve oxygen delivery.[93,94] Studies have generally demonstrated that exercise, as administered in a supervised program, increases maximal walking time by 120% to 150% (Fig. 19.12).[95,96] Current AHA/ACC PAD guidelines and the ESC guidelines recommended supervised exercise for patients with PAD.[2,4]

Home-based (unsupervised) exercise may be beneficial when supervised programs are not available, although they are generally less effective than supervised programs. A home-based exercise program including cognitive behavioral intervention was tested in a trial of approximately 200 patients with PAD (see Fig. 19.12).[97] At 6 months, the intervention resulted in increased 6-minute walk distance, as well as increased maximal walking time, overall physical activity, and Walking Impairment Questionnaire (WIQ) scores.[97] The results supported the benefit of home-based exercise in patients with PAD who are unwilling or unable to participate in supervised exercise.[97] Benefits of the intervention were sustained at 12 months.[98] Although studies of home-based interventions have shown mixed results, a meta-analysis including 547 patients concluded that structured home-based exercise improved function in patients with PAD.[99–102]

There has been controversy about the relative efficacy of exercise compared with revascularization for functional improvement. This was tested in the CLEVER study, which compared supervised exercise training with endovascular intervention as a treatment strategy for patients with claudication.[103] A total of 111 patients were randomized to optimal medical care (OMC), OMC plus supervised exercise, or OMC and endovascular therapy. Supervised exercise showed the greatest improvement in peak walking time (PWT) during follow-up.[103]

A meta-analysis comparing functional improvement with supervised exercise, supervised exercise combined with endovascular therapy, and endovascular therapy alone, found that optimal outcomes were achieved with the combination of both supervised exercise and endovascular therapy and that there was no improvement in outcomes with endovascular therapy alone.[104] In practice, exercise and endovascular therapy are not competing strategies, but rather all patients should exercise and selected patients should also undergo revascularization. The Revascularization and Supervised Exercise (ERASE) trial tested this strategy versus exercise alone in 212 patients with aortoiliac or femoral-popliteal artery disease.[9] The combination of exercise and endovascular therapy was superior to exercise alone at 1 month, 6 months, and 12 months (mean difference, 282 m), with consistent benefits in pain-free walking distance, ABI, and quality of life.[9]

Recommendations

Supervised exercise training is recommended as an initial treatment modality for patients with intermittent claudication, and improvements in coverage are hoped to improve access. Exercise programs should use a treadmill and last 45 to 60 minutes at least 3 times a week for a minimum of 12 weeks. Prior to beginning exercise rehabilitation,

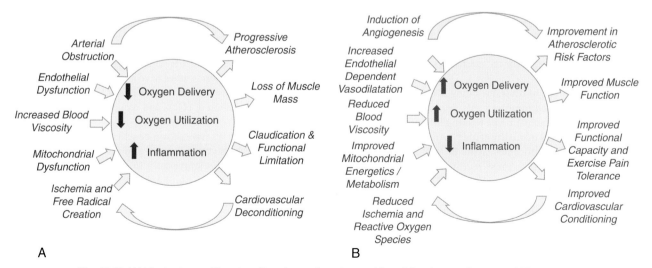

Fig. 19.11 (A) Mechanisms of functional impairment in patients with peripheral artery disease and (B) potential mechanisms of exercise in improving function. (From Bonaca MP, Creager MA. Pharmacological treatment and current management of peripheral artery disease. *Circ Res*. 2015;116:1579–1598.)

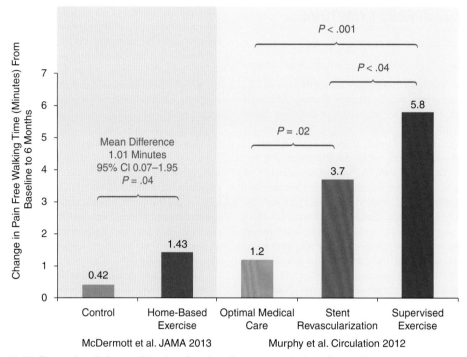

Fig. 19.12 Change in pain-free walking time from baseline to 6 months in patients with symptomatic peripheral artery disease with control or optimal medical therapy alone, home-based exercise, stent revascularization without exercise, and structured exercise. (From Bonaca MP, Creager MA. Pharmacological treatment and current management of peripheral artery disease. *Circ Res.* 2015;116:1579–1598.)

patients should undergo a comprehensive risk assessment that includes a history and examination. During the training session, patients should be encouraged to walk until symptoms of moderate severity develop. Following a rest period and resolution of symptoms, walking should resume until symptoms recur. This cycle should be repeated as many times as possible during the 45- to 60-minute period. For patients unable to participate in a supervised exercise training program, a home-based walking program is recommended.

Pharmacologic Therapies

Cilostazol is an effective pharmacotherapy directed solely at symptom improvement. It inhibits phosphodiesterase-3 (PDE-3). Randomized trials have shown that cilostazol improves symptoms of claudication and function. PDE-3 inhibitors reduce platelet aggregation and smooth muscle proliferation and cause vasodilation, but it is not known whether these effects account for the mechanism by which cilostazol improves claudication.[105,106]

A meta-analysis of eight trials, including 2702 patients with stable claudication, reported improvements in maximal walking distance (MWD) by 50% and pain-free walking distance by 67%, with associated improvements in quality of life.[107] Another meta-analysis of seven trials found significant benefits in MWD with cilostazol compared with placebo.[108] A more recent meta-analysis, including nine randomized controlled trials and 1258 patients, observed improvements in MWD with cilostazol by 50.7% compared with a 24.3% improvement with placebo and an absolute increase of 42.1 m.[109]

Cilostazol is contraindicated in patients with heart failure, although risk has not been seen in trials of cilostazol. The contraindication is derived from adverse events observed in trials with other PDE-3 inhibitors, such as milrinone.[110] Patients may experience gastrointestinal side effects, as well as headache and dizziness, and these symptoms may

limit tolerability. Overall, use of cilostazol is low, approximating 10% of patients with symptomatic PAD.

Pentoxifylline is a theophylline that has been hypothesized to reduce blood viscosity by improving deformability of erythrocytes.[111] Some, but not all, studies demonstrate a modest improvement in symptoms with pentoxifylline.[112,113]

The efficacy of cilostazol and pentoxifylline was compared in a trial of 922 patients with claudication.[113] Overall mean MWD was significantly greater with cilostazol than with pentoxifylline or placebo. At 24 weeks of treatment, cilostazol was significantly better than both pentoxifylline and placebo; however, pentoxifylline showed no significant benefit relative to placebo.

Statin Therapy

Statins are indicated in all patients with PAD based on lowering risk of MACE. Additional benefits with regard to functional status have been investigated. These studies have largely been driven by observations that statins have a broad range of effects beyond LDL-C lowering, including upregulation of eNOS and reductions in oxidant stress and inflammation.[114]

Several small trials have shown benefits in reducing severity of intermittent claudication and improving function. One trial randomized 354 patients to placebo, atorvastatin 10 mg daily, or atorvastatin 80 mg daily and demonstrated a significant improvement in pain-free walking time with atorvastatin 80 mg.[115] Another study found benefits in exercise time with simvastatin compared with placebo.[116] A third randomized study found an increase in mean pain-free walking distance with simvastatin compared with placebo.[117] A comprehensive review of therapies to reduce claudication symptoms and improve function found that lipid-lowering therapies demonstrated benefit, with mean increase in MWD of 160 m, whereas the other classes of therapies showed modest improvement (50 m).[118] The benefits of statin therapies described are supported by the observations of reductions in the need for peripheral revascularization seen in the observational REACH Registry and in the randomized HPS previously described in the section on lipid lowering.

Recommendations

Pharmacotherapy with cilostazol is effective in improving function and reducing symptoms in patients with claudication. AHA/ACC PAD guidelines recommend a therapeutic trial of cilostazol in patients with claudication.[2] Cilostazol should not be used in patients with heart failure and may have limiting side effects including gastrointestinal symptoms. Pentoxifylline is not clinically effective and is not recommended for treatment of symptomatic PAD.

Statin therapy is recommended for all patients with PAD to reduce MACE. Potential benefits include improvements in symptoms and functional status.

Investigational Therapies

Vasodilator Drugs

Vasodilator drugs have undergone extensive investigation for treatment of patients with claudication and CLI. It is intuitive to assume that treatment with a medication that reduces arteriolar resistance would be as effective for patients with PAD as nitrates and calcium channel blockers are for patients with angina. However, in general, vasodilator drug therapy has been disappointing for relief of intermittent claudication. Differences in the pathophysiology of limb and myocardial ischemia may promote insight into the disparate efficiency of vasodilator drugs. Vasodilator therapy may decrease myocardial oxygen demand but is not likely to affect skeletal muscle oxygen demand. Therefore, to be effective, vasodilators would have to improve the blood supply to exercising muscle.

Vasodilator prostaglandins have undergone somewhat extensive investigation for the treatment of patients with intermittent claudication or CLI. This class of drugs includes prostaglandin E1 (PGE1), prostacyclin (PGI2), and its analogs beraprost and iloprost. The efficacy of vasodilator prostaglandins administered intra-arterially (IA) or intravenously (IV) has been assessed in patients with intermittent claudication and in patients with CLI.[119] Two placebo-controlled trials of oral beraprost administered for 6 months had conflicting results, one showing improvement and one showing no change in pain-free or MWD.[120,121] In one multicenter placebo-controlled trial, iloprost administered for 6 months was no more effective than placebo in improving pain-free or MWD among patients with intermittent claudication.[112]

Short-term (i.e., 3 to 4 days) IA or IV administration of PGE1, iloprost, or ciprostene is not effective in ameliorating CLI, but when administered parenterally for longer periods of time (7 to 28 days) may reduce pain, ulcer size, or risk of amputation. The Ischemia Cronica degli Arti Inferiori study assessed the efficacy of IV PGE1 or placebo in 1560 patients with CLI.[122] The relative risk of death, major amputation or persistence of CLI, acute MI, or stroke was significantly reduced by 13% at the time of hospital discharge but not at 6 months. After 6 months of treatment, there was no difference between groups in death or amputation, but there was a greater chance of resolution of CLI in those survivors who did not have amputation. Two randomized placebo-controlled studies assessed the effect of oral iloprost on CLI.[123,124] There was no apparent benefit of iloprost in terms of

reducing the risk of the primary end point of amputation or death, but there was a modest benefit in terms of resolution of ulcers and rest pain in those who survived without amputation. In a recent trial of patients with CLI, twice-daily infusion of taprostene compared with placebo did not improve pain control, wound healing, or amputation rates. Side effects of prostaglandins include flushing, headache, and gastrointestinal distress. A review of prostanoids for CLI including 33 randomized controlled trials and 4477 patients found high-quality evidence that prostanoids had no effect on total amputations, moderate-quality evidence that there may be small beneficial effects on rest pain and ulcer healing compared with placebo, and higher rates of adverse events.[119]

Metabolic Agents

Symptoms of intermittent claudication may be related in part to abnormalities in skeletal muscle metabolism (see Chapter 17). Therefore drugs that favorably affect oxidative metabolism may confer benefit by enhancing skeletal muscle function even without improving blood supply. For example, L-carnitine and its derivative propionyl-L-carnitine enhance glucose oxidation and oxidative metabolism via the Krebs cycle by providing a source of carnitine. Three placebo-controlled trials have assessed the efficacy of propionyl-L-carnitine in patients with intermittent claudication. In these studies, propionyl-L-carnitine administered as a 1-g oral dose twice daily improved MWD by 54% to 73%, whereas those randomized to placebo increased MWD 25% to 46%. Propionyl-L-carnitine improved physical function, walking speed, and distance as assessed by quality-of-life questionnaires. Propionyl-L-carnitine was not associated with any significant adverse side effects.[125]

One trial assessed the potential benefit of propionyl-L-carnitine therapy (vs. placebo) as adjunctive treatment to home-based monitored exercise training for patients with intermittent claudication.[125] In this trial, maximal walking time increased in both the propionyl-L-carnitine and placebo groups after 6 months of exercise training, with a nonsignificant trend toward improved walking in the propionyl-L-carnitine group. Propionyl-L-carnitine has potential merit for treating intermittent claudication but should be considered investigational at this time.

Ranolazine is a piperazine derivative that inhibits fatty acid oxidation, activates pyruvate dehydrogenase, and shifts metabolism toward carbohydrate oxidation, thereby increasing efficiency of oxygen use. Ranolazine improves exercise capacity and decreases angina frequency in patients with CAD. It was associated with improvement in pain-free walking time (vs. placebo) among patients with intermittent claudication in a single-center pilot study.[126]

Cell-Based Therapy

Administration of stem cells (hematopoietic or bone marrow) is an investigational therapy for symptomatic PAD, particularly CLI, with possible mechanisms of benefit that include growth or stimulation of new blood vessel formation. Bone marrow mononuclear cells include endothelial progenitor cells.[127,128]

Intramuscular injection of autologous bone marrow–derived mononuclear cells improves collateral blood vessel formation in animal models of myocardial and hind limb ischemia.[127] The effect of autologous implantation of bone marrow–derived mononuclear cells has been studied in patients with PAD, including those with limb ischemia. Injection of bone marrow mononuclear cells has been associated with improvements in rest pain, improved pain-free walking time, and lower rates of amputation.[127-130] Angiographic evidence of collateral blood vessel formation has also been described in patients who have received bone marrow–derived mononuclear cells.[131] Additional data supporting potential angiogenic benefit of intramuscular injection or IA infusion of bone marrow–derived mononuclear cells or bone marrow–derived mesenchymal cells for patients with CLI and limited revascularization options have been reported in multiple small single-center early phase trials.[3,105,106] Many of these studies used noninvasive measures of pressure or flow (e.g., ABI, toe-brachial index [TBI], plethysmography) rather than angiography to document evidence of angiogenesis.

A Cochrane review focused on intramuscular administration of mononuclear cells included two small trials and a total of 57 patients. Stem cell therapy was associated with lower rates of amputation, with the individual studies suggesting benefits including increased ABI, improved function, and improved rate of healing of ischemic ulcers.[132,133] A more recent meta-analysis including observational and randomized studies of autologous stem cells in patients with severe PAD (CLI or anatomy not amenable to revascularization) found that stem cell therapy was associated with reduced pain and amputation risk.[127] This association was not significant after excluding observational studies.

The PACE trial evaluated the efficacy of ALDH-bright cells versus placebo in 82 patients with PAD.[134] Overall there was no difference in the primary end point of PWT or secondary end points (collaterals, hyperemic popliteal flow, capillary perfusion by MRI). A post hoc exploratory analysis suggested that ALDH-bright cell administration might be associated with an increase in the number of collateral arteries in participants with completely occluded femoral arteries. The MOBILE trial evaluated autologous concentrated bone marrow aspirate (cBMA) in patients with PAD.[135] The cell therapy showed an excellent safety profile, as well as trends for reductions in amputation-free survival. Post hoc analyses showed significant reductions in major amputations in Rutherford 4 and nondiabetic Rutherford 5 CLI patients. In addition, significant increases in TcPO2 were interpreted as demonstrating improvements in microvascular function.

Cell-based therapy in PAD remains an area of intensive research particularly in patients with CLI, with several studies investigating this strategy recently completed or ongoing; however, results continue to be mixed.[136,137]

Angiogenic Growth Factors

Angiogenic growth factors have undergone investigation for treatment of PAD with the goal of forming new vessels. This class of drugs includes vascular endothelial growth factor (VEGF), fibroblast growth factor (FGF), hepatocyte growth factor (HGF), and hypoxia-inducible factor-1α (HIF-1α).[138] They may be administered as recombinant proteins or by gene transfer using plasmid deoxyribonucleic acid (DNA) or an adenoviral vector that encodes the angiogenic growth factor. VEGF, FGF, and HIF-1α increase collateral blood vessels and improve blood flow in animal models of hind limb ischemia.[139] Therefore angiogenic growth factors have the potential to promote collateral blood vessel formation and thereby increase blood flow to the ischemic limbs of patients with PAD. To date, trials investigating these therapies have had mixed results.[138]

Several nonrandomized open-label studies found that IA gene transfer therapy of pHVEGF165 increased collateral blood vessels, as assessed by MRI or digital subtraction angiography in patients with PAD. In addition, pHVEGF165 administration improved blood flow and increased ABI in some patients who participated in these trials.

Recombinant FGF2 administered directly into the femoral artery was evaluated in a placebo-controlled study.[140] Patients were randomized to receive FGF2 on one occasion only, on two occasions 30 days apart, or placebo. One-time administration of FGF2 increased PWT at 90 days by 34% compared with 14% for placebo. Yet, there was no significant improvement in PWT compared with placebo when FGF2 was administered on two occasions. A nonrandomized study of patients with CLI observed that intramuscular injection of plasmid DNA encoding FGF1 reduced pain and ulcer size and increased the ABI.[141] In a phase 2 placebo-controlled study of patients with CLI, intramuscular administration of FGF1 using a plasmid vector did not improve ulcer healing, the primary end point, but did decrease secondary end points including all amputations and the composite of major amputation and death.[142] However, in a follow-up phase 3 study of patients with CLI, FGF1 did not decrease amputation-free survival.[139]

HGF using a plasmid vector and given as an intramuscular injection increased TcPO2 but did not improve pain, heal ulcers, or decrease amputations in a placebo-controlled trial of patients with CLI.[143]

HIF-1α is an inducible transcriptional regulatory factor. In conditions of low oxygen tension, HIF-1α binds to hypoxia-responsive elements in the promoter/enhancer region of target genes, inducing those encoding VEGF-A, platelet-derived growth factor (PDGF), angiotensin 1, and inducible nitric oxide synthase (iNOS). A trial randomized patients with intermittent claudication to placebo or one of three doses of the adenovirus encoding HIF-1α and found no benefit of HIF-1α on PWT, claudication onset time, or ABI up to 1 year after randomization.[144]

A systemic review and meta-analysis evaluating a variety of angiogenic factors in patients with claudication or CLI found no significant benefit of these therapies for amputation, wound healing, or broader outcomes such as mortality.[139,144,145]

SUMMARY AND CONCLUSION

Patients with PAD are at heightened risk of MACE and MALE and suffer from functional impairment. Exercise therapy is highly effective at addressing symptoms of claudication and improving functional capacity. Available pharmacotherapies, including blood pressure–lowering, glucose-lowering, and LDL-C–lowering drugs, antithrombotic therapy, and potentially antiinflammatory therapy, modify axes of risk (Fig. 19.13). In addition, therapies such as cilostazol improve symptoms of claudication. Identifying patients with PAD is critical to initiating education and broad interventions to reduce risk such as dietary interventions, smoking cessation, and blood pressure optimization. Assessment of the individual patient, including understanding his or her relative risk of MACE and MALE and the impacts on quality of life, may be helpful in determining a personalized approach, including the use of intensive antithrombotic and lipid-lowering therapies (Fig. 19.14). Efforts are needed to intensify prevention in patients with PAD because observational studies demonstrate underutilization of available effective therapies.

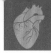

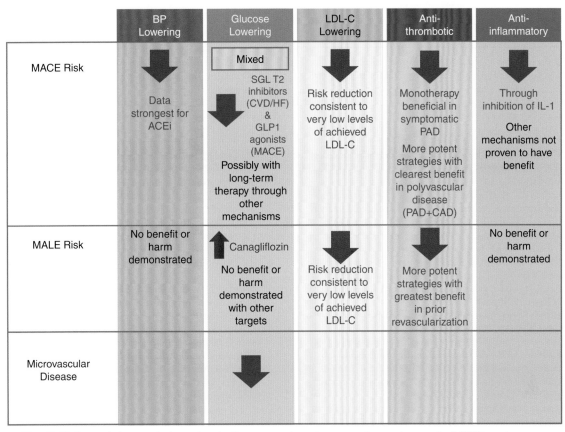

Fig. 19.13 Axes of therapy *(columns)* and effects on major adverse cardiovascular events *(MACE)*, major adverse limb events *(MALE),* and microvascular disease in patients with peripheral artery disease *(PAD)* with or without diabetes (glucose lowering therapies relevant for patients with diabetes). *ACEi,* Angiotensin-converting enzyme inhibitor; *BP,* blood pressure; *CAD,* coronary artery disease; *CVD/HF,* cardiovascular death/heart failure; *IL-1,* interleukin-1; *LCL-C,* low-density lipoprotein cholesterol.

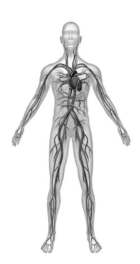

Therapies for MACE Reduction in All Patients
- Lifestyle Modification
- Tobacco Cessation Therapies
- Targeting blood pressure goals with preference for ACEi
- LDL-C lowering with statin ± ezetimibe and/or PCSK9i
- Antiplatelet monotherapy (symptomatic), preference for $P2Y_{12}$ inhibition

Therapies for Cardiac Risk Reduction in Selected Patients
Diabetes
- Glucose lowering to reduce microvascular risk
- GLP-1, SGLT2 inhibitors but caution with canagliflozin

Prior MI or CAD (Polyvascular Disease) and low bleeding risk
- ASA + rivaroxaban 2.5 BID (broad polyvascular definition)
- ASA + ticagrelor 60 mg BID (prior MI or other need for DAPT)
- ASA and/or clopidogrel with vorapaxar (prior MI or diabetes)

Therapies for MALE Reduction in All Patients
- LDL-C lowering with statin ± ezetimibe and/or PCSK9i

Therapies for MALE Reduction in Selected Patients
Prior peripheral revascularization & low bleeding risk
- ASA + rivaroxaban 2.5 BID
- ASA + ticagrelor 60 mg BID (prior MI or other need for DAPT)
- ASA and/or clopidogrel with vorapaxar

Therapies for Claudication
Symptomatic Patients
- Cilostazol 100 mg BID (only if no history of heart failure)

Fig. 19.14 An overview of risk reduction medical therapies in patients with peripheral artery disease in all patients or in selected populations based on risk. *ACEi,* Angiotensin-converting enzyme inhibitor; *ASA,* aspirin; *BID,* twice a day; *CAD,* coronary artery disease; *DAPT,* dual antiplatelet therapy; *LDL-C,* low-density lipoprotein cholesterol; *MACE,* major adverse cardiovascular events; *MALE,* major adverse limb events; *MI,* myocardial infarction.

REFERENCES

1. Bonaca MP, Creager MA. Pharmacological treatment and current management of peripheral artery disease. *Circ Res.* 2015;116:1579–1598.

2. Gerhard-Herman MD, Gornik HL, Barrett C, et al. 2016 AHA/ACC guideline on the management of patients with lower extremity peripheral artery disease: a report of the American College of Cardiology/American Heart Association Task Force on Clinical Practice Guidelines. *Circulation.* 2017;135(12):e726–e779.

3. Bonaca MP, Creager MA. Antithrombotic therapy and major adverse limb events in peripheral artery disease: a step forward. *J Am Coll Cardiol.* 2018;71:2316–2318.

4. Aboyans V, Ricco JB, MEL Bartelink, et al. 2017 ESC guidelines on the diagnosis and treatment of peripheral arterial diseases, in collaboration with the European Society for Vascular Surgery (ESVS): document covering atherosclerotic disease of extracranial carotid and vertebral, mesenteric, renal, upper and lower extremity arteries. Endorsed by: the European Stroke Organization (ESO), The Task Force for the Diagnosis and Treatment of Peripheral Arterial Diseases of the European Society of Cardiology (ESC) and of the European Society for Vascular Surgery (ESVS). *Eur Heart J.* 2018;39(9):763–816.

5. Hess CN, Hiatt WR. Antithrombotic therapy for peripheral artery disease in 2018. *JAMA.* 2018;319:2329–2330.

6. Bonaca MP, Nault P, Giugliano RP, et al. Low-density lipoprotein cholesterol lowering with evolocumab and outcomes in patients with peripheral artery disease: insights from the FOURIER Trial (Further Cardiovascular Outcomes Research With PCSK9 Inhibition in Subjects With Elevated Risk). *Circulation.* 2018;137:338–350.

7. Gutierrez A, Bonaca M, Cannon C, et al. Polyvascular disease, diabetes mellitus and long-term vascular risk: insights from the IMPROVE-IT TIMI 40 Trial. *J Am Coll Cardiol.* 2016;67(13 Suppl):2264.

8. Suarez C, Zeymer U, Limbourg T, et al. Influence of polyvascular disease on cardiovascular event rates. Insights from the REACH Registry. *Vasc Med.* 2010;15:259–265.

9. Fakhry F, Hunink MG. Randomized comparison of endovascular revascularization plus supervised exercise therapy versus supervised exercise therapy only in patients with peripheral artery disease and intermittent claudication: results of the Endovascular Revascularization and Supervised Exercise (ERASE) Trial. *Circulation.* 2013;128:2704–2722.

10. Secemsky EA, Yeh RW, Kereiakes DJ, et al. Extended duration dual antiplatelet therapy after coronary stenting among patients with peripheral arterial disease: a subanalysis of the Dual Antiplatelet Therapy Study. *JACC Cardiovasc Interv.* 2017;10:942–954.

11. Anand SS, Caron F, Eikelboom JW, et al. Major adverse limb events and mortality in patients with peripheral artery disease: the COMPASS Trial. *J Am Coll Cardiol.* 2018;71:2306–2315.

12. Bonaca MP, Gutierrez JA, Creager MA, et al. Acute limb ischemia and outcomes with vorapaxar in patients with peripheral artery disease: results from the trial to assess the effects of vorapaxar in preventing heart attack and stroke in patients with atherosclerosis-thrombolysis in myocardial infarction 50 (TRA2 degrees P-TIMI 50). *Circulation.* 2016;133:997–1005.

13. Bonaca MP, Bhatt DL, Storey RF, et al. Ticagrelor for prevention of ischemic events after myocardial infarction in patients with peripheral artery disease. *J Am Coll Cardiol.* 2016;67:2719–2728.

14. Jones WS, Baumgartner I, Hiatt WR, et al. Ticagrelor compared with clopidogrel in patients with prior lower extremity revascularization for peripheral artery disease. *Circulation.* 2017;135:241–250.

15. Eckel RH, Jakicic JM, Ard JD, et al. 2013 AHA/ACC guideline on lifestyle management to reduce cardiovascular risk: a report of the American College of Cardiology/American Heart Association Task Force on Practice Guidelines. *Circulation.* 2014;129:S76–S99.

16. Grundy SM, Stone NJ, Bailey AL, et al. AHA/ACC/AACVPR/AAPA/ABC/ACPM/ADA/AGS/APhA/ASPC/NLA/PCNA guideline on the management of blood cholesterol: a report of the American College of Cardiology/American Heart Association Task Force on Clinical Practice Guidelines. *Circulation.* 2018; Nov 10; [Epub ahead of print].

17. Gornik HL, Creager MA. Medical treatment of peripheral artery disease. In: Creager MA, Beckman JA, Loscalzo J, eds. *Vascular Medicine: A Companion to Braunwald's Heart Disease.* 2nd ed. Philadelphia: Elsevier; 2013:242–248.

18. Alvarez LR, Balibrea JM, Surinach JM, et al. Smoking cessation and outcome in stable outpatients with coronary, cerebrovascular, or peripheral artery disease. *Eur J Prev Cardiol.* 2013;20:486–495.

19. Hennrikus D, Joseph AM, Lando HA, et al. Effectiveness of a smoking cessation program for peripheral artery disease patients: a randomized controlled trial. *J Am Coll Cardiol.* 2010;56:2105–2112.

20. Rigotti NA, Pipe AL, Benowitz NL, et al. Efficacy and safety of varenicline for smoking cessation in patients with cardiovascular disease: a randomized trial. *Circulation.* 2010;121:221–229.

21. Fiore MC, Jaen CR. A clinical blueprint to accelerate the elimination of tobacco use. *JAMA.* 2008;299:2083–2085.

22. Whelton PK, Carey RM, Aronow WS, et al. 2017 ACC/AHA/AAPA/ABC/ACPM/AGS/APhA/ASH/ASPC/NMA/PCNA guideline for the prevention, detection, evaluation, and management of high blood pressure in adults: a report of the American College of Cardiology/American Heart Association Task Force on Clinical Practice Guidelines. *Hypertension.* 2018;71.

23. Wright Jr JT, Williamson JD, Whelton PK, et al. A randomized trial of intensive versus standard blood-pressure control. *N Engl J Med.* 2015;373:2103–2116.

24. Mehler PS, Coll JR, Estacio R, et al. Intensive blood pressure control reduces the risk of cardiovascular events in patients with peripheral arterial disease and type 2 diabetes. *Circulation.* 2003;107:753–756.

25. Bavry AA, Anderson RD, Gong Y, et al. Outcomes among hypertensive patients with concomitant peripheral and coronary artery disease: findings from the INternational VErapamil-SR/Trandolapril STudy. *Hypertension.* 2010;55:48–53.

26. Yusuf S, Sleight P, Pogue J, et al. Effects of an angiotensin-converting-enzyme inhibitor, ramipril, on cardiovascular events in high-risk patients. The Heart Outcomes Prevention Evaluation Study Investigators. *N Engl J Med.* 2000;342:145–153.

27. Fox KM. EURopean trial On reduction of cardiac events with Perindopril in stable coronary Artery disease investigators. Efficacy of perindopril in reduction of cardiovascular events among patients with stable coronary artery disease: randomised, double-blind, placebo-controlled, multicentre trial (the EUROPA study). *Lancet.* 2003;362:782–788.

28. Yusuf S, Teo KK, Pogue J, et al. Telmisartan, ramipril, or both in patients at high risk for vascular events. *N Engl J Med.* 2008;358:1547–1559.

29. Paravastu SC, Mendonca DA, Da Silva A. Beta blockers for peripheral arterial disease. *Cochrane Database Syst Rev.* 2013;9:CD005508.

30. Lane DA, Lip GY. Treatment of hypertension in peripheral arterial disease. *Cochrane Database Syst Rev.* 2013;12:CD003075.

31. Diehm C, Pittrow D, Lawall H. Effect of nebivolol vs. hydrochlorothiazide on the walking capacity in hypertensive patients with intermittent claudication. *J Hypertens.* 2011;29:1448–1456.

32. Sarwar N, Gao P, Seshasai SR, et al. Diabetes mellitus, fasting blood glucose concentration, and risk of vascular disease: a collaborative meta-analysis of 102 prospective studies. *Lancet.* 2010;375:2215–2222.

33. Singh S, Armstrong EJ, Sherif W, et al. Association of elevated fasting glucose with lower patency and increased major adverse limb events among patients with diabetes undergoing infrapopliteal balloon angioplasty. *Vasc Med.* 2014;19:307–314.

34. Boyko EJ, Ahroni JH, Cohen V, et al. Prediction of diabetic foot ulcer occurrence using commonly available clinical information: the Seattle Diabetic Foot Study. *Diabetes Care.* 2006;29:1202–1207.

35. Bonaca MP, Beckman JA. Sodium glucose cotransporter 2 inhibitors and amputation risk: Achilles' heel or opportunity for discovery? *Circulation.* 2018;137:1460–1462.

36. Gerstein HC, Miller ME, Byington RP, et al. Effects of intensive glucose lowering in type 2 diabetes. *N Engl J Med.* 2008;358:2545–2559.

37. Duckworth W, Abraira C, Moritz T, et al. Glucose control and vascular complications in veterans with type 2 diabetes. *N Engl J Med.* 2009;360:129–139.

38. Wing RR, Bolin P, Brancati FL, et al. Cardiovascular effects of intensive lifestyle intervention in type 2 diabetes. *N Engl J Med.* 2013;369:145–154.

39. Holman RR, Paul SK, Bethel MA, et al. 10-year follow-up of intensive glucose control in type 2 diabetes. *N Engl J Med*. 2008;359:1577–1589.

40. Scirica BM, Bhatt DL, Braunwald E, et al. Saxagliptin and cardiovascular outcomes in patients with type 2 diabetes mellitus. *N Engl J Med*. 2013;369:1317–1326.

41. White WB, Cannon CP, Heller SR, et al. Alogliptin after acute coronary syndrome in patients with type 2 diabetes. *N Engl J Med*. 2013;369:1327–1335.

42. Dormandy JA, Charbonnel B, Eckland DJ, et al. Secondary prevention of macrovascular events in patients with type 2 diabetes in the PROactive Study (PROspective pioglitAzone Clinical Trial In macroVascular Events): a randomised controlled trial. *Lancet*. 2005;366:1279–1289.

43. Zinman B, Lachin JM, Inzucchi SE. Empagliflozin, cardiovascular outcomes, and mortality in type 2 diabetes. *N Engl J Med*. 2016;374:1094.

44. Wanner C, Lachin JM, Inzucchi SE, et al. Empagliflozin and clinical outcomes in patients with type 2 diabetes, established cardiovascular disease and chronic kidney disease. *Circulation*. 2018;137(2):119–129.

45. Verma S, Mazer CD, Al-Omran M, et al. Cardiovascular outcomes and safety of empagliflozin in patients with type 2 diabetes mellitus and peripheral artery disease: a subanalysis of EMPA-REG OUTCOME. *Circulation*. 2018;137(4):405–407.

46. Inzucchi SE, Iliev H, Pfarr E, Zinman B. Empagliflozin and assessment of lower-limb amputations in the EMPA-REG OUTCOME Trial. *Diabetes Care*. 2018;41:e4–e5.

47. Neal B, Perkovic V, Matthews DR. Canagliflozin and cardiovascular and renal events in type 2 diabetes. *N Engl J Med*. 2017;377:2099.

48. Kosiborod M, Cavender MA, Fu AZ, et al. Lower risk of heart failure and death in patients initiated on sodium-glucose cotransporter-2 inhibitors versus other glucose-lowering drugs: the CVD-REAL Study (Comparative Effectiveness of Cardiovascular Outcomes in New Users of Sodium-Glucose Cotransporter-2 Inhibitors). *Circulation*. 2017;136:249–259.

49. United States Food and Drug Administration. *FDA drug safety communication: interim clinical trial results find increased risk of leg and foot amputations, mostly affecting the toes, with the diabetes medicine canagliflozin (Invokana, Invokamet); FDA to investigate*. http://www.fda.gov/Drugs/DrugSafety/ucm500965.htm; 2016. (Accessed August 27, 2018).

50. Udell JA, Zhong Y, Rush T, et al. Cardiovascular outcomes and risks after initiation of a sodium glucose co-transporter 2 inhibitor: results from the EASEL population-based cohort study (Evidence for Cardiovascular Outcomes With Sodium Glucose Cotransporter 2 Inhibitors in the Real World). *Circulation*. 2018;137(14):1450–1459.

51. Raz I, Mosenzon O, Bonaca MP, et al. DECLARE-TIMI 58: Participants' baseline characteristics. *Diabetes Obes Metab*. 2018;20(5):1102–1110.

52. Wiviott SD, Raz I, Bonaca MP, et al. The design and rationale for the Dapagliflozin Effect on Cardiovascular Events (DECLARE)-TIMI 58 Trial. *Am Heart J*. 2018;200:83–89.

53. Marso SP, Bain SC, Consoli A, et al. Semaglutide and cardiovascular outcomes in patients with type 2 diabetes. *N Engl J Med*. 2016;375:1834–1844.

54. Marso SP, Daniels GH, Brown-Frandsen K, et al. Liraglutide and cardiovascular outcomes in type 2 diabetes. *N Engl J Med*. 2016;375:311–322.

55. Randomised trial of cholesterol lowering in 4444 patients with coronary heart disease. the Scandinavian Simvastatin Survival Study (4S). *Lancet*. 1994;344:1383–1389.

56. Bulbulia R, Bowman L, Wallendszus K, et al. Randomized trial of the effects of cholesterol-lowering with simvastatin on peripheral vascular and other major vascular outcomes in 20,536 people with peripheral arterial disease and other high-risk conditions. *J Vasc Surg*. 2007;45:645–654. discussion 653-654.

57. Cannon CP, Blazing MA, Giugliano RP, et al. Ezetimibe added to statin therapy after acute coronary syndromes. *N Engl J Med*. 2015;372:2387–2397.

58. Sabatine MS, Giugliano RP, Pedersen TR. Evolocumab in patients with cardiovascular disease. *N Engl J Med*. 2017;377:787–788.

59. Ridker PM, Revkin J, Amarenco P, et al. Cardiovascular efficacy and safety of bococizumab in high-risk patients. *N Engl J Med*. 2017;376(16):1527–1539.

60. Schwartz GG, Bessac L, Berdan LG, et al. Effect of alirocumab, a monoclonal antibody to PCSK9, on long-term cardiovascular outcomes following acute coronary syndromes: rationale and design of the ODYSSEY outcomes trial. *Am Heart J*. 2014;168:682–689.

61. Giugliano RP, Pedersen TR, Park JG, et al. Clinical efficacy and safety of achieving very low LDL-cholesterol concentrations with the PCSK9 inhibitor evolocumab: a prespecified secondary analysis of the FOURIER trial. *Lancet*. 2017;390(10106):1962–1971.

62. BodenWE, Probstfield JL, Anderson T, et al. Niacin in patients with low HDL cholesterol levels receiving intensive statin therapy. *N Engl J Med*. 2011;365:2255–2267.

63. Kumbhani DJ, Steg PG, Cannon CP, et al. Statin therapy and long-term adverse limb outcomes in patients with peripheral artery disease: insights from the REACH registry. *Eur Heart J*. 2014;35:2864–2872.

64. Dosluoglu HH, Davari-Farid S, Pourafkari L, et al. Statin use is associated with improved overall survival without affecting patency and limb salvage rates following open or endovascular revascularization. *Vasc Med*. 2014;19:86–93.

65. Feringa HH, Karagiannis SE, van Waning VH, et al. The effect of intensified lipid-lowering therapy on long-term prognosis in patients with peripheral arterial disease. *J Vasc Surg*. 2007;45:936–943.

66. Aiello FA, Khan AA, Meltzer AJ, et al. Statin therapy is associated with superior clinical outcomes after endovascular treatment of critical limb ischemia. *J Vasc Surg*. 2012;55:371–379. discussion 380.

67. Stavroulakis K, Borowski M, Torsello G, et al. Association between statin therapy and amputation-free survival in patients with critical limb ischemia in the CRITISCH registry. *J Vasc Surg*. 2017;66(5):1534–1542.

68. Westin GG, Armstrong EJ, Bang H, et al. Association between statin medications and mortality, major adverse cardiovascular event, and amputation-free survival in patients with critical limb ischemia. *J Am Coll Cardiol*. 2014;63:682–690.

69. Rajamani K, Colman PG, Li LP, et al. Effect of fenofibrate on amputation events in people with type 2 diabetes mellitus (FIELD study): a prespecified analysis of a randomised controlled trial. *Lancet*. 2009;373:1780–1788.

70. Baigent C, Sudlow C, Collins R, Peto R. Collaborative meta-analysis of randomised trials of antiplatelet therapy for prevention of death, myocardial infarction, and stroke in high risk patients. *BMJ*. 2002;324:71–86.

71. Baigent C, Blackwell L, Collins R, et al. Aspirin in the primary and secondary prevention of vascular disease: collaborative meta-analysis of individual participant data from randomised trials. *Lancet*. 2009;373:1849–1860.

72. Berger JS, Krantz MJ, Kittelson JM, Hiatt WR. Aspirin for the prevention of cardiovascular events in patients with peripheral artery disease: a meta-analysis of randomized trials. *JAMA*. 2009;301:1909–1919.

73. Belch J, MacCuish A, Campbell I, et al. The prevention of progression of arterial disease and diabetes (POPADAD) trial: factorial randomised placebo controlled trial of aspirin and antioxidants in patients with diabetes and asymptomatic peripheral arterial disease. *BMJ*. 2008;337:a1840.

74. Fowkes FG, Price JF, Stewart MC, et al. Aspirin for prevention of cardiovascular events in a general population screened for a low ankle brachial index: a randomized controlled trial. *JAMA*. 2010;303:841–848.

75. Janzon L, Bergqvist D, Boberg J, et al. Prevention of myocardial infarction and stroke in patients with intermittent claudication; effects of ticlopidine. Results from STIMS, the Swedish Ticlopidine Multicentre Study. *J Intern Med*. 1990;227:301–308.

76. Bergqvist D, Almgren B, Dickinson JP. Reduction of requirement for leg vascular surgery during long-term treatment of claudicant patients with ticlopidine: results from the Swedish Ticlopidine Multicentre Study (STIMS). *Eur J Vasc Endovasc Surg*. 1995;10:69–76.

77. Gent M, Beaumont D, Blanchard J, et al. A randomised, blinded, trial of clopidogrel versus aspirin in patients at risk of ischaemic events (CAPRIE). CAPRIE Steering Committee. *Lancet*. 1996;348:1329–1339.

78. Hiatt WR, Fowkes FG, Heizer G, et al. Ticagrelor versus clopidogrel in symptomatic peripheral artery disease. *N Engl J Med*. 2017;376:32–40.

79. Bhatt DL, Fox KA, Hacke W, et al. Clopidogrel and aspirin versus aspirin alone for the prevention of atherothrombotic events. *N Engl J Med*. 2006;354:1706–1717.

80. Cacoub PP, Bhatt DL, Steg PG, et al. Patients with peripheral arterial disease in the CHARISMA trial. *Eur Heart J*. 2009;30:192–201.

81. Belch JJ, Dormandy J, Biasi GM, et al. Results of the randomized, placebo-controlled clopidogrel and acetylsalicylic acid in bypass surgery for peripheral arterial disease (CASPAR) trial. *J Vasc Surg.* 2010;52:825–833. 833.e1-2.

82. Morrow DA, Braunwald E, Bonaca MP, et al. Vorapaxar in the secondary prevention of atherothrombotic events. *N Engl J Med.* 2012;366:1404–1413.

83. Magnani G, Bonaca MP, Braunwald E, et al. Efficacy and safety of vorapaxar as approved for clinical use in the United States. *J Am Heart Assoc.* 2015;4:e001505.

84. Bonaca MP, Scirica BM, Creager MA, et al. Vorapaxar in patients with peripheral artery disease: results from TRA2{degrees}P-TIMI 50. *Circulation.* 2013;127:1522–1529. 1529e1-6.

85. Bonaca MP, Creager MA, Olin J, et al. Peripheral revascularization in patients with peripheral artery disease with vorapaxar: insights from the TRA 2 degrees P-TIMI 50 Trial. *JACC Cardiovasc Interv.* 2016;9:2157–2164.

86. Anand S, Yusuf S, Xie C, et al. Oral anticoagulant and antiplatelet therapy and peripheral arterial disease. *N Engl J Med.* 2007;357:217–227.

87. Mega JL, Braunwald E, Mohanavelu S, et al. Rivaroxaban versus placebo in patients with acute coronary syndromes (ATLAS ACS-TIMI 46): a randomised, double-blind, phase II trial. *Lancet.* 2009;374:29–38.

88. Mega JL, Braunwald E, Wiviott SD, et al. Rivaroxaban in patients with a recent acute coronary syndrome. *N Engl J Med.* 2012;366:9–19.

89. Eikelboom JW, Connolly SJ, Bosch J, et al. Rivaroxaban with or without aspirin in stable cardiovascular disease. *N Engl J Med.* 2017;377:1319–1330.

90. Anand SS, Bosch J, Eikelboom JW, et al. Rivaroxaban with or without aspirin in patients with stable peripheral or carotid artery disease: an international, randomised, double-blind, placebo-controlled trial. *Lancet.* 2018;391(10117):20–26.

91. Bonaca MP, Bhatt DL, Cohen M, et al. Long-term use of ticagrelor in patients with prior myocardial infarction. *N Engl J Med.* 2015;372:1791–1800.

92. Franzone A, Piccolo R, Gargiulo G, et al. Prolonged vs short duration of dual antiplatelet therapy after percutaneous coronary intervention in patients with or without peripheral artery disease: a subgroup analysis of the PRODIGY randomized clinical trial. *JAMA Cardiol.* 2016;1(7):795–803.

93. Hamburg NM, Balady GJ. Exercise rehabilitation in peripheral artery disease: functional impact and mechanisms of benefits. *Circulation.* 2011;123:87–97.

94. Stewart KJ, Hiatt WR, Regensteiner JG, Hirsch AT. Exercise training for claudication. *N Engl J Med.* 2002;347:1941–1951.

95. Fokkenrood HJ, Bendermacher BL, Lauret GJ, et al. Supervised exercise therapy versus non-supervised exercise therapy for intermittent claudication. *Cochrane Database Syst Rev.* 2013;8:CD005263.

96. Watson L, Ellis B, Leng GC. Exercise for intermittent claudication. *Cochrane Database Syst Rev.* 2008;4:CD000990.

97. McDermott MM, Liu K, Guralnik JM, et al. Home-based walking exercise intervention in peripheral artery disease: a randomized clinical trial. *JAMA.* 2013;310:57–65.

98. McDermott MM, Guralnik JM, Criqui MH, et al. Home-based walking exercise in peripheral artery disease: 12-month follow-up of the goals randomized trial. *J Am Heart Assoc.* 2014;3:e000711.

99. Gardner AW, Parker DE, Montgomery PS, Blevins SM. Step-monitored home exercise improves ambulation, vascular function, and inflammation in symptomatic patients with peripheral artery disease: a randomized controlled trial. *J Am Heart Assoc.* 2014;3:e001107.

100. McDermott MM, Kibbe M, Guralnik JM, et al. Comparative effectiveness study of self-directed walking exercise, lower extremity revascularization, and functional decline in peripheral artery disease. *J Vasc Surg.* 2013;57:990–996. e1.

101. Collins TC, Lunos S, Carlson T, et al. Effects of a home-based walking intervention on mobility and quality of life in people with diabetes and peripheral arterial disease: a randomized controlled trial. *Diabetes Care.* 2011;34:2174–2179.

102. Li Y, Li Z, Chang G, et al. Effect of structured home-based exercise on walking ability in patients with peripheral arterial disease: a meta-analysis. *Ann Vasc Surg.* 2015;29:597–606.

103. Murphy TP, Cutlip DE, Regensteiner JG, et al. Supervised exercise versus primary stenting for claudication resulting from aortoiliac peripheral artery disease: six-month outcomes from the claudication: exercise versus endoluminal revascularization (CLEVER) study. *Circulation.* 2012;125:130–139.

104. Pandey A, Banerjee S, Ngo C, et al. Comparative efficacy of endovascular revascularization versus supervised exercise training in patients with intermittent claudication: meta-analysis of randomized controlled trials. *JACC Cardiovasc Interv.* 2017;10:712–724.

105. Kohda N, Tani T, Nakayama S, et al. Effect of cilostazol, a phosphodiesterase III inhibitor, on experimental thrombosis in the porcine carotid artery. *Thromb Res.* 1999;96:261–268.

106. Reilly MP, Mohler 3rd ER. Cilostazol: treatment of intermittent claudication. *Ann Pharmacother.* 2001;35:48–56.

107. Thompson PD, Zimet R, Forbes WP, Zhang P. Meta-analysis of results from eight randomized, placebo-controlled trials on the effect of cilostazol on patients with intermittent claudication. *Am J Cardiol.* 2002;90:1314–1319.

108. Robless P, Mikhailidis DP, Stansby GP. Cilostazol for peripheral arterial disease. *Cochrane Database Syst Rev.* 2008;1:CD003748.

109. Pande RL, Hiatt WR, Zhang P, et al. A pooled analysis of the durability and predictors of treatment response of cilostazol in patients with intermittent claudication. *Vasc Med.* 2010;15:181–188.

110. Hiatt WR, Money SR, Brass EP. Long-term safety of cilostazol in patients with peripheral artery disease: the CASTLE study (Cilostazol: A Study in Long-term Effects). *J Vasc Surg.* 2008;47:330–336.

111. Rao KM, Simel DL, Cohen HJ, et al. Effects of pentoxifylline administration on blood viscosity and leukocyte cytoskeletal function in patients with intermittent claudication. *J Lab Clin Med.* 1990;115:738–744.

112. Creager MA, Pande RL, Hiatt WR. A randomized trial of iloprost in patients with intermittent claudication. *Vasc Med.* 2008;13:5–13.

113. Dawson DL, Cutler BS, Hiatt WR, et al. A comparison of cilostazol and pentoxifylline for treating intermittent claudication. *Am J Med.* 2000;109:523–530.

114. Oesterle A, Laufs U, Liao JK. Pleiotropic effects of statins on the cardiovascular system. *Circ Res.* 2017;120:229–243.

115. Mohler 3rd ER, Hiatt WR, Creager MA. Cholesterol reduction with atorvastatin improves walking distance in patients with peripheral arterial disease. *Circulation.* 2003;108:1481–1486.

116. Aronow WS, Nayak D, Woodworth S, Ahn C. Effect of simvastatin versus placebo on treadmill exercise time until the onset of intermittent claudication in older patients with peripheral arterial disease at six months and at one year after treatment. *Am J Cardiol.* 2003;92:711–712.

117. Mondillo S, Ballo P, Barbati R, et al. Effects of simvastatin on walking performance and symptoms of intermittent claudication in hypercholesterolemic patients with peripheral vascular disease. *Am J Med.* 2003;114:359–364.

118. Momsen AH, Jensen MB, Norager CB, et al. Drug therapy for improving walking distance in intermittent claudication: a systematic review and meta-analysis of robust randomised controlled studies. *Eur J Vasc Endovasc Surg.* 2009;38:463–474.

119. Vietto V, Franco JV, Saenz V, et al. Prostanoids for critical limb ischaemia. *Cochrane Database Syst Rev.* 2018;1:CD006544.

120. Mohler 3rd ER, Hiatt WR, Olin JW, et al. Treatment of intermittent claudication with beraprost sodium, an orally active prostaglandin I2 analogue: a double-blinded, randomized, controlled trial. *J Am Coll Cardiol.* 2003;41:1679–1686.

121. Lievre M, Morand S, Besse B, et al. Oral beraprost sodium, a prostaglandin I(2) analogue, for intermittent claudication: a double-blind, randomized, multicenter controlled trial. Beraprost et Claudication Intermittente (BERCI) Research Group. *Circulation.* 2000;102:426–431.

122. Prostanoids for chronic critical leg ischemia. A randomized, controlled, open-label trial with prostaglandin E1. The ICAI Study Group. Ischemia Cronica degli Arti Inferiori. *Ann Intern Med.* 1999;130:412–421.

123. Mazzone A, Di Salvo M, Mazzuca S, et al. Effects of iloprost on pain-free walking distance and clinical outcome in patients with severe stage IIb peripheral arterial disease: the FADOI 2bPILOT Study. *Eur J Clin Invest.* 2013;43:1163–1170.

124. Vitale V, Monami M, Mannucci E. Prostanoids in patients with peripheral arterial disease: a meta-analysis of placebo-controlled randomized clinical trials. *J Diabetes Complications.* 2016;30:161–166.

125. Hiatt WR, Creager MA, Amato A, Brass EP. Effect of propionyl-L-carnitine on a background of monitored exercise in patients with claudication secondary to peripheral artery disease. *J Cardiopulm Rehabil Prev.* 2011;31:125–132.

126. Ma A, Garland WT, Smith WB, et al. A pilot study of ranolazine in patients with intermittent claudication. *Int Angiol.* 2006;25:361–369.

127. Rigato M, Monami M, Fadini GP. Autologous cell therapy for peripheral arterial disease: systematic review and meta-analysis of randomized, nonrandomized, and noncontrolled studies. *Circ Res.* 2017;120:1326–1340.

128. Lasala GP, Minguell JJ. Vascular disease and stem cell therapies. *Br Med Bull.* 2011;98:187–197.

129. Idei N, Soga J, Hata T, et al. Autologous bone-marrow mononuclear cell implantation reduces long-term major amputation risk in patients with critical limb ischemia: a comparison of atherosclerotic peripheral arterial disease and Buerger disease. *Circ Cardiovasc Interv.* 2011;4:15–25.

130. Lasala GP, Silva JA, Minguell JJ. Therapeutic angiogenesis in patients with severe limb ischemia by transplantation of a combination stem cell product. *J Thorac Cardiovasc Surg.* 2012;144:377–382.

131. Ruiz-Salmeron R, de la Cuesta-Diaz A, Constantino-Bermejo M, et al. Angiographic demonstration of neoangiogenesis after intra-arterial infusion of autologous bone marrow mononuclear cells in diabetic patients with critical limb ischemia. *Cell Transplant.* 2011;20:1629–1639.

132. Moazzami K, Majdzadeh R, Nedjat S. Local intramuscular transplantation of autologous mononuclear cells for critical lower limb ischaemia. *Cochrane Database Syst Rev.* 2011;12:CD008347.

133. Moazzami K, Moazzami B, Roohi A, et al. Local intramuscular transplantation of autologous mononuclear cells for critical lower limb ischaemia. *Cochrane Database Syst Rev.* 2014;12:CD008347.

134. Perin EC, Murphy MP, March KL, et al. Evaluation of cell therapy on exercise performance and limb perfusion in peripheral artery disease: the CCTRN PACE Trial (Patients With Intermittent Claudication Injected With ALDH Bright Cells). *Circulation.* 2017;135:1417–1428.

135. Wang SK, Green LA, Motaganahalli RL, et al. Rationale and design of the MarrowStim PAD Kit for the Treatment of Critical Limb Ischemia in Subjects with Severe Peripheral Arterial Disease (MOBILE) trial investigating autologous bone marrow cell therapy for critical limb ischemia. *J Vasc Surg.* 2017;65:1850–1857. e2.

136. McDermott MM, Ferrucci L, Tian L, et al. Effect of granulocyte-macrophage colony-stimulating factor with or without supervised exercise on walking performance in patients with peripheral artery disease: the PROPEL randomized clinical trial. *JAMA.* 2017;318:2089–2098.

137. Lindeman JHN, Zwaginga JJ, Kallenberg-Lantrua G, et al. No clinical benefit of intramuscular delivery of bone marrow-derived mononuclear cells in nonreconstructable peripheral arterial disease: results of a phase-III randomized-controlled trial. *Ann Surg.* 2018;268:756–761.

138. Shimamura M, Nakagami H, Taniyama Y, Morishita R. Gene therapy for peripheral arterial disease. *Expert Opin Biol Ther.* 2014;14:1175–1184.

139. Belch J, Hiatt WR, Baumgartner I, et al. Effect of fibroblast growth factor NV1FGF on amputation and death: a randomised placebo-controlled trial of gene therapy in critical limb ischaemia. *Lancet.* 2011;377:1929–1937.

140. Lederman RJ, Mendelsohn FO, Anderson RD, et al. Therapeutic angiogenesis with recombinant fibroblast growth factor-2 for intermittent claudication (the TRAFFIC study): a randomised trial. *Lancet.* 2002;359:2053–2058.

141. Comerota AJ, Throm RC, Miller KA, et al. Naked plasmid DNA encoding fibroblast growth factor type 1 for the treatment of end-stage unreconstructible lower extremity ischemia: preliminary results of a phase I trial. *J Vasc Surg.* 2002;35:930–936.

142. Nikol S, Baumgartner I, Van Belle E, et al. Therapeutic angiogenesis with intramuscular NV1FGF improves amputation-free survival in patients with critical limb ischemia. *Mol Ther.* 2008;16:972–978.

143. Powell RJ, Simons M, Mendelsohn FO, et al. Results of a double-blind, placebo-controlled study to assess the safety of intramuscular injection of hepatocyte growth factor plasmid to improve limb perfusion in patients with critical limb ischemia. *Circulation.* 2008;118:58–65.

144. Creager MA, Olin JW, Belch JJ, et al. Effect of hypoxia-inducible factor-1alpha gene therapy on walking performance in patients with intermittent claudication. *Circulation.* 2011;124:1765–1773.

145. Hammer A, Steiner S. Gene therapy for therapeutic angiogenesis in peripheral arterial disease—a systematic review and meta-analysis of randomized, controlled trials. *Vasa.* 2013;42:331–339.

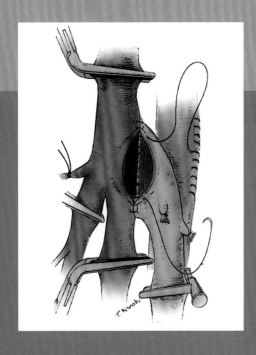

第20章
外周动脉疾病的腔内治疗

　　患者和病变的选择标准包括解剖标准和功能标准，解剖标准涉及病变的形态、器械通过的难易度和入路的选择。功能标准主要是患者的临床症状，如间歇性跛行、严重肢体缺血（静息痛、溃疡、坏疽）或急性肢体缺血。腔内治疗的技术考量：术前需对患者全身状况和病变进行全面评估，术前用药主要是阿司匹林；术中技术要点包括抗凝、血管入路和导丝、球囊、支架等器械的选择和准备。腔内治疗的临床结果：主髂动脉病变推荐一期支架植入，其中球囊扩张式支架适用于髂动脉开口病变或有明显弹性回缩的病变，自膨式支架更适用于髂动脉直径差较大和扭曲的病变。覆膜支架对于泛大西洋学会联盟（Trans-Atlantic Inter-Society Consensus，TASC）分级C、D级复杂病变的长期疗效较金属裸支架更有优势。股腘动脉的腔内治疗方式有球囊扩张、金属裸支架、覆膜支架、药物涂层球囊、药物洗脱支架、腔内照射、斑块切除、激光、切割球囊、冷冻疗法等，应根据病变的性质、长度、部位、通过方式等因素进行综合考量。膝下动脉的腔内治疗主要针对重症肢体缺血患者，以缓解疼痛、促进溃疡愈合、预防大截肢、改善生活质量、提高生存率。治疗方法主要是球囊扩张加补救支架。膝下动脉支架主要选择药物洗脱支架，其疗效已为多个临床研究数据所证实。血管再生治疗在不具备腔内治疗条件时可作为膝下严重缺血患者的一种治疗选择。

包俊敏

Endovascular Treatment of Peripheral Artery Disease

Christopher J. White

The concept of percutaneous catheter-based peripheral vascular intervention (PVI) was first described by Charles Dotter and further advanced with the development of balloon dilation catheters by Andreas Gruentzig. Catheter-based revascularization has largely replaced conventional open surgery as the treatment of first choice in selected patients treated for lower-extremity ischemia.[1]

No single specialty program (cardiology, radiology, or surgery) offered training that satisfied the entire skill set needed to perform peripheral endovascular intervention (Table 20.1). Recognition of this unmet need for a trained cadre of clinicians to care for patients with peripheral artery disease (PAD) prompted the development of a core cardiology training symposium (COCATS-4) to codify the necessary cardiology fellowship training.[2,3]

The Society for Cardiovascular Angiography and Interventions (SCAI) published revised Appropriate Use Criteria (AUC) for endovascular therapy (EVT) for atherosclerotic PAD.[4] The peripheral AUC were developed to assist clinicians' decision making, to improve patients' understanding regarding relative risks and benefits of a procedure, and to guide future research. Clinical scenarios were described in which catheter-based intervention was classified as "appropriate," "may be appropriate," or "rarely appropriate," incorporating the best clinical and scientific evidence, cost-effectiveness data, and the consensus of experts.

PATIENT AND LESION SELECTION CRITERIA

Indications

Anatomical and Functional Criteria

Patient selection for catheter-based vascular intervention depends upon both anatomical and functional criteria (Table 20.2). Anatomical lesion criteria include the ability to gain vascular access, a reasonable likelihood of crossing the lesion with a guidewire, and the expectation that a therapeutic catheter can be advanced across the target lesion. Vascular access site complications following catheter-based procedures are preferentially treated with percutaneous therapy (Fig. 20.1).[5] Patients with hypotension and a high suspicion of bleeding after common femoral artery (CFA) access require urgent diagnostic angiography from the contralateral femoral artery to determine the bleeding site. Rapid identification of the bleeding site may provide an opportunity for lifesaving hemostasis with balloon tamponade.

Functional criteria to select patients for peripheral endovascular revascularization typically include lifestyle or vocation-limiting symptoms of claudication, critical limb ischemia (CLI; rest pain, non-healing ulcers, or gangrene), or acute limb ischemia. Asymptomatic patients with anatomically suitable iliac artery lesions are not considered candidates for PVI unless it is to facilitate vascular access, such as for intra-aortic counterpulsation balloon placement or for vascular access to perform coronary intervention.

Patients with lifestyle-limiting symptoms of claudication, and without heart failure, should first be treated with pharmacological therapy, cilostazol 100 mg bid, and structured exercise training before revascularization is attempted. If exercise training and pharmacotherapy are not effective, if patients are intolerant of cilostazol or cannot be treated with the drug because of heart failure (black box warning), or if a supervised exercise program is unavailable, an attempt at endovascular intervention is appropriate. In general, patients with claudication rarely progress to limb loss, so endovascular revascularization is reserved for those patients with favorable anatomy who either fail conservative therapy and have lifestyle-limiting symptoms, or who have vocation-limiting symptoms. The therapeutic goals for claudicants are symptom relief, increased walking distance, plus improved functionality and quality of life (QOL). For this reason, the durability of patency after the procedure is performed becomes important.

Patients with CLI or limb-threatening ischemia (gangrene, non-healing ulcer, or rest pain) are candidates for urgent revascularization. When considering a patient with CLI for revascularization, it is important to remember that multilevel disease (iliac, femoral, and tibial) is likely to be present and that simply improving "inflow" without addressing the more distal vascular lesions or runoff vessels may fail to solve the clinical problem. Patients with CLI typically have more extensive disease than claudicants and require urgent revascularization to prevent tissue loss (see Table 20.2).[1,6]

The prognosis for patients presenting with CLI is poor.[1] Those with tobacco abuse and/or diabetes are 10 times more likely to require amputation. Patients with CLI tend to be older, with almost 50% of patients older than 80 years undergoing amputations. Within 3 months of presentation, 12% will require an amputation, and 9% will die; the 1-year mortality rate is 22%. Anatomy suitable for EVT is often present in one or more below-knee vessels. Therapy should be designed to restore pulsatile straight-line flow to the distal part of the limb, with as low a procedural morbidity as possible. The guiding principle is that less blood flow is required to maintain tissue integrity than to heal a wound, so restenosis does not usually result in recurrent CLI unless there has been repeated injury to the limb. Therefore, the emphasis is less on long-term vessel patency and more on limb salvage.

TABLE 20.1   Required Skill Elements for Optimal Peripheral Vascular Intervention

Skill Element	Description
Cognitive	Extensive knowledge of vascular disease, including natural history, pathophysiology, diagnostic methods, and treatment alternatives
Technical	Competence in both diagnostic angiography and interventional techniques, such as the use and selection of balloons, guidewires, stents, and emboli protection devices
Clinical	Ability to manage inpatients, interpret laboratory tests, obtain informed consent, assess risk/benefit ratio, and admitting privileges

TABLE 20.2   Classification of Peripheral Arterial Disease: Fontaine's Stages and Rutherford's Categories

FONTAINE		RUTHERFORD		
Stage	Clinical	Grade	Category	Clinical
I	Asymptomatic	0	0	Asymptomatic
IIa	Mild claudication	I	1	Mild claudication
IIb	Moderate to severe claudication	I	2	Moderate claudication
		I	3	Severe claudication
III	Rest pain	II	4	Rest pain
IV	Ulceration or gangrene	III	5	Minor tissue loss
		IV	6	Ulceration or gangrene

Modified from Norgren L, Hiatt WR, Dormandy JA, et al. Inter-Society Consensus for the management of peripheral arterial disease (TASC II). *J Vasc Surg.* 2007;45 Suppl S:S5–S67.

The Bypass versus Angioplasty in Severe Ischaemia of the Leg (BASIL) trial was a multicenter randomized trial comparing an initial strategy of balloon angioplasty (percutaneous transluminal angioplasty [PTA]) to open surgery in 452 patients with CLI.[7] The primary outcome was time to amputation or death (amputation-free survival). Surgery had significantly greater length of stay and needed significantly more intensive care unit (ICU) care than did those allocated angioplasty. The cost was about one-third lower for patients assigned an angioplasty-first strategy. Beyond 2 years there was a significantly reduced hazard in amputation-free survival (adjusted hazard ratio [HR] 0.37 [95% confidence interval [CI]: 0.17–0.77], $P = .008$) and all-cause mortality (HR 0.34 [95% CI: 0.17–0.71], $P = .004$) for surgery relative to angioplasty. For patients with limb-threatening lower extremity ischemia and an estimated life expectancy of **<2 years**, or in patients in whom an autogenous vein conduit is not available, balloon angioplasty is reasonable to perform (when possible) as the initial procedure to improve distal blood flow. For patients with limb-threatening ischemia and an estimated life expectancy of **>2 years**, bypass surgery (when possible) if an autogenous vein conduit is available, is reasonable to perform as the initial treatment to improve distal blood flow.

It is very likely that major advances in endovascular technology, including drug-coated balloons (DCB) and drug-eluting stents (DES) will have further improved the outcomes of endo-first treated patients relative to conventional bypass surgery. The ongoing BEST-CLI trial is expected to help inform our decision making.[8]

Contraindications

Relative contraindications to catheter-based PVI include lesions likely to generate atheroemboli, and lesions that are not dilatable. Other relative contraindications include any other instances in which risks of the procedure seem to outweigh the potential benefits. For example, patients unlikely to be independent or ambulatory, and the risk of contrast-induced nephropathy in a patient with severe renal impairment, must be weighed against expected functional improvement.

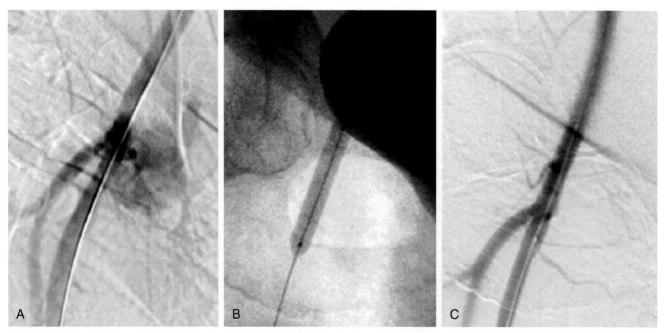

Fig. 20.1 Access site complication with bleeding (A) successfully tamponaded with balloon inflation (B), and final angiogram showing hemostasis (C).

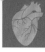

TECHNICAL AND PROCEDURAL CONSIDERATIONS

Pre-procedure
General Measures

Prior to performing peripheral endovascular intervention, the patient should have a complete cardiovascular evaluation, with specific attention directed to the status of atherosclerotic risk factors. Atherosclerosis is a systemic disease, and appropriate risk-factor modification (tobacco-cessation counseling, treatment of lipids to target values), screening tests for cardiovascular diseases, and optimization of medical therapy should be performed.

Prior to performing lower-extremity endovascular intervention, it is necessary to objectively determine the patient's functional status. A history, physical examination, and appropriate noninvasive testing should be obtained prior to planning peripheral endovascular revascularization. If the patient is ambulatory, a rest and exercise ankle-brachial index (ABI) should be measured, and pulse volume recordings (PVRs) should be performed. Other noninvasive modalities, such as vascular ultrasound, or alternative imaging modalities, such as magnetic resonance angiography (MRA) or computed tomographic angiography (CTA), may be helpful to resolve conflicting data and are used at the discretion of the physician (Fig. 20.2). When planning lower-extremity revascularization, status of the inflow and outflow vessels relative to the target lesion must be visualized angiographically. This is usually done with invasive diagnostic angiography, but in selected patients, MRA or CTA may be very useful.

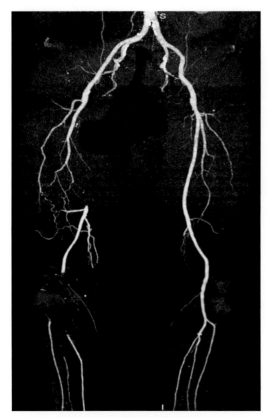

Fig. 20.2 Computed Tomographic Angiogram of Lower-Extremity Vasculature. There is occlusion of arterial segments of the right femoral, popliteal, and tibial segments.

Premedication

The only premedication requirement for peripheral endovascular intervention is aspirin therapy (81 to 325 mg daily). The use of other antiplatelet agents is optional since there is no evidence that their use improves procedural success or decreases complications. If the patient is intolerant to aspirin, a thienopyridine drug would be appropriate.[1] There is no objective evidence supporting the benefit of dual antiplatelet therapy after EVT or following peripheral vascular stent placement.

Procedure
Anticoagulation

There is no standard for anticoagulation therapy, except to state that intravenous unfractionated heparin (UFH), in a dose up to 5000 International Units, is commonly used to achieve an activated clotting time (ACT) of 250 to 300 seconds. At present, there is no evidence that the use of glycoprotein (GP)-IIb/IIIa platelet receptor antagonists, low-molecular-weight heparins, or antithrombins improve procedural efficacy or safety for PVI.

Vascular Access

The first step to ensure a successful procedure is to select the most appropriate vascular access. The majority of peripheral endovascular interventions can be performed from multiple arterial access sites (i.e., radial, brachial, femoral, or popliteal arteries). However, cases occasionally require a specific access to achieve a successful result. Consequently, familiarity with a variety of vascular access sites and techniques is one of the most important components of the basic skill set. The ability to gain both retrograde and antegrade common femoral access is a required skill for the peripheral vascular interventionalist. An infrapopliteal target lesion may be best approached with antegrade femoral access, whereas a proximal superficial femoral artery (SFA) lesion may require a contralateral retrograde femoral approach. Occasionally, bilateral retrograde femoral artery access is desirable—for example, when treating a common iliac bifurcation lesion. Finally, there will be times when the antegrade approach fails and distal tibial access is required for a retrograde approach to an occlusion.

Equipment Choices
Guidewires

Smaller catheters with lower crossing profiles, smaller sheath sizes, and increased flexibility for the smallest 0.014-inch systems, are balanced against the increased support and pushability of the larger-profile 0.035-inch systems. It is most common that 0.014-inch systems are used for below-knee intervention where the vessels are smaller, compared to the 0.035-inch systems used for the larger balloons and stents placed in the iliac vessels. It is recommended that the interventional laboratory be stocked with several redundant lines of equipment to allow for flexibility in the approach to difficult or complex lesions. In general, the lowest profile system within the smallest vascular access sheath should be used.

The use of coated "glidewires" should be carefully restricted to instances when their unique properties are necessary because these wires are more difficult to control than conventional guidewires and are prone to vascular perforation. Their lack of a "transition point" makes them ideal for negotiating abrupt angles and crossing occlusions. Ideally, once they have crossed the occlusion it is wise to exchange this wire, which is more difficult to manage, for a safer and more controllable wire.

Balloon Catheters

A wide variety of monorail and over-the-wire balloon catheters are available that are suitable for dilating lower-extremity lesions. A pressure manometer is recommended to monitor balloon inflation pressure. Although no optimal inflation pressure or duration has been determined, it is generally recommended that the balloon be inflated with adequate pressure to ensure full expansion of the lesion.

Stents

The two primary categories of stents are balloon expandable (BE) and self-expanding (SE). Both types may be covered with material. BE stents can be deployed with more precision than SE stents, although there is some shortening associated with their expansion. SE stents resist permanent deformation and are elastic. Their flexible nature allows them to be delivered in longer lengths, and they will fit themselves to a tapering artery. SE stents may be made of nitinol or a stainless steel alloy. At this time, there is no evidence that either material is associated with any safety or efficacy advantage.[9]

Adjunctive Devices

Other adjunctive devices, such as laser catheters, atherectomy catheters (rotational and directional), brachytherapy catheters, cryotherapy balloons, and cutting balloons have been developed, tested, and aggressively marketed. With the possible exception of the brachytherapy devices and laser angioplasty for managing in-stent restenosis (see below), there is no comparative evidence that these adjunctive devices bring any added value, efficacy, or increased safety over balloons and stents.

CLINICAL OUTCOMES

Aortoiliac Vessels

The CLEVER (Claudication: Exercise Versus Endoluminal Revascularization) trial randomized EVT, optimal medical therapy (OMT), and supervised exercise therapy (SET).[10,11] The change in peak walking time at the 6-month follow-up (the primary endpoint)

was greatest for SET, intermediate for EVT, and least with OMT, whereas patient-reported QOL was better with EVT than SET, and was least with OMT. However, at 18 months the improvement in both peak-walking time and patient-reported QOL and was not different between SET and EVT.

The Endovascular Revascularization and Supervised Exercise (ERASE) for Peripheral Artery Disease and Intermittent Claudication trialed randomized patients with aortoiliac and/or femoral-popliteal artery disease to receive EVT plus SET, or SET alone.[12] Those who received both had greater improvement in walking distance and health-related QOL compared with those who received only SET. These trials support SET as an effective alternative to revascularization, but indicate that combining SET with EVT, in the presence of guideline-directed medical therapy, may represent the best option overall.

The current best practice for iliac revascularization favors an endovascular first strategy (Fig. 20.3). This recommendation is based upon the morbidity and mortality associated with open surgery in patients with significant comorbidity, and the excellent outcomes available with current endovascular techniques. In a large single-center registry of 505 iliac stent procedures, the technical success rate was 98%, the 8-year primary stent patency rate was 74%, and the secondary patency rate was 84%.[13] In a 10-year iliac stent patency study, common iliac artery (CIA) lesions had greater long-term patency than external iliac artery (EIA) lesions.[14]

There is uncertainty regarding the most efficacious method of EVT between "provisional stent placement," which is the selective use of stents only when balloon dilation has failed or is suboptimal, and "primary stent placement," which is the practice of deploying a stent regardless of the balloon result. The Dutch Iliac Stent Trial demonstrated that selective iliac artery stenting achieved an equivalent hemodynamic result compared to primary stenting. Translesional pressure gradients after primary stent placement (5.8 ± 4.7 mm Hg) were significantly lower than after balloon angioplasty alone (8.9 ± 6.8 mm Hg), but not after provisional stenting (5.9 ± 3.6 mm Hg) in the PTA group.[15]

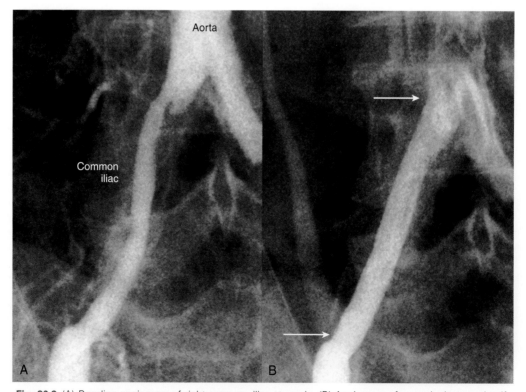

Fig. 20.3 (A) Baseline angiogram of right common iliac stenosis. (B) Angiogram after angioplasty and self-expanding stent *(arrows)*.

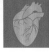

The procedural success rate, defined as a postprocedural gradient less than 10 mm Hg, revealed no difference between the two treatment strategies, (primary stenting = 81% vs. PTA plus provisional stenting = 89%). By employing a provisional stenting strategy in the iliac artery, stent placement was avoided in 63% of lesions. After 5 years of follow-up, the selective stent placement strategy had greater symptomatic improvement compared with primary stent placement, but there was no difference in patency rates, ABI, and QOL between groups.[16,17]

Aortoiliac artery primary stent placement is supported by a meta-analysis, which looked at more than 2000 patients.[18] Procedural success was higher in the primary stent group, and there was a 43% reduction in 4-year failures for aortoiliac stent placement compared to balloon angioplasty alone. Advantages of primary stent placement include efficient and reliable vascular reconstruction, minimizing concern over abrupt occlusion. Direct stenting minimizes the technical challenges of determining translesional pressure gradients and the need to administer vasodilator medications. The current American College of Cardiology/American Heart Association (ACC/AHA) guideline document supports primary stenting of the common and EIAs with a class I recommendation (Level of Evidence B).[1]

BE or SE stents were compared in a study of 660 patients with Rutherford Classification 1–4, which demonstrated that the 1-year primary stent restenosis rate was 6.1% after SE versus 14.9% after BE stents (P = .006).[19] Usually, BE stents are chosen for ostial lesions where precise placement is a priority, or when significant recoil is anticipated, while SE stents more readily contour to tapering and tortuous vessels. While DES and DCB have not been evaluated in iliac arteries, in highly selected cases, they may be useful in an appropriately sized vessel with in-stent restenosis.[20]

The COvered versus Balloon Expandable Stent Trial (COBEST) trial did not find a difference for binary restenosis or freedom from occlusion at 18 months between covered and bare-metal stents (BMS).[21] However, outcomes up to 5 years were more favorable for covered stents in complex lesions (TASC C and D).[22] Yet, a meta-analysis did not show a patency advantage for iliac artery covered stents, but there was a higher ABI and a lower reintervention rate.[23]

Femoral-Popliteal Vessels

Angioplasty and Bare-Metal Stent Placement

Comparative outcomes data in femoral-popliteal (FP) artery disease are available for guideline-directed medical therapy, exercise, balloon angioplasty, stents, brachytherapy, and laser angioplasty. SE stents are preferred in this location because of the risk of stent compression and the torsion and flexion of the vessels. As mentioned above, the ERASE for Peripheral Artery Disease and Intermittent Claudication trial demonstrated greater improvement in walking distance and health-related QOL for combined SET plus EVT compared with SET alone.[12]

The goals of therapy for patients with PAD are driven by the severity of the patient's clinical condition, and by the anatomic features and distribution of the vascular disease.

All PAD patients should be treated with guideline-directed medical therapy, including smoking cessation, lipid lowering, diabetes and hypertension treatment according to current national treatment guidelines, and antiplatelet therapy.[3] The clinical objective in treating a patient who is functionally impaired due to chronic stable limb ischemia, claudication, after failing cilostazol and exercise therapy, is durable relief of vocation or lifestyle limiting symptoms. For patients with chronic CLI, the goal is limb salvage with urgent revascularization of the affected extremity. Comparative data are notably absent for debulking devices (e.g., directional atherectomy, orbital atherectomy) and specialty catheters (e.g., cutting balloons and cryoplasty) despite their prominent position in the marketplace.

For CFA lesions, surgical endarterectomy has historically been the treatment of choice.[24] However a large pooled analysis (n = 1014) of CFA procedures from the Vascular Quality Initiative, demonstrate low procedural morbidity with EVT.[25] The Endovascular Versus Open Repair of the Common Femoral Artery (TECCO) trial compared surgery versus EVT in de novo CFA lesions, showing a significant advantage of EVT with a lower rate of 30-day morbid events and a similar 2-year patency rate.[26]

There have been three randomized controlled trials comparing primary stenting to balloon angioplasty with bailout stenting (provisional stenting).[27-29] Lesion length and complexity accounted for increased restenosis rates for the balloon angioplasty groups, but not for stent placement (Fig. 20.4). Synthesizing these results, the data suggest that longer FP lesions (≥7 cm) are better approached with a strategy of primary stenting, whereas more discrete lesions (<4 cm) do well with a provisional stenting strategy in which balloon angioplasty is given an opportunity to stand alone (Table 20.3).

Covered Stents

The Viabahn stent graft (W.L. Gore, Flagstaff, AZ) has demonstrated satisfactory results for longer FP lesions and higher complexity.[30] A 1-year follow-up of randomized PAD patients with long FP lesions failed to show a significantly better primary patency rate for covered stents (HR 70.9% [95% CI: 0.58–0.80]) versus BMS (HR 55.1% [95% CI: 0.41–0.67] (log-rank test P = .11); however, for lesions >20 cm the patency rate was significantly better in covered stent patients 71.3% vs. BMS 36.8%; P = .01). The 24-month primary patency rates were significantly better in the covered stent (63.1%, 95 % CI: 0.52–0.76) compared to the BMS group (41.2 %, 95 % CI: 0.29–0.57; log rank P = .04); however, clinical outcomes, such as improvement according to Rutherford categories, ABI, and walking distance—according to the Walking Impairment Questionnaire—were not different.[31]

Drug-Eluting Balloons

There have been multiple randomized trials published with three commercially available DCB (Lutonix [Bard Lutonix, New Hope, MN]; IN.PACT [Medtronic Vascular, Santa Rosa, CA]; and Stellarex [Spectranetics Corp., Colorado Springs, CO]) demonstrating superior patency compared to conventional devices. It is unlikely there is a "class effect" due to the different characteristics of the individual DCB devices with paclitaxel coating densities from 2 to 3.5 µg/mm^2 and diverse excipients—polysorbate and sorbitol, urea and polyethylene glycol—so that each device must be considered on its own merits.[32]

The IN.PACT SFA (Randomized Trial of IN.PACT Admiral Drug Eluting Balloon vs. Standard PTA for the Treatment of SFA and Proximal Popliteal Arterial Disease) trial randomized a DCB to an uncoated PTA balloon in patients with FP PAD (mean lesion length of 8.94 ± 4.89 cm). The DCB group had higher primary patency (82.2% vs. 52.4%; P < .001) at 12 months and a very low rate of clinically driven target lesion revascularization (TLR) (2.4% in the DCB arm vs. 20.6% in the PTA arm; P < .001).[33] The patency advantage without a safety signal has persisted to the 2-year follow-up for the DCB compared with PTA (78.9% vs. 50.1%; P < .001) and with lower rates of clinically driven TLR (9.1% vs. 28.3% (P < .001), respectively.[34]

The LEVANT (Lutonix Paclitaxel-Coated Balloon for the Prevention of Femoropopliteal Restenosis) I and II trials, used a different, lower-dose, paclitaxel DCB. Both LEVANT studies confirmed the safety profile of this DCB and demonstrated improved patency at 12 months compared to PTA alone (65.2% vs. 52.6%; P = .02). The proportion of patients free from primary safety events was 83.9% with the DCB and 79.0% with uncoated PTA (P = .005 for noninferiority).[35]

331

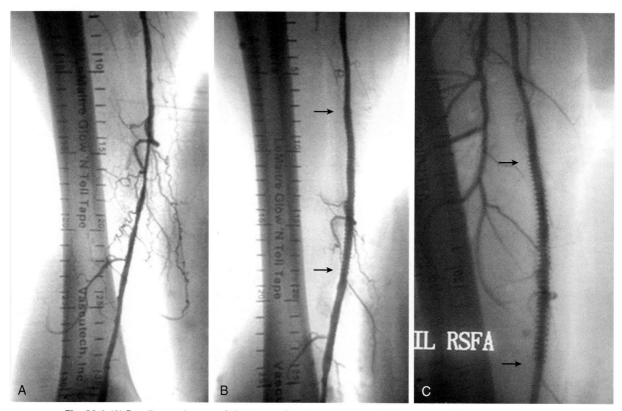

Fig. 20.4 (A) Baseline angiogram of distal superficial femoral artery *(SFA)* stenosis. (B) Post-stent placement *(between arrows)*. (C) Six-month follow-up with patent SFA stent segment.

TABLE 20.3 Relationship of Lesion Length to Restenosis with Stents and Balloons

	Schillinger	Krankenberg
Stent	Guidant	Bard
Lesion length	101 mm	45 mm
Stent restenosis	36.7%	31.7%
PTA restenosis	63.5%	38.6%[a]

[a]$P = .004$.

PTA, Percutaneous transluminal angioplasty.
Data from Schillinger M, Sabeti S, Loewe C, et al. Balloon angioplasty versus implantation of nitinol stents in the superficial femoral artery. *N Engl J Med.* 2006;354:1879–1888; and Krankenberg H, Schluter M, Steinkamp HJ, et al. Nitinol stent implantation versus percutaneous transluminal angioplasty in superficial femoral artery lesions up to 10 cm in length: the Femoral Artery Stenting Trial (FAST). *Circulation.* 2007;116:285–292.

The third DCB to achieve US Food and Drug Administration approval for use in de novo and restenotic FP lesions was the Stellarex DCB,[36] which has a paclitaxel dose of 2 μg/mm² and a proprietary polyethylene glycol excipient. A U.S.-based trial compared this DCB to PTA in 300 patients. Restenosis rates (23.7% vs. 42.2%, $P = .003$) and clinically driven TLR were lower (7.9% vs. 16.8%, $P = .023$) in the DCB group compared with the PTA group at 12 months.[37]

The 5-year follow-up of the THUNDER (Local Taxan With Short Time Contact for Reduction of Restenosis in Distal Arteries) trial demonstrated a TLR rate (21% vs. 56%; $P = .0005$) favoring DCB treatment over PTA alone, with no signs of drug-related local vessel abnormalities.[38] The current data suggest that DCB are cost-effective therapy. A formal analysis based on the 2-year results suggests a 70% to 80% likelihood that the DCB is an economically attractive strategy.[39,40]

Drug-Eluting Stents

The Zilver PTX (Cook Medical, Bloomington, IN) continues to show promise for the SE DES with 5-year data from the randomized trial demonstrating continued safety and clinical durability in comparison with PTA.[41] This trial had a two-stage randomization with initial randomization to DES ($n = 236$) or PTA ($n = 238$). Patients who were initially randomized to PTA ($n = 238$) and experienced flow-limiting dissections and/or recoil requiring stenting were then secondarily randomized to provisional BMS ($n = 59$) or DES ($n = 61$). The remaining 118 patients (not randomized to DES or BMS) were in the standard care group. At 5 years, DES showed a significant clinical benefit compared to PTA alone for freedom from persistent or worsening symptoms of ischemia (79.8% vs. 59.3%, $P < .01$), patency (66.4% vs. 43.4%, $P < .01$), and freedom from TLR (83.1% vs. 67.6%, $P < .01$).

In patients who did undergo a second randomization to either DES or BMS, there was a sustained benefit of DES. At 5 years, the provisional DES recipients, when compared to the BMS group, had improved clinical benefit (81.8% vs. 63.8%, $P = .02$), patency (72.4% vs. 53.0%, $P = .03$), and freedom from TLR (84.9% vs. 71.6%, $P = .06$). These results represent a >40% relative risk reduction in restenosis and TLR through 5 years for the DES group overall in comparison with standard care, and for provisional DES in comparison with provisional BMS.

Brachytherapy

Adjunctive endovascular brachytherapy (EBT) with an iridium-192 source, with a prescribed dose of 12 to 14 Gy, compared to PTA alone for the treatment of de novo long-segment stenoses of the femoral artery, has a delaying effect on the occurrence of restenosis.[42,43] In one study, there appeared to be an early restenosis benefit for the EBT plus PTA group; however, at the 5-year follow-up, there was "catch-up," and the recurrence rate was equal (72.5%) in both groups.[43] Brachytherapy has greater efficacy in restenotic lesions compared with de novo lesions.[44-46] A novel approach has been to deliver external beam irradiation to de novo femoral artery lesions after PTA. At the 1-year follow-up, there was a significant benefit for patients treated with 14 Gy in a single treatment session compared with a control group and a group who received lower Gy doses; however, in a study following BMS stenting of de novo lesions the 2-year patency results after external beam delivery of 24 Gy showed no benefit for brachytherapy in reducing restenosis.[47,48]

Atherectomy

Successive generations of atherectomy catheters have failed to demonstrate any consistent clinical benefit over less-expensive conventional therapies.[49-51] Comparative studies are very few and generally they are small, inconclusive trials, thereby leaving us with noncomparative data from self-reported registries that are subject to bias. There are safety concerns regarding the incidence of distal embolization and perforation.[52] Despite the lack of objective evidence of superior efficacy, there is evidence that the generous reimbursement for in-office atherectomy is driving increased utilization.[53]

Laser-Assisted Angioplasty

Laser-assisted angioplasty does not appear to add any benefit to conventional EVT for de novo peripheral arterial lesions.[54,55] The Peripheral Excimer Laser Angioplasty (PELA) trial randomized 251 patients to either PTA or laser-assisted PTA in patients with claudication and a total femoral occlusion. There was no difference in clinical events or patency rates at 1-year follow-up.[56]

The Excimer Laser Randomized Controlled Study for Treatment of Femoropopliteal In-Stent Restenosis (EXCITE-ISR) trial randomized 250 patients to excimer laser atherectomy (ELA) plus PTA versus PTA alone for FP ISR.[57] The 6-month freedom from TLR of 73.5% (ELA-PTA) versus 51.8% (PTA) ($P < .005$), and 30-day major adverse event rates were 5.8% versus 20.5% ($P < .001$), respectively. Overall, ELA+PTA was associated with a 52% reduction in TLR for the treatment of FP ISR. A randomized controlled trial of 48 patients with femoral occlusion and ISR treated with ELA-DCB compared to DCB alone for the treatment of FP ISR in CLI patients demonstrated that 1-year patency rates in the ELA-DCB group (66.7%) were significantly higher than in the DCB only group (37.5%, $P = .01$).[58] The benefit of a strategy of debulking for ISR with devices such as ELA will need to be confirmed in larger populations and with longer than a 6-month follow-up before it can be adopted as standard of care.

Cutting Balloon

The cutting balloon is useful in arteries that have "undilatable" lesions. There is limited evidence that would support extending the indications for this device beyond this narrow indication in the peripheral arteries,[59] and there is no evidence that a cutting balloon is an efficacious treatment for in-stent restenosis.

Cryoplasty

Clinical trials have failed to demonstrate any advantage for cryoplasty over conventional angioplasty in peripheral arterial intervention.[60] In a diabetic population with FP artery lesions, cryoplasty was associated with lower primary patency rates and more clinically driven repeat procedures after long-term follow-up than conventional balloon angioplasty.[61]

Infrapopliteal Intervention

Revascularization of infrapopliteal PAD is generally limited to those patients presenting with CLI where in-line flow to the foot is the standard of care for wound healing and/or resolution of rest pain. In general, nonambulatory patients with a shortened life expectancy and extensive lower extremity tissue necrosis should undergo primary amputation at the lowest level possible to ensure healing of the surgical site. Patients who have the opportunity to regain ambulatory function should undergo noninvasive testing with an ABI, toe-brachial index (TBI), or other modalities such as $TcPO_2$ or skin perfusion pressure. However, the ABI may be normal or noncompressible in approximately 30% of patients with isolated infrageniculate disease. In these individuals, noninvasive modalities, such as MRA or CTA, may be necessary. However, in most cases digital subtraction angiography is the gold standard to visualize the extent of lower extremity arterial disease, including foot and pedal arch.

The goals of therapy for CLI patients (Rutherford 4–6) with infrapopliteal arterial disease include: relieving pain, healing ulcerations, preventing major amputation, improving the patient's QOL, and prolonging survival. Infrapopliteal intervention procedural success is commonly defined as the re-establishment of direct "in-line" pulsatile flow to the foot. It is currently unknown whether healing rates are improved when in-line flow to the foot is established through more than one artery, but maximizing blood flow through more than one artery is particularly attractive in patients with inadequate collateral circulation, disease of the plantar arch vessels, or limb-threatening ischemia.

Balloon Angioplasty with Bailout-Stenting

Two clinical trials have demonstrated the efficacy and attractiveness of an initial percutaneous approach to selected patients with CLI and below-knee vascular disease (Fig. 20.5).[62,63] The limb salvage rate in these patients treated with PTA ranged from 85% to 91% after 2 to 5 years. This evidence supports the contention that angioplasty of the tibioperoneal vessels should not necessarily be reserved for limb salvage situations. However, caution is still advised in patient selection, since the surgical options are limited if angioplasty fails.

Infrapopliteal Drug-Eluting Stents

There have been five randomized trials[64-68] describing the outcomes of infrapopliteal DES versus either PTA, BMS, or DCB. The DESTINY (Drug-Eluting Stents in the Critically Ischemic Lower Leg) study randomized 140 CLI patients (Rutherford Classification [RC] 4,5) with infrapopliteal disease and compared BMS to DES (Xience V, Abbott Laboratories, Abbott Park, IL). At 1 year there was no difference regarding good functional outcomes (RC 0 to 1) between DES (60%) and BMS (56%), and there were very few amputations. The DES group demonstrated superior patency (DES 85% vs. BMS 54%, $P = .0001$) and freedom from TLR (DES 91% vs. BMS 66%, $P = .001$).[64]

The ACHILLES (Comparing Angioplasty and DES in the Treatment of Subjects with Ischemic Infrapopliteal Arterial Disease) trial compared 200 patients treated with PTA or DES (Cypher Select Sirolimus Eluting Stent, Cordis, Bridgewater, NJ) and found superior patency rates at 1 year for the DES group (DES 75% vs. PTA 57.1%, $P = .025$). At 6 months, there was better wound healing with DES versus PTA (95% healing vs. 60% healing, $P = .048$). The QOL score improved significantly up to 1 year in the DES cohort ($P < .0001$), but not with the PTA group.[65]

The Infrapopliteal Drug-Eluting Angioplasty Versus Stenting (IDEAS) trial compared a paclitaxel DCB (IN.PACT Amphirion, Medtronic) to DES in long (>70 mm) infrapopliteal lesions in 50 RC 3 to 6 patients. At 6 months, the angiographic restenosis rate was significantly lower in DES (28% vs. 57.9% in DCB; $P = .046$). There were no significant differences with regard to TLR (7.7% in DES vs. 13.6% in DCB; $P = .65$).[66]

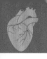

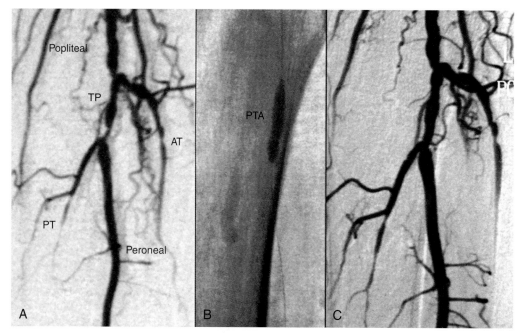

Fig. 20.5 (A) Baseline angiogram of severe stenosis (70%) of tibioperoneal *(TP)* artery. (B) Balloon angioplasty of TP trunk. (C) Final angiogram with less than 30% stenosis. *AT,* Anterior tibial artery; *PT,* posterior tibial artery; *PTA,* percutaneous transluminal angioplasty.

The YUKON-BTX (YUKON-Drug-Eluting Stent Below the Knee) trial randomized 161 patients with severe claudication and CLI to infrapopliteal treatment with BMS or DES (Sirolimus eluting YUKON stent, Translumina, Hechingen, Germany). The primary patency at 1 year for the DES group was 80.6% versus 55.6% with BMS (*P* = .004). At 3 years of follow-up there was a significant clinical benefit for the DES group for event-free survival (DES 65.8% vs. 44.6% for BMS, *P* = .02), reduced amputation rates (DES 2.6% vs. BMS 12.2%, *P* = .03) and TLR rates (DES 9.2% vs. BMS 20% (*P* = .06).[67]

The Percutaneous transluminal Angioplasty versus Drug eluting stents for Infrapopliteal lesions (PADI) trial compared paclitaxel-eluting DES to PTA-BMS of infrapopliteal lesions in CLI patients.[68] The 5-year clinical outcomes of amputation and event-free survival (survival free from major amputation or reintervention) showed that the DES arm was superior to the PTA-BMS group (31.8% vs. 20.4%, *P* = .043; and 26.2% vs. 15.3%, *P* = .041, respectively). These data, including meta-analyses, provide convincing evidence favoring infra-popliteal DES over PTA and BMS for (1) improved patency, (2) reduced re-interventions, (3) reduced amputation, and (4) improved event-free survival.[69]

Angiogenesis

Often, the severity of infrapopliteal disease abolishes most, if not all, of the named vasculature, and percutaneous mechanical revascularization is not possible. Therapeutic angiogenesis using growth factors as agents (e.g., vascular endothelial growth factor [VEGF], fibroblast growth factor [FGF]), genes, and cellular therapies have been proposed as a means of maintaining limb viability. At present, there have been no clinical break-throughs, but ongoing basic science activity appears to be promising.[70]

CONCLUSIONS

Percutaneous revascularization therapies are rapidly replacing open surgery as the treatment of choice for lower-extremity PAD. Stents appear to improve the outcomes for iliac and FP artery lesions. However,

their role in infrainguinal revascularization is not established so their use should be limited to bailout situations after failed or failing angioplasty. Adjunctive high-cost niche devices, such as atherectomy, lasers, cryotherapy, and cutting balloons, have a very limited role, if any, in the treatment of lower-extremity ischemic lesions.

The successful development of antirestenosis therapies, including DES and drug-coated balloons for peripheral arteries, will launch a new era of percutaneous revascularization, with efficacy and durability similar to that seen for coronary DES. The primacy of EVT for the treatment of PAD will be established if antirestenosis therapies prove as effective in preserving late patency as they have in coronary arteries.

REFERENCES

1   Gerhard-Herman MD, Gornik HL, Barrett C, et al.: 2016 AHA/ACC Guideline on the management of patients with lower extremity peripheral artery disease: executive summary: a report of the American College of Cardiology/American Heart Association Task Force on Clinical Practice Guidelines. *J Am Coll Cardiol* 69:1465-1508, 2017.

2. Creager MA, Gornik HL, Gray BH, et al. COCATS 4 Task Force 9: training in vascular medicine. *J Am Coll Cardiol.* 2015;65:1832–1843.

3. King SB, Babb JD, Bates ER, et al. COCATS 4 Task Force 10: training in cardiac catheterization. *J Am Coll Cardiol.* 2015;65:1844.

4. Klein AJ, Jaff MR, Gray BH, et al. SCAI appropriate use criteria for peripheral arterial interventions: an update. *Catheter Cardiovasc Interv.* 2017;90:E90–E110.

5. Samal AK, White CJ. Percutaneous management of access site complications. *Catheter Cardiovasc Interv.* 2002;57:12–23.

6. Norgren L, Hiatt WR, Dormandy JA, et al. Inter-Society Consensus for the management of peripheral arterial disease (TASC II). *J Vasc Surg.* 2007;45(Suppl S):S5–S67.

7. Adam DJ, Beard JD, Cleveland T, et al. Bypass versus Angioplasty in Severe Ischaemia of the Leg (BASIL): multicentre, randomised controlled trial. *Lancet.* 2005;366:1925–1934.

8. Menard MT, Farber A, Assmann SF, et al. Design and rationale of the best endovascular versus best surgical therapy for patients with critical limb ischemia (BEST-CLI) trial. *J Am Heart Assoc.* 2016;5. pii: e003219.

9. Ponec D, Jaff MR, Swischuk J, et al. The Nitinol SMART stent vs. Wallstent for suboptimal iliac artery angioplasty: CRISP-US trial results. *J Vasc Interv Radiol*. 2004;15:911–918.

10. Murphy TP, Cutlip DE, Regensteiner JG, et al. Supervised exercise versus primary stenting for claudication resulting from aortoiliac peripheral artery disease: six-month outcomes from the claudication: exercise versus endoluminal revascularization (CLEVER) study. *Circulation*. 2012;125:130–139.

11. Murphy TP, Cutlip DE, Regensteiner JG, et al. Supervised exercise, stent revascularization, or medical therapy for claudication due to aortoiliac peripheral artery disease: the CLEVER study. *J Am Coll Cardiol*. 2015;65:999–1009.

12. Fakhry F, Spronk S, van der Laan L, et al. Endovascular revascularization and supervised exercise for peripheral artery disease and intermittent claudication: a randomized clinical trial. *JAMA*. 2015;314:1936–1944.

13. Murphy TP, Ariaratnam NS, Carney Jr WI, et al. Aortoiliac insufficiency: long-term experience with stent placement for treatment. *Radiology*. 2004;231:243–249.

14. Park KB, Do YS, Kim JH, et al. Stent placement for chronic iliac arterial occlusive disease: the results of 10 years experience in a single institution. *Korean J Radiol*. 2005;6:256–266.

15. Tetteroo E, Haaring C, van der Graaf Y, et al. Intraarterial pressure gradients after randomized angioplasty or stenting of iliac artery lesions. Dutch Iliac Stent Trial Study Group. *Cardiovasc Intervent Radiol*. 1996;19:411–417.

16. Klein WM, van der Graaf Y, Seegers J, et al. Long-term cardiovascular morbidity, mortality, and reintervention after endovascular treatment in patients with iliac artery disease: the Dutch Iliac Stent Trial Study. *Radiology*. 2004;232:491–498.

17. Klein WM, van der Graaf Y, Seegers J, et al. Dutch Iliac Stent Trial: long-term results in patients randomized for primary or selective stent placement. *Radiology*. 2006;238:734–744.

18. Bosch JL, Hunink MG. Meta-analysis of the results of percutaneous transluminal angioplasty and stent placement for aortoiliac occlusive disease. *Radiology*. 1997;204:87–96.

19. Krankenberg H, Zeller T, Ingwersen M, et al. Self-expanding versus balloon-expandable stents for iliac artery occlusive disease: the randomized ICE trial. *JACC Cardiovasc Interv*. 2017;10:1694–1704.

20. Stahlhoff S, Donas KP, Torsello G, et al. Drug-eluting vs standard balloon angioplasty for iliac stent restenosis. *J Endovasc Ther*. 2015;22:314–318.

21. Mwipatayi BP, Thomas S, Wong J, et al. A comparison of covered vs bare expandable stents for the treatment of aortoiliac occlusive disease. *J Vasc Surg*. 2011;54:1561–1570.

22. Mwipatayi BP, Sharma S, Daneshmand A, et al. Durability of the balloon-expandable covered versus bare-metal stents in the Covered versus Balloon Expandable Stent Trial (COBEST) for the treatment of aortoiliac occlusive disease. *J Vasc Surg*. 2016;64:83–94. e81.

23. Hajibandeh S, Hajibandeh S, Antoniou SA, et al. Covered vs uncovered stents for aortoiliac and femoropopliteal arterial disease. *J Endovasc Ther*. 2016;23:442–452.

24. Heo S, Soukas P, Aronow HD. Is common femoral artery stenosis still a surgical disease? *Interv Cardiol Clin*. 2017;6:181–187.

25. Siracuse JJ, Van Orden K, Kalish JA, et al. Endovascular treatment of the common femoral artery in the Vascular Quality Initiative. *J Vasc Surg*. 2017;65:1039–1046.

26. Goueffic Y, Della Schiava N, Thaveau F, et al. Stenting or surgery for de novo common femoral artery stenosis. *JACC Cardiovasc Interv*. 2017;10:1344–1354.

27. Krankenberg H, Schluter M, Steinkamp HJ, et al. Nitinol stent implantation versus percutaneous transluminal angioplasty in superficial femoral artery lesions up to 10 cm in length: The Femoral Artery Stenting Trial (FAST). *Circulation*. 2007;116:285–292.

28. Laird JR, Katzen BT, Scheinert D, et al. Nitinol stent implantation versus balloon angioplasty for lesions in the superficial femoral artery and proximal popliteal artery: twelve-month results from the RESILIENT randomized trial. *Circ Cardiovasc Interv*. 2010;3:267–276.

29. Schillinger M, Sabeti S, Loewe C, et al. Balloon angioplasty versus implantation of nitinol stents in the superficial femoral artery. *N Engl J Med*. 2006;354:1879–1888.

30. Lammer J, Zeller T, Hausegger KA, et al. Heparin-bonded covered stents versus bare-metal stents for complex femoropopliteal artery lesions: the randomized VIASTAR trial (Viabahn endoprosthesis with PROPATEN bioactive surface [VIA] versus bare nitinol stent in the treatment of long lesions in superficial femoral artery occlusive disease). *J Am Coll Cardiol*. 2013;62:1320–1327.

31. Lammer J, Zeller T, Hausegger KA, et al. Sustained benefit at 2 years for covered stents versus bare-metal stents in long SFA lesions: the VIASTAR trial. *Cardiovasc Intervent Radiol*. 2015;38:25–32.

32. Katsanos K. Paclitaxel-coated balloons in the femoropopliteal artery: it is all about the pharmacokinetic profile and vessel tissue bioavailability. *JACC Cardiovasc Interv*. 2016;9:1743–1745.

33. Tepe G, Laird J, Schneider P, et al. Drug-coated balloon versus standard percutaneous transluminal angioplasty for the treatment of superficial femoral and popliteal peripheral artery disease: 12-month results from the IN.PACT SFA randomized trial. *Circulation*. 2015;131:495–502.

34. Laird JR, Schneider PA, Tepe G, et al. Durability of treatment effect using a drug-coated balloon for femoropopliteal lesions: 24-month results of IN.PACT SFA. *J Am Coll Cardiol*. 2015;66:2329–2338.

35. Rosenfield K, Jaff MR, White CJ, et al. Trial of a paclitaxel-coated balloon for femoropopliteal artery disease. *N Engl J Med*. 2015;373:145–153.

36. Schroeder H, Werner M, Meyer DR, et al. Low-dose paclitaxel-coated versus uncoated percutaneous transluminal balloon angioplasty for femoropopliteal peripheral artery disease: one-year results of the ILLUMENATE European randomized clinical trial (randomized trial of a novel paclitaxel-coated percutaneous angioplasty balloon). *Circulation*. 2017;135:2227–2236.

37. Krishnan P, Faries P, Niazi K, et al. Stellarex drug-coated balloon for treatment of femoropopliteal disease: 12-month outcomes from the randomized ILLUMENATE pivotal and pharmacokinetic studies. *Circulation*. 2017;136:1102–1113.

38. Tepe G, Schnorr B, Albrecht T, et al. Angioplasty of femoral-popliteal arteries with drug-coated balloons: 5-year follow-up of the THUNDER trial. *JACC Cardiovasc Interv*. 2015;8:102–108.

39. Katsanos K, Geisler BP, Garner AM, et al. Economic analysis of endovascular drug-eluting treatments for femoropopliteal artery disease in the UK. *BMJ Open*. 2016;6:e011245.

40. Salisbury AC, Li H, Vilain KR, et al. Cost-effectiveness of endovascular femoropopliteal intervention using drug-coated balloons versus standard percutaneous transluminal angioplasty: results from the IN.PACT SFA II trial. *JACC Cardiovasc Interv*. 2016;9:2343–2352.

41. Dake MD, Ansel GM, Jaff MR, et al. Durable clinical effectiveness with paclitaxel-eluting stents in the femoropopliteal artery: 5-year results of the Zilver PTX randomized trial. *Circulation*. 2016;133:1472–1483.

42. Diehm N, Silvestro A, Do DD, et al. Endovascular brachytherapy after femoropopliteal balloon angioplasty fails to show robust clinical benefit over time. *J Endovasc Ther*. 2005;12:723–730.

43. Wolfram RM, Budinsky AC, Pokrajac B, et al. Endovascular brachytherapy for prophylaxis of restenosis after femoropopliteal angioplasty: five-year follow-up–prospective randomized study. *Radiology*. 2006;240:878–884.

44. Wolfram RM, Budinsky AC, Pokrajac B, et al. Endovascular brachytherapy: restenosis in de novo versus recurrent lesions of femoropopliteal artery–the Vienna experience. *Radiology*. 2005;236:338–342.

45. Pokrajac B, Kirisits C, Rainer S, et al. Beta endovascular brachytherapy using CO2-filled centering catheter for treatment of recurrent superficial femoropopliteal artery disease. *Cardiovasc Revasc Med*. 2009;10:162–165.

46. Ho KJ, Devlin PM, Madenci AL, et al. High dose-rate brachytherapy for the treatment of lower extremity in-stent restenosis. *J Vasc Surg*. 2017;65:734–743.

47. Therasse E, Donath D, Lesperance J, et al. External beam radiation to prevent restenosis after superficial femoral artery balloon angioplasty. *Circulation*. 2005;111:3310–3315.

335

48. Therasse E, Donath D, Elkouri S, et al. Results of a randomized clinical trial of external beam radiation to prevent restenosis after superficial femoral artery stenting. *J Vasc Surg.* 2016;63:1531–1540.

49. Vroegindeweij D, Tielbeek AV, Buth J, et al. Directional atherectomy versus balloon angioplasty in segmental femoropopliteal artery disease: two-year follow-up with color-flow duplex scanning. *J Vasc Surg.* 1995;21:255–268. discussion 268–9.

50. Indes JE, Shah HJ, Jonker FHW, et al. Subintimal angioplasty is superior to Silverhawk atherectomy for the treatment of occlusive lesions of the lower extremities. *J Endovasc Ther.* 2010;17:243–250.

51. Ambler GK, Radwan R, Hayes PD, et al. Atherectomy for peripheral arterial disease. *Cochrane Database Syst Rev.* 2014;3:CD006680.

52. Suri R, Wholey MH, Postoak D, et al. Distal embolic protection during femoropopliteal atherectomy. *Catheter Cardiovasc Interv.* 2006;67:417–422.

53. Mukherjee D, Hashemi H, Contos B. The disproportionate growth of office-based atherectomy. *J Vasc Surg.* 2017;65:495–500.

54. Scheinert D, Laird Jr. JR, Schroder M, et al. Excimer laser-assisted recanalization of long, chronic superficial femoral artery occlusions. *J Endovasc Ther.* 2001;8:156–166.

55. Steinkamp HJ, Rademaker J, Wissgott C, et al. Percutaneous transluminal laser angioplasty versus balloon dilation for treatment of popliteal artery occlusions. *J Endovasc Ther.* 2002;9:882–888.

56. Tan JWC, Yeo KK, Laird JR. Excimer laser assisted angioplasty for complex infrainguinal peripheral artery disease: a 2008 update. *J Cardiovasc Surg.* 2008;49:329.

57. Dippel EJ, Makam P, Kovach R, et al. Randomized controlled study of excimer laser atherectomy for treatment of femoropopliteal in-stent restenosis: initial results from the EXCITE ISR trial (EXCImer Laser Randomized Controlled Study for Treatment of FemoropopliTEal In-Stent Restenosis). *JACC Cardiovasc Interv.* 2015;8:92–101.

58. Gandini R, Del Giudice C, Merolla S, et al. Treatment of chronic SFA in-stent occlusion with combined laser atherectomy and drug-eluting balloon angioplasty in patients with critical limb ischemia: a single-center, prospective, randomized study. *J Endovasc Ther.* 2013;20:805–814.

59. Engelke C, Sandhu C, Morgan RA, et al. Using 6-mm cutting balloon angioplasty in patients with resistant peripheral artery stenosis: preliminary results. *AJR Am J Roentgenol.* 2002;179:619–623.

60. Wildgruber M, Berger H. Cryoplasty for the prevention of arterial restenosis. *Cardiovasc Intervent Radiol.* 2008;31:1050–1058.

61. Spiliopoulos S, Katsanos K, Karnabatidis D, et al. Cryoplasty versus conventional balloon angioplasty of the femoropopliteal artery in diabetic patients: long-term results from a prospective randomized single-center controlled trial. *Cardiovasc Intervent Radiol.* 2010;33: 929–938.

62. Krankenberg H, Sorge I, Zeller T, et al. Percutaneous transluminal angioplasty of infrapopliteal arteries in patients with intermittent claudication: acute and one-year results. *Catheter Cardiovasc Interv.* 2005;64:12–17.

63. Soder HK, Manninen HI, Jaakkola P, et al. Prospective trial of infrapopliteal artery balloon angioplasty for critical limb ischemia: angiographic and clinical results. *J Vasc Interv Radiol.* 2000;11: 1021–1031.

64. Bosiers M, Scheinert D, Peeters P, et al. Randomized comparison of everolimus-eluting versus bare-metal stents in patients with critical limb ischemia and infrapopliteal arterial occlusive disease. *J Vasc Surg.* 2012;55:390–398.

65. Scheinert D, Katsanos K, Zeller T, et al. ACHILLES Investigators. A prospective randomized multicenter comparison of balloon angioplasty and infrapopliteal stenting with the sirolimus-eluting stent in patients with ischemic peripheral arterial disease: 1-year results from the ACHILLES trial. *J Am Coll Cardiol.* 2012;60:2290–2295.

66. Siablis D, Kitrou P, Spiliopoulos S, et al. Paclitaxel-coated balloon angioplasty versus drug-eluting stenting for the treatment of infrapopliteal long-segment arterial occlusive disease: the IDEAS randomized controlled trial. *JACC Cardiovasc Interv.* 2014;7:1048–1056.

67. Rastan A, Brechtel K, Krankenberg H, et al. Sirolimus-eluting stents for treatment of infrapopliteal arteries reduce clinical event rate compared to bare-metal stents: long-term results from a randomized trial. *J Am Coll Cardiol.* 2012;60:587–591.

68. Spreen MI, Martens JM, Knippenberg B, et al. Long-term follow-up of the PADI trial: percutaneous transluminal angioplasty versus drug-eluting stents for infrapopliteal lesions in critical limb ischemia. *J Am Heart Assoc.* 2017;6. pii: e004877.

69. Cassese S, Ndrepepa G, Liistro F, et al. Drug-coated balloons for revascularization of infrapopliteal arteries: a meta-analysis of randomized trials. *JACC Cardiovasc Interv.* 2016;9:1072–1080.

70. Briquez PS, Clegg LE, Martino MM, et al. Design principles for therapeutic angiogenic materials. *Nat Rev Mater.* 2016;1:15006.

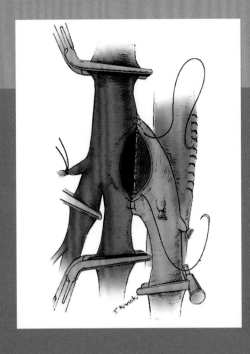

第21章
外周动脉疾病的重建手术

本章主要阐述外科重建手术在主髂动脉和腹股沟韧带以下动脉闭塞性疾病中的作用。

1.主髂动脉闭塞症：对于药物治疗无效或腔内治疗不成功者，外科手术重建仍是必要的。手术方式包括以下几种。

（1）主髂动脉内膜剥脱术：多适用于局限于腹主动脉远端和髂动脉近端的病变，具有避免使用人工血管、长期通畅率高等优点，但在腔内治疗时代已经很少有合适的患者需要进行此类手术了。主动脉-双股动脉旁路术已取代内膜剥脱术和主髂动脉旁路术成为主髂动脉闭塞的主要手术方式。因股总动脉更易于显露和吻合，也便于必要时行股动脉分叉部的内膜剥脱术以改善重要的股深动脉血流。近端腹主动脉吻合方式有"端-端"和"端-侧"两种，前者建立的线性血流更符合生理，产生的湍流少，在伴有腹主动脉瘤或闭塞延至肾动脉水平时尤为适合。但在髂外动脉完全闭塞时，为避免髂内动脉或肠系膜下动脉缺血，可采用"端-侧"吻合方式。

（2）解剖外旁路术：当主髂动脉闭塞症患者因各种原因不适合行主动脉显露和吻合时，可以选择一些替代性的手术方式，如腋-双股动脉旁路术、股-股动脉旁路术、髂-股动脉旁路术、胸主动脉-股动脉旁路术和腹腔镜下动脉重建术。

2.腹股沟韧带以下动脉闭塞性疾病：此类疾病是最为常见的动脉闭塞性疾病，重建手术的指征主要是间歇性跛行和威胁肢体的重症缺血，动脉旁路术是最主要的手术重建方式，近端吻合部位最常选择股总动脉，远端吻合口可选择膝上腘动脉、膝下腘动脉、胫腓干动脉及胫后动脉、胫前动脉或腓动脉。自体静脉旁路术：获取自体静脉倒转后行旁路术，其通畅率明显优于人工血管旁路术，尤其是远端吻合口位于膝下动脉时。静脉原位旁路术：此术可减少长切口获取静脉移植物带来的创面愈合并发症，动、静脉直径也更为匹配，但需注意瓣膜破坏和分支结扎。人工血管旁路术：主要采用聚酯或聚四氟乙烯人工血管，适合于远端吻合口位于膝上腘动脉者。同种异体移植物：仅适用于伴有局部感染，又无自体静脉移植物可用者。生物工程同种异体移植物：仍在临床试验阶段。再次旁路手术：此手术涉及瘢痕动脉显露和自体移植移植物缺乏等难题。

3.重建术后的管理：主要涉及坏疽或感染创面的换药、清创及截肢等。术后药物治疗主要是抗血小板治疗，必要时可加用华法林等抗凝药物。

4.移植物失败和管理：依据术后不同的闭塞时间分为早期、中期、晚期移植物失败。

包俊敏

Reconstructive Surgery for Peripheral Artery Disease

Matthew T. Menard, Christine E. Lotto, and Michael Belkin

The clinical manifestations and complications of atherosclerosis are the most common therapeutic challenges encountered by vascular surgeons. The tendency for lesions to develop at specific anatomic sites and to follow recognizable patterns of progression was appreciated as long ago as the late 1700s by the extraordinary British anatomist and surgeon John Hunter. Considered one of the forefathers of vascular surgery, his dissections of atherosclerotic aortic bifurcations remain on view at the Hunterian Museum in London and presage the disease process that Leriche would give name to 150 years later.[1]

The modern era of surgical reconstruction for complex atherosclerotic occlusive disease began in earnest in 1947, when the Portuguese surgeon J. Cid dos Santos successfully endarterectomized a heavily diseased common femoral artery.[2] Four years later, Wylie and coworkers in San Francisco extended this new technique to the aortoiliac level.[3] At the same time, and building on the pioneering work of Alexis Carrel,[4] Kunlin[5] would report the first long segment vein bypass in the lower extremity, in 1948. It would be another 10 years before synthetic grafts were being regularly used for aortic bypass grafting and the first efforts to extend vein grafting to the tibial level were described by McCaughan.[6] Tremendous advances in both the understanding of atherosclerosis biology and the ability to treat arterial occlusive disease percutaneously have dramatically impacted the treatment algorithms for arterial insufficiency in recent years. This chapter will review the current role for the surgical management of aortoiliac and infrainguinal arterial occlusive disease.

AORTOILIAC OCCLUSIVE DISEASE

Chronic obliterative atherosclerosis of the distal aorta and iliac arteries commonly manifests as symptomatic arterial insufficiency of the lower extremities. Disease in this location is seen often in combination with occlusive disease of the femoropopliteal arteries, producing a range of symptoms from mild claudication to more severe levels of tissue loss and critical ischemia. Patients with hemodynamic impairment limited to the aortoiliac system may have intermittent claudication of the calf muscles alone or involvement of the thigh, hip, and/or buttocks. If the disease distribution also targets the hypogastric vessels, patients may additionally suffer from difficulty in achieving and maintaining an erection, resulting from inadequate perfusion of the internal pudendal arteries. A well-characterized constellation of symptoms and signs, known as the Leriche syndrome, which is associated with aortoiliac occlusive disease in the male, includes thigh, hip, or buttock claudication, atrophy of the leg muscles, impotence, and reduced femoral pulses.[7] While vasculogenic female sexual dysfunction has been described,[8,9] the equivalent impact of impaired pelvic perfusion in women remains poorly understood and more research is needed to discern the true incidence and the

appropriate treatment. A meta-analysis did demonstrate fewer complications in women compared to men when one or more hypogastric arteries was disrupted by embolization, coverage, or ligation. The authors attributed this to the fact that most of the female patients in the study had obstetric-related pathologies, while more men had trauma, vascular, or oncologic indications for treatment. The authors further speculated that the younger age and the increased levels of estrogen in the female cohort may have contributed to the gender-related differences that were seen.[10]

While atherosclerotic disease limited to the aortoiliac region commonly gives rise to claudication of varying degrees, it is rarely associated with lower extremity ischemic rest pain or ischemic tissue loss. This is largely the result of adequate collateralization around the point of obstruction via lumbar, sacral, and circumflex iliac vessels that serves to reconstitute the infrainguinal system with enough well-perfused arterial blood to ensure sufficient resting tissue perfusion (Fig. 21.1). A well-recognized exception to this general observation arises in the situation of embolic disease. The so-called blue toe syndrome represents a situation where atherosclerotic debris breaks free from an aortic or iliac plaque and embolizes to the distal vessels (see Chapter 45).[11,12] Wire manipulation during coronary or peripheral angiographic procedures and cross-clamping across a calcific aortic plaque during cardiac surgery are common sources of such emboli. The terminal target of the microembolic particles, be they cholesterol crystals, calcified plaque, thrombus, or platelet aggregates, is typically the small vessels of the toes.

If, on the other hand, aortoiliac occlusive disease is found in combination with femoropopliteal occlusive disease, ischemic rest pain, or even more severe perfusion impairment leading to ischemic tissue loss or gangrene is not uncommon.[13] Such progressive disease, affecting multiple levels of the peripheral vasculature tree, is most frequently encountered in the elderly. Approximately one-third of patients operated on for symptomatic aortoiliac occlusive disease have orificial profunda femoris occlusive disease, and more than 40% have superficial femoral artery occlusions. Aortoiliac disease typically begins at the distal aorta and common iliac artery origins, and slowly progresses proximally and distally over time.[14] This progression is quite variable, but may ultimately extend to the level of the renal arteries or result in total aortic occlusion.

A particularly virulent form of atherosclerotic arterial disease is often found in young women smokers.[15] Radiographic imaging in this subset of patients typically reveals atretic, narrowed vasculature with diffusely calcific atherosclerotic changes. Frequently, a focal stenosis is found posteriorly near the aortic bifurcation. This particular distribution of disease and the characteristic patient profile have been referred to as the small aortic syndrome (Fig. 21.2).[16] Such patients invariably have an extensive smoking history, with or without other typical factors for

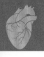

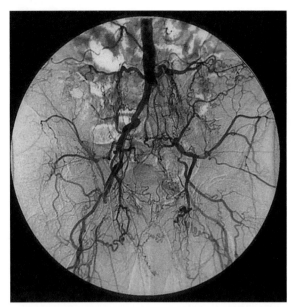

Fig. 21.1 Aortoiliac occlusive disease results in a variable degree of collateralization. Here the left hypogastric artry is reconstituted via prominent distal lumbar collaterals and the right hypogastric artery. Hypogastric collaterals are, in turn, perfusing the femoral circumflex vessels.

atherosclerosis. While the diminutive size of the aorta and iliac vessels has led to compromised durability when treated endovascularly, ongoing improvements in percutaneous technology have resulted in better outcomes in this patient population in more recent years.[17,18]

The diagnosis of aortoiliac occlusive disease is generally made based on patient symptomatology, physical examination, and non-

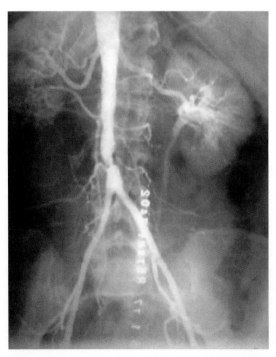

Fig. 21.2 Aortoiliac occlusive disease may consist of a short segment stenosis localized to the distal aorta, a lesion particularly common in young female smokers. Such a lesion may be amenable to endarterectomy.

invasive tests such as segmental pressure measurements and pulse volume recordings (see Chapter 18). Following the diagnosis of aortoiliac disease and the decision to pursue intervention, further imaging is warranted. In many centers, magnetic resonance angiography (MRA) (see Chapter 13) or computed tomographic angiography (CTA) (see Chapter 14) has supplanted catheter-based angiography (see Chapter 15) as the initial imaging study of choice. Should a lesion amenable to percutaneous therapy be identified, catheter-based angiography is then pursued. In cases in which a good quality roadmap is obtained with MRA or CTA and the clinical situation or anatomic pattern is unfavorable to a percutaneous approach, surgery can, in most instances, be planned directly from the MRA, obviating the need for traditional subtraction angiography.

In the minority of cases necessitating digital subtraction angiography for preoperative planning, a retrograde femoral approach is typically utilized, while the transbrachial approach serves as a useful alternative in patients with particularly challenging anatomy (see Chapter 15).[19] Additional lateral and oblique views of the abdominal aorta are advised if concomitant mesenteric or renal occlusive disease is present and multiple projections of the iliac and femoral bifurcations are essential in clarifying the extent of disease in these regions (see Chapter 15). Finally, full runoff views of the lower extremities are needed to assess the presence or absence of femoropopliteal or crural disease. In ambiguous cases, pullback pressure measurements, both before and after the administration of a systemic vasodilator, such as papaverine or nitroglycerine, or the application of a tourniquet to induce reactive hyperemia, can be useful in documenting the hemodynamic significance of a particular stenotic zone.[20] Finally, the use of gadolinium[21] or carbon dioxide[22] as contrast agents in patients with compromised renal function can minimize or eliminate the nephrotoxic effects associated with standard iodinated contrast medium.

Management Considerations

Risk factor modification remains a cornerstone of the management of aortoiliac occlusive disease (see Chapter 19). Smoking cessation, blood pressure control, and aggressive efforts at cholesterol lowering should be addressed with every patient with atherosclerotic disease. Strong evidence exists supporting the benefit of a structured walking program[23] in increasing the walking distance of patients with claudication; it is hoped that utilization of this important treatment strategy will increase now that it is a reimbursable therapeutic option. Interestingly, studies have failed to identify any exercise components; for example, intensity, duration, or content, which independently predict improvements in maximum walking distance and pain-free walking distance.[23] The benefit of walking outside of a structured regimen with close follow-up is more debatable.[24] Medical management with cilostazol has benefit in a subset of patients and is a reasonable first line approach to improve claudication symptoms.[25] Recent studies have found lower rates of restenosis, amputation, and target lesion revascularization in claudicants treated with cilostazol.[26–28]

There has been a considerable change in the management approach to claudication in recent years. Anyone suffering from disabling claudication, rest pain, or ischemia-related tissue loss continues to warrant serious consideration for arteriography and either percutaneous or surgical intervention. Previously, such aggressive treatment would have been considered inappropriate for claudication that was not clearly disabling. However, as percutaneous treatment has become increasingly safer and more effective, and its application has spread to increasingly more arterial beds, the indications for transluminal angioplasty have correspondingly increased (see Chapter 20). Such a sea change in the overall management approach to aortoiliac disease has had a dramatic impact on the numbers of patients now proceeding to open surgery. The rising popularity and success of aortic and iliac balloon angioplasty and stenting as first-line therapy has noticeably reduced the volume of aortoiliac reconstructive procedures performed in this country.

When medical therapy or percutaneous treatment has proven inadequate or is technically inadvisable, open surgical revascularization remains indicated for those patients with aortoiliac disease and disabling claudication, ischemic rest pain, and ischemic ulceration or gangrene. Patients with nighttime foot rest pain or tissue loss usually have multisegment disease and the decision whether to perform both supra- and infra-inguinal revascularization procedures or to perform only an inflow procedure is guided by the severity of the ischemia.[13,29-31] In general, patients presenting with significant tissue loss or gangrene are much more likely to require simultaneous or staged inflow and outflow procedures.

The numerous surgical options available to the trained vascular surgeon allow tailoring of the approach to the particular overall and anatomic situation of each patient. Historically, the reconstructive options for aortoiliac occlusive disease include aortoiliac endarterectomy, aortobifemoral bypass, and so-called extra-anatomic revascularization in the form of iliofemoral, femorofemoral, or axillofemoral grafting.

Endarterectomy

Aortic endarterectomy was commonly performed in the early era of aortoiliac reconstruction.[32,33] While it is particularly suited to localized disease limited to the distal aorta or proximal iliac arteries, it has proven to be less reliable for disease involving the entire infrarenal aorta and extending into the external iliac arteries.[34,35] The obvious benefit of endarterectomy is the elimination of the need for a prosthetic graft, removing the possibility of the myriad late graft-related complications. The long-term patency of limited endarterectomy is excellent and on par with bypass procedures.[36] However, the number of patients suitable for this reconstructive approach is small and continues to diminish in the era of endoluminal reconstruction. Experience with endarterectomy during one's training or early surgical career is another important factor influencing the choice of therapy offered, as significant technical expertise is required and many surgeons in the current era have limited familiarity with this approach.

Aortobifemoral Bypass

Aortobifemoral bypass remains the mainstay of operative treatment for aortoiliac occlusive disease. During the last 20 years, the procedure has supplanted both aortic endarterectomy and aortoiliac bypass procedures. In the latter case, this change was largely driven by the recognition of subsequent graft failure due to progression of native iliac arterial disease.[34,37] Early experience with aortobifemoral grafting in the 1970s was associated with a 5% to 8% 30-day operative mortality rate.[35,36,38] Over recent decades, mortality rates of 1% have been reported, on par with that of elective abdominal aortic aneurysm repair.[39,40]

Typically, half of patients proceeding to surgery for aortoiliac occlusive disease will have significant coronary artery disease, while even more will have hypertension and almost 80% will be current or prior cigarette smokers.[39] The reduced mortality and morbidity seen in recent years is in large part due to advances in the management of concomitant coronary disease. Specifically, the importance and benefit of better preoperative identification of patients in need of initial coronary revascularization, awareness of the benefit of waiting an interval period following coronary stenting prior to proceeding with major

noncoronary vascular surgery, improved perioperative pharmacologic management of patients with impaired myocardium, and more focused efforts to tailor operative and postoperative fluid administration to the individual patient's myocardial reserve are all well-recognized.[41,42] General advances in postoperative intensive care unit management, including pulmonary care, infection control, and blood product utilization, have further contributed to the progress seen.

Current early patency rates for aortobifemoral bypass grafting are excellent, approaching 100% in many reporting institutions. Five-year patency rates are greater than 80%[36,38,39,43] while 10-year rates are near 75%.[36] There are multiple reasons for the improved patency. The current graft material used by most surgeons for aortoiliac reconstruction is a knitted Dacron prosthesis, which has enhanced hemostatic properties and which tends to have a more stable pseudointima than the earlier used woven grafts.[44,45] More attention is paid to avoiding graft redundancy and to ensuring a good size match between the graft and the recipient vessels. Grafts are more routinely extended beyond the iliac level to the femoral vessels, which not only improves exposure and makes for a technically easier distal anastomosis, but is also associated with less graft thrombosis from unanticipated progression of atherosclerotic disease in the external iliac vessels.[37] With meticulous skin preparation, close attention to draping, careful surgical technique, and judicious use of a short course of intravenous antibiotic therapy, the feared higher rate of graft infection from placing the distal dissection at the groin has not materialized.[46] However, an exception to this general practice is recommended in certain circumstances. For example, patients with hostile groin creases from prior surgery or radiation therapy, or obese, diabetic patients with an intertriginous rash at the inguinal crease will all likely be better served by performing the distal anastomosis at the external iliac level if their anatomy for such a procedure is suitable.

The increased awareness of the critical role played by the deep femoral artery in preserving the long-term patency of aortobifemoral grafts[36,47,48] has also undoubtedly contributed to the better results seen. This awareness parallels a better overall appreciation for the importance of establishing adequate outflow at the femoral level in achieving higher early and late graft patency rates and sustained symptom relief. The true impact of concomitant superficial femoral artery disease is unclear from the literature. Some reports have indicated similar patency rates between those patients with and without superficial femoral artery occlusion,[29,31] while others have suggested that late patency rates are reduced in this setting.[46,49] What has definitely been shown is the benefit of a profundaplasty in the presence of significant superficial and profunda femoral occlusive disease.[47,50] Some authors have even recommended that a profundaplasty should be carried out in every case of superficial femoral artery occlusion, even in the absence of orificial profunda disease, arguing that a "functional" obstruction on the order of 50% stenosis is present in these patients.[51] While this position has not been universally adopted, it is now common practice to extend the hood of the distal anastomosis over the origin of the profunda femoral artery to enhance the graft outflow, especially in situations in which the superficial femoral artery is occluded or severely diseased. In the presence of significant common femoral or profunda femoral origin plaque, an extensive endarterectomy and/or profundaplasty is indicated (Fig. 21.3). In these circumstances, it is preferable to close the endarterectomized recipient bed with a vein, bovine pericardial or Dacron patch, onto which the distal anastomosis can then be attached, rather than creating a long femoris patch with the graft limb.[47]

There are several technical considerations related to aortobifemoral bypass grafting, which are the subject of considerable and passionate debate. The first involves the manner of the proximal anastomotic

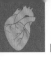

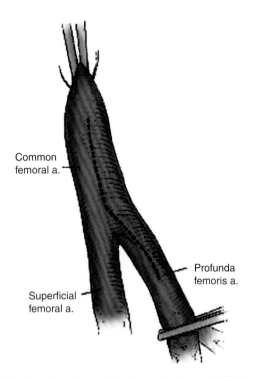

Common femoral a.

Profunda femoris a.

Superficial femoral a.

Fig. 21.3 In the setting of superficial femoral artery and orificial profunda femoral artery disease, extending the common femoral arteriotomy into the origin of the profunda and performing a profundaplasty prior to completing the distal anastomosis of the aortobifemoral bypass will improve outflow and maximize graft patency.

creation. Advocates of an end-to-end configuration claim that it facilitates a more comprehensive thromboendarterectomy of the proximal stump and allows for a direct, more in-line flow pattern, with less turbulence and more favorable flow characteristics.[52] The obviation of competitive flow through the excluded iliac vessels with this approach is likely more of theoretical rather than real benefit. Certainly, with concomitant aneurysmal disease or complete aortic occlusion extending up to the level of the renal arteries, end-to-end grafting is indicated. Creation of an end-to-side anastomosis can, at times, be technically challenging in a heavily diseased aorta partially occluded by a side-biting clamp. A lower rate of proximal suture line pseudoaneurysms and better long-term patency rates have been found in some series.[53] Stapling or over-sewing of the distal aorta with the end-to-end technique minimizes the immediate risk of clamp-induced emboli to the lower extremities following release of the distal clamp. Finally, those in favor of this approach claim that the ability to more effectively close the retroperitoneum, particularly after resection of a short segment of the infrarenal aorta, results in a lower rate of late graft infection and aortoenteric fistulae, although there is no direct evidence to support this assertion.

There are certain circumstances, on the other hand, when an end-to-side proximal anastomotic configuration is advantageous. The most common indication involves those patients with occluded external iliac arteries, in whom interruption of forward aortic flow may result in loss of perfusion to an important hypogastric or inferior mesenteric artery and consequent significant pelvic ischemia. Colon ischemia (1% to 2%),[54] or even more rarely, paraplegia secondary to cauda equina syndrome (<1%),[55] are additional complications that can be avoided by an end-to-side configuration. Although advocated by some,[52] routine preservation of a patent inferior mesenteric artery is not universally practiced.

Operative Management

The operative procedure is performed under general endotracheal anesthesia, with an epidural catheter placed for postoperative pain control. The patient is sterilely prepped and draped from the mid chest to the mid thighs. The femoral vessels are first exposed through bilateral longitudinal, oblique incisions, thereby reducing the time in which the abdomen is open and the viscera exposed. The extent of exposure of the femoral vessels necessary is dictated by the severity of disease and the level of reconstruction planned of the common femoral artery and its bifurcation. Next, the inferior aspect of the retroperitoneal tunnel through which the graft will course to reach the femoral region is begun with digital manipulation posterior to the inguinal ligament and tracking along the anterior aspect of the external iliac artery. Antibiotic-soaked sponges are then placed in the groin wounds and attention is turned to the aortic dissection.

The proximal reconstruction is performed via a midline laparotomy. In general, the aortic dissection is limited to the region between the renal arteries and the inferior mesenteric artery. This allows avoidance of extensive dissection anterior to the aortic bifurcation, where the autonomic nerve plexus regulating erection and ejaculation in men sweeps over the aorta. It is interesting to note that several studies have found a similar rate of male sexual dysfunction with endovascular aortic aneurysm repair as with open surgical repair.[56] This would suggest the effects of aortic dissection in this area are perhaps less important than historically believed.

In situations where significant aortic calcification extends up to the level of the renal arteries, it may be necessary to continue the aortic dissection to the suprarenal or even the supraceliac level to allow for safe proximal clamp placement. Alternatively, proximal control may be obtained by intralumenal balloon deployment. If end-to-side repair is planned, circumferential dissection of the aortic segment to be clamped is recommended, as gaining control of any lumbar or accessory renal vessels encountered prior to performing the aortotomy helps to avoid troublesome backbleeding. The superior aspect of the graft limb tunnels is then completed, taking care to maintain a course anterior to the common iliac vessels but posterior to the ureters. Between 5000 and 7000 units of heparin are administered, with additional heparin given throughout the procedure to maintain the activated clotting time near the target range of 250 to 300 seconds. After allowing sufficient time for the heparin to circulate, atraumatic vascular clamps are placed above the inferior mesenteric artery and just below the renal arteries. The distal clamp is applied first to avoid any distal embolization of plaque dislodged with placement of the proximal clamp. If an end-to-end anastomosis is planned, the aorta is transected 1 to 2 cm below the proximal clamp and a short segment of the distal aortic cuff is excised (Fig. 21.4A). This results both in better exposure of the aortic neck and a more precise proximal reconstruction and also allows the graft to lie flat against the vertebral column rather than being anteriorly oriented, facilitating later retroperitoneal coverage. If necessary, a thromboendarterectomy of the infrarenal neck is carried out at this point (see Fig. 21.4B). The anastomosis is performed with a running suture of #3-0 polypropylene (see Fig. 21.4C). The distal aorta is then oversewn with two layers of a running monofilament suture, or stapled with a surgical stapler. If an end-to-side anastomosis is performed, an anterior longitudinal arteriotomy is carried out after placement of proximal and distal transaortic clamps. If necessary, an endarterectomy is performed and the anastomosis carried out after the graft is beveled appropriately (see Fig. 21.4D). If there is minimal plaque present, the distal anastomosis is performed to the common femoral artery, and individual dissection of the superficial femoral and profunda femoral arteries is not necessary.

Another point of some debate concerns the optimal management of patients with multilevel occlusive disease. The question frequently

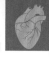

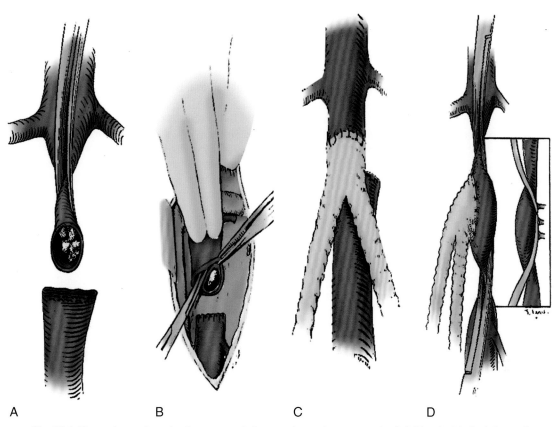

A   B   C   D

Fig. 21.4 The end-to-end proximal anastomosis for aortofemoral reconstruction is initiated with the infrarenal aorta cross clamp placed in anterior/posterior direction as close to the origin of the renal arteries as possible. The aorta is transected 1 to 2 cm below the proximal clamp. A short segment of distal aortic cuff is excised and the aorta is stapled or oversewn just proximal to the origin of the inferior mesenteric artery (A). If necessary, a thromboendarterectomy of the aortic cuff is carried out (B). The end-to-end configuration allows the graft to lie flat against the vertebral column and results in less turbulent flow (C). An end-to-side configuration is required to preserve antegrade pelvic perfusion in situations where retrograde flow would be compromised due to heavily diseased or occluded external iliac arteries (D).

arises as to whether, or under what circumstances, a concomitant or staged outflow procedure should be performed. It is generally believed that up to 80% of patients with both inflow and outflow disease will be substantially improved following aortofemoral bypass grafting.[13,30] However, other reports have suggested that between as many as one-quarter to one-third of such patients will not have significant symptomatic relief with an inflow procedure alone.[31] While no single parameter exists to reliably guide the surgeon to know in which circumstances a combined procedure is optimal, the severity of distal ischemia is probably the most important factor to be considered. The overall medical condition of the patient and their ability to tolerate a prolonged operative procedure is also clearly important. Finally, the status of the profunda femoral artery must be taken into consideration. In the presence of superficial femoral artery occlusion, a profunda that is atretic or extensively diseased may well be unable to provide sufficient collateral runoff to the foot.

If the bypass procedure is undertaken for claudication alone or mild rest pain, restoring adequate inflow may provide sufficient and relatively durable symptomatic relief. If, on the other hand, significant tissue loss is present, a combined inflow and outflow procedure is likely warranted if limb salvage is to be achieved. If several operating teams are utilized, performing both procedures at the same time can be done in an acceptably timely fashion and has been found to be safe. Indeed, several recent reports found no significant differences in operative mortality or perioperative morbidity in patients undergoing concurrent inflow and outflow procedures compared with those having major inflow reconstruction alone.[55,57,58] While staged revascularization may be preferable in certain circumstances, both the risk of wound and graft infection resulting from re-dissection in the groin and the risk of progressive tissue loss during the initial recuperative period must be considered with this approach.

Another solution to multilevel disease has been the utilization of hybrid approaches, which combine elements of both open surgical and endovascular therapy and which have been shown to have high technical success rates and long-term patency. Many retrospective and prospective series have indicated good limb salvage, and morbidity and mortality rates equal to or better than open bypass procedures with a hybrid approach.[59–62] As iliac stenting is now the first line for treatment of amenable TASC C/D iliac lesions, a combined approach using endovascular and open techniques can often fully address both inflow and outflow simultaneously.[59–61] This can offer an alternative to open approaches in medically high risk patients and significantly shorten hospital and intensive care unit lengths of stay.[60]

Outcomes

Aortobifemoral bypass grafting is associated with patency rates that are among the highest reported for any major arterial reconstruction. As indicated earlier, 5-year primary patency rates of 70% to 88% and 10-year rates of 66% to 79% have been described.[36,38,39] Better rates have been realized in those patients with good infrainguinal outflow operated on for claudication compared to those with limb-threatening ischemia and associated infrainguinal occlusive disease. In general, patients with disease limited to the aortoiliac region have excellent relief of symptoms following aortobifemoral grafting, while those with multilevel disease have less complete levels of symptom diminution. Perioperative mortality rates average 4%, while 5-year survival rates between 70% and 75% have been reported.[38,62,63] This latter rate is notably less than the 5-year survival of the age-matched control population but is on par with that typically seen for patients with claudication in general.

While the early and late mortality rates are similar across different age groups, the 5-year primary and secondary patency rates are significantly increased with each increase in age group. Reed and colleagues reported that primary patency rates were 66%, 87%, and 96%, and secondary patency rates were 79%, 91%, and 98% (Fig. 21.5), respectively, for those <50 years, those 50 to 59 years of age, and those >60 years of age.[39] Based on these findings, it seems prudent to apply caution in the application of aortobifemoral bypass grafting for younger patients with virulent aortoiliac disease. The potential impact of graft failure and the need for subsequent complex interventions should be considered, especially given the longer life expectancy of younger patients. Full utilization of all medical and endovascular options appears to be the best first-line option for younger patients with severe aortoiliac occlusive disease.

Extra-anatomic Bypass

When comorbid disease renders a patient with aortoiliac occlusive disease particularly unsuitable for major vascular surgery and aortic cross clamping, or when sepsis, prior surgery or the presence of a stoma presents a hostile surgical environment for abdominal exploration, there are several alternatives available to the vascular surgeon. Such reconstructive options, in which the thoracic aorta, axillary, iliac, or femoral arteries serve as the donor vessels, are generally referred to as extra-anatomic to distinguish them from the in-line flow represented by an aortobifemoral procedure. The concept of extra-anatomic arterial reconstruction emerged in the 1950s at a time of many new developments in the field of vascular surgery. Freeman and Leeds provided one of the first descriptions in 1952 in their report of

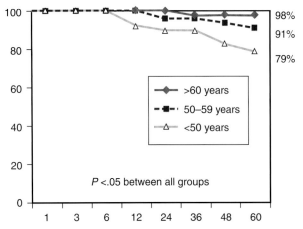

Fig. 21.5 Overall 5-year cumulative secondary patency rates in a cohort of patients undergoing aortobifemoral bypass grafting, indicating an inverse relationship between age and graft patency. (From Reed AB, Conte MS, Donaldson MC, et al. The impact of patient age and aortic size on the results of aortobifemoral bypass grafting. *J Vasc Surg.* 2003;37:1219–1225.)

the use of the superficial femoral artery as the conduit for a crossover femorofemoral bypass graft.[64] These approaches are also called upon in desperate situations represented by the infection of a previously placed aortic graft.

Axillobifemoral Bypass

Axillobifemoral bypass grafting was introduced by Blaisdell and Hall[65] in the early 1960s and has since enjoyed increasing popularity as an alternative to aortobifemoral bypass. This is largely due to the reliability of the axillary artery as a donor vessel and the minimal morbidity incurred, making it a particularly appealing option for patients with significant operative risk from comorbid disease. It is also appropriate in patients with significant aortoiliac occlusive disease of the distal aorta and the iliac arteries in the setting of intraabdominal sepsis, a history of multiple prior abdominal operations, intraabdominal adhesions or prior pelvic irradiation. Of note, LoGerfo and colleagues[66] have shown that axillobifemoral grafting has improved long-term patency compared with axillounifemoral grafting, presumably due to the increased flow afforded by the second outflow limb.

Although usually performed under general anesthesia, it is possible to carry out the procedure using a combination of local anesthesia and intravenous conscious sedation. In the event that one arm has a higher blood pressure or a stronger pulse, that side should be selected as the donor site. If both sides are equal, the right axillary artery is chosen as evidence suggests there is a lower risk of arterial occlusive disease developing in the right subclavian artery compared with the left. The right side is also preferable in cases of aortic infection, as subsequent operations may require a left flank incision or left thoracotomy. In cases of groin infection, bilateral axillounifemoral artery bypass may be necessary to avoid infected wounds.

The axillary artery is exposed through a short infraclavicular incision parallel to the clavicle in the deltopectoral groove. The pectoralis major muscle is then bluntly separated between the clavicular and sternal heads, and the pectoralis minor muscle is identified and typically divided, enhancing exposure and allowing more space for the graft as it courses from the axilla to the subcutaneous space. The axillary artery medial to the pectoralis minor is then isolated as the proximal anastomosis is optimally placed as close to the chest as possible to minimize the risk of kinking or graft avulsion during rotational shoulder movement. Avoiding more lateral dissection further reduces the risk of injuring the medial and lateral cords of the brachial plexus as they emerge anteriorly to form the median nerve. A tunnel is created between the axillary and femoral arteries in the subcutaneous space, tracking deep to the pectoralis major muscle and inferiorly along the mid-axillary line before coursing medial to the anterior superior iliac spine; this latter orientation is important to avoid kinking of the conduit in the sitting position. Long, rigid tunneling devices with a removable central obturator are specifically designed for this step and have helped to lower the incidence of graft infection by obviating the need for counter incisions.

The common femoral arteries are then dissected through standard bilateral short groin incisions and a second subcutaneous tunnel is fashioned between them in an extrafascial, suprapubic plane. A Dacron or polytetrafluoroethylene graft, typically 8 mm in diameter, is then drawn through the tunnel. While there is no convincing evidence that one graft material is superior to the other, several reports support the common practice of using an externally reinforced graft.[67,68] Newer grafts are available that are prefigured in an axillobifemoral configuration, thereby reducing from four to three the number of anastomoses needed. As in aortobifemoral bypass grafting, unrestricted outflow should be ensured by carrying the hood of the femoral grafts down over the profunda orifice and performing an endarterectomy or profundaplasty when necessary. If a prefigured graft is unavailable, the origin of the cross-femoral graft can be tailored to the body habitus of the patient. In most cases, the graft is taken off the distal hood of the descending axillofemoral graft. However, in particularly obese individuals, it may be preferable to move the takeoff more proximally to prevent kinking at the level of the inguinal ligament. Orienting the takeoff of the crossover graft at an acute angle to give an "S-shaped" final configuration has been associated with higher patency rates in some studies.[69]

Many of the complications following axillofemoral grafting are directly related to the graft and are potentially avoidable. Disruption of the proximal anastomosis can be minimized by proper orientation of the proximal hood and ensuring that the descending limb of the graft is free from undue tension.[70] Kinking and subsequent thrombosis of the graft can be reduced by strict attention to tunnel position and use of a reinforced conduit.

Given the minimal physiologic insult, most patients undergoing axillofemoral grafting are ambulatory and able to tolerate a regular diet on the first postoperative day.

The reported long-term patency rates of axillofemoral grafts have varied significantly, ranging from as low as 29% to as high as 85%.[71–73] Favorable results were reported by Passman and colleagues,[74] who achieved 5-year patency rates of 74% and a long-term limb salvage rate of 89% and who are advocates of a wider use for this approach. More recently, Liedenbaum et al. reported 3-year primary and secondary patency rates of 49% and 86%, respectively.[75] In general, axillobifemoral grafting should be reserved for high-risk patients with significant tissue loss in danger of limb loss, and not be used for the treatment of claudication.

Femorofemoral Bypass

Femorofemoral bypass grafts are ideally suited to those patients with preserved flow in both the aorta and one iliac branch, but occlusion or severe stenosis of the contralateral iliac is not amenable to percutaneous treatment (Figs. 21.6 and 21.7A). Although a femorofemoral artery bypass graft is possible to perform under local anesthesia in high-risk patients, it is best carried out under regional or general anesthesia. On occasion, it has been performed in an intensive care unit setting in the particular instance of a leg rendered acutely ischemic by the placement of an intraaortic balloon pump. The technical details are identical to that of the crossover component of the axillobifemoral grafting discussed above. The suprapubic tunnel is created in a gentle C-curve just superficial to the deep fascia and can, in most instances, be completed by blunt finger dissection approaching from both groin incisions. While some surgeons advocate the placement of the tunnel beneath the rectus sheath, this is a minority view. Again, if warranted by the presence of significant concomitant femoral disease, an endarterectomy or profundaplasty is indicated prior to completion of the proximal or distal anastomosis.

Graft failure due to progression of inflow disease following femorofemoral grafting is less problematic than one might predict. Some investigators have argued that the increased flow through the donor iliac artery following the restoration of bilateral outflow, in essence shifting the aortic bifurcation to a more distal point, serves to impede the further development of atherosclerotic disease. Animal studies correlating blood flow and shear stress with intimal hyperplasia lend support to this explanation.[76] Maini and Mannick reported a 5-year cumulative patency rate of 80%.[77] This is similar to other reports in the literature[78–80] and compares favorably to the 85% rate seen with conventional aortobifemoral bypass grafting.[47]

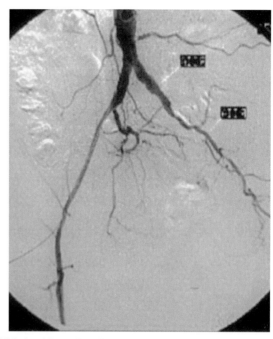

Fig. 21.6 An oblique view digital subtraction angiogram indicating a long segment total occlusion of the left external iliac artery. Extra-anatomic left-to-right femorofemoral or iliofemoral bypass grafting would be appropriate options for this anatomic disease distribution (see Fig. 21.7).

With its high patency rates and low associated morbidity, cross-femoral grafting is an excellent option in patients with favorable anatomy. Given the risk of late graft failure from progression of inflow disease and the potential need to reintervene on previously dissected femoral beds should a later aortobifemoral graft be needed, it has traditionally been advised to proceed directly to aortobifemoral grafting in good-risk patients with any evidence of atherosclerotic disease in the aorta or patent iliac vessels. In the current era, aortic or iliac angioplasty and/or stenting in combination with cross-femoral grafting is a viable alternative in this setting, particularly for those patients at increased operative risk.

Iliofemoral Bypass

Iliofemoral grafting is another alternative to aortobifemoral grafting for a select group of patients with hemodynamically significant disease limited to the external iliac artery (see Fig. 21.6). Currently, most patients with this anatomic pattern of disease would typically undergo an attempt at percutaneous recanalization of a tightly stenotic or long segment external iliac occlusion. Indeed, as the success rates with such efforts increase, the number of iliofemoral bypass grafts performed has continued to fall. However, if the percutaneous approach is unsuccessful, an iliofemoral bypass remains an excellent surgical option as it can be performed with minimal morbidity and cardiopulmonary insult, and avoids the long descending limb necessitated by an axillofemoral graft (see Fig. 21.7B, C). As the grafts are situated within the pelvis, they are also better protected from kinking, infection, and thrombosis than either axillofemoral or femorofemoral grafts. Less disturbance of inguinal lymph nodes and lymphatic channels typically occurs with the more limited dissection necessary. Either the ipsilateral common iliac or proximal external iliac artery can serve as the donor site, and if need be, a bifurcated graft can be used and taken to both femoral vessels. Alternatively, bilateral iliofemoral grafts or an ilio-iliac graft can be fashioned as appropriate. Iliac exposure can be achieved through an oblique

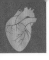

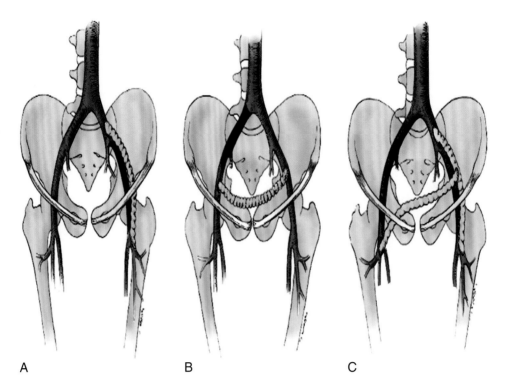

Fig. 21.7 A patent common or external iliac artery may be used as a donor vessel for the (A) ilioiliac, (B) iliofemoral, or (C) iliofemoral bypass grafts depicted. The lesions depicted in (A) and (B) would also be appropriate for femorofemoral grafts, while the lesion in (C) would be appropriate for aortobifemoral or axillobifemoral grafting.

suprainguinal "transplant" incision and development of the retroperitoneal plane, which affords excellent proximal exposure even in the obese patient. Care must be taken in isolating the donor vessel and tunneling the graft to avoid injury to the ureter coursing over the iliac bifurcation. If a crossover graft is used, it can be tunneled retroperitoneally in the iliac fossa or across the preperitoneum deep to the rectus sheath.

In early experience with iliac origin grafts reported by Couch and colleagues, there were no operative deaths and a 77% 4-year patency rate.[81] Nearly half of these patients were operated on for limb salvage in the face of critical ischemia. In those patients undergoing revascularization with bilateral iliofemoral grafts, the 4-year patency rate was 92%, while an 85% patency rate was seen if both the superficial and the deep femoral vessels were patent.[81] Other reported series of iliofemoral bypass grafting have indicated similar patency rates.[82]

Thoracic Aorto-to-Femoral Artery Bypass

As early as 1961, Blaisdell and colleagues reported on a novel extra-anatomic bypass from the descending thoracic aorta to the femoral artery, followed by a femorofemoral bypass.[83] Although carried out in the setting of sepsis after a ruptured aneurysm repair and not for occlusive disease, it provided a new alternative when the infrarenal aorta is inaccessible or inappropriate as a donor vessel. The procedure is performed through a thoracotomy incision, typically entering the chest through the eighth or ninth interspace. A muscle-sparing technique in which the latissimus dorsi muscle is not divided aids in postoperative pain management. The distal descending thoracic aorta is circumferentially dissected enough to allow for clamp control, with care taken to avoid injury to the adjacently positioned esophagus. A tunnel is fashioned by separating the diaphragm from the posterior chest wall over a distance of two-finger breadths. Both Dacron and PTFE grafts have been used with success,[84,85] although Dacron is much more commonly used in this anatomic

location. Hughes et al. have described a thoracofemoral reconstruction using femoral vein in a patient with multiple prior graft infections.[86] In 1994, Criado and Keagy reviewed the literature and summarized 193 reconstructions taken off the descending thoracic aorta. Not unexpectedly, the majority were performed for thrombosis or infection of a previously placed aortic graft, although some primary procedures undertaken in the setting of a "hostile" abdomen were included. Cumulative 5-year primary and secondary patency rates of 73% and 83%, respectively, were obtained, and the operative mortality rate was 6%.[87]

Laparoscopic Revascularization

There has been some historic interest in applying laparoscopic techniques to the treatment of aortic occlusive disease over the last several decades, reflected in a small body of literature of individual cases series.[88,89] Some surgeons have favored a more limited approach using hand-assisted techniques and smaller incisions,[90] while others have championed the use of complete laparoscopic or robot-assisted revascularization.[88,91] Several studies have documented shorter hospital stays, less perioperative pain and postoperative complications, but longer operative times and high conversion rates.[92–94] A series published in 2016 demonstrated 5-year primary, primary assisted, and secondary patency rates 83%, 92%, and 97%, respectively.[94] At present, it remains a technically challenging procedure with a significant learning curve. As both laparoscopic and robotic technology continues to advance, the role of both of these modalities for aortic reconstruction may expand or become more defined.

INFRAINGUINAL ARTERIAL OCCLUSIVE DISEASE

Infrainguinal arterial occlusive disease is the most prevalent manifestation of chronic arterial occlusive disease encountered and treated by the vascular surgeon. Isolated disease of the superficial femoral artery

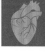

typically presents as calf muscle claudication, while patients with multilevel disease involving the superficial femoral, popliteal, and tibial arteries generally have rest pain or ischemic tissue loss. Ischemic ulcerations usually begin as small, dry ulcers of the toes or heel area, and progress to frankly gangrenous changes of the forefoot or heel with greater degrees of arterial insufficiency (see Chapter 61). Several identifiable patterns of disease are recognized, with smokers typically having disease limited to the superficial femoral artery and corresponding symptoms of claudication. Diabetes, on the other hand, most often targets the popliteal and tibial vessels, and patients may present with frank tissue necrosis with no prior history of claudication.

Infrainguinal reconstruction for the treatment of peripheral vascular occlusive disease has been increasingly successful for both the long-term palliation of intermittent claudication and the salvage of limbs threatened by critical ischemia. While there are certainly times when primary amputation represents the safest and most advisable solution in the face of irreversible ischemia—particularly in cases where extensive infection or tissue necrosis is present—an attempt at reconstruction is almost always indicated when a limb is threatened by severe ischemia. Improvements in perioperative management and surgical technique have allowed progressively more distal reconstructions to be successfully completed in an older, sicker, and challenging patient population. In general, high rates of relief for claudication and up to an 80% to 90% limb salvage rate may be anticipated for patients with critical ischemia at institutions devoted to peripheral bypass surgery.

The two major indications for surgical intervention of infrainguinal arterial occlusive disease are claudication and limb-threatening critical ischemia. Claudication is a relative indication given the natural history of the disease; of patients with claudication, only 1% per year will ultimately progress to limb loss.[95,96] As such, it remains a subjective assessment on the part of both patient and surgeon as to the relative degree of disability a given level of claudication pain represents.

Role of Percutaneous Transluminal Angioplasty

There has been significant shift in the indications for percutaneous intervention for infrainguinal occlusive disease in recent years. As the associated risks of balloon angioplasty and stenting have fallen and the relative success rates have risen, the threshold for offering endovascular treatment to both claudicants and patients with critical limb ischemia has considerably decreased. Patients once considered appropriate only for risk factor modification, exercise therapy, and medical treatment are now increasingly being offered percutaneous revascularization as a primary treatment option (see Chapter 20).

Similarly, occlusive disease of the tibial vessels, once thought to be the exclusive domain of operative bypass, is now readily being treated percutaneously. The impact of these trends on the natural history of the disease, and to what extent the expanding reach of percutaneous therapy will affect subsequent operative management in a given patient remains undefined. Certainly, as the enthusiasm for less-invasive options has spread to include the infrapopliteal and even pedal level, the relative roles of surgical and percutaneous intervention are further being tested. Newer generation atherectomy devices, better and more flexible stents designed to withstand the unique torsional forces of the leg and drug-eluting angioplasty balloons and stents, have all led to improved patency and durability rates.[97,98] However, until the longer term results of infrainguinal percutaneous intervention are better understood, surgical revascularization will remain the gold standard for most patients with critical limb ischemia. For patients with favorable anatomy and significant operative risk, and for the treatment of claudication in general, percutaneous therapy has assumed a more primary role.

Duplex ultrasonography, CTA, and MRA are increasingly being utilized as first-line modalities in the assessment of patients with infrainguinal occlusive disease (see Chapters 12 to 14). Although a growing collection of literature supports the use of duplex scanning as a stand-alone preoperative mapping modality,[99] this requires a highly dedicated vascular lab, and to date has not gained wide acceptance. CTA and MRA can be particularly useful as noninvasive screening tests to determine the suitability for percutaneous therapy. Operative planning based solely on CTA or MRA scanning with high-quality time of flight, gadolinium-enhanced images is now being performed with increasing frequency,[100,101] as imaging technology continues to improve at delineating tibial- and pedal-level arterial occlusive disease.[102] Newer, less nephrotoxic MR contrast agents, such as the iron-based ferumoxytol, also have been used with greater regularity and with good diagnostic accuracy in patients with renal insufficiency.[103,104]

Operative Management

Infrainguinal bypass can be performed under general anesthesia, or in the appropriate patient, regional spinal or epidural anesthesia. The multiple sites of dissection and the harvesting of saphenous vein or an alternative vein conduit make these procedures particularly suited to a two-team approach. The time saved, particularly in cases involving potentially more tedious arm vein or lesser saphenous vein harvesting, has direct benefit in minimizing the total anesthetic load and physiologic insult to the patient. Typically, the site proposed for the distal anastomosis is explored first to ascertain whether the preoperative imaging was accurate in predicting the suitability of the target vessel. On occasion, the operation is begun with an on-table angiogram to clarify the anatomy if preoperative imaging was deferred or ambiguous.

The above-knee popliteal vessel is easily exposed through a medial thigh incision, with subsequent posterolateral retraction of the sartorius muscle. The popliteal artery with its accompanying vein and nerve is found just posterior to the femur. The vessel is palpated to determine the presence of atherosclerotic plaque, which will guide the extent of dissection and the optimal bypass target site. The below-knee popliteal artery is also exposed through a medial incision in the proximal calf (Fig. 21.8). If the saphenous vein is to be harvested, the incision is made directly over the vein to minimize the creation of devascularized skin flaps. With the exposed vein carefully protected, the incision is carried through the deep muscular fascia and the medial head of the gastrocnemius is reflected posterolaterally to expose the below-knee popliteal fossa. The distal popliteal artery is then dissected free from the adjacent tibial nerve posteriorly and the popliteal vein medially. If the distal target is the tibioperoneal trunk, the dissection is continued along the anteromedial surface of the distal popliteal artery after dividing the origin of the soleus muscle from the tibia (Fig. 21.9). In instances in which the below-knee popliteal artery has been previously exposed or where sepsis is involved, a lateral approach with the excision of a segment of proximal fibula is a useful alternative approach.

While exposure of the proximal posterior and peroneal vessels can be gained by extending the tibioperoneal trunk dissection distally, more distal exposure of these vessels is best gained through targeted medial incisions. The posterior tibial artery is found more medially on the reflected soleus muscle, while the peroneal artery is deeper and more lateral. The posterior tibial artery at the level of the ankle is a relatively easier target given the proximity of the vessel to the skin surface. The initial incision is made just posterior to the medial malleolus, and the artery exposed by division of the overlying retinaculum. Further distal dissection allows access to the bifurcation and medial and lateral plantar branches.[105] The anterior tibial artery is typically approached from the anterolateral aspect of the calf (see Fig. 21.9) and is found

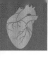

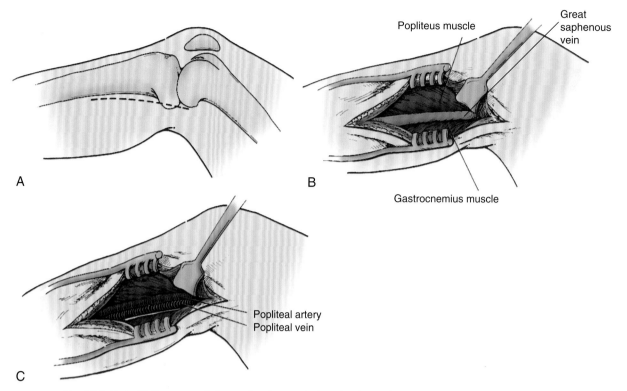

Fig. 21.8 (A to C) Exposure of the popliteal artery below the knee. The medial incision is made directly overlying the course of the greater saphenous vein.

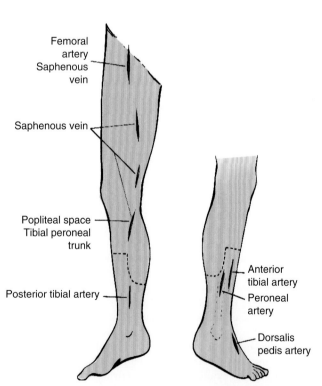

Fig. 21.9 Placement of incisions for femoropopliteal and femorotibial bypass and for greater saphenous vein harvest. These should avoid the incision lines for a below-knee amputation.

deep within the anterior compartment with the adjacent deep peroneal nerve and anterior tibial veins. The dorsalis pedis artery is easily exposed through an axial incision on the dorsum of the foot just lateral to the extensor hallucis longus tendon (see Fig. 21.9).

Following exposure of the distal anastomotic target vessel, the site of the proximal anastomosis is dissected. For patients with superficial femoral artery disease, this will most commonly be at the level of the common femoral artery. The artery is mobilized as described above, from the level of the inguinal ligament to its terminal bifurcation. The distal extent of this dissection is dictated by the presence of concomitant femoral plaque. Lymphatic tissue overlying the femoral vessels is best ligated and divided to prevent the postoperative development of lymph fistulas or lymphoceles. If an extensive endarterectomy or profundaplasty is required, the proximal profunda femoral artery is dissected along its proximal length accordingly.

If all or part of the superficial femoral artery is spared of significant atherosclerotic involvement, the proximal anastomosis can be moved distally as dictated by the particular anatomic pattern of disease, and a so-called "distal origin graft" can be fashioned (Fig. 21.10).[106] This situation is particularly applicable to the diabetic population, where infrapopliteal disease is the rule and sparing of the superficial femoral and popliteal arteries is not uncommon. It is also used in situations where conduit is sparse, and a moderately diseased proximal vessel is accepted as an inflow source for a more distal origin bypass graft in the interests of performing a fully autologous vein graft rather than utilizing prosthetic material. An increasingly popular approach when only limited conduit is available is to combine, either concurrently in the operating room or as a staged preoperative procedure, catheter-based treatment of the superficial femoral or popliteal artery inflow with more distal bypass.[106]

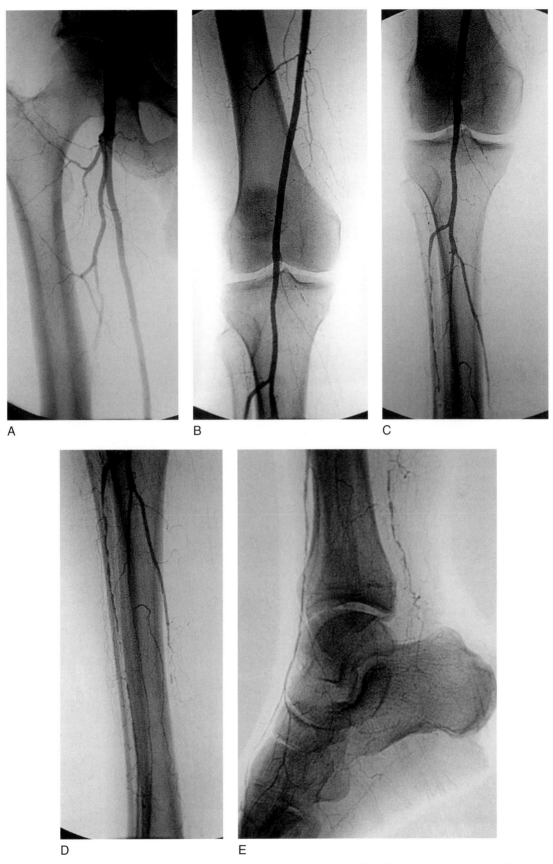

A   B   C

D   E

Fig. 21.10 (A to E) Arteriogram indicating the preservation of the superficial femoral artery and the popliteal arteries with mid-calf occlusions of all three infrageniculate vessels. This anatomic pattern of disease is amenable to "distal origin" vein grafting from the below-knee popliteal or proximal posterior tibial artery to the dorsalis pedis artery.

Autogenous Vein Bypass

In general, infrainguinal bypass surgery is best performed with autogenous vein conduit, preferably the ipsilateral greater saphenous vein if available.[107] This is particularly true for grafts extending below the knee, where prosthetic conduits of Dacron or PTFE have significantly poorer patency rates. The first report of a femoropopliteal bypass graft using the autogenous greater saphenous vein in a reversed orientation was by Kunlin in 1951.[5] Given the orientation of the vein valves, the vein is reversed such that the distal end of the vein is sewn to the proximal inflow artery and the larger proximal end of the vein is sewn to the distal outflow artery. The vein is harvested through a long incision overlying the course of the vein or by more tedious but less invasive sequential skip incisions with intervening cutaneous skin bridges (see Fig. 21.9). All side branches are ligated and after harvest, the vein is cannulated and gently dilated with a solution containing heparin and papaverine to assess its suitability. Veins with chronic fibrosis or that fail to dilate to a diameter of 3 mm or greater will likely have poor long-term function.

For prosthetic grafts, a tunnel is usually fashioned through the sub-sartorial plane between the groin incision and the above-knee popliteal space in the interests of protecting the graft from subsequent infection. For vein conduits, it remains the surgeon's preference as to whether the graft is tunneled deeply or in a superficial location in the subcutaneous space. The more superficial configuration greatly facilitates ongoing clinical examination and ultrasonographic surveillance as well as later surgical revision, but carries a risk of graft exposure should there be wound healing problems. Occlusion from trauma to grafts placed superficially has been of theoretic, not practical, concern.

The order of anastomoses is surgeon dependent, with strong feelings expressed in each camp. Prior to occluding the target vessel, the patient is systemically anticoagulated with 5000 to 10,000 units of heparin. The artery is then clamped proximally and distally and incised; the vein spatulated; and a beveled anastomosis is carried out. Typically, a 5-0 monofilament suture of Prolene is used for the femoral anastomosis, a 6-0 used at the popliteal level, and a very fine 7-0 suture used at the tibial or pedal level. If the target tibial vessel is deep within the calf and visibility is challenging, a technique of "parachuting" the heel of the distal anastomosis is often employed. After completing the first anastomosis, the graft is carefully marked to ensure against mechanical twisting or kinking of the graft during the tunneling process. One of the benefits of performing the proximal anastomosis first is that following release of the clamps, the adequacy of flow through the graft can be assessed.

Occasionally, such extensive calcification of the target vessel is encountered that the risk of a significant injury from clamping, even with the minimally traumatic clamps in use today, is prohibitively high. In such cases, proximal inflow and distal artery backbleeding can be controlled by occlusion balloons placed intraluminally. For distal anastomoses at the knee or more distal level, another alternative technique is the use of a proximally placed sterile pneumatic tourniquet. This is particularly advantageous when sewing to diminutive distal tibial or pedal targets, where the impact of a crush injury or plaque dislodgement on graft function could be considerable. Removing the need for clamps by using the tourniquet has two further advantages. First, it improves the operative visibility. Second, and more importantly, given that less longitudinal and circumferential dissection is needed, the degree of vessel spasm and venous bleeding that frequently accompanies vessel exposure at this level is kept to a minimum.

Flow through the graft and the outflow arteries should be evaluated following completion of the bypass by manual pulse assessment and with a continuous-wave Doppler. Two additional intraoperative completion studies that are considerably more sensitive to screen for hemodynamically significant abnormalities within the graft are duplex ultrasonography and contrast angiography (Fig. 21.11)[108,109]; both allow for immediate repair of any identified technical defects; for example, twisting or kinking of the graft, a retained valve cusp, or thrombus formation within the graft (Fig. 21.12).[110] Current reports of the 5-year results of reversed saphenous vein graft using modern techniques have been excellent, with primary and secondary patency rates of 75% and 80%, respectively, and limb salvage rates of 90%.[111,112]

In Situ Grafting

There has been ongoing enthusiasm in some circles for in situ vein bypass grafting, whereby—except for its proximal and distal extent— the greater saphenous vein is left undisturbed in its native bed. This technique was first described in 1962[113] but was later popularized by Leather and Karmody in the late 1970s.[114] Recent reports of in situ saphenous vein grafting have indicated 5-year graft patency rates approaching 80%, and limb salvage rates of 84% to 90%.[112,114–117]

The approach minimizes trauma to the vein during excision and handling, and in theory enhances preservation of the vasovasorum and endothelium. It further lowers the considerable risk of wound healing complications seen with traditional vein harvesting, and facilitates the creation of more technically precise anastomoses as the proximal and distal vein diameters are more closely matched to those of the inflow and outflow target vessels (Fig. 21.13). The extent of the proximal vein mobilization is dictated by the location of the saphenofemoral junction relative to the proposed site of the proximal anastomosis. At times it may be necessary to perform an endarterectomy of the superficial femoral artery if the length of proximal vein is insufficient. Lysis of the valve cusps is obligatory given the nonreversed configuration, and is facilitated by newer, less traumatic valvulotomes that function safely through the blinded segments of undissected graft. Critics of this technique argue that the advantages listed above have not translated into improved graft function or patency. They further argue that the time required and the dissection involved in finding and ligating substantial side branches that can develop into physiologically important arteriovenous fistulae that "steal" distal flow obviates the stated benefits of this approach. Techniques utilizing angioscopy and endoluminal coiling[118] of larger side branches may help to minimize these concerns.

Angioscopic-assisted valve lysis has been employed by some enthusiasts but has never gained widespread favor. While there is a significant learning curve with this technology, and operative times—at least initially—are significantly prolonged, advocates site fewer wound complications, shorter hospital stays, and decreased recuperative periods as potential benefits. Proponents of routine angioscopy for direct visualization of valve lysis stress its particular utility in demonstrating such unsuspected endoluminal venous pathology as phlebitic strictures, webs, and fibrotic valve cusps.[119] This adjunct may be particularly useful in cases where an arm vein is used, when endoluminal pathology is more frequently encountered and is presumably responsible, in part, for suboptimal results.[120]

Nonreversed saphenous vein grafts. Recognizing the many practical advantages inherent to the in situ technique, Belkin and colleagues and others have modified the approach to infrainguinal bypass grafting with venous conduit to incorporate several of the same principles.[121] In particular, if the harvested vein is tapered to any significant extent, it is used in a nonreversed fashion. By optimizing the size matching between the artery and vein at both the proximal and distal anastomosis sites as discussed above, one can often accept smaller veins for use than would be suitable for reversed vein grafting. The nonreversed configuration also allows the preservation of the saphenous vein hood, which

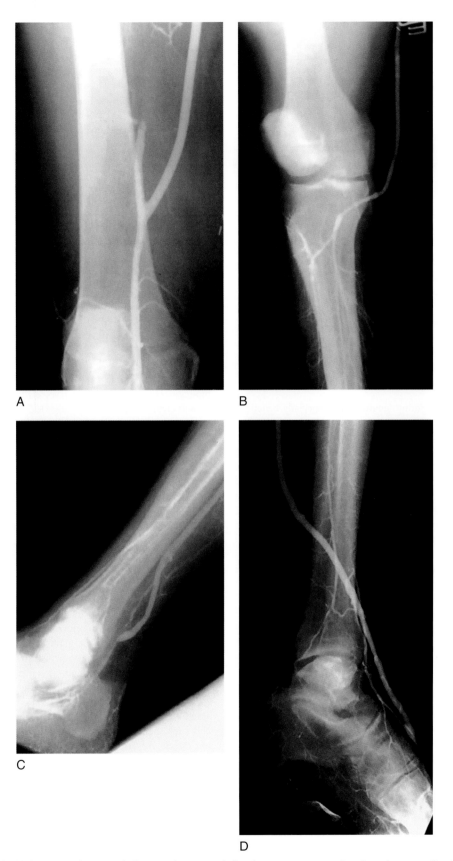

Fig. 21.11 Intraoperative completion arteriograms of distal anastomoses to the above-knee popliteal (A), below-knee popliteal (B), distal posterior tibial (C), and dorsalis pedis (D) arteries.

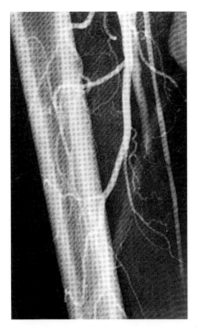

Fig. 21.12 Intraoperative completion arteriogram of an in situ femoropopliteal vein graft indicating a retained valve, visualized as a filling defect in the graft, and a persistent arteriovenous fistula.

both extends the available conduit length and is especially beneficial when the femoral artery is thick-walled and diseased.

The vein is harvested and dilated in a similar fashion to reversed vein grafts, and the cusps of the proximal valve of the greater saphenous vein are excised under direct vision with fine Potts scissors. There are currently two main types of valvulotomes available. The modified Mills valvulotome is a short, metal, hockey-stick–shaped cutter that can be introduced through the distal end of the vein or through the side branches. After the proximal anastomosis is performed and with the perfused conduit on gentle stretch, the valves are carefully lysed in a sequential fashion by pulling the valvulotome inferiorly. An alternative, recently designed self-centering valvulotome allows lysis of all valves in a single pass and is thought by some to be less traumatic. Once acceptable pulsatile flow is ensured, the distal anastomosis is performed in the standard fashion.

It is important to note that similar patency rates have consistently been demonstrated regardless of which technique is applied,[116,117] so surgeon preference and comfort level is an acceptable reason for choosing one method over another.

Prosthetic Bypass

It is recommended that infrainguinal bypass surgery be performed with the saphenous vein or an autologous substitute whenever feasible given the clearly demonstrated enhanced patency rates.[107,122] Some institutions more frequently rely on prosthetic grafts. When the distal target is the above-knee popliteal artery and the tibial outflow is relatively well preserved, this is an acceptable approach, as patency rates in this situation approach those of vein grafts.[123] A variety of surgical adjunctive procedures, from patching the distal anastomotic target vessel to the creation of a distal arteriovenous fistula, or various autogenous vein cuffs interposed between the distal prosthetic and the target artery, have all been attempted as a means of improving the patency rates of grafts extending below the knee.[124] Flared grafts designed to minimize turbulence and shear stress between the prosthetic and native vessel have also gained some popularity. Distaflo (Bard Medical, Covington, GA), a precuffed expanded PTFE graft, has similar pri-

mary and secondary patency and limb salvage rates compared to other noncuffed PTFE grafts[125] but patency rates are low in comparison to the autogenous saphenous vein.[126,127] Polyester (Dacron) and PTFE grafts are the two main types of prosthetic available and, as in other anatomic positions, available data show generally equal results with either choice. The entire procedure is carried out through two small proximal and distal incisions between which the graft is tunneled anatomically. The selection of a 6- or 8-mm graft is dictated by the size of the native vessels.

Cadaveric Allografts

Cryopreserved cadaver vein allografts are an additional, typically last resort, option for lower extremity revascularization. Currently, they are primarily used for limb salvage in infected fields in patients without autogenous veins, as they are more resistant to subsequent reinfection than other options.[128–130] Their limited use is due to consistently poor patency rates; one typical series reported 1- and 3-year primary patency rates of 37% and 24%, respectively.[130] Of note, there is some evidence to suggest that donor-recipient blood type compatibility can significantly improve limb salvage when cryopreserved allografts are used.[131] More recently, cryopreserved cadaveric femoral artery grafts have become available, but there is, as yet, no literature to support their use.

Bioengineered Allografts

Phase II clinical trials are currently underway assessing the use of bioengineered human acellular vessels for lower extremity bypass in patients with peripheral artery disease. These conduits have lower infection rates than prosthetic grafts and have shown acceptable patency rates when used in hemodialysis access.[132] At present, data clarifying their role in peripheral vascular reconstruction are lacking.

Reoperative Bypass Surgery

As the patient population treated by vascular surgeons has increased in age, and an increasing number of challenging cases are accepted for primary treatment, there has been a corresponding increase in the incidence of reoperative bypass surgery performed for infrainguinal arterial occlusive disease. Such reoperative procedures are particularly challenging, both because of the scarring present at the inflow and outflow target sites and because there is typically a lack of the ipsilateral greater saphenous vein. Whenever possible, the first problem is addressed by choosing anastomotic sites just above or below the previous touchdown points, thereby avoiding dissection through often densely scarred tissue planes. When the ipsilateral greater saphenous vein is absent due to prior infrainguinal or coronary artery bypass surgery or prior saphenous vein stripping, there are a number of alternative conduit sites available. Chew and colleagues studied the consequence of using the contralateral greater saphenous vein in these situations and found it to be the optimal conduit; despite the presumably high incidence of contralateral lower extremity as well as coronary occlusive disease in this population, the short- and long-term impact was found to be minimal.[133]

In the absence of any greater saphenous vein, preoperative venous duplex ultrasonography is employed to evaluate the cephalic and basilic veins of the arms and the lesser saphenous veins of the legs in an effort to determine the best conduit available. Often the veins distal to the antecubital crease are scarred and of small caliber, but their more proximal counterparts are often of excellent size and quality. The use of arm veins in general can be extremely technically challenging and for that reason has not been universally adopted. The dissection of the basilic vein can be particularly tedious as it has multiple side branches and lies adjacent to several important nerves. As arm veins are often relatively short, a venovenostomy is often required to create composite

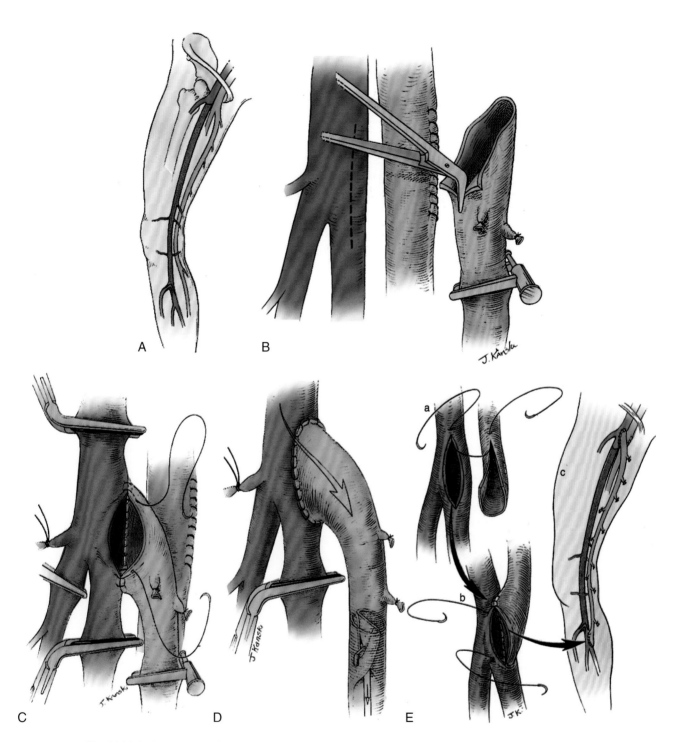

Fig. 21.13 In the in situ method of infrainguinal reconstruction, the saphenous vein is left undisturbed in its native bed except at the proximal and distal anastomotic sites—in this case the common femoral artery and the tibioperoneal trunk, respectively (A). The saphenofemoral junction is transected in the groin, the venotomy in the femoral vein is oversewn, and the proximal end of the saphenous vein spatulated in preparation for anastomosis (B). After the first venous valve is excised under direct vision, the graft is anastomosed end-to-side to the femoral artery (C). Flow is then restored through the vein graft and the valvulotome passed from the distal end to lyse the residual valves (D) before the distal anastomosis is performed (E).

grafts long enough to complete the arterial reconstruction (Fig. 21.14). This is performed with generous spatulation of each vein hood to create a widely patent vein to vein anastomosis. Given their thin-walled nature, arm vein grafts are also quite prone to twisting and kinking, and special care must be taken during the tunneling process to avoid these problems. The more proximal arm veins can be relatively large,

and it is often advantageous to use one or more of the segments in a nonreversed fashion to better match the graft to the inflow vessel size.

Not surprisingly, the results of reoperative infrainguinal bypass surgery do not match those of primary reconstruction. With autogenous vein, 5-year patency rates of 60% and limb salvage rates of 70% to 80% have been reported.[133,134] Warfarin may improve long-term patency in

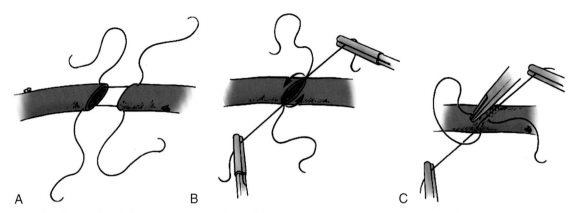

Fig. 21.14 (A to C) Creation of a composite graft from two or more segments of arm vein or lesser saphenous vein is sometimes necessary to obtain the desired length of fully autogenous conduit for an infrainguinal bypass. A widely spatulated venovenostomy is optimal.

patients with compromised outflow or in whom the conduit is of marginal quality.[135,136] However, this remains controversial as other studies have failed to demonstrate improvement in outcomes.[137]

Post-Reconstruction Management

Many of the patients undergoing surgical reconstruction for arterial insufficiency will require one or more adjunctive operative procedures of their foot. Small, uninfected ulcerations of the toe or foot often can be safely managed conservatively. However, larger, gangrenous lesions of the toe, forefoot, or heel usually require debridement of all necrotic tissue at the completion of the revascularization procedure. If the ischemia is particularly severe or infection is present, toe or transmetatarsal amputation may be necessary in order to achieve a margin of healthy tissue. This is particularly important in patients with diabetes or end-stage renal disease, in whom persistent infection or necrosis can result in limb loss despite the presence of a well-revascularized extremity. The wounds are usually left open and treated with saline wet-to-dry dressings or newer, vacuum sponge dressings. Serial debridement on the ward or in the operating room are often necessary for the larger wounds, which can then be surgically closed after an interval healing period, or allowed to slowly close via secondary intention over time.

Unless otherwise contraindicated, all patients should be maintained indefinitely on an antiplatelet regimen with either aspirin or clopidogrel following surgical bypass.[138] In cases in which a graft is at increased risk of failure, such as in the redo setting or when compromised outflow or a marginal conduit was accepted, the antiplatelet agent may be supplemented with warfarin.[135,139] Aggressive risk factor modification in the form of smoking cessation, lipid reduction, exercise, blood pressure management, and diabetic blood sugar control is of further paramount importance in minimizing the risk of disease progression or recurrence.[138] More immediately, aggressive rehabilitation maximizes the chances of, and shortens the time to, a return to full function after extensive reconstructive surgery.

Graft Failure and Surveillance

Postoperative graft failures are typically classified according to the time interval from surgery as early, intermediate or late. Graft thrombosis occurring within 30 days, so-called early graft failures, are generally thought to be due to technical or judgement errors by the surgeon. Included in this list would be such technical errors as twists, kinks, incompletely lysed valves or anastomotic defects, as well as judgment errors in using a poor quality vein or targeting an outflow vessel with inadequate runoff to support the graft. Intermediate graft failures include those between 30 days and 2 years and are generally attributed

to the proliferation of intimal hyperplasia at the anastomoses or prior valve sites within the graft (Fig. 21.15). Late graft failures occurring beyond 2 years are typically due to the progression of atherosclerotic occlusive disease within the inflow or outflow arteries.

Given the known incidence of graft failure and the potentially dire consequence in terms of limb salvage or preservation of limb function in a patient with limited options for secondary or tertiary bypass, the ability to maintain graft patency through early identification and prompt correction of graft stenoses is of paramount importance.[138] Serial postoperative surveillance scanning with a duplex ultrasound has proven an excellent means of accurately identifying hemodynamically significant stenoses within an autologous or cadaveric vein graft or a prosthetic bypass that may threaten graft patency.[140] Subsequent confirmation by angiography and prophylactic treatment by percutaneous balloon angioplasty and/or stenting, surgical patch angioplasty, or the interposition grafting of significant lesions, minimize the risk of graft thrombosis and ensure optimal long-term graft patency.

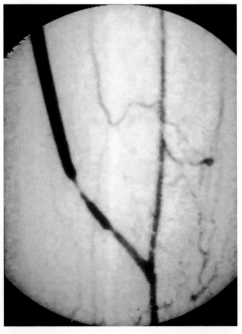

Fig. 21.15 Arteriogram demonstrating severe stenosis of distal graft from intimal hyperplasia, likely at a prior valve site.

REFERENCES

1. Gray EA. *Portrait of a Surgeon: A Biography of John Hunter*. London: Robert Hale; 1952.
2. dos Santos JC. Sur la desobstion des thromboses arterielles anciennes. *Mem Acad Chir*. 1947;73:409–411.
3. Wylie EJ, Kerr E, Davies O. Experimental and clinical experiences with the use of fascia lata applied as a graft about major arteries after thromboendarterectomy and aneurysmorrhaphy. *Surg Gynecol Obstet*. 1951;93:257–272.
4. Carrel A. The surgery of blood vessels, etc. *Johns Hopkins Hosp Bull*. 1907;190:18.
5. Kunlin J. Le traitement de l'ischemie arteritique par la greffe veineuse longue. *Rev Chir*. 1951;70:206–235.
6. McCaughan Jr JJ. Surgical exposure of the distal popliteal artery. *Surgery*. 1958;44:536–539.
7. Leriche R, Morel A. The syndrome of thrombotic obliteration of the aortic bifurcation. *Ann Surg*. 1948;127:193–206.
8. Berman JR, Berman LA, Goldstein I. Female sexual dysfunction: incidence, pathophysiology, evaluation, and treatment options. *Urology*. 1999;54:385–391.
9. Goldstein I, Berman JR. Vasculogenic female sexual dysfunction: vaginal engorgement and clitoral erectile insufficiency syndromes. *Int J Impot Res*. 1998;10(Suppl 2):S84–S90.
10. Chitragari G, Schlosser FJ, Ochoa Chaar CI, Sumpio BE. Consequences of hypogastric artery ligation, embolization, or coverage. *J Vasc Surg*. 2015;62:1340–1347.
11. Wingo JP, Nix ML, Greenfield LJ, Barnes RW. The blue toe syndrome: hemodynamic and therapeutic correlates of outcome. *J Vasc Surg*. 1986;3:475–480.
12. Karmody AM, Powers SR, Monaco VJ, Leather RP. "Blue toe" syndrome. *Arch Surg*. 1976;111:1263–1268.
13. Brewster DC, Perler BA, Robison JG, Darling RC. Aortofemoral graft for multilevel occlusive disease: predictors of success and need for distal bypass. *Arch Surg*. 1982;117:1593–1600.
14. Imparata AM, Kim G, Davidson T, Crowley JG. Intermittent claudication: its natural course. *Surgery*. 1975;78:795–799.
15. Cronenwett JL, Davis Jr JT, Gooch JB, Garrett HE. Aortoiliac occlusive disease in women. *Surgery*. 1980;88:775–784.
16. Caes F, Cham B, Van den Brande P, Welch W. Small artery syndrome in women. *Surg Gynecol Obstet*. 1985;161:165–170.
17. Walton BL, Dougherty K, Mortazavi A, et al. Percutaneous intervention for the treatment of hypoplastic aortoiliac syndrome. *Catheter Cardiovasc Interv*. 2003;60:329–334.
18. Domanin M, Bissaco D, Romagnoli S, Buora A. Acute pseudoaneurysm after endarterectomy for small aorta syndrome. *Int J Surg Case Rep*. 2017;39:98–101.
19. Seldinger SI. Catheter replacement of the needle in percutaneous arteriography: a new technique. *Acta Radiol*. 1953;39:368–376.
20. Udoff EJ, Barth KH, Harrington DP, et al. Hemodynamic significance of iliac artery stenosis: pressure measurements during angiography. *Radiology*. 1979;132:289–293.
21. Spinosa DJ, Kaufmann JA, Hartwell GD. Gadolinium chelates in angiography and interventional radiology: a useful alternative to iodinated contrast media for angiography. *Radiology*. 2002;223:319–325. discussion 326-7.
22. Back MR, Caridi JG, Hawkins Jr IF, Seeger JM. Angiography with carbon dioxide (CO2). *Surg Clin North Am*. 1998;78:575–591.
23. Fakhry F, van de Luijtgaarden KM, Bax L, et al. Supervised walking therapy in patients with intermittent claudication. *J Vasc Surg*. 2012;56:1132–1142.
24. Regensteiner JG, Meyer TJ, Krupski WC, et al. Hospital vs home-based exercise rehabilitation for patients with peripheral arterial occlusive disease. *Angiology*. 1997;48:291–300.
25. Dawson DL, Cutler BS, Hiatt WR, et al. A comparison of cilostazol and pentoxifylline for treating intermittent claudication. *Am J Med*. 2000;109:523–530.
26. Warner CJ, Greaves SW, Larson RJ, et al. Cilostazol is associated with improved outcomes after peripheral endovascular interventions. *J Vasc Surg*. 2014;59:1607–1614.
27. Iida O, Yokol H, Soga Y, et al. Cilostazol reduces angiographic restenosis after endovascular therapy for femoropopliteal lesions in the Sufficient Treatment of Peripheral Intervention by Cilostazol study. *Circulation*. 2013;127:2307–2315.
28. Zen K, Takahara M, Iida O, et al. Drug-eluting stenting for femoropopliteal lesions, followed by cilostazol treatment, reduces stent restenosis in patients with symptomatic peripheral artery disease. *J Vasc Surg*. 2017;65:720–725.
29. Martinez BD, Hertzer NR, Beven EG. Influence of distal arterial occlusive disease on prognosis following aortobifemoral bypass. *Surgery*. 1980;88:795–805.
30. Malgor RD, Ricotta JJ, Bower TC, et al. Common femoral artery endarterectomy for lower extremity ischemia: evaluating the need for distal limb revascularization. *Ann Vasc Surg*. 2012;26(7):946–956.
31. Harris PL, Bigley DJ, McSweeney L. Aortofemoral bypass and the role of concomitant femorodistal reconstruction. *Br J Surg*. 1985;72:317–320.
32. Darling RC, Linton RR. Aortoiliofemoral endarterectomy for atherosclerotic occlusive disease. *Surgery*. 1964;55:184–194.
33. Barker WF, Cannon JA. An evaluation of endarterectomy. *Arch Surg*. 1953;66:488–495.
34. Crawford ES, Manning LG, Kelly TF. "Redo" surgery after operations for aneurysm and occlusion of the abdominal aorta. *Surgery*. 1977;81:41–52.
35. Perdue GD, Long WD, Smith 3rd RB. Perspective concerning aortofemoral arterial reconstruction. *Ann Surg*. 1971;173:940–944.
36. Pearce FB, Yang S, Shi R, et al. Circumferential aortic endarterectomy followed with immediate infrarenal clamping obviates suprarenal clamping for juxtarenal aortic occlusion. *Ann Vasc Surg*. 2016;34:48–53.
37. Baird RJ, Feldman P, Miles JT, et al. Subsequent downstream repair after aorta-iliac and aorta-femoral bypass operations. *Surgery*. 1977;82:785–793.
38. Garcia-Fernandez F, Marchena Gomez J, Cabrera Moran V, et al. Chronic infrarenal aortic occlusion: predictors of surgical outcome in patients undergoing aortobifemoral bypass reconstruction. *J Cardiovasc Surg*. 2011;52(3):371–380.
39. Reed AB, Conte MS, Donaldson MC, et al. The impact of patient age and aortic size on the results of aortobifemoral bypass grafting. *J Vasc Surg*. 2003;37:1219–1225.
40. Menard MT, Chew DK, Chan RK, et al. Outcome in patients at high risk after open surgical repair of abdominal aortic aneurysm. *J Vasc Surg*. 2003;37:285–292.
41. Whittemore AD, Clowes AW, Hechtman HB, Mannick JA. Aortic aneurysm repair: reduced operative mortality associated with maintenance of optimal cardiac performance. *Surgery*. 1980;192(3):414–421.
42. Kaluza GL, Joseph J, Lee JR, et al. Catastrophic outcomes of noncardiac surgery soon after coronary stenting. *J Am Coll Cardiol*. 2000;35:1288–1294.
43. Garcia-Fernandez F, Marchena Gomez J, Moran Cabrera, et al. Chronic infrarenal aortic occlusion: predictors of surgical outcome in patients undergoing aortobifemoral bypass reconstruction. *J Cardiovasc Surg*. 2011;52(3):371–380.
44. Cooley DA, Wukasch DC, Bennett JG, et al: Double velour knitted Dacron grafts for aortoiliac vascular replacements. Paper presented at Vascular Graft Symposium, National Institutes of Health, Bethesda, MD, November 5, 1976.
45. Yates SG, AA Barros D'Sa, Berger K, et al. The preclotting of porous arterial prosthesis. *Ann Surg*. 1978;188:611–622.
46. Nevelsteen A, Wouters L, Suy R. Aorto-femoral dacron reconstruction for aortoiliac occlusive disease: a 25-year survey. *Eur J Vasc Surg*. 1991;5:179–186.
47. Malone JM, Goldstone J, Moore WS. Autogenous profundaplasty: the key to long-term patency in secondary repair of aortofemoral graft occlusion. *Ann Surg*. 1978;188:817–823.
48. Morris Jr GC, Edwards E, Cooley DA, et al. Surgical importance of profunda femoris artery. *Arch Surg*. 1961;82:32–37.
49. Rutherford RB, Jones DN, Martin MS, et al. Serial hemodynamic assessment of aortobifemoral bypass. *J Vasc Surg*. 1986;4:428–435.
50. Bernhard VM, Ray LI, Militello JP. The role of angioplasty in the profunda femoris artery in revascularization of the ischemic limb. *Surg Gynecol Obstet*. 1976;142:840–844.

51. Berguer R, Higgins RF, Cotton LT. Geometry, blood flow, and reconstruction of the deep femoral artery. *Am J Surg.* 1975;130:68–73.

52. Seegar JM, Coe DA, Kaelin LD, Flynn TC. Routine reimplantation of patent inferior mesenteric arteries limits colon infarction after aortic reconstructions. *J Vasc Surg.* 1992;15:635–641.

53. Pierce GE, Turrentine M, Stringfield S, et al. Evaluation of end-to-side v end-to-end proximal anastomosis in aortobifemoral bypass. *Arch Surg.* 1982;117:1580–1588.

54. Brewster DC, Franklin DP, Cambria RP, et al. Intestinal ischemia complicating abdominal aortic surgery. *Surgery.* 1991;109:447–454.

55. Patel SD, Donatl T, Zayed H. Hybrid revascularization of multilevel disease: a paradigm shift in critical limb ischemia treatment. *J Cardiovasc Surg.* 2014;55(5):613–623.

56. Prinssen M, Buskens E, Blankensteijn JD. *Sexual dysfunction after conventional or endovascular AAA repair: results of a randomized trial.* In: *Paper presented at 17th International Congress of Endovascular Interventions,* Phoenix, Arizona, February 12; 2004.

57. Nypaver TJ, Ellenby MI, Mendoza O, et al. A comparison of operative approaches and parameters of success in multilevel arterial occlusive disease. *J Am Coll Surg.* 1994;179:449–456.

58. Sharples A, Kay M, Sykes T, et al. Multilevel bypass grafting: is it worth it? *Ann Vasc Surg.* 2014;28:1697–1702.

59. Dosluoglu HH, Lall P, Cherr GS, et al. Role of simple and complex hybrid revascularization procedures for symptomatic lower extremity occlusive disease. *J Vasc Surg.* 2010;51:1425–1435.

60. Piazza M, Ricotta 2nd JJ, Bower TC, et al. Iliac artery stenting combined with open femoral endarterectomy is as effective as open surgical reconstruction for severe iliac and common femoral occlusive disease. *J Vasc Surg.* 2011;54:402–411.

61. Patel SD, Donati T, Zayed H. Hybrid revascularization of complex multilevel disease: a paradigm shift in critical limb ischemia treatment. *J Cardiovasc Surg.* 2014;55:613–623.

62. Oral K, Ezelsoy M, Ayalp K, Kayabali M. Hybrid vascular surgery approaches for multilevel arterial occlusive disease. *Heart Surg Forum.* 2015;18:E28–E30.

63. Malone JM, Moore WS, Goldstone J. Life expectancy following aortofemoral arterial grafting. *Surgery.* 1977;81:551–555.

64. Freeman NE, Leeds FH. Operations on large arteries. *Calif Med.* 1952;77:229–233.

65. Blaisdell FW, Hall AD. Axillary-femoral artery bypass for lower extremity ischemia. *Surgery.* 1963;54:563–568.

66. LoGerfo FW, Johnson WC, Corson JD, et al. A comparison of the late patency rates of axillo-bilateral femoral and axillo-unilateral femoral grafts. *Surgery.* 1977;81:33–38. discussion 38-40.

67. Mii S, Morl A, Sakata H, et al. Fifteen year experience in axillofemoral bypass with externally supported knitted Dacron prosthesis in a Japanese hospital. *J Am Coll Surg.* 1998;186(5):581–588.

68. el-Massry S, Saad E, Sauvage LR, et al. Axillofemoral bypass using externally-supported, knitted Dacron grafts: a follow-up through twelve years. *J Vasc Surg.* 1993;17:107–114. discussion 114-115.

69. Broomé A, Christenson JT, Eklöff B, Norgren L. Axillofemoral bypass reconstructions in sixty-one patients with leg ischemia. *Surgery.* 1980;88:673–676.

70. Taylor Jr LM, Park TC, Edwards JM, et al. Acute disruption of polytetrafluoroethylene grafts adjacent to axillary anastomoses: A complication of axillofemoral grafting. *J Vasc Surg.* 1994;20:520–526. discussion 526-528.

71. Dickas D, Verrel F, Kalff J, et al. Axillobifemoral bypass: reappraisal of an extra anatomic bypass by analysis and results and prognostic factors. *World J Surg.* 2018;42(1):283–294.

72. Ascer E, Veith FJ, Gupta SK, et al. Comparison of axillounifemoral and axillobifemoral bypass operations. *Surgery.* 1985;97:169–175.

73. Rutherford RB, Patt A, Pearce WH. Extra-anatomic bypass: a closer look. *J Vasc Surg.* 1987;6:437–446.

74. Passman MA, Taylor LM, Moneta GL, et al. Comparison of axillofemoral and aortofemoral bypass for aortoiliac occlusive disease. *J Vasc Surg.* 1996;23:263–269. discussion 269-271.

75. Liedenbaum MH, Verdam FJ, Spelt D, et al. The outcome of the axillofemoral bypass: a retrospective review of 45 patients. *World J Surg.* 2009;33:2490–2496.

76. Berguer R, Higgins RJ, Reddy DJ. Intimal hyperplasia: an experimental study. *Arch Surg.* 1980;115:332–335.

77. Maini BS, Mannick JA. Effect of arterial reconstruction on limb salvage. *Arch Surg.* 1978;113:1297–1304.

78. Plecha FR, Plecha FM. Femorofemoral bypass grafts: ten years experience. *J Vasc Surg.* 1984;1:555–561.

79. Park KM, Park YJ, Kim YW, et al. Long term outcomes of femorofemoral crossover bypass grafts. *Vasc Specialist Int.* 2017;33(2):55–58.

80. Rinckenbach S, Guelle N, Lillaz J, et al. Femorofemoral bypass as an alternative to direct aortic approach in daily practice: appraisal of its current indications. *Ann Vasc Surg.* 2012;26(3):359–364.

81. Couch NP, Clowes AW, Whittemore AD, et al. The iliac-origin arterial graft: a useful alternative for iliac occlusive disease. *Surgery.* 1985;97:83–87.

82. Schneider JR, Besso SR, Walsh DB, et al. Femorofemoral versus aortobifemoral bypass: outcome and hemodynamic results. *J Vasc Surg.* 1994;19:43–55. discussion 55-7.

83. Blaisdell FW, DeMattei GA, Gauder PJ. Extraperitoneal thoracic aorta to femoral bypass grafts as replacement for an infected aortic bifurcation prosthesis. *Am J Surg.* 1961;102:583–585.

84. Nunn DB, Kamal MA. Bypass grafting from the thoracic aorta to femoral arteries for high aortoiliac occlusive disease. *Surgery.* 1972;72:749–755.

85. Dimuzio PJ, Reilly LM, Stoney RJ. Redo aortic grafting after treatment of aortic graft infection. *J Vasc Surg.* 1996;24:328–335. discussion 336-337.

86. Hughes R, Moawad M, Harvey JS, et al. Thoracofemoral bypass using spliced femoral vein with removal of an infected axillobifemoral bypass graft. *Eur J Vasc Endovasc Surg.* 2005;29:429–432.

87. Criado E, Keagy BA. Use of the descending thoracic aorta as an inflow source in aortoiliac reconstruction: indications and long term results. *Ann Vasc Surg.* 1994;8:38–47.

88. Dion YM, Gracia CR. A new technique for laparoscopic aortobifemoral grafting in occlusive aortoiliac disease. *J Vasc Surg.* 1997;26:685–692.

89. Ahn SS, Hiyama DT, Rudkin GH, et al. Laparoscopic aortobifemoral bypass. *J Vasc Surg.* 1997;26:128–132.

90. Kelly JJ, Kercher KW, Gallagher KA, et al. Hand-assisted laparoscopic aortobifemoral bypass versus open bypass for occlusive disease. *J Laparoendosc Adv Surg Tech A.* 2002;12:339–343.

91. Wisselink W, Cuesta MA, Gracia C, Rauwerda JA. Robot-assisted laparoscopic aortobifemoral bypass for aortoiliac occlusive disease: A report of two cases. *J Vasc Surg.* 2002;36:1079–1082.

92. Ghammad K, Dupuis A, Amond L, et al. Total laparoscopic bypass is safe and effective for aortoiliac occlusive disease. *J Vasc Surg.* 2015;61:698–702.

93. Segers B, Horn D, Lemaitre J, et al. Preliminary results from a prospective study of laparoscopic aortobifemoral bypass using a clampless and sutureless aortic anastomotic technique. *Eur J Vasc Endovasc Surg.* 2014;48:400–406.

94. Lecot F, Sabbe T, Houthoofd S, et al. Long-term results of totally laparoscopic aortobifemoral bypass. *Eur J Vasc Endovasc Surg.* 2016;52:581–587.

95. McAllister FF. The fate of patients with intermittent claudication managed non-operatively. *Am J Surg.* 1976;132:593–595.

96. Walsh DB, Gilbertson JJ, Zwolak RM, et al. The natural history of superficial femoral artery stenoses. *J Vasc Surg.* 1991;14:299–304.

97. Faries PF, Morrisey NJ, Teodorescu V, et al. Recent advances in peripheral angioplasty and stenting. *Angiology.* 2002;53:617–626.

98. Duda SH, Poerner TC, Wiesenger B, et al. Drug-eluting stents: potential applications for peripheral arterial occlusive disease. *J Vasc Interv Radiol.* 2003;14:291–301.

99. Grassbaugh JA, Nelson PR, Rzucidlo EM, et al. Blinded comparison of preoperative duplex ultrasound scanning and contrast arteriography for planning revascularization at the level of the tibia. *J Vasc Surg.* 2003;37:1186–1190.

100. Baum RA, Rutter CM, Sunshine JH, et al. Multicenter trial to evaluate vascular magnetic resonance angiography of the lower extremity. *JAMA.* 1995;274:875–880.

101. Koelemay MJ, Lijmer JG, Stoker J, et al. Magnetic resonance angiography for the evaluation of lower extremity arterial disease: a meta-analysis. *JAMA*. 2001;285:1338–1345.

102. Hansmann J, Michaely HJ, Morelli JN, et al. Impact of time-resolved MRA on diagnostic accuracy in patients with symptomatic peripheral artery disease of the calf station. *AJR Am J Roentgenol*. 2013;201: 1368–1375.

103. Walker JP, Nosova E, Sigovan M, et al. Ferumoxytol-enhanced magnetic resonance angiography is a feasible method for the clinical evaluation of lower extremity arterial disease. *Ann Vasc Surg*. 2015;29:63–68.

104. Schwein A, Chinnadurai P, Shah DJ, et al. Feasibility of three-dimensional magnetic resonance angiography-fluoroscopy image fusion technique in guiding complex endovascular aortic procedures in patients with renal insufficiency. *J Vasc Surg*. 2017;65:1440–1452.

105. Ascer E, Veith FJ, Gupta SK. Bypasses to plantar arteries and other tibial branches: an extended approach to limb salvage. *J Vasc Surg*. 1988;8: 434–441.

106. Reed AB, Conte MS, Belkin M, et al. Usefulness of autogenous bypass grafts originating distal to the groin. *J Vasc Surg*. 2002;35:48–54. discussion 54-55.

107. Vieth FJ, Gupta SK, Ascer E, et al. Six-year prospective multicenter randomized comparison of autologous saphenous vein and expanded polytetrafluoroethylene grafts in infrainguinal arterial reconstructions. *J Vasc Surg*. 1986;3:104–114.

108. Gilbertson JJ, Walsh DB, Zwolak RM, et al. A blinded comparison of angiography, angioscopy, and duplex scanning in the intraoperative evaluation of in situ saphenous vein bypass grafts. *J Vasc Surg*. 1992;15:121–127. discussion 127-129.

109. Bandyk DF, Johnson BL, Gupta AK, Esses GE. Nature and management of duplex abnormalities encountered during infrainguinal vein bypass grafting. *J Vasc Surg*. 1996;24:430–436. discussion 437-438.

110. Baxter BT, Rizzo RJ, Flinn WR, et al. A comparative study of intraoperative angioscopy and completion arteriography following femorodistal bypass. *Arch Surg*. 1990;125:997–1002.

111. Taylor Jr LM, Edwards JM, Porter JM. Present status of reversed vein bypass grafting: five-year results of a modern series. *J Vasc Surg*. 1990;11:193–205. discussion 205-206.

112. Khan SZ, Rivero M, McCralth M, et al. Endoscopic vein harvest does not negatively affect patency of great saphenous vein lower extremity bypass. *J Vasc Surg*. 2015;63(6):1546–1554.

113. Hall KV. The great saphenous vein used in situ as an arterial shunt after extirpation of vein valves. A preliminary report. *Surgery*. 1962;51:492–495.

114. Leather RP, Powers SR, Karmody AM. A reappraisal of the in situ saphenous vein arterial bypass: its use in limb salvage. *Surgery*. 1979;86:453–461.

115. Donaldson MC, Mannick JA, Whittemore AD. Femoral-distal bypass with in situ greater saphenous vein: long term results using Mills valvulotome. *Ann Surg*. 1991;213:457–464. discussion 464-465.

116. Moody AP, Edwards PR, Harris PL. In situ versus reversed femoropopliteal vein grafts: long-term follow-up of a prospective, randomized trial. *Br J Surg*. 1992;79:750–752.

117. Wengerter KR, Veith FJ, Gupta SK, et al. Prospective randomized multicenter comparison of in situ and reversed vein infrapopliteal bypasses. *J Vasc Surg*. 1991;13:189–197. discussion 197-199.

118. Rosenthal D, Dickson C, Rodriquez FJ, et al. Infrainguinal endovascular in situ saphenous vein bypass: ongoing results. *J Vasc Surg*. 1994;20:389–394. discussion 394-395.

119. Panetta TF, Marin ML, Veith FJ, et al. Unsuspected pre-existing saphenous vein disease: an unrecognized cause of vein bypass failure. *J Vasc Surg*. 1992;15:102–110. discussion 110-112.

120. Marcaccio EJ, Miller A, Tannenbaum GA, et al. Angioscopically directed interventions improve arm vein bypass grafts. *J Vasc Surg*. 1993;17:994–1002. discussion 1003-1004.

121. Belkin M, Knox J, Donaldson MC, et al. Infrainguinal arterial reconstruction with nonreversed greater saphenous vein. *J Vasc Surg*. 1996;24:957–962.

122. Whittemore AD, Kent KC, Donaldson MC, et al. What is the proper role of polytetrafluoroethylene grafts in infrainguinal reconstruction? *J Vasc Surg*. 1989;10:299–305.

123. Quiñones-Baldrich WJ, Prego AA, Ucelay-Gomez R, et al. Long-term results of infrainguinal revascularization with polytetrafluoroethylene: a ten-year experience. *J Vasc Surg*. 1992;16:209–217.

124. Miller JH, Foreman RK, Ferguson L, Faris I. Interposition vein cuff for anastomosis of prosthesis to small artery. *Aust NZ J Surg*. 1984;54:283–285.

125. Bellosta R, Natalini G, Luzzani L, et al. Comparison of precuffed expanded polytetrafluorothylene and heparin-bonded polytetrafluorothylene graft in crural bypass. *Ann Vasc Surg*. 2013;27:218–224.

126. Loh SA, Howell BS, Rockman CB, et al. Mid- and long-term results of the treatment of infrainguinal arterial occlusive disease with precuffed expanded polytetrafluoroethylene grafts compared with vein grafts. *Ann Vasc Surg*. 2013;27:208–217.

127. Van der Slegt J, Steunenberg SL, Donker JM, et al. The current position of precuffed expanded polytetrafluoroethylene bypass grafts in peripheral vascular surgery. *J Vasc Surg*. 2014;60:120–128.

128. Bannazadeh M, Sarac TP, Bena J, et al. Reoperative lower extremity revascularization with cadaver vein for limb salvage. *Ann Vasc Surg*. 2009;23:24–31.

129. Brown KE, Heyer K, Rodriguez H, et al. Arterial reconstruction with cryopreserved human allografts in the setting of infection: a single-center experience with midterm follow up. *J Vasc Surg*. 2009;49:660–666.

130. Harris L, O'Brien-Irr M, Ricotta JJ. Long-term assessment of cryopreserved vein bypass grafting success. *J Vasc Surg*. 2001;33:528–532.

131. Zehr BP, Niblick CJ, Downey H, Ladowski JS. Limb salvage with CryoVein cadaver saphenous vein allografts used for peripheral arterial bypass: role of blood compatibility. *Ann Vasc Surg*. 2011;25:177–181.

132. Lawson JH, Glickman MH, Ilzecki M, et al. Bioengineered human acellular vessels for dialysis access in patients with end-stage renal disease: two phase 2 single arm trials. *Lancet*. 2016;387:2026–2034.

133. Chew DK, Owens CD, Belkin M, et al. Bypass in the absence of ipsilateral greater saphenous vein: safe superiority of the contralateral greater saphenous vein. *J Vasc Surg*. 2002;35:1085–1092.

134. Belkin M, Conte MS, Donaldson MC, et al. Preferred strategies for secondary infrainguinal bypass: lessons learned from 300 consecutive reoperations. *J Vasc Surg*. 1995;21:282–293.

135. Sarac TP, Huber TS, Back MR, et al. Warfarin improves the outcome of infrainguinal vein bypass grafting at high risk for failure. *J Vasc Surg*. 1998;28:446–457.

136. Creager MA. Medical management of peripheral arterial disease. *Cardiol Rev*. 2001;9:238–245.

137. Geraghty AJ, Welch K. Antithrombotic agents for preventing thrombosis after infrainguinal arterial bypass surgery. *Cochrane Database Syst Rev*. 2011;6:CD000536.

138. Veith FJ, Weiser RK, Gupta SK, et al. Diagnosis and management of failing lower extremity arterial reconstructions prior to graft occlusion. *J Cardiovasc Surg*. 1984;25:381–384.

139. Liang NL, Baril DT, Avgerinos ED, et al. Comparative effectiveness of anticoagulation on midterm infrainguinal bypass graft patency. *J Vasc Surg*. 2017;66(2):499–505.

140. Bandyk DF, Schmitt DD, Seabrook GR, et al. Monitoring functional patency of in situ saphenous vein bypasses: the impact of a surveillance protocol and elective revision. *J Vasc Surg*. 1989;9:286–296.

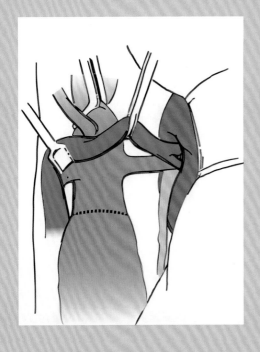

PART V

第五部分

Renal Artery Disease

肾动脉疾病

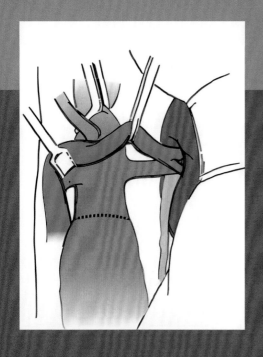

中文导读

第22章
肾动脉疾病的病理生理学

　　本章重点阐述肾动脉狭窄的病理生理学，对肾动脉狭窄病理生理学方面的一些基本概念进行了定义，介绍了关键性和非关键性肾动脉狭窄与肾损害的关系，对关键性肾动脉狭窄缺血引起肾内血管的病理变化和肾组织损伤进行了深入阐述。如果只强调肾动脉狭窄程度，往往只关注到血流动力学的改变，实际上问题的关键是狭窄缺血后引起的肾微血管病理变化，低灌注缺氧引发一系列病理效应，包括肾素–血管紧张素–醛固酮系统激活、氧化应激、炎症反应，导致间质小管线粒体损伤、肾小球纤维化等，最终发生不可逆的肾组织损伤和肾功能丧失。本章强调肾动脉狭窄有不同类型，包括单侧狭窄、双侧狭窄，还有单功能肾肾动脉狭窄，其有各自的病理生理学特点，所表现的相关临床症状或临床综合征也有所差异。希望通过对肾动脉狭窄病理机制的深刻认识，合理解释临床表现的差异，识别干预肾动脉狭窄的合适时间窗，达到比较理想的血管重建临床疗效。如果错失良机，肾已经发生了不可逆的组织损伤，功能难以恢复，血管重建治疗无效。

蒋雄京

Pathophysiology of Renal Artery Disease

Alfonso Eirin, Lilach O. Lerman, and Stephen C. Textor

Vascular disease affecting the renal arteries presents complex challenges to clinicians. Partly due to advances in vascular imaging, more patients than ever before are being identified with some degree of atherosclerotic or fibromuscular renovascular disease. Many of these lesions are of minor hemodynamic importance at the time of detection. Some reach a degree at which perfusion pressures and intrarenal hemodynamics are altered, leading to changes in blood pressure regulation and renal function. Such hemodynamic changes can produce a variety of recognizable clinical syndromes illustrated in Fig. 22.1. These range from modest changes in systemic arterial pressure to impaired volume control associated with congestive cardiac failure to threatened viability of the kidney, sometimes designated "ischemic nephropathy." Understanding the pathways by which renovascular disease affects cardiovascular and renal disease is important both for diagnosis and for defining optimal management using tools to control blood pressure, to block the renin-angiotensin system, and to restore the circulation.

Most renovascular lesions are the result of atherosclerosis. With the aging of the US and other Western populations and reduced mortality from stroke and coronary disease, the prevalence of vascular disease in other vascular beds reaching clinically "critical" levels appears to be increasing.[1] Understanding the variety of clinical manifestations of these lesions, the potential for disease progression, and the benefits and limitations of vascular repair are essential for vascular medicine specialists. This chapter will examine the pathophysiology of renovascular lesions regarding blood pressure control, ischemic nephropathy, and clinical syndromes such as "flash" pulmonary edema. Specific aspects regarding diagnostic evaluation and management will be addressed elsewhere (see Chapters 23 and 24).

A wide range of vascular lesions can affect the renal blood supply, some of which are summarized in Box 22.1. Historically, recognition of renovascular disease resulted from searching for underlying causes of hypertension. This followed the seminal observations of Goldblatt more than 80 years ago that renal artery constriction produced an increase in arterial pressure in the dog. These studies were among the first to establish a primary role of the kidney in overall blood pressure regulation. Renovascular hypertension produced by a "clipped" or constricted renal artery remains among the most widely studied experimental forms of angiotensin-dependent hypertension.[2]

EPIDEMIOLOGY OF RENAL ARTERY DISEASE

Fibromuscular dysplasia may be identified in 1% to 3% of normal kidney donors subjected to angiography before donor nephrectomy.[3]

Of those developing clinical hypertension and referred for revascularization, more than 85% are females with a predilection for disease in the right renal artery. The location of these lesions is most commonly in the midportion and distal segments of the renal artery. A variety of fibromuscular lesions have been described, but the most common is medial fibroplasia (also see Chapter 58). Occasionally, such lesions may be found in the carotid and other vascular beds, but most commonly they are limited to the renal arteries. Most do not progress to impair renal function, although some lead to arterial dissection and/or thrombosis with loss of the kidney.

Atherosclerosis is the most common cause of renal artery disease. Its presence and severity are related to age and the presence of other atherosclerotic disease of the abdominal aorta and arteries of the lower extremities. In population-based studies in the United States, up to 6.8% of healthy people older than 65 years were found to have significant renal artery stenosis (defined as Doppler peak systolic velocity greater than 1.8 m/s).[2] Renal arterial occlusive disease commonly represents an incidental finding in patients with widespread atherosclerosis undergoing carotid, coronary, or peripheral angiography. Peripheral artery and aortic disease is associated with higher prevalence (25% to 33%). As expected, risk factors predicting the presence of renal artery stenosis include smoking, hyperlipidemia, hypertension, and diabetes. A corollary observation is that renovascular hypertension resulting from these lesions is now most commonly superimposed gradually upon preexisting "essential" hypertension. Hence the blood pressure response and "cure" rates after successful restoration of blood flows to the kidney are limited by preexisting conditions.

PATHOPHYSIOLOGIC CONSEQUENCES OF RENOVASCULAR DISEASE

Under basal conditions, renal blood flow is among the highest of all organs. This feature reflects the kidney's filtration function, and less than 10% of delivered oxygen is sufficient to maintain renal metabolic needs. The renal cortex receives more blood flow than the medullary segments, but the latter consume more oxygen as a result of active tubular solute transport. Hence the kidney normally functions with a gradient of tissue oxygenation that decreases to overtly hypoxic ranges in deeper medullary areas. Reductions in renal blood flow are accompanied initially by decreased glomerular filtration and oxygen consumption, partly due to reduced metabolic demands of filtration

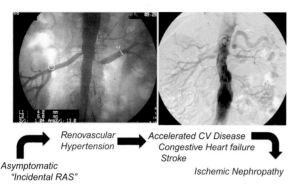

Fig. 22.1 Renal artery stenosis produces a broad range of manifestations, ranging from "incidental" disease with no hemodynamic effect to deteriorating kidney function and accelerating cardiovascular morbidity. *RAS*, Renal artery stenosis. (Modified from Herrmann SM, Saad A, Textor SC. Management of atherosclerotic renovascular disease after Cardiovascular Outcomes in Renal Atherosclerotic Lesions [CORAL]. *Nephrol Dial Transplant*. 2015;30:366–375.)

BOX 22.1 Vascular Lesions That Produce Renal Hypoperfusion and Renovascular Hypertension Syndrome

Unilateral Disease (Analogous to One-clip, Two-kidney Hypertension)
- Unilateral atherosclerotic renal artery stenosis
- Unilateral fibromuscular dysplasia (FMD)
  - Medial fibroplasia
  - Perimedial fibroplasia
  - Intimal fibroplasia
  - Medial hyperplasia
- Renal artery aneurysm
- Arterial embolus
- Arteriovenous fistula (congenital/traumatic)
- Segmental arterial occlusion (posttraumatic)
- Extrinsic compression of renal artery (e.g., pheochromocytoma)
- Renal compression (e.g., metastatic tumor)

Bilateral Disease or Solitary Functioning Kidney (Analogous to One-clip, One-kidney Model)
- Stenosis to a solitary functioning kidney
- Bilateral renal arterial stenosis
- Aortic coarctation
- Systemic vasculitis (e.g., Takayasu arteritis, polyarteritis)
- Atheroembolic disease
- Vascular occlusion due to endovascular aortic stent graft

---

and tubular solute reabsorption. As a result, moderately reduced renal blood flow can be sustained without measurable change in total kidney oxygen levels (as assessed by renal vein oxygen tension)[4] or reduced medullary and cortical tissue oxygenation as measured in human subjects using blood oxygen level–dependent (BOLD) magnetic resonance (Fig. 22.2).[5] These observations argue against an overall lack of oxygen as an initial stimulus for either hypertension or renal tissue injury in moderate renal artery stenosis and underscore the tolerance of normal kidneys to tolerate moderately reduced perfusion pressures beyond the stenotic lesions. Nonetheless, increasingly severe vascular stenosis leading to diminished renal perfusion eventually does lead to renal hypoxia,[6] tissue injury, and interstitial fibrosis (see Fig. 22.2, left).

Subcritical Levels of Stenosis

The majority of renal arterial lesions that compromise renal function are caused by gradually developing atherosclerosis of the renal vascular bed. As noted previously, some patients undergoing cardiac catheterization have "incidental" renal lesions producing more than 50% cross-sectional stenosis for whom the presence of renal artery stenosis is a strong independent predictor of mortality. Moreover, nonobstructive renal artery stenosis (20% to 50% decrease in renal arterial luminal diameter) can be found in almost one-third of patients undergoing cardiac catheterization and half of those undergoing aortography for peripheral vascular disease.[1] Although lesions producing less than 50% arterial luminal diameter are not considered hemodynamically significant, the relationships between resting pressure gradients and angiographic degree of stenosis are curvilinear and only approximate at best. As a predictor of mortality, even low-grade atherosclerotic lesions denote a hazard nearly equal to more advanced disease.[7] Estimating severity of vascular occlusion from angiographic images is notoriously unreliable. It should be emphasized that activation of pressor mechanisms depends upon the presence of a pressure gradient between the aorta and distal renal vasculature (Fig. 22.3). Although there is a general relationship between estimated diameter stenosis and peak translesional pressure gradients, the relationship is not linear. In some instances, an abrupt decrease in poststenotic pressure develops beyond a subcritical range of stenosis. Moderate stenosis, especially when superimposed on intrarenal microvascular disease, may contribute to adverse renal outcomes. Even relatively minor stenosis in the renal artery might have long-term functional implications, including renal artery disease progression and atrophy (defined radiologically as a loss of kidney size), especially in the presence of additional risk factors or coexisting renal disease.

Renal Microvascular Disease

Lesions in the main renal artery may be superimposed upon or confused with other causes for ischemic renal injury. Intrarenal vascular lesions are commonly observed in the course of various nephropathies, many of which have an ischemic component. Risk factors including diabetes, hypertension, atherosclerosis, and aging elicit vasoconstriction and/or structural changes leading to intrarenal small vessel disease and ischemic injury similar to that observed in large vessel disease. The loss of microvessels and impaired capillary repair correlate with the development of glomerular and tubulointerstitial scarring[8] and may lead to end-stage renal failure. Renal microvascular disease distal to a stenosis in the renal artery may perpetuate and exacerbate renal parenchymal injury and may blunt renal recovery. The presence of small microvessel injury is difficult to verify in human subjects but may account for changes in diastolic blood flow, such as that producing changes in renal resistance index. Elevations of renal resistance index tend to predict poor outcomes in many renal diseases, including renovascular disease.[9]

Critical Renal Artery Stenosis

High-grade vascular stenosis eventually leads to a decrease in renal perfusion pressure. "Critical" stenosis is identified when it produces a decrease in renal blood flow and glomerular filtration rate. During experimental renal artery occlusion, the kidney sustains autoregulation of blood flow through a range of perfusion pressures from 200 mm Hg to approximately 80 mm Hg. Mechanisms underlying autoregulation include myogenic responses to changes in wall tension, release of vasoactive substances, and the tubuloglomerular feedback. The latter responds to decreased renal perfusion pressure and salt delivery by decreasing vascular resistance distal to the obstruction. In addition, during a decrease in renal perfusion pressure, the kidney

Tissue Oxygenation (BOLD MR) in Occlusive Renovascular Disease

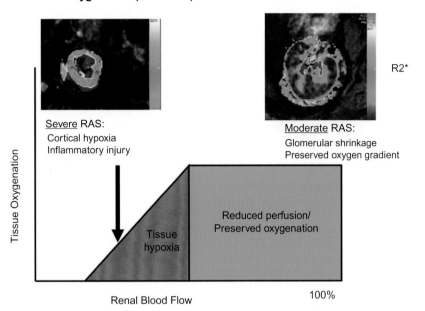

Fig. 22.2 Adaptation of Tissue Oxygenation Within the Kidney to Renovascular Disease. Axial blood oxygen level–dependent magnetic resonance *(BOLD-MR)* imaging of a kidney with moderate renal artery stenosis *(RAS)* leading to renal blood flow reductions of 30% to 40% is associated with a normal oxygen gradient between cortex and medulla and preserved tubular structures. More severe and prolonged stenosis ultimately leads to overt tissue hypoxia in cortical tissue and widening fractions of medullary hypoxia with activation of inflammatory injury and irreversible fibrosis (see text). (Modified from Textor SC. Renal arterial disease and hypertension. *Med Clin North Am.* 2017;101:65–79, with permission.)

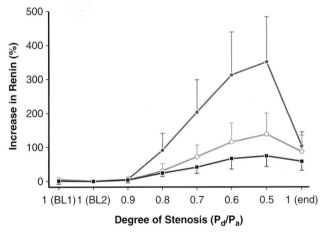

Fig. 22.3 Relationship Between Developed Pressure Gradient Between Aorta *(Pa)* and Distal Renal Artery *(Pd)* and Activation of the Renin-Angiotensin System in Human Subjects. Progressive gradients were developed by expanding a catheter balloon. These data indicate that activation of renal venous renin activity occurred only after a translesional gradient between 10 and 20 mm Hg was created. Such a gradient usually requires advanced occlusive disease, usually more than 70% lumen occlusion. (Reproduced with permission from De Bruyne B, Manoharan G, Pijls NH, et al. Assessment of renal artery stenosis severity by pressure gradient measurements. *J Am Coll Cardiol.* 2006;48:1851–1855.)

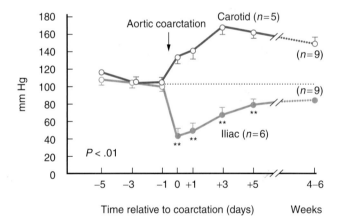

Fig. 22.4 Development of Arterial Hypertension After Placement of a Renal Artery Clip Lesion in a Conscious Rat Aortic Coarct Model. Poststenotic pressures (iliac artery) increase to near baseline levels at the expense of systemic arterial pressures *(Carotid)*. Despite a significant pressure gradient, renal perfusion is maintained. However, reduction of systemic pressures lowers renal perfusion and activates pressor systems, including the renin-angiotensin system (see text). (Reproduced with permission from Textor SC, Smith-Powell L. Post-stenotic arterial pressure, renal haemodynamics and sodium excretion during graded pressure reduction in conscious rats with one- and two-kidney coarctation hypertension. *J Hypertens.* 1988;6:311–319.)

activates multiple pathways that elevate systemic blood pressure, an effect which tends to restore renal perfusion pressure and sustain renal blood flow at the expense of systemic arterial hypertension (Fig. 22.4). Consequently, as long as systemic arterial pressure is allowed to increase, a decrease in renal blood flow does not occur until renal arterial diameter is reduced by 65% to 75%.

Noninvasive radiologic imaging commonly overstates the degree of stenosis. Measurement of physiologic stimuli, such as the release of renin, indicates that a translesion gradient of at least 10% to 20% reduction is necessary for biologic responses to occur in humans. To achieve such a gradient, luminal occlusion may need to exceed 80% stenosis. Under some conditions, gradients ≥20 mm

Hg that develop during intrarenal hyperemic challenge with dopamine may disclose hemodynamic significance of lesions under 60% in severity.[10]

When the renal perfusion pressure decreases gradually, additional mechanisms are recruited that protect the kidney from the functional and morphologic consequences observed after acute ischemic injury. These include development of collateral vessels and redistribution of intrarenal blood flow from the cortex to the medulla. Renal cortical blood flow autoregulates more efficiently than the outer medulla, which is continuously at the verge of hypoxia. During chronic reduction of renal blood flow, medullary perfusion and oxygenation are relatively maintained by adaptive mechanisms at the expense of cortical blood flow. When poststenotic renal artery pressures eventually decrease further, either due to progressive vascular occlusion or to reduction of systemic blood pressures by drug therapy, renal volume decreases.

In clinical terms, renal "atrophy" can be defined as a loss of renal length by at least 1 cm, and a difference in size between the two kidneys is suggestive of unilateral renal artery stenosis (or a higher grade of stenosis in one of the kidneys). A decrease in renal volume results from a decrease in filling pressure, filtrate, and blood content of the kidney, as well as structural atrophy of the renal tubules due to apoptosis and necrosis. Apoptosis is an active, preprogrammed form of cell death, which is intricately regulated and distinct from cellular necrosis and likely serves as a protective mechanism to allow renal "hibernation." These changes may be reversible, because tubular cells show vigorous potential for regeneration. Loss of intrarenal microvessels that accompanies the ongoing scarring process may also contribute to renal shrinkage (Fig. 22.5) but might be partly reversible upon enhancement of angiogenic signaling.[11] However, if a blood flow deficit persists, permanent damage to the kidney may occur. As mentioned previously, decreased renal blood flow is often accompanied by a decline in GFR and inhibition of tubular epithelial transport that limit renal oxygen consumption and maintain oxygen saturation. Hence the kidney does not actually develop tissue hypoxia until an extreme decrease in renal blood flow develops.

Renovascular Hypertension

Goldblatt et al. and Loesch showed in the 1930s that obstruction of the renal artery is followed by an increase in systemic blood pressure. The characteristics of renovascular hypertension depend to a large extent on the status of the kidneys. Unilateral renal artery stenosis may be present with an intact contralateral renal artery (the experimental form is termed two-kidney, one-clip [2K1C]). This model is characterized by counterregulatory processes in the contralateral kidney leading to sodium excretion in response to elevated arterial pressure ("pressure natriuresis") (Fig. 22.6). Alternatively,

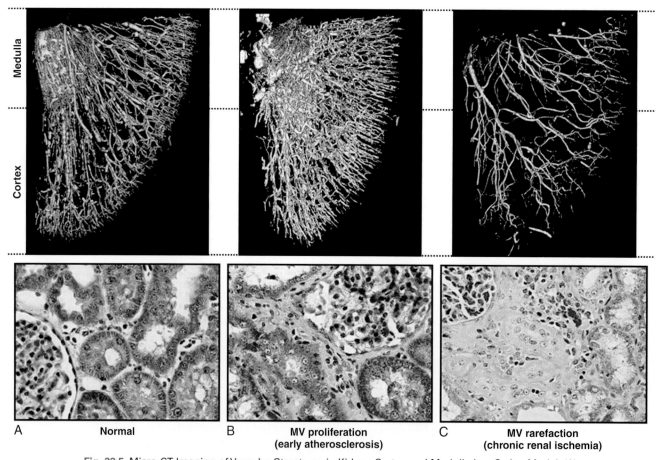

A   **Normal**   B   **MV proliferation (early atherosclerosis)**   C   **MV rarefaction (chronic renal ischemia)**

Fig. 22.5 Micro-CT Imaging of Vascular Structures in Kidney Cortex and Medulla in a Swine Model. (A) Normal vascular density, (B) vascular proliferation observed after cholesterol feeding, and (C) microvascular (MV) rarefication and interstitial fibrosis observed beyond a high-grade renal artery stenosis. (Reproduced with permission from Lerman LO, Chade AR. Angiogenesis in the kidney: a new therapeutic target? *Curr Opin Nephrol Hypertens.* 2009;18:160–165.)

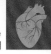

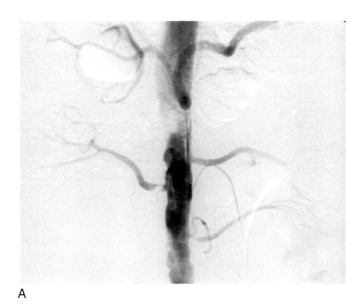

A

Unilateral Renal Artery Stenosis

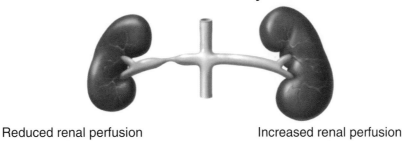

Reduced renal perfusion　　　　　　　　Increased renal perfusion

↑ Renin-angiotensin system (RAS)　　　Suppressed RAS　Increased Na+ excretion
↑ Renin　　　　　　　　　　　　　　　　　　　　　　　　　　　(pressure natriuresis)
↑ Ang II
↑ Aldosterone

Ang II-dependent hypertension

Effect of blockade of RAS
Reduced arterial pressure
Enhanced lateralization of diagnostic tests
GFR in stenotic kidney may fall

Diagnostic tests
Plasma renin activity elevated
Lateralized features (e.g., renin levels in renal veins, captopril-enhanced renography)

B

Fig. 22.6 (A) Angiogram of unilateral renal arterial stenosis with well-preserved vascular supply to the contralateral kidney. (B) Schematic illustrating the pathophysiology of unilateral renovascular hypertension (two-kidney, one-clip). The stenotic kidney responds to reduced perfusion with activation of the renin-angiotensin system producing widespread effects, including an increase in arterial pressure. However, elevated pressures subject the nonstenotic kidney to "pressure natriuresis," leading to asymmetric sodium excretion, a decrease in blood pressure, and continued stimuli to the stenotic kidney. Such asymmetry is the basis for diagnostic testing, such as captopril renography and renal vein renin measurements. *Ang*, Angiotensin; *GFR*, glomerular filtration rate.

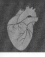

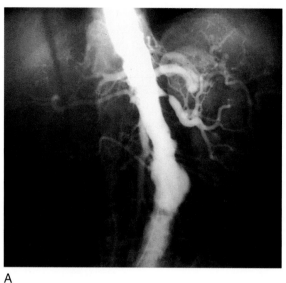

A

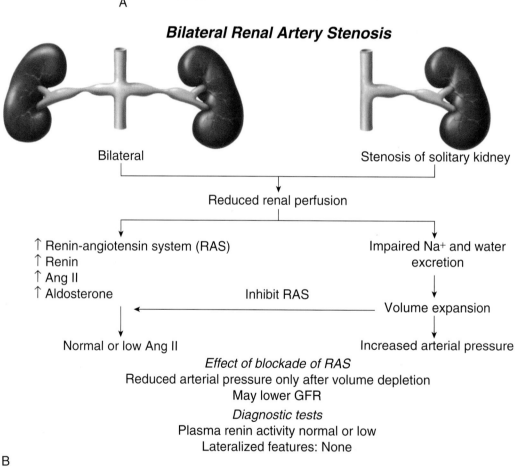

Bilateral Renal Artery Stenosis

Bilateral   Stenosis of solitary kidney

Reduced renal perfusion

↑ Renin-angiotensin system (RAS)   Impaired Na+ and water
↑ Renin   excretion
↑ Ang II
↑ Aldosterone   Inhibit RAS   Volume expansion

Normal or low Ang II   Increased arterial pressure

Effect of blockade of RAS
Reduced arterial pressure only after volume depletion
May lower GFR

Diagnostic tests
Plasma renin activity normal or low
Lateralized features: None

B

Fig. 22.7 (A) Angiogram illustrating renal artery stenosis affecting the entire renal mass, in this case a solitary functioning kidney. The contralateral kidney is occluded. (B) Schematic illustrating the pathophysiology of renovascular hypertension in which stenosis affects the entire renal mass. In the absence of a normal contralateral kidney, sodium retention occurs and hypertension is heavily dependent upon volume mechanisms. *Ang*, Angiotensin; *GFR*, glomerular filtration rate.

renal artery stenosis may affect a solitary kidney (one-kidney, one-clip [1K1C]) (Fig. 22.7). Bilateral renal artery stenosis and 1K1C lead to more severe renovascular hypertension, although bilateral renal artery stenosis may behave similar to 2K1C if one kidney is significantly less ischemic than the other. Patients with this constellation of findings have higher mortality, are more prone to circulatory congestion, and are more likely to experience deterioration of kidney function during administration of antihypertensive agents, including angiotensin-converting enzyme (ACE) inhibitors or angiotensin II receptor blockers (ARBs).

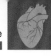

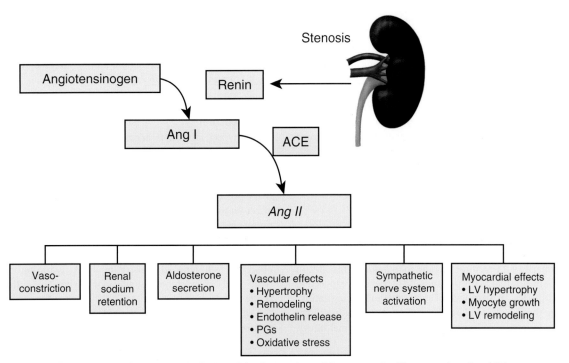

Fig. 22.8 Actions of Angiotensin II *(Ang II)* in Generation of Renovascular Hypertension. In addition to direct effects on vascular tone and sodium homeostasis, angiotensin II modulates and induces vasoconstriction by several independent mechanisms, including oxidative stress. Induction of "slow pressor" responses are associated with reduction of circulating levels of plasma renin activity and loss of demonstrable pressure dependence upon angiotensin II (see text). *ACE,* Angiotensin-converting enzyme; *LV,* left ventricular; *PG,* prostaglandin.

The exact mechanisms responsible for renovascular hypertension have long been debated. The immediate increase in blood pressure in renal artery stenosis results from release of renin from the stenotic kidney. This leads to increased formation of angiotensin II, which increases peripheral vascular resistance, plasma aldosterone, sodium retention, extracellular volume, and cardiac output (Fig. 22.8).[12] Blockade of angiotensin action in experimental models prevents the initial series of events and delays the development of renovascular hypertension indefinitely.[13] Activation of the sympathetic nervous system also plays an important role in the pathogenesis of renovascular hypertension primarily via the renal afferent nerves. Both the peripheral and central aspects of the autonomic system are also under the influence of angiotensin II. If the increase in pressure restores renal perfusion pressure distal to the stenosis, most of these alterations return to baseline levels, with the exception of peripheral vascular resistance.

After the initial increase in activity from the renin-angiotensin system, maintenance of renovascular hypertension in 1K1C models depends mainly on volume expansion. In 2K1C models the interplay between plasma renin activity and extracellular volume is more complex. The contralateral kidney responds to the elevated systemic pressure by increasing sodium excretion (pressure natriuresis), an effect that tends to drive the blood pressure down and decrease perfusion pressure of the stenotic kidney. This effect again leads to an increase in renin release, which in turn elevates systemic blood pressure, and so forth. In high-grade renal artery stenosis, this cycle of events may induce extracellular volume depletion and renal failure. Although these features are consistently demonstrated in experimental models, human renovascular hypertension frequently has elements of both 1K and 2K pathophysiology, particularly when the function of the contralateral kidney is compromised.

It is important to recognize that activation of the systemic renin-angiotensin system is transient in renovascular hypertension. Circulating levels of plasma renin activity and angiotensin decrease after some time, despite sustained elevation of peripheral vascular resistance. This may be the result of both a "slow-response" to angiotensin II through which low levels of angiotensin have pressor actions and recruitment of additional mechanisms of vasoconstriction. The latter includes activation of vasoconstrictor lipoxygenase products, oxidative stress, and endothelin. Further increments in pressure result from an imbalance between vasoconstrictors and vasodilators, including decreased bioavailability of nitric oxide (NO). An important role is ascribed to dissociation between systemic blood pressure, extracellular volume, and inappropriate levels of angiotensin II. The complexity of these relationships partly explains the failure of measuring any single clinical pathway to predict blood pressure responses to renal revascularization.

Accelerated Hypertension and Pulmonary Edema

Series of patients referred for renal revascularization in recent decades have included older patients with more widespread atherosclerotic disease than ever before.[14] This reflects both improved medical care leading to better blood pressure control and reduced mortality from coronary and cerebrovascular disease. Patient demographics commonly include more women than men and a high prevalence of coronary disease, congestive cardiac failure, and known cerebrovascular disease. In some cases, suspicion arises regarding renal artery stenosis because of rapid acceleration of these processes, particularly the rapid increase in arterial pressure in a previously stable patient. When untreated, a cycle of malignant-phase hypertension and hyponatremia (attributed to the dipsogenic action of angiotensin II) may ensue. In other cases, presenting symptoms include recent progression of hypertension followed by neurologic symptoms of an acute stroke.

Some patients develop cycles of worsening congestive cardiac failure out of proportion to left ventricular dysfunction. This sometimes has been designated "flash" pulmonary edema.[15] Many of these patients have bilateral disease or stenosis to a solitary functioning kidney. When volume expanded, renal function may improve slightly at the price of hypertension and circulatory congestion. Sudden pulmonary edema partly reflects diastolic dysfunction precipitated by a rapid increase in afterload in addition to impaired sodium excretion as a result of renal hypoperfusion. During volume depletion, serum creatinine commonly rises with evidence of "prerenal" azotemia. This condition warrants recognition because several series indicate that cycles of symptomatic exacerbation, hospitalization, and mortality can be improved with successful renal revascularization.[16,17]

Renal Hypoperfusion Injury: "Ischemic Nephropathy"

Negative results from prospective clinical trials of revascularization for atherosclerotic renovascular disease have led to more patients being treated primarily with medical therapy than before. This shift in clinical practice means that many poststenotic kidneys are exposed to perfusion pressures less than the level of autoregulation during antihypertensive drug therapy. A corollary observation is an increased likelihood of those kidneys developing irreversible parenchymal injury.

The precise mechanisms responsible for irreversible renal scarring in "ischemic" nephropathy have not been fully elucidated. They are likely related to both components of "hypoperfusion" and "recurrent local ischemia," resulting in interactions among several systems activated in the kidney, as proposed in Fig. 22.9.

Renal Vasoactive Hormonal Systems
Angiotensin II

Renal hypoperfusion is accompanied by activation of the renin-angiotensin system, a mechanism normally designed to regulate volume homeostasis and maintain GFR during a transient decrease in renal perfusion pressure. Angiotensin II maintains glomerular capillary pressure and GFR by way of its predominant vasoconstrictor effect on the efferent arteriole. The importance of angiotensin II for preserving GFR is most evident under conditions of reduced preglomerular arterial pressures, particularly under conditions of volume depletion. This feature underlies the decrease in GFR sometimes observed following administration of ACE inhibitors to patients with renal artery stenosis, particularly when the entire renal mass is affected.

Angiotensin II effects in the kidney include induction of cell hypertrophy and hyperplasia, and stimulation of hormone synthesis

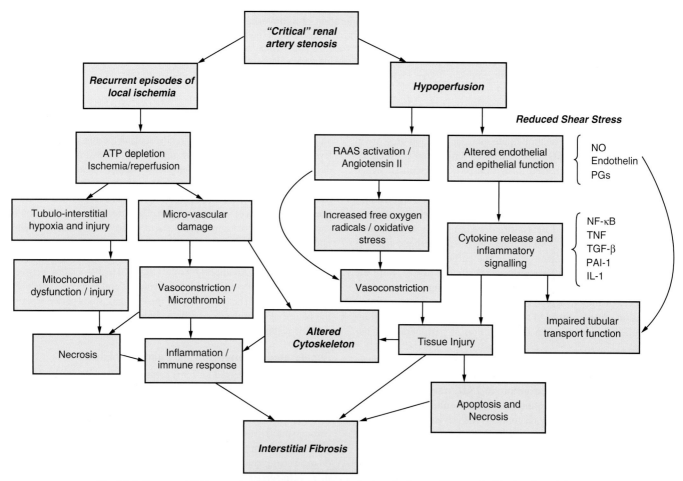

Fig. 22.9 Proposed Pathways by Which Renal Hypoperfusion Activates Fibrogenic Mechanisms Within the Kidney and Ultimately Produces Irreversible Parenchymal Injury and Interstitial Fibrosis. Both intermittent local ischemia *(shown on the left)* and vasoconstrictor-mediated cytokine-mediated pathways *(right)* participate in this process. *ATP*, Adenosine triphosphate; *IL-1*, interleukin 1; *NO*, nitric oxide; *NF-κB*, nuclear factor κB; *PAI-1*, plasminogen activator inhibitor 1; *PG*, prostaglandin; *RAAS*, renin-angiotensin-aldosterone system; *TGF-β*, transforming growth factor β; *TNF*, tumor necrosis factor. (Modified with permission from Lerman L, Textor SC. Pathophysiology of ischemic nephropathy. *Urol Clin North Am.* 2001;28:793–803.)

and ion transport. It also contributes to renal fibrosis by recruiting bone marrow–derived fibrocytes, circulating cells that contribute to the pathogenesis of fibrotic diseases.[18] Its renal actions are mediated primarily through AT1 receptors expressed on endothelial, epithelial, and vascular cells. Chronic activation of AT1 receptors in renal ischemic injury may elicit local inflammatory and fibrogenic responses. Angiotensin II has been implicated in stimulation of vascular smooth muscle and mesangial cell growth, platelet aggregation, generation of superoxide, activation of adhesion molecules and macrophages, infiltration of inflammatory cells, increased expression of extracellular matrix proteins, and induction of proto-oncogenes.

The intrarenal effects of angiotensin II during renal ischemia are modulated by interactions with other humoral systems (see Fig. 22.8). Vasodilator prostaglandins attenuate vasoconstriction caused by angiotensin II and may limit ischemia caused by elevated levels of this hormone. NO negates many actions of angiotensin II, modulates the effects of angiotensin II on the afferent arteriole and the proximal tubule, and downregulates ACE and AT1 gene expression. Conversely, endothelin-1 regulates and amplifies renal ACE expression, mediates some of the vascular effects of angiotensin II and amplifies its pressor effects, and activates a similar signal transduction pathway for growth- and differentiation-related genes.[19] Thromboxane A_2, a vasoconstrictor metabolite of arachidonic acid, is also released within the kidney by angiotensin II and mediates much of the pressor and renal hemodynamic responses to angiotensin II.

Therefore angiotensin II participates in short-term renal adaptive response to hypoperfusion and ischemia, but long-term activation of the renin-angiotensin system and its interaction with other humoral systems can lead to progressive destruction of renal tissue.

Nitric Oxide

NO is synthesized from L-arginine within the kidney by a family of nitric oxide synthases (NOSs), and plays a crucial role in the regulation of renal hemodynamics and excretory function. The differential expression, localization, and regulation of three isoforms of NOS expressed in the kidney, namely neuronal (nNOS), inducible (iNOS), and endothelial (eNOS) isoforms, contribute to diverse intrarenal actions.[20] Consequently, NO reduces vascular tone, increases sodium excretion, modulates tubuloglomerular feedback, has antithrombotic protection, inhibits growth-related responses to injury, and modulates the aforementioned renal actions of angiotensin II. NO further buffers many processes implicated in the pathogenesis of tissue injury in renovascular disease, including growth of vascular smooth muscle cells, mesangial cell hypertrophy and hyperplasia, and synthesis of extracellular matrix. However, regulation of renal blood flow becomes less dependent on eNOS-derived NO and more dependent on prostaglandins as renal artery stenosis progresses, in part due to decreased renal perfusion pressure and vascular shear stress distal to the stenosis, which are primary stimuli to eNOS. On the other hand, the contralateral kidney continues to rely on NO to buffer the actions of angiotensin II.

However, the role of NO in renal tissue ischemia is complex. The iNOS isoform is upregulated during renal ischemia and generates NO that can be cytotoxic to renal epithelial cells and contributes to tubular injury, both by decreasing the activity of the eNOS isoform and by formation of the oxidant peroxynitrite (ONOO⁻).

Endothelins

The *endothelin* peptides comprise a family of peptides produced and released from endothelial cells, which have potent and long-lasting vasoconstrictor effects on the renal microcirculation and modify tubular function. Endothelin release can be stimulated by angiotensin

II, thrombin, transforming growth factor (TGF)-β, and other cytokines (e.g., tumor necrosis factor-α, interleukin-1β). Tissue levels of endothelin-1 are increased in the stenotic kidney,[21] and in fact in most forms of renal failure, and may persist for days after resolution of the initial injury. Its involvement in renal ischemic injury is underscored by the observation that ET-1 blockade is more efficient in improving the early course of postischemic renal injury than inhibition of angiotensin II. Chronic blockade of the endothelin A-receptor directly inhibits cellular growth and gene expression and, in ischemic acute renal failure, provides long-term functional and morphological benefits in experimental models. Renal blood flow, glomerular filtration rate, and redox status significantly improve in the swine stenotic kidney after endothelin A-receptor but not endothelin B-receptor blockade, implying that the former ameliorate renal injury in pigs with advanced renovascular disease.[22] These effects are greater than those observed during simultaneous blockade of both the A and B receptor, likely due to the role of the latter in eliminating salt, although the endothelin B-receptor has also been implicated in inflammation and fibrosis in progressive renal injury.

Prostaglandins

Prostaglandins are cyclooxygenase (COX) derivatives of arachidonic acid, which have important roles in maintaining renal blood flow and glomerular filtration. Biosynthesis of vasodilator prostaglandins, including prostacyclin and prostaglandin E2, protects the kidney against the effects of prolonged ischemia and angiotensin II and limits hypoxic tissue injury.[23] In renal artery stenosis, they selectively prevent preglomerular constriction and thus limit a decrease in GFR in the stenotic kidney, potentially through regulatory interactions with NO. Conversely, thromboxane A_2 is an endothelium-derived vasoconstrictor prostaglandin that is upregulated in kidneys with renovascular disease. It is released within the kidney by reactive oxygen species or angiotensin II, modulates some of the deleterious effects of angiotensin II and endothelin-1, and contributes to kidney disease. Blockade of thromboxane A_2 receptors thus improves urine volume, glomerular filtration rate, and renal plasma flow in ischemic kidneys and exerts a variety of beneficial effects that reduce the severity of ischemic damage. Furthermore, vascular expression of COX-2 is upregulated in kidneys with arterial stenosis, and COX-2–derived prostaglandin I2 regulates renin release and renovascular hypertension in severe and moderate renal artery stenoses.

Oxidative Stress and Fibrosis

A growing body of evidence implicates increased generation of reactive radical species as a mechanism for renal injury in renovascular disease.[24] Angiotensin II is a potent stimulus for superoxide production via the membrane NADH/NADPH oxidase system, and xanthine oxidase is an important source of oxygen free radicals during renal ischemia. Increased oxidative stress can promote the formation of a variety of vasoactive mediators including endothelin-1, leukotrienes, and prostaglandin $F_2\alpha$ isoprostanes, endogenous products of lipid peroxidation. In addition, a chemical reaction between superoxide anion and NO not only decreases the bioavailability of NO but also leads to the production of toxic species (e.g., ONOO⁻). Functionally, reactive oxygen species have been implicated in decreasing stenotic kidney blood flow and sustaining renovascular hypertension.[25,26]

Furthermore, oxidative stress contributes to progressive tissue damage in the stenotic kidney. In mesangial cells, superoxide promotes hypertrophy and extracellular matrix production, by both interaction with NO and by acting as an intracellular signal for growth related responses, which may lead to microvascular and tissue remodeling. In addition, reactive oxygen species are implicated in the pathogenesis of ischemic renal injury by causing lipid peroxidation of cell and organelle membranes and disrupting the structural integrity and capacity for cell transport and energy production, especially in the proximal tubule. Activation of growth factors and cytokines such as nuclear factor κB may also play an important role in the mechanism of action of angiotensin II and reactive oxygen species. Studies in humans confirm that oxidative stress contributes to the impairment in endothelium-dependent vasodilatation observed in patients with renovascular hypertension, which can be reversed with successful renal revascularization.[16]

The fibrogenic factors TGF-β, tissue inhibitor of metalloproteinases (TIMP)-1, and plasminogen activator inhibitor (PAI)-1, which are upregulated in stenotic kidneys, are important mediators of extracellular matrix synthesis that characterizes progression of renal tissue injury. Early induction of TGF-β via the AT1 receptor plays a major role in tissue fibrosis[27] by increasing type IV collagen deposition and may play a role in interstitial scarring observed in chronic renal injury characterized by increased activity of intrarenal angiotensin II. It interacts with endothelin and several growth factors and cytokines in promoting progressive interstitial fibrosis primarily via its downstream effectors from the Smad family. In line with this, abrogation of TGF-β/Smad3 signaling confers protection against the development of fibrosis and atrophy in the clipped mice kidney, suggesting that signaling through Smad3 is essential for the development of renal atrophy in the stenotic kidney.[28]

Mitochondrial Injury

Emerging evidence suggests that mitochondrial structural abnormalities and dysfunction might play an important role in the development and progression of renovascular disease.[29] Renal mitochondrial damage in renovascular disease might result from either chronic hypoperfusion or acute insults, such as reperfusion of an ischemic kidney during angioplasty. In patients with chronic renovascular disease, elevated urinary levels of mitochondrial DNA, which are surrogate markers of mitochondrial injury, correlate with markers of renal injury and dysfunction.[30] Furthermore, in patients treated with medical therapy or revascularization, urinary mitochondrial DNA varies as a function of serum creatinine and estimated glomerular filtration rate, implicating mitochondrial injury in renal damage in human renovascular disease.

Rapid restoration of blood flow to a poststenotic kidney can trigger "ischemia-reperfusion injury," characterized by apoptosis, oxidative stress, inflammation, and calcium overload. This in turn favors formation of the mitochondrial permeability transition pore, a high conductance channel formed in the inner mitochondrial membrane. Opening of this pore facilitates release of cytochrome c and mitochondrial reactive oxygen species to the cytoplasm, initiating apoptosis and contributing to cellular oxidative stress. Studies in pigs with atherosclerotic renovascular disease demonstrate that renal reperfusion is associated with acute increments in plasma levels of the proinflammatory cytokine monocyte chemoattractant protein (MCP)-1.[31] Adjunctive targeted mitochondrial protection during renal revascularization does not immediately alter MCP-1 levels but improves stenotic kidney renal blood flow and glomerular filtration rate 4 weeks later, suggesting that functional mitochondrial injury during renal reperfusion may limit kidney recovery after renal angioplasty. A prospective pilot study in patients with atherosclerotic renal artery stenosis undergoing renal revascularization demonstrated that infusion of mitochondria-targeted peptides immediately before and during renal revascularization increased renal blood flow and cortical perfusion, and estimated GFR by 3 months later.[32]

Taken together, these observations suggest that mitochondrial protection has the potential to reduce procedure-associated ischemic injury and improve outcomes of revascularization in human atherosclerotic renal artery stenosis.

Inflammation

Accumulating evidence indicates that inflammatory pathways are an important mediator of deleterious processes in the stenotic kidney. Experimental studies have shown that angiotensin II triggers Th-1 lymphocyte activation and macrophage infiltration.[33] Biopsies obtained from the stenotic kidneys of patients with subtotal atherosclerotic vascular occlusion are characterized by increased inflammatory cellular infiltrates, particularly CD68+ macrophages, associated with reduced blood flow.[34] Importantly, macrophage infiltration can aggravate kidney injury by secreting proinflammatory and profibrotic cytokines, leading to tubulointerstitial fibrosis and glomerulosclerosis. The poststenotic human kidney releases multiple markers reflecting active inflammation that translate to kidney injury and reduced function.[35] Importantly, these inflammation-related pathways may serve as homing signals to recruit endothelial progenitor cells that participate in reparative processes. Renal vein levels of the injury marker neutrophil gelatinase-associated lipocalin (NGAL) are elevated in patients with atherosclerotic renovascular disease, likely due to ongoing kidney and systemic inflammation and ischemia[36] and soluble CD40 ligand (sCD40L) plasma levels are elevated, suggesting platelet activation.[37] Therefore these inflammation-related pathways may serve as novel therapeutic targets to repair the poststenotic kidney.

Tubular Cells

Acute ischemic renal failure is characterized by a rapid decline in adenosine triphosphate (ATP) that leads to secondary cascades of cellular injury, including increases in intracellular calcium, activation of phospholipases, and generation of oxygen radicals, which cause significant surface membrane damage. Susceptible proximal tubule cells are primarily responsible for the pathophysiologic and clinical aspects of ischemic acute renal failure. Of central importance is disruption and dissociation of the actin cytoskeleton and associated surface membrane structures that occur rapidly and depend upon the severity and duration of ischemic injury. These alterations may be secondary to activation and relocation of the actin-associated protein actin depolymerizing factor/cofilin and β1 integrin to the apical membrane. ATP depletion also induces necrotic cell death by inducing opening of a plasma membrane "death channel," normally kept closed in ischemic tissue, by tissue glycine and decreased pH. The epithelial brush border may disappear, in association with apical membrane blebbing, interruption of cell-to-cell junctions, and subsequently epithelial desquamation. Detachment of tubule cells and microvilli contributes to backleak of glomerular filtrate and formation of intraluminal aggregations of exfoliated cells, proteins, and glycoproteins like fibronectin, resulting in tubular obstruction. The functional ramifications of these changes are substantial in terms of tubular reabsorption, function of the intercellular tight junction, impaired cell-substrate adhesion, and integral membrane protein function.

Tubulointerstitial Injury

The severity of pathological tissue damage in the kidney beyond an atherosclerotic renal artery stenosis is an important determinant and predictor of renal functional outcome. The earliest and most prominent pathologic feature in renal ischemia is tubulointerstitial injury. The early phase of tubulointerstitial injury involves cellular activation, migration of mononuclear cells into the interstitium, leukocyte-endothelial interactions, and release of inflammatory products by myofibroblasts/activated-fibroblasts. Altered antigenic profile of the tubular epithelium may initiate a cell-mediated immune response, and be accompanied by interstitial inflammatory infiltrates composed of B lymphocytes, T helper lymphocytes, and macrophages.[34] Subsequently, immunosuppressive regulatory T cells (Tregs) promote repair during the healing process, possibly by regulating proinflammatory cytokine production of other T cell subsets. Although the tubular lesions are initially reversible, tubulointerstitial injury may lead to irreversible fibrosis. A plethora of fibrogenic factors have been implicated in development of renal fibrosis following ischemic injury, such as TGF-β1, PAI-1, TIMP-1, α1(IV) collagen, fibronectin-EIIIA (FN-EIIIA), tissue transglutaminase, and others, which may increase synthesis of extracellular matrix. Recent evidence suggests that, in the context of atherosclerosis, matrix degradation is also impaired, so that the overall matrix turnover balance favors fibrosis.

Glomerulosclerosis

In human atherosclerotic renal artery stenosis, glomerulosclerosis is a relatively late sequela and exacerbated by long duration, preexisting renal injury, and comorbid clinical conditions. In experimental models of chronic moderate renal artery stenosis, glomerular lesions are initially minimal. Ischemia may elicit global or focal segmental glomerulosclerosis, manifested as segmental collapse or sclerosis, with or without reactive podocyte hypertrophy and proliferation. Initiation of glomerular cell apoptosis, thickening of the basement membrane, and expansion of the mesangium, lead to progression of glomerulosclerosis. The presence of glomeruli that are not connected to normal tubule segments correlates with the concomitant decrease in GFR.

Cellular Death and Repair

Reactive oxygen species produced in renal proximal tubule epithelium under conditions of ischemia/reperfusion or hypoxia/reoxygenation are partly responsible for the apoptotic death of these cells. This process is partly mitigated by autophagy, a process of degradation and recycling of cytoplasmic constituents that may either contribute to cell death or ameliorate further cellular damage. During hypoxic and ischemic renal injury, autophagy seems to provide a protective mechanism and enhance cell survival.[38]

Despite multiple and varied defense mechanisms that are activated during an ischemic insult, cell loss by apoptosis or necrosis does occur when renal hypoxia is severe. For reconstitution of its function, successful repair of the kidney requires rapid replacement of injured cells.[39] Cell loss during kidney injury is followed by dedifferentiation and proliferation of adjacent surviving tubular cells, which are the chief contributors to tubular repair, and to a lesser degree interstitial kidney stem cells are stimulated to divide, migrate, and undergo phenotypic changes that allow them to replace lost cells. Bone marrow–derived cells likely contribute relatively little to this process. Nevertheless, exogenous administration of progenitor cells has been shown to improve renal function and attenuate renal damage in the chronic renal artery stenosis in swine[40] and ischemia/reperfusion injury in mice,[41] suggesting a potential therapeutic utility for this experimental approach to preserve the ischemic kidney. Furthermore, a single intraarterial infusion of autologous adipose tissue-derived mesenchymal stem cells increased renal tissue oxygenation and cortical blood flow in patients with atherosclerotic renovascular disease, supporting a potential role for stem cell–based strategies to improve and/or recover renal function in renovascular disease.[42]

RENAL ARTERY DISEASE AND MORTALITY

Role of Disease Progression

In patients with incidentally identified renal artery disease, renal artery stenosis independently predicts subsequent mortality. Rarely is this risk due to progressive renal disease alone, but more commonly to associated cardiovascular events. Mortality is remarkably similar in those treated either with medical management or renal revascularization. Progression of renal dysfunction is relatively uncommon. Death is most commonly related to cardiovascular events and only infrequently is progressive renal failure the primary cause of death. Some authors suggest that atherosclerotic disease affecting the kidney is a general marker of the degree of "atherosclerotic burden."[43] Others argue that renovascular disease augments these conditions and accelerates cardiovascular mortality directly. Available data from the Cardiovascular Outcomes in Renal Atherosclerotic Lesions (CORAL) study do not support an added benefit from renal revascularization to improve overall survival over that observed during optimal medical therapy for moderate renovascular disease.[44] Numerous observational series from patients with high-risk clinical syndromes and severe stenoses indicate that patients experiencing an improvement in GFR after successful revascularization do, in fact, have reduced cardiovascular mortality over several years of follow-up.[45,46]

Survival is reduced in patients with bilateral renal artery disease or stenosis to a solitary functioning kidney. Prospective studies using Doppler ultrasound indicate that atherosclerotic lesions commonly progress in severity over periods of 3 to 5 years. The risks of progression are related to initial severity of the stenotic lesion and systolic blood pressure levels. It must be emphasized that clinical manifestations of renal artery disease within an individual patient may change over time. It is important that clinicians identify these transitions to consider interventions timed to when they are most likely to be effective.

Specific decisions regarding management of patients with renovascular disease depend heavily upon recognizing the clinical syndromes developing as a result of these lesions. As with many other forms of peripheral vascular disease, the opportunity to benefit patients is greatest in those with overt clinical manifestations of the disease. Understanding the pathophysiology underlying the clinical syndromes identified here will assist the clinician in choosing patients most likely to benefit from intervention.

REFERENCES

1. Textor SC. Renal arterial disease and hypertension. *Med Clin North Am*. 2017;101(1):65–79.
2. Goldblatt H, Lynch J, Hanzal RE, Summerville WW. Studies on experimental hypertension I: the production of persistent elevation of systolic blood pressure by means of renal ischemia. *J Exp Med*. 1934;59:347–379.
3. Lorenz EC, Vrtiska TJ, Lieske JC, et al. Prevalence of renal artery and kidney abnormalities by computed tomography among healthy adults. *Clin J Am Soc Nephrol*. 2010;5:431–438.
4. Gloviczki ML, Glockner JF, Lerman LO, et al. Preserved oxygenation despite reduced blood flow in poststenotic kidneys in human atherosclerotic renal artery stenosis. *Hypertension*. 2010;55:961–966.
5. Gloviczki ML, Saad A, Textor SC. Blood oxygen level-dependent (BOLD) MRI analysis in atherosclerotic renal artery stenosis. *Curr Opin Nephrol Hypertens*. 2013;22:519–524.
6. Gloviczki ML, Glockner JF, Crane JA, et al. Blood oxygen level-dependent magnetic resonance imaging identifies cortical hypoxia in severe renovascular disease. *Hypertension*. 2011;58:1066–1072.
7. Dechering DG, Kruis HM, Adiyaman A, et al. Clinical significance of low-grade renal artery stenosis. *J Intern Med*. 2010;267:305–315.

8. Urbieta-Caceres VH, Lavi R, Zhu XY, et al. Early atherosclerosis aggravates the effect of renal artery stenosis on the swine kidney. *Am J Physiol Renal Physiol*. 2010;299:F135–F140.

9. Bige N, Levy PP, Callard P, et al. Renal arterial resistive index is associated with severe histological changes and poor renal outcome during chronic kidney disease. *BMC Nephrol*. 2012;13:139.

10. Mangiacapra F, Trana C, Sarno G, et al. Translesional pressure gradients to predict blood pressure response after renal artery stenting in patients with renovascular hypertension. *Circ Cardiovasc Interv*. 2010;3:537–542.

11. Chade AR. Renal vascular structure and rarefaction. *Compr Physiol*. 2013;3:817–831.

12. Textor SC, Lerman L. Renovascular hypertension and ischemic nephropathy. *Am J Hypertens*. 2010;23:1159–1169.

13. Evans KL, Tuttle KR, Folt DA, et al. Use of renin-angiotensin inhibitors in people with renal artery stenosis. *Clin J Am Soc Nephrol*. 2014;9:1199–1206.

14. Textor SC, Misra S, Oderich GS. Percutaneous revascularization for ischemic nephropathy: the past, present, and future. *Kidney Int*. 2013;83:28–40.

15. Kawarada O, Yasuda S, Noguchi T, et al. Renovascular heart failure: heart failure in patients with atherosclerotic renal artery disease. *Cardiovasc Interv Ther*. 2016;31:171–182.

16. Textor SC, Lerman LO. Renal artery stenosis: medical versus interventional therapy. *Curr Cardiol Rep*. 2013;15:409.

17. Ritchie J, Green D, Chrysochou C, et al. High-risk clinical presentations in atherosclerotic renovascular disease: prognosis and response to renal artery revascularization. *Am J Kidney Dis*. 2014;63(2):186–197.

18. Reich B, Schmidbauer K, Rodriguez Gomez M, et al. Fibrocytes develop outside the kidney but contribute to renal fibrosis in a mouse model. *Kidney Int*. 2013;84:78–89.

19. Kohan DE, Barton M. Endothelin and endothelin antagonists in chronic kidney disease. *Kidney Int*. 2014;86:896–904.

20. Tessari P. Nitric oxide in the normal kidney and in patients with diabetic nephropathy. *J Nephrol*. 2015;28:257–268.

21. Saeed A, Herlitz H, Nowakowska-Fortuna E, et al. Oxidative stress and endothelin-1 in atherosclerotic renal artery stenosis and effects of renal angioplasty. *Kidney Blood Press Res*. 2011;34:396–403.

22. Chade AR, Stewart NJ, Peavy PR. Disparate effects of single endothelin-A and -B receptor blocker therapy on the progression of renal injury in advanced renovascular disease. *Kidney Int*. 2014;85:833–844.

23. Rahman S, Malcoun A. Nonsteroidal antiinflammatory drugs, cyclooxygenase-2, and the kidneys. *Prim Care*. 2014;41:803–821.

24. Kwon SH, Lerman LO. Atherosclerotic renal artery stenosis: current status. *Adv Chronic Kidney Dis*. 2015;22:224–231.

25. Chade AR, Krier JD, Rodriguez-Porcel M, et al. Comparison of acute and chronic antioxidant interventions in experimental renovascular disease. *Am J Physiol Renal Physiol*. 2004;286:F1079–F1086.

26. Palm F, Onozato M, Welch WJ, Wilcox CS. Blood pressure, blood flow, and oxygenation in the clipped kidney of chronic 2-kidney, 1-clip rats: effects of tempol and angiotensin blockade. *Hypertension*. 2010;55:298–304.

27. Leask A. Potential therapeutic targets for cardiac fibrosis: TGFbeta, angiotensin, endothelin, CCN2, and PDGF, partners in fibroblast activation. *Circ Res*. 2010;106:1675–1680.

28. Warner GM, Cheng J, Knudsen BE, et al. Genetic deficiency of Smad3 protects the kidneys from atrophy and interstitial fibrosis in 2K1C hypertension. *Am J Physiol Renal Physiol*. 2012;302:F1455–F1464.

29. Eirin A, Lerman A, Lerman LO. Mitochondria: a pathogenic paradigm in hypertensive renal disease. *Hypertension*. 2015;65:264–270.

30. Eirin A, Saad A, Tang H, et al. Urinary mitochondrial DNA copy number identifies chronic renal injury in hypertensive patients. *Hypertension*. 2016;68:401–410.

31. Eirin A, Li Z, Zhang X, et al. A mitochondrial permeability transition pore inhibitor improves renal outcomes after revascularization in experimental atherosclerotic renal artery stenosis. *Hypertension*. 2012;60:1242–1249.

32. Saad A, Herrmann SMS, Eirin A, et al. Phase 2a clinical trial of mitochondrial protection (elamipretide) during stent revascularization in patients with atherosclerotic renal artery stenosis. *Circ Cardiovasc Interv*. 2017;10(9):e005487.

33. Stouffer GA, Pathak A, Rojas M. Unilateral renal artery stenosis causes a chronic vascular inflammatory response in ApoE-/- mice. *Trans Am Clin Climatol Assoc*. 2010;121:252–264.

34. Gloviczki ML, Keddis MT, Garovic VD, et al. TGF expression and macrophage accumulation in atherosclerotic renal artery stenosis. *Clin J Am Soc Nephrol*. 2013;8:546–553.

35. Eirin A, Gloviczki ML, Tang H, et al. Inflammatory and injury signals released from the post-stenotic human kidney. *Eur Heart J*. 2013;34:540–548a.

36. Eirin A, Gloviczki ML, Tang H, et al. Chronic renovascular hypertension is associated with elevated levels of neutrophil gelatinase-associated lipocalin. *Nephrol Dial Transplant*. 2012;27:4153–4161.

37. Haller S, Adlakha S, Reed G, et al. Platelet activation in patients with atherosclerotic renal artery stenosis undergoing stent revascularization. *Clin J Am Soc Nephrol*. 2011;6:2185–2191.

38. Jiang M, Liu K, Luo J, Dong Z. Autophagy is a renoprotective mechanism during in vitro hypoxia and in vivo ischemia-reperfusion injury. *Am J Pathol*. 2010;176:1181–1192.

39. Guo JK, Cantley LG. Cellular maintenance and repair of the kidney. *Annu Rev Physiol*. 2010;72:357–376.

40. Chade AR, Zhu XY, Krier JD, et al. Endothelial progenitor cells homing and renal repair in experimental renovascular disease. *Stem Cells*. 2010;28:1039–1047.

41. Li B, Cohen A, Hudson TE, et al. Mobilized human hematopoietic stem/progenitor cells promote kidney repair after ischemia/reperfusion injury. *Circulation*. 2010;121:2211–2220.

42. Saad A, Dietz AB, Herrmann SMS, et al. Autologous mesenchymal stem cells increase cortical perfusion in renovascular disease. *J Am Soc Nephrol*. 2017;28:2777–2785.

43. Khangura KK, Eirin A, Kane GC, et al. Extrarenal atherosclerotic disease blunts renal recovery in patients with renovascular hypertension. *J Hypertens*. 2014;32:1300–1306.

44. Cooper CJ, Murphy TP, Cutlip DE, et al. Stenting and medical therapy for atherosclerotic renal-artery stenosis. *N Engl J Med*. 2014;370:13–22.

45. Kennedy DJ, Colyer WR, Brewster PS, et al. Renal insufficiency as a predictor of adverse events and mortality after renal artery stent placement. *Am J Kidney Dis*. 2003;42:926–935.

46. Kalra PA, Chrysochou C, Green D, et al. The benefit of renal artery stenting in patients with atheromatous renovascular disease and advanced chronic kidney disease. *Catheter Cardiovasc Interv*. 2010;75:1–10.

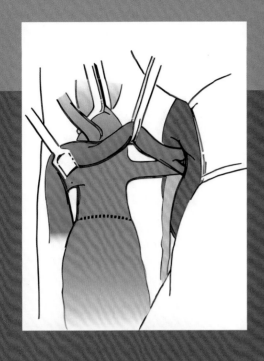

第23章
肾动脉疾病的临床评估

　　本章节详细讲述了肾动脉疾病的临床影像学评估方法，以及具体各种方法的优势和临床应用价值。本章在开始时，对肾动脉狭窄的临床病因学进行了简单的描述，指出动脉粥样硬化是其主要的原因，占比90%以上，其次，导致肾动脉狭窄的第二位原因在西方国家是纤维肌发育不良，在我国则是多发性大动脉炎。接着，本章节讲述了肾动脉狭窄导致的一系列临床表现，从而为临床对本病的识别提供很好的帮助，如继发性高血压、肾功能不全和萎缩、对心脏和肺水肿的影响等。同时，肾动脉疾病往往合并其他的外周血管疾病，包括动脉瘤、主髂动脉狭窄、下肢动脉缺血等。因此，尽管常规的体格检查不能提示有肾动脉疾病的存在，但临床的表现结合相应的影像学检查，就可以很好地评估肾动脉疾病的存在。本章节的重点内容就是通过各种影像方式对肾动脉狭窄进行诊断。以动脉粥样硬化为例，本章详细讲述了超声、磁共振血管成像、CT血管造影、数字减影肠系膜血管成像对狭窄的评估及其各自的优势。尤其强调了超声检查的重要性，不光是在初始病变中的判断，对于介入治疗放置支架后，因超声可以穿透支架，而不会产生其他影像学检查的伪影，在随访中具有独特的作用和优势。本章还针对纤维肌发育不良的影像学特点进行了专门的讲述，比较了数字减影肠系膜血管成像和光学相干断层扫描术（optical coherence tomography，OCT）的影像，再次揭示了纤维肌发育不良（fibromuscular dysplasia，FMD）不仅是内膜病变，也可以累及中膜甚至全层。尽管尚存争议，但鉴于肾动脉疾病往往是心脏事件的重要危险因素，因此在冠状动脉造影检查的同时进行肾动脉造影，及时发现病变也是可以考虑的检查手段。

李拥军

23

Clinical Evaluation of Renal Artery Disease

Jeffrey W. Olin

Approximately 46% of individuals age 20 and older have high blood pressure.[1] In those age 75 and older, 79% of men and 85% of women have hypertension. Most have primary (essential) hypertension; however, there are a number of different causes of secondary hypertension, including those related to lifestyle or medications, such as obesity, excess alcohol ingestion, drug abuse, and oral contraceptive agents. Among other secondary causes, renovascular disease and renal parenchymal disease are the most common. Notably, there is a difference between hypertension that is associated with atherosclerotic renal artery stenosis (RAS) and hypertension caused by RAS (renovascular hypertension). Incidentally discovered RAS is quite common, whereas atherosclerotic renovascular hypertension occurs much less frequently.[2] More than 90% of all renovascular disease is caused by atherosclerosis.[3] Fibromuscular dysplasia (FMD) is the second most common cause of RAS.[4] Patients with atherosclerotic RAS are typically older than age 65 and have the usual risk factors for atherosclerosis. FMD predominately occurs in women (94%) with a mean age at diagnosis of 54, but it may occur at any age.[5] The most common clinical manifestation of FMD is hypertension, whereas atherosclerotic RAS may present with hypertension, acute and chronic kidney disease (CKD), and/or recurrent episodes of heart failure and "flash" pulmonary edema.[6-9] FMD and atherosclerotic RAS may also be incidental findings when imaging is performed for another reason. Atherosclerotic RAS most often occurs at the ostium or proximal portion of the renal artery, while FMD usually occurs in the mid- to distal renal artery and its primary branches (Figs. 23.1 and 23.2).

In addition to the sequelae of RAS (hypertension, CKD), patients with atherosclerotic RAS succumb prematurely from myocardial infarction (MI) and stroke.[9] It is therefore important to treat patients with atherosclerotic RAS with optimal medical therapy similar to those with coronary and carotid artery disease (antiplatelet agent, statin, and management of other cardiovascular [CV] risk factors).

When considering the diagnosis of RAS, it is useful to think in terms of the circumstances in which RAS is likely to occur (Box 23.1).

CONSEQUENCES OF RENAL ARTERY STENOSIS

Hypertension

Individuals who develop hypertension between the ages of 30 and 64 usually have primary hypertension. If the initial diagnosis of hypertension is made before the age of 30, it is usually due to FMD if other known secondary causes (obesity, oral contraceptive use, drug abuse, and parenchymal renal disease) have been excluded. Because atherosclerosis occurs in older individuals, it is usually the cause of RAS in individuals aged 65 or older. There is no recent data regarding the prevalence of RAS in patients older than 65 years. In an older population-based study of Medicare patients aged 65 or older, the

prevalence of atherosclerotic RAS was 6.8%.[10] In this cohort, RAS was found in nearly twice as many men as women (9.1% vs. 5.5%); no significant differences were identified between Caucasian and African American subjects (6.9% vs. 6.7%).[10] It is not uncommon for patients to have primary hypertension for many years, and as they age, develop atherosclerotic RAS. Under those circumstances, the patient may have had well-controlled blood pressure that suddenly becomes more difficult to control.

Patients may have anatomically significant RAS and no hypertension at all. In a systematic review of 40 studies that evaluated a total of 15,879 patients, the mean prevalence of RAS among patients with suspected renovascular hypertension was 14.1%.[3] On further analysis of the patients who were incidentally found to have RAS on imaging studies, 65.5% were hypertensive and 27.5% had renal failure.[3] Therefore the mere presence of RAS and hypertension does not necessarily mean that one is causing the other.[11] Accelerated or malignant hypertension has also been associated with a very high prevalence of RAS. Resistant hypertension is defined as the failure to normalize blood pressure to less than 140/90 mm Hg despite an optimal medical regimen consisting of at least three drugs with different mechanisms of action, including a diuretic.[1] The diagnosis of renovascular disease should be strongly considered in patients with true drug-resistant hypertension.

Renal Abnormalities

The presence of RAS may lead to an atrophic kidney, or a discrepancy in size between the two kidneys. An investigation for the presence of renovascular disease should be undertaken if either are present. Additionally, it has long been recognized that patients who develop azotemia while receiving angiotensin-converting enzyme (ACE) inhibitors or angiotensin II receptor blocking (ARB) agents may have bilateral RAS, RAS to a single functioning kidney, or decompensated congestive heart failure (CHF) in the sodium-depleted state.[12,13] These clinical scenarios are absolute indications for investigation, because they usually reflect the presence of severe RAS to the entire functioning renal mass, thus placing the patient in jeopardy of renal failure.[14] The pathophysiologic mechanisms of acute and chronic renal failure in patients with renal artery disease are discussed in detail in Chapter 22.

There are no prospective studies evaluating how often atherosclerotic renovascular disease leads to end-stage renal disease (ESRD). A retrospective cohort study was conducted using data from the National Health Insurance Research Database of Taiwan for the years 1999 through 2011.[15] A total of 2184 patients with atherosclerotic RAS were enrolled and of these, 840 had ESRD. Using multivariable logistic regression analysis, they showed that the occurrence of ESRD was more likely with a higher Charleson comorbidity index (CCI) (odds ratio [OR] 6.69 for CCI = 2; OR 20.0 for CCI ≥ 3), diabetes (OR 1.55), hypertension (OR 3.66), and age 20 to 49 years old (OR 2.14). Those

377 «««

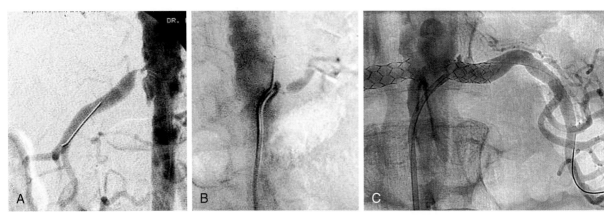

Fig. 23.1 (A) and (B) Digital subtraction angiogram showing typical features of atherosclerotic renal artery stenosis (RAS). There is severe bilateral ostial RAS. (C) Angiogram after stents were placed in right and left renal arteries.

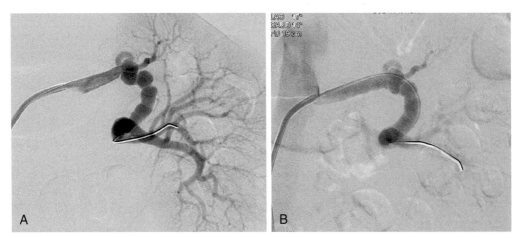

Fig. 23.2 (A) Digital subtraction angiogram demonstrating multifocal fibromuscular dysplasia located in the mid to distal part of the left renal artery. Note "beading," with beads larger than the normal caliber of the artery, typical of multifocal fibromuscular dysplasia. (B) Angiogram of the left renal artery after percutaneous balloon angioplasty. Angiographic appearance is improved, and there was resolution of the pressure gradient.

undergoing renal artery revascularization for atherosclerotic RAS had a lower risk (OR 0.64) of ESRD.[15] Data from the older literature found that atherosclerotic renovascular disease was the cause of ESRD in 12% to 14% of patients starting dialysis therapy.[16] De Mast and Beutler reported that 41% of patients with ESRD had at least one renal artery with more than 50% stenosis.[3] RAS must be excluded in every patient starting dialysis if a clear-cut etiology for the ESRD is not known because the mortality in this patient population is extremely high. The presence of ESRD secondary to atherosclerotic RAS portends a poor prognosis. In the series by Mailloux et al., median survival in patients with ESRD secondary to RAS was 25 months, while 2-, 5-, and 10-year survival was 56%, 18%, and 5%, respectively.[16,17] This may be an overestimation of poor survival, because these studies were conducted prior to the routine use of statins and other medical therapies proven to decrease the risk of MI, stroke, and cardiovascular death.

Effects of Renal Artery Stenosis on the Heart

Recurrent heart failure and flash pulmonary edema unrelated to ischemic heart disease can result from bilateral RAS (or unilateral RAS to a single functioning kidney).[6,14] In one renal artery stent series, 39 patients (19% of all patients undergoing renal artery stent implantation from 1991 to 1997) had recurrent episodes of heart failure or flash pul-

monary edema as the primary indication for renal artery stenting.[14] Nineteen of 39 patients had moderate to severe left ventricular (LV) systolic function. Although not completely understood, the mechanism of heart failure may be related in part to the inability to use ACE inhibitors or ARBs in patients with bilateral RAS or RAS to a single functioning kidney, to the direct adverse effects of angiotensin II (Ang II) on myocardial function, to severe hypertension and the related increase in afterload, or to the inability to control volume adequately. If coronary ischemia has been excluded as a cause of heart failure, renal artery stent implantation is a very effective method of treatment in these individuals.[14]

Presence of Atherosclerosis in Other Vascular Beds

Several series have examined the prevalence of renovascular disease in patients who have atherosclerotic disease elsewhere. To determine the prevalence of atherosclerotic RAS, Olin et al. studied 395 consecutive patients who underwent catheter-based arteriography as part of an evaluation for an abdominal aortic aneurysm, aortoiliac occlusive disease, or peripheral artery disease (PAD; Table 23.1).[18] These patients did not have the usual clinical clues to suggest RAS. Severe bilateral renal artery disease was present in approximately 13% of patients. In addition, 76 patients had an aortogram performed for suspected RAS, and RAS was

BOX 23.1 Clinical Clues That Suggest Presence of Renal Artery Stenosis

Hypertension
- Hypertension onset age <30 or >65 years
- Malignant or accelerated hypertension
- Resistant hypertension (blood pressure >140/90 mm Hg despite appropriate three-drug regimen, including a diuretic)
- Loss of blood pressure control in a previously well-controlled patient

Renal Abnormalities
- Acute renal failure precipitated by an angiotensin-converting enzyme (ACE) inhibitor or angiotensin receptor blocking (ARB) agent
- Unexplained azotemia
- Patient receiving renal replacement therapy (dialysis) without a definite known cause of end-stage renal disease (ESRD)
- Atrophic or small kidney

Cardiac Disease
- Recurrent congestive heart failure (CHF) or flash pulmonary edema
- Angina disproportionate to coronary anatomy

Presence of Atherosclerosis in Other Vascular Beds
- Peripheral artery disease (PAD)
- Aortoiliac occlusive disease
- Aortic aneurysm
- Multivessel coronary artery disease (CAD)

TABLE 23.1 Prevalence of Atherosclerotic Renal Artery Stenosis

≥50% Stenosis	Abdominal Aortic Aneurysm (n = 109)	Aortoiliac Occlusive Disease (n = 21)	Peripheral Artery Disease (n = 189)	Renal Artery Stenosis (n = 76)
All patients	41 (38%)	7 (33%)	74 (39%)	53 (70%)[a]
Diabetic patients	6 (50%)	1 (33%)	34 (50%)[b]	10 (71%)
Nondiabetic patients	35 (36%)	6 (33%)	40 (33%)	43 (69%)[a]

[a] P < .001, [b] P < .02.
From Olin JW, Melia M, Young JR, et al. Prevalence of atherosclerotic renal artery stenosis in patients with atherosclerosis elsewhere. *Am J Med.* 1990;88:46N–51N.

present in 70% of these subjects. In a more contemporary series of 400 consecutive patients undergoing catheter-based angiography for PAD, incidental RAS was found in 14% of patients. Because two-thirds of the patients had critical limb ischemia, this was a cohort of patients with severe PAD. The reason for the low prevalence of RAS in this contemporary series compared to many other studies (in which 22% to 59% of PAD patients had RAS) is not clear.[19]

It has also been established that RAS is common in patients with coronary artery disease (CAD). Of 7758 patients undergoing cardiac catheterization during a 78-month period of time, 3987 underwent aortography at the time of catheterization to screen for RAS[20]; 191 (4.8%) had more than 75% RAS, and 0.8% had severe bilateral disease. In a Mayo Clinic series, renal arteries were studied at the time of cardiac catheterization in patients with hypertension.[21] Ninety percent of the renal arteries were adequately visualized, and no complications occurred

from the aortogram. More than 50% RAS was present in 19.2%, more than 70% stenosis in 7%, and bilateral RAS was present in 3.7% of patients. The likelihood of significant RAS is markedly increased in patients with disease in two or more coronary arteries. It is important to recognize that atherosclerotic RAS is a manifestation of systemic atherosclerosis and thus supports the concept of treating the entire patient with optimal medical management rather than focusing on the circulatory bed involved at a given point in time.

The presence of RAS even prior to development of ESRD portends a poor prognosis. All of the studies reported occurred prior to the routine use of statins and less stringent guidelines for the maximal medical therapy for patients with atherosclerosis. Therefore, the contemporary mortality rates are not known. It is however known that the mortality is higher in patients with RAS compared to those without RAS.[20]

PHYSICAL EXAMINATION

The physical examination is generally not helpful in the diagnosis of RAS. Evidence of coronary, cerebral, or PAD is associated with a higher likelihood of renal artery disease because of the systemic nature of atherosclerosis. An abdominal bruit is common and nonspecific and may arise from any of the visceral vessels in the abdomen or from the iliac arteries. An abdominal bruit with a systolic and diastolic component occurs more often in patients with FMD than in patients who have atherosclerotic disease.[22] The presence of a bruit may be helpful, but absence does not exclude the diagnosis of either atherosclerotic renovascular disease or FMD.

DIAGNOSIS OF RENOVASCULAR DISEASE

In the past, indirect methods of assessing the renal arteries were commonly used to diagnose RAS. Most of these tests as described below are no longer used because of limited sensitivity and specificity and because of the availability of duplex renal artery ultrasound, magnetic resonance angiography (MRA), and computed tomographic angiography (CTA), each of which can directly visualize the renal arteries and are accurate diagnosing significant RAS.[11,23–26] Intravenous urography is obsolete as a screening tool, owing to its poor sensitivity and specificity. Plasma renin activity as a standalone screening test is not reliable for diagnosing or excluding renal artery disease. Elevated plasma renin activity may be present in approximately 15% of patients with essential hypertension. In addition, patients with bilateral disease or disease to a solitary functioning kidney may have normal or low plasma renin activity due to extracellular volume expansion, position of the patient during the test, or medication use. The captopril test (plasma renin measurement before and after administration of captopril) is not an ideal screening test and is rarely used. Renal vein renin measurement is not a useful test to screen for RAS; in addition, it has little value in determining who will benefit from revascularization. Except under unusual circumstances, this test is rarely used to make clinical decisions. Captopril scintigraphy involves measuring renal blood flow and excretory function before and after the administration of an ACE inhibitor such as captopril. This test is rarely used because of the poor sensitivity and specificity (especially in those with bilateral renal artery disease, and in those with renal artery disease affecting a single functioning kidney or CKD).

Imaging Modalities to Detect Renal Artery Stenosis

Although catheter-based renal angiography with pressure gradient measurements is the definitive gold standard of RAS assessment, several noninvasive imaging modalities such as duplex ultrasound, CTA, and MRA, have become more practical first-line tests for the diagnosis of RAS. Imaging has become so sophisticated and accurate, that it is seldom necessary to perform catheter-based angiography for the *diagnosis* of renal artery disease; it is usually reserved for imaging at the time of percutaneous revascularization. The ideal imaging procedure should do the following[23]:

1. Identify the main renal arteries and the accessory or polar vessels.
2. Localize the site of stenosis or disease.
3. Determine the type of disease present (e.g., atherosclerosis, FMD).
4. Provide evidence for the hemodynamic significance of the lesion.
5. Determine the likelihood of a favorable response to revascularization.
6. Identify associated pathology (i.e., abdominal aortic aneurysm, renal mass, etc.) that may have an impact on the treatment of the renal artery disease.
7. Detect restenosis after percutaneous or surgical revascularization.

Duplex ultrasonography, CTA, and MRA do not, by themselves, fulfill all these criteria. Local expertise and availability, as well as economic costs, often dictate the preferred imaging modality used (Table 23.2). Factors that may play a role in determining the optimal screening test include the patient's renal function, body habitus, and personal preference (e.g., claustrophobia).

Duplex Renal Artery Ultrasonography

Duplex renal artery ultrasonography (also see Chapter 12), which is composed of real-time brightness (B-mode/gray scale) imaging and color pulsed-wave Doppler, has the advantages of being noninvasive, and is the least expensive of the imaging modalities. It provides both anatomical and functional information about the arterial segments being evaluated. Duplex ultrasonography also does not require the use of potentially nephrotoxic agents. Overall, when compared to angiography, duplex renal artery ultrasonography has a sensitivity and specificity of 84% to 98% and 62% to 99%, respectively, when used to

diagnose RAS.[24,25,27] In a prospective blinded study, there was a very good correlation between duplex ultrasonography and angiography (Table 23.3). In addition, it was determined that if the end-diastolic velocity (EDV) was 150 cm/s or greater, the degree of stenosis was likely to be 80% or more.[27]

Renal artery ultrasound should be performed from both an anterior and oblique (or posterior [flank]) approach (Fig. 23.3). In the longitudinal view, the peak systolic flow velocity in the aorta is recorded at the level of the renal arteries. The renal-to-aortic ratio (RAR), which is the ratio of the highest peak systolic velocity (PSV) in the renal arteries to the PSV in the aorta, can then be calculated to help classify the degree of stenosis (Table 23.4).[23,27] The renal arteries are best visualized in a transverse (short-axis) view. Using the B-mode image and a 60-degree angle of insonation, the arteries are interrogated with pulsed-wave Doppler. The Doppler should be swept through the artery from its origin to the renal hilum, which will allow the examiner to survey the artery for velocity shifts along the entire course of the renal artery. Velocities should be recorded at the origin, proximal, mid-, and distal arterial segments. The best way to visualize the renal artery in its entirely, from the origin until it enters the kidney, is a subcostal view. From an oblique approach, the renal artery can be visualized at the renal hilum and followed to the aorta. By studying the patient from an anterior, subcostal, and an oblique approach, Doppler velocity measurements are obtained in multiple views, assuring that a focal stenosis is not missed and that the angle of insonation is correct. Because multifocal fibroplasia most often occurs in the mid to distal renal artery, the subcostal and oblique approaches are particularly good for detecting this type of stenosis. It is important to note that segmental Doppler interrogation (spot-checking) of the renal artery velocities is inadequate and often leads to an inaccurate result. When there is a discrepancy in kidney size

TABLE 23.2 Utility of the Various Noninvasive Diagnostic Tests

	Duplex Ultrasound	CT Angiography	MR Angiography
Identify main renal artery	+++	+++	+++
Identify accessory renal artery	+	+++	++
Determine type of disease	++	+++	++
Provide evidence of hemodynamic significance	+++	–	–
Determine likelihood of favorable response to stenting	+	–	–
Identify associated pathology (AAA, renal mass)	+	+++	+++
Detect restenosis after percutaneous or surgical revascularization	+++	+	–

+++, Most useful; +, least useful; –, not useful at all. *AAA*, Abdominal aortic aneurysm; *CT*, computed tomography; *MR*, magnetic resonance.

TABLE 23.3 Comparison of Duplex Ultrasound with Arteriography

	STENOSIS BY ARTERIOGRAPHY				
Stenosis by Ultrasound	0%–59%	60%–79%	80%–99%	100%	Total
0%–59%	62	0	1	1	64
60%–99%	1	31	67	0	99
100%	0	1	1	22	24
Total	63	32	69	23	187
Sensitivity	0.98				
Specificity	0.98				
Positive predictive value	0.99				
Negative predictive value	0.97				

From Olin JW, Piedmonte MR, Young JR, DeAnna S, Grubb M, Childs MB. The utility of duplex ultrasound scanning of the renal arteries for diagnosing significant renal artery stenosis. *Ann Intern Med.* 1995;122(1):833–838.

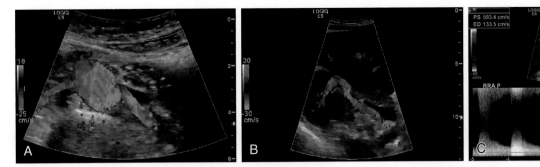

Fig. 23.3 (A) Color duplex ultrasound of renal arteries from an anterior approach. The right renal artery takes off at approximately 9 to 10 o'clock and the left renal artery at 3 to 4 o'clock. (B) Color duplex ultrasound from oblique view imaging from kidney to proximal renal artery. Note how the entire renal artery is visualized from this approach. (C) Duplex ultrasound from the anterior view. There is turbulence to flow on the color Doppler and markedly increased velocities of blood flow (peak systolic velocity 593 cm/s and end-diastolic velocity 134 cm/s), indicating severe stenosis.

TABLE 23.4   Duplex Criteria for Diagnosis of Renal Artery Stenosis

RAR <3.5 and PSV <200 cm/s	0%–59%
RAR ≥3.5 and PSV >200 cm/s	60%–99%
RAR >3.5 and EDV ≥150 cm/s	80%–99%
Absent flow, low-amplitude parenchymal signal	Occluded

EDV, End-diastolic velocity; *PSV,* peak systolic velocity; *RAR,* renal-to-aortic ratio.

of 1.5 cm or greater, the ultrasonographer should search very carefully for the presence of severe RAS or an occluded renal artery.

A three-category classification scheme based on the peak systolic velocity (PSV) within the proximal segment of the renal arteries is commonly used: 0% to 59% stenosis; 60% to 99% stenosis, and total occlusion. If the RAR of the PSV is ≥3.5, the PSV is greater than 200 cm/s, and turbulence is present in the color Doppler flow, the stenosis would be classified as 60% to 99% (also see Chapter 12). In the presence of a severe stenosis, there may be characteristic spectral broadening of the Doppler arterial waveform or parvus-tardus waveform just distal to the lesion (see Table 23.3). The RAR is not an accurate representation of the degree of stenosis when the aortic velocity is less than 40 cm/s or greater than 100 cm/s, or when an abdominal aortic aneurysm or aortic stent graft is present.

Indirect assessment using the acceleration time (AT), acceleration index (AI), and resistive index (RI) have been used by some investigators to *diagnose* RAS. However, direct measurement of blood flow velocities in the visualized segments of the renal arteries is the most accurate method of determining whether significant RAS is present.

There are two other important advantages of duplex ultrasonography. Though controversial, duplex ultrasonography may help identify patients who will have a favorable clinical outcome after surgical or catheter-based renal revascularization.[28] The RI is calculated as follows: [1-(EDV/PSV)] (Fig. 23.4). Using a zero-degree angle of insonation, the PSV and EDV are measured within the parenchyma of the kidney. Two studies help support use of the RI. A prospective study followed 138 patients with more than 50% RAS who underwent renal artery angioplasty or surgery for blood pressure control or preservation of renal function.[28] A renal RI of 0.80 or greater identified patients in whom angioplasty or surgery was not associated with improved blood pressure, renal function, or kidney survival. Ninety-seven percent of patients with an increased renal RI demonstrated no improvement in blood pressure, and 80% had no improvement in renal function. The

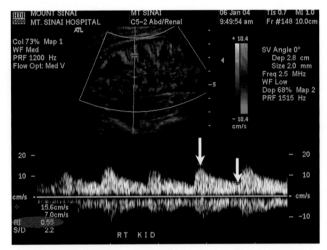

Fig. 23.4 Measurement of Resistive Index (RI) ([1-(End-Diastolic Velocity/Peak Systolic Velocity)]). Parenchyma of the kidney is visualized. Note blood flow within kidney. Doppler angle is zero degrees to optimize Doppler waveform. Color velocity scale is set low to optimize color flow. By measuring peak systolic velocity *(arrow)* and end-diastolic velocity *(arrow),* the ultrasound machine calculates the RI *(shown in the gray area at bottom left portion of this image).* RI = 0.55.

authors suggested that the increased RI identifies structural abnormalities in the small vessels of the kidney. Such small-vessel disease is typical of long-standing hypertension associated with nephrosclerosis or glomerulosclerosis. Similar conclusions were drawn from a second study that retrospectively evaluated the significance of associating pre-procedural RI with postintervention outcomes (endovascular or open surgical repair for RAS treatment). This study found that a preprocedural RI of 0.8 or higher was highly associated with a postprocedural decline in renal function, and that the RI was also highly predictive of all-cause mortality.[29] Not all investigators, however, believe that RI is an accurate predictor of the response to renal artery revascularization. A prospective study of renal stent placement in 241 patients demonstrated that individuals with an elevated RI (0.80) achieved a favorable blood pressure response and renal functional improvement a year after renal arterial intervention.[30] Zeller et al. demonstrated that patients with the most abnormal RI values experienced the greatest magnitude of benefit.[30,31] Until more information becomes available, an elevated RI should not be considered a contraindication to performing renal artery revascularization.

The second major advantage of duplex ultrasonography is its ability to detect restenosis after percutaneous therapy or surgical bypass (Fig. 23.5).[32] Unlike MRA (which may be affected by artifact or scatter produced by the stent), ultrasound transmission through the stent is not a problem. CTA has not been adequately studied in this respect. In a series of 134 patients with renal artery stents, velocity-derived criteria were developed. All patients with a PSV of less than 241 cm/s were free of in-stent restenosis, whereas all patients with a PSV of 300 cm/s or greater had in-stent restenosis as confirmed by CTA or catheter-based angiogram. If the PSV was between 241 and 299 cm/s, a judgment was required involving assessment of the degree of turbulence and appearance on grayscale and color Doppler. Using these criteria, the sensitivity was 91%, specificity was 97%, positive predictive value was 91%, negative predictive value was 96%, and accuracy was 95%.[32]

All patients who have undergone percutaneous intervention should be in a surveillance program to identify restenosis and treat it before the artery occludes. Following percutaneous transluminal angioplasty (PTA) and stent implantation, a renal artery duplex ultrasound should be obtained at the first office visit, and 6 months, 12 months, and yearly thereafter.[33]

There are several limitations of duplex ultrasonography. It is technically demanding, there is a steep learning curve, and it is particularly challenging in the obese individual. The sensitivity of identifying accessory renal arteries is only about 67%. In addition, approximately 5% of renal artery duplex ultrasound studies are of suboptimal quality because of the presence of bowel gas. All patients should fast for 12 hours prior to renal artery duplex ultrasound examination.

Magnetic Resonance Angiography

MRA (also see Chapter 13) of the renal arteries can be performed rapidly with excellent image quality. It does not involve ionizing radiation, and it allows for direct visualization of the aorta and renal arteries. Although there are studies suggesting that MRA can provide functional assessment of blood flow via absolute blood flow rate and glomerular filtration rate (GFR) measurements, this is rarely if ever done in the clinical setting. Also, functional renal perfusion can be assessed by MRA.

Compared to conventional catheter angiography as the reference standard, three-dimensional (3D) contrast-enhanced gadolinium MRA has a mean sensitivity of 96% and mean specificity of 93% for RAS (Table 23.5 and Fig. 23.6).[34–48]

TABLE 23.5   Accuracy of Three-Dimensional Gadolinium Magnetic Resonance Angiography for Renal Artery Stenosis

Author	Year	Patients	Sensitivity	Specificity
Snidow[46]	1996	47	100	89
Hany[42]	1997	39	93	98
De Cobelli[38]	1997	55	100	97
Rieumont[45]	1997	30	100	71
Bakker[37]	1998	54	97	92
Schoenberg[48]	1999	50	94	100
Hahn[41]	1999	22	91	79
Fain[40]	2001	25	97	92
Hood[43]	2002	21	100	74
Willmann[47]	2003	46	93	100
Patel[44]	2005	68	87	69
Eklöf[39]	2005	58	93	91
Bicakci[34]	2006	84	69–100	86–96
Rountas[35]	2007	58	90	94
Stacul[36]	2008	35	83	73–78

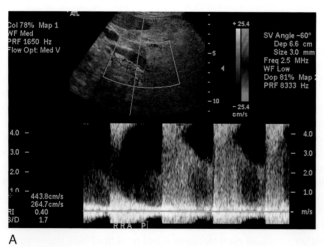

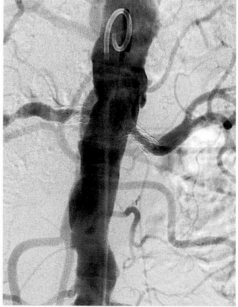

Fig. 23.5 (A) Duplex ultrasound demonstrating severe stenosis on first surveillance ultrasound 6 months after bilateral renal artery stent implantation. There is turbulence on the color image. Peak systolic velocity in the right renal artery is 444 cm/s, and end-diastolic velocity is 265 cm/s, with a renal-to-aortic ratio of 7:4. This is consistent with an 80% to 99% stenosis. (B) Digital subtraction angiogram of the same patient demonstrating severe bilateral in-stent restenosis; the right is more severe than left.

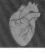

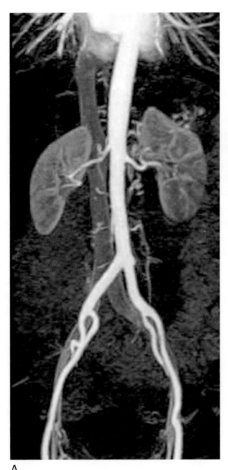

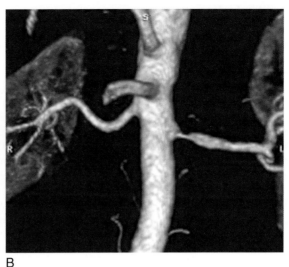

Fig. 23.6 (A) Three-dimensional gadolinium-enhanced magnetic resonance angiogram demonstrating normal renal arteries bilaterally. There is an excellent view of the aorta from the diaphragm to the inguinal ligament. By imaging a large field of view, one can be certain not to miss an accessory renal artery. Kidneys are also well seen with this technology. Inferior vena cava can be seen in the background. (B) Severe atherosclerotic renal artery stenosis of the left renal artery. Right renal artery is normal.

Contrast-enhanced 3D MRA is a commonly used modality for renal artery imaging because of its ability to produce 3D angiographic images with excellent image quality and improved speed of acquisition.[24,49,50] Contrast-enhanced 3D MRA exploits the T1-shortening effects of gadolinium-based contrast agents. Blood appears bright, and stationary tissues have a dark appearance. Use of gadolinium shortens image acquisition times, significantly limiting artifact due to patient movement and respiration. Because signal intensity with gadolinium is concentration dependent and not flow based, low-flow related artifacts are reduced, and visualization of small vessels is improved compared to other MRI techniques. Contrast-enhanced MRA is performed using fast 3D gradient echo pulse sequences. These pulse sequences are available primarily at higher magnetic field strengths (1.5 Tesla and 3.0 Tesla). Because hundreds of images are acquired, 3D image processing is subsequently performed to project vessels in views of high diagnostic interest.

Kidneys, adrenal glands, and surrounding soft tissues are evaluated by T1- and T2-weighted image acquisition. Time-of-flight (high-velocity jet within stenosis appears black because of signal loss), phase contrast (gadolinium injection allows phase shift difference detection and rendering of renal arterial blood flow), and maximal intensity projection are the most widely applied MRA imaging techniques. After 20 minutes of source image acquisition, additional time is required for 3D reconstruction, which increases diagnostic yield. Proper equipment, software, and technical expertise are critical for optimal renal MRA and account for significant variability of study quality between institutions.

Despite all of the advances, MRA is still limited by several factors, including high cost, imaging artifacts such as those attributed to patient movement, and difficulty resolving highly tortuous vessels and the smaller accessory renal arteries. MRA acquisition times are longer than those for CTA, and patients must therefore be able to remain motionless for minutes at a time. The image resolution is not as good as it is in CTA.[26] Moreover, MRA may not be possible for patients with claustrophobia and those with metal clips, pacemakers, or other metallic devices. MRA is also not useful for monitoring patients after renal artery angioplasty and stenting because of artifact produced by the stent. It also has a tendency to overestimate stenosis severity and may miss accessory renal arteries if the field of view is too narrow.

Exposure to gadolinium-based contrast agents in the setting of renal failure has been associated with nephrogenic systemic fibrosis (NSF), an exceedingly rare condition that involves fibrosis of the skin, joints, eyes, and internal organs.[51] Current recommendations advise against administering gadolinium contrast to individuals with a GFR below 30 mL/min/1.73 m^2 or those with acute renal failure or acute deterioration of chronic renal failure.[51]

Computed Tomographic Angiography

CTA (also see Chapter 14) can be performed rapidly and safely for assessment of renal artery disease. Multidetector-row CTA provides excellent image quality with higher resolution than could be obtained previously with single-detector-row technology. Most clinical imaging centers currently use 64- to 256-multidetector-row scanners, with 320-multidetector-row scanners available in some centers, to study the coronary arteries and bypass grafts.[52,53] The advantages of CTA over catheter-based angiography are[24-26] its volumetric acquisition, better visualization of the anatomy from multiple angles and in multiple planes after a single acquisition; improved visualization of soft tissues and other adjacent anatomical structures; less invasive process and thus fewer complications; and lower cost.

CTA has several advantages over MRA, such as higher spatial and temporal resolution, absence of flow-related phenomena that may distort MRA images, and the ability to visualize calcification and metallic implants such as endovascular stents or stent grafts. CTA also markedly decreases total examination time, with most 64-multidetector scanners currently performing a complete vascular examination of the abdominal aorta, mesenteric, renal, and iliac arteries in 5 to 10 seconds with submillimeter spatial resolution. When exposure to ionizing radiation is a concern (e.g., in younger patients), MRA may be the preferred imaging modality.

The increased speed of acquisitions coupled with subsecond gantry rotations obtained with multidetector-row CTA allows for greater longitudinal coverage for a given scan duration and greater spatial resolution. This may not be of as much importance for assessing renal artery disease, but it has great advantages when assessing the thoracoabdominal, aortoiliac, and lower-extremity inflow and runoff, which may require up to 1400 mm of coverage.[26] Rapid acquisition of images allows

for reduction in the amount of iodinated contrast material needed while maintaining excellent and uniform vascular enhancement.[26] Thin beam collimation (<1 mm), rotational speed of the tube, and rate of table feed are key parameters in determining imaging protocols. The first set of images produced are sequential or overlapping axial images, which should be interpreted with attention to all nonvascular structures, including bones, bowel, visceral organs, and lung. To create angiographic representations, postprocessing of the volumetric data is necessary (Fig. 23.7).

Over the past several years, more complex postprocessing algorithms have been formulated to display volumetric data, including maximum intensity projection (MIP), shaded surface display (SSD), and volumetric rendering (VR). These techniques allow manipulation of raw data to optimize visualization of relevant lesions or disease processes. An important common pitfall is selective visualization of the maximally opacified vascular lumen. Both automated and manual creation of postprocessed images risk inadvertent rejection of critical vascular and nonvascular information. The sensitivity of CTA for RAS ranges from 89% to 100%, and specificity ranges from 82% to 100%.[25,26] The area of acquisition should include the area from just proximal to the celiac artery to and including the iliac arteries. This will ensure that accessory renal arteries are detected and associated aortic and visceral artery pathology is not overlooked.

Noninvasive Imaging for Renal Fibromuscular Dysplasia

The most accurate diagnostic test for diagnosing FMD is catheter-based angiography. However, duplex ultrasound and CTA can accurately identify FMD most of the time (see Fig. 23.7B). MRA may lead to both false positives and false negatives due to body movement and poorer image resolution.[4,5]

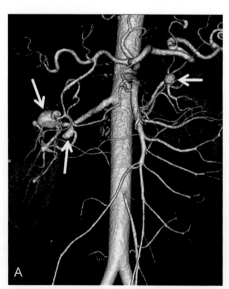
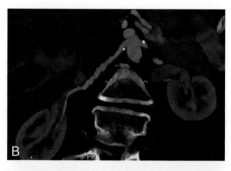
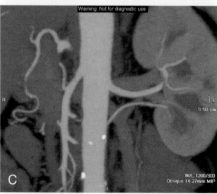

Fig. 23.7 Three-Dimensional Computed Tomographic Angiogram of Renal Arteries With 250 Multidetector Computed Tomography (CT) Scanner. (A) Volume rendering shows multiple renal artery aneurysms (arrows) on the right and left sides. (B) Axial slice of a CT angiogram demonstrating the classic "string of beads" appearance in multifocal fibromuscular dysplasia. (C) Normal left main and accessory renal artery.

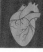

Catheter-Based Angiography

Although duplex ultrasonography, MRA, and CTA have replaced catheter-based angiography for the diagnosis of RAS in most circumstances, catheter-based angiography remains the gold standard and is usually performed following noninvasive imaging during a planned intervention (also see Chapter 15). It is the most accurate test to diagnose RAS secondary to both atherosclerosis and FMD. It can visualize branch vessels and cortical blood flow clearly and is excellent for identifying accessory renal arteries.[54]

Digital subtraction angiography (DSA) has replaced screen-film or cut film angiography in nearly all institutions for vascular applications. The standard imaging matrix is now 1024 × 1024, but 2048 × 2048 are available with image intensifiers that have viewing capability up to 48 cm in diameter. Flat-panel image intensifiers have become standard in nearly all commercially available configurations. A recent advancement in detector technology advancement is the use of low-dose fluoroscopy to create high-resolution images. Current radiation doses are up to 80% lower for imaging studies as compared to studies performed a decade ago, while maintaining the same image quality (see Fig. 23.1).

The renal arteries often come off the aorta posteriorly, and therefore oblique views of the aorta may be needed to adequately visualize the origin of the renal arteries. Pressure gradients should be obtained to confirm the physiological significance of a given lesion. Advantages of DSA are the high resolution compared to current cross-sectional imaging techniques, the ability to selectively evaluate individual vessels, acquisition of direct physiological information such as pressure gradients, and its utilization as a platform for intervention. During a planned intervention, other imaging techniques such as intravascular ultrasound (IVUS) and optical coherence tomography (OCT) may be used to assess the degree of stenosis, or to determine whether a dissection or intramural hematoma is present or if the stent is positioned correctly and fully expanded (Fig. 23.8). Disadvantages are exposure to ionizing radiation, use of iodinated contrast agents (contrast-induced nephropathy), and risks related to vascular access (pseudoaneurysm, hematoma, retroperitoneal bleed) and catheterization (atheromatous embolization). Nevertheless, until an alternative platform is developed for intervention or completely MR-compatible devices become available, DSA will have a central role in the management of patients with vascular disease.

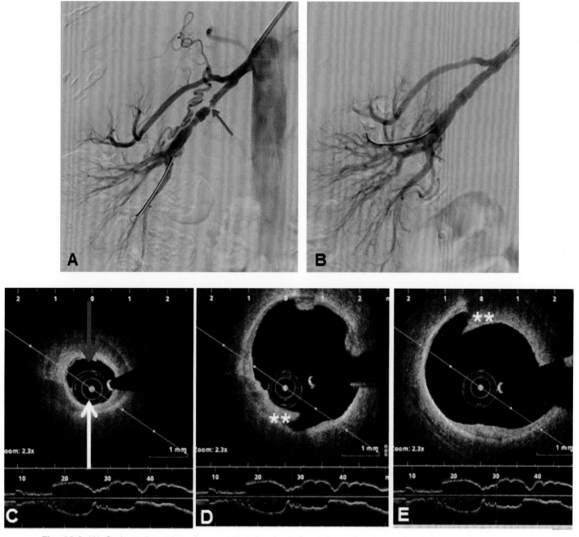

Fig. 23.8 (A) Catheter-based angiogram showing both focal *(arrow)* and multifocal fibromuscular dysplasia (FMD) in the same artery. (B) Post balloon angioplasty showing a nearly normal appearing artery. (C) Optimal coherence tomography (OCT) demonstrated the catheter inside the renal artery *(white arrow)* and the extremely narrow lumen *(red arrow)*. (D) and (E) OCT. Note the large lumen immediately distal to the stenosis seen in (C). The stenosis alternating with the enlargement gives the appearance of the "string of beads." Asterisks in (D) and (E) represent the webs that are present in the artery of a patient with FMD.

Renal Angiography at the Time of Cardiac Catheterization

This controversial subject has led to numerous debates over the most appropriate management strategy for patients with CAD and possible RAS. Patients with CAD have a higher prevalence of RAS than the general population. Proponents of angiography at the time of catheterization state that the procedure can be performed accurately with no added risk and provide the cardiologist with knowledge that the patient has RAS so that the patient can then be followed serially and treated with optimal secondary preventive measures.[21] Those against routine angiography claim that knowing that the patient has RAS adds nothing to the patient's overall management other than to tempt the angiographer to stent the stenotic lesion in the absence of accepted clinical indications.[55] It is appropriate to perform renal angiography at the time of cardiac catheterization if acceptable indications for renal artery intervention are present.[55] Further prospective natural history studies in this population are needed, however, to answer the question of whether routine renal artery angiographic screening should be performed at the time of cardiac catheterization.

REFERENCES

1. Whelton PK, Carey RM, Aronow WS, et al. 2017 ACC/AHA/AAPA/ABC/ACPM/AGS/APhA/ASH/ASPC/NMA/PCNA Guideline for the prevention, detection, evaluation, and management of high blood pressure in adults: a Report of the American College of Cardiology/American Heart Association Task Force on Clinical Practice Guidelines. *J Am Coll Cardiol*. 2018;71(19):e127–e248.
2. Bavishi C, de Leeuw PW, Messerli FH. Atherosclerotic renal artery stenosis and hypertension: pragmatism, pitfalls, and perspectives. *Am J Med*. 2016;129(6):635. e5-635 e14.
3. de Mast Q, Beutler JJ. The prevalence of atherosclerotic renal artery stenosis in risk groups: a systematic literature review. *J Hypertens*. 2009;27(7):1333–1340.
4. Narula N, Kadian-Dodov D, Olin JW. Fibromuscular dysplasia: contemporary concepts and future directions. *Prog Cardiovasc Dis*. 2018;60(6):580–585.
5. Olin JW, Gornik HL, Bacharach JM, et al. Fibromuscular dysplasia: state of the science and critical unanswered questions: a scientific statement from the American Heart Association. *Circulation*. 2014;129(9):1048–1078.
6. Messerli FH, Bangalore S, Makani H, et al. Flash pulmonary oedema and bilateral renal artery stenosis: the Pickering syndrome. *Eur Heart J*. 2011;32(18):2231–2235.
7. Green D, Ritchie JP, Chrysochou C, Kalra PA. Revascularization of atherosclerotic renal artery stenosis for chronic heart failure versus acute pulmonary oedema. *Nephrology (Carlton)*. 2018;23(5):411–417.
8. Green D, Ritchie JP, Chrysochou C, Kalra PA. Revascularisation of renal artery stenosis as a therapy for heart failure: an observational cohort study. *Lancet*. 2015;385(Suppl 1):S11.
9. Ritchie J, Green D, Chrysochou C, et al. High-risk clinical presentations in atherosclerotic renovascular disease: prognosis and response to renal artery revascularization. *Am J Kidney Dis*. 2014;63(2):186–197.
10. Hansen KJ, Edwards MS, Craven TE, et al. Prevalence of renovascular disease in the elderly: a population-based study. *J Vasc Surg*. 2002;36(3):443–451.
11. Textor SC. Renal arterial disease and hypertension. *Med Clin North Am*. 2017;101(1):65–79.
12. Herrmann SM, Saad A, Textor SC. Management of atherosclerotic renovascular disease after Cardiovascular Outcomes in Renal Atherosclerotic Lesions (CORAL). *Nephrol Dial Transplant*. 2015;30(3):366–375.
13. Herrmann SM, Textor SC. Diagnostic criteria for renovascular disease: where are we now? *Nephrol Dial Transplant*. 2012;27(7):2657–2663.
14. Gray BH, Olin JW, Childs MB, et al. Clinical benefit of renal artery angioplasty with stenting for the control of recurrent and refractory congestive heart failure. *Vasc Med*. 2002;7(4):275–279.
15. Yu TM, Sun CS, Lin CL, et al. Risk factors associated with end-stage renal disease (ESRD) in patients with atherosclerotic renal artery stenosis: a nationwide population-based analysis. *Medicine (Baltimore)*. 2015;94(21):e912.
16. Mailloux LU, Napolitano B, Bellucci AG, et al. Renal vascular disease causing end-stage renal disease, incidence, clinical correlates, and outcomes: a 20-year clinical experience. *Am J Kidney Dis*. 1994;24(4):622–629.
17. Mailloux LU, Bellucci AG, Napolitano B, et al. Survival estimates for 683 patients starting dialysis from 1970 through 1989: identification of risk factors for survival. *Clin Nephrol*. 1994;42(2):127–135.
18. Olin JW, Melia M, Young JR, et al. Prevalence of atherosclerotic renal artery stenosis in patients with atherosclerosis elsewhere. *Am J Med*. 1990;88(1N):46N–51N.
19. Aboyans V, Desormais I, Magne J, et al. Renal artery stenosis in patients with peripheral artery disease: prevalence, risk factors and long-term prognosis. *Eur J Vasc Endovasc Surg*. 2017;53(3):380–385.
20. Conlon PJ, Little MA, Pieper K, Mark DB. Severity of renal vascular disease predicts mortality in patients undergoing coronary angiography. *Kidney Int*. 2001;60(4):1490–1497.
21. Rihal CS, Textor SC, Breen JF, et al. Incidental renal artery stenosis among a prospective cohort of hypertensive patients undergoing coronary angiography. *Mayo Clin Proc*. 2002;77(4):309–316.
22. Olin JW. Evaluation of the peripheral circulation. In: Izzo JL, Black HR, eds. *Hypertension Primer*. Dallas: American Heart Association; 2007:374–378.
23. Carman TL, Olin JW, Czum J. Noninvasive imaging of the renal arteries. *Urol Clin North Am*. 2001;28(4):815–826.
24. AbuRahma AF, Yacoub M. Renal imaging: duplex ultrasound, computed tomography angiography, magnetic resonance angiography, and angiography. *Semin Vasc Surg*. 2013;26(4):134–143.
25. Al-Katib S, Shetty M, Jafri SM, Jafri SZ. Radiologic assessment of native renal vasculature: a multimodality review. *Radiographics*. 2017;37(1):136–156.
26. Falesch LA, Foley WD. Computed tomograpy angiography of the renal circulation. *Radiol Clin North Am*. 2016;54(1):71–86.
27. Olin JW, Piedmonte MR, Young JR, et al. The utility of duplex ultrasound scanning of the renal arteries for diagnosing significant renal artery stenosis. *Ann Intern Med*. 1995;122(11):833–838.
28. Radermacher J, Chavan A, Bleck J, et al. Use of Doppler ultrasonography to predict the outcome of therapy for renal-artery stenosis. *N Engl J Med*. 2001;344(6):410–417.
29. Crutchley TA, Pearce JD, Craven TE, et al. Clinical utility of the resistive index in atherosclerotic renovascular disease. *J Vasc Surg*. 2009;49(1):148–155. 155.e1-3; discussion 155.
30. Zeller T, Müller C, Frank U, et al. Stent angioplasty of severe atherosclerotic ostial renal artery stenosis in patients with diabetes mellitus and nephrosclerosis. *Catheter Cardiovasc Interv*. 2003;58(4):510–515.
31. Zeller T, Frank U, Müller C, et al. Predictors of improved renal function after percutaneous stent-supported angioplasty of severe atherosclerotic ostial renal artery stenosis. *Circulation*. 2003;108(18):2244–2249.
32. Del Conde I, Galin ID, Trost B, et al. Renal artery duplex ultrasound criteria for the detection of significant in-stent restenosis. *Catheter Cardiovasc Interv*. 2014;83(4):612–618.
33. White CJ, Olin JW. Diagnosis and management of atherosclerotic renal artery stenosis: improving patient selection and outcomes. *Nat Clin Pract Cardiovasc Med*. 2009;6(3):176–190.
34. Bicakci K, Soker G, Binokay F, et al. Estimation of the ratio of renal artery stenosis with magnetic resonance angiography using parallel imaging technique in suspected renovascular hypertension. *Nephron Clin Pract*. 2006;104(4):c169–c175.
35. Rountas C, Vlychou M, Vassiou K, et al. Imaging modalities for renal artery stenosis in suspected renovascular hypertension: prospective intraindividual comparison of color Doppler US, CT angiography, GD-enhanced MR angiography, and digital substraction angiography. *Ren Fail*. 2007;29(3):295–302.
36. Stacul F, Gava S, Belgrano M, et al. Renal artery stenosis: comparative evaluation of gadolinium-enhanced MRA and DSA. *Radiol Med*. 2008;113(4):529–546.

37. Bakker J, Beek FJ, Beutler JJ, et al. Renal artery stenosis and accessory renal arteries: accuracy of detection and visualization with gadolinium-enhanced breath-hold MR angiography. *Radiology*. 1998;207(2):497–504.

38. De Cobelli F, Vanzulli A, Sironi S, et al. Renal artery stenosis: evaluation with breath-hold, three-dimensional, dynamic, gadolinium-enhanced versus three-dimensional, phase-contrast MR angiography. *Radiology*. 1997;205(3):689–695.

39. Eklöf H, Ahlstrom H, Bostrom A, et al. Renal artery stenosis evaluated with 3D-Gd-magnetic resonance angiography using transstenotic pressure gradient as the standard of reference. A multireader study. *Acta Radiol*. 2005;46(8):802–809.

40. Fain SB, King BF, Breen JF, et al. High-spatial-resolution contrast-enhanced MR angiography of the renal arteries: a prospective comparison with digital subtraction angiography. *Radiology*. 2001;218(2):481–490.

41. Hahn U, Miller S, Nägele T, et al. Renal MR angiography at 1.0 T: three-dimensional (3D) phase-contrast techniques versus gadolinium-enhanced 3D fast low-angle shot breath-hold imaging. *AJR Am J Roentgenol*. 1999;172(6):1501–1508.

42. Hany TF, Debatin JF, Leung DA, Pfammatter T. Evaluation of the aortoiliac and renal arteries: comparison of breath-hold, contrast-enhanced, three-dimensional MR angiography with conventional catheter angioraphy. *Radiology*. 1997;204(2):357–362.

43. Hood MN, Ho VB, Corse WR. Three-dimensional phase-contrast magnetic resonance angiography: a useful clinical adjunct to gadolinium-enhanced three-dimensional renal magnetic resonance angiography. *Mil Med*. 2002;167(4):343–349.

44. Patel ST, Mills Sr JL, Tynan-Cuisinier G, et al. The limitations of magnetic resonance angiography in the diagnosis of renal artery stenosis: comparative analysis with conventional arteriography. *J Vasc Surg*. 2005;41(3):462–468.

45. Rieumont MJ, Kaufman JA, Geller SC, et al. Evaluation of renal artery stenosis with dynamic gadolinium-enhanced MR angiography. *AJR Am J Roentgenol*. 1997;169(1):39–44.

46. Snidow JJ, Johnson MS, Harris VJ, et al. Three-dimensional gadolinium-enhanced MR angiography for aortoiliac inflow assessment plus renal artery screening in a single breath hold. *Radiology*. 1996;198(3):725–732.

47. Willmann JK, Wildermuth S, Pfammatter T, et al. Aortoiliac and renal arteries: prospective intraindividual comparison of contrast-enhanced three-dimensional MR angiography and multi-detector row CT angiography. *Radiology*. 2003;226(3):798–811.

48. Schoenberg SO, Essig M, Bock M, et al. Comprehensive MR evaluation of renovascular disease in five breath holds. *J Magn Reson Imaging*. 1999;10(3):347–356.

49. Albert TS, Akahane M, Parienty I, et al. An international multicenter comparison of time-SLIP unenhanced MR angiography and contrast-enhanced CT angiography for assessing renal artery stenosis: the renal artery contrast-free trial. *AJR Am J Roentgenol*. 2015;204(1):182–188.

50. Zhang HL, Schoenberg SO, Resnick LM, Prince MR. Diagnosis of renal artery stenosis: combining gadolinimum-enhanced three-dimensional magnetic resonance angiography with functional magnetic resonance pulse sequences. *Am J Hypertens*. 2003;16(12):1079–1082.

51. Schieda N, Blaichman JI, Costa AF, et al. Gadolinium-based contrast agents in kidney disease: comprehensive review and clinical practice guideline issued by the Canadian Association of Radiologists. *Can Assoc Radiol J*. 2018;69(2):136–150.

52. van Velzen JE, Schuijf JD, de Graaf FR, et al. Diagnostic performance of non-invasive multidetector computed tomography coronary angiography to detect coronary artery disease using different endpoints: detection of significant stenosis vs. detection of atherosclerosis. *Eur Heart J*. 2011;32(5):637–645.

53. de Graaf FR, van Velzen JE, Witkowska AJ, et al. Diagnostic performance of 320-slice multidetector computed tomography coronary angiography in patients after coronary artery bypass grafting. *Eur Radiol*. 2011;21(11):2285–2296.

54. Kaufman JA. Renal arteries. In: Kaufman JA, Lee MJ, eds. *Vascular and Interventional Radiology: The Requisites*. 2nd ed. Philadelphia: Elsevier; 2014:265–286.

55. White CJ, Jaff MR, Haskal ZJ, et al. Indications for renal arteriography at the time of coronary arteriography: a science advisory from the American Heart Association Committee on Diagnostic and Interventional Cardiac Catheterization, Council on Clinical Cardiology, and the Councils on Cardiovascular Radiology and Intervention and on Kidney in Cardiovascular Disease. *Circulation*. 2006;114(17):1892–1895.

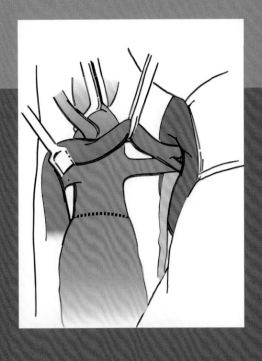

第24章
肾动脉狭窄的治疗

　　本章节的重点是肾动脉狭窄的治疗，分为3部分内容，包括纤维肌发育不良的治疗选择，动脉粥样硬化性肾动脉狭窄的治疗，不常见的肾动脉狭窄（如多发性大动脉炎、Williams综合征等），以及肾动脉瘤的治疗情况。其中动脉粥样硬化性肾动脉狭窄的治疗是重点。本章节以2017年ACC/AHA指南为标准，讲述了肾动脉狭窄介入治疗的进展和临床研究脉络，指出对于动脉粥样硬化性肾动脉狭窄，药物治疗仍然是Ⅰa级推荐；而对于药物治疗失败（难治性高血压、持续性肾功能恶化、难治性心力衰竭），非动脉粥样硬化性疾病（包括纤维肌发育不良），或考虑血运重建对患者有利的情形，专家们给出了Ⅱb级的建议，进行积极外科干预治疗。本章节还重点叙述了外科治疗的应用场景、术前准备及外科手术的技术和技巧，包括外科旁路手术、血栓和内膜剥脱手术、肾动脉间位移植手术、解剖外的内脏动脉旁路肾动脉手术，尤其详细讲述了原位肾自体移植手术。书中详细描述外科操作内容，清晰明了，难能可贵，值得阅读。同时，本章节还讲述了术中超声检查进行即刻血流评估对预后的影响，以及肾动脉狭窄外科治疗后的长期预后。

李拥军

Treatment of Renal Artery Disease

Christopher J. Cooper and Matthew S. Edwards

The treatment of renal artery disease should be guided by the cause of the arterial obstruction and the health consequence(s) of the obstruction. A renal artery stenosis (RAS) of any cause that has no sequelae, such as hypertension or functional kidney impairment, generally requires no treatment. Although this circumstance might seem unusual, it is becoming more commonplace as imaging of the abdominal aorta becomes more frequent and incidental stenoses are identified. In children with congenital stenosis, surgical revascularization may be optimal. In patients with fibromuscular dysplasia, balloon angioplasty is the treatment of choice. In patients with atherosclerotic RAS, medical therapy that addresses the systemic nature of atherosclerosis is the ideal treatment; endovascular stenting is reserved for those who have failed medical therapy. In this chapter we review key concepts in the treatment of renal artery disease.

CRITICAL FUNCTIONS OF THE KIDNEY

The kidneys have several critical functions, including filtration of blood and regulation of salt, water, and blood pressure. Disorders of the arterial circulation of the kidney may have an adverse impact on some or all of these functions (see Chapter 22). As early as the 1930s, Goldblatt determined that stenosis of a renal artery resulted in increases in systemic blood pressure.[1] From this critical observation, it would seem intuitive that in the presence of RAS, the approach should be "find it, fix it." Simply put, if the blockage can cause problems, then fix the blockage. Importantly though, the circulation of the kidney is somewhat more complex than many other vascular beds. Control of cortical renal blood flow is under the influence of both the afferent and efferent arterioles of the glomerulus. Generally, cortical blood flow extracts minimal amounts of oxygen and is mostly related to autoregulation of the filtering glomerulus.[2] In addition, there is a separate circulation for the medulla of the kidney. As a consequence, the straightforward concept that "a blockage of a renal artery decreases function of the kidney" is often not correct. Due to the ability of the kidney to autoregulate, it is undoubtedly true that even a hemodynamically significant stenosis may not result in a decrement of excretory renal function. Finally, the renal circulation responds to vasoactive agents independently of other circulations. As an example, adenosine is a vasodilator in the coronary circulation and can cause vasoconstriction in the kidney.[3]

MEDICAL THERAPY FOR RENAL ARTERY DISEASE

Generally, medical therapy is directed at the pathophysiology of the ischemic kidney and biologically, to block the activity of the renin-angiotensin system. Thus, for all patients with RAS and hypertension, consideration should be given to the use of a long-acting angiotensin receptor blocker or angiotensin converting enzyme inhibitor that has a high trough-to-peak ratio to provide consistent blood pressure lowering and biologic effects. In some patients, additional treatment with a long-acting thiazide-type diuretic, such as chlorthalidone, can be quite useful.[4] In patients with more advanced renal dysfunction, loop diuretics may play a role. Long-acting calcium channel antagonists can be quite useful, and on occasion the use of β-blockers or α-β blockers can provide an added benefit. Importantly, for many patients with RAS, hypertension control can often be achieved with current modern medical therapy and with few if any side effects.

When a patient fails to respond to medical therapy, there are several considerations that arise, first of which is noncompliance with treatment. This may be due to limited financial resources, drug-related side effects, and symptoms attributed to the medication(s) that are unrelated, among others. In some individuals, the lack of blood pressure control may be due to other concomitant issues such as sodium noncompliance, the presence of hyperaldosteronism, or excess alcohol consumption. Thus it is critical to carefully evaluate patients for other causes of drug-resistant hypertension when they appear to be failing medical therapy for blood pressure control.[5] There are some patients that can be difficult to manage; these are principally patients with (1) advanced kidney disease, (2) severe global ischemia, or (3) both. However, these situations should not be used as a reason to avoid a trial of medical therapy, because many if not most patients will tolerate antihypertensive medications, including the use of angiotensin receptor blockers or angiotensin converting enzyme inhibitors. In some individuals there will be a modest rise in serum creatinine with blood pressure lowering and/or the use of renin-angiotensin inhibition, however, it most often stabilizes and remains stable for very long periods. Only patients who experience a rapid and significant worsening of kidney function should have treatment withdrawn. As will be discussed later in this chapter, for patients with atherosclerotic RAS, medical therapy should also address atherosclerosis risk *per se*, including lipid-lowering therapy, antiplatelet medication, smoking cessation, and diabetes control if indicated.

FIBROMUSCULAR DYSPLASIA

Fibromuscular dysplasia (FMD) is an important cause of hypertension in young adults and in middle-aged individuals (see Chapter 58).[6] A common presentation would be a young female with unexpected hypertension that is moderate to severe, and may be accompanied by an abdominal bruit. Importantly, FMD may be unilateral or bilateral, and may occur in other vascular beds including the carotid and iliac arteries. FMD is infrequently associated with renal dysfunction, and commonly associated with hypertension. It is interesting that it has also now been associated with spontaneous arterial dissections in a variety of vascular beds, including the carotid and coronary arteries.

FMD can present in a variety of forms, which have been described pathologically as intimal, medial, and periadventitial. More recently, an angiographic classification has been used to characterize the stenosis as uni- or multifocal. The most common type is the multifocal medial type, which has the appearance of a string of beads. In contrast to atherosclerotic stenosis, which is typically ostial in location, FMD most often occurs in mid-artery or beyond. This is important during diagnostic imaging because a complete assessment of the mid- and distal renal artery is necessary when FMD is suspected. Furthermore, because of the web-like nature of some FMD lesions, conventional angiographic or axial anatomic imaging may not be sufficient to gauge the severity of the stenosis. Oftentimes function assessment is needed, such as duplex ultrasonography or the use of a pressure guidewire when invasive imaging is performed. Additionally, intravascular ultrasound offers another adjunct to examine the luminal anatomy of the renal artery in FMD patients, which may offer considerable insight as to the location and severity of areas of flow restriction, which are often difficult to visualize. FMD may be familial or sporadic, with no known gene yet identified as causative. Likely, there is a genetic predilection, because the disorder is far more common in women than men.

Treatment of Fibromuscular Dysplasia

Most of the information regarding treatment of FMD is derived from single or small case series, but this is starting to change. Trinquart and colleagues performed a metaregression analysis that used a number of case series to demonstrate several important findings.[7] First, they demonstrated that the likelihood of a hypertension cure with angioplasty declined with age (Fig. 24.1). Second, they also showed that more contemporary angioplasty case series were associated with lower cure rates. This is almost certainly related to the fact that the thresholds for hypertension cure have become more stringent with lower and lower blood pressure values. Experienced operators now recognize that hypertension cures may be less common, but it is not uncommon for patients undergoing revacularization to experience an improvement in blood pressure along with a lessened need for antihypertensive therapy. Patients who are younger often have a better response to revascularization of FMD than do older patients. Whether this is due to vascular remodeling, the presence of concomitant essential hypertension, aging itself, or some other factor is unknown.

For normotensive patients with incidental FMD noted on imaging studies, observation alone is indicated. For hypertensive patients, antihypertensive medical therapy is important. As stated above, treatment should be with a long-acting angiotensin receptor blocker or angiotensin converting enzyme inhibitor that has a high trough-to-peak ratio. In younger women who are planning pregnancy or who are pregnant, other antihypertensive agents should be used due to the potential of harm to a fetus with the use of drugs that interrupt the renin-angiotensin system. Although there is little data to support this approach, some experts recommend the use of daily aspirin for patients with FMD.[6]

If the blood pressure is elevated, or less commonly, if there is renal insufficiency, revascularization should be considered. In general, in these young patients, stenting should be avoided because it is unnecessary and the long-term presence of metallic stents in the mid- or distal artery may lead to stent fracture over years. The renal artery is often mobile during the respirophasic cycle, and may cause an implanted stent to bend during inspiration/expiration. The repetitive stress may cause tissue injury at the ends of the stent, or cause fracture(s) of the stent that result in adverse occurrences such as restenosis.[8] Surgical revascularization may be reasonable for some complex cases of FMD or in those cases that cannot be treated with an endovascular approach. Patients with FMD and concomitant aneurysms may be quite challenging to treat adequately from an endovascular approach and as a consequence some may benefit from surgical repair.

The dominant strategy for treatment of FMD is balloon angioplasty, also referred to as percutaneous transluminal angioplasty (PTA). The goal of PTA is to sufficiently dilate the vessel and tear intimal webs to relieve the hemodynamic obstruction and postobstructive pressure

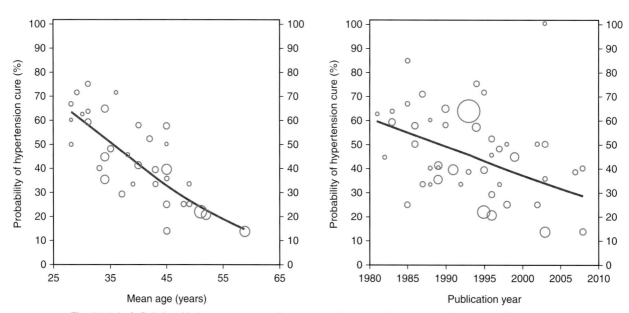

Fig. 24.1 *Left,* Relationship between age at diagnosis and hypertension cure in patients with fibromuscular dysplasia. *Right,* Relationship between publication year and hypertension cure in patients with fibromuscular dysplasia. (From Trinquart L, Mounier-Vehier C, Sapoval M, et al. Efficacy of revascularization for renal artery stenosis caused by fibromuscular dysplasia: a systematic review and meta-analysis. *Hypertension.* 2010;56:525–532.)

decline that are associated with these lesions. As stated previously, the severity of the lesions, and as an extension, the anatomic completeness of PTA, are difficult to ascertain angiographically. Addition of intravascular ultrasound can provide significant information to assist in localizing lesions for treatment in cases where the culprit lesion is difficult to visualize. The use of 0.014-inch diameter pressure-sensing guidewires that can be left in during the procedure, and that can be used for delivery of the PTA balloons, have made the decision(s) of when to continue to use larger balloons and when to conclude the procedure more objective and easier. As a general approach, the lesion is sequentially dilated with balloons. In general, the balloon's size should match the normal diameter of the vessel. If the stenosis is not adequately relieved, then a higher pressure can be used to more fully expand the initial balloon, or a slightly larger balloon can be used to achieve a larger diameter. Importantly, the index balloon should never be selected to match the diameter of poststenotic dilation, because such treatment may result in the dreaded complication of vessel rupture. In general, a successful procedure results in the reduction of the translesional gradient to less than 10 mm Hg. It is also important to note that the angiographic appearance after balloon dilation may not be markedly different than the pretreatment angiogram and is often still quite abnormal in appearance due to the continued presence of the disrupted or torn webs. However, if the lesion has been adequately dilated and the pressure gradient is significantly improved, then the angiographic appearance is of minimal significance.

ATHEROSCLEROTIC RENAL ARTERY STENOSIS

Ostial lesions of the renal artery, especially in middle-aged and older individuals, are most often due to atherosclerosis. Many, if not most of these likely represent the encroachment of aortic plaque into the renal artery, thus the presence of RAS is often accompanied by moderate or even severe atherosclerotic plaquing of the abdominal aorta or at times, aneurysms of the abdominal aorta. As a consequence, the aorta may represent a minefield of risk in these individuals, especially related to atheroembolization.

The occurrence of atherosclerotic RAS has certain features that are similar and different from atherosclerosis in other vascular beds. First, atherosclerotic RAS tends to occur in older individuals, with a mean age of 70 years, which is about a decade older than the mean age of a first myocardial infarction. Tobacco use is a very important risk factor for atherosclerotic RAS, and is associated with an occurrence that is about 9-years prior to nonsmokers. Atherosclerotic RAS affects men and women equally. This is in sharp contrast to coronary artery disease, which tends to occur more often in men, and with FMD, which occurs more often in women. Why atherosclerotic RAS equally affects men and women is not known.

Atherosclerotic RAS often is diagnosed incidentally during imaging of the abdominal aorta for other indications. When it is identified, irrespective of other issues, it is certainly a marker of advanced atherosclerosis and the risk for atherosclerotic events. Several groups have developed prediction models to understand who is likely to have atherosclerotic RAS. Factors that are important include advanced age, atherosclerosis in other beds, presence of renal dysfunction, and hypertension.[9]

There are several ways to establish a diagnosis when atherosclerotic RAS is suspected. The least invasive and least expensive is duplex ultrasonography (see Chapter 12). For many patients this is possible, however, certain measures should be taken to improve the likelihood of a definitive study. Foremost among these are measures to minimize bowel gas that can interfere with imaging. Steps that are helpful include withholding food the morning of the procedure,

avoiding gassy foods for 24 hours prior to the study, and ingestion of simethicone the night before and morning of the procedure. When these steps are taken, and an experienced technician performs the study, the likelihood of a conclusive study is improved. Several duplex ultrasound criteria can be used to identify a significant stenosis, including peak systolic velocity, renal aortic ratio, and other indirect criteria that suggest the potential presence of a stenosis.[10] The peak systolic velocity is quite helpful and the range for determining a positive result ranges from 150 to 300 cm/s. Generally, the higher the velocity threshold used, the better the specificity at the cost of a lower sensitivity. Importantly, however, with a positive study demonstrating high velocity, poststenotic turbulence, and vessel expansion, the diagnosis is made and the functional significance is established. Despite enhanced recognition of multiple arteries by color Doppler flow, only 40% of accessory renal vessels are currently identified by renal duplex ultrasound examination.

Other tools for diagnosis include computerized tomographic angiography (CTA) (see Chapter 14) and magnetic resonance angiography (MRA) (see Chapter 13). CTA has the advantage of rapid scan time, and good spatial and temporal resolution. However, the need for iodinated contrast makes it impractical for some patients with moderate or advanced chronic kidney disease who have a risk for contrast-induced nephropathy. MRA can be an excellent alternative, especially when a noncontrast imaging strategy is used. In some patients, gadolinium-based MRA contrast may pose the risk of progressive systemic sclerosis. Importantly, when tomographic imaging is performed, the assessment of stenosis severity should be based on the lumen of the stenosis compared to the lumen of the normal distal vessel. Comparisons made to the overall vessel diameter at the site of the stenosis will exaggerate the stenosis severity due to the Glagov phenomenon of positive vascular remodeling. Similarly, comparisons of lumen dimension to areas of poststenotic dilation will also potentially overestimate stenosis severity. Finally, with any imaging modality, the characteristics of the downstream kidney provide important clues to the lesion severity, including the size of the kidney. Generally, when the downstream kidney is less than 8 cm, it is often nonfunctional.

Treatment of Atherosclerotic Renal Artery Stenosis

Over the past two decades there has been considerable debate about the appropriate treatments for patients with atherosclerotic RAS. What has become clear is that medical therapy is the cornerstone for all patients (Table 24.1). Patients with atherosclerotic RAS have systemic atherosclerosis, and thus are in need of treatment for this systemic disorder. The indicated therapies include effective cholesterol lowering therapy, antiplatelet medication, smoking cessation, and diabetes management to goal for those with diabetes. In addition, reducing blood pressure with effective, long-acting agents is critically important, because nearly all patients with significant atherosclerotic RAS also have systolic hypertension. A key component of reducing blood pressure in these individuals is the use of potent, long-acting agents to interrupt the renin-angiotensin system, such as angiotensin receptor blockers or angiotensin converting enzyme inhibitors.[11] The purpose of medical therapy is to prevent progression of atherosclerosis generally, and of the renal artery specifically, prevent thromboembolic complications, and minimize the deleterious effects of systemic hypertension on the heart and vascular system.

Several important trials were completed in the last decade that addressed whether revascularization with endovascular stenting conferred significant benefits when added to a background of medical therapy. These trials, including CORAL[12] and ASTRAL,[13] demonstrated

TABLE 24.1	ACC/AHA 2017 High Blood Pressure Clinical Practice Guideline Recommendation for the Treatment of Atherosclerotic Renal Artery Stenosis	
Class of Recommendation	Level of Evidence	Recommendations
I	A	1. Medical therapy is recommended for adults with atherosclerotic renal artery stenosis.
IIb	C-EO	2. In adults with renal artery stenosis for whom medical management has failed (refractory hypertension, worsening renal function, and/or intractable HF) and those with nonatherosclerotic disease, including fibromuscular dysplasia, it may be reasonable to refer the patient for consideration of revascularization (percutaneous renal artery angioplasty and/or stent placement).

ACC/AHA, American College of Cardiology/American Heart Association.
From Whelton PK, Carey RM, Aronow WS, et al. 2017 ACC/AHA/AAPA/ABC/ACPM/AGS/APhA/ASH/ASPC/NMA/PCNA guideline for the prevention, detection, evaluation, and management of high blood pressure in adults: a report of the American College of Cardiology/American Heart Association Task Force on Clinical Practice Guidelines. *Hypertension.* 2018;71(6):e13–e115.

that medical therapy was as effective as medical therapy with stenting (Fig. 24.2). CORAL addressed this in patients with hypertension on medical treatment or with chronic kidney disease and ASTRAL did so in patients in whom the decision to revascularize was unclear. From these two studies it can be concluded that for most patients with atherosclerotic RAS, medical therapy is the preferred treatment strategy. This point was made clear in the recent American College of Cardiology/American Heart Association (ACC/AHA) Hypertension Guidelines of 2017 (see Table 24.1).

A controversial issue is whether there are some patients who should still be considered for revascularization, and if so, how are these individuals identified for treatment. Fundamentally, the kidneys require arterial blood flow to function, so presumably there must be a threshold at which a stenosis becomes significant enough to warrant treatment. Experienced operators may encounter occasional patients with nearly occluded renal arteries (or, rarely, occluded renal arteries) that, upon opening of the vessel, observe a marked and immediate beneficial effect that can be indicated by diuresis, a substantial drop in blood pressure, or a marked improvement in kidney function. However, these cases tend to be exceptional, and unfortunately, it is often difficult to predict those individuals who will experience such a benefit. Some authors have suggested a more detailed use of renal scintigraphy, combined with arterial imaging, to assess the function of the stenotic kidney and to predict its likelihood of improvement. An alternative approach is to discount treatment in patients with severe stenosis that are unlikely to benefit, because of factors such as a high resistive index, proteinuria, or a small distal kidney. Unfortunately, some patients are not well represented in the comparative clinical trials; thus, a decision to treat may be based on operator judgment and careful consent from the affected person. In the 2017 AHA/ACC Hypertension Guidelines, the use of revascularization for RAS was categorized as a Class of Recommendation IIb (weak), and Level of Evidence C-EO, (Consensus of Expert Opinion based on clinical experience) (see Table 24.1).

Recent work suggests a limited role for surgical revascularization, due to the associated high morbidity and mortality in this population. PTA alone is also of limited utility due to the high rates of restenosis, presumably due to recoil of aortic plaque into the ostium of the vessel. As a consequence, stenting is the dominant strategy when revascularization is planned for atherosclerotic RAS. When stenting is

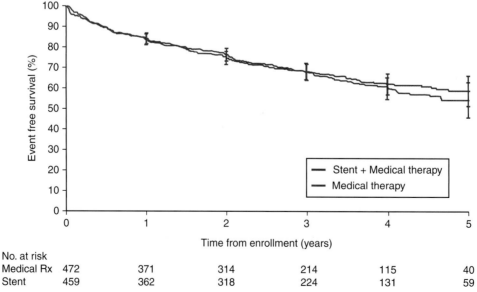

No. at risk
Medical Rx	472	371	314	214	115	40
Stent	459	362	318	224	131	59

Fig. 24.2 Kaplan Meier curve demonstrating survival of patients with atherosclerotic renal artery stenosis treated with optimal medical therapy or optimal medical therapy and renal artery stenting in the CORAL trial. (Modified from Cooper CJ, Murphy TP, Cutlip DE, et al. Stenting and medical therapy for atherosclerotic renal-artery stenosis. *N Engl J Med.* 2014;370:13–22.)

contemplated, careful attention must be given to the approach, to maximize the likelihood of success and minimize the risk for aorta-induced complications such as atheroembolization.

When endovascular revascularization of atherosclerotic RAS is planned, the approach requires careful consideration. Generally, there are two approaches, from above using upper extremity access, and from below using femoral access. Femoral access provides a shorter route and often better torque control on the guiding catheter. In contrast, upper extremity access can be easier in the setting of a downward directed renal artery. From the upper extremity, left arm access may be easier because the leftward placement of that subclavian artery may pose fewer challenges in manipulating into and down the thoracic aorta. From the femoral approach, depending upon the geometry of the aorta and iliac vessels, the femoral artery ipsilateral or contralateral to the side of the renal artery may impact the procedural success. This is especially critical in the presence of significant aortic tortuosity or an abdominal aortic aneurysm that can markedly change the ideal approach.

The use of effective antiplatelet therapy(s) should be strongly considered prior to treatment with an endovascular stent.[14] In addition, there are a number of technical details that can impact the ease and success of renal artery stenting. First, the origin of the renal artery must be clearly identified with the fewest catheter manipulations and using the least amount of contrast. Consideration should be given for a nonselective aortogram, given in low volume and at a high rate, to outline all the renal arteries and their relationship(s) to the aorta and other visible structures such as the underlying vertebrae. From this, the origin can be carefully selected with a diagnostic catheter, or using a "no touch technique," to minimize aortic wall contact.[15] This is critical to avoid atheroembolization and other complications. Once the renal artery is engaged, a guiding catheter or sheath can be telescoped into the treatment site. An experienced operator should be able to accomplish these steps in most cases using minimal contrast media.

Once a guidewire is positioned in the renal artery, treatment may proceed with direct stenting or balloon predilation. Although predilation introduces another step in the procedure, it does have several potential benefits. First, it is an opportunity to demonstrate that the lesion can actually be dilated. Although infrequent, there are rare cases where the ostial stenosis does not respond to balloon dilation, and this becomes far more complex if the first step is to deploy a stent that cannot be adequately inflated. Second, the balloon dilation can be angiographically recorded with the balloon partially inflated. This gives an excellent outline of the lesion and can be quite useful for detailing the landing site of the stent. The stent, once advanced into the lesion, should be deployed with 1 to 2 mm of strut outside the ostium to ensure that the aortic plaque is adequately covered. Unfortunately, restenosis is sometimes related to overlooked lesions when the stent is deployed too far into the lesion. During dilation of the stent, the goal is to safely expand the stent to match the diameter of the distal normal vessel. Achieving a larger lumen area is clearly tied to improved rates of long-term in-stent restenosis. In contrast, the stent should not be deployed to match the diameter of poststenotic dilation, because this overexpansion can lead to vessel rupture. Finally, when the stent is being deployed, the patient should be asked about back pain, because this can be a sign of impending vessel rupture. Should vessel rupture occur, immediate balloon tamponade is helpful, often with the stent delivery balloon or an oversized balloon at low pressures. If the rupture does not seal with balloon inflation, then use of a covered stent or surgical repair may be necessary. At no time should vessel rupture be left without definitive repair.

Similarly, careful attention to the details of technique are necessary to avoid other complications such as kidney perforation, side branch

occlusion with renal infarction, and contrast nephropathy. Perforation of the kidney typically occurs with the use of either hydrophilic guide wires or when careful attention is not placed on the distal end of the wire and it perforates the kidney parenchyma. Unfortunately, when the kidney is perforated, and a subcapsular hematoma develops, the subsequent pressure on the kidney can lead to the loss of the kidney. Side branch occlusion typically occurs with early branching renal arteries when side-branch vessels are jailed by a stent. Again, lesion selection and careful attention to treatment planning are critical because these side branch occlusions may result in loss of kidney function or persistent hypertension. Finally, contrast nephropathy is a real concern. Many patients who require treatment have advanced kidney disease and are intolerant of large or even moderate doses of contrast media. Careful planning, along with meticulous attention to detail, can markedly reduce contrast use; in some instances, alternative contrast media, such as CO_2, can be of use.

After a successful revascularization procedure, the late complications of stent treatment can include restenosis within the stent, progression to end-stage kidney disease, and stent fracture. Fortunately, these complications are infrequent when experienced operators use careful technique. Alternatively, the cavalier use of stents, poorly placed and deployed, can result in significant early and late complications.

TREATMENT OF UNUSUAL CAUSES OF RENAL ARTERY STENOSIS

There are occasional unusual causes of RAS that require treatment. These include iatrogenic stenosis caused by the placement of aortic endografts with suprarenal fixation. Although treatment through the interstices of the endograft are possible, this can be technically demanding, and the concomitant performance of renal artery interventions during aortic endograft procedures may be associated with worsened clinical outcomes.[16] In addition, descending aortic dissections will at times result in the disruption of blood flow to one or both kidneys and may require treatment of the dissection *per se*, or the renal artery specifically. Cardiac emboli rarely cause acute renal ischemia when they include the renal artery.

Other potential causes of RAS that may require revascularization include Takayasu arteritis, Williams syndrome, Kawasaki disease, and neurofibromatosis. When a child or adolescent presents with a clinical syndrome compatible with renovascular disease and has an anatomic lesion, these are the more common causes. For several of these conditions, including Takayasu arteritis and neurofibromatosis, balloon angioplasty may be sufficient to relieve the obstruction and improve the clinical syndrome. When possible, stents should be avoided in children due to the unknown long-term consequences. In some patients, the lesions can be difficult to dilate adequately and then very careful consideration can be given to more aggressive strategies to dilate the vessel, or alternatively, referring the patient for surgical revascularization at a center with pediatric renal revascularization experience.

TREATMENT OF RENAL ARTERY ANEURYSMS

Aneurysms of the renal artery are an unusual finding that typically presents in later life and are more common in women, often presenting in conjunction with fibromuscular dysplasia.[17] Typically, the indications for treatment include diameter ≥2.5 cm, occurrence in a woman planning for pregnancy, symptoms of pain or hematuria, and hypertension not responsive to medical treatment. For patients requiring definitive treatment, the options include surgical repair or endovascular treatment.

Surgical repair is ideally suited to aneurysms at major branch points and for complex aneurysms. Endovascular treatment includes coiling or embolization of saccular aneurysms and stent exclusion of main renal artery aneurysms. Importantly, when planning treatment, especially of more distal aneurysms, there is often concomitant stenosis, vessel coiling, and kinking at or near the site of the aneurysm. Thus, each aneurysm should be carefully evaluated for significance and treatment options prior to endovascular or surgical treatment attempts. Poorly planned or executed treatment may result in vessel dissection, perforation, arterial occlusion, or unplanned embolization within the kidney.

SURGICAL MANAGEMENT OF ATHEROSCLEROTIC RENAL ARTERY DISEASE

Surgical revascularization of the renal arteries is now reserved for highly selective cases of atherosclerotic renovascular disease with truly refractory hypertension, observed rapidly declining renal function, and/or cardiac complications such as refractory heart failure or unstable angina, when these cases cannot be managed effectively via medical therapy or endovascular means.[18] Although there are several operative techniques for surgical revascularization, no single technique is clearly superior. Optimal methods of operative renal reconstruction vary with the patient, pattern of renal artery disease, and clinical significance of associated aortic lesions.

In planning open operative therapy, high-quality CTA is the most versatile single imaging technique, providing important details regarding perivisceral venous anatomy, other visceral arterial disease, and definitive information regarding aortic occlusive and aneurysmal disease. Concurrent mesenteric artery disease is identified in 50% of patients with significant RAS,[19] which can alter or validate plans to use the splenic or hepatic arteries as inflow for renal revascularization. Detailed understanding of any concomitant aortic disease is also essential in appropriate selection of revascularization technique to maximize safety and expected durability of the reconstruction.

Complete renal artery repair after a rapid decline in excretory renal function is associated with the best opportunity for recovery of renal function. Most importantly, improved renal function after operation has been demonstrated to be the primary determinant of dialysis-free survival among patients with preoperative ischemic nephropathy.[20]

Surgical repair of unilateral renal artery disease may be appropriate as a combined aortic procedure when hypertension is severe, the patient does not have significant risk factors for operation, and the probability of technical success is high. In these circumstances, correction of a renal artery lesion may be justified to eliminate all possible causes of hypertension and renal dysfunction. Because the probability of blood pressure benefit is lower in such a patient, morbidity from the procedure must also be predictably low.

When a patient has bilateral RAS and hypertension, the surgical decision to intervene is based on severity of the renovascular lesions and degree of hypertension. If the pattern of renal artery disease consists of severe stenosis on one side and only mild or moderate disease on the contralateral side, the patient is treated as though only a unilateral lesion exists. If both renal arteries have only moderately severe disease (65% to 80% diameter-reducing stenosis), renal revascularization is undertaken only if hypertension is severe. In contrast, if both renal artery lesions are severe (>80% stenosis) and the patient has resistant hypertension despite medical therapy, bilateral simultaneous renal revascularization is performed.

It is important to note that surgical revascularization for atherosclerotic renovascular disease is rarely performed in contemporary practice. Furthermore, those procedures carry significant incidences of morbidity and mortality, even in higher-volume centers with expertise in the area. Referral to high-volume centers is recommended if surgical revascularization is considered.

Management Options

Surgical management for atherosclerotic renovascular disease has become a rarely performed procedure. Surgical reconstruction of the renal arteries is now actually more commonly performed for nonatherosclerotic conditions including cases of FMD in which angioplasty fails, renal artery aneurysms involving the renal artery branches, and congenital lesions; such lesions are usually hypoplastic lesions in pediatric patients or young adults and respond very poorly to endovascular techniques.

Operative Management

With the exception of disease requiring bilateral *ex vivo* reconstructions that are staged, all hemodynamically significant renal artery disease is corrected in a single operation. Having observed beneficial blood pressure and renal function response regardless of kidney size or histological pattern on renal biopsy, nephrectomy is reserved for unreconstructable renal artery disease to a nonfunctioning kidney (i.e., <10% function by renography). Direct aortorenal reconstructions are preferred over extraanatomical methods (i.e., splanchnorenal bypass) because concomitant disease of the celiac axis is present in 40% to 50% of patients, and bilateral renal artery repair is required in 50% of patients. Failed surgical repair is associated with a significant and independent increased risk of eventual dialysis dependence. To minimize these failures, intraoperative duplex ultrasound is used to evaluate the technical results of surgical repair.[21]

Preoperative Preparation

Antihypertensive medications are reduced during the preoperative period to the minimum necessary for blood pressure control. Patients requiring large doses of multiple medications will often have reduced requirements while hospitalized on bed rest. If continued therapy is required, vasodilators and selective β-adrenergic blocking agents are the drugs of choice. Due to potential disturbance in the kidney's capacity for autoregulation following warm ischemia during repair, it is recommended that renin-angiotensin axis-based antihypertensive agents be held for up to a week after revascularization, and longer if significant acute kidney injury occurs in the perioperative period.

Operative Techniques

A variety of operative techniques have been used to treat renal artery atherosclerosis. From a practical standpoint, the three basic operations that have been most frequently used are *aortorenal bypass*, *renal artery thromboendarterectomy*, and *renal artery reimplantation*. Although each method may have its proponents, no single approach provides optimal repair for all types of renal artery disease. Aortorenal bypass is probably the most versatile technique. However, thromboendarterectomy is especially useful for ostial atherosclerosis involving multiple renal arteries. When the artery is sufficiently redundant and the aorta healthy, reimplantation is probably the simplest technique and one particularly appropriate for combined repairs of aortic and renal pathology.

Certain measures are used in almost all renal artery operations. Mannitol is administered IV in 12.5-g doses early, and repeated before and after periods of renal ischemia, up to a total dose of 1 g/kg body weight but not exceeding 50 g in total administered dose. Just prior to renal artery occlusion, a bolus of 100 units of heparin per kilogram body weight is given intravenously, and systemic anticoagulation is verified by activated clotting time.

Aortorenal bypass. The most common method of revascularization is aortorenal bypass (Fig. 24.3). Three types of material are available for conduit: autologous saphenous vein, autologous hypogastric artery, and prosthetic grafts. No data exist to demonstrate superiority of any conduit over others for reconstruction of atherosclerotic disease. The choice of conduit can be affected by numerous factors. Small renal arteries are probably best suited to bypass with saphenous vein. If the vein is small or unavailable, internal iliac artery or a synthetic graft can be used. A 6-mm, thin-walled polytetrafluoroethylene (PTFE) graft is satisfactory when the distal renal artery is of large caliber (≥4 mm) and provides long-term patency equivalent to that of saphenous vein. For more normal, larger renal arteries, 6-mm Dacron or PTFE represent our conduits of choice.

For renal bypass procedures performed in young patients and children, an important additional point must be made in terms of conduit choice. Prosthetic bypasses are an excellent choice for reconstructions of the main renal artery, but many of these cases involve the branches or small renal arteries. In these cases, use of the internal iliac artery is preferable for two reasons. First, saphenous vein will almost uniformly become aneurysmal during follow-up due to the low resistance, high-volume flow of the kidney. Second, autogenous conduit offers the potential for growth with the patient. For this reason interrupted anastomotic techniques are employed in pediatric reconstructions.

Thromboendarterectomy. Thromboendarterectomy is another versatile technique and one particularly well suited to the management of cases involving multiple renal arteries with orificial disease. In cases of bilateral atherosclerosis of the renal artery origins, simultaneous bilateral endarterectomy may be the most appropriate procedure. Although endarterectomy may be performed in a transrenal fashion, the transaortic technique is used in most instances. Transaortic endarterectomy is performed through a longitudinal aortotomy, with sleeve endarterectomy of the aorta and eversion endarterectomies of the renal arteries (Fig. 24.4). When aortic replacement is planned, and there is concomitant RAS, the transaortic endarterectomy is performed through the transected aorta (Fig. 24.5). When using the transaortic technique, it is important to mobilize the renal arteries extensively to allow eversion of the vessel into the aorta. This allows the distal endpoint to be completed under direct vision.

Renal artery reimplantation. Reimplantation is most commonly used for nonatherosclerotic disease and requires healthy aorta and short segment ostial disease to function as a definitive and durable reconstruction. After the renal artery has been dissected from the surrounding retroperitoneal tissue, the vessel may be somewhat redundant. When the RAS is ostial and there is sufficient vessel length, the renal artery can be transected and reimplanted into the aorta at a slightly lower level. The renal artery must be spatulated and a portion of the aortic wall removed, as in renal artery bypass.

Splanchnorenal bypass. Splanchnorenal bypass and other extraanatomic procedures are also used as alternative methods for renal revascularization.[22] Most commonly, these bypasses employ the common hepatic and splenic artery as inflow sources for the right and left kidney, respectively. In general, the authors do not believe these procedures

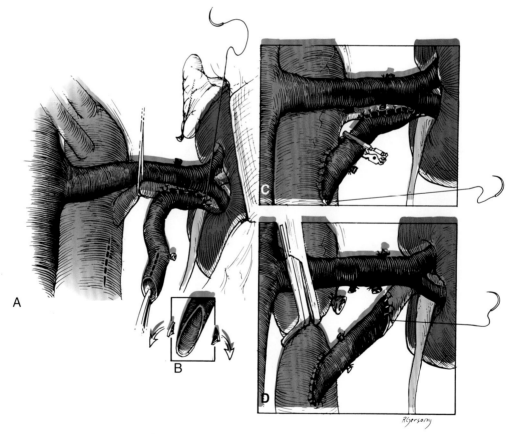

Fig. 24.3 Technique for end-to-side (A to C) and end-to-end (D) aortorenal bypass grafting. The length of the arteriotomy is at least three times the diameter of the artery to prevent recurrent anastomotic stenosis. For the anastomosis, 6-0 or 7-0 monofilament polypropylene sutures are used in continuous fashion under loupe magnification. If apex sutures are placed too deeply or with excess advancement, stenosis can be created, posing risk of late graft thrombosis. (From Benjamin ME, Dean RH. Techniques in renal artery reconstruction: part I. *Ann Vasc Surg.* 1996;10:306–314.)

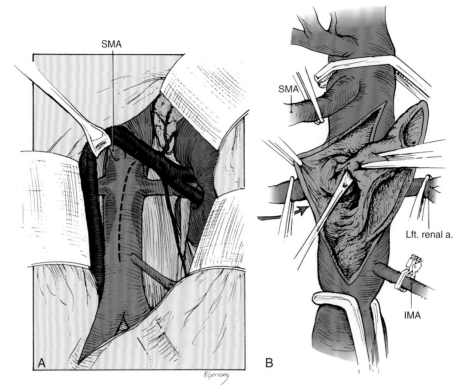

Fig. 24.4 Exposure for longitudinal transaortic endarterectomy is through the standard transperitoneal approach. The duodenum is mobilized from the aorta laterally in standard fashion or, for more complete exposure, ascending colon and small bowel are mobilized. (A) The dotted line shows the location of the aortotomy. (B) Plaque is transected proximally and distally, and with eversion of renal arteries, atherosclerotic plaque is removed from each renal ostium. Aortotomy is typically closed with a running 4-0 or 5-0 polypropylene suture. *IMA,* Inferior mesenteric artery; *SMA,* superior mesenteric artery. (From Benjamin ME, Dean RH. Techniques in renal artery reconstruction: part I. *Ann Vasc Surg.* 1996;10:306–314.)

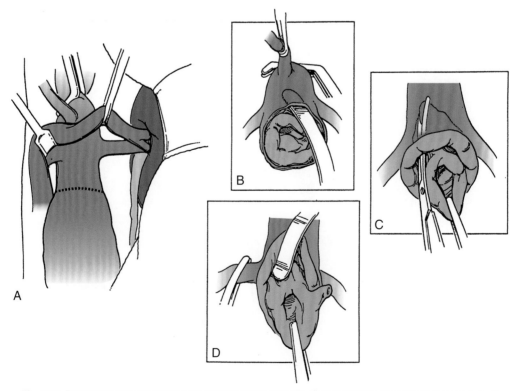

Fig. 24.5 For aortic repair combined with bilateral ostial stenosis of renal arteries, thromboendarterectomy is most commonly performed through the divided aorta. (From Edwards MS, Cherr GS, Hansen KJ. Treatment of renovascular disease: surgical therapy. In: Hallet JW, Mills JL, Earnshaw J, Reekers JA, eds. *Comprehensive Vascular and Endovascular Surgery.* Edinburgh: Mosby; 2004.)

demonstrate long-term patency equivalent to direct aortorenal reconstructions, but they are useful in a selected subgroup of high-risk patients in whom a proximal aortic clamp should be avoided. Subcostal incisions are used to perform splanchnorenal bypass. The right and left renal arteries are exposed through medial visceral rotation. A great saphenous vein (GSV) graft is typically used to construct the bypass. Occasionally the gastroduodenal artery on the right and splenic artery on the left can be transected and anastomosed directly to the renal artery.

Ex vivo reconstruction. Ex vivo reconstructions are rarely used for atherosclerotic disease, and much more commonly used in the treatment of complex cases of FMD and aneurysmal disease. Operative strategy for renal artery branch vessel repair is determined by the required exposure and anticipated period of renal ischemia. When reconstruction can be accomplished with less than 30 minutes of ischemia, an *in situ* repair is undertaken without special measures for renal preservation (Fig. 24.6). When longer periods of ischemia are anticipated, one of two techniques for hypothermic preservation of the kidney are considered. These techniques include renal mobilization without renal vein transection and *ex vivo* repair and anatomical replacement in the renal fossa. *Ex vivo* management is necessary when extensive exposure will be required for extended periods.

Intraoperative Duplex Ultrasonography

Provided the best method of reconstruction is chosen for renal artery repair, the short course and high blood flow rates characteristic of renal reconstruction favor long-term patency. Consequently, flawless technical repair plays a dominant role in determining postoperative success. Intraoperative duplex ultrasonography provides a rapid, safe method of verifying technically flawless repair.[21] Because the ultrasound probe can be placed immediately adjacent to the vascular repair, high carrying frequencies may be used that provide excellent B-scan detail sensitive to less than 1-mm anatomical defects. Once imaged, defects can be viewed in multiple projections during conditions of uninterrupted pulsatile blood flow. Intimal flaps not apparent during static conditions are easily imaged while avoiding the adverse effects of additional renal ischemia. In addition to excellent anatomical detail, important hemodynamic information is obtained from spectral analysis of the Doppler-shifted signal proximal and distal to the imaged defect.[20] In general, approximately 10% of completion studies will demonstrate major defects mandating revision. At 12-month follow-up, renal artery patency free of critical stenosis was demonstrated in 97% of normal studies, 100% of minor defects, and 88% of revised major defects, providing an overall patency of 97%.

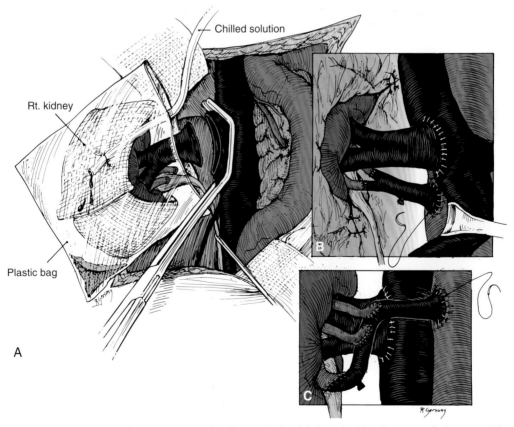

Fig. 24.6 (A) An ellipse of vena cava containing the renal vein origin is excised by placement of a large, partially occluding clamp. After *ex vivo* branch repair, renal vein can then be reattached without risk of anastomotic stricture. (B) Kidney is repositioned in its native bed after *ex vivo* repair. Gerota fascia is reattached to provide stability to replaced kidney. Arterial reconstruction can be accomplished via end-to-end anastomoses (as here) or occasionally with a combination of end-to-end and end-to-side anastomoses (C). (From Benjamin ME, Dean RH. Techniques in renal artery reconstruction: part II. *Ann Vasc Surg.* 1996;10:409–414.)

Results of Surgical Management

Marone et al. reported on operative management for ischemic nephropathy due to atherosclerotic RAS with a perioperative mortality and morbidity of 4.1% and 5%, respectively.[23] Their patients demonstrated improved early renal function in 42%, worsened in 17%, and 41% exhibited no significant change. Improved renal function was durable among surgical survivors at a mean follow-up of 46 months, whereas 28% developed worsened function, and 39% remained unchanged. These authors noted that early renal function response was an accurate predictor of long-term survival. Perioperative mortality was significantly and independently associated with advanced age and congestive heart failure (CHF).

In a series of patients with ischemic nephropathy by Hansen and colleagues, blood pressure measurements and medication requirements at least 1 month after operative intervention were used to define blood pressure response. Among all surgical survivors, 85% were cured or had improved blood pressure, and 15% did not. Renal function improved significantly after operation from an estimated glomerular filtration rate of 41 to 48 mL/min/m^2 [$P < .0001$].[20] Among the subgroup of 27 dialysis-dependent patients, 70% were permanently removed from dialysis. Preoperative factors significantly and independently associated with death or dialysis included diabetes mellitus, severe aortic occlusive disease, and poor preoperative renal function. An increased risk of death or dialysis was also observed if there was no improvement in postoperative renal function.

Surgical management for renal artery disease remains an important tool in our treatment armamentarium, but one that is becoming infrequently applied for atherosclerotic disease. Nonetheless, in highly selected patients, open operative repair of bilateral ostial atherosclerosis and renal artery occlusion associated with refractory hypertension and renal insufficiency and/or cardiac disturbance may be useful. Surgical reconstruction is performed much more commonly for congenital and complex nonatherosclerotic conditions including branch level aneurysms and FMD. These repairs are frequently complex and likely should be performed at referral centers with considerable experience and expertise to maximize patient outcomes.

REFERENCES

1. Goldblatt H, Lynch J, Hanzal RF, Summerville WW. Studies on experimental hypertension; production of persistent elevation of systolic blood pressure by means of renal ischemia. *J Exper Med.* 1934;59:347–379.
2. Textor SC. Renal arterial disease and hypertension. *Med Clin North Am.* 2017;101(1):65–79.
3. Lu Y, Zhang R, Ge Y, et al. Identification and function of adenosine A3 receptor in afferent arterioles. *Am J Physiol Renal Physiol.* 2015;308(9):F1020–F1025.
4. Whelton PK, Carey RM, Aronow WS, et al. 2017 ACC/AHA/AAPA/ABC/ACPM/AGS/APhA/ASH/ASPC/NMA/PCNA guideline for the prevention, detection, evaluation, and management of high blood pressure in adults: a report of the American College of Cardiology/American Heart Association Task Force on Clinical Practice Guidelines. *Hypertension.* 2018;71(6):e13–e115.
5. Calhoun DA, Jones D, Textor S, et al. Resistant hypertension: diagnosis, evaluation, and treatment. *Circulation.* 2008;117:e510–e526.
6. O'Connor SC, Gornik HL. Recent developments in the understanding and management of fibromuscular dysplasia. *J Am Heart Assoc.* 2014;3(6):e001259.
7. Trinquart L, Mounier-Vehier C, Sapoval M, et al. Efficacy of revascularization for renal artery stenosis caused by fibromuscular dysplasia: a systematic review and meta-analysis. *Hypertension.* 2010;56:525–532.
8. Raju MG, Bajzer CT, Clair DG, et al. Renal artery stent fracture in patients with fibromuscular dysplasia. *Circ Cardiovasc Interv.* 2013;6:e30–e31.
9. Colyer WR, Eltahawy E, Cooper CJ. Renal artery stenosis: optimizing diagnosis and treatment. *Prog Cardiovasc Dis.* 2011;54(1):29–35.
10. Schäberle W, Leyerer L, Schierling W, Pfister K. Ultrasound diagnostics of renal artery stenosis: stenosis criteria, CEUS and recurrent in-stent stenosis. *Gefasschirurgie.* 2016;21:4–13.
11. Chrysouchou C, Foley RN, Young JF, et al. Dispelling the myth; the use of renin-angiotensin blockade in atheromatous renovascular disease. *Nephrol Dial Transplant.* 2012;27:1403–1409.
12. Cooper CJ, Murphy TP, Cutlip DE, et al. Stenting and medical therapy for atherosclerotic renal-artery stenosis. *N Engl J Med.* 2014;370(1):13–22.
13. ASTRAL Investigators, Wheatley K, Ives N, et al. Revascularization versus medical therapy for renal-artery stenosis. *N Engl J Med.* 2009;361:1953–1962.
14. Haller S, Adlakha S, Reed G, et al. Platelet activation in patients with atherosclerotic renal artery stenosis undergoing stent revascularization. *Clin J Am Soc Nephrol.* 2011;6(9):2185–2191.
15. Feldman RL, Wargovich TJ, Bittl JA. No-touch technique for reducing aortic wall trauma during renal artery stenting. *Catheter Cardiovasc Interv.* 1999;46(2):245–248.
16. Ultee KHJ, Zettervall SL, Soden PA, et al. The impact of concomitant procedures during endovascular abdominal aortic aneurysm repair on perioperative outcomes. *J Vasc Surg.* 2016;63(6):1411–1419. e2.
17. Coleman DM, Stanley JC. Renal artery aneurysms. *J Vasc Surg.* 2015;62:779–785.
18. Edwards MS, Corriere MA. Contemporary management of atherosclerotic renovascular disease. *J Vasc Surg.* 2009;50:1197–1210.
19. Valentine RJ, Martin JD, Myers SI, et al. Asymptomatic celiac and superior mesenteric artery stenoses are more prevalent among patients with unsuspected renal artery stenoses. *J Vasc Surg.* 1991;14:195–199.
20. Hansen KJ, Cherr GS, Craven TE, et al. Management of ischemic nephropathy: dialysis-free survival after surgical repair. *J Vasc Surg.* 2000;32:472–481.
21. Hansen KJ, O'Neil EA, Reavis SW, et al. Intraoperative duplex sonography during renal artery reconstruction. *J Vasc Surg.* 1991;14:364–374.
22. Moncure AC, Brewster DC, Darling RC, et al. Use of the splenic and hepatic arteries for renal revascularization. *J Vasc Surg.* 1986;3:196–203.
23. Marone LK, Clouse WD, Dorer DJ, et al. Preservation of renal function with surgical revascularization in patients with atherosclerotic renovascular disease. *J Vasc Surg.* 2004;39:322–329.

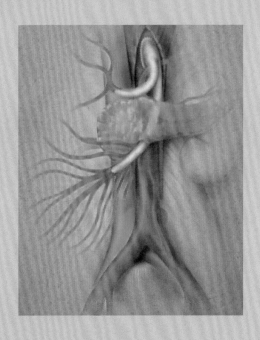

Mesenteric Vascular
Disease

肠系膜血管疾病

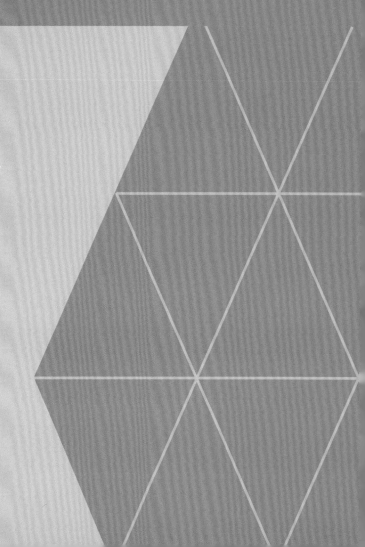

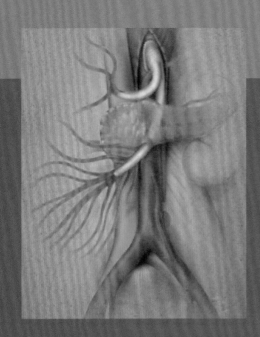

第25章
肠系膜血管疾病的流行病学和病理生理学

　　肠系膜血管疾病是较常见的一种血管疾病，严重者因大面积肠坏死可致死亡。本章节通过对其流行病学的调查及病理生理学的全面分析，对及时诊断和精准治疗具有较大的临床指导意义。与其他器官的血管疾病一样，肠系膜血管疾病分动脉性疾病和静脉性疾病，形态上总体分为扩张性、闭塞性和血管畸形3类。但病种较多，病情也较为复杂。在流行病学上，男女比例、各年龄段发病均不同。病理生理学上的改变各病种也千差万别，尽管随着当代科技的发展，诊断设备愈加先进，但对其理论知识的掌握还是相当重要。例如，非闭塞性的肠系膜血管缺血（non-occlusive mesenteric ischemia，NOMI）是由微血管痉挛引起，占急性肠缺血病因的25%，病因复杂，临床上常被误诊，本章全面而系统地描述了其流行病学和病理生理学，为我们及时诊断和治疗本病提供了依据。急性广泛的肠系膜静脉血栓形成死亡率较高，如果能在发病初期准确诊断，及时溶栓和抗凝，阻断血栓进展，就能挽救生命。通过对本章节的仔细阅读、思考，并回顾多年的临床工作，相信对肠系膜常见血管疾病的流行病学和病理生理学会有更深刻的体会。

陈学明

Epidemiology and Pathophysiology of Mesenteric Vascular Disease

Olamide Alabi, Matthew C. Koopmann, and Gregory L. Moneta

Mesenteric vascular disease can be characterized as acute or chronic, symptomatic or asymptomatic. Severe acute intestinal ischemia results from sudden symptomatic reduction in intestinal blood flow of sufficient magnitude to result potentially in intestinal infarction. Acute ischemia of the small bowel, colon, and liver may result from mesenteric arterial occlusion (embolus or thrombosis), mesenteric venous occlusion, and/or nonocclusive processes, particularly vasospasm.[1] Dissections of the superior mesenteric artery (SMA) or celiac artery, either in association with cystic medial degeneration of the arteries or as a complication of an aortic dissection, may also result in acute intestinal ischemia.

ACUTE ARTERIAL OCCLUSIVE MESENTERIC ISCHEMIA

Epidemiology

Approximately 25% of all cases of acute mesenteric ischemia are due to emboli to the SMA, 25% of cases are due to thrombosis of preexisting atherosclerotic lesions, and the remaining 50% are due to a variety of other etiologies (Fig. 25.1).

Mesenteric emboli can originate from left atrial or ventricular mural thrombi or from cardiac valvular lesions. Mesenteric artery embolism is most often associated with cardiac dysrhythmias such as atrial fibrillation, global myocardial dysfunction with poor ejection fraction, or discrete hypokinetic regions produced by previous myocardial infarction (MI).[1] About 15% of SMA emboli lodge at the origin of the SMA, however, the majority lodge 3 to 10 cm distally in the tapered segment of the SMA just past the origin of the middle colic artery (Fig. 25.2). More than 20% of emboli to the SMA are associated with concurrent emboli to another arterial bed. Intestinal ischemia due to embolic arterial occlusion can be compounded by reactive mesenteric vasospasm, further reducing collateral flow and exacerbating the ischemic insult.[2]

Thrombosis of the SMA or the celiac artery is usually associated with preexisting high-grade stenoses. Many of these patients have histories consistent with chronic mesenteric ischemia (CMI), including postprandial pain, weight loss, and "food fear."[1] SMA thrombosis can be regarded as a complication of untreated chronic intestinal ischemia.[1] The SMA plaque likely progresses slowly to a critical stenosis over years until thrombosis occurs. Unlike embolic occlusions, thrombosis of the SMA generally occurs flush with the aortic origin of the vessel. Acute mesenteric ischemia or thrombosis is also an uncommon (<1%) but serious complication of cardiac surgery, with a reported mortality rate of greater than 50% in most series.[2] Presumably, the nonpulsatile perfusion delivered by most extracorporeal circuits allows severely stenotic visceral vessels to occlude while the patient is on cardiopulmonary bypass. Identified risk factors for this complication include prolonged cross-clamp times, use of intraaortic balloon counterpulsation, low cardiac output syndromes, blood transfusion, triple-vessel disease, coronary artery disease (CAD), and peripheral artery disease (PAD).

Pathophysiology

Acute mesenteric ischemia, whether the underlying cause is embolic or thrombotic, may eventually lead to intestinal infarction while isolated mesenteric artery dissection rarely results in intestinal infarction (Fig. 25.3). Hypoxia and hypercarbia that occur during flow interruption, and reperfusion injury once intestinal blood flow is restored, all contribute to tissue loss.[3]

Reperfusion injury is believed to be mediated principally by activation of the enzyme xanthine oxidase, and recruitment and activation of circulating polymorphonuclear leukocytes (PMNs). The mechanism of injury likely involves production of oxygen-derived free radicals by xanthine oxidase, which then causes profound local tissue injury through lipid peroxidation, membrane disruption, and increased microvascular permeability.[2] The ischemic endothelium recruits PMNs in an autocrine and paracrine manner by secreting chemotactic cytokines (such as tumor necrosis factor [TNF]-α, interleukin [IL]-1, and platelet-derived growth factor [PDGF]) that perpetuate further damage to the reperfused tissue. Once activated, PMNs degranulate, releasing myeloperoxidase, collagenases, and elastases that further injure already ischemic and vulnerable tissue.[2] Activation of this endogenous inflammatory cascade is not restricted to the injured organ and may also have deleterious systemic effects, with cardiac, pulmonary, and other organ system dysfunction.[2]

Natural History

The mortality rate for occlusive acute mesenteric ischemia generally exceeds 70% in most series.[1,2] Occlusive acute intestinal ischemia resulting from SMA embolism has a more favorable prognosis than that resulting from SMA thrombosis.[1] Survival following acute intestinal ischemia due to SMA thrombosis is rare. The more favorable prognosis associated with embolism is attributable to the location at which most emboli lodge in the SMA (distal to the origin of the middle colic

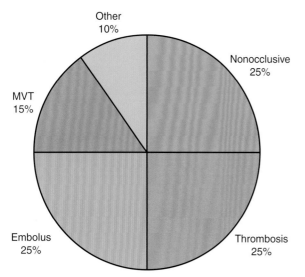

Fig. 25.1 Etiology of Acute Mesenteric Ischemia. *MVT,* Mesenteric venous thrombosis.

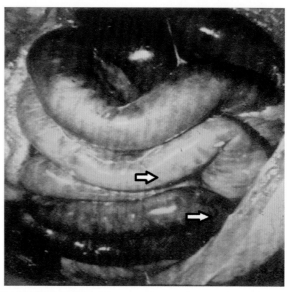

Fig. 25.3 Ischemic Bowel. Arrows indicate segments of clearly infarcted intestine.

Epidemiology

Although SMADs are infrequent, they are recognized more frequently with the increased use of modern cross-sectional imaging. As of 2017, there were approximately 200 cases of isolated celiac artery dissection and 250 cases of SMAD reported in the English-language literature[4] with an additional 622 cases of SMAD reported in the Chinese literature.[5] SMAD patients are predominantly male (>80%), have a mean age of 50 to 60 years, and often suffer from comorbid conditions, including hypertension and hyperlipidemia.[4,5]

Pathophysiology

The etiology of isolated dissection of the SMA and isolated dissection of the celiac artery is unclear. Hypertension is the most common risk factor for SMAD, particularly involving the SMA, but is not regarded as a distinct etiology.[5] Isolated dissection of the SMA may primarily be caused by abnormal mechanical stress exerted on the anterior wall of the SMA due to the hemodynamic forces associated with the convex curvature of the vessel.[6] Indeed, this hypothesis is supported by the fact that the majority of entry sites for isolated dissection of the SMA occur in the anterior wall of the artery between 1 cm proximal to and 1 cm distal to the SMA curvature.[7] This hypothesis does not apply to the celiac artery.

Two major vascular disorders are implicated in the pathogenesis of up to 13% of SMAD: fibromuscular dysplasia (FMD) and segmental arterial mediolysis (SAM).[4] FMD can affect nearly all medium-sized arteries, with the renal, extracranial carotid, and vertebral arteries most commonly affected. The mesenteric arteries are involved in 22% to 26% of FMD cases, but only 8% of mesenteric involvement is due to arterial dissection (2% overall incidence in FMD patients).[8]

In 1976, Slavin et al.[9] first described what was originally termed "segmental mediolytic arteriopathy." The name was eventually changed to SAM given no consistent pathologic or clinical findings to suggest inflammation.[10] It is a rare, nonatherosclerotic, noninflammatory vascular disorder that targets the mesenteric arteries, extramural coronary arteries, and posterior basilar cerebral arteries, and may lead to dissection, stenosis, occlusion, and aneurysm formation.[11,12] The hallmark of SAM is a lytic process that destroys the arterial media leading to separation of the layers of the arterial wall and dissection. There are four distinct pathologic lesions in SAM: (1) mediolysis, the cardinal

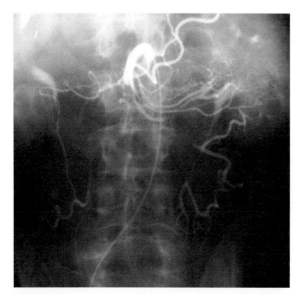

Fig. 25.2 Mesenteric Angiography Demonstrating Acute Mesenteric Emboli. Note the abrupt cutoff of the superior mesenteric artery (SMA), distal to the middle colic artery takeoff, consistent with SMA embolism.

artery). This allows perfusion of the proximal intestine via the middle colic and jejunal artery branches.[1] Thrombotic occlusion of the SMA, however, usually occurs proximal to the middle colic artery, and therefore completely interrupts midgut arterial perfusion in patients with a poorly developed celiac artery or inferior mesenteric artery (IMA) collateral flow.[1]

MESENTERIC ARTERY DISSECTION

Spontaneous mesenteric artery dissections (SMADs) are distinct from nonspontaneous dissections because there is no inciting event (e.g., trauma, aortic dissection). Isolated dissection of the SMA or celiac artery occur when a SMAD is not caused by an underlying diagnosed vascular disorder.

lesion of SAM; (2) separation of the outer media from the adventitia; (3) arterial gaps; and (4) proliferative repair.[11] The underlying cause of SAM is unknown but may be related to vasospasm with endothelin-1 (ET-1) hypothesized to play an indirect role.[11]

Natural History

Isolated dissection of the SMA is symptomatic in the majority of patients (65% to 93%) and abdominal pain is the most common presenting symptom.[4,5,13] Repeat imaging after 1 week of conservative treatment shows worsening stenosis of the true lumen in up to 59% of patients (and occlusion in up to 22%), primarily in patients with a partial or complete thrombosis of the false lumen on their initial imaging.[14] However, even with early radiographic deterioration, symptoms resolve within 11 to 14 days in up to 90% of patients treated conservatively.[14,15] Clinical deterioration is uncommon and delayed imaging (>6 months) demonstrates improved true lumen diameter in 89%[14] and complete remodeling in 42% of patients.[15] For patients treated conservatively, early intervention is required for persistent symptoms in only 5% to 7.7% and late intervention for symptom recurrence or aneurysmal formation in patients treated conservatively is rare.[4,15] Mortality rates in large isolated dissection of the SMA series range from 0% to 2.2%.[4,5,14,15] The natural history of isolated dissection of the celiac artery is not as well characterized. However, one small series suggests a higher need for early and late intervention and a higher rate of aneurysm formation in isolated dissection of the celiac artery compared to isolated dissection of the SMA.[16] SMAD related to SAM has a more severe natural history compared to isolated dissection of the SMA, with a higher rate of hemodynamic shock at presentation (25%), greater need for intervention (24% endovascular, 41% open surgery) (see Fig. 25.3), lower rate of successful conservative management (14%), and a higher mortality rate (22%).[13]

NONOCCLUSIVE MESENTERIC ISCHEMIA

Epidemiology

Nonocclusive mesenteric ischemia (NOMI) is likely declining in incidence but can account for up to 25% of all episodes of acute intestinal ischemia.[1,2] In NOMI, arterial blood flow is inadequate to supply perfusion to the bowel, resulting in intestinal ischemia and infarction in the presence of patent macroscopic vasculature. Previous reports have identified multiple risk factors for development of NOMI (Box 25.1). Mesenteric arterial vasoconstriction may occur in a setting of a severe concurrent illness, particularly sepsis or cardiac failure, and may also follow elective revascularization procedures for chronic SMA occlusion. In such cases, vasoconstriction of small and medium-sized vessels

---

BOX 25.1 Risk Factors for Development of Nonocclusive Mesenteric Ischemia

- Age >50 years
- Atherosclerotic mesenteric arterial disease
- Digitalis use
- Sepsis
- Prior hypotensive episodes
- Congestive heart failure (CHF)
- Coronary artery disease (CAD)
- Vasoconstrictive drugs
- Recent myocardial infarction (MI)
- Cardiac arrhythmias

---

is precipitated by early enteral feeding. Without prompt intervention, NOMI may progress from localized intestinal ischemia to transmural infarction, peritonitis, and death. Mortality is high, regardless of treatment, as a result of the underlying medical conditions that precipitate NOMI and frequent delays in diagnosis.[2]

Pathophysiology

NOMI was first recognized in autopsies of patients with small-intestinal gangrene in the absence of arterial or venous occlusion. Investigation of the regulatory mechanisms of mesenteric circulation has demonstrated that the pathophysiology of NOMI is multifactorial. Virtually all patients with NOMI have a severe coexisting illness, such as cardiac failure.[17] It is postulated that hypoperfusion from cardiac failure results in peripheral hypoxemia and splanchnic vasoconstriction, which then precipitates intestinal ischemia. Mesenteric vasoconstriction, intestinal hypoxia, and ischemia-reperfusion injury all contribute to development of NOMI.

Mesenteric vasoconstriction, the hallmark of NOMI, can be considered an exaggerated homeostatic mechanism induced by excessive sympathetic activity during cardiogenic shock or hypovolemia. The body attempts to maintain cardiac and cerebral perfusion at the expense of the splanchnic and peripheral circulations. Experimental evidence suggests mediators of this response are ET-1, nitric oxide (NO), vasopressin, and angiotensin. ET-1 is a potent vasoconstrictor secreted from endothelial cells. In concert with other vasoactive peptides, ET-1 regulates myogenic cells in the vascular wall. NO can have paradoxical effects on vascular tone, depending on local concentration. At low concentrations, NO acts as a vasodilator; whereas, at higher concentrations, it acts as an oxygen-derived free radical, impairing mitochondrial energy production.

The splanchnic autoregulatory system is affected by local arteriolar smooth muscle relaxation and vasodilation, as well as increased cellular oxygen extraction. Adequate oxygen delivery (Do_2) may be maintained despite declining perfusion pressures until a critical threshold is reached. In experimental models, maximal extraction is reached at a pressure of 40 mm Hg, but beyond this point, oxygen consumption (Vo_2) declines, and ischemia ensues. Postoperative cardiac surgery patients who develop NOMI have persistent deficits between Do_2 and Vo_2 secondary to poor circulatory reserve. In contrast, postoperative cardiac patients who do not develop NOMI are able to normalize their Do_2:Vo_2 ratio by optimizing their cardiac output. In the presence of impaired perfusion, blood flow is not evenly distributed in the bowel wall. The mucosa retains its perfusion at the expense of the serosal layers through mucosal production of NO, prostaglandins, and stimulation of dopamine-I receptors. Histologic damage is therefore first observed at the villous tip and progresses to the deeper muscularis, submucosa, and mucosa within a few hours.

Once set in motion, mesenteric vasospasm may persist despite correction of the precipitating event or underlying illness. The etiology of persistent vasoconstriction once adequate blood flow is restored is unknown, but it may respond to direct intraarterial papaverine infusion or other vasodilators, including iloprost (Fig. 25.4). This phenomenon of protracted vasoconstriction, however, plays an important role in development and maintenance of occlusive and nonocclusive intestinal ischemia, and may also complicate mesenteric revascularization.

Use of vasoconstrictor agents and digitalis are associated with the majority of cases of NOMI. Vasoactive agents, including α-adrenergic drugs and vasopressin, produce splanchnic vasoconstriction directly, whereas digoxin preparations alter mesenteric vasoreactivity by stimulating arterial and venous smooth muscle cell contraction. This may enhance mesenteric arteriolar vasoconstriction in the setting of acute venous hypertension.

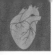

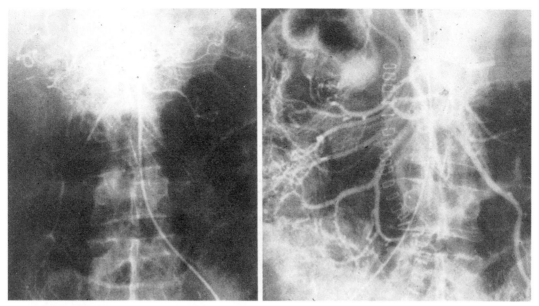

Fig. 25.4 Nonocclusive mesenteric ischemia pre- and post-vasodilator administration.

Restoration of blood flow to the ischemic intestine may also be complicated by reperfusion injury. During critical ischemia, adenosine triphosphate (ATP) levels are depleted, causing distortion of ATP-dependent cell membrane systems. This results in loss of cellular homeostasis, with cellular swelling and electrolyte imbalances. Reduction in ATP levels also generates large amounts of adenosine, a precursor of hypoxanthine. Within the swollen cells, calcium accumulates and triggers hydrolysis of the enzyme xanthine dehydrogenase into xanthine oxidase, which reacts with intracellular hypoxanthine to produce uric acid and toxic oxygen free radicals.[2] Free radicals directly damage cellular membranes, causing capillary leak syndrome, and incite endogenous inflammatory cascades that cause widespread tissue injury. The deleterious effects of free radicals are usually limited by endogenous scavengers such as glutathione, catalase, superoxide dismutase, and NO. However, in cases of prolonged ischemia, the capacity of this scavenger system to eliminate reactive oxygen species is exceeded, and damage continues. The degree of reperfusion injury is thus related to the frequency and duration of the ischemic episodes. Clark and Gewertz demonstrated that two short 15-minute periods of low flow followed by reperfusion resulted in a more severe histological injury than a single 30-minute period of ischemia.

In NOMI, a similar scenario exists: hypoperfusion may be partial and, occasionally, repetitive. It is believed that episodic reperfusion creates a local environment replete with primed neutrophils within the ischemic bed that are capable of degranulating and releasing superoxide. This concept is substantiated by experimental evidence that reperfusion injury may be attenuated by reperfusion with leuko-depleted blood or by blockade of endothelial cell surface receptors for leukocyte adherence.[18] Several compounds, including *N*-acetylcysteine and vitamin E, have been shown in animal models to reduce tissue damage caused by reactive oxygen species. Application of these novel approaches in human NOMI awaits further translational study.

MESENTERIC VENOUS THROMBOSIS

Mesenteric venous thrombosis (MVT) refers to thrombosis of the veins draining the intestine (inferior mesenteric, superior mesenteric, splenic, and portal veins). This venous outflow obstruction leads to edema, intestinal distention, and in some cases, infarction of the affected segments of bowel.[1,2]

Epidemiology

MVT is a comparatively rare form of mesenteric ischemia. The clinical presentation may vary from asymptomatic to fulminant with intestinal infarction and hemodynamic collapse. MVT was first described by Elliot in 1895 as "thrombosis of the portomesenteric venous system" and was further characterized as a distinct clinical entity in 1935 by Warren and Eberhard.

MVT currently constitutes up to 16% of all cases of acute mesenteric ischemia. Abdu et al. found 372 patients with MVT reported between 1911 and 1984. The Mayo Clinic reviewed their experience from 1972 to 1993 and found that MVT accounted for only 6.2% of 1167 patients treated for mesenteric ischemia. Ottinger and Austen found that MVT represented 0.006% of hospital admissions. It is estimated that intestinal infarction due to MVT is encountered in less than 1 in 1000 laparotomies for acute abdomen.[19]

Pathophysiology

MVT can be classified as primary or secondary. Primary MVT is defined as spontaneous idiopathic thrombosis of mesenteric veins not associated with any other disease or determined etiology.[1,2] The number of patients in this group has decreased substantially in the past decade because of increased recognition of inherited thrombotic disorders and hypercoagulable states.

Patients in whom an etiology can be identified are classified as secondary MVT. Causative factors can be identified in 35% to 90% of patients with MVT.[20] Known causes of secondary MVT are shown in Box 25.2. Oral contraceptive use accounts for 9% to 18% of episodes of MVT in young women. Factor V Leiden mutation, protein C and S deficiency, antithrombin III deficiency, dysfibrinogenemia, abnormal plasminogen, JAK 2 V617F mutation, polycythemia vera, essential thrombocytosis, and sickle cell disease (SCD), have all been associated with MVT.[1,2] Localized secondary MVT has also been reported, most commonly secondary to volvulus, intussusception, or mechanical bowel strangulation.

Location of the thrombus may be predicted by etiology. Thrombosis due to an intraabdominal cause such as inflammatory

BOX 25.2 Causes of Secondary Mesenteric Venous Thrombosis

- Trauma
- Surgery
- Cancer
- Cirrhosis
- Portal hypertension
- Inflammatory bowel disease
- Oral contraceptive use
- Splenomegaly
- Pancreatitis
- Dehydration
- Infection
- Diverticular disease
- Hypercoagulable states
  - Factor V Leiden mutation, protein C and S deficiency, antithrombin III deficiency, dysfibrinogenemia, abnormal plasminogen
- Myeloproliferative disorders
  - Polycythemia vera (PCV), essential thrombocytosis (ET), JAK 2 mutation (may precede PCV and ET)
- Sickle cell disease

conditions or surgery starts in the larger vessels at a site of venous compression resulting from these processes and propagates distally to involve the smaller venous arcades and arcuate channels. In contrast, thrombosis due to an underlying hypercoagulable state is thought to usually begin in the small vessels and later involves the larger vessels. Occlusion of the venae rectae and the intramural vessels interferes with adequate venous drainage, with eventual hemorrhagic infarction of the involved bowel segment. The transition from normal to ischemic bowel is usually gradual, unlike that seen with acute embolic or thrombotic occlusion.

Natural History

The natural history of MVT varies based on the etiology. In most cases, it does not result in gangrenous bowel.[1,2] Similarly, symptomatic manifestations are diverse. Patients may present with a benign abdominal examination and few symptoms or with profound hemodynamic collapse. Most patients have abdominal pain. Although it can be sudden in onset, more frequently, it begins insidiously and worsens over time. Approximately 50% of patients have pain from 5 to 30 days before seeking medical attention, and 27% report abdominal pain for more than 1 month. Harward et al. reviewed 16 patients with MVT at a single institution and found that 31% were offered an exploratory laparotomy and all of those patients required bowel resection. Despite improved diagnostic modalities and more aggressive treatment regimens, symptomatic acute MVT is an indicator of poor prognosis, with an approximate 10% to 20% 30-day mortality rate and a 3-year survival rate of 35%.[19] Patients with evidence of chronic thrombosis fare somewhat better because collateral venous channels form, and thereby augment intestinal venous drainage.

CHRONIC MESENTERIC ISCHEMIA

Symptomatic chronic mesenteric arterial insufficiency is a well-described but infrequently encountered clinical problem. The earliest report of chronic intestinal ischemia was by Councilman in 1894. However, in 1918, Goodman credited Baccelli as the first to correctly

associate postprandial pain with CMI. Eighteen years later, Dunphy suggested that the abdominal pain associated with chronic mesenteric arterial occlusion was a possible precursor of later intestinal infarction.

Epidemiology

CMI results from atherosclerosis of the mesenteric arteries in 90% of cases.[1,2,21,22] Nonatherosclerotic causes of CMI are listed in Box 25.3. Nonatherosclerotic etiologies have been described in young adults and children as young as 30 months of age.[21,22] In general, risk factors for atherosclerotic-associated CMI are similar to those of other atherosclerotic conditions, including a positive family history, sedentary lifestyle, hypertension, hypercholesterolemia, and smoking.[1,2,21,22] In contrast to other atherosclerotic vascular diseases, approximately 60% of patients with CMI are female, and nearly 50% of patients have a history of prior cardiovascular surgery.[22] Symptomatic CMI generally manifests at a mean age of 58 years.[1,2,22] More than one-third of patients have hypertension, CAD, and/or cerebrovascular disease.[1,2] Nearly 20% have evidence of chronic renal insufficiency, and 10% have diabetes mellitus.[21]

Although there is a high prevalence of mesenteric artery atherosclerosis, the clinical syndrome of symptomatic mesenteric ischemia is uncommon.[1] In a Finnish series of 120 consecutive autopsies, rates of significant stenoses in the celiac, SMA, and IMA were 22%, 16%, and 10%, respectively. The prevalence of potentially flow-limiting stenosis within the mesenteric vessels increases with age, with up to 67% of those older than 80 years of age having more than 50% stenosis in some mesenteric artery. Aortograms performed for aortic aneurysmal or aortic occlusive disease demonstrate significant stenosis of the celiac artery in 33% of cases and SMA lesions in nearly 20%.

Pathophysiology

CMI occurs when the blood supply is insufficient to meet the metabolic demands of the bowel, resulting from increased motility, secretion, and absorption induced by meals. The infrequent occurrence of symptomatic disease may be explained in part by the extensive

BOX 25.3 Nonatherosclerotic Conditions Associated With Chronic Mesenteric Ischemia

- Neurofibromatosis
- Middle aortic syndrome
- Median arcuate ligament compression
- Visceral artery dissection
- Thromboangiitis obliterans
- Vasculitides
- Rheumatoid arthritis
- Systemic lupus erythematosus (SLE)
- Polyarteritis nodosa
- Mesenteric arteritis
- Cogan's syndrome
- Thoracic aortic aneurysm (TAA)
  - Thrombosis associated with TAA repair
- Aortic coarctation repair
- Radiation injury
- Congenital afibrinogenemia
- Vasoconstrictive agents
  - Ergot poisoning
  - Cocaine abuse

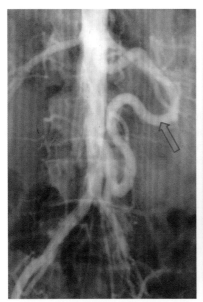
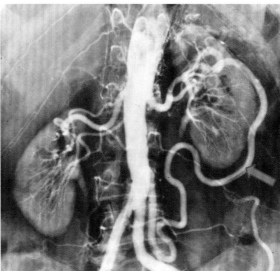

Fig. 25.5 Viscero-visceral collateral pathways in chronic mesenteric ischemia: arc of Riolan *(arrows)*, also referred to as the meandering artery (of Moskowitz), is a collateral pathway between the superior mesenteric artery (SMA) and inferior mesenteric artery (IMA) (classically described as connecting the middle colic branch of the SMA to the left colic branch of the IMA).

mesenteric collateral circulation, which includes both viscerovisceral (celiac artery-SMA-IMA), and parietovisceral (hypogastric-IMA) blood flow (Fig. 25.5).[1,2] The slow development of a chronic high-grade stenosis or occlusion of one or more of the major mesenteric vessels may thus be fully compensated by collateral blood flow. In addition, recent evidence suggests that preexisting significant stenoses in even remote arterial beds may provide protective effects through the mechanism of ischemic preconditioning.

It has been proposed that the pathophysiology of symptomatic CMI involves a regional vascular steal phenomenon. Investigators have used tonometric assessment of splanchnic blood flow in dogs with 50% stenoses of both the celiac artery and SMA to show that food intake reduced intestinal perfusion by 50%. This reduction was associated with a significant decrease in intestinal intramural pH that was attributed to steal from the intestinal to the gastric circulation stimulated by a food bolus within the stomach. Rarely, single-vessel disease of the SMA may produce symptoms characteristic of CMI. The vast majority of patients who present with symptomatic CMI, however, have arteriographic evidence of multivessel visceral artery disease virtually always including the SMA.[1,2,21,22]

Natural History

A variety of pain syndromes characterize patients with CMI. In general, the symptoms consist of upper abdominal cramping or aching pain beginning 20 to 30 minutes after eating. At first the pain may be of short duration, but later it may become more persistent and last for 3 to 4 hours after eating. As the disease progresses, the amount of food that precipitates abdominal pain may decrease. Patients avoid eating to prevent the resulting abdominal pain. Most patients with CMI suffer weight loss secondary to diminished nutritional intake; malabsorption is not the primary mechanism of weight loss in patients with CMI. No form of bowel activity is "classic" for CMI. Patients may have diarrhea (which can potentially exacerbate their nutritional depletion), constipation, or normal bowel habits. Without intervention, patients may develop severe protein-calorie malnutrition and/or progress to bowel infarction.[21]

Most fatal cases of CMI occur in patients with a prolonged history of chronic abdominal complaints.[1] Such cases are frequently characterized by months of abdominal complaints and multiple negative endoscopies, computed tomography scans, and other diagnostic tests. In retrospect, the diagnosis is usually obvious. A high index of suspicion and prompt intervention are clearly indicated in cases of unexplained abdominal pain and weight loss. Early diagnosis may prevent acute thrombosis of stenotic vessels and the often fatal complication of intestinal infarction.[1,21,22]

REFERENCES

1. Martin MC, Wyers MC. Mesenteric vascular disease: acute ischemia. In: Cronenwett JL, Johnston KW, eds. *Rutherford's Vascular Surgery*. 8th ed. Philadelphia: Elsevier; 2014:2398–2413.
2. Schwartz LB, Ng TT, McKinsey JF, et al. Diagnosis and surgical management of visceral ischemic syndromes. In: Moore WS, ed. *Vascular and Endovascular Surgery: A Comprehensive Review*. 8th ed. Philadelphia: Elsevier; 2013:423–435.
3. Wyers MC. Acute mesenteric ischemia: diagnostic approach and surgical treatment. *Semin Vasc Surg*. 2010;23(1):9–20.
4. Morgan CE, Mansukhani NA, Eskandari MK, Rodriguez HE. Ten-year review of isolated spontaneous mesenteric arterial dissections. *J Vasc Surg*. 2018;67:1134–1142.
5. Luan JY, Guan X, Li X, et al. Isolated superior mesenteric artery dissection in China. *J Vasc Surg*. 2016;63(2):530–536.
6. Park YJ, Park CW, Park KB, et al. Inference from clinical and fluid dynamic studies about underlying cause of spontaneous isolated superior mesenteric artery dissection. *J Vasc Surg*. 2011;53(1):80–86.
7. Li DL, He YY, Alkalei AM, et al. Management strategy for spontaneous isolated dissection of the superior mesenteric artery based on morphologic classification. *J Vasc Surg*. 2014;59(1):165–172.
8. Bolen MA, Brinza E, Renapurkar RD, et al. Screening CT angiography of the aorta, visceral branch vessels, and pelvic arteries in fibromuscular dysplasia. *JACC Cardiovasc Imaging*. 2017;10(5):554–561.
9. Slavin RE, Gonzalez-Vitale JC. Segmental mediolytic arteritis: a clinical pathologic study. *Lab Invest*. 1976;35(1):23–29.
10. Slavin RE, Saeki K, Bhagavan B, Maas AE. Segmental arterial mediolysis: a precursor to fibromuscular dysplasia? *Mod Pathol*. 1995;8(3):287–294.

11. Slavin RE, Inada K. Segmental arterial mediolysis with accompanying venous angiopathy: a clinical pathologic review, report of 3 new cases, and comments on the role of endothelin-1 in its pathogenesis. *Int J Surg Pathol.* 2007;15(2):121–134.

12. Shenouda M, Riga C, Naji Y, Renton S. Segmental arterial mediolysis: a systematic review of 85 cases. *Ann Vasc Surg.* 2014;28(1):269–277.

13. Kim HS, Min SI, Han A, et al. Longitudinal evaluation of segmental arterial mediolysis in splanchnic arteries: case series and systematic review. *PLoS One.* 2016;11(8):e0161182.

14. Kim HK, Jung HK, Cho J, et al. Clinical and radiologic course of symptomatic spontaneous isolated dissection of the superior mesenteric artery treated with conservative management. *J Vasc Surg.* 2014;59(2):465–472.

15. Han Y, Cho YP, Ko GY, et al. Clinical outcomes of anticoagulation therapy in patients with symptomatic spontaneous isolated dissection of the superior mesenteric artery. *Medicine (Baltimore).* 2016;95(16):e3480.

16. Sun J, Li DL, Wu ZH, et al. Morphologic findings and management strategy of spontaneous isolated dissection of the celiac artery. *J Vasc Surg.* 2016;64(2):389–394.

17. Bourcier S, Oudjit A, Goudard G, et al. Diagnosis of non-occlusive acute mesenteric ischemia in the intensive care unit. *Ann Intensive Care.* 2016;6(1):112.

18. Toledo-Pereyra LH. Leukocyte depletion, ischemic injury, and organ preservation. *J Surg Res.* 2011;169(2):188–189.

19. Harnik IG, Brandt LJ. Mesenteric venous thrombosis. *Vasc Med.* 2010;15(5):407–418.

20. Clair DG, Beach JM. Mesenteric ischemia. *N Engl J Med.* 2016;374(10):959–968.

21. White CJ. Chronic mesenteric ischemia: diagnosis and management. *Prog Cardiovasc Dis.* 2011;54(1):36–40.

22. Zeller T, Rastan A, Sixt S. Chronic atherosclerotic mesenteric ischemia (CMI). *Vasc Med.* 2010;15(4):333–338.

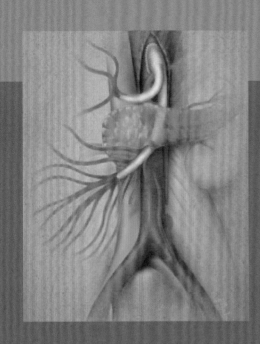

第26章
肠系膜血管疾病的临床评估和治疗

肠系膜动脉缺血的主要类别包括慢性肠系膜缺血（chronic mesenteric ischemia，CMI）、急性闭塞性肠系膜缺血（acute occlusive mesenteric ischemia，AMI）、非闭塞性肠系膜缺血（non-occlusive mesenteric ischemia，NOMI）和肠系膜静脉血栓形成（mesenteric vein thrombosis，MVT）、自发性肠系膜动脉夹层（spontaneous mesenteric artery dissection，SMAD）。尽管各种病因的潜在病理和发生的临床环境不同，但其临床表现可能存在一致，最关键的一点是了解可能导致肠缺血的各种临床因素，并将肠系膜缺血纳入腹痛患者的鉴别诊断中。其目标是在肠梗死和脓毒血症发生之前实现快速有效的诊断。慢性肠系膜缺血最常见的原因是动脉粥样硬化，其典型表现是餐后腹痛，在进食后15～30分钟开始，持续4小时，通常没有腹膜炎的迹象，疼痛的程度与进食的量相关。腹泻、恶心和呕吐可能与疼痛有关。其辅助诊断方式包括双功能超声、CT血管造影、数字减影肠系膜血管成像和磁共振血管成像。传统上，慢性肠系膜缺血的首选治疗方法是开放搭桥术。然而，在大多数情况中，手术修复与显著的并发症率和死亡率相关，所以血管内介入治疗现已超过开放性旁路治疗，成为慢性肠系膜缺血最常用的治疗方法。目前还没有随机研究比较开放式外科血管重建术和血管内介入治疗。普遍的共识是，血管内途径与较低的发病率和死亡率及良好的即刻技术成功率相关，对所有年龄段的人来说都更具成本效益。急性闭塞性肠系膜缺血最常见的原因是动脉粥样硬化性栓塞或急性血栓闭塞。急性闭塞性肠系膜缺血的发病率和死亡率为60%～70%，尽管早期积极治疗，但发病率和死亡率并没有随着时间的推移而改变。严重的急性发作腹痛是急性闭塞性肠系膜缺血患者最常见的症状，典型的急性剧烈腹痛与体检结果不成比例，强烈提示肠缺血。实验室数值通常是非特定的，腹部X线片也是非特异性的，双功能超声在诊断急性闭塞性肠系膜缺血中的作用有限。如果患者的临床状况允许，腹部CT血管造影是准确和实用的，可以迅速识别动脉和静脉阻塞。无论CT结果如何，有反跳痛、压痛、肌紧张、中毒或休克迹象的患者都应接受急诊剖腹探查。急性闭塞性肠系膜缺血的治疗取决于疾病的病因和患者的临床状态，肠道活力的评估是至关重要的。血管腔内治疗对急性闭塞性肠系膜缺血的作用仍存在争议。急性非闭塞性肠系膜缺血的发生是由于严重和持续的肠系膜动脉血管痉挛，没有动脉或静脉阻塞的证据。早期明确诊断和治疗对患者的生存至关重要。20%~25%的非闭塞性肠系膜缺血患者没有腹痛，可能出现腹胀，伴有隐匿性或明显的胃肠道出血。非闭塞性肠系膜缺血患者的放射学评估类似于闭塞性急性闭塞性肠系膜缺血，怀疑患有非闭塞性肠系膜缺血的患者应该进行紧急肠系膜血管造影术以确认诊断，Siegelman等描述了诊断肠系膜血管痉挛的4个可靠的血管造影标准：①肠系膜动脉多支起始处狭窄；②肠分支交替扩张和狭窄——"香肠串征"；③肠系膜弓痉挛；④肠壁内血管充盈受损。高死亡率与延迟诊断有关。非闭塞性肠系膜缺血的主要治疗方法是内科治疗，并辅以危重护理支持，以纠正导致全身性低灌流的全身状况。对于腹膜炎患者，需要手术探查以充分评估肠道存活率。

毕　伟

Clinical Evaluation and Treatment of Mesenteric Vascular Disease

Enjae Jung, Cherrie Abraham, Gregory J. Landry, and Gregory L. Moneta

Clinical evaluation of possible mesenteric ischemia begins with an appropriate index of suspicion for the diagnosis followed by a careful history and physical examination. The major categories of mesenteric ischemia include chronic mesenteric ischemia (CMI), acute occlusive mesenteric ischemia (AMI), nonocclusive mesenteric ischemia (NOMI), and mesenteric venous thrombosis (MVT) (also see Chapter 25). Spontaneous mesenteric artery dissections (SMADs) are infrequent causes of abdominal pain that are becoming increasingly recognized due to the routine use of modern cross-sectional imaging. Although the various etiologies differ in their underlying pathologies and the clinical settings in which they occur, there may be significant overlap in their clinical presentation. The most crucial point is to understand the variety of clinical settings in which intestinal ischemia can occur and to include mesenteric ischemia in the differential diagnosis of patients presenting with abdominal pain. The goal is to achieve a rapid and efficient diagnosis prior to the onset of bowel infarction and resulting sepsis.

CHRONIC MESENTERIC ISCHEMIA

Clinical Presentation

The most common cause of CMI is atherosclerosis, and CMI therefore predominantly affects an older patient population, but with a slight female predominance. Most patients with atherosclerotic mesenteric vascular disease are asymptomatic and at low risk for bowel infarction due to only mild to moderate stenosis of the mesenteric arteries and a robust collateral network that may compensate for reduced flow through one mesenteric artery. On the other hand, patients who have symptomatic CMI generally have high-grade stenosis or occlusion of both the celiac and superior mesenteric arteries (SMAs). Though uncommon, single-vessel mesenteric artery disease can result in symptomatic CMI in the presence of insufficient collateral reserve. The inferior mesenteric artery (IMA) may not be a source of collateral flow in most cases due to proximal atherosclerotic disease, but occasionally can be a vital collateral preventing ischemic catastrophe.

The classic presentation of CMI is postprandial pain described as colicky or a dull intense ache that generally begins 15 to 30 minutes after eating and lasts up to 4 hours. There are no signs of peritonitis, and the degree of pain may reflect the volume of the ingested meal. Diarrhea, nausea, and vomiting may be associated with the pain. Early in the course of CMI, some meals may be ingested without pain, so symptoms may be mistakenly attributed to other potential causes such as cholelithiasis, peptic ulcer disease, or malignancy. Patients often undergo extensive evaluation with endoscopy, computed tomography (CT), barium studies, and abdominal ultrasonography prior to reaching a diagnosis of CMI. As the disease progresses, patients experience pain with each meal and may develop a fear of food, termed sitophobia.[1] Weight loss, one of the hallmarks of CMI, results from limited nutritional intake, not malabsorption. Patients with CMI generally have normal testing for gastrointestinal malabsorption.

Evaluation

CMI is a clinical diagnosis and patients should have suggestive clinical symptoms. Confirmatory studies to identify mesenteric artery lesions associated with CMI include duplex ultrasonography, computed tomography angiography (CTA), digital subtraction mesenteric angiography (DSA) and, less commonly, magnetic resonance angiography (MRA).

Duplex Ultrasonography

Duplex ultrasonography can serve as a valuable noninvasive screening test for mesenteric artery stenosis and for follow-up in patients with mesenteric artery reconstructions. Duplex ultrasound examination of the mesenteric arteries can be technically difficult and should be performed by vascular technologists with extensive experience in abdominal ultrasound techniques (Fig. 26.1).

Duplex ultrasound can detect hemodynamically significant stenoses in splanchnic vessels. In 1986, investigators at the University of Washington found that flow velocities in stenotic SMAs and celiac arteries were increased when compared with normal SMAs and celiac arteries.[2] Quantitative criteria for splanchnic artery stenosis were first developed and validated at Oregon Health and Science University.[3] In a blinded prospective study of 100 patients who underwent mesenteric artery duplex scanning and lateral aortography, a peak systolic velocity (PSV) in the SMA of 275 cm/s or more indicated 70% or greater stenosis, and a PSV of 200 cm/s or higher in the celiac artery indicated a 70% or greater stenosis (Fig. 26.2), both with high sensitivity and specificity (Table 26.1).[4] Criteria were developed to detect $\geq$70% stenosis, as symptomatic mesenteric ischemia is unusual with lesser degrees of mesenteric artery stenosis.

Although the initial diagnosis of significant visceral artery stenosis can be made using duplex ultrasound, cross-sectional imaging, or in some cases, DSA, is crucial for preprocedure planning.

Computed Tomography Angiography

Multidetector CTA is a noninvasive modality with high sensitivity for detection of stenosis of the mesenteric arteries.[5] In most cases, CTA has replaced other modalities as the imaging study of choice for evaluation of CMI because it can accurately identify significant stenosis in the celiac artery and SMA, identify significant visceral collaterals, and exclude other potential intraabdominal processes. There is not a set guideline to define significant stenosis on CTA. Some studies have used 50% luminal narrowing as a cutoff for significant stenosis, and others have delineated 70% luminal narrowing as significant stenosis in keeping with the Doppler criterion for significant stenosis.[6]

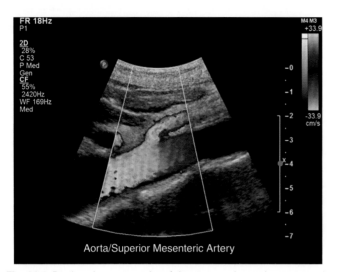

Fig. 26.1 Duplex ultrasonography of the aorta and superior mesenteric artery.

Together with noncontrast images, CTA, in many cases, offers enough anatomic detail to plan open and endovascular procedures. Preprocedure CTA is used to evaluate the angle of origin of the mesenteric vessels in relation to the aortic axis, the presence of calcium and thrombus as well as the length of the stenotic lesion, and the presence of important collaterals or unusual anatomy in proximity to the target lesion (Fig. 26.3). Limitations include contrast-related nephropathy, hypersensitivity reaction, and ionizing radiation exposure.

Mesenteric Angiography

Mesenteric angiography has traditionally been the gold standard for diagnosis of hemodynamically significant mesenteric artery stenosis. Lateral and anteroposterior views of the aorta are required for full evaluation of the severity of visceral stenosis, occlusion of a mesenteric artery, and the extent of collateral development (Fig. 26.4). With the improved image quality of CTA and MRA, mesenteric angiography is currently reserved primarily for treatment if the patient, based on axial imaging, is felt to be a candidate for endovascular intervention or is used in cases when noninvasive imaging is inconclusive.

Treatment

Traditionally, the preferred treatment of CMI was open surgical bypass. Operative repair, however, is associated with significant morbidity and mortality in most series. Given the expected morbidity in this patient population with significant weight loss, advanced age, malnutrition, and low albumin levels, all of which are predictors of increased morbidity and mortality after any major surgery, endovascular intervention has now surpassed open bypass as the most frequently utilized treatment for CMI. Endovascular treatment has high technical and early clinical success rates, with decreased morbidity and mortality compared to surgical intervention.[7] It is, however, associated with lower long-term patency and a greater likelihood of the need for repeat interventions.[8] There are no randomized controlled trials comparing treatment modalities for CMI. Therefore, treatment decisions must be based on large case series in which a variety of procedures have been used. Although endovascular intervention is the first-line treatment for most patients with CMI, certain patients remain more appropriate for surgery, including those with concomitant aneurysmal disease in need of repair, and those with flush occlusions of the culprit mesenteric vessel(s) (Fig. 26.5).

Indications for Operation

Revascularization is indicated for symptomatic intestinal ischemia. Revascularization for asymptomatic high-grade SMA obstruction is recommended only in patients undergoing otherwise indicated aortic surgery for aneurysmal or occlusive disease. In this group of patients, acute intestinal ischemia following aortic surgery has been well documented, and SMA reconstruction prior to or at the time of aortic repair seems prudent.

Techniques of Superior Mesenteric Artery Bypass

Retrograde bypass. The distal infrarenal aorta as an origin for an SMA bypass graft has advantages and disadvantages. The exposure is familiar, and risks of dissection and clamping are less than with more proximal aortic exposures. In addition, the procedure can be readily

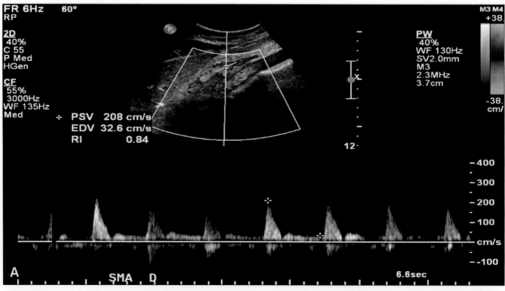

Fig. 26.2 (A) Duplex ultrasonography of the superior mesenteric artery *(SMA)*, with peak systolic velocity *(PSV)* of 208 cm/s signifying a normal SMA.

Continued

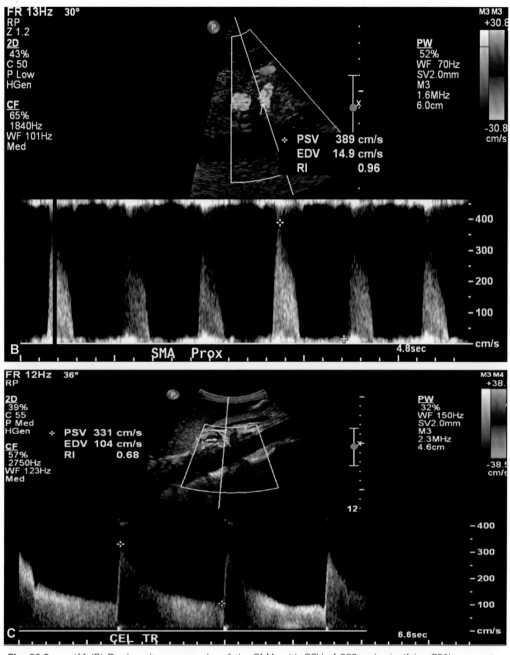

Fig. 26.2, cont'd (B) Duplex ultrasonography of the SMA with PSV of 389 cm/s signifying 70% or greater SMA stenosis. (C) Duplex ultrasonography of the celiac artery, with PSV of 331 cm/s signifying 70% or greater celiac artery stenosis.

TABLE 26.1   Oregon Health and Science University Criteria for Mesenteric Artery Stenoses

	>70% stenosis	Sensitivity	Specificity	PPV	NPV	Accuracy
SMA	PSV ≥ 275 cm/s	92%	96%	80%	99%	96%
CA	PSV ≥ 200 cm/s	87%	80%	63%	94%	82%

CA, Celiac artery; *NPV,* negative predictive value; *PPV,* positive predictive value; *PSV,* peak systolic velocity; *SMA,* superior mesenteric artery. From Moneta GL, Lee RW, Yeager RA, et al. Mesenteric duplex scanning: a blinded prospective study. *J Vasc Surg.* 1993;17(1):79–84.

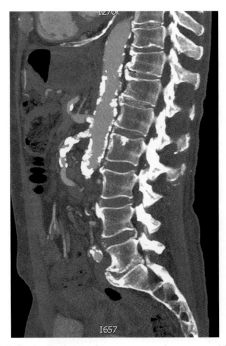

Fig. 26.3 Sagittal view of a computed tomographic angiogram demonstrating severe atherosclerotic disease of the proximal and mid-superior mesenteric artery.

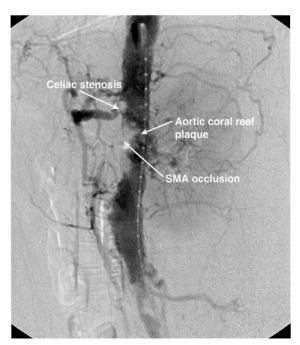

Fig. 26.5 Lateral aortogram demonstrating "coral reef" atherosclerotic plaque in aorta, with associated superior mesenteric artery *(SMA)* occlusion and celiac artery stenosis.

combined with other intraabdominal vascular procedures. The primary disadvantage is that the infrarenal aorta and iliac arteries are frequently calcified, increasing the technical difficulty of the proximal anastomosis.

Prosthetic grafts are used most often in cases of mesenteric revascularization. Exceptions are cases complicated by bowel necrosis. For these patients, vein grafts are preferred to minimize the possibility of

graft infection. Special attention must be paid to graft configuration to avoid graft kinking when the graft is placed in a retrograde configuration. A preference for the origin of the graft is the area of the junction of the aorta and right common iliac artery (CIA), although any suitable site on the infrarenal aorta or either CIA is satisfactory. A single limb is cut from a bifurcated graft in the manner described by Wylie and colleagues, which provides a "flange" for sewing and prevents anastomotic

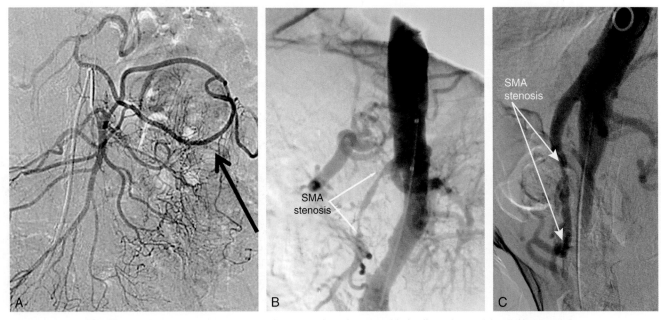

Fig. 26.4 (A) Anteroposterior aortogram demonstrating a hypertrophied collateral vessel *(arrow)* between the celiac artery and the superior mesenteric artery *(SMA)*. (B) Lateral aortogram demonstrating long-segment stenosis of the SMA. (C) Lateral aortogram demonstrating long-segment stenosis of the middle SMA.

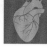

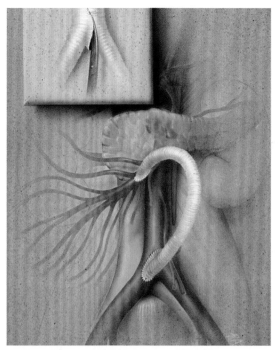

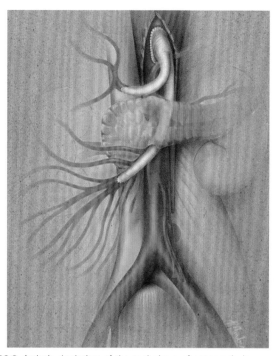

Fig. 26.6 Artist's depiction of the infrarenal aorta–to–superior mesenteric artery bypass technique. Graft is fashioned using one limb of a bifurcated graft. After the inflow anastomosis is performed, the graft is arranged in an inverse "c" configuration.

Fig. 26.8 Artist's depiction of the technique of antegrade bypass from the supraceliac aorta to the celiac and superior mesenteric arteries.

stricture (Fig. 26.6).[9] The ligament of Treitz is dissected. The proximal (inflow) anastomosis is completed first. The graft is then arranged first cephalad, then turning anteriorly and inferiorly a full 180 degrees to terminate in an antegrade anastomosis to the anterior wall of the SMA, just beyond the inferior border of the pancreas. The graft is excluded from the peritoneal cavity by closing the mesenteric peritoneum, approximating the ligament of Treitz, and closing the posterior parietal peritoneum.

Antegrade bypass. Antegrade bypasses originate from the anterior surface of the supraceliac aorta. The proximal aorta is exposed through the upper midline (Fig. 26.7) or, when the intraabdominal supraceliac

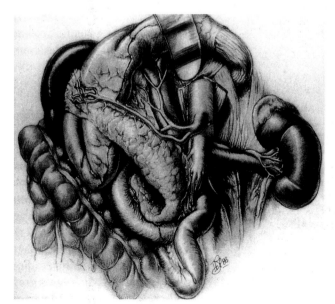

Fig. 26.7 Artist's depiction of exposure of the supraceliac aorta.

aorta is calcified, using a low thoracoabdominal incision. Antegrade bypass provides prograde flow to the mesenteric vessels and is clearly the preferred approach in patients with contraindications to use of the infrarenal aorta or an iliac artery as a bypass origin. Visceral bypass grafts can be constructed with a partial-occlusion clamping of the aorta in many cases, although in most cases, the "partial" occlusion is actually near-total occlusion. Transient hepatic and renal ischemia is usually well tolerated, but is a potential disadvantage to the antegrade approach, particularly in patients with significant preexisting renal insufficiency.

Antegrade grafts to the SMA are normally tunneled behind the pancreas and anastomosed to the anterior wall of the SMA in an end-to-side fashion (Fig. 26.8). A disadvantage of the antegrade bypass is that the retropancreatic space is limited, and great care is necessary when tunneling the graft. Some surgeons advocate prepancreatic tunneling to avoid compression of the graft within the tunnel. A prepancreatic tunnel, however, places the graft in apposition to the posterior wall of the stomach and theoretically increases the possibility of graft infection. Occasionally, in the setting of very focal SMA origin disease and an easily mobilized pancreas, the antegrade bypass can be constructed entirely superior to the pancreas, obviating the need for a retropancreatic tunnel.

Multiple-Vessel Revascularization Versus Single-Vessel Revascularization

One debated issue is the optimal number of vessels to revascularize. Multiple-vessel revascularization implies repair or bypass of all diseased or occluded vessels (Fig. 26.9), most often the celiac artery and SMA. Bypass to the IMA is usually unnecessary for successful revascularization, except in unusual cases. Proponents of multiple-vessel, or "complete" revascularization suggest that this approach makes recurrent symptomatic ischemia less likely should one graft or graft limb thrombose.[10,11] In a 1992 study, overall graft patency and survival were better in patients who underwent multiple-vessel bypass than in those

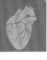

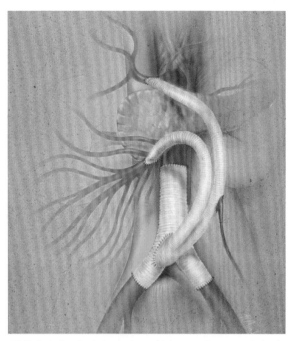

Fig. 26.9 Artist's depiction of multiple-vessel revascularization. A retrograde mesenteric bypass to the celiac and superior mesenteric arteries, with reimplantation of the inferior mesenteric artery performed from the proximal right common iliac artery.

who underwent single-vessel bypass.[10] The investigators concluded that multiple-vessel bypass patients were likely to remain asymptomatic because of the presence of additional grafts or graft limbs that remained patent. Others maintain that the critical vessel involved in CMI is the SMA and argue that bypass to the SMA alone is a relatively simple procedure that relieves symptoms of mesenteric ischemia. More recent data also suggest that the rate of symptomatic recurrence, graft patency, and patient survival are unaffected by the number of revascularized vessels.[12–15] Foley et al. evaluated 49 patients who underwent bypass to the SMA alone and reported a 9-year primary-assisted graft patency rate of 79% and a 5-year survival rate of 61%[12]—results equivalent to those noted in contemporary studies of multiple-vessel revascularization for CMI.[13]

Postoperative Care

Patients with chronic visceral ischemia often have significant ischemic bowel injury that requires time for recovery. Sitophobia may persist temporarily after revascularization and some are unable to achieve adequate oral nutrition following visceral revascularization for a prolonged period. For this reason, total parenteral nutrition is used liberally. Some patients with severe preoperative ischemia develop postoperative revascularization syndrome, which consists of abdominal pain, tachycardia, leukocytosis, and intestinal edema. Any departure from a normal postoperative course should prompt CTA, arteriography, or exploration as delayed diagnosis of graft occlusion or intestinal necrosis is usually fatal.

Endovascular Therapy for Mesenteric Occlusive Disease

Mesenteric angiography and intervention can be performed via femoral or brachial arterial access. The brachial artery approach is preferred by many for patients with an angulated target mesenteric vessel or in those with occlusion or long-segment lesions due to the coaxial alignment of diagnostic and guiding catheters with the downward takeoff of the mesenteric vessels. The disadvantage of brachial arterial access

is the relative inability to use larger sheaths in patients with small brachial arteries. In general, 4-5 Fr sheaths are sufficient for diagnostic angiography, but 6-7 Fr sheaths are generally required for mesenteric stenting. In patients with two- or three-vessel disease including the SMA, the preferred target vessel for treatment is the SMA. The risks of dissection, stent fractures, and residual stenosis are higher with treatment of the celiac artery and the patency rates are lower than for SMA interventions.[16] This may be due to the short length of the celiac artery, angulation of the artery, the presence of fibromuscular tissue investing the celiac axis, or the presence of significant median arcuate ligament compression. However, in high-risk patients where SMA recanalization is not possible, celiac artery intervention can be undertaken and is preferred to a low-yield attempt at SMA intervention. Though uncommon, for patients with occluded celiac and SMA not amenable to intervention, stenting of a stenotic IMA can result in relief of CMI symptoms.[17]

Following intraluminal access through a femoral or brachial artery approach, a nonselective abdominal aortogram is performed. Systemic heparin is administered intravenously. A hydrophilic guiding sheath or guiding catheter is positioned in the abdominal aorta near the vessel origin for better visualization and improved support and a diagnostic catheter is used to select the mesenteric artery. The choice of catheter shape depends on access site, angle of origin, institutional availability, and individual preference. The initial selective angiography should demonstrate the origin of the vessel from the aortic wall and the severity of the stenosis. It should also document the distal branches for comparison with postintervention views. A soft, hydrophilic guidewire is advanced past the lesion, which is followed by the catheter. A low-volume contrast injection is performed through the catheter to confirm intraluminal position and the initial guidewire is then exchanged for a stiffer wire. The tip of the wire should be visualized within the field and positioned within the main trunk of the SMA and not within a small jejunal branch.

Although there are no data comparing angioplasty alone with primary stenting, angioplasty is rarely performed alone for atherosclerotic disease in CMI, as mesenteric artery lesions are typically heavily calcified and do not respond adequately to balloon dilation alone. When treating an ostial lesion, the length of the angioplasty balloon should be approximately 2 mm longer than the length of the stenotic lesion so that the balloon protrudes into the aorta to ensure complete treatment of the ostium. Stenting is strongly considered for residual stenosis >30% or a residual pressure gradient across the lesion >15 mm Hg, calcified ostial or high-grade eccentric stenoses, chronic occlusions, or in the presence of dissection after angioplasty. If performing primary stenting, predilation is recommended for tight stenoses, occlusions, and severe calcification. The stent is positioned across the lesion within the sheath, protecting the stent from dislodging while traversing an irregular stenotic lesion. The stent should cover slightly more than the entire length of the lesion and extend 1 to 2 mm into the aortic lumen for ostial lesions to ensure complete treatment of the ostium. Ideally, the stent should be flared gently into the aorta. A follow-up selective angiogram is performed of the treated vessel to look for residual stenosis, distal emboli, or dissection (Fig. 26.10).

Outcome Evaluation and Surveillance

There are no randomized studies comparing open surgical revascularization to endovascular intervention. Most of the data are derived from case series and case reports. There is general consensus that the endovascular approach is associated with lower morbidity and mortality rates with good immediate technical success rates. However, endovascular interventions may be less durable than surgical intervention with higher rates of restenosis and recurrent symptoms. In a systematic

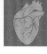

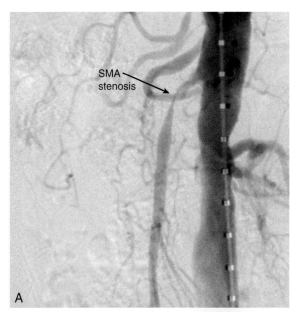

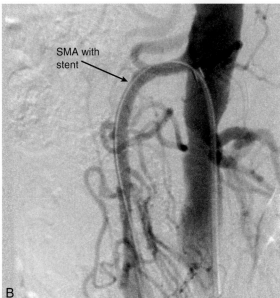

Fig. 26.10 (A) Lateral aortogram demonstrating stenosis of the superior mesenteric artery *(SMA)* just prior to stent placement. (B) Lateral aortogram demonstrating patency of the SMA just after stent placement.

with endovascular intervention, a recent meta-analysis evaluating the comparative effectiveness and cost-effectiveness of endovascular repair versus open revascularization found that endovascular intervention was more cost-effective for all age groups.[20]

Although there is controversy surrounding the ideal type of stent (balloon vs. self-expandable, covered vs. bare metal), most interventions currently use bare metal balloon-expandable stents to treat ostial lesions, and self-expandable stents for distal lesions affecting tortuous segments. Covered stents for mesenteric artery origin stenting however, may provide improved patency rates, but there is limited data regarding covered stents for treatment of mesenteric artery disease. Schoch et al. first reported favorable results in 14 patients treated by covered stents with no reinterventions after 2 years of follow-up.[21] Oderich et al. more recently reported a nonrandomized comparison of covered versus bare metal stents in 225 patients treated for CMI. Covered stents outperformed bare metal stents with lower rates of restenosis, symptom recurrence, and reintervention, and improved patency rates. At 3-year follow-up, primary patency was 92% and secondary patency was 100%.[22] Lower restenosis rates observed with covered stents may be explained by barriers to tissue ingrowth with coverage of the stent. Other potential benefits of covered stents include precise deployment, excellent radial force, prevention of embolism by debris entrapment, and potentially less risk of arterial disruption. However, the cost of a covered stent is 3 to 5 times more than a bare metal stent, and these stents require 7 Fr sheaths, a major limitation compared with smaller-profile stents that can be introduced through a smaller sheath over a 0.014- or 0.018-inch platform.

There are well-established duplex criteria for identifying high-grade stenosis in the native SMA, but there are no standardized ultrasound criteria for the detection of high-grade stenosis in stented SMAs. We have previously shown that angiographic pressure gradients in stented SMAs are affected by the presence or absence of high-grade celiac artery stenoses.[23] In addition, although fasting duplex measurement of SMA peak systolic velocities are reduced after stenting, they remain greater than the criteria predicting high-grade native artery SMA stenosis. Duplex ultrasound criteria applied to assess the presence of stenosis in native arteries cannot be applied to stented SMAs. This is consistent with a growing body of literature showing that current duplex ultrasound criteria for defining stenosis in native mesenteric arteries overestimate the degree of in-stent restenosis.[24,25] Soult et al. performed a retrospective review of patients who underwent SMA or celiac stenting and reviewed 103 paired duplex ultrasounds with angiograms. Based on their data, they proposed an SMA PSV of ≥445 cm/s and a celiac artery PSV of ≥289 cm/s to define in-stent restenosis of ≥70% (Table 26.2).[25] It is our practice to obtain a postprocedure mesenteric duplex to serve as a baseline for future comparison. Patients are followed with history, clinical examination, and duplex ultrasound every 3 months for the first year, every 6 months for the second year, then annually thereafter. Markedly elevated focal peak systolic velocities within the stented regions, especially if increasing on serial examinations, should lead to an angiogram to confirm in-stent or distal native arterial stenosis.

review by van Petersen et al., endovascular treatment was associated with more restenosis (37% vs. 15%), recurrent symptoms (30% vs. 13%) and reinterventions (20% vs. 9%) compared to open surgical bypass.[18] In comparison, open surgical bypass has a reported 5-year primary patency of 80% to 90%.[19] Despite the higher reintervention rates

TABLE 26.2	Mesenteric Artery In-stent Restenosis Criteria				
	>70% Stenosis	Sensitivity	Specificity	PPV	NPV
SMA	PSV ≥ 445 cm/s	83%	83%	81%	86%
CA	PSV ≥ 289 cm/s	100%	57%	79%	100%

CA, Celiac artery; *NPV,* negative predictive value; *PPV,* positive predictive value; *PSV,* peak systolic velocity; *SMA,* superior mesenteric artery. From Soult MC, Wuammett JC, Ahanchi SS, et al. Duplex ultrasound criteria for in-stent restenosis of mesenteric arteries. *J Vasc Surg.* 2016;64(5):1366–1372.

Similarly, duplex ultrasonography has been used for postoperative graft surveillance after mesenteric artery bypasses. Although duplex ultrasound examination is difficult in the early postoperative period because of incisional tenderness and postoperative ileus, it has proven to be a valuable tool in later surveillance of mesenteric bypass grafts. A retrospective study at our institution defined normal duplex ultrasonography-derived velocity characteristics of mesenteric artery bypass grafts. The anastomotic and midgraft peak systolic velocities are not affected by the orientation of the graft. Mean peak systolic velocities for most grafts are between 140 and 200 cm/s and remain relatively stable on repeat examinations. Serial duplex ultrasound examinations can be used to assess the patency of bypass grafts to mesenteric arteries.[26] We routinely use postoperative duplex ultrasound scanning to establish baseline values and permit comparisons for follow-up evaluation of graft patency. If markedly elevated focal peak systolic velocities (>300 cm/s) are recorded, especially if they increase on serial examinations, secondary imaging (CT or conventional angiography) should be obtained to confirm graft stenosis and to possibly plan intervention.

ACUTE OCCLUSIVE MESENTERIC ISCHEMIA

Clinical Presentation

AMI is most commonly caused by embolism to the SMA or acute thrombotic occlusion of an atherosclerotic SMA. Arterial embolism to the visceral vessels, most commonly from a cardiac source, was thought to be the most common etiology. More recent data, however, suggest that arterial thrombosis is the most common cause.[27] Aneurysms, vasculitis, and mesenteric artery dissection, either spontaneous or as a complication of aortic dissection and trauma, can be another infrequent cause of AMI. AMI carries a 60% to 70% morbidity and mortality rate that has not changed over time despite early aggressive treatment.

Severe acute onset abdominal pain is the most common presenting symptom in patients with AMI, and physical examination findings can range from nonspecific tenderness to an acute abdomen. The classic presentation of acute, severe abdominal pain out of proportion to the physical examination findings is strongly suggestive of intestinal ischemia. The duration of symptoms does not necessarily correlate with the degree of intestinal infarction. Peritonitis is initially absent, but vomiting and diarrhea may be present and occult gastric or rectal bleeding can be identified in up to 25% of patients. Patients with embolism tend to present with an acute onset of abdominal pain, whereas patients with thrombosis of a stenotic SMA may have a more delayed presentation due to developed collaterals.

Evaluation

Laboratory values are typically nonspecific. The majority of patients will have moderate to marked leukocytosis, but about 10% of patients will have a normal white blood cell count. Elevated serum amylase and metabolic acidosis may occur in patients with necrotic bowel, but an absence of these findings does not exclude bowel necrosis.

Plain abdominal radiographs are usually nonspecific and 25% of patients may have normal findings. Duplex ultrasound has a limited role in diagnosing AMI due to technical limitations from gaseous visceral distention that is frequently associated with AMI.

Abdominal CTA is an accurate and practical diagnostic test, if the patient's clinical status allows. In addition to detecting other abdominal pathologies causing abdominal pain, CTA can promptly identify arterial and venous obstruction, and evaluate changes in the bowel wall indicative of intestinal ischemia such as bowel luminal dilation, bowel wall thickening, submucosal edema or hemorrhage, pneumatosis

intestinalis, and portal venous gas. A meta-analysis looking at the diagnostic accuracy of multidetector CT in AMI found a pooled sensitivity and specificity of 93% and 96%, respectively.[28] Regardless of CT findings, patients with rebound tenderness, rigidity, or evidence of toxicity or shock, should undergo emergent exploratory laparotomy, and as appropriate, resection of necrotic bowel and revascularization.

Mesenteric angiography was once considered the gold standard in diagnostic evaluation due to its high sensitivity and specificity for detecting mesenteric artery occlusion or high-grade stenosis. Today, angiography is used primarily as a confirmatory tool in stable patients when noninvasive radiologic studies do not provide conclusive results, or in select patients in whom a therapeutic endovascular approach is chosen. The typical CTA or angiographic finding of AMI due to embolism is occlusion just distal to the middle colic artery of the SMA (Fig. 26.11). In contrast, arterial in situ thrombosis usually occurs at the ostium of the SMA, superimposed on a preexisting atherosclerotic lesion (Fig. 26.12).

Treatment

Treatment of AMI is determined by the etiology of the disease and the clinical status of the patient. The role of endovascular therapy in AMI remains controversial. In cases of AMI, assessment of intestinal viability is crucial and can be achieved only with abdominal exploration and direct bowel inspection. The role of diagnostic laparoscopy has not been described extensively and may be underutilized. Endovascular treatment modalities are usually reserved for patients without peritoneal signs on physical examination in whom it is felt safe to defer surgical exploration for necrotic bowel.

The choice of operation for revascularizing the bowel depends on the underlying etiology. Embolectomy is indicated for arterial embolism. If the suspected etiology is thrombotic occlusion, bypass or a hybrid approach with open exploration combined with retrograde stenting at the time of the laparotomy are options. Bypass options are similar to bypasses for CMI as previously discussed. SMAD is discussed in depth in Chapter 25. Patients with SMAD usually improve with conservative management, with only 5% to 7% of patients requiring intervention for persistent symptoms.[29]

Operative Embolectomy

Following a midline abdominal incision, a thorough examination of the abdominal contents is performed. The small bowel may be deeply cyanotic yet still viable and in most cases, bowel resection should not be performed until after revascularization. The transverse colon is reflected cephalad and the ligament of Treitz is divided. The SMA is exposed at the root of the small bowel mesentery. The SMA should be readily palpable in this location because it crosses over the third portion of the duodenum. The dissection is continued to obtain sufficient proximal and distal control of the vessel. Embolectomy is performed through a transverse arteriotomy using standard balloon catheters, and the embolus is extracted. If there is any possibility that a bypass graft may be needed, then a longitudinal arteriotomy is made. The arteriotomy is then closed and the intestines are again inspected for viability and any clearly nonviable bowel is resected. A Doppler probe can be used to assess the antimesenteric border for intestinal arterial flow. If the bowel viability is equivocal, a second-look operation can be planned in the following 24 to 48 hours to reassess the bowel and resect if necessary.

Endovascular Thrombolysis and Embolectomy

Catheter-directed thrombolysis is a potentially useful treatment modality for AMI,[30,31] but should only be considered in highly selected patients under close supervision. It has a high probability of restoring

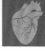

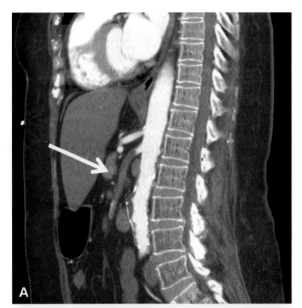

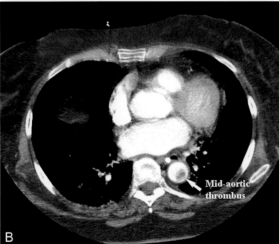

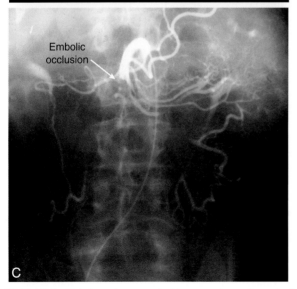

Fig. 26.11 (A) Sagittal view of a computed tomography angiography from a patient with atrial fibrillation and an acute distal superior mesenteric artery (SMA) embolus *(arrow)*. (B) Axial computed tomography scan demonstrating a mid-aortic thrombus that caused embolic occlusion of the SMA. (C) Anteroposterior angiogram of the SMA demonstrating embolic occlusion of the distal SMA just distal to the middle colic artery origin.

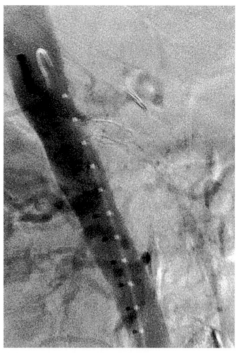

Fig. 26.12 Mesenteric angiogram demonstrating acute stent occlusion in a patient with a prior superior mesenteric artery stent placed for chronic mesenteric ischemia.

perfusion when performed within 12 hours of symptom onset. Successful resolution of the mesenteric thrombus will facilitate identification of a possible underlying mesenteric occlusive lesion and allow for definitive angioplasty and stenting of the offending lesion. The drawbacks to catheter-directed thrombolysis are the inability to inspect the bowel following restoration of mesenteric flow and the potentially prolonged period of time necessary to achieve successful revascularization. An incomplete or unsuccessful thrombolysis may lead to delayed operative revascularization, which in turn, may necessitate more bowel resection for irreversible intestinal necrosis than would have been needed with more prompt revascularization. Catheter thrombectomy or suction embolectomy is an adjunct to catheter-directed thrombolysis and can be employed in treatment of AMI due to SMA thromboembolism.

Endovascular access is commonly from the femoral artery, although a brachial approach is sometimes used. After positioning the guiding sheath in the abdominal aorta near the vessel origin, a soft, hydrophilic guidewire is used to recanalize the SMA. Once the lesion is crossed, an infusion catheter is advanced into the SMA and the patient is given 2 to 4 mg of intraarterial bolus of tissue plasminogen-activator (TPA) followed by an infusion started at 0.25 to 1 mg/h. A flat rate of heparin (500 units/h) through the sheath should be maintained. The patient's complete blood counts and fibrinogen levels are followed serially. Repeat angiogram is performed every 12 hours. Once the distal clot clears, any underlying stenotic lesion should have definitive angioplasty and stenting. If the patient demonstrates an increase in abdominal pain, rising lactic acidosis, or clinical deterioration, lysis is stopped and the patient is taken to the operating room for immediate open exploration and revascularization.

If suction embolectomy is performed, the occluded SMA is recanalized and an aspiration or guiding catheter is advanced over the wire. The wire is then removed and the catheter is slowly withdrawn while manually aspirating from the catheter. This process is repeated multiple times as needed until the embolus is completely removed or further removal of the embolus is not possible. This method can be supplemented with bolus of TPA into the SMA prior to and during the embolectomy. There should be a low threshold to perform abdominal exploration even after successful percutaneous intervention.

Hybrid Technique: Retrograde Open Mesenteric Stenting

Hybrid vascular techniques combine the attributes of both endovascular and open procedures. A hybrid approach for mesenteric revascularization allows for both endovascular treatment of mesenteric vessels and thorough assessment of bowel viability. Initial results show a 100% initial success and a lower in-hospital mortality rate of 17% compared with surgical bypass or endovascular treatment.[32] If Retrograde Open Mesenteric Stenting (ROMS) is anticipated, use of a hybrid operating room with fixed angiographic imaging capabilities is preferred. Similar to operative embolectomy, the abdominal contents are carefully inspected through a midline abdominal incision. The SMA is identified and dissected out at the root of the mesentery. The artery is incised longitudinally and a local thromboendarterectomy with patch angioplasty is performed with either bovine pericardium or saphenous vein. Through the distal patch, a sheath is placed into the SMA in a retrograde fashion. The occlusive lesion is crossed with a guidewire and the lesion is stented. After confirming technical success and flow restoration through a completion angiogram, the sheath is removed and the puncture site in the patch is repaired.

ACUTE NONOCCLUSIVE MESENTERIC ISCHEMIA

Clinical Presentation

Acute NOMI occurs as a result of severe and prolonged mesenteric arterial vasospasm, usually in the distribution of the SMA, without evidence of arterial or venous obstruction. This form of AMI occurs in up to 25% of patients with AMI and carries the highest mortality rates because of its frequent association with multisystem organ failure.[33] Although a hypoperfusion state is present in most patients with NOMI, some have NOMI due to visceral vasoconstriction alone, as is the case with cocaine or ergot intoxication. Early definitive diagnosis and treatment are essential for patient survival. A patient with NOMI may have an insidious onset and protracted clinical course that may complicate diagnosis. Furthermore, they are least able to offer any history because they are often critically ill. Therefore, recognition of factors associated with NOMI is necessary for its prompt diagnosis. These include acute myocardial infarction, congestive heart failure, valvular heart disease, aortic dissection, cardiopulmonary bypass, renal failure requiring hemodialysis, sepsis, and the use of vasopressors and digitalis. Findings on physical examination are varied and do not confirm or exclude the diagnosis of NOMI. Abdominal pain may be present and can vary widely in character, location, and intensity, but is absent in 20% to 25% of patients with NOMI. Abdominal distention with occult or frank gastrointestinal bleeding may be present. As in occlusive AMI, laboratory values are nonspecific.

Evaluation

Radiological evaluation of patients with NOMI is in many ways similar to that of patients with occlusive AMI. However, although CTA supplants diagnostic angiography in the diagnostic algorithm for occlusive AMI, patients suspected to have NOMI should undergo urgent mesenteric angiography to confirm the diagnosis. Significant mortality is associated with a delayed diagnosis. The angiographic appearance of NOMI can be subtle, but Siegelman et al. described four reliable angiographic criteria for the diagnosis of mesenteric vasospasm: (1)

narrowing of the origins of multiple branches of the SMA, (2) alternating dilatation and narrowing of the intestinal branches—the "string of sausages" sign, (3) spasm of the mesenteric arcades, and (4) impaired filling of the intramural vessels.[34]

Treatment

The primary treatment of NOMI is medical, with critical care support to correct the systemic condition leading to generalized hypoperfusion. Once NOMI is diagnosed through mesenteric angiogram, intraarterial vasodilators can be infused through an infusion catheter in the SMA. The most common intraarterial agent used is papaverine, a phosphodiesterase inhibitor, but other vasodilators such as prostaglandin E_1 and nitroglycerin are also used.[35,36] Papaverine is initiated at a dose of 30 to 60 mg/h, and often continued for several days as long as the patient's condition remains stable or until there is improvement. Papaverine is metabolized primarily by the liver, so systemic hypotension is uncommon as long as the catheter remains in the SMA. Heparin is chemically incompatible with papaverine and should not be infused simultaneously through the same catheter.

In patients with peritonitis, an operative exploration is required to adequately evaluate bowel viability. For this reason, catheter-based therapy alone is insufficient in patients with peritoneal findings. At the operation, the bowel is inspected for viability and necrotic intestine resected. A handheld Doppler instrument is used to assess the mesenteric vessels proximally and distally. Intravenous fluorescein is also used to evaluate areas of possible ischemia; absent perivascular, or patchy fluorescein patterns represent areas of ischemia.[37] A second-look laparotomy within 24 to 48 hours allows for reassessment of bowel viability, and additional bowel resection can be performed if necessary.

MESENTERIC VENOUS THROMBOSIS

Clinical Presentation

The symptomatic presentation of patients with MVT range from asymptomatic to an acute abdomen with peritoneal signs on physical examination. MVT accounts for 10% to 15% of AMI.[38] Abdominal pain is the most common symptom, but it is typically less severe and more insidious pain than in patients with arterial occlusion. Most patients present after more than 24 hours of symptoms, and many patients may experience pain for 1 month before diagnosis. With transmural bowel infarction, peritoneal findings may be present, in addition to other symptoms. These include nausea, vomiting, and/or gastrointestinal bleeding, which can be present in 20% to 30% of patients. Leukocytosis and metabolic acidosis may accompany MVT that has resulted in bowel infarction.

Predisposing risk factors include malignancy, oral contraceptive usage, sepsis, liver disease or portal hypertension, sickle cell disease, and pancreatitis.[39] Many patients have heritable hematologic disorders including factor V Leiden mutations and deficiencies in proteins C, S, and antithrombin III.

Evaluation

Plain abdominal radiographs can rule out free air suggestive of perforated viscus, but will usually demonstrate a nonspecific bowel gas pattern and are generally nondiagnostic. Currently, contrast-enhanced CT with a portal venous phase is the diagnostic study of choice in patients suspected of having MVT. In addition to MVT, CT can accurately detect portal and ovarian vein thrombosis. Other suggestive findings include bowel-wall thickening, pneumatosis intestinalis, or mesenteric edema.

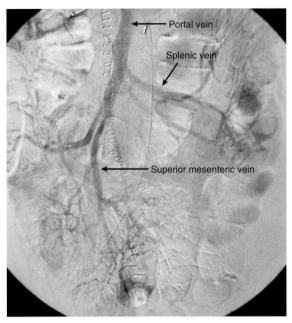

Fig. 26.13 Aortoportography demonstrating patent portal vein, superior mesenteric vein, and splenic vein.

In patients who have minimal abdominal pain or are asymptomatic, duplex ultrasonography may be used to evaluate patency of the mesenteric veins. The examination is performed after a period of fasting, and blood flow velocities within the aorta, inferior vena cava, hepatic veins, portal vein, hepatic artery, splenic vein, and superior mesenteric vein are evaluated. Additional information that can be obtained from duplex ultrasonography includes the presence or absence of ascites, recanalized umbilical vein, and/or liver mass. Duplex ultrasonography is limited in the evaluation of the mesenteric veins when there is severe ascites, recent surgery or liver biopsy, and obesity.

Mesenteric angiography is indicated when associated arterial ischemia is suspected or when findings on abdominal CT are equivocal. The mesenteric venous system cannot be directly punctured, but is visualized indirectly through catheter-directed contrast injections into the SMA and celiac artery, followed by delayed filming (Fig. 26.13). MVT is demonstrated by a filling defect within the mesenteric veins.

Treatment

A mainstay of MVT treatment is to prevent intestinal infarction, or minimize the extent of bowel resection if bowel infarction is present. In patients with peritoneal findings, urgent laparotomy is required. These patients generally have reduced intravascular volume as a result of fluid third-spacing. In addition to urgent anticoagulation, they often need aggressive fluid resuscitation. Findings at laparotomy consist of edema and cyanotic discoloration of the mesentery and bowel wall with thrombus involving the distal mesenteric veins. Complete thrombosis of the superior mesenteric vein is rare, occurring in only 12% of patients undergoing laparotomy for suspected MVT. The arterial supply to the involved bowel is usually intact. Nonviable bowel is resected and primary anastomosis performed. If viability of the remaining bowel is in question, a repeat second-look operation is performed in 24 to 48 hours.

There are reports of successful systemic thrombolysis treatment for extensive MVT with TPA.[40] In recent years, endovascular procedures for the treatment of MVT have been developed and described. These include percutaneous transfemoral or transjugular intrahepatic portosystemic shunting (TIPS) with mechanical aspiration thrombectomy and catheter-directed thrombolysis, percutaneous transhepatic mechanical thrombectomy or thrombolysis, percutaneous thrombolysis via the SMA, and thrombolysis via an operatively placed mesenteric vein catheter.[41-43] Patients should be anticoagulated with heparin following endovascular treatment. Patency of the portal system after TIPS can be evaluated by follow-up Doppler ultrasound. Clearance of the thrombus can be evaluated with CT, but there is not a clear correlation between radiologic findings and clinical symptoms.

There are no large or well-controlled studies to guide recommendations and establish the indication for endovascular treatment of MVT. Most of the endovascular treatments are described in case reports and small series with variable results. Most report success in terms of survival, patency of the portomesenteric veins, lower rates of portal hypertension, and avoidance of bowel resection in selected patients, but endovascular intervention for MVT can be associated with high complication rates.[43]

Most patients are treated successfully with medical treatment alone. In the minority of patients that deteriorate during medical treatment, or in centers where there are sufficient technical expertise and experience, aggressive endovascular therapy can be considered as an adjunct to anticoagulation in patients with acute MVT without infarction.[44]

In patients without peritoneal findings, anticoagulation with intravenous heparin is promptly initiated and the patient is observed with serial abdominal examinations while maintaining bowel rest. Ileus is usually present, and bowel rest and decompression with nasogastric suction is required. Ileus may be prolonged, so total parenteral nutrition should be considered early. Once the patient's clinical status improves, oral intake can be cautiously introduced. A search for a predisposing primary or secondary hypercoagulable condition is required. In the interim, the patient is transitioned to oral anticoagulation over 3 to 4 days once intestinal function has returned. Lifelong anticoagulation is usually maintained, especially in cases of idiopathic MVT or when an uncorrectable hypercoagulable state has been identified.

REFERENCES

1. Biolato M, Miele L, Gasbarrini G, et al. Abdominal angina. *Am J Med Sci.* 2009;338:389–395.
2. Nicholls SC, Kohler TR, Martin RL, et al. Use of hemodynamic parameters in the diagnosis of mesenteric insufficiency. *J Vasc Surg.* 1986;3:507–510.
3. Moneta GL, Yeager RA, Dalman R, et al. Duplex ultrasound criteria for diagnosis of splanchnic artery stenosis or occlusion. *J Vasc Surg.* 1991;14:511–518.
4. Moneta GL, Lee RW, Yeager RA, et al. Mesenteric duplex scanning: a blinded prospective study. *J Vasc Surg.* 1993;17:79–84.
5. Schaefer PJ, Pfarr J, Trentmann J, et al. Comparison of noninvasive imaging modalities for stenosis grading in mesenteric arteries. *Rofo.* 2013;185:628–634.
6. Jaster A, Choudhery S, Ahn R, et al. Anatomic and radiologic review of chronic mesenteric ischemia and its treatment. *Clin Imaging.* 2016;40:961–969.
7. Schermerhorn ML, Giles KA, Hamdan AD, et al. Mesenteric revascularization: management and outcomes in the United States. *J Vasc Surg.* 2009;50:341–348. e1.
8. Atkins MD, Kwolek CJ, LaMuraglia GM, et al. Surgical revascularization versus endovascular therapy for chornic mesenteric ischemia: a comparative experience. *J Vasc Surg.* 2007;45:1162–1171.
9. Wylie EJ, Stoney RJ, Ehrenfeld WK. *Manual of Vascular Surgery.* New York: Springer-Verlag; 1980.
10. McAfee MK, Cherry KJ, Naessens JM, et al. Influence of complete revascularization on chronic mesenteric ischemia. *Am J Surg.* 1992;164:220–224.

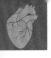
11. Hollier LH, Bernatz PE, Pairolero PC, et al. Surgical management of chronic intestinal ischemia: a reappraisal. *Surgery*. 1991;90:940–946.

12. Foley MI, Moneta GL, Abou-Zamza AM, et al. Revascularization of the superior mesenteric artery alone for treatment of intestinal ischemia. *J Vasc Surg*. 2000;32:37–47.

13. Park WM, Cherry KJ, Chua HK, et al. Current results of open revascularization for chronic mesenteric ischemia: a standard for comparison. *J Vasc Surg*. 2002;35:853–859.

14. White CJ. Chronic mesenteric ischemia: diagnosis and management. *Prog Cardiovasc Dis*. 2011;54:36–40.

15. Gentile AT, Moneta GL, Taylor Jr LM, et al. Isolated bypass to the superior mesenteric artery for intestinal ischemia. *Arch Surg*. 1994;129:926–931.

16. Ahanchi SS, Stout CL, Dahl TJ, et al. Comparative analysis of celiac versus mesenteric artery outcomes after angioplasty and stenting. *J Vasc Surg*. 2013;57:1062–1066.

17. Wohlauer M, Kobeiter H, Desgranges P, et al. Inferior mesenteric artery stenting as a novel treatment for chronic mesenteric ischemia in patients with an occluded superior mesenteric artery and celiac trunk. *Eur J Vasc Endovasc Surg*. 2014;27:e21–e23.

18. van Petersen AS, Kolkman JJ, Beuk RJ, et al. Open or percutaneous revascularization for chronic splanchnic syndrome. *J Vasc Surg*. 2010;51:1309–1316.

19. Ryer EJ, Oderich GS, Bower TC, et al. Differences in anatomy and outcomes in patients treated with open mesenteric revascularization before and after the endovascular era. *J Vasc Surg*. 2011;53:1611–1618. e2.

20. Hogendoorn W, Hunink MG, Schlösser FJ, et al. A comparison of open and endovascular revascularization for chronic mesenteric ischemia in a clinical decision model. *J Vasc Surg*. 2014;60:715–725. e2.

21. Schoch DM, LeSar CJ, Joels CS, et al. Management of chronic mesenteric vascular insufficiency: an endovascular approach. *J Am Coll Surg*. 2011;212:668–675.

22. Oderich GS, Erodes LS, Lesar C, et al. Comparison of covered stents versus bare metal stents for treatment of chronic atherosclerotic mesenteric arterial disease. *J Vasc Surg*. 2013;58:1316–1323.

23. Mitchell EL, Chang EY, Landry GJ, et al. Duplex criteria for native superior mesenteric artery stenosis overestimates stenosis in stented superior mesenteric arteries. *J Vasc Surg*. 2009;50:335–340.

24. Aburahma AF, Mousa AY, Stone PA, et al. Duplex velocity criteria for native celiac/superior mesenteric artery stenosis vs in-stent stenosis. *J Vasc Surg*. 2012;55:730–738.

25. Soult MC, Wuamett JC, Ahanchi SS, et al. Duplex ultrasound criteria for in-stent restenosis of mesenteric arteries. *J Vasc Surg*. 2016;64:1366–1372.

26. Liem TK, Segall JA, Wei W, et al. Duplex scan characteristics of bypass grafts to mesenteric arteries. *J Vasc Surg*. 2007;45:922–927.

27. Ryer EJ, Kalra M, Oderich GS, et al. Revascularization for acute mesenteric ischemia. *J Vasc Surg*. 2012;55:1682–1699.

28. Menke J. Diagnostic accuracy of multidetector CT in acute mesenteric ischemia: systematic review and meta-analysis. *Radiology*. 2010;256: 93–101.

29. Morgan CE, Mansukhani NA, Eskandari MK, Rodriguez HE. Ten-year review of isolated spontaneous mesenteric arterial dissections. *J Vasc Surg*. 2018;67:1134–1142.

30. Calin GA, Calin S, Ionescu R, et al. Successful local fibrinolytic treatment and balloon angioplasty in superior mesenteric arterial embolism: a case report and literature review. *Hepatogastroenterology*. 2003;50:732–734.

31. Michel C, Laffy P, Leblanc G, et al. Intra-arterial fibrinolytic therapy for acute mesenteric ischemia. *J Radiol*. 2001;82:55–58.

32. Wyers MC, Powell RJ, Nolan BW, Cronenwett JL. Retrograde mesenteric stenting during laparotomy for acute occlusive mesenteric ischemia. *J Vasc Surg*. 2007;45:269–275.

33. Bassiouny HS. Nonocclusive mesenteric ischemia. *Surg Clin North Am*. 1997;7:319–326.

34. Siegelman SS, Sprayregen S, Boley SJ. Angiographic diagnosis of mesenteric arterial vasoconstriction. *Radiology*. 1974;112:533–542.

35. Luckner G, Jochberger S, Mayr VD, et al. Vasopressiin as adjunct vasopressor for vasodilatory shock due to non-occlusive mesenteric ischemia. *Anaesthesist*. 2006;55:283–286.

36. Niederhäuser U, Genoni M, von Segesser LK, et al. Mesenteric ischemia after a cardiac operation: conservative treatment with local vasodilation. *Ann Thorac Surg*. 1996;61:1817–1819.

37. Bergman R, Gloviczki P, Welch T, et al. The role of intravenous fluorescein in the detection of colon ischemia during aortic reconstruction. *Ann Vasc Surg*. 1992;6:74–79.

38. Singh M, Long B, Koyfman A. Mesenteric ischemia: a deadly miss. *Emerg Med Clin North Am*. 2017;35:879–888.

39. Lewiss R, Egan D, Shreves A. Vascular abdominal emergencies. *Emerg Med Cliun North Am*. 2011;29:253–272.

40. Hrstic I, Kalauz M, Cukovic-Cavka S, et al. Treatment of extensive subacute portal, mesenteric and ileocolic vein thrombosis with recombinant tissue plasminogen activator. *Blood Coagul Fibrinolysis*. 2007;18:581–583.

41. Wang MQ, Liu FY, Duan F, et al. Acute symptomatic mesenteric venous thrombosis: treatment by catheter-directed thrombolysis with transjugular intrahepatic route. *Abd Imaging*. 2011;36:390–398.

42. Takahashi N, Kuroki K, Yanaga K. Percutaneous transhepatic mechanical thrombectomy for acute mesenteric venous thrombosis. *J Endovasc Ther*. 2005;12:508–511.

43. Di Minno M, Milone F, Milone M, et al. Endovascular thrombolysis in acute mesenteric vein thrombosis: a 3-year follow-up with the rate of short and long-term sequaelae in 32 patients. *Thromb Res*. 2010;126: 295–598.

44. Harnik IG, Brandt LJ. Mesenteric venous thrombosis. *Vasc Med*. 2010;15:407–418.

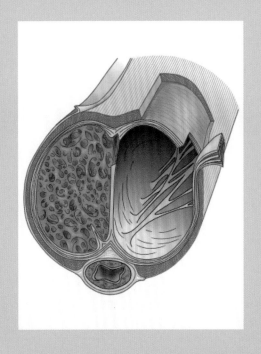

PART VII

第七部分

Vasculogenic Erectile
Dysfunction

血管源性勃起功能障碍

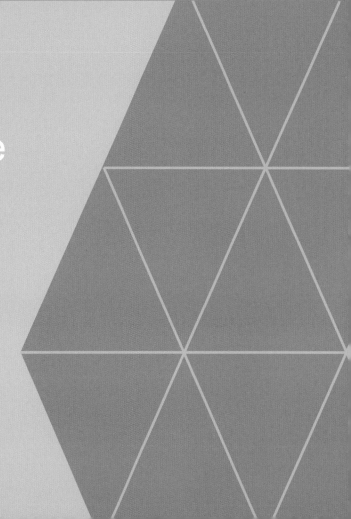

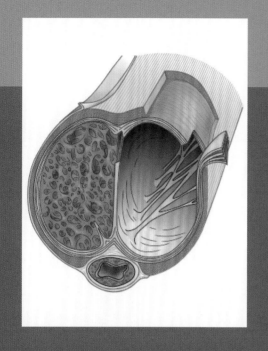

第27章
血管源性勃起功能障碍

　　第一次对勃起功能障碍的描述可以追溯到4000多年前埃及金字塔时代，那个时代的埃及学者将勃起功能障碍分为2种形式，一种是"自然"的男性不能进行性生活，另一种是"超自然"的勃起功能障碍，即来自诅咒。第一次对阴茎解剖等的准确描述是1585年，当时认为阴茎是由神经、静脉、动脉、两层白膜"韧带"和尿道等组成的。经过数个世纪对男性勃起在血流动力学和解剖机制方面的研究，才在过去30年中确定了现代阴茎勃起的生理学定义。该理论关于阴茎勃起生理学的中心意义是平滑肌作用在其中起到至关重要的作用，而平滑肌作用受动脉和静脉血流、白膜结构、作为主要神经递质的一氧化氮（NO）等因素的调节可使阴茎勃起，受磷酸二酯酶的调节可使勃起消退。近年来有专家对内皮细胞对平滑肌作用的调节、离子通道和内皮细胞缝隙连接的完整性进行研究，使我们对勃起生理功能的理解进一步加深。该章节对以上这些新发现，以及勃起功能障碍的患病率、临床评估、诊断试验、药物和外科治疗、公共卫生可能的影响及关于血管源性勃起功能障碍的最新指南进行了详细的论述。

张小明

Vasculogenic Erectile Dysfunction

Annie L. Darves-Bornoz, Kirk A. Keegan, and David F. Penson

The first historical descriptions of erectile dysfunction (ED) date back to Egyptian papyrus, nearly 4000 years ago. Egyptian scholars described two types of ED: a "natural" form in which the man was not capable of performing the sex act and a "supernatural" form rooted in evil charms and spells.[1] Ancient thinkers, such as Hippocrates and Aristotle, also theorized on the etiology of ED. However, the first accurate depiction of penile anatomy and rudimentary analysis of erection was not published until 1585, when Ambroise Paré described it in his *Ten Books on Surgery* and the *Book of Reproduction*.[2] In these texts, Paré portrayed the penis as a tube with concentric coats of nerves, veins, arteries, two "ligaments" composed of the corpora cavernosa, and the urinary tract.

Over the succeeding centuries, there has been considerable investigation into the hemodynamic and anatomic mechanisms of the male erection. The modern understanding of erectile physiology has been delineated only in the past 30 years. Central to our current theories of erectile physiology is the role of smooth muscle in control of arterial and venous flow, the architecture of the tunica albuginea, the role of nitric oxide (NO) as the principal neurotransmitter regulating tumescence, and the function of phosphodiesterases (PDEs) for detumescence. Recent research on the role of endothelial regulation of smooth muscle, the influence of ion channels, and the integral function of endothelial gap junctions has furthered our understanding. This chapter will review these findings, as well as the prevalence, clinical evaluation, diagnostic testing, medical and surgical management, public health implications, and current guidelines regarding vasculogenic ED in detail.

DEFINITION AND CLASSIFICATIONS

In 1992 the National Institutes of Health convened a Consensus Development Conference on Impotence. The group renamed impotence as "male erectile dysfunction" and defined it as "the inability to achieve or maintain an erection sufficient for satisfactory sexual performance."[3] Furthermore, they noted that ED represents the most appropriate term, given that sexual desire, orgasm, and ejaculation may be intact, despite the inability to achieve or maintain erection.

Multiple schema have been proposed to classify the different types of ED. Broadly, ED can be described in terms of organic and psychogenic dysfunction (Box 27.1). The main thrust of this chapter will center on vasculogenic ED, which is composed of impaired endothelial function, arterial occlusive disease, veno-occlusive dysfunction, and structural changes to the corpora cavernosa.

EPIDEMIOLOGY

Prevalence and Incidence

ED is quite common, affecting approximately 30 million men in the United States.[4] Several population-based studies have been performed to address male sexual function and specifically the prevalence and incidence of ED in the American male population. The National Health Social and Life Survey (NHSLS) was a national cross-sectional interview survey in 1992 of 1410 American men between the ages of 18 and 59 years. In the study group, the prevalence of ED in men aged 18 to 29 years was 7%, aged 30 to 39 was 9%, aged 40 to 49 was 11%, and aged 50 to 59 was 18%.[5] The Massachusetts Male Aging Study (MMAS), a longitudinal population-based study, evaluated 1709 men between the ages of 40 and 70 years who returned questionnaires about a broad range of physiologic measures, demographic information, and self-reported sexual function. The participants were surveyed between the years 1987 and 1989 and then reevaluated between 1995 and 1997. In this series, the age-adjusted prevalence of significant ED was 39% in men with coronary artery disease, 25% in men with diabetes mellitus, and 15% in men with hypertension. The incidence of ED on reevaluation was 25.9 cases per 1000 men per year (95% confidence interval [CI], 22.5 to 29.9).[6] Using these data, it was estimated that for white men, 617,715 new cases of ED would present in the 40 to 69 age group each year.[7] Data from European and Brazilian researchers suggest a similar incidence of ED in their respective countries.[8,9]

PUBLIC HEALTH AND CLINICAL IMPLICATIONS

The prevalence of ED is expected to increase as the incidence of obesity and cardiovascular and metabolic disease increase. As of 1995 an estimated 152 million men worldwide had ED, and this is predicted to increase to 322 million men by 2025.[10] ED is often referred to as a "canary in a coal mine" because it can be an indication of underlying systemic vascular disease. The National Health and Nutritional Examination Survey (NHANES) cross-sectional study revealed that 90% of men with ED had at least one major cardiovascular risk factor (diabetes mellitus, hypercholesterolemia, hypertension, smoking).[11] Furthermore, several longitudinal studies have shown that men with ED are at an increased risk for serious cardiac events and mortality compared with men without ED.[11,12] A recent follow-up to the NHANES cohort found that the men who reported ED at the time

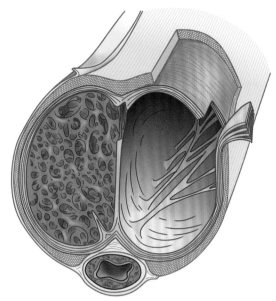

Fig. 27.1 Drawing of three-dimensional anatomy of human penis, demonstrating inner circular layers and outer longitudinal layers of the tunica albuginea, intervening supports, sinusoidal tissue in corpora cavernosa, corpus spongiosum, and urethra.

of the initial study were found to have a 70% increased risk of premature all-cause mortality over the duration of the study.[13] This led the Princeton Consensus Conference (PCC), a multispecialty collaborative tradition dedicated to optimizing sexual function and preserving cardiovascular health, to issue new recommendations concerning the work-up of ED. Held in 2010, the third PCC added recommendations for stringent evaluation and management of cardiovascular risk in men with ED and no known cardiovascular disease (CVD).[14] These recommendations will be discussed further when discussing management of ED.

Although ED has traditionally been thought of as a disease of the older man, the global epidemic of obesity and associated comorbidities has led to an increase in the rate of ED in younger men.[15] Obesity is an independent risk factor for ED, with a recent study revealing rates of ED in 22.4% versus 13.4% of men with a body mass index $>30 \text{ kg/m}^2$ and $<25 \text{ kg/m}^2$, respectively.[16] Diabetes mellitus is a major risk factor of ED given its vascular, neurologic, and endocrine disturbances; and we have likewise seen increased prevalence of diabetes in the younger population.[17]

FUNCTIONAL ANATOMY

The functional anatomy of the human penis is composed of several key components. Principally, these are three cylindrical structures—two corpora cavernosa surrounded by a tough tunica albuginea and the solitary corpus spongiosum, which contains the urethra. The vascular components include arteries and arterioles, highly compliant sinusoids within the corpora cavernosa, and compressible venules and veins.

Corporal Bodies, Sinusoids, and Glans

The corpora cavernosa are paired, spongy cylinders that lie on the superior aspect of the penis. They are enveloped by the tunica albuginea. The proximal ends of the corpora are separate structures anchored at the ischial ramus. The corpora then fuse underneath the pubic ramus and share a common septum distally towards the glans.

Within the corpora, interconnected sinusoids are enveloped by trabeculae of smooth muscle, collagen, and elastin (Fig. 27.1). The sinusoidal smooth muscle is in intimate association with the cavernous nerves and the helicine arteries within the penis. The sinusoids are tonically constricted during the flaccid state. Arterial blood flow diffuses

through larger central sinusoids to smaller peripheral sinusoids. In the flaccid state, this slow diffusion of arterial blood results in blood gas values similar to venous blood. During sexual stimulation, a release of neurotransmitters causes the smooth muscle around the sinusoids to relax. This results in the rapid influx of arterial blood, subsequent entrapment of blood within these expanding sinusoids, and occlusion of veins traversing the tunica albuginea. Subsequent tumescence results in pressure increases of several hundred millimeters of mercury and blood gas values approaching arterial levels.[18]

The interior of the glans and corpus spongiosum share a similar sinusoidal architecture as the corpora cavernosa. However, the tunica surrounding the spongiosum is thinner and is completely absent around the glans. The corpus spongiosum is a highly compliant body that houses the urethra and facilitates the expulsion of semen. The glans is exquisitely sensitive and conical in shape, eases intromission, and forms a cushion for the rigid corporal bodies. These areas engorge in a similar fashion as the corpora cavernosa, however to a lesser degree, largely due to an absence of the tunica albuginea and diminished venous trapping.

Tunica Albuginea

The tunica albuginea is composed primarily of tough type 1 collagen with a minority component of more flexible type III collagen and elastin. It is arranged in a bilayer, with inner circular layers and outer longitudinal layers (see Fig. 27.1). Intervening struts traverse the body of the corpora cavernosa and provide further support.[19] The longitudinal layers of the tunica are present from the glans to the proximal crura, where each corporal body inserts into its ischial ramus to form a foundation for support of the erect penis. Emissary veins (Fig. 27.2) pierce the tunica albuginea. During engorgement, these veins become compressed and allow entrapment of blood within the penis.

Arterial System

The internal pudendal artery, a branch of the internal iliac artery, is the principal source of blood flow to the penis. Up to 70% of men may have

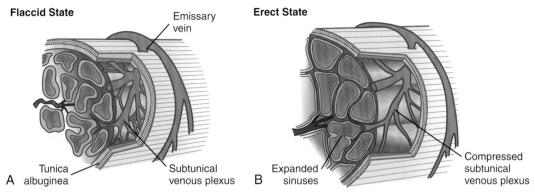

Fig. 27.2 Penile Erection. (A) When flaccid, the corpora cavernosa, including arterioles, sinusoids, and arteries, are contracted. This allows free flow of blood through intervening sinusoidal spaces. Blood exits the corpora cavernosa via emissary veins. (B) During erection, arterioles, sinusoids, and arteries relax. This constricts venules and veins and effectively compresses emissary veins under the tunica albuginea. Vascular inflow exceeds outflow, effectively creating an erection.

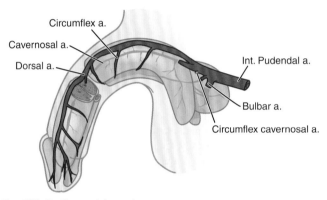

Fig. 27.3 Penile arterial supply.

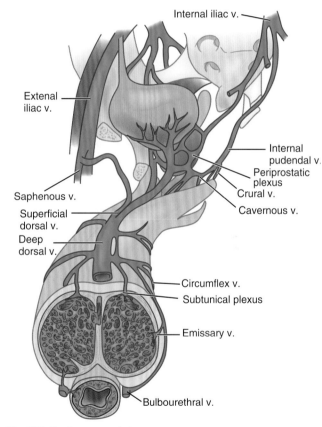

Fig. 27.4 Penile venous drainage.

accessory pudendal branches that originate from the external iliac, obturator, or vesical arteries.[20] The internal pudendal artery gives rise to the penile artery, which in turn branches into the dorsal, bulbourethral, and cavernous arteries (Fig. 27.3). The cavernous artery supplies the corpus cavernosum via helicine arteries, which lie in close approximation to the sinusoidal tissue. During erection, these vessels dilate, resulting in engorgement.

Venous System

The venous drainage originates from the three corporal bodies. Venules interdigitate through the cavernosal sinusoids and coalesce below the tunica albuginea into a subtunical plexus. The plexi then form emissary veins that penetrate the tunica albuginea. From there, numerous subcutaneous veins course along the shaft of the penis to form the superficial dorsal vein and a deep dorsal venous system, which in turn drain into the saphenous vein and retropubic venous plexus, respectively (Fig. 27.4; see Fig. 27.2).[21]

Nervous System

Penile innervation occurs via both autonomic (parasympathetic and sympathetic) and somatic (motor and sensory) pathways. Erection and detumescence are largely regulated via the autonomic system. Sympathetic and parasympathetic nerves coalesce to form the cavernous nerve, which penetrates the corpora cavernosa to exert its effect on erection (Fig. 27.5). Sensation and contraction of penile musculature occurs via the somatic nerves.

Autonomic Pathways

Between the 11th thoracic and 2nd lumbar spinal segments, the sympathetic trunk begins. These fibers then form the sympathetic chain ganglia, which continue caudally to the inferior mesenteric and superior hypogastric plexi. Further sympathetic fibers exit to form the hypogastric nerves and ultimately the sympathetic portions of the pelvic plexus.[22]

Between the second, third, and fourth sacral spinal cord segments, the parasympathetic pathway originates. These fibers also continue caudally to the pelvic plexus (see Fig. 27.5), where they join

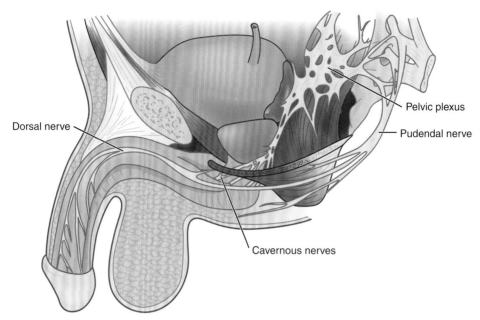

Fig. 27.5 Penile nerves.

the aforementioned sympathetic nerves. Together, these nerves then join to form a network of nervous tissue that passes along the lateral and posterior aspect of the prostate, to create the cavernous nerves.[23] Stimulation of the sympathetic trunk, via the cavernous nerves, results in detumescence. Excitation of the parasympathetic aspects of the pelvic plexus and cavernous nerves is responsible for erection. A clear understanding of the location of these nerves is critical during pelvic surgery, such as radical prostatectomy or abdominal perineal resection, to avoid iatrogenic ED.

Somatic Pathways

The sensory receptors in the penile skin and glans are unique in the human body.[24] They are composed of free nerve endings composed of unmyelinated C fibers and thin myelinated A-lamba fibers. These nerve fibers coalesce into the dorsal nerve of the penis, which ultimately forms the pudendal nerve. The pudendal nerve then enters the S2 to S4 nerve roots at the spinal cord. Via spinothalamic and spinoreticular pathways, sensations such as touch, pain, and temperature are perceived.[25] Interestingly, research by Burnett and colleagues[26] suggests that the dorsal nerve of the penis carries both autonomic and somatic signals and therefore contributes to penile sensation, erection, and ejaculation.

PATHOPHYSIOLOGY OF ERECTILE DYSFUNCTION

Vasculogenic Erectile Dysfunction

As noted in Box 27.1, ED often represents a multifactorial disease state. Although the focus of this chapter is on the vasculogenic determinants of ED, it is worth noting that within an individual patient, neurologic, hormonal, or psychological etiologies of ED may be of contributory or even primary importance. With that said, it is clear that the vascular system is responsible for providing blood flow to the erectile tissues of the penis. Therefore any dysfunction within the vascular system, may affect erectile function.

Arteriogenic Erectile Dysfunction

Arteriogenic ED can be the result of atherosclerotic or traumatic arterial occlusive disease. Michal and Ruzbarsky[27] noted that

impaired penile perfusion is an indicator of generalized atherosclerotic disease and that the age of onset of ED and coronary artery disease is often similar. As discussed previously, ED has been shown to be a bellwether for the development of coronary artery disease in asymptomatic men,[28] and both diseases share the same risk factors, specifically, smoking, diabetes, hypercholesterolemia, and hypertension.[29] In arteriogenic ED, the corpora cavernosa demonstrate lower oxygen tension,[30] which may result in a decreased volume of sinusoidal smooth muscle and subsequent venous leak.[31] In an experimental animal model, rabbits with iatrogenic iliac atherosclerotic disease demonstrated alterations in their downstream penile arteries and a reduction in cavernosal smooth muscle content.[32] These alterations were associated with decreased nitric oxide synthase (NOS) and NO-mediated relaxation of corpora cavernosal tissue.[33] ED due to traumatic stenosis of cavernous or pudendal arteries has been noted in young men with pelvic trauma[34] and in long distance cyclists.[35]

Venogenic Erectile Dysfunction

Not only can diabetes, hypertension, hypercholesterolemia, and penile injury result in penile arterial disease, but these disorders can result in a loss of elastic fibers within the cavernosal venules and sinusoids. This loss of compliance results in diminished venous trapping and subsequent veno-occlusive dysfunction.[36] In fact, diminished venous occlusion may represent the most common form of vasculogenic ED.[37] The loss of smooth muscle relaxation due to heightened adrenergic tone or decreased NO release may exacerbate already poor compliance in these fibrotic sinusoids.[38] Finally, fibrosis leading to increased collagen deposition between cell membranes may abolish critical signaling and intercellular transmission via disrupted gap junctions.[39]

Drug-Induced (Iatrogenic) Erectile Dysfunction

The data are clear that diabetes, hypercholesterolemia, and hypertension have strong influence on ED. Not surprisingly, some of the medications used to treat these disorders have been implicated as contributing factors in the development of ED. However, it is often difficult to ascertain the direction of causation in medication-induced ED.

Of the cardiovascular medications, thiazide diuretics have the strongest association with the development of ED. Chang and colleagues[40] demonstrated that men treated with thiazide diuretics showed a significant increase in ED relative to those men prescribed placebo medication. Further evidence of the role of thiazides in ED was noted in the Treatment of Mild Hypertension Study (TOMHS). This study demonstrated that the prevalence of ED was twofold higher in men taking a thiazide versus placebo or other agent.[41] Curiously, after 4 years of treatment in this study, the prevalence of ED within the placebo group approached that of those receiving thiazide. The significance of this finding is not clear but may be related to the early unmasking of clinically undetected ED in those men receiving thiazides. Nonselective β-blockers such as propranolol have been shown to inhibit erection compared with placebo, but this has not been demonstrated in the selective β₁-antagonists.[42] In clinical series, there does not appear to be a deleterious influence of angiotensin-converting enzyme inhibitors nor calcium channel blockers on erection.[33,43] Interestingly, in clinical series, angiotensin receptor antagonists and some statins, such as atorvastatin, appear to improve erectile function.[44,45] Of note, some α-blockers such as terazosin have occasionally been implicated in the development of priapism, or pathologic erection, likely related to the α-adrenergic blockade of the sympathetic outflow necessary for detumescence.[46] Other medications implicated in the development of ED include: spironolactone, some antipsychotics, selective serotonin reuptake inhibitors, opiates, and antiandrogens.[47] One of the most common drug offenders causing ED and decreased libido in younger males is finasteride (i.e., proprecia, proscar), which is commonly used for hair loss and prostatic hyperplasia.[48]

EVALUATION OF ERECTILE DYSFUNCTION

The evaluation and treatment of a man presenting with ED have changed considerably over the past 30 years. This shift is largely due to the influence of oral therapies for treatment and a transition to a more patient-centered and evidence-based treatment plan. The evaluation of a man with ED should begin with an in-person and detailed medical, sexual, and psychosocial history (Fig. 27.6). In addition, the use of a quantifiable questionnaire such as the International Index of Erectile Function (IIEF)[49] may be useful to establish baseline sexual function and to assess future treatment efficacy.

History

The history should begin with a thorough discussion of the patient's medical history, with particular attention to medical comorbidities. As previously mentioned, ED is an early marker for systemic atherosclerotic disease and all patients should be questioned about their cardiovascular health.[50] In particular, a detailed discussion regarding any chest pain, palpitations, dyspnea, and limb pain may reveal occult coronary artery disease, congestive heart failure, or peripheral artery disease. In addition, querying the patient about his medication use may elucidate medications that contribute to ED or that may be a contraindication to oral PDE therapy, such as nitrates. A sexual history should focus on the timing, duration, and severity of the patient's ED, as well as the occurrence of other associated problems, such as premature ejaculation, desire, or anorgasmia. To complete the sexual history, a psychosocial evaluation may be relevant because sexual dysfunction may affect self-esteem and coping. Both depression and treatment for depression may be associated with ED.

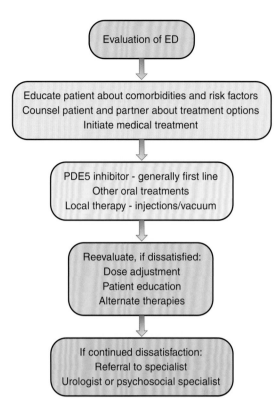

Fig. 27.6 Algorithm for evaluation of erectile dysfunction *(ED)*. *PDE5*, Phosphodiesterase 5. (Modified from Lue TF, Giuliano F, Montorsi F, et al. Summary of the recommendations on sexual dysfunctions in men. *J Sex Med.* 2004;1:6–23; and Lue TF, Broderick GA. Evaluation and nonsurgical management of erectile dysfunction and premature ejaculation. In: Wein AJ, Kavoussi LR, Nocik AC, et al, eds. *Campbell-Walsh Urology.* 9th ed. Philadelphia: Saunders; 2007:751–752.)

Physical Examination

The physical examination may be equally revealing. The general appearance of the patient may alert the physician to serious underlying CVD if the patient is cyanotic, dyspneic, emaciated, or plethoric. Additional pertinent findings on physical examination include general body habitus, secondary sex characteristics, staining of fingers associated with smoking, nail clubbing, lower extremity ulcers, or edema. A thorough cardiopulmonary examination is required. Finally, an examination of the genitalia may demonstrate chordee, Peyronie disease, or signs of hypogonadism such as Kallman or Klinefelter syndrome.

Laboratory Assessments

Laboratory testing for men with sexual dysfunction may include fasting glucose, lipid levels, and sex hormone values (including morning free and total testosterone levels) and other endocrine tests, such as thyroid function tests and prolactin levels. Again, this testing may reveal comorbid conditions such as diabetes, hyperlipidemia, or hypogonadism that may contribute to ED. Although controversial, the most recent PCC recommended checking testosterone levels in all men with ED, especially those who have failed medical therapy, because low testosterone levels have been correlated with increased CVD.[14]

Education and Referral

Due to the advent of oral PDE inhibitors, the majority of initial ED consultations occur in the primary care physician's office, with referrals made as indicated. It is important to review with the patient the likely etiologies, pertinent anatomy and physiology, and potential treatment options. Given the strong correlation between ED and CVD noted in many recent studies, providers may wish to consider further evaluation of CVD in the patient with ED and no known CVD. The Framingham Risk Score (FRS) may be used as a starting point for risk stratification and estimating likelihood of subclinical atherosclerosis in men with ED. However, the FRS may underestimate the presence of CVD, especially in the younger man, given the small number of younger males in the initial longitudinal studies from Framingham. To this end, it is important to consider other risk factors of CVD not included in the FRS (e.g., family history, fasting glucose level, creatinine, and potentially, testosterone level).[14] Further cardiac evaluation may be warranted at the discretion of the patient's primary care physician.

Regardless of whether a patient initially elects to try medical therapy for ED, it is imperative to discuss modifiable risk factors with patients presenting with ED. These include weight loss, exercise, smoking cessation, alcohol abuse, and medication use—all of which may contribute to ED. Recent studies have shown a demonstrable and independent improvement in erectile function when patients undertake smoking cessation or weight loss or increase in physical activity.[51] The promise of improved erectile function may provide a tangible motivator for patients to implement these positive health behaviors.

If focal vascular injury is suspected for the etiology of a patient's ED, further evaluation of the penile vascular system may be undertaken. Although rarely performed and usually only after an empiric trial of oral PDE-5 inhibitors, first-line urologic evaluation of penile blood flow consists of a combined intracavernous injection of a single or combination of vasodilators and some form of penile stimulation. This testing allows the urologist to evaluate the specific mechanics of the erectile response and to avoid the confounding influence of neurologic or hormonal factors. Second line urologic evaluation includes intracavernous injection of a vasodilator and blood flow measurement with duplex ultrasonography, possibly Doppler waveform analysis, and peak systolic velocity calculations. Third-line evaluations may include calculations of cavernous arterial systolic occlusion pressures (CASOP), pharmacologic arteriography, pharmacologic cavernosometry, or cavernosography with injection of contrast dye to localize lesion.[52] These increasingly invasive procedures are often reserved for young men who have failed medical therapy and with traumatic pelvic or penile arterial injuries that are considered candidates for arterial revascularization.

TREATMENT

As noted previously, the initial step in penile tumescence is arousal and subsequent release of NO into vascular and cavernous smooth muscle cells. This causes stimulation of guanylyl cyclase with a concomitant rise in cyclic guanosine monophosphate (cGMP) and a resultant reduction of cytoplasmic calcium. This leads to smooth muscle relaxation, increased arterial inflow, venous trapping, and subsequent erection.[53] With the discovery that PDE inhibitors prevent the breakdown of cGMP[54] and ensuing US Food and Drug Administration (FDA) approval of sildenafil in 1998, a new era in ED treatment was born.

Oral Agents

Sildenafil was the first specific PDE inhibitor to be approved for the treatment of ED. Vardenafil and tadalafil have since followed

suit. Multiple PDE subtypes have been identified; however, PDE-5 is present in high concentrations in corpora cavernosal tissues. As such, sildenafil, vardenafil, and tadalafil represent specific PDE-5 inhibitors. The three medications appear to have equivalent efficacy and are generally well tolerated. Primary side effects include visual disturbances, flushing, and dyspepsia. Vardenafil should be avoided in patients who take type-1A antiarrhythmics such as quinidine or procainamide, type-3 antiarrhythmics such as sotalol or amiodarone, or in patients with congenital prolonged QT syndrome. All three medications should be avoided in patients taking nitrates. Each medication requires approximately 15 minutes to 1 hour to be effective. The half-lives of sildenafil and vardenafil are shorter, at approximately 5 hours, whereas the half-life of tadalafil is approximately 18 hours. For those patients who do not respond to oral treatment or who are not candidates for oral PDE-5 inhibitors, there are a number of other options available, although all are more invasive.

Alprostadil (Prostaglandin E1)

Prostaglandin E1 (PGE1) mediates relaxation of corporal cavernosal tissue by the activation of prostaglandin receptors and subsequent increased cyclic adenosine monophosphate (cAMP) levels in the corporal smooth muscle. Elevated cAMP results in a reduction of cytosolic calcium and subsequent smooth muscle relaxation. Alprostadil is formulated for both intraurethral placement and intracavernosal injection. The intraurethral administration occurs via a pellet approximately 3 mm in size and is placed 2 to 3 cm within the distal urethra. The medication is absorbed via the urethral mucosa and passes through the corpus spongiosum and then via the emissary veins. The medication passes in to the corpora cavernosa to exert its vasodilatory effects. The efficacy of intraurethral alprostadil is approximately 66% in office placement and approximately 50% in home placement.[55] Penile pain is often a significant side effect of alprostadil treatment.

Intracavernous injection of alprostadil works by the same mechanism as intraurethral placement. Researchers have noted higher efficacy with intracavernosal placement. However, alprostadil is still limited by pain during erections in 16.8% of patients, penile fibrosis in 2%, hematoma at the injection site in 1.5%, and priapism in 1.3% of patients.[56] Alprostadil is formulated in a powder and must be reconstituted and refrigerated.

Papaverine and Phentolamine

Other injectable agents include papaverine and phentolamine. Papaverine exerts its effect on penile erectile tissue by an inhibitory action on PDE resulting in increased cAMP and cGMP, as well as inhibition of voltage-gated calcium channels. These mechanisms each result in cavernosal smooth muscle relaxation and subsequent erection. Its efficacy is approximately 50%, although it has not been expressly approved by the FDA for use in ED therapy. The incidence of priapism may be as high as 33% in patients receiving solitary papaverine treatment. In addition, there is high incidence of penile fibrosis with this form of treatment.[43] Phentolamine is also used for injection therapy but works by a different mechanism. It functions as a competitive α-adrenergic antagonist. It is postulated to induce erection by releasing sympathetic tone and thereby increasing corporal blood flow. Systemic hypotension, reflex tachycardia, and nasal congestion are its principal side effects.[57]

Typically, these drugs are used in two or three drug combinations, which allow dose reductions of each medication, increased efficacy approaching 90%, and decreased rates of pain, fibrosis, and priapism.

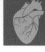

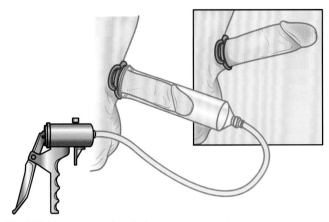

Fig. 27.7 Vacuum erection device.

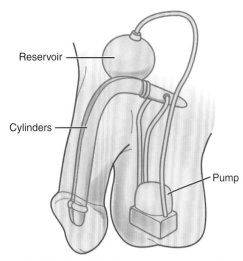

Reservoir

Cylinders

Pump

Fig. 27.8 Surgically implanted inflatable penile prosthesis.

For those men unwilling or unable to inject themselves to induce erections, several other options exist.

Vacuum Erection Devices

In 1917 Otto Lederer was awarded the first patent for a surgical device to induce and maintain erection.[58] Since then, the vacuum erection device (VED) has been modified and perfected, yet the principal remains the same. The VED consists of a cylinder and suction pump that induces erection by negative pressure and subsequent increased corporal flow. A compression band is then placed at the base of the penis to trap the engorged blood (Fig. 27.7). The erection is different than a physiologic erection, in that girth is increased and the penis is cooler and less rigid than a natural erection. However, success rates are good, and patient and partner satisfaction are high. Cookson and Nadig noted a 90% chance of achieving a good-quality erection, with satisfaction rates greater than 80%.[59] For those patients failing the aforementioned treatments, surgery is typically reserved as the final treatment option.

Surgery

In 1936 a Russian surgeon named Bogoraz was the first person to create a functional autologous penile implant. He used rib cartilage in an attempt to correct ED. Although innovative, his success with this treatment was limited largely due to resorption of the cartilage.[60] In 1973 Scott ushered in the modern era of penile implantation with the development of the three-piece inflatable penile prosthesis.[61] Penile prostheses are typically reserved for those men with organic ED who have failed or rejected treatments such as oral medications, VEDs, intraurethral alprostadil, or injection therapy. Three classes of penile implants exist: malleable, semirigid, and inflatable. Malleable and semirigid prostheses are typically placed via a distal penile approach. The inflatable prosthesis comes either as a two-piece or three-piece model that is composed of inflatable cylinders, tubing, a pump mechanism, and a reservoir (Fig. 27.8). Typically these are placed under general anesthetic, via a penoscrotal or infraumbilical incision. Infection rates vary from 3% to 8%.[62] Patient and partner satisfaction is greater than 90%, and freedom from mechanical failure ranges between 80% and 95% at 5 years.[63]

Vascular Surgery

During the 1970s and 1980s, surgery for arteriogenic ED was performed routinely. However, a more contemporary understanding of the pathophysiology of ED has limited the use of vascular surgery for ED. We now understand that ED often represents a systemic disruption of vascular smooth muscle. Currently, the only group where penile revascularization surgery is likely to be successful is in nonsmoking, nondiabetic, young men who have no demonstrable venous leak and have stenosis of the internal pudendal artery due to trauma or congenital causes. As noted previously, these patients should undergo dynamic infusion cavernosography and cavernosometry (DICC) to rule out veno-occlusive dysfunction before embarking on surgical treatment.

LONGITUDNAL PSYCHOLOGICAL OUTCOMES

There is significant interplay between psychological health and ED. However, the direction of that relationship is not always clear. Few studies have evaluated the psychological benefit from ED treatment or baseline psychological characteristics of men with ED. In 2006 we evaluated 153 men in an observational ED registry and collected clinical and psychosocial data at baseline and during follow-up. Of those patients who responded to treatment, these men reported significant improvements in sexual self-efficacy, whereas nonresponders reported small decrements. Surprisingly, nearly 42% of the patients describing ED were not offered treatment by their physicians.[64] Given the benefits in psychologic health suggested by this study and the high incidence of occult CVD noted in previous studies, this should be a call to all healthcare providers to actively diagnose and treat ED in their patients.

GUIDELINES

In 2005 the American Urologic Association convened a consensus group of experts within the discipline of ED.[55] These guidelines were again validated in 2011. The committee created a set of guidelines to help clarify the standard of care, recommended treatments, and expert opinion in the treatment of ED. The primary findings of these guidelines are presented in Box 27.2 and form the basis of current standard practice.

BOX 27.2 American Urological Association Management Guidelines for Erectile Dysfunction

Standards of Care

- Oral phosphodiesterase type 5 (PDE5) inhibitors, unless contraindicated, should be offered as a first line of therapy for erectile dysfunction.
- PDE5 inhibitors are contraindicated in patients who are taking organic nitrates.
- The initial trial dose of alprostadil intraurethral suppositories should be administered under healthcare provider supervision due to the risk of syncope.
- The initial trial dose of intracavernous injection therapy should be administered under healthcare provider supervision.
- Physicians who prescribe intracavernous injection therapy should (1) inform patients of the potential occurrence of prolonged erections, (2) have a plan for the urgent treatment of prolonged erections, and (3) inform the patient of the plan.
- The patient considering prosthesis implantation and, when possible, his partner should be informed of the following: types of prostheses available; possibility and consequences of infection and erosion, mechanical failure, and resulting reoperation; differences from the normal flaccid and erect penis, including penile shortening; and potential reduction of the effectiveness of other therapies if the device is subsequently removed.
- Prosthetic surgery should not be performed in the presence of systemic, cutaneous, or urinary tract infection.
- Antibiotics providing gram-negative and gram-positive coverage should be administered preoperatively.

Recommendations

- The monitoring of patients receiving continuing PDE5 inhibitor therapy should include a periodic follow-up of efficacy, side effects, and any significant change in health status including medications.
- Prior to proceeding to other therapies, patients reporting failure of PDE5 inhibitor therapy should be evaluated to determine whether the trial of PDE5 inhibition was adequate.
- Patients who have failed a trial with PDE5 inhibitor therapy should be informed of the benefits and risks of other therapies, including the use of a different PDE5 inhibitor, alprostadil intraurethral suppositories, intracavernous drug injection, vacuum constriction devices, and penile prostheses.
- Only vacuum constriction devices containing a vacuum limiter should be used, whether purchased over the counter or procured with a prescription.
- The use of trazodone in the treatment of erectile dysfunction is not recommended.
- Testosterone therapy is not indicated for the treatment of erectile dysfunction in the patient with a normal serum testosterone level.
- Yohimbine is not recommended for the treatment of erectile dysfunction.
- Herbal therapies are not recommended for the treatment of erectile dysfunction.
- Surgeries performed with the intent to limit the venous outflow of the penis are not recommended.

Opinion

- Arterial reconstructive surgery is a treatment option only in healthy individuals with recently acquired erectile dysfunction secondary to a focal arterial occlusion and in the absence of any evidence of generalized vascular disease.

Data from https://www.auanet.org/guidelines/male-sexual-dysfunction-erectile-dysfunction-(2018). Accessed January 2018.

REFERENCES

1. Lue TF. Physiology of penile erection and pathophysiology of erectile dysfunction. In: Wein AJ, Kavoussi LR, Novick AC, et al., eds. *Campbell-Walsh Urology*. 9th ed. Philadelphia: Elsevier; 2007.
2. Brenot P. *Male Impotence- A Historical Perspective, L' Esprit du Temps*; 1994.
3. Impotence. NIH Consensus Statement, 1992;10:1.
4. Sun P, Cameron A, Seftel A, et al. Erectile dysfunction- an observable marker of diabetes mellitus? A large national epidemiological study. *J Urol*. 2006;176:1081–1085.
5. Laumann E, Paik A, Rosen R. Sexual dysfunction in the United States: prevalence and predictors. *JAMA*. 1999;281:537–544.
6. Johannes CB, Araujo AB, Feldman HA, et al. Incidence of erectile dysfunction in men 40 to 69 years old: longitudinal results from the Massachusetts Male Aging Study. *J Urol*. 2000;163:460–463.
7. Lewis RW, Hatzchistou D, Laumann E, et al. Epidemiology and natural history of erectile dysfunction: risk factors including iatrogenic and aging. Proceedings of the 1st International Consultation on Erectile Dysfunction. *Health Publication*. 2000;21–51.
8. Schouten BW, Bosch JL, Bernsen RM, et al. Incidence rates of erectile dysfunction in the Dutch general population. Effects of definition, clinical relevance, and duration of follow-up in the Krimpen study. *Int J Impot Res*. 2005;17:58–62.
9. Moreira ED, Lbo CR, Diament A, et al. Incidence of erectile dysfunction in men 40–69 years old: results from a population based cohort in Brazil. *Urology*. 2003;61:431–436.
10. Aytac IA, McKinlay JB, Krane RJ. The likely worldwide increase in erectile dysfunction between 1995 and 2025 and some possible policy consequences. *BJU Int*. 1999;84:50–56.
11. Selvin E, Burnett AL, Platz EA. Prevalence and risk factors for erectile dysfunction in the US. *Am J Med*. 2007;120:151–157.
12. Marumo K, Murai M. Aging and erectile dysfunction: the role of aging and concomitant chronic illness. *Int J Urol*. 2001;8:S50–S57.
13. Loprinzi PD, Nooe A. Erectile dysfunction and mortality in a national prospective cohort study. *J Sex Med*. 2015;12(11):2130–2133.
14. Nehra A, Jackson G, Miner M, et al. The Princeton III Consensus recommendations for the management of erectile dysfunction and cardiovascular disease. *Mayo Clin Proc*. 2012;87(8):766–778.
15. Kappus RM, Fahs CA, Smith D, et al. Obesity and overweight associated with increased carotid diameter and decreased arterial function in young otherwise healthy men. *Am J Hypertens*. 2014;27:628–634.
16. Mialon A, Berchtold A, Michaud PA, et al. Sexual dysfunctions among young men: prevalence and associated factors. *J Adolesc Health*. 2012;51:25–31.
17. Dabelea D, Mayer-Davis EJ, Saydah S, et al. Prevalence of type 1 and type 2 diabetes among children and adolescents from 2001 to 2009. *JAMA*. 2014;311:1778–1786.
18. Sattar AA, Haot J, Schulman CC, et al. Relationship between intrapenile O2 level and quantity of intracavernous smooth muscle fibers: current physiopathological concept. *Acta Urol Belg*. 195; 63:53-59.
19. Hsu GL, Brock G, Martinez-Pineiro L, et al. The three dimensional structure of the human tunica albuginea: anatomical and ultrastructural levels. *Int J Impot Res*. 1992;4:117–129.
20. Droupy S, Benoit G, Giuliano F, et al. Penile arteries in humans. *Surg Radiol Anat*. 1997;19:161–167.
21. Hsu GL, Hsieh CH, Wen HS, et al. Penile venous anatomy: an additional description and its clinical implication. *J Androl*. 2003;24:921–927.
22. de Groat WC, Booth A. Neural control of penile erection. In: Maggi CA, ed. *The Autonomic Nervous System*. London: Harwood; 1993:465–513.
23. Walsh PC, Brendler CB, Chang T, et al. Preservation of sexual function in men during radical pelvic surgery. *Md Med J*. 1990;39:389–393.
24. Halata Z, Munger BL. The neuroanatomical basis for the protopathic sensibility of the human glans penis. *Brain Res*. 1986;371:205–230.
25. McKenna KE. Central control of penile erection. *Int J Impot Res*. 1998;10(Suppl):S25–S34.
26. Burnett AL, Tillman SL, Chang TS, et al. Immunohistochemical localization of nitric oxide synthase in the autonomic innervation of the human penis. *J Urol*. 1993;150:73–76.

27. Michal V, Ruzbarsky V. Histological changes in the penile arterial bed with aging and diabetes. In: Zorgniotti AW, Rossi G, eds. *Vasculogenic Impotence: Proceedings of the 1st International Conference on Corpus Cavernosum Revascularization*; 1980:113–119.

28. Vlachopoulos C, Rokkas K, Ioakeimidis N, et al. Prevalence of asymptomatic coronary artery disease in men with vasculogenic erectile dysfunction: a prospective angiographic study. *Eur Urol*. 2005;48:996–1003.

29. Gratzke C, Angulo J, Chitaley K, et al. Anatomy, physiology, and pathophysiology of erectile dysfunction. *J Sex Med*. 2010;7:445–475.

30. Tarhan F, Kuyumcuoglu U, Kolsuz A, et al. Cavernous oxygen tension in the patients with erectile dysfunction. *Int J Impot Res*. 1997;9:149–153.

31. Nehra A, Azadoi KM, Moreland RB, et al. Cavernosal expandability is an erectile tissue mechanical property which predicts trabecular histology in an animal model of vasculogenic erectile dysfunction. *J Urol*. 1998;159:2229–2236.

32. Azadzoi KM, Park K, Andry C, et al. Relationship between cavernosal ischemia and corporal veno-occlusive dysfunction in an animal model. *J Urol*. 1997;157:1011–1017.

33. Azadzoi KM, Krane RJ, Saenz de Tejada I, et al. Endothelium-derived nitric oxide and cyclooxygenase products modulate corpus cavernosum smooth muscle tone. *J Urol*. 1992;147:220–225.

34. Levine FJ, Greenfield AJ, Goldstein I. Arteriographically determined occlusive disease within the hypogastric-cavernous bed in impotent patients following blunt perineal and pelvic trauma. *J Urol*. 1990;144:11147–11153.

35. Richiuti VS, Haas CA, Seftel AD, et al. Pudendal nerve injury associated with avid bicycling. *J Urol*. 1999;162:2099–2100.

36. Sattar AA, Wespes E, Schulman CC. Computerized measurement of penile elastic fibers in potent and impotent men. *Eur Urol*. 1994;25:142–144.

37. Rajfer J, Rosciszewski A, Mehringer M. Prevalence of corporeal venous leakage in impotent men. *J Urol*. 1988;140:69–71.

38. Christ GJ, Maayani S, Valcic M, et al. Pharmacological studies of human erectile tissue: characteristics of spontaneous contractions and alterations in alpha-adrenorecptor responsiveness with age and disease in isolated tissues. *Br J Pharmacol*. 1990;101:375–381.

39. Christ GJ, Moreno AP, Parker ME, et al. Intercellular communication through gap junctions: a potential role in pharmacomechanical coupling and synctial tissue contraction in vascular smooth muscle isolated from the human corpus cavernosum. *Life Sci*. 1991;49:PL195–PL200.

40. Chang SW, Fine R, Siegel D, et al. The impact of diuretic therapy on reported sexual function. *Arch Intern Med*. 1991;151:2402–2408.

41. Grimm Jr RH, Grandits GA, Prineas RJ, et al. Long term effects on sexual function of five anti-hypertensive drugs and nutritional hygienic treatment in hypertensive men and women. Treatment of Mild Hypertension Study (TOMHS). *Hypertension*. 1997;29:8–14.

42. Franzen D, Metha A, Seifert N, et al. Effects of beta-blockers on sexual performance in men with coronary artery disease. A prospective, randomized, and double blinded study. *Int J Impot Res*. 2001;13:348–351.

43. Fogari R, Zoppi A, Corradi L, et al. Sexual function in hypertensive males treated with lisinopril or atenolol: a crossover study. *Am J Hypertens*. 1998;11:1244–1247.

44. Llisteri JL, Lozano JV, Aznar VJ, et al. Sexual dysfunction in hypertensive patients treated with losartan. *Am J Med Sci*. 2001;321:336–341.

45. Salzman EA, Guay AT, Jacobson J. Improvement in erectile function in men with organic erectile dysfunction by correction of elevated cholesterol levels: a clinical observation. *J Urol*. 2004;172:255–258.

46. Sadeghi-Nejah H, Jackson I. New onset priapism associated with ingestion of terazosin in an otherwise healthy man. *J Sex Med*. 2007;6:1766–1768.

47. Gratzke C, Angulo J, Chitaley K, et al. Anatomy, physiology, and pathophysiology of erectile dysfunction. *J Sex Med*. 2010;7:445–475.

48. Traish AM, Hassani J, Guay AT, et al. Adverse side effects of 5- alpha reductase inhibitors therapy: persistent diminished libido and erectile dysfunction and depression in a subset of patients. *J Sex Med*. 2011;8:872–874.

49. Rosen RC, Riley A, Wagner G, et al. The International Index of Erectile Function (IIEF): a multidimensional scale for assessment of erectile dysfunction. *Urology*. 1997;49:822–830.

50. Schwartz BG, Kloner RA. How to save a life during a clinic visit for erectile dysfunction by modifying cardiovascular risk factors. *Int J Impot Res*. 2009;21:327–335.

51. Hehemann MC, Kashanian JA. Can lifestyle modification affect men's erectile function? *Translational Andrology and Urology*. 2016;5(2):187–194.

52. Lue TF, Broderick GA. Evaluation and nonsurgical management of erectile dysfunction and premature ejaculation. In: Wein AJ, Kavoussi LR, Novick AC, et al., eds. *Campbell-Walsh Urology*. 9th ed. Philadelphia: Elsevier; 2007.

53. Prieto D. Physiological regulation of penile ateries and veins. *Int J of Imp Res*. 2008;20:17–29.

54. Lincoln TM, Hall CL, Park CR, Corbin JD. Guanosine 3':5' cyclic monophosphate binding proteins in rat tissues. *Proc Natl Acad Sci USA*. 1976;73:2559–2563.

55. Hellastrom WJ, Bennett AH, Gesundheit N, et al. A double blind, placebo controlled evaluation of the erectile response to transurethral alprostadil. *Urology*. 1996;48:851–856.

56. Linet OL, Neff LL. Intracavernous prostaglandin E1 in erectile dysfunction. *Clin Invest*. 1994;72:139–149.

57. Padma-Nathan H, Christ G, Adaikan G, et al. Pharmacotherapy for erectile dysfunction. *J Sex Med*. 2004;1:128–140.

58. Earle CM, Seah M, Coulden SE, et al. The use of the vacuum erection device in the management of erectile impotence. *In J Impot Res*. 1996;8:237–240.

59. Cookson MS, Nadig PW. Long term results with vacuum constriction device. *J Urol*. 1993;149:290–294.

60. Mulcahy JJ, Austoni E, Barada JH, et al. The penile implant for erectile dysfunction. *J Sex Med*. 2004;1:98–109.

61. Subrini L. Subrini penile implants: surgical, sexual, and psychological results. *Eur Urol*. 1982;8:222–226.

62. Hellstrom JG, Montague DK, Moncada I, et al. Implants, mechanical devices, and vascular surgery for erectile dysfunction. *J Sex Med*. 2010;7:501–523.

63. Montorsi F, Rigatti P, Carmignani G, et al. AMS three-piece inflatable implants for erectile dysfunction: a long term multi-institutional study in 200 consecutive patients. *Eur Urol*. 2000;37:50–55.

64. Latini DM, Penson DF, Wallace KL, et al. Longitudinal differences in psychological outcomes for men with erectile dysfunction. *Results from ExCEED*. 2006;3:1068–1076.

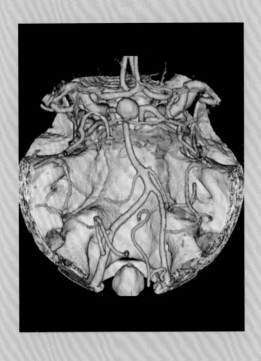

PART **VIII**

第八部分

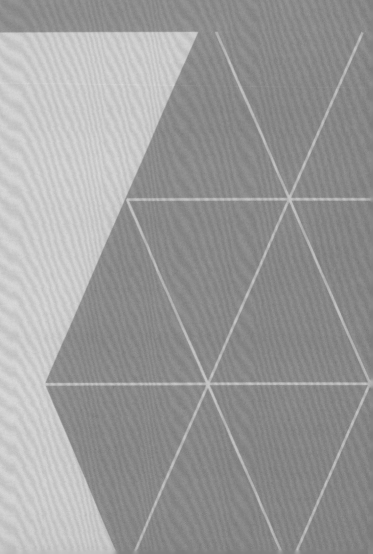

Cerebrovascular
Ischemia

脑血管缺血

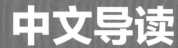
中文导读

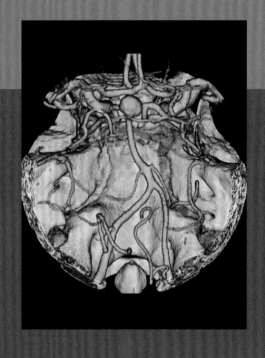

第28章
脑血管疾病的流行病学

  卒中是一种常见病、多发病。在世界范围内，卒中每年至少影响着1600万人口，是全世界第二大死亡原因。可将卒中大致分为缺血性卒中和出血性卒中，前者是由于脑血管闭塞所致，占全部卒中患者的80%左右；而出血性卒中则是由于脑血管破裂所致，占比约20%。鉴于卒中具有高发病率、高致残率、高复发率及高致死率的特点，积极预防、早期确诊、主动干预显得尤为重要。卒中的临床表现多样，发病机制及病因也各不相同，在某些情况下，上述特点为明确诊断设立了障碍；然而，在多数情况下，基于明确诊断的早期干预有助于提升卒中患者的神经功能预后。本章将聚焦于各种卒中类型的临床表现及诊断方法，希望借此提升读者对于卒中的理解，为进一步改善患者潜在的神经功能预后提供帮助。

吉训明

Epidemiology of Cerebrovascular Disease

Larry B. Goldstein

OVERVIEW

Stroke is the second leading cause of death worldwide, accounting for 4 million deaths in 2004.[1] Cerebrovascular disease is currently the fifth most common cause of death in the United States behind diseases of the heart, cancer, chronic lower respiratory diseases, and unintentional accidents.[2] On average, every 40 seconds someone in the United States has a stroke and every 4 minutes, someone dies.[2] Stroke is also a leading cause of long-term disability in adults, ranking third worldwide in 2015.[3] There are a variety of nonmodifiable and modifiable stroke risk factors (Box 28.1).[4] Worldwide, a group of 10 modifiable risk factors (hypertension, current smoking, physical inactivity, high apolipoprotein ApoB/ApoA1 ratio, poor diet, high waist-to-hip ratio, psychosocial factors, cardiac disease, excessive alcohol consumption, and diabetes mellitus) account for 90.7% of population attributable stroke risk.[5]

Stroke Burden

An estimated 795,000 people have a stroke in the United States each year, with an estimated 7.2 million people aged 20 years or older who have had a stroke living in the country.[2] Ischemic strokes account for 87% of all strokes, with 10% due to parenchymal intracerebral hemorrhages (ICHs) and 3% occurring because of aneurysmal subarachnoid hemorrhages (SAHs).[2] About 610,000 of these strokes are first events with 185,000 occurring in persons who had a prior stroke.[2] The risk of first ischemic stroke varies by race-ethnicity. Based on data from 2005, age-adjusted ischemic stroke incidence was lower in whites (179/100,000) than blacks (294/100,000); incidence rates for ICH were 30 versus 56 and for SAH 8 versus 20 per 100,000 in whites compared to blacks, respectively).[2] Approximately 55,000 more women than men had a stroke in the United States that year.[2] In 2012, there were over 1 million hospital discharges for stroke and approximately 2.4 million physician office visits attributable to cerebrovascular disease.[2] Likely an underestimate, about 5 million people in the United States report a physician-diagnosed transient ischemic attack (TIA).[2] Two-thirds of patients hospitalized for stroke are over age 65.[6] Among those over age 65 years, the rate of hospitalization for stroke is nearly three times higher for those over age 85 years (288/100,000) compared to those aged 65 to 74 years (108/100,000).[6] Importantly, the population over age 85 years is anticipated to more than double from 6.3 million in 2015 to 14.6 million in 2040.[7]

A TIA precedes approximately 15% to 23% of ischemic strokes, carries a 90-day stroke risk of 9% to 17%,[8] and a 25% risk of death over the ensuing year.[9] However, another study found lower 1-year rates of recurrent stroke or TIA (12%) or death (1.8%).[10] About 20% of patients with symptoms of TIA or minor stroke are undiagnosed,[11] and about half of all patients who have a TIA fail to report their symptoms to a healthcare provider.[12] With an estimated 5 million people in the United States with a physician-diagnosed TIA, it is an important target for secondary stroke prevention.[2]

Mortality from stroke accounted for 1 out of every 20 deaths in the United States in 2014 (133,000 deaths).[2] Data on long-term survivorship following ischemic stroke reflect wide ranges of estimated mortality: 13% to 45% at 1 year, 36% to 69% at 5 years, and 31% to 87% at 10 years.[13–33] In a recent population-based study, the cumulative mortality rates following stroke were 10.5% at 30 days, 21.2% at 1 year, 39.8% at 5 years, and 58.42% at 24 years.[34] These estimates are primarily obtained from international studies or single regions within the United States. Women and minority populations may have higher long-term mortality following stroke, although the evidence is limited and more research is needed to evaluate differences by patient characteristics.[16,19,21]

Disability and quality of life can be as important as mortality as stroke outcomes. Living with a major stroke can be considered as being worse than death by patients at high risk of stroke.[35] Twenty percent of stroke survivors still require institutional care after 3 months, and 15% to 30% are permanently disabled.[36] Given the large number of stroke survivors in the United States, effective rehabilitation and secondary prevention are important targets for public health interventions.

Cost

Acute stroke was among the 10 highest contributors to Medicare hospital costs in 2011, and was the 11th most costly for payers.[37] In 2012 to 2013, the total annual cost of stroke in the United States was estimated at $33.9 billion with $17.9 billion attributed to direct costs.[2] Total direct stroke-related medical costs are projected to increase to $184 billion by 2030.[38] The mean lifetime cost of stroke was estimated to be $90,981 for ischemic stroke, $123,565 for ICH, $228,030 for SAH, and $103,576 averaged across all stroke subtypes.[39]

Regional Patterns of Stroke

Stroke mortality has varied regionally in the United States over the past 50 years, with the highest mortality rates in the southeast United States, a region of the country termed the "Stroke Belt" (Fig. 28.1).[40–44] The Stroke Belt is usually defined as including the eight southern states of North Carolina, South Carolina, Georgia, Tennessee, Mississippi,

BOX 28.1   Stroke Risk Factors (Partial List)

Demographic Factors
Age
Sex
Race-ethnicity

Lifestyle Factors
Diet/nutrition
Physical inactivity
Overweight/obesity
Environmental factors
Cigarette smoking
Alcohol consumption

Medically Treatable Risk Factors
Hypertension
Lipids
Diabetes
Atrial fibrillation
Sickle cell disease
Sleep disordered breathing

Other Risk Factors
Fibrinogen, clotting factors, and inflammation
Blood homocysteine levels
Migraine

Alabama, Louisiana, and Arkansas. These geographic differences have been documented since at least 1940,[43] and despite some minor shifts,[44] they still persist.[41,42] The reason for the existence of the Stroke Belt remains uncertain. Within the Stroke Belt, a "buckle" region along the coastal plain of North Carolina, South Carolina, and Georgia was identified with even higher stroke mortality rates than the remainder of the Stroke Belt.[45] Average stroke mortality is ≈20% higher in the Stroke Belt than in the rest of the nation and ≈40% higher in the stroke buckle. Overall, individuals living in the southeast United States have a 50% greater risk of dying from a stroke compared to residents of other regions.[45] Higher stroke mortality rates are now also being noted in the Pacific northwest regions of the United States.[46,47]

Total mortality reflects a combination of incidence and case-fatality rates. Stroke incidence is higher in the southeast,[40,48,49] whereas case-fatality rates vary little across the country.[40] Maps published by the Centers for Disease Control and Prevention (CDC) show geographic patterns in age-adjusted stroke hospitalization rates by county, which coincide with stroke mortality patterns (Fig. 28.2).[50] There are also regional differences in the rates of recurrent stroke events within the year after a stroke hospitalization, even after adjusting for common risk factors.[51,52] The causes for these disparities remain unclear. National data are needed to monitor incident and prevalent stroke patterns over time, particularly by age, race-ethnicity, and sex subgroups.

STROKE RISK FACTORS: DEMOGRAPHIC FACTORS

Age

Age is a major risk factor for stroke (the risk doubles with every decade of age over 55 years) and is relatively uncommon in children. The prevalence of perinatal strokes in the United States is 29/100,000

live births.[2] Because of the lack of uniform case definitions, the true prevalence in likely higher. The overall annual incidence of stroke in US children aged 0 to 15 years is 6.4/100,000 children and for those aged 0 to 19 years is 4.6/100,000 children.[2] Unlike adults, about half of all incident childhood strokes are hemorrhagic.[2]

The rate of adverse outcomes and complications associated with stroke increase with advancing age.[53] As reported by the CDC, 30-day stroke mortality rates increase with age from 9% in patients 65 to 74 years of age, to 13.1% in those 74 to 84 years of age, and 23% in those ≥85 years of age.[54] The mean age of stroke patients in the United States is currently 70 years. The population aged >65 years increased from 36.6 million in 2005 to 47.8 million in 2015 (a 30% increase) and is projected to more than double to 98 million in 2060; the population age >85 years is expected to increase threefold, from 6.3 million in 2015 to 14.6 million in 2040.[7] This will increase the proportions of the population at high risk of stroke, stroke mortality, and stroke-related complications based on age alone. Because stroke is so strongly age-dependent, understanding the epidemiology of stroke in the elderly is critical for both clinicians and policy makers.

Sex

Women are older at stroke onset compared with men (75 years compared with 71 years, respectively).[2] Women have a lower age-adjusted stroke incidence than men; however, women have a higher lifetime risk of stroke, and sex-related differences in stroke risk are modified by age.[2] Compared with white men, white women aged 45 to 84 years have a lower stroke risk than men, but this association is reversed in older ages with women over 85 years of age having a higher risk compared with men.[2]

The absolute number of strokes in the population is also greater for women because of the increasing risk of stroke with advancing age, combined with women's longer life expectancy (about 55,000 more women than men have a stroke each year).[2] About 55% of all strokes occur in women who have approximately 60% of stroke-related deaths. The relatively higher number of stroke-related deaths in women result from a higher mortality in women and their disproportionate representation in the population. Not only do more strokes occur in women, but also the majority are in women over the age of 70 years; these women are more likely to be socially isolated, live alone, have fiscal constraints, and higher rates of comorbid disease. The greater burden of stroke deaths in women is predicted to be even greater in the future based on population projections. An excess of 32,000 stroke deaths in women in 2000 is anticipated to increase to nearly 68,000 by 2050.[55]

The risk of stroke increases in association with pregnancy, with the majority occurring during the postpartum period.[56] The rate of stroke is estimated at being between 11 and 26/100,000 deliveries.[56] Risk factors for stroke in pregnancy include advanced maternal age, African American race-ethnicity, migraines, preeclampsia, and gestational hypertension.[57]

Meta-analyses indicate that oral contraceptive users have about twice the risk of stroke compared with nonusers.[57] Hypertension, cigarette smoking, and migraine further increase stroke risk in women taking oral contraceptives. Women under the age of 50 years are generally considered to be at lower stroke risk than men, although women aged 35 to 64 years are almost three times more likely than men to report a history of stroke, largely because of higher rates in 45- to 54-year olds.[58,59] The prevalence of stroke increases as women reach the menopausal transition. Studies suggest that women are protected by endogenous estrogens; however, clinical trials have not found a lower risk of either stroke or cardiac events in postmenopausal women treated with exogenous estrogen and progesterone.[55]

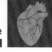

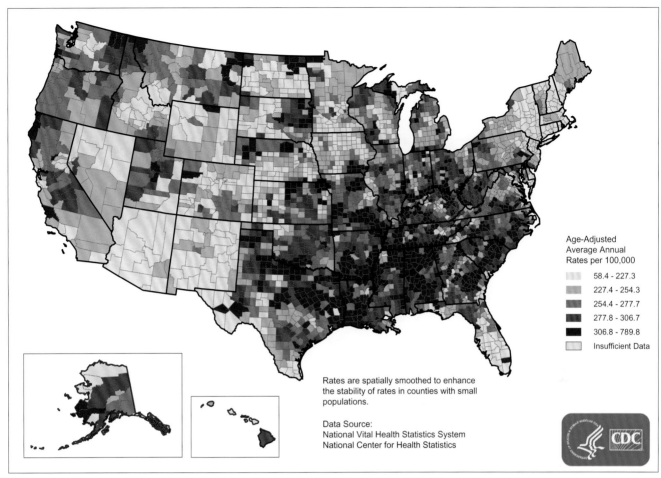

Fig. 28.1 Stroke death rates, 2013 to 2015, for adults aged 65 and over by county. (From Centers for Disease Control and Prevention, National Center for Chronic Disease Prevention and Health Promotion, Division for Heart Disease and Stroke Prevention: Stroke maps and data sources, 2017. https://www.cdc.gov/stroke/maps_data.htm. Accessed May 15, 2018.)

Race-ethnicity

There are prominent race-ethnic disparities in stroke in the United States with blacks and American Indian/Alaska Natives being at particularly high risk. In 2005, the age-adjusted incidence of ischemic stroke was 179/100,000 versus 294/100,000; and for ICH 30/100,000 versus 56/100,000 for whites and blacks, respectively.[2] Approximately 2.5% of non-Hispanic whites, 2.4% of Hispanics (of any race), 4.5% of non-Hispanic blacks, and 5.4% of American Indian/Alaska Natives reported a history of stroke.[2] Although differences may be more prominent in the young,[60] race-ethnic differences remain among the older age groups.[61] Stroke incidence is actually higher in white men aged ≥85 years than similarly aged black men (32.1/100,000 vs. 14.7/100,000, respectively),[2] which is possibly due to a survivor effect with higher stroke-related mortality among younger blacks.

STROKE RISK FACTORS: LIFESTYLE

Diet/Nutrition

Numerous studies implicate dietary factors in the risk for stroke. Aspects of diet that have received attention include consumption of omega-3 fatty acids, vitamins C and E, potassium, calcium, fatty acids, homocysteine, sodium, and fruits and vegetables. Greater adherence to the Dietary Approaches to Stop Hypertension (DASH) diet and

the Mediterranean-type diets has been associated with a lower risk of stroke.[62,63] Although some evidence suggests higher total fat intake increases stroke risk,[64] higher fish consumption—a marker for omega-3 fatty acid intake—was associated with a reduced stroke risk in the Nurses' Health Study and the Health Professionals Follow-up study.[65,66] Those adhering to a Mediterranean-type diet had a lower stroke risk compared to those following a low-fat diet.[62] A meta-analysis of cohort studies reported a 26% reduction in stroke risk associated with consumption of >5 servings/day of fruits and vegetables compared with consumption of <3 servings/day,[67] a finding consistent with the results of a clinical trial.[68]

Reduced sodium and increased potassium intake are also associated with decreased stroke risk.[69–72] The effects are likely in part due to the impact of low dietary sodium and high potassium in lowering blood pressure (BP). The DASH diet, which is low in sodium, high in potassium, and includes a high intake of fruits and vegetables, consumption of low-fat dairy products, and low intake of saturated and total fat, effectively lowers BP,[73] and was associated with an 18% lower risk of stroke in the Nurses' Health Study (highest quintile vs. lowest quintile).[74] As noted above, the Mediterranean-type diet is also associated with cardiovascular benefits, including a reduction in stroke. Women in the Nurses' Health Study at the highest versus lowest quintiles of the Alternate Mediterranean Diet Score had a lower risk of stroke (relative risk [RR] = 0.87, 95% confidence interval [CI] 0.73 to 1.02) after

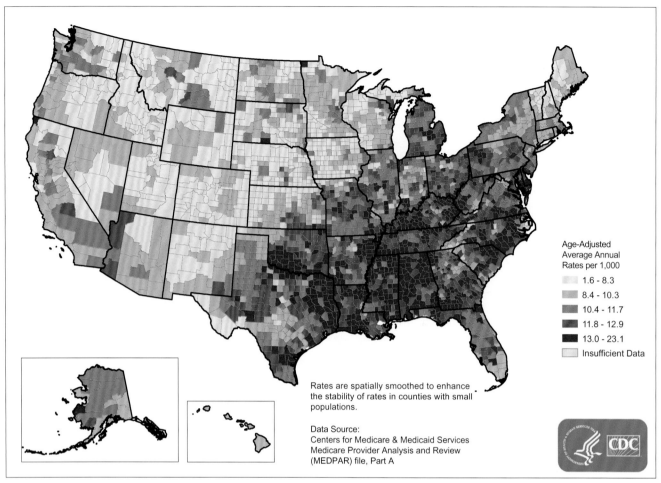

Fig. 28.2 Stroke hospitalization rates, 2012 to 2014, for Medicare recipients aged 65+ by county. (From Centers for Disease Control and Prevention, National Center for Chronic Disease Prevention and Health Promotion, Division for Heart Disease and Stroke Prevention: Stroke maps and data sources, 2017. https://www.cdc.gov/stroke/maps_data.htm. Accessed May 15, 2018.)

20 years of follow-up.[75] Analyses in the same group of women evaluating consumption of a "prudent" diet (i.e., high in vegetable, fruit, legume, fish, and whole grain intake) and a "Western" diet (i.e., high in red and processed meats, refined grains, sweets, and desserts) found a 58% increased risk of stroke in the highest versus lowest quintile of a "Western" diet and a 22% lower risk of stroke in the highest versus lowest quintile of a "prudent" diet.[76] Dietary guidelines for the prevention of stroke recommend reduced sodium intake and increased potassium intake, a diet rich in fruits and vegetables, as well as the DASH or Mediterranean-type diet.[4] Unfortunately, according to national surveys conducted in 2011 to 2012, 91% of US children aged 12 to 19 years, 82% of adults aged 20 to 49 years, and 69% of those ≥50 years consume an unhealthy diet.[2]

Physical Inactivity

Lack of regular physical activity is a well-established predictor of early mortality and cardiovascular disease, and regular exercise is associated with a lower risk of stroke in prospective and case-control studies.[77–84] The effects of physical activity may be mediated through reductions in BP, improvements in glucose tolerance, reductions in body weight, reductions in plasma fibrinogen and platelet activity, elevations in high-density lipoprotein cholesterol (HDL) concentration, and control of other cardiovascular risk factors.[84–90] Stroke prevention guidelines recommend that healthy adults should perform at least moderate

to vigorous intensity aerobic physical activity at least 40 min/day 3 to 4 days each week.[4] In the 2011 to 2012 NHANES survey, 42% of those aged 20 to 49 years and 55% of those age ≥50 years did not meet minimal physical activity recommendations.[2] Physical inactivity accounts for 6% and 8% of stroke deaths worldwide in middle- to low-income and high-income countries, respectively.[91] Participants in the Physicians' Health Study engaging in vigorous exercise ≥5-times/week had a 14% lower risk of stroke compared with those engaging in vigorous activity <1 time/week.[90] The Framingham Heart Study and the Honolulu Heart Program have found similar effects in men.[77,78] Studies in women including the Nurses' Health Study and the Copenhagen City Heart Study also report reductions in stroke incidence with increased physical activity.[83,84] Among women aged ≥45 years in the Women's Health Study, higher levels of physical activity (measured in kcal per week) were associated with a 20% to 40% reduction in stroke risk.[92] Finally, in the Northern Manhattan Stroke Study, there was a 63% reduction in stroke risk associated with increased physical activity regardless of age, sex, and race-ethnicity (white, black, Hispanic) subgroups.[82] This analysis also suggested that heavy physical activity was more beneficial than low-to-moderate activity.[82] However, other evidence supports the beneficial effect of light exercise. For example, the intensity of physical activity was not related to stroke risk among participants in the Women's Health Study, although walking time and pace were inversely related to stroke risk.[92]

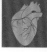

Overweight/Obesity

Obesity likely increases stroke risk through multiple mechanisms including increased BP, impaired glucose tolerance, and more frequent atherogenic serum lipid level profiles. Traditionally, weight categorization is defined according to the body mass index (BMI; weight [kg] divided by the square of height [m]), with 25 and $30 kg/m^2$ used as cut-points defining overweight and obesity, respectively. In the Framingham cohort, BMI was related to first cerebrovascular events after adjustment for traditional stroke risk factors.[93] RRs for stroke in an analysis of women aged 30 to 55 years in the Nurses' Health Study ranged from 1.75 for a BMI of 27 to $28.9 kg/m^2$ to 2.37 for a BMI $>32 kg/m^2$ and were independent of other risk factors including age, smoking, hormone use, and menopausal status.[94] Obesity was also identified as an independent stroke risk factor in the Honolulu Heart Study.[95] Abdominal obesity has emerged as an even stronger risk factor for stroke than BMI. In a study of 28,643 male health professionals, the RR of stroke was 2.3-times higher in the upper compared with the lower quintiles of waist-to-hip ratio.[96] Obesity is a major public health problem worldwide. According to data from the National Health and Nutrition Examination Survey 2013 to 2014, 37.7% of US adults were obese (35.0% of men and 40.4% of women).[2] The prevalence among children aged 2 to 19 years was 33.4%. As the US population ages, the impact of obesity on stroke risk is likely to increase owing to the high prevalence of obesity in the young.

Environmental Factors

The components of air pollution include a heterogenous combination of gases, liquids, and particulate matter (PM). A 2004 American Heart Association (AHA) Scientific Statement on the relationship between PM, air pollution, and cardiovascular disease concluded that both short- and long-term exposure to ambient PM increases the risk of acute cardiovascular events.[97] A subsequent update reflected several additional studies.[98] The majority of epidemiologic studies report an increased risk of cardiovascular events associated with exposure to fine PM $<2.5 \mu m$ in aerodynamic diameter ($PM_{2.5}$) for susceptible individuals (e.g., the elderly or those with existing cardiovascular conditions). The risk of stroke also may be related to long-term exposure to $PM_{2.5}$.[99] Ultrafine particulates ($<0.1 \mu m$), copollutants, such as ozone and nitrogen oxides, and specific sources of pollution, such as motor vehicle traffic, also contribute to cardiovascular risk.

The strength of evidence for an association between air pollution and cerebrovascular disease is less than that for heart disease. Among $>60,000$ postmenopausal women initially free of cardiovascular disease in the Women's Health Initiative, each $10 \mu m/m^3$ increase in annual $PM_{2.5}$ exposure was associated with a 28% increased risk of stroke, a 35% increased risk of stroke or fatal cerebrovascular disease, and an 83% increased risk of fatal cerebrovascular disease.[100] In contrast, there was no association between fatal cerebrovascular and long-term $PM_{2.5}$ exposure in a cohort of $>300,000$ adults derived from the American Cancer Society's Cancer Prevention Study-II.[101]

Several studies have reported small but statistically significant associations between short-term pollutant exposure and stroke. Studies using surveillance data from Dijon, France[102] and Corpus Christi, TX[103] have linked certain types of air pollutants with the risk of ischemic stroke and TIA. Others include daily time-series studies from Korea (Seoul),[104,105] China (Shanghai),[106] and Finland (Helsinki)[107] that each reported an association between elevated levels of air pollution and stroke mortality; however, the associations were found for ischemic but not hemorrhagic stroke mortality in one of the studies,[106] and in the warm but not cold seasons in another.[107] These complexities and other unmeasured confounders may underlie some of the disparities among studies.

In addition to acute cardiovascular events, air pollutants potentially contribute to subclinical physiologic changes including increasing systemic inflammation and oxidative stress, coagulation/thrombosis, systemic and pulmonary arterial BP, atherosclerosis, heart rate variability and conduction abnormalities, cardiac ischemia, epigenetic changes, and traditional cardiovascular risk factors.[98] Such associations provide further support for a causal relationship between air pollution and cardiovascular disease. As a potentially avoidable risk factor for acute events, it may be prudent for those at high stroke and cardiovascular risk to limit outdoor air exposure on high pollution days.

Cigarette Smoking

Cigarette smoking is consistently identified as a major independent risk factor for ischemic stroke in epidemiologic studies including the Framingham study,[108] the Cardiovascular Health Study,[109] the Honolulu Heart Study[110] and INTERSTROKE.[111] Cigarette smoking leads to an approximate twofold increase in stroke risk.[110] Smoking is also associated with a two- to fourfold increase in risk of SAH.[112-115] Studies of the relationship between smoking and the risk of parenchymal ICH are less consistent. Analyses of data from the Hemorrhagic Stroke Project,[116] Physicians' Health Study,[113] and the Women's Health Study[112] found an association between smoking and increased ICH risk, whereas analyses from other studies, including a pooled analysis of data from the Atherosclerosis Risk in Communities (ARIC) Study and the Cardiovascular Health Study, found no relationship.[117] One meta-analysis even reported a paradoxical protective effect of smoking for ICH risk,[118] although a subsequent review found an approximate 30% increase in smoking-associated ICH risk.[119] Based on data from 2005 to 2009, the CDC estimated that 15,300 cerebrovascular deaths annually could be attributed to smoking in the United States.[120]

Environmental tobacco smoke (also known as passive or secondhand smoke) is also thought to increase the risk of stroke for lifelong nonsmokers. A meta-analysis of 24 sex-specific estimates from 15 studies found an overall 25% (95% CI 16% to 36%) increased risk of stroke if the spouse (or nearest equivalent) currently smoked.[121] There was no heterogeneity by sex, publication year, or outcome; however, risk estimates tended to be lower for prospective studies and those studies with United States or European cohorts. The risk of SAH was not increased, and overall risk estimates were similar if the spouse ever smoked or using total exposure rather than current spousal exposure. There was a 56% (95% CI 34% to 82%) increased risk of stroke for the highest level of spousal exposure. The CDC estimates that environmental tobacco smoke causes 41,000 deaths each year among adults in the United States, although the specific contribution of stroke deaths was not included in the calculation.[120]

Whether there is a linear dose effect for smoking and stroke risk is uncertain. Some studies suggest a nonlinear effect, with the stroke risk attributable to smoking increasing sharply at lower cigarette consumption levels and then plateauing as the number of cigarettes smoked per day increase.[122] The similarities between stroke risk estimates and changes in biomarkers of cardiovascular risk for active and passive smokers further support a nonlinear relationship between cigarette smoking and cardiovascular risk, suggesting a low threshold of increased risk associated with tobacco smoke exposure.[4,123,124] Clinical and experimental studies suggest that both the acute and chronic effects of cigarette smoking likely contribute to stroke risk.[122] Cigarette smoking causes endothelial injury and dysfunction in both coronary and peripheral arteries. It increases the risk of thrombus generation associated with atherosclerotic plaque and leads to chronic inflammation that promotes atherosclerosis. Smoking also promotes an atherogenic lipid profile with higher triglycerides and lower HDL-cholesterol, and may increase insulin resistance that along with chronic inflammation, can accelerate macrovascular and microvascular-related diseases such as nephropathy. Smoking even one cigarette increases heart rate, mean BP, and cardiac index, and decreases arterial distensibility.[125,126] There is also a synergistic detrimental effect of smoking with other cardiovascular risk factors including systolic BP (SBP),[127] vital exhaustion,[128] and oral contraceptives.[129]

Smoking cessation is an essential component of primary and secondary stroke prevention.[4,130] Stroke risk declines rapidly with smoking cessation with considerable reductions in risk apparent within 5 years in both men and women.[118,131–135] Although stroke risk is lower for former compared to current smokers, whether the risk with cessation completely reverts to that of never smokers is not clear. Data from the Framingham Study[132] and the Nurses' Health Study[133] found that risk returned to never-smoker levels, whereas data from the Honolulu Heart Program,[131] the British Regional Heart Study,[134] and others[118,135] report a small residual excess risk for former heavy smokers that may persist for up to two decades after quitting.[134,135]

Alcohol Consumption

The effects of alcohol consumption on stroke risk is dependent on the amount of consumption and varies with stroke type. In the Honolulu Heart Study, there was a very strong dose-response relationship between alcohol intake and both ICH and SAH.[136] Alcohol intake also appears to confer risk for ischemic stroke, although low to moderate consumption may be associated with a reduction in risk. A study of male health professionals reported an increased risk of stroke with an intake >2 drinks/day, but no clear association with lower levels of consumption.[137] Other studies support a J-shaped relationship between alcohol intake and the risk of ischemic stroke with low-to-moderate intake associated with reduced risk, and heavy consumption associated with higher risk.[138–144] A meta-analysis of the effects of alcohol (1 drink defined as 12 g of alcohol) and stroke risk reported a 20% to 28% reduced risk of stroke among those consuming <1 or 1 to 2 drinks/day relative to abstainers, with heavy drinking associated with a 69% increased risk.[145] The population attributable risk associated with alcohol use for stroke mortality in middle- and low-income countries and high-income countries is estimated as 5% and 11%, respectively.[91] Heavy alcohol use may affect other stroke risk factors leading to increases in BP, higher rates of atrial fibrillation, coagulation disorders, and reductions in cerebral blood flow. However, at moderate levels of intake alcohol may have beneficial effects through reductions in platelet aggregation and plasma fibrinogen concentration, and improvements in HDL-cholesterol levels and endothelial function. Guidelines endorse no more than moderate alcohol consumption (≤2 drinks/day for men and ≤1 drink/day for nonpregnant women) who consume alcohol.[4]

MEDICALLY TREATABLE RISK FACTORS

Hypertension

High BP, defined as SBP ≥140 mm Hg, diastolic BP (DBP) ≥90 mm Hg, or being told at least twice by a health professional that one has hypertension, affects 85.7 million adults in the United States ≥20 years of age.[2] In 2011 to 2014, the prevalence of hypertension was 11.6% among those 20 to 39 years of age, 37.3% among those 40 to 59 years of age, and 67.2% among those ≥60 years of age.[2] The prevalence of hypertension in the United States is highest among non-Hispanic black women (46.3%) followed by non-Hispanic black men (45%), non-Hispanic white men (34.5%), non-Hispanic white women (32.3%), Hispanic women (30.7%) and Hispanic men (28.9%).[2] Data from 2011 to 2014 found that of those with hypertension who were ≥20 years of age, 15.9% were unaware of their condition, 24% were not being treated, and 45.6% did not have

their hypertension under control.[2] Data from 2007 to 2014 indicate that BP control is lowest in Mexican-American men (37.0%) followed by non-Hispanic black men (41.6%), Mexican-American women (49.2%), non-Hispanic black women (53.4%), non-Hispanic white men (53.9%), and is best in non-Hispanic white women (58.0%).[2]

High BP is one of the most important treatable risk factors for both ischemic and hemorrhagic stroke. Individuals with BP <120/80 mm Hg have approximately half the lifetime risk of stroke of persons with hypertension.[2] There is a 38% increased RR of stroke for every 10 to 20 mm Hg increase in SBP and a 34% increased RR for every 5 mm Hg increase in DBP.[146] This increased risk is graded with no specific threshold for increased risk, even within the normal range. The risk is increased even among those with pre-hypertension.[147] Lowering BP reduces the incidence of stroke.[146]

Control of hypertension begins with lifestyle. As discussed above, adherence to the DASH diet lowers BP.[68,73] Weight loss is also strongly related to improved BP. A meta-analysis found that a 5.1 kg loss of body weight is associated with an average lowering of systolic BP by 4.4 mm Hg and of DBP by 3.6 mm Hg.[148] Treatment with β-blockers lowers the risk for stroke by 29% (RR = 0.71, 95% CI 0.59 to 0.86) and diuretics are estimated to reduce the risk by 51% (RR = 0.49, 95% CI 0.39 to 0.62).[149] The overall reduction in incident stroke with antihypertensive therapy is estimated at 35% to 44%.[150] Reductions in stroke risk may also be related to the type of antihypertensive used based on their relative effects on BP variability.[151–154]

The Systolic Blood Pressure Intervention Trial (SPRINT) assigned 9361 persons with an SBP ≥130 mm Hg and an increased cardiovascular risk, but without diabetes, to an SBP target of <120 mm Hg (intensive treatment) or <140 mm Hg (standard treatment).[155] Intensive treatment led to a lower rate of the primary composite outcome (myocardial infarction, other acute coronary syndromes, stroke, heart failure, or death from cardiovascular causes; 1.65%/year versus 2.19%/year; hazard ratio [HR] = 0.75; 95% CI 0.64 to 0.89, P < .001), all-cause mortality (HR = 0.73, 95% CI 0.60 to 0.90, P = 0.003), but not stroke alone (0.41%/year vs. 0.47%/year, HR = 0.89, 95% CI 0.63 to 1.25, P = .50). However, SPRINT was not powered to detect differences in the components of its composite primary endpoint. Rates of serious adverse events (hypotension, syncope, electrolyte abnormalities, and acute kidney injury or failure) were higher in the intensive-treatment group. Intensive SBP treatment was projected to prevent ≈107,500 deaths/year (95% CI, 93,300 to 121,200) but cause 56,100 (95% CI 50,800 to 61,400) episodes of hypotension, 34,400 (95% CI 31,200 to 37,600) episodes of syncope, 43,400 (95% CI 39,400 to 47,500) serious electrolyte disorders, and 88,700 (95% CI 80,400 to 97,000) cases of acute kidney injury per year if adopted nationally in the United States.[156]

Lipids

A clear linear relationship exists between serum cholesterol levels and coronary heart disease; the relationship between serum cholesterol and stroke is more complex. The totality of evidence from large epidemiologic studies suggests, at best, a minimal association between increasing usual total cholesterol levels and stroke.[157] A meta-analysis of 45 prospective cohorts involving 450,000 people and 13,000 incident strokes found no relationship between total cholesterol and stroke.[158] The cohorts upon which the analyses were based included many middle-aged participants, and the stroke subtypes were not specified. Other studies found a small association between higher total or low-density lipoprotein (LDL) cholesterol levels and increasing ischemic stroke risk; paradoxically, lower total or LDL-cholesterol has generally been associated with an increased risk of hemorrhagic stroke.[157] These competing risks may in part explain the lack of a relationship between cholesterol levels and overall stroke rates.

An individual-data meta-analysis of nearly 900,000 patients from 61 studies worldwide found only a weak positive association between total cholesterol and total stroke mortality at ages 40 to 59 years, with no association at older ages.[159] A weak positive association was also found between total cholesterol and ischemic stroke with a negative association with hemorrhagic stroke. For both total and ischemic stroke mortality, associations were larger with a baseline SBP <145 mm Hg.

HDL cholesterol protects against atherosclerosis through reverse cholesterol transport, improvement of endothelial function, and antioxidant, anti-inflammatory, and antithrombotic effects.[160,161] Numerous large cohort studies have evaluated the relationship between serum HDL-cholesterol and stroke risk.[161] Despite using different HDL-cholesterol cut-points and including cohorts of different ages and geography, most of these studies find either a strong and statistically significant inverse relationship between HDL-cholesterol and stroke risk[162–166] or a trend toward such a relationship.[167,168] The risk of atherosclerotic stroke in particular may be most strongly related to low HDL-cholesterol levels.[169–171] However, a large meta-analysis found no evidence for a significant association between HDL-cholesterol and stroke mortality, and only a weak positive association between the ratio total/HDL-cholesterol and stroke mortality for those aged 40 to 69 years.[159] There have been no studies showing that pharmacologically raising HDL cholesterol levels decreases stroke risk.

The relationship between triglycerides and ischemic stroke is conflicting. Fasting levels were not associated with ischemic stroke in the ARIC Study,[168] but a meta-analysis of prospective studies in the Asia–Pacific region showed a 50% increase in ischemic stroke risk for those with the highest versus the lowest fasting levels.[172] In the Copenhagen City Heart Study[173] and the Women's Health Study,[174] higher nonfasting triglycerides were associated with increased risk of ischemic stroke. The Women's Health Study also evaluated fasting triglycerides and found no association with ischemic stroke.[174]

Although no large, consistent association between cholesterol and total stroke has been observed in epidemiologic cohorts, data from randomized trials show that statin therapy reduces the risk of stroke among patients with established coronary heart disease and in those at increased vascular risk.[175,176] One meta-analysis of data from 14 trials including more than 90,000 patients found an approximate 17% to 21% reduction in the RR of incident stroke per mmol/L decrease in LDL-cholesterol.[175] A significant trend with greater proportional reductions in stroke were associated with greater mean absolute LDL-cholesterol reductions. Another meta-analysis including nearly 166,000 participants in trials of statins in combination with other preventive interventions also found an approximate 21% decrease in stroke for each mmol/L decrease in LDL-cholesterol.[176] Incidence of all strokes was reduced by 18%, and a reduction in the risk of recurrent stroke and major cardiovascular events among persons with noncardioembolic stroke was found with a trend toward a lower incidence of fatal stroke. Use of statin therapy to reduce cholesterol did not lead to an increased risk of hemorrhagic stroke in primary stroke prevention populations. Among those with prior stroke or TIA, statins may be associated with an increased risk of hemorrhagic stroke that partially attenuates their overall benefit. Other lipid-modification therapies—including niacin, fibric acid derivatives, bile acid sequestrants, and ezetimibe—also have favorable effects on lipid parameters, but the evidence in support of such strategies for stroke prevention is not well established.[4]

Diabetes

Diabetes is a complex metabolic condition with both microvascular and macrovascular complications. In 2017, the CDC estimated that 30.2 million adults in the United States had diabetes, 7.2 million of whom were unaware or did not report they had the condition.[177] The prevalence of diabetes among those aged 45 to 64 years or older was estimated at 17%, and for those aged 60 years or older, 25%. Diabetes is overrepresented among patients who present with ischemic stroke, with prevalence estimates of 15% to 33%.[178] Diabetic patients are more susceptible to the development of atherosclerosis and often have other cardiovascular risk factors such as hypertension, dyslipidemia, atrial fibrillation, heart failure, and prior myocardial infarction (MI). Epidemiologic studies show the relationship between diabetes and stroke is independent of such other risk factors.

An individual-data meta-analysis based on 97 studies involving nearly 600,000 people worldwide without prior vascular disease found a more than twofold excess risk of incident fatal or first-ever nonfatal ischemic stroke among people with diabetes, even after adjusting for other vascular risk factors.[179] The excess risk with diabetes was similar for unclassified stroke (84% increased risk), but slightly lower for hemorrhagic stroke (56% increased risk). Although diabetes was consistently associated with increased ischemic stroke risk across clinically relevant strata, risks tended to be higher for women, younger adults (aged 40 to 59 years), and those within the highest tertile of BMI. Much more moderate and nonlinear associations with stroke risk were observed for fasting blood glucose concentration.

Diabetes is a strong predictor of stroke outcomes.[178] diabetes doubles the risk of recurrent stroke, and an estimated 9% of recurrent strokes can be attributed to diabetes. Diabetic patients have higher stroke mortality rates, greater residual disability, and slower recovery after stroke.[179,180]

Evidence that tight control of glycemic levels lowers stroke (or cardiovascular risk) is lacking.[4] However, stroke risk can be modified among diabetic patients.[4] A comprehensive cardiovascular program that includes hypertension control with an angiotensin converting enzyme inhibitor or angiotensin receptor blocker reduces stroke risk. Statin treatment, especially among diabetic patients with additional risk factors, decreases the risk of a first or a recurrent stroke. Monotherapy with a fibrate may be helpful in reducing stroke risk, but data are conflicting; the addition of a fibrate to statin therapy does not lower stroke risk among diabetic patients.

Atrial Fibrillation

Atrial fibrillation is a major risk factor for ischemic stroke. The prevalence of atrial fibrillation in the United States increases from 0.5% in those aged 50 to 59 years to 1.8% for those aged 60 to 69 years, 4.8% for those aged 70 to 79 years, and 8.8% for those aged 80 to 89 years.[181] The population attributable stroke risk for atrial fibrillation increases from 1.5% to 2.8%, 9.9%, and 23.5% over these same age groups, respectively. Estimates of the prevalence of atrial fibrillation in the United States varies from 2.7 to 6.1 million.[2] In a US national biracial sample of adult men and women, among those with confirmed atrial fibrillation, blacks were approximately one-third as likely to be aware that they had the arrythmia as whites.[182]

In addition to age, a variety of other patient characteristics can affect atrial fibrillation-related stroke risk. A review of seven studies including six independent cohorts found the strongest, most consistent risk factors for stroke in persons with atrial fibrillation were a history of prior stroke or TIA (RR = 2.5, 95% CI 1.8 to 3.5), increasing age (RR = 1.5/decade, 95% CI 1.3 to 1.7), a history of hypertension (RR = 2.0, 95% CI 1.6 to 2.5), and diabetes mellitus (RR = 1.7, 95% CI 1.4 to 2.0).[183] Stroke rates for single independent risk factors were 1.5% to 3%/year for age >75 years, 6% to 9%/year for prior stroke/TIA, 1.5% to 3%/year for history of hypertension, and 2.0% to 3.5%/year for diabetes.

Several published schemes are available to stratify an individual patient's atrial fibrillation-related stroke risk. A comparison of 12 of these schemes found that they varied considerably.[184] Of these, 7 were based on extant data and 5 on expert consensus. Factors most commonly included were previous stroke/TIA (all schemes), patient age (83%), hypertension (83%), and diabetes (83%), with 8 additional variables included in 1 or more schemes. When applied to the same cohort, the fractions of patients categorized by the different schemes varied considerably (the proportions of patients categorized as "low risk" varied from 9% to 49%, and the proportions categorized as "high-risk" varied from 11% to 77%). The predictive capacity of these various schemes is limited.[185] The differences in the schemes are not trivial and have important public health and clinical implications.

The CHADS2 scheme is the most commonly used for stroke risk stratification in patients with atrial fibrillation.[186] One point is given for congestive heart failure (C), hypertension (H), age over 75 years (A), and diabetes mellitus (D), and 2 points for a history of prior stroke or TIA. A validation study found that a score of 0 points reflected low risk (0.5% to 1.7%/year); 1 point, moderate risk (1.2% to 2.2%/year); and 2 points or more, high risk (1.9% to 7.6%/year).[186] However, it should be noted that a history of prior stroke or TIA in a patient with atrial fibrillation alone is associated with a high risk of recurrent cerebrovascular events (6% to 10%/year).[183]

Patients with paroxysmal or chronic atrial fibrillation at moderate or high stroke risk are candidates for treatment with an anticoagulant for prevention of stroke (see Chapter 30). Novel anticoagulants including direct thrombin inhibitors and oral Factor Xa inhibitors are now available for treatment of this population of patients. Yet, many people with atrial fibrillation are not adequately anticoagulated.[187]

Sickle Cell Disease

The prevalence of sickle cell disease (SCD), an autosomal recessive inherited disorder, is 0.25% in blacks and confers a 200- to 400-fold increased RR of stroke compared to black children without the condition.[181] The prevalence of stroke by age 20-years is approximately 11% in persons homozygous for SCD.[188] Transcranial Doppler (TCD) ultrasonography is useful in identifying children with SCD who are at high and low stroke risk. Children with a timed mean TCD velocity in the middle cerebral artery >200 cm/sec have a stroke rate in excess of 10%/year whereas those with velocities below this level have stroke rates of about 1%/year.[189] Although a variety of treatments are available, regular red blood cell transfusion is the only preventive intervention proven in randomized trials to prevent stroke in children with SCD.[190] Transfusion therapy reduced the risk of stroke from 10% to less than 1% annually.

Sleep-Disordered Breathing

Sleep-disordered breathing (SDB) is highly prevalent in patients with established cardiovascular disease. Obstructive sleep apnea (OSA), one form of SDB, affects an estimated 15 million adult Americans, and is present in a large proportion of patients with hypertension and those with other cardiovascular conditions, including coronary artery disease, atrial fibrillation, and stroke.[191–197] OSA is characterized by repetitive interruption of ventilation during sleep caused by collapse of the pharyngeal airway. A meta-analysis suggests that nearly three-quarters of stroke and TIA patients have SDB, with the predominate form being OSA.[197] In this review, SDB was more common among men and those with recurrent strokes or strokes of unknown etiology; SDB was less common among patients whose strokes were of cardioembolic etiology. An observational study of consecutive patients who underwent polysomnography who had subsequent verified events (strokes and deaths) found that even after adjusting for age, sex, race-ethnicity, and comorbid conditions, OSA increased the risk of stroke or death from any cause (adjusted hazard ratio [aHR] = 1.97, 95% CI 1.12 to 3.48).[191] In a trend analy-

sis, increased severity of sleep apnea at baseline was associated with an increased risk of this composite end point.[191] Patients who had a stroke and OSA who were followed for 10 years had an increased risk of death (aHR = 1.76, 95% CI 1.05 to 2.95), which is independent of age, sex, and other common cardiovascular risk factors.[192] Whether patients with stroke and OSA have cardiovascular benefit from treatment with continuous positive airway pressure ventilation remains to be determined.

OTHER RISK FACTORS

Fibrinogen, Clotting Factors, and Inflammation

Inflammation has a role in the initiation, progression, and complications of atherosclerosis and is a contributor to the destabilization of atherosclerotic lesions.[198] The measurement of a diverse set of proinflammatory factors adds prognostic information beyond that already provided by traditional cardiovascular risk factors. High-sensitivity C-reactive protein (CRP) is one of the most widely studied of these biomarkers. CRP is an acute-phase reactant, which is released predominately by hepatocytes in response to inflammatory cytokine stimulation; it is also released in response to systemic inflammation such as in connective tissue disease and infections. Despite the lack of specificity for the cause of the inflammation, a multitude of epidemiologic studies, including the Physicians' Health Study, the Women's Health Study, and the Framingham Study, found an association between elevated CRP and the risk of incident and recurrent vascular events, including stroke.[4] Risks for those in the highest tertiles/quartiles of CRP concentration are between 1.5 and 2 times higher than those in the lowest tertiles/quartiles. A meta-analysis of individual records from over 50 prospective studies involving over 160,000 participants without preexisting vascular disease found log-transformed CRP concentrations linearly related to the risk of ischemic stroke with no apparent risk threshold.[199] One standard deviation increase in log-transformed CRP concentration (threefold increase) was associated with a 27% to 44% increased risk of ischemic stroke and a 55% to 71% increased risk of vascular mortality, depending upon risk-adjustment factors. Although somewhat controversial, guidelines have tended to suggest that CRP measurement be limited to persons with intermediate cardiovascular risk (10% to 20% 10-year risk based upon the Framingham Risk Score) to help guide clinical decision making.[181,200] Guidelines indicate that measurement of inflammatory markers, such as hs-CRP in patients without cardiovascular disease, may be considered to identify those who may be at increased risk of stroke, although its usefulness in routine clinical practice is not well established.[4] Other markers of inflammation, such as lipoprotein-associated phospholipase A2 (LpPLA2), also may be considered with the same caveate.[4]

In addition to examining the relationship between inflammation and stroke based on the measurement of proinflammatory factors, patients with systemic chronic inflammatory conditions, such as rheumatoid arthritis and systemic lupus erythematosus, generally have an excess risk for cardiovascular events and stroke.[4] Chronic infection with *Helicobacter pylori* might promote atherosclerosis, but randomized trials of antibiotics have not shown a benefit for the prevention of vascular events. Acute infectious diseases might trigger a TIA or stroke via possible induction of clotting factors, such as fibrinogen, or the destabilization of atherosclerotic plaques. Influenza has been associated with increased cardiovascular mortality, and antiviral treatment of influenza within a few days of onset decreases the 6-month risk of stroke or TIA. A relationship between influenza vaccination and reduced risk for stroke has also been found.[200a]

Fibrinogen, a clotting factor thought to accelerate the thrombotic process, is another potentially useful marker of inflammation for use in

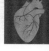

vascular disease prediction and prevention.[201] An individual-data meta-analysis of 31 prospective studies involving over 150,000 participants without preexisting vascular disease found an approximate log-linear association of usual fibrinogen level and the risk of a first nonfatal or fatal stroke.[201] The association was present within each age group (40 to 59, 60 to 69, and ≥70 years) with no risk threshold. In analyses adjusted for age, sex, and other established vascular risk factors, the risk of stroke was nearly double with each 1 g/L increase in usual fibrinogen level. When stroke was categorized into subtypes, the magnitude of the association with fibrinogen was present for ischemic stroke and stroke attributed to unspecified causes, but was somewhat lower for hemorrhagic stroke. The usefulness of screening specific treatments for primary stroke prevention in asymptomatic patients with a hereditary or acquired thrombophilia factors (e.g., Factor V Leiden, prothrombin 20210a mutations, protein C and protein S deficiencies, lupus anticoagulants and anticardiolipin antibodies) is not well established.[4]

Blood Homocysteine Levels

Homocysteine is an intermediary amino acid that is formed during the metabolism of the essential amino acid methionine. Normal plasma levels of homocysteine are 5 to 15 μmol/L. Elevated homocysteine levels, or hyperhomocysteinemia, may result from genetic defects that reduce enzymatic activity in homocysteine metabolism (e.g., homozygosity for the thermolabile variant of methylene tetrahydrofolate reductase [MTHFR; TT genotype]), nutritional deficiencies in vitamin cofactors (e.g., vitamin B_6, vitamin B_{12}, folic acid), chronic medical conditions (e.g., chronic renal failure, which retards renal clearance of homocysteine), certain medications (e.g., fibrates and nicotinic acid, which are used in the treatment of hypercholesterolemia), or lifestyle behaviors (e.g., smoking).[202–206] Numerous studies support a modest association between elevated homocysteine levels and atherosclerotic vascular diseases.[207–216] One meta-analysis involving 463 nonfatal or fatal stroke or TIA events from 12 prospective studies found a 25% lower usual homocysteine level (~3 μmol/L) was associated with a 19% (95% CI 5% to 31%) lower risk of stroke after adjustment for known cardiovascular risk factors and regression dilution bias.[207] Another meta-analysis, which involved 676 stroke events from eight prospective studies and adjusted for similar factors, found a 59% increased risk of stroke for a 5 μmol/L increase in homocysteine.[208] On this basis, a 3 μmol/L decrease in current homocysteine concentrations would be expected to reduce the risk of stroke by 24% (95% CI 15% to 33%). This meta-analysis did not find a significant relationship of the MTHFR TT polymorphism (compared to wildtype CC) with stroke (odds ratio 1.65, 95% CI 0.66 to 4.13), although the seven included MTHFR studies yielded relatively few data. Later studies continue to report a relationship between hyperhomocysteinemia and stroke, recurrent stroke, and silent brain infarction.[209–215] A subsequent meta-analysis including data from over 15,000 persons initially free of cardiovascular disease found that homozygotes for the T allele of the MTHFR polymorphism had a greater mean homocysteine level and a 26% (95% CI 1.14 to 1.40) greater risk of stroke.[216] Cohort restrictions by age, race, and geographic location yielded similar results.

Laboratory findings and genetic association studies support the biologic plausibility of a causal role for elevated homocysteine in stroke pathogenesis; however, the results of randomized clinical trials have not established the efficacy of homocysteine-lowering therapies for the reduction of stroke risk.[68] Clinical trials confirm that vitamins B_6, B_{12}, and folic acid lower homocysteine levels, but several large trials of supplementation with these vitamins as a means of lowering homocysteine levels in patients with established cardiovascular disease have generally found no reduction in major vascular events or death. The largest of such trials to date, VITamins TO Prevent Stroke (VITATOPS), was a

double-blind, placebo-controlled trial including over 8000 patients with recent TIA or stroke from 20 countries who were followed for a median duration of 3.4 years.[217] Although VITATOPS found daily administration of B vitamins was safe and lowered homocysteine levels, it was not more effective than placebo in reducing the risk of the primary combined endpoint of stroke, MI, or vascular death (RR = 0.91, 95% CI 0.82 to 1.00). Secondary analyses by outcome revealed similar results except for a reduction in vascular death (RR = 0.86, 95% CI 0.75 to 0.99). When the VITATOPS findings were included in a meta-analysis with other clinical trials of homocysteine-lowering therapy in patients with and without preexisting cerebrovascular disease, B vitamin supplementation led to no reductions in the risks of a first (RR 0.94, 95% CI 0.83-1.06) or recurrent (RR 0.96, 95% CI 0.85-1.07) stroke.[218] Despite negative individual trial results for B vitamins in the prevention of stroke, a clinically beneficial effect of homocysteine-lowering therapies cannot be excluded. Interventions that are powered to detect smaller risk reductions, which can achieve and sustain larger reductions in homocysteine, or that are focused on certain subgroups such as those with lacunar infarction or ICH caused by small-vessel disease, could produce clinically beneficial results. The above referenced meta-analysis, which included 14 randomized, controlled trials with 54,913 participants, found an overall 7% reduction in stroke from lowering homocysteine with B vitamin supplementation (RR = 0.93, 95% CI 0.86–1.00, $P = .04$).[218]

Migraine

Accumulating evidence suggests a relationship between migraine headache and an increased risk of ischemic stroke. A meta-analysis of 14 studies published through June 2004 reported a pooled RR of 2.16 (95% CI 1.89 to 2.48); results were similar for analyses restricted to persons age <45 years and were consistent among those having migraine with and without aura.[219] A later meta-analysis incorporating nine studies published through January 2009 also reported an increased risk of ischemic stroke among persons with any type of migraine compared to those without migraine (pooled RR = 1.73, 95% CI 1.31 to 2.29).[220] However, stratification by migraine aura status showed that the higher risk of stroke was largely confined to those having migraine with aura (pooled RR = 2.16, 95% CI 1.53 to 3.03 for those with aura vs. pooled RR = 1.23, 95% CI 0.90 to 1.69 for those without aura). Additional stratified analyses suggested a greater risk of ischemic stroke for women with migraine (pooled RR 2.08, 95% CI 1.13 to 3.84) but not men (pooled RR = 1.37, 95% CI 0.89 to 2.11), persons age <45 years (pooled RR = 2.65, 95% CI 1.41 to 4.97), particularly women (pooled RR = 3.65, 95% CI 2.21 to 6.04), smokers (pooled RR = 9.03, 95% CI 4.22 to 19.34) and women also using oral contraceptives (pooled RR = 7.02, 95% CI 1.51 to 32.68). Three studies each examined the relationship of any migraine to TIA and hemorrhagic stroke; higher risk was found for TIA (pooled RR = 2.34, 95% CI 1.90 to 2.88) but not for hemorrhagic stroke (pooled RR = 1.18, 95% CI 0.87 to 1.60). Several studies find an association between migraine headache and nonspecific white matter hyperintensities on MRI, localized predominately in the posterior circulation white matter or cerebellum.[221–224] The clinical significance of these MRI findings is uncertain. There is no evidence that migraine control lowers stroke risk, but as noted above, the risk of migraine-associated stroke is higher among women who smoke and use oral contraceptives.[4]

AWARENESS OF STROKE WARNING SIGNS AND ACUTE TREATMENT

The recognition of stroke symptoms is higher in women compared to men, among whites versus blacks and Hispanics-Latinos, and among people with higher versus lower educational attainment.[225] Although the awareness of stroke warning signs has improved over time, the recognition of multiple warning signs remains low, as does people's ability to identify tissue plasminogen activator (tPA) as an available drug therapy, or the importance of presenting for treatment as soon as possible after symptom onset.[226] Symptoms associated with increased likelihood of calling "9-1-1" include weakness, confusion/decreased level of consciousness, speech/language deficits, and dizziness/coordination/vertigo; however, numbness and headache were not associated with the decision to call.[227] The administration of intravenous tissue plasminogen activator (IV-tPA) improves the likelihood that selected patients with acute ischemic stroke will have an excellent outcome when administered within 4.5 hours of symptom onset. Despite this benefit, only about 2% of ischemic stroke patients in the United States are treated with IV-tPA.[228]

THE FUTURE

Driven primarily by ischemic stroke, stroke incidence had decreased in US whites between the 1990s and 2005, but not in US blacks.[229] Between 2004 and 2014, the age-adjusted stroke death rate in the United States fell by 28.7% (from 51.2/100,000 to 36.5/100,000), and the actual number of stroke deaths decreased by 11.3% (from 150,074 deaths to 133,103 deaths).[2] Much of the decline is attributed to more effective prevention.[230] However, the improvement failed to continue in 38 states between 2013 and 2015 with rates now increasing in some populations.[231] Part of this reversal may be related to an increase in stroke risk factors in the population such as diabetes and obesity.[232] A harbinger of the future, ischemic stroke hospitalization rates increased for both men and women and for certain race/ethnic groups among younger adults aged 18 to 54 years between 2003 and 2004, and 2011 and 2012, almost doubling for men aged 18 to 34 and 35 to 44 years since 1995 to 1996 with a 41.5% increase among men aged 35 to 44 years from 2003 to 2004, to 2011 to 2012.[233] These increasing hospitalization rates occurred on a background of higher prevalences of traditional stroke risk factors in young adults (hypertension increased from 4% to 11%, lipid disorders 12% to 21%, diabetes 4% to 7%, tobacco use 5% to 16%, and obesity 4% to 9%).[233] If these trends continue, the burden of stroke in the United States will dramatically increase in the years ahead. Other potential or emerging risk factors not addressed in this chapter are available for review in the AHA Primary Stroke Guidelines.[4]

REFERENCES

1. Feigin VL, Forouzanfar MH, Krishnamurthi R, et al. Global and regional burden of stroke during 1990-2010: findings from the Global Burden of Disease Study 2010. *Lancet.* 2014;383:245–254.
2. Benjamin EJ, Blaha MJ, Chiuve SE, et al. Heart Disease and Stroke Statistics—2017 Update. *Circulation.* 2017;135:e146–e603.
3. World Health Organization. *Global Health Estimates 2015 Summary Tables: Global DALYs by Cause, Age and Sex, 2000-2015.* Geneva, Switzerland; 2016.
4. Meschia JF, Bushnell C, Boden-Albala B, et al. Guidelines for the primary prevention of stroke. *Stroke.* 2014;45:3754–3832.
5. O'Donnell MJ, Chin SL, Rangarajan S, et al. Global and regional effects of potentially modifiable risk factors associated with acute stroke in 32 countries (INTERSTROKE): a case-control study. *Lancet.* 2016;388:761–765.
6. Hall MJ, Levant S, DeFrances CJ. Hospitalization for stroke in U.S. hospitals, 1989-2009. *NCHS data brief.* 2012;(95):1–8.
7. Administration on Aging, Administration for Community Living, and US Department of Health and Human Services. A profile of older Americans: 2016. https://acl.gov/sites/default/files/Aging%20and%20Disability%20in%20America/2016-Profile.pdf.
8. Wu CM, McLaughlin K, Lorenzetti DL, et al. Early risk of stroke after transient ischemic attack: a systematic review and meta-analysis. *Arch Intern Med.* 2007;167:2417–2422.
9. Kleindorfer D, Panagos P, Pancioli A, et al. Incidence and short-term prognosis of transient ischemic attack in a population-based study. *Stroke.* 2005;36:720–723.
10. Amarenco P, Lavallee PC, Labreuche J, et al. One-year risk of stroke after transient ischemic attack or minor stroke. *N Engl J Med.* 2016;374:1533–1542.
11. Howard G, Safford MM, Meschia JF, et al. Stroke symptoms in individuals reporting no prior stroke or transient ischemic attack are associated with a decrease in indices of mental and physical functioning. *Stroke.* 2007;38:2446–2452.
12. Johnston SC, Fayad PB, Gorelick PB, et al. Prevalence and knowledge of transient ischemic attack among US adults. *Neurology.* 2003;60:1429–1434.
13. Bravata DM, Ho SY, Brass LM, et al. Long-term mortality in cerebrovascular disease. *Stroke.* 2003;34:699–704.
14. Bronnum-Hansen H, Davidsen M, Thorvaldsen P. Long-term survival and causes of death after stroke. *Stroke.* 2001;32:2131–2136.
15. Collins TC, Petersen NJ, Menke TJ, et al. Short-term, intermediate-term, and long-term mortality in patients hospitalized for stroke. *J Clin Epidemiol.* 2003;56:81–87.
16. Eriksson M, Norrving B, Terent A, Stegmayr B. Functional outcome 3 months after stroke predicts long-term survival. *Cerebrovasc Dis.* 2008;25:423–429.
17. Hallstrom B, Jonsson AC, Nerbrand C, et al. Stroke incidence and survival in the beginning of the 21st century in southern Sweden: comparisons with the late 20th century and projections into the future. *Stroke.* 2008;39:10–15.
18. Sacco RL, Shi T, Zamanillo MC, Kargman DE. Predictors of mortality and recurrence after hospitalized cerebral infarction in an urban community: the Northern Manhattan Stroke Study. *Neurology.* 1994;44:626–634.
19. Sacco RL, Wolf PA, Kannel WB, McNamara PM. Survival and recurrence following stroke: The Framingham Study. *Stroke.* 1982;13:290–295.
20. von Arbin M, Britton M, De Faire U. Mortality and recurrences during eight years following stroke. *J Intern Med.* 1992;231:43–48.
21. Qureshi AI, Suri MF, Zhou J, Divani AA. African American women have poor long-term survival following ischemic stroke. *Neurology.* 2006;67:1623–1629.
22. Hankey GJ, Jamrozik K, Broadhurst RJ, et al. Long-term risk of first recurrent stroke in the Perth Community Stroke Study. *Stroke.* 1998;29:2491–2500.
23. Hankey GJ, Jamrozik K, Broadhurst RJ, et al. Five-year survival after first-ever stroke and related prognostic factors in the Perth Community Stroke Study. *Stroke.* 2000;31(9):2080–2086.
24. Lai SM, Alter M, Friday G, Sobel E. Prognosis for survival after an initial stroke. *Stroke.* 1995;26:2011–2015.
25. Prencipe M, Culasso F, Rasura M, et al. Long-term prognosis after a minor stroke: 10-year mortality and major stroke recurrence rates in a hospital-based cohort. *Stroke.* 1998;29:126–132.
26. Hartmann A, Rundek T, Mast H, et al. Mortality and causes of death after first ischemic stroke: the Northern Manhattan Stroke Study. *Neurology.* 2001;57:2000–2005.
27. Terent A. Trends in stroke incidence and 10-year survival in Soderhamn, Sweden, 1975-2001. *Stroke.* 2003;34:1353–1358.
28. Kammersgaard LP, Olsen TS. Cardiovascular risk factors and 5-year mortality in the Copenhagen Stroke Study. *Cerebrovasc Dis.* 2006;21:187–193.
29. Qureshi AI, Suri MF, Zhou J, Divani AA. African American women have poor long-term survival following ischemic stroke. *Neurology.* 2006;67:1623–1629.
30. La Spina P, Savica R, Serra S, et al. Long-term survival and outcome after first stroke in the Sicilian Aeolian Island Archipelago population. *Neurol Sci.* 2008;29:153–156.
31. Andersen KK, Olsen TS. One-month to 10-year survival in the Copenhagen stroke study: interactions between stroke severity and other prognostic indicators. *J Stroke Cerebrovasc Dis.* 2011;20:117–123.

32. Tu JV, Gong Y. Trends in treatment and outcomes for acute stroke patients in Ontario, 1992-1998. *Arch Intern Med*. 2003;163:293–297.

33. Hardie K, Hankey GJ, Jamrozik K, et al. Ten-year survival after first-ever stroke in the Perth Community Stroke Study. *Stroke*. 2003;34:1842–1846.

34. Koton S, Schneider AL, Rosamond WD, et al. Stroke incidence and mortality trends in US communities, 1987 to 2011. *JAMA*. 2014;312:259–268.

35. Matchar DB, Samsa GP, Goldstein LB, et al. Is major stroke worse than death? Results from a survey of preferences among persons at increased risk for stroke. *Neurology*. 1998;50:A326–A327.

36. Asplund K, Stegmayr B, Peltonen M. From the twentieth to the twenty-first century: a public health perspective on stroke. In: Ginsberg MD, Bogousslavsky J, eds. *Cerebrovascular Disease Pathophysiology, Diagnosis, and Management*. Malden, MA: Blackwell Science; 1998; 2.

37. Torio CM, Andrews RM. National inpatient hospital costs: the most expensive conditions by payer, 2011. In: *Healthcare Cost and Utilization Project (HCUP) Statistical Briefs*. Rockville (MD): Agency for Healthcare Research and Quality (US); 2006.

38. Ovbiagele B, Goldstein LB, Higashida RT, et al. Forecasting the future of stroke in the United States: a policy statement from the American Heart Association and American Stroke Association. *Stroke*. 2013;44:2361–2375.

39. Taylor TN, Davis PH, Torner JC, et al. Lifetime cost of stroke in the United States. *Stroke*. 1996;27:1459–1466.

40. Lanska DJ, Kryscio R. Geographic distribution of hospitalization rates, case fatality, and mortality from stroke in the United States. *Neurology*. 1994;44:1541–1550.

41. Lanska DJ. Geographic distribution of stroke mortality in the United States: 1939-1941 to 1979-1981. *Neurology*. 1993;43:1839–1851.

42. Pickle LW, Mungiole M, Gillum RF. Geographic variation in stroke mortality in blacks and whites in the United States. *Stroke*. 1997;28:1639–1647.

43. Borhani NO. Changes and geographic distribution of mortality from cerebrovascular disease. *Am J Public Health Nations Health*. 1965;55:673–681.

44. El-Saed A, Kuller LH, Newman AB, et al. Geographic variations in stroke incidence and mortality among older populations in four US communities. *Stroke*. 2006;37:1975–1979.

45. Howard G. Why do we have a stroke belt in the Southeastern United States? A review of unlikely and uninvestigated potential causes. *Am J Med Sci*. 1999;317:160–167.

46. Howard G, Evans GW, Pearce K, et al. Is the stroke belt disappearing? An analysis of racial, temporal, and age effects. *Stroke*. 1995;26:1153–1158.

47. Howard G, Howard VJ, Katholi C, et al. Decline in US stroke mortality. An analysis of temporal patterns by sex, race, and geographic region. *Stroke*. 2001;32:2213–2218.

48. Gillum RF, Ingram DD. Relation between residence in the southeast region of the United States and stroke incidence. The NHANES I Epidemiologic Followup Study. *Am J Epidemiol*. 1996;144:665–673.

49. Howard G. Why do we have a stroke belt in the southeastern United States? A review of unlikely and uninvestigated potential causes. *Am J Med Sci*. 1999;317:160–167.

50. Centers for Disease Control and Prevention. *Stroke hospitalization rates 2012-2014, Medicare Beneficiaries, Ages 65 +, by County*. https://www.cdc.gov/dhdsp/maps/national_maps/stroke_hospitalization_all.htm; 2017. (Accessed October 8, 2017).

51. Allen NB, Holford TR, Bracken MB, et al. Geographic variation in 1-year recurrent ischemic stroke rates for elderly Medicare beneficiaries in the USA. *Neuroepidemiology*. 2010;34:123–129.

52. Allen NB, Holford TR, Bracken MB, et al. Trends in one-year recurrent ischemic stroke among the elderly in the USA: 1994-2002. *Cerebrovasc Dis*. 2010;30:525–532.

53. Davenport RJ, Dennis MS, Wellwood I, Warlow CP. Complications after acute stroke. *Stroke*. 1996;27:415–420.

54. Casper ML, Nwaise IA, Croft JB, Nilasena DS. *Atlas of Stroke Hospitalizations Among Medicare Beneficiaries*. Atlanta: U.S. Department of Health and Human Services, Centers for Disease Control and Prevention; 2008.

55. Reeves MJ, Bushnell CD, Howard G, et al. Sex differences in stroke: epidemiology, clinical presentation, medical care, and outcomes. *Lancet Neurol*. 2008;7:915–926.

56. Davie CA, O'Brien P. Stroke and pregnancy. *J Neurol Neurosurg Psychiatry*. 2008;79:240–245.

57. Bushnell CD. Stroke in women: risk and prevention throughout the lifespan. *Neurol Clin*. 2008;26:1161–1176.

58. Towfighi A, Saver JL, Engelhardt R, Ovbiagele B. A midlife stroke surge among women in the United States. *Neurology*. 2007;69:1898–1904.

59. Towfighi A, Markovic D, Ovbiagele B. Persistent sex disparity in midlife stroke prevalence in the United States. *Cerebrovasc Dis*. 2011;31:322–328.

60. Lackland DT, Bachman DL, Carter TD, et al. The geographic variation in stroke incidence in two areas of the Southeastern Stroke Belt - The Anderson and Pee Dee Stroke Study. *Stroke*. 1998;29:2061–2068.

61. Bian J, Oddone EZ, Samsa GP, et al. Racial differences in survival post cerebral infarction among the elderly. *Neurology*. 2003;60:285–290.

62. Estruch R, Ros E, Salas-Salvado J, et al. Primary prevention of cardiovascular disease with a Mediterranean diet. *N Engl J Med*. 2013;368:1279–1290.

63. Larsson SC, Wallin A, Wolk A. Dietary approaches to stop hypertension diet and incidence of stroke: results from 2 prospective cohorts. *Stroke*. 2016;47:986–990.

64. Boden-Albala B, Elkind MS, White H, et al. Dietary total fat intake and ischemic stroke risk: the Northern Manhattan Study. *Neuroepidemiology*. 2009;32:296–301.

65. Iso H, Rexrode KM, Stampfer MJ, et al. Intake of fish and omega-3 fatty acids and risk of stroke in women. *JAMA*. 2001;285:304–312.

66. Gillum RF, Mussolino ME, Madans JH. The relationship between fish consumption and stroke incidence. The NHANES I Epidemiologic Follow-up Study (National Health and Nutrition Examination Survey). *Arch Intern Med*. 1996;156:537–542.

67. He FJ, Nowson CA, MacGregor GA. Fruit and vegetable consumption and stroke: meta-analysis of cohort studies. *Lancet*. 2006;367:320–326.

68. John JH, Ziebland S, Yudkin P, et al. Effects of fruit and vegetable consumption on plasma antioxidant concentrations and blood pressure: a randomised controlled trial. *Lancet*. 2002;359:1969–1974.

69. He J, Ogden LG, Vupputuri S, et al. Dietary sodium intake and subsequent risk of cardiovascular disease in overweight adults. *JAMA*. 1999;282:2027–2034.

70. Nagata C, Takatsuka N, Shimizu N, Shimizu H. Sodium intake and risk of death from stroke in Japanese men and women. *Stroke*. 2004;35:1543–1547.

71. Khaw KT, Barrett-Connor E. Dietary potassium and stroke-associated mortality. A 12-year prospective population study. *N Engl J Med*. 1987;316:235–240.

72. Ascherio A, Rimm EB, Hernan MA, et al. Intake of potassium, magnesium, calcium, and fiber and risk of stroke among US men. *Circulation*. 1998;98:1198–1204.

73. Appel LJ, Moore TJ, Obarzanek E, et al. A clinical trial of the effects of dietary patterns on blood pressure. DASH Collaborative Research Group. *N Engl J Med*. 1997;336:1117–1124.

74. Fung TT, Chiuve SE, McCullough ML, et al. Adherence to a DASH-style diet and risk of coronary heart disease and stroke in women. *Arch Intern Med*. 2008;168:713–720.

75. Fung TT, Rexrode KM, Mantzoros CS, et al. Mediterranean diet and incidence of and mortality from coronary heart disease and stroke in women. *Circulation*. 2009;119:1093–1100.

76. Fung TT, Stampfer MJ, Manson JE, et al. Prospective study of major dietary patterns and stroke risk in women. *Stroke*. 2004;35:2014–2019.

77. Abbott RD, Rodriguez BL, Burchfiel CM, Curb JD. Physical activity in older middle-aged men and reduced risk of stroke: The Honolulu Heart Program. *Am J Epidemiol*. 1994;139:881–893.

78. Kiely DK, Wolf PA, Cupples LA, et al. Physical activity and stroke risk: The Framingham Study. *Am J Epidemiol*. 1994;140:608–620.

79. Haheim LL, Holme I, Hjermann I, Leren P. Risk factors of stroke incidence and mortality. A 12-year follow-up of the Oslo Study. *Stroke*. 1993;24:1484–1489.

80. Gillum RF, Mussolino ME, Ingram DD. Physical activity and stroke incidence in women and men. The NHANES I Epidemiologic Follow-up Study. *Am J Epidemiol*. 1996;143:860–869.

81. Wannamethee G, Shaper AG. Physical activity and stroke in British middle aged men. *BMJ*. 1992;304:597–601.

82. Sacco RL, Gan R, Boden-Albala B, et al. Leisure-time physical activity and ischemic stroke risk: the Northern Manhattan Stroke Study. *Stroke*. 1998;29:380–387.

83. Lindenstrom E, Boysen G, Nyboe J. Lifestyle factors and risk of cerebrovascular disease in women. The Copenhagen City Heart Study. *Stroke*. 1993;24:1468–1472.

84. Manson JE, Rimm EB, Stampfer MJ, et al. Physical activity and incidence of non-insulin-dependent diabetes mellitus in women. *Lancet*. 1991;338:774–778.

85. Blair SN, Kampert JB, Kohl 3rd HW, et al. Influences of cardiorespiratory fitness and other precursors on cardiovascular disease and all-cause mortality in men and women. *JAMA*. 1996;276:205–210.

86. Kokkinos PF, Narayan P, Colleran JA, et al. Effects of regular exercise on blood pressure and left ventricular hypertrophy in African-American men with severe hypertension. *N Engl J Med*. 1995;333:1462–1467.

87. Lakka TA, Salonen JT. Moderate to high intensity conditioning leisure time physical activity and high cardiorespirtory fitness are associated with reduced plasma fibrinogen in eastern Finnish men. *J Clin Epidemiol*. 1993;46:1119–1127.

88. Williams PT. High-density lipoprotein cholesterol and other risk factors for coronary heart disease in female runners. *N Engl J Med*. 1996;334:1298–1303.

89. Wang JS, Jen CJ, Chen HI. Effects of exercise training and deconditioning on platelet function in men. *Arterioscler Thromb Vasc Biol*. 1995;15:1668–1674.

90. Lee IM, Hennekens CH, Berger K, et al. Exercise and risk of stroke in male physicians. *Stroke*. 1999;30:1–6.

91. Ezzati M, Hoorn SV, Lopez AD, et al. Comparative quantification of mortality and burden of disease attributable to selected risk factors. In: Lopez AD, Mathers CD, Ezzati M, et al., eds. *Global Burden of Disease and Risk Factors*. Washington DC: World Bank; 2006.

92. Sattelmair JR, Kurth T, Buring JE, Lee IM. Physical activity and risk of stroke in women. *Stroke*. 2010;41:1243–1250.

93. Wilson PW, Bozeman SR, Burton TM, et al. Prediction of first events of coronary heart disease and stroke with consideration of adiposity. *Circulation*. 2008;118:124–130.

94. Rexrode KM, Hennekens CH, Willett WC, et al. A prospective study of body mass index, weight change, and risk of stroke in women. *JAMA*. 1997;277:1539–1545.

95. Burchfiel CM, Curb JD, Arakaki R, et al. Cardiovascular risk factors and hyperinsulinemia in elderly men: the Honolulu Heart Program. *Ann Epidemiol*. 1996;6:490–497.

96. Walker SP, Rimm EB, Ascherio A, et al. Body size and fat distribution as predictors of stroke among US men. *Am J Epidemiol*. 1996;144:1143–1150.

97. Brook RD, Franklin B, Cascio W, et al. Air pollution and cardiovascular disease. *Circulation*. 2004;109:2655–2671.

98. Brook RD, Rajagopalan S, Pope CA, et al. Particulate matter air pollution and cardiovascular disease. *Circulation*. 2010;121:2331–2378.

99. Qiu H, Sun S, Tsang H, et al. Fine particulate matter exposure and incidence of stroke: a cohort study in Hong Kong. *Neurology*. 2017;88:1709–1717.

100. Miller KA, Siscovick DS, Sheppard L, et al. Long-term exposure to air pollution and incidence of cardiovascular events in women. *N Engl J Med*. 2007;356:447–458.

101. Pope III CA, Burnett RT, Thurston GD, et al. Cardiovascular mortality and long-term exposure to particulate air pollution: epidemiological evidence of general pathophysiological pathways of disease. *Circulation*. 2004;109:71–77.

102. Henrotin JB, Besancenot JP, Bejot Y, Giroud M. Short-term effects of ozone air pollution on ischaemic stroke occurrence: a case-crossover analysis from a 10-year population-based study in Dijon, France. *Occup Environ Med*. 2007;64:439–445.

103. Lisabeth LD, Escobar JD, Dvonch JT, et al. Ambient air pollution and risk for ischemic stroke and transient ischemic attack. *Ann Neurol*. 2008;64:53–59.

104. Hong Y-C, Lee J-T, Kim H, et al. Effects of air pollutants on acute stroke mortality. *Environ Health Perspect*. 2002;110:.

105. Hong Y-C, Lee J-T, Kim H, Kwon H-J. Air pollution: a new risk factor in ischemic stroke mortality. *Stroke*. 2002;33:2165–2169.

106. Kan H, Jia J, Chen B. Acute stroke mortality and air pollution: new evidence from Shanghai. *China J Occup Health*. 2003;45:321–323.

107. Kettunen J, Lanki T, Tiittanen P, et al. Associations of fine and ultrafine particulate air pollution with stroke mortality in an area of low air pollution levels. *Stroke*. 2007;38:918–922.

108. Wolf PA, D'Agostino RB, Belanger AJ, Kannel WN. Probability of stroke: a risk profile from the Framingham study. *Stroke*. 1991;22:312–318.

109. Manolio TA, Kronmal RA, Burke GL, et al. Short-term predictors of incident stroke in older adults: the Cardiovascular Health Study. *Stroke*. 1996;27:1479–1486.

110. Rodriguez BL, D'Agostino R, Abbott RD, et al. Risk of hospitalized stroke in men enrolled in the Honolulu Heart Program and the Framingham Study: a comparison of incidence and risk factor effects. *Stroke*. 2002;33:230–236.

111. O'Donnell MJ, Xavier D, Liu L, et al. Risk factors for ischaemic and intracerebral haemorrhagic stroke in 22 countries (the INTERSTROKE study): a case-control study. *Lancet*. 2010;376:112–123.

112. Kurth T, Kase CS, Berger K, et al. Smoking and risk of hemorrhagic stroke in women. *Stroke*. 2003;34:2792–2795.

113. Kurth T, Kase CS, Berger K, et al. Smoking and the risk of hemorrhagic stroke in men. *Stroke*. 2003;34:1151–1155.

114. Feigin V, Parag V, Lawes CMM, et al. Smoking and elevated blood pressure are the most important risk factors for subarachnoid hemorrhage in the Asia-Pacific Region: an overview of 26 cohorts involving 306,620 participants. *Stroke*. 2005;36:1360–1365.

115. Feigin VL, Rinkel GJE, Lawes CMM, et al. Risk factors for subarachnoid hemorrhage: an updated systematic review of epidemiological studies. *Stroke*. 2005;36:2773–2780.

116. Feldmann E, Broderick JP, Kernan WN, et al. Major risk factors for intracerebral hemorrhage in the young are modifiable. *Stroke*. 2005;36:1881–1885.

117. Sturgeon JD, Folsom AR, Longstreth Jr WT, et al. Risk factors for intracerebral hemorrhage in a pooled prospective study. *Stroke*. 2007;38:2718–2725.

118. Shinton R, Beevers G. Meta-analysis of relation between cigarette smoking and stroke. *BMJ*. 1989;298:789–794.

119. Ariesen MJ, Claus SP, Rinkel GJ, Algra A. Risk factors for intracerebral hemorrhage in the general population: a systematic review. *Stroke*. 2003;34:2060–2065.

120. Centers for Disease Control and Prevention. *Tobacco-related mortality*. https://www.cdc.gov/tobacco/data_statistics/fact_sheets/health_effects/tobacco_related_mortality/index.htm; 2016. (Accessed October 14, 2017).

121. Lee PN, Forey BA. Environmental tobacco smoke exposure and risk of stroke in nonsmokers: a review with meta-analysis. *J Stroke Cerebrovasc Dis*. 2006;15:190–201.

122. U.S. Department of Health and Human Services. *How Tobacco Smoke Causes Disease: The Biology and Behavioral Basis for Smoking-Attributable Disease: A Report of the Surgeon General*. Atlanta: GA: Department of Health and Human Services, Centers for Disease Control and Prevention, National Center for Chronic Disease Prevention and Health Promotion, Office on Smoking and Health; 2010.

123. Howard G, Thun MJ. Why is environmental tobacco smoke more strongly associated with coronary heart disease than expected? A review of potential biases and experimental data. *Environ Health Perspect*. 1999;107:853–858.

124. Ambrose JA, Barua RS. The pathophysiology of cigarette smoking and cardiovascular disease: an update. *J Am Coll Cardiol*. 2004;43:1731–1737.

125. Kool MJ, Hoeks AP, Struijker Boudier HA, et al. Short- and long-term effects of smoking on arterial wall properties in habitual smokers. *J Am Coll Cardiol*. 1993;22:1881–1886.

126. Silvestrini M, Troisi E, Matteis M, et al. Effect of smoking on cerebrovascular reactivity. *J Cereb Blood Flow Metab*. 1996;16:746–749.

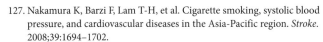

127. Nakamura K, Barzi F, Lam T-H, et al. Cigarette smoking, systolic blood pressure, and cardiovascular diseases in the Asia-Pacific region. *Stroke.* 2008;39:1694–1702.

128. Schwartz SW, Carlucci C, Chambless LE, Rosamond WD. Synergism between smoking and vital exhaustion in the risk of ischemic stroke: evidence from the ARIC study. *Ann Epidemiol.* 2004;14:416–424.

129. World Health Organization. Ischaemic stroke and combined oral contraceptives: results of an international, multicentre, case-control study. WHO Collaborative Study of Cardiovascular Disease and Steroid Hormone Contraception. *Lancet.* 1996;348:498–505.

130. Kernan WN, Ovbiagele B, Black HR, et al. Guidelines for the prevention of stroke in patients with stroke and Transient Ischemic Attack: a guideline for healthcare professionals from the American Heart Association/American Stroke Association. *Stroke.* 2014;45:2160–2236.

131. Abbott RD, Yin Y, Reed DM, Yano K. Risk of stroke in male cigarette smokers. *N Engl J Med.* 1986;315:717–720.

132. Wolf PA, D'Agostino RB, Kannel WB, et al. Cigarette smoking as a risk factor for stroke. The Framingham Study. *JAMA.* 1988;259:1025–1029.

133. Kawachi I, Colditz GA, Stampfer MJ, et al. Smoking cessation and decreased risk of stroke in women. *JAMA.* 1993;269:232–236.

134. Wannamethee SG, Shaper AG, Whincup PH, Walker M. Smoking cessation and the risk of stroke in middle-aged men. *JAMA.* 1995;274(2):155–160.

135. Shinton R. Lifelong exposures and the potential for stroke prevention: the contribution of cigarette smoking, exercise, and body fat. *J Epidemiol Community Health.* 1997;51:138–143.

136. Donahue RP, Abbott RD, Reed DM, Yano K. Alcohol and hemorrhagic stroke. The Honolulu Heart Program. *JAMA.* 1986;255:2311–2314.

137. Mukamal KJ, Ascherio A, Mittleman MA, et al. Alcohol and risk for ischemic stroke in men: the role of drinking patterns and usual beverage. *Ann Intern Med.* 2005;142:11–19.

138. Gill JS, Zezulka AV, Shipley MJ, et al. Stroke and alchol consumption. *N Engl J Med.* 1986;315:1041–1046.

139. Stampfer MJ, Colditz GA, Willett WC, et al. A prospective study of moderate alcohol consumption and the risk of coronary disease and stroke in women. *N Engl J Med.* 1988;319:267–273.

140. Berger K, Ajani UA, Kase CS, et al. Light-to-moderate alcohol consumption and risk of stroke among U.S. male physicians. *N Engl J Med.* 1999;341:1557–1564.

141. Sacco RL, Elkind M, Boden-Albala B, et al. The protective effect of moderate alcohol consumption on ischemic stroke. *JAMA.* 1999;281: 53–60.

142. Hillbom M, Numminen H, Juvela S. Recent heavy drinking of alcohol and embolic stroke. *Stroke.* 1999;30:2307–2312.

143. Malarcher AM, Giles WH, Croft JB, et al. Alcohol intake, type of beverage, and the risk of cerebral infarction in young women. *Stroke.* 2001;32:77–83.

144. Iso H, Baba S, Mannami T, et al. Alcohol consumption and risk of stroke among middle-aged men: the JPHC Study Cohort I. *Stroke.* 2004;35: 1124–1129.

145. Reynolds K, Lewis B, Nolen JD, et al. Alcohol consumption and risk of stroke: a meta-analysis. *JAMA.* 2003;289:579–588.

146. Law M, Wald N, Morris J. Lowering blood pressure to prevent myocardial infarction and stroke: a new preventive strategy. *Health Technol Assess.* 2003;7:1–94.

147. Huang Y, Cai X, Li Y, et al. Prehypertension and the risk of stroke: a meta-analysis. *Neurology.* 2014;82:1153–1161.

148. Neter JE, Stam BE, Kok FJ, et al. Influence of weight reduction on blood pressure: a meta-analysis of randomized controlled trials. *Hypertension.* 2003;42:878–884.

149. Psaty BM, Smith NL, Siscovick DS, et al. Health outcomes associated with antihypertensive therapies used as first-line agents. A systematic review and meta-analysis. *JAMA.* 1997;277(9):739–745.

150. Neal B, MacMahon S, Chapman N. Effects of ACE inhibitors, calcium antagonists, and other blood-pressure-lowering drugs: results of prospectively designed overviews of randomised trials. Blood Pressure Lowering Treatment Trialists' Collaboration. *Lancet.* 2000;356: 1955–1964.

151. Webb AJS, Fischer U, Mehta Z, Rothwell PM. Effects of antihypertensive-drug class on interindividual variation in blood pressure and risk of stroke: a systematic review and meta-analysis. *Lancet.* 2010;375:906–915.

152. Rothwell PM. Limitations of the usual blood-pressure hypothesis and importance of variability, instability, and episodic hypertension. *Lancet.* 2010;375:938–948.

153. Rothwell PM, Howard SC, Dolan E, et al. Prognostic significance of visit-to-visit variability, maximum systolic blood pressure, and episodic hypertension. *Lancet.* 2010;375:895–905.

154. Rothwell PM, Howard SC, Dolan E, et al. Effects of β blockers and calcium-channel blockers on within-individual variability in blood pressure and risk of stroke. *Lancet Neurol.* 2010;9:469–480.

155. Wright Jr JT, Williamson JD, Whelton PK, et al. A randomized trial of intensive versus standard blood-pressure control. *N Engl J Med.* 2015;373:2103–2116.

156. Bress AP, Kramer H, Khatib R, et al. Potential deaths averted and serious adverse events incurred from adoption of the SPRINT intensive blood pressure regimen in the U.S.: projections from NHANES. *Circulation.* 2017;135:1617–1628.

157. Amarenco P, Lavallee P, Touboul PJ. Stroke prevention, blood cholesterol, and statins. *Lancet Neurol.* 2004;3:271–278.

158. Prospective Studies Collaboration. Cholesterol, diastolic blood pressure, and stroke: 13 000 strokes in 450 000 people in 45 prospective cohorts. *Lancet.* 1995;346:1647–1653.

159. Prospective Studies Collaboration. Blood cholesterol and vascular mortality by age, sex, and blood pressure: a meta-analysis of individual data from 61 prospective studies with 55,000 vascular deaths. *Lancet.* 2007;370:1829–1839.

160. Brewer HB. Increasing HDL cholesterol levels. *N Engl J Med.* 2004;350:1491–1494.

161. Sanossian N, Saver JL, Navab M, Ovbiagele B. High-density lipoprotein cholesterol: an emerging target for stroke treatment. *Stroke.* 2007;38: 1104–1109.

162. Lindenstrom E, Boysen G, Nyboe J. Influence of total cholesterol, high density lipoprotein cholesterol, and triglycerides on risk of cerebrovascular disease: The Copenhagen City Heart Study. *BMJ.* 1994;309:11–15.

163. Tanne D, Yaari S, Goldbourt U. High-density lipoprotein cholesterol and the risk of ischemic stroke mortality. A 21-year follow-up of 8,586 men from the Israeli Ischemic Heart Disease Study. *Stroke.* 1997;28:83–87.

164. Simons LA, McCallum J, Friedlander Y, Simons J. Risk factors for ischemic stroke: Dubbo Study of the Elderly. *Stroke.* 1998;29: 1341–1346.

165. Soyama Y, Miura K, Morikawa Y, et al. High-density lipoprotein cholesterol and risk of stroke in Japanese men and women: the Oyabe Study. *Stroke.* 2003;34:863–868.

166. Curb JD, Abbott RD, Rodriguez BL, et al. High density lipoprotein cholesterol and the risk of stroke in elderly men: the Honolulu Heart Program. *Am J Epidemiol.* 2004;160:150–157.

167. Wannamethee SG, Shaper AG, Ebrahim S. HDL-cholesterol, total cholesterol, and the risk of stroke in middle-aged British men. *Stroke.* 2000;31:1882–1888.

168. Shahar E, Chambless LE, Rosamond WD, et al. Plasma lipid profile and incident ischemic stroke. The Atherosclerosis Risk in Communities (ARIC) Study. *Stroke.* 2003;34:623–631.

169. Sacco RL, Benson RT, Kargman DE, et al. High-density lipoprotein cholesterol and ischemic stroke in the elderly - The Northern Manhattan Stroke Study. *JAMA.* 2001;285:2729–2735.

170. Tirschwell DL, Smith NL, Heckbert SR, et al. Association of cholesterol with stroke risk varies in stroke subtypes and patient subgroups. *Neurology.* 2004;63:1868–1875.

171. Johnsen SH, Mathiesen EB, Fosse E, et al. Elevated high-density lipoprotein cholesterol levels are protective against plaque progression: a follow-up study of 1952 persons with carotid atherosclerosis: the Tromso Study. *Circulation.* 2005;112:498–504.

172. Asia Pacific Cohort Studies Collaboration. Serum triglycerides as a risk factor for cardiovascular diseases in the Asia-Pacific region. *Circulation.* 2004;110:2678–2686.

173. Freiberg JJ, Tybjaerg-Hansen A, et al. Nonfasting triglycerides and risk of ischemic stroke in the general population. *JAMA.* 2008;300(18): 2142–2152.

174. Bansal S, Buring JE, Rifai N, et al. Fasting compared with nonfasting triglycerides and risk of cardiovascular events in women. *JAMA.* 2007;298(3):309–316.

175. Baigent C, Keech A, Kearney PM, et al. Efficacy and safety of cholesterol-lowering treatment: prospective meta-analysis of data from 90,056 participants in 14 randomised trials of statins. *Lancet.* 2005;366:1267–1278.

176. Amarenco P, Labreuche J. Lipid management in the prevention of stroke: review and updated meta-analysis of statins for stroke prevention. *Lancet Neurol.* 2009;8:453–463.

177. Centers for Disease Control and Prevention. *National Diabetes Statistics Report, 2017.* Atlanta, GA; 2017.

178. Furie KL, Kasner SE, Adams RJ, et al. Guidelines for the prevention of stroke in patients with stroke or transient ischemic attack. *Stroke.* 2011;42:227–276.

179. The Emerging Risk Factors Collaboration. Diabetes mellitus, fasting blood glucose concentration, and risk of vascular disease: a collaborative meta-analysis of 102 prospective studies. *Lancet.* 2010;375:2215–2222.

180. Mankovsky BN, Ziegler D. Stroke in patients with diabetes mellitus. *Diabetes Metab Res Rev.* 2004;20:268–287.

181. Goldstein LB, Bushnell CD, Adams RJ, et al. Guidelines for the primary prevention of stroke. A Guideline for Healthcare Professionals From the American Heart Association/American Stroke Association. *Stroke.* 2011;42:517–584.

182. Meschia JF, Merrill P, Soliman EZ, et al. Racial disparities in awareness and treatment of atrial fibrillation: the REasons for Geographic and Racial Differences in Stroke (REGARDS) Study. *Stroke.* 2010;41:581–587.

183. Hart RG, Pearce LA, Albers GW, et al. Independent predictors of stroke in patients with atrial fibrillation: a systematic review. *Neurology.* 2007;69:546–554.

184. Hart RG, Pearce LA, Halperin JL, et al. Comparison of 12 risk stratification schemes to predict stroke in patients with nonvalvular atrial fibrillation. *Stroke.* 2008;39(6):1901–1910.

185. Goldstein LB. Anticoagulation in patients with atrial fibrillation in the setting of prior hemorrhage: an ongoing dilemma. *Stroke.* 2017;48: 2654–2659.

186. Gage BF, Waterman AD, Shannon W, et al. Validation of clinical classification schemes for predicting stroke: results from the National Registry of Atrial Fibrillation. *JAMA.* 2001;285:2864–2870.

187. Gladstone DJ, Bui E, Fang J, et al. Potentially preventable strokes in high-risk patients with atrial fibrillation who are not adequately anticoagulated. *Stroke.* 2009;40:235–240.

188. Ohene-Frempong K, Weiner SJ, Sleeper LA, et al. Cerebrovascular accidents in sickle cell disease: rates and risk factors. *Blood.* 1998;91: 288–294.

189. Adams RJ, McKie VC, Carl EM, et al. Long-term stroke risk in children with sickle cell disease screened with transcranial Doppler. *Ann Neurol.* 1997;42:699–704.

190. Adams RJ, McKie VC, Hsu L, et al. Prevention of a first stroke by transfusions in children with sickle cell anemia and abnormal results on transcranial Doppler ultrasonography. *N Engl J Med.* 1998;339:5–11.

191. Yaggi H, Mohsenin V. Sleep apnea and stroke: a risk factor or an association. *Sleep Med Clin.* 2007;2:583–591.

192. Somers VK, White DP, Amin R, et al. Sleep apnea and cardiovascular disease. *J Am Coll Cardiol.* 2008;52:686–717.

193. Hermann DM, Bassetti CL. Sleep-related breathing and sleep-wake disturbances in ischemic stroke. *Neurology.* 2009;73:1313–1322.

194. Dyken ME, Im KB. Obstructive sleep apnea and stroke. *Chest.* 2009;136(6):1668–1677.

195. Bagai K. Obstructive sleep apnea, stroke, and cardiovascular diseases. *Neurologist.* 2010;16:329–339.

196. Budhiraja R, Budhiraja P, Quan SF. Sleep-disordered breathing and cardiovascular disorders. *Respir Care.* 2010;55:1322–1330.

197. Johnson KG, Johnson DC. Frequency of sleep apnea in stroke and TIA patients: a meta-analysis. *J Clin Sleep Med.* 2010;6:131–137.

198. Libby P, Ridker PM. Inflammation and atherothrombosis: from population biology and bench research to clinical practice. *J Am Coll Cardiol.* 2006;48(Suppl A):A33–A46.

199. The Emerging Risk Factors Collaboration. C-reactive protein concentration and risk of coronary heart disease, stroke, and mortality: an individual participant meta-analysis. *Lancet.* 2010;375:132–140.

200. Pearson TA, Mensah GA, Alexander RW, et al. Markers of inflammation and cardiovascular disease: application to clinical and public health practice. *Circulation.* 2003;107:499–511.

200a. Lavallee P, Perchaud V, Gautier-Bertrand M, et al. Association between influenza vaccination and reduced risk of brain infarction. *Stroke.* 2002;33:513–518.

201. Fibrinogen Studies Collaboration. Plasma fibrinogen level and the risk of major cardiovascular diseases and nonvascular mortality. *JAMA.* 2005;294:1799–1809.

202. Selhub J, Jacques PF, Wilson PWF, et al. Vitamin status and intake as primary determinants of homocysteinemia in an elderly population. *JAMA.* 1993;270:2693–2698.

203. Welch GN, Loscalzo J. Homocysteine and atherothrombosis. *N Engl J Med.* 1998;338(15):1042–1050.

204. Rosenson RS. Antiatherothrombotic effects of nicotinic acid. *Atherosclerosis.* 2003;171:87–96.

205. Bazzano LA, Jiang H, Munter P, et al. Relationship between cigarette smoking and novel risk factors for cardiovascular disease in the United States. *Ann Intern Med.* 2003;138:891–897.

206. Dierkes J, Westphal S, Luley C. The effect of fibrates and other lipid-lowering drugs on plasma homocysteine levels. *Expert Opin Drug Saf.* 2004;3:101–111.

207. Homocysteine Studies Collaboration. Homocysteine and risk of ischemic heart disease and stroke: a meta-analysis. *JAMA.* 2002;288:2015–2022.

208. Wald DS, Law M, Morris JK. Homocysteine and cardiovascular disease: evidence on causality from a meta-analysis. *BMJ.* 2002;325:1202–1206.

209. Kelly PJ, Rosand J, Kistler JP, et al. Homocysteine, MTHFR 677C-->T polymorphism, and risk of ischemic stroke - results of a meta-analysis. *Neurology.* 2002;59:529–536.

210. McIlroy SP, Dynan KB, Lawson JT, et al. Moderately elevated plasma homocysteine, methylenetetrahydrofolate reductase genotype, and risk for stroke, vascular dementia, and Alzheimer Disease in Northern Ireland. *Stroke.* 2002;33:2351–2356.

211. Boysen G, Brander T, Christensen H, et al. Homocysteine and risk of recurrent stroke. *Stroke.* 2003;34:1258–1261.

212. Kim NK, Choi BO, Jung WS, et al. Hyperhomocysteinemia as an independent risk factor for silent brain infarction. *Neurology.* 2003;61:1595–1599.

213. Li Z, Sun L, Zhang H, et al. Elevated plasma homocysteine was associated with hemorrhagic and ischemic stroke, but methylenetetrahydrofolate reductase gene C677T polymorphism was a risk factor for thrombotic stroke: a multicenter case-control study in China. *Stroke.* 2003;34: 2085–2090.

214. Tanne D, Haim M, Goldbourt U, et al. Prospective study of serum homocysteine and risk of ischemic stroke among patients with preexisting coronary heart disease. *Stroke.* 2003;34:632–636.

215. Iso H, Moriyama Y, Sato S, et al. Serum total homocysteine concentrations and risk of stroke and its subtypes in Japanese. *Circulation.* 2004;109:2766–2772.

216. Casas JP, Bautista LE, Smeeth L, et al. Homocysteine and stroke: evidence on a causal link from Mendelian randomisation. *Lancet.* 2005;365: 224–232.

217. Hankey GJ, Eikelboom JW, Baker RI, et al. B vitamins in patients with recent transient ischaemic attack or stroke in the VITAmins TO Prevent Stroke (VITATOPS) trial: a randomised, double-blind, parallel, placebo-controlled trial. *Lancet Neurol.* 2010;9:855–865.

218. Ji Y, Tan T, Xu Y, et al. Vitamin supplementation, homocysteine levels, and the risk of cerebrovascular disease. A meta-analysis. *Neurology.* 2013;81:1–10.

219. Etminan M, Takkouche B, Isorna FC, Samii A. Risk of ischaemic stroke in people with migraine: systematic review and meta-analysis of observational studies. *BMJ.* 2005;330:63.

220. Schurks M, Rist PM, Bigal ME, et al. Migraine and cardiovascular disease: systematic review and meta-analysis. *BMJ*. 2009;339:b3914.

221. Kruit MC, van Buchem MA, Hofman PAM, et al. Migraine as a risk factor for subclinical brain lesions. *JAMA*. 2004;291:427–434.

222. Swartz RH, Kern RZ. Migraine is associated with magnetic resonance imaging white matter abnormalities - a meta-analysis. *Arch Neurol*. 2004;61:1366–1368.

223. Kruit MC, Launer LJ, Ferrari MD, van Buchem MA. Infarcts in the posterior circulation territory in migraine. The population-based MRI CAMERA study. *Brain*. 2005;128:2068–2077.

224. Scher AI, Gudmundsson LS, Sigurdsson S, et al. Migraine headache in middle age and late-life brain infarcts. *JAMA*. 2009;301:2563–2570.

225. Centers for Disease Control and Prevention. Awareness of stroke warning symptoms—13 States and the District of Columbia, 2005. *MMWR Morb Mortal Wkly Rep*. 2008;57:481–485.

226. Kleindorfer D, Khoury J, Broderick JP, et al. Temporal trends in public awareness of stroke: warning signs, risk factors, and treatment. *Stroke*. 2009;40:2502–2506.

227. Kleindorfer D, Lindsell CJ, Moomaw CJ, et al. Which stroke symptoms prompt a 911 call? A population-based study. *Am J Emerg Med*. 2010;28:607–612.

228. Kleindorfer D, Lindsell CJ, Brass L, et al. National US estimates of recombinant tissue plasminogen activator use: ICD-9 codes substantially underestimate. *Stroke*. 2008;39:924–928.

229. Kleindorfer DO, Khoury J, Moomaw CJ, et al. Stroke incidence is decreasing in whites but not in blacks: a population-based estimate of temporal trends in stroke incidence from the Greater Cincinnati/Northern Kentucky Stroke Study. *Stroke*. 2010;41:1326–1331.

230. Lackland DT, Roccella EJ, Deutsch AF, et al. Factors influencing the decline in stroke mortality: a Statement From the American Heart Association/American Stroke Association. *Stroke*. 2014;45:315–353.

231. Yang Q, Tong X, Schieb L, et al. Vital Signs: recent trends in stroke death rates - United States, 2000-2015. *MMWR Morb Mortal Wkly Rep*. 2017;66:933–939.

232. Otite FO, Liaw N, Khandelwal P, et al. Increasing prevalence of vascular risk factors in patients with stroke: a call to action. *Neurology*. 2017;89:1985–1994.

233. George MG, Tong X, Bowman BA. Prevalence of cardiovascular risk factors and strokes in younger adults. *JAMA Neurol*. 2017;74:695–703.

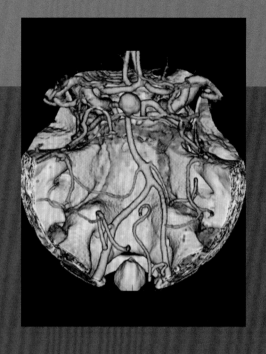

中文导读

第29章
脑血管疾病的临床表现和诊断

　　卒中管理的涵盖范围较广，主要包括急性期管理及对卒中复发的预防。由于缺血性卒中是最常见的卒中类型，因此这将是本章介绍的重点，我们对脑出血的急性期管理与二级预防仅做简要介绍。急性缺血性卒中是由于动脉闭塞导致脑血流量下降进而引起的中枢神经系统急性局灶性损伤性病变。血管闭塞将引起一系列损伤性级联反应，最终导致脑组织产生不可逆性坏死，即梗死。然而，脑梗死并非在血管闭塞后即刻发生，部分缺血区脑组织在血管闭塞后的数小时内仍未完全坏死，及时采取干预措施有望使其存活，这种有可能被挽救的脑组织被称为缺血性半暗带，也是急性缺血性卒中救治的关键。一些影像学检查手段可协助判断缺血性半暗带的范围，从而为接下来的治疗提供契机。急性缺血性卒中的治疗主要包括旨在提升缺血区脑组织血流量的血管再通治疗及旨在阻止缺血细胞死亡的神经保护治疗。由于神经保护治疗的有效性尚未被充分证实，因此前者将是本章介绍的重点。本章还将讨论缺血性脑卒中的一级预防与二级预防。

吉训明

Clinical Presentation and Diagnosis of Cerebrovascular Disease

Mark J. Alberts

Stroke is a common and serious disorder. Each year stroke affects almost 800,000 people in the United States, at least 16 million people globally, and is the second leading cause of death in the world (see Chapter 28).[1,2] The associated high morbidity and mortality of stroke, combined with its high cost for acute and chronic care, provide impetus for improving the diagnosis, acute management, and prevention of strokes. A full understanding of how patients with stroke and cerebrovascular disease come to medical attention, along with a logical approach for defining the mechanism of stroke, is needed for safe and effective implementation of acute therapies and prevention strategies. This chapter will focus on clinical manifestations of all types of cerebrovascular disease and how clinicians can approach diagnostic evaluation.

OVERVIEW OF CLINICAL STROKE

Stroke and cerebrovascular disease are caused by a disturbance of the cerebral vessels and/or cerebral blood flow in almost all cases. In simple terms, we can divide stroke into two major types: ischemic and hemorrhagic. Ischemic stroke is the most common variety and is responsible for 80% to 85% of all strokes; hemorrhagic stroke accounts for the remainder.[3–5] On occasion, an ischemic stroke can undergo secondary hemorrhagic transformation; likewise, a cerebral hemorrhage (particularly a subarachnoid hemorrhage [SAH]) can cause a secondary ischemic stroke via vasospasm.

Ischemic stroke occurs when a blood vessel in or around the brain becomes occluded or has a high-grade stenosis that reduces the perfusion of distal cerebral tissue. A variety of mechanisms and processes can lead to such occlusions and will be discussed later in more detail. On rare occasions, thrombosis and occlusion of a cerebral vein can lead to ischemic as well as hemorrhagic strokes (venous infarction).

A hemorrhagic stroke (intracerebral hemorrhage [ICH] and SAH) occurs when a blood vessel in or around the brain ruptures or leaks blood into the brain parenchyma (ICH) or into the subarachnoid space (SAH). It is not uncommon for there to be some overlap, such as an ICH also causing some degree of SAH and/or an intraventricular hemorrhage. Likewise, an SAH can produce some elements of an ICH if the aneurysmal rupture directs blood into the brain parenchyma. As with ischemic stroke, a variety of processes and lesions can produce ICH and SAH, but most affect the integrity of the vessel wall in some way.

CLINICAL MANIFESTATIONS OF STROKE AND CEREBROVASCULAR DISEASE

Stroke is similar to real estate in that much of its presentation and prognosis depend on size and location. The area of brain involved by the stroke typically dictates the presenting symptoms. Furthermore,

blood vessels that supply different parts of the brain are affected by different types of cerebrovascular disease and have different mechanisms (pathophysiology) for the stroke. This concept greatly influences and defines the approach a vascular neurologist or neurosurgeon uses when assessing patients with a known or suspected stroke or cerebrovascular disease.[6–8]

For example, a patient with evidence of involvement of the left hemispheric cortex (e.g., aphasia, visual field defect, weakness of contralateral face and arm) is likely to have a process involving the left middle cerebral artery (MCA). If head computed tomography (CT) does not show evidence of a hemorrhage, likely etiologies would include an embolic event from the heart (e.g., atrial fibrillation) or an artery-to-artery embolism (as might be seen with a high-grade lesion at the carotid bifurcation in the neck). Another patient with a pure motor hemiparesis but no other deficits is likely to have a lesion affecting the motor pathways in the internal capsule, often due to occlusion of a small penetrating artery (lenticulostriate vessel) deep in the brain. Most ischemic strokes will respect the vascular territory of one or more arteries.[9] Indeed, lesions that do not respect typical arterial territories lead to concern for a nonvascular process (e.g., tumor, infection), or an atypical vascular process (i.e., venous infarction, vasculitis). Common ischemic stroke syndromes can be found in Tables 29.1 and 29.2.

Evaluation of a patient with a hemorrhagic stroke follows a similar logical assessment but is further complicated by spread of the initial bleed, the effects of increased intracranial pressure, and other secondary effects that lead to neurological manifestations beyond the original injury. In this case, detailed cerebral imaging is vital for understanding the mechanism of the stroke and reasons for secondary worsening. The discussions that follow offer more detailed descriptions of common hemorrhagic stroke syndromes correlated with their likely anatomy and most likely etiology and pathophysiology.

Besides the location of the stroke, the tempo of onset and progression of symptoms often provide valuable information about stroke etiology and mechanism. Stroke symptoms that progress in a casual manner with gradual onset and worsening over many minutes or longer often suggest a thrombotic process or hypoperfusion due to occlusion or stenosis of a larger proximal vessel. Such a leisurely progression can also be seen with stroke mimics such as complicated migraines or partial seizures. The converse is a stroke syndrome with sudden onset of maximal symptoms that remain stable; this suggests an embolic process such as a cardioembolic stroke due to atrial fibrillation or an artery-to-artery process (although a thrombotic occlusion is still a possibility).

Similar reasoning holds true for most cases of hemorrhagic stroke. ICH often presents with the apparent abrupt onset of symptoms, but close questioning may reveal that symptoms actually progressed over 15 to 30 minutes as the hematoma grew and expanded.[10] SAH is often characterized by sudden onset of the worst headache of one's life, with significant nausea, vomiting, and stiff neck in many cases. The phrase "worst headache of my life" is so characteristic of SAH that a patient

TABLE 29.1   Common Large-Vessel Ischemic Stroke Syndromes

Syndrome	Anatomy Involved	Major Symptoms	Vessels Involved	Etiology
Left MCA	Left frontal/parietal cortex and subcortical structures	Aphasia, right visual field cut, right motor/sensory deficits; face > arm > leg weakness; left gaze preference	Left MCA or major branch; could also be left ICA or siphon	Emboli from heart or proximal lesion; intrinsic atherothrombosis
Right MCA	Right frontal/parietal cortex and subcortical structures	Neglect syndrome, agnosia, apraxia, left motor/sensory deficits, visual field deficit; right gaze preference	Right MCA or major branch; right ICA or siphon	Same as left MCA
Left ACA	Left frontal and parasagittal areas	Speech disturbance, behavioral changes, leg > arm weakness	Left ACA	Intrinsic atherothrombosis, embolic
Right ACA	Right frontal and parasagittal areas	Behavioral changes, leg > arm weakness	Right ACA	Same as left ACA
Brainstem	Pons, midbrain, medulla, cerebellum	Ophthalmoplegia, bilateral motor deficits, ataxia/dysmetria; nausea/vomiting/vertigo, coma/altered mentation	Basilar artery	Intrinsic atherothrombosis, embolism from heart or proximal vessel
PCA	Upper midbrain, occipital cortex/subcortex, thalamus, medial temporal lobes	Visual field cut, motor/sensory loss, seizures, gaze problems; third nerve deficits	Posterior cerebral artery, thalamic perforators	Embolism from proximal lesion, intrinsic atherothrombosis

ACA, Anterior cerebral artery; *ICA*, internal carotid artery; *MCA*, middle cerebral artery; *PCA*, posterior cerebral artery.

TABLE 29.2   Common Lacunar Stroke Syndromes

Syndrome	Vessel Typically Involved	Brain Location	Symptoms
Pure motor hemiparesis	Lenticulostriate or basilar/pontine perforator	Internal capsule, pons	Unilateral weakness only
Mixed motor/sensory	Lenticulostriate or thalamic perforator or deep white matter vessel	Internal capsule, deep white matter, thalamus	Motor and sensory deficits
Pure sensory	Thalamic perforator	Posterior thalamus	Loss of contralateral sensory modalities
Ataxic hemiparesis	Lenticulostriate or basilar/pontine perforator	Internal capsule, basis pontis	Unilateral weakness with prominent ataxia, leg > arm
Dysarthria/clumsy hand	Lenticulostriate or deep white matter vessel	Internal capsule, deep white matter	Prominent dysarthria with isolated hand weakness

who presents with that symptom complex is assumed to have a SAH until proven otherwise.[11,12]

Transient Ischemic Attack

A transient ischemic attack (TIA) can be a prodrome to an ischemic stroke. Symptoms of a TIA are identical to those of a stroke but with resolution within 24 hours (according to the old definition of a TIA). In reality, most TIA syndromes last just a few minutes, not many hours. In fact, modern brain imaging using magnetic resonance imaging (MRI) with diffusion-weighted sequences has shown that 25% to 30% of patients with a TIA lasting 30 minutes to 2 hours will have a new diffusion-weighted imaging (DWI) lesion on MRI, indicating a stroke (based on a tissue definition).[13–15] TIA symptoms lasting 6 hours or longer have a 50% likelihood of having a new stroke on MRI with DWI techniques. Therefore the perceived distinction between a TIA and a stroke should be viewed more as a continuum from minor transient neuronal dysfunction to actual brain infarction with permanent symptoms.

Although it was once thought that the risk of stroke after a TIA was low, new imaging studies and epidemiological studies have proven this is not the case. Based on purely clinical criteria (not MRI results), several recent studies have shown that after a TIA, 10% of patients will have a stroke within 3 months and half those strokes (5%) will occur within 48 hours of the initial TIA. Approximately 25% of patients with a TIA will have a stroke, myocardial infarction (MI), death, or recurrent TIA or be hospitalized within the next 3 months.[9,16,17] Based on these poor outcomes, recently published guidelines recommend hospital admission for patients with a recent TIA.[13,15,18]

Further studies have attempted to better define those patients with a TIA who are at higher risk of having a stroke within the next 2 to 7 days. Several scoring systems have been developed (Table 29.3) that may be useful for assessing such risks.[19] Of course, any such assessment tool must be tempered by good clinical judgment and consideration of all clinical factors.

Several types of TIAs deserve special mention because of their unique presentations and symptom complex. One is sudden blindness in one eye, which typically occurs as a "shade coming down" over the eye. Some patients report a graying out of vision in the eye, like looking through a gray haze or cloud. This type of TIA is often referred to as *amaurosis fugax*. This symptom complex typically resolves in a few minutes, although it can last for several hours. There is sometimes pain in or around the eye, globe, and orbit, but patients usually do not have any other focal neurological complaints at the same time. Some cases of amaurosis are due to emboli to the retinal circulation from an ulcerated plaque in or near the carotid bifurcation in the neck. Other cases can be due to local disease in the ophthalmic artery or in the posterior ciliary artery that supplies the optic nerve.[20] A process such as temporal arteritis can produce headaches, eye pain, and sudden loss of vision.[21]

Another unique type of TIA is the *limb-shaking TIA*. This typically involves the arm or leg on one side of the body. Patients report uncontrollable shaking of a limb that can be precipitated by movement. These spells can last seconds to minutes. They are not epileptic in origin; the electroencephalogram (EEG) is unremarkable. These TIAs are associated with severe stenosis of the contralateral internal or common carotid artery.[22] Once the carotid artery is opened (usually with an endarterectomy), the spells cease.

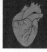

TABLE 29.3	**Transient Ischemic Attack Scoring Systems**
ABCD	Age, blood pressure, clinical symptoms, duration
ABCD2	Age, blood pressure, clinical symptoms, duration, diabetes
ABCD2I	Age, blood pressure, clinical symptoms, duration, diabetes, infarction
ABCD3	Age, blood pressure, clinical symptoms, duration, diabetes, dual TIAs
ABCD3-I	Age, blood pressure, clinical symptoms, duration, diabetes, dual TIAs, imaging

Age: 60 years or greater = 1 point
Blood pressure: systolic 140 mm Hg or greater = 1 point or diastolic 90 mm Hg or greater = 1 point
Clinical symptoms: unilateral weakness = 2 points; speech disturbance without weakness = 1 point
Duration: 60 min or more = 2 points; 10–59 min = 1 point
Diabetes: 1 point (on antidiabetic medications)
Dual TIA: One TIA prompting medical attention plus another TIA in preceding 7 days
Imaging: evidence for acute ischemic stroke on CT or MRI or >50% ipsilateral ICA stenosis (ABCD3-I only)

CT, Computed tomography; *ICA*, internal carotid artery; *MRI*, magnetic resonance imaging; *TIA*, transient ischemic attack.
Data from Johnston SC, Rothwell PM, Nguyen-Huynh MN, et al. Validation and refinement of scores to predict very early stroke risk after transient ischaemic attack. *Lancet.* 2007;369(9558):283–292; and Kiyohara T, Kamouchi M, Kumai Y, et al. ABCD3 and ABCD3-I scores are superior to ABCD2 score in the prediction of short- and long-term risks of stroke after transient ischemic attack. *Stroke.* 2014;45(2):418–425.

Lastly is the topic of *crescendo TIAs*. This refers to a pattern where TIAs are recurrent, last longer, and/or are progressive or more severe in nature. This is a very worrisome type of TIA and is associated with a risk of stroke as high as 25% to 50% over the next few weeks.[23,24] This presentation is very worrisome for high-grade ipsilateral carotid disease that might need urgent therapy.

It is important to understand that many patients have transient episodes of apparent neurological dysfunction (disturbed speech, motor symptoms, numbness, visual changes) from nonvascular etiologies. Causes can range from metabolic disturbances to seizures, atypical migraines to hysteria. Often a detailed evaluation, including brain and vessel imaging studies, is needed to establish a correct diagnosis.

Some hemorrhagic strokes may also have a TIA equivalent, namely the *sentinel headache* before a SAH. The sentinel headache presents as an acute headache that is unusual in terms of its nature, severity, and onset. It typically lasts more than an hour but does not have other impressive focal neurological findings and resolves prior to the definitive SAH presentation. Sentinel headaches occur in 25% to 50% of patients with a subsequent aneurysmal SAH and typically antedate the SAH by days to weeks (average 2 weeks).[25,26] It is thought that most of these headaches are due to either minor leakage from a fragile aneurysm or enlargement of the aneurysm, resulting in pressure on a nearby structure that produces pain.

Ischemic Stroke Syndromes

There are numerous manifestations of ischemic stroke, and they can be classified based on affected brain region, affected artery, disease process, or symptoms. Although modern diagnostic techniques (MRI) have altered some of the clinical rules of stroke symptoms and etiology, there are still some useful concepts that can guide us in terms of

stroke location and mechanism. Tables 29.1 and 29.2 list some classic ischemic stroke syndromes with their major clinical manifestations, vascular territory, and underlying pathophysiology.[5,9]

Broadly speaking, ischemic strokes typically involve one or more vessels or vascular territories and produce a focal neurological deficit. Typically, clinicians look for unilateral weakness or sensory deficits, unilateral visual field abnormalities, speech disturbance (aphasia or dysarthria), neglect syndromes, unilateral ataxia, ophthalmoplegias, gaze abnormalities, or a specific behavioral syndrome as clues of a stroke. Vague or nonfocal symptoms such as diffuse weakness alone, headaches alone, long-term memory loss, abnormal behavior, or isolated dizziness are rarely caused by an ischemic stroke. The appearance of a lesion in a typical vascular territory (based on brain imaging) is a key feature of almost all stroke syndromes.[6]

The presence of cortical deficits (aphasia, visual field cuts, neglect syndromes) often indicates involvement of a major vessel in the cerebral hemispheres. The presence of ataxia, bilateral motor or sensory deficits, Horner syndrome, ophthalmoplegias, and crossed sensory findings (one side of the face and the other side of the body) often indicates a stroke in the posterior fossa and vertebral-basilar territory. There are specific syndromes that indicate small-vessel involvement deep in the brain. These so-called lacunar strokes are due to occlusion of small penetrating arteries that arise directly from larger parent vessels. Favored locations include the deep basal ganglia structures, thalamus, and brainstem (especially the pons). A listing of common large-vessel and lacunar syndromes appears in Tables 29.1 and 29.2.

Atherothrombosis accounts for the majority of ischemic strokes. These lesions can occur anywhere in the cerebral vasculature, but they tend to have a preference for specific locations such as the bifurcation of the carotid artery in the neck, intracranial carotid siphons, proximal portion of the MCA, midportion of the basilar artery, and aortic arch. An atherosclerotic plaque forms over many years then ruptures, causing formation of a superimposed thrombus.[27,28] This atherothrombotic lesion can totally occlude the vessel, produce severe narrowing (leading to watershed ischemia), or be a source of embolic material that embolizes to more distal parts of the cerebral vasculature (artery-to-artery emboli).

Cardiac embolism accounts for 15% to 20% of all ischemic strokes. A variety of conditions such as atrial fibrillation, endocarditis, prior MI, valvular disease, and cardiomyopathy often lead to formation of intracardiac thrombi that subsequently embolize to the brain (and other organs).[4,6,8,15,29] Most lacunar strokes are due to either lipohyalinosis or microatheromata occluding a small penetrating artery.

Special Cases
Ischemic Stroke in Young Adults

It is not uncommon to see young adults (often defined as ≤45 years of age) with ischemic strokes. Such cases often entail a special evaluation because of the unique processes and conditions that can produce strokes in this age group, as well as the long-term consequences of a stroke in a young patient. Many case series have examined the diseases leading to ischemic strokes in the young, and in general they fall into a few major categories: (1) premature atherosclerosis, (2) unusual vascular pathologies, (3) cardiac etiologies, (4) coagulopathies, and (5) a variety of other diseases common in the young (Table 29.4).[30,31]

Premature atherosclerosis typically occurs in patients with risk factors for atherosclerosis; in some cases these have not been diagnosed or not properly treated. Examples include hypertension, hyperlipidemia (often familial), diabetes, smoking, and obesity. Such patients often have a family history of vascular disease or events (MI, coronary artery bypass grafting, stroke) at a young age. The types of uncommon vascular pathologies sometimes seen in young adults with a stroke include dissection of a vessel (often not related to any obvious trauma), fibromuscular dysplasia, moyamoya disease, or a vasculitis related to an inflammatory condition or drug abuse.[32,33] Numerous cardiac processes can lead to strokes in the young, such as congenital heart disease, a patent foramen ovale (particularly with evidence of venous thrombi in the legs or pelvis), valvular disease (infectious or inflammatory), cardiomyopathy (inherited or acquired), atrial myxoma, papillary fibroelastoma, and many others.[34]

Myriad clotting disorders have been associated with strokes in young adults, the most common being lupus anticoagulants, anticardiolipin (antiphospholipid) antibodies, factor V Leiden mutation, and protein C and protein S deficiency.[35] In general, these coagulopathies are more likely to cause venous thrombosis than arterial thrombosis. Clotting disorders related to hematological malignancies can cause both ischemic and hemorrhagic strokes.[36] Various systemic diseases are also associated with hypercoagulable states such as inflammatory bowel disease, hemoglobinopathies, elevated homocysteine, and cancer.[37,38]

The "other" category covers a host of conditions, some rare and some common, that cause strokes in young adults. Migraine headaches and pregnancy are the most common of these. Patients with complex or complicated migraines, with prolonged auras, or taking contraceptives or hormone therapy have a higher risk of stroke.[39] Pregnancy, particularly in the third trimester and up to 3 months postpartum, is associated with increased stroke risk, particularly venous thrombosis and cerebral hemorrhage.[40–42] Drug abuse is another common cause of ischemic and hemorrhagic strokes in young adults.[43] Other rare conditions include CADASIL (cerebral autosomal dominant arteriopathy with subcortical infarcts and leukoencephalopathy), MELAS (mitochondrial encephalomyopathy, lactic acidosis, and stroke), isolated central nervous system (CNS) vasculitis, Sneddon syndrome (combination of a livedo reticularis rash, antiphospholipid antibodies, and ischemic stroke), Marfan syndrome, and a host of others (especially connective tissue disorders) have been known to cause strokes in this population.[32,33]

Brain inflammatory conditions such as meningitis (bacterial, fungal, viral, others) can lead to strokes due to vessel inflammation or invasion by pathogenic organisms. A meningitis caused by cancer can also lead to strokes due to vessel invasion by cancer cells that lead to vessel occlusion.[44–47]

Strokes Related to Systemic Disease

Numerous systemic disorders are important and potent risk factors for stroke: hypertension, diabetes, hyperlipidemia, smoking, heart disease (atrial fibrillation, MI, valvular disease, etc.), drug abuse, and others. These have been covered in other chapters of this book

(see Chapter 28). Our focus here is on specific systemic disorders that lead to specific or unusual types of strokes.

Autoimmune diseases, such as lupus, can produce strokes through a variety of mechanisms that include advanced or premature atherosclerosis, vasculitis, hypercoagulable states, and cardioembolic events.[48] Sickle cell disease (SCD) also leads to ischemic strokes and hemorrhagic strokes due to myriad processes, including a large-vessel arteriopathy, small-vessel occlusion, rupture of moyamoya vessels (producing ICH and/or SAH), and accelerated atherosclerosis due to hypertension and renal failure.[49–51] These disorders tend to affect younger patients in many cases.

Drug abuse, particularly cocaine, can produce ischemic strokes via a number of processes including vasospasm, cardiac emboli (due to cardiomyopathy), hypertension, and endocarditis.[52,53] Drug abuse can produce an ICH or SAH due to extreme hypertension and a necrotizing vasculitis. It is a fallacy to assume that drug abuse occurs only in young patients or those from certain demographic groups. All patients admitted with a stroke should be tested for drug abuse with urine toxicology screens, not excluding those older than 50 years and white-collar professionals.

Human immunodeficiency virus/acquired immunodeficiency syndrome (HIV/AIDS) is currently recognized as increasing the risk of stroke. This is partially because patients with HIV/AIDS are living longer, and some are having strokes as a result of accelerated development of typical stroke risk factors. It is also clear that modern drug therapy for AIDS can increase the risk of stroke (particularly ischemic stroke).[54–56]

Systemic cancer is a commonly overlooked cause of strokes. Sometimes the stroke diagnosis precedes diagnosis of the underlying cancer. Mechanisms for strokes related to cancer include a hypercoagulable state and nonbacterial thrombotic endocarditis. Oftentimes these strokes are multiple, variable in size, and in different vascular territories.[57–59] Such patients may also have deep venous thrombosis (DVT). Strokes due to local vessel involvement with neoplastic cells are discussed earlier. Renal failure and liver disease appear to increase the risk of ischemic and hemorrhagic stroke.[60–62]

Intracerebral Hemorrhage

In broad terms, ICH can be divided into traumatic and nontraumatic etiologies. This chapter will focus on nontraumatic ICH because ICH related to trauma is not routinely considered a stroke. ICH is typically caused by rupture of a blood vessel within the brain parenchyma. Patients typically develop a focal neurological deficit suddenly, but symptoms often evolve over 10 to 30 minutes as the hematoma gradually expands. Headache is commonly present, and the vast majority of patients have markedly elevated blood pressure (often in

TABLE 29.4 Common Causes of Ischemic Strokes in Young Adults				
Disease Process	**Details**	**Risk Factors**	**Work-Up**	**Treatment**
Premature atherosclerosis	Occurs in typical atherothrombotic locations	Hypertension, smoking, hyperlipidemia	Vascular and cardiac imaging, assessment for risk factors	Antithrombotic therapy, risk factor control
Vascular pathologies	Dissections, fibromuscular dysplasia, vasculitis, moyamoya	Neck trauma, autoimmune disease	Detailed vessel imaging	Antithrombotic therapy, steroids
Cardiac disease	PFO, valve lesions, myxoma, myopathy, congenital heart disease, endocarditis	Underlying heart disease	TTE, TEE, cardiac MRI	Anticoagulation, PFO closure, antibiotics
Clotting disorders	Sporadic or inherited; may cause cerebral venous thrombosis	Hypercoagulable states, Positive family history	Laboratory testing; genetic analysis; check for DVT	Anticoagulation
Other diseases	Pregnancy, migraines, genetic disorders, drug abuse, sickle cell disease	Various	Variable	Variable

DVT, Deep vein thrombosis; *MRI,* magnetic resonance imaging; *PFO,* patent foramen ovale; *TEE,* transesophageal echocardiogram; *TTE,* transthoracic echocardiogram.

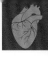

excess of 180 mm Hg systolic) even without a prior history of hypertension. Nausea and vomiting can also occur, particularly with an ICH that involves the brainstem and/or cerebellum.

Chronic or acute hypertension is the most common etiology for nontraumatic ICH, and this type of bleed typically occurs in specific brain locations (Table 29.5). As with ischemic stroke, the location of the ICH is highly correlated with the type of symptoms produced. Recent studies using serial brain scans have shown that 30% to 40% of ICHs will expand over the first 24 hours after admission; such expansion is almost always associated with clinical worsening.[63-65] High blood pressure was once thought to be a major risk factor for ICH expansion, although recent studies have not found a clear association between acutely elevated BP and ICH expansion.[66-68]

Another increasingly common etiology for ICH is cerebral amyloid angiopathy (CAA), which typically affects patients older than 70 years. CAA is caused by deposition of one or more amyloid proteins within the wall of cerebral small arterioles. A typical CAA bleed occurs in a lobar region (junction of the gray matter and white matter), most commonly in the parietal, temporal, and occipital lobes. ICHs due to CAA can be multiple and recurrent.[69-72] There is a clear association between CAA, ICH, dementia, and Alzheimer disease.[73] Bleeds due to CAA can recur in 20% or more of cases.[74]

Sometimes an ischemic stroke can undergo hemorrhagic transformation and become an ICH. This occurs in up to 15% of cases of ischemic stroke and is associated with larger size, cardioembolic etiology, and the use of anticoagulants and thrombolytic agents.

A variety of vascular malformations can cause an ICH, particularly arteriovenous malformations (AVMs) and cavernous malformations (less commonly, capillary telangiectasias and developmental venous anomalies). AVMs are the most common and serious type of vascular malformation that cause an ICH and recurrent ICHs, as well as producing seizures and local neurological deficits.[75,76] The characteristics and hemorrhagic risk of each of these lesions is shown in Table 29.6.

ICH can occur as a consequence of anticoagulation use, the administration of thrombolytic therapy (either for a stroke or another systemic condition), other coagulopathies, hematological disorders, endocarditis, infections (fungal, bacterial, viral), drug abuse (cocaine, heroin, amphetamines), brain tumors (typically metastases), and venous thrombosis.[63] Iatrogenic causes of ICH deserve special mention because there is now extensive use of powerful antiplatelet agents and anticoagulants for a variety of conditions. Using dual antiplatelet therapy or combining anticoagulants with antiplatelet agents can increase the risk of an ICH.[77-81] The use of tissue plasminogen activator (tPA), as well as endovascular therapies (thrombectomy, stenting), as therapies for acute ischemic stroke can lead to ICH (and less commonly SAH).[82,83]

Subarachnoid Hemorrhage

Most cases of nontraumatic SAH are due to rupture of a saccular aneurysm that typically occurs at the bifurcation of blood vessels at the base of the brain around the circle of Willis. However, using modern imaging techniques, we can image aneurysms that occur more distally in the arterial tree. Such lesions are often due to an underlying infec-

TABLE 29.5 Location and Symptoms for Common Types of Intracerebral Hemorrhage

ICH Location	Likely Etiology	Common Symptoms
Basal ganglia	Hypertension	Contralateral hemiparesis, speech changes, gaze deviation, altered mentation if large
Lobar	Hypertension, CAA	Cortical syndromes, weakness, visual field lesions, altered mentation if large
Thalamus	Hypertension	Altered mentation, sensory changes, gaze abnormalities
Pons	Hypertension	Coma, gaze and pupil abnormalities, quadriparesis
Cerebellum	Hypertension, AVM	Ipsilateral ataxia, dizziness, vertigo, nausea/vomiting
Hemispheric cortex	AVM, extreme hypertension, mycotic aneurysm	Headaches, seizures, cortical syndromes

AVM, Arteriovenous malformation; *CAA*, cerebral amyloid angiopathy; *ICH*, intracerebral hemorrhage.

TABLE 29.6 Common Types of Central Nervous System Vascular Lesions That Lead to Cerebral Hemorrhage

Lesion Type	Typical Location	Anatomy	Pressure Characteristics	Typical Hemorrhage Type	Risk of Bleeding/ Other Events
Aneurysm	Arterial bifurcations around circle of Willis	Degeneration of parts of vessel wall leads to outpouching of vessel	High	SAH	Depends on size; approximately 1% or less in general population
AVM	Anywhere in CNS	Arteries draining directly into veins; abnormal intervening brain tissue	High	ICH and/or SAH	High; may also cause seizures
Cavernous angioma	Anywhere is CNS	Collection of enlarged capillaries; no intervening brain tissue	Low	ICH most common	Low in most cases; may cause seizures
Telangiectasia (capillary)	Anywhere; brainstem and white matter most common	Dilated capillaries with normal intervening brain	Low	Pontine ICH	Low
Venous angioma	Hemisphere, cerebellum	Collection of small veins; radial pattern; draining vein; normal brain tissue	Low	Deep white matter, cerebellum	Very low

AVM, Arteriovenous malformation; *CNS*, central nervous system; *ICH*, intracerebral hemorrhage; *SAH*, subarachnoid hemorrhage.

tion (most commonly endocarditis), although they can be seen as a complication of vasculitis or an inherited condition (polycystic kidney disease, Marfan syndrome).[84,85]

SAH typically produces a severe and sudden headache along with nausea/vomiting, nuchal rigidity, and elevated blood pressure. Depending on the location of the ruptured aneurysm, some patients may have additional focal neurological findings. For example, an aneurysm involving the posterior communicating artery can produce an ipsilateral third nerve palsy that involves the pupil. Rupture of an aneurysm of the anterior communicating artery can produce speech and behavioral changes. Aneurysmal rupture that leads to extensive bleeding around the brain and into the ventricles can lead to altered mental status, coma, and sometimes early or sudden death due to dramatic increases in intracranial pressure. A listing of common aneurysm locations and symptoms can be found in Table 29.7.

Following an aneurysmal SAH, patients are at high risk for a number of complications, including rebleeding (if the aneurysm is not secured by surgery or coiling), vasospasm causing ischemic stroke, seizures, hydrocephalus, SIADH (syndrome of inappropriate antidiuretic hormone secretion), and central fever, among others.[86,87]

An ICH or SAH that causes extensive hemorrhage into the ventricular system can produce an acute or subacute hydrocephalus syndrome with worsening headaches, nausea/vomiting, and altered mental status, potentially leading to coma. All strokes, but particularly ICH or SAH, can produce seizures, particularly if the blood involves parts of the cortex or epileptogenic deep structures such as the hippocampus. In the long term, some patients may develop cognitive impairment, along with behavioral and personality changes.

Stroke Mimics

It is incumbent upon the clinician to ensure that a patient with a presumed stroke is in fact having a cerebrovascular event. Many medical conditions can present with stroke-like symptoms and even physical findings but with a different etiology. This has obvious implications in terms of acute therapy, ongoing care, and secondary prevention. Table 29.8 lists some common stroke mimics and diagnostic tests that may be helpful for confirming the diagnosis.

CLINICAL ASSESSMENT TOOLS

History and Physical

Any assessment of a patient with suspected stroke or TIA begins with a focused history and physical. Factors of key concern include prior medical history with assessment of stroke risk factors (hypertension, diabetes, heart disease, etc.), prior stroke or TIA, the presenting symptoms, their mode of onset, precipitating factors, and time course (stable, improving, getting worse). We are particularly concerned about symptoms such as disturbances of speech, language, and mentation; evidence of cranial nerve dysfunction (diplopia, vision loss in one eye or sector, dysarthria, dysphagia, facial weakness); focal motor weakness or coordination problems; gait abnormalities; and sensory symptoms. A particular challenge for stroke patients is that often their ability to sense or report these various symptoms may be affected by the very stroke causing the symptoms. This makes obtaining historical details from family, friends, or caregivers very important.

TABLE 29.7   Common Locations for Saccular Aneurysms and Related Symptoms in Subarachnoid Hemorrhage

Location	Clinical Symptoms
Anterior communicating artery	Leg weakness, speech disturbance, personality changes, seizures, memory loss
Posterior communicating artery/ internal carotid artery junction	Ipsilateral third nerve palsy
Bifurcation of middle cerebral artery	Contralateral weakness, sensory changes, speech changes
Basilar artery tip	Altered mentation, pupil and gaze abnormalities

TABLE 29.8   Common Stroke Mimics: Diagnosis and Treatment

Stroke Mimic	Diagnostic Clues	Confirmatory Tests	Treatment
Hypoglycemia/ hyperglycemia	Hx of diabetes, taking glycemic medications	Blood glucose; serial testing	Correct underlying disease
Electrolyte disturbance	Predisposing condition, taking medications	Electrolyte monitoring	Correct underlying condition
Migraine	Gradual Sx onset; prior Hx of headaches; family Hx of migraine	Rule out other conditions; identify precipitating factors	Avoid triggers; prophylactic medications if frequent migraines, discontinue hormone therapies
Seizures	Aura at beginning; preexisting illness; postictal lethargy	EEG; may require serial monitoring	Antiepileptic medications
Conversion reaction	Nonphysiological neurological examination; prior psychiatric events; secondary gain	Rule out other conditions; repeated examinations with inconsistent findings	Psychiatric evaluation
Demyelinating disease (MS)	Young age; gradual Sx onset	MRI findings; LP results	Treat MS with immunotherapy
CNS tumor	Lesion in nonvascular territory; risk factors for cancer	MRI findings; serial scans evaluate for systemic neoplasm	Treat tumor
Subdural hematoma	Head trauma; bleeding risk factors	Head CT or MRI	Correct coagulopathy; surgical drainage
Medication side effects	Sx associated with medication ingestion	Rule out other conditions	Change/discontinue medications
Infection	Fever, high white count	Brain imaging, LP, blood cultures	Antibiotics, antiviral medications

CNS, Central nervous system; CT, computed tomography; EEG, electroencephalogram; Hx, history; LP, lumbar puncture; MRI, magnetic resonance imaging; MS, multiple sclerosis; Sx, symptom(s).

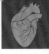

Another key aspect is time of onset of stroke symptoms because this will determine whether the patient is a candidate for acute intervention (this is of particular importance for ischemic stroke).[88] Time of stroke onset is often (and incorrectly) assumed to be when the patient is found with evidence of a stroke. The correct definition of time of onset is when stroke symptoms first began. If a patient has been under constant observation, the time of onset will be when the patient was first noticed to have stroke symptoms. But if a patient has been home alone and discovered with stroke symptoms by a family member, the time of onset has to be when the patient was last known to be normal (assuming the patient cannot determine the time of onset). Therefore, in the case of a patient who awakens in the morning unable to speak at 7 am, time of onset is assumed to be when the patient went to bed normal the night before, unless there is clear documentation otherwise. This strict definition essentially rules out many patients with so-called wake-up strokes from receiving acute therapies such as tPA.[89] However, the recent finding that thrombectomy up to 24 hours after stroke onset is safe and effective in selected patients allows for treatment in many patients with a presumed wake-up stroke.[90,91]

The physical examination will provide valuable information about the likely location of the stroke and suggest the vascular territory and blood vessel or vessels most likely to be involved. As already noted, this is a key step in determining the stroke mechanism and etiology. Besides vital signs and a thorough neurological examination, there are particular aspects of the general medical examination that provide important diagnostic information to the clinician. These include an assessment for cervical bruits, a complete cardiac examination, checking blood pressure and pulses in both arms, a skin examination, and evidence of trauma to the head and neck. Examination of the skin is particularly important because lesions such as rashes, purpura, or digital ischemia might provide important clues about a systemic disorder (i.e., endocarditis, syphilis) that could cause a stroke. Table 29.9 offers an outline of a neurological assessment for patients with known or suspected cerebrovascular disease.

Clinicians often use a variety of scales or scoring systems to assess severity of various types of stroke. These scoring systems can provide guidance about treatment options and overall prognosis. The National Institutes of Health Stroke Scale (NIHSS) is often used to assess patients with an ischemic stroke.[88] The NIHSS is a formalized neurological examination, and scores can range from 0 to 42 (0 being normal, higher score being more severe). The Glasgow Coma Scale (GCS) is often used in patients with ICH and SAH. It measures a patient's responses to a variety of stimuli. The GCS can range from 0 to 15, with 15 being normal. The Hunt and Hess Scale is used to assess severity of SAH, with 1 being a patient with only a headache and 5 being deep coma. The Fisher Grade is used to measure the amount of subarachnoid blood seen on the head CT. Scores range from 1 (no blood seen) to 4 (intraventricular or parenchymal blood).

In recent years, the identification of patients in the field with a suspected stroke has assumed importance for determining transportation destination. A variety of assessment tools and scales are being used in the field by EMS personnel and in the emergency department by medical personnel. Some of these various scales are listed in Table 29.10.

Brain Imaging

Our ability to rapidly and accurately image the brain and cerebral vasculature has been a key factor in our capability to determine the type of stroke, its locations, and likely mechanism.[92] Almost every hospital in the United States is able to perform a head CT scan on patients in the emergency department. On-site personnel or remote radiology reading services can provide a reading within 30 to 60 minutes. The ability to rapidly perform and interpret brain imaging is a key component of a primary and comprehensive stroke center.[93,94]

A head CT scan can easily, rapidly, and safely be used to diagnose an acute stroke, especially if it is a hemorrhagic stroke. In some cases when a patient with an ischemic stroke is imaged very soon after symptom onset, the head CT may be negative or show only subtle changes. In such cases, a repeat head CT in 12 to 24 hours will almost certainly show changes indicative of a large- or medium-sized ischemic stroke (Fig. 29.1). However, a head CT can miss small and acute strokes, particularly if they are in the brainstem or posterior fossa.

TABLE 29.9 Typical Components of a Neurological Examination Pertinent to Stroke

Testing Domain	Specific Functions Tested
Mentation and cognition	Level of alertness, orientation, speech, naming/repetition, memory, personality, apraxia, agnosia, neglect syndromes
Cranial nerves	Testing of nerves II–XII typically performed, including visual acuity and funduscopic examination
Motor function	Tone, bulk, abnormal movements; strength, fine movements
Cerebellar function	Coordination, rapid movements, balance
Gait	Ability to walk, balance, tandem gait
Sensory	Pain/pin prick, light touch, vibration/proprioception
Reflexes	Deep tendon reflexes, plantar response (Babinski); cutaneous reflexes, primitive reflexes (snout, suck, grasp, palmomental)
Vascular system	Auscultation of neck and heart; blood pressure measurements in both arms; check pulses in hands and feet; consider ankle-brachial index (ABI)

TABLE 29.10 Some Scales Used for EMS and Emergency Department Assessment of Patients with a Possible Stroke

Common Name	Definition	Domains Tested	Comments
FAST	Face, arm, speech test	Face, arm, speech	High sensitivity; fair specificity
LAPSS	Los Angeles Pre-hospital Stroke Screen	Face, arm, grip	Good specificity, fair sensitivity
CPSSS	Cincinnati Prehospital Stroke Severity Scale	Consciousness, head/gaze, arm	Fair sensitivity and specificity
RACE	Rapid Arterial Occlusion Evaluation	Head/gaze deviation, face, arm, leg, aphasia, neglect	Gaining acceptance for identification of large vessel occlusion

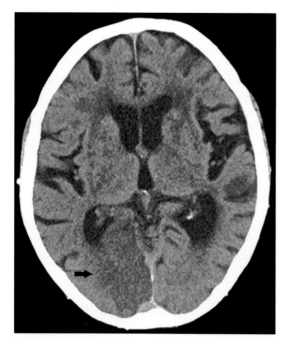

Fig. 29.1 Head Computed Tomography Scan Without Contrast. Arrow indicates a subacute stroke *(darker gray area)* in right occipital lobe in a patient with a new visual field deficit present for approximately 24 hours.

Head CT is very sensitive for imaging hemorrhagic strokes, particularly ICH. ICHs appear as white lesions in the brain parenchyma that represent the actual hematoma (Fig. 29.2A). Often there is early evidence of edema around the ICH, which can worsen over several hours and days. In 30% to 40% of ICH cases, the actual hematoma will expand and lead to clinical worsening. In patients with a large SAH, the head CT will show bright signal (blood) at the base of the brain and within some cortical sulci (see Fig. 29.2B). However, a small SAH or sentinel bleed rarely may be missed by CT and even MRI.[95] Hence a lumbar puncture is needed to definitively rule out a small SAH.

Numerous studies, as well as recent guidelines, have supported use of brain MRI for the work-up of patients with known or suspected strokes.[88,93,96] MRI using diffusion techniques (DWI) is extremely sensitive and accurate for diagnosing essentially all types of ischemic strokes (and some types of hemorrhagic stroke). MRI is particularly useful for imaging small strokes, acute strokes, and those in the posterior fossa (Fig. 29.3). In addition to DWI sequences, use of gradient echo (GRE) sequences or susceptibility-weighted images (SWIs) allow detection of small amounts of blood. Using these techniques, studies have shown that up to 40% of ischemic strokes may have microhemorrhages within the area of ischemia.[97,98] This is especially true for strokes due to a cardioembolic mechanism (i.e., atrial fibrillation, endocarditis).

MRI results will often provide invaluable information about stroke etiology, even if the patient's symptoms and presentation suggest an alternative etiology. For example, a patient may present with symptoms pointing to a small-vessel stroke deep in the brain. In the proper setting, this type of stroke might be caused by typical vascular risk factors such as hypertension or diabetes. However, if the MRI showed evidence of other small acute strokes in other vascular territories, this would shift focus away from an isolated small-vessel stroke to alternative mechanisms such as cardioembolic strokes due to atrial fibrillation, a hypercoagulable state, or even a vasculitis.

Another advantage of MRI is that it can accurately distinguish acute strokes from subacute strokes using lesion characteristics. An acute ischemic stroke will be bright on DWI, dark on apparent diffusion coefficients (ADCs) and not show enhancement with gadolinium (Fig. 29.4A and B). A stroke that is 7 to 10 days old will be less bright on DWI and less dark on ADC and show enhancement with gadolinium (see Fig. 29.4C). A chronic stroke may be bright on DWI (due to T2 shine through) and bright on ADC and show no enhancement.

Advanced MRI techniques are currently available that can identify potentially salvageable brain from infarcted brain based on comparing DWI lesions with magnetic resonance (MR) perfusion lesions (Fig. 29.5). Patients with an acute stroke who have a large area of perfusion abnormality on an MR perfusion study but a smaller area of ischemia (DWI lesion) may benefit from reperfusion therapy using lytic or endovascular therapies even 6 to 8 hours after stroke onset. Use

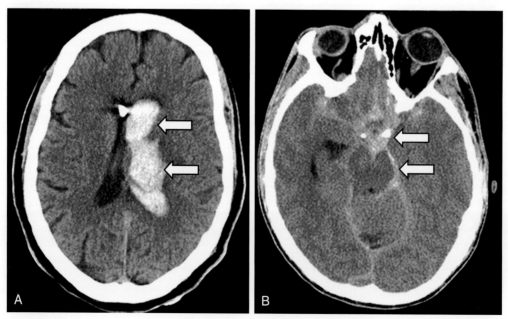

Fig. 29.2 (A) Head computed tomography (CT) scan without contrast. Arrows indicate a deep intracerebral hemorrhage with rupture into the ventricular system *(white area)*. (B) Head CT scan without contrast. Arrows indicate a subarachnoid hemorrhage *(white areas)* at the base of the brain filling the basal cisterns.

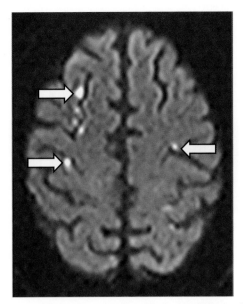

Fig. 29.3 Magnetic Resonance Imaging of Brain with Diffusion-Weighted Sequence. White dots *(arrows)* show areas of acute ischemic or infarction consistent with several acute strokes in a patient with atrial fibrillation.

of these advanced MRI techniques to select patients with an apparent "ischemic penumbra" is an area of active research.[96,99–101]

The recently published DAWN and DEFUSE 3 studies used a similar imaging paradigm but with CT perfusion as the main technique (see Fig. 29.5B). This new paradigm (sometimes referred to as RAPID) can extend the window for reperfusion therapy up to 24 hours after stroke onset in select patients.[90,91] The premise is to select patients with relatively small areas of infarcted brain but larger areas of ischemic but salvageable brain.

MRI of an ICH is more complex, owing to signal changes caused by the metabolism of various blood constituents. Approximately 48 to 72 hours after an ICH, the hemoglobin (Hb) in the hematoma is metabolized into intracellular methemoglobin, which appears bright on the MRI using T1 sequences and dark on T2 sequences. After a week or more, methemoglobin becomes extracellular and becomes bright on T1 and T2 sequences. Hemosiderin is then formed in the hematoma and produces a dark signal in GRE (Fig. 29.6).[102]

Imaging Cerebral Vasculature

Of equal importance to imaging the brain parenchyma is detailed imaging of the cerebral vasculature, both extracranial (aorta, carotid and vertebral arteries) and intracranial.[103] Although in most cases we are

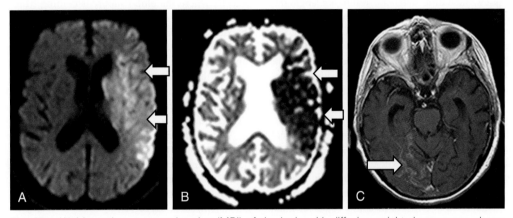

Fig. 29.4 (A) Magnetic resonance imaging (MRI) of the brain with diffusion-weighted sequences shows evidence of a large left hemispheric stroke *(white areas with arrows)*. (B) Apparent diffusion coefficient of same region; dark area is abnormal and indicates ischemia/infarction consistent with an acute stroke. (C) Brain MRI after infusion of gadolinium showing enhancement of a right occipital stroke consistent with a subacute infarction (at least 5 to 7 days old).

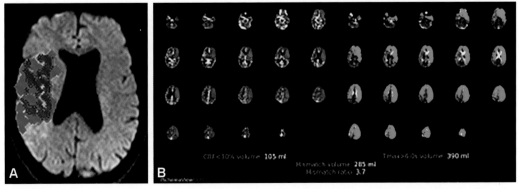

Fig. 29.5 (A) Magnetic resonance imaging of brain with superimposed perfusion and diffusion images showing areas of "mismatch" indicating existence of an apparent ischemic penumbra. Perfusion defect is blue; infarcted brain is pink/purple. (B) Typical computed tomography perfusion image from a DAWN study eligible patient using the RAPID software package.

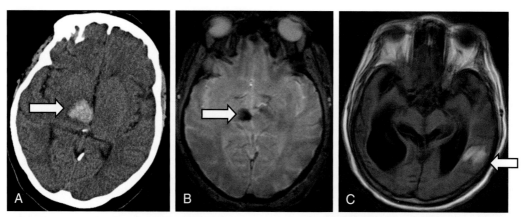

Fig. 29.6 (A) Head computed tomography showing right thalamic intracerebral hemorrhage (ICH) *(white area with arrow)*. (B) Brain magnetic resonance imaging with gradient echo sequences showing same stroke *(arrow)*. Dark area represents iron deposition caused by the bleed. (C) Subacute ICH white area *(arrow)* is methemoglobin formed from a recent cerebral hemorrhage.

focusing on the arterial vasculature, in certain cases it is also important to image the cerebral veins (so-called sinuses) to rule out a cerebral venous thrombosis.

There are several noninvasive modalities available for imaging the cerebral vessels, including magnetic resonance angiography (MRA) (see Chapter 13), computed tomographic angiography (CTA) (see Chapter 14), duplex ultrasonography (see Chapter 12), MR venography, and transcranial Doppler (TCD) (Figs. 29.7 and 29.8).[92] Each method has certain advantages and some limitations (Table 29.11). We typically use either MRA or CTA because they are capable of imaging the entire cerebral vasculature (from the great vessels in the chest to medium-sized intracranial vessels), with a single study lasting only 5 to 10 minutes for CTA and 25 to 30 minutes for MRA. CTA requires intravenous contrast agents, whereas MRA can be done either with intravenous gadolinium or without (using a time-of-flight [TOF] protocol). MRA with contrast (vs. no contrast) provides better images, permitting visualization of small lesions such as dissections or a vasculitis. CTA provides modestly more precise anatomical detail in terms of its ability to detect small aneurysms and small dissection flaps and to accurately determine the degree of arterial stenoses. However, CTA does expose patients to ionizing radiation.

High-resolution CTA or MRA of the intracranial vessel wall can detect areas of acute plaque rupture (seen in atherothrombotic disease) or inflammation (seen with a vasculitis). Such findings can pinpoint the location and type of vessel pathology, which can be used to determine therapeutic options (Fig. 29.9).

Carotid duplex ultrasound is a safe and noninvasive method to image selected segments of the large vessels in the neck. TCD is another safe and noninvasive technique to assess blood flow velocity segments of the intracranial vasculature. Both techniques can provide information about direction and velocity of blood flow. Carotid ultrasound can be performed serially over the course of months and years to assess changes in the degree of stenosis of a neck artery, and it can determine plaque size and composition. TCD is often performed daily after SAH to determine whether there is development of cerebral vasospasm that may cause an ischemic stroke.

The "gold standard" imaging modality for cerebral vessels remains the digital subtraction angiogram (DSA) (also see Chapter 15). In cases where CTA and MRA show different degrees of stenosis, we may do a DSA to determine the exact degree of stenosis (often before doing a carotid endarterectomy or carotid artery

stent). Besides offering precise imaging of small, medium, and large vessels, a DSA also provides invaluable information about cerebral hemodynamics. By injecting the various cerebral vessels, an angiogram can determine (in cases of a vessel stenosis or occlusion) exactly where the blood supply is coming from and going to. The angiogram can detect collateral vessels (or lack thereof) that may be supplying a region of brain thought to be poorly perfused due to occlusion of a proximal vessel. We commonly see patients with apparent lack of flow through a severely diseased basilar artery, only to find that there is still some flow, or collaterals are supplying the brainstem with adequate perfusion (Fig. 29.10). A DSA is also very important when planning surgical treatment for an AVM, aneurysm, and other vascular lesions.

Using computer reconstruction algorithms, images from all the aforementioned techniques can be assembled into three-dimensional (3D) pictures to provide a comprehensive view of the cerebral vessels. These images can be rotated and flipped as needed to aid the clinician in determining the type, location, and severity of the lesion (stenosis, aneurysm, etc.) (Fig. 29.11).

Laboratory Tests

All patients with a stroke (ischemic or hemorrhagic) require standard testing that should include a complete blood cell count (CBC), chemistry panel, coagulation studies, chest x-ray, electrocardiogram (ECG), urinalysis, and the brain imaging already detailed.[88,104] Again, *all* patients should undergo toxicology screening for drug use because this is a common condition and patients are often not forthcoming about drug abuse. The Centers for Disease Control and Prevention (CDC) recommends HIV testing for most adults who are hospitalized, and this would include patients with an acute stroke.[105–107] A listing of routine laboratory testing recommended for patients with ischemic stroke is in Table 29.12.

Special blood tests are warranted if a hypercoagulable state is suspected based on the patient's age or lack of other risk factors or if another condition is suspected.[108] An elevated D dimer may indicate ongoing thrombosis or the presence of a DVT. Blood cultures may be obtained to rule out endocarditis in patients with multiple embolic strokes. In patients with suspected vasculitis or a possible autoimmune disorder, tests for inflammatory conditions, such as a sedimentation rate, antinuclear antibody (ANA) titers, and other serologies, may be performed. Hb electrophoresis can rule out SCD or trait, as well as thalassemia.

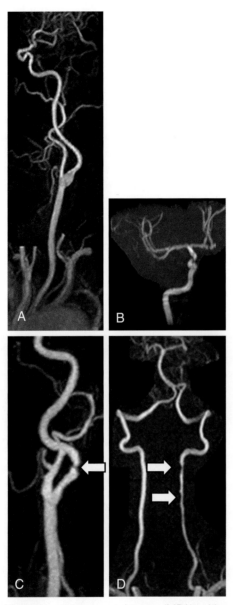

Fig. 29.7 Magnetic resonance angiogram (MRA) with gadolinium, showing normal extracranial common, internal, and external carotid arteries (A) and intracranial vessels (B). (C) Stenosis due to atherosclerosis in proximal internal carotid artery (arrow). (D) MRA of vertebral-basilar system showing irregularity of left vertebral artery due to either fibromuscular dysplasia or dissection (arrows).

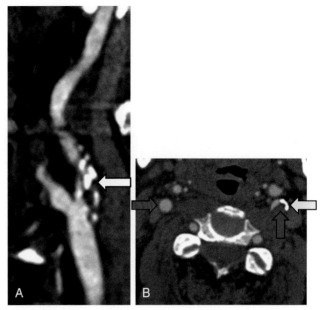

Fig. 29.8 Computed Tomographic Angiogram of Neck Vessels. (A) Side oblique view shows severe calcification of distal common carotid artery and proximal internal carotid artery (ICA) (white arrow). (B) Axial images show a normal right carotid artery (blue arrow) and calcified left ICA. Calcified region is depicted with yellow arrow; soft plaque is shown by the red arrow.

Because the heart can be the cause of up to 25% of all ischemic strokes, a thorough cardiac assessment is needed in most cases. Beyond the standard clinical cardiac examination and an ECG, all patients with an ischemic stroke should receive at least 48 hours of cardiac monitoring (using computerized telemetry) to detect rhythm changes that could cause a stroke (e.g., atrial fibrillation), as well as dysrhythmia that could indicate underlying coronary artery disease (CAD) or cardiomyopathy (e.g., ventricular tachycardia).[20] In some cases, more prolonged monitoring using a Holter device or a subcutaneous device is warranted to further assess for paroxysmal atrial fibrillation. Cardiac imaging including a transthoracic echocardiogram (TTE) or a transesophageal echocardiogram (TEE) is often performed to evaluate cardiac function and assess for the presence of a cardiac clot or other structural lesion (i.e., patent foramen ovale). Typically we begin with a TTE and, if negative, then proceed to the TEE.[109,110] On occasion, a cardiac CT or MRI may be warranted.

Monitoring a patient's respiratory status and oxygen saturation is important in the acute setting because changes may indicate an increase in intracranial pressure or presence of obstructive sleep apnea (OSA) (which is an underrecognized risk factor for stroke).

Duplex venous ultrasound examination of the lower and upper extremities is commonly performed to detect DVT when this is considered a possible source of stroke (in patients with a patent foramen ovale) or a complication of stroke (in patients who are obese, sedentary, or were found down at home after many hours or days). Presence of DVT can also be an indicator of an underlying hypercoagulable state or cancer.[111] A thorough evaluation for underlying malignancy should be considered in patients with a stroke and DVT, as well as patients with cryptogenic strokes or strokes in different vascular territories.

A lumbar puncture is warranted in patients with suspected vasculitis or if a small SAH is suspected but not proven based on brain CT or MRI. Special genetic testing is performed in cases of suspected disorders such as CADASIL or Marfan syndrome. Apolipoprotein E genotype analysis in patients with suspected CAA may be appropriate because the e2 and e4 alleles are strongly associated with Alzheimer disease and CAA-related ICH.

The utility of these tests is greatest in patients with strokes of unusual type, size, and location, particularly if there are no risk factors for atherothrombosis and cerebrovascular disease. A typical patient with one or more risk factors who has an uncomplicated ischemic stroke of known mechanism does not require the special testing listed (in most cases).

TABLE 29.11 Vascular Imaging Techniques

Test Name	Imaging Technique	Vasculature Imaged	Advantages	Disadvantages
Carotid Doppler	Ultrasound	Extracranial carotid and vertebral arteries	Safe, noninvasive, no radiation, inexpensive; provides some anatomical and physiological data	Limited to extracranial vasculature in the neck
TCD	Ultrasound	Intracranial arteries	Safe, noninvasive, no radiation, inexpensive; provides some physiological data	Limited to mostly intracranial vasculature; limited anatomical detail
MRA	Magnetic resonance	Large and medium extracranial and intracranial arteries and veins; great vessels in chest	Safe, noninvasive, no radiation; some anatomical details; can image most vessels; can evaluate cerebral perfusion; some aneurysm detection	Cannot be used with some pacemakers or metal; limited in severe claustrophobia; contrast often needed; expensive
CTA	X-ray	Extracranial and intracranial arteries and veins; great vessels in chest; can detect some small vessels	Significant anatomical detail; can evaluate cerebral perfusion; can image most vessels; accurate stenosis and aneurysm measurements	Radiation exposure; requires contrast; cautious use with renal dysfunction; expensive
Digital cerebral angiography	X-ray	All arteries and veins, including small vessels	Significant anatomical detail; can evaluate cerebral perfusion and collateral flow; accurate stenosis and aneurysm measurement	Invasive procedure; radiation exposure; requires contrast; limited use with renal dysfunction; expensive

CTA, Computed tomographic angiography; *MRA,* magnetic resonance angiography; *TCD,* transcranial Doppler.
Some data derived from Latchaw RE, Alberts MJ, Lev MH, et al. Recommendations for imaging of acute ischemic stroke: a scientific statement from the American Heart Association. *Stroke.* 2009;40(11):3646–3678.

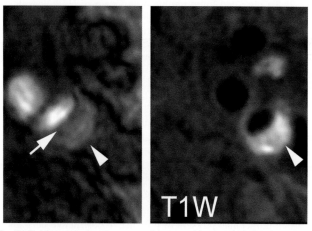

Fig. 29.9 Magnetic resonance angiogram with contrast showing vessel wall abnormalities consistent with plaque rupture with bleeding *(white areas).* Arrow represents a thin fibrous cap on the plaque. Arrowheads represent areas of hemorrhage within the plaque. (From Demarco JK, Ota H, Underhill HR, et al. MR carotid plaque imaging and contrast-enhanced MR angiography identifies lesions associated with recent ipsilateral thromboembolic symptoms: an in vivo study at 3T. *AJNR Am J Neuroradiol.* 2010;31:1395–402.)

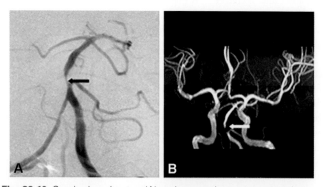

Fig. 29.10 Cerebral angiogram (A) and magnetic resonance angiogram (B) showing high-grade basilar artery stenosis *(arrows).* (From Lou X, Ma N, Ma L, Jiang WJ. Contrast-enhanced 3T high-resolution MR imaging in symptomatic atherosclerotic basilar artery stenosis. *AJNR Am J Neuroradiol.* 2013;34:513–517.)

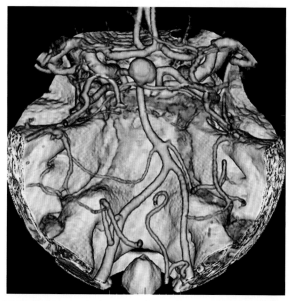

Fig. 29.11 Brain computed tomography angiogram with 3D reconstruction showing basilar tip aneurysm. (From Machida H, Takeuchi H, Tanaka I, et al. Improved delineation of arteries in the posterior fossa of the brain by model-based iterative reconstruction in volume-rendered 3D CT angiography. *AJNR Am J Neuroradiol.* 2013;34:971–975.)

CONCLUSIONS

Stroke is a complex and heterogeneous disease that is the culmination of a variety of medical factors and cerebral vascular anatomy. Based on results of the history, physical, and blood and imaging tests, the clinician can make an accurate assessment as to the location, type, mechanism, and cause of the stroke. Based upon this formulation, an approach for acute therapy can be planned, along with interventions to avoid secondary complications and prevent a recurrent stroke. A better understanding of the basics of stroke in terms of type, cause, presentation, and diagnosis will lead to improved therapies and increase the chance that the patient will have a better outcome.

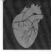

TABLE 29.12 Suggested Laboratory Testing for Patients with Stroke

Routine Tests	Tests for Special Cases[a]	Comments (for Special Tests)
CBC with differential	Hgb electrophoresis	Useful if SCD or thalassemia suspected
Comprehensive chemistry profile	Vasculitis screen (ANA, rheumatoid factor, etc.)	Useful if arteries show beading
APTT, PT, INR	Hypercoagulable screen: lupus anticoagulant, anticardiolipin antibodies, protein C and S activity); factor V Leiden and prothrombin gene mutations; cryoglobulin screen; antithrombin III level	Useful for ischemic strokes in young adults; postpartum; cryptogenic strokes
Sedimentation rate	Fibrinogen, DIC screen	Detects ongoing thrombosis
Fasting lipid profile	CADASIL gene mutation	Characteristic MRI and positive family history
Hb A$_{1C}$	Apolipoprotein E genotype	CAA with recurrent ICH, dementia, MRI changes
Homocysteine	Fabry disease test	Positive family history; skin changes; renal disease
Vitamins B$_{12}$ and folate	Blood cultures	Suspected endocarditis; multiple strokes
Thyroid panel	Assay of clotting factors	Recurrent cerebral hemorrhages
HIV	CT of chest/abdomen/pelvis	Look for cancer in patient with recurrent stroke
Urine toxicology screen (drug abuse)	Tests for specific toxins based on clinical scenario	Possible poisoning
Platelet function tests[b]	Tests for specific platelet disorders	Atypical clinical picture; patient refractory to usual therapy

[a] *Special cases* refer to unusual or atypical presentations or stroke syndromes, including cryptogenic etiologies.
[b] Benefits of platelet function testing for improving efficacy and safety of stroke therapy remain experimental; however, such testing may be important for detecting platelet dysfunction in patients with hemorrhagic stroke.
ANA, Antinuclear antibody; *APTT*, activated partial thromboplastin time; *CAA*, cerebral amyloid angiopathy; *CADASIL*, cerebral autosomal dominant arteriopathy with subcortical infarcts and leukoencephalopathy; *CBC*, complete blood cell count; *CT*, computed tomography; *DIC*, disseminated intravascular coagulopathy; *Hb*, hemoglobin; *HIV*, human immunodeficiency virus; *ICH*, intracerebral hemorrhage; *INR*, International Normalized Ratio; *MRI*, magnetic resonance imaging; *PT*, prothrombin time; *SCD*, sickle cell disease.

REFERENCES

1. Lloyd-Jones D, Adams RJ, Brown TM, et al. Executive summary: heart disease and stroke statistics--2010 update: a report from the American Heart Association. *Circulation.* 2010;121:948–954.
2. Roger VL, Go AS, Lloyd-Jones DM, et al. Heart disease and stroke statistics--2011 update: a report from the American Heart Association. *Circulation.* 2011;123:e18–e209.
3. Broderick J, Brott T, Kothari R, et al. The Greater Cincinnati/Northern Kentucky Stroke Study: preliminary first-ever and total incidence rates of stroke among blacks. *Stroke.* 1998;29:415–421.
4. Benjamin EJ, Blaha MJ, Chiuve SE, et al. Heart disease and stroke statistics—2017 update: a report from the American Heart Association. *Circulation.* 2017;135:e146–e603.
5. Ojaghihaghighi S, Vahdati SS, Mikaeilpour A, Ramouz A. Comparison of neurological clinical manifestation in patients with hemorrhagic and ischemic stroke. *World J Emerg Med.* 2017;8:34–38.
6. Caplan LR. Diagnosis and treatment of ischemic stroke. *JAMA.* 1991;266:2413–2418.
7. Brott T, Bogousslavsky J. Treatment of acute ischemic stroke. *N Engl J Med.* 2000;343:710–722.
8. Caplan LR, Furlan AJ, Hacke W. Acute ischemic stroke therapy: the way forward. *JAMA Neurol.* 2015;72:1405–1406.
9. Kumar S, Caplan LR. Why identification of stroke syndromes is still important. *Curr Opin Neurol.* 2007;20:78–82.
10. Aguilar MI, Freeman WD. Spontaneous intracerebral hemorrhage. *Semin Neurol.* 2010;30:555–564.
11. Edlow JA, Caplan LR. Avoiding pitfalls in the diagnosis of subarachnoid hemorrhage. *N Engl J Med.* 2000;342:29–36.
12. Suarez JI, Tarr RW, Selman WR. Aneurysmal subarachnoid hemorrhage. *N Engl J Med.* 2006;354:387–396.
13. Lee J, Inoue M, Mlynash M, et al. MR perfusion lesions after TIA or minor stroke are associated with new infarction at 7 days. *Neurology.* 2017;88:2254–2259.
14. Shono K, Satomi J, Tada Y, et al. Optimal timing of diffusion-weighted imaging to avoid false-negative findings in patients with transient ischemic attack. *Stroke.* 2017;48:1990–1992.
15. Easton JD, Saver JL, Albers GW, et al. Definition and evaluation of transient ischemic attack: a scientific statement for healthcare professionals from the American Heart Association/American Stroke Association Stroke Council; Council on Cardiovascular Surgery and Anesthesia; Council on Cardiovascular Radiology and Intervention; Council on Cardiovascular Nursing; and the Interdisciplinary Council on Peripheral Vascular Disease. The American Academy of Neurology affirms the value of this statement as an educational tool for neurologists. *Stroke.* 2009;40:2276–2293.
16. Johnston SC, Gress DR, Browner WS, Sidney S. Short-term prognosis after emergency department diagnosis of TIA. *JAMA.* 2000;284:2901–2906.
17. Valls J, Peiro-Chamarro M, Cambray S, et al. A current estimation of the early risk of stroke after transient ischemic attack: a systematic review and meta-analysis of recent intervention studies. *Cerebrovasc Dis.* 2017;43:90–98.
18. Degan D, Ornello R, Tiseo C, et al. Epidemiology of transient ischemic attacks using time- or tissue-based definitions: a population-based study. *Stroke.* 2017;48:530–536.
19. Kiyohara T, Kamouchi M, Kumai Y, et al. ABCD3 and ABCD3-I scores are superior to ABCD2 score in the prediction of short- and long-term risks of stroke after transient ischemic attack. *Stroke.* 2014;45:418–425.
20. Adams RJ, Albers G, Alberts MJ, et al. Update to the AHA/ASA recommendations for the prevention of stroke in patients with stroke and transient ischemic attack. *Stroke.* 2008;39:1647–1652.
21. Nesher G. The diagnosis and classification of giant cell arteritis. *J Autoimmun.* 2014;48-49:73–75.
22. Baquis GD, Pessin MS, Scott RM. Limb shaking--a carotid TIA. *Stroke.* 1985;16:444–448.
23. Donnan GA, O'Malley HM, Quang L, et al. The capsular warning syndrome: pathogenesis and clinical features. *Neurology.* 1993;43:957–962.
24. Camps-Renom P, Delgado-Mederos R, Martinez-Domeno A, et al. Clinical characteristics and outcome of the capsular warning syndrome: a multicenter study. *Int J Stroke.* 2015;10:571–575.
25. Beck J, Raabe A, Szelenyi A, et al. Sentinel headache and the risk of rebleeding after aneurysmal subarachnoid hemorrhage. *Stroke.* 2006;37:2733–2737.

26. de Falco FA. Sentinel headache. *Neurol Sci.* 2004;25(Suppl 3). S215-7.

27. Kannel WB, Wolf PA. Peripheral and cerebral atherothrombosis and cardiovascular events in different vascular territories: insights from the Framingham Study. *Curr Atheroscler Rep.* 2006;8:317–323.

28. Schnabel RB, Sullivan LM, Levy D, et al. Development of a risk score for atrial fibrillation (Framingham Heart Study): a community-based cohort study. *Lancet.* 2009;373:739–745.

29. White H, Boden-Albala B, Wang C, et al. Ischemic stroke subtype incidence among whites, blacks, and Hispanics: the Northern Manhattan Study. *Circulation.* 2005;111:1327–1331.

30. Adams Jr HP, Kappelle LJ, Biller J, et al. Ischemic stroke in young adults. Experience in 329 patients enrolled in the Iowa Registry of Stroke in young adults. *Arch Neurol.* 1995;52:491–495.

31. Varona JF, Guerra JM, Bermejo F, et al. Causes of ischemic stroke in young adults, and evolution of the etiological diagnosis over the long term. *Eur Neurol.* 2007;57:212–218.

32. Ferro JM, Massaro AR, Mas JL. Aetiological diagnosis of ischaemic stroke in young adults. *Lancet Neurol.* 2010;9:1085–1096.

33. Larrue V, Berhoune N, Massabuau P, et al. Etiologic investigation of ischemic stroke in young adults. *Neurology.* 2011;76:1983–1988.

34. Ji R, Schwamm LH, Pervez MA, Singhal AB. Ischemic stroke and transient ischemic attack in young adults: risk factors, diagnostic yield, neuroimaging, and thrombolysis. *JAMA Neurol.* 2013;70:51–57.

35. Urbanus RT, Siegerink B, Roest M, et al. Antiphospholipid antibodies and risk of myocardial infarction and ischaemic stroke in young women in the RATIO study: a case-control study. *Lancet Neurol.* 2009;8:998–1005.

36. Hart RG, Kanter MC. Hematologic disorders and ischemic stroke. A selective review. *Stroke.* 1990;21:1111–1121.

37. Lee MJ, Chung JW, Ahn MJ, et al. Hypercoagulability and mortality of patients with stroke and active cancer: The OASIS-CANCER Study. *J Stroke.* 2017;19:77–87.

38. Katsanos AH, Kosmidou M, Giannopoulos S, et al. Cerebral arterial infarction in inflammatory bowel diseases. *Eur J Intern Med.* 2014;25:37–44.

39. Chen M. Stroke as a complication of medical disease. *Semin Neurol.* 2009;29:154–162.

40. Feske SK. Stroke in pregnancy. *Semin Neurol.* 2007;27:442–452.

41. Sells CM, Feske SK. Stroke in pregnancy. *Semin Neurol.* 2017;37:669–678.

42. Skidmore FM, Williams LS, Fradkin KD, et al. Presentation, etiology, and outcome of stroke in pregnancy and puerperium. *J Stroke Cerebrovasc Dis.* 2001;10:1–10.

43. Sloan MA. Illicit drug use/abuse and stroke. *Handb Clin Neurol.* 2009;93:823–840.

44. Chan KH, Cheung RT, Lee R, et al. Cerebral infarcts complicating tuberculous meningitis. *Cerebrovasc Dis.* 2005;19:391–395.

45. Mishra AK, Arvind VH, Muliyil D, et al. Cerebrovascular injury in cryptococcal meningitis. *Int J Stroke.* 2018;13:57–65.

46. Kastenbauer S, Wiesmann M, Pfister HW. Cerebral vasculopathy and multiple infarctions in a woman with carcinomatous meningitis while on treatment with intrathecal methotrexate. *J Neurooncol.* 2000;48:41–45.

47. Bodilsen J, Dalager-Pedersen M, Schonheyder HC, Nielsen H. Stroke in community-acquired bacterial meningitis: a Danish population-based study. *Int J Infect Dis.* 2014;20:18–22.

48. Kitagawa Y, Gotoh F, Koto A, Okayasu H. Stroke in systemic lupus erythematosus. *Stroke.* 1990;21:1533–1539.

49. Earley CJ, Kittner SJ, Feeser BR, et al. Stroke in children and sickle-cell disease: Baltimore-Washington Cooperative Young Stroke Study. *Neurology.* 1998;51:169–176.

50. Ware RE, de Montalembert M, Tshilolo L, Abboud MR. Sickle cell disease. *Lancet.* 2017;390:311–323.

51. Roach ES, Golomb MR, Adams R, et al. Management of stroke in infants and children: a scientific statement from a Special Writing Group of the American Heart Association Stroke Council and the Council on Cardiovascular Disease in the Young. *Stroke.* 2008;39:2644–2691.

52. Caplan LR, Hier DB, Banks G. Current concepts of cerebrovascular disease--stroke: stroke and drug abuse. *Stroke.* 1982;13:869–872.

53. Sordo L, Indave BI, Barrio G, et al. Cocaine use and risk of stroke: a systematic review. *Drug Alcohol Depend.* 2014;142:1–13.

54. Dobbs MR, Berger JR. Stroke in HIV infection and AIDS. *Expert Rev Cardiovasc Ther.* 2009;7:1263–1271.

55. Sen S, Rabinstein AA, Elkind MS, Powers WJ. Recent developments regarding human immunodeficiency virus infection and stroke. *Cerebrovasc Dis.* 2012;33:209–218.

56. Ortiz G, Koch S, Romano JG, et al. Mechanisms of ischemic stroke in HIV-infected patients. *Neurology.* 2007;68:1257–1261.

57. Cestari DM, Weine DM, Panageas KS, et al. Stroke in patients with cancer: incidence and etiology. *Neurology.* 2004;62:2025–2030.

58. Kreisl TN, Toothaker T, Karimi S, DeAngelis LM. Ischemic stroke in patients with primary brain tumors. *Neurology.* 2008;70:2314–2320.

59. Kwon HM, Kang BS, Yoon BW. Stroke as the first manifestation of concealed cancer. *J Neurol Sci.* 2007;258:80–83.

60. Han E, Lee YH. Non-alcoholic fatty liver disease: the emerging burden in cardiometabolic and renal diseases. *Diabetes Metab J.* 2017;41:430–437.

61. Tsukamoto Y, Takahashi W, Takizawa S, et al. Chronic kidney disease in patients with ischemic stroke. *J Stroke Cerebrovasc Dis.* 2012;21:547–550.

62. Hilkens NA, Algra A, Greving JP. Predicting major bleeding in ischemic stroke patients with atrial fibrillation. *Stroke.* 2017;48:3142–3144.

63. Fewel ME, Thompson Jr BG, Hoff JT. Spontaneous intracerebral hemorrhage: a review. *Neurosurg Focus.* 2003;15:E1.

64. Broderick J, Connolly S, Feldmann E, et al. Guidelines for the management of spontaneous intracerebral hemorrhage in adults: 2007 update: a guideline from the American Heart Association/American Stroke Association Stroke Council, High Blood Pressure Research Council, and the Quality of Care and Outcomes in Research Interdisciplinary Working Group. *Circulation.* 2007;116:e391–e413.

65. Hemphill 3rd JC, Greenberg SM, Anderson CS, et al. Guidelines for the management of spontaneous intracerebral hemorrhage: a guideline for healthcare professionals from the American Heart Association/American Stroke Association. *Stroke.* 2015;46:2032–2060.

66. Morotti A, Boulouis G, Romero JM, et al. Blood pressure reduction and noncontrast CT markers of intracerebral hemorrhage expansion. *Neurology.* 2017;89:548–554.

67. Morotti A, Brouwers HB, Romero JM, et al. Intensive blood pressure reduction and spot sign in intracerebral hemorrhage: a secondary analysis of a randomized clinical trial. *JAMA Neurol.* 2017;74:950–960.

68. Majidi S, Suarez JI, Qureshi AI. Management of acute hypertensive response in intracerebral hemorrhage patients after ATACH-2 trial. *Neurocrit Care.* 2017;27:249–258.

69. Towfighi A, Greenberg SM, Rosand J. Treatment and prevention of primary intracerebral hemorrhage. *Semin Neurol.* 2005;25:445–452.

70. Smith EE, Gurol ME, Eng JA, et al. White matter lesions, cognition, and recurrent hemorrhage in lobar intracerebral hemorrhage. *Neurology.* 2004;63:1606–1612.

71. Greenberg SM, Eng JA, Ning M, et al. Hemorrhage burden predicts recurrent intracerebral hemorrhage after lobar hemorrhage. *Stroke.* 2004;35:1415–1420.

72. Banerjee G, Carare R, Cordonnier C, et al. The increasing impact of cerebral amyloid angiopathy: essential new insights for clinical practice. *J Neurol Neurosurg Psychiatry.* 2017;88:982–994.

73. Weller RO, Nicoll JA. Cerebral amyloid angiopathy: pathogenesis and effects on the ageing and Alzheimer brain. *Neurol Res.* 2003;25:611–616.

74. van Etten ES, Gurol ME, van der Grond J, et al. Recurrent hemorrhage risk and mortality in hereditary and sporadic cerebral amyloid angiopathy. *Neurology.* 2016;87:1482–1487.

75. Wilkins RH. Natural history of intracranial vascular malformations: a review. *Neurosurgery.* 1985;16:421–430.

76. Derdeyn CP, Zipfel GJ, Albuquerque FC, et al. Management of brain arteriovenous malformations: a scientific statement for healthcare professionals from the American Heart Association/American Stroke Association. *Stroke.* 2017;48:e200–e224.

77. Hokari M, Shimbo D, Asaoka K, et al. Impact of antiplatelets and anticoagulants on the prognosis of intracerebral hemorrhage. *J Stroke Cerebrovasc Dis.* 2018;27:53–60.

78. Khan NI, Siddiqui FM, Goldstein JN, et al. Association between previous use of antiplatelet therapy and intracerebral hemorrhage outcomes. *Stroke.* 2017;48:1810–1817.

79. McDonald MM, Almaghrabi TS, Saenz DM, et al. Dual antiplatelet therapy is associated with coagulopathy detectable by thrombelastography in acute stroke. *J Intensive Care Med*. 2017. 885066617729644.

80. Easton JD, Aunes M, Albers GW, et al. Risk for major bleeding in patients receiving ticagrelor compared with aspirin after transient ischemic attack or acute ischemic stroke in the SOCRATES study (acute stroke or transient ischemic attack treated with aspirin or ticagrelor and patient outcomes). *Circulation*. 2017;136:907–916.

81. James SK, Storey RF, Khurmi NS, et al. Ticagrelor versus clopidogrel in patients with acute coronary syndromes and a history of stroke or transient ischemic attack. *Circulation*. 2012;125:2914–2921.

82. Flaherty ML, Woo D, Kissela B, et al. Combined IV and intra-arterial thrombolysis for acute ischemic stroke. *Neurology*. 2005;64:386–388.

83. Bansal S, Sangha KS, Khatri P. Drug treatment of acute ischemic stroke. *Am J Cardiovasc Drugs*. 2013;13:57–69.

84. Schuknecht B. High-concentration contrast media (HCCM) in CT angiography of the carotid system: impact on therapeutic decision making. *Neuroradiology*. 2007;49(Suppl 1). S15–S26.

85. Debette S, Germain DP. Neurologic manifestations of inherited disorders of connective tissue. *Handb Clin Neurol*. 2014;119:565–576.

86. Fernandez A, Schmidt JM, Claassen J, et al. Fever after subarachnoid hemorrhage: risk factors and impact on outcome. *Neurology*. 2007;68:1013–1019.

87. Flemming KD, Brown Jr RD, Wiebers DO. Subarachnoid hemorrhage. *Curr Treat Options Neurol*. 1999;1:97–112.

88. Jauch EC, Saver JL, Adams Jr HP, et al. Guidelines for the early management of patients with acute ischemic stroke: a guideline for healthcare professionals from the American Heart Association/American Stroke Association. *Stroke*. 2013;44:870–947.

89. Hills NK, Johnston SC. Why are eligible thrombolysis candidates left untreated? *Am J Prev Med*. 2006;31:S210–S216.

90. Nogueira RG, Jadhav AP, Haussen DC, et al. Thrombectomy 6 to 24 hours after stroke with a mismatch between deficit and infarct. *N Engl J Med*. 2018;378:11–21.

91. Albers GW, Marks MP, Kemp S, et al. Thrombectomy for stroke at 6 to 16 hours with selection by perfusion imaging. *N Engl J Med*. 2018;378:708–718.

92. Latchaw RE, Alberts MJ, Lev MH, et al. Recommendations for imaging of acute ischemic stroke: a scientific statement from the American Heart Association. *Stroke*. 2009;40:3646–3678.

93. Alberts MJ, Latchaw RE, Jagoda A, et al. Revised and updated recommendations for the establishment of primary stroke centers: a summary statement from the Brain Attack Coalition. *Stroke*. 2011;42: 2651–2665.

94. Alberts MJ, Latchaw RE, Selman WR, et al. Recommendations for comprehensive stroke centers: a consensus statement from the Brain Attack Coalition. *Stroke*. 2005;36:1597–1616.

95. Dubosh NM, Bellolio MF, Rabinstein AA, Edlow JA. Sensitivity of early brain computed tomography to exclude aneurysmal subarachnoid hemorrhage: a systematic review and meta-analysis. *Stroke*. 2016;47: 750–755.

96. Schellinger PD, Bryan RN, Caplan LR, et al. Evidence-based guideline: the role of diffusion and perfusion MRI for the diagnosis of acute ischemic stroke: report of the Therapeutics and Technology Assessment Subcommittee of the American Academy of Neurology. *Neurology*. 2010;75:177–185.

97. Koennecke HC. Cerebral microbleeds on MRI: prevalence, associations, and potential clinical implications. *Neurology*. 2006;66:165–171.

98. Kleinig TJ. Associations and implications of cerebral microbleeds. *J Clin Neurosci*. 2013;20:919–927.

99. Latchaw RE, Yonas H, Hunter GJ, et al. Guidelines and recommendations for perfusion imaging in cerebral ischemia: a scientific statement for healthcare professionals by the writing group on perfusion imaging, from the Council on Cardiovascular Radiology of the American Heart Association. *Stroke*. 2003;34:1084–1104.

100. Seiler A, Blockley NP, Deichmann R, et al. The relationship between blood flow impairment and oxygen depletion in acute ischemic stroke imaged with magnetic resonance imaging. *J Cereb Blood Flow Metab*. 2017; 271678x17732448.

101. Vilela P, Rowley HA. Brain ischemia: CT and MRI techniques in acute ischemic stroke. *Eur J Radiol*. 2017;96:162–172.

102. Anzalone N, Scotti R, Riva R. Neuroradiologic differential diagnosis of cerebral intraparenchymal hemorrhage. *Neurol Sci*. 2004;25(Suppl 1). S3–S5.

103. Latchaw RE, Alberts MJ, Lev MH, et al. Recommendations for imaging of acute ischemic stroke: a scientific statement from the American Heart Association. *Stroke*. 2009;40:3646–3678.

104. Adams Jr HP, del Zoppo G, Alberts MJ, et al. Guidelines for the early management of adults with ischemic stroke: a guideline from the American Heart Association/American Stroke Association Stroke Council, Clinical Cardiology Council, Cardiovascular Radiology and Intervention Council, and the Atherosclerotic Peripheral Vascular Disease and Quality of Care Outcomes in Research Interdisciplinary Working Groups: the American Academy of Neurology affirms the value of this guideline as an educational tool for neurologists. *Circulation*. 2007;115. e478–e534.

105. Branson BM, Handsfield HH, Lampe MA, et al. Revised recommendations for HIV testing of adults, adolescents, and pregnant women in health-care settings. *MMWR Recomm Rep*. 2006;55:1–17. quiz CE1–4.

106. Chow FC, Price RW, Hsue PY, Kim AS. Greater risk of stroke of undetermined etiology in a contemporary HIV-infected cohort compared with uninfected individuals. *J Stroke Cerebrovasc Dis*. 2017;26:1154–1160.

107. Haukoos JS, Hopkins E, Byyny RL. Denver Emergency Department HIV Testing Study Group. Patient acceptance of rapid HIV testing practices in an urban emergency department: assessment of the 2006 CDC recommendations for HIV screening in health care settings. *Ann Emerg Med*. 2008;51:303–309. 309 e1.

108. Bushnell CD, Goldstein LB. Diagnostic testing for coagulopathies in patients with ischemic stroke. *Stroke*. 2000;31:3067–3078.

109. de Bruijn SF, Agema WR, Lammers GJ, et al. Transesophageal echocardiography is superior to transthoracic echocardiography in management of patients of any age with transient ischemic attack or stroke. *Stroke*. 2006;37:2531–2534.

110. Anaissie J, Monlezun D, Seelochan A, et al. Left atrial enlargement on transthoracic echocardiography predicts left atrial thrombus on transesophageal echocardiography in ischemic stroke patients. *Biomed Res Int*. 2016;2016. 7194676.

111. Bentsen L, Christensen A, Havsteen I, et al. Frequency of new pulmonary neoplasm incidentally detected by computed tomography angiography in acute stroke patients—a single-center study. *J Stroke Cerebrovasc Dis*. 2015;24:1008–1012.

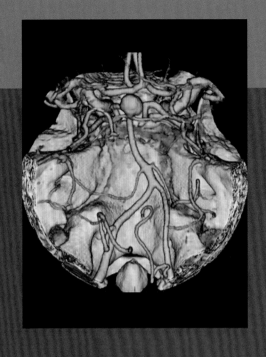

第30章
脑卒中的预防和治疗

　　卒中的治疗包括在急性期管理各生理指标、减轻急性损伤程度和预防复发。缺血性卒中是最常见的一类脑血管疾病。本章将主要讨论缺血性卒中，并对原发性颅内出血（primary intracerebral hemorrhage，ICH）及其急性期处理和二级预防做简要介绍。心脏或其他来源的血栓栓塞颅内或颅外血管时便会导致急性缺血性卒中（acute ischemic stroke，AIS）。除非合并有颅内大动脉粥样硬化，因原位血栓形成导致的急性缺血性卒中并不常见。动脉急性栓塞引发的一系列血管内事件会最终造成梗死等不可逆的组织损伤。但是，血管阻塞后数小时内，被称作缺血性半暗带（ischemic penumbra，IP）的部分脑区仍可能保持活性并可通过及时治疗挽救。而预测缺血脑组织转归的最重要因子为脑血流（cerebral blood flow，CBF）减少程度。急性缺血性卒中后少或无脑血流的脑区会迅速进展为梗死区，不具备治疗价值。而缺血性半暗带的脑血流减少较少，进展为梗死的速度较慢，为挽救脑组织提供了时间窗，目前认为及早进行血流重建治疗可使患者获益。其他影响缺血性脑损伤的因素包括侧支循环、体温、血糖水平、血压水平及其他代谢因素。急性缺血性卒中的治疗方法主要包括两大类：通过血运重建增加缺血区脑血流，以及通过神经保护减轻缺血性卒中的损伤后果。本章将对急性缺血性卒中的临床诊疗途径展开介绍。

吉训明

Prevention and Treatment of Stroke

Marc Fisher, Bharti Manwani, and Meg VanNostrand

The medical management of stroke encompasses a wide range of therapies that include managing physiological parameters in the acute phase, reducing the extent of acute injury, and preventing recurrent strokes. Ischemic stroke is the most common form of cerebrovascular disease and will be the focus of this chapter. Only a brief mention of primary intracerebral hemorrhage (ICH) with regard to acute management and secondary prevention will be included.

Acute ischemic stroke (AIS) occurs after occlusion of an intracranial or extracranial vessel by a thrombus that has embolized from the heart or a more proximal artery, for large artery ischemic strokes, and small, intracranial vessels for lacunar strokes. Unlike acute myocardial infarction (AMI), in situ thrombosis is uncommon in large artery strokes, except in Asian populations in whom large vessel intracranial atherosclerosis is relatively common. As a consequence of acute vascular occlusion, a cascade of intracellular events (Fig. 30.1) is initiated leading to irreversible tissue injury (i.e., infarction).[1] The temporal development of infarction within the ischemic brain region is quite variable, and portions of the ischemic brain tissue may not be irreversibly injured for many hours after the initial vascular occlusion.[2] Ischemic brain tissue that remains viable and amenable to salvage with the timely initiation of therapeutic interventions is called the *ischemic penumbra*, and this potentially salvageable tissue is the target of AIS therapies.[3,4] The basic concept underlying AIS therapy is that reducing the extent of brain infarction should translate into improved clinical outcome, as measured by commonly used outcome scales such as the modified Rankin Scale (mRS) or Barthel Index.[5]

The most important factor predisposing ischemic brain tissue to infarction is the severity of cerebral blood flow (CBF) decline.[6] Regions with little or no residual CBF will evolve into infarction rapidly and are not the target of AIS therapies because reperfusion cannot, in most cases, be performed rapidly enough to salvage this ischemic core region. In the ischemic penumbra, CBF decline is more modest, and this ischemic tissue progresses more slowly toward infarction, providing a time window for intervention that can salvage tissue to some extent. The recently published thrombectomy trials demonstrated that treated selected patients with a large ischemic penumbra and small ischemic core up to 24 hours after stroke onset may derive benefit from invasive therapy.[7] A variety of definitions for the ischemic penumbra have been suggested over time and are outlined in Box 30.1. Other factors that affect evolution of ischemic injury include collateral blood flow, temperature, glucose, blood pressure (BP), and other metabolic factors.[8,9] The implication of the diversity of the factors that contribute to the evolution of ischemic injury is that individual AIS patients have quite variable therapeutic time windows for successful therapeutic intervention. Earlier therapy initiation is more likely to be beneficial. Additionally, advanced imaging techniques can discern individual variation in the amount of viable tissue. These techniques, including diffusion/perfusion magnetic resonance imaging (MRI) and computed tomography (CT) perfusion imaging, characterize the extent of the ischemic core and penumbra, revealing potentially viable ischemic tissue that may be salvaged (Figs. 30.2 and 30.3).

AIS therapy can be divided into two broad areas: (1) recanalization/reperfusion approaches directed at improving altered CBF within ischemic tissue; and (2) neuroprotection or cytoprotection designed to impede the cellular consequences of ischemic injury. The focus of this chapter will be on the former because no neuroprotection strategies have been demonstrated to have significant benefit. Recanalization/reperfusion can be accomplished with intravenous (IV) or intra-arterial (IA) thrombolytics as well as mechanical devices. These approaches comprise the currently available AIS treatments. This chapter will also discuss secondary and primary prevention of ischemic stroke.

PREHOSPITAL AND EMERGENCY DEPARTMENT MANAGEMENT OF ISCHEMIC STROKE

Prehospital management is critically important to increasing the survival rates of stroke patients. This phase starts with the emergency medical services (EMS) call and continues in the hospital emergency department (ED) (Table 30.1). Many ischemic stroke patients do not reach the hospital soon enough, owing to lack of local services and facilities, and for social reasons. When a stroke is first suspected, the patient should be rapidly transported to an appropriate facility for diagnostic evaluation and treatment initiation.[10] Stroke patients who present within 3 to 4.5 hours or less of symptom onset are eligible for IV thrombolysis.[11-15] EMS use is strongly associated with a decreased time to initial physician examination, initial CT imaging, and neurological evaluation.[14,16-18] The benefits of EMS contact are superior to contacting the family physician or hospital directly, and were confirmed with several studies.[19,20] Stroke should be given a priority dispatch like myocardial infarction (MI) and trauma.[21] Patients who show signs and symptoms of hyperacute stroke must be treated as time-sensitive emergency cases and transported without delay to the closest institution that provides emergency stroke care. With the demonstration that thrombectomy is a highly effective treatment for patients with proximal, large vessel, intracranial occlusion, patients should be transported to hospitals that perform thrombectomy, as long as bypassing primary stroke centers that only give tissue plasminogen activator (tPA) does not result in an excessive delay. The precise paradigm for primary stroke center bypass remains to be elucidated. One approximation would approve the bypass of a primary stroke center if the delay to reaching a thrombectomy-capable center is 30 minutes or less.[22]

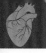
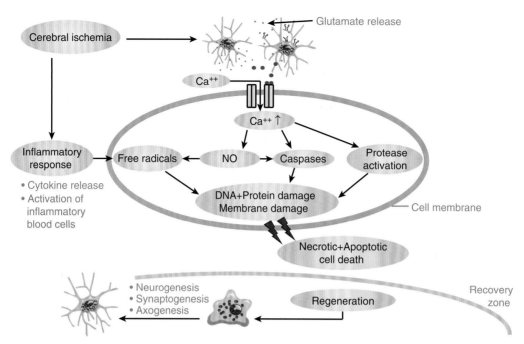

Fig. 30.1 Depiction of the major events that encompass the ischemic cascade of cellular injury. *DNA,* Deoxyribonucleic acid; *NO,* nitric oxide. (Courtesy Dr. Wolf-Rudiger Schaebitz.)

BOX 30.1   Definitions of the Ischemic Penumbra Over Time

- A region of reduced CBF with absent electrical activity but preserved ion homeostasis and transmembrane electrical potentials
- A region with reduced CBF and preserved energy metabolism
- A region with impaired protein synthesis but preserved ATP levels
- A region that is potentially salvageable with timely intervention[a]

[a]This definition is the most clinically relevant one and relates directly to imaging identification.
ATP, Adenosine triphosphate; *CBF,* cerebral blood flow.

To facilitate this process, medical authorities and media sources should encourage the recognition of stroke signs by providing public education about this condition.[23] All members of the public should be able to recognize and identify the signs and symptoms of stroke. These include sudden localized weakness, difficulty speaking, loss of vision, headache, and dizziness.[24] Patient, family, and caregiver education is an integral part of stroke care that should be addressed at all stages across the continuum of stroke care for both adult and pediatric patients.[24] Currently, thrombolytic treatment with tPA and thrombectomy are the only approved treatment options for AIS. The National Institute of Neurological Disorders and Stroke (NINDS) and Advanced Cardiac Life Support Resources (ACLSR) recommend the possible timing sequences shown in Table 30.2 for the potential recanalization candidate.

Data from the Thomas Lewis Latané (TLL) Temple Foundation Stroke Project controlled trial showed the benefits of educational interventions on stroke identification and management targeting patients, EMS, hospitals, and community physicians. This approach increased thrombolytic use in patients with ischemic stroke from 2.21% to 8.65% compared with communities that did not have such programs, which saw only a 0.06% increase. For patients with ischemic stroke who were eligible for thrombolytic therapy, rates of tPA usage increased from 14% to 52% in intervention communities.[25,26] Prehospital delays continue to contribute the largest proportion of time to late initiation of therapy.[27]

EMS arrival starts the diagnostic and management process. The EMS crew transfers the patient to a medical center able to provide appropriate diagnostic and treatment modalities to stroke patients.[10] After the ambulance arrives on the scene, EMS providers should obtain a brief history and patient examination, stabilize vital signs, and rapidly transport the patient to the closest, most appropriate facility for either IV thrombolysis or thrombectomy in appropriate patients (Table 30.3). Several prehospital assessment scales have been developed with varying degrees of accuracy to identify acute stroke patients with a likely large vessel occlusion (LVO) because patients with a likely LVO should be transported to a thrombectomy ready center, if the transport time is not unreasonable compared to transport to a primary stroke center. Prehospital evaluation is helpful for ED physicians and the inpatient care team for planning treatment options. Critical medical interventions in the ED should focus on the need for intubation, BP control, and determining risk/benefit for thrombolysis or thrombectomy.[28] General ED stroke care issues are outlined in Table 30.4.[29,30]

Acute stroke patients urgently need IV access and cardiac monitoring in the ED, preferably initiated in the transporting ambulance. These patients also are at risk for acute cardiac diseases such as arrhythmias and MI. In addition, atrial fibrillation may be associated with acute stroke as either the etiology (embolic disease) or as a result.[31,32] Acute stroke patient evaluation in the ED should include a rapid assessment by obtaining a relevant history, physical examination, neurological examination, stroke scale scores (National Institutes of Health Stroke Scale [NIHSS]), and appropriate diagnostic tests (Box 30.2).[10]

Patients presenting with compromised ventilation require emergent airway control via nasal oxygenation or rapid sequence intubation. Adequate tissue oxygenation is important in the management of acute cerebral ischemia to prevent hypoxia and further brain damage. The most common causes of hypoxia in the patient with acute stroke are partial airway obstruction, hypoventilation, atelectasis, or aspiration pneumonia.[10,28,29,33] Oxygen requirements should be monitored with pulse oximetry, with a target oxygen saturation level ≥92%.[34]

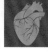

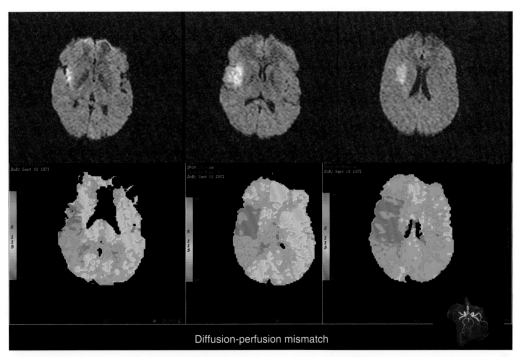

Diffusion-perfusion mismatch

Fig. 30.2 Example of a diffusion and perfusion mismatch on an acute magnetic resonance imaging scan. Yellow to blue indicates decreasing level of perfusion. Blue area indicates the hypoperfused brain tissue.

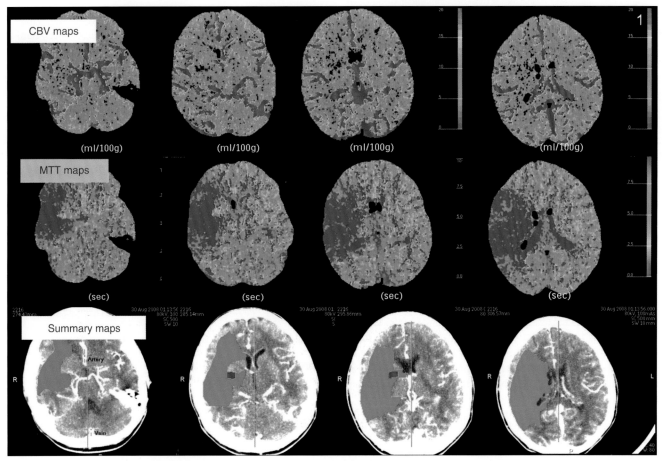

Fig. 30.3 Perfusion computed tomography scan of an acute ischemic stroke patient, demonstrating a very small basal ganglial abnormality on the cerebral blood volume *(CBV)* map and a large area of hypoperfusion on the mean transit time *(MTT)* map of brain perfusion. Summary maps are integrated CBV and MTT maps.

TABLE 30.1   Stroke Chain of Survival

Detection	Recognition of Stroke Signs and Symptoms
Dispatch	Call 911 (emergency phone number) and priority EMS dispatch
Delivery	Prompt transport and prehospital notification to hospital
Door	Immediate ED triage
Data	ED evaluation, prompt laboratory studies, and CT imaging
Decision	Diagnosis and decision about appropriate therapy
Drug	Administration of appropriate drugs or other interventions

CT, Computed tomography; ED, emergency department; EMS, emergency medical services.
Modified from Adams HP Jr, del Zoppo G, Alberts MJ, et al. Guidelines for the early management of adults with ischemic stroke: a guideline from the American Heart Association/American Stroke Association Stroke Council, Clinical Cardiology Council, Cardiovascular Radiology and Intervention Council, and the Atherosclerotic Peripheral Vascular Disease and Quality of Care Outcomes in Research Interdisciplinary Working Groups: the American Academy of Neurology affirms the value of this guideline as an educational tool for neurologists. Stroke. 2007;38(5):1655–1711.

TABLE 30.2   Stroke Evaluation Time Benchmarks for Potential Thrombolysis Candidate

Time Interval	Time Target
Door to doctor	10 min
Access to neurological expertise	15 min
Door to CT scan completion	25 min
Door to CT scan interpretation	45 min
Door to treatment	60 min
Admission to monitored bed	3 h

CT, Computed tomography.

Endotracheal intubation and supplemental nasal oxygen may be used as needed. If brain herniation is present, hyperventilation using mechanical ventilation (to decrease intracranial pressure [ICP]) by decreasing CBF) is recommended. An arterial partial pressure of carbon dioxide (Pco_2) of 32 to 36 mm Hg should be targeted. IV mannitol may be considered to reduce increased ICP. Oxygen supplementation should be guided by a pulse oximeter.[28,29,34]

ACUTE STROKE THERAPY

The only AIS pharmacotherapy currently approved by the US Food and Drug Administration (FDA) is IV tPA initiated within 3 hours after symptom onset. Approval of this treatment is based on the results of the NINDS tPA trial in 1995.[35] The NINDS tPA trial used two primary outcome measures: improvement over 24 hours after tPA and improvement at 90 days. The trial demonstrated a significant improvement in 90-day outcome on multiple outcome measures (mRS, Barthel Index, and NIHSS), with a number needed to treat of 8. However, the trial did not show a statistically significant early improvement with tPA (within 24 hours), which is a point worth noting when discussing this treatment with patients.

The benefit in functional status was observed in different stroke subtypes and in patients with various ranges of baseline stroke severity,

TABLE 30.3   Guidelines for Emergency Medical Services Management of Patients with Suspected Stroke

Recommended	Not Recommended
Manage ABCs	Dextrose-containing fluids in nonhypoglycemic patients
Cardiac monitoring	Hypotension/excessive blood pressure reduction
IV access	Excessive IV fluids
Oxygen (as required for O_2 saturation <92%)	
Assess for hypoglycemia	
Nil per os (NPO)	
Alert receiving emergency department	
Rapid transport to closest appropriate facility capable of treating acute stroke	

ABCs, Airway, breathing, circulation; IV, intravenous.
Modified from Adams HP Jr, del Zoppo G, Alberts MJ, et al. Guidelines for the early management of adults with ischemic stroke: a guideline from the American Heart Association/American Stroke Association Stroke Council, Clinical Cardiology Council, Cardiovascular Radiology and Intervention Council, and the Atherosclerotic Peripheral Vascular Disease and Quality of Care Outcomes in Research Interdisciplinary Working Groups: the American Academy of Neurology affirms the value of this guideline as an educational tool for neurologists. Stroke. 2007;38(5):1655–1711.

TABLE 30.4   Acute Stroke Management

Parameter	Management
Blood glucose	Treat hypoglycemia with D_{50}
Blood pressure	Evaluate recommendations for thrombolysis candidates and noncandidates
Cardiac monitor	Continuous monitoring for ischemic changes and atrial fibrillation
IV fluids	Avoid D_5W and excessive fluid administration; IV isotonic sodium chloride solution at 50 mL/h unless otherwise indicated
Oral intake	NPO initially; aspiration risk is great; avoid oral intake until swallowing assessed
Oxygen	Supplement if indicated (Sao_2 <93%, hypotensive, etc.)
Temperature	Avoid hyperthermia; oral or rectal acetaminophen and cooling blankets as needed

IV, Intravenous; NPO, nil per os; Sao_2, arterial blood oxygen saturation.
Modified from Krieger D, Hacke W. The intensive care of the stroke patient. In: Barnett HJ, Mohr JP, Stein BM, eds. Stroke: Pathophysiology, Diagnosis and Management, 3rd ed. New York: Churchill Livingstone: 1998; and Albers GW, Diener HC, Frison L. Ximelagatran vs warfarin for stroke prevention in patients with nonvalvular atrial fibrillation: a randomized trial. JAMA. 2005;293(6):690–698.

ranging from mild to severe.[36] Despite a 6.4% risk of symptomatic intracranial hemorrhage, the overall treatment benefit remained significant. Following the NINDS trial, several other trials attempted to extend the therapeutic time window of tPA to 6 hours after stroke

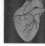

BOX 30.2   Immediate Diagnostic Studies for Patients with Suspected Acute Ischemic Stroke

All Patients
Noncontrast brain CT or brain MRI
Blood glucose
Serum electrolytes/renal function
ECG
Markers of cardiac ischemia
CBC, including platelet count
Prothrombin time/INR
APTT
Oxygen saturation

Selected Patients
Hepatic function tests
Toxicology screen
Blood alcohol level
Pregnancy test
Arterial blood gas tests (if hypoxia is suspected)
Chest radiography (if lung disease is suspected)
Lumbar puncture (if SAH is suspected and CT scan is negative for blood)
EEG (if seizures are suspected)

Although it is desirable to know the results of these tests before giving rtPA, thrombolytic therapy should not be delayed while awaiting the results unless (1) there is clinical suspicion of a bleeding abnormality or thrombocytopenia, (2) the patient has received heparin or warfarin, or (3) the use of anticoagulants is not known.
APTT, Activated partial thromboplastin time; *CBC*, complete blood cell count; *CT*, computed tomography; *ECG*, electrocardiogram; *EEG*, electroencephalogram; *INR*, International Normalized Ratio; *MRI*, magnetic resonance imaging; *rtPA*, recombinant tissue plasminogen activator; *SAH*, subarachnoid hemorrhage.
Modified from Adams HP Jr, del Zoppo G, Alberts MJ, et al. Guidelines for the early management of adults with ischemic stroke: a guideline from the American Heart Association/American Stroke Association Stroke Council, Clinical Cardiology Council, Cardiovascular Radiology and Intervention Council, and the Atherosclerotic Peripheral Vascular Disease and Quality of Care Outcomes in Research Interdisciplinary Working Groups: the American Academy of Neurology affirms the value of this guideline as an educational tool for neurologists. *Stroke.* 2007;38(5):1655–1711.

BOX 30.3   Subgroup Analysis of the European Cooperative Acute Stroke Studies III Trial of Intravenous Tissue Plasminogen Activator in the 3- to 4.5-Hour Time Window

Patient Characteristics Associated With Modest or No Benefit With Tissue Plasminogen Activator
- Female
- Age >65[a]
- Moderate baseline stroke severity[a]
- Diabetes mellitus
- Hypertension[a]
- Atrial fibrillation[a]

Modified from Bluhmki E, Chamorro A, Dávalos A, et al. Stroke treatment with alteplase given 3.0-4.5 h after onset of ischaemic stroke (ECASS III): additional outcomes and subgroup analysis of a randomised controlled trial. *Lancet Neurol.* 2009;8(12):1095–1102.
[a]Denotes patients with an increased risk for symptomatic intracerebral hemorrhage.

onset.[37–39] None of these trials demonstrated a significant benefit on the pre-specified primary outcome measures. However, a combined analysis of the European Cooperative Acute Stroke Studies (ECASS) I & II and ATLANTIS trials demonstrated a significant treatment effect with IV tPA out to 4.5 hours after stroke onset.[40] The ECASS III trial evaluated AIS patients between 3 and 4.5 hours after onset of stroke and reflected the European license for tPA: excluding patients over 80, those with very severe strokes with an NIHSS score >25, history of prior stroke, diabetes, and use of anticoagulants prior to stroke.[41] The ECASS III study demonstrated that 52.4% of tPA-treated patients achieved a favorable outcome of 0 to 1 on the mRS, compared to 45.2% with placebo treatment (odds ratio [OR], 1.34; 95% confidence interval [CI], 1.02–1.76; P = .04). The results of ECASS III led to recommendations from the American Heart Association (AHA) and others that the use of IV tPA be extended to 4.5 hours in selected AIS patients.[42] A subgroup analysis of the ECASS III data suggested that patients older than 65 and those with more severe strokes had less benefit than younger patients or those with milder deficits (Box 30.3).[43]

In 2016, the ENCHANTED trial compared low-dose versus standard-dose IV tPA in the treatment of AIS.[44] The trial was developed to address the concern that some subpopulations, particularly Asians, may be at increased risk of symptomatic intracranial hemorrhage with standard dose IV tPA. Trials in Japan have shown similar efficacy using low-dose tPA with a decreased risk of intracranial hemorrhage. The ENCHANTED trial randomized 3310 patients who met guideline-recommended criteria for treatment with thrombolysis to management with standard dose (0.9 mg/kg) or low dose (0.6 mg/kg) IV tPA. The trial did not show that lower dose IV tPA was noninferior to standard dose IV tPA for the primary outcome of death or disability. There was a weak trend that patients with prior antiplatelet therapy may be at increased risk for spontaneous ICH and therefore benefit from treatment with lower dose tPA. Subsequent subgroup analysis of the ENCHANTED data showed that there appeared to be a trend toward more favorable outcomes in patients on prior antiplatelet therapy who received treatment with low dose tPA.[45] Further study in this area is needed.

Though IV tPA remains the only FDA-approved drug for the treatment of AIS, other thrombolytic agents have been investigated. In 2012, a phase 2B clinical trial compared IV tPA with two different doses of IV tenecteplase on the coprimary endpoints of reperfusion and clinical improvement at 24 hours.[46] Tenecteplase is a genetically engineered mutant tPA with a higher specificity for fibrin and longer half-life. Tenecteplase can be administered as a bolus dose and is approved for the treatment of AMI. The 2012 study enrolled 75 patients and treated patients within 6 hours of symptom onset. Patients were required to have an NIHSS ≥4, computed tomographic angiography (CTA) confirmed LVO, and CT perfusion imaging showing a mismatch between core infarct and penumbra of at least 20% for study enrollment. The study reported that tenecteplase was associated with a statistically significant improvement in clinical outcomes and rates of reperfusion with no increased risk of symptomatic ICH. Based on these promising results, a 2017 phase 3 superiority trial compared treatment with higher dose tenecteplase compared to standard treatment with IV tPA.[47] While there was again no statistically significant difference in the safety outcomes between the two treatments, tenecteplase was not superior to tPA for the primary outcome measure of mRS 0 to 1 ("excellent clinical outcome") at 3 months. One important critique of the study was that it was underpowered to detect a large

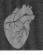

treatment effect, compounded by the fact that the majority of the patients enrolled suffered minor strokes (median NIHSS of 6 vs. NIHSS ~14 in the 2012 study). Given the promising nature of this drug, there are multiple ongoing studies which continue to compare it with tPA (ATTEST-2, TASTE) and to examine its roll in specific patient populations (prior to thrombectomy EXTEND-IA TNK, minor strokes with proven occlusion TEMPO-2, wake-up strokes TWIST).

In 2016, the efficacy of IV desmoteplase was examined in an extended time window.[48,49] Patients were eligible for inclusion if they presented with ischemic stroke between 3 and 9 hours from symptom onset, had an NIHSS between 4 and 24, and had imaging confirmation of an LVO. Patients with infarcts >1/3 of the middle cerebral artery (MCA) territory were excluded. The pooled data from DIAS-3/4/J did demonstrate a significant increase in the recanalization rate of LVOs by ~11% with no increase in rates of symptomatic ICH. However, this benefit did not translate into improved clinical outcomes, and it failed to reach significance for its primary outcome measure of mRS 0 to 2 at 90 days.

In addition to IV tPA treatment, multiple recent studies have now shown a clear benefit of endovascular thrombus retrieval among carefully selected patients. Several studies in 2013 (IMS III, SYNTHESIS, and MR RESCUE) failed to show a benefit of endovascular treatments on the primary outcome of mRS score at 90 days.[50-52] There have been multiple critiques of these studies, the most salient of which include: failure to systematically identify LVOs radiographically (IMS III and SYNTHESIS) and the low recanalization rates achieved with older devices (41% in IMS III, 27% in MR RESCUE, not reported for SYNTHESIS).

In 2015, several high-quality randomized, controlled trials were published showing significantly improved functional outcomes with endovascular clot retrieval (MR CLEAN, EXTEND-IA, ESCAPE, SWIFT PRIME, REVASCAT).[53-57] The first significant difference between these studies and prior negative trials was the use of advanced imaging to identify patients more likely to benefit from endovascular clot retrieval. To this end, all of the newer studies required radiographic evidence of LVO with either CTA or magnetic resonance angiography (MRA) as part of their inclusion criteria. Additionally, the majority of the studies sought to exclude patients with large core infarcts on presentation. ESCAPE, REVASCAT, EXTEND-IA, and SWIFT PRIME all required an ASPECTS score of ≥6 (REVASCAT ≥7) for enrollment. EXTEND-IA (and some SWIFT PRIME sites) utilized diffusion-weighted MRI of CT perfusion imaging to identify patients with small core infarcts (<70 cc) and at least some area of salvageable brain tissue.

The second significant difference was the widespread use of stent retriever (stentreiver) devices; all patients in EXTEND-IA, SWIFT PRIME, and REVASCAT were treated with stent retriever devices. This resulted in markedly improved recanalization rates (TICI IIb or III) in comparison to prior trials. While MR CLEAN and REVASCAT reported recanalization rates of 58.7% and 65.7%, respectively, EXTEND-IA and SWIFT PRIME were able to achieve rates of 86.2% and 88.0%, respectively.

Finally, emphasis was placed on timely intervention. Though the time window for intervention ranged from up to 6 to 12 hours after symptom onset, groin puncture for endovascular procedure happened within 4.5 hours after symptom onset in the majority of patients.

The HERMES collaboration pooled data from these five studies, analyzing individual patient data from 1287 patients (634 treated with thrombectomy, 653 treated with best medical management).[57] HERMES reported a clear reduced chance of disability at 90 days (mRS >2) in the intervention group ($P < .0001$). They state: "The degree of benefit conferred by endovascular thrombectomy is substantial: for every 100 patients treated, 38 will have a less disabled outcome than with best medical management, and 20 more achieve functional independence (mRS 0-2) as a result of the treatment." This benefit was preserved across all analyzed subgroups including groups stratified by age, sex, NIHSS, occlusion site, whether or not patient was eligible and received IV tPA, ASPECTS (6 to 8 vs. 9 to 10), presence of tandem occlusions, and time to randomization (0 to 300 minutes vs. 300 to 420 minutes). There was no significant difference in mortality between the two treatments and no significant difference in the risk of symptomatic intracranial hemorrhage.

The AHA/American Stroke Association (ASA) guidelines reflect the findings of these studies with Class I/Level of Evidence A recommendations that endovascular thrombectomy should be the standard of care for patients who meet the following criteria: "(a) prestroke mRS 0–1, (b) acute ischemic stroke receiving IV tPA within 4.5 hours according to treatment guidelines, (c) causative occlusion of the internal carotid artery or proximal MCA (M1), (d) age ≥18 years, (e) NIHSS ≥6, (f) ASPECTS ≥6, and (g) treatment can be initiated (groin puncture) within 6 hours of symptom onset."[58] These guidelines also stress that all patients should still be treated with IV tPA if they are eligible, but that observation for improvement post-tPA is not indicated and should not delay endovascular treatment. As with IV tPA, timely reperfusion is stressed, with earlier recanalization being associated with improved outcomes. IA tPA remains a possible treatment modality. However, the fact that current practice guidelines now recommend endovascular thrombectomy as the first-line treatment renders many previous IA tPA studies moot. The use of IA tPA as an adjunctive or second-line treatment for reperfusion is often left to the discretion of the physician performing the endovascular procedure. Finally, the guidelines specifically recommend the use of stent retrievers over other devices, with final discretion being again left to the physician performing the procedure.

Recently, the DAWN trial examined extended window thrombectomy in carefully selected patients.[59] Patients presenting within 6 to 24 hours were eligible for treatment with thrombectomy if they met the following criteria: NIHSS ≥10, evidence of LVO on CTA or MRA, and core infarct below a threshold size. Core infarct was measured with CT perfusion or diffusion-weighted imaging (DWI), and had to be less than 21 cc in patients over 80 with an NIHSS score between 10 and 19, less than 31 cc in patients under 80 with an NIHSS score between 10 and 19, or less than 51 cc in patients under 80 with an NIHSS ≥20. The selection criteria were chosen to target patients with a small core and large amount of tissue at risk ("clinical-imaging mismatch"). The trial was positive and stopped at interim analysis. The authors report a number needed to treat of just 2.8 for one additional patient to achieve functional independence (mRS 0 to 2) at 90 days. There were no differences in the safety outcomes of stroke-related death, death from any cause, and symptomatic intracranial hemorrhage. The design and results of the five trials included in the HERMES collaboration as well as the DAWN trial are summarized in Table 30.5.

The results of the DAWN trial suggest that dichotomizing patients by time of presentation (i.e., "in the window" or "out of the window") may be an oversimplification. Increasingly, perfusion-weighted imaging is being used to select for a subset of patients with slow progressing strokes who may be eligible for interventions beyond the currently accepted time windows. Indeed, trials (EXTEND) are underway to apply this concept to extending the IV thrombolytic time window.

In addition to recanalization therapies, the only other acute intervention with a documented significant improvement in outcome is the use of specialized stroke care units. In acute coronary care, specialized units have a long-standing history and proven track record. For AIS, the development and use of specialized care units is much

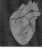

TABLE 30.5   Summary of Endovascular Thrombectomy Trials

Trial, Publication Year	Study Design	Clinical Inclusion Criteria	Radiographic Inclusion Criteria	Outcome Measure	Absolute Difference in mRS 0–2 at 90 Days	NNT
MR CLEAN, 2015	Standard medical care vs. standard medical care + thrombectomy	Age ≥18 No premorbid condition specified NIHSS ≥2 Initiation of thrombectomy within 6 h of last known well	Occlusion of intracranial ICA, MCA (M1 or M2), or ACA (A1 or A2) confirmed by CTA or MRA	mRS at 90 days	13.50%	7.4
ESCAPE, 2015	Standard medical care vs. standard medical care + thrombectomy	Age ≥18 Prestroke Barthel index >90 NIHSS >5 Randomization within 12 h of last known well	Occlusion of intracranial ICA or MCA-M1 confirmed by CTA or MRA ASPECTS score >5	mRS at 90 days	23.70%	4
REVASCAT, 2015	Standard medical care vs. standard medical care + thrombectomy	Age ≥ 18 and ≤85 Prestroke mRS <2 Baseline NIHSS >6 Initiation of thrombectomy within 8 h of last known well	Occlusion of intracranial ICA or MCA-M1 confirmed by CTA or MRA ASPECTS score >6	mRS at 90 days	15.50%	6.5
EXTEND-IA, 2015	IV tPA vs. IV tPA + thrombectomy	Age ≥18 Prestroke mRS <2 Any NIHSS Initiation of IV tPA within 4.5 h of symptom onset Initiation of thrombectomy within 6 h of last known well	Occlusion of carotid terminus or M1 segment confirmed by CTA or MRA Perfusion imaging (CT or MR) meeting the following criteria: Mismatch ratio >1.2 Absolute mismatch volume >10 cc Ischemic core volume < 70 cc	Reperfusion at 24 h and early neurologic improvement Secondary endpoint: mRS at 90 days	31%	3.2
SWIFT PRIME, 2015	IV tPA vs. IV tPA + thrombectomy	Age 18–80 Prestroke mRS ≤1 NIHSS ≥8, <30 Initiation of IV tPA within 4.5 h of symptom onset Initiation of thrombectomy within 6 h of last known well	Occlusion of carotid terminus or MCA-M1 confirmed by CTA or MRA Baseline CT with ASPECTS ≥6 or MRI or CTP core infarct ≤50 cc, penumbra ≥15 cc, and mismatch ratio >1.8	mRS at 90 days	25%	4
DAWN, 2017	Standard medical care vs. standard medical care + thrombectomy	Age ≥18 Prestroke mRS <2 NIHSS ≥10 Randomization between 6 and 24 h after last known well	Occlusion of intracranial ICA or MCA-M1 confirmed by CTA or MRA Perfusion imaging (CT or MR) showing clinical-imaging mismatch defined: 0–20 cc core infarct and NIHSS ≥10 (and age ≥80 years) 0–30 cc core infarct and NIHSS ≥10 (and age <80 years) 0–50 cc core infarct and NIHSS ≥20 (and age <80 years)	mRS at 90 days and UW mRS at 90 days	36%	2.8

ACA, Anterior cerebral artery; *CT,* computed tomography; *CTA,* computed tomographic angiography; *CTP,* computed tomography perfusion; *ICA,* internal carotid artery; *IV,* intravenous; *MR,* magnetic resonance; *MRI,* magnetic resonance imaging; *mRS,* modified Rankin Scale; *NIHSS,* National Institutes of Health Stroke Scale; *NNT,* number needed to treat; *tPA,* tissue plasminogen activator; *UW,* utility-weighted.

more recent, and efficacy was documented later than for coronary care units. Several studies found that the admission of AIS patients to stroke care units reduces mortality and disability when compared to care on general medical units with stroke team consultation.[60,61] The precise reasons for these benefits are uncertain but likely relate to stricter adherence to care guidelines, better BP and glucose management, and earlier mobilization.[62] Additionally, it is now apparent that management guidelines recommendations, such as the AHA "Get with the Guidelines," reduce complications after AIS, and that these guidelines should be implemented both in stroke units and in general hospital units if at all possible.[63]

The other approach to AIS treatment besides recanalization/reperfusion is neuroprotection, or reduction of infarction by treatments targeting the manifold cellular consequences of focal brain ischemia, which has a long and undistinguished track record. In animal stroke models, many categories of neuroprotective drugs reduce infarct size, and some also improve functional outcome (Box 30.4).[64,65] The reduction of infarct size for many neuroprotective drugs occurred without reperfusion, implying that enough of the drug reached the ischemic penumbra in sufficient concentration to impede development of the infarction. This can occur because there is sufficient residual CBF in the penumbral region to deliver the neuroprotective drug and to allow this tissue to survive.

Based on preclinical data of varying quality and extensiveness, many neuroprotective drugs went into clinical development, including phase III trials in some cases.[66] None of the neuroprotective drugs demonstrated significant efficacy, and currently no neuroprotective drug is available for AIS treatment. Many reasons for the multitude of failures of neuroprotective drug development programs were proposed regarding both the preclinical assessment of these agents and the clinical development programs (Box 30.5).[67] Neuroprotection as an AIS treatment strategy remains appealing, primarily in combination with reperfusion. Combining neuroprotection with reperfusion therapy can be envisioned in several ways. Very early initiation of a neuroprotectant could potentially extend survival of the ischemic penumbra, allowing for later deployment of an IV or IA reperfusion therapy.[68] In animals, both high-flow 100% oxygen delivery and granulocyte colony stimulating factor (GCSF) have the capability to extend penumbral survival, but this approach has not yet been tested in clinical trials.[69,70] Another

---

BOX 30.4   Types of Neuroprotective Drugs That Have Been Evaluated as Potential Treatments for Acute Ischemic Stroke

- NMDA antagonists
- AMPA antagonists
- Free radical scavengers
- Growth factors
- Calcium channel antagonists
- GABA agonists
- Serotonin antagonists
- Potassium channel activator
- Antiinflammatory agents

Modified from Schäbitz WR, Fisher M. Perspectives on neuroprotective stroke therapy. *Biochem Soc Trans.* 2006;34(Pt 6):1271–1276; and Donnan GA. A new road map for neuroprotection. *Stroke.* 2008;39:242–248.
AMPA, α-Amino-3-hydroxy-5-methyl-4-isoxazolepropionate; *GABA,* γ-aminobutyric acid; *NMDA,* N-methyl-D-aspartate.

BOX 30.5   Potential Preclinical and Clinical Trials Flaws That May Have Hampered Neuroprotective Drug Development

Preclinical Testing Flaws

- Inadequate sample sizes in treatment experiments
- Lack of adequate physiological monitoring
- Lack of blinding to treatment outcomes
- Not testing the drug in animals that were female, aged, or had relevant comorbidities
- Only testing the study drug in rodents
- Only evaluating histological endpoints and not behavioral outcomes
- Lack of determining effects on both ischemic gray and white matter

Clinical Trial Flaws

- Treating patients too long after stroke onset
- Including stroke subtypes not likely to respond to treatment, such as lacunar stroke patients
- Moving to phase III trials without adequate assessment of the study drug's pharmacology
- Side effects precluded reaching the therapeutic blood level shown to be effective in animals
- Inadequately powered phase III trials to detect a modest but clinically meaningful treatment effect
- Using an insensitive or flawed primary outcome measure

Modified from Gladstone DJ, Black SE, Hakim AM. Toward wisdom from failure: lessons from neuroprotective stroke trials and new directions. *Stroke.* 2002;33(8):2123–2136.

---

potential combination of neuroprotection with reperfusion would be to use an appropriate agent to reduce potential deleterious tissue consequences of successful reperfusion (i.e., reperfusion injury).[70] Neuroprotective drugs that affect free radicals or reduce the recruitment of inflammatory white blood cells (WBCs) may be particularly suited to reduce reperfusion injury, and clinical development programs with such agents after successful reperfusion should be considered.

A final consideration for future neuroprotection development programs would be to use agents that reduce infarct size when given early after AIS, but also enhance the natural recovery processes that occur weeks and months later.[71] This combination approach is appealing because both the reduction of infarct size engendered by the neuroprotective effect and the recovery-enhancing effect will contribute to improved stroke outcome. Current pessimism for neuroprotection in AIS may be replaced by guarded optimism, but the organization and conduct of clinical trials in combination with reperfusion will be more complex and difficult than in the past.[72]

General Medical Management of Acute Stroke Patients

Hypoglycemia should be corrected with rapid IV administration of concentrated glucose solution. Hypoglycemia is detrimental to the ischemic process. At the opposite end of the spectrum, a blood glucose of 200 mg/dL (10 mmol/L) or higher justifies insulin administration. Hyperglycemia is found in nearly 20% to 50% of stroke patients.[73–75] Severe hyperglycemia is independently associated with stroke progression and increase in infarct size. Moreover, admission hyperglycemia is independently associated with the risk of spontaneous ICH and poor outcomes in acute stroke patients treated with IV tPA.[76,77] Increased blood glucose causes reduced reperfusion in thrombolysis, as well as extension of the infarcted territory.[78–81] Glucose-containing IV fluids should not be given to normoglycemic stroke patients because this may lead to hyperglycemia and may worsen ischemic cerebral injury. Blood sugar control should be tightly maintained to establish normoglycemia (90 to 140 mg/dL).

Core temperature is elevated in up to 50% of patients within 48 hours after stroke onset. High temperature is an alarming sign whether or not there is infection. Management of fever may have both favorable or unfavorable consequences. Pyrogens can enhance the effects of interferons (molecules involved in the immune response), inhibit growth of some microorganisms, enhance the activity of WBCs, and enhance tissue repair. The presence of fever has been found to correlate with poorer outcome in stroke, mostly resulting from increased metabolic demand, enhanced release of neurotransmitters, and increased free radical production.[35,82–86] Fever has been shown experimentally to increase infarct size, and high body temperature may favor stroke progression and poor long-term outcome. Antipyretics are indicated for febrile stroke patients because hyperthermia accelerates ischemic neuronal injury.

The Paracetamol (Acetaminophen) in Stroke (PAIS) trial assessed whether early treatment with paracetamol improves functional outcome in patients with acute stroke by reducing body temperature and preventing fever. Patients ($n = 1400$) were randomly assigned to receive acetaminophen (6 g daily) or placebo within 12 hours of symptom onset. After 3 months, improvement on the mRS with acetaminophen was not greater than expected. These results do not support routine use of high-dose acetaminophen in patients with acute stroke.[87] Antipyretics are recommended early in the management of acute stroke until the temperature is lowered to 37.5°C. Antibiotics should be used early in cases of apparent bacterial infection.

Hypothermia is currently being evaluated in clinical trials as a neuroprotective approach.[88,89] It has been shown to be neuroprotective in experimental stroke models. A large meta-analysis of preclinical studies shows that mild therapeutic hypothermia during AIS reduces infarct size and causes better functional outcomes.[90] The ICTuS (Intravascular Cooling in the Treatment of Stroke), ICTuS-L, and ICTuS-2 trials were designed to test the safety and feasibility of therapeutic hypothermia by using an endovascular cooling device in combination with the administration of a tPA in acute stroke patients.[91] Therapeutic hypothermia was well tolerated, although there was an increased incidence of pneumonia among the hypothermia cohort. Nonetheless, despite preclinical evidence, there are little data about the utility of induced hypothermia for treatment of patients with stroke.[92–96]

Cerebral perfusion pressure is high when patients are maintained in a supine position. However, lying flat may serve to increase ICP and thus it is not recommended in cases of subarachnoid or other ICH. This information is applicable during transportation of stroke patients for enhancing favorable outcome.[97] Life-threatening space-occupying brain edema occurs in up to 10% of patients with supratentorial infarcts and is associated with an increased mortality rate of nearly 80%. Ischemic stroke patients develop maximal cerebral edema 48 to 72 hours after onset.[9] In patients with ischemic stroke, a recent study, The Head Positioning in Acute Stroke Trial (HeadPoST) the lying-flat head position, as compared to the sitting-up position, initiated early after presentation and maintained for 24 hours, did not change disability/mortality outcomes.[98] Hyperventilation and mannitol are used routinely to decrease ICP quickly and temporarily but are of uncertain long-term value. Both approaches require careful monitoring of blood chemistry. There is no evidence supporting the use of corticosteroids to decrease cerebral edema in AIS. Many patients who develop hemorrhagic transformation or progressive cerebral edema will demonstrate acute clinical decline. In cases of evolving large MCA infarction, the malignant MCA syndrome, early surgical decompression is now the "antiedema" therapy of first choice for patients younger than 60 years, independent of the affected hemisphere. Over the past decade, it has

been shown that early decompressive hemicraniectomy for malignant MCA infarction lowers mortality and prevents severe disability.[99–103] In patients older than 60 years of age with malignant middle-cerebral-artery infarction, early hemicraniectomy does significantly increase survival but most survivors have substantial disability, so patient and family choices about the quality of life should be considered in this patient population before making surgical decisions.[104]

Maintaining electrolyte balance is also important during the acute stages of stroke, especially to avoid plasma volume contraction. Disturbance of fluid balance could worsen brain perfusion pressure. Patients should be adequately hydrated. All stroke patients should receive IV fluid therapy, with a slightly positive fluid balance according to the level of dehydration, as indicated by the hematocrit and serum osmolality. A careful approach should be employed in patients having possible cerebral edema. Therefore, all stroke patients need daily electrolyte monitoring.

Although patients with heart disease are at high risk for ischemic stroke, both myocardial ischemia and cardiac arrhythmias are potential complications of acute cerebrovascular diseases.[105] The most common arrhythmia detected in the setting of acute stroke is atrial fibrillation, which may be either the cause or a complication of stroke.[9] Other potentially life-threatening cardiac arrhythmias are uncommon, but sudden death may occur.[31,106] No clinical trials have tested the utility of cardiac monitoring for patients with ischemic stroke or the use of cardioprotective agents or medications to prevent cardiac arrhythmias. Still, a consensus exists that patients with AIS should have cardiac monitoring for at least the first 24 hours and that any significant cardiac arrhythmia should be treated. The utility of prophylactic administration of medications to prevent cardiac arrhythmias among patients with stroke is unclear.[9]

Hypertension has a devastating effect on the brain and is a major risk factor for ischemic and hemorrhagic stroke. Hypertension alters the structure of cerebral blood vessels and disrupts intricate vasoregulatory mechanisms that ensure adequate blood supply to the brain. These alterations threaten cerebral blood supply and increase susceptibility of the brain to ischemic injury.[107] High BP is often detected in the first hours after stroke. BP monitoring and treatment are critical in stroke treatment. Hypotension and hypertension are both dangerous for stroke patients because these conditions disturb cerebral perfusion. Hypotension and abnormalities in cardiac rhythm must be corrected as quickly as possible to ensure adequate cerebral perfusion.[108] However, elevated BP should be managed according to suggested guidelines. Aggressive efforts to lower BP may decrease cerebral perfusion pressure and worsen the ischemic process.

Both elevated and low BPs are associated with poor outcomes in patients with acute stroke.[109,110] BP normalization may acutely reduce the hemorrhagic transformation risk of ischemic stroke and reduce the risk of stroke recurrence and brain edema. Aggressive antihypertensive therapy should be used in stroke patients with hypertensive encephalopathy, aortic dissection, acute renal failure, acute pulmonary edema, or AMI.[110,111] Unfortunately, aggressive treatment of BP may lead to neurological worsening by reducing perfusion pressure to ischemic brain regions.[110,112] Excessive lowering of BP acutely in ischemic stroke patients has been associated with neurological worsening. When the BP must be lowered, titratable short-acting IV medication is preferred to minimize the risk of cerebral hypoperfusion. Typically, during the first hours after stroke onset, but sometimes not until 24 hours later, BP drops spontaneously, which is unrelated to any specific medication.[113]

Precise recommendations for control of hypertension in the setting of acute stroke are controversial owing to results of several studies related to acute BP control.[110] Systolic blood pressure (SBP) greater than 185 mm Hg or diastolic pressure of greater than 110 mm Hg are contraindications to thrombolysis; emergency BP control is indicated to allow for thrombolytic administration.[114] Outside of the consideration of thrombolytic administration, in the absence of hypertension-related complications, no data support the administration of emergency antihypertensive drugs in acute stroke. Many clinical trials have now shown that BP reduction in the acute phase of stroke with antihypertensive medications does not reduce death or disability compared with the absence of hypertensive medication.[115] The consensus recommendation is to lower BP only if systolic pressure is in excess of 220 mm Hg or if diastolic pressure is greater than 120 mm Hg.[9] However, rapid reduction of BP, no matter the degree of hypertension, may in fact be harmful.

The management of BP in patients with AIS is divided into those who are candidates for thrombolytic therapy and those who are not. For patients who are not tPA candidates and whose SBP is less than 220 mm Hg and diastolic BP is less than 120 mm Hg in the absence of evidence of end-organ involvement (i.e., pulmonary edema, aortic dissection, hypertensive encephalopathy), BP should be monitored (without acute intervention), and stroke symptoms and complications should be treated (increased ICP, seizures). For patients with SBPs elevated above 220 mm Hg or diastolic BPs between 120 and 140 mm Hg, labetalol (10 to 20 mg IV for 1 to 2 minutes) should be the initial drug of choice unless a contraindication to its use exists.[114] Dosing may be repeated or doubled every 10 minutes to a maximum dose of 300 mg. Alternatively, nicardipine (5 mg/h IV initial infusion) titrated to effect via increasing 2.5 mg/h every 5 minutes to a maximum dose of 15 mg/h may be used for BP control. Lastly, nitroprusside at 0.5 μg/kg/min IV infusion may be used in the setting of continuous BP monitoring. The goal of intervention is a reduction of 10% to 15% of BP.[9]

For patients who will be receiving tPA, SBP should be lower than 185 mm Hg and diastolic BP lower than 110 mm Hg. Monitoring and control of BP during and after thrombolytic administration are vital because uncontrolled hypertension is associated with hemorrhagic complications.[35] For the first 2 hours after IV thrombolysis, BP should be checked every 15 minutes, then every 30 minutes for 6 hours, and finally every hour for 16 hours. If BP levels are in the ranges of 180 to 230 mm Hg systolic or 105 to 120 mm Hg diastolic, it is appropriate to administer labetalol 10 mg IV over 1 to 2 minutes or enalaprilat 1.25 mg IV push. This may be repeated every 10 to 20 minutes to a maximum dose of 300 mg. If BP is not controlled, sodium nitroprusside may be considered (Table 30.6).[116]

Anticoagulation and Antiplatelet Therapy

IV anticoagulation therapy is used by some physicians, even though there are no data demonstrating its benefit. It is unknown whether IV heparin prevents recurrent cardioembolic stroke in the subacute phase, and it is unlikely this therapy inhibits progression of stroke deficits. Current guidelines do not recommend IV anticoagulation for any stroke subgroup.[117–122] Immobilized stroke patients who are not receiving anticoagulants (e.g., IV heparin, an oral anticoagulant) may benefit from low-dose subcutaneous unfractionated heparin (UFH) or low-molecular-weight heparin (LMWH), which reduce the risk of deep vein thrombosis (DVT).[9] Multiple past studies of LMWH failed to show beneficial effects for AIS. Although trials of anticoagulants in the treatment of AIS are ongoing, no data exist to support their use in AIS.[9]

Published guidelines for the prevention of stroke in patients with ischemic stroke or transient ischemic attack (TIA) due to atrial fibrillation recommend anticoagulation with adjusted-dose warfarin for secondary prevention (target international normalized ratio [INR] 2.5, range 2.0 to 3.0) or DOACs (direct oral anticoagulants).[116,123] Oral anticoagulation with warfarin is also recommended for patients

with ischemic stroke due to AMI in whom left ventricular (LV) mural thrombus is identified, patients with dilated cardiomyopathy, and patients with valvular heart disease for secondary prevention.[116]

For patients with noncardioembolic ischemic stroke or TIA, including strokes caused by large-artery atherosclerosis, small penetrating artery disease, and cryptogenic infarcts, antiplatelet agents rather than oral anticoagulation are recommended to reduce the risk of recurrent stroke and other cardiovascular events.

The DOACs, dabigatran, rivaroxaban, apixaban, and edoxaban have demonstrated safety and efficacy compared with warfarin in recent clinical trials for the reduction of risk of stroke in patients with nonvalvular atrial fibrillation.[124] Dabigatran etexilate 110 mg given twice daily was associated with rates of stroke and systemic embolism similar to those associated with warfarin, but with lower rates of

TABLE 30.6 Blood Pressure Management in Patients With Stroke

Patient	Blood Pressure	Treatment
Candidates for fibrinolysis	*Pretreatment:* SBP >185 mm Hg or DBP >110 mm Hg	Labetalol 10–20 mg IVP 1–2 doses *or* Enalaprilat 1.25 mg IVP
	Posttreatment: DBP >140 mm Hg SBP >230 mm Hg or DBP 121–140 mm Hg SBP 180–230 mm Hg or DBP 105–120 mm Hg	Sodium nitroprusside (0.5 μg/kg/min) Labetalol 10–20 mg IVP, and consider labetalol infusion at 1–2 mg/min or nicardipine 5 mg/h IV infusion and titrate Labetalol 10 mg IVP, may repeat and double every 10 min up to maximum dose of 150 mg
Noncandidates for fibrinolysis	DBP >140 mm Hg	Sodium nitroprusside 0.5 μg/kg/min
	SBP >220 mm Hg or DBP 121–140 mm Hg or MAP >130 mm Hg	Labetalol 10–20 mg IVP over 1–2 min; may repeat and double every 10 min up to maximum dose of 150 mg *or* Nicardipine 5 mg/h IV infusion and titrate
	SBP >220 mm Hg or DBP 105–120 mm Hg or MAP <130 mm Hg	Antihypertensive therapy indicated only if AMI, aortic dissection, severe CHF, or hypertensive encephalopathy present

AMI, Acute myocardial infarction; *CHF*, congestive heart failure; *DBP*, diastolic blood pressure; *IV*, intravenous; *IVP*, IV push; *MAP*, mean arterial pressure; *SBP*, systolic blood pressure.
Modified from Krieger D, Hacke W. The intensive care of the stroke patient. In: Barnett HJ, Mohr JP, Stein BM, eds. *Stroke: Pathophysiology, Diagnosis and Management.* 3rd ed. New York: Churchill Livingstone; 1998; and Sacco RL, Adams R, Albers G, et al. Guidelines for prevention of stroke in patients with ischemic stroke or transient ischemic attack: a statement for healthcare professionals from the American Heart Association/American Stroke Association Council on Stroke: co-sponsored by the Council on Cardiovascular Radiology and Intervention: the American Academy of Neurology affirms the value of this guideline. *Stroke.* 2006;37(2):577–617.

hemorrhagic side effects. Dabigatran 150 mg twice daily, compared with warfarin, was associated with lower rates of stroke and systemic embolism, but with similar rates of major hemorrhage.[125] Dabigatran is primarily cleared by the kidney. Patients with a creatinine clearance (CrCl) of 15 to 30 mL/min should receive a dose of 75 mg twice daily. Patients with CrCl <15 mL/min or on dialysis should not be given dabigatran. The direct factor Xa inhibitors are rivaroxaban, apixaban, and edoxaban. Rivaroxaban has been shown to be noninferior to warfarin for the prevention of stroke.[126] In patients with a CrCl >50 mL/min, a dose of 20 mg once daily is given, while patients with a CrCl of 15 to 50 mL/min are given a reduced dose of 15 mg once daily. Apixaban, had similar risk of ischemic stroke when compared to warfarin, but was found to have a significant reduction in the risk of intracranial hemorrhage and major bleeding.[127] Apixaban is recommended at a dose of 5 mg twice daily, but reduced oral dose of 2.5 mg twice daily is given to patients in whom two of the three following criteria are met: age ≥80 years, weight ≤60 kg, or serum creatinine ≥1.5 mg/dL. Apixaban has been given a class 1, level A evidence classification from the AHA/ASA guidelines as it appears to have a good combination of safety and efficacy.[128]

Heparin or LMWH in AIS are associated with increased risk of bleeding complications and symptomatic hemorrhagic transformation. Although antiplatelet agents were shown to be useful for preventing recurrent stroke or stroke after TIA, their use should be regarded as a preventive measure, not an acute stroke treatment.[26]

The International Stroke Trial (IST) and the Chinese Acute Stroke Trial (CAST) demonstrated that the use of aspirin started within 48 hours of stroke results in a 1% absolute reduction in risk of stroke and death over the first 2 weeks after stroke.[129,130] Early aspirin therapy is therefore recommended within 48 hours of the onset of symptoms, but should be delayed for at least 24 hours after recombinant tPA administration. Aspirin should not be considered as an alternative to IV thrombolysis or other therapies aimed at improving outcomes after stroke.[9]

Other antiplatelet agents were evaluated for use in the acute phase of ischemic stroke. The platelet glycoprotein IIb/IIIa inhibitors were evaluated in the treatment of AIS because they may increase the rate of spontaneous recanalization and improve microvascular patency.[131] The Abciximab in Emergent Stroke Treatment Trial (AbESTT) was a randomized double-blinded placebo-controlled phase IIb study that involved 400 patients with AIS who were treated 3 to 6 hours after symptom onset.[132] Results demonstrated significant improvements in outcomes of abciximab-treated patients, measured by mRS, Barthel Index, and NIHSS.[133] A subsequent phase III trial evaluating the safety and efficacy of abciximab in patients with AIS was halted because of an increased rate of bleeding and lack of efficacy.[132] The use of ticlopidine, clopidogrel, or dipyridamole in the setting of AIS has not been evaluated.

Viscosity and Hemodilution

AIS patients have a variety of abnormalities that may increase blood viscosity. Accordingly, hemodilution could improve CBF to hyperperfuse potentially viable brain tissue supplied by leptomeningeal collaterals in an attempt to salvage the ischemic penumbra.[134] In all trials, and in the Multicenter Austrian Hemodilution Stroke Trial study in particular, hemodilution did not reduce deaths within the first 4 weeks.[135] Hemodilution also had no significant influence on death, dependency, or institutionalization/long-term care. In several trials, hemodilution was associated with a tendency toward reduction in DVT and pulmonary embolism (PE) at 3 to 6 months. Despite volume expansion and hemodilution, the risk of significant cardiac events did not increase.[9] Maintenance of a normal circulating blood volume with regulation of metabolic parameters within physiological ranges is desirable.[9]

SECONDARY PREVENTION OF ISCHEMIC STROKE

Secondary stroke prevention includes measures that prevent stroke in patients with TIAs and treatments that prevent recurrent stroke in patients who have had an ischemic stroke. A TIA is defined as a transient episode of neurological dysfunction caused by focal ischemia, initially lasting up to 24 hours but now modified to 1 hour in duration.[136] The overall risk for stroke after a TIA is approximately 10% over the subsequent 90 days, with the greatest risk within the first week after the event.[137] Patients with a transient focal neurological deficit lasting less than 24 hours who have an ischemic lesion on DWI have higher risk for subsequent stroke than those who do not have this MRI abnormality, especially if they have evidence of vessel narrowing on MRA.[138] This substantial stroke risk with TIA is why TIA should be considered a medical emergency and requires urgent evaluation and treatment.[139] The history, physical, and laboratory examinations should help exclude less frequent causes of transient focal neurological symptoms, such as pressure-related or positionally related peripheral nerve or nerve root compression, peripheral vestibulopathy, and metabolic abnormalities (also see Chapter 29). The initial evaluation should also exclude other possible causes of focal neurological symptoms such as seizures, migraine auras, and syncope.[140]

Patients who have had a TIA should have an evaluation that includes basic blood work studies (e.g., electrolytes, glucose, complete blood cell count [CBC]), an electrocardiogram, brain imaging, and neurovascular imaging. Brain imaging can be performed with either CT or MRI scans, although the latter is preferable because DWI can detect abnormalities not seen on CT scans that can predict a higher risk of subsequent stroke. In the past, carotid ultrasound was the initial study employed to evaluate the carotid arteries. Currently, both CT and contrast-enhanced MRA have distinct advantages over carotid ultrasound. Both of these imaging modalities accurately image the vessels in the neck and brain, providing information about the occlusive status in both locations, as well as the presence of an occult aneurysm or vascular malformation. The accuracy of both CT and contrast-enhanced MRA allow for their use in planning a procedure such as carotid endarterectomy (CEA) or carotid artery stenting (CAS). In rare cases, digital subtraction angiography (DSA) may be needed. If a cardiac source for the TIA is a consideration, echocardiography and electrocardiographic monitoring should be performed.

Treatment decisions should be made rapidly in TIA patients after information from the workup has been obtained. Evaluation and treatment of TIA patients can be performed in the hospital or an urgent-access outpatient clinic. Urgent-access TIA evaluation clinics were shown to substantially reduce the incidence of subsequent stroke, and highlight the appropriateness of considering TIA a medical emergency.[141] The basic consideration for deciding upon the treatment for a TIA patient is whether a procedure, such as CEA or carotid stenting, is appropriate, or whether the patient should be treated with medical therapy alone (also see Chapter 31). Carotid artery procedures are not appropriate for patients with TIA symptoms in the posterior circulation; such patients should receive appropriate medical therapy. For patients with anterior circulation TIA symptoms, the degree of carotid stenosis is the primary factor for deciding whether a procedure is needed. For symptomatic patients with greater than 70% stenosis of the proximal internal carotid artery (ICA), the North American Symptomatic Carotid Endarterectomy Trial (NASCET) demonstrated clear evidence that CEA was superior to medical therapy, and this procedure is recommended for most such patients.[142] For patients with 50% to 70% carotid artery stenosis, an extension of this trial demonstrated significant benefit of CEA for men but not for women overall, which is likely related to the lower subsequent stroke risk in women.[143]

In women with 50% to 70% stenosis and a TIA, high-risk subgroups were shown to have significant benefit. Patients with less than 50% stenosis were not shown to benefit from CEA. In the NASCET trial, the degree of carotid artery stenosis was confirmed by DSA. Currently, this invasive procedure is performed infrequently, and decisions about the percentage of stenosis can be reliably made by CTA or contrast MRA.

Another procedure for treating carotid artery stenosis is carotid stenting (see Chapter 31). The benefits and side effects of CAS and CEA were compared directly in the Carotid Revascularization Endarterectomy versus Stenting Trial (CREST). No significant difference between the two procedures on the primary outcome measure of stroke, death, or nonfatal MI was observed.[144] However, the risk of periprocedural stroke was significantly lower in the CEA group, and the risk of MI was significantly lower in the stenting group. A relationship between age and the effects of treatment was observed, with patients younger than 60 years of age benefiting more from stenting, and those older than 70 doing better with CEA. The CREST trial included more asymptomatic patients with carotid stenosis than TIA patients, so generalizing the results to TIA patients is problematic. In choosing which procedure to recommend to patients, the clinician must be aware of complication rates of the operators who will be doing the procedure, the aortic arch anatomy, and the level of carotid artery bifurcation. It is our practice to recommend CEA to most patients and to reserve the use of stenting for high-risk patients, such as those with radiation-induced stenosis and after a failed prior CEA (see Chapter 31).

Risk factor modification and antiplatelet therapy for patients who have had a TIA or ischemic stroke is indicated. Underlying risk factors should be managed as in poststroke patients. Patients should be started on an antiplatelet agent; choices include aspirin, clopidogrel, or extended-release dipyridamole/low-dose aspirin. Low-dose aspirin (50 to 81 mg) is usually recommended as the initial approach. In patients who have a TIA on aspirin, one of the other antiplatelet drugs may be substituted, or they may be used initially in high-risk patients with multiple vascular risk factors. The combination of extended-release dipyridamole/low-dose aspirin was shown to be superior to aspirin in two large clinical trials, but when this combination was compared to clopidogrel, no significant difference in subsequent stroke outcome was observed.[145,146] The combination therapy group had a significantly greater risk for major bleeding side effects and drug discontinuation because of headaches. Clopidogrel, which is an irreversible inhibitor of the $P2Y_{12}$ subtype of the adenosine diphosphate receptor and inhibits platelet aggregation, has also attained recent widespread usage. The clopidogrel versus aspirin in patients at Risk of Ischemic Events (CAPRIE) trial demonstrated that in patients with atherosclerotic vascular disease, clopidogrel is more effective than aspirin in reducing the combined risk of ischemic stroke, MI, or vascular death.[147] However, the effect was mostly driven by a decreased rate of complications in peripheral artery disease patients. The MATCH trial (Management of ATherothrombosis with Clopidogrel in High-risk patients) showed that aspirin and clopidogrel combination treatment is no more effective than clopidogrel alone in high-risk patients with recent ischemic stroke/TIA.[148] The risk of major and minor hemorrhage was significantly increased in the dual antiplatelet group. Similarly, the effects of aspirin plus clopidogrel versus aspirin alone was evaluated in the CHARISMA trial (Clopidogrel for High Atherothrombotic Risk and Ischemic Stabilization, Management, and Avoidance) and there was no benefit of dual antiplatelet therapy over aspirin alone, although there was a suggestion of benefit with clopidogrel treatment in patients with previously symptomatic atherothrombosis.[149] The CHANCE (Clopidogrel in High-Risk Patients with Acute Nondisabling Cerebrovascular Events) trial showed superiority of combination therapy of aspirin and clopidogrel for 90 days compared to aspirin monotherapy in patients

with TIA or minor stroke.[150] However, the trial was done in the Chinese population where the predominant mechanism of stroke is intracranial atherosclerosis, and it has been established that dual antiplatelet therapy is beneficial in patients with intracranial atherosclerosis.[151] In addition, patients should be treated with statins to reduce low-density lipoprotein (LDL) cholesterol.[152,153]

Antihypertensive therapy is indicated to prevent recurrent stroke. A meta-analysis of 15,257 patients with previous stroke or TIA demonstrated that antihypertensive therapy with a variety of agents (β-adrenergic blockers, diuretics, angiotensin-converting enzyme [ACE] inhibitors) resulted in a 24% reduction in recurrent stroke.[154] In the Morbidity and Mortality After Stroke, Eprosartan Compared with Nitrendipine for Secondary Prevention (MOSES) study, 1405 subjects with a stroke or TIA and hypertension were randomized to the angiotensin receptor blocker (ARB) eprosartan, or the calcium channel blocker nitrendipine. Despite similar reductions in BP, total strokes and TIAs were reduced by 25% among those randomized to eprosartan. It should be noted that the reduction in TIAs accounted for most of the cerebrovascular benefit, with no significant difference in ischemic strokes noted.[155] In the Perindopril Protection Against Recurrent Stroke (PROGRESS) Study of 6105 subjects with a history of stroke or TIA, those randomized to perindopril had a significant reduction in recurrent stroke.[156] In this trial, the thiazide diuretic indapamide could be used at the discretion of the treating physician. Patients treated with the combination of perindopril and indapamide had the greatest stroke reduction (43%). Interestingly, in the Prevention Regimen for Effectively Avoiding Second Strokes (PRoFESS) study of 20,332 patients with ischemic stroke, telmisartan did not significantly reduce the rate of stroke compared to placebo.[157] The negative findings have been ascribed to aggressive antihypertensive management in the placebo group and a minimal difference in BP between groups.

Until the advent of the statin era, the impact of lipids on cerebrovascular disease was thought to be modest, with reductions in ischemic stroke offset by increases in hemorrhagic stroke with decreasing levels of LDL. In the Stroke Prevention by Aggressive Reduction in Cholesterol Levels (SPARCL) study, 4731 patients with stroke or TIA and LDL-cholesterol levels between 100 and 190 mg/dL were randomized to atorvastatin 80 mg or placebo.[158] Over 5 years of follow-up, there was a 16% risk reduction of recurrent stroke. The trial was positive, despite only a 78% adherence to trial-allocated therapies by the end of the trial. In a post hoc analysis of SPARCL, patients with the greatest reduction in LDL also enjoyed the most impressive stroke reduction.[153] Patients with a 50% or greater reduction in LDL saw a 31% reduction in stroke risk and a 33% decrease in ischemic stroke.

PRIMARY PREVENTION OF ISCHEMIC STROKE

The effect of risk factor modification in asymptomatic carotid disease has yet to be studied directly. The AHA/ASA guidelines for the primary prevention of stroke suggest aggressive risk-factor modification, as recommended for coronary heart disease (CHD), CHD risk equivalents, and diabetes mellitus.[159]

The management of patients with asymptomatic carotid stenosis is controversial. Two large earlier randomized trials that compared CEA to medical therapy in patients with more than 60% stenosis demonstrated a significant reduction in stroke occurrence with CEA. The absolute risk reduction was about 1% per year.[160,161] With the improvement in medical management of patients with asymptomatic carotid stenosis, it has been suggested that in many cases the previously confirmed benefit for CEA may no longer be applicable.[162] It may be possible to identify higher- and lower-risk asymptomatic carotid stenosis patients based on a more sophisticated ultrasound evaluation of plaque characteristics and/or the detection of intracranial emboli on a transcranial Doppler (TCD) ultrasound study.[163] Based on results of the CREST trial, both CEA and carotid stenting could be considered if a procedure is deemed appropriate for an individual patient. The recent ACT1 (Asymptomatic Carotid Trial) showed that stenting was noninferior to CEA in asymptomatic patients with severe carotid stenosis who were not at high risk for surgical complications.[164] The acceptable rate of periprocedural complications in asymptomatic patients undergoing a procedure is usually considered lower than for symptomatic patients because of the lower stroke risk in asymptomatic patients. The CREST-2 trial comparing both stenting and CEA to aggressive medical therapy in patients with high-grade asymptomatic carotid stenosis is ongoing.

Management of Primary Intracerebral Hemorrhage

Extravasation of blood into the brain occurs when blood vessels within the parenchyma rupture, leading to the development of ICH. Hypertension and cerebral amyloid angiopathy, particularly in older patients, are the most common causes of spontaneous ICH. ICH can also occur with the use of oral or IV anticoagulants and is then termed *secondary to anticoagulant use*, although in many cases, blood vessel rupture is also the likely cause. ICH accounts for 10% to 15% of the acute cerebrovascular events and is more common among Asians, African Americans, and Latin Americans than the US Caucasian population.[165] The pathophysiology of tissue injury is distinctly different than that observed with ischemic stroke. The developing hematoma not only causes local cellular injury by direct mechanical effects, but also may secondarily induce cellular injury due to toxic and inflammatory effects of hemoglobin degradation products, edema development, mitochondrial dysfunction, and neurotransmitter release.[166] It is well established that the majority of ICH patients experience hematoma enlargement during the first few hours after onset, and that ICH growth is associated with a poorer prognosis (Fig. 30.4).[167] Imaging with CT/CTA or MRI/MRA can readily illustrate the presence of ICH,

distinguish this condition from ischemic stroke, and identify the cause of ICH.[168] In ICH cases of undetermined etiology, additional imaging with catheter angiography and/or CT/MR venography should be performed to look for the presence of an underlying arteriovenous malformation (AVM), aneurysm, or dural venous thrombosis.

Initial management of ICH includes airway assessment, BP control, reversal of coagulopathy (if present), and treatment of elevated ICP if warranted. ICH patients should be managed in an intensive care unit or specialized stroke care unit. Patients with respiratory compromise or at high risk for aspiration may require intubation. Many ICH patients have elevated BP initially, and this may associate with hematoma expansion. The precise BP target in ICH patients remains uncertain. A phase III, randomized, placebo-controlled trial investigating the safety and efficacy of early intensive BP lowering after ICH in 2839 patients found that intensive lowering of SBP to <140 mm Hg compared to a target SBP <180 mm Hg was safe and associated with a modest reduction in disability at 90 days.[169] However, a similar trial in 1000 patients, intensive SBP lowering to 110 to 139 mm Hg versus 140 to 179 mm Hg did not result in improved functional outcome or reduced mortality after ICH.[170] Furthermore, the rate of renal adverse events, including renal failure, was significantly higher in the intensive-treatment group. Therefore, lowering SBP to 140 mm Hg may be reasonable based on the latest AHA/ASA guidelines for the management of ICH.[171] Many antihypertensive agents are used (see Table 30.6).[172] The optimal approach for treating elevated ICP in ICH patients remains contentious. Osmotic agents such as mannitol or hypertonic saline are widely used in ICH patients, but clear evidence of efficacy remains lacking.[173] Mannitol may induce hypovolemia and a hyperosmotic state, so when it is used, serum osmolality should be monitored regularly and maintained in the range of 300 to 320 mOsm/kg. The use of steroids to decrease brain swelling or ICP after ICH should be avoided because these agents increase infection risk without other benefit.[174] If the ICH patient is febrile, their temperature should be lowered with parenteral acetaminophen to normothermia. It is unclear whether induction of hypothermia is beneficial. Similarly, hyperglycemia should be avoided, and insulin sliding scale should be used to maintain euglycemia. If

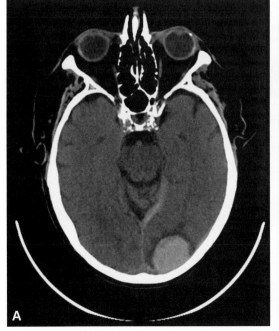
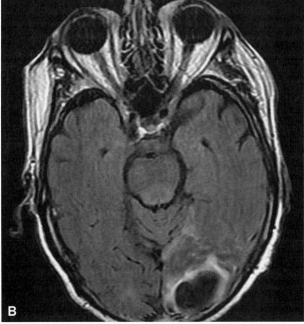

Fig. 30.4 (A) Acute intracerebral hemorrhage in the left occipital lobe on computed tomography scan. (B) Same hemorrhage on T1-weighted magnetic resonance imaging. (Courtesy Dr. Magdy Selim.)

clinical seizures occur, an anticonvulsant should be initiated, but anticonvulsant prophylaxis may be avoided.[171] Most ICH patients will be immobilized for a period of time and are at risk for developing DVT and PE. Intermittent pneumatic compression should be initiated at admission, and subcutaneous LMWH or UFH may be started days later if the patient remains immobilized and if imaging supports the stability of ICH.[175] Gastric ulceration is common in ICH patients. Prophylaxis is often warranted before the initiation of feeding; and prophylaxis with H2 blockers may be preferred over proton pump inhibitors, which have been associated with an increased incidence of pneumonia in some studies.

Approximately 20% of ICH patients are receiving an oral anticoagulant at the time of ICH onset. Anticoagulation is associated with a poorer prognosis than in patients who are not receiving such treatment.[176–178] Early reversal of the anticoagulant effect should be initiated, and several options are available. Patients with warfarin-related ICH should (1) have their warfarin withheld, (2) receive therapy to replace vitamin K–dependent factors and correct the INR, and (3) receive IV vitamin K.[171] Either fresh frozen plasma (FFP) or prothrombin complex concentrates (PCCs) can be used to replenish all vitamin K-dependent factors. However, FFP may take a long time to reverse the anticoagulant effect, and the large fluid load associated with its use may be problematic in cardiac patients. Because PCCs may have fewer complications and correct the INR more rapidly than FFP, they might be considered over FFP. Neither FFP nor PCCs have been shown to improve outcomes after warfarin-related ICH. The use of recombinant activated factor VII (rFVIIa) is not indicated in warfarin-related ICH because it does not replenish all clotting factors and clotting may not be restored in vivo. The monoclonal antibody, idarucizumab, should be used for reversal of coagulopathy in dabigatran-related ICH.[179] The first factor Xa inhibitor, andexanet alfa, has been recently FDA approved for reversal of apixaban and rivaroxaban. Until then, potential reversal strategies include the use of activated charcoal, PCCs, or factor eight inhibitor bypassing activity (FEIBA).

No specific therapy directed at the underlying pathophysiology of ICH-induced injury is available, although several trials targeting the secondary injury caused by the blood and its degradation products are currently underway or in planning. Since the appreciation of the role of hematoma expansion as a predictor of worse outcome, treatment directed at reducing this mechanism of injury was proposed. rFVIIa in nonanticoagulated ICH patients was tested in two clinical trials. In the phase II trial, three doses of rFVIIa (40, 80, or 160 µg/kg) or vehicle were given to ICH patients within 3 hours of onset.[180] Hematoma expansion was reduced, as was mortality with rFVIIa. In a phase III trial that used 20 or 80 µg/kg of rFVIIa compared to vehicle,[181] hematoma expansion was again reduced with both rFVIIa doses, but no clinical benefit was observed. The 80 µg/kg dose had an increased risk of thrombotic events when compared to vehicle. A recent small study using CTA to select patients at risk for hematoma expansion also did not show a benefit from using rFVIIa.

Surgical evacuation of the hematoma has an inherent appeal for the treatment of ICH, but aside from cerebellar hemorrhages, it remains of unproven value.[182] Many randomized trials comparing surgical evacuation of ICH to medical therapy were performed and failed to show a benefit. The use of minimally invasive endoscopic techniques for hematoma evacuation or hemicraniectomy in patients at risk for herniation to improve outcomes is promising. These alternatives are currently being examined in randomized, controlled trials. Early surgical evacuation is recommended for larger cerebellar hemorrhages, especially if neurological deterioration occurs or hydrocephalus is developing.

REFERENCES

1. Hossman KA. Pathophysiology and therapy of experimental stroke. *Cell Mol Neurobiol.* 2006;26:1055–1081.
2. Baron J. Mapping the ischaemic penumbra with PET: implications for acute stroke treatment. *Cerebrovasc Dis.* 1999;9:193–201.
3. Fisher M. The ischemic penumbra: a new opportunity for neuroprotection. *Cerebrovasc Dis.* 2006;21(Suppl 2):64–70.
4. Heiss W. Ischemic penumbra: evidence from functional imaging in man. *J Cereb Blood Flow Metab.* 2000;20:1276–1293.
5. Fisher M. Characterizing the target of acute stroke treatment. *Stroke.* 1997;28:866–872.
6. Bang OY, Saver JL, Buck BH, et al. Impact of collateral flow on tissue fate in acute ischaemic stroke. *J Neurol Neurosurg Psychiatry.* 2008;79:625–629.
7. Goyal M, Menon BK, van Zwam WH, et al. Endovascular thrombectomy after large-vessel ischaemic stroke: a meta-analysis of individual patient data from five randomised trials. *Lancet.* 2016;387:1723–1731.
8. Martini SR, Kent TA. Hyperglycemia in acute ischemic stroke: a vascular perspective. *J Cereb Blood Flow Metab.* 2007;27:435–451.
9. Ntaios G, Bath P, Michel P. Blood pressure treatment in acute ischemic stroke: a review of studies and recommendations. *Curr Opin Neurol.* 2010;23:46–52.
10. Adams Jr HP, del Zoppo G, Alberts MJ, et al. Guidelines for the early management of adults with ischemic stroke: a guideline from the American Heart Association/American Stroke Association Stroke Council, Clinical Cardiology Council, Cardiovascular Radiology and Intervention Council, and the Atherosclerotic Peripheral Vascular Disease and Quality of Care Outcomes in Research Interdisciplinary Working Groups: the American Academy of Neurology affirms the value of this guideline as an educational tool for neurologists. *Stroke.* 2007;38:1655–1711.
11. Handschu R, Poppe R, Rauss J, et al. Emergency calls in acute stroke. *Stroke.* 2003;34:1005–1009.
12. Williams JE, Rosamond WD, Morris DL. Stroke symptom attribution and time to emergency department arrival: the delay in accessing stroke healthcare study. *Acad Emerg Med.* 2000;7:93–96.
13. Zweifler RM, Mendizabal JE, Cunningham S, et al. Hospital presentation after stroke in a community sample: the Mobile Stroke Project. *South Med J.* 2002;95:1263–1268.
14. Lacy CR, Suh DC, Bueno M, et al. Delay in presentation and evaluation for acute stroke: Stroke Time Registry for Outcomes Knowledge and Epidemiology (S.T.R.O.K.E.). *Stroke.* 2001;32:63–69.
15. De Luca A, Toni D, Lauria L, et al. An emergency clinical pathway for stroke patients – results of a cluster randomised trial (isrctn41456865). *BMC Health Serv Res.* 2009;9:14.
16. Schroeder EB, Rosamond WD, Morris DL, et al. Determinants of use of emergency medical services in a population with stroke symptoms: the Second Delay in Accessing Stroke Healthcare (DASH II) Study. *Stroke.* 2000;31:2591–2596.
17. Morris DL, Rosamond WD, Hinn AR, et al. Time delays in accessing stroke care in the emergency department. *Acad Emerg Med.* 1999;6:218–223.
18. Menon SC, Pandey DK, Morgenstern LB. Critical factors determining access to acute stroke care. *Neurology.* 1998;51:427–432.
19. Barsan WG, Brott TG, Broderick JP, et al. Time of hospital presentation in patients with acute stroke. *Arch Intern Med.* 1993;153:2558–2561.
20. Wester P, Rådberg J, Lundgren B, Peltonen M. Factors associated with delayed admission to hospital and in-hospital delays in acute stroke and TIA: a prospective, multicenter study. *Stroke.* 1999;30:40–48.
21. Committee ECC. Subcommittees and Task Forces of the American Heart Association: American Heart Association Guidelines for Cardiopulmonary Resuscitation and Emergency Cardiovascular Care. *Circulation.* 2005;112(24 Suppl):IV1–IV203.
22. Goyal M, Wilson AT, Kamal N, et al. Amartya Sen and the organization of endovascular stroke treatment. *Stroke.* 2017;48:2310–2312.
23. Schwamm L, Fayad P, Acker 3rd JE, et al. Translating evidence into practice: a decade of efforts by the American Heart Association/American

Stroke Association to reduce death and disability due to stroke: a presidential advisory from the American Heart Association/American Stroke Association. *Stroke*. 2010;41:1051–1065.

24. Lindsay P, Bayley M, Hellings C, et al. (Canadian Stroke Strategy Best Practices and Standards Writing Group, on behalf of the Canadian Stroke Strategy, a joint initiative of the Canadian Stroke Network and the Heart and Stroke Foundation of Canada*): Canadian best practice recommendations for stroke care (updated 2008). *CMAJ*. 2008;179(12 Suppl):S1–S25.

25. Morgenstern LB, Bartholomew LK, Grotta JC, et al. Sustained benefit of a community and professional intervention to increase acute stroke therapy. *Arch Intern Med*. 2003;163:2198–2202.

26. Morgenstern LB, Staub L, Chan W, et al. Improving delivery of acute stroke therapy: the TLL Temple Foundation Stroke Project. *Stroke*. 2002;33:160–166.

27. Evenson KR, Foraker R, Morris DL, Rosamond WD. A comprehensive review of prehospital and in-hospital delay times in acute stroke care. *Int J Stroke*. 2009;4:187–199.

28. Becker JU, Wira CR, Arnold JL. *Stroke, ischemic eMedicine Specialties Emergency Medicine*. June 4, 2010. Neurology.

29. Krieger D, Hacke W. The intensive care of the stroke patient. In: Barnett HJ, Mohr JP, Stein BM, eds. *Stroke: Pathophysiology, Diagnosis and Management*. ed 3. New York: Churchill Livingstone; 1998.

30. Albers GW, Diener HC, Frison L, et al. Ximelagatran vs. warfarin for stroke prevention in patients with nonvalvular atrial fibrillation: a randomized trial. *JAMA*. 2005;293:690–698.

31. Oppenheimer SM, Hachinski VC. The cardiac consequences of stroke. *Neurol Clin*. 1992;10(1):167–176.

32. Kolin A, Norris JW. Myocardial damage from acute cerebral lesions. *Stroke*. 1984;15:990–993.

33. Milhaud D, Popp J, Thouvenot E, et al. Mechanical ventilation in ischemic stroke. *J Stroke Cerebrovasc Dis*. 2004;13:183–188.

34. Treib J, Grauer MT, Woessner R, Morgenthaler M. Treatment of stroke on an intensive stroke unit: a novel concept. *Intensive Care Med*. 2000;26:1598–1611.

35. National Institute of Neurological Disorders and Stroke rt-PA Stroke Study Group. Tissue plasminogen activator for acute ischemic stroke. *N Engl J Med*. 1995;333:1581–1587.

36. The National Institute of Neurological Disorders and Stroke rt-PA Stroke Study Group. Generalized efficacy of t-PA for acute stroke: subgroup analysis of the NINDS t-PA Stroke Trial. *Stroke*. 1997;28:2119–2125.

37. Hacke W, Kaste M, Fieschi C, et al. Intravenous thrombolysis with recombinant tissue plasminogen activator for acute hemispheric stroke. The European Cooperative Acute Stroke Study (ECASS). *JAMA*. 1995;274:1017–1025.

38. Hacke W, Kaste M, Fieschi C, et al. Randomised double-blind placebo-controlled trial of thrombolytic therapy with intravenous alteplase in acute ischaemic stroke (ECASS II). Second European-Australasian Acute Stroke Study Investigators. *Lancet*. 1998;352:1245–1251.

39. Clark WM, Wissman S, Albers GW, et al. Recombinant tissue type plasminogen activator (alteplase) for ischemic stroke 3 to 5 hours after symptom onset. The ATLANTIS Study: a randomized controlled trial, Alteplase Thrombolysis for Acute Noninterventional Therapy in Ischemic Stroke. *JAMA*. 1999;282:2019–2026.

40. Hacke W, Donnan G, Fieschi C, et al. Association of outcome with early stroke treatment: pooled analysis of ATLANTIS, ECASS, and NINDS rt-PA stroke trials. *Lancet*. 2004;363:768–774.

41. Hacke W, Kaste M, Bluhrnki E, et al. Thrombolysis with alteplase 3 to 4.5 hours after acute ischemic stroke. *N Engl J Med*. 2008;359:1317–1329.

42. Del Zoppo GJ, Saver JL, Jauch EC, et al. Expansion of the time window for treatment of acute ischemic stroke with intravenous tissue plasminogen activator: a science advisory from the American Heart Association/American Stroke Association. *Stroke*. 2009;40:2945–2948.

43. Bluhmki E, Chamorro A, Dávalos A, et al. Stroke treatment with alteplase given 3.0–4.5 h after onset of ischaemic stroke (ECASS III): additional outcomes and subgroup analysis of a randomised controlled trial. *Lancet Neurol*. 2009;8:1095–1102.

44. Anderson C, Robinson T, Lindley RI, et al. Low-dose versus standard-dose intravenous alteplase in acute ischemic stroke. *N Engl J Med*. 2016;374:2313–2323.

45. Robinson TG, Wang X, Arima H, et al. Low-versus standard dose alteplase in patients on prior antiplatelet therapy: the ENCHANTED Trial (Enhanced Control of Hypertension and Thrombolysis Stroke Study). *Stroke*. 2017;48:1877–1883.

46. Parsons M, Spratt N, Bivard A, et al. A randomized trial of tenecteplase versus alteplase for acute ischemic stroke. *N Engl J Med*. 2012;366:1099–1107.

47. Logallo N, Novotny V, Assmus J, et al. Tenecteplase versus alteplase for management of acute ischaemic stroke (NOR-TEST): a phase 3, randomised, open-label, blinded endpoint trial. *Lancet Neurol*. 2017;16:781–788.

48. Albers GW, von Kummer R, Truelsen T, et al. Safety and efficacy of desmoteplase given 3–9 h after ischaemic stroke in patients with occlusion or high-grade stenosis in major cerebral arteries (DIAS-3): a double-blind, randomised, placebo-controlled phase 3 trial. *Lancet Neurol*. 2015;14:575–584.

49. von Kummer R, Mori E, Truelsen T, et al. Desmoteplase 3 to 9 hours after major artery occlusion stroke: the DIAS-4 Trial (Efficacy and Safety Study of Desmoteplase to Treat Acute Ischemic Stroke). *Stroke*. 2016;47:2880–2887.

50. Broderick JP, Palesch YY, Demchuk AM, et al. Endovascular therapy after intravenous t-PA versus t-PA alone for stroke. *N Engl J Med*. 2013;368:893–903.

51. Ciccone A, Valvassori L, Nichelatti M, et al. Endovascular treatment for acute ischemic stroke. *N Engl J Med*. 2013;368:904–913.

52. Kidwell CS, Jahan R, Gornbein J, et al. A trial of imaging selection and endovascular treatment for ischemic stroke. *N Engl J Med*. 2013;368:914–923.

53. Berkhemer OA, Fransen PS, Beumer D, et al. A randomized trial of intraarterial treatment for acute ischemic stroke. *N Engl J Med*. 2015;372:11–20.

54. Campbell BC, Mitchell PJ, Kleinig TJ, et al. Endovascular therapy for ischemic stroke with perfusion-imaging selection. *N Engl J Med*. 2015;372:1009–1018.

55. Goyal M, Demchuk AM, Menon BK, et al. Randomized assessment of rapid endovascular treatment of ischemic stroke. *N Engl J Med*. 2015;372:1019–1030.

56. Saver JL, Goyal M, Bonafe A, et al. Stent-retriever thrombectomy after intravenous t-PA vs. t-PA alone in stroke. *N Engl J Med*. 2015;372:2285–2295.

57. Jovin TG, Chamorro A, Cobo E, et al. Thrombectomy within 8 hours after symptom onset in ischemic stroke. *N Engl J Med*. 2015;372:2296–2306.

58. Powers WJ, Derdeyn CP, Biller J, et al. AHA/ASA focused update of the 2013 guidelines for the early management of patients with acute ischemic stroke regarding endovascular treatment. *Stroke*. 2015;2015. http://stroke.ahajournals.org/content/early/2015/06/26/STR.0000000000000074.abstract. Accessed April 19, 2018.

59. Nogueira RG, Jadhav AP, Haussen DC, et al. Thrombectomy 6 to 24 hours after stroke with a mismatch between deficit and infarct. *N Engl J Med*. 2018;378:11–21.

60. Indredavik B, Bakke F, Slordahl SA, et al. Treatment in a combined acute and rehabilitation stroke unit: which aspects are most important? *Stroke*. 1999;30:917–923.

61. Gilligan AK, Thrift AG, Sturm JW, et al. Stroke units, tissue plasminogen activator, aspirin and neuroprotection: which stroke intervention could provide the greatest community benefit? *Cerebrovasc Dis*. 2005;20:239–244.

62. Cadilhac DA, Ibrahim J, Pearce DC, et al. Multicenter comparison of processes of care between stroke units and conventional care wards in Australia. *Stroke*. 2004;35:1035–1040.

63. Schwamm LH, Fonarow GC, Reeves MJ, et al. Get with the guidelines—stroke is associated with sustained improvement in care for patients with stroke or transient ischemic attack. *Circulation*. 2009;119:107–115.

64. Schabitz WR, Fisher M. Perspectives on neuroprotective stroke therapy. *Biochem Soc Trans*. 2006;34:1271–1276.

65. Donnan GA. A new road map for neuroprotection. *Stroke*. 2008;39: 242–248.

66. O'Collins VE, Macleod MR, Donnan GA, et al. 1,026 experimental treatments in acute stroke. *Ann Neurol*. 2006;59:467–477.

67. Gladstone DJ, Black SE, Hakim AM. Toward wisdom from failure: lessons from neuroprotective stroke trials and new directions. *Stroke*. 2002;33:2123–2136.

68. Savitz SI, Baron JC, Yenari M, et al. Reconsidering neuroprotection in the reperfusion era. *Stroke*. 2017;48:3413–3419.

69. Henninger N, Bratane BT, Bastan B, et al. Normobaric hyperoxia and delayed tPA treatment in a rat embolic stroke model. *J Cereb Blood Flow Metab*. 2009;29:119–129.

70. Bråtane B, Bouley J, Schneider A, et al. Granulocyte-colony stimulating factor delays PWI/DWI mismatch evolution and reduces final infarct volume in permanent-suture and embolic focal cerebral ischemia models in the rat. *Stroke*. 2009;40:3102–3106.

71. Warach SW, Latour LL. Evidence of reperfusion injury, exacerbated by thrombolytic therapy, in human focal brain ischemia using a novel imaging marker of early blood–brain barrier disruption. *Stroke*. 2004;35:2559–2661.

72. Fisher M. New approaches to neuroprotective drug development. *Stroke*. 2012;42:S24–S27.

73. Williams LS, Rotich J, Qi R, et al. Effects of admission hyperglycemia on mortality and costs in acute ischemic stroke. *Neurology*. 2002;59:67–71.

74. Scott JF, Robinson GM, French JM, et al. Prevalence of admission hyperglycaemia across clinical subtypes of acute stroke. *Lancet*. 1999;353:376–377.

75. Baird TA, Parsons MW, Barber PA, et al. The influence of diabetes mellitus and hyperglycaemia on stroke incidence and outcome. *J Clin Neurosci*. 2002;9:618–626.

76. Baird TA, Parsons MW, Phanh T, et al. Persistent poststroke hyperglycemia is independently associated with infarct expansion and worse clinical outcome. *Stroke*. 2003;34:2208–2214.

77. Poppe AY, Majumdar SR, Jeerakathil T, et al. Admission hyperglycemia predicts a worse outcome in stroke patients treated with intravenous thrombolysis. *Diabetes Care*. 2009;32:617–622.

78. Bruno A, Levine SR, Frankel MR, et al. Admission glucose level and clinical outcomes in the NINDS rt-PA Stroke Trial. *Neurology*. 2002;59:669–674.

79. Bruno A, Biller J, Adams Jr HP, et al. Acute blood glucose level and outcome from ischemic stroke. Trial of ORG 10172 in Acute Stroke Treatment (TOAST) Investigators. *Neurology*. 1999;52:280–284.

80. Toni D, Chamorro A, Kaste M, et al. Acute treatment of ischaemic stroke. European Stroke Initiative. *Cerebrovasc Dis*. 2004;17(Suppl 2):30–46.

81. Bruno A, Kent TA, Coull BM, et al. Treatment of hyperglycemia in ischemic stroke (THIS): a randomized pilot trial. *Stroke*. 2008;39:384–389.

82. Azzimondi G, Bassein L, Nonino F, et al. Fever in acute stroke worsens prognosis. A prospective study. *Stroke*. 1995;26:2040–2043.

83. Castillo J, Dávalos A, Marrugat J, Noya M. Timing for fever-related brain damage in acute ischemic stroke. *Stroke*. 1998;29:2455–2460.

84. Ginsberg MD, Busto R. Combating hyperthermia in acute stroke: a significant clinical concern. *Stroke*. 1998;29:529–534.

85. Wang Y, Lim LL, Levi C, et al. Influence of admission body temperature on stroke mortality. *Stroke*. 2000;31:404–409.

86. Kammersgaard LP, Jorgensen HS, Rungby JA, et al. Admission body temperature predicts long-term mortality after acute stroke: the Copenhagen Stroke Study. *Stroke*. 2002;33:1759–1762.

87. den Hertog HM, van der Worp HB, van Gemert HM, et al. The Paracetamol (Acetaminophen) In Stroke (PAIS) trial: a multicentre, randomised, placebo-controlled, phase III trial. *Lancet Neurol*. 2009;8:434–440.

88. Marion DW. Controlled normothermia in neurologic intensive care. *Crit Care Med*. 2004;32(Suppl):S43–S45.

89. Olsen TS, Weber UJ, Kammersgaard LP. Therapeutic hypothermia for acute stroke. *Lancet Neurol*. 2003;2:410–416.

90. van der Worp HB, Sena ES, Donnan GA, et al. Hypothermia in animal models of acute ischaemic stroke: a systematic review and meta-analysis. *Brain*. 2007;130:3063–3074.

91. Lyden P, Hemmen T, Grotta J, et al. Results of the ICTuS 2 Trial (Intravascular Cooling in the Treatment of Stroke 2). *Stroke*. 2016;47:2888–2895.

92. Hammer MD, Krieger DW. Hypothermia for acute ischemic stroke: not just another neuroprotectant. *Neurologist*. 2003;9:280–289.

93. Georgiadis D, Schwarz S, Kollmar R, Schwab S. Endovascular cooling for moderate hypothermia in patients with acute stroke: first results of a novel approach. *Stroke*. 2001;32:2550–2553.

94. Krieger DW, De Georgia MA, Abou-Chebl A, et al. Cooling for acute ischemic brain damage (COOL AID): an open pilot study of induced hypothermia in acute ischemic stroke. *Stroke*. 2001;32:1847–1854.

95. Milhaud D, Thouvenot E, Heroum C, Escuret E. Prolonged moderate hypothermia in massive hemispheric infarction: clinical experience. *J Neurosurg Anesthesiol*. 2005;17:49–53.

96. Correia M, Silva M, Veloso M. Cooling therapy for acute stroke. *Cochrane Database Syst Rev*. 2000;2:CD001247.

97. Paula WK. Heads down: flat positioning improves blood flow velocity in acute ischemic stroke. *Neurology*. 2005;65:1514.

98. Anderson CS, Arima H, Lavados P, et al. Cluster-randomized, crossover trial of head positioning in acute stroke. *N Engl J Med*. 2017;376:2437–2447.

99. Vahedi K, Hofmeijer J, Juettler E, et al. Early decompressive surgery in malignant infarction of the middle cerebral artery: a pooled analysis of three randomised controlled trials. *Lancet Neurol*. 2007;6:215–222.

100. Juttler E, Schwab S, Schmiedek P, et al. Decompressive surgery for the treatment of malignant infarction of the middle cerebral artery (DESTINY)—outcome results [abstract]. *Int J Stroke*. 2006;s38:1.

101. Vahedi K, Vicaut E, Mateau J, et al. Decimal trial: a sequential design, multicenter, randomized, controlled trial of decompressive craniectomy in malignant middle cerebral artery (MCA) infarction [abstract]. *Int J Stroke*. 2006;1:s38.

102. Hofmeijer J, Amelink GJ, Algra A, et al. Hemicraniectomy after middle cerebral artery infarction with life-threatening edema trial (HAMLET). Protocol for a randomised controlled trial of decompressive surgery in space-occupying hemispheric infarction. *Trials*. 2006;7:29.

103. Vahedi K, Vicaut E, Mateo J, et al. Sequential-design, multicenter, randomized, controlled trial of early decompressive craniectomy in malignant middle cerebral artery infarction (DECIMAL Trial). *Stroke*. 2007;38:2506–2517.

104. Jüttler E, Unterberg A, Woitzik J, et al. Hemicraniectomy in older patients with extensive middle-cerebral-artery stroke. *N Engl J Med*. 2014;370:1091–1100.

105. Kocan MJ. Cardiovascular effects of acute stroke. *Prog Cardiovasc Nurs*. 1999;14:61–67.

106. Britton M, de Faire U, Helmers C, et al. Arrhythmias in patients with acute cerebrovascular disease. *Acta Med Scand*. 1979;205:425–428.

107. Iadecola C, Davisson RL. Hypertension and cerebrovascular dysfunction. *Cell Metab*. 2008;7:476–484.

108. Castillo J, Leira R, García MM, et al. Blood pressure decrease during the acute phase of ischemic stroke is associated with brain injury and poor stroke outcome. *Stroke*. 2004;35:520–526.

109. Johnston KC, Mayer SA. Blood pressure reduction in ischemic stroke: a two-edged sword. *Neurology*. 2003;61:1030–1031.

110. Kaplan NM. Management of hypertensive emergencies. *Lancet*. 1994;344:1335–1338.

111. Powers WJ. Acute hypertension after stroke: the scientific basis for treatment decisions. *Neurology*. 1993;43(pt 1):461–467.

112. Goldstein LB. Blood pressure management in patients with acute ischemic stroke. *Hypertension*. 2004;43:137–141.

113. Phillips SJ. Pathophysiology and management of hypertension in acute ischemic stroke. *Hypertension*. 1994;23:131–136.

114. Adams Jr HP, Brott TG, Furlan AJ, et al. Guidelines for thrombolytic therapy for acute stroke: a supplement to the guidelines for the management of patients with acute ischemic stroke. A statement for healthcare professionals from a Special Writing Group of the Stroke Council, American Heart Association. *Circulation*. 1996;94:1167–1174.

115. He J, Zhang Y, Xu T, et al. Effects of immediate blood pressure reduction on death and major disability in patients with acute ischemic stroke: the CATIS randomized clinical trial. *JAMA*. 2014;311:479–489.

116. Sacco RL, Adams R, Albers G, et al. Guidelines for prevention of stroke in patients with ischemic stroke or transient ischemic attack: a statement for healthcare professionals from the American Heart Association/American Stroke Association Council on Stroke: co-sponsored by the Council on Cardiovascular Radiology and Intervention: the American Academy of Neurology affirms the value of this guideline. *Stroke.* 2006;37:577–617.

117. Al-Sadat A, Sunbulli M, Chaturvedi S. Use of intravenous heparin by North American neurologists: do the data matter. *Stroke.* 2002;33:1574–1577.

118. Adams Jr HP. Emergency use of anticoagulation for treatment of patients with ischemic stroke. *Stroke.* 2002;33:856–861.

119. Caplan LR. Resolved: heparin may be useful in selected patients with brain ischemia. *Stroke.* 2003;34:230–231.

120. Donnan GA, Davis SM. Heparin in stroke: not for most, but the controversy lingers. *Stroke.* 2003;34:232–233.

121. Moonis M, Fisher M. Considering the role of heparin and low molecular-weight heparins in acute ischemic stroke. *Stroke.* 2002;33:1927–1933.

122. Sandercock P. Full heparin anticoagulation should not be used in acute ischemic stroke. *Stroke.* 2003;34:231–232.

123. January CT, Wann LS, Alpert JS, et al. 2014 AHA/ACC/HRS guideline for the management of patients with atrial fibrillation: executive summary: a report of the American College of Cardiology/American Heart Association Task Force on practice guidelines and the Heart Rhythm Society. *Circulation.* 2014;130:2071–2104.

124. Gonzalez-Quesada CJ, Giugliano RP. Comparison of the phase III clinical trial designs of novel oral anticoagulants versus warfarin for the treatment of nonvalvular atrial fibrillation: implications for clinical practice. *Am J Cardiovasc Drugs.* 2014;14:111–127.

125. Maegdefessel L, Spin JM, Azuma J, Tsao PS. New options with dabigatran etexilate in anticoagulant therapy. *Vasc Health Risk Manag.* 2010;6:339–349.

126. Patel MR, Mahaffey KW, Garg J, et al. Rivaroxaban versus warfarin in nonvalvular atrial fibrillation. *N Engl J Med.* 2011;365:883–891.

127. Granger CB, Alexander JH, McMurray JJ, et al. Apixaban versus warfarin in patients with atrial fibrillation. *N Engl J Med.* 2011;365:981–992.

128. Kernan WN, Ovbiagele B, Black HR, et al. Guidelines for the prevention of stroke in patients with stroke and transient ischemic attack: a guideline for healthcare professionals from the American Heart Association/American Stroke Association. *Stroke.* 2014;45:2160–2236.

129. The International Stroke Trial (IST): a randomised trial of aspirin, subcutaneous heparin, both, or neither among 19435 patients with acute ischaemic stroke. International Stroke Trial Collaborative Group. *Lancet.* 1997;349:1569–1581.

130. Tan LB. Interpretation of IST and CAST stroke trials. International Stroke Trial. Chinese Acute Stroke Trial. *Lancet.* 1997;350:443.

131. Lapchak PA, Araujo DM. Therapeutic potential of platelet glycoprotein IIb/IIIa receptor antagonists in the management of ischemic stroke. *Am J Cardiovasc Drugs.* 2003;3:87–94.

132. Abciximab Emergent Stroke Treatment Trial (AbESTT) Investigators. Emergency administration of abciximab for treatment of patients with acute ischemic stroke: results of a randomized phase 2 trial. *Stroke.* 2005;36:880–890.

133. Mitsias PD, Lu M, Morris D, et al. Treatment of acute supratentorial ischemic stroke with abciximab is safe and may result in early neurological improvement. A preliminary report. *Cerebrovasc Dis.* 2004;18:249–250.

134. Stocchetti N, Maas AI, Chieregato A, Plas AA. Hyperventilation in head injury. *Chest.* 2005;127:1812–1827.

135. Aichner FT, Fazekas F, Brainin M, et al. Hypervolemic hemodilution in acute ischemic stroke: the Multicenter Austrian Hemodilution Stroke Trial (MAHST). *Stroke.* 1998;29:743–749.

136. Easton JD, Saver JL, Albers GW, et al. Definition and evaluation of transient ischemic attack: a scientific statement for healthcare professionals from the American Heart Association/American Stroke Association Stroke Council; Council on Cardiovascular Surgery and Anesthesia; Council on Cardiovascular Radiology and Intervention; Council on Cardiovascular Nursing; and Interdisciplinary Council on Peripheral Vascular Disease. The American Academy of Neurology affirms the value of this statement as an educational tool for neurologists. *Stroke.* 2009;40:2276–2293.

137. Kleindorfer D, Panagos P, Pancioli A, et al. Incidence and short-term prognosis of transient ischemic attack in a population-based study. *Stroke.* 2005;36:720–723.

138. Mlynash M, Olivot JM, Tong DC, et al. Yield of combined perfusion and diffusion MR imaging in hemispheric TIA. *Neurology.* 2009;72:1127–1133.

139. Donnan GA, Davis SM, Hill MD, Gladstone DJ. Patients with transient ischemic attack or minor stroke should be admitted to hospital. *Stroke.* 2006;37:1137–1138.

140. Johnston SC, Nguyen-Huynh MN, Schwarz ME, et al. National Stroke Association guidelines for the management of transient ischemic attacks. *Ann Neurol.* 2006;60:301–313.

141. Rothwell PM, Giles MF, Chandratheva A, et al. Effect of urgent treatment on transient ischaemic attack and minor stroke on early recurrent stroke (EXPRESS study): a prospective population-based sequential comparison. *Lancet.* 2007;370:1432–1442.

142. Barnett HJM, Taylor DW, Haynes RB, et al. Beneficial effects of carotid endarterectomy in symptomatic patients with high-grade carotid stenosis. *N Engl J Med.* 1991;325:445–452.

143. Barnett HJM, Taylor DW, Eliasziw M, et al. Benefit of carotid endarterectomy in symptomatic patients with moderate and severe stenosis. *N Engl J Med.* 1998;339:1415–1425.

144. Brott TG, Hobson 2nd RW, Howard G, et al. Stenting versus endarterectomy for treatment of carotid stenosis. *N Engl J Med.* 2010;363:11–23.

145. Sacco RL, Diener CH, Yusuf S, et al. Aspirin and extended-release dipyridamole versus clopidogrel for recurrent stroke. *N Engl J Med.* 2008;359:1238–1251.

146. Halkes PH, van Gijn J, Kappelle LJ, et al. Medium intensity oral anticoagulation versus aspirin after cerebral ischaemia of arterial origin. *Lancet Neurol.* 2007;6:115–124.

147. Gent M, Beaumont D, Blanchard J, et al. A randomised, blinded, trial of clopidogrel versus aspirin in patients at risk of ischaemic events (CAPRIE). CAPRIE Steering Committee. *Lancet.* 1996;348:1329–1339.

148. Diener HC, Bogousslavsky J, Brass LM, et al. Aspirin and clopidogrel compared with clopidogrel alone after recent ischaemic stroke or transient ischaemic attack in high-risk patients (MATCH): randomised, double-blind, placebo-controlled trial. *Lancet.* 2004;364:331–337.

149. Bhatt DL, Fox KA, Hacke W, et al. Clopidogrel and aspirin versus aspirin alone for the prevention of atherothrombotic events. *N Engl J Med.* 2006;354:1706–1717.

150. Wang Y, Wang Y, Zhao X, et al. Clopidogrel with aspirin in acute minor stroke or transient ischemic attack. *N Engl J Med.* 2013;369:11–19.

151. Chimowitz MI, Lynn MJ, Derdeyn CP, et al. Stenting versus aggressive medical therapy for intracranial arterial stenosis. *N Engl J Med.* 2011;365:993–1003.

152. Amarenco P, Goldstein LB, Szarek M, et al. Effects of intense low-density lipoprotein cholesterol reduction in patients with stroke or transient ischemic attack: the Stroke Prevention by Aggressive Reduction in Cholesterol Levels (SPARCL) trial. *Stroke.* 2007;38:3198–3204.

153. Amarenco P, Labreuche J. Lipid management in the prevention of stroke: review and updated meta-analysis of statins for stroke prevention. *Lancet Neurol.* 2009;8:453–463.

154. Rashid P, Leonardi-Bee J, Bath P. Blood pressure reduction and secondary prevention of stroke and other vascular events: a systematic review. *Stroke.* 2003;34:2741–2748.

155. Schrader J, Lüders S, Kulschewski A, et al. Morbidity and mortality after stroke, eprosartan compared with nitrendipine for secondary prevention: principal results of a prospective randomized controlled study (MOSES). *Stroke.* 2005;36:1218–1226.

156. PROGRESS Collaborative Group. Randomised trial of a perindopril-based blood-pressure-lowering regimen among 6,105 individuals with previous stroke or transient ischaemic attack. *Lancet.* 2001;358:1033–1041.

157. Yusuf S, Diener HC, Sacco RL, et al. Telmisartan to prevent recurrent stroke and cardiovascular events. *N Engl J Med.* 2008;359:1225–1237.

158. Amarenco P, Bogousslavsky J, Callahan 3rd A, et al. High-dose atorvastatin after stroke or transient ischemic attack. *N Engl J Med.* 2006;355:549–559.

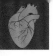
159. Goldstein LB, Bushnell CD, Adams RJ, et al. Guidelines for the primary prevention of stroke: a guideline for healthcare professionals from the American Heart Association/American Stroke Association. *Stroke*. 2011;42:517–584.

160. Endarterectomy for asymptomatic carotid artery stenosis. Executive Committee for the Asymptomatic Carotid Atherosclerosis Study. *JAMA*. 1995;273:1421–1428.

161. Halliday A, Mansfield A, Marro J, et al. Prevention of disabling and fatal strokes by successful carotid endarterectomy in patients without recent neurological symptoms: randomized controlled trial. *Lancet*. 2004;363:1491–1502.

162. Spence JD, Coates V, Li H, et al. Effects of intensive medical therapy on microemboli and cardiovascular risk in asymptomatic carotid stenosis. *Arch Neurol*. 2010;67:180–186.

163. Madani A, Beletsky V, Tamayo A, et al. High-risk asymptomatic carotid stenosis: ulceration on 3D ultrasound versus TCD microemboli. *Neurology*. 2011;77:744–750.

164. Rosenfield K, Matsumura JS, Chaturvedi S. Randomized trial of stent versus surgery for asymptomatic carotid stenosis. *J Vasc Surg*. 2016;64:536.

165. Labovitz DL, Halim A, Boden-Albala B, et al. The incidence of deep and lobar intracerebral hemorrhage in whites, blacks and Hispanics. *Neurology*. 2005;65:518–522.

166. Manno EM, Atkinson JL, Fulgham JR, Wijdicks EF. Emergency medical and surgical management strategies in the evaluation and treatment of intracerebral hemorrhage. *Mayo Clin Proc*. 2005;80:420–433.

167. Brott T, Broderick J, Kothari R, et al. Early hemorrhage growth in patients with intracerebral hemorrhage. *Stroke*. 1997;28:1–5.

168. Kidwell CS, Chalela JA, Saver JL, et al. Comparison of MRI and CT for detection of intracerebral hemorrhage. *JAMA*. 2004;292:1823–1830.

169. Anderson CS, Heeley E, Huang Y, et al. Rapid blood-pressure lowering in patients with acute intracerebral hemorrhage. *N Engl J Med*. 2013;368:2355–2365.

170. Qureshi A, Palesch Y, Barsan W, et al. Intensive blood-pressure lowering in patients with acute cerebral hemorrhage. *N Engl J Med*. 2016;375:1033–1043.

171. Hemphill 3rd JC, Greenberg SM, Anderson CS, et al. Guidelines for the management of spontaneous intracerebral hemorrhage: a guideline for healthcare professionals from the American Heart Association/American Stroke Association. *Stroke*. 2015;46:2032–2060.

172. Anderson CS, Huang Y, Wang JG, et al. Intensive blood pressure reduction in acute cerebral haemorrhage trial (INTERACT): a randomised pilot trial. *Lancet Neurol*. 2008;7:391–399.

173. Misra UK, Kalita J, Ranjan P, Mandal SK. Mannitol in intracerebral hemorrhage: a randomized controlled study. *J Neurol Sci*. 2005;234:41–45.

174. Poungvarin N, Bhoopat W, Viriyavejakul A, et al. Effects of dexamethasone in primary supratentorial intracerebral hemorrhage. *N Engl J Med*. 1987;316:1229–1233.

175. Lacut K, Bressollee L, Le Gal G, et al. Prevention of venous thrombosis in patients with acute intracerebral hemorrhage. *Neurology*. 2005;65:865–869.

176. Flaherty ML, Kissela B, Woo D, et al. The increasing incidence of anticoagulation-associated intracerebral hemorrhage. *Neurology*. 2007;68:116–121.

177. Flibotte JJ, Hagan N, O'Donnell J, et al. Warfarin, hematoma expansion and outcome of intracerebral hemorrhage. *Neurology*. 2004;63:1059–1064.

178. Huttner HB, Schellinger PD, Hartmann M, et al. Hematoma growth and outcome in treated neurocritical care patients with intracerebral hemorrhage related to oral anticoagulant therapy: comparison of acute treatment strategies using vitamin K, fresh frozen plasma, and prothrombin complex concentrates. *Stroke*. 2006;37:1465–1470.

179. Pollock Jr CV, Reilly PA, van Ryn J, et al. Idarucizumab for dabigtan reversal: full cohort analysis. *N Engl J Med*. 2017;377:431–441.

180. Mayer SA, Brun NC, Begtrup K, et al. Recombinant activated factor VII for acute intracerebral hemorrhage. *N Engl J Med*. 2005;352:777–785.

181. Mayer SA, Brun NC, Begtrup K, et al. Efficacy and safety of recombinant activated factor VII for acute intracerebral hemorrhage. *N Engl J Med*. 2008;358:2127–2137.

182. Qureshi AI, Mendelow AD, Hanley DF. Intracerebral hemorrhage. *Lancet*. 2009;373:1632–1644.

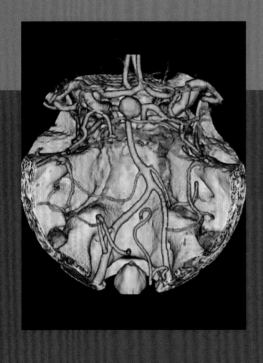

第31章
颈动脉血管重建

颈动脉内膜切除术（carotid endarterectomy，CEA）、颈动脉支架植入术（carotid artery stenting，CAS）及最佳药物治疗（best medical therapy，BMT）是颈动脉疾病的主要治疗方式，如何选择是当前的热点与争议焦点。

颈动脉内膜剥脱术仍是症状性患者的一线治疗方式，需要在症状出现48小时内尽早手术，如发现大面积脑梗死、严重神经功能障碍或梗死后再出血，则延迟2～14天手术。颈动脉内膜剥脱术高风险患者采用颈动脉支架植入术，<50%的症状性患者建议最佳药物治疗。对于无症状性患者则应在围手术期中风和死亡率低于3%且预期寿命为3～5年的条件下行颈动脉内膜剥脱术治疗，手术高风险时采用颈动脉支架植入术治疗。颈动脉内膜剥脱术术中脑监测患者5%～15%需用转流管，如不监测则需所有患者放置转流管。患者选择是提高颈动脉支架植入术手术安全性的关键。增加颈动脉支架植入术风险的因素包括Ⅱ～Ⅲ型主动脉弓、严重扭曲、斑块负荷重，颈总动脉（common carotid artery，CCA）/颈内动脉（internal carotid artery，ICA）迂曲；颈内动脉病变严重钙化、环形钙化，存在软血栓。为避免传统颈动脉支架植入术弓部操作和远端保护装置（embolic protection devices，EPD）穿过病变时引发栓塞风险，经颈动脉血运重建（transcarotid artery revascularization，TCAR）技术应用于临床，早期结果显示卒中和死亡总体发生率为1.4%。围手术期不建议使用β受体阻滞剂，如已服可不停药，术前颈动脉内膜剥脱术需单抗治疗，颈动脉支架植入术需双抗治疗，同时尽早使用他汀类药物。血压控制和神经系统监测是颈动脉内膜剥脱术/颈动脉支架植入术术后管理的关键。一旦患者出现神经功能缺损症状，则必须行床旁超声或头颈部CT血管造影评估颈内动脉的通畅性。5%～22%的患者会出现术后再狭窄，大多为无症状性；术后2年内出现与内膜增生相关，2年以上则与动脉硬化进展相关。颈动脉支架植入术是颈动脉内膜剥脱术术后再狭窄的首选治疗方法。

刘　鹏　叶志东

31

Carotid Artery Revascularization

Richard J. Powell and Nikolaos Zacharias

The management of carotid artery disease remains a topic of current investigation and vigorous debate regarding optimal treatments. Multiple prospective randomized controlled trials have compared the standard therapies, which include carotid endarterectomy (CEA), carotid artery stenting (CAS), and best medical therapy (BMT). In addition, hybrid procedures to treat carotid artery stenosis have been added to the therapeutic armamentarium. This chapter focuses on the evidence base, clinical decision making, and outcomes of the carotid revascularization techniques.

INDICATIONS FOR CAROTID REVASCULARIZATION

Symptomatic Patients

Based on the latest multisociety evidence-based guidelines, CEA is recommended as first-line treatment for most symptomatic patients with 50% to 99% internal carotid artery (ICA) stenosis.[1] CAS is recommended for symptomatic patients with 50% to 99% stenosis who, for anatomic or medical reasons, are at high risk for CEA (Box 31.1).[1] BMT alone is recommended for patients with symptomatic ICA stenosis <50%.[1] The timing of carotid revascularization in symptomatic patients remains controversial. Concern over recurrent stroke following the initial event has resulted in a push toward early revascularization within 48 hours following initiation of symptoms. This is especially true for patients with stroke or profound symptoms of a transient ischemic attack (TIA). In contrast, the natural history of amaurosis fugax appears to be more benign. Patients who present with large infarcts on cerebral imaging, profound neurological impairment, or hemorrhage within the infarct should be considered for delayed revascularization between 2 and 14 days following initial presentation.

Asymptomatic Patients

CEA is recommended for patients with 70% to 99% asymptomatic ICA stenosis if the patient's perioperative stroke and death rate is less than 3% and if the patient has at least a 3- to 5-year life expectancy.[1] The use of CAS to treat asymptomatic patients is controversial.[2] Currently CAS for asymptomatic patients is not reimbursed by Medicare outside of an Investigational Device Exemption (IDE)–approved clinical trial. However, CAS is frequently performed for asymptomatic patients at high anatomic risk for CEA. In addition, there are several large randomized trials demonstrating that CAS can be performed with a stroke and death rate of <3% in standard-risk asymptomatic patients. The most representative is the Carotid Revascularization Endarterectomy Versus Stenting Trial (CREST) (Table 31.1). BMT

alone is recommended for patients with asymptomatic stenosis of <70% who are at high risk for intervention or with a life expectancy of <3 years.[1]

Last, the current data that inform decision making regarding the treatment of asymptomatic patients is dated and do not include rigorous BMT——using statins, improved blood pressure control, and antiplatelet therapy——which would be considered the current standard of care. Indications for when to perform CEA and when to perform carotid stent placement are discussed in greater detail below.

PREOPERATIVE MANAGEMENT

The perioperative guidelines of the American Heart Association (AHA) classify CEA as an intermediate-risk procedure.[3] Preoperative cardiac assessment in patients undergoing CEA commonly includes a 12-lead electrocardiogram (EKG). Additional testing, such as a nuclear perfusion scans or dobutamine stress echocardiography, is based on the patient's clinical profile, including the lesion's risk for cardiovascular complications and stroke. It is recommended if the patient has three or more clinical risk factors (coronary artery disease [CAD], history of heart failure, diabetes mellitus, renal insufficiency), more in-depth cardiac risk assessment be considered. This is especially true for asymptomatic patients with critical carotid stenosis where the absolute risk reduction of stroke is lower than that in symptomatic patients. In a prospective trial, no medications have been shown to reduce perioperative outcomes. The preoperative medical management of patients undergoing CEA should include the chronic treatment for atherosclerosis, such as a statin. Interestingly in the PeriOperative ISchemic Evaluation-2 (POISE-2) trial, the addition of aspirin did not reduce adverse cardiovascular events in patients undergoing vascular surgery. Initiation of β-adrenergic blocking agents is not recommended either. However, if a patient is taking these agents they should not be discontinued, because withdrawal of a β-blocker is associated with an increase in cardiovascular events.

β-Blockers

According to the 2014 Clinical Practice Guidelines of the AHA and the American College of Cardiology, including data from 17 studies (16 randomized controlled trials), perioperative β-blockade started within 1 day or less before noncardiac surgery decreases nonfatal myocardial infarction (MI) but increases the risks of stroke, death, hypotension, and bradycardia.[4] The current recommendation is to continue β-blockade in patients who are already on a β-blocker. There is a weak recommendation to start β-blockade in patients with a history of CAD or more than one clinical risk factor.[2]

BOX 31.1 High-Surgical-Risk Criteria for Carotid Endarterectomy

Previous carotid endarterectomy
Previous neck dissection
Radiation therapy
Presence of stoma (tracheostomy/esophagostomy)
Lesion above second cervical vertebra (C2)
Contralateral cranial nerve injury

TABLE 31.1 CREST Study Results for Asymptomatic Patients

	CAS	CEA	P
MI	7 (1.2%)	13 (2.2%)	.2
All stroke	15 (2.5%)	8 (1.4%)	.15
Major stroke	3 (0.5%)	2 (0.3%)	.66
Minor stroke	12 (2.0%)	6 (1.0%)	.15
Stroke + death	15 (2.5%)	8 (1.4%)	.15
Stroke/death/MI	21 (3.5%)	21 (3.5%)	.96

CAS, Carotid artery stenting; *CEA*, carotid endarterectomy; *CREST*, Carotid Revascularization Endarterectomy Versus Stenting Trial; *MI*, myocardial infarction.

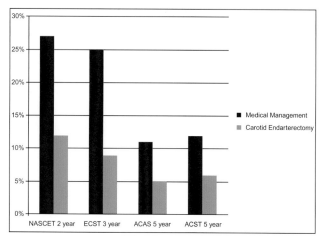

Fig. 31.1 Proven benefits of carotid endarterectomy over medical management for 30-day stroke, myocardial infarction, death, and late ipsilateral stroke.

Statins

Statins are highly effective in reducing perioperative cardiovascular morbidity as well as perioperative stroke.[5] In a large retrospective single-center study, McGirt et al. demonstrated a post-CEA reduction in perioperative strokes associated with statin use (1.2% vs. 4.5%, P < .01) as well as a reduction in all-cause mortality and hospital length of stay.[6] Similar results for patients undergoing CAS have been published.[5] The guidelines of the AHA include the observation that statin use is reasonable in patients undergoing major vascular surgery. Medications should be started as early as possible before the surgery date, and liver function tests and creatinine kinase levels monitored throughout the perioperative period.[7]

Antiplatelet Therapy

The Society for Vascular Surgery's guidelines for the management of carotid artery disease recommend that all patients undergoing CEA receive aspirin (81 to 325 mg) perioperatively.[2] Jones et al. reviewed patients undergoing CEA in the Vascular Quality Initiative (2003 to 2014) and compared patients on dual antiplatelet therapy (DAPT) versus aspirin alone.[9] Preoperative DAPT was associated with a 40% risk reduction for neurological events but was also associated with a significantly increased risk of reoperation for bleeding.[9]

Patients undergoing CAS should receive DAPT, which includes aspirin (81 to 325 mg/day) and clopidogrel (75 mg/day) prior to the procedure and for at least 30 days thereafter.[10] In patients who have not received DAPT prior to CAS, a loading dose of 300 mg the day prior or 600 mg of clopidogrel immediately prior to the procedure is recommended in addition to aspirin. In patients who cannot receive clopidogrel, the platelet adenosine diphosphate receptor P2Y12 inhibitor ticagrelor may be used. DAPT is recommended for 30 days following CAS, after which aspirin or clopidogrel alone can be continued.

CAROTID ENDARTERECTOMY

The era of CEA began in 1954, when Eastcott and Robb reported the first successful reconstruction to treat symptomatic carotid artery disease in a woman with TIAs.[11] DeBakey et al. had performed a successful CEA the year before and published their experience in 1963, documenting numerous approaches to carotid, vertebral, and aortic arch reconstruction including patch angioplasty, CEA, and shunting.[12]

Landmark studies such as the North American Symptomatic Carotid Endarterectomy Trial (NASCET), the European Carotid Surgery Trial (ECST) for symptomatic disease, the Asymptomatic Carotid Atherosclerosis Study (ACAS), and the Asymptomatic Carotid Surgery Trial (ACST) for asymptomatic disease confirmed the benefits of CEA over BMT (Fig. 31.1).[13–16] The most commonly used CEA technique is CEA with patch angioplasty. CEA with eversion is an alternative technique that has been shown to have shorter procedure times and decreased cost as well as similar freedom from neurological morbidity, mortality, and reintervention compared with conventional CEA with patch angioplasty.[17]

Carotid Endarterectomy with Patch Angioplasty

This is the most commonly used technique for CEA and consists of a vertical arteriotomy starting on the common carotid artery (CCA) and extending into the ICA. An incision is performed along the anterior border of the sternocleidomastoid muscle and the subcutaneous tissue and platysma muscle are divided with electrocautery. The sternocleidomastoid muscle is mobilized laterally and the fascial vein is identified and ligated. The internal jugular vein is mobilized laterally. The carotid sheath is entered and the vagus nerve is identified and preserved. The CCA, ICA, and external carotid artery (ECA) are exposed proximally and distally until healthy artery is exposed for clamping. The hypoglossal nerve is carefully mobilized if needed and preserved cephalad to the bifurcation. The patient is heparinized. Subsequently the ICA is clamped first, followed by the ECA and CCA. The patient's neurological status can be monitored by measuring a stump pressure (a mean pressure of 60 mm Hg is considered adequate), EEG, or awake neurological monitoring if the procedure is performed under cervical plexus block. With changes on EEG monitoring in patients with low carotid stump pressure as well as changes in mental status in awake patients, a shunt is placed to maintain cerebral perfusion while the endarterectomy is completed. In general, 5% to 15% of patients will require a shunt using these techniques. An alternative to cerebral monitoring is to shunt all patients during CEA. An endarterectomy is performed and the plaque excised (Fig. 31.2). Studies have shown that carotid artery patch angioplasty at completion of the CEA decreases the rate of neurological events and restenosis. This finding is largely limited to women and patients with

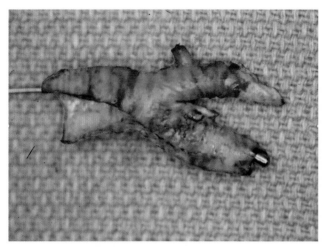

Fig. 31.2 Carotid endarterectomy plaque.

small ICAs. Hemostasis is obtained by reversing the heparin with protamine. To ensure a technically satisfactory procedure, intraoperative carotid artery duplex may be performed to verify patency and flow and exclude the presence of flaps causing hemodynamic compromise.

Eversion Carotid Endarterectomy Technique

The surgical exposure is identical to the technique for conventional CEA with patch angioplasty. After exposure of the ICA, CCA, and ECA is completed, the bifurcation is completely transected. The endarterectomy is performed by mobilizing the entire circumference of the carotid wall of the plaque. Subsequently the ICA wall is mobilized cephalad while gentle caudal traction is applied to the plaque. The same maneuver is performed on the CCA and ECA. Once the endarterectomy is complete, the divided bifurcation is reunited with an end-to-side anastomosis. This can be performed rapidly and the vessel is not prone to restenosis; therefore a patch is not required.[18] This technique is extremely useful with ICA coils and kinks. The redundant portion can be excised and the ICA pulled down and straightened.

CAROTID ARTERY STENTING

CAS for symptomatic carotid artery stenosis was introduced in the early 1980s. CAS use has increased dramatically over the past 30 years.

In 2005, CAS received Center for Medicare and Medicaid Services coverage for symptomatic patients who are at high risk for CEA.[19,20] There has been a general agreement that CAS is appropriate in symptomatic patients who are at high anatomic risk for CEA. These criteria include previous ipsilateral CEA, other neck surgery or radiation, lesions extending proximal to the clavicle or distal to the C2 vertebral body, the presence of significant radiation to the neck, or a tracheal stoma (see Box 31.1).[2,21] The medically high-risk criteria are controversial, particularly for asymptomatic patients who do not have a life expectancy long enough to make treating an asymptomatic carotid lesion beneficial.[2,19–23]

Carotid Artery Stenting Technique

In CAS planning, it is important to recognize the type of aortic arch and the variant anatomy of the arch vessels. A preprocedural computed tomography angiogram (CTA) of the neck and aortic arch is commonly used to define the type of aortic arch in question (I to III). The femoral artery approach has been preferred for conventional CAS, although brachial and transradial approaches may be used. After access is obtained under ultrasound guidance, a 5-Fr sheath is inserted into the common femoral artery; the patient receives a bolus of heparin;

and a flush catheter is advanced to the ascending thoracic aorta over a J-wire. An arch angiogram is performed to verify the location of the carotid artery ostium. A 6-Fr 90- to 100-cm sheath is advanced to the aortic arch and the CCA is selected with a stiff Glidewire and a selective catheter. A long sheath is then advanced into the CCA. An embolic protection device is used to cross the stenotic carotid lesion. A road map guidance image can often be useful to navigate the wire. Once the lesion has been crossed, the filter is deployed in the distal ICA. The lesion may also be predilated before a stent is placed. If there is significant recoil within the stent, then poststenting balloon angioplasty may be performed. A completion angiogram is then obtained and the embolic protection filter is retrieved. Technology related to carotid stenting is rapidly evolving. More flexible stents with tighter cell patterns can provide better coverage of the carotid lesion and have the potential to decrease the acute postprocedural embolic events seen with earlier open-cell stent designs. In addition, more advanced lower-profile embolic protection devices and flow reversal systems are in development, which may make CAS safer.

Patient selection for CAS is the most important variable for improving CAS safety. There are several anatomic and lesion-specific variables that increase the risk of CAS. This includes a hostile aortic arch (defined by the tortuosity and type II–III arch anatomy), significant atherosclerosis burden in the arch, and finally tortuous common and/or internal carotid arteries. Unfavorable lesion characteristics include heavily calcified or circumferentially calcified ICA lesions or the presence of soft thrombus within the lesion (Fig. 31.3). These unfavorable anatomic and lesion variants can be identified prior to considering intervention through the use of three-dimensional CTA of the aortic arch, carotid arteries, and circle of Willis.

POSTOPERATIVE MANAGEMENT

Blood pressure control and neurological monitoring are the cornerstones of postoperative management for patients undergoing CEA or CAS. A systolic blood pressure ≤140 mm Hg, and diastolic blood pressure <80 mm Hg is generally recommended.[2] Frequent neurological examinations are also performed.

If a patient develops neurological deficits postoperatively, assessment of the patency of the ICA must be performed emergently with a bedside duplex ultrasound or CTA of the head and neck. If the ICA appears occluded soon after a CEA, urgent return to the operating room for an exploration is appropriate. Technical issues such as intimal flaps, clamp injuries, and residual plaque must be addressed. The presence of in situ thrombosis and platelet aggregation can be managed with an interposition bypass with saphenous vein or prosthetic graft. If the patient's ICA is patent postoperatively and embolic material is identified in the proximal intracranial circulation, a carotid angiogram is recommended to investigate intracerebral vessel occlusion/embolization and consider neurological rescue treatment.

Cerebral hyperperfusion syndrome is a rare but devastating complication of carotid revascularization and has been reported to occur in 0.4% to 7.7% after CEA. This complication has also been reported after CAS procedures.[24] Symptoms include severe frontal headache associated with severe hypertension and acute neurological deficits. Intracerebral hemorrhagic stroke is the most severe manifestation.[24] Diagnosis can be made in the setting of clinical symptoms and evidence of elevated ipsilateral velocities of the intracranial vessels as determined by transcranial duplex (TCD) measurements. Strict blood pressure control and neurological monitoring is recommended. TCD can be used to follow the efficacy of therapy. A study by Ascher et al. reported that hyperperfusion syndrome can be predicted by a significant drop in pressure across the carotid

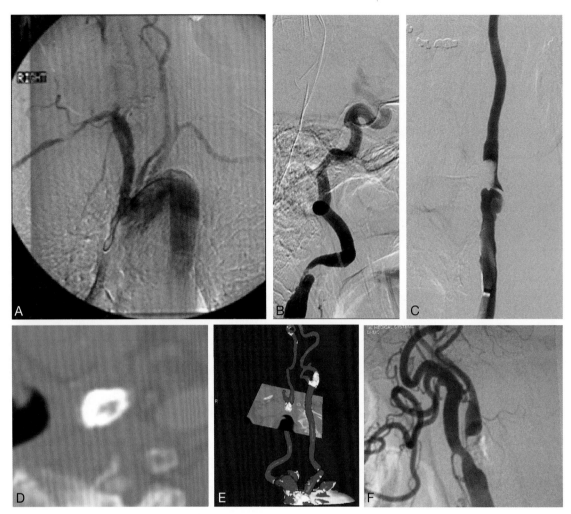

Fig. 31.3 (A) Type 3 aortic arch. (B) Tortuous internal carotid artery. (C–D) Fresh thrombus in internal carotid artery. (E) Three-dimensional computed tomography angiogram of an internal carotid artery demonstrating circumferential calcification. (F) Calcified complex internal carotid artery stenosis.

stenosis leading to temporary loss of cerebral autoregulation in the middle cerebral artery.[25] This study also found that CEA performed ≤3 months after contralateral CEA was associated with a higher risk of hyperperfusion syndrome.[25]

OUTCOMES FOR CAROTID ENDARTERECTOMY AND CAROTID ARTERY STENTING

Several recently completed trials compared the outcomes of CEA and CAS. The CREST was conducted to evaluate the safety of CAS and CEA.[26] CREST enrolled 1321 symptomatic and 1181 asymptomatic patients. The overall aggregate risk of periprocedural stroke, MI, death, and 1-year ipsilateral stroke did not differ between CAS and CEA (5.2% versus 4.5%, P = .38) (Fig. 31.4). When the individual end points comprising the composite end point were examined, there was a trend toward decreased neurological events in patients undergoing CEA compared with a trend toward decreased cardiac events in patients undergoing CAS. Whether each of these end points carried equal impact on the patient's quality of life and long-term survival has been a topic of intense debate. For patients

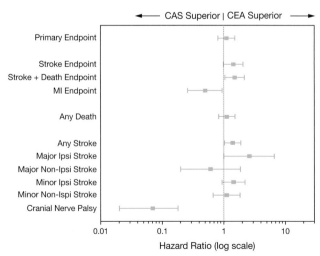

Fig. 31.4 CREST study findings based on calculation of hazard ratio for the end points of early and late stroke, myocardial infarction *(MI)*, death, and cranial nerve palsy. *CAS,* Carotid artery stenting; *CEA,* carotid endarterectomy.

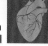

TABLE 31.2 Comparison of ACT I and CREST Study Findings for Patients With Asymptomatic Carotid Artery Stenosis			
	CAS	**CEA**	***P***
ACT I——primary end point	3.8%	3.4%	.011
CREST——primary end point	5.6%	4.9%	.562
ACT I——30-day stroke, MI, death	3.3%	2.6%	.60
CREST——30-day stroke, MI, death	3.5%	3.6%	.96
ACT I——30-day stroke, death	2.9%	1.7%	.33
CREST——30-day stroke, death	2.5%	1.4%	.15

ACT I, Asymptomatic Carotid Trial I; *CREST*, Carotid Revascularization Endarterectomy Versus Stenting Trial; *MI*, myocardial infarction.

with symptomatic carotid stenosis, the periprocedural stroke and death rates were 6.0% for CAS and 3.2% for CEA (*P* = .02). The authors conclude that both CAS and CEA are safe, with a stroke and death rate <6% in symptomatic patients and <3% in asymptomatic patients (Table 31.2).

In long term follow-up of patients enrolled in the CREST trial (10 years) there was no significant difference between CAS and CEA with respect to the risk of late restenosis or ipsilateral stroke.[27]

A comparison of periprocedural stroke death and MI in asymptomatic normal-risk patients has shown similar results to that of the asymptomatic patients in CREST. In the Asymptomatic Carotid Trial I (ACT I), asymptomatic patients with average operative risk were randomized to CAS versus CEA.[28] The rate of stroke or death within 30 days was 2.9% in CAS patients versus 1.7% in patients undergoing CEA (*P* = .33). There was no difference between the groups in outcome and the event rate was less than the 3% that would be anticipated to be beneficial in stroke prevention in asymptomatic patients. The cumulative 5-year rate of stroke-free survival was 93.1% in CAS versus 94.7% in the endarterectomy group (*P* = .44). A comparison of the findings of CREST and ACT I for patients with asymptomatic carotid artery stenosis is presented in Table 31.2.

TRANSCERVICAL CAROTID STENTING WITH FLOW REVERSAL

Previous studies have demonstrated that in CAS, patients are at greatest risk of major stroke during catheter manipulation within the aortic arch and while crossing the lesion with the embolic protection device.[10] In 2012 a novel method of CAS was introduced using the principle of flow reversal, which may have advantages in the avoidance of embolization and perioperative stroke that is inherent with the use of filter devices during CAS.[29] The device (ENROUTE Transcarotid NPS, from Silk Road Medical Inc., Sunnyvale, CA) consists of two proprietary 8-Fr sheaths connected by a large-bore regulated flow line to create an arteriovenous shunt (Fig. 31.5). One sheath is placed in the CCA after cervical exposure is performed and the other is placed in the femoral vein. A flow regulator allows the clinician to modify the flow to induce retrograde flow within the ICA. This allows for the carotid lesion to be crossed with a wire without a significant risk of embolization. The carotid stent is delivered through a transcervical approach after flow reversal has been applied (Fig. 31.6). In the pivotal trial, early results reported an overall stroke and death rate of 1.4%.[29]

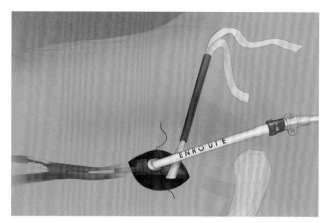

Fig. 31.5 Artist's rendering showing how, after the common carotid artery has been exposed through a transverse incision, an 8-Fr sheath is inserted. (Courtesy Silk Road Medical, Sunnyvale, CA.)

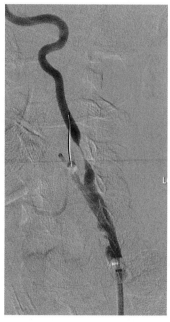

Fig. 31.6 Flow reversal is applied, creating a standing contrast column distal to the internal carotid artery stenosis, thus preventing embolic debris from reaching the brain.

MANAGEMENT OF POSTCAROTID ENDARTERECTOMY STENOSIS

An important complication of both CAS and CEA is the development of recurrent stenosis.[30] Generally the development of recurrent carotid stenosis occurs within 2 years after intervention and is related to intimal hyperplasia, whereas the development of recurrent stenosis after 2 years is related to the development of recurrent atherosclerotic disease. Recurrent stenosis is estimated to occur in 5% to 22% of patients and is mostly asymptomatic. In the CREST trial, at 2 years the rate of significant restenosis or occlusion following CEA was 6.3%.[25] AbuRahma et al. compared patients undergoing primary CAS with patients undergoing CAS for recurrent stenosis after CEA. CAS for CEA restenosis carried a lower risk of early and late neurological events than primary CAS (10.8% versus 1.8%, *P* = .275).[30] In many institutions CAS is the preferred treatment for patients developing significant restenosis after CEA.

REFERENCES

1. Brott TG, Halperin JL, Abbara S, et al. 2011. ASA/ACCF/AHA/AANN/AANS/ACR/ASNR/CNS/SAIP/SCAI/SIR/SNIS/SVM/SVS. Guideline on the Management of Patients with Extracranial Carotid and Vertebral Artery Disease, A Report of the American College of Cardiology Foundation/American Heart Association Task Force on Practise Guidelines, and the American Stroke Association, American Association of Neuroscience Nurses, American Association of Neurological Surgeons, American College of Radiology, American Society of Neuroradiology, Congress of Neurological Surgeons, Society of Atherosclerosis Imaging and Prevention, Society for Cardiovascular Angiography and interventions, Society of Interventional Radiology, Society of Neurointerventional Surgery, Society for Vascular Medicine, and Society for Vascular Surgery Developed in Collaboration With the American Academy of Neurology and Society of Cardiovascular Computed Tomography. *J Am Coll Cardiol*. 2011;57:e16–e94.

2. Ricotta JJ, Aburahma A, Ascher E, et al. Updated Society for Vascular Surgery guidelines for management of extracranial carotid artery disease. *J Vasc Surg*. 2011;54(3):e1–e31.

3. Fleisher LA, Beckman JA, Brown KA, et al. 2009 ACCF/AHA focused update on perioperative beta blockade incorporated into the ACC/AHA 2007 guidelines on perioperative cardiovascular evaluation and care for noncardiac surgery: a report of the American College of Cardiology Foundation/American Heart Association task force on practice guidelines. *Circulation*. 2009;120(21):e169–e276.

4. Wijeysundera DN, Duncan D, Nkonde-Price C, et al. Perioperative beta-blockade in noncardiac surgery: a systematic review for the 2014 ACC/AHA guideline on perioperative cardiovascular evaluation and management of patients undergoing noncardiac surgery. *J Am Coll Cardiol*. 2014;64(22):2406–2425.

5. Perler BA. The effect of statin medications on perioperative and long-term outcomes following carotid endarterectomy or stenting. *Semin Vasc Surg*. 2007;20(4):252–258.

6. McGirt MJ, Perler BA, Brooke BS, et al. 3-hydroxyl-3-methylglutaryl coenzyme A reductase inhibitors reduce the risk of perioperative stroke and mortality after carotid endarterectomy. *J Vacs Surg*. 2005;42(5):829–836.

7. Hirsch AT, Haskal ZJ, Hertzer NR, et al. ACC/AHA Guidelines for the management of patients with peripheral arterial disease (lower extremity, renal, mesenteric, and abdominal aortic): a collaborative report from the American Associations for Vascular Surgery/Society for Vascular Surgery, Society for Cardiovascular Angiography and Interventions, Society for Vascular Medicine and Biology, Society of Interventional Radiology, and the ACC/AHA Task Force on Practice Guidelines (writing committee to develop guidelines for the management of patients with peripheral arterial disease)-summary of recommendations. *J Am Coll Cardiol*. 2006;47(6):1239–1312.

8. Deleted in review.

9. Jones DW, Goodney PP, Conrad MF, et al. Dual antiplatelet therapy reduces stroke but increased bleeding at the time of carotid endarterectomy. *J Vasc Surg*. 2016;63(5):1262–1270.

10. Bonati LH, Jongen LM, Haller S, et al. New ischemic brain lesions on MRI after stenting or endarterectomy for symptomatic carotid stenosis: a substudy of International Carotid Stenting Study (ICSS). *Lancet Neurol*. 2010;9(4):353–362.

11. Tallarita T, Gerbino M, Gurrieri C, Lanzino G. History of carotid artery surgery: from ancient Greeks to the modern era. *Perspect Vasc Surg Endovasc Ther*. 2013;25(3-4):57–64.

12. Crawford ES, DeBakey ME. Surgical treatment of stroke by arterial reconstructive operation. *Clin Neurosurg*. 1963;9:150–162.

13. North American Symptomatic Carotid Endarterectomy Trial Collaborators, Barnett HJM, Taylor DW, et al. Beneficial effect of carotid endarterectomy in symptomatic patients with high-grade carotid stenosis. *N Engl J Med*. 1991;325(7):445–453.

14. Randomised trial of endarterectomy for recently symptomatic carotid stenosis: final results of the MRC European Carotid Surgery Trial (ECST). *Lancet*. 1998;351(9113):1379–1387.

15. Endarterectomy for asymptomatic carotid artery stenosis. Executive Committee for the Asymptomatic Carotid Atherosclerosis Study. *JAMA*. 1995;273(18):1421–1428.

16. Halliday AW, Thomas DJ, Mansfield AO. The Asymptomatic Carotid Surgery Trial (ACST). *Int Angiol*. 1995;14(1):18–20.

17. Schneider JR, Helenowski IB, Jackson CR, et al. A comparison of results with eversion versus conventional carotid endarterectomy from the Vascular Quality Initiative and Mid-America Vascular Study Group. *J Vasc Surg*. 2015;61(5):1216–1222.

18. Shah DM, Darling 3rd RC, Chang BB, et al. Carotid endarterectomy by eversion technique: its safety and durability. *Ann Surg*. 1998;228(4):471–478.

19. Spangler EL, Goodney PP, Schanzer A, et al. Outcomes of carotid endarterectomy versus stenting in comparable medical risk patients. *J Vasc Surg*. 2014;60(5):1227–1231.

20. Centers for Medicare and Medicaid Services. *Decision memo for CAROTID artery stenting (CAG-00085R)*. https://www.cms.gov/medicare-coverage-database/details/nca-decision-memo.aspx?NCAId=157&NcaName=Carotid+Artery+Stenting+(1st+Recon)&fromdb=true; 2005. Accessed August 23, 2018.

21. Yadav JS, Wholey MH, Kuntz RE, et al. Protected carotid-artery stenting versus endarterectomy in high-risk patients. *N Engl J Med*. 2004;351(15):1493–1501.

22. Bertges DJ, Goodney PP, Zhao Y, et al. The Vascular Study Group of New England Cardiac Risk Index (VSG-CRI) predicts cardiac complications more accurately than the Revised Cardiac Risk Index in vascular surgery patients. *J Vasc Surg*. 2010;52(3):674–683. 683.el-683.e3.

23. Schermerhorn ML, Fokkema M, Goodney P, et al. The impact of Centers for Medicare and Medicaid Services high-risk criteria on outcome after carotid endarterectomy and carotid artery stenting in the SVS Vascular Registry. *J Vasc Surg*. 2013;57:1318–1324.

24. Galyfos S, Sianou A, Filis K. Cerebral hyperperfusion syndrome and intracranial hemorrhage after carotid endarterectomy or carotid stenting: a meta-analysis. *J Neurol Sci*. 2017;381:74–82.

25. Ascher E, Markevich N, Schutzer RW, et al. Cerebral hyperperfusion syndrome after carotid endarterectomy: predictive factors and hemodynamic changes. *J Vasc Surg*. 2003;37(4):769–777.

26. Silver FL, Mackey A, Clark WM, et al. Safety of stenting and endarterectomy by symptomatic status in the Carotid Revascularization Endarterectomy Versus Stenting Trial (CREST). *Stroke*. 2011;42(3):675–680.

27. Brott TG, Howard G, Roubin GS, et al. Long-term results of stenting versus endarterectomy for carotid-artery stenosis. *N Engl J Med*. 2016;374(11):1021–1031.

28. Rosenfield K, Matsumura JS, Chaturvedi S, et al. Randomized trial of stent versus surgery for asymptomatic carotid stenosis. *N Engl J Med*. 2016;374(11):1011–1020.

29. Kwolek CJ, Jaff MR, Ignacio Leal J, et al. Results of the ROADSTER multicenter trial of the transcarotid stenting with dynamic flow reversal. *J Vasc Surg*. 2015;62(5):1227–1234.

30. AbuRahma AF, Abu-Halimah S, Bensenhaver J, et al. Primary carotid artery stenting versus carotid artery stenting for postcarotid endarterectomy stenosis. *J Vasc Surg*. 2009;50(5):1031–1039.

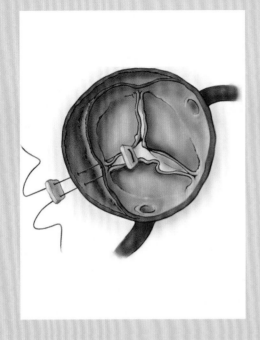

PART IX

第九部分

Aortic Dissection

主动脉夹层

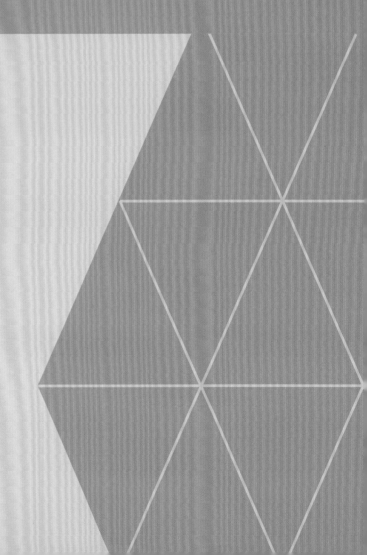

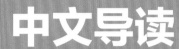

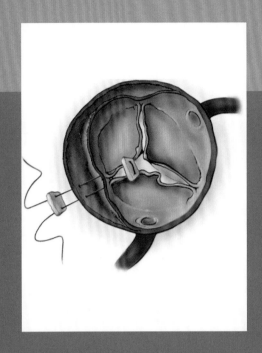

第32章
主动脉夹层的病理生理学、临床评估和药物治疗

　　急性主动脉夹层有较高的死亡率和并发症发生率，且疾病进展迅速，常需快速识别并及时药物和手术治疗以减少夹层所带来的灾难性后果。经临床多中心、内外科医师、科学家的共同努力，为主动脉夹层建立了分型和临床治疗策略，并描述和总结了主动脉夹层的临床特点、治疗方案、发病机制及遗传学特点，随着临床实践和科学研究进展，对于主动脉夹层的致病机制研究和治疗将进一步深入。鉴于主动脉夹层的严重危害及发病症状的多样性，对临床医师诊断的准确性和治疗及时性提出了更高要求，也对相关致病因素的科学认识和治疗提出了要求。本章将重点介绍夹层的分类、分期、诊断手段、临床表现、相应治疗措施和预后，并对主动脉夹层的临床流行病学特点、致病机制进行概述。

董念国

Pathophysiology, Clinical Evaluation, and Medical Management of Aortic Dissection

Brett J. Carroll, Bradley A. Maron, and Patrick T. O'Gara

Acute aortic dissection is an uncommon but life-threatening emergency that requires prompt diagnosis, rapid triage, and immediate treatment. A unified effort across several international centers over the past 20 years has resulted in the establishment of a detailed, prospective registry that describes the major aspects of the presentation, management, and outcomes of patients with acute aortic dissection.[1] This longitudinal experience has led to important clinical insights into an old disease and generated additional efforts to explore its genetics and pathobiology.[2]

Despite advancements in diagnostic and treatment modalities for acute aortic dissection, in-hospital mortality rates remain significantly elevated at 20%, with little change over the past decade.[3] Thus high-quality, prospective data to guide clinical management for acute aortic dissection are needed. In addition, enhanced awareness among practitioners regarding risk factors, presentation, diagnostic pathways, and treatment options for aortic dissection is a critical first step towards improving patient outcomes.[4]

EPIDEMIOLOGY

Published figures on the incidence of aortic dissection likely underestimate the actual occurrence rate because misdiagnosis is common and the percentage of acute aortic dissection patients who expire before hospital presentation is not known. Nonetheless, acute aortic dissection may, by conservative estimates, constitute 7% of all out-of-hospital cardiac arrests.[5,6] However, overall, acute aortic dissection is a rare event, which, in turn, may be responsible partly for its underrecognition in clinical practice. For example, analysis of the Swedish National Cause of Death Register between 1987 and 2002 estimated the incidence of thoracic aortic aneurysm or dissection to be 16.3 per 100,000 men and 9.1 per 100,000 women.[7] A population-based study in the United Kingdom reported an incidence of acute aortic dissection of 6 per 100,000 people per year among the general population.[8] More recently, a prospective cohort of patients with an average age of 58 years was longitudinally followed for a median of 16 years in Sweden.[9] The incidence of acute dissection was 15 per 100,000 patient years; others have reported acute aortic dissection affecting 30 per million individuals per year.[1] Acute myocardial infarction is 140-fold more common than aortic dissection, even by conservative estimates.[1] Data from the International Registry of Aortic Dissection (IRAD) support these epidemiological trends and show that the mean age of patients at presentation with aortic dissection is 62 years, with men accounting for 67% of cases.[3]

CLASSIFICATION

Classifying aortic dissection according to anatomic location and time from onset of symptoms helps to stratify risk and guide selection of initial treatment strategy (Fig. 32.1). The Stanford classification system designates dissections that involve the aorta proximal to the brachiocephalic artery (i.e., root and ascending aorta) as type A and those that do not as type B.[10] This distinction is clinically important because dissection involving the ascending aorta is a key determinate of early death and major morbidity. The location of the intimal tear does not influence Stanford dissection type. In the older DeBakey classification, a type I dissection *originates* within the ascending aorta and extends for a variable distance beyond the take-off of the innominate artery. A DeBakey type II dissection is confined to the ascending aorta, whereas a type III dissection originates in the descending thoracic aorta beyond the origin of the left subclavian artery and either terminates above (type IIIA) or extends below (type IIIB) the level of the diaphragm.[11] Although there is no single universally accepted classification system, the Stanford classification scheme is most often used currently in practice and will be used throughout this chapter. The terms "communicating" and "noncommunicating" refer to the presence or absence, respectively, of blood flow between the true and false lumens of the aorta.

Traditionally, aortic dissection was considered *acute* or *chronic* if presentation occurs within or after 14 days, respectively, of symptom onset. However, adverse remodeling of the aorta is evident 2 to 12 weeks following presentation, which is also a time frame associated with increased risk of complications and mortality (Fig. 32.2).[12-14] For this reason, a European interdisciplinary consensus group has proposed a subacute phase, defined as 2 to 6 weeks after presentation.[15] Based on data from IRAD, postaortic dissection chronology was refined further as follows: hyperacute (<24 hours), acute (2 to 7 days), subacute (8 to 30 days), and chronic (>30 days).[12]

In clinical practice, aortic dissection is diagnosed by imaging data that demonstrate an intimal flap with separation of true and false lumens. In type A dissection, the true lumen is usually displaced along the inner curvature of the aortic arch and continues caudally along the medial aspect of the descending thoracic aorta. Aortic branch vessel blood flow may derive from either the true or false lumen. Alternatively, flow may be sluggish or absent within the false lumen, or branch vessels may be completely occluded at or near their origins.

DeBakey Type I	Type II	Type III

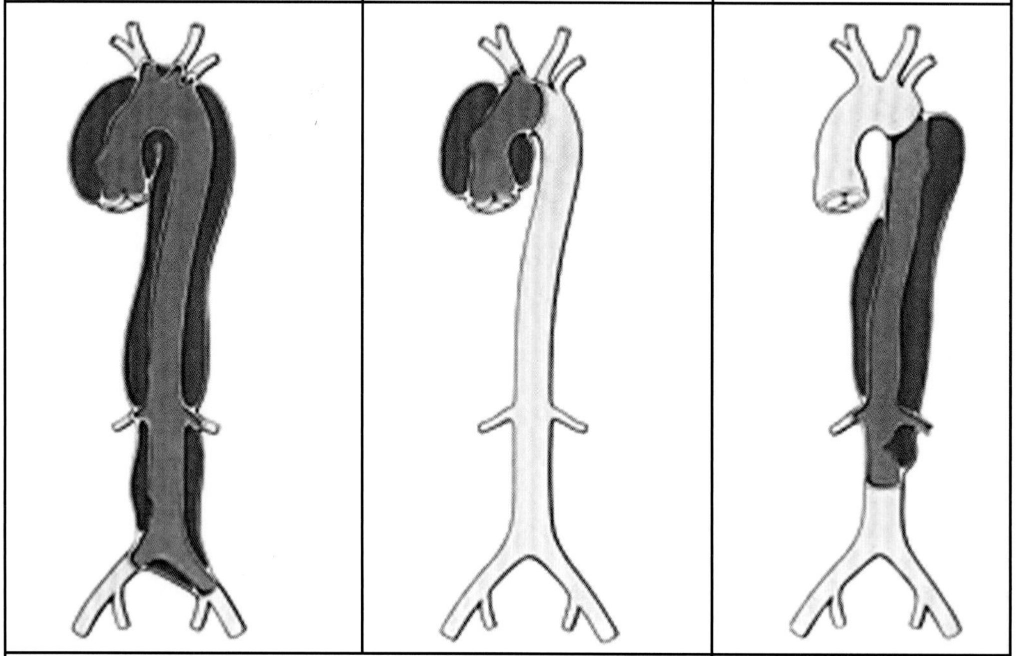

Stanford	Type A	Type B

DeBakey

Type I   Originates in the ascending aorta, propagates at least to the aortic arch and often beyond it distally

Type II   Originates in and is confined to the ascending aorta

Type III   Originates in the descending aorta and extends distally down the aorta or, rarely, retrograde into the aortic arch and ascending aorta

Stanford

Type A   All dissections involving the ascending aorta, regardless of the site of origin

Type B   All dissections not involving the ascending aorta

Hyperacute: Presentation within 24 hours of symptom onset

Acute: Presentation 2-7 days after symptom onset

Subacute: Presentation 8-30 days after symptom onset

Chronic: Presentation >30 days after symptom onset

Fig. 32.1 Aortic dissection type according to the DeBakey and Stanford classification systems. (From Nienaber CA, Eagle KA. Aortic dissection: new frontiers in diagnosis and management: Part I: from etiology to diagnostic strategies. *Circulation.* 2003;108:628–635.)

PATHOGENESIS

Forces that weaken the medial layer of the aorta increase the probability of dilation, aneurysm formation, and dissection (Box 32.1). Acquired and genetic diseases that mediate this process are discussed next. In classic aortic dissection, the initiating event is an intimal tear through which blood rapidly surges into the media under systolic pressure, splitting the layers of the aortic wall and creating an intimal flap that separates the true from the false lumen. The dissecting hematoma most commonly propagates distally (anterograde), although proximal (retrograde) or bidirectional migration is also observed.

Intimal Tear

Contemporary imaging modalities or autopsy findings identify the primary entry tear in approximately 90% of cases. The entry tear is most frequently located a few centimeters above the level of the aortic valve along the greater curvature of the aorta in cases of type A dissection and accounts for nearly 60% of all cases. Compared with other locations in the ascending aorta, the proximal few centimeters of the greater curvature are exposed to relatively greater hemodynamic, shear, and torsional forces. A pivot region located in the descending thoracic aorta just beyond the insertion of the ligamentum arteriosum, where the relatively mobile arch meets the fixed descending thoracic aorta, is the second most common entry site for intimal tears, which will then propagate as a type B dissection (30% of cases). Arch entry occurs in 7% of cases. The abdominal aorta is the least common site for entry (3% of cases) despite the high prevalence of intimal-medial ulcers in patients with atherosclerotic disease in this segment.[16–18]

The dissecting hematoma usually propagates in an anterograde direction, although retrograde extension can occur. By this mechanism,

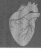

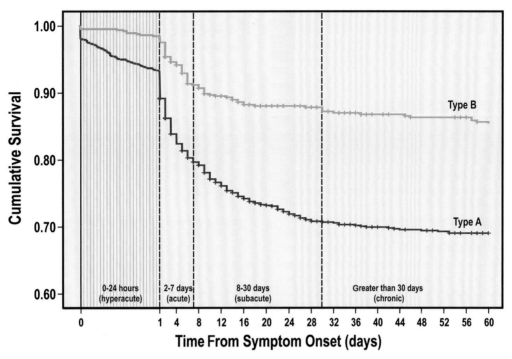

Fig. 32.2 60-day Kaplan-Meier survival curves for type A and type B acute aortic dissection from the International Registry of Aortic Dissection. (From Booher AM, Isselbacher EM, Nienaber CA, et al. The IRAD classification system for characterizing survival after aortic dissection. *Am J Med.* 2013;126:730.e19–e24.)

BOX 32.1 Aortic Dissection Predisposing Factors

Genetic

Marfan syndrome
Ehlers-Danlos syndrome
Familial thoracic aortic aneurysm disease
Bicuspid aortic valve disease
Aberrant right subclavian artery
Aortic coarctation
Noonan syndrome
Turner syndrome
Polycystic kidney disease
Loeys-Dietz syndrome

Acquired

Hypertension
Iatrogenic
Pregnancy
Inflammatory aortitis
Cocaine, chronic amphetamine use

as many as 20% of dissections that originate in the distal arch or descending thoracic aorta may involve the ascending aorta through retrograde extension.[19] Such dissections appear to have a comparable 5-year survival rate to those type B dissection without retrograde extension.[20] In rare cases, a second tear may occur, resulting in a three-channel dissection.[21]

Blood within the false lumen may reenter the true lumen anywhere along the length of the dissection. Reentry may be protective because of spontaneous decompression of the false lumen, which, in turn, may reduce the risks of rupture and/or the development of malperfusion syndromes.

Aortic Rupture and End-Organ Malperfusion

Aortic rupture, defined as a tearing in the vessel wall that results in extravascular hemorrhage, most commonly occurs with trauma and aortic transection but may occur secondary to dissection.[22] Rupture into the pericardial space resulting in cardiac tamponade may occur in type A dissection, whereas rupture into the left pleural space can be encountered with type B dissection. Dissection-mediated end-organ ischemia or infarction occurs from (i) mechanical compression of aortic branch vessels by false lumen hematoma, (ii) extension of the dissection plane across the ostium of the branch vessel, or (iii) dynamic vessel inlet obstruction caused by an oscillating intimal flap. Compromise of the coronary, brachiocephalic, mesenteric, renal, spinal, and iliac circulations can occur and result in a myriad of clinical presentations. Occlusion of the left ventricular (LV) outflow tract by an intimal flap has also been reported.

False Lumen Thrombosis

Thrombosis of blood within the false lumen may seal the entry tear, thus eliminating communication with the true lumen and preventing false lumen expansion. However, partial thrombosis of the false lumen has been identified as a risk factor for long-term death in patients with type B dissection.[23,24] Elevation of pressure within the false lumen with partial thrombosis may lead to further extrinsic compression of the true lumen and impairment of blood flow to critical organs. Alternatively, it has been proposed that partial thrombosis of the false lumen is associated with worse clinical outcomes via the promotion of vascular inflammation, tissue hypoxia, and/or neovascularization with weakening of adjacent vascular structures and an increased risk for aortic rupture.[24–28]

Persistent patency of the false lumen is also associated with a higher risk of long-term complications, such as late rupture or false aneurysm formation requiring operative intervention.[23,26–28] Although native aortic aneurysm disease is often a risk factor for dissection, a dissection need not result in aneurysm formation. The term "dissecting aneurysm" is an inaccurate anachronism because these diseases are not synonymous, a distinction that is particularly important when considering their natural histories and treatments.

PREDISPOSING GENETIC FACTORS

As is true for aneurysms, any process that leads to the destruction or degeneration of the major supporting elements of the aortic media (elastin, collagen, smooth muscle cells) can predispose to the development of dissection. The histopathologic term *medial degeneration* refers to the noninflammatory destruction or fragmentation of elastic lamellar units, dropout of vascular smooth muscle cells (VSMCs), and accumulation of mucopolysaccharide ground substances (not always in distinct cystic spaces), which characterize the final common pathway for a variety of processes that affect the integrity of the aortic media (Fig. 32.3). Although such changes predispose to aneurysm development, dissection may occur prior to significant aneurysm enlargement. In the GenTac registry of patients with a genetically associated thoracic aortic aneurysm, only 4 of the 31 patients (13%) with acute aortic dissection met criteria for intervention on predissection imaging.[2]

Marfan syndrome (MFS) is the most common inherited connective tissue disorder, with an estimated prevalence of 1 case per 3000 to 5000 individuals irrespective of racial, ethnic, or geographic considerations.[29–32] If untreated, aortic disease in MFS is progressive and incompatible with normal longevity. Of patients with aortic dissection younger than 40 years of age, half have a history of MFS.[33] However, medial degeneration is not pathognomonic of MFS and may be present in numerous other conditions.[34]

The clinical spectrum of MFS is heterogenous, although the presence of an aortic root aneurysm (aortic diameter z score ≥2) and ectopia lentis is sufficient to make the diagnosis even in the absence of a family history.[35] Conversely, in the absence of either of these two clinical features, the current Ghent nosology for MFS provides a scoring system based on the presence of an *FBN1* mutation and/or other key systemic features of MFS that can be used to make the diagnosis (Boxes 32.2 and 32.3). Systemic features that are suggestive of MFS include:

[a]Caveat: without discriminating features of Shprintzen-Goldberg syndrome, Loeys-Dietz syndrome, or vascular Ehlers-Danlos syndrome *and* after TGFBA1/2, collagen biochemistry, COL3A1 testing if indicated. Other conditions/genes will emerge with time.
In general, MFS is diagnosed in the presence of aortic root dilation/dissection and ectopia lentis; aortic root dilation/dissection plus *FBN1* mutation; aortic root dilation plus sufficient systemic findings (Box 32.3, ≥7 points); ectopia lentis plus a *FBN1* mutation previously associated with aortic disease; or, in an individual with a positive family history of MFS, the diagnosis is made in the presence of ectopia lentis, or a systemic score ≥7 points or aortic root dilation.
Ao, Aortic diameter at the sinuses of Valsalva above indicated *z* score or aortic root dissection; *EL*, ectopia lentis; *ELS*, ectopia lentis syndrome; *FBN1*, fibrillin-1 mutation; *FBN1 not known with Ao*, FBN1 mutation that has not previously been associated with aortic root aneurysm/dissection; *FBN1 with known Ao*, FBN1 mutation that has been identified in an individual with aortic aneurysm; *MASS*, myopia, mitral valve prolapse, borderline (z < 2) aortic root dilation, striae, skeletal findings phenotype; *MFS*, Marfan syndrome; *MVPS*, mitral valve prolapse syndrome; *Syst*, systemic score (see Box 32.3); *z*, z score.

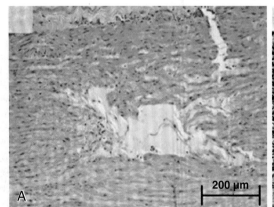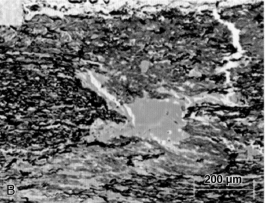

Fig. 32.3 Cystic Medial Degeneration. In (A), hematoxylin and eosin microscopic section of an aorta reveals fragmentation and loss of elastin fibers with cyst-like structures present within the media. In (B), Movat pentachrome stain emphasis medial interlamellar cystic "drop out." (From Maleszewski JJ, Miller DV, Lu J, et al. Histopathologic findings in ascending aortas from individuals with Loeys-Dietz Syndrome (LDS). *Am J Surg Pathol.* 2009;33:194–201.)

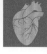

BOX 32.3 Scoring of Systemic Features of Marfan Syndrome

Wrist and thumb sign: 3 (wrist or thumb sign: 1)
Pectus carinatum deformity: 2 (pectus excavatum or chest asymmetry: 1)
Hindfoot deformity: 2 (plain pes planus: 1)
Pneumothorax: 2
Dural ectasia: 2
Protrusio acetabuli: 2
Reduced US/LS and increased arm/height and no severe scoliosis: 1
Scoliosis or thoracolumbar kyphosis: 1
Reduced elbow extension: 1
Facial features (3/5): 1 (dolichocephaly, enophthalmos, downslanting palpebral fissures, malar hypoplasia, retrognathia)
Skin striae: 1
Myopia > 3 diopters: 1
Mitral valve prolapse (all types): 1

Maximum total: 20 points; ≥7 indicates systemic involvement.
US/LS, Upper segment/lower segment ratio.
From Loeys BL, Dietz HC, Braverman AC, et al. The revised Ghent nosology for the Marfan syndrome. *J Med Genet.* 2010;47:476–485.

positive wrist sign (i.e., entire distal phalanx of the adducted thumb extends beyond the ulnar border of the palm); positive thumb sign (i.e., the tip of the thumb covers the entire fingernail of the fifth finger when wrapped around the contralateral wrist); pectus excavatum; pneumothorax; dural ectasia; hindfoot deformity; and protrusio acetabuli. Other clinical features less strongly associated with MFS include mitral valve prolapse, various abnormal facial features, and thoracolumbar kyphosis.

Limited forms (i.e., forme frustes) of MFS that feature cardiovascular manifestations include mitral valve prolapse syndrome (MVPS) (mitral valve prolapse, pectus excavatum, scoliosis, and mild arachnodactyly) and the MASS phenotype (myopia, mitral valve prolapse, borderline and nonprogressive aortic root dilation, skeletal findings and striae). There is increasing awareness of familial thoracic aortic aneurysm and dissection (FTAAD), although candidate genes affecting both matrix and smooth muscle cell components have been identified in only 20% of such patients. Vascular-type Ehlers-Danlos syndrome (EDS) is associated with arterial rupture and dissection, including of the aorta.[35,36]

MFS is a monogenic disorder caused by a variety of mutations in the *FBN1* gene, which encodes fibrillin-1, an extracellular matrix protein that is associated with elastic fibers. It was initially believed that loss of function of the *FBN1* gene directly affected the structural integrity of the extracellular matrix. Additional investigations have demonstrated that abnormal cell-signaling plays an important role.[37] Using an in vivo murine model of MFS, Dietz and colleagues demonstrated that fibrillin-1 is a key target for binding of latent transforming growth factor (TGF)-β by cytokines that acts as a "master-switch" regulator of inflammatory, profibrotic, and metalloproteinase signaling pathways in vascular endothelial cells and VSMCs.[38] Thus deficiency in fibrillin-1 leads to reduced TGF-β binding and the potential for enhanced activation of numerous cell-signaling pathways with alteration of the extracellular matrix.

Angiotensin I (AT-1)-mediated TGF-β activation has been studied as a pharmacologic target to inhibit or reverse aortic dilation in MFS. Habashi and colleagues studied the effects of losartan, an AT-1 receptor antagonist, on aortic aneurysm formation in transgenic mice encoding a cysteine to glutamine substitution at position 1039 in the *FBN-1* gene (Fbn1^C1039G/-). Mice expressing this particular fibrillin-1

mutation, the most common mutation with MFS, demonstrate significant and progressive aortic root dilation compared with control mice.[39] Treatment with losartan attenuated TGF-β signaling in the aortic wall and resulted in full normalization of aortic wall thickness, marked by improvement in aortic wall architecture (i.e., a decrease in elastin fiber disruption), compared with treatment with placebo or with the β-adrenergic receptor antagonist, propranolol.

In one small clinical trial of young MFS patients, losartan decreased the rate of aortic root growth significantly (mean change 0.46 ± 0.62 mm/year vs. 3.5 ± 2.8 mm/year prior to treatment, P < .001).[40] These findings were supported by the results of a randomized trial of losartan versus placebo in 116 adults with MFS, which demonstrated a decreased rate of aortic root dilatation in the losartan group, including those with prior aortic surgery. Notably, more than 70% of patients in both groups were also using β-adrenergic receptor antagonist therapy, raising the possibility that these two complimentary therapies may be synergistically effective.[41,42] Indeed, one small study of 28 patients with MFS found losartan added to a β-adrenergic receptor antagonist was associated with a slower rate of dilatation compared with the use of a β-adrenergic receptor antagonist alone.[43] The comparative efficacy of losartan versus atenolol was assessed in a larger randomized trial of 608 children and young adults with MFS. Contrary to expectations, neither the 3-year primary end points (rate of change in aortic root z scores) nor secondary end points of the trial differed between treatment groups. Both strategies resulted in a decrease in the rate of aortic root growth over time. In clinical practice, and in the absence of more effective therapies, MFS patients are frequently placed on maximally tolerated doses of both an angiotensin II type 1 receptor antagonist and a β-adrenergic receptor antagonist.

MFS is associated with a sixfold increased risk of dissection compared with the other monogenic causes of thoracic aneurysms.[2] In a Dutch review of 600 patients with MFS, risk factors for type B dissection included prior prophylactic aortic aneurysm surgery and proximal descending aortic diameter ≥27 mm. In this nonrandomized study, use of angiotensin II receptor blockade therapy was associated with a decrease in type B dissection of (HR 0.3; 95% CI: 0.1 to 0.9; P = .03) compared with patients not receiving angiotensin II receptor blockade.[44]

The Loeys-Dietz syndrome (LDS) is a related disorder caused by mutations in *TGFBR1* and *TGFBR2*, which regulate signal transduction of the TGF-β ligand. Phenotypical features of LDS include chest wall deformity, high-arched palate, bifid uvula, and hypertelorism. LDS is a diffuse arteriopathy that can cause tortuosity, dissection, and aneurysm disease of the peripheral arteries and aorta, and is a particularly aggressive form of arteriopathy with a mean age of death of 26 years.[45,46] It is recommended that aortic repair be considered at an internal diameter of ≥4.2 cm measured by echocardiography or ≥4.4 cm measured by computed tomography or magnetic resonance imaging (MRI) (external diameter),[6] because dissection in these patients frequently occurs at a diameter <5.0 cm.[45]

The EDS (1:5000 births) comprises a heterogeneous group of disorders characterized clinically by hypermobile joints, hyperextensile skin, and tissue fragility. Vascular-type EDS (type IV) is associated with spontaneous vascular rupture and dissection. Aortic involvement occurs in EDS type IV, an autosomal dominant disorder attributed to structural defects in the pro-α1 (III) chain of type III collagen, encoded by the *COL3A1* gene on chromosome 2q31.[47] Associated clinical features of EDS type IV include thin skin, easy bruising, and visceral and uterine rupture. Median survival is 48 years, and the most common cause of death is arterial dissection or rupture.[48]

The FTAAD phenotype is specific for aortic pathology and does not involve extra-aortic disease. FTAAD has been mapped to several genetic loci, including 16p13.11 (*MYH11* gene), 5q13-14, and

11q23.2-q24, which are not associated with abnormalities of fibrillin or collagen.[49,50] More than five mutations in the *FBN-1* gene have been identified in patients with familial or spontaneous thoracic aortic aneurysm and dissection, with histopathologic changes characteristic of medial degeneration, yet with no demonstrable abnormalities of collagen or fibrillin in fibroblast culture.[51,52]

Polymorphisms encoding vitamin K epoxide reductase complex subunit 1 (*VKORC1*) result in undercarboxylation of specific matrix proteins and are associated with calcification of the arterial wall. In patients carrying the C allele (CT or CC), a relative twofold increase in the probability of developing aortic dissection has been observed.[53] A missense mutation in the *ACTA2* gene that encodes for actin filaments in VSMCs is linked to 14% of patients with FTAAD.[54] As a consequence of this mutation, intracellular actin filament assembly is disrupted, promoting focal areas of VSMC disarray, decreased VSMC contraction, and medial degeneration of the aorta. This phenotype is believed to be associated with weakening of the aortic wall and increased predisposition to dissection.

More recently, defects in the *MYLK* and *PRKG1* genes have been implicated in the development of thoracic aortic aneurysm via disruption of normal actin-myosin interaction. *MYLK* encodes myosin light chain kinase, and *PRKG1* disinhibits activity of the type 1 cGMP-dependent protein kinase, which is an inhibitor of myosin light chain phosphatase and thus a negative regulator of actin-myosin physical associations.[37,55]

Bicuspid aortic valve (BAV) disease is the most common congenital cardiac anomaly in adults (4:1000 live births) and is often accompanied by an aortopathy that is histologically similar to but less severe than that observed in patients with MFS. Dilatation of the root and more commonly of the ascending aorta is present in up to 40% of patients with BAV disease and is a risk factor for dissection or rupture. It appears to be inherited in an autosomal dominant pattern with incomplete penetrance.[56] Pathogenesis of aortic dissection in BAV patients is possibly due to interplay between hemodynamic and histologic processes that weaken the aortic wall. In particular, some reports indicate that BAV patients have a thinner intima and decreased smooth muscle actin expression.[57,58]

Although BAV is associated with aortic aneurysm and dissection, recent guidelines have increased the recommended size threshold for prophylactic surgical intervention from 5.0 to 5.5 cm in the absence of a family history of acute aortic syndrome, an annual increase in size of ≥0.5 cm, or the need for surgical aortic valve replacement for severe valve disease. This is the same size criterion applied to patients with ascending aortic aneurysm disease without BAV.[59] Single-center observational data of patients with acute dissection have demonstrated that BAV patients have larger aortic diameters at presentation than patients with trileaflet aortic valves.[60]

Similar histopathological changes have been described in patients with aortic coarctation (many of whom have BAV disease), Noonan syndrome, Turner syndrome, and polycystic kidney disease.

ACQUIRED DISORDERS

There are numerous acquired disorders that contribute to aortic dissection. The incidence of aortic dissection increases with age (27 per 100,000 for 65 to 75 years old and 35 per 100,000 for ≥75 years old).[8] Dissection is also more common in men; women tend to be older with more atypical symptoms, delayed diagnosis, and an overall higher mortality (30% vs. 21%).[61] Systemic hypertension is the most common modifiable risk factor for aortic dissection and is present in approximately 75% of patients.[3,62] Hypertension accelerates the normal aging process and leads to intimal thickening, VSMC apoptosis, vascular fibrosis, loss of elasticity, and compromise of nutritive blood supply (see Chapter 3). Decreased aortic compliance and vulnerability to pulsatile

forces predispose to injury and create a substrate for dissection. In one report, ambulatory blood pressure was higher in those who did not survive to hospital admission with aortic dissection.[8] However, aortic diameter is the strongest predictor of dissection in patients without an underlying genetic predisposing disorder.[62,63]

Iatrogenic Dissection

In the IRAD registry, iatrogenic aortic dissection after cardiac surgery or catheterization accounted for 5% of the total reported, although the association of dissection with prior cardiac surgery may be even more frequent, because 16% of those in the registry had a history of cardiac surgery.[3,64] Older age, hypertension, and severe peripheral vascular disease are risk factors associated with procedure-related dissection.[65] Pain may be absent in iatrogenic dissection. In one review of three European hospitals, aortic dissection complicated 0.06% of the 108,083 cardiac catheterizations. Short- and long-term outcomes following iatrogenic dissection were good, with stent implantation when a coronary artery was involved and conservative therapy in the majority of the remainder. Need for cardiac surgery was rare, with an overall low mortality and long-term complication rate.[66] Retrograde dissections created at the time of catheterization usually seal spontaneously on withdrawal of the catheter. Aortic atherosclerotic plaques may prevent the longitudinal propagation of a dissection. Dissections arising from sites where the aorta has been incised or cross-clamped may occur intraoperatively or at any time following surgery.

Deceleration injury from high-speed accidents results in aortic transection with false aneurysm formation and rupture, most commonly in the region of the aortic isthmus just beyond the origin of the left subclavian artery. Transection results in a transmural tear that is different both pathologically and etiologically from aortic dissection.

Dissection in Pregnancy

Risk of aortic dissection is fourfold higher during pregnancy but is a rare complication with an estimated incidence of 5.5 per 1 million.[67] However, by some estimates, 50% of all dissections in women younger than the age of 40 occur during labor, delivery, or early following birth.[68] Histopathologic changes affecting the aortic media of pregnant women have been described, including alterations in elastic fibers and VSMCs.[69] Both estrogen and relaxin are associated with alterations in matrix metalloproteinase (MMP) homeostasis and contribute to vascular remodeling and a susceptibility to injury, independent of the hemodynamic stress of labor and delivery. In many cases, pregnancy "unmasks" primary conditions that predispose to aortic dissection (e.g., MFS). In those patients with preexisting MFS or BAV disease, aortic root size >4.0 cm is a contraindication to pregnancy due to the increased risk for spontaneous rupture or dissection.[6]

Drug Use and Other Acquired Conditions

Recent cocaine use, particularly among young men who smoke tobacco, is an additional risk factor for aortic dissection.[70] Among 38 patients with acute aortic dissection occurring over a 20-year period in an urban center, 37% reported cocaine (in particular, crack cocaine) use within the preceding 24 hours (mean, 12 hours). Chronic amphetamine use and/or dependence appears to increase the probability of developing a thoracoabdominal aortic dissection in those aged 18 to 49 years.[71] The presumed mechanisms for aortic injury from cocaine and amphetamine use involve oxidant stress–mediated endothelial dysfunction and extreme catecholamine-induced shear forces with abrupt hypertension and tachycardia, which collectively lead to weakening of the aortic media and predisposition to tearing. Current or past use of fluoroquinolones has also been associated with increased risk of aortic aneurysm or dissection.[72]

Inflammatory diseases of the aorta can lead to destruction of extracellular matrix proteins and VSMCs, with subsequent aneurysm formation and/or dissection. Aortic dissection has been reported in patients with Takayasu arteritis, giant cell aortitis, Behçet disease, relapsing polychondritis, systemic lupus erythematosus, and the aortitis associated with inflammatory bowel disease.[6] In contrast, syphilitic aortitis does not predispose to dissection, perhaps because of intense, reactive medial scarring and fibrosis that occur in response to the spirochetal infection. Pheochromocytoma and weight lifting (believed due to intense or repetitious Valsalva maneuvers) also predispose to aortic dissection.

CLINICAL PRESENTATION

The most important element of any diagnostic algorithm for a suspected acute aortic syndrome is a high clinical index of suspicion, based foremost on the presenting history and physical examination (Box 32.4). Absent an appreciation of the cardinal features of dissection, the diagnosis can be missed in a substantial number of patients. Simple clinical prediction rules have been developed to estimate the probability of acute aortic dissection.[73] The IRAD investigators have confirmed the sensitivity of 12 clinical risk markers proposed in the 2010 Thoracic ACCF/AHA Aortic Disease Guidelines.[6] These markers, assessed at the bedside, can be divided into three distinct categories: predisposing factors, characteristics of the pain at time of presentation, and key physical examination findings.[74,75] The presence of risk factors from at least one category identified 95.7% of acute aortic dissection patients in the IRAD database. Utilization of the risk score in two clinical centers found a sensitivity and specificity of 91% and 40%, respectively, when any one risk marker was present. However, specificity increased to 86% when >1 risk marker was present.[76]

History

The diagnosis of aortic dissection may be missed on initial clinical evaluation in approximately one-third of cases, and an equal number are detected only at autopsy.[77] Chest pain is the dominant feature of the clinical presentation and occurs in 85% of type A and 67% of type B dissections.[3] It is qualitatively severe and may in many cases be distinguished from coronary ischemia by *abrupt* onset and maximal intensity at inception. More than 84% of aortic dissection patients described chest pain as "worst ever" in the IRAD registry.[2,78] The pain is characterized as sharp more often than tearing or ripping in nature and may radiate or be sensed anteriorly (suggestive of type A dissection) or in the interscapular, lower back, or abdominal area (suggestive of type B dissection). Back pain is more common in type B dissection (occurring in 70%), although not infrequent in type A dissections (occurring in 43%).[3] Visceral discomfort or limb pain may be indicative of aortic branch vessel ischemia from malperfusion.

BOX 32.4	Acute Aortic Syndromes

Aortic dissection
Intramural hematoma
Penetrating aortic ulcer
Rapid aneurysm expansion
Trauma

Modified from Hiratzka LF, Bakris GL, Beckman JA, et al. 2010 ACCF/AHA/AATS/ACR/ASA/SCA/SCAI/SIR/STS/SVM guidelines for the diagnosis and management of patients with thoracic aortic disease. *J Am Coll Cardiol.* 2010;55:e27–e129.

Syncope is a particularly ominous presenting symptom and may reflect cardiac tamponade from intrapericardial aortic rupture, cerebral malperfusion, and/or neurally mediated hypotension in response to the intense pain of the dissection and occurs in almost 20% of those with a type A dissection.[3] In the IRAD registry, patients with syncope were more likely to die in the hospital or suffer stroke. Neurologic complications are noted in up to 20% of aortic dissection patients. For example, paraplegia may develop when critical impairment of flow to the anterior spinal artery, thoracic intercostals, or the artery of Adamkiewicz occurs. Abdominal pain is an underrecognized symptom of acute aortic dissection; when present, it is associated with elevated in-hospital mortality and increased frequency of malperfusion syndromes.[6,73,74]

Numerous other less common clinical manifestations of aortic dissection may be evident on initial evaluation and include Horner syndrome (compression of the superior cervical ganglion), hoarseness (pressure against the recurrent laryngeal nerve), hemoptysis (rupture into a bronchus), hematemesis (perforation into the esophagus), ischemic enterocolitis (mesenteric artery compromise), and fever of undetermined source (pyrogens released from the false lumen).

Physical Examination

Patients with acute aortic dissection appear ill, uncomfortable, and apprehensive.

Hypertension is present in more than two-thirds of type B dissection patients and in approximately one-third of type A patients.[1,6] A murmur of aortic regurgitation can be heard in approximately 40% of patients with type A dissection.[64] Due to rapid equilibration of aortic and LV diastolic pressure, the murmur is usually of shorter duration, lower in pitch, and of lesser intensity than the diastolic murmur of chronic severe aortic regurgitation. Additional auscultatory findings include a soft first heart sound and a grade 1 or 2 midsystolic murmur at the base or along the left sternal border.

Pulse deficits occur in 31% of patients with a type A and 19% with a type B dissection.[3] An inverse correlation between the presence of pulse deficits and mortality is observed in acute aortic dissection.[79] Furthermore, pulse deficits may obscure accurate blood pressure assessment, which arises from an inability to measure the central aortic pressure when bilateral subclavian and/or femoral artery compromise is present. Thus invasive intraarterial monitoring may be necessary in some aortic dissection patients.

Elevation of the jugular venous pressure, especially with pulsus paradoxus, may indicate pericardial involvement with tamponade. Superior vena cava syndrome can rarely occur with compression by an expanding false aneurysm along the greater curvature of the ascending aorta. Thoracic dullness to percussion with decreased breath sounds suggests pleural effusion, which is more common in the left chest and is not necessarily indicative of rupture. In fact, pleural effusions are quite frequent with both type A and B dissections and are usually sympathetic in nature, reflective of the intense inflammation associated with the acute tear.

LABORATORY TESTING

Biomarkers

Plasma smooth muscle myosin heavy chain protein, D dimer, and high-sensitivity C-reactive protein (CRP) have been proposed as potentially useful biomarkers to assist with diagnosis of aortic dissection. In one study of 95 patients with acute aortic dissection, elevated levels of circulating smooth muscle myosin heavy chain protein (>2.5 μg/L) had a sensitivity of 90% and a specificity of 98% when measured within 3 hours of presentation.[80] In this analysis, smooth muscle myosin heavy chain protein levels were elevated in all patients presenting with a proximal or type A dissection.

Soluble elastin fragment (sELAF) levels have also been proposed to be a useful biomarker for the early detection of acute aortic dissection. Despite a natural rise with age in plasma concentration sELAF levels, a level >3 standard deviations above normal for age is associated with a 64% positivity rate in acute aortic dissection compared with 2% for patients with acute myocardial infarction. Interestingly, patients with complete false lumen thrombosis, which is associated with improved prognosis in chronic type B dissections, appear to have no detectable sELAF.[81,82]

Suzuki and colleagues conducted a multicenter study of 220 patients with suspected acute aortic dissection.[83] A D-dimer level of <500 ng/mL when drawn within 24 hours of symptom onset was associated with a negative likelihood ratio for aortic dissection of 0.07. D dimer may be most helpful when incorporated within the context of a patient's presentation. A recent large meta-analysis of 1557 patients found a sensitivity of 98% and negative likelihood ratio of 0.05; however, specificity was low at 42% with a positive likelihood ratio of 2.11. A negative D dimer used in a low-risk population had a posttest probability of acute aortic dissection of 0.3%.[84] Consistent with these findings, a recent prospective, multicenter trial evaluated D dimer and the aortic dissection detection risk score and demonstrated a false negative rate of 0.3% when patients had a negative D dimer and a risk score of ≤1.[85] Plasma MMP-8 and MMP-9 are also increased in patients with acute aortic dissection but are of uncertain diagnostic relevance. In one small study, normal MMP-8, MMP-9, and D dimer had a negative predictive value of 100%, although additional data are needed to characterize the role of this approach.[86]

An early, rapid increase in CRP levels following acute aortic dissection has been observed, with levels falling rapidly 24 hours following symptom onset.[87] Calponin, a counterpart protein to troponin in VSMCs, may provide enhanced specificity for early detection of type A aortic dissection but requires future comprehensive testing in advance of clinical application.[88]

Other Point-of-Care Tests

The chest x-ray is abnormal in 80% to 90% of patients with aortic dissection but is an insufficient tool to "rule out" this condition, particularly when pathology is confined to the ascending aorta.[89] Findings suggestive of aortic dissection include: mediastinal widening, which is present in more than 50% of type A dissections[3]; disparity in the caliber of the ascending and descending thoracic aortic segments; localized bulge or angulation along the normally smooth border of the aorta; displacement of intimal calcium (especially in the region of the aortic knob); and a double aortic contour. Associated findings may include cardiomegaly (pericardial effusion) and pleural effusion (left > right). Effusions that occupy more than 50% of the chest cavity may be indicative of rupture with hemothorax.

Nonspecific electrocardiographic (ECG) repolarization abnormalities are present in approximately 40% of dissection patients.[64] Changes indicative of active ischemia may be found in 15% of patients, and findings suggestive of acute myocardial infarction (new Q waves, ST segment elevation) are present in a small minority (3%) of cases.[64] A thorough assessment is critical to avoid the initiation of acute reperfusion therapy in this setting.

DIAGNOSTIC IMAGING

Retrograde aortography, the original diagnostic "gold standard" for aortic dissection, has been replaced by transesophageal echocardiography (TEE) and computed tomographic angiography (CTA). A re-view of temporal trends in diagnostic testing in IRAD showed CT has become the initial diagnostic modality in almost 75% of patients. By contrast, TEE is used less frequently, with only 25% of type A dissections diagnosed initially through this modality.[3] MRI/magnetic resonance angiography (MRA) is performed much less frequently in the acute setting. The sensitivity and specificity of these three noninvasive techniques are essentially equivalent and exceed 90% in most series.[6] The choice of imaging technique depends chiefly on availability, speed, safety, and local expertise in performance and interpretation. A second test is frequently needed for clarification when the first study is abnormal but nondiagnostic. Regardless of the diagnostic sequence used, an institutional commitment to rapid imaging of critically ill patients is key. The essential features to be defined for both treatment and prognosis include: the presence or absence of ascending aortic involvement, entry and reentry sites, pericardial and aortic valve involvement, the extent of the dissection, major branch vessel compromise, and the anatomic substrate for potential malperfusion syndrome(s).

Transesophageal Echocardiography (Fig. 32.4)

A surface transthoracic echocardiogram (TTE) alone is not sufficient for diagnosis and characterization of aortic dissection in most cases.[90] However, when combined with TEE, the sensitivity and specificity of these tests reaches 99% and 89%, respectively.[90] With increasing use of bedside ultrasonography in the emergency department, TTE may be helpful in the initial evaluation for pericardial effusion or severity of aortic regurgitation. However, TTE should not delay performing TEE, which can be accomplished at the bedside in the emergency department or in the operating room within 15 to 20 minutes in many centers. Oropharyngeal anesthesia and conscious sedation are required with simultaneous monitoring of the heart rate and rhythm, blood pressure, and oxygen saturation. Orthogonal and longitudinal scan planes combined with M-mode, two-dimensional, and Doppler profile interrogation provide information regarding: (1) entry and reentry sites; (2) the longitudinal extent and oscillation of the intimal flap; (3) flow velocity and direction within the true and false lumens; (4) spontaneous contrast or thrombus within the false lumen; (5) aortic valve competence and the mechanism of regurgitation; (6) ostial coronary artery involvement; (7) pericardial effusion; and (8) global and

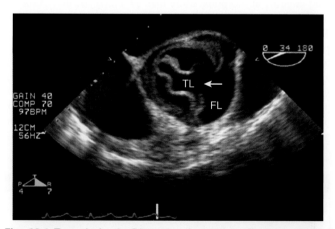

Fig. 32.4 Type A Aortic Dissection Imaged by Transesophageal Echocardiography. Horizontal plane transesophageal echocardiographic image of Stanford type A aortic dissection reveals a true lumen *(TL)* diminished in size and false lumen *(FL)* extending circumferentially. A communication through the dissection flap that joins the TL and FL is present *(arrow)*. (From Meredith EL, Masani ND. Echocardiography in the emergency assessment of acute aortic syndromes. *Eur J Echocardiogr.* 2009;10:i31–i39.)

regional LV function. In most cases the true lumen is differentiated from the false lumen by observing systolic expansion and diastolic collapse, absence or minimal spontaneous echo contrast, and/or an antegrade Doppler signal. However, vessel diameter alone is *not* sufficient for making this determination. In ambiguous cases (e.g., with a large false lumen), a pressure gradient between true and false lumen between 10 and 25 mm Hg may be observed by continuous wave Doppler interrogation.[91,92]

A series of TEE "blind spots" lie in the distal portion of the ascending aorta, anterior portion of the aortic arch, and anterior to the trachea and left main stem bronchus. Signal dropout may occur in the presence of free fluid around the aorta or pericardium, present in some cases of traumatic aortic penetration.

Computed Tomographic Angiography (Fig. 32.5)

Multislice CTA using rapid acquisition protocols and postprocessing of the volumetric data (multiplanar reformatting, maximum intensity pro-

jection, shaded surface display, volumetric rendering) provides highly detailed and visually familiar anatomic images (see Chapter 14). The diagnostic accuracy of 64-slice CTA approaches 100% for aortic dissection.[93] The intimal flap appears as a thin, low-attenuation, linear or spiral structure that separates the true and false lumens. Additional findings include displacement of intimal calcium, delayed contrast enhancement of the false lumen, and aortic widening. Branch vessel involvement anywhere along the course of the aorta to the level of the iliac arteries can be precisely displayed. In addition, CTA can visualize the proximal third of the coronary arteries. Limitations to CTA include exposure to intravenous (IV) contrast and ionizing radiation. In addition, CTA is an anatomic study; neither aortic valve nor LV function can be rapidly assessed. Motion artifact, mural thrombi, and image artifacts may negatively affect study accuracy.[93] Dedicated emergency department scanners are now widespread, and studies can be obtained, reconstructed, and interpreted within 15 to 20 minutes. CTA has several advantages relative to MRA, including wider availability, quicker throughput,

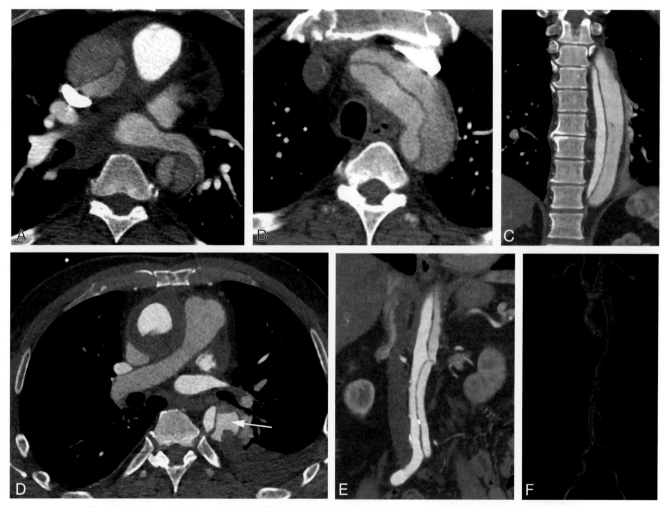

Fig. 32.5 Computed Tomographic (CT) of a Type A Dissection Prerepair and Post Repair With Residual Descending Aortic Dissection. A 64-year-old man presented with chest pain for which CT angiography was performed to evaluate for pulmonary embolism. He was found to have a type A dissection (A, axial image; B, axial image of aortic arch; C, coronal image of descending aortic dissection) and underwent ascending aortic repair. One month follow-up CT angiography: (D) Axial image of intact ascending aortic repair with a residual postoperative hematoma surrounding the graft and a residual dissection flap in the descending aorta with partial thrombosis of the false lumen *(arrow)*. There is also a residual left pleural effusion. (E) Sagittal image of residual dissection involving the origin of the left renal artery and continuing into the abdominal aorta and iliac arteries. (F) Three-dimensional reconstruction demonstrating the ascending repair with dilation of the arch and residual dissection flap.

higher spatial resolution, absence of arterial flow-related artifacts, and the capability to visualize calcification and metallic implants.

Magnetic Resonance Imaging/Angiography (Fig. 32.6) (Also See Chapter 13)

Contemporary MRI technology affords rapid scanning with the ability to cover a wide field of view and a comprehensive analysis of dissection anatomy and extra-aortic involvement.[93,94] MRI allows for the assessment of pericardial involvement, aortic regurgitation, proximal coronary artery involvement, and LV function. ECG-gating software allow for expedited scanning across multiple levels during a single breath hold. Despite these advances, MRI is infrequently used as the initial imaging study in patients with suspected acute aortic syndromes. Reasons for its limited use in the acute setting include lack of widespread availability, difficulties with patient transport to and monitoring within MRI scanners, and the presence of implanted cardiac devices or metallic clips. Nevertheless, MRI can provide excellent imaging of false lumen thrombus, intramural hematoma (IMH), and penetrating atherosclerotic ulcers.[93,94]

Invasive Aortography

The risk for catheter-related injury, length of time required to assemble the necessary personnel in an emergency situation, use of contrast and ionizing radiation, low sensitivity (77%), and availability of highly accurate noninvasive imaging techniques have eliminated the use of invasive aortography as an initial diagnostic test for acute aortic dissection.[95,96] Aortography is particularly limited in diagnosing non-communicating aortic dissections, IMHs, and penetrating ulcers.[95,97] Inadvertent injection into the false lumen or equal and rapid opacification of true and false lumens without obvious aortic dilatation may make the correct diagnosis of aortic dissection difficult. Invasive angiography is a feature of any catheter-based intervention.

Intravascular Ultrasound

Low-frequency (<20 MHz) intravascular ultrasound (IVUS) affords maximal signal penetration of the aortic wall and nearly 100% diagnostic accuracy for aortic dissection with a procedure that can be completed in less than 10 minutes, and it allows for better evaluation of the descending and abdominal aorta than does TEE.[96,98] This method provides clear delineation of several key findings, including: entry points, longitudinal and circumferential extent, luminal dimensions and contour, and thrombus if present. IVUS can be used as a second imaging technique for diagnosis in patients in whom false negative results on invasive aortography are suspected and femoral access has been obtained. IVUS may also have a role during performance of endovascular procedures.

Coronary Angiography

Selective coronary angiography is neither indicated nor advisable in anticipation of emergency surgery for type A dissection.[99] Operative mortality is generally not related to myocardial ischemia but rather to aortic rupture, and the performance of angiography consumes valuable time before life-saving surgery. Routine preoperative coronary angiography for hemodynamically stable, chronic type A dissection patients is a subject of debate.[92,99] Preoperative coronary angiography is reasonable in select type A dissection patients who have a history of previous coronary artery bypass graft surgery or in type B patients with acute coronary syndrome prior to planned aortic and/or coronary intervention. Other clinical exigencies may pertain that require surgical judgment, but these are infrequent.

DIFFERENTIAL DIAGNOSIS

Other Acute Aortic Syndromes

Aortic transection from deceleration injury and traumatic aortic valve disruption with acute severe aortic regurgitation occur in the setting of high-speed motor vehicle accidents or vertical falls. However, the nontraumatic acute aortic syndromes are often *not* distinguishable from classic dissection on clinical grounds alone but rather are delineated with cross-sectional imaging.

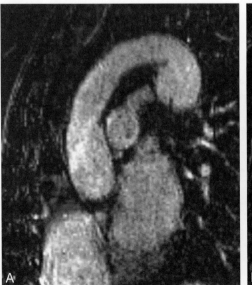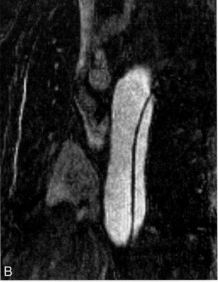

Fig. 32.6 Magnetic Resonance Angiography After Aneurysm Repair With Type B Dissection. A 50-year-old woman with Marfan syndrome underwent magnetic resonance angiography in follow-up of prior ascending aortic aneurysm repair with subsequent type B aortic dissection and graft to segment of infrarenal aorta. Sagittal images of prior ascending aortic repair (A) with descending aortic dissection flap (B).

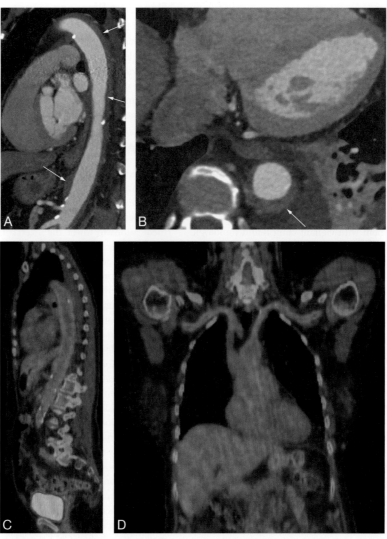

Fig. 32.7 Computed Tomographic Angiography and Positron Emission Tomography of Type B Intramural Hematoma (IMH). An 81-year-old woman with history of giant cell arteritis presented with type B intramural hematoma *(arrows)* from left subclavian artery to infrarenal aorta on computed tomographic angiography (A, sagittal image; B, axial image). Positron emission tomography (PET) was performed to evaluate for evidence of active inflammation after vascular duplex ultrasound demonstrated subclavian and axillary artery wall thickening. PET scan demonstrated FDG avidity in the aorta as expected with acute IMH (C, sagittal image) but also in the subclavian arteries and iliac arteries (D, coronal image). The patient was initiated on tocilizumab in addition to prednisone for increased immunosuppression.

Aortic Intramural Hematoma (Fig. 32.7)

IMH is defined as a contained collection of blood within the wall of the aorta without evidence of an intimal flap, entry tear, or double lumen. Mechanisms to account for IMH include primary rupture of the nutrient vasa vasorum or a limited intimal tear that cannot be detected with imaging.[100–102] IMH is observed clinically in 6% to 20% of cases of suspected acute aortic dissection and is discovered at autopsy in 5% to 13% of acute aortic syndrome cases.[6,101,103] It is believed the inciting event in IMH is rupture of the vasa vasorum causing bleeding into the aortic media; however, it can progress to dissection if the intimal layer ruptures.[104] In IRAD, IMH more frequently involved the descending aorta (58%) than the ascending aorta (42%).[103] Approximately 10% of aortic IMHs undergo spontaneous resorption.

Predicting evolution of IMH to dissection, rupture, aneurysm formation, or false aneurysm development is difficult. Type A IMH thickness >11 mm is an independent risk factor for death, surgery, or progression to dissection.[102,105] Likewise, an ascending aortic diameter >4.8 cm is a high-risk feature.[6,100–102,105] Lack of β-adrenergic receptor antagonist use may also be associated with lesion progression.[103]

Aortic IMH is generally managed with the same principles that pertain to aortic dissection. In IRAD, medical management was more frequently pursued in patients with type B IMH compared with classic aortic dissection (89% vs. 64%). There was no difference in rate of operative management for type A IMH and classic dissection. In-hospital and 1-year mortality rates were similar between IMH and classic dissection. Observations suggest thoracic endovascular repair in type B IMH with high-risk features should be considered.[106]

Diagnosis of IMH by TEE requires visualization of crescentic or circumferential wall thickening >0.7 cm or the identification of fresh thrombus within the aortic wall. CTA and MRA are more accurate than TEE for distinguishing IMH from aortic aneurysm with mural thrombus, severe atherosclerosis, or aortitis with medial inflammation and edema.

Penetrating Aortic Ulcer (Fig. 32.8)

An inflamed atherosclerotic plaque that disrupts the normal architecture of the aortic wall may result in erosion of the internal elastic membrane, thus allowing luminal blood to burrow into the media of the aorta and beyond. Penetrating aortic ulcers (PAUs) are most commonly seen in the mid-\to-distal descending thoracic aorta in older persons with a heavy burden of atherosclerotic disease and appear as irregular craters or outpouchings of contrast. They may result in IMH formation or frank dissection. Ganaha and colleagues observed in a retrospective analysis of 65 symptomatic IMH patients with PAU that ulcer depth (>1.0 cm) and diameter (>2.0 cm) positively correlated with disease progression (i.e., IMH expansion, aortic rupture, propagation of dissection).[107] Others suggest that PAU location in the proximal segment of the descending thoracic aorta and refractory symptoms rather than the presence of an ulcer per se is most worrisome.[108] Medical management with vigilant clinical and radiologic follow-up is advised for the initially uncomplicated descending thoracic PAU. Such a strategy appears to be associated with low rates of rupture and complications in asymptomatic patients.[109] Surgery or endovascular stent grafting when feasible can be undertaken for failed medical therapy, pseudoaneurysm formation, or rupture, and in observational studies has shown good procedural success and results in midterm follow-up.[110]

Acute Aneurysm Expansion

Acute, painful expansion of a previously established aortic aneurysm may herald impending rupture. Aortic aneurysm due to atherosclerosis (especially abdominal or descending thoracic in location) is particularly susceptible to sudden expansion, although this phenomenon can also occur with aortitis and other aortopathies such as MFS. Imaging studies in patients with atherosclerotic or inflammatory aortic disease may reveal wall thickening and periaortic stranding or hematoma, as well as a measurable increase in aortic dimensions when compared with available past studies. Although rapid expansion of the aorta in MFS is not related to inflammation, it is particularly concerning given risk of further progression and warrants urgent surgical referral.

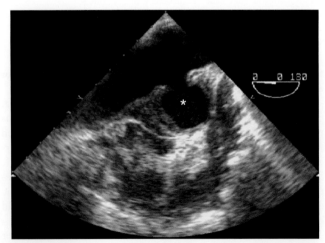

Fig. 32.8 Penetrating Atherosclerotic Ulcer. Transesophageal echocardiographic image of the anterior aortic arch wall demonstrates an outpouching from an ulcer-like crater *(asterisk)*. (From Firschke C, Orban M, Andrássy P, et al. Penetrating atherosclerotic ulcer of the aortic arch. *Circulation.* 2003;108:e14–e15.)

Nonaortic Diseases

Chest or back pain may be the presenting symptom of a variety of conditions, including acute coronary syndrome, pericarditis, musculoskeletal pain, pulmonary embolism, pneumonia, pleuritis, and cholecystitis. Attention to the patient's description of the nature and quality of the pain, the presence of predisposing factors, the physical examination, and the initial laboratory studies should allow early differentiation.

INITIAL MEDICAL TREATMENT (Fig. 32.9)

It is estimated that half of patients with acute type A dissection will die prior to arrival to the hospital. Those patients who do survive to the hospital are often ill and at high risk for rapid clinical decompensation.[5,8]

Patients with acute aortic syndromes should be treated with IV medications to lower the arterial blood pressure as expeditiously as possible. Because aortic wall strain is a function of LV contraction velocity (expressed mathematically as change in pressure divided by change in time, [dP/dT]), β-adrenergic receptor antagonists, given to attenuate LV systolic contractile force *and* decrease heart rate, are first line therapeutic agents (Table 32.1). In patients with a contraindication or intolerance to β-adrenergic receptor antagonists, a heart rate–slowing nondihydropyridine calcium channel blocker, such as diltiazem or verapamil, may be substituted.

Targets for systolic blood pressure and heart rate are 110 mm Hg and ≤60 beats/min, respectively, but medications may require titration according to clinical evidence of impaired end-organ perfusion. β-Adrenergic receptor antagonists alone are often insufficient for achieving blood pressure control. Therefore administration of a direct vasodilator may be necessary. Sodium nitroprusside is the agent of first choice in aortic dissection patients with hypertension refractory to initial β-blocker therapy but should not be initiated without adequate heart rate control because reflex tachycardia unfavorably influences the dP/dT response. The starting dose is 25 μg/min by continuous infusion, and adjustments are usually made in increments of 10 to 25 μg. At infusion rates greater than 2 μg/kg/min, the circulating concentration of the metabolite cyanide (CN^-) exceeds the rate of excretion by the kidneys. After a total nitroprusside load of 500 μg/kg, endogenous molecular CN^- buffers are depleted, increasing the probability of drug toxicity. In clinical practice, measuring levels of thiocyanate, a by-product of CN^- metabolism, is critical to prevent drug-induced CN^- toxicity, particularly in patients with renal insufficiency. Alternative IV vasodilators available for use in the acute setting include enalaprilat, hydralazine, and nicardipine.[111] Labetalol is also used for its α- and β-adrenergic receptor antagonism. Concomitant analgesia for pain control is essential and may favorably influence blood pressure and heart rate.

For acute aortic dissection patients with hypotension, tamponade from hemopericardium should be considered. Volume resuscitation or pressor therapy may be necessary to maintain vital organ perfusion, but these are merely temporizing measures. Pericardiocentesis for relief of tamponade is not recommended, and surgery should be performed emergently.

For patients who survive to hospital discharge, prescription of a β-adrenergic receptor antagonist is associated with improved survival, including among those patients who undergo surgical repair for type A dissection. Calcium channel antagonists have been associated with improved survival in type B patients.[112] There is no mortality benefit associated with the use of angiotensin-converting enzyme inhibitors.[112] Optimal heart rate control (<60 beats/min) is predictive of negative or limited aortic growth.[82] Statins have been associated with decreased rates of rupture in atherosclerotic abdominal aortic aneurysms, but there is no evidence of benefit in the setting of aortic dissection.[113]

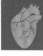

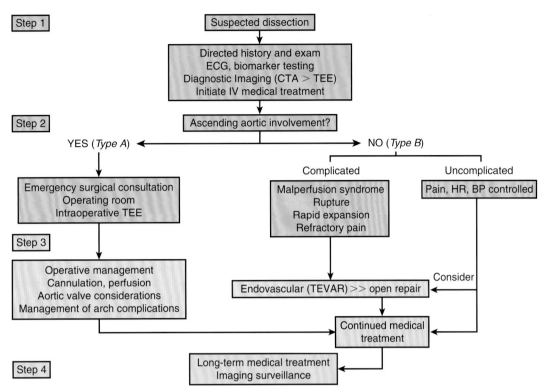

Fig. 32.9 Proposed Management Pathway for Acute Aortic Dissection. In Step 1, a high index of clinical suspicion for acute aortic dissection should prompt early diagnostic testing while medical therapy is initiated. Step 2 involves the determination of ascending aortic involvement, which influences significantly the importance of emergent surgical consultation. In Step 3, patients with type A aortic dissection are referred for surgery and patients with complicated type B aortic dissection are referred for endovascular therapy or surgery. Patients with uncomplicated type B aortic dissection are continued on medical therapy and monitored for changes in clinical status. There is growing use of thoracic endovascular aortic repair *(TEVAR)* for uncomplicated type B dissection. In Step 4, a care plan is established that emphasizes the importance of long-term medical therapy, imaging surveillance, and lifestyle modifications to decrease the risk of postdissection complications. Long-term medical therapy should include β-receptor antagonists and angiotensin receptor blockers or angiotensin-converting enzyme inhibitors to achieve a resting heart rate *(HR)* of <60 beats/min and blood pressure *(BP)* of <120/80 mm Hg, respectively. *CTA,* Computed tomographic angiography; *ECG,* electrocardiogram; *IV,* intravenous; *TEE,* transesophageal echocardiography. (Modified from Hiratzka LF, Bakris GL, Beckman JA, et al. 2010 ACCF/AHA/AATS/ACR/ASA/SCA/SCAI/SIR/STS/SVM guidelines for the diagnosis and management of patients with thoracic aortic disease. *J Am Coll Cardiol.* 2010;55:e27–e129.)

TABLE 32.1 Intravenous β-Adrenergic Receptor Antagonists for the Management of Acute Aortic Dissection

Therapy	Dose	Receptor Selectivity and Half-Life
Metoprolol	5-mg bolus every 5 min for 3 doses; additional doses of 5–10 mg every 4–6 h as needed	$\beta_1 > \beta_2$ 3–6 h
Labetolol	10–20-mg bolus, repeat 20–40-mg bolus every 10–15 min as needed. Maintenance infusion 1–2 mg/min; maximum total dose of 300 mg	α_1-, β_1-, and β_2 ~5.5 h
Esmolol	0.5-mg/kg bolus, then 50 µg/kg/min infusion	β_1 9 min
Propranolol	0.05–0.15 mg/kg every 4–6 h as needed	$\beta_1 \approx \beta_2$ 5–7 h

INDICATIONS FOR INTERVENTION (Box 32.5)

Anatomic location of disease, patient comorbidities, initial complications, and acuity of presentation (i.e., acute vs. chronic) are key factors influencing treatment decisions (Fig. 32.10). There is evolving evidence suggesting a relationship between clinical outcome and surgeon experience and a multidisciplinary team (MDT) approach to care.[114] Increasing hospital volume for open abdominal aortic aneurysm repair is associated with improved survival, particularly at centers that perform >50 abdominal aortic aneurysm repairs annually.[115] Less well established are clinically useful parameters for referral of patients with thoracic aortic disease. *Centers of excellence* for surgical repair of thoracic aortic disease might be defined by procedural volumes (surgeon and facility), outcomes, time to diagnosis and intervention, and logistical measures including distance to nearest referral center and services available.[6,116]

Type A Aortic Dissection

Recommendations pertaining to patient selection for surgical, endovascular, or medical treatment of acute aortic dissection are derived from

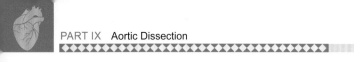

BOX 32.5 Indications for Intervention

Acute Dissection

Type A: All patients
Type B: With Complications
Rupture
Extension
Rapid aneurysm expansion
Malperfusion syndrome
Marfan syndrome

Chronic Dissection

Type A:
Maximal dimension ≥5.5 cm
Marfan syndrome with maximum dimension ≥4.5–5 cm
Increase in dimension ≥1 cm/yr
Severe aortic regurgitation
Symptoms suggestive of expansion or compression
Type B:
Maximal dimension ≥6 cm
Increase in dimension ≥1 cm/yr
  Symptoms suggestive of expansion or compression

consensus expert opinion (level of evidence C) as randomized trials are limited.[6,117] Emergency surgery is indicated for all acute type A dissections, regardless of the site of entry, because medical therapy alone is associated with a rate of in-hospital mortality exceeding 50%.[3,6,118] Over the past 20 years, there has been a trend toward decreased mortality in patients with type A dissections undergoing surgical repair.[119] There is an observed doubling of surgical mortality in patients older than 70 years.[120] Nevertheless, given the high rate of death in those with type A disease managed with medical therapy alone, surgical repair remains the treatment of choice also in this population.

Surgery is performed to prevent rupture with exsanguination or tamponade and to relieve aortic regurgitation when present. The extent and complexity of surgery (resection/grafting of the ascending aorta, valve resuspension or replacement, coronary artery reimplantation) are determined on a case-by-case basis. Incorporation of the aortic arch in the primary repair is indicated when the tear traverses this segment of the aorta or when it has become acutely aneurysmal. Single-center results suggest favorable short-term outcomes in patients undergoing total arch replacement in acute type A dissection in patients with primary or secondary arch tear, arch aneurysm, circumferential arch dissection, or concomitant carotid artery dissection.[121] Patients with MFS have a lower rate of reoperation when initial type A dissection surgery includes aortic root replacement or repair, which should be performed when feasible.[117,122]

The indications for and timing of surgical repair for the unusual case of chronic, stable type A aortic dissection are unresolved. In this situation, surgeon preference and patient comorbidities weigh heavily in decision-making, as does any information related to aortic enlargement over time. Outcomes with conservative management may not be inferior to surgical repair in the chronic phase, as suggested by limited single center experiences and retrospective data.[23,123] Thoracic endovascular aortic repair (TEVAR) has been used in acute and chronic type A dissection, although experience is very limited and endovascular repair is considered off-label. Evidence is limited to small case series that have shown decreased false lumen size after stent grafting but with a significant rate of complications.[124,125] Additional studies and device modifi-

cations are required before TEVAR can be considered a valid treatment option for type A dissections. Although more commonly used for aneurysmal disease, hybrid approaches that involve both open and endovascular intervention ("elephant trunk") can also be performed in patients with acute dissection with complex anatomy, particularly with involvement of the aortic arch and proximal descending aorta.[117,126]

Surgery for chronic type A aortic dissection is indicated for the treatment of severe aortic regurgitation associated with symptoms or LV systolic dysfunction or for aneurysmal disease according to conventional size criteria (≥5.5 cm for ascending aortic aneurysm, ≥5.5 to 6.0 cm for descending thoracic aneurysm, ≥5.5 cm for thoracoabdominal aortic aneurysm or increase in size >0.5 to 1.0 cm/year).[6] Of note, in high-risk patients, such as those with MFS or EDS, elective aortic repair is recommended at smaller aortic diameters.

Type B Aortic Dissection

Uncomplicated type B dissection is treated medically with emphasis on tight heart rate and blood pressure control. Serial imaging is performed to monitor disease evolution. Lifestyle modifications, including the possibility of job change, may be necessary to avoid strenuous lifting, pushing, or straining that requires intense or repetitive Valsalva maneuvers.[6]

Surgery or endovascular treatment for acute type B dissection is generally reserved for those patients who have failed initial conservative therapy and have a complicated course as indicated by refractory or recurrent pain, continued extension, early aneurysmal expansion, rupture, malperfusion syndrome, dissection location within a previously known aneurysmal aortic segment, and for patients with MFS. A prediction model for in-hospital mortality has been developed based on review of patients in IRAD with acute type B dissection. Independent predictors include increasing age, hypotension/shock, periaortic hematoma, descending aortic diameter ≥5.5 cm, mesenteric ischemia, acute renal failure, and limb ischemia. Although not externally validated, such prediction models might be helpful in risk stratifying and estimating prognosis early in a patient's course (Fig. 32.11).[127] The importance of refractory pain in otherwise *uncomplicated* type B dissection has been recognized. In a prospective analysis of 365 type B dissection patients without conventional high-risk features, the presence of pain or persistent hypertension despite medical therapy was associated with a 35-fold increase in mortality compared with the absence of these clinical features.[128]

There has been increasing adoption of endovascular stent graft treatment for complicated type B dissection, although randomized trial data are lacking (Fig. 32.12; see Chapter 34). Most high-volume centers have moved in this direction, and it is unlikely that a pivotal trial versus surgery will be conducted in patients with traditional indications for surgery (Table 32.2).[117] In a review of 1129 patients in IRAD with type B dissection, 24.4% underwent TEVAR. Patients with TEVAR were more likely to present with a complicated dissection and had similar in-hospital mortality, 1-year mortality, and recurrent or new dissection compared with those who received medical therapy alone; however, survival at 5 years was higher in those who received TEVAR.[15]

Although medical therapy is the initial treatment option for uncomplicated type B dissection, a single-center study reported a 6-year intervention-free survival rate of only 41% using such a strategy.[129] Data remain limited, but there are suggestions of improved aortic remodeling and the potential for long-term benefit in patients with uncomplicated type B dissection managed with TEVAR. The Investigation of STEnt Grafts in Aortic Dissection (INSTEAD) trial randomized 140 *stable* type B patients between 2 and 52 weeks following dissection to optimal medical therapy versus optimal medical therapy plus endovascular stent grafting.[130] Although this trial was underpowered

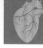

Type A Acute Aortic Dissection

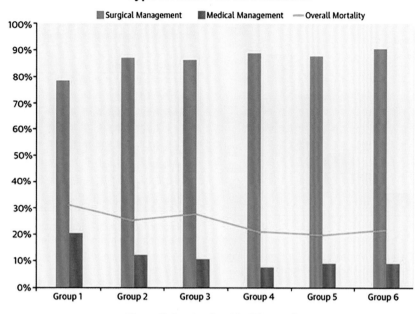

Type B Acute Aortic Dissection

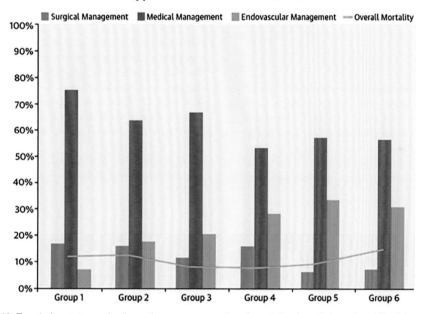

Fig. 32.10 Trends in acute aortic dissection management and mortality from International Registry of Aortic Dissection registry from 1996 to 2013. Group 1: 12/1995-2/1999; Group 2: 2/1999-3/2002; Group 3: 3/2002-8/2005; Group 4: 8/2005-11/2007; Group 5: 11/2007-2/2010; Group 6: 2/2010-2/2013. (From Pape LA, Awais M, Woznicki EM, et al. Presentation, diagnosis, and outcomes of acute aortic dissection: 17-year trends from the International Registry of Acute Aortic Dissection. *J Am Coll Cardiol.* 2015;66:350–358.)

for the primary end point of aorta-related death at 2 years, a substantially greater number of patients who underwent stent grafting demonstrated recovery of true lumen size and contour and the development of false lumen thrombosis (91%), compared with those who received optimal medical therapy alone (19%, *P* < .001). Five-year follow-up data from the INSTEAD trial showed improved aorta-specific survival and delayed disease progression in those who received TEVAR.[61] A larger retrospective analysis of uncomplicated acute type B dissection showed no difference in early mortality in patients who received

TEVAR versus medical therapy; however, during a mean follow-up of 34 months, patients who received TEVAR had a lower rate of aortic complications, aortic-related mortality, and all-cause mortality.[131] In a small trial evaluating 61 patients with type B dissection randomized to best medical therapy versus stent graft placement within 14 days of acute dissection, the stent graft group had a 97% rate of false lumen thrombosis (compared with 43% for the medical therapy group), reduced false lumen size, increased true lumen size, and decreased overall transverse aortic diameter at 1-year follow-up.[132]

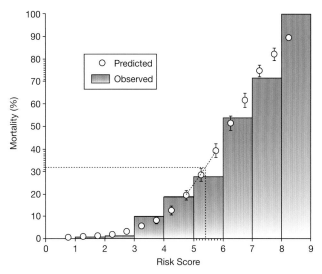

Fig. 32.11 Observed Versus Predicted Mortality Rate for Patients With Acute Type B Dissection in the International Registry of Aortic Dissection. The equation to derive risk score is: ln (risk/(1 − risk)) = −6.0 + 0.3 × (female) + 0.3 × (age in decades) + 1.9 × (hypotension/shock) + 1.1 × (periaortic hematoma) + 1.8 (aortic diameter ≥5.5 cm) + 2.2 × (mesenteric ischemia) + 1.3 × (acute renal failure) + 1.1 × (limb ischemia). (Modified from Tolenaar JL, Froehlich W, Jonker FH, et al. Predicting in-hospital mortality in acute type B aortic dissection: evidence from International Registry of Acute Aortic Dissection. *Circulation* 2014;130[11 Suppl. 1]:S45–S50.)

TABLE 32.2   European Society of Cardiology Class I and II Recommendations for Thoracic Stent Graft Insertion

Patient Subgroup	Classification	Level of Evidence
Type A AD with organ malperfusion (hybrid approach)	IIa	B
Uncomplicated Type B AD	IIa	B
Complicated Type B AD	I	C
Complicated Type B IMH	IIa	C
Complicated Type B PAU	IIa	C
Contained Aortic Aneurysm Rupture[a]	I	C
Traumatic Aortic Injury[a]	IIa	C

[a]Thoracic endovascular aortic repair preferred to surgery when appropriate anatomy and expertise available.

AD, Aortic dissection; *IMH*, intramural hematoma; *PAU*, penetrating aortic ulcer.

Data from Erbel R, Aboyans V, Boileau C, et al. 2014 ESC Guidelines on the diagnosis and treatment of aortic diseases. *Eur Heart J.* 2014;35(41):2873–2926.

There appears to be a greater degree of remodeling in TEVAR patients in the acute phase compared with chronic phase, with higher rates of false lumen thrombosis and aortic diameter.[133] However, there may also be an increased rate of retrograde dissection when performed within the first 14 days of dissection presentation. In patients with dissection and underlying connective tissue disorders, open repair is still recommended due to increased rates of endoleak and mortality with stent grafting compared with historical data for open repair.[117,134] Endoleak is the most frequently encountered complication of TEVAR and was reported at a rate of 8% in a systematic review but can be higher in individual centers.[135,136] Endoleaks are often asymptomatic, thus TEVAR patients require regular follow-up imaging. Other complications include stent migration, thrombosis, and stroke, with a reported average reintervention rate of 16% in a systematic review of 17 studies and 567 patients.[135,137]

Indications for percutaneous balloon fenestration include false lumen-compression of the true lumen with end-organ hypoperfusion

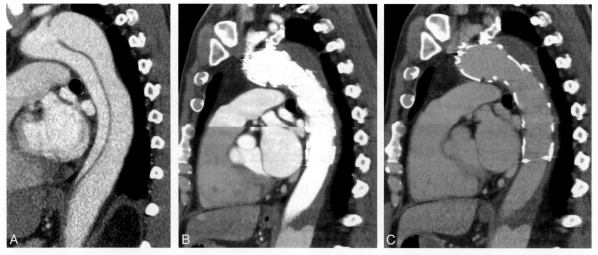

Fig. 32.12 Computed Tomographic Angiography of a Type B Dissection Before and After Thoracic Endovascular Aortic Repair. A 58-year-old man presented with acute type B aortic dissection. On follow-up imaging (A, sagittal image), the aortic diameter was larger than it was at baseline and he was referred for thoracic endovascular aortic repair (sagittal image with [B] and without contrast [C]). Left subclavian artery coil embolization with subsequent left common carotid–left subclavian artery bypass was required in this instance prior to thoracic endograft placement.

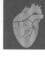

BOX 32.6 Predictors of Aortic Growth in Uncomplicated Type B Aortic Dissection

Patient Characteristics

Age <60 years
White race
Heart rate ≥60 beats/min
Marfan syndrome

Aortic Dissection Characteristics

Aortic diameter ≥40 mm on initial imaging
Patent or partially thrombosed false lumen
Proximal descending false lumen diameter ≥22 mm on initial imaging
Sac formation in partially thrombosed false lumen
One entry tear
Large entry tear (≥10 mm)
Intimal tear at inner curvature of aorta
Elliptical configuration of true lumen/round configuration of false lumen
Fusiform dilatation of proximal descending aorta (fusiform index ≥0.64)[a]
Fibrinogen-fibrin degradation product ≥20 µg/mL on presentation

[a]Fusiform index = (maximum diameter of proximal descending aorta) / (diameter of distal aortic arch + diameter of descending aorta at level of origin of main pulmonary artery).
Modified from van Bogerijen GH, Tolenaar JL, Rampoldi V, et al. Predictors of aortic growth in uncomplicated type B aortic dissection. *J Vasc Surg.* 2014;59(4):1134–1143.

(see Chapter 34). In this procedure, a balloon catheter is used to create a transverse tear across the dissection flap to attenuate the compressive forces on the true lumen and improve flow to compromised organs. Placement of a stent into side branch vessels to restore blood flow may be performed to enhance regional perfusion.[17] There is growing use of branched and fenestrated endovascular graft repairs, which can be customized for each patient to decrease the risks of malperfusion and endoleak, and expand treatment options to patients with complex anatomy. There are limited data, but small observational studies suggest potential utility and safety in appropriate patients.[138,139]

Appropriate patient selection is critical in assessing who may benefit from TEVAR. Recent studies have evaluated a variety of features that predict a higher risk of an increase in aortic diameter after dissection (Box 32.6). One such high-risk feature includes long-term patency or partial thrombosis of the false lumen.[6,140] It has been proposed that partial thrombosis of the false lumen confers a worse outcome on patients with type B aortic dissection due to associated increases in pressure within the false lumen that may compromise true lumen blood flow to critical organs.[26–28] Nonetheless, it remains unclear how to use this and other information to determine which patients with uncomplicated type B dissection would best benefit from TEVAR.

PROGNOSIS

The European Cooperative study group reported 1- and 2-year mortality rates for patients with type A dissection of 60% and 50%, respectively.[141] Approximately one-third of aortic dissection survivors will experience rupture or extension or require surgery for aneurysm formation within 5 years of recovery from the initial event.[17] Outcome in acute type A dissection is heavily influenced by treatment strategy: in-hospital mortality rate is 20% in those with surgical repair and 57% with medical

therapy alone.[3] Mortality increases further at 60 days: 26% after surgical repair and 62% with medical therapy (Fig. 32.13).[12] Surgical outcomes are poor in patients demonstrating signs of malperfusion prior to dissection repair, with an increasing risk of death as a function of the number of compromised organ systems.[17,142] A bedside risk prediction tool for in-hospital mortality incorporating these variables offers clinicians, patients, and families a useful method by which to understand the complexities and hazards of the acute dissection process.[118]

For type B dissection, current in-hospital mortality rates approach 11%.[3] For patients with type B dissection managed medically, in-hospital survival is 91%, whereas for higher risk patients who require surgical intervention for the indications listed previously, in-hospital survival is only 83%. Those undergoing endovascular repair have an 88% survival rate.[3] Unlike patients with type A dissection, there is minimal increased mortality after hospital discharge up to 60 days in those with type B dissection, regardless of treatment modality.[12]

Analysis of IRAD showed that in contrast to type A dissection outcome, which has improved since the 1990s, there has been no significant change in mortality for type B dissections despite an increase in surgical and endovascular management strategies.[3]

LONG-TERM SURVEILLANCE

Because of the life-long risk of subsequent aortic and cardiovascular complications, vigilant clinical and radiographic follow-up is mandatory for all hospital survivors. Medical management remains targeted to strict blood pressure (≤120/80 mm Hg) and heart rate (≤60 beats/min) goals. Statin therapy is indicated for the treatment of atherosclerosis. Although routine exercise remains important to overall health, certain activities should be avoided post dissection, including lifting of heavy objects at or near maximal effort, weight lifting to failure, or interval training.[143]

Patients need to be educated regarding the chronic nature of this disease, awareness of dissection-associated symptoms, and the importance of medication adherence. Imaging of the entire aorta is recommended predischarge, at 1 month, and at 3, 6, and 12 months, then annually thereafter, although it should vary based on individual risk and aortic diameter.[117,144] Follow-up imaging is critical in patients who have undergone endovascular stent graft placement to monitor for development of complications, particularly endoleak development.[117] Studies show poor follow-up rates; an assessment of likelihood of patient adherence should be included when selecting patients for intervention.[77] Patients who do not follow up have been shown to have a lower survival rate.[145] Preliminary data suggest there may be a role for positron emission tomography imaging of chronic dissections to evaluate ongoing inflammation, which may warrant intervention or closer monitoring in those with fluorodeoxyglucose avidity.[146]

Aortic imaging is recommended for first-degree relatives of patients with thoracic aortic dissection to aid in the identification of asymptomatic disease.[6] Given the variability of age of onset, screening every 5 years in at-risk relatives is also recommended.[117] Genetic screening should be offered to patients with aortic dissection and syndromic features. Genetic screening can also be considered in patients without known risk factors for dissection who have a concerning family history.

The continued high rates of death and disability from acute aortic dissection reinforce the urgent need for improvements in the treatment of identifiable risk factors (notably, hypertension), genetic and biomarker screening, clinical awareness, regional referral networks, standardized care protocols both during and after hospitalization, and, possibly, the designation of surgical centers of excellence in aortic repair.

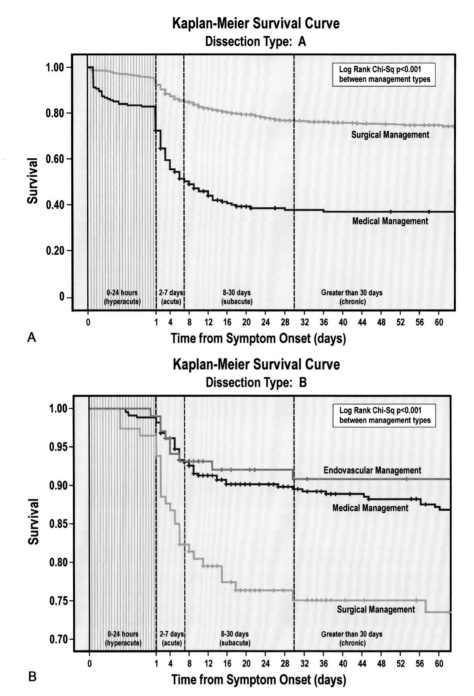

Fig. 32.13 60-day Kaplan-Meier survival curves from the International Registry of Aortic Dissection based on type of dissection and treatment approach. (From Booher AM, Isselbacher EM, Nienaber CA, et al. The IRAD classification system for characterizing survival after aortic dissection. *Am J Med.* 2013;126:730:e19–e24.)

REFERENCES

1. Hagan PG, Nienaber CA, Isselbacher EM, et al. The International Registry of Acute Aortic Dissection (IRAD). *JAMA*. 2000;283(7):897–903.
2. Weinsaft JW, Devereux RB, Preiss LR, et al. Aortic dissection in patients with genetically mediated aneurysms: Incidence and predictors in the GenTAC registry. *J Am Coll Cardiol*. 2016;67(23):2744–2754.
3. Pape LA, Awais M, Woznicki EM, et al. Presentation, diagnosis, and outcomes of acute aortic dissection: 17-year trends from the International Registry of Acute Aortic Dissection. *J Am Coll Cardiol*. 2015;66(4):350–358.
4. Mussa FF, Horton JD, Moridzadeh R, et al. Acute aortic dissection and intramural hematoma: a systematic review. *JAMA*. 2016;316(7): 754–763.
5. Tanaka Y, Sakata K, Sakurai Y, et al. Prevalence of type A acute aortic dissection in patients with out-of-hospital cardiopulmonary arrest. *Am J Cardiol*. 2016;117(11):1826–1830.
6. Hiratzka LF, Bakris GL, Beckman JA, et al. 2010 ACCF/AHA/AATS/ACR/ASA/SCA/SCAI/SIR/STS/SVM guidelines for the diagnosis and management of patients with thoracic aortic disease. *J Am Coll Cardiol*. 2010;55(14):e27–e29.

7. Olson C, Thelin S, Ståhle E, et al. Thoracic aortic aneurysm and dissection. Increasing prevalence and improved outcomes reported in a nationwide population-based study of more than 14,000 cases from 1987 to 2002. *Circulation.* 2006;114(24):2611–2618.

8. Howard DP, Banerjee A, Fairhead JF, et al. Population-based study of incidence and outcome of acute aortic dissection and premorbid risk factor control: 10-year results from the Oxford vascular study. *Circulation.* 2013;127(20):2031–2037.

9. Landenhed M, Engstrom G, Gottsater A, et al. Risk profiles for aortic dissection and ruptured or surgically treated aneurysms: a prospective cohort study. *J Am Heart Assoc.* 2015;4(1):e001513.

10. Daily PO, Trueblood HW, Stinson EB, et al. Management of acute aortic dissections. *Ann Thorac Surg.* 1970;10(3):237–247.

11. DeBakey ME, Beall Jr AC, Cooley DA, et al. Dissecting aneurysms of the aorta. *Surg Clin North Am.* 1966;46(4):1045–1055.

12. Booher AM, Isselbacher EM, Nienaber CA, et al. The IRAD classification system for characterizing survival after aortic dissection. *Am J Med.* 2013;126(8): 730.e19–24.

13. Steuer J, Bjorck M, Mayer D, et al. Distinction between acute and chronic type B aortic dissection: is there a sub-acute phase? *Eur J Vasc Endovasc Surg.* 2013;45(6):627–631.

14. VIRTUE Registry Investigators. Mid-term outcomes and aortic remodelling after thoracic endovascular repair for acute, subacute, and chronic aortic dissection: the VIRTUE registry. *Eur J Vasc Endovasc Surg.* 2014;48(4):363–371.

15. Fattori R, Cao P, De Rango P, et al. Interdisciplinary expert consensus document on management of type B aortic dissection. *J Am Coll Cardiol.* 2013;61(16):1661–1678.

16. Ganaha F, Miller DC, Sugimoto K, et al. Prognosis of aortic intramural hematoma with and without penetrating atherosclerotic ulcer: a clinical and radiological analysis. *Circulation.* 2002;106(3):342–348.

17. Nienaber C, Eagle KA. Aortic dissection: new frontiers in diagnosis and management: Part I: from etiology to diagnostic strategies. *Circulation.* 2003;108(5):628–635.

18. Hirst AE, Johns VJ, Kime SW. Dissecting aneurysm of the aorta: a review of 505 cases. *Medicine (Baltimore).* 1958;37(3):217–279.

19. Lansman SL, McCullough JN, Nguyen KH, et al. Subtypes of acute aortic dissection. *Ann Thorac Surg.* 1999;67(6):1975–1978.

20. Nauta FJ, Tolenaar JL, Patel HJ, et al. Impact of retrograde arch extension in acute type B aortic dissection on management and outcomes. *Ann Thorac Surg.* 2016;102(6):2036–2043.

21. Ando M, Okita Y, Tangusari O, et al. Surgery in three-channeled aortic dissection. A 31-patient review. *Jpn J Thorac Cardiovasc Surg.* 2000;48(6):339–343.

22. Richens D, Kotidis K, Neale M, et al. Rupture of the aorta following road traffic accidents in the United Kingdom 1992-1990. The results of the co-operative crash injury study. *Eur J Cardiothroac Surg.* 2003;23(2):143–148.

23. Trimarchi S, Nienaber CA, Rampoldi V, et al. Results of surgery in acute type B aortic dissection: insights from the International Registry of Acute Aortic Dissection (IRAD). *Circulation.* 2006;114(1 Suppl):I357–I364.

24. Tsai TT, Evangelista A, Nienaber CA, et al. Partial thrombosis of the false lumen in patients with acute type B aortic dissection. *N Engl J Med.* 2007;357(4):349–359.

25. Satta J, Laara E, Juvonen T. Intraluminal thrombus predicts rupture of an abdominal aortic aneurysm. *J Vasc Surg.* 1996;23(4):737–739.

26. Wolf YG, Thoas WS, Brennan FJ, et al. Computed tomography scanning findings associated with rapid expansion of abdominal aortic aneurysms. *J Vasc Surg.* 1994;20(4):529–535.

27. Kazi M, Thyberg J, Religa P, et al. Influence of intraluminal thrombus on structural and cellular composition of abdominal aortic aneurysm wall. *J Vasc Surg.* 2003;38(6):1283–1292.

28. Vorp DA, Lee PC, Wang DH, et al. Association of intraluminal thrombus in abdominal aortic aneurysm with local hypoxia and wall weakening. *J Vasc Surg.* 2001;34(2):291–299.

29. Nataatmadja M, West M, West J, et al. Abnormal extracellular matrix protein transport associated with increased apoptosis of vascular smooth muscle cells in Marfan syndrome and bicuspid aortic valve thoracic aortic aneurysm. *Circulation.* 2003;108(Suppl 1):II329–34.

30. De Paepe A, Devereux RB, Dietz HC, et al. Revised diagnostic criteria for the Marfan syndrome. *Am J Med Genet.* 1996;62(4):417–426.

31. Judge DP, Dietz HC. Marfan's syndrome. *Lancet.* 2005;366(9501):1965–1976.

32. Keane MG, Pyeritz RE. Medical management of Marfan syndrome. *Circulation.* 2008;117(21):2802–2813.

33. Januzzi JL, Isselbacher EM, Fattori R, et al. Characterizing the young patient with aortic dissection: results from the International Registry of Aortic Dissection (IRAD). *J Am Coll Cardiol.* 2004;43(4):665–669.

34. Larson ED, Edwards WD. Risk factors for aortic dissection: a necroscopy study of 161 cases. *Am J Cardiol.* 1984;53(6):849–855.

35. Loeys BL, Dietz HC, Braverman AC, et al. The revised Ghent nosology for the Marfan syndrome. *J Med Genet.* 2010;47(7):476–485.

36. Roman MJ, Devereux RB, Kramer-Fox R, et al. Comparison of cardiovascular and skeletal features of primary mitral valve prolapse and Marfan syndrome. *Am J Cardiol.* 1989;63(5):317–321.

37. Isselbacher EM, Lino Cardenas CL, Lindsay ME. Hereditary influence in thoracic aortic aneurysm and dissection. *Circulation.* 2016;133(24):2516–2528.

38. Dietz HC, Cutting GR, Pyeritz RE, et al. Marfan syndrome caused by a recurrent de novo missense mutation in the fibrillin gene. *Nature.* 1991;352(6333):337–339.

39. Habashi JP, Judge DP, Holm TM, et al. Losartan, an AT1 antagonist, prevents aortic aneurysm in a mouse model of Marfan syndrome. *Science.* 2006;312(5770):117–121.

40. Brooke BS, Habashi JP, Judge DP, et al. Angiotensin II blockade and aortic-root dilation in Marfan's syndrome. *N Engl J Med.* 2008;358(26):2787–2795.

41. Groenink M, den Hartog AW, Franken R, et al. Losartan reduces aortic dilatation rate in adults with Marfan syndrome: a randomized controlled trial. *Eur Heart J.* 2013;34(45):3491–3500.

42. Lacro RV, Dietz HC, Sleeper LA, et al. Atenolol versus losartan in children and young adults with Marfan's syndrome. *N Engl J Med.* 2014;371(22):2061–2071.

43. Chiu HH, Wu MH, Wang JK, et al. Losartan added to beta-blockade therapy for aortic root dilation in Marfan syndrome: a randomized, open-label pilot study. *Mayo Clin Proc.* 2013;88(3):271–276.

44. den Hartog AW, Franken R, Zwinderman AH, et al. The risk for type B aortic dissection in Marfan syndrome. *J Am Coll Cardiol.* 2015;65(3):246–254.

45. Loeys BL, Schwarze U, Holm T, et al. Aneurysm syndromes caused by mutations in the TGF-β receptor. *N Engl J Med.* 2006;355(8):788–798.

46. Loeys BL, Chen J, Neptune ER, et al. A syndrome of altered cardiovascular, craniofacial, neurocognitive and skeletal development caused by mutations in TGFBR1 or TGFBR. *Nat Genet.* 2005;37(3):275–281.

47. Smith LB, Hadoke PW, Dyer E, et al. Haploinsufficiency of the murine Col3a1 locus causes aortic dissection: a novel model of the vascular type of Ehlers-Danlos syndrome. *Cardiovasc Res.* 2011;90(1):182–190.

48. Pepin ME, Chwarze U, Uperti-Furga AS, et al. Clinical and genetic features of Ehlers-Danlos syndrome type IV, the vascular type. *N Engl J Med.* 2000;342(10):673–680.

49. Guo D, Hasham S, Kuang SQ, et al. Familial thoracic aortic aneurysms and dissections: genetic heterogeneity with a major locus mapping to 5q13-14. *Circulation.* 2001;103(20):2461–2468.

50. Vaughan CJ, Casey M, He J, et al. Identification of a chromosome 11q23.2-q24 locus for familial aortic aneurysm disease, a genetically heterogeneous disorder. *Circulation.* 2001;103(20):2469–2475.

51. Furthmayr H, Francke U. Ascending aortic aneurysm with or without features of Marfan syndrome and other fibrillinopathies: new insights. *Semin Thorac Cardiovasc Surg.* 1997;9(3):191–205.

52. Pereira L, Lee SY, Gayraud B, et al. Pathogenetic sequence for aneurysm revealed in mice underexpressing fibrillin-1. *Proc Natl Acad Sci U S A.* 1999;96(7):3819–3823.

53. Wang Y, Zhang W, Zhang Y, et al. VKORC1 haplotypes are associated with arterial vascular diseases (stroke, coronary heart disease, and aortic disease). *Circulation.* 2006;113(12):1615–1621.

54. Guo DC, Pannu H, Tran-Fadulu V, et al. Mutations in smooth muscle α-actin (ACTA2) lead to thoracic aortic aneurysms and dissections. *Nat Genet.* 2007;39(12):1488–1493.

55. Guo DC, Regalado E, Casteel DE, et al. Recurrent gain-of-function mutation in PRKG1 causes thoracic aortic aneurysms and acute aortic dissections. *Am J Hum Genet.* 2013;93(2):398–404.

56. Cripe L, Andelfinger G, Martin LJ, et al. Bicuspid aortic valve is heritable. *J Am Coll Cardiol.* 2004;44(1):138–143.

57. Grewal N, Gittenberger-de Groot AC, Poelmann RE, et al. Ascending aorta dilation in association with bicuspid aortic valve: a maturation defect of the aortic wall. *J Thorac Cardiovasc Surg.* 2014;148(4):1583–1590.

58. Pasta S, Phillippi JA, Gleason TG, et al. Effect of aneurysm on the mechanical dissection properties of the human ascending thoracic aorta. *J Thorac Cardiovasc Surg.* 2012;143(2):460–467.

59. Hiratzka LF, Creager MA, Isselbacher EM, et al. Surgery for aortic dilatation in patients with bicuspid aortic valves: a statement of clarification from the American College of Cardiology/American Heart Association task force on clinical practice guidelines. *Circulation.* 2016;133(7):680–686.

60. Eleid MF, Forde I, Edwards WD, et al. Type A aortic dissection in patients with bicuspid aortic valves: Clinical and pathological comparison with tricuspid aortic valves. *Heart.* 2013;99(22):1668–1674.

61. Nienaber CA, Fattori R, Mehta RH, et al. Gender-related differences in acute aortic dissection. *Circulation.* 2004;109(24):3014–3021.

62. Kim JB, Spotnitz M, Lindsay ME, et al. Risk of aortic dissection in the moderately dilated ascending aorta. *J Am Coll Cardiol.* 2016;68(11):1209–1219.

63. Kim JB, Kim K, Lindsay ME, et al. Risk of rupture or dissection in descending thoracic aortic aneurysm. *Circulation.* 2015;132(17):1620–1629.

64. Januzzi JL, Sabatine MS, Eagle KA, et al. Iatrogenic aortic dissection. *Am J Cardiol.* 2002;89(5):623–626.

65. Ketenci B, Enc Y, Ozay B, et al. Perioperative type I aortic dissection during conventional coronary artery bypass surgery: risk factors and management. *Heart Surg Forum.* 2008;11(4):E231–E236.

66. Nunez-Gil IJ, Bautista D, Cerrato E, et al. Incidence, management, and immediate- and long-term outcomes after iatrogenic aortic dissection during diagnostic or interventional coronary procedures. *Circulation.* 2015;131(24):2114–2119.

67. Kamel H, Roman MJ, Pitcher A, et al. Pregnancy and the risk of aortic dissection or rupture: a cohort-crossover analysis. *Circulation.* 2016;134(7):527–533.

68. Braverman AC. Acute aortic dissection: clinician update. *Circulation.* 2010;122(2):184–188.

69. Manalo-Estrella P, Barker AE. Histopathologic findings in human aortic media associated with pregnancy. *Arch Pathol.* 1967;83(4):336–341.

70. Hsue PY, Salinas CL, Bolger AF, et al. Acute aortic dissection related to crack cocaine. *Circulation.* 2002;105(13):1592–1595.

71. Westover AN, Nakonezny PA. Aortic dissection in young adults who abuse amphetamines. *Am Heart J.* 2010;160(2):315–321.

72. Lee CC, Lee MT, Chen YS, et al. Risk of aortic dissection and aortic aneurysm in patients taking oral fluoroquinolone. *JAMA Intern Med.* 2015;175(11):1839–1847.

73. von Kodolitsch Y, Schwartz AG, Nienaber CA. Clinical prediction of acute aortic dissection. *Arch Intern Med.* 2000;160(19):2977–2982.

74. Bickerstaff LK, Pairolero PC, Hollier LH, et al. Thoracic aortic aneurysms: a population-based study. *Surgery.* 1982;92(6):1103–1108.

75. Rogers AM, Hermann LK, Booher AM, et al. Sensitivity of the aortic dissection detection risk score, a novel guideline-based tool for identification of acute aortic dissection at initial presentation: results from the International Registry of Acute Aortic Dissection. *Circulation.* 2011;123(20):2213–2218.

76. Nazerian P, Giachino F, Vanni S, et al. Diagnostic performance of the aortic dissection detection risk score in patients with suspected acute aortic dissection. *Eur Heart J Acute Cardiovasc Care.* 2014;3(4):373–381.

77. Kret MR, Azarbal AF, Mitchell EL, et al. Compliance with long-term surveillance recommendations following endovascular aneurysm repair or type B aortic dissection. *J Vasc Surg.* 2013;58(1):25–31.

78. Tsai TT, Trimarchi S, Nienaber CA. Acute aortic dissection: perspectives from the International Registry of Acute Aortic Dissection (IRAD). *Euro J Vasc Endovasc Surg.* 2009;37(2):149–159.

79. Bossone E, Rampoldi V, Nienaber CA, et al. Usefulness of pulse deficit to predict in-hospital complications and mortality in patients with acute type A aortic dissection. *Am J Cardiol.* 2002;89(7):851–855.

80. Suzuki T, Katoh H, Tsuchio Y, et al. Diagnostic implications of elevated levels of smooth-muscle myosin heavy-chain protein in acute aortic dissection. The smooth muscle myosin heavy chain study. *Ann Intern Med.* 2000;133(7):537–541.

81. Shinohara T, Suzuki K, Okada M, et al. Soluble elastin fragments in serum are elevated in acute aortic dissection. *Atheroscler Thromb Vasc Biol.* 2003;23(10):1839–1844.

82. van Bogerijen GH, Tolenaar JL, Rampoldi V, et al. Predictors of aortic growth in uncomplicated type B aortic dissection. *J Vasc Surg.* 2014;59(4):1134–1143.

83. Suzuki T, Distante A, Zizza A, et al. Diagnosis of acute aortic dissection by D-dimer: the International Registry of Acute Aortic Dissection substudy on biomarkers (IRAD-Bio) experience. *Circulation.* 2009;119(20):2702–2707.

84. Asha SE, Miers JW. A systematic review and meta-analysis of D-dimer as a rule-out test for suspected acute aortic dissection. *Ann Emerg Med.* 2015;66(4):368–378.

85. Nazerian P, Mueller C, Soeiro A, et al. Diagnostic accuracy of the aortic dissection detection risk score plus d-dimer for acute aortic syndromes: the ADvISED prospective multicenter study. *Circulation.* 2018;137(3):250–258.

86. Giachino F, Loiacono M, Lucchiari M, et al. Rule out of acute aortic dissection with plasma matrix metalloproteinase 8 in the emergency department. *Crit Care.* 2013;17(1):R33.

87. Schillinger M, Domanovits H, Bayegan K, et al. C-reactive protein and mortality in patients with acute aortic disease. *Intensive Care Med.* 2002;28(6):740–745.

88. Ranasinghe AM, Bonser RS. Biomarkers in acute aortic dissection and other aortic syndromes. *J Am Coll Cardiol.* 2010;56(19):1535–1541.

89. von Kodolitsch Y, Nienaber CA, Dieckmann C, et al. Chest radiography for the diagnosis of acute aortic syndrome. *Am J Med.* 2004;116(2):73–77.

90. Erbel R, Alfonso F, Boileau C, et al. Diagnosis and management of aortic dissection. *Eur Heart J.* 2001;22(18):1642–1681.

91. Mohr-Kahaly S, Erbel R, Rennollet H, et al. Ambulatory follow-up of aortic dissection by transesophageal two-dimensional and color-coded Doppler echocardiography. *Circulation.* 1989;80(1):24–33.

92. Erbel R, Oelert H, Meyer J, et al. Effect of medical and surgical therapy on aortic dissection evaluated by transesophageal echocardiography. Implications for prognosis and therapy. The European Cooperative Study Group on Echocardiography. *Circulation.* 1993;87(5):1604–1615.

93. Macura KJ, Szarf G, Fishman EK, et al. Role of computed tomography and magnetic resonance imaging in assessment of acute aortic syndromes. *Semin Ultrasound CT MR.* 2003;24(4):232–254.

94. Clough RE, Schaeffter T, Taylor PR. Magnetic resonance imaging for aortic dissection. *Eur J Endovasc Surg.* 2010;39(4):514.

95. Bansal RC, Chandrasekaran K, Ayala K, et al. Frequency and explanation of false negative diagnosis of aortic dissection by aortography and transesophageal echocariography. *J Am Coll Cardiol.* 1995;25(6):1393–1401.

96. Weintraub AR, Erbel R, Gorge G, et al. Intravascular ultrasound imaging in acute aortic dissection. *J Am Coll Cardiol.* 1994;24(2):495–503.

97. Sommer T, Fehske W, Holzknecht N, et al. Aortic dissection: a comparative study of diagnosis with spiral CT, multiplanar transesophageal echocardiography, and MR imaging. *Radiology.* 1996;199(2):347–352.

98. Alfonso F, Goicolea J, Aragoncillo P, et al. Diagnosis of aortic intramural hematoma by intravascular ultrasound imaging. *Am J Cardiol.* 1995;76(10):735–738.

99. Creswell LL, Kouchoukos NT, Cox JL, et al. Coronary artery disease in patients with type A aortic dissection. *Ann Thorac Surg.* 1995;59:585–590.

100. Kang DH, Song JK, Song MG, et al. Clinical and echocardiographic outcomes of aortic intramural hemorrhage compared with acute aortic dissection. *Am J Cardiol.* 1998;81(2):202–206.

101. Nienaber CA, von Kodolitsch Y, Petersen B, et al. Intramural hemorrhage of the thoracic aorta. Diagnostic and therapeutic implications. *Circulation.* 1995;92(6):1465–1472.

102. Song JK, Kim HS, Kang DH, et al. Different clinical features of aortic intramural hematoma versus dissection involving the ascending aorta. *J Am Coll Cardiol.* 2001;37(6):1604–1610.

103. Harris KM, Braverman AC, Eagle KA, et al. Acute aortic intramural hematoma: an analysis from the International Registry of Acute Aortic Dissection. *Circulation.* 2012;126(11 Suppl 1):S91–S96.

104. Tsai TT, Nienaber CA, Eagle KA. Acute aortic syndromes. *Circulation*. 2005;112(24):3802–3813.

105. Song JK, Yim JH, Ahn JM, et al. Outcomes of patients with acute type A aortic intramural hematoma. *Circulation*. 2009;120(21):2046–2052.

106. Li D, Zhang H, Cai Y, et al. Acute type B aortic intramural hematoma: treatment strategy and the role of endovascular repair. *J Endovasc Ther*. 2010;17(5):617–621.

107. Ganaha F, Miller C, Sugimoto K, et al. Prognosis of aortic intramural hematoma with and without penetrating atherosclerotic ulcer. *Circulation*. 2002;106(3):342–348.

108. Robbins RC, McMamus RP, Mitchell RS, et al. Management of patients with intramural hematoma of the thoracic aorta. *Circulation*. 1993;88(5 P 2):II1–10.

109. Gifford SM, Duncan AA, Greiten LE, et al. The natural history and outcomes for thoracic and abdominal penetrating aortic ulcers. *J Vasc Surg*. 106;63(5):1182-1188.

110. D'Annoville T, Ozdemir BA, Alric P, et al. Thoracic endovascular aortic repair for penetrating aortic ulcer: literature review. *Ann Thorac Surg*. 2016;101(6):2272–2278.

111. Kim KH, Moon IS, Park JS, et al. Nicardipine hydrochloride injectable phase IV open-label clinical trial: study on the anti-hypertensive effect and safety of nicardipine for acute aortic dissection. *J Int Med Res*. 2002;30(3):337–345.

112. Suzuki T, Isselbacher EM, Nienaber CA, et al. Type-selective benefits of medications in treatment of acute aortic dissection (from the International Registry of Acute Aortic Dissection [IRAD]). *Am J Cardiol*. 2012;109(1):122–127.

113. Wemmelund H, Hogh A, Hundborg HH, et al. Statin use and rupture of abdominal aortic aneurysm. *Br J Surg*. 2014;101(8):966–975.

114. Andersen ND, Ganapathi AM, Hanna JM, et al. Outcomes of acute type A dissection repair before and after implementation of a multidisciplinary thoracic aortic surgery program. *J Am Coll Cardiol*. 2014;63(17):1796–1803.

115. Landon BE, O'Malley JA, Giles K, et al. Volume-outcome relationships and abdominal aortic aneurysm repair. *Circulation*. 2010;122(13):1290–1297.

116. Luft HS, Bunker JP, Enthoven AC. Should operations be regionalized? The empirical relation between surgical volume and mortality. *N Engl J Med*. 1979;301(25):1364–1369.

117. Erbel R, Aboyans V, Boileau C, et al. 2014 ESC guidelines on the diagnosis and treatment of aortic diseases: document covering acute and chronic aortic diseases of the thoracic and abdominal aorta of the adult. The task force for the diagnosis and treatment of aortic diseases of the European Society of Cardiology (ESC). *Eur Heart J*. 2014;35(41):2873–2926.

118. Mehta RH, Suzuki T, Hagan PG, et al. Predicting death in patients with acute type A aortic dissection. *Circulation*. 2002;105(2):200–206.

119. Parikh N, Trimarchi S, Gleason TG, et al. Changes in operative strategy for patients enrolled in the International Registry of Acute Aortic Dissection interventional cohort program. *J Thorac Cardiovasc Surg*. 2017;153(4):S74–S79.

120. Bruno VD, Chivasso P, Guida G, et al. Surgical repair of Stanford type A aortic dissection in elderly patients: a contemporary systematic review and meta-analysis. *Ann Cardiothorac Surg*. 2016;5(4):257–264.

121. Trivedi D, Navid F, Balzer JR, et al. Aggressive aortic arch and carotid replacement strategy for type A aortic dissection improves neurologic outcomes. *Ann Thorac Surg*. 2016;101(3):896–903.

122. Rylski B, Bavaria JE, Beyersdorf F, et al. Type A aortic dissection in Marfan syndrome: extent of initial surgery determines long-term outcome. *Circulation*. 2014;129(13):1381–1386.

123. Sun L, Qi R, Zhu J, et al. Total arch replacement combined with stented elephant trunk implantation: a new "standard" therapy for type A dissection involving repair of the aortic arch. *Circulation*. 2011;123(9):971–978.

124. Li Z, Lu Q, Feng R, et al. Outcomes of endovascular repair of ascending aortic dissection in patients unsuitable for direct surgical repair. *J Am Coll Cardiol*. 2016;68(18):1944–1954.

125. Muetterties CE, Menon R, Wheatley GH. A systematic review of primary endovascular repair of the ascending aorta. *J Vasc Surg*. 2017;67(1):332–342.

126. Martin G, Riga C, Gibbs R, et al. Short- and long-term results of hybrid arch and proximal descending thoracic aortic repair: a benchmark for new technologies. *J Endovasc Ther*. 2016;23(5):783–790.

127. Tolenaar JL, Froehlich W, Jonker FH, et al. Predicting in-hospital mortality in acute type B aortic dissection: evidence from International Registry of Acute Aortic Dissection. *Circulation*. 2014;130(Suppl 1):S45–S50.

128. Trimarchi S, Eagle KA, Nienaber CA, et al. Importance of refractory pain and hypertension in acute type B aortic dissection: insights from the International Registry of Acute Aortic Dissection (IRAD). *Circulation*. 2010;122(13):1283–1289.

129. Durham CA, Cambria RP, Wang LJ, et al. The natural history of medically managed acute type B aortic dissection. *J Vasc Surg*. 2015;61(5):1192–1198.

130. Nienaber CA, Rousseau H, Eggebrecht H, et al. Randomized comparison of strategies for type B aortic dissection: the INvestigation of STEnt Grafts in Aortic Dissection (INSTEAD) trial. *Circulation*. 2009;120(25):2519–2528.

131. Qin YL, Wang F, Li TX, et al. Endovascular repair compared with medical management of patients with uncomplicated type B acute aortic dissection. *J Am Coll Cardiol*. 2016;67(24):2835–2842.

132. Brunkwall J, Kasprzak P, Verhoeven E, et al. Endovascular repair of acute uncomplicated aortic type B dissection promotes aortic remodelling: 1 year results of the ADSORB trial. *Eur J Vasc Endovasc Surg*. 2104;48(3):285-291.

133. Fanelli F, Cannavale A, O'Sullivan GJ, et al. Endovascular repair of acute and chronic aortic type B dissections: main factors affecting aortic remodeling and clinical outcome. *JACC Cardiovasc Interv*. 2016;9(2):183–191.

134. Pacini D, Parolari A, Berretta P, et al. Endovascular treatment for type B dissection in marfan syndrome: is it worthwhile? *Ann Thorac Surg*. 2013;95(2):737–749.

135. Thrumurthy SG, Karthikesalingam A, Patterson BO, et al. A systematic review of mid-term outcomes of thoracic endovascular repair (TEVAR) of chronic type B aortic dissection. *Eur J Vasc Endovasc Surg*. 2011;42(5):632–647.

136. Andersen ND, Keenan JE, Ganapathi AM, et al. Current management and outcome of chronic type B aortic dissection: results with open and endovascular repair since the advent of thoracic endografting. *Ann Cardiothorac Surg*. 2014;3(3):264–274.

137. Cambria RP, Crawford RS, Cho JS, et al. A multicenter clinical trial of endovascular stent graft repair of acute catastrophes of the descending thoracic aorta. *J Vasc Surg*. 2009;50(6):1255–1264.

138. Schanzer A, Simons JP, Flahive J, et al. Outcomes of fenestrated and branched endovascular repair of complex abdominal and thoracoabdominal aortic aneurysms. *J Vasc Surg*. 2017;66(3):687–694.

139. Tsilimparis N, Debus ES, von Kodolitsch Y, et al. Branched versus fenestrated endografts for endovascular repair of aortic arch lesions. *J Vasc Surg*. 2016;64(3):592–599.

140. Grommes J, Greiner A, Bendermacher B, et al. Risk factors for mortality and failure of conservative treatment after aortic type B dissection. *J Thorac Cardiovasc Surg*. 2014;148(5):2155–2160.

141. Erbel R, Alfonso F, Boileau C, et al. Diagnosis and management of aortic dissection. *Eur Heart J*. 2011;22(18):1642–1681.

142. Czerny M, Schoenhoff F, Etz C, et al. The impact of pre-operative malperfusion on outcome in acute type A aortic dissection: results from the GERAADA registry. *J Am Coll Cardiol*. 2015;65(24):2628–2635.

143. Chaddha A, Kline-Rogers E, Woznicki EM, et al. Activity recommendations for postaortic dissection patients. *Circulation*. 2014;130(16):e140–e142.

144. Yeh CH, Chen MC, Wu YC, et al. Risk factors for descending aortic aneurysm formation in medium-term follow-up of patients with type A aortic dissection. *Chest*. 2003;124:989.

145. Hicks CW, Zarkowsky DS, Bostock IC, et al. Endovascular aneurysm repair patients who are lost to follow-up have worse outcomes. *J Vasc Surg*. 2017;65(6):1625–1635.

146. Sakalihasan N, Nienaber CA, Hustinx R, et al. (Tissue PET) Vascular metabolic imaging and peripheral plasma biomarkers in the evolution of chronic aortic dissections. *Eur Heart J Cardiovasc Imaging*. 2015;16(6):626–633.

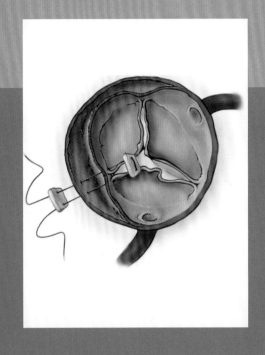

中文导读

第33章
主动脉夹层的手术治疗

　　人类首次描述主动脉夹层这一疾病距今已有250年，但这一疾病能被外科医师治疗的历史仅短短70年。鉴于主动脉夹层的突发性和凶险性，以往医师面对这一棘手的疾病时，都显得力不从心。随着现代体外循环技术和人造血管材料的不断进步，这一疾病逐渐有了治疗的可能。尽管如此，外科治疗主动脉夹层对于医师来说依然是个挑战，这一挑战源于主动脉夹层所累及组织器官速度之快、范围之广、问题之多、程度之严重，都是其他疾病所不及的。因此在面对主动脉夹层时，有3个方面问题需要医师首先明确，即夹层累及的范围、夹层出现的时间及夹层继发了哪些病理生理学问题。从这3个方面出发，医师就可以抉择恰当的介入或手术方案。众所周知，主动脉夹层的整体治疗原则是防止破裂、打开真腔、消灭假腔、恢复灌注。围绕这个原则，按照Stanford分型，A型夹层的治疗重点在于恰当处理主动脉弓部及主动脉根部。比较国内外的处理理念，在主动脉弓部，国外更倾向半弓置换和头臂血管岛状吻合技术，国内更多使用全弓置换加冰冻象鼻技术；在主动脉根部，无论使用哪种技术，都要以充分消灭根窦部假腔、保证冠状动脉血流、恢复主动脉瓣功能为治疗目标。急性且不稳定的B型夹层需要积极干预；而慢性B型夹层，病情高度个体化，外科干预的方向是防止破裂及解决脏器缺血。

于存涛

Surgical Therapy for Aortic Dissection

George J. Arnaoutakis and Joseph E. Bavaria

Morgagni described the first cases of aortic dissection in 1773, and Maunoir coined the entity "aortic dissection."[1] Despite these early reports of thoracic aortic disease, it was not until 1952 that Drs. De Bakey and Cooley first successfully operated on a patient with a descending thoracic aortic aneurysm using a lateral resection. In 1956 De Bakey and Cooley replaced the ascending aorta using cardiopulmonary bypass and homograft for conduit.[2] Grafts manufactured from polyester cloth were later used as the preferred conduit for aortic replacement. The hemostatic qualities of synthetic grafts have been improved by modifications in textile engineering through the impregnation of collagen or gelatin. The routine use of cardiopulmonary bypass and widespread availability of synthetic graft material ushered in the modern era of surgical treatment for aortic dissection. Nevertheless, surgical management of aortic dissection remains a formidable challenge to surgeons. In addition to the inherent weak nature of the aortic tissues, patients may present with a wide spectrum of anatomic and physiologic derangements. Surgical decision making hinges on three primary considerations: (1) anatomic location of the dissection, (2) the time course in respect to onset of symptoms, and (3) the presence of complications related to the dissection.

The DeBakey and Stanford classifications define dissections according to their anatomical location; both systems place significance on involvement of the ascending aorta (Fig. 33.1).[3] DeBakey type I dissection originates in the ascending aorta and extends for a varying distance into the thoracoabdominal aorta, often reaching the aortic bifurcation. DeBakey type II dissection is limited to the ascending aorta. Type IIIa includes dissections with an origin in the descending thoracic aorta and no abdominal involvement. Type IIIb has origin in the descending thoracic aorta but includes abdominal extension. The Stanford system categorizes aortic dissection in two functional groups and is widely incorporated in clinical practice due to its simplicity. Any dissection involving the ascending aorta is categorized as type A, irrespective of the entry tear site or distal extent.

Timing of the operation in relation to onset of symptoms is important because surgical repair becomes safer as the dissection becomes older and the aorta less fragile. Risks posed by tissue fragility must be weighed against the competing risk of acute complications, which include rupture, severe aortic regurgitation, heart failure, and malperfusion. Although somewhat arbitrary, the Society of Thoracic Surgeons has differentiated timing of aortic dissection into the following categories: hyperacute (<48 hours), acute (48 hours to 2 weeks), subacute (>2 weeks to 90 days), and chronic (>90 days).

Aortic dissections can cause numerous potentially lethal complications that warrant emergent surgical intervention. Aortic rupture can occur anywhere along the dissected aorta. Life-threatening proximal aortic complications include pericardial tamponade, acute aortic valve regurgitation, and myocardial infarction (MI) from coronary artery malperfusion. In more distal segments of the aorta, branch vessel malperfusion may lead to stroke, paraplegia, mesenteric ischemia, kidney failure, and limb-threatening ischemia (Fig. 33.2). The combination of these potential complications with severe physiological derangements and extreme tissue fragility make aortic dissection one of the most formidable conditions treated by cardiovascular surgeons.

The three previously listed considerations form the basis for surgical intervention and operative strategies for aortic dissection. Surgical procedures to address proximal aortic dissections involving the ascending aorta and transverse aortic arch differ distinctly from strategies for treating distal aortic dissections involving the descending thoracic and thoracoabdominal aorta. Accordingly, type A and type B aortic dissection will be discussed independently.

TYPE A AORTIC DISSECTION

Natural History

Elective aortic replacement in patients with ascending aortic aneurysm may prophylactically prevent aortic catastrophes such as acute type A aortic dissection, which harbors a very high mortality. The grim natural history of untreated acute type A aortic dissection is underscored by data reporting 50% mortality at 48 hours.[4] However, recent studies have questioned the "1% mortality per hour" that has been previously associated with missed diagnoses or delayed treatment. In a study involving only octogenarians, 25% of patients were unfit to undergo surgery and successfully managed medically.[5] Nevertheless, the extensive morbidity associated with acute type A dissection highlights the importance of prompt diagnosis and expedient surgical intervention in patients determined to be surgical candidates.

Indications for Operation

Aortic repairs for type A aortic dissection undertaken in the chronic phase invariably have superior results compared to those performed in the acute timeframe. Unfortunately, the high risk associated with early operation is outweighed by the even greater risk of a patient suffering a fatal complication (e.g., aortic rupture, coronary malperfusion) while undergoing medical management. Therefore, the presence of an acute type A aortic dissection has traditionally been considered an absolute indication for emergency surgical repair and remains the standard approach.[6] Although controversial, delayed operative management of acute type A aortic dissection has been suggested for the following scenarios: elderly patients, patients with severe malperfusion, dissection occurring after prior cardiac surgery, and to enable transport to a specialized center.

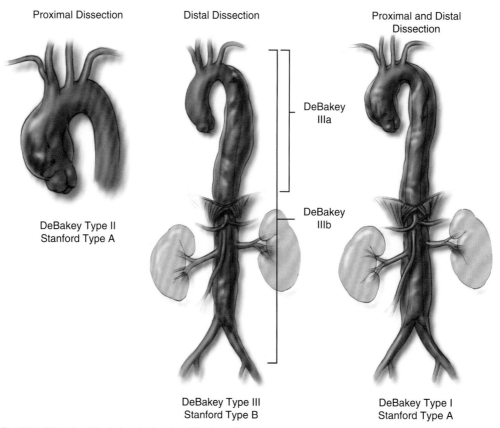

Proximal Dissection

Distal Dissection

Proximal and Distal Dissection

DeBakey IIIa

DeBakey IIIb

DeBakey Type II
Stanford Type A

DeBakey Type III
Stanford Type B

DeBakey Type I
Stanford Type A

Fig. 33.1 This simplified, descriptive classification scheme categorizes aortic dissection based on involvement of proximal aorta, distal aorta, or both segments. Corresponding Debakey classifications are included for comparison. The primary limitation of the Stanford classification is that it is based solely on the presence (type A) or absence (type B) of ascending aortic involvement; it does not provide information about distal aortic involvement, a factor that has important management and prognostic implications.

Elderly Patients

Emergent repair of type A dissection in patients with advanced age greater than 80 years remains controversial. In recent literature, operative mortalities of nearly 50% have been reported for octogenarian patients. One may argue that surgical treatment is not warranted in the elderly because it does not alter the unfavorable natural history of the disease. In addition, while not reaching significance, an International Registry of Aortic Dissection (IRAD) study revealed an absolute survival benefit of 20% among elderly patients who underwent surgical repair of acute type A aortic dissection compared with medical management.[7]

Surgical results of institutions and communities should be considered to optimize best outcomes. Extensive operations such as total arch or aortic root replacement should be weighed against the mortality risk associated with these prolonged and technically challenging operations. In patients whose compromised physiological reserve makes them poor candidates for emergency aortic repair, initial medical optimization followed by semielective surgery may be a reasonable treatment strategy.

Severe Malperfusion

Branch-vessel obstruction due to dissection may cause a wide spectrum of malperfusion syndromes ranging from mild (e.g., weakened distal extremity pulse) to severe (e.g., frank stroke or bowel infarction with necrosis) (Box 33.1). In many cases of mild malperfusion, repair of the proximal aorta restores predominant flow through the true lumen and corrects distal malperfusion. However, patients in

whom ischemia has caused severe end-organ dysfunction are unlikely to benefit from immediate ascending aortic repair. Stroke with resulting coma and bowel infarction with frank peritonitis remain ominous conditions in the setting of type A aortic dissection. Due to these observations, some centers advocate a strategy of delayed surgical treatment in patients with severe malperfusion. These strategies involve aggressive pharmacological treatment to reduce dP/dt (rate of rise of left ventricular [LV] pressure), diagnostic angiography, and percutaneous fenestration or stenting to augment true lumen flow to compromised branch vessels. Delayed proximal aortic operation is undertaken once the patient has recovered from the malperfusion. The optimal treatment strategy in these critically ill patients remains a topic of debate.

Type A Dissection After Prior Cardiac Surgery

Delayed management with elective operation has been proposed for patients who have had previous cardiac surgery. The presence of prosthetic aortic valves, aortic suture lines, coronary bypass grafts, and mediastinal adhesions surrounding the aortic wall are theoretically considered protective. Their presence can potentially prevent rupture, avoid valvular insufficiency, and minimize coronary malperfusion. In one study by the IRAD investigators, patients with type A aortic dissection and a history of previous cardiac operations were less likely to present with chest pain and cardiac tamponade than those without a history of previous cardiac operations.[8] It should be emphasized that the perceived reduced rupture risk has not been conclusively supported by the available literature and does not apply to dissections occurring

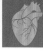

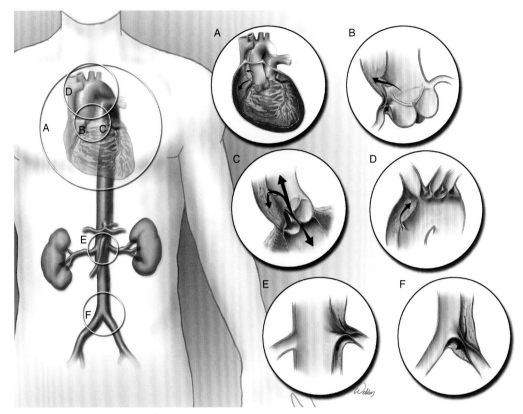

Fig. 33.2 Life-Threatening Complications of Aortic Dissection. Weakened aortic wall can rupture at any location and often results in fatal exsanguination. Rupture of ascending aorta into pericardial space (A) causes cardiac tamponade. Aortic dissection can lead to acute cardiac failure via (B) extension into coronary ostia, causing myocardial ischemia, and (C) disruption of aortic valve commissures, causing acute valvular insufficiency. Complications of branch vessel malperfusion include (D) stroke or upper-extremity ischemia when brachiocephalic branches are involved, paraplegia when segmental intercostal and lumbar arteries are compromised, (E) renal failure or mesenteric ischemia when visceral vessels are disrupted, and (F) lower-limb ischemia when iliac arteries are occluded.

BOX 33.1 Definitions of Severe Malperfusion

Severe Myocardial Malperfusion
Acute infarction diagnosed by electrocardiographic changes or elevated myocardial-specific enzyme levels associated with new-onset ventricular dysfunction

Severe Cerebral Malperfusion
Generalized nonresponsiveness or severe localized neurological deficit lasting >48 h

Severe Visceral Malperfusion
Abdominal pain, physical findings consistent with an acute abdomen, and associated abnormal laboratory findings including lactic acidosis

Severe Extremity Malperfusion
New-onset absence of pulse for more than 4 h associated with pain, neurological symptoms, and physical findings consistent with threatened limb function

Modified from Deeb GM, Williams DM, Bolling SF, et al. Surgical delay for acute type A dissection with malperfusion. *Ann Thorac Surg.* 1997;64:1669–1675.

during the initial several weeks after cardiac surgery. Acute type A aortic dissection during the early postoperative period carries a high risk of rupture and tamponade; these patients should undergo early reoperation. Patients with ongoing chest pain should also undergo prompt surgical repair as well.

Transport to Specialized Centers

Patients with type A aortic dissections frequently require transport to centers where cardiac surgery services are available. Even in centers that offer cardiac surgery, transfer to high-volume centers may be considered in hemodynamically stable patients. There is evidence of improved outcomes in patients transferred to specialized centers. Prior to initiating transport, the patient's condition must be stabilized. Aggressive pharmacological management should be initiated and metabolic derangements addressed. Consistent administration and titration of vasoactive infusions during transport can be facilitated by central venous and arterial catheters. Inotropic agents and diuretic therapy can be given to patients presenting with low cardiac output and acute ventricular distention due to aortic valvular insufficiency and volume overload. If patients with pericardial tamponade must be transferred, a pericardial drain should be placed to allow intermittent drainage during transport. Whenever possible, patients with limb-threatening ischemia should undergo revascularization—usually via femoral-to-femoral artery bypass—before transport to minimize the severe metabolic derangements that result from prolonged limb ischemia and improve chances of survival. Standardized treatment protocols have been developed to optimize the hemodynamic management of patients with type A aortic dissection during transport.

Surgical Repair

Preoperative Considerations

There are several important considerations that may influence conduct of the operation, including the presence of connective tissue disorder, preexisting aortic root or arch aneurysm, and presence of severe malperfusion. A dissection that occurs in the setting of a preexisting aneurysm will likely require complete replacement of that segment. Preoperative computed tomography (CT) scans provide information about true lumen compression and existing malperfusion. Identification of which femoral vessel will provide access to the true lumen has implications for hemodynamic monitoring, cannulation for CPB, and subsequent access for revascularization procedures such as femoral-femoral bypass. The extent of aortic valve incompetence on preoperative echocardiography and any contraindications to anticoagulation will also dictate the need for aortic valve replacement and prosthesis type (mechanical vs. biological).

Cardiopulmonary Bypass

Median sternotomy provides access to the heart and proximal aorta. There are numerous options for arterial access to safely establish cardiopulmonary bypass. Peripheral options in cannulation for arterial inflow include the femoral artery and axillary artery. The femoral artery is a reliable option, which can provide rapid access in patients who are in extremis, although malperfusion and retrograde atheroembolization can occur. The axillary artery usually allows perfusion of true lumen and simplifies antegrade cerebral perfusion.[9] Occasionally dissection may involve the innominate artery and extend into the axillary artery, and one should exercise extreme caution if deciding to cannulate this vessel. Central aortic cannulation, either via direct ascending aortic cannulation or advancement of the cannula into the ascending aorta via the LV apex, is a feasible alternative.[10] Direct ascending cannulation is performed using Seldinger technique and is reliant on echocardiographic imaging to ensure wire access in the true lumen. Venous drainage is accomplished using a dual-stage cannula placed in the inferior vena cava (IVC) via the right atrium. Standard LV venting is performed with a vent catheter placed in the left ventricle via the right superior pulmonary vein.

Most surgeons perform type A aortic dissection repair utilizing a period of hypothermic circulatory arrest.[11] This permits an open distal aortic anastomosis and the opportunity for visual inspection of the entire arch to ensure no additional intimal tears are present. Furthermore, this strategy avoids additional intima tears that may occur from an aortic clamp positioned across the fragile aorta.

Neuroprotection Strategies

Two fundamental concepts in neuroprotection are hypothermia and cerebral perfusion. Hypothermia decreases the body's metabolic demands and permits safe periods of circulatory arrest. Surgeons must be cognizant of time periods of circulatory arrest in order to ensure satisfactory outcomes. Ample literature has shown that longer periods of circulatory arrest are associated with worse outcomes.[12] Traditionally, circulatory arrest was initiated with deep hypothermia at 18°C, but this extent of hypothermia is associated with longer CPB duration due to longer rewarming periods and worse coagulopathy. There is recent

experience that supports the safe use of moderate hypothermia (20°C to 24°C) during circulatory arrest.[13] If the anticipated circulatory arrest time will approach 60 minutes, a standard approach is to use deep hypothermia. Ongoing research trials are underway to determine the optimal core body temperature for performing complex aortic reconstructions utilizing circulatory arrest.

The two commonly employed cerebral perfusion strategies include retrograde cerebral perfusion (RCP) and antegrade cerebral perfusion.[14,15] RCP delivers cold oxygenated blood from the pump into a cannula placed in the superior vena cava. Accumulating evidence suggests that this technique does not provide cerebral oxygenation, but rather provides benefit by maintaining cerebral hypothermia and flushing the cerebral circulation of air and loose debris.[16] Many centers have adopted use of selective antegrade cerebral perfusion to provide oxygenated arterial blood flow to the brain during the period of circulatory arrest. There are multiple techniques for accomplishing this, but a widely adopted approach is via the right axillary artery. An atraumatic vascular clamp or snare is placed at the base of the innominate artery upon initiating circulatory arrest with antegrade cerebral perfusion via a cannula in the axillary artery. Flow is maintained at 8 to 10 mL/kg/min at 10°C, and this provides unilateral antegrade cerebral perfusion. If left-sided cerebral saturations drop upon initiation of ACP and there is copious back bleeding out the ostium of the left common carotid, a vascular occlusion clamp should be placed across the base of the left carotid to pressurize the left-sided circulation. This maneuver often corrects the situation if there is an intact circle of Willis. Alternatively, with the aorta open, selective use of left carotid perfusion by a separate balloon-tipped catheter can be performed, depending on the anticipated length of circulatory arrest. Furthermore, cerebral oximetry, near-infrared spectroscopy (NIRS) cerebral monitoring, and electroencephalography (EEG) are useful monitoring adjuncts during deep hypothermia when cerebral electrical silence is desired. However, with moderate hypothermia, EEG silence is usually not achieved.

Distal Reconstruction

Once the ascending aorta is resected and circulatory arrest established, the transverse aortic arch can be carefully inspected, and decisions made regarding the extent of aortic arch resection (Box 33.2). Most patients will require replacement of the segment of the ascending aorta between the sinotubular junction and the origin of the innominate artery. In the setting of emergent operation for acute dissection, more extensive total arch replacement has been associated with increased early morbidity and mortality, although recent studies have shown equivalent results.[17,18] Therefore, the repair is generally only extended into the arch if there is arch aneurysm or a primary tear located within the arch. When only the proximal portion of the arch has an intimal tear, a beveled graft replacement of the lesser curvature is performed in

---

BOX 33.2   Options for Managing the Aortic Arch During Proximal Aortic Dissection Repair

Ascending replacement only
Beveled hemi-arch replacement
Total arch replacement with island reattachment of brachiocephalic branches
Total arch replacement with separate reimplantation to brachiocephalic branches
Elephant trunk or "Frozen elephant trunk" technique

open hemi-arch fashion (Fig. 33.3). If malperfusion was preoperatively owing to true lumen compression in the descending thoracic aorta, true lumen expansion can be improved by open antegrade deployment of an endovascular stent-graft in the descending thoracic aorta. Whether this intervention influences the natural history of the residual dissected thoracoabdominal aorta is currently a matter of intensive research.[19]

The dissecting membrane that separates the true and false lumens is excised to the distal aortic cuff (see Fig. 33.3B). There are multiple described techniques for performing a hemostatic suture line to dissected aorta. The aorta may be prepared by tacking the inner and outer walls together using surgical adhesive to obliterate the false lumen and strengthen the tissue (see Fig. 33.3C). A felt "sandwich" technique has been described whereby a felt buttress is applied on both the inner and outer layer of the aortic wall, thus leading to a robust suture line. We favor the felt "neomedia" technique.[20] Teflon felt is placed between the

dissected media and adventitia layers to create a reinforced "neomedia." This strengthened tissue can better withstand suture placement. An appropriate size graft is then anastomosed to the distal aorta with 4-0 or 3-0 polypropylene in an "onlay" type anastomosis with the graft invaginated into the distal aorta. This drives the prosthetic graft material into the native aorta when pressurized and prevention against leaks (see Fig. 33.3D). Restoration of true lumen flow often alleviates any mild distal malperfusion that was present preoperatively. The graft is de-aired and clamped, and full CPB is resumed with the release of the innominate snare. Rewarming is initiated, and attention returned to the proximal portion of the repair (see Fig. 33.3E).

Total Aortic Arch Replacement

Extensive aneurysms involving the entire arch usually require total arch replacement. Primary tears affecting the greater curvature or any of the brachiocephalic branch vessels should be resected. The distal

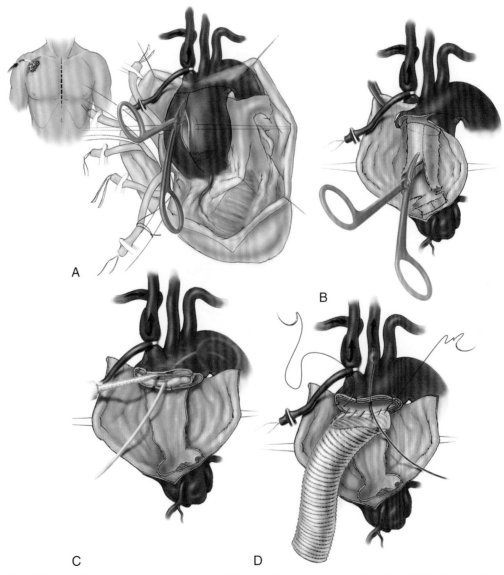

Fig. 33.3 Graft Repair of Ascending Aorta and Proximal Transverse Aortic Hemi-Arch With Concomitant Aortic Valve Resuspension. (A) Operation is performed via median sternotomy. Cardiopulmonary bypass inflow is established via the right axillary artery. (B) After initiating circulatory arrest and antegrade cerebral perfusion, ascending aorta is opened, and dissecting membrane is excised. (C) Distal aortic cuff is prepared using surgical adhesive; balloon catheter in descending aorta prevents distal migration of adhesive. (D) Open distal anastomosis between graft and aorta is completed and reinforced with additional adhesive.

Continued

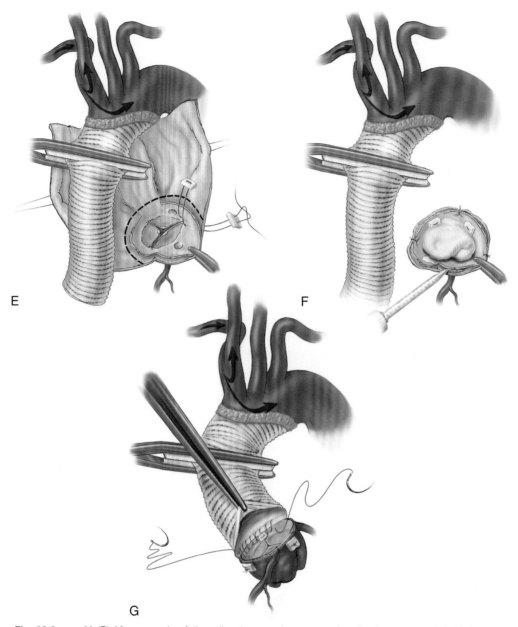

Fig. 33.3, cont'd (E) After resuming full cardiopulmonary bypass, aortic valve is resuspended. (F) Proximal aortic cuff is repaired with adhesive. (G) Proximal anastomosis is performed.

anastomosis is created beyond the primary tear at the transverse arch or at the proximal descending thoracic aorta, using a tube graft. While island patch inclusion of the great vessels has been described, the preferred approach currently is for reattachment of the arch vessels individually, using a trifurcated or bifurcated graft (Fig. 33.4). There are prefabricated aortic grafts with three separate limbs for great vessel reimplantation. Alternatively, each of the three limbs of a trifurcated arch graft can be separately anastomosed to the individual arch vessels and the main limb anastomosed to the ascending graft. In extreme cases, the aneurysm extends past the arch and into the descending thoracic aorta. This can be managed using the elephant trunk technique described by Borst for total arch replacement.[21] The distal anastomosis is constructed so that a portion of the graft is left suspended within the true lumen of the proximal descending thoracic aorta. In addition to directing flow into the true lumen, this "trunk" can be used to facilitate repair of the descending thoracic aorta during a subsequent thoracotomy approach to repair the descending aorta.

Due to patient body habitus or significant arch aneurysm, exposure for the anastomosis to the left subclavian artery can be difficult in certain cases and prolong circulatory arrest times. The concept of zone 2 arch replacement involves a distal anastomosis in zone 2 of the aortic arch (between left common carotid and left subclavian arteries), with reimplantation of the left common carotid and innominate arteries in similar fashion to total arch replacement. Reimplanting the two arch vessels proximal enough on the ascending graft permits ample landing zone for subsequent thoracic endovascular aortic repair (TEVAR) in the future either with a branched endograft into the left subclavian artery or with a concomitant carotid-subclavian bypass.

Antegrade Thoracic Endovascular Aortic Repair

Despite efforts to aggressively resect the primary intimal tear and elimination of the false lumen at the distal aortic suture line, the false lumen often persists at the level of the descending thoracic aorta and into the thoracoabdominal aorta. Persistence of false lumen flow after type A

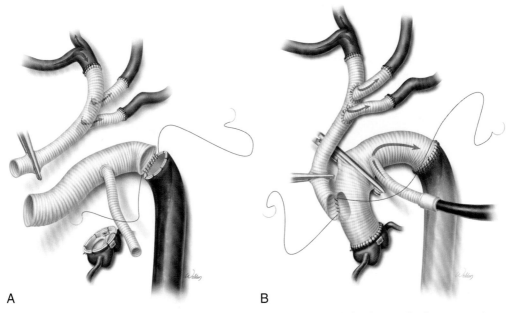

Fig. 33.4 (A and B) Graft replacement of entire transverse aortic arch involves a distal anastomosis to descending thoracic aorta and separate reattachment of brachiocephalic branches. This approach is generally reserved for patients with primary tears within the arch or large aortic arch aneurysms. (Courtesy Baylor College of Medicine.)

dissection repair is a risk factor for late aortic degeneration and aneurysm formation, need for reoperation, and death. Furthermore, in the acute setting, true lumen compression in the descending thoracic aorta can cause malperfusion in the mesenteric vessels, renal vessels, and lower extremities. To address both concerns, concomitant antegrade TEVAR in the descending thoracic aorta combined with either standard ascending or hemi-arch reconstruction or in an extended total arch reconstruction in a "frozen elephant trunk" are surgical options. The outcomes with these surgical techniques are the subject of much ongoing current research.

We employ antegrade TEVAR if the patient presents with clinically significant malperfusion (e.g., ischemia in the lower extremities, paraplegia, renal compromise) preoperatively and evidence of true lumen compression on CT imaging. The endograft is sized to the true lumen. Caution should be exercised not to oversize an endograft within the friable dissected aorta. A guidewire is advanced into the true lumen of the open descending aorta under direct vision during circulatory arrest. The stent-graft is deployed in an antegrade fashion, with the proximal landing zone just distal to the left subclavian artery. One or two tacking sutures can be placed to fix the stent-graft to the distal arch to prevent migration and endoleak.[22] The objective of an antegrade TEVAR is to direct flow into the true lumen, eliminate malperfusion, and potentially affect positive aortic remodeling in the descending thoracic aorta by promoting false lumen thrombosis. Addition of an antegrade TEVAR is well tolerated and adds minimal time to the period of circulatory arrest, although long-term outcomes have not been widely reproduced as of yet.[23] Recently designed hybrid arch grafts have a prefabricated branched frozen elephant trunk to facilitate antegrade TEVAR at the time of total arch replacement (Fig. 33.5).[24] These hybrid arch grafts are not yet FDA approved for widespread use in the United States at the present time.

Aortic Root Considerations

A preexisting aortic root aneurysm or connective tissue disorder, the degree to which the dissection flap extends into the root, and the degree of aortic valve distortion are factors for consideration when evaluating

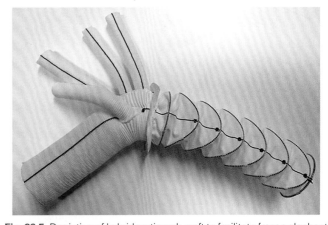

Fig. 33.5 Depiction of hybrid aortic arch graft to facilitate frozen elephant trunk procedures.

the aortic root during Type A aortic dissection. Potential strategies to address the aortic valve are listed in Box 33.3.

Supracommissural Anastomosis with Aortic Valve Repair

When there is no significant aortic root pathology nor significant aortic valve disease, the aortic valve and root can be preserved. Many patients have detachment of one or more commissures from the outer aortic wall, with resulting aortic valve regurgitation. Normal aortic valve function can be restored by resuspending the commissures into their normal position (Fig. 33.6).[25] This can be performed with three separate 4-0 Prolene pledgeted horizontal mattress sutures placed at the top of each commissure and through all three layers of the aortic wall. Some surgeons use surgical adhesive within the false channel to strengthen this aortic root reconstruction. The proximal aortic cuff can be prepared in similar fashion to the distal aorta using a felt "neomedia" technique (Fig. 33.7). Alternatively, a felt sandwich technique with

BOX 33.3   Options for Managing the Aortic Valve During Proximal Aortic Dissection Repair

Aortic valve repair: commissural resuspension
    Commissural plication annuloplasty
    Resuspension and annuloplasty
Aortic valve replacement with mechanical or biological prosthesis
Aortic root replacement:
    Composite valve graft
    Aortic homograft
    Stentless porcine root
    Valve-sparing techniques (controversial)

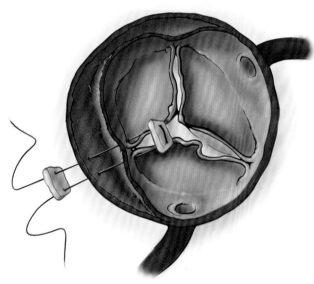

Fig. 33.6 Cross-section of aortic root illustrates dehiscence of two aortic valve commissures, which causes acute valvular regurgitation. Resuspending commissures onto outer aortic wall restores valve competency.

felt buttress on the inner and outer layer of the aortic walls can be used as well. Once the root and valve repairs are complete, the proximal aortic anastomosis is completed at the sinotubular junction.

By preserving the aortic valve, long-term anticoagulation is often avoided; this theoretically may help with thrombosis of the false lumen and prevent subsequent dilation of the thoracoabdominal aorta. Another advantage of a valve-sparing approach is that it requires fewer stitches and can be performed quickly. Limiting the extent of repair reduces cardiac ischemia, CPB, and overall operative times, and may translate into lower postoperative morbidity and mortality. Therefore, although more extensive procedures can reduce risk of reoperation, limited repairs are performed whenever possible to increase the chance of survival after the initial operation. In a recent report of 210 patients who were discharged from the hospital after aortic valve repair for type A dissection, freedom from reoperation for aortic valve insufficiency was 97%, 92%, and 82% at 5, 10, and 23 years, respectively.[26] The rapid evolution of transcatheter therapies may also permit a less invasive manner to address any subsequent aortic valve pathology in the future.

Aortic Valve Replacement

Some patients with acute type A dissection require concomitant correction of aortic valve pathology. Occasionally the valvular damage

caused by the dissection is too severe to repair. In this case, separate replacement of the valve and graft replacement of the tubular segment of the ascending aorta are performed. This is also an option for patients who have significant preexisting aortic valvular disease such as aortic stenosis. Separate aortic valve replacement with ascending graft replacement is generally not a preferred option for patients with annuloaortic ectasia or Marfan syndrome (MFS) because progressive dilation of the remaining sinus segment eventually leads to complications requiring reoperation.

Aortic Root Replacement

Full aortic root replacement entails a mechanical or biological graft that has both valve and aortic conduit components. Three commercially available graft options are (1) composite valve grafts, which comprise a mechanical or biological stented prosthesis attached to a polyester tube graft; (2) aortic root homografts, which are harvested from cadavers and cryopreserved; and (3) stentless porcine aortic root grafts. Valve-sparing aortic root reimplantation is an option for full root replacement and involves excision of the aortic sinuses, attachment of a prosthetic graft to the native annulus, and resuspension of the native aortic valve inside the graft. Superior hemodynamics of the native valve and avoidance of anticoagulation are major advantages to this approach. Experienced centers have performed valve-sparing root replacements in patients with acute dissection and have obtained mixed results.[27] Because of the substantial technical demands and lack of long-term outcome data, the role of valve-sparing root replacement in patients with acute aortic dissection remains controversial, especially in patients with MFS.

Ascending Thoracic Endovascular Aortic Repair

The standard approach to ascending aorta pathology remains open surgical repair. However, some patients present with such extreme comorbidities, rendering them prohibitive risk for open surgical repair.[28,29] These patients may still benefit from a minimally invasive endograft option. Currently, there are no FDA-approved endografts designed for application in the ascending aorta. There is a single device accessible in Europe produced by Cook Medical.[30] Reports from European and US centers describe outcomes with ascending TEVAR for acute Type A aortic dissection in patients not deemed open surgical candidates.[31] Refinements in technology are necessary to overcome the complex anatomic considerations, including the coronary ostia, innominate artery origin, and discrepant diameters between the sinuses of Valsalva and ascending aorta.

Chronic Proximal Dissection

Occasionally, patients with type A aortic dissection are identified in the chronic setting. With certain exceptions, the presence of chronic type A dissection warrants surgical repair to prevent aortic rupture. These surgical repairs are undertaken in similar fashion to those performed in the acute setting. There is often improved tissue strength in the chronic setting, allowing for more hemostatic suture lines. In addition, instead of obliterating the false lumen at the distal anastomosis, the dissecting membrane is fenestrated or resected into the arch to ensure blood flow in both lumens and to prevent postoperative peripheral ischemia. The absence of both acute inflammation and malperfusion simplifies perioperative management. These factors partially account for substantial differences in outcomes between patients who undergo surgery in the acute setting and those who undergo repair in the chronic phase. Compared with patients who undergo repairs in the acute phase, those who undergo repair of chronic dissection have lower incidences of death and stroke. Contemporary series report both early mortality and stroke rates below 8%.[32,33]

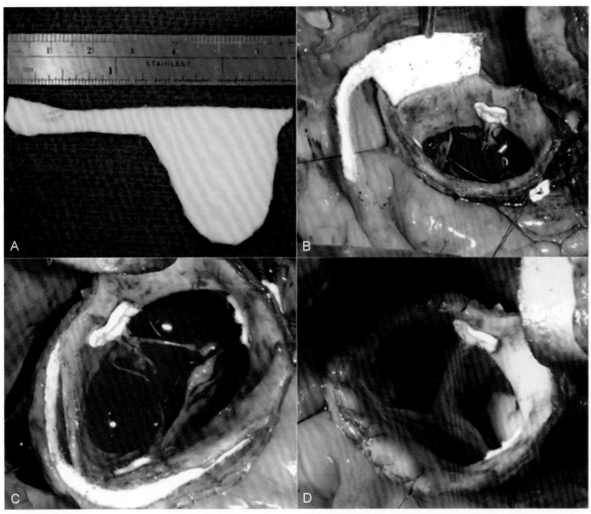

Fig. 33.7 (A–D) Felt "neomedia" technique whereby felt is placed between adventitia and intima/media layers and secured in place with running 5-0 Prolene suture. Proximal or distal suture line is strengthened by this reinforced aortic wall.

Outcomes

According to recent data from the IRAD, the risk for mortality ranges between 17% and 26%.[12] As operative techniques and critical care have improved, so has mortality at most centers. At one center, mortality improved in a stepwise fashion from 21% during their first quartile (1979 to 1980) to just 4% during their last quartile (2000 to 2003).[34] Published risk factors for operative mortality include increasing patient age, pericardial tamponade, preoperative shock, preoperative neurological deficits, delay in diagnosis, repair of the aortic arch, coronary artery disease (CAD), acute myocardial infarction (AMI), concomitant coronary artery bypass, and malperfusion. Despite the substantial risks involved with surgical treatment, contemporary results are excellent compared with the high mortality rates of unrepaired acute type A aortic dissection. In the IRAD registry, 155 patients (17%) were managed nonoperatively, with an observed in-hospital mortality of 59% compared with 24% in those treated surgically.[7] Causes of late mortality are multifactorial, with most deaths being related to nonaortic causes such as stroke, heart failure, and malignancy. The most common aorta-related late deaths result from complications related to the residual dissected aortic arch and thoracoabdominal aorta. In recent studies focusing on long-term survival after proximal aortic dissection repair, persistent false lumen patency has been noted as a risk factor for late aorta-related mortality and the need for intervention. The incidence of persistent false lumen flow varies significantly in the literature, from 20% to 90%. Instances of partial thrombosis have been observed, with a higher incidence of persistent false lumen patency in the abdomen. Long-term implications of persistent false lumen flow have been the motivation for concurrent intervention at the distal segment of the initial proximal repair; however, outcomes for this strategy remain an intense topic of current research. Patients with residual dissection in the distal aortic segments require careful surveillance and aggressive blood pressure management to avoid long-term complications, including aneurysmal degeneration.

ACUTE TYPE B AORTIC DISSECTION

The standard treatment approach for acute type B aortic dissection without complicating features remains nonoperative management (see Chapter 32). Medical therapy focuses on blood pressure and heart rate control, which is referred to as anti-impulse therapy, and close observation for the development of complicating features. Monitoring entails frequent clinical assessment in an intensive care unit (ICU) setting, continuous arterial line blood pressure measurement, and interval imaging at 48 to 72 hours to assess for acute changes in the dissected aorta. Traditionally surgical intervention in the acute period has been reserved for aneurysmal changes, impending or contained rupture, or

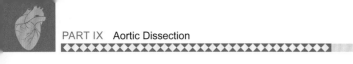

malperfusion. Whether surgical intervention for acute uncomplicated type B dissection alters the natural history of the disease process and avoids late aorta-related deaths remains an area of active debate.

Indications for Operation

Aortic rupture and end-organ ischemia are the most common causes of death in acute type B dissection, and therefore surgical intervention is indicated to correct these complications. Specific complications that indicate need for operative treatment include aortic rupture or mediastinal hematoma, rapid aortic expansion, uncontrolled hypertension, malperfusion, or refractory pain despite aggressive pharmacological therapy. Acute dissection superimposed on a preexisting aneurysm is considered a life-threatening condition and is also an indication for operation. Many patients with acute type B dissection will develop a reactive left pleural effusion; this finding does not necessarily indicate impending rupture and alone is not an indication for surgery. However, increasing periaortic or pleural fluid associated with other worrisome findings, such as aortic expansion or mediastinal hematoma, warrants surgical intervention. Finally, surgical treatment should be considered in patients who are noncompliant with medical therapy, provided they are otherwise satisfactory operative candidates.

Surgical Repair

Operative Techniques

A wide range of surgical techniques are potentially applicable for treating complications of acute type B dissection. Therapy should be tailored to the goals of treatment, condition of the patient, anatomical considerations, and capabilities of the institution. Malperfusion of the extremities can be treated by peripheral extra-anatomical bypass. A femoral-femoral bypass or carotid-subclavian bypass can perfuse an ischemic extremity and allow continued nonoperative management of the dissected aorta.

Endovascular techniques have recently expanded surgical alternatives and are the mainstay of surgical treatment for acute type B dissection. Visceral and renal malperfusion can ideally be addressed by endovascular intervention. Endovascular fenestration of the dissecting membrane or placement of stents into obstructed branch vessels can reestablish organ perfusion. In compromised patients with mesenteric ischemia or renal failure, endovascular reperfusion may allow clinical stabilization for other subsequent therapies or decision making. TEVAR has been adopted widely, with the goal of sealing large entry tears, treating distal aortic malperfusion, excluding a dilated thoracic aorta, or promoting long-term remodeling to prevent the late sequela of aneurysm formation (also see Chapter 34).[35] TEVAR may perhaps be ideal to treat acute dilations of limited thoracic dissections. The introduction of branched TEVAR technology permits more proximal fixation in potentially nondissected aorta of the distal arch. When performing TEVAR for acute complicated type B dissection, intravascular ultrasound should be used to confirm wire access in the true lumen. In addition, the endograft should not be oversized, with a target of 10% or less oversizing to the overall normal aorta diameter. Oversizing risks retrograde type A dissection, endograft-induced new entry tears, and proximal neck dilation with endograft migration.

When the endovascular approach is unavailable or unsuccessful in treating complications of the acute type B dissection, open surgical options such as graft replacement of the aorta, open aortic fenestration, and branch artery bypass should be considered.[36] In the acute phase, the primary surgical objectives are to prevent fatal rupture and restore branch artery blood flow. A limited graft repair of the life-threatening segment can achieve these objectives while minimizing risks. Because the most common site of rupture is in the upper third of the descending thoracic aorta, replacement usually extends from the level of the left subclavian artery to the middescending level. The distal portion of the descending thoracic aorta is also replaced if it is aneurysmal. Graft replacement of the entire thoracoabdominal aorta is only considered in the acute setting if there is a large coexisting aneurysm, but this is an exceedingly rare clinical scenario. Similarly, the repair is not extended proximally into the arch, even if the primary tear is located there, unless the arch is substantially dilated.

Because surgery for acute type B dissection carries an increased risk of postoperative paraplegia, adjuncts that provide spinal cord protection are used liberally. Cerebrospinal fluid drainage and left heart bypass are often used, even when the planned repair is limited to the upper descending thoracic aorta. Proximal control is usually obtained by placing a clamp between the left common carotid and left subclavian arteries. Manipulation of mediastinal hematoma around the proximal descending thoracic aorta is avoided until proximal control is established. The aorta is opened, and the dissecting membrane is removed from the segment being replaced. The proximal and distal anastomoses incorporate all layers of the aortic wall, thereby obliterating the false lumen with the suture lines and directing all blood flow into the true lumen. Although there are usually multiple patent intercostal arteries, the extreme tissue fragility often precludes their reattachment.

Outcomes

Aggressive pharmacological management has led to a substantial decrease in mortality for patients with acute distal aortic dissection. Still, some 10% to 20% of medically treated patients without acute complications at the time of presentation die during the initial treatment phase.[37] Primary causes of death during nonoperative management include rupture, malperfusion, and cardiac failure. Risk factors associated with medical treatment failure include a large entry tear, enlarged aorta, persistent hypertension despite maximal treatment, oliguria, and peripheral ischemia.

Patients undergoing surgery for acute type B dissection are a high-risk group that includes patients with rupture, neurological dysfunction, renal failure, and peripheral ischemia. Therefore, it is not surprising that results after surgery for acute complicated type B dissection are often worse than those of medical therapy. Results from the IRAD registry show a mortality of 11% for endovascular operations, compared with 34% after open operations for acute type B dissections.[38] Long-term data are currently lacking regarding the fate of the false lumen and the implications of late aneurysm formation after endovascular treatment of long thoracoabdominal dissections and uncomplicated dissections. Despite the early survival advantage with nonoperative management compared with surgical treatment, long-term results are similar in patients in both groups. The reported actuarial survival rates with nonoperative management are 76% at 5 years and 56% at 10 years.[39] Five- and 10-year survival rates after repair range from 80% to 55%, respectively.[40]

Results from the only randomized prospective trial of uncomplicated chronic type B dissections for which TEVAR was performed between 2 and 52 weeks after dissection show no significant differences in mortality or adverse event rates at 2 years.[41] However, recent publication of 5-year follow-up revealed that TEVAR plus optimal medical management leads to improved aorta-specific survival and delayed disease progression compared with optimal medical management alone.[42]

CHRONIC TYPE B AORTIC DISSECTION

Chronic aortic dissection is a progressive disease that requires lifelong management. The rationale for careful surveillance lies in the natural history of the disease. Rupture and ischemic events related to the dissection are responsible for most late deaths, and therefore surgical intervention is eventually required in approximately one-third of patients.

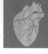

Indications for Operation

Operative repair for a chronic type B aortic dissection is required in the setting of those patients for whom medical management was initially successful but who subsequently develop an indication for surgery. Patients who underwent successful type A dissection but have residual descending dissection also frequently require intervention. Although subsequent malperfusion or ischemic events can occur in a chronically dissected aorta, the majority of patients will require operative intervention for aneurysmal degeneration of chronic dissection. Interval surveillance is critical in monitoring the growth of the aneurysm. Although the entire thoracoabdominal aorta may be dissected, the mere presence of dissection in the descending aorta is not an indication for surgical intervention. In asymptomatic patients, an elective operation is considered when the aneurysmal segment has reached 5.5 to 6 cm, or when it has enlarged more than 1 cm during a 1-year period. A lower threshold is reserved for patients with connective tissue disorders, including Marfan, Loeys-Dietz, and other familial aortic syndromes.

Urgent operation is considered if the aneurysm becomes symptomatic. Patients with symptomatic aneurysms are at increased risk of rupture and deserve expeditious evaluation and treatment. The onset of new pain in a patient with a known aneurysm is particularly concerning and may herald significant expansion, leakage, or impending rupture. Emergent surgery is reserved for patients with clinical signs or imaging findings of rupture.

Operative strategies are considerably different in emergent versus elective procedures. Patients with chronic dissection who require emergency open surgical repair because of acute pain or rupture undergo limited graft replacement of the symptomatic segment. Although the entire thoracoabdominal aorta may be dissected and aneurysmal, typically a relatively localized segment is the cause of the symptoms. Limited repair minimizes early postoperative morbidity. In appropriate surgical candidates, elective repairs replace the entire descending thoracic aorta and often extend to include the thoracoabdominal aorta (Fig. 33.8).

Preoperative Assessment

A detailed preoperative assessment of physiological reserve is critical. All patients should undergo a thorough evaluation before undergoing elective operation, with a focus on baseline cardiovascular, pulmonary, and renal function.

Cardiovascular Status

Ischemic heart disease is common in patients with thoracic aortic disease and contributes to a substantial proportion of early and late postoperative deaths. In addition, valvular pathology and ventricular dysfunction have important implications when planning anesthetic management and strategies for aortic repair. Transthoracic echocardiography (TTE) is routinely performed to evaluate both valvular and ventricular function. Nuclear stress tests or myocardial perfusion studies are used selectively to identify reversible myocardial ischemia. Cardiac catheterization with coronary arteriography should be considered in patients who have evidence of coronary disease or a depressed ejection fraction. Patients who are asymptomatic and have severe CAD may undergo percutaneous angioplasty or surgical revascularization before aneurysm repair.

The hemodynamic changes that occur during thoracic aortic repair can precipitate stroke in patients with significant cerebrovascular

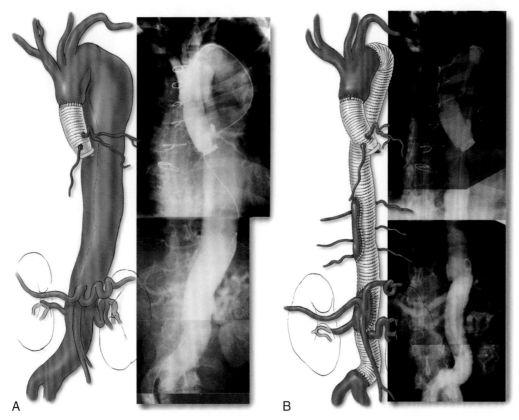

Fig. 33.8 Presentation (A) and repair (B) of an Extent II thoracoabdominal aortic aneurysm that developed secondary to chronic distal aortic dissection. Patient had previously undergone repair of a proximal aortic dissection.

disease. Therefore, carotid duplex ultrasound studies are also routinely obtained to detect occult carotid artery stenosis. It is recommended that significant carotid artery stenosis be corrected with an endarterectomy before proceeding with the aortic operation.

Pulmonary Status

The most common complication after descending thoracic and thoracoabdominal aortic repairs is pulmonary dysfunction, with prolonged ventilator dependence and the need for tracheostomy. Therefore, pulmonary function testing, including arterial blood gases and spirometry, is also routinely obtained before surgery to assess risk and allow optimization of the patient's pulmonary status. Patients with a forced expiratory volume in the first second of expiration (FEV_1) exceeding 1 L and a partial pressure of carbon dioxide (Pco_2) below 45 mm Hg are considered reasonable candidates for elective surgery. In selected patients, borderline pulmonary function can be improved with a 1- to 3-month regimen that includes smoking cessation, exercise, weight loss, and treatment of bronchitis. In most cases, operation is not withheld in patients with symptomatic aneurysms and poor pulmonary reserve. Surgical techniques, however, can be modified to improve the chance of recovery in these high-risk patients. For example, precautions can be taken to ensure preservation of the left recurrent laryngeal and phrenic nerves. Diaphragm-sparing techniques may also be helpful in such patients.

Renal Status

Preoperative renal status is evaluated on the basis of serum electrolytes, blood urea nitrogen (BUN), and creatinine (Cr) measurements. The CT or magnetic resonance imaging (MRI) studies obtained to evaluate the aorta also provide information regarding kidney size and perfusion. Patients with severely impaired renal function frequently require at least temporary hemodialysis after operation; these patients are also at increased risk of death.[43,44] In addition, perfusion strategies and perioperative medications are adjusted on the basis of renal function. Finally, patients with poor renal function due to renal malperfusion from a dissection flap or from occlusive disease can undergo renal endarterectomy, stenting, or bypass grafting during thoracoabdominal aortic aneurysm (TAAA) repair.

Surgical Repair

Operative Techniques

Surgical strategies are determined on the basis of the extent of the aneurysm being repaired.[45] Descending TAAs are confined to the chest and are therefore repaired through a left thoracotomy. Extent of the thoracoabdominal replacement is defined by the Crawford classification of TAAAs (Fig. 33.9). In patients with TAAAs, this incision is extended across the costal margin and into the abdomen (Fig. 33.10A). A double-lumen endobronchial tube is used to allow selective single lung ventilation. Retroperitoneal exposure of the thoracoabdominal aorta is achieved by dividing the diaphragm and retracting the peritoneal contents medially.

Aortic repair requires a period of aortic clamping. The clamp is ideally applied distal to the left subclavian artery but is often required between the left common carotid artery (CCA) and left subclavian artery because of the anatomy of the aneurysm. In patients who have undergone previous coronary artery bypass surgery using the left

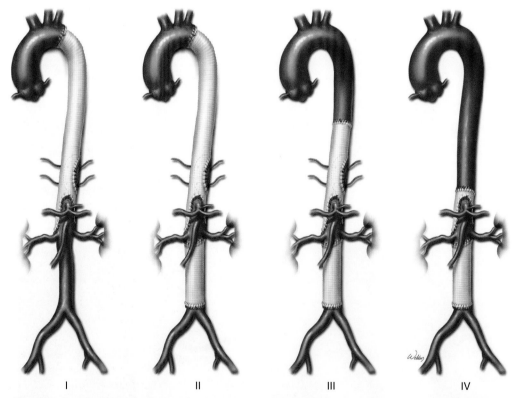

Fig. 33.9 Crawford classification categorizes thoracoabdominal aortic aneurysms based on the extent of aortic repair. Extent I repairs begin in upper descending thoracic aorta, often near left subclavian artery, and extend to region of visceral and renal arteries. Extent II repairs also involve upper descending thoracic aorta but extend distally beyond renal arteries, often to aortic bifurcation. Extent III repairs begin in lower descending thoracic aorta (below sixth rib) and extend into abdominal segment. Extent IV repairs begin at diaphragmatic crura and extend distally, often involving entire abdominal aorta. (From Coselli JS, Bozinovski J, LeMaire SA. Open surgical repair of 2286 thoracoabdominal aortic aneurysms. *Ann Thorac Surg.* 2007;83:S862–S864.)

internal thoracic artery, clamping proximal to the left subclavian artery can induce severe myocardial ischemia. When clamping at this location is anticipated, a left common carotid-to-subclavian bypass is performed preoperatively to avoid cardiac complications. In certain situations, such as contained rupture, an extremely large aneurysm, or extension into the distal transverse arch, there is no suitable proximal clamp site, and hypothermic circulatory arrest is required. Once proximal control is established whether via a clamp site or hypothermic circulatory arrest, the aneurysmal segment of aorta is replaced with a polyester tube graft (see Fig. 33.10B–J).

Because of the periaortic inflammation caused by the dissection, the vagus and left recurrent laryngeal nerves are often adherent to the aortic wall and susceptible to injury during repair of the proximal descending segment. Careful dissection of the proximal descending thoracic aorta from the underlying esophagus before performing the proximal anastomosis minimizes the risk of esophageal injury and development of aortoesophageal fistula. The aortic branch vessels—including the intercostal, celiac, superior mesenteric, renal, and lumbar arteries—are reattached to the prosthetic graft, either via patch anastomosis or individual vessel reimplantation.

When dissection extends into the visceral or renal arteries, the membrane can be fenestrated or the false lumen can be obliterated using sutures or intraluminal stents. Asymmetrical expansion of the false lumen often displaces the left renal artery laterally enough to require separate reattachment or use of a side branch graft. If the dissection stops at the level of the visceral vessels, the distal anastomosis can be beveled to include the abdominal branches. Although it is tempting to resect as much of the dissected aorta as possible, risks of the operation, including paraplegia, are incrementally increased with the greater extent of aortic replacement. Adjacent dissected aorta that is not aneurysmal is fenestrated by resecting wedges of the dissecting membrane proximally and distally from within the aortic cuffs, allowing blood to flow through both true and false channels after the reconstruction is completed. The distal anastomosis is performed at the proximal most level of non-aneurysmal aorta.

Organ Protection

Clamping the descending thoracic aorta creates ischemia of the spinal cord and abdominal viscera. Clinically significant postoperative manifestations of hepatic, pancreatic, and bowel ischemia are

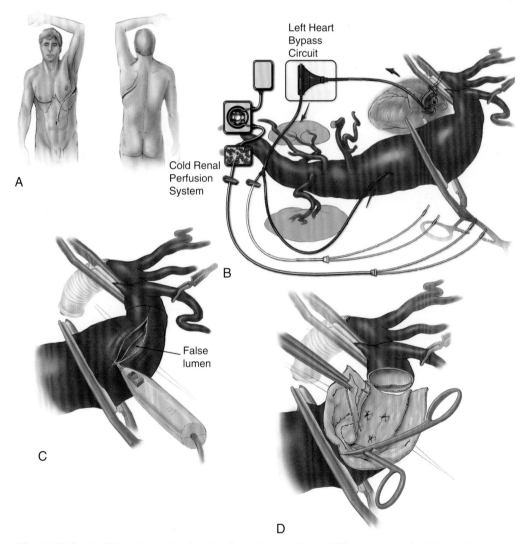

Fig. 33.10 Surgical Techniques Involved in Repairing an Extent II Thoracoabdominal Aortic Aneurysm Related to Chronic Aortic Dissection. (A) Repair is performed through left thoracoabdominal incision. (B) Aortic clamps are applied after establishing distal aortic perfusion via a left heart bypass circuit. (C) The segment of aorta isolated between clamps is opened. (D) Dissecting membrane is excised, and intercostal arteries are ligated.
Continued

547

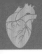
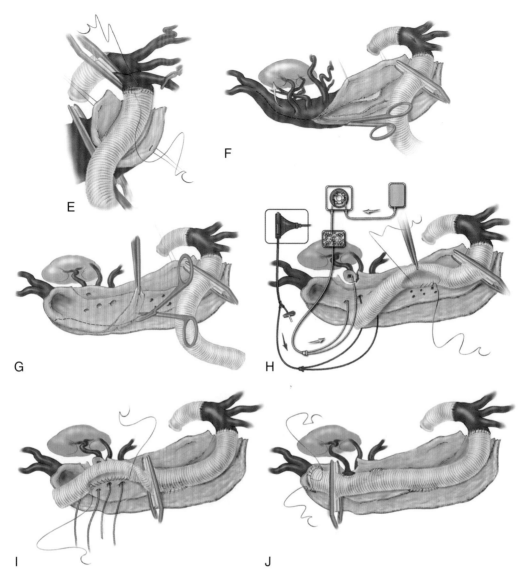

Fig. 33.10, cont'd (E) Graft is sutured to proximal descending thoracic aorta. (F) Clamps are repositioned to restore perfusion of left subclavian artery, left heart bypass is stopped, and the remainder of the aneurysm is opened. (G) Dissecting membrane is removed to allow identification of patent segmental arteries and origins of visceral and renal arteries. (H) Blood from left heart bypass circuit is delivered to celiac axis and superior mesenteric artery via balloon perfusion catheters. Cold perfusion is delivered to kidneys through catheters placed in renal arterial ostia. Critical intercostal arteries are attached to an opening in graft. (I) Reattachment of visceral branches and (J) the distal aortic anastomosis complete the repair.

relatively uncommon. Acute kidney injury and spinal cord injury, however, are the main causes of morbidity and mortality after these operations. Therefore, several aspects of the operation are devoted to minimizing spinal and renal ischemia (Box 33.4).[45] A multimodality approach to spinal cord protection includes cerebrospinal fluid drainage, mild permissive hypothermia (32°C to 34°C, nasopharyngeal), steroid administration, moderate systemic heparinization to prevent small-vessel thrombosis, distal aortic perfusion with left heart bypass during proximal anastomosis, sequential clamping of the lower aortic segments to reestablish flow to proximal organs as the proximal anastomoses are completed, and reattachment of the segmental intercostal and lumbar arteries. Cerebrospinal fluid drainage is used in extensive thoracoabdominal repairs (i.e., Crawford I and II) and in selected redo operations. Cerebrospinal fluid drainage improves spinal perfusion by reducing cerebrospinal fluid pressure and has been shown to be beneficial by a randomized clinical trial.[46] There is some evidence

that staging replacement of the entire thoracoabdominal aorta may minimize paraplegia rates.[47] Left heart bypass or full cardiopulmonary bypass are employed to provide perfusion of the distal aorta and its branches during the proximal clamp period. Left heart bypass is employed by placing an angled-tip cannula in the left atrium via the inferior pulmonary vein. Oxygenated blood is returned to the patient via an arterial cannula placed in either the femoral artery or distal aorta. Alternatively, full cardiopulmonary bypass can be established using the femoral vein and artery. In instances where hypothermic circulatory arrest will be necessary, it is important to ascertain any baseline aortic valve insufficiency. Because the patient will fibrillate, it is important to avoid LV distention and often a LV vent is necessary. The visceral and distal aortic anastomoses are completed sequentially. During this time, balloon perfusion cannulas connected to the left heart bypass circuit can be used to deliver blood directly to the celiac axis and superior mesenteric artery (SMA) during their reattachment. Potential benefits

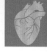

> **BOX 33.4 Strategies for Spinal Cord, Visceral, and Renal Protection During Repair of Distal Thoracic Aortic Dissection**
>
> **All Extents**
> Permissive mild hypothermia (32°C–34°C, nasopharyngeal)
> Moderate heparinization
> Aggressive reattachment of segmental arteries (especially T8–L1)
> Sequential aortic clamping when possible
> Perfusion of renal arteries with 4°C perfusate when possible
>
> **Extent I and II Thoracoabdominal Repairs**
> Cerebrospinal fluid drainage
> Left heart bypass during proximal anastomosis
> Selective perfusion of celiac axis and superior mesenteric artery during intercostal and visceral/renal anastomoses

of reducing hepatic and bowel ischemia include reduced risks of postoperative coagulopathy and bacterial translocation, respectively. Renal protection is performed using cold renal perfusion (4°C).[48]

Outcomes

When performed in specialized centers, these operations achieve excellent survival with acceptable morbidity. Early mortality for chronic distal dissection repair ranges from 6% to 10%.[49] Predictors of operative mortality include increasing age, congestive heart failure (CHF), aortic rupture (contained or free), and preoperative renal failure. Risk of paraplegia or paraparesis is 3% to 9%. These outcomes are significantly better than those obtained in patients who undergo surgery during the acute phase. For example, comparative results in patients who require replacement of the entire thoracoabdominal aorta (Crawford type II repairs) in chronic versus acute settings include early mortality in 5% versus 10%, paraplegia/paraparesis in 5% versus 11%, and renal failure in 13% versus 20%, respectively.[43]

Postoperative Considerations

Excellent postoperative management is critical to optimize organ perfusion and prevent morbidity. Optimizing organ perfusion, especially to the spinal cord, requires appropriate oxygen delivery. Therefore, careful invasive monitoring of blood pressure, cardiac output, and hemoglobin levels is necessary. Mean arterial blood pressure is targeted at 80 to 90 mm Hg; however, optimal organ perfusion must be balanced against the risk of bleeding. Aortic tissue in the setting of dissection is extremely thin and fragile, and bleeding risk is significant. Excess postoperative hypertension can precipitate severe bleeding or pseudoaneurysm formation. Therefore, during the initial postoperative phase, aggressive blood pressure regulation is maintained with infusion of short-acting vasoactive agents. Drugs such as nitroprusside, clevidipine, or intravenous (IV) β-adrenoreceptor antagonists are used to treat hypertension. Appropriate volume resuscitation is usually required to address hypotension, with inotropes and vasopressors used judiciously. In patients with extremely friable aortic tissue, such as those with acute dissection or MFS, a lower target (70 to 80 mm Hg) is used.

While preventing hypertensive episodes, maintaining adequate blood pressure, preload, and cardiac inotropic state are important in preventing delayed paraplegia and postoperative renal failure. In the absence of postoperative bleeding, blood pressure should be kept near its preoperative baseline level. Delayed paraplegia can arise hours to days after aortic surgery. In the postoperative period, strategies to reverse paraplegia include inducing systemic hypertension, decreasing

cerebrospinal pressure by cerebrospinal fluid drainage, correcting anemia, preventing fever, and administering cardiac inotropes, mannitol, and steroids. Atrial tachyarrhythmias are common after extensive aortic reconstruction and may precipitate acute hypotension.[50] Pharmacologic interventions such as amiodarone and beta blockade are effective therapies. However, synchronized cardioversion should be used liberally and expeditiously to restore sinus rhythm promptly and correct hypotension. Recovery from paraplegia is possible, but if cord function does not return promptly after these measures are taken, such a recovery is not likely.

Aortic graft infections are a threat to anastomotic integrity and are associated with extremely high morbidity and mortality. Definitive treatment often requires complete removal of the graft and complex vascular reconstruction. To prevent this complication, administration of perioperative IV antibiotic prophylaxis is necessary, and early but appropriate withdrawal of all indwelling catheters should be performed. Similarly, all postoperative infections are treated aggressively with IV antibiotics to minimize the risk of bacteremia and secondary graft infection.

Vocal cord paresis is not uncommon after dissection at the distal arch. Resulting hoarseness is a concern that affects both voice and postoperative pulmonary toilet. Vocal fold medialization with silicon injection can improve functional status and should be performed early before discharge. An exception would be in the event of anticipated reintubation for a planned subsequent operation, such as completion of an elephant trunk. Thyroplasty can be definitive treatment; however, reintubation can potentially disrupt the thyroplasty. Therefore, this treatment is reserved for the outpatient setting when the patient has recovered from the operation yet remains hoarse.

FUTURE THERAPIES

Treatment paradigms for aortic dissection continue to evolve. Newer prophylactic therapies are being explored to lessen the risk of patients developing paraplegia after thoracic aortic replacement. Targeted stem cell therapy may offer hope for those patients who suffer this dreaded complication. In the setting of rapidly evolving endovascular technology, previously untreatable patient conditions can be addressed with innovative treatment strategies that involve hybrid approaches to complex aortic arch and thoracoabdominal aortic pathology. As further experience is gained with branched and fenestrated aortic endografts, more complex aortic pathology will be treatable with endovascular approaches, obviating the need for open aortic replacement. The ascending aorta and aortic root represent the next frontier in endovascular therapy. Furthermore, greater understanding of the molecular pathways that underlie aortic dissection may uncover novel medical treatments that reduce the rate of aortic expansion and the risk of fatal rupture.

REFERENCES

1. Bergqvist D. Historical aspects on aneurysmal disease. *Scand J Surg.* 2008;97:90–99.
2. Cooley DA, De Bakey ME. Resection of entire ascending aorta in fusiform aneurysm using cardiac bypass. *JAMA.* 1956;162:1158–1159.
3. Hiratzka LF, Bakris GL, Beckman JA, et al. 2010 ACCF/AHA/AATS/ACR/ASA/SCA/SCAI/SIR/STS/SVM guidelines for the diagnosis and management of patients with thoracic aortic disease: a report of the American College of Cardiology Foundation/American Heart Association Task Force on Practice Guidelines, American Association for Thoracic Surgery, American College of Radiology, American Stroke Association, Society of Cardiovascular Anesthesiologists, Society for Cardiovascular Angiography and Interventions, Society of Interventional Radiology, Society of Thoracic Surgeons, and Society for Vascular Medicine. *Circulation.* 2010;121:e266–e369.

4. Fann JI, Miller DC. Aortic dissection. *Ann Vasc Surg*. 1995;9:311–323.

5. Dumfarth J, Peterss S, Luehr M, et al. Acute type A dissection in octogenarians: does emergency surgery impact in-hospital outcome or long-term survival? *Eur J Cardiothorac Surg*. 2017;51:472–477.

6. Estrera AL, Huynh TT, Porat EE, et al. Is acute type A aortic dissection a true surgical emergency? *Semin Vasc Surg*. 2002;15:75–82.

7. Trimarchi S, Eagle KA, Nienaber CA, et al. Role of age in acute type A aortic dissection outcome: report from the International Registry of Acute Aortic Dissection (IRAD). *J Thorac Cardiovasc Surg*. 2010;140:784–789.

8. Collins JS, Evangelista A, Nienaber CA, et al. Differences in clinical presentation, management, and outcomes of acute type A aortic dissection in patients with and without previous cardiac surgery. *Circulation*. 2004;110:II237–42.

9. Wong DR, Coselli JS, Palmero L, et al. Axillary artery cannulation in surgery for acute or subacute ascending aortic dissections. *Annals Thorac Surg*. 2010;90:731–737.

10. Frederick JR, Yang E, Trubelja A, et al. Ascending aortic cannulation in acute type a dissection repair. *Ann Thorac Surg*. 2013;95:1808–1811.

11. Rylski B, Milewski RK, Bavaria JE, et al. Long-term results of aggressive hemiarch replacement in 534 patients with type A aortic dissection. *J Thorac Cardiovasc Surg*. 2014;148:2981–2985.

12. Berretta P, Patel HJ, Gleason TG, et al. IRAD experience on surgical type A acute dissection patients: results and predictors of mortality. *Ann Cardiothorac Surg*. 2016;5:346–351.

13. Arnaoutakis GJ, Vallabhajosyula P, Bavaria JE, et al. The impact of deep versus moderate hypothermia on postoperative kidney function after elective aortic hemiarch repair. *Ann Thorac Surg*. 2016;102:1313–1321.

14. De Paulis R, Czerny M, Weltert L, et al. Current trends in cannulation and neuroprotection during surgery of the aortic arch in Europe. *Eur J Cardiothorac Surg*. 2015;47:917–923.

15. Bergeron EJ, Mosca MS, Aftab M, et al. Neuroprotection strategies in aortic surgery. *Cardiol Clin*. 2017;35:453–465.

16. Girardi LN, Shavladze N, Sedrakyan A, Neragi-Miandoab S. Safety and efficacy of retrograde cerebral perfusion as an adjunct for cerebral protection during surgery on the aortic arch. *J Thorac Cardiovasc Surg*. 2014;148:2927–2933.

17. Rice RD, Sandhu HK, Leake SS, et al. Is total arch replacement associated with worse outcomes during repair of acute type A aortic dissection? *Ann Thorac Surg*. 2015;100:2159–2165. discussion 2165-6.

18. Trivedi D, Navid F, Balzer JR, et al. Aggressive aortic arch and carotid replacement strategy for type A aortic dissection improves neurologic outcomes. *Ann Thorac Surg*. 2016;101:896–903. discussion 903-5.

19. Sultan I, Wallen TJ, Habertheuer A, et al. Concomitant antegrade stent grafting of the descending thoracic aorta during transverse hemiarch reconstruction for acute DeBakey I aortic dissection repair improves aortic remodeling. *J Card Surg*. 2017;32:581–592.

20. Rylski B, Bavaria JE, Milewski RK, et al. Long-term results of neomedia sinus valsalva repair in 489 patients with type A aortic dissection. *Ann Thorac Surg*. 2014;98:582–588. discussion 588-9.

21. Borst HG. The birth of the elephant trunk technique. *J Thorac Cardiovasc Surg*. 2013;145:44.

22. Roselli EE, Idrees JJ, Bakaeen FG, et al. Evolution of simplified frozen elephant trunk repair for acute DeBakey type I dissection: midterm outcomes. *Ann Thorac Surg*. 2018;105:749–755.

23. Vallabhajosyula P, Gottret JP, Menon R, et al. Central repair with antegrade TEVAR for malperfusion syndromes in acute Debakey I aortic dissection. *Ann Thorac Surg*. 2017;103:748–755.

24. Shrestha M, Martens A, Kaufeld T, et al. Single-centre experience with the frozen elephant trunk technique in 251 patients over 15 years. *Eur J Cardiothorac Surg*. 2017;52:858–866.

25. Bavaria JE, Pochettino A, Brinster DR, et al. New paradigms and improved results for the surgical treatment of acute type A dissection. *Ann Surg*. 2001;234:336–342. discussion 342-3.

26. Dell'Aquila AM, Concistre G, Gallo A, et al. Fate of the preserved aortic root after treatment of acute type A aortic dissection: 23-year follow-up. *J Thorac Cardiovasc Surg*. 2013;146:1456–1460.

27. Leshnower BG, Myung RJ, McPherson L, Chen EP. Midterm results of David V valve-sparing aortic root replacement in acute type A aortic dissection. *Ann Thorac Surg*. 2015;99:795–800. discussion 800-1.

28. Roselli EE, Idrees J, Greenberg RK, et al. Endovascular stent grafting for ascending aorta repair in high-risk patients. *J Thorac Cardiovasc Surg*. 2015;149:144–151.

29. Vallabhajosyula P, Gottret JP, Bavaria JE, et al. Endovascular repair of the ascending aorta in patients at high risk for open repair. *J Thorac Cardiovasc Surg*. 2015;149:S144–S150.

30. Tsilimparis N, Debus ES, Oderich GS, et al. International experience with endovascular therapy of the ascending aorta with a dedicated endograft. *J Vasc Surg*. 2016;63:1476–1482.

31. Horton JD, Kolbel T, Haulon S, et al. Endovascular repair of type A aortic dissection: current experience and technical considerations. *Semin Thorac Cardiovasc Surg*. 2016;28:312–317.

32. Kazui T, Yamashita K, Washiyama N, et al. Impact of an aggressive surgical approach on surgical outcome in type A aortic dissection. *Ann Thorac Surg*. 2002;74:S1844–S1847. discussion S1857-63.

33. Safi HJ, Miller 3rd CC, Reardon MJ, et al. Operation for acute and chronic aortic dissection: recent outcome with regard to neurologic deficit and early death. *Ann Thorac Surg*. 1998;66:402–411.

34. Stevens LM, Madsen JC, Isselbacher EM, et al. Surgical management and long-term outcomes for acute ascending aortic dissection. *J Thorac Cardiovasc Surg*. 2009;138:1349. 57.e1.

35. Kische S, Ehrlich MP, Nienaber CA, et al. Endovascular treatment of acute and chronic aortic dissection: midterm results from the Talent Thoracic Retrospective Registry. *J Thorac Cardiovasc Surg*. 2009;138:115–124.

36. Panneton JM, Teh SH, Cherry Jr KJ, et al. Aortic fenestration for acute or chronic aortic dissection: an uncommon but effective procedure. *J Vasc Surg*. 2000;32:711–721.

37. Hagan PG, Nienaber CA, Isselbacher EM, et al. The International Registry of Acute Aortic Dissection (IRAD): new insights into an old disease. *JAMA*. 2000;283:897–903.

38. Fattori R, Tsai TT, Myrmel T, et al. Complicated acute type B dissection: is surgery still the best option?: a report from the International Registry of Acute Aortic Dissection. *JACC Cardiovasc Interv*. 2008;1:395–402.

39. Masuda Y, Yamada Z, Morooka N, et al. Prognosis of patients with medically treated aortic dissections. *Circulation*. 1991;84:III7–13.

40. Lansman SL, Hagl C, Fink D, et al. Acute type B aortic dissection: surgical therapy. *Ann Thorac Surg*. 2002;74:S1833–S1835. discussion S1857-63.

41. Nienaber CA, Rousseau H, Eggebrecht H, et al. Randomized comparison of strategies for type B aortic dissection: the INvestigation of STEnt Grafts in Aortic Dissection (INSTEAD) trial. *Circulation*. 2009;120:2519–2528.

42. Nienaber CA, Kische S, Rousseau H, et al. Endovascular repair of type B aortic dissection: long-term results of the randomized investigation of stent grafts in aortic dissection trial. *Circ Cardiovasc Interv*. 2013;6:407–416.

43. Coselli JS, LeMaire SA, Preventza O, et al. Outcomes of 3309 thoracoabdominal aortic aneurysm repairs. *J Thorac Cardiovasc Surg*. 2016;151:1323–1337.

44. LeMaire SA, Miller 3rd CC, Conklin LD, et al. A new predictive model for adverse outcomes after elective thoracoabdominal aortic aneurysm repair. *Ann Thorac Surg*. 2001;71:1233–1238.

45. Coselli JS, de la Cruz KI, Preventza O, et al. Extent II thoracoabdominal aortic aneurysm repair: how I do it. *Semin Thorac Cardiovasc Surg*. 2016;28:221–237.

46. Coselli JS, LeMaire SA, Koksoy C, et al. Cerebrospinal fluid drainage reduces paraplegia after thoracoabdominal aortic aneurysm repair: results of a randomized clinical trial. *J Vasc Surg*. 2002;35:631–639.

47. Etz CD, Zoli S, Mueller CS, et al. Staged repair significantly reduces paraplegia rate after extensive thoracoabdominal aortic aneurysm repair. *J Thorac Cardiovasc Surg*. 2010;139:1464–1472.

48. Lemaire SA, Jones MM, Conklin LD, et al. Randomized comparison of cold blood and cold crystalloid renal perfusion for renal protection during thoracoabdominal aortic aneurysm repair. *J Vasc Surg*. 2009;49:11–19. discussion 19.

49. Corvera J, Copeland H, Blitzer D, et al. Open repair of chronic thoracic and thoracoabdominal aortic dissection using deep hypothermia and circulatory arrest. *J Thorac Cardiovasc Surg*. 2017;154:389–395.

50. Dolapoglu A, Volguina IV, Price MD, et al. Cardiac arrhythmia after open thoracoabdominal aortic aneurysm repair. *Ann Thorac Surg*. 2017;104:854–860.

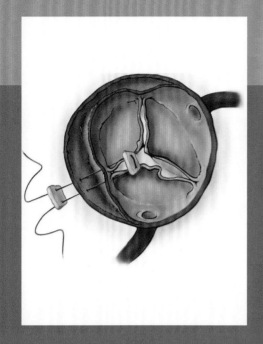

中文导读

第34章
主动脉夹层的腔内治疗

　　本章主要介绍主动脉夹层的腔内修复，包括使用覆膜支架对无并发症夹层进行修复的指征和对有并发症夹层进行修复的要点。对于涉及内脏分支动脉受累的各种情况和其机制也进行了分析并介绍不同情况下进行腔内修复的注意要点。此外，对于合并假腔破裂的主动脉夹层的胸主动脉腔内修复（thoracicendovascularaortic repair，TEVAR）及其并发症处理（主要是外科处理）也进行了介绍。合并有马方综合征的患者在特定情况下是可以进行腔内治疗的，但马方综合征患者发生急性主动脉夹层时仍然首先选择外科手术治疗。对于大多数的具有并发症的Stanford B型主动脉夹层，胸主动脉腔内修复目前已成为一线治疗方式。基于影像学分析后所得到的结果显示，约1/3的Stanford A型夹层在现有的腔内技术基础上可以进行覆膜支架治疗。但需要对于主动脉弓上三分支做出相应的特殊处理而保留。对于年龄较大、手术风险大的患者值得使用，但需要特别注意诸如脑梗死等严重并发症的风险。目前这类手术的报道例数和研究均不多，还需要进一步循证医学证据予以支持。

舒 畅

Endovascular Therapy for Aortic Dissection

Benjamin D. Colvard and Michael D. Dake

Acute aortic dissection (AAD) is a precipitous event associated with a wide range of outcomes from uncomplicated to catastrophic. Current endovascular strategies are based on identifying features that portend increased risk of death or other poor outcome, and applying interventional techniques to prevent the life-threatening complications of the dissection.[1-3]

During the last 2 decades, there has been increasing interest in exploring endovascular procedures for management of aortic dissection.[4-13] Initially, endovascular approaches focused on addressing branch vessel involvement and ischemic complications associated with the dissection process (Fig. 34.1).[8,9] Subsequently, endovascular aortic stent grafts (initially developed to repair aortic aneurysms) were applied in type B aortic dissection to cover the primary entry tear of the dissection and promote thrombosis of the thoracic aortic false lumen (Fig. 34.2).[4,5] These basic endovascular tactics are now routine in the contemporary armamentarium for treatment of aortic dissection and its myriad manifestations.

Endovascular approaches are complementary to the two traditional therapeutic paradigms of open surgical repair for type A dissection and medical treatment for uncomplicated type B disease. Invasive interventional procedures fit between the existing operative and noninvasive alternatives to provide effective options for type A dissection with severe branch vessel compromise (before or after ascending aortic repair), complicated type B dissection (branch vessel involvement, descending aortic rupture, extension of disease, or early aortic dilation, etc.), arch involvement, and ascending aortic intramural hematoma associated with an intimal tear distal to the left subclavian artery.

This chapter will review the specific endovascular procedures currently in use to manage aortic dissection, the patient subgroups in which these techniques are commonly employed, and the outcomes of these interventions.

BRANCH VESSEL INTERVENTIONS

Branch vessel involvement accompanying aortic dissection is a well-recognized complication occurring in more than 30% of cases.[7,8,14] For appropriate intervention selection, the pathoanatomical concepts of static and dynamic branch involvement are crucial to selection of the endovascular option for reperfusion of an affected vascular bed.[15-17] As the dissection process extends distally from the primary entry tear, the dissection septum may engage the ostia of branch vessels. If the aortic flap, which consists of the intima and portion of the media shorn away from the wall, engages a branch orifice as it extends, two pathophysiological situations referred to respectively as *static* and *dynamic branch involvement* may occur (Fig. 34.3).

Static Branch Involvement

One manifestation that may arise when the advancing dissection septum intersects an aortic branch is static branch vessel involvement (Fig. 34.4). In static involvement, the aortic dissection flap extends directly into the branch for a variable distance. In this case, orientation of the septal trajectory is such that the branch ostium is incompletely engaged by the edge of the dissection plane. Rather than being circumferentially shorn by the septum, there is only partial circumferential involvement of the branch by the dissection. The aortic flap extends into the branch, creating a false lumen within the artery. As a result, the individual branch has both a true and false lumen, like the aorta.

Also similar to the aorta, a branch affected by static involvement may have multiple fates. At the end of the dissection where the flap terminates in the branch, a *reentry tear* in the false lumen may or may not occur. If a reentry tear occurs at the end of the false lumen, branch perfusion results from blood flow in both the true and false lumens. In many such cases, dual lumen perfusion is not associated with ischemic branch vessel symptoms. If reentry does not occur in cases of static branch vessel involvement, however, the false lumen within the branch has no outflow. The absence of a distal tear to allow communication with the vascular bed beyond the dissection may impair blood flow significantly. This *no reentry* state within the branch's false lumen renders perfusion limited to that contributed by the true lumen. Unfortunately, the true lumen may be compromised by the engorged false lumen. The blind pouch of the false lumen, without outflow, swells to a maximum dimension at its distal end. The pressure exerted by the false lumen severely distorts and compresses the true lumen to markedly reduce branch vessel flow. Commonly, the degree of ischemia experienced by the involved vascular bed may be significant and can lead to irreversible tissue necrosis if not relieved quickly.

In no-reentry situations, a local solution directed at improving flow within the affected artery is required because the problem is localized within the specific branch. Two options for endovascular treatment are possible. Resistance to outflow within the false lumen may be decreased by creating a distal tear or fenestration within the blind channel. This can be accomplished with the end of a guidewire or other endovascular probe placed within the false lumen through the aortic false lumen. This approach is associated with practical challenges, including the avoidance of distal extension of the dissection process, safe penetration of the false lumen wall to create an effective outflow tear, and determination of the presence of thrombus within the blind sac of stagnant false lumen blood to avoid its distal embolization.

In most cases, the preferred strategy involves increasing branch flow by decreasing the resistance to true lumen blood flow. This is performed by placing a stent in the true lumen of the branch through catheterization from the aortic true lumen. The stent is typically placed from beyond the end of the false lumen in the branch back to the aortic true lumen. A self-expanding nitinol stent is commonly employed because this distance is frequently greater than 2 cm and because there is a risk of squeezing any existing clot out of the false lumen with a

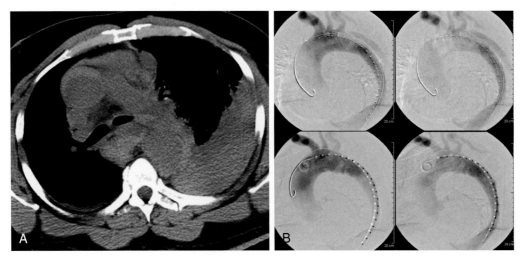

Fig. 34.1 Type B Aortic Dissection with Proximal Entry Tear Distal to Left Subclavian Artery, Retrograde Extension, Ascending Intramural Hematoma, and Rupture into Left Chest. (A) Non–contrast-enhanced axial computed tomography image through the aorta demonstrates an ascending aortic mural-based ring with increased density, indicative of intramural hematoma. Also apparent is abnormal extravascular tissue surrounding aorta, with characteristic appearance of a rupture with clot. (B) Series of images from a thoracic aortogram demonstrate entry tear just beyond left subclavian artery, with contrast media opacifying both the true and false lumens. Precise point of rupture is not identified.

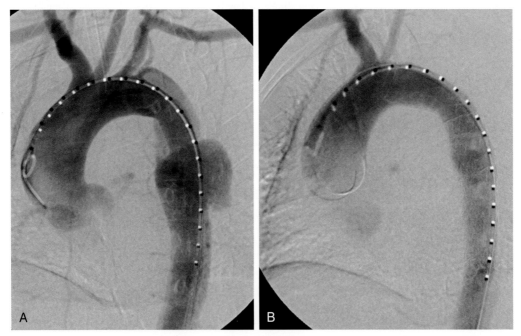

Fig. 34.2 Aortic Dissection with Rupture. (A) Thoracic aortogram demonstrates type B aortic dissection with mid-descending aortic rupture. (B) Repeat aortogram following placement of thoracic endograft over proximal entry tear just above the site of rupture, without evidence of residual contrast extravasation.

balloon-expandable stent. These stents are sized to the total transarterial diameter of the branch and allowed to progressively expand on their own (post deployment) without supplemental balloon dilation. There are many successful reports of this approach in mesenteric, renal, and iliac arteries affected by no-reentry or static involvement.[8,9,18,19]

Occasionally, static branch vessel involvement with reentry anatomy and double-barrel flow may require endovascular intervention. The most common indication for stent placement in this setting occurs with involvement of a renal artery (Fig. 34.5). The kidney supplied by a dissected renal artery may be affected by the physical presence of a flap within the branch. The variable flow reduction caused by the

flap, and resultant disrupted pattern of true and false lumen perfusion, may contribute to an exacerbation of hypertension. In cases where high blood pressure is sustained and recalcitrant to numerous intravenous (IV) medications, endovascular intervention may be warranted to restore a single lumen without flap. The approach to treatment involves placement of a balloon-expandable renal stent within the true lumen of the renal artery through the aortic true lumen. In most cases, this type of reentry involvement does not extend into the branch as far as the no-reentry extension. Thus stents less than 2 cm long are typically implanted. This technique is well established at most centers that manage cases of aortic dissection frequently.

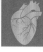

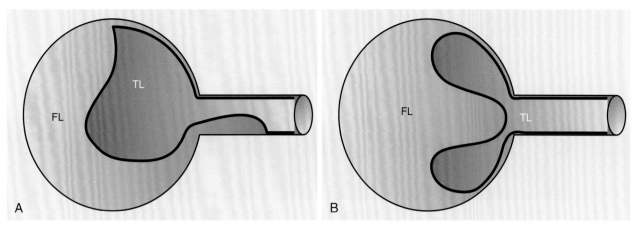

Fig. 34.3 (A) Static obstruction. Dissection has extended into a branch vessel. (B) Dynamic obstruction. Membrane is lying across and obstructing origin of branch vessel. *FL,* False lumen; *TL,* true lumen.

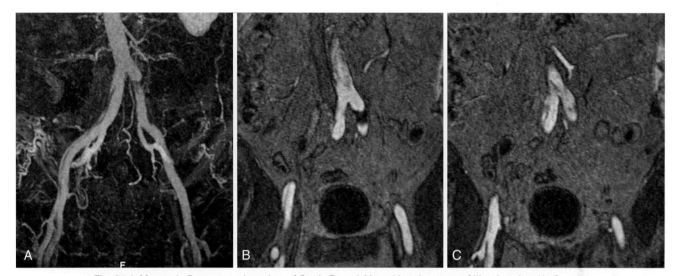

Fig. 34.4 Magnetic Resonance Imaging of Static Branch Vessel Involvement of Iliac Arteries. (A) Coronal image of pelvis identifies a flap extending into right common iliac artery (CIA) and down to distal external iliac artery (EIA). Flow is evident in both true and false lumens within the right iliac artery. This is an example of static involvement with direct flap extension from the aorta into a branch. At the end of the dissection within the EIA, there is a distal reentry tear. This terminal tear establishes double-barrel flow within the iliac artery, which is rarely associated with ischemic symptoms. (B and C) Similar coronal views show flap extension into left iliac system, but a segmental flow void *(black segment)* within false lumen of left CIA. This is associated with a no-reentry situation at distal extent of false lumen. No reentry within a branch is typically associated with obstruction of true lumen by a dilated false lumen cul-de-sac. The flow void noted may represent thrombosis in a blind channel or simply no blood flow. The usual consequence of this phenomenon of no reentry is branch vessel ischemia due to a lack of false lumen perfusion and compromised true lumen branch flow.

Dynamic Branch Involvement

In addition to primary branch pathology that occurs as a complication of aortic dissection, another mechanism, dynamic branch vessel involvement, may be responsible for organ ischemia. Dynamic branch involvement is a phenomenon associated with obstruction to branch vessel flow by an aortic septum that has prolapsed over the branch ostia like a curtain. In contrast to static involvement, where the aortic flap extends directly into a branch, dynamic obstruction occurs as an aortic process exclusively without an associated branch lesion. Propagation of the aortic flap may create a circumferential cleavage of the aortic wall surrounding the branch ostium (Fig. 34.6). Factors associated with this event include the flap trajectory, the resultant orientation of the septal plane proximal to the branch, and the inclusion of the ostium by the cleaved flap as it extends past. In this situation, the dissection septum surrounds the branch

ostium as it tears distally. The cleavage plane extends 1 to 2 mm into the branch, and then circumferentially reenters, creating a cylindrical tear, coring out a short segment of the intimal/medial lining of the most proximal aspect of the branch. The septum retracts into the aortic lumen with a fenestration corresponding to the branch orifice. This gives the flap a stencil-like appearance when viewed en face, with the number of holes related to the number of branch vessels involved in this phenomenon. When imaged in an axial plane, the affected artery appears to originate exclusively from the aortic false lumen. Closer inspection usually allows the identification of a tear in the flap at the level of or adjacent to the level of the branch. The flap often displays small projections angled from the edge of the tear, giving its outline on axial imaging an appearance similar to the contour of a metal rivet, the short-legged extensions corresponding to the amputated proximal lining of the branch.

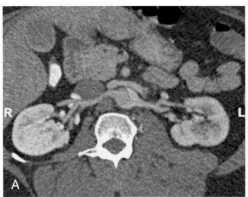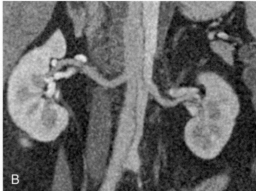

Fig. 34.5 Computed Tomography (CT) Images of True and False Lumen Relationships to Renal Arteries. Axial (A) and coronal (B) CT images at level of left renal artery show that left renal artery is supplied by the false lumen (left aortic lumen). True lumen is located along right wall of aorta, and flap shows a characteristic natural fenestration or defect corresponding to left renal ostium. Flap around fenestration has small tail-like extensions pointing to the left that represent the initial few millimeters of left renal intimal lining that were torn away with the retracted aortic septum.

In dynamic branch obstruction, hemodynamic flow patterns result in a large aortic false lumen with a diminutive or collapsed true lumen. There is variability, however, in the degree of true lumen obliteration related to the dynamic compromise.

In the majority of aortic dissection cases with true and false lumen aortic flow (often called *double-barrel flow*), the process described does *not* cause critical branch perfusion abnormalities. Flow to the branch originates primarily from the false lumen, with a small contribution from the true lumen through the corresponding fenestration in the aortic septum. Most of the false lumen flow usually occurs in diastole. During systole, the small contribution from the true lumen arrives through the septal window into the false lumen and branch. If the proximal primary tear is very large or the entry tear is in close proximity to the branch, the dominant flow pattern supplying branch perfusion may be in systole. In general, a branch that originates exclusively from the aortic false lumen is rarely affected by an ischemic complication.

Consistently, the aortic septum prolapses with a convex contour toward a compromised crescent-shaped true lumen. Consequently, all branches originating from the true lumen are at risk of obstruction. In this regard, the aortic septum in a dynamic obstructive process often assumes a coronal position, oriented across the aorta from left to right, in the distal descending thoracic proximal abdominal aortic segments. Thus the anteriorly oriented mesenteric vessels are in peril of ischemia because they frequently originate exclusively from a miniscule aortic true lumen. The likelihood of developing clinically relevant dynamic branch vessel compromise appears related in part to the area of the proximal entry tear. Although the process of dynamic involvement is dependent on multiple factors, as a general rule, the more severe the true lumen collapse, the larger or more circumferential the size of the proximal primary entry tear. Management of more than one ischemic vascular bed related to dynamic branch involvement and an obliterated aortic true lumen that supplies the compromised branches is most expeditiously and effectively approached by an endovascular aortic procedure rather than a strategy directed at the individual branches.

More than one mechanism of branch involvement can coexist in any given patient. The clinical manifestations and the analysis of imaging for any patient requires an individualized approach that must synthesize information and aortic and branch vessel involvement to customize an optimal treatment strategy that will safely, successfully, and durably address the most compelling effects of the dissection.

AORTIC INTERVENTIONS

Endovascular aortic stent grafting is a less invasive alternative to open surgery for selected patients with both thoracic and abdominal aneurysms. Recently, the application of similar technology for management of acute aortic syndromes, including aortic dissection, has emerged as a focus of interest and study.[7,10–13,20,21] As with any new procedure, the key question is the determination of specific patient populations who may benefit from the new technique. In this regard, the use of traditional classification parameters for risk stratification of aortic dissection patients has advanced evaluation of the possible benefits and risks of endograft management.

Nearly all experience in endograft management of aortic dissection has been with type B disease when there is exclusive involvement of the descending thoracic aorta. Experience with endograft applications in type A dissection is limited to isolated case reports. In the United States, type B aortic dissections constitute approximately 30% to 35% of all dissections. The initial risk stratification of the type B dissection is made with the determination of the presence or absence of complications.

Medical management is the traditional treatment strategy for uncomplicated AAD. Current reports cite a 30-day mortality rate of approximately 10%.[22,23] Use of stent grafting for stable uncomplicated patients with type B aortic dissection has yet to realize any improvement in survival compared with traditional medical therapy. Indeed, current conservative noninterventional management of uncomplicated cases is associated with 1-year survival rates of around 80%. Such results may be hard to improve upon with endograft therapy.[23,24]

Stent Grafts for Uncomplicated Type B Dissection

The Investigation of Stent Grafts in Patients with Type B Aortic Dissection (INSTEAD) trial observed that elective stent graft placement in survivors of uncomplicated chronic (>2 weeks from onset) type B dissection does not improve 1-year survival and adverse event rates compared with medical therapy. Among the 140 patients randomized in this prospective trial, 1-year survival was 91% compared with 97% in patients randomized to medical therapy.[25,26] Moreover, aorta-related mortality was not different, and the risk for the combined endpoint of aorta-related death (rupture) and progression (including conversion or additional endovascular or open surgical intervention) was similar. However, patients who underwent thoracic endovascular aortic

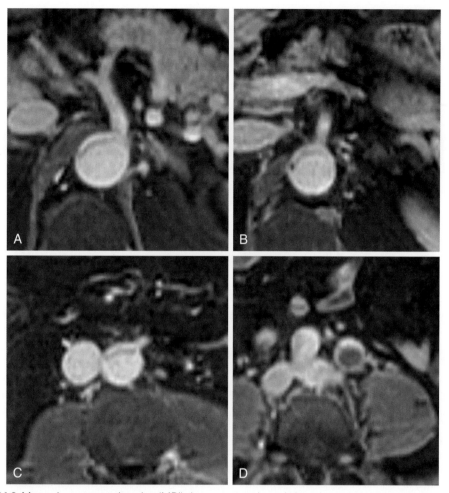

Fig. 34.6 Magnetic resonance imaging (MRI) demonstrates dynamic branch vessel involvement, with aortic true lumen collapse and accompanying static no-reentry obstruction of left common iliac artery (CIA). (A–C) Axial MRI shows wafer-thin crescent-shaped true lumen collapsed against anterior aortic wall at level of visceral arteries. Aortic septum prolapses like a curtain across the origins of branches originating from true lumen, with resultant malperfusion and multiorgan ischemia. (D) At the level just below aortic bifurcation, there is marked asymmetry in appearance of CIAs. Lumen of left CIA has a flow void *(black circle)* due to static involvement without reentry that coexists with the dynamic process observed more proximally.

repair (TEVAR) demonstrated significantly more aortic remodeling, including true-lumen recovery and false lumen thrombosis (91.3% vs. 19.4%). The ongoing ADSORB trial is the first randomized study of TEVAR versus medical therapy for uncomplicated acute type B aortic dissection.[27] Early results indicate that TEVAR is significantly more effective at reducing false lumen size, inducing false lumen thrombosis, and increasing true lumen diameter.[28] More recently, in a retrospective analysis of patients undergoing TEVAR or medical therapy for uncomplicated type B dissection, Qin et al. showed that patients in the TEVAR group had significantly fewer late aortic-related adverse events (23.9% vs. 38.3%, $P = .005$), and significantly lower all-cause mortality rate (10.2% vs. 20.1%, $P = .03$).[29] These studies indicate that a shift may be underway in the paradigm of uncomplicated type B dissection management. Until definitive results emerge, however, medical management remains the treatment of choice for uncomplicated type B aortic dissections in both the acute and chronic phases.

Monitoring of the medically managed patient with type B aortic dissection is typically performed with serial CT angiograms. The goal of this imaging regimen is to identify patients who may develop complications of chronic type B dissection such as degenerative aneurysm formation. Current data suggest that up to 38% of medically managed

patients will eventually require an aortic intervention for aneurysmal degeneration.[30] Identifying imaging-based risk factors may allow for earlier interventions to be performed to prevent catastrophic events, or to decrease the number of imaging procedures in those who are low risk. Current literature suggests that an increased number of entry tears (>2) is associated with a lower risk of aneurysmal degeneration.[31,32] This may be attributable to a lower perfusion pressure in the false lumen in the presence of multiple fenestrations. Indeed, a number of aorta-specific risk factors for aneurysmal degeneration can be seen as markers of high false lumen pressure, including the presence of a saccular or circular false lumen with an elliptical true lumen (indicating a compressed true lumen). These morphologic findings are frequently associated with a patent or partially thrombosed false lumen.[33] In patients managed with TEVAR in the acute setting, favorable aortic remodeling can be expected, with up to 84% having complete false lumen obliteration, which appears to be critical for the prevention of late aneurysmal degeneration.[34] Monitoring of the dissected visceral and infrarenal aortic segments is mandatory for the early detection of aneurysmal degeneration.

In the setting of complicated aortic dissection, medical management is associated with a high mortality rate, such that most patients

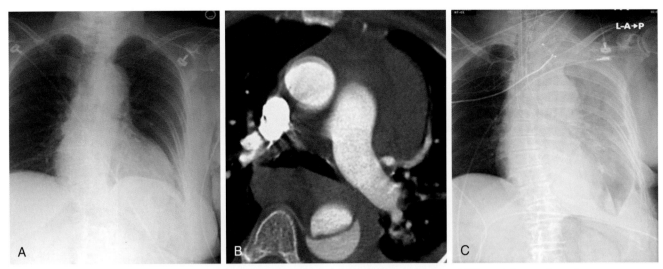

Fig. 34.7 Acute Type B Aortic Dissection with Rupture in a 68-Year-Old Woman. (A) Frontal chest radiograph upon presentation to emergency room with severe back pain and hypertension that occurred while gardening. (B) Axial computed tomography scan after contrast media administration shows typical appearance of aortic dissection in mid-descending aorta. (C) Repeat chest radiograph performed after transfer to referral facility 4 hours after initial study, with marked interval change including opacification of left hemithorax from leaking blood.

will only undergo surgery to address life-threatening complications.[2,4] Depending on the patient's underlying medical conditions and the nature of the complication(s), surgical mortality rates range between 30% and 60% or higher.[35,36] It is in these high-risk scenarios that an opportunity exists to establish a role for interventional management. Thus the question becomes, *What constitutes complicated type B aortic dissection?* There is no strict definition for this category of disease, but traditionally it is relegated to two unambiguous disease manifestations: *aortic rupture* (Fig. 34.7) and *symptomatic branch vessel involvement.* These conditions are clear and their diagnosis unequivocal. Other adverse effects of the dissection process, such as uncontrollable hypertension, unrelenting pain, and increasing pleural fluid, defy easy classification and do not have uniform criteria for comparative assessment. These so-called softer indications for intervention are commonly included as a surgical indication in most published series of acute complicated dissection.[8,37]

Endograft Treatment of Complicated Type B Dissection

The procedural goal for endovascular stent grafting in patients with complicated acute type B aortic dissection is endograft elimination of blood flow entry into the proximal entry tear. Obliterating the primary communication between the true lumen and the false redirects pulsatile flow into the true lumen, promotes false lumen thrombosis, and ultimately improves remodeling of the aorta by increasing the dimensions of the true lumen while shrinking the false lumen (Fig. 34.8).

Specific procedural techniques vary, depending on the precise complication. Faced with dynamic branch vessel involvement and clinically relevant obstruction compromising flow to one or multiple branches, the procedural strategy focuses on unloading the aortic false lumen by increasing resistance to false lumen inflow or decreasing resistance to its outflow. The former is attempted by deploying an endograft over the proximal primary entry tear and rechanneling all flow into the true lumen. Logistically, this typically involves placement of a 15-cm-long (range 12 to 20 cm) stent graft from the nondissected segment of aorta proximal to the primary intimal tear, commonly between the origins of the left carotid and left subclavian arteries. This may require intentional partial or complete coverage of the left subclavian origin. The

distal extent of the device usually remains above the diaphragm. The diameter of the implant selected is based on the transaortic dimension of the nondissected aorta just proximal to the dissection, rather than the size of the true lumen or transaortic diameter of the dissected segment.

Endovascular Treatment of Branch Vessel Involvement

The outcomes of stent graft therapy for reversal of dynamic branch vessel involvement are excellent, with procedural success in up to 95% of cases and complete false lumen thrombosis in 85% of patients.[7–9] These procedures are associated with 67.7% 5-year freedom from aortic rupture and open repair.[9] In addition, static branch involvement remote from the covered proximal aortic entry tear may require separate targeted intervention to manage residual ischemic compromise. This is especially important in cases with no-reentry anatomy complicating static branch involvement. In these situations, endovascular branch intervention should be provided emergently.

An alternative to endograft placement in dynamic branch compromise is distal flap fenestration.[9,38] Percutaneous balloon fenestration of the aortic septum has replaced the operative procedure. Balloon fenestration of the septum is designed to unload the aortic false lumen by decreasing the resistance to outflow. Technically, initial transgression of the aortic flap with a small cardiac transseptal TIPS needle and cannula usually is performed from the small true lumen into the larger target of the false channel. The site of the needle puncture commonly lies within the infrarenal aorta at the level of the aortic bifurcation. Once successful transgression of the septum is confirmed, a wire is advanced across the flap and well into the targeted lumen. Sequentially larger balloon dilation of the flap is performed until a final size of between 20 and 25 mm is obtained.

Balloon fenestration causes a linear transverse tear in the flap that allows greater mixture of blood between the two aortic channels and decompresses the true lumen. These effects must be confirmed by aortography or intravascular ultrasound (IVUS) to ensure relief of the dynamic pattern of branch obstruction. After these two endovascular (endograft or fenestration) procedures, imaging comparisons of the anatomical effects (with computed tomography [CT], magnetic

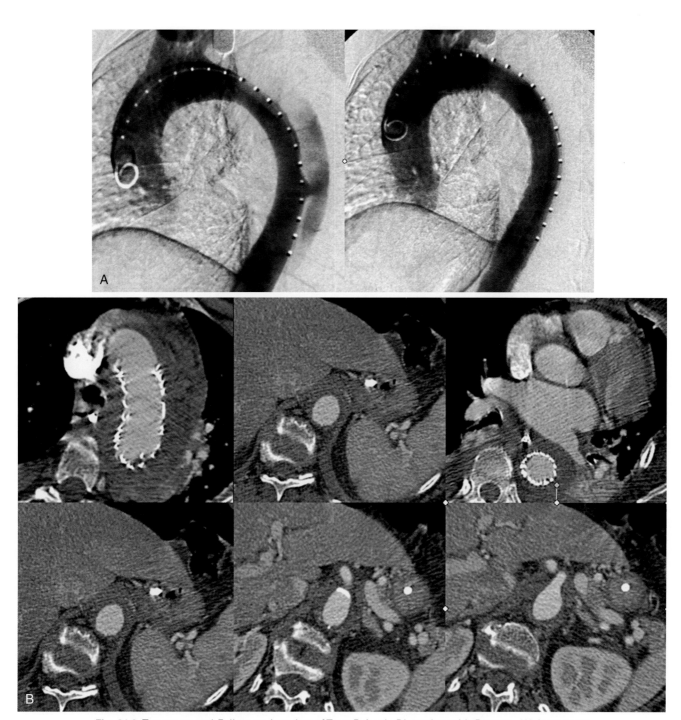

Fig. 34.8 Treatment and Follow-up Imaging of Type B Aortic Dissection with Rupture. (A) Aortograms pre- and postplacement of a thoracic endograft across middescending aorta entry tear of a type B dissection in the 68-year-old woman described in Fig. 34.7. (B) Series of axial computed tomography images obtained 1 week postendograft management of a type B dissection with rupture. Stent graft is in good position, and false lumen is thrombosed. Residual extravascular blood and hematoma are evident.

resonance imaging [MRI], or IVUS), including changes in the size of the aortic lumens, typically demonstrate a more dramatic result following endograft management. Specifically, the magnitude of true lumen expansion with stent grafting is greater than that observed after distal flap fenestration. Because false lumen fenestration promotes flow in the false lumen, whereas endograft placement promotes false lumen thrombosis, the latter is thought to be a superior method to minimize late aneurysm formation. Consequently, the opportunities for percutaneous balloon fenestration are decreasing now that thoracic endograft availability has improved. Fenestration is typically limited to situations when stent grafts are unavailable or when the specific aortic anatomy is unsuitable for endograft placement.

Aortic Rupture and Open Surgery for Complicated Dissections

Rupture that complicates aortic dissection is an interventional imperative.[39,40] The procedural considerations for aortic rupture focus on preventing exsanguination. Both open surgical and endovascular therapies are associated with high mortality and morbidity rates in the presence of aortic rupture. Recent reports suggest that endovascular approaches permit treatment of more patients, including older and less fit individuals whose operative risk in this setting is prohibitive.[21,39,40]

Open surgical repair for acute complicated type B aortic dissection has largely been replaced by TEVAR. TEVAR has been found to be superior to open repair in short- and mid-term mortality, procedure related complications, and cost.[41–44] Even in the case of rupture, TEVAR has been shown to have equivalent or better outcomes than open surgery.[45,46] In the modern era of type B aortic dissection management, open repair should be reserved for patients with complicated dissections whose anatomy is unsuitable for endovascular repair.

Localizing the precise site of rupture noninvasively is not always possible. The point of rupture through the false lumen wall may be evident by the presence of contrast enhancement beyond the anticipated aortic border, though this occurs typically in the setting of severe hemodynamic instability or shock (Fig. 34.9). More commonly, a periaortic, mediastinal, and/or pleural collection is evident on CT imaging, which has an appearance and attenuation value consistent with hematoma or complex fluid. This abnormality may be most prominent around a focal aortic segment or extend diffusely over a wider zone.

The goal of endograft management for aortic rupture is coverage of the proximal entry tear, with isolation of the false lumen, to ensure false lumen obliteration and expeditious thrombosis. It is thrombosis of the false lumen that prevents aortic leakage of blood. To facilitate rapid false lumen thrombosis, the overall endograft coverage of the aorta is often longer than that used for other thoracic pathologies. By extending the length of coverage (20 to 30 cm) to at least the level of the diaphragm or celiac trunk, the aortic septum is braced by the stent in the true lumen, and the thoracic false lumen is converted to a long,

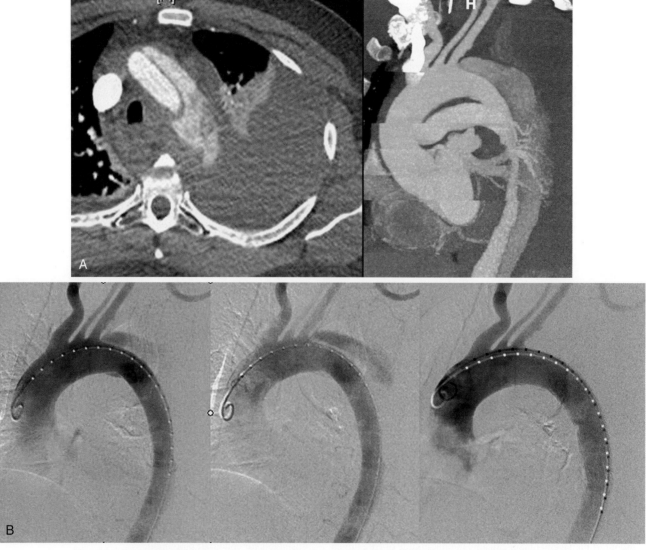

Fig. 34.9 Endograft Management of Aortic Dissection with Rupture. (A) Axial and sagittal computed tomography images of 59-year-old man with acute type B dissection with primary tear distal to left subclavian artery and retrograde extension into the proximal arch (DeBakey class IIID) complicated by rupture. Axial projection shows a large quantity of extravascular fluid, and sagittal image shows a faint wisp of contrast extravasation above aorta, just distal to subclavian artery. (B) Three views from the stent graft procedure, with the left and middle panels before device placement, and the right panel after deployment. A good result is evident, with contrast opacification of the true lumen only.

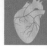

inverted cul-de-sac, or blind pouch. Then with flap pulsation limited by the buttressing stent, blood in the false lumen becomes stagnant and prone to thrombosis.[47–49]

False lumen thrombosis is critical because the precise rupture point in any individual patient is frequently unknown, and the breech may exist well below the entry tear. Simple coverage of the proximal entry may then eliminate direct flow into the false lumen, but if distal retrograde flow from abdominal sources persists, the risk of a continued leak exists and morbidity remains. Although this strategy is associated with considerable mortality and procedural complications, it represents an addition to the existing treatment armamentarium.

Other Indications for Aortic Endografts

The question of unidentified patient subgroup(s) who present with uncomplicated acute type B aortic dissection and may benefit from endograft placement remains. Some investigators have identified certain high-risk features in patients with acute uncomplicated type B dissection that may portend an increased risk of early aneurysm formation and increased mortality. These features include measurements of various aortic dimensions at the time of initial diagnosis. Initial attempts to propose high-risk criteria from CT imaging considered descriptive features associated with a poor prognosis and disease progression, such as a patent false lumen, a gaping and circumferential entry tear with resultant small true lumen, and a dominant false lumen with early fusiform expansion of the proximal descending aorta within 3 months of initial symptoms.

Marui et al. proposed that patients with uncomplicated aortic dissection and transaortic diameter greater than 40 mm were at high risk of rapid aortic expansion.[50] When applied to larger groups of patients with dissection, this benchmark provided modest prognostic value. The poor results encouraged others to focus on the issues and pursue more in-depth imaging analysis. Thereafter, Marui et al. offered an improved prognostic factor that was based on the extent of proximal descending aorta dilation at the time of initial diagnosis[51]: the *fusiform index*. This index is defined as the maximum transaortic diameter of the distal aortic arch divided by the sum of the minimum diameter of the proximal aortic arch plus the aortic diameter at the level of the pulmonary artery. A value greater than 0.64 anticipates late aortic events in patients with uncomplicated type B aortic dissection. The investigators recommended that patients with these predictors should undergo early intervention with open surgery or stent graft implantation.

Immer et al. analyzed imaging studies (CT or MRI) over the initial 18 months after diagnosis in 84 patients with acute type A aortic dissection.[52] They concluded that a large false lumen at the time of the initial diagnostic scan is the strongest predictor of subsequent downstream aortic enlargement. This was especially true if the true lumen was less than 30% of the overall transaortic area 6 months after aortic surgery for repair of type A dissection.

This concept of the initial false lumen diameter as a determinant of late clinical deterioration was evaluated for type B disease in 2007 by Song et al.[53] These authors studied 100 consecutive patients with AAD, including 51 with type A dissection and 49 with type B dissection. More than half of the patients underwent CT imaging follow-up through 24 months. Of these, an aneurysm (diameter > 60 mm) was diagnosed in 28%, with the maximal aortic diameter located in the proximal descending segment. A greater than 22-mm initial false lumen diameter of the upper thoracic segment of the descending aorta predicted late aneurysm formation with a sensitivity of 100% and a specificity of 76%. The 42 patients with an initial false lumen diameter greater than 22 mm had a higher event rate than the 58 with smaller false lumen aortic diameters (aneurysm, 42% vs. 5%; or death, 12% vs. 5%).

More recently, another predictive feature for early complication and clinical deterioration was described by Tsai et al. after reviewing data from the International Registry of Aortic Dissection (IRAD).[54] They reviewed 201 cases of type B AAD. During the index hospitalization, 114 patients (56.7%) had a patent false lumen, 68 patients (33.8%) had partial thrombosis of the false lumen, and 19 (9.5%) had complete thrombosis of the false lumen. The mean 3-year mortality rate for patients with a patent false lumen was 13.7%; for those with partial thrombosis it was 31.6%, and for those with complete thrombosis it was 22.6%. Although postdischarge mortality was high among patients with acute type B aortic dissection, partial thrombosis, as compared with complete patency, is a significant independent predictor of postdischarge mortality (relative risk, 2.69; 95% confidence interval [CI], 1.45–4.98; P = .002).

In the future, it is likely that more sophisticated analysis will identify additional factors beyond simple dimensional aortic measurements to better predict patients with acute type B aortic dissection who are at increased risk of disease progression, rapid deterioration, or acute rupture. As prognostic evaluation of aortic dissection improves, the use of endovascular approaches will better target and improve outcomes of this disease.

Management of Aortic Dissection in the Patient with Connective Tissue Disease

Aortic pathologies are a major cause of death in patients with connective tissue disorders such as Marfan syndrome. These patients often present with aortic dissection at a much younger age than the general population, and they may require multiple operations for sequential degeneration of the aorta. Open surgical repair remains the gold standard of treatment for the sequelae of aortic degeneration in this population; however, endovascular treatments may have a role in a small subset of high-risk patients. Reports of TEVAR in patients with Marfan syndrome have demonstrated a higher incidence of reintervention and open surgical conversion (both early and late) as compared with the non-Marfan TEVAR literature, primarily for type I endoleak.[55] Of particular concern is the risk of retrograde type A dissection resulting from endovascular instrumentation in the fragile Marfan aorta. One subset of patients in whom TEVAR may be more readily considered is those who have previously undergone open surgical replacement of the aorta proximal and distal to the descending thoracic aorta, and thus have prosthetic landing zones that are unsusceptible to further degeneration. The majority of patients with connective tissue disorders and acute or chronic type B dissection, however, should be considered for open surgical repair.

New Developments for TEVAR Management of Type A and Ascending Disease

While TEVAR is widely accepted as the first-line treatment modality for acute complicated type B aortic dissection, open surgical repair is the gold standard for treatment of acute type A dissection. Immediate surgical repair has long been recommended for patients presenting with this pathology because of the excessively high mortality associated with medical management. TEVAR has been proposed as an adjunctive or alternative procedure in select patients who are high-risk for open surgical repair of the ascending aorta. Imaging based studies have demonstrated that about one-third of patients with type A aortic dissection may be suitable candidates for endovascular stent grafting, with up to half becoming candidates if a hybrid approach (including carotid-carotid bypass or other debranching procedures) is considered.[56,57] Evidence to support the safety and efficacy of stent graft placement in the ascending aorta is limited, however, and significant technical challenges with the available stent graft systems make this an option reserved for very high-risk patients. Most reports are limited to less than 20 patients, and while technical success is high, complication rates such as stroke and reintervention vary so widely as to not be generalizable.[58]

REFERENCES

1. Erbel R, Alfonso F, Boileau C, et al. Diagnosis and management of aortic dissection. *Eur Heart J.* 2001;22:1642–1681.
2. Glower DD, Speier RH, White WD, et al. Management and long-term outcome of aortic dissection. *Ann Surg.* 1991;214:21–41.
3. Wong DR, Lemaire SA, Coselli JS. Managing dissections of the thoracic aorta. *Am Surg.* 2008;74:364–380.
4. Dake MD, Kato N, Mitchell RS, et al. Endovascular stent graft placement for the treatment of acute aortic dissection. *N Engl J Med.* 1999;340:1546–1552.
5. Neinaber CA, Fattori R, Lund G, et al. Nonsurgical reconstruction of thoracic aortic dissection by stent-graft placement. *N Engl J Med.* 1999;340:1539–1545.
6. Mukherjee D, Eafle KA. Aortic dissection—an update. *Curr Probl Cardiol.* 2005;30:287–325.
7. Parker JD, Golledge J. Outcome of endovascular treatment of acute type B aortic dissection. *Ann Thorac Surg.* 2008;86:1707–1712.
8. Fattori R, Botta L, Lovato L, et al. Malperfusion syndrome in type B aortic dissection: role of the endovascular procedures. *Acta Chir Belg.* 2008;108:192–197.
9. Patel HJ, Williams DM, Meekov M, et al. Long-term results of percutaneous management of malperfusion in acute type B aortic dissection: implications for thoracic aortic endovascular repair. *J Thorac Cardiovasc Surg.* 2009;138:300–308.
10. Czermak BV, Waldenberger P, Fraedrich G, et al. Treatment of Stanford type B aortic dissection with stent grafts: preliminary results. *Radiology.* 2000;217:544–550.
11. Feezor RJ, Martin TD, Hess PJ, et al. Early outcomes after endovascular management of acute, complicated type B aortic dissection. *J Vasc Surg.* 2009;49:561–566.
12. Pearce BJ, Passman MA, Patterson MA, et al. Early outcomes of thoracic endovascular stent-graft repair for acute complicated type B dissections using the gore TAG endoprosthesis. *Ann Vasc Surg.* 2008;22:742–749.
13. Parsa CJ, Schroder JN, Daneshmand MA, et al. Midterm results for endovascular repair of complicated acute and chronic type B aortic dissection. *Ann Thorac Surg.* 2010;89:97–104.
14. Oderich GS, Panneton JM, Bower TC, et al. Aortic dissection with aortic side branch compromise: impact of malperfusion on patient outcome. *Perspect Vasc Surg Endovasc Ther.* 2008;20:190–200.
15. Apostolakis E, Baikoussis NG, Georgiopoulos M. Acute type-B aortic dissection: the treatment strategy. *Hellenic J Cardiol.* 2010;51:338–347.
16. Williams DM, Lee DY, Hamilton BH, et al. The dissected aorta: part III. Anatomy and radiological diagnosis of branch-vessel compromise. *Radiology.* 1997;203:37–44.
17. Williams DM, Lee DY, Hamilton BH, et al. The dissected aorta: percutaneous treatment of ischemic complications-principles and results. *J Vasc Interv Radiol.* 1997;8:605–625.
18. Shiiya N, Matsuzaki K, Kunihara T, et al. Management of vital organ malperfusion in acute aortic dissection: proposal of a mechanism-specific approach. *Gen Thorac Cardiovasc Surg.* 2007;55:85–90.
19. Deeb GM, Patel HJ, Williams DM. Treatment for malperfusion syndrome in acute type A and B aortic dissection: a long-term analysis. *J Thorac Cardiovasc Surg.* 2010;140:98–100.
20. Kische S, Ehrlich MP, Nienaber CA, et al. Endovascular treatment of acute and chronic aortic dissection: midterm results from the talent thoracic retrospective registry. *J Thorac Cardiovasc Surg.* 2009;138:115–124.
21. Fattori R, Tsai TT, Myrmel T, et al. Complicated acute type B dissection: is surgery still the best option? A report from the international registry of acute aortic dissection. *JACC Cardiovasc Interv.* 2008;1:395–402.
22. Tefera G, Acher CW, Hoch JR, et al. Effectiveness of intensive medical therapy in type B aortic dissection: a single-center experience. *J Vasc Surg.* 2007;45:1114–1118.
23. Estrera AL, Miller CC, Safi HJ, et al. Outcomes of medical management of acute type B aortic dissection. *Circulation.* 2006;114:384–389.
24. Tsai TT, Fattori R, Trimarchi S, et al. Long-term survival in patients presenting with type B acute aortic dissection: insights from the International Registry of Acute Aortic Dissections. *Circulation.* 2006;114:2226–2231.
25. Nienaber CA, Rousseau H, Eggebrecht H, et al. Randomized comparison of strategies for type B aortic dissection. The Investigation of Stent Grafts in Aortic Dissection (INSTEAD) trial. *Circulation.* 2009;120:2519–2528.
26. Nienaber CA, Kische S, Akin I, et al. Strategies for subacute/chronic type B aortic dissection: the Investigation of Stent Grafts in Patients with Type B Aortic Dissection (INSTEAD) trial 1-year outcome. *J Thorac Cardiovasc Surg.* 2010;140(6 Suppl):S101–S108.
27. Brunkwall J, Lammer J, Verhoeven E, Taylor P. ADSORB: a study on the efficacy of endovascular grafting in uncomplicated acute dissection of the descending aorta. *Eur J Vasc Endovasc Surg.* 2012;44(1):31–36.
28. Brunkwall J, Kasprzak P, Verhoeven E, et al. Endovascular repair of acute uncomplicated aortic type B dissection promotes aortic remodelling: 1 year results of the ADSORB trial. *Eur J Vasc Endovasc Surg.* 2014;48(3):285–291.
29. Qin YL, Wang F, Li TX, et al. Endovascular repair compared with medical management of patients with uncomplicated type B acute aortic dissection. *J Am Coll Cardiol.* 2016;67(24):2835–2842.
30. Schwartz SI, Durham C, Clouse WD, et al. Predictors of late aortic intervention in patients with medically treated type B aortic dissection. *J Vasc Surg.* 2018;67(1):78–84.
31. Tolenaar JL, van Keulen JW, Jonker FHW, et al. Morphologic predictors of aortic dilatation in type B aortic dissection. *J Vasc Surg.* 2013;58(5):1220–1225.
32. Kotelis D, Grebe G, Kraus P, et al. Morphologic predictors of aortic expansion in chronic type B aortic dissection. *Vascular.* 2016;24(2):187–193.
33. van Bogerijen GHW, Tolenaar JL, Rampoldi V, et al. Predictors of aortic growth in uncomplicated type B aortic dissection. *J Vasc Surg.* 2014;59(4):1134–1143.
34. Conrad MF, Carvalho S, Ergul E, et al. Late aortic remodeling persists in the stented segment after endovascular repair of acute complicated type B aortic dissection. *J Vasc Surg.* 2015;62(3):600–605.
35. Giersson A, Szeto WY, Pochettino A, et al. Significance of malperfusion syndromes prior to contemporary surgical repair for acute type A dissection: outcomes and need for additional revascularizations. *Eur J Cardiothorac Surg.* 2007;32:255–262.
36. Hagan PG, Nienaber CA, Isselbacher EM, et al. The International Registry of Acute Aortic Dissection (IRAD): new insight into an old disease. *JAMA.* 2000;283:897–903.
37. Trimarchi S, Eagle KA, Neinaber CA, et al. Importance of refractory pain and hypertension in acute type B aortic dissection: insights from the International Registry of Acute Aortic Dissection (IRAD). *Circulation.* 2010;122:1283–1289.
38. Slonim SM, Miller DC, Mitchell RS, et al. Percutaneous balloon fenestration and stenting for life-threatening ischemic complications in patients with acute aortic dissections. *J Thorac Cardiovasc Surg.* 1999;117:1118–1127.
39. Xenos ES, Minion DJ, Davenport DL, et al. Endovascular versus open repair for descending thoracic aortic rupture: institutional experience and meta-analysis. *Eur J Cardiothorac Surg.* 2009;35:282–286.
40. Patel HJ, Williams DM, Upchurch GR, et al. A comparative analysis of open and endovascular repair for the ruptured descending thoracic aorta. *J Vasc Surg.* 2009;50:1265–1270.
41. Luebke T, Brunkwall J. Cost-effectiveness of endovascular versus open repair of acute complicated type B aortic dissections. *J Vasc Surg.* 2014;59(5):1247–1255.
42. Hogendoorn W, Hunink MGM, Schlösser FJV, et al. Endovascular vs. open repair of complicated acute type B aortic dissections. *J Endovasc Ther.* 2014;21(4):503–514.
43. Sachs T, Pomposelli F, Hagberg R, et al. Open and endovascular repair of type B aortic dissection in the Nationwide Inpatient Sample. *J Vasc Surg.* 2010;52(4):860–866. discussion 866.

44. Chou HP, Chang HT, Chen CK, et al. Outcome comparison between thoracic endovascular and open repair for type B aortic dissection: a population-based longitudinal study. *J Chin Med Assoc.* 2015;78(4):241–248.

45. Minami T, Imoto K, Uchida K, et al. Clinical outcomes of emergency surgery for acute type B aortic dissection with rupture. *Eur J Cardiothorac Surg.* 2013;44(2):360–364. discussion 364-365.

46. Wilkinson DA, Patel HJ, Williams DM, et al. Early open and endovascular thoracic aortic repair for complicated type B aortic dissection. *Ann Thorac Surg.* 2013;96(1):23–30. discussion 230.

47. Resch TA, Delle M, Falkenberg M, et al. Remodeling of the thoracic aorta after stent grafting of type B dissection: a Swedish multicenter study. *J Cardiovasc Surg (Torino).* 2006;47:503–508.

48. Kusagawa H, Shimono T, Ishida M, et al. Changes in false lumen after transluminal stent-graft placement in aortic dissections: six years' experience. *Circulation.* 2005;111:2951–2957.

49. Sayer D, Bratby M, Brooks M, et al. Aortic morphology following endovascular repair of acute and chronic type B aortic dissection: implications for management. *Eur J Vasc Endovasc Surg.* 2008;36:522–529.

50. Marui A, Mochizuki T, Mitsui N, et al. Toward the best treatment for uncomplicated patients with type B acute aortic dissection: a consideration for sound surgical indication. *Circulation.* 1999;100(Suppl II):II275–II280.

51. Marui A, Mochizuki T, Koyama T, Mitsui N. Degree of fusiform dilation of the proximal descending aorta in type B acute aortic dissection can predict late events. *J Thorax Cardiovasc Surg.* 2007;134:1163–1170.

52. Immer F, Krähenbühl E, Hagan U, et al. Large area of false lumen favors secondary dilation of the aorta after acute type A aortic dissection. *Circulation.* 2005;112(Suppl I): I249–I252.

53. Song JM, Kim JH, Kang DH, et al. Long-term predictors of descending aorta aneurismal change in patients with aortic dissection. *J Am Coll Cardiol.* 2007;50:799–804.

54. Tsai TT, Evangelista A, Nienaber CA, et al. Partial thrombosis of the false lumen in patients with acute type B aortic dissection. *N Engl J Med.* 2007;357:349–359.

55. Pacini D, Parolari A, Berretta P, et al. Endovascular treatment for type B dissection in Marfan syndrome: is it worthwhile? *Ann Thorac Surg.* 2013;95(2):737–749.

56. Sobocinski J, O'Brien N, Maurel B, et al. Endovascular approaches to acute aortic type A dissection: a CT-based feasibility study. *Eur J Vasc Endovasc Surg.* 2011;42(4):442–447.

57. Huang C, Zhou M, Liu Z, et al. Computed tomography-based study exploring the feasibility of endovascular treatment of type A aortic dissection in the Chinese population. *J Endovasc Ther.* 2014;21(5): 707–713.

58. Horton JD, Kölbel T, Haulon S, et al. Endovascular repair of type A aortic dissection: current experience and technical considerations. *Semin Thorac Cardiovasc Surg.* 2016;28(2):312–317.

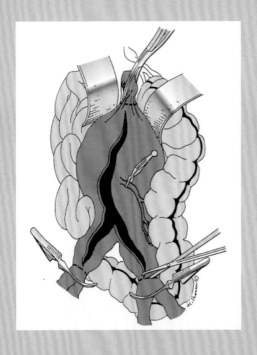

PART X
第十部分

Aortic Aneurysm

主动脉瘤

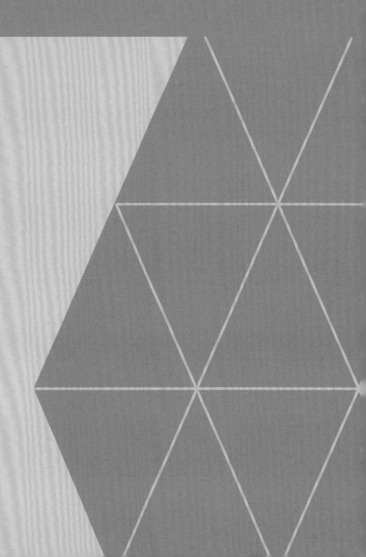

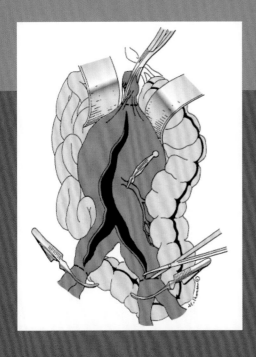

第35章
主动脉瘤的流行病学与预后

　　主动脉瘤是一类致死率和致残率均很高的疾病，在美国每年导致将近10 000人死亡和69 000人住院。主动脉瘤根据病变累及部位的不同，可以分为腹主动脉瘤、胸主动脉瘤和胸腹主动脉瘤，这3类主动脉瘤在疾病诊断、发病率、高危致病因素、干预时机和疾病预后等方面都有各自的特点，本章节将分别给予详细介绍。主动脉瘤根据病理类型的不同，可以分为退行性病变、遗传性病变、感染性病变、炎性病变和创伤性病变。退行性病变主要指主动脉的囊状中层坏死，该病理过程与年龄、高血压及其他主动脉遗传性病变有关。遗传性病变主要包括一系列累及主动脉的遗传性结缔组织病（如马方综合征、Ehlers-Danlos综合征和Loeys-Dietz综合征等）和部分先天性心脏病（如主动脉瓣二叶畸形和主动脉缩窄）。感染性病变包括霉菌性主动脉瘤、结核性主动脉瘤和梅毒性主动脉瘤等。炎性病变包括巨细胞动脉炎、Takayasu动脉炎、白塞综合征和血清阴性脊柱关节病等。不同病理类型的主动脉瘤在发病率、干预时机和疾病预后等方面存在着巨大的差异，而针对不同病因做出及时有效的干预往往能有效改善疾病的预后，本章将对上述内容进行详细介绍。

范瑞新

Epidemiology and Prognosis of Aortic Aneurysms

Aaron W. Aday and Joshua A. Beckman

Aortic aneurysms result in significant morbidity and mortality, accounting for nearly 10,000 deaths and 69,000 hospital discharges per year in the United States.[1] A wide variety of pathological states are associated with aortic aneurysms, including degenerative diseases, genetic disorders, infections, inflammatory conditions, and trauma. Although aneurysms may affect any part of the aorta from the aortic root to the abdominal aorta, the prognosis and outcome in patients with aortic aneurysms vary based on location, etiology, and comorbidities. Timely and appropriate intervention may improve the natural history of the disease process. This chapter reviews the epidemiology and prognosis of aortic aneurysms.

THE NORMAL AORTA

The aorta is the primary conduit vessel through which the heart delivers blood to the entire body. It courses from the heart through the thorax and abdomen, and ultimately bifurcates into the common iliac arteries (CIAs) in the lower abdomen. In the thorax, the aorta can be subdivided into three segments: ascending aorta (from the aortic valve to the innominate artery), transverse aorta or aortic arch (including the great vessels and extending to the left subclavian artery), and descending aorta (from the distal edge of the subclavian artery to the level of the diaphragm) (Fig. 35.1). The abdominal aorta consists of the segment between the diaphragm and the iliac bifurcation.

Like other arterial structures, the aorta is composed of three layers: *tunica intima, tunica media,* and *adventitia.* The innermost surface of the tunica intima is lined by a single-cell-thick layer of endothelial cells (ECs). The intima is bound by the internal elastic lamina. The tunica media is composed of vascular smooth muscle cells (VSMCs) intertwined with collagen, fibroblasts, and elastin fibers, which together control vessel tone. The presence of elastin fibers in the media defines the aorta as an elastic artery and provides the tensile strength that permits the aorta to withstand high-pressure, pulsatile blood flow from the heart. Elastin content gradually decreases with greater distance from the heart.[2] The outermost layer, the adventitia, is a thin layer that contains collagen fibers and fibroblasts, and the nutritive vasa vasorum. In addition to the vasa vasorum, nutrients are delivers to the vessel wall layers via trans-intimal diffusion.

DEFINITION OF AORTIC ANEURYSM

In adults, the normal diameter of the aorta is approximately 3.5 to 4.0 cm in the aortic root to 3 cm in the ascending aorta, 2.5 cm in the descending thoracic aorta, and 1.8 to 2 cm in the abdominal aorta. *Aortic aneurysm* is defined as 50% increase in size compared with the normal proximal segment and varies by location in the aorta. Mild expansion that does not meet these criteria may be referred to as *aortic ectasia.* True aneurysms are classified into two major groups on the basis of morphology: (1) *fusiform* (Fig. 35.2), defined as a circumferential expansion of the aorta, and (2) *saccular,* representing a focal outpouching of a segment of the aorta (Fig. 35.3). Fusiform aneurysms are the most common form of aneurysmal disease. In contrast to true aneurysms, which involve expansion of all three layers of the aortic wall, a *pseudoaneurysm,* also known as a *false aneurysm,* results from a disruption of the aortic wall and essentially represents a contained aortic rupture.

EPIDEMIOLOGY AND PROGNOSIS OF AORTIC ANEURYSMS

Abdominal Aortic Aneurysms

Aortic aneurysms (Fig. 35.4) are typically defined as an increase in diameter of 50% compared with the adjacent normal segment of the aorta; the upper limit of normal for the abdominal aorta is 3 cm. The absolute size definition for abdominal aortic aneurysms (AAAs) is preferable, given that body size and baseline diameter may vary on the basis of height, sex, weight, and presence of a thoracoabdominal aortic aneurysm (TAAA). However, all these factors should be taken into consideration when considering risk in any given individual.

Prevalence

The prevalence of aneurysms of the abdominal aorta has been determined on the basis of several large screening studies and autopsy series (Table 35.1). In an early series of 24,000 consecutive autopsies performed over 23 years, 1.97% of the subjects were found to have an AAA.[3] Of the 473 aneurysms found, 58% were larger than 4 cm in diameter, nearly three quarters of the patients were men, and one-fourth of the aneurysms had ruptured. More recent large screening programs in targeted populations have further evaluated the prevalence of AAA. The largest screening program performed was the Aneurysm Detection and Management (ADAM) Study Screening Program, which studied 126,196 veterans 50 to 79 years of age.[4] In this cohort of predominantly male American veterans, 3.6% of subjects had an infrarenal aortic diameter greater than 3 cm, and an AAA 4 cm or larger was found in 1.2%. The Multicentre Aneurysm Screening Study (MASS) also screened 27,147 of 33,830 invited men aged 65 to 74 and reported a 4.9% prevalence of AAA 3 cm or larger.[5]

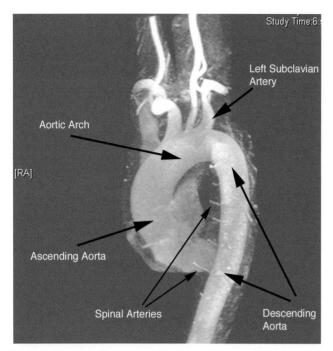

Fig. 35.1 Magnetic Resonance Angiography of the Thoracic Aorta. Note the different aortic segments: ascending aorta, aortic arch, and descending aorta. Left subclavian artery separates the aortic arch from the descending aorta.

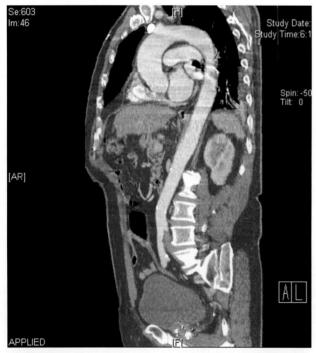

Fig. 35.2 Magnetic Resonance Angiogram of Ascending Aortic Aneurysm. Aneurysm involves entire circumference of the ascending aorta and is thus fusiform. Normal ascending aorta size is less than 3 cm.

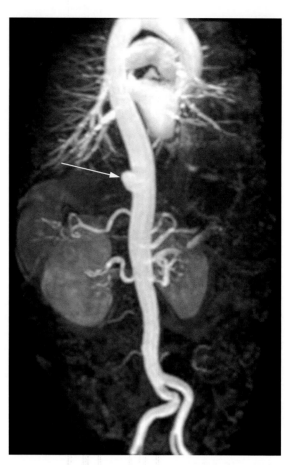

Fig. 35.3 Maximal Intensity Projection of Magnetic Resonance Image of Saccular Aneurysm. Note outpouching of an otherwise normal descending aorta (arrow). This pattern of aneurysm is more common in infectious aneurysms.

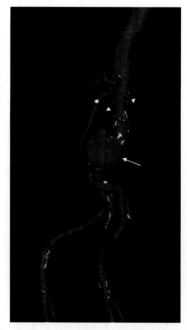

Fig. 35.4 3-D Reconstruction of Computed Tomographic Angiogram of Infrarenal Abdominal Aortic Aneurysm. Aneurysm measures 5.1 cm in maximal dimension. Nearby structures include the superior mesenteric artery (asterisk) and renal arteries (arrowheads).

Several studies have demonstrated a lower prevalence of AAA in women. The largest of these studies screened nearly 10,012 women (mean age, 69.6 years) and found an AAA prevalence rate of 0.7%, with only 4 of 74 detected aneurysms measuring larger than 5 cm.[6] These low prevalence rates were consistent with findings from earlier studies.

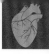

TABLE 35.1 Prevalence of Aortic Aneurysm in Large Epidemiological Studies

Author	No.	Gender	Age (Years)	Aneurysm Frequency (%)	Nation
Pleumeekers[14]	5,419	42% M	>55	4.1 M, 0.7 F	Netherlands
Lederle[4]	126,196	97% M	50–79	1.3	United States
Ashton[5]	27,147	M	65–74	4.9	United Kingdom
Singh[8]	2,998	F	25–84	2.2	Norway
Lederle[9]	3,450	F	50–79	1.0	United States
Scott[16]	9,342	F	65–80	1.3	United Kingdom

F, Female; *M*, male.

Among 4237 subjects aged 65 to 80 who participated in a screening study among general practitioners in West Sussex, United Kingdom, 2290 women agreed to undergo abdominal ultrasonography.[7] Only 1.4% of the women had an AAA 3 cm or larger, and only 0.3% had an AAA 4 cm or larger. This dramatically lower prevalence in women has been confirmed in subsequent studies. In the Norwegian Tromso study, 2% of 2943 women aged 55 to 84 had an AAA 3 cm or larger, and 0.5% had an abdominal aneurysm 4 cm or larger.[8] Finally, among female American veterans, the prevalence of an AAA 3 cm or larger was just 1%.[9] However, an increasing number of cardiovascular risk factors does increase the risk of AAA in women, with a prevalence rate as high as 6.4% in this higher-risk group.[6]

Risk Factors

Three risk factors predict the vast majority of AAAs: age, sex, and cigarette smoking. Aneurysms usually affect the elderly, seldom occurring in those younger than 60 years of age, and there is a clear increase in incidence with increasing age, even when limiting the studies to older individuals.[10–12] In a Norwegian population-based study of 6386 men and women aged 25 to 84, the incidence of AAA in men increased from 0% in those aged 25 to 44, to 6% in those aged 55 to 64, and to 18.5% in those aged 75 to 84.[8] Large North American epidemiological studies have demonstrated an increase in AAA risk ranging from 58% to 300% with each additional decade of life.[13] Sex is also an important predictor of AAA formation; in all age groups, risk of AAA is two- to sixfold higher in men than in women.[8,9,14–17] Cigarette smoking is the most potent modifiable risk factor and increases the risk of AAA by 60% to 850%.[18–25] In the ADAM study and the Edinburgh Artery Study, risk of an aneurysm increased threefold with any smoking history.[4,26] Risk of AAA development further increases with number of cigarettes smoked, duration of smoking, and lack of filtration, indicating a dose-response relationship.[27] In the Whitehall study of 18,403 male civil servants examined at age 40 to 64 years, aneurysm frequency increased from sixfold with manufactured cigarettes with filters to 25-fold with hand-rolled cigarettes.[28] Smoking cessation can reduce the risk of aneurysm formation, with former smokers having a lower AAA risk than current smokers.[13,28,29]

Risk factors for cardiovascular disease in general (e.g., hypertension, hyperlipidemia) also increase the risk of AAA formation but are less potent risk factors than age, gender, and smoking.[4,13,30–32] In the REACH registry, there was a clear but modest association of both hypertension and hyperlipidemia with AAA.[33] Earlier studies suggested a less consistent relationship with hypertension,[15,34] but aneurysm formation seems to correlate best with diastolic blood pressure[35] or use of an antihypertensive medication.[17] Some data suggest that hypertension may be a greater risk factor for aneurysm rupture than for initial aneurysm formation.[36] The association between cholesterol and AAA is clear, although hyperlipidemia is a less potent risk factor

than those mentioned previously.[12,14,25,37] Risk of AAA formation increased 30% per 40 mg/dL total cholesterol in the Chicago Heart Association Detection Project in Industry cohort.[15] For specific components of the lipid profile, higher levels of low-density lipoprotein cholesterol (LDL-C) and lower levels of high-density lipoprotein cholesterol (HDL-C) are both associated with aneurysm formation.[10,37] Similarly, the presence of atherosclerosis increases risk of aneurysm formation.[10,11,14] In the ADAM study of more than 100,000 subjects, hypertension, elevated cholesterol, and presence of other vascular disease increased risk of aneurysm formation by 15%, 44%, and 66%, respectively.[4] In contrast, diabetes and black race appear protective against formation of an aneurysm.[4,9,13,38,39] Diabetes decreases risk of aneurysm formation by 30% to 50%.[13,35]

A dramatic increase in frequency of AAA formation in relatives of patients with aortic aneurysm suggests a genetic component to the disease. Although cigarette smoking numerically accounts for the vast majority of AAAs in the population,[13] the most potent risk factor for aneurysm formation is a history of aneurysm in a first-degree relative. Norrgård et al.[40] identified an 18% incidence of aneurysms in first-degree relatives of patients with AAA. In the ADAM study, a family history doubled the risk of AAA, but was reported in only 5.1% of more than 100,000 participants.[41] Investigations specific to the impact of family history demonstrate a larger risk. Several studies have demonstrated that a family history of AAA increases the risk of AAA four- to fivefold.[35,42] Frydman et al.[43] screened the siblings of 400 AAA patients and found an AAA in 43% of male siblings and 16% of female siblings. More specifically, the risk of AAA formation consistently rises above 20% for men older than 50 who have a first-degree relative with AAA.[40,44–47] Using segregation analysis, Majumder et al.[48] reported that the relative risk of developing an AAA is 3.97 and 4.03 with paternal and maternal history, respectively. Risk increases to nearly 10-fold with an affected male sibling and 23-fold when a female sibling is affected.[48] In the Liege AAA Family Study, investigators found a lifetime prevalence of AAA of 32% among brothers.[49] Twin studies further support a genetic component to AAA formation, with one study reporting an odds ratio (OR) of 71 (95% confidence interval [CI], 27–183) for monozygotic twins and 7.6 (95% CI, 3.0–19) for dizygotic twins.[50] Overall estimates for the heritability of AAA are as high as 77%.[51] Family history of AAA was also related to earlier AAA formation and rupture by nearly a decade.[42] Rate of rupture was nearly fourfold higher in patients with a family history than in sporadic AAA patients.[49] Similarly, in a study of 374 Japanese individuals with AAA, family history was an independent predictor of accelerated aneurysm expansion.[52]

Despite the wealth of data supporting a genetic component to AAA formation, no clear mode of inheritance and no single candidate gene have been identified. Early studies suggested evidence of both sex-linked and autosomal dominant patterns of inheritance. Associations have been made with blood types, haptoglobin variations, α_1-antitrypsin, and human leukocyte antigen class II (HLA-II) immune response genes.[53-55] More than 100 reports on genetic associations with AAA have appeared in the literature.[56] One study suggested an association between reduced AAA growth and five single-nucleotide polymorphisms (SNPs) in latent TGF-β binding protein (LTBP4), as well as an allelic variant of TGFB3.[57] However, another study showed no association between genetic polymorphisms in the main receptors for TGF-β and AAA formation.[58] Two genome-wide association studies (GWAS) have suggested an association between AAA and a SNP located on chromosome 3p12.3 in a region near the gene encoding contactin-3 (CNTN3), a lipid-anchored cell adhesion molecule.[59] Another GWAS in a population from Iceland and the Netherlands found an SNP on 9q33 associated with AAA with an OR of 1.21. The same SNP has been associated with coronary artery disease (CAD), peripheral artery disease (PAD), and pulmonary embolism (PE).[60] The SNP resides in the gene encoding DAB2IP, a cell growth and survival inhibitor. In addition, the same gene variant associated with myocardial infarction (MI) at locus 9p21 has been associated with AAA.[61,62] Additional GWAS and candidate gene studies have implicated genes involved in lipid pathways (LDLR and SORT1),[63,64] vascular integrity (LRP1),[65,66] and inflammation (IL6R).[67] More recently, a meta-analysis of GWAS results including 10,204 AAA cases identified four new loci that were not associated with CAD or other traditional cardiovascular risk factors.[68] Finally, of interest but of unclear significance, is the association between telomere length and AAA in a small cohort in the United Kingdom.[69] This may represent the association of aging, telomere length, and aneurysm formation, but the direct pathophysiological link remains unclear.

Prognosis

The natural history of AAA is one of silent, progressive expansion followed by sudden lethal rupture. In a large autopsy study performed over a quarter of a century, one-fourth of abdominal aneurysms were ruptured on postmortem examination.[3] The frequency of rupture was dependent largely on size in this study population, ranging from 9.5% in aneurysms smaller than 4 cm to 45.6% in aneurysms 7.1 to 10 cm in diameter. In a comparison of patients with aortic aneurysms divided into two groups at a cutoff point of 6 cm, survival was markedly decreased in the patients with larger aneurysms.[70] In a single-center study that included 60 ruptured AAAs over a 30-year period, only two occurred in patients with an aneurysm diameter smaller than 5 cm.[71] Similarly, in a study in Rochester, Minnesota, no ruptures occurred in aneurysms smaller than 5 cm, whereas rupture occurred in 25% of AAAs larger than 5 cm.[72] In 198 patients with aneurysms 5.5 cm in diameter or larger, but who were deemed too risky for surgery, 23% had presumed rupture over a mean follow-up of 1.6 years.[73] Mortality rates as high as 53% to 66% are observed in patients who present with a ruptured aortic aneurysm.[74,75]

On the basis of these data, two large trials have been conducted to determine whether early recognition and treatment can alter the natural history of AAA. The UK Small Aneurysm Trial randomized 1090 patients aged 60 to 76 years with asymptomatic AAAs 4 to 5.5 cm in diameter to undergo early elective open surgery or ultrasonographic surveillance.[76] In the surveillance group, surgery was performed when the aneurysm reached 5.5 cm. Early surgery did not affect overall mortality. At 3 years, nearly 20% of both groups had died, although abdominal aneurysms accounted for only a quarter of the deaths in both groups. Cardiovascular mortality unrelated to the aneurysm accounted for 40% of total mortality, and cancer caused slightly more than 20% of the deaths. Even among the lowest risk individuals within the trial, there was no benefit to early intervention,[77] and there was no long-term benefit seen after 12 years of follow-up.[78] In a similar study performed by the US Veterans Administration, 1136 subjects aged 50 to 79 years with asymptomatic AAA 4 to 5.5 cm in diameter were randomized to undergo either early elective open surgery or ultrasonographic surveillance.[31] After 5 years, there was no significant difference in survival between the groups, each with

a near 25% mortality rate. In this study, aneurysm-related deaths accounted for only 3% of total mortality. More recently, the PIVOTAL study demonstrated no difference between surveillance and early endovascular repair in patients with small aneurysms (measuring 4 to 5 cm), and no difference in aneurysm-related death in the two groups after 3 years of follow-up.[79] Together, these data suggest that early repair of small aneurysms does not alter outcomes.

Several factors can predict the likelihood of expansion and rupture of AAAs and can help identify which patients require intervention. The factor most predictive of rupture is initial size of the aneurysm. In one study of patients too ill for surgery, aneurysm rupture rates ranged from 9.4% for AAA of 5.5 to 5.9 cm to 32.5% for AAA of 7 cm or more.[73] In the UK Small Aneurysm Study, the rate of rupture was 0.9% in aneurysms 3 to 3.9 cm, 2.7% in aneurysms 4 to 5.5 cm, and 27.8% in aneurysms 5.6 cm and larger.[36] Larger aneurysm size also predicted a more rapid increase in diameter.[80] Similar to factors that predispose to initial development of AAA, cigarette smoking and higher blood pressure increase the risks of rapid expansion and rupture. In contrast to the decreased risk of AAA development in women, being female actually increases risk of rupture and death after rupture in those with established AAA.[36,81-83] In the UK Small Aneurysm Study, women had a threefold higher risk of AAA rupture than men.[36] As mentioned previously, some have advocated use of biomechanical factors (wall stress, wall strength) to help with risk prediction. Prospective studies will be required to determine whether these factors can improve assessment of patients at high risk for aneurysm rupture and can improve selection of patients for aneurysm repair.

Thoracic and Thoracoabdominal Aortic Aneurysms
Prevalence

The most common location of involvement of thoracic aortic aneurysms (TAAs) is the ascending aorta and/or aortic root (noted in 60%), with the descending aorta affected in approximately 40% of cases and the aortic arch in 10%.[84] The diagnosis of an aneurysm in the thoracic aorta depends on its location. At the aortic root, an aortic diameter of greater than 4.0 cm would be considered an aortic aneurysm. TAAAs are defined by contiguous involvement of the descending thoracic aorta and abdominal aorta, and account for 5% to 10% of all aortic aneurysms.[84,85] The prevalence of isolated TAA is poorly defined but estimated at 6 persons per 100,000 per year.[86] In autopsy records reported from 63% of 70,368 deaths between 1958 and 1985 in the city of Malmo, Sweden, TAAs were diagnosed in 205 of the deceased, 53% of whom were men.[87] Of the 44,332 autopsies performed, 63 individuals (0.14%) had died of a ruptured TAA. The relative infrequency of TAA is confirmed by a retrospective analysis in Rochester, Minnesota.[88] Over 30 years, of approximately 45,000 residents, 72 (0.16%) were diagnosed with a TAA; 61% were women, and 67 patients had thoracic aortic involvement only. Most studies, however, suggest that men are twice as likely to develop a TAA as women.[88,89] TAAAs occur even more infrequently. Of the 44,332 people to undergo necropsy in Malmo, Sweden, a mere 10 had TAAA.[87] In the Rochester, Minnesota, experience the incidence was 0.37 per 100,000 person-years of follow-up.[88] Because of the relatively small sample sizes reported in the literature, risk factors for TAAA development are less well defined. Risk factors currently associated with development of TAAA include smoking, hypertension, and atherosclerotic vascular disease.[84]

Etiology and Pathophysiology

Aneurysms involving the thoracic aorta commonly develop as a result of cystic medial necrosis, a degenerative process that histologically involves degeneration of elastic fibers and VSMCs. Cystic medial degeneration can arise as an isolated abnormality or as a result of an underlying connective tissue disease, such as Marfan syndrome (MFS) or vascular

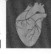

Ehlers-Danlos syndrome (EDS). Degeneration of the media within the arterial wall results in impaired structural integrity of the aorta, leading to eventual aortic dilation, aneurysm formation, and risk of rupture.

As with AAA, age is a significant risk factor for development of TAA; median age for presentation varies from 64 to 69 years.[84] Cystic medial necrosis develops to some degree as a natural consequence of aging and may be accelerated by comorbid conditions such as hypertension.[90] Although a degenerative aneurysmal process is found in the majority of patients with TAAA, several other etiologies should be considered, including inherited collagen vascular disorders (e.g., MFS), bicuspid aortic valve (BAV) disease, aortic dissection, infection, and vasculitis (e.g., giant cell or Takayasu arteritis [TA]). Rarer causes of TAA include coarctation of the aorta and trauma. Finally, some aneurysms develop because of a familial predisposition termed *familial thoracic aortic syndrome.*

Natural History and Prognosis

The natural history and prognosis for TAAs and TAAAs remain poor but incompletely defined, partly because modern imaging techniques now allow for early detection and intervention of aneurysm before rupture, and because the natural history is dependent in large part on underlying etiology. However, in a study accumulated over 25 years that followed 94 patients with TAAAs who did not undergo operative repair, 76% died within 2 years of follow-up, with half of the deaths resulting from aneurysm rupture.[91] A more recent experience with 57 TAAA patients managed without operation revealed a 69% 2-year survival, with aneurysm rupture as the cause of death in 19%.[92] Features associated with aneurysm expansion and rupture include smoking, chronic obstructive pulmonary disease (COPD), and renal insufficiency.[93] Dissection as an underlying cause of aneurysm formation is also associated with a greater risk of rupture compared with degenerative causes.[94] Extension of a TAA into the abdomen is associated with a 50% relative increase in risk of rupture, compared with those limited to the thoracic aorta alone.[95]

The natural history of TAA depends in large part on rate of expansion. Initial aneurysm size at the time of diagnosis is the most important predictor of both thoracic aneurysm growth and rupture.[84,96] Longitudinal data have suggested that the mean rate of growth of thoracic aneurysms averages 0.1 cm/year.[97] Several factors also contribute to the rate of growth. Growth rate is increased in the setting of an aortic dissection. In one study, the presence of a chronic aortic dissection was associated with a 0.37 cm/year rate of growth.[97] Descending TAAs tend to increase in size more rapidly than ascending TAAs.[97,98] Those who smoke have a twofold increased rate of growth over nonsmokers.[99]

Survival rates for TAA range from 39% to 87% at 1 year and from 13% to 46% at 5 years.[92,99,100] In a study of 67 patients with TAA (mean age, 65 years), those with an aortic diameter less than 5 cm had a 90% 3-year survival rate, compared with 60% for patients with a TAA larger than 5 cm.[99] Similarly, in two other studies, patients with TAAs 6 cm or larger had a higher mortality rate than those with smaller aneurysms.[98] Based on these data, referral for surgery is recommended when the aneurysm reaches 5.5 cm or greater in the ascending aorta and 6 cm in the descending aorta.[101]

However, several factors increase risk of aneurysm rupture and may prompt earlier referral for intervention. Guidelines recommend that patients with MFS or other genetic disorders (e.g., vascular EDS, Loeys-Dietz, and Turner syndromes, or familial aortic aneurysm) may require intervention at smaller diameters, such as 4.0 cm to 5.0 cm, depending on clinical circumstances.[98,101–106] In addition, those with a more rapid rate of growth than expected (i.e., ≥0.5 cm/year) may be at increased risk of rupture and require repair at diameters less than 5.5 cm.[101] For individuals with BAV and an additional risk factor for dissection, such as family history, ascending aortic aneurysm repair may be warranted at a threshold of 5.0 cm.[107] Finally, repair should be

considered in patients with ascending aortic diameter greater than 4.5 cm if undergoing aortic valve surgery.[101]

For aneurysms involving the aortic arch, surgery should be considered when the diameter reaches 5.5 cm or greater.[101] For degenerative descending TAAs, repair is recommended when the diameter exceeds 5.5 cm, although in individuals with TAAAs or those with high surgical risk, elective surgery is recommended when the diameter exceeds 6.0 cm.[101] Other factors reported to significantly increase rate of rupture or need for surgery include older age, history of COPD, pain possibly related to the aneurysm, higher blood pressure, and extension of the aneurysm into the abdomen.[93,95]

INHERITED AND DEVELOPMENTAL DISORDERS

Marfan Syndrome

MFS is an autosomal dominant inherited disorder of connective tissue arising from mutations in *FBN1*, a gene on chromosome 15 encoding the extracellular matrix (ECM) protein fibrillin-1 (FBN1). Abnormalities in fibrillin synthesis affect multiple tissues in patients with MFS, including the cardiovascular, skeletal, and ocular systems.[108] Excessive signaling through the TGF-β cascade has been shown to be a contributing factor.[109] This is additionally supported by experiments showing that TGF-β-neutralizing antibodies reverse aortic disease in a mouse model of MFS, and by the demonstration that losartan, an angiotensin receptor blocker (ARB) with anti-TGF-β properties, can partially reverse aortic wall defects in these mice.[110] Clinical manifestations of MFS include ectopia lentis, hyperelasticity and ligamentous redundancy, valvular heart disease, and abnormalities in skin, fascia, skeletal muscle, and adipose tissue.[108]

However, potentially the most lethal complication in MFS is disease of the ascending aorta resulting in aneurysm, dissection, and rupture. Dilation of the aortic root has been demonstrated early in childhood in patients with MFS. Histologically, changes in the media seen in patients with MFS include cystic medial necrosis with fragmentation and disarray of elastic fibers, a paucity of smooth muscle cells, and separation of muscle fibers by collagen and glycosaminoglycans.[111]

Ehlers-Danlos Syndrome

Ehlers-Danlos syndrome type 4 (vascular EDS) is a rare congenital defect in the synthesis of type 3 collagen resulting from a mutation in the COL3A1 gene.[112] Patients with vascular EDS typically present with acrogeria (distinctive facial appearance), bruising, thin skin, and vascular or visceral rupture.[108] Histological examination reveals a thinned, fragmented internal elastic lamina.[113] Moreover, deposition of glycosaminoglycans in the media of major arteries and intima of smaller arteries, with intimal thickening, has been noted.[114] Abnormalities in type 3 collagen fiber formation reduce stability or prevent formation of collagen, decreasing vascular wall stability.[113] In a study of 199 patients with confirmed vascular EDS, 25% of patients suffered a ruptured vessel or viscus by age 20 and 80% by age 40.[115] Mean survival was 48 years. There were 131 deaths, 103 of which were due to vascular rupture. Complications of pregnancy caused the death of 15% of the women who became pregnant. Outcomes differ based on the specific COL3A1 mutation involved. Mutations leading to minimal type III collagen formation are associated with a lower incidence of aortic pathology but overall higher mortality due to arterial complications than mutations associated with a 50% production of normal collagen.[116]

Loeys-Dietz Syndrome

Loeys-Dietz syndrome is an autosomal dominant condition arising from mutations in either the type I or type II receptor for TGF-β (TGFBR1 or TGFBR2). Individuals with Loeys-Dietz syndrome have several characteristic features, including abnormal uvula, hyper-telorism (increased space between the eyes), and arterial aneurysms, among other abnormalities, some of which are similar to MFS.[106,108] The syndrome is characterized by particularly aggressive arterial disease manifested as aortic aneurysm with high risk of aortic dissection and rupture. As such, the average age of death is 26 years. Because of the high morbidity and mortality and the high rate of aortic dissection, even with aneurysms of less than 5.0 cm in size, early repair at smaller diameters is recommended.[101,106]

Bicuspid Aortic Valve

Presence of a BAV increases the risk of ascending aortic aneurysm formation.[84] Although it was once thought that the aneurysmal dilation was a "poststenotic" phenomenon arising secondary to abnormal flow through a diseased aortic valve, more recent data support the notion that aortic expansion occurs independently of valvular dysfunction, severity, age, and body size.[117] Further evidence that aortic dilation is not dependent on valve dysfunction is found in a study of 118 consecutive patients with BAV in whom the diameter of the ascending aorta was not correlated with severity of aortic stenosis.[118] Moreover, abnormalities in the aortic wall can arise even when there is no hemodynamically significant aortic valve disease, in part due to abnormal helical flow in the proximal aorta,[119] and replacement of a diseased valve does not change the rate of aortic expansion.[120]

In one study comparing aorta and pulmonary artery specimens in patients with BAV and tricuspid aortic valve disease, those with BAV had decreased FBN1 concentrations in both the aortic and pulmonary specimens, suggesting a systemic disorder.[121] Additional studies have identified FBN1 mutations in individuals with BAV but no evidence of MFS.[122] VSMCs from patients with BAV show intracellular accumulation and reduction of extracellular distribution of several ECM structural elements, including fibrillin, fibronectin, and tenascin.[123] Surgical specimens demonstrate greater amounts of inflammation and increased expression of matrix metalloproteinase (MMP)-2 and MMP-9, both of which are endopeptidases that degrade ECM components, in patients with BAV compared with those with tricuspid aortic valve disease.[124,125] Patients with Turner syndrome, who are at increased risk of developing BAV, also exhibit an increased rate of aneurysm formation.[126]

Aortic Coarctation

Coarctation of the aorta represents 5% of congenital heart disease. The clinical consequences of aortic coarctation are varied, ranging from being life-threatening in infancy to remaining unappreciated until adulthood.[127] Coarctation has long been associated with de novo aortic aneurysm development, and aneurysms can also develop at the site of coarctation repair—specifically patch angioplasty repair—in up to 20% of patients.[128–130] Some reports indicate aneurysm formation can even occur several decades after initial repair.[131] Intermediate follow-up studies suggest that percutaneous balloon angioplasty repair results in a 2% to 5% rate of repair-site aortic aneurysm formation.[132,133] More recent data on thoracic endovascular aortic repair in adult patients with coarctation found a 1-year freedom from intervention rate of 78%.[134] A potential explanation for the relationship between coarctation and aortic aneurysm is the common link with the presence of BAV in approximately 15% of patients with aortic coarctation.[104]

OTHER CONDITIONS ASSOCIATED WITH AORTIC ANEURYSM

Although most aortic aneurysms occur as a result of degenerative processes in the aortic wall as described earlier, certain disease states

> ### BOX 35.1   Disorders Associated with Aortic Aneurysms
>
> Degenerative
> Cystic medial necrosis
> Aortic dissection
> Developmental
> Marfan syndrome (MFS)
> Loeys-Dietz syndrome
> Ehlers-Danlos syndrome (EDS)
> Bicuspid aortic valve (BAV)
> Turner syndrome
> Aortic coarctation
> Infectious
> Tuberculosis
> Syphilis
> *Staphylococcus*
> *Salmonella*
> Vasculitis
> Takayasu arteritis (TA)
> Giant cell arteritis (GCA)
> Behçet disease
> Rheumatoid arthritis
> Systemic lupus erythematosus (SLE)
> Sarcoidosis
> Ankylosing spondylitis
> Reiter syndrome
> Relapsing polychondritis
> Cogan syndrome
> Trauma

including vasculitis, infection, and inherited abnormalities of structural proteins predispose patients to aortic aneurysm formation (Box 35.1).

Vasculitides
Giant Cell Arteritis

Giant cell arteritis (GCA; see Chapter 40) is a medium-vessel chronic inflammatory vasculitis that affects the aorta and its branch vessels. It most commonly occurs in patients older than 55 years of age and is twice as common in women as in men.[135] Between 1% and 33% of GCA patients develop aneurysms, most commonly in the thoracic aorta, with the highest incidence in the first 5 years following diagnosis.[136,137] In a study of 6999 individuals with GCA, there was a twofold increase in the risk of aortic aneurysm compared with age- and sex-match controls.[138] In a series of 41 patients with GCA-related TAAs, 16 developed aortic dissection, 15 had aortic annular expansion causing symptomatic aortic valve insufficiency, and 18 required surgery.[139] In a series of 168 patients with GCA, 18% developed aortic aneurysm or dissection, and these occurrences were inversely associated with development of intracranial disease manifestations.[136] The presence of an aortic aneurysm itself was not associated with increased mortality; however, the nine individuals who developed aortic dissection had significantly increased mortality.[140] The mechanism of aneurysm formation seems to be similar to patients without GCA, with increases in MMP-2- and MMP-9-associated destruction of the vessel wall.[141,142]

Takayasu Arteritis

Named for a Japanese professor of ophthalmology, TA (see Chapter 40) is a large-vessel vasculitis that typically has its onset between the age of 10 and 30 years. The most common vascular

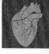

presentation is occlusive disease, found in 80% to 94% of patients; however, aortic aneurysms may be found in up to one-fourth of patients with TA.[143,144] Development of aneurysmal disease has been associated with worse outcome in a series of 120 Japanese patients followed for 13 years.[145] Blood levels of MMP-2 and MMP-9 are elevated in TA, but the mechanism of aneurysm formation remains unknown.[146]

Behçet Disease

Behçet disease (see Chapter 41) is a small-vessel vasculitis originally characterized by a set of three symptoms: aphthous stomatitis, genital ulcers, and uveitis.[147] Involvement of medium-sized and large arteries, as well as veins, arises not from direct vascular inflammation but rather due to vasculitis of the small arteries of the vasa vasorum that supply the vessel wall.[148] Vascular involvement, including aortic and pulmonary artery aneurysms, can be found in 7% to 38% of patients.[147,149] Management of aneurysmal disease in Behçet disease depends in large part on the location of the abnormality and clinical circumstances. First-line therapy includes an antiinflammatory regimen with corticosteroids. As with other vasculitides, risk of intervention is greatest during the state of active inflammation, and there is an increased risk of rupture, dissection, and/or future aneurysmal dilation at the site of revascularization.

Seronegative Spondyloarthropathies

The spondyloarthropathies (see Chapter 39) are characterized by inflammation of the spine and sacroiliac joints, association with HLA-B27, and absence of circulating rheumatoid factor (RF). These disorders are known to be associated with an increased risk of aortic aneurysm formation. Specific spondyloarthropathies include ankylosing spondylitis, Reiter syndrome, and relapsing polychondritis.

Ankylosing spondylitis is an HLA-B27 disease that requires the presence of four of the five following features: onset younger than 40 years of age, back pain for more than 3 months, insidious onset of symptoms, morning stiffness, and improvement with exercise. In a series of 44 outpatients, aortic root disease and valve disease were found in 82%; thickening of the aortic valve was noted in 41% of patients, and aortic dilation in 25%.[150] Aortic valve thickening manifested as nodularities of the aortic cusps, forming a characteristic subaortic bump. Valve regurgitation was seen in almost half of patients, and 40% had moderate lesions.

Reiter syndrome is a reactive arthritis that affects the lower limbs, causing an asymmetrical oligoarthritis. To make the diagnosis, patients must have evidence of an antecedent infection, diarrhea, or urethritis 4 weeks preceding the syndrome.[151] Less than 1% of Reiter syndrome patients develop cardiovascular complications. Among this group, aortic insufficiency is a late finding.

Relapsing polychondritis is a paroxysmal and progressive inflammatory disease of the cartilaginous structures, affecting the ear, nose, and hyaline cartilage of the tracheobronchial tree. Cardiovascular disease, including aortic aneurysms, is found in 25% to 50% of patients.[152]

Infectious Aortic Aneurysms
Mycotic Aneurysms

Also known as *infective endarteritis* (see Chapter 59), mycotic aneurysms are rare phenomena. Two large necropsy studies including 22,000 and 20,000 patients, respectively, revealed a combined incidence of 0.03% in the United States.[153,154] The average age of patients with mycotic aneurysms is 65, and men are threefold more likely to develop mycotic aneurysms than women.[155,156] Hematogenous seeding,

such as occurs in patients with endocarditis, affects a vessel that may be "at risk" because of preexisting atherosclerosis or previous damage and represents the most common cause of mycotic aneurysms.[157] Indeed, as many as 15% of patients with endocarditis developed mycotic aneurysm before the antibiotic era.[158] Other etiologies include septic microemboli, contiguous extension, and trauma with direct contamination. In contrast to the typical degenerative or vasculitic fusiform expansion, mycotic aneurysms are more likely to be saccular (see Fig. 35.3). The outpouching may range in size from 1 mm to 10 cm and include components of acute and chronic inflammation, hemorrhage, abscess formation, and necrosis.

Clinical manifestations of mycotic aneurysm most commonly include pain and fever and, if related to a new aneurysm, should prompt directed investigation. The organisms that most commonly cause mycotic aneurysms include *Staphylococcus* and *Salmonella* species, which cause 40% and 20% of mycotic aneurysms, respectively.[159,160] Surgery should be prompt, since rupture occurs in up to 80%.[161,162] Prognosis for cerebral vascular infection is dire, with 1-year mortality for patients who have cerebrovascular mycotic aneurysms reaching as high as 90%.[162]

Tuberculous Aneurysms

Aortic aneurysm due to tuberculosis is quite rare. In a series of more than 22,000 autopsies performed at one urban medical center in the first half of the 20th century, only 1 of 308 aortic aneurysms had tuberculous aneurysms,[153] whereas there were no tuberculous aneurysms among 20,000 autopsies performed in a rural setting.[154] Three mechanisms have been postulated to facilitate tuberculous adhesion and endarteritis. It is thought that direct extension from a contiguous source, such as the spine or lung, may cause 75% of tuberculous aneurysms.[163] Other possibilities include adhesion to a vessel damaged by atherosclerosis or infiltration of the inner layers of the aorta via the vasa vasorum.[163] The abdominal and thoracic portions of the aorta are affected similarly. The presentation of the patient with a tuberculous aneurysm varies significantly. The patient may be asymptomatic, have a palpable or radiologically visible paraaortic mass, complain of chest or abdominal pain, or present with aortic rupture and hypovolemic shock. Tuberculous aneurysms that are symptomatic or rapidly expanding, as well as tuberculous pseudoaneurysms, typically require surgical repair.

Syphilitic Aneurysms

Although syphilis may once have been a common cause of aortic disease, antibiotics have greatly diminished the incidence of syphilitic aortic aneurysm (luetic aneurysm), such that fewer than 50 cases have been reported in the antibiotic era.[164] Central nervous system (CNS) and cardiovascular complications denote the tertiary stage of syphilis. Classically, this arises after a latent phase of approximately 10 to 30 years from initial spirochete infection. Syphilitic aortitis may occur in up to 10% of patients with tertiary syphilis (Fig. 35.5). Destruction of the elastic lamina occurs as a consequence of lymphoplasmacytic infiltrate around the vasa vasorum, owing to direct spirochete infection of the aortic media. This ultimately leads to expansion but also fibrosis and calcification, producing the classic "tree bark" radiographic pattern. Luetic aortic aneurysms commonly involve the ascending aorta and are saccular. Involvement of the coronary ostia may result in coronary stenosis and resultant anginal symptoms. Survival with syphilitic aortic aneurysm is worse than in the general population.

Trauma

Aneurysms related to trauma are discussed in Chapter 62.

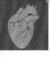

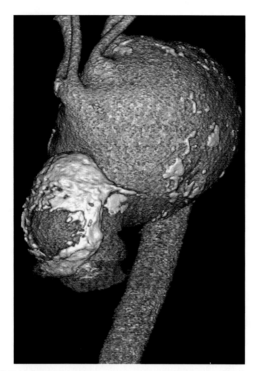

Fig. 35.5 Volume-rendered maximum intensity projections from computed tomographic angiography of chest of patient with tertiary syphilis, showing extensively calcified thoracic aortic aneurysm measuring 11.5 cm × 11.4 cm in short axis and 18 cm in length. (From Tomey MI, Murthy VL, Beckman JA. Giant syphilitic aortic aneurysm: a case report and review of the literature. *Vasc Med.* 2011;16:360–364.)

REFERENCES

1. Benjamin EJ, Virani SS, Callaway CW, et al. Heart disease and stroke statistics—2018 update: a report from the American Heart Association. *Circulation.* 2018;137(12):e67–e492.
2. Wolinsky H, Glagov S. A lamellar unit of aortic medial structure and function in mammals. *Circ Res.* 1967;20(1):99–111.
3. Darling RC, Messina CR, Brewster DC, Ottinger LW. Autopsy study of unoperated abdominal aortic aneurysms. The case for early resection. *Circulation.* 1977;56(3 Suppl):II161–II164.
4. Lederle FA, Johnson GR, Wilson SE, et al. The aneurysm detection and management study screening program: validation cohort and final results. Aneurysm Detection and Management Veterans Affairs Cooperative Study Investigators. *Arch Intern Med.* 2000;160(10):1425–1430.
5. Ashton HA, Buxton MJ, Day NE, et al. The Multicentre Aneurysm Screening Study (MASS) into the effect of abdominal aortic aneurysm screening on mortality in men: a randomised controlled trial. *Lancet.* 2002;360(9345):1531–1539.
6. Derubertis BG, Trocciola SM, Ryer EJ, et al. Abdominal aortic aneurysm in women: prevalence, risk factors, and implications for screening. *J Vasc Surg.* 2007;46(4):630–635.
7. Scott RA, Ashton HA, Kay DN. Abdominal aortic aneurysm in 4237 screened patients: prevalence, development and management over 6 years [see comments]. *Br J Surg.* 1991;78(9):1122–1125.
8. Singh K, Bønaa KH, Jacobsen BK, et al. Prevalence of and risk factors for abdominal aortic aneurysms in a population-based study: the Tromso Study. *Am J Epidemiol.* 2001;154(3):236–244.
9. Lederle FA, Johnson GR, Wilson SE. Abdominal aortic aneurysm in women. *J Vasc Surg.* 2001;34(1):122–126.
10. Alcorn HG, Wolfson Jr SK, Sutton-Tyrrell K, et al. Risk factors for abdominal aortic aneurysms in older adults enrolled in the Cardiovascular Health Study. *Arterioscler Thromb Vasc Biol.* 1996;16(8):963–970.
11. Kurvers HA, van der Graaf Y, Blankensteijn JD, et al. Screening for asymptomatic internal carotid artery stenosis and aneurysm of the abdominal aorta: comparing the yield between patients with manifest atherosclerosis and patients with risk factors for atherosclerosis only. *J Vasc Surg.* 2003;37(6):1226–1233.
12. Tornwall ME, Virtamo J, Haukka JK, et al. Life-style factors and risk for abdominal aortic aneurysm in a cohort of Finnish male smokers. *Epidemiology.* 2001;12(1):94–100.
13. Lederle FA, Johnson GR, Wilson SE, et al. Prevalence and associations of abdominal aortic aneurysm detected through screening. Aneurysm Detection and Management (ADAM) Veterans Affairs Cooperative Study Group. *Ann Intern Med.* 1997;126(6):441–449.
14. Pleumeekers HJ, Hoes AW, van der Does E, et al. Aneurysms of the abdominal aorta in older adults. The Rotterdam Study. *Am J Epidemiol.* 1995;142(12):1291–1299.
15. Rodin MB, Daviglus ML, Wong GC, et al. Middle age cardiovascular risk factors and abdominal aortic aneurysm in older age. *Hypertension.* 2003;42(1):61–68.
16. Scott RA, Bridgewater SG, Ashton HA. Randomized clinical trial of screening for abdominal aortic aneurysm in women. *Br J Surg.* 2002;89(3):283–285.
17. Vardulaki KA, Walker NM, Day NE, et al. Quantifying the risks of hypertension, age, sex and smoking in patients with abdominal aortic aneurysm. *Br J Surg.* 2000;87(2):195–200.
18. Doll R, Peto R, Wheatley K, et al. Mortality in relation to smoking: 40 years' observations on male British doctors. *BMJ.* 1994;309(6959):901–911.
19. Goldberg RJ, Burchfiel CM, Benfante R, et al. Lifestyle and biologic factors associated with atherosclerotic disease in middle-aged men. 20-year findings from the Honolulu Heart Program. *Arch Intern Med.* 1995;155(7):686–694.
20. Hammond EC. Smoking in relation to the death rates of one million men and women. *Natl Cancer Inst Monogr.* 1966;19:127–204.
21. Nilsson S, Carstensen JM, Pershagen G. Mortality among male and female smokers in Sweden: a 33-year follow-up. *J Epidemiol Community Health.* 2001;55(11):825–830.
22. Rogot E, Murray JL. Smoking and causes of death among U.S. veterans: 16 years of observation. *Public Health Rep.* 1980;95(3):213–222.
23. Tang JL, Morris JK, Wald NJ, et al. Mortality in relation to tar yield of cigarettes: a prospective study of four cohorts. *BMJ.* 1995;311(7019): 1530–1533.
24. Weir JM, Dunn Jr JE. Smoking and mortality: a prospective study. *Cancer.* 1970;25(1):105–112.
25. Tang W, Yao L, Roetker NS, et al. Lifetime risk and risk factors for abdominal aortic aneurysm in a 24-year prospective study: the ARIC study (Atherosclerosis Risk in Communities). *Arterioscler Thromb Vasc Biol.* 2016;36(12):2468–2477.
26. Lee AJ, Fowkes FG, Carson MN, et al. Smoking, atherosclerosis and risk of abdominal aortic aneurysm. *Eur Heart J.* 1997;18(4):671–676.
27. Wilmink TB, Quick CR, Day NE. The association between cigarette smoking and abdominal aortic aneurysms. *J Vasc Surg.* 1999;30(6):1099–1105.
28. Strachan DP. Predictors of death from aortic aneurysm among middle-aged men: the Whitehall study. *Br J Surg.* 1991;78(4):401–404.
29. Lederle FA, Nelson DB, Joseph AM. Smokers' relative risk for aortic aneurysm compared with other smoking-related diseases: a systematic review. *J Vasc Surg.* 2003;38(2):329–334.
30. Powell JT, Greenhalgh RM. Clinical practice. Small abdominal aortic aneurysms. *N Engl J Med.* 2003;348(19):1895–1901.
31. Lederle FA, Wilson SE, Johnson GR, et al. Immediate repair compared with surveillance of small abdominal aortic aneurysms. *N Engl J Med.* 2002;346(19):1437–1444.
32. Brady AR, Thompson SG, Fowkes FG, et al. Abdominal aortic aneurysm expansion: risk factors and time intervals for surveillance. *Circulation.* 2004;110(1):16–21.
33. Baumgartner I, Hirsch AT, Abola MT, et al. Cardiovascular risk profile and outcome of patients with abdominal aortic aneurysm in out-patients with atherothrombosis: data from the Reduction of Atherothrombosis for Continued Health (REACH) Registry. *J Vasc Surg.* 2008;48(4):808–814.

34. Franks PJ, Edwards RJ, Greenhalgh RM, Powell JT. Risk factors for abdominal aortic aneurysms in smokers. *Eur J Vasc Endovasc Surg.* 1996;11(4):487–492.

35. Blanchard JF, Armenian HK, Friesen PP. Risk factors for abdominal aortic aneurysm: results of a case-control study. *Am J Epidemiol.* 2000;151(6):575–583.

36. Brown LC, Powell JT. Risk factors for aneurysm rupture in patients kept under ultrasound surveillance. UK Small Aneurysm Trial Participants. *Ann Surg.* 1999;230(3):289–296.

37. Hobbs SD, Claridge MW, Quick CR, et al. LDL cholesterol is associated with small abdominal aortic aneurysms. *Eur J Vasc Endovasc Surg.* 2003;26(6):618–622.

38. Gillum RF. Epidemiology of aortic aneurysm in the United States. *J Clin Epidemiol.* 1995;48(11):1289–1298.

39. Lederle FA. The strange relationship between diabetes and abdominal aortic aneurysm. *Eur J Vasc Endovasc Surg.* 2012;43(3):254–256.

40. Norrgård O, Rais O, Angquist KA. Familial occurrence of abdominal aortic aneurysms. *Surgery.* 1984;95(6):650–656.

41. Baird PA, Sadovnick AD, Yee IM, et al. Sibling risks of abdominal aortic aneurysm. *Lancet.* 1995;346(8975):601–604.

42. Verloes A, Sakalihasan N, Koulischer L, Limet R. Aneurysms of the abdominal aorta: familial and genetic aspects in three hundred thirteen pedigrees. *J Vasc Surg.* 1995;21(4):646–655.

43. Frydman G, Walker PJ, Summers K, et al. The value of screening in siblings of patients with abdominal aortic aneurysm. *Eur J Vasc Endovasc Surg.* 2003;26(4):396–400.

44. Adams DC, Tulloh BR, Galloway SW, et al. Familial abdominal aortic aneurysm: prevalence and implications for screening. *Eur J Vasc Surg.* 1993;7(6):709–712.

45. Cole CW, Barber GG, Bouchard AG, et al. Abdominal aortic aneurysm: consequences of a positive family history. *Can J Surg.* 1989;32(2):117–120.

46. Webster MW, Ferrell RE, St. Jean PL, et al. Ultrasound screening of first-degree relatives of patients with an abdominal aortic aneurysm. *J Vasc Surg.* 1991;13(1):9–13.

47. Webster MW, St. Jean PL, Steed DL, et al. Abdominal aortic aneurysm: results of a family study. *J Vasc Surg.* 1991;13(3):366–372.

48. Majumder PP, St Jean PL, Ferrell RE, et al. On the inheritance of abdominal aortic aneurysm. *Am J Hum Genet.* 1991;48(1):164–170.

49. Sakalihasan N, Defraigne J, Kerstenne M, et al. Family members of patients with abdominal aortic aneurysms are at increased risk for aneurysms: analysis of 618 probands and their families from the Liège AAA Family Study. *Ann Vasc Surg.* 2014;28(4):787–797.

50. Wahlgren CM, Larsson E, Magnusson PK, et al. Genetic and environmental contributions to abdominal aortic aneurysm development in a twin population. *J Vasc Surg.* 2010;51(1):3–7.

51. Joergensen TM, Christensen K, Lindholt JS, et al. Editor's choice – High heritability of liability to abdominal aortic aneurysm: a population based twin study. *J Vasc Surg.* 2016;64(2):537.

52. Akai A, Watanabe Y, Hoshina K, et al. Family history of aortic aneurysm is an independent risk factor for more rapid growth of small abdominal aortic aneurysms in Japan. *J Vasc Surg.* 2015;61(2):287–290.

53. Wiernicki I, Gutowski P, Ciechanowski K, et al. Abdominal aortic aneurysm: association between haptoglobin phenotypes, elastase activity, and neutrophil count in the peripheral blood. *Vasc Surg.* 2001;35(5):345–350.

54. St Jean P, Hart B, Webster M, et al. Alpha-1-antitrypsin deficiency in aneurysmal disease. *Hum Hered.* 1996;46(2):92–97.

55. Schardey HM, Hernandez-Richter T, Klueppelberg U, et al. Alleles of the alpha-1-antitrypsin phenotype in patients with aortic aneurysms. *J Cardiovasc Surg (Torino).* 1998;39(5):535–539.

56. Hinterseher I, Tromp G, Kuivaniemi H. Genes and abdominal aortic aneurysm. *Ann Vasc Surg.* 2011;25(3):388–412.

57. Thompson AR, Cooper JA, Jones GT, et al. Assessment of the association between genetic polymorphisms in transforming growth factor beta, and its binding protein (LTBP), and the presence, and expansion, of abdominal aortic aneurysm. *Atherosclerosis.* 2010;209(2):367–373.

58. Golledge J, Clancy P, Jones GT, et al. Possible association between genetic polymorphisms in transforming growth factor beta receptors, serum transforming growth factor beta1 concentration and abdominal aortic aneurysm. *Br J Surg.* 2009;96(6):628–632.

59. Elmore JR, Obmann MA, Kuivaniemi H, et al. Identification of a genetic variant associated with abdominal aortic aneurysms on chromosome 3p12.3 by genome wide association. *J Vasc Surg.* 2009;49(6):1525–1531.

60. Gretarsdottir S, Baas AF, Thorleifsson G, et al. Genome-wide association study identifies a sequence variant within the DAB2IP gene conferring susceptibility to abdominal aortic aneurysm. *Nat Genet.* 2010;42(8):692–697.

61. Helgadottir A, Thorleifsson G, Magnusson KP, et al. The same sequence variant on 9p21 associates with myocardial infarction, abdominal aortic aneurysm and intracranial aneurysm. *Nat Genet.* 2008;40(2):217–224.

62. Thompson AR, Golledge J, Cooper JA, et al. Sequence variant on 9p21 is associated with the presence of abdominal aortic aneurysm disease but does not have an impact on aneurysmal expansion. *Eur J Hum Genet.* 2009;17(3):391–394.

63. Bradley DT, Hughes AE, Badger SA, et al. A variant in LDLR is associated with abdominal aortic aneurysm. *Circ Cardiovasc Genet.* 2013;6(5):498–504.

64. Jones GT, Brown MJ, Gretarsdottir S, et al. A sequence variant associated with sortilin-1 (SORT1) on 1p13.3 is independently associated with abdominal aortic aneurysm. *Hum Mol Genet.* 2013;22(14):2941–2947.

65. Brown MJ, Jones GT, Harrison SC, et al. Abdominal aortic aneurysm is associated with a variant in low-density lipoprotein receptor-related protein 1. *Am J Hum Genet.* 2011;89(5):619–627.

66. Boucher P, Gotthardt M, Li WP, et al. LRP: role in vascular wall integrity and protection from atherosclerosis. *Science.* 2003;300(5617):329–332.

67. Harrison SC, Smith AJ, Jones GT, et al. Interleukin-6 receptor pathways in abdominal aortic aneurysm. *Eur Heart J.* 2013;34(48):3707–3716.

68. Jones GT, Tromp G, Kuivaniemi H, et al. Meta-analysis of genome-wide association studies for abdominal aortic aneurysm identifies four new disease-specific risk loci. *Circ Res.* 2017;120(2):341–353.

69. Atturu G, Brouilette S, Samani NJ, et al. Short leukocyte telomere length is associated with abdominal aortic aneurysm (AAA). *Eur J Vasc Endovasc Surg.* 2010;39(5):559–564.

70. Szilagyi DE, Elliott JP, Smith RF. Clinical fate of the patient with asymptomatic abdominal aortic aneurysm and unfit for surgical treatment. *Arch Surg.* 1972;104(4):600–606.

71. Bickerstaff LK, Hollier LH, Van Peenen HJ, et al. Abdominal aortic aneurysms: the changing natural history. *J Vasc Surg.* 1984;1(1):6–12.

72. Nevitt MP, Ballard DJ, Hallett Jr JW. Prognosis of abdominal aortic aneurysms. A population-based study. *N Engl J Med.* 1989;321(15):1009–1014.

73. Lederle FA, Johnson GR, Wilson SE, et al. Rupture rate of large abdominal aortic aneurysms in patients refusing or unfit for elective repair. *JAMA.* 2002;287(22):2968–2972.

74. Harris LM, Faggioli GL, Fiedler R, et al. Ruptured abdominal aortic aneurysms: factors affecting mortality rates. *J Vasc Surg.* 1991;14(6):812–818.

75. Karthikesalingam A, Holt PJ, Vidal-Diez A, et al. Mortality from ruptured abdominal aortic aneurysms: clinical lessons from a comparison of outcomes in England and the USA. *Lancet.* 2014;383(9921):963–969.

76. Mortality results for randomised controlled trial of early elective surgery or ultrasonographic surveillance for small abdominal aortic aneurysms. The UK Small Aneurysm Trial Participants. *Lancet.* 1998;352(9141):1649–1655.

77. Brown LC, Thompson SG, Greenhalgh RM, et al. Fit patients with small abdominal aortic aneurysms (AAAs) do not benefit from early intervention. *J Vasc Surg.* 2008;48(6):1375–1381.

78. Powell JT, Brown LC, Forbes JF, et al. Final 12-year follow-up of surgery versus surveillance in the UK Small Aneurysm Trial. *Br J Surg.* 2007;94(6):702–708.

79. Ouriel K, Clair DG, Kent KC, et al. Endovascular repair compared with surveillance for patients with small abdominal aortic aneurysms. *J Vasc Surg.* 2010;51(5):1081–1087.

80. Brown PM, Sobolev B, Zelt DT. Selective management of abdominal aortic aneurysms smaller than 5.0 cm in a prospective sizing program with gender-specific analysis. *J Vasc Surg.* 2003;38(4):762–765.

81. Powell JT, Brown LC. The natural history of abdominal aortic aneurysms and their risk of rupture. *Acta Chir Belg.* 2001;101(1):11–16.

82. Evans SM, Adam DJ, Bradbury AW. The influence of gender on outcome after ruptured abdominal aortic aneurysm. *J Vasc Surg.* 2000;32(2):258–262.

83. Lo RC, Bensley RP, Hamdan AD, et al. Gender differences in abdominal aortic aneurysm presentation, repair, and mortality in the Vascular Study Group of New England. *J Vasc Surg.* 2013;57(5):1261–1268.

84. Isselbacher EM. Thoracic and abdominal aortic aneurysms. *Circulation.* 2005;111(6):816–828.

85. Svensson LG. Natural history of aneurysms of the descending and thoracoabdominal aorta. *J Card Surg.* 1997;12(2 Suppl):279–284.

86. Ince H, Nienaber CA. Etiology, pathogenesis and management of thoracic aortic aneurysm. *Nat Clin Pract Cardiovasc Med.* 2007;4(8):418–427.

87. Svensjo S, Bengtsson H, Bergqvist D. Thoracic and thoracoabdominal aortic aneurysm and dissection: an investigation based on autopsy. *Br J Surg.* 1996;83(1):68–71.

88. Bickerstaff L, Pairolero P, Hollier L, et al. Thoracic aortic aneurysms: a population-based study. *Surgery.* 1982;92(6):1103–1108.

89. Svensson LG, Crawford ES, Hess KR, et al. Experience with 1509 patients undergoing thoracoabdominal aortic operations. *J Vasc Surg.* 1993;17(2):357–368.

90. Guo D, Hasham S, Kuang SQ, et al. Familial thoracic aortic aneurysms and dissections: genetic heterogeneity with a major locus mapping to 5q13–14. *Circulation.* 2001;103(20):2461–2468.

91. Crawford ES, DeNatale RW. Thoracoabdominal aortic aneurysm: observations regarding the natural course of the disease. *J Vasc Surg.* 1986;3(4):578–582.

92. Cambria RA, Gloviczki P, Stanson AW, et al. Outcome and expansion rate of 57 thoracoabdominal aortic aneurysms managed nonoperatively. *Am J Surg.* 1995;170(2):213–217.

93. Griepp RB, Ergin MA, Galla JD, et al. Natural history of descending thoracic and thoracoabdominal aneurysms. *Ann Thorac Surg.* 1999;67(6):1927–1930.

94. Pitt MP, Bonser RS. The natural history of thoracic aortic aneurysm disease: an overview. *J Card Surg.* 1997;12(2 Suppl):270–278.

95. Juvonen T, Ergin MA, Galla JD, et al. Prospective study of the natural history of thoracic aortic aneurysms. *Ann Thorac Surg.* 1997;63(6):1533–1545.

96. Kim JB, Kim K, Lindsay ME, et al. Risk of rupture or dissection in descending thoracic aortic aneurysm. *Circulation.* 2015;132(17):1620–1629.

97. Davies RR, Goldstein LJ, Coady MA, et al. Yearly rupture or dissection rates for thoracic aortic aneurysms: simple prediction based on size. *Ann Thorac Surg.* 2002;73(1):17–27.

98. Elefteriades JA. Natural history of thoracic aortic aneurysms: indications for surgery, and surgical versus nonsurgical risks. *Ann Thorac Surg.* 2002;74(5):S1877–S1880.

99. Dapunt OE, Galla JD, Sadeghi AM, et al. The natural history of thoracic aortic aneurysms. *J Thorac Cardiovasc Surg.* 1994;107(5):1323–1332.

100. Pressler V, McNamara JJ. Aneurysm of the thoracic aorta. Review of 260 cases. *J Thorac Cardiovasc Surg.* 1985;89(1):50–54.

101. Hiratzka LF, Bakris GL, Beckman JA, et al. 2010 ACCF/AHA/AATS/ACR/ASA/SCA/SCAI/SIR/STS/SVM guidelines for the diagnosis and management of patients with thoracic aortic disease: a report of the American College of Cardiology Foundation/American Heart Association Task Force on Practice Guidelines, American Association for Thoracic Surgery, American College of Radiology, American Stroke Association, Society of Cardiovascular Anesthesiologists, Society for Cardiovascular Angiography and Interventions, Society of Interventional Radiology, Society of Thoracic Surgeons, and Society for Vascular Medicine. *Circulation.* 2010;121(13):e266–e369.

102. Gott VL, Greene PS, Alejo DE, et al. Replacement of the aortic root in patients with Marfan's syndrome. *N Engl J Med.* 1999;340(17):1307–1313.

103. Svensson LG, Kouchoukos NT, Miller DC, et al. Expert consensus document on the treatment of descending thoracic aortic disease using endovascular stent-grafts. *Ann Thorac Surg.* 2008;85(1 Suppl):S1–S41.

104. Tzemos N, Therrien J, Yip J, et al. Outcomes in adults with bicuspid aortic valves. *JAMA.* 2008;300(11):1317–1325.

105. Vallely MP, Semsarian C, Bannon PG. Management of the ascending aorta in patients with bicuspid aortic valve disease. *Heart Lung Circ.* 2008;17(5):357–363.

106. Loeys BL, Schwarze U, Holm T, et al. Aneurysm syndromes caused by mutations in the TGF-beta receptor. *N Engl J Med.* 2006;355(8):788–798.

107. Hiratzka LF, Creager MA, Isselbacher EM, Svensson LG. 2010 ACCF/AHA/AATS/ACR/ASA/SCA/SCAI/SIR/STS/SVM Guideline for the Diagnosis and Management of Patients with Thoracic Aortic Disease Surgery for aortic dilatation in patients with bicuspid aortic valves: a statement of clarification from the American College of Cardiology/American Heart Association Task Force on Clinical Practice Guidelines. *Circulation.* 2016;133(7):680–686.

108. Meester JAN, Verstraeten A, Schepers D, et al. Differences in manifestation of Marfan syndrome, Ehlers-Danlos syndrome, and Loeys-Dietz syndrome. *Ann Cardiothorac Surg.* 2017;6(6):582–594.

109. Holm TM, Habashi JP, Doyle JJ, et al. Noncanonical TGFβ signaling contributes to aortic aneurysm progression in Marfan syndrome mice. *Science.* 2011;332(6027):358–361.

110. Habashi JP, Judge DP, Holm TM, et al. Losartan, an AT1 antagonist, prevents aortic aneurysm in a mouse model of Marfan syndrome. *Science.* 2006;312(5770):117–121.

111. El-Hamamsy I, Yacoub MH. Cellular and molecular mechanisms of thoracic aortic aneurysms. *Nat Rev Cardiol.* 2009;6(12):771–786.

112. Germain DP. Clinical and genetic features of vascular Ehlers-Danlos syndrome. *Ann Vasc Surg.* 2002;16(3):391–397.

113. Arteaga-Solis E, Gayraud B, Ramirez F. Elastic and collagenous networks in vascular diseases. *Cell Struct Funct.* 2000;25(2):69–72.

114. Nishiyama Y, Manabe N, Ooshima A, et al. A sporadic case of Ehlers-Danlos syndrome type IV: diagnosed by a morphometric study of collagen content. *Pathol Int.* 1995;45(7):524–529.

115. Pepin M, Schwarze U, Superti-Furga A, Byers PH. Clinical and genetic features of Ehlers-Danlos syndrome type IV, the vascular type. *N Engl J Med.* 2000;342(10):673–680.

116. Shalhub S, Black 3rd JH, Cecchi AC, et al. Molecular diagnosis in vascular Ehlers-Danlos syndrome predicts pattern of arterial involvement and outcomes. *J Vasc Surg.* 2014;60(1):160–169.

117. Nistri S, Sorbo MD, Marin M, et al. Aortic root dilatation in young men with normally functioning bicuspid aortic valves. *Heart.* 1999;82(1):19–22.

118. Keane MG, Wiegers SE, Plappert T, et al. Bicuspid aortic valves are associated with aortic dilatation out of proportion to coexistent valvular lesions. *Circulation.* 2000;102(19 Suppl 3):III35–III39.

119. Hope MD, Hope TA, Meadows AK, et al. Bicuspid aortic valve: four-dimensional MR evaluation of ascending aortic systolic flow patterns. *Radiology.* 2010;255(1):53–61.

120. Yasuda H, Nakatani S, Stugaard M, et al. Failure to prevent progressive dilation of ascending aorta by aortic valve replacement in patients with bicuspid aortic valve: comparison with tricuspid aortic valve. *Circulation.* 2003;108(Suppl 1):II291–II294.

121. Fedak PW, de Sa MP, Verma S, et al. Vascular matrix remodeling in patients with bicuspid aortic valve malformations: implications for aortic dilatation. *J Thorac Cardiovasc Surg.* 2003;126(3):797–806.

122. Pepe G, Nistri S, Giusti B, et al. Identification of fibrillin 1 gene mutations in patients with bicuspid aortic valve (BAV) without Marfan syndrome. *BMC Med Genet.* 2014;15:23.

123. Nataatmadja M, West M, West J, et al. Abnormal extracellular matrix protein transport associated with increased apoptosis of vascular smooth muscle cells in Marfan syndrome and bicuspid aortic valve thoracic aortic aneurysm. *Circulation.* 2003;108(Suppl 1):II329–II334.

124. Schmid FX, Bielenberg K, Holmer S, et al. Structural and biomolecular changes in aorta and pulmonary trunk of patients with aortic aneurysm and valve disease: implications for the Ross procedure. *Eur J Cardiothorac Surg.* 2004;25(5):748–753.

125. Boyum J, Fellinger EK, Schmoker JD, et al. Matrix metalloproteinase activity in thoracic aortic aneurysms associated with bicuspid and tricuspid aortic valves. *J Thorac Cardiovasc Surg.* 2004;127(3):686–691.

126. Sybert VP. Cardiovascular malformations and complications in Turner syndrome. *Pediatrics.* 1998;101(1):E11.

127. Jenkins NP, Ward C. Coarctation of the aorta: natural history and outcome after surgical treatment. *QJM.* 1999;92(7):365–371.

128. Knyshov GV, Sitar LL, Glagola MD, Atamanyuk MY. Aortic aneurysms at the site of the repair of coarctation of the aorta: a review of 48 patients. *Ann Thorac Surg.* 1996;61(3):935–939.

129. Benzaquen BS, Therrien J. Thoracic aortic aneurysm occurring at a coarctation repair site. *Can J Cardiol.* 2003;19(5):561–562.

130. Vriend JW, Mulder BJ. Late complications in patients after repair of aortic coarctation: implications for management. *Int J Cardiol.* 2005;101(3): 399–406.

131. Walhout RJ, Braam RL, Schepens MA, et al. Aortic aneurysm formation following coarctation repair by Dacron patch aortoplasty. *Neth Heart J.* 2010;18(7-8):376–377.

132. Rao PS, Galal O, Smith PA, Wilson AD. Five- to nine-year follow-up results of balloon angioplasty of native aortic coarctation in infants and children. *J Am Coll Cardiol.* 1996;27(2):462–470.

133. Fletcher SE, Nihill MR, Grifka RG, et al. Balloon angioplasty of native coarctation of the aorta: midterm follow-up and prognostic factors. *J Am Coll Cardiol.* 1995;25(3):730–734.

134. Lala S, Scali ST, Freezor RJ, et al. Outcomes of thoracic endovascular aortic repair in adult coarctation patients. *J Vasc Surg.* 2018;67(2): 369–381.

135. Beckman JA. Giant cell arteritis. *Curr Treat Options Cardiovasc Med.* 2000;2(3):213–218.

136. Nuenninghoff DM, Hunder GG, Christianson TJ, et al. Incidence and predictors of large-artery complication (aortic aneurysm, aortic dissection, and/or large-artery stenosis) in patients with giant cell arteritis: a population-based study over 50 years. *Arthritis Rheum.* 2003;48(12):3522–3531.

137. García-Martínez A, Arguis P, Prieto-González S, et al. Prospective long term follow-up of a cohort of patients with giant cell arteritis screened for aortic structural damage (aneurysm or dilatation). *Ann Rheum Dis.* 2014;73(10):1826–1832.

138. Robson JC, Kiran A, Maskell J, et al. The relative risk of aortic aneurysm in patients with giant cell arteritis compared with the general population of the UK. *Ann Rheum Dis.* 2015;74(1):129–135.

139. Evans JM, Bowles CA, Bjornsson J, et al. Thoracic aortic aneurysm and rupture in giant cell arteritis. A descriptive study of 41 cases, [published erratum appears in Arthritis Rheum 38(2):290, 1995]. *Arthritis Rheum.* 1994;37(10):1539–1547.

140. Nuenninghoff DM, Hunder GG, Christianson TJ, et al. Mortality of large-artery complication (aortic aneurysm, aortic dissection, and/or large-artery stenosis) in patients with giant cell arteritis: a population-based study over 50 years. *Arthritis Rheum.* 2003;48(12):3532–3537.

141. Nikkari ST, Höyhtyä M, Isola J, Nikkari T. Macrophages contain 92-kd gelatinase (MMP-9) at the site of degenerated internal elastic lamina in temporal arteritis. *Am J Pathol.* 1996;149(5):1427–1433.

142. Tomita T, Imakawa K. Matrix metalloproteinases and tissue inhibitors of metalloproteinases in giant cell arteritis: an immunocytochemical study. *Pathology.* 1998;30(1):40–50.

143. Subramanyan R, Joy J, Balakrishnan KG. Natural history of aortoarteritis (Takayasu's disease). *Circulation.* 1989;80(3):429–437.

144. Kerr GS, Hallahan CW, Giordano J, et al. Takayasu arteritis. *Ann Intern Med.* 1994;120(11):919–929.

145. Ishikawa K, Maetani S. Long-term outcome for 120 Japanese patients with Takayasu's disease. Clinical and statistical analyses of related prognostic factors. *Circulation.* 1994;90(4):1855–1860.

146. Matsuyama A, Sakai N, Ishigami M, et al. Matrix metalloproteinases as novel disease markers in Takayasu arteritis. *Circulation.* 2003;108(12):1469–1473.

147. Sakane T, Takeno M, Suzuki N, Inaba G. Behçet's disease. *N Engl J Med.* 1999;341(17):1284–1291.

148. Yazici H, Yurdakul S, Hamuryudan V. Behçet disease. *Curr Opin Rheumatol.* 2001;13(1):18–22.

149. Ehrlich GE. Vasculitis in Behçet's disease. *Int Rev Immunol.* 1997;14(1):81–88.

150. Roldan CA, Chavez J, Wiest PW, et al. Aortic root disease and valve disease associated with ankylosing spondylitis. *J Am Coll Cardiol.* 1998;32(5):1397–1404.

151. Amor B. Reiter's syndrome. Diagnosis and clinical features. *Rheum Dis Clin North Am.* 1998;24(4):677–695. vii.

152. Letko E, Zafirakis P, Baltatzis S, et al. Relapsing polychondritis: a clinical review. *Semin Arthritis Rheum.* 2002;31(6):384–395.

153. Parkhurst GF, Dekcer JP. Bacterial aortitis and mycotic aneurysm of the aorta; a report of twelve cases. *Am J Pathol.* 1955;31(5):821–835.

154. Sommerville RL, Allen EV, Edwards JE. Bland and infected arteriosclerotic abdominal aortic aneurysms: a clinicopathologic study. *Medicine (Baltimore).* 1959;38:207–221.

155. Bennett DE, Cherry JK. Bacterial infection of aortic aneurysms. A clinicopathologic study. *Am J Surg.* 1967;113(3):321–326.

156. Sedwitz MM, Hye RJ, Stabile BE. The changing epidemiology of pseudoaneurysm. Therapeutic implications. *Arch Surg.* 1988;123(4): 473–476.

157. Mansur AJ, Grinberg M, Leão PP, et al. Extracranial mycotic aneurysms in infective endocarditis. *Clin Cardiol.* 1986;9(2):65–72.

158. Anderson CB, Butcher Jr HR, Ballinger WF. Mycotic aneurysms. *Arch Surg.* 1974;109(5):712–717.

159. Jarrett F, Darling RC, Mundth ED, Austen WG. The management of infected arterial aneurysms. *J Cardiovasc Surg (Torino).* 1977;18(4): 361–366.

160. Vogelzang RL, Sohaey R. Infected aortic aneurysms: CT appearance. *J Comput Assist Tomogr.* 1988;12(1):109–112.

161. Taylor Jr LM, Deitz DM, McConnell DB, Porter JM. Treatment of infected abdominal aneurysms by extraanatomic bypass, aneurysm excision, and drainage. *Am J Surg.* 1988;155(5):655–658.

162. Johansen K, Devin J. Mycotic aortic aneurysms. A reappraisal. *Arch Surg.* 1983;118(5):583–588.

163. Long R, Guzman R, Greenberg H, et al. Tuberculous mycotic aneurysm of the aorta: review of published medical and surgical experience. *Chest.* 1999;115(2):522–531.

164. Pugh PJ, Grech ED. Syphilitic aortitis. *N Engl J Med.* 2002;346(9):676.

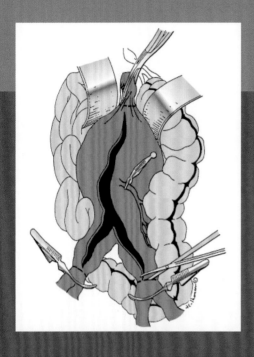

第36章
主动脉瘤的临床评估

    主动脉瘤是大血管外科中最为重要的一类疾病。主要包括胸主动脉瘤、胸腹主动脉瘤和腹主动脉瘤。其具有起病隐匿，临床表现不典型，漏诊率、死亡率高等特点。本章分别介绍了不同部位主动脉瘤的临床症状，还介绍了各类主动脉瘤的临床评估方法。本章从病史入手，从体格检查出发，到具有筛查或诊断意义的各种影像学检查，如超声、CT、MRI和血管造影，从不同角度较为全面地介绍了主动脉瘤临床评估的各个方法，并对比了不同方法之间的优劣势。同时，还引用了各类研究报道，评价了不同检查手段的敏感度和特异度。

钱向阳

Clinical Evaluation of Aortic Aneurysms

Joshua A. Beckman and Mark A. Creager

The vast majority of aortic aneurysms are asymptomatic, accounting for a much higher disease prevalence than hospitalization and mortality statistics would suggest (see Chapter 35). These data underscore the central challenge in aortic aneurysmal disease: a common clinical problem that is silent until rupture and death. Aortic aneurysms typically increase in size slowly over years or decades, with few warning signs. The management of aortic aneurysmal disease, therefore, requires suspicion and diligence to avoid adverse outcomes. This chapter will focus on the history, physical examination, and diagnostic tests important to clinical evaluation of aortic aneurysms.

CLINICAL HISTORY

Thoracic Aortic Aneurysms

Thoracic aortic aneurysms (TAA) typically produce no symptoms, but a variety of symptom complexes may arise related to aneurysm size and location within the thorax.

Patients with aneurysmal dilation of the ascending thoracic aorta may develop clinical manifestations of congestive heart failure (CHF) as a consequence of aortic valvular regurgitation. Enlargement of the sinuses of Valsalva may cause myocardial ischemia or infarction due to direct compression of the coronary arteries or coronary arterial thromboembolism. Right ventricular (RV) outflow tract obstruction and tricuspid regurgitation may result from aneurysmal deformation of the noncoronary sinus. Aneurysms of the sinuses of Valsalva may rupture directly into the RV cavity, right atrium, or pulmonary artery, causing heart failure associated with a continuous murmur. Chest pain may occur when the aneurysm compresses surrounding structures or erodes into adjacent bone such as the ribs or sternum. Compression of the superior vena cava may produce venous congestion of the head, neck, and upper extremities. Symptoms are frequently a harbinger of rupture or death. Rupture may occur into the left pleural space, pericardium, pulmonary artery, or superior vena cava.

Aneurysms of the aortic arch may produce symptoms by compression of contiguous structures, but most are asymptomatic. Dyspnea or cough may be caused by compression of the trachea or mainstem bronchi, dysphagia by compression of the esophagus, or hoarseness secondary to left vocal cord paralysis related to compression of the left recurrent laryngeal nerve. The superior vena cava syndrome and pulmonary artery stenosis result when these vessels are compressed.[1,2] Chest pain, related either to compression of adjacent structures or to erosion of ribs or vertebrae, is typically positional. Aneurysms of the aortic arch may rupture into the mediastinum, pleural space, tracheobronchial tree (causing hemoptysis), or esophagus (causing hematemesis). Arteriovenous fistulas (AVFs) may result from rupture into the superior vena cava or pulmonary artery. Tuberculous aneurysms, akin to other causes of TAA, may present with pain but are commonly asymptomatic or may present with hypovolemic shock as a consequence of rupture.

Symptoms of descending TAAs include chest pain from compression of surrounding soft tissues or erosion of vertebrae. Irritation of the recurrent laryngeal nerve may produce hoarseness. Dyspnea may result from bronchial compression, and hemoptysis from direct erosion into the lung parenchyma. Dysphagia and hematemesis are features of esophageal compression or erosion. Rupture may occur into the mediastinum or left pleural space.

Thoracoabdominal Aortic Aneurysms

Although most patients with thoracoabdominal aortic aneurysms (TAAA) are asymptomatic, discomfort occasionally develops in the epigastrium or left upper quadrant of the abdomen. Back or flank pain may occur when the patient lies in left lateral decubitus position. Erosion of the anterior surfaces of the vertebral bodies may occur, leading to radiculopathy. Visceral artery occlusion may occur, but frank ischemia and infarction are infrequent. Patients who complain of claudication also may have occlusive atherosclerotic disease of the aorta, iliac, or more distal arteries. Because mural thrombosis is so common in atherosclerotic aneurysms, they may be the source of peripheral atheroembolism, causing occlusion of distal vessels. Rupture of the thoracic component of these aneurysms generally occurs into the left pleural space, producing a hemothorax; the abdominal component may rupture into the retroperitoneum, inferior vena cava, or duodenum.

Abdominal Aortic Aneurysms

Most patients with abdominal aortic aneurysms (AAAs) are asymptomatic, yet symptoms may take the form of abdominal discomfort or back pain; some patients become aware of abdominal pulsation. Less frequently, pain may occur in the legs, chest, or groin; anorexia, nausea, vomiting, constipation, or dyspnea may develop. Compression of the left iliac vein may cause left leg swelling, just as compression of the left ureter may cause hydronephrosis, or compression of testicular veins may cause varicocele. As the aneurysm expands and compresses vertebrae and lumbar nerve roots, pain may develop in the lower back and radiate to the posterior aspects of the legs. Flank pain radiating to the anterior left thigh or scrotum may reflect compression of the left genitofemoral nerve. Nausea and vomiting may occur as the aneurysm compresses the duodenum. Bladder compression may cause urinary frequency or urgency.

Occasionally, nascent or frank rupture occurs and causes symptoms indicating a life-threatening emergency. The mortality of patients with AAA rupture is 60%; patients with symptoms suggestive of rupture require emergent surgical referral. The classical triad associated with AAA rupture includes hypotension, back pain, and a pulsatile abdominal mass; however, fewer than 50% of patients have all components of this triad. Diverticulitis, renal colic, and gastrointestinal hemorrhage represent common disorders in the differential diagnosis in these patients.

In the absence of patient complaints, physicians must intuit the presence of aneurysm based on the clinical characteristics of the patient. Risk factors for aortic aneurysm disease (see Chapter 35) can be used to guide directed physical examination and, if necessary, diagnostic testing.

PHYSICAL EXAMINATION

Physical examination is usually unhelpful in diagnosing TAAs because the rib cage precludes palpation of the aorta. Physical examination may demonstrate right sternoclavicular lift or tracheal deviation. Dilation of the aortic root may cause aortic valve regurgitation.

The key physical finding for an AAA is a pulsatile abdominal mass. The patient should be positioned supine with the knees flexed. A pulsatile epigastric or periumbilical mass may be visible as well as palpable. To distinguish an AAA from paraaortic masses requires that the examiner's hands address the lateral borders (Fig. 36.1). *An aneurysm expands laterally with each systole.* This technique also permits estimation of the transverse diameter of the aneurysm. Auscultation may reveal a bruit over the mass, but abdominal bruits are not specific for aneurysm formation, and only about 40% of such aneurysms are associated with bruits. Proper physical examination of the abdomen may detect the presence of an AAA in 30% to 48% of patients with AAA.[3,4] In a review of 15 studies, the sensitivity of abdominal examination for aneurysm detection was 49% (Table 36.1).[4]

Several factors limit the potential for AAA diagnosis. First, palpation for an aneurysm requires consideration of the diagnosis prior to examination. The sensitivity of routine physical examination for AAA detection is poor. A directed vascular examination increases the

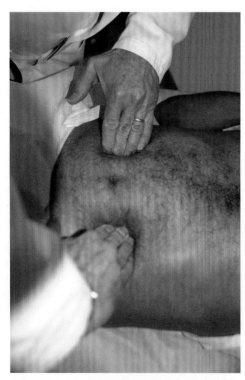

Fig. 36.1 Examination to detect lateral borders of an aortic aneurysm should be performed with fingertips of both hands. An aneurysm should expand laterally with each heartbeat. Aortic aneurysm transverse diameter may be estimated as distance between closest fingers.

likelihood of AAA detection (see Chapter 11). Second, size matters; as the size of an aneurysm increases, so does the likelihood of making the diagnosis. Sensitivity of palpation increases to 75% in patients with aneurysms greater than 5 cm in diameter.[4] Third, increasing abdominal girth reduces the likelihood of discovery. In one study of 201 patients, all 6 aneurysms present were diagnosed in patients with an abdominal girth less than 100 cm, but only 3 of 12 were detected when the abdominal girth exceeded 100 cm.[5] So although the directed physical examination has moderate sensitivity and specificity for AAA diagnosis, routine examination misses the diagnosis more commonly than making it.

The finding of a pulsatile mass in the groin, suggesting an iliac artery aneurysm, or in the popliteal fossa, suggesting a popliteal artery aneurysm, should raise the index of suspicion that an AAA may be present, since multiple aneurysms often coexist. Physical signs such as carotid bruits or diminished arterial pulses in the lower extremities may reflect atherosclerosis of other vessels.

Rupture of an AAA usually produces the clinical picture of extreme distress as a result of abdominal catastrophe. Despite surgical advances, mortality is still the rule because the abrupt nature of circulatory collapse prevents timely intervention in most cases. Patients frequently have severe abdominal or back pain, but the pattern of pain varies considerably and may be either persistent or intermittent, sharp or dull, constricting or burning. The aneurysm may rupture into the retroperitoneum or into the peritoneal or pleural cavities. Patients may develop hypotension, tachycardia, pallor, diaphoresis, or shock, depending on the extent of rupture and associated blood loss into the extravascular space. On occasion, rupture occurs directly into the duodenum, causing an aortoduodenal fistula and acute gastrointestinal bleeding. This possibility should be considered when gastrointestinal bleeding is evident, along with signs of an aneurysm on physical examination. Rupture may also occur into the inferior vena cava or iliac veins, producing an AVF; this is suggested by rapid development of leg swelling or so-called high-output CHF in the presence of an AAA.

SCREENING OF AORTIC ANEURYSMS

Several trials have evaluated the possibility of reducing AAA event rates as a result of screening. In a study from Chichester, United Kingdom, 15,775 men and women aged 65 to 80 years were divided into two groups, and half were invited for an abdominal ultrasound screening.[6] Nearly 70% of those offered screening accepted the invitation, and aneurysm was detected in 4%. A 55% reduction in rate of aneurysm rupture (2.8 per 1000 vs. 6.2 per 1000 subjects) and a 42% reduction in AAA-related mortality in men only (3 per 1000 vs. 5.3 per 1000 male subjects) were noted in the screening group compared with controls. Only one trial has assessed the impact of screening on total mortality. The Multicentre Aneurysm Screening Study (MASS) assessed the impact of AAA screening in 67,800 men aged 65 to 74 years.[7] Half were invited for AAA screening, and the others were not. Long-term mortality was monitored in both groups. In the screened group, there was a 42% relative risk reduction in aneurysm-related mortality from 0.33% to 0.19%, representing 48 fewer deaths over a mean of 4.1 years. Total mortality was not significantly decreased in this time period. After 13 years, there remained a 42% relative risk reduction in aneurysm-related mortality, from 1.12% to 0.66%, and a modest but significant overall reduction in all-cause mortality of 3%.[8]

Some clinical features exist to suggest which patients should definitely undergo screening for aortic aneurysm, and AAA in particular. These include patients with a family history for aneurysm and inherited disorders of connective tissue (e.g., Marfan syndrome [MFS])

TABLE 36.1	Sensitivity and Specificity of Physical Examination for Abdominal Aortic Aneurysm							
Source	Age Range	No. Screened	All AAA	Sensitivity	4–4.9 cm AAA	Sensitivity	≥5 cm AAA	Sensitivity
Cabellon[38]	43–79	73	9	22%	NA	NA	NA	NA
Ohman[39]	50–88	50	3	0%	1	0%	0	NA
Twomey[40]	>50	200	14	64%	3	100%	4	75%
Allen[41]	>65	168	3	0%	0	NA	1	0%
Allardice[42]	39–90	100	15	33%	3	100%	2	100%
Lederle[5]	60–75	201	20	45%	5	20%	5	80%
Collin[43]	65–74	426	23	35%	NA	NA	NA	NA
Shapira[44]	31–83	101	4	0%	0	NA	2	0%
Andersson[45]	38–86	288	14	29%	NA	NA	NA	NA
Spiridonov[46]	17–67	163	10	70%	4	100%	3	100%
MacSweeney[47]	NA	200	55	24%	16	44%	6	100%
Karanjia[48]	55–82	89	9	100%	5	100%	2	100%
Molnar[49]	65–83	411	7	43%	3	33%	2	50%
al-Zahrani[50]	60–80	392	7	57%	4	50%	2	100%
Arnell[51]	55–81	96	1	100%	0	NA	0	NA
Fink[52]	51–88	200	99	68%	44	69%	14	82%
SUMMARY		3158	293	49%				

AAA, Abdominal aortic aneurysm; *NA*, not available.
Modified from Lederle FA, Simel DL. The rational clinical examination. Does this patient have abdominal aortic aneurysm? *JAMA.* 1999;281(1):77–82.

and those with arteritis (e.g., Takayasu and giant cell arteritis [GCA]). First-degree relatives of patients with an AAA have an approximate twofold increased risk of having an aneurysm.[9]

On the basis of these data, the American College of Cardiology/American Heart Association (ACC/AHA) Practice Guidelines for the Management of Peripheral Arterial Disease recommend that "Men 60 years of age or older who are either the siblings or offspring of patients with AAAs" and "men who are 65 to 75 years of age who have ever smoked should undergo a physical examination and one-time ultrasound screening for detection of AAAs."[10] The US Preventive Services Task Force recommends one-time screening for AAA by ultrasonography in men aged 65 to 75 who have ever smoked, but does not recommend routine screening in women.[11] Medicare will pay for a one-time screening if the patient has a family history of AAA or is a man aged 65 to 75 who has smoked at least 100 cigarettes in his lifetime.

Screening for TAAs is less well established. Recent data have shown that bicuspid aortic valve (BAV) disease is an autosomal dominant condition that may be associated with TAA formation. Interestingly, patients with this condition may manifest the valvular or aneurysmal findings alone or in tandem.[12] Thus the ACC/AHA thoracic aortic disease guidelines recommend that all patients with a BAV should have both the aortic root and ascending thoracic aorta evaluated for evidence of aortic dilatation. In pedigree analysis of more than 500 patients with TAA, Albornoz et al. have shown that one in five non-MFS patients have an inherited pattern of disease.[13]

Because of the frequency of both known and unknown genetic conditions associated with TAA, the ACC/AHA thoracic aortic disease guidelines recommend that first-degree relatives of patients with a BAV, premature onset of thoracic aortic disease with minimal risk factors, and/or a familial form of TAA and dissection should be evaluated for the presence of a BAV and asymptomatic thoracic aortic disease.[14]

SURVEILLANCE OF AORTIC ANEURYSMS

Upon diagnosis of an AAA, the recommended surveillance intervals are 3 years for aneurysms 3.0 to 3.9 cm, 12 months for aneurysm 4.0 to 4.9 cm, and 6 months for aneurysms 5.0 to 5.4 cm.[15] Serial imaging studies should be performed until the rate of expansion is 0.5 cm or more per year, or the diameter increases to a point that merits surgical or endovascular repair (see Chapters 37 and 38). There are no specific recommendations for TAA; however, these same intervals are reasonable for TAA that are not of Marfan or Loeys-Dietz origin. Surveillance of patients with either of the latter two syndromes should be more frequent to detect aneurysm growth, as repair is recommended at smaller diameters.[14]

DIAGNOSTIC TESTING

Major objectives of imaging studies include identifying the aorta and its branches, diagnosing and characterizing the type of aneurysm (fusiform or saccular), determining the transverse and longitudinal dimensions of the aneurysm, and detecting associated pathology that may affect treatment. Imaging studies are also indicated for longitudinal surveillance of known aneurysms, or for anatomical definition before endovascular or surgical repairs. An understanding of the benefits and limitations of the several imaging modalities will enable appropriate test selection (Table 36.2).

Chest roentgenography may provide the first indication of a TAA (Fig. 36.2). Aneurysms of the ascending thoracic aorta are usually evident on the right side of the mediastinum. Aneurysms of the aortic arch widen the mediastinal shadow and may project more toward the left. These aneurysms may displace or compress the trachea or left mainstem bronchus. Descending TAAs typically appear as mediastinal masses extending into the left hemithorax. Assessment of the aorta by chest roentgenography requires both posteroanterior and lateral

TABLE 36.2   Abdominal Aortic Aneurysm Imaging Modalities: Strengths and Weaknesses

Modality	Advantages	Disadvantages	Optimal Use
Ultrasound	Highly accurate sizing	Unable to discern longitudinal extent	Initial diagnosis
	Inexpensive	Cannot define branch artery anatomy	Follow-up until repair
CT	Highly accurate sizing	Ionizing radiation	Pre-repair assessment
	Defines branch artery involvement well	Contrast required	Stent graft follow-up
MRA	Highly accurate sizing	Cannot image some stent grafts	Pre-repair assessment
	No ionizing radiation		
	Defines branch artery involvement well		
Contrast angiography	Defines branch artery involvement well	Cannot size aneurysm	Stent graft implantation
		Invasive	
		Ionizing radiation	
		Contrast required	

Note: Sensitivity and specificity of each examination exceed 95% for diagnosis of abdominal aortic aneurysm. *CT*, Computed tomography; *MRA*, magnetic resonance angiography.

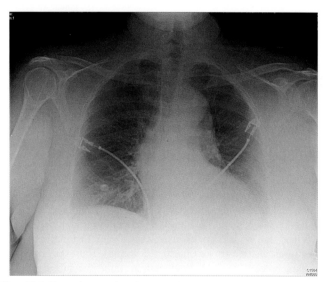

Fig. 36.2 Posterior-anterior chest radiograph demonstrating widened mediastinum in patient with a 5-cm ascending thoracic aortic aneurysm.

projections. Failure to detect TAA roentgenographically, however, does not exclude the diagnosis, since aneurysms may not become apparent until considerable dilation has occurred.

Similarly, plain abdominal roentgenography frequently discloses an unsuspected AAA. Anteroposterior and lateral views of the abdomen may disclose a curvilinear rim of calcification in the wall of the aneurysm, and the diameter of the aneurysm may be estimated when such calcification is visible in two opposing walls. In 25% to 50% of suspected cases, however, the walls of the aneurysm are not sufficiently calcified to permit radiographic identification. Furthermore, it may underestimate anteroposterior aneurysm size by 15%.

Ultrasound

Ultrasonography is the most commonly used method for identification and characterization of AAA. It is the least expensive modality, does not expose the patient to ionizing radiation, and can accurately determine the anteroposterior, transverse, and longitudinal dimensions of an AAA (Fig. 36.3). Sensitivity for diagnosis of an AAA 3 cm or larger approaches 100%.[10] The examination is rapid and easily

performed. The abdominal aorta is subject to anteroposterior, transverse, and longitudinal evaluation. Sonographic classification of AAA begins when the maximum diameter exceeds 3 cm in either anteroposterior or transverse dimensions. Care must be taken to image the aorta perpendicular to its longitudinal axis to avoid eccentricity, which may lead to overestimating its true diameter. Thrombus is frequently identified within the lumen, and echo-dense calcification may be present in or adjacent to the aortic wall. Beyond determining the size of an aneurysm, ultrasound imaging may help define the relation of major arterial branches and adjacent organs. Certain ultrasound characteristics have potential value in predicting rupture. Intramural hematoma, appearing as a hypoechoic soft-tissue mass surrounding the aorta that may silhouette the psoas muscle, appears to represent such a sign.[16] This may be indistinguishable from periaortic fibrosis, which appears on ultrasound examination as a hypoechoic mantle surrounding the aortic wall in patients with inflammatory aortic aneurysms.

Several groups have recently demonstrated the reliability of a "quick screen" in emergency departments.[17] In a prospective study of 125 emergency department patients, quick evaluations did not miss an AAA. Emergency department testing had 100% sensitivity and 98% specificity.[18] Indeed, accuracy is maintained at 100% when the "quick screen" and classical ultrasound examination approaches are compared within a noninvasive vascular laboratory.[19] Recent work has also demonstrated that urgent ultrasonography in the emergency department may be a viable mechanism to exclude ruptured AAA in patients who present with abdominal pain.[20]

Accuracy of ultrasonography should be considered in respect to other imaging modalities (see later discussion). In the Abdominal Aortic Aneurysm Detection and Management (ADAM) Veterans Administration Cooperative Study Group study, computed tomography (CT) and ultrasound were compared. Although both techniques demonstrated sizing variability between local and central reading sites,[21] in a third of subjects, the variation between ultrasound and CT was 0.5 cm or more. Ultrasonographic evaluation undersized the aneurysm by a mean of 0.27 cm compared with CT measurements. Similarly, in 334 patients participating in an aneurysm endograft study, CT reported a greater aneurysm diameter than ultrasound 95% of the time.[21] The correlation between the two measurements was strong at 0.7, but in nearly half the patients, aortic diameter varied by a centimeter or more between the ultrasound and CT studies. Smaller studies confirm both the high sensitivity yet consistent undersizing by ultrasound.

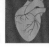

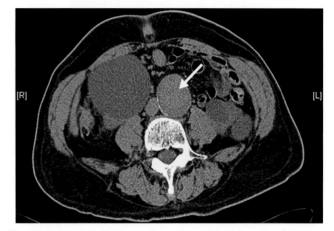

Fig. 36.3 (A) Transverse B-mode ultrasound image of widest portion of abdominal aorta. Electronic calipers have been applied and demonstrate a 5.6-cm transverse diameter and 5.2-cm anteroposterior diameter. (B) Sagittal view of same vessel demonstrating transition from normal to aneurysmal aorta.

Despite these observations, two large surgical trials have shown that ultrasonography is an appropriate method to evaluate and follow AAA. The UK Small Aneurysm Trial[22] and the Aneurysm Detection and Management Trial[23] used ultrasonographic monitoring to determine the time of surgical repair in the group of patients randomized to surveillance. Also, in the Comparison of Surveillance versus Aortic Endografting for Small Aneurysm Repair (CAESAR) trial, which compared early endovascular repair to watchful waiting, ultrasonographic monitoring was used similarly for monitoring.[24] In the absence of any clinical data suggesting the inadequacy of ultrasound, it remains the primary tool for diagnosis and follow-up. Postrepair, ultrasound, with contrast or color Doppler imaging, is now recommended as the primary modality for surgical and endovascular surveillance if the 1-year CT scan does not show an endoleak or enlarging sac size.[15]

Ultrasound can also be employed to diagnose and monitor TAA. Transthoracic echocardiography visualizes the aortic root and a portion of the ascending aorta. Transesophageal echocardiography (TEE) images much of the thoracic aorta well, with sensitivity and specificity both above 95%,[25] except where obscured by the trachea. The limitation of TEE for routine diagnostic purposes is that it requires sedation and is relatively invasive compared with other techniques to evaluate TAA, such as CT and magnetic resonance imaging (MRI) examinations (see later discussion).

Computed Tomography

Rapid advances in technology have put computed tomographic angiography (CTA) in the forefront of aortic imaging (see Chapter 14). Contemporary multidetector-row CTA can acquire 320 simultaneous helices, creating high-resolution images and providing better sensitivity and specificity than could be obtained previously (Figs. 36.4 and 36.5).[26] Yet even with single-detector scanners, CT was able to determine aortic aneurysm size to within 0.2 mm.[27]

CTA is now a preferred imaging modality for preoperative definition of aortic aneurysms because of its accuracy.[15] CTA has replaced angiography as the primary presurgical examination because it is noninvasive and provides detailed information about the vessel walls, such as inflammation, mural thrombus, and vascular calcification. Moreover, CTA creates better anatomical definition with various 3D visualization techniques (Fig. 36.6).[28] Also, it can diagnose abnormalities in adjacent structures. Recent data suggest that multidetector CTA has similar image quality and diagnostic accuracy as magnetic resonance angiography (MRA), with 91% sensitivity and 98% specificity.[29]

CTA also can demonstrate mural calcification and aortic angulation. Placement of aortic stent grafts for AAA requires acquisition

Fig. 36.4 Coronal Section of an X-ray Multidetector Computed Tomographic Scan of Abdomen. Arrow indicates the abdominal aortic aneurysm.

of specific anatomical information prior to the procedure. The most important parameter measured prior to placement of an endograft is the diameter of the neck. Modalities that create a cross-sectional image, including CT, can accurately determine vessel diameter.[30] Currently, 3D CTA reconstruction is now routinely used and may provide even better anatomic assessment than 2D images.[31] CTA also has been used to create a three-dimensional model of the aneurysm to be repaired using a three-dimensional printer.[32]

Postoperatively, CT imaging is directed at the primary complications of stent grafts: endoleaks, device failure, aneurysm expansion, and aneurysm rupture. The standard surveillance intervals after endovascular aneurysm repair are 1 month, 6 months, and 12 months, but the 6 month study may be eliminated in the absence of endoleak or sac enlargement.[15] Determining the type of endoleak has important prognostic implications. In a study of 40 aortic stent graft patients, CTA was superior to digital subtraction angiography (DSA) in determining the presence of endoleak, with a sensitivity of 92% for CTA and only 63% for DSA. CTA also is effective in detecting stent graft migration, distortion, and destruction. Thus CT imaging is indicated for preprocedural planning and postendograft surveillance.

CTA also is useful to image the thoracic aorta for diagnosis, follow-up, and perioperative management of TAA (Fig. 36.7). Computed tomography can be used to follow aneurysm growth,[33] detecting changes as small as a millimeter. Use of contrast permits evaluation of aneurysms from any angle and the creation of

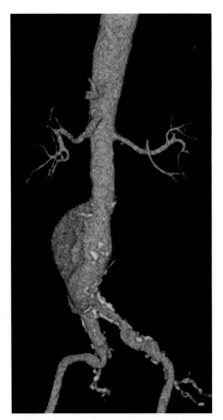

Fig. 36.5 Three-dimensional Reconstruction of Abdominal Aortic Aneurysm From a Multidetector Computer Tomography Angiographic Scan. Note infrarenal location of aneurysm, vascular calcification in white, and tortuosity of iliac arteries.

3D images. Computed tomography may also play an important role in the follow-up of thoracic endovascular grafts by demonstrating volumetric changes in the aneurysm, and thrombus suggestive of a successful repair.[34] CTA can be used to accurately assess the thoracic aorta prior to operation, assists in operative planning, and is the standard imaging modality for follow-up.

Magnetic Resonance Imaging

MRI and angiography are also used to image and characterize aortic aneurysms (see Chapter 13). The technique has been used for diagnosis of AAA for more than 20 years and is quite acceptable for preoperative evaluation. MRA can determine aneurysm diameter, longitudinal extent, involvement of branch vessels, and proximity to renal arteries (Fig. 36.8). Both MRI and gadolinium-enhanced MRA have better than 90% sensitivity and specificity for determination of TAA.[35] Moreover, MRA has better than 90% sensitivity and specificity for detecting concordant stenoses in splanchnic, renal, or iliac branches.[35]

MRA is an accurate method for defining aortic anatomy, required prior to aortic endograft, and is superior to duplex ultrasonography.[30,36] MRA is at least as good as CTA for postprocedural surveillance of stent grafts. In a study of 108 patients, MRA diagnosed endoleaks with sensitivity and specificity of 96% and 100%, respectively, compared with 83% and 100% for CTA.[30] Cine-MRA can show the pulsatility of the aneurysm and quantify AAA wall motion before and after endovascular graft placement to help identify endoleaks.

One of the more important issues associated with repair of the thoracic aorta is identifying the artery of Adamkiewicz. This artery arises most commonly from the left side of the aorta between T8 and L4 and supplies perfusion to the lower two-thirds of the spinal cord. Both CT and MR, with their high spatial resolution, visualize the artery well.

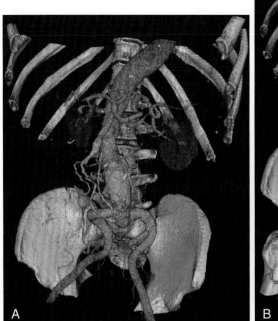
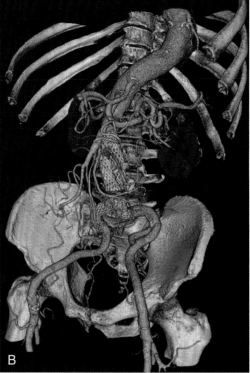

Fig. 36.6 A 62-year-old man with abdominal aortic aneurysm before (A) and after (B) placement of aortic stent. (A) Patient underwent contrast-enhanced computed tomography (CT) for preinterventional evaluation of abdominal aorta and aneurysm, and for planning. (B) After successful placement of stent, CT scan demonstrates effective exclusion of aneurysm and restitution of aortic lumen.

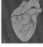

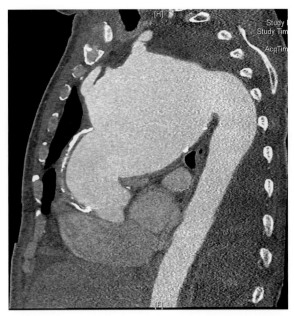

Fig. 36.7 Sagittal view of computed tomographic image of thorax, demonstrating aneurysm involving ascending aorta and aortic arch, measuring more than 10 cm in diameter. (From Tomey MI, Murthy VL, Beckman JA. Giant syphilitic aortic aneurysm: a case report and review of the literature. *Vasc Med.* 2011;16:360–364.)

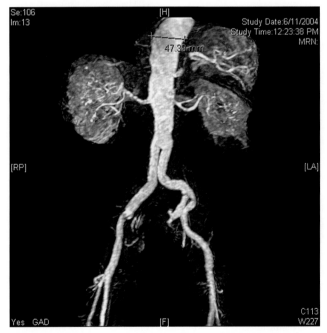

Fig. 36.8 Maximal intensity projection of magnetic resonance angiogram demonstrating a 4.7-cm suprarenal abdominal aortic aneurysm.

In a series of 30 patients with TAA, both MRA and CTA visualized the artery of Adamkiewicz via a clear identification of the vascular anatomy.[37]

Contrast Angiography

Contrast angiography is useful to define branch vessel anatomy and the longitudinal extent of aortic aneurysms (Fig. 36.9). Angiography, which provides information about the aortic lumen, cannot accurately size an aneurysm because it does not visualize the vessel wall or

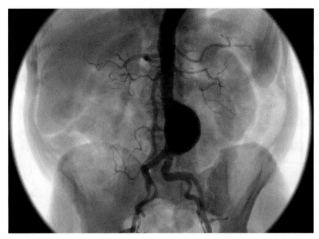

Fig. 36.9 Contrast Abdominal Aortography Revealing Infrarenal Abdominal Aortic Aneurysm. Note that angiogram cannot determine aneurysm size, but can show that renal arteries are not involved.

aneurysm thrombus. DSA has similar accuracy to MRA and CTA in defining aneurysm length and aortic anatomy prior to endograft placement. In a study of 20 patients prior to endograft placement, length and diameter measurements were similar between MRA and CT, but superior to DSA.[36] Contrast angiography is less commonly performed than noninvasive imaging studies because of its invasive nature, the nephrotoxicity of contrast, and the lack of diagnostic superiority.

REFERENCES

1. Tomey MI, Murthy VL, Beckman JA. Giant syphilitic aortic aneurysm: a case report and review of the literature. *Vasc Med.* 2011;16:360–364.
2. Boulia SP, Metaxas E, Augoulea M, Krassas AI, Balis E, Tatsis G. Superior vena cava syndrome due to giant aortic aneurysm. *Asian Cardiovasc Thorac Ann.* 2010;18:396–397.
3. Karkos CD, Mukhopadhyay U, Papakostas I, Ghosh J, Thomson GJ, Hughes R. Abdominal aortic aneurysm: the role of clinical examination and opportunistic detection. *Eur J Vasc Endovasc Surg.* 2000;19:299–303.
4. Lederle FA, Simel DL. The rational clinical examination. Does this patient have abdominal aortic aneurysm? *JAMA.* 1999;281:77–82.
5. Lederle FA, Walker JM, Reinke DB. Selective screening for abdominal aortic aneurysms with physical examination and ultrasound. *Arch Intern Med.* 1988;148:1753–1756.
6. Scott RA, Wilson NM, Ashton HA, Kay DN. Influence of screening on the incidence of ruptured abdominal aortic aneurysm: 5-year results of a randomized controlled study. *Br J Surg.* 1995;82:1066–1070.
7. Ashton HA, Buxton MJ, Day NE, et al. The Multicentre Aneurysm Screening Study (MASS) into the effect of abdominal aortic aneurysm screening on mortality in men: a randomised controlled trial. *Lancet.* 2002;360:1531–1539.
8. Thompson SG, Ashton HA, Gao L, et al. Final follow-up of the Multicentre Aneurysm Screening Study (MASS) randomized trial of abdominal aortic aneurysm screening. *Br J Surg.* 2012;99:1649–1656.
9. Joergensen TM, Houlind K, Green A, Lindholt JS. Abdominal aortic diameter is increased in males with a family history of abdominal aortic aneurysms: results from the Danish VIVA-trial. *Eur J Vasc Endovasc Surg.* 2014;48:669–675.
10. Hirsch AT, Haskal ZJ, Hertzer NR, et al. ACC/AHA 2005 Practice Guidelines for the management of patients with peripheral arterial disease (lower extremity, renal, mesenteric, and abdominal aortic): a collaborative report from the American Association for Vascular Surgery/Society for Vascular Surgery, Society for Cardiovascular Angiography and Interventions, Society for Vascular Medicine and Biology, Society of Interventional Radiology, and the ACC/AHA Task Force on Practice Guidelines (Writing Committee to Develop

Guidelines for the Management of Patients With Peripheral Arterial Disease): endorsed by the American Association of Cardiovascular and Pulmonary Rehabilitation; National Heart, Lung, and Blood Institute; Society for Vascular Nursing; TransAtlantic Inter-Society Consensus; and Vascular Disease Foundation. *Circulation* 2006;113:e463-654.

11. Guirguis-Blake JM, Beil TL, Senger CA, Whitlock EP. Ultrasonography screening for abdominal aortic aneurysms: a systematic evidence review for the U.S. Preventive Services Task Force. *Ann Intern Med.* 2014;160:321–329.

12. Loscalzo ML, Goh DL, Loeys B, Kent KC, Spevak PJ, Dietz HC. Familial thoracic aortic dilation and bicommissural aortic valve: a prospective analysis of natural history and inheritance. *Am J Med Genet A.* 2007;143A:1960–1967.

13. Albornoz G, Coady MA, Roberts M, et al. Familial thoracic aortic aneurysms and dissections--incidence, modes of inheritance, and phenotypic patterns. *Ann Thorac Surg.* 2006;82:1400–1405.

14. Hiratzka LF, Bakris GL, Beckman JA, et al. 2010 ACCF/AHA/AATS/ACR/ASA/SCA/SCAI/SIR/STS/SVM guidelines for the diagnosis and management of patients with Thoracic Aortic Disease: a report of the American College of Cardiology Foundation/American Heart Association Task Force on Practice Guidelines, American Association for Thoracic Surgery, American College of Radiology, American Stroke Association, Society of Cardiovascular Anesthesiologists, Society for Cardiovascular Angiography and Interventions, Society of Interventional Radiology, Society of Thoracic Surgeons, and Society for Vascular Medicine. *Circulation.* 2010;121:e266–e369.

15. Chaikof EL, Dalman RL, Eskandari MK, et al. The Society for Vascular Surgery practice guidelines on the care of patients with an abdominal aortic aneurysm. *J Vasc Surg.* 2018;67:2–77. e2.

16. Cumming MJ, Hall AJ, Burbridge BE. Psoas muscle hematoma secondary to a ruptured abdominal aortic aneurysm: case report. *Can Assoc Radiol J.* 2000;51:279–280.

17. Salen P, Melanson S, Buro D. ED screening to identify abdominal aortic aneurysms in asymptomatic geriatric patients. *Am J Emerg Med.* 2003;21:133–135.

18. Tayal VS, Graf CD, Gibbs MA. Prospective study of accuracy and outcome of emergency ultrasound for abdominal aortic aneurysm over two years. *Acad Emerg Med.* 2003;10:867–871.

19. Blois B. Office-based ultrasound screening for abdominal aortic aneurysm. *Can Fam Physician.* 2012;58:e172–e178.

20. Hahn B, Bonhomme K, Finnie J, Adwar S, Lesser M, Hirschorn D. Does a normal screening ultrasound of the abdominal aorta reduce the likelihood of rupture in emergency department patients? *Clin Imaging.* 2016;40:398–401.

21. Lederle FA, Wilson SE, Johnson GR, et al. Variability in measurement of abdominal aortic aneurysms. Abdominal Aortic Aneurysm Detection and Management Veterans Administration Cooperative Study Group. *J Vasc Surg.* 1995;21:945–952.

22. Mortality results for randomised controlled trial of early elective surgery or ultrasonographic surveillance for small abdominal aortic aneurysms. The UK Small Aneurysm Trial Participants. *Lancet.* 1998;352:1649–1655.

23. Lederle FA, Wilson SE, Johnson GR, et al. Immediate repair compared with surveillance of small abdominal aortic aneurysms. *N Engl J Med.* 2002;346:1437–1444.

24. Cao P, De Rango P, Verzini F, et al. Comparison of Surveillance Versus Aortic Endografting for Small Aneurysm Repair (CAESAR): results from a randomised trial. *Eur J Vasc Endovasc Surg.* 2011;41:13–25.

25. Chirillo F, Cavallini C, Longhini C, et al. Comparative diagnostic value of transesophageal echocardiography and retrograde aortography in the evaluation of thoracic aortic dissection. *Am J Cardiol.* 1994;74:590–595.

26. Hein PA, Romano VC, Lembcke A, May J, Rogalla P. Initial experience with a chest pain protocol using 320-slice volume MDCT. *Eur Radiol.* 2009;19:1148–1155.

27. Todd GJ, Nowygrod R, Benvenisty A, Buda J, Reemtsma K. The accuracy of CT scanning in the diagnosis of abdominal and thoracoabdominal aortic aneurysms. *J Vasc Surg.* 1991;13:302–310.

28. Filis KA, Arko FR, Rubin GD, Zarins CK. Three-dimensional CT evaluation for endovascular abdominal aortic aneurysm repair.

29. Willmann JK, Wildermuth S, Pfammatter T, et al. Aortoiliac and renal arteries: prospective intraindividual comparison of contrast-enhanced three-dimensional MR angiography and multi-detector row CT angiography. *Radiology.* 2003;226:798–811.

30. Lutz AM, Willmann JK, Pfammatter T, et al. Evaluation of aortoiliac aneurysm before endovascular repair: comparison of contrast-enhanced magnetic resonance angiography with multidetector row computed tomographic angiography with an automated analysis software tool. *J Vasc Surg.* 2003;37:619–627.

31. Pitoulias GA, Donas KP, Schulte S, Aslanidou EA, Papadimitriou DK. Two-dimensional versus three-dimensional CT angiography in analysis of anatomical suitability for stentgraft repair of abdominal aortic aneurysms. *Acta Radiol.* 2011;52:317–323.

32. Meess KM, Izzo RL, Dryjski ML, et al. 3D printed abdominal aortic aneurysm phantom for image guided surgical planning with a patient specific fenestrated endovascular graft system. *Proc SPIE Int Soc Opt Eng.* 2017;10138.

33. Masuda Y, Takanashi K, Takasu J, Morooka N, Inagaki Y. Expansion rate of thoracic aortic aneurysms and influencing factors. *Chest.* 1992;102:461–466.

34. Czermak BV, Fraedrich G, Schocke MF, et al. Serial CT volume measurements after endovascular aortic aneurysm repair. *J Endovasc Ther.* 2001;8:380–389.

35. Backes WH, Nijenhuis RJ, Mess WH, Wilmink FA, Schurink GW, Jacobs MJ. Magnetic resonance angiography of collateral blood supply to spinal cord in thoracic and thoracoabdominal aortic aneurysm patients. *J Vasc Surg.* 2008;48:261–271.

36. Engellau L, Albrechtsson U, Dahlstrom N, Norgren L, Persson A, Larsson EM. Measurements before endovascular repair of abdominal aortic aneurysms. MR imaging with MRA vs. angiography and CT. *Acta Radiol.* 2003;44:177–184.

37. Yoshioka K, Niinuma H, Ohira A, et al. MR angiography and CT angiography of the artery of Adamkiewicz: noninvasive preoperative assessment of thoracoabdominal aortic aneurysm. *Radiographics.* 2003;23:1215–1225.

38. Cabellon Jr S, Moncrief CL, Pierre DR, Cavanaugh DG. Incidence of abdominal aortic aneurysms in patients with atheromatous arterial disease. *Am J Surg.* 1983;146:575–576.

39. Ohman EM, Fitzsimons P, Butler F, Bouchier-Hayes D. The value of ultrasonography in the screening for asymptomatic abdominal aortic aneurysm. *Ir Med J.* 1985;78:127–129.

40. Twomey A, Twomey E, Wilkins RA, Lewis JD. Unrecognised aneurysmal disease in male hypertensive patients. *Int Angiol.* 1986;5:269–273.

41. Allen PI, Gourevitch D, McKinley J, Tudway D, Goldman M. Population screening for aortic aneurysms. *Lancet.* 1987;2:736.

42. Allardice JT, Allwright GJ, Wafula JM, Wyatt AP. High prevalence of abdominal aortic aneurysm in men with peripheral vascular disease: screening by ultrasonography. *Br J Surg.* 1988;75:240–242.

43. Collin J, Araujo L, Walton J, Lindsell D. Oxford screening programme for abdominal aortic aneurysm in men aged 65 to 74 years. *Lancet.* 1988;2:613–615.

44. Shapira OM, Pasik S, Wassermann JP, Barzilai N, Mashiah A. Ultrasound screening for abdominal aortic aneurysms in patients with atherosclerotic peripheral vascular disease. *J Cardiovasc Surg (Torino).* 1990;31:170–172.

45. Andersson AP, Ellitsgaard N, Jorgensen B, et al. Screening for abdominal aortic aneurysm in 295 outpatients with intermittent claudication. *Vascular Surgery.* 1991;25:516–520.

46. Spiridonov AA, Omirov ShR. Selective screening for abdominal aortic aneurysms by using the clinical examination and ultrasonic scanning. *Grud Serdechnososudistaia Khir.* 1992;33–36.

47. MacSweeney ST, O'Meara M, Alexander C, O'Malley MK, Powell JT, Greenhalgh RM. High prevalence of unsuspected abdominal aortic aneurysm in patients with confirmed symptomatic peripheral or cerebral arterial disease. *Br J Surg.* 1993;80:582–584.

48. Karanjia PN, Madden KP, Lobner S. Coexistence of abdominal aortic aneurysm in patients with carotid stenosis. *Stroke.* 1994;25:627–630.

49. Molnar LJ, Langer B, Serro-Azul J, Wanjgarten M, Cerri GG, Lucarelli CL. Prevalence of intraabdominal aneurysm in elderly patients. *Rev Assoc Med Bras*. 1995;41:43–46.

50. al-Zahrani HA, Rawas M, Maimani A, Gasab M, Aba al Khail BA. Screening for abdominal aortic aneurysm in the Jeddah area, western Saudi Arabia. *Cardiovasc Surg*. 1996;4:87–92.

51. Arnell TD, de Virgilio C, Donayre C, Grant E, Baker JD, White R. Abdominal aortic aneurysm screening in elderly males with atherosclerosis: the value of physical exam. *Am Surg*. 1996;62:861–864.

52. Fink HA, Lederle FA, Roth CS, Bowles CA, Nelson DB, Haas MA. The accuracy of physical examination to detect abdominal aortic aneurysm. *Arch Intern Med*. 2000;160:833–836.

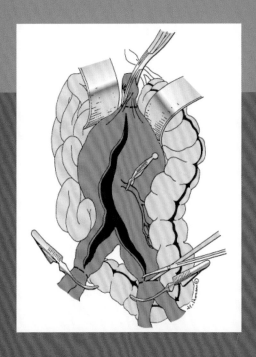

中文导读

第37章
腹主动脉瘤的手术治疗

    腹主动脉瘤（abdominal aortic aneurysm，AAA）仍然是老年人死亡的主要原因之一。在美国，腹主动脉瘤破裂是排在第15位的死因，是55岁以上男性第10位的死亡病因。绝大多数的腹主动脉瘤位于肾动脉平面以下。该章节内容首先紧紧围绕着腹主动脉瘤的定义、手术决策的制定、破裂风险预测、动脉瘤增长率、择期手术的风险及生存预期等诸多方面进行了剖析。开放手术修复腹主动脉瘤是复杂且具有挑战性的。有效的术前评估、缜密的围手术期管理、合理的麻醉及术后镇痛的选择等因素，对于患者的预后都至关重要。通过经腹或经腹膜后入路的手术方式，均可以充分显露腹主动脉瘤，并达到手术目的。不同的入路方式各有千秋，本章内容也将详细评述两种经典手术的有关细节差异。尽管手术技术和围手术期管理水平不断提高，将腹主动脉瘤术后死亡率降至5%以下，但是如何预防术后并发症始终是临床工作中最为关切的问题，对于术后心脏事件的监测、胃肠道缺血情况的判断及较少关注的男性性功能受损等并发症，本章内容将给出详细的答案。

郭　伟

Surgical Treatment of Abdominal Aortic Aneurysms

Bjoern D. Suckow and David H. Stone

Abdominal aortic aneurysms (AAAs) remain a leading cause of death in the elderly. In the United States, ruptured AAAs are the 15th leading cause of death overall and the 10th leading cause of death in men older than age 55.[1] AAAs account for more than 5500 hospital deaths in the United States,[2] which likely underestimates their true number because 30% to 50% of all patients with ruptured AAAs die before they reach a hospital.[3] In addition, 30% to 40% of patients with ruptured AAAs die after reaching a hospital but without operation.[3] When combined with an operative mortality rate of 40% to 50%,[4-8] this results in an overall mortality rate of 80% to 90% for AAA rupture.[3,9-11] Unfortunately, this high mortality rate for ruptured AAAs has not changed over the past 20 years despite improvements in operative technique and perioperative critical care management that have reduced the elective surgical mortality rate to less than 5% in most series.[4] Ruptured aneurysms also impose a substantial financial burden on overall healthcare costs. One report estimated that as much as $50 million and 2000 lives could have been saved in 1 year if AAAs had been repaired prior to rupture.[12] Another study showed that emergency operations for AAAs resulted in a mean financial loss to the hospital of $24,655 per patient.[13] These data have significant implications in an era of healthcare cost containment. For all of these reasons, AAAs remain a central focus for vascular surgeons and an important healthcare problem for all physicians.

DEFINITION

Most aortic aneurysms are true aneurysms, involving all layers of the aortic wall, and are infrarenal in location. As shown by Pearce and colleagues,[14] normal aortic diameter gradually decreases from the thorax (28 mm in men) to the infrarenal location (20 mm in men). At all anatomic levels, normal aortic diameter is approximately 2 mm larger in men than in women and increases with age and increased body surface area.[14] Because the average infrarenal aortic diameter was 2 cm for these patients, using a 3-cm definition for an infrarenal AAA was recommended, without the need to consider a more complicated definition based on factors such as gender or body surface area. Although such definitions are useful for large patient groups, in clinical practice with individual patients it is more common to define an aneurysm based on a greater than or equal to 50% diameter enlargement compared with the adjacent, nonaneurysmal aorta.[15] This is particularly true for patients with unusually small arteries, in whom even a 2.5-cm local dilation of the infrarenal aorta might be aneurysmal if the adjacent aorta were only 1.5 cm in diameter.

DECISION-MAKING FOR ELECTIVE ABDOMINAL AORTIC ANEURYSM REPAIR

The choice between observation and elective surgical repair of an AAA for an individual patient at any given point should take into account (1) the rupture risk under observation, (2) the operative risk of repair, (3) the patient's life expectancy, and (4) the personal preferences of the patient.[16,17] Two randomized trials have provided substantial information to assist with this decision-making process. The United Kingdom (UK) Small Aneurysm Trial was the first randomized trial to compare early surgery with surveillance of 4- to 5.5-cm diameter AAAs in 1090 patients aged 60 to 76.[18] Those undergoing surveillance underwent repeat ultrasound every 6 months for AAAs 4 to 4.9 in diameter cm and every 3 months for those 5 to 5.5 cm. If AAA diameter exceeded 5.5 cm, the expansion rate was more than 1 cm per year, the AAA became tender, or repair of an iliac or thoracic aneurysm was necessary, elective surgical repair was recommended. At the initial report in 1998, after a mean 4.6 years of follow-up, there was no difference in survival between the two groups. After 3 years, patients who had undergone early surgery had better late survival, but the difference was not significant. It was notable that more than 60% of patients randomized to surveillance eventually underwent surgery at a median time of 2.9 years. The rupture risk among those undergoing careful surveillance was 1% per year.

In 2002 the UK trial participants published results of long-term follow-up.[19] At 8 years there was a small survival advantage in the early surgery group (7.2% improved survival). However, the proportion of deaths caused by rupture of an unrepaired AAA was low (6%). The early surgery group had a higher rate of smoking cessation, which may have contributed to a reduction in overall mortality. An additional 12% of surveillance patients underwent surgical repair during extended follow-up, to bring the total to 74%. Fatal rupture occurred in only 5% of men but 14% of women in the surveillance group. Risk of rupture was more than four times higher for women than for men. This prompted the participants to recommend a lower diameter threshold for elective AAA repair in women.

The Aneurysm Detection and Management (ADAM) study conducted at US Department of Veterans Affairs (VA) hospitals was published in 2002.[20] In this trial 1163 veterans (99% male) aged 50 to 79 with AAAs 4- to 5.4-cm diameter were randomized to surveillance versus early surgery. Surveillance entailed ultrasound or CT scan every 6 months with elective surgery for expansion to 5.5 cm, expansion of greater than 0.7 cm in 6 months or greater than 1 cm in 1 year, or development of symptoms attributable to the AAA. CT was used for the initial evaluation with AAA diameter defined as the maximal cross-sectional measurement in any plane that was perpendicular to the aorta. Ultrasound was used for the majority of surveillance visits, but CT was used when the diameter reached 5.3 cm. Patients with severe heart or lung disease were excluded, as were those who were not likely to comply with surveillance. As in the UK trial, there was no survival difference between the two strategies after a mean follow-up of 4.9 years. Similarly, greater than 60% of patients in the surveillance arm underwent repair. Initial AAA diameter predicted subsequent surgical repair in the surveillance group, because 27% of those with AAAs initially 4 to 4.4 cm underwent repair during follow-up, compared with 53% of those with 4.5 to 4.9 cm and 81% of those with 5- to 5.4-cm diameter AAAs. Operative mortality was 2.7% in the early surgery group and 2.1% in the surveillance group. Rupture risk in those undergoing surveillance was 0.6% per year. This trial confirmed the results of the UK trial, demonstrating the lack of benefit of early surgery for AAAs 4 to 5.5 cm even if operative mortality is low. Compliance with surveillance was high in both trials. Furthermore, Ouriel and colleagues reported results of 728 patients who were randomized to either ultrasound surveillance or early endovascular aneurysm repair (EVAR). Mean follow-up of 20 ± 12 months demonstrated no difference in AAA rupture, aneurysm-related death, or overall mortality between groups.[21]

Taken together, these two large randomized studies indicate that it is generally safe to wait for AAA diameter to reach 5.5 cm before performing surgery in select men who are compliant with surveillance, even if their operative mortality is predicted to be low, even in the endovascular era. However, compliance in these carefully monitored trials of select patients was high. In another VA population, Valentine and colleagues[22] reported that 32 of 101 patients undergoing AAA surveillance were not compliant despite several appointment reminders, and 3 or 4 of these 32 patients experienced rupture. In addition, the increased rupture risk for women seen in the UK trial highlights the need to individualize treatment on the basis of a careful assessment of individual patient characteristics (rupture risk, operative risk, life expectancy, and patient preferences).

RUPTURE RISK

The importance of diameter in determining AAA rupture risk is universally accepted, initially on the basis of a pivotal study reported by Szilagyi and associates in 1966.[23] These authors compared the outcome of patients with large (>6 cm by physical examination) and small (<6 cm) AAAs who were managed nonoperatively, even though at least one-half were considered fit for surgery in that era. During follow-up, 43% of the larger AAAs ruptured, compared with only 20% of the small AAAs, although the actual size at the time of rupture is unknown. This difference in rupture rate contributed to a 5-year survival of only 6% for patients with large AAAs compared with 48% for patients with small AAAs. These results were confirmed by Foster and colleagues in 1969,[24] who reported rupture in 16% of AAAs less than 6 cm in diameter, compared with 51% for AAAs greater than 6 cm in patients managed nonoperatively. Modern imaging techniques were not available to accurately measure these aneurysms. Therefore it is likely that diameter was overestimated by physical examination, such that the "large" 6-cm AAAs in these studies were closer to 5 cm by current standards, although exact dimensions remain unknown. Nonetheless, the influence of size on AAA rupture risk was firmly established and has provided a sound basis for recommending elective repair for large AAAs, especially because both these studies demonstrated a marked improvement in survival after operative repair.[23,24]

Autopsy studies have also demonstrated that larger AAAs are more prone to rupture. In an influential study from 1977, Darling and colleagues[25] analyzed 473 consecutive patients who had an AAA at autopsy, of which 25% had ruptured. Probability of rupture increased with diameter: less than 4 cm, 10%; 4 to 7 cm, 25%; 7 to 10 cm, 46%; and greater than 10 cm, 61%. Sterpetti and associates[26] confirmed these results in a more recent autopsy series of 297 patients with AAAs in which rupture had occurred in 5% of AAAs less than or equal to 5 cm in diameter; in 39% of 5- to 7-cm diameter AAAs; and in 65% of greater than or equal to 7-cm diameter AAAs.[26] Although these autopsy studies have clearly shown the impact of relative AAA size on rupture rate, absolute diameter measurements at autopsy likely underestimate actual size because the aorta is no longer pressurized. Following rupture, size

measurement is even more difficult because the AAA is no longer intact. Furthermore, autopsy series are biased toward patients with larger AAAs that rupture and more likely lead to autopsy than smaller AAAs in asymptomatic patients who die of other causes. Thus the rupture rates assigned to specific aneurysm diameters by autopsy studies likely overestimate true aneurysm rupture risk.

Further data regarding rupture risk were obtained from high-risk patients who were deemed too fragile to undergo elective repair. Lederle et al.[27] published on a cohort ($n = 198$) of VA patients who had AAAs of at least 5.5-cm diameter but were medically unfit for or refused operative repair. They were followed for a mean of 1.5 years during which 57% died. Aneurysm-related mortality was determined postmortem and reaffirmed once more that rupture risk correlates with aneurysm size and exponentially increased with increasing aortic diameter. The reported 1-year incidence of rupture was 9.4% for AAA diameter of 5.5 to 5.9 cm, 10.2% for AAA of 6.0 to 6.9 cm (19.1% for the subgroup of 6.5 to 6.9 cm), and 32.5% for AAA of 7.0 cm or greater, and 25.7% over 6 months only for AAA measuring 8.0 cm or larger.

The simple observation that not all AAAs rupture at a specific diameter indicates that other patient-specific and aneurysm-specific variables must also influence rupture. Several studies have used multivariate analyses to examine the predictive value of various clinical parameters on AAA rupture risk. The UK Small Aneurysm Trialists followed 2257 patients over the 7-year period of the trial, including 1090 randomized patients and an additional 1167 patients who were ineligible for randomization.[18] There were 103 documented ruptures. Predictors of rupture using proportional hazards modeling (adjusted hazard ratio in parentheses) were: female sex (3), initial AAA diameter (2.9 per cm), smoking status (never smokers 0.65, former smokers 0.59—both vs. current smokers), mean blood pressure (1.02 per mm Hg), and lower forced expiratory volume in 1 second (FEV_1) (0.62 per L). The mean diameter for ruptures was 1 cm lower for women (5 cm) compared with men (6 cm). By comparing patients with ruptured and intact AAAs at autopsy, Sterpetti and colleagues also concluded that larger initial AAA size, hypertension, and bronchiectasis were independently associated with AAA rupture.[26] Patients with ruptured AAAs had significantly larger aneurysms (8 vs. 5.1 cm), more frequently had hypertension (54% vs. 28%), and more frequently had both emphysema (67% vs. 42%) and bronchiectasis (29% vs. 15%). Thus, in addition to AAA size, these reports strongly implicate hypertension, chronic pulmonary disease, female gender, and current smoking status as important risk factors for AAA rupture. Adding to these findings is a recent analysis of the Atherosclerosis Risk in Communities (ARIC) study, which recruited 15,792 participants between 1987 and 1989 and followed them through 2013.[28] The authors noted that smoking, white race, sex, greater height, and greater low-density lipoprotein were associated with increased risk of clinically symptomatic or ruptured AAA.

Women are known to have smaller aortas than men.[29] Intuitively, a 4-cm AAA in a small woman with a 1.5-cm diameter native aorta would be at greater rupture risk than a comparable 4-cm AAA in a large man with a native aortic diameter of 2.5 cm. However, the validity of this concept has not been proven. Ouriel and colleagues[30] have suggested that a relative comparison between aortic diameter and the diameter of the third lumbar vertebra may increase the accuracy for predicting rupture risk, by adjusting for differences in body size. However, the improvement in prediction potential was minimal when compared with absolute AAA diameter and the relative risk of gender. A recent analysis[31] of 23,245 patients with AAA in the UK National Vascular Registry found no sex-based difference in mortality from rupture. However, when checked against the UK Hospital Episode Statistics dataset, there was a slightly higher rate of in-hospital mortality following ruptured open AAA repair for women (33.6%) compared with men (27.1%, $P < .001$).

Because AAA diameter size by itself and other patient biochemical parameters remain unreliable in predicting AAA rupture, there is evolving work using computer-assisted biomechanical profiling of AAAs in an attempt to better predict AAA expansion and rupture. Wall stress measurements using finite element analysis, computational analysis, rupture index, rupture potential index, severity parameter, and geometric factors all may offer improved prediction of AAA expansion and rupture. However, to date, these novel predictive tools remain difficult to validate in vivo and are still some time away from widespread clinical use.[32,33] Furthermore, the amount of aortic mural thrombus and the presence of aortoiliac outflow occlusive disease may raise the risk of aortic rupture, as evidenced by small series compiled by Moneta et al.[34,35]; however, more conclusive evidence yet remains elusive in this regard.

Although a positive family history of AAA is known to increase the prevalence of AAAs in other first-degree relatives (FDRs), it also appears that familial AAAs have a higher rupture risk. Darling and colleagues[36] reported that the frequency of ruptured AAAs increased with the number of FDRs who have AAAs: 15% with two FDRs, 29% with three FDRs, and 36% with greater than or equal to four FDRs. Women with familial aneurysms were more likely (30%) to present with rupture than men with familial AAAs (17%). Verloes and colleagues[37] found that the rupture rate was 32% in patients with familial versus 9% in patients with sporadic aneurysms and that familial AAAs ruptured 10 years earlier (65 vs. 75 years of age). These observations suggest that patients with a strong family history of AAA may have an individually higher risk of rupture, especially if they are female. However, these studies did not consider other potentially confounding factors, such as AAA size, which might have been different in the familial group. Thus further epidemiologic research is required to determine whether a positive family history is an independent risk factor for AAA rupture in addition to a risk factor for increased AAA prevalence.

In summary, AAA rupture risk requires more precise definition. Currently available data suggest the following estimates for rupture risk as a function of diameter: less than 4-cm AAAs, 0% per year; 4- to 5-cm AAAs, 0.5% to 5% per year; 5- to 6-cm AAAs, 3% to 15% per year; 6- to 7-cm AAAs, 10% to 20% per year; 7- to 8-cm AAAs, 20% to 40% per year; and greater than 8-cm AAAs, 30% to 50% over 6 months (Table 37.1). For a given-sized AAA, sex, hypertension, chronic obstructive pulmonary disease (COPD), current smoking status, and wall stress appear to be independent risk factors for rupture. Family history and rapid expansion are probably risk factors for rupture, whereas the influences of thrombus content and diameter ratio remain less certain.

EXPANSION RATE

Estimating expected AAA expansion rate is important to predict the likely time when a given AAA will reach the individual threshold diameter for elective repair. Expansion rate is most accurately represented as an exponential rather than a linear function of initial AAA size. Limet

TABLE 37.1 Risk of Abdominal Aortic Aneurysm Rupture by Diameter

AAA Diameter	Risk of Rupture
Less than 4 cm	0.5% per year or less
4–5 cm	0.5%–5% per year
5–6 cm	3%–15% per year
6–7 cm	10%–20% per year
7–8 cm	20%–40 % per year
Greater than 8 cm	30%–50% per 6 months

AAA, Abdominal aortic aneurysm.

and colleagues[38] calculated the median expansion rate of small AAAs to be $e^{0.106t}$, where t equals years. For a 1-year time interval, this formula predicts an 11% increase in diameter per year, nearly identical to the 10% per year calculation reported by Cronenwett and colleagues[39] in 1990. Several more recent studies have confirmed this estimate of approximately 10% per year for clinically relevant AAAs in the size range of 4 to 6 cm in diameter.[6,40–42] In particular, a literature review by Hallin and colleagues[6] found mean expansion rates of 0.33 cm/year for AAAs 3 to 3.9 cm, 0.41 cm/year for AAAs 4 to 5 cm, and 0.51 cm/year for AAAs greater than 5 cm. Studies that have identified small AAAs, usually through screening, suggest that the expansion rate may be less than 10% a year for AAAs smaller than 4 cm.[6,43–45]

Although average AAA expansion rate can be estimated for a large population, it is important to realize that individual AAAs behave in a more erratic fashion. Periods of rapid expansion may be interspersed with periods of slower expansion.[46,47] Chang and colleagues[47] found that in addition to large initial AAA diameter, rapid expansion is independently associated with advanced age, smoking, severe cardiac disease, and stroke. The influence of smoking has been confirmed by others.[48–50] The UK trialists showed that current smoking is predictive of more rapid expansion, whereas former smoking is not.[51] In addition to these factors, hypertension and pulse pressure have been identified as independent predictors of a more rapid expansion rate.[6,39,44,52,53] In the VA ADAM trial, 567 patients were randomized with small AAA to surveillance and followed. Risk factors for expansion specifically included elevated diastolic blood pressure and active smoking, whereas diabetes mellitus was protective of aneurysm expansion.[53] Finally, Krupski and others[54,55] have shown that increased thrombus content within an AAA and the extent of the aneurysm wall in contact with the thrombus are associated with more rapid expansion.

β-Blockade has been postulated to decrease the rate of AAA expansion. This was first demonstrated in animal models.[56–60] Subsequent retrospective analyses in humans appeared to corroborate this.[41,61,62] However, two subsequent randomized trials failed to demonstrate any reduction in growth rate with β-blockade.[63,64] Furthermore, the randomized trial from Toronto demonstrated that patients taking β-blockers had worse quality of life and did not tolerate the drug well.[63] Even when they analyzed only those who tolerated their medication, there was no effect of propranolol on AAA expansion rate.

The role of statin therapy in preventing AAA expansion and rupture has been the subject of ongoing work. Multiple studies have previously correlated dyslipidemia with coronary disease and peripheral vascular disease alike. Interestingly, it appears that the clinical salutary effects of statin therapy persist irrespective of their effect on lipid lowering. These presumptive "pleiotropic" effects appear to involve numerous events at the cellular level which may impact vascular wall biology and hence their potential benefit on AAA expansion and/or rupture. These effects may involve endothelial cells, smooth muscle cells, platelets, monocytes and macrophages, and finally inflammation. A meta-analysis by Takagi et al. collectively pooled 697 patients from five large observational studies in which patients with small AAA were grouped by statin therapy versus no statin therapy. Accordingly, the authors documented that the patients undergoing statin therapy demonstrated significantly diminished AAA expansion compared to the untreated group.[65,66]

Doxycycline, 150 mg daily, was shown to slow the rate of AAA expansion in one small randomized trial, whereas roxithromycin, 30 mg daily, was shown to reduce expansion rate in another.[67,68] These antibiotics have activity against *Chlamydia pneumoniae*, which has been shown to be present in many AAAs.[69,70] Vammen and colleagues[71] showed that antibodies to *C. pneumoniae* predicted expansion in small AAAs and suggested that antibody-positive patients may benefit from anti–*C. pneumoniae* treatment. Doxycycline has also been shown to suppress matrix metalloproteinase expression and to improve proteolytic balance in human AAAs and to reduce aneurysm formation in animal models.[72-74] A pharmacologic systematic literature review of eight human studies concluded that the existing literature remains sparse (<300 patients total) with multiple confounding variables that were uncontrolled, varying drug dosages, lack of compliance, and lack of sufficient follow-up to determine safety and efficacy of doxycycline in AAA patients and thus cannot recommend it for treatment.[75] Further research in this area remains necessary before routine treatment with these antibiotics can be recommended routinely.

ELECTIVE OPERATIVE RISK

As expected, considerable variation in operative risk occurs among individual patients and depends on specific risk factors. A meta-analysis by Steyerberg and colleagues[76] identified seven prognostic factors that were independently predictive of operative mortality after elective AAA repair and calculated the relative risk for these factors (Table 37.2). The most important risk factors for increased operative mortality were renal dysfunction (creatinine >1.8 mg/dL), congestive heart failure (CHF) (cardiogenic pulmonary edema, jugular vein distension, or the presence of a gallop rhythm), and ischemic changes on resting electrocardiogram (ECG) (ST depression >2 mm). Age had a limited effect on mortality when corrected for the highly associated comorbidities of cardiac, renal, and pulmonary dysfunction (mortality increased only 1.5-fold per decade). This explains the excellent results reported in multiple series in which select octogenarians have undergone elective AAA repair with mortality comparable with younger patients.[77]

On the basis of their analysis, Steyerberg and colleagues[76] developed a clinical prediction rule to estimate the operative mortality for individual patients undergoing elective AAA repair (Box 37.1). This scoring system takes into account the seven independent risk factors plus the average overall elective mortality for a specific center. To demonstrate the impact of the risk factors on a hypothetical patient, it can be seen that the predicted operative mortality for a 70-year-old man in a center with an average operative mortality of 5% could range from 2% if no risk factors were present to more than 40% if cardiac, renal, and pulmonary comorbidities were all present. Obviously, this would have a substantial impact on the decision to perform elective AAA repair. A similar Bayesian model for perioperative cardiac risk assessment in vascular patients has been reported by L'Italien and colleagues,[78]

TABLE 37.2 Independent Risk Factors for Operative Mortality After Elective Abdominal Aortic Aneurysm Repair

Risk Factor	Odds Ratio[a]	95% CI
Creatinine >1.8 mg/dL	3.3	1.5–7.5
Congestive heart failure	2.3	1.1–5.2
ECG ischemia	2.2	1–5.1
Pulmonary dysfunction	1.9	1–3.8
Older age (per decade)	1.5	1.2–1.8
Female gender	1.5	0.7–3

[a]Indicates relative risk compared with patients without that risk factor.
CI, Confidence interval; ECG, electrocardiogram.
From Steyerberg EW, Klevit J, de mol Van Otterloo JC, et al. Perioperative mortality of elective abdominal aortic aneurysm surgery. A clinical prediction rule based on literature and individual patient data. Arch Intern Med. 1995;155:1998–2004.

BOX 37.1 Predicting Operative Mortality After Elective Abdominal Aortic Aneurysm Repair

1. Surgeon-specific Average Operative Mortality:

Mortality (%):	3	4	5	6	8	12
Score:	−5	−2	0	+2	+5	+10___

2. Individual Patient Risk Factors:

Age (yrs):	60	70	80
Score:	−4	0	+4

Gender:	Female	Male
Score:	+4	0

Cardiac comorbidity:	MI	CHF	ECG ischemia
Score:	+3	+8	+8

Renal comorbidity: Creatinine >1.8 mg/dL
Score: +12

Pulmonary comorbidity: COPD, dyspnea
Score: +7

3. Estimated Individual Surgical Mortality: Total Score: _____

Total score:	−5	0	5	10	15	20	25	30	35	40
Mortality (%):	1	2	3	5	8	12	19	28	39	51

Based on total score from sum of scores for each risk factor (line 2), including surgeon-specific average mortality for elective AAA repair (line 1), estimate patient-specific mortality from the table (line 3). AAA, Abdominal aortic aneurysm; CHF, congestive heart failure; COPD, chronic obstructive pulmonary disease; ECG, electrocardiogram; MI, myocardial infarction.
Steyerberg EW, Kievit J, de Mol Van Otterloo JC, et al. Perioperative mortality of elective abdominal aortic aneurysm surgery. A clinical prediction rule based on literature and individual patient data. Arch Intern Med. 1995;155(18):1998–2004.

which demonstrated the added predictive value of dipyridamole-thallium studies in patients with intermediate risk for cardiac death. This study also demonstrated the protective effect of coronary artery bypass surgery within the previous 5 years, which reduced the risk of myocardial infarction or death following AAA repair by 2.2-fold. Although this type of statistical modeling cannot substitute for experienced clinical judgment, it helps to identify high-risk patients who might benefit from further evaluation, risk factor reduction, or medical management instead of surgery if AAA rupture risk is not high.

The review of Hallin and colleagues[6] supports the findings of Steyerberg that renal failure is the strongest predictor of mortality with a fourfold to ninefold increased mortality risk. Cardiac disease (a history of either coronary artery disease [CAD], CHF, or prior myocardial infarction) was associated with a 2.6- to 5.3-fold greater operative mortality risk. Older age and female gender appeared to be associated with increased risk, but the evidence was not as strong. Valuable data regarding predictors of operative risk have been generated by prospective trials. In the Canadian Aneurysm Study, overall operative mortality was 4.8%.[79] Preoperative predictors of death were ECG evidence of ischemia, chronic pulmonary disease, and renal insufficiency. The randomized UK Small Aneurysm Trial found older age, lower FEV_1, and higher creatinine to be associated with mortality on univariate analysis.[80] With multivariate analysis the effect of age was diminished, whereas renal disease and pulmonary disease remained strong predictors of operative mortality. The predicted mortality ranged from 2.7% for younger patients with below-average creatinine and above-average FEV_1 to 7.8% in older patients with above-average creatinine and below-average FEV_1. The UK trial participants noted that the Steyerberg prediction rule did not work well for the UK trial patients. However, they did not gather information on a history of CHF (one of the strongest predictors in Steyerberg's analysis) in the randomized UK trial. Female gender has also been found to be associated with higher operative risk in several population-based studies using administrative data.[4,76,81,82] However, these databases may suffer from inaccurate coding of comorbidities and thereby lack of ability to fully adjust for comorbid conditions.[83] Gender has not been found to be associated with operative mortality in prospective trials.[80,84]

A study by Beck et al., from the Vascular Study Group of New England, assessed risk factors associated with 1-year mortality following open AAA repair and EVAR. In this study, 1387 consecutive patients underwent elective AAA repair in whom 748 underwent open repair and 639 underwent EVAR between 2003 and 2007. Consistent with other studies, factors independently associated with 1-year mortality following open AAA repair included age (>70), COPD, chronic renal insufficiency (Cr>1.8 mg/dL), and suprarenal aortic clamp site. Likewise, factors associated with 1-year mortality following EVAR included CHF and AAA diameter. One-year mortality correlated linearly with the number of risk factors present and, accordingly, should likely be factored into decision-making when considering elective AAA repair.[85] This predictive model has since been externally validated and shown to be more sensitive and robust (C-statistic = 0.82) than other predictive models derived from Medicare or center-based datasets and is now widely available on handheld device applications and electronic medical records for real-time assessment of mortality risk for AAA patients at the time of decision-making regarding AAA repair.[86]

LIFE EXPECTANCY

Assessment of life expectancy is crucial to determine if an individual patient will benefit from prophylactic repair of an AAA. Many patients with AAAs have been long-term smokers. Most AAA patients also have extensive comorbid disease, particularly CAD, COPD, hypertension, hyperlipidemia, cerebrovascular disease, and cancer.[87–92] Many of these chronic conditions increase operative risk, as noted earlier. In addition, these factors impact life expectancy. Patients who survive elective AAA repair have a reduced life expectancy compared with age- and gender-matched populations.[93–95] In 2001 Norman and colleagues[96] reviewed 32 publications over 20 years that described long-term survival after AAA repair. They found that the mean 5-year survival after AAA repair was 70%, compared with 80% in the age- and gender-matched population without AAA. Predictors of late death after successful AAA repair include age, cardiac disease, chronic pulmonary disease, renal insufficiency, and continued smoking.[93,97,98] The UK trial participants found (after adjustment for age, gender, and AAA diameter but not cardiac disease) that both FEV_1 and current smoking status (plasma cotinine) predicted late death.[98] Table 37.3 shows US census data that have been adjusted to reflect the life expectancy of an average patient surviving elective AAA repair.[99] These numbers should be adjusted according to the relative severity of comorbid disease but may be used to guide clinical decision-making.

SURGICAL DECISION-MAKING

In patients with symptomatic AAAs, operative repair is nearly always appropriate because of the high mortality associated with rupture or

TABLE 37.3 Life Expectancy (Years) for Patients Following Abdominal Aortic Aneurysm Repair by Age, Gender, and Race

Age (yr)	Total	MALE White	MALE Black	FEMALE White	FEMALE Black
60	13	12	11	14	13
65	11	11	10	12	11
70	10	9	8	10	10
75	8	8	7	9	8
80	6	6	6	7	6
85 and older	5	4	4	5	5

thrombosis and the high likelihood of limb loss associated with peripheral embolism. Occasionally, high-risk patients or those with short life expectancies may choose to forego emergency repair of symptomatic AAAs, but in general, surgical decision-making for symptomatic AAAs is straightforward. A contemporary analysis of outcomes of symptomatic AAAs by De Martino et al. from the Vascular Study Group of New England assessed 2386 AAA repairs in whom 1959 were elective, 156 were symptomatic, and 271 were ruptured. EVAR was successfully performed in 945 elective patients, 60 symptomatic patients, and 33 ruptured AAA patients, respectively. The hospital mortality was 1.7% for elective AAA as compared with 1.3% for the symptomatic cohort. One- and 4-year survival was determined to be 83% and 68%, respectively, among the symptomatic group which compared favorably to the elective group with 89% and 73% 1- and 4-year survival.[100]

For those with asymptomatic AAAs, randomized trials have provided assurance that the typical male patient can generally be safely monitored with careful ultrasound surveillance until the AAA reaches 5.5 cm, at which time elective repair can be performed. However, decision analyses and cost-effectiveness modeling have previously demonstrated that individual patient rupture risk, operative risk, and life expectancy need to be considered to determine the optimal threshold for intervention.[16,17,101,102] Both the UK and ADAM trials excluded patients who were considered "unfit" for repair, highlighting the fact that those with high operative risk and short life expectancy should have a threshold diameter greater than 5.5 cm. In the UK trial, the rupture risk for women was 4.5-fold higher than for men, prompting the authors to recommend a lower threshold for women than men. It seems logical to consider other factors that may make rupture more likely during surveillance as well. In both randomized trials, 60% to 75% of patients undergoing surveillance eventually underwent AAA repair.[20,103] In the UK trial, 81% of those with initial diameters 5 to 5.4 cm eventually underwent repair. Clearly, for many patients with this size AAA, the question is not whether to perform AAA repair but when. Therefore, in patients with AAA diameters approaching 5.5 cm whose life expectancy is expected to be more than 5 years and whose operative risk is estimated to be low, the patient should be informed that AAA repair would likely be required within the next few years. This subgroup of patients could be offered surgery at a time when it is convenient for them, with the understanding that waiting for expansion to 5.5 cm has little risk. In these cases, patient preference should weigh heavily in the decision-making process. For those with multiple risk factors for rupture, long life expectancy, and low operative risk, it would seem prudent to recommend AAA repair at less than 5.5 cm. In addition, the ability of the patient to comply with careful surveillance should be considered.

Although the recent randomized trials have provided a great deal of information to guide decision-making, clinicians should not adopt a "one-size-fits-all" policy for treating patients with AAA. Moreover, with a progressively aging population in mind, quality-of-life assessments should likely also be factored into decision-making analyses. Suckow et al. recently developed and validated a disease-specific quality-of-life instrument to assess the impact of aneurysm surveillance and repair on AAA patient quality of life.[104] The instrument was found to be both sensitive and specific to determine quality of life in patients under surveillance for small AAA and for those who had undergone repair. Validation of the instrument, which is a patient survey, highlighted that few AAA patients are adequately educated about their pathology and thus lack insight into the natural history and subsequent treatment options. Furthermore, physicians play a critical role in educating patients and remain the primary source of information for them. With improved knowledge about AAA, a patient's quality of life appears improved with regards to worry and stress. Furthermore, this work may implicate that the effect of AAA on patient quality of life could potentially be a factor to play into the shared decision-making process as it relates to how and when to repair a AAA. A prospective trial (Preferences for Open versus Endovascular Repair for Aortic Abdominal Aneurysm [PROVE-AAA] trial) is currently underway to investigate how education about aneurysm repair options affects patient preference for type of repair, and whether patient and physician preferences for the type of repair better align with patient education.[105]

PREOPERATIVE ASSESSMENT

Patient Evaluation

A careful history, physical examination, and basic laboratory data are the most important factors for estimating perioperative risk and subsequent life expectancy. These factors may not only influence the decision to perform elective AAA repair, but they may focus preoperative management to reduce modifiable risk. Assessments of activity level, stamina, and stability of health are important and can be translated into metabolic equivalents to help assess both cardiac and pulmonary risks.[106] Because COPD is an independent predictor of operative mortality,[80,84] it should be assessed by pulmonary function studies, as well as room air arterial blood gas measurement, in patients who have apparent pulmonary disease. In some cases, preoperative treatment with bronchodilators and pulmonary toilet can reduce operative risk.[107] In more extreme cases, pulmonary risk may substantially reduce life expectancy, and in these cases, formal pulmonary consultation may be helpful to estimate survival. Serum creatinine is one of the most important predictors of operative mortality[79] and must be assessed. The impact of other diseases, such as malignancy, on expected survival should also be carefully considered.

It is well established that patients with AAAs have a high prevalence of CAD. By performing routine preoperative coronary arteriography at the Cleveland Clinic, Hertzer and colleagues,[108] in 1979, reported that only 6% of patients with AAAs had normal arteries; 29% had mild to moderate CAD; 29% had advanced compensated CAD; 31% had severe correctable CAD; and 5% had severe uncorrectable CAD. Furthermore, this study established that clinical prediction of the severity of CAD was imperfect, because 18% of patients without clinically apparent CAD had severe correctable CAD on arteriography, compared with 44% of patients whose CAD was clinically apparent. This pivotal study has led to intense efforts to identify risk factors and algorithms that more accurately predict the presence of severe CAD that would justify its correction before AAA repair or would lead to avoiding AAA repair. A number of clinical parameters, such as angina, history of myocardial infarction, Q wave on ECG, ventricular arrhythmia, CHF, diabetes, and increasing age, have been reported to increase

the risk of postoperative cardiac events.[109] Various combinations of these risk factors have been used to generate prediction algorithms for perioperative cardiac morbidity.[106] In general, these algorithms identify low-risk, high-risk, or intermediate-risk patients. For high-risk patients, such as those with unstable angina, more sophisticated cardiac evaluation is required, whereas low-risk patients may undergo elective AAA repair without further testing. For intermediate-risk patients, who comprise the vast majority with AAAs, decision-making is more difficult and may be assisted by additional cardiac testing.[109]

Aneurysm Evaluation

Most surgeons recommend a preoperative imaging study using either CT scanning, magnetic resonance imaging (MRI) or magnetic resonance angiography (MRA), or arteriography. Contrast-enhanced CT scanning appears to be the most useful study for preoperative AAA evaluation when considering information obtained, invasiveness, and cost. This is particularly true for spiral CT scanning, with thin "slices" in the region of interest. This allows not only accurate size measurements but also accurate definition of the relationship of an AAA to visceral and renal arteries. Furthermore, CT scanning aids in the identification of venous anatomic anomalies, such as a retroaortic left renal vein or a duplicated vena cava, or renal abnormalities, such as horseshoe or pelvic kidney, which would influence operative techniques and approach. CT scanning is the technique of choice to identify suspected inflammatory aneurysms and may reveal unsuspected abdominal pathology, such as associated malignancy or gallbladder disease. Given the widespread availability of this imaging modality, CT angiography has made percutaneous intraarterial angiography virtually unnecessary in the vast majority of AAA patients. Moreover, in the EVAR era, CT scanning is of vital importance for case planning and accurate detailed anatomic assessment of aortic neck anatomy, iliac anatomy and tortuosity, and perirenal mural thrombus burden, among other factors. In addition, three-dimensional modeling of contemporary CT scanning is profoundly useful prior to EVAR and even open AAA repair and has largely supplanted the role of conventional angiography.

MRI is comparable with CT scanning in terms of AAA measurement accuracy and other preoperative planning issues. It avoids nephrotoxic contrast, which may represent an advantage over CT scanning for select patients. Because it is more expensive and time consuming, it also is not as widely used as CT scanning. However, when MRA is included with this technique, it can significantly increase the value in patients for whom additional imaging would otherwise be required.

SURGICAL TREATMENT

For the past 40 years, AAAs have been repaired using the technique of endoaneurysmorrhaphy with intraluminal graft placement, as described by Creech.[110] This procedure is described later in the section on transperitoneal approach. The development of this technique was based in part on the failure of previous "nonresective" operations, now of historical interest, including aneurysm ligation, wrapping, and attempts at inducing aneurysm thrombosis that yielded uniformly dismal results. AAA thrombosis by iliac ligation combined with axillobifemoral bypass enjoyed a brief resurgence in popularity for high-risk patients but demonstrated a high complication rate, including late aneurysm rupture, and an operative mortality rate comparable with conventional repair in similar patients.[111–115] Thus this technique was similarly abandoned. As an alternative to standard open AAA repair, Shah and Leather and colleagues[116] proposed exclusion of an AAA with bypass to reduce operative blood loss. However, this group has since published long-term follow-up and no longer recommends this procedure due to persistent flow in the excluded AAA sac and rupture in rare cases.[117] In another attempt to reduce the invasiveness of open AAA repair, the use of laparoscopy as an adjunct has been suggested to assist AAA repair. This approach uses laparoscopic techniques to dissect the aneurysm neck and iliac arteries followed by a standard endoaneurysmorrhaphy through a mini-laparotomy. Cohen and colleagues[118] have reported their results in 20 patients to demonstrate the feasibility of this approach, but a clear benefit has not been shown, because the intraoperative, intensive care unit, and total hospital duration were comparable with conventional AAA repair. Furthermore, two publications describe early experiences with robotic aortic aneurysm repair with comparable hospital stay, complications, and mortality rates.[119,120] However, the lack of demonstrable benefit and the increased associated equipment cost appears to limit the widespread adaptation of this modality for repair.

EVAR was introduced by Parodi in 1991 and has rapidly gained in popularity in the United States after reports of clinical trials and subsequent FDA approval.[121] EVAR has been shown to reduce operative morbidity, mortality, length of stay, and disability after surgery.[122–125] Recovery time is shorter after endovascular repair than open repair.[123,126] However, endovascular repair may not be as durable as open repair.[127–134] Frequent and lifelong surveillance is required after endovascular repair along with reintervention or conversion to open repair in some. There also appears to be a small ongoing risk of rupture after endografting. Decision analysis suggests that there is little difference between open and endovascular repair for most patients.[132] However, EVAR is usually recommended for those with suitable anatomy for EVAR or those with marginal anatomy but high operative risk for open surgery. Open surgery may be preferred for younger, healthier patients in whom there is little difference in operative risk between the two strategies, and for whom long-term durability is a concern, although contemporary stent grafts appear to have improved durability from their initial constructs and are currently recommended for most patients with reasonable anatomy.

Since the advent of EVAR, the rate of EVAR performed for AAA repair has dramatically increased and the rate of open AAA repairs has declined. A recent review of Medicare claims data by Suckow et al. demonstrates the rate of EVAR versus open repair over the past decade.[135] As shown in Fig. 37.1, the number of EVAR surpassed the number of open AAA repairs in 2006. Since then, the number of EVAR has appeared to plateau while the number of open repairs has

continued to decline. In 2013, approximately 25,000 total AAA repairs were performed among Medicare patients, nearly 80% of which were done via endovascular approach.

To date, there are several important randomized trials comparing open AAA repair with endovascular repair. Specifically, in EVAR I and the DREAM trials, patients were randomized to either open repair versus EVAR. The EVAR I study demonstrated a 3% lower initial mortality associated with endovascular treatment, with a persistent associated reduction in AAA-related death at 4 years. However, there was no overall improvement in all-cause mortality between groups. Likewise, the DREAM trial demonstrated an operative mortality advantage associated with EVAR compared with open surgical repair, but 1-year survival was similar between groups. The EVAR II study randomized patients unfit for open AAA repair to either EVAR or no surgical therapy. This trial failed to demonstrate a survival advantage for the EVAR treatment group compared with the no-treatment group. However, it should be noted that most ruptures in the EVAR group occurred during a prolonged delay before surgery, making the results in this group appear worse. In addition, 27% of patients in EVAR II crossed over from the no-treatment group to the EVAR group, potentially limiting the study's findings.[131,136–138] Likewise, the VA Open vs. Endovascular AAA Repair (OVER) study randomized patients to either open AAA repair and EVAR. Results demonstrated diminished perioperative mortality in the EVAR group compared with the open repair group (0.5% vs. 3.0%). However, there was no observed difference in mortality at 2 years between groups. This study also demonstrated diminished median procedure times, blood loss, transfusion requirement, duration of mechanical ventilation, hospital length of stay, and intensive care unit length of stay in the EVAR group.[139] Lastly, Schermerhorn et al. reviewed long-term survival in nearly 80,000 matched Medicare patients who underwent open repair versus EVAR.[140] Similar to the randomized trials described previously, there was an early survival advantage for EVAR patients but no significant long-term survival advantage between repair types over 8 years. These trials illustrate many of the advantages of EVAR therapy versus open surgery. However, the ultimate treatment needs to be individually tailored to specific patients, especially those with high associated surgical risk. Ongoing rapid advances in stent graft technology will need to be considered in the future because device applicability and accompanying morbidity may change.

Perioperative Management

Preoperative intravenous (IV) antibiotics are administered to reduce the risk of prosthetic graft infection.[141] Ample IV access, intraarterial pressure recording, and Foley catheter monitoring of urine output are routine. For patients with significant cardiac disease, transesophageal echocardiography (TEE) can be useful to monitor ventricular volume and cardiac wall motion abnormalities and to guide fluid administration and the use of vasoactive drugs. The use of TEE has become nearly routine during open AAA repair these days. In select patients, pulmonary artery catheters may be used to guide volume replacement and vasodilator or inotropic drug therapy in the early postoperative period and the intensive care unit. Mixed venous oxygen tension measuring, available with these catheters, can provide an additional estimate of global circulatory function. However, studies have concluded no demonstrable benefit is derived from these catheters with regards to patient-level outcome,[142,143] and therefore selective use is probably more appropriate than routine application, especially given the associated risk profile.

The volume of blood lost during AAA repair often requires blood replacement. Therefore intraoperative autotransfusion, as well as

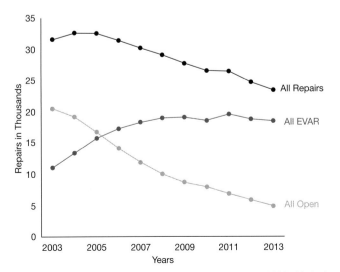

Fig. 37.1 Abdominal aortic aneurysm repair rates 2003–2013 in Medicare patients. *EVAR*, Endovascular aneurysm repair.

preoperative autologous blood donation, has become popular, primarily to avoid the infection risk associated with allogeneic transfusion. However, studies of the cost-effectiveness of such procedures question their routine use.[144-146] Autologous blood donation is less important for elderly patients in whom life expectancy is shorter than the usual time for development of transfusion-associated viral illness. Autologous blood donation does not appear to be cost-effective in elderly cardiovascular patients because the allogenic blood pool has become safer and the transfusion requirement for elective AAA repairs lower.[144] Intraoperative autotransfusion during AAA repair is widely used because of the documented safety of this technique.[147] Because it is usually difficult to predict the volume of blood loss during AAA repair, most surgeons use autotransfusion in case blood loss becomes extensive. Optimizing oxygen delivery to patients with reduced cardiac output by maintaining an adequate hematocrit appears beneficial in patients undergoing AAA repair. One study has shown that a postoperative hematocrit of less than 28% was associated with significant cardiac morbidity in vascular surgery patients.[148]

Maintenance of normal body temperature during aortic surgery is important to prevent coagulopathy, allow extubation, and maintain normal metabolic function. In a review of patients undergoing elective AAA repair, Bush and colleagues[149] noted significantly more organ dysfunction (53% vs. 29%) and higher mortality (12% vs. 1.5%) in hypothermic patients (temperature <34.5°C) compared with normothermic patients. The only predictor of intraoperative hypothermia was female gender, whereas prolonged hypothermia was related to initial hypothermia, indicating the difficulty in rewarming cold patients. A recent randomized trial found significantly reduced cardiac morbidity (1.4% vs. 6.3%) in patients who were normothermic (36.7°C) versus hypothermic (35.4°C) intraoperatively.[150] To prevent hypothermia, a warm forced-air blanket should be placed in contact with the patient. IV fluids, including any blood returned from an autotransfusion device, should be warmed before administration.

The role of ischemic preconditioning in lowering the incidence of perioperative myocardial infarction during open AAA repair remains somewhat undefined, although there are some data to support its potential benefit. In the largest study to date, Ali et al. randomized 82 patients undergoing elective open AAA repair to receive remote ischemic preconditioning or not. The technique involves sequential clamping of each common iliac artery for 10 minutes followed by 10 minutes of respective reperfusion. The authors demonstrated that patients undergoing remote ischemic preconditioning had both diminished rates of postoperative myocardial infarction and diminished critical care length of stay compared with the control groups.[151]

Anesthesia

Nearly all patients undergo general anesthesia for AAA repair. The supplemental use of continuous epidural anesthesia, begun immediately preoperatively and continued for postoperative pain control, is increasing in popularity.[152] This technique allows a lighter level of general anesthesia to be maintained, while controlling pain through the epidural blockade. Additional benefits may include a reduction in the sympathetic-catecholamine stress response, which might decrease cardiac complications. One randomized trial comparing general anesthesia with combined general-epidural anesthesia demonstrated decreased deaths, cardiac events, infection, and overall complications.[153] However, these benefits were not observed in another randomized trial,[154] suggesting that the details of perioperative management and patient selection may determine the impact of epidural anesthesia. Furthermore, it is possible that the major benefit of

epidural anesthesia accrues in the postoperative period, rather than intraoperatively.[155]

Preoperative β-adrenergic blockade remains controversial given findings of randomized controlled trials.[156] Earlier studies by Pasternack and colleagues[157] demonstrated that patients who underwent vascular surgery and received metoprolol immediately before operation had significantly lower heart rates and less intraoperative myocardial ischemia than untreated controls. Mangano and colleagues[158] performed the first randomized, placebo-controlled trial to assess the effect of atenolol (given intravenously immediately before and after surgery and orally during that hospitalization) in patients at risk for CAD who underwent noncardiac surgery. A significant reduction in mortality extending 2 years after discharge was observed in the atenolol-treated patients (3% vs. 14% 1-year mortality) due to a reduction in death from cardiac causes. In a separate analysis, they noted that atenolol-treated patients had a 50% lower incidence of myocardial ischemia during the first 48 hours after surgery and a 40% lower incidence during postoperative days 0 to 7.[159] Patients with perioperative myocardial ischemia were significantly more likely to die within 2 years after surgery.

More recently however, results from the POISE trial, a randomized controlled trial reflecting 190 hospitals, 23 countries, and an enrollment of 8351 patients, provided different results. This study compared the effects of perioperative extended-release metoprolol succinate to placebo among patients undergoing noncardiac surgery. Results demonstrated that there was a significant reduction in the composite end point of cardiovascular death, nonfatal myocardial infarction, and nonfatal cardiac arrest among patients receiving perioperative β-blocker therapy. However, the study also revealed that there were more deaths and strokes among the treated group compared with placebo.[156] A regional quality improvement initiative by the Vascular Study Group of New England was able to increase compliance with preoperative β-blocker administration in patients undergoing AAA repair from 68% to 88% over the time period from 2005 to 2008. However, the authors found no significant change in the rate of postoperative myocardial infarctions despite the increase in β-blocker use during this time period.[162] Given these conflicting findings, perioperative β-blocker usage, when used, should at least be titrated to heart rate and reserved for medically high-risk patients. It should be continued in patients routinely taking them, whereas the benefit of starting a new β-blocker on a β-blocker–naïve patient remains arguable.

Given this knowledge, it has been suggested that β-blockers are underused, likely due to fears about use in patients with COPD or prior heart failure. However, chronic β-blocker use is now known to improve outcomes in patients with heart failure.[163,164] In addition, Gottlieb and colleagues[163] demonstrated that COPD should not be considered a contraindication for β-blockade. They found a 40% reduction in risk of death after myocardial infarction in patients with COPD who were taking β-blockers compared with those who were not. In Mangano's trial, the only exclusion criteria were preexisting ECG abnormalities that would preclude detection of new ischemic events. β-Blockers were withheld during the trial only for a heart rate of less than 55 beats/min, systolic blood pressure less than 100 mm Hg, acute bronchospasm, current evidence of CHF, or third degree heart block. The weight of evidence supports the routine use of β-blockers for nearly all patients undergoing AAA repair.

Choice of Incision

AAA repair can be accomplished through an anterior transperitoneal incision (midline or transverse) (Fig. 37.2) or through a retroperitoneal approach (Fig. 37.3). Midline, transperitoneal incisions can be

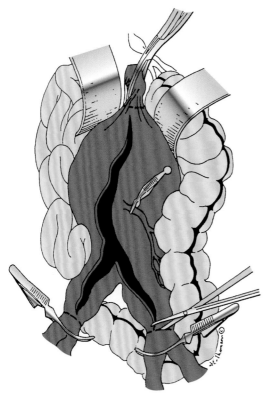

Fig. 37.2 Transperitoneal abdominal aortic aneurysm exposure, vascular clamps in place, incising the aneurysm.

performed rapidly and provide wide access to the abdomen, but they may be associated with more pulmonary complications due to postoperative splinting from upper abdominal pain. Transverse abdominal incisions, just above or below the umbilicus, require more time to open and close but may be associated with fewer pulmonary complications and late incisional hernias, although this has not yet been proven. Retroperitoneal incisions, from the lateral rectus margin extending

into the 10th or 11th intercostal space, afford good exposure of both the infrarenal and suprarenal aorta but limit exposure of the contralateral renal and iliac arteries. In addition, this exposure does not allow access to intraabdominal organs unless the peritoneum is purposely opened. The left retroperitoneal approach is usually favored over the right for exposure of the upper abdominal aorta because the spleen is easier to mobilize and retract than the liver. The right retroperitoneal approach is used when specific abdominal problems, such as a stoma, preclude the left-sided approach.[165]

In recent years the left retroperitoneal approach has enjoyed a resurgence in popularity due to suggestions that pulmonary morbidity, ileus, and IV fluid requirements are decreased postoperatively. However, randomized trials have reached different conclusions about the potential advantages of retroperitoneal over transabdominal incisions. In one randomized trial, Sieunarine and colleagues[166] found no differences in operating time, cross-clamp time, blood loss, fluid requirement, analgesia requirement, gastrointestinal function, intensive care unit stay, or hospital stay for transperitoneal versus retroperitoneal approaches for aortic surgery. However, in long-term follow-up, there were significantly more wound problems (hernias, bulging, and pain) in the retroperitoneal group. A more recent review of the National Surgical Quality Improvement Program (NSQIP) dataset comparing the two incisions demonstrated that patients with a retroperitoneal approach more commonly had suprarenal clamp placement, concomitant revascularization of the renal, visceral, or distal arteries, but that postoperative mortality and reoperation rates were comparable. Transperitoneal incision patients had a higher likelihood of wound dehiscence while the retroperitoneal patients had a slightly higher rate of postoperative pneumonia. However, after adjusting for confounding, the only significant difference was a slightly higher rate of reintubation for pulmonary complications in the retroperitoneal patients.[167]

These results suggest that in most cases the choice of incision for AAA repair is a matter of personal preference, as well as potentially dictated by the anatomy for clamp placement or concomitant visceral revascularization. However, both the transperitoneal and retroperitoneal approaches have advantages in certain patients. Relative indications for retroperitoneal exposure include a "hostile" abdomen due

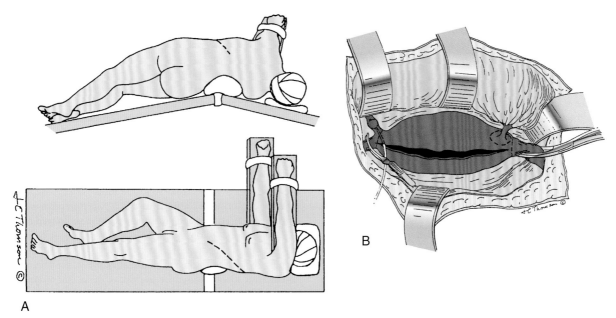

Fig. 37.3 (A) Positioning and skin incision for retroperitoneal approach for abdominal aortic aneurysm repair. (B) Retroperitoneal aortic exposure with left kidney retracted anteriorly for repair of suprarenal abdominal aortic aneurysm. Left renal artery will be reimplanted as a Karrel patch. Right iliac artery is controlled with a balloon catheter.

to multiple previous transperitoneal operations, an abdominal wall stoma, a horseshoe kidney, an inflammatory aneurysm, or anticipated need for suprarenal endarterectomy or anastomosis, mindful that the retroperitoneal approach provides facilitated access to the visceral aorta or even supraceliac aortic segments. Relative indications for a transperitoneal approach include a ruptured AAA, coexistent intra-abdominal pathology, uncertain diagnosis, left-sided vena cava, large bilateral iliac aneurysms, or need for access to both renal arteries. The advantages of each approach make it advisable for surgeons to become proficient with both techniques.

Transperitoneal Approach

After entering the abdomen through a transperitoneal incision, the abdomen is thoroughly explored to exclude other pathology and to assess the extent of the aneurysm. The transverse colon is then retracted superiorly, and the ligament of Treitz is divided to allow retraction of the small bowel to the right. Exposure is greatly assisted using a fixed, self-retaining retractor. A longitudinal incision is made in the peritoneum just to the left of the base of the small bowel mesentery to expose the aneurysm. This incision extends from the inferior border of the pancreas proximally to the level of normal iliac arteries distally. Care must be taken to avoid the ureters, especially if exposure includes the iliac bifurcation where the ureters normally cross. Autonomic nerves to the pelvis course anterior to the proximal left common iliac artery and should be retracted with associated retroperitoneal tissue rather than incised, to prevent sexual dysfunction in men. The left renal vein should be identified and retracted superiorly, if necessary, to fully expose the neck of the aneurysm. Care must be taken not to avulse renal vein tributaries, particularly a descending lumbar vein, frequently encountered to the left of the aorta, which must be divided before the left renal vein is mobile enough to allow upward retraction. Rarely, proximal exposure cannot be obtained without division of the left renal vein. In such cases, this should be done at its junction with the vena cava to maintain patency of collateral drainage via adrenal and gonadal branches. Multiple studies demonstrate that the left renal vein can be safely ligated without any long-term renal function complications.[168,169] If necessary, reanastomosis can be performed if renal vein engorgement suggests inadequate collateral drainage.

After obtaining adequate aortoiliac exposure, the normal aorta and iliac arteries are dissected sufficiently to place a vascular clamp proximal and distal to the aneurysm. Regardless of the proximal extent of an infrarenal AAA, it is desirable to construct the proximal aortic anastomosis near the renal arteries, to avoid subsequent aneurysmal degeneration of residual infrarenal aorta. When an AAA approaches or involves the renal arteries, it can be safer to apply the cross-clamp proximal to the celiac artery rather than between the renal arteries and the superior mesenteric artery (SMA). Green and colleagues[170] demonstrated much higher operative mortality (32% vs. 3%) and renal failure requiring dialysis (23% vs. 3%) after infrarenal AAA repair when clamping was performed between the SMA and renal arteries versus proximal to the celiac artery. They attributed this to the greater likelihood of dislodging atherosclerotic debris in the pararenal aorta as opposed to the supraceliac aorta, which is usually less diseased. Complications resulted from atheroembolization to the kidneys, legs, and intestine, or injury to the aorta or renal arteries. Others have also noted the relative safety of clamping the supraceliac aorta, which can easily be accessed by dividing the gastrohepatic ligament and the diaphragmatic crus.[171] However, aortic clamping between the renal arteries and the SMA is also safe when performed in properly selected patients without extensive plaque in this region.[172] In patients for whom clamp placement is not possible due to lack of healthy tissue or in emergent situations, such as a rupture, an aortic occlusion balloon

may be used for temporary proximal control. This can be placed at the outset of the operation via endovascular approach from the femoral or sometimes high axillary artery or directly via the open aneurysm with a styletted occlusion balloon.

Occasionally it is possible to obtain distal control of an AAA on the aorta, but usually aneurysmal changes or calcification in this location make iliac clamping preferred. A disease-free area of proximal aorta and iliac arteries should be identified for clamping to minimize the possibility of clamp injury or embolization of arterial debris. Some iliac arteries may be so diffusely calcified that clamping without injury is impossible. In such cases, internal occlusion with a balloon catheter or extension of the graft to the femoral arteries is required. In most cases, it is unnecessary to completely encircle the aorta and iliac arteries, because vascular clamps can be placed in the anterior-posterior direction, leaving the back wall undissected. This minimizes the likelihood of injury to both lumbar and iliac veins. Sometimes posterior arterial plaque necessitates placement of a vascular clamp transversely on either the aorta or iliac arteries, which then require careful posterior dissection precisely on the plane of the artery to avoid venous injury.

AAA repair can be accomplished with a straight ("tube") graft in 40% to 50% of patients, without extension onto the iliac arteries.[84,173] Although concern has been raised about the potential for future aneurysm development in the iliac arteries after tube graft repair of AAAs, late follow-up has shown that this is not clinically significant if the iliac arteries were not aneurysmal at the time of AAA repair.[174] Extension to the iliac arteries with a bifurcated graft for AAA repair is necessary in the remaining 50% to 60% of patients due to aneurysmal involvement of the iliac arteries or to severe calcification of the aortic bifurcation. Extension of the graft to the femoral level is indicated for severe concomitant iliac occlusive disease or rarely because of technical difficulties associated with a deep pelvic anastomosis. However, iliac anastomoses are preferred due to decreased infection and pseudoaneurysm complications compared with femoral anastomoses. Prosthetic grafts available for AAA repair include knitted or woven polyester (Hemashield or Dacron) and polytetrafluoroethylene (PTFE). There is no clear evidence that any of these graft types provide superior outcome. In a prospective randomized comparison of PTFE and woven polyester, long-term patency was equivalent, but PTFE had a higher incidence of early graft failure and graft sepsis.[175] Another advantage of these graft materials compared with older materials, such as nylon or vinyon N-cloth, is their impervious nature precluding the need for preclotting. This allows for graft selection to be delayed until the aneurysm is opened so that a graft diameter corresponding to the inner diameter of the normal proximal aorta can be selected, as well as delaying the selection of a straight versus bifurcated graft that may not always be obvious before the aneurysm is open and the distal aorta can be carefully inspected.

Most surgeons use heparin anticoagulation during aortic cross-clamping to reduce lower-extremity thrombotic complications. Heparin dosage varies from 50 to 150 units per kg, based on personal preference. Activated clotting time (ACT) measurement is useful to determine the need for supplemental heparin in prolonged cases and the appropriate dose of protamine sulfate to reverse anticoagulation after declamping.[176] The sequence for applying proximal and distal vascular clamps is selected to apply the initial clamp in the area of least atherosclerotic disease to reduce the risk of distal embolization. The aneurysm is opened longitudinally along its anterior surface, away from the inferior mesenteric artery (IMA) in case this requires later reimplantation. The proximal aorta is then incised horizontally at the level selected for proximal anastomosis (see Fig. 37.2). To avoid potential injury to posterior veins, this incision does not need to extend through the back wall of the aorta, although some surgeons prefer complete transection for better exposure. Intraluminal thrombotic material and atherosclerotic debris are extracted from the aneurysm sac, which usually discloses several back-bleeding lumbar artery orifices that require suture ligation. If the IMA is patent, it should be controlled temporarily with a small vascular clamp (see Fig. 37.2) so that its need for reimplantation can be assessed after the revascularization is completed. IMA revascularization may be advised if the hypogastric arteries are diseased or as discussed later.

Once hemostasis within the opened aneurysm sac has been achieved, the proximal anastomosis is performed. There is often a distinct ring at the aneurysm neck that defines the appropriate level for this anastomosis. Usually 3-0 polypropylene suture is used, taking large aortic "bites" and incorporating a double thickness of posterior aortic wall for added strength. If the aortic wall is friable, pledgets of Teflon or woven polyester can be incorporated into the suture line. After completing the proximal anastomosis, the graft is clamped and the proximal aortic clamp is released briefly to check for and correct any suture line bleeding. If the distal anastomosis is to the aorta, a similar technique is used just above its bifurcation, suturing from within the lumen and encompassing both iliac artery orifices within the suture line. If iliac artery aneurysms exist, these are incised anteriorly so that the limbs of a bifurcated graft can be sutured to the normal iliac artery beyond these aneurysms (Fig. 37.4). Often this requires graft extension to the common iliac bifurcation, including the orifices of both the internal and external iliac arteries within the distal anastomosis. In rare instances, aneurysmal involvement of the distal common iliac artery may preclude anastomosis to both the internal and external iliac artery orifices because these are widely separated. In such cases, an external iliac artery anastomosis can be constructed, but care must be taken to preserve adequate pelvic blood flow, which may mean direct revascularization of at least one internal iliac artery. The need for internal iliac revascularization is usually assessed by the extent of back-bleeding, as discussed later in this chapter (isolated iliac aneurysms). For large aneurysms of the left iliac artery, medial reflection of the sigmoid mesocolon assists a retroperitoneal approach to the distal common iliac artery and external iliac artery and prevents unnecessary dissection of autonomic nerves crossing the proximal left common iliac artery. Before completing the distal anastomoses, arterial clamps are carefully removed and vigorous irrigation is used to flush out any thrombus or debris.

When the first iliac (or distal aortic) anastomosis is completed, flow into that extremity should be restored, releasing the clamp slowly to minimize "declamping" hypotension. Declamping shock is rare if adequate IV fluid replacement has been administered. However, sudden restoration of blood flow into a dilated distal vascular bed and the associated venous return of vasoactive substances that have accumulated in the ischemic limbs usually causes some hypotension. Declamping should therefore be gradual and carefully coordinated with the anesthesia team, because additional volume administration and temporary vasoactive medication administration can be required. This is often modulated with partial finger compression of the graft as blood pressure is maintained. In some cases the clamp must be intermittently reapplied to allow adequate volume resuscitation and prevent hypotension. After restoration of lower-extremity and pelvic blood flow, the IMA and sigmoid colon are inspected.

The IMA can be ligated with a transfixing suture applied to its internal orifice if it is small and not associated with known SMA occlusive disease; if it has good backflow on release of its vascular clamp; if the sigmoid colon and arterial pulsations are good; and if at least one internal iliac artery is patent. In questionable cases, Doppler signals from the sigmoid colon or an assessment of IMA stump pressure[177] may be necessary to determine the need for IMA reimplantation. In the rare circumstances when sigmoid colon perfusion appears marginal, a circular cuff of the aortic wall around the IMA orifice is excised (Karrel patch) and anastomosed to the left side of the graft (Fig. 37.5). Next, the adequacy of lower-extremity blood flow is determined by visual inspection of the feet, palpation of distal pulses, or more sophisticated Doppler or pulse volume recording. If reduced blood flow is detected, intraoperative arteriography can differentiate thrombosis or embolism from peripheral vasoconstriction, which is relatively common if the procedure is prolonged and the patient is hypothermic. Embolism or thrombosis requires prompt surgical correction, whereas vasoconstriction requires

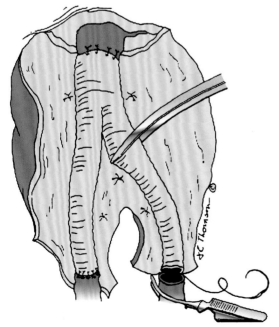

Fig. 37.4 Completing the Iliac Anastomosis of an Abdominal Aortic Aneurysm Repair. Lumbar artery orifices have been suture ligated. Flow has already been established through the right graft limb.

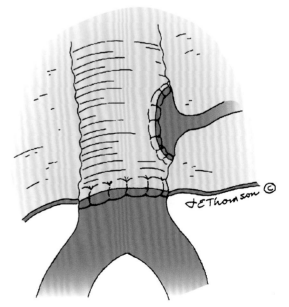

Fig. 37.5 Reimplanting inferior mesenteric artery with a Karrel patch technique after abdominal aortic aneurysm repair with tube graft.

correction of any volume deficit and rewarming. After assuring adequate intestinal and lower-extremity circulation, heparin is reversed with protamine sulfate if sufficient heparin has been given to justify reversal, and hemostasis is achieved. The aneurysm wall and retroperitoneum are then closed over the graft with dissolvable suture to provide a tissue barrier between the prosthesis and the adjacent intestine (Fig. 37.6). The aortic prosthesis and upper anastomosis must be isolated from the overlying duodenum during closure; if necessary, a pedicle of greater omentum can be interposed to achieve this purpose. The small bowel should be inspected carefully and replaced in its normal position before abdominal closure.

Retroperitoneal Approach

Proper patient positioning is essential to achieve optimal exposure using the retroperitoneal approach. For most infrarenal AAAs a left retroperitoneal incision centered on the 11th or 12th rib is used. The patient's left shoulder is elevated at a 45- to 60-degree angle relative to the table while the pelvis is positioned relatively flat. The table is flexed with the break positioned at a level midway between the iliac crest and the costal margin (see Fig. 37.3A). An air-evacuating "bean bag" is helpful to maintain proper positioning. Beginning at the lateral border of the left rectus muscle midway between the pubis and umbilicus, the skin incision is carried superiorly and then curved laterally up to the tip of the 11th or 12th rib. If extensive exposure of the right iliac artery is required, the incision can be extended inferolaterally into the right lower quadrant, or a separate right lower quadrant retroperitoneal incision can be used. The underlying lateral abdominal wall muscles are divided, exposing the underlying peritoneum and the anterior edge of the properitoneal fat layer at the lateral aspect of this exposure. Dissection in the retroperitoneal plane is then developed, either anterior or posterior to the left kidney, until the aorta is encountered.

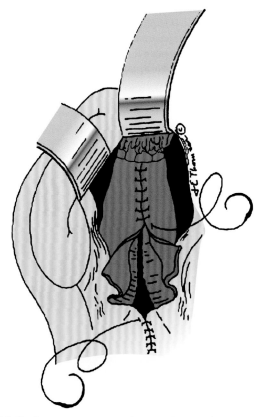

Fig. 37.6 Closing aneurysm sac and retroperitoneum between graft and duodenum.

For infrarenal aneurysm exposure, it is often sufficient to proceed anteriorly and leave the left kidney in its normal position. For juxtarenal or suprarenal aneurysms that require more cephalad exposure, the kidney is mobilized anteriorly to approach the aorta from behind the left renal artery (see Fig. 37.3B). If the need for higher exposure is anticipated, the incision should be directed more cephalad over the 9th or 10th rib and the shoulders positioned as perpendicularly as possible to the table. In this case, more table flexion is required to open the space between the pelvis and ribs, and the trunk is twisted so that the angle between the pelvis and the table is approximately 30 degrees. When approaching the aorta from behind the left renal artery, it is necessary to divide a large lumbar branch of the left renal vein to mobilize the kidney and renal vein anteriorly. The ureter must be identified and retracted medially with the kidney, taking care to separate it from the iliac bifurcation distally.

Medial mobilization of the peritoneal contents exposes the IMA, which usually is divided for more complete exposure of the aortic bifurcation and right renal artery, depending on the size of the AAA. Exposure is greatly assisted by using a fixed, self-retaining retractor. If necessary, exposure of the right iliac artery and right renal artery is easier after opening and decompressing the AAA. Right iliac artery control is often best accomplished by using a balloon occlusion catheter after entering the aneurysm (see Fig. 37.3B). After achieving adequate exposure, repair of the AAAs is usually carried out as described earlier for the transperitoneal approach. The retroperitoneal technique does not normally afford an opportunity to inspect colonic and intestinal viability, but the peritoneum can be opened to accomplish this if any concern exists.

Associated Arterial Disease

Indications for concomitant mesenteric or renal artery revascularization during elective AAA repair are comparable with those used for isolated disease in these arteries. Occasionally, patients with asymptomatic, high-grade stenoses of these arteries warrant "prophylactic" concomitant reconstruction, if the patient is at low operative risk and the AAA repair proceeds uneventfully. Although the natural history of asymptomatic mesenteric artery stenosis is not well characterized, it appears that patients with critical disease of all three mesenteric arteries are at sufficiently high risk for future complications of mesenteric ischemia that concomitant revascularization is justified.[178] Progression of renal artery stenosis has been better documented,[179,180] but the ultimate clinical impact of such progression appears minimal in nonhypertensive patients with normal renal function.[180] The adjacency of the renal arteries to the operative field for AAA repair has led some to recommend prophylactic repair of critical but asymptomatic renal artery stenoses.[182] Although this may be appropriate in younger, good-risk patients, it adds morbidity and mortality to the AAA repair, leading others to recommend the combined procedure only for standard indications of hypertension or ischemic nephropathy.[183,184]

COMPLICATIONS OF ABDOMINAL AORTIC ANEURYSM REPAIR

Despite improvements in the outcome of elective AAA repair, major complications occur and must be correctly managed or avoided to maintain the low mortality necessary to justify prophylactic AAA repair. Myocardial infarction is the leading single-organ cause of both early and late mortality in patients undergoing AAA repair[79] and must be carefully assessed and managed to reduce mortality. However, in a review of patients undergoing elective AAA repair, Huber and colleagues[146] found that multisystem organ failure (MSOF) caused more deaths (57%) than cardiac events (25%). Visceral organ dysfunction, specifically renal failure, was the most common cause of MSOF,

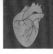

followed by postoperative pneumonia. However, most patients with MSOF had associated cardiac dysfunction, which may have aggravated visceral ischemic injury. Several factors may be responsible for the emergence of MSOF as a more prominent cause of death following elective AAA repair. First, with modern techniques of intensive care, it is uncommon for patients to die with single-system failure (even cardiac) following AAA repair. Second, strict attention to cardiac risk in these patients may have reduced the relative impact of cardiac complications. Finally, in Huber's series, older patients with more associated visceral and renal artery disease underwent AAA repair and had the highest likelihood of MSOF postoperatively. The relative frequency of single system complications following elective AAA repair based on a cumulative literature review is listed in Table 37.4.

Cardiac Complications

The majority of cardiac ischemic events occur within the first 2 days following surgery, during which time intensive care monitoring is appropriate for high-risk patients. Maximizing myocardial function with adequate preload, controlling oxygen consumption by the reduced heart rate and blood-pressure product, ensuring adequate oxygenation,

TABLE 37.4 Early (30-Day) Complications After Elective Open Abdominal Aortic Aneurysm Repair

Complication	Frequency
Death	<5%
All cardiac	15%
Myocardial infarction	2%–8%
All pulmonary	8%–12%
Pneumonia	5%
Renal insufficiency	5%–12%
Dialysis dependent	1%–6%
Deep vein thrombosis	8%
Bleeding	2%–5%
Ureteral injury	<1%
Stroke	1%
Leg ischemia	1%–4%
Colon ischemia	1%
Spinal cord ischemia	<1%
Wound infection	<5%
Graft infection	<1%
Graft thrombosis	<1%

Estimated from the following surgical series: Johnston KW. Multicenter prospective study of nonruptured abdominal aortic aneurysm. Part II. Variables predicting morbidity and mortality. *J Vasc Surg.* 1989;9:437–447; Johnston KW, Scobie TK. Multicenter prospective study of nonruptured abdominal aortic aneurysm. I. Population and operative management. *J Vasc Surg.* 1988;7:69–81; Olsen PS, Schroeder T, Agerskov K, et al. Surgery for abdominal aortic aneurysms. A survey of 656 patients. *J Cardiovasc Surg.* 1991;32:636–642; AbuRahma AF, Robinson PA, Boland JP, et al. Elective resection of 332 abdominal aortic aneurysms in a southern West Virginia community during a recent five-year period. *Surgery.* 1991;109:244–251; Diehl JT, Cali RF, Hertzer NR, Beven EG. Complications of abdominal aortic reconstruction. An analysis of perioperative risk factors in 557 patients. *Ann Surg.* 1983;197:49–56; and Richardson JD, Main KA. Repair of abdominal aortic aneurysms. A statewide experience. *Arch Surg.* 1991;126:614–616.

and establishing effective analgesia are important techniques for preventing myocardial ischemia postoperatively. Patients with cardiac dysfunction have a greater risk of myocardial infarction when the postoperative hematocrit is less than 28%, even though this is well tolerated by normal individuals.[185] Postoperative epidural analgesia, in addition to providing excellent pain control, may reduce myocardial complications by decreasing the catecholamine stress response.[153]

Hemorrhage

Intraoperative or postoperative hemorrhage usually results from difficulties with the proximal aortic anastomosis or from iatrogenic venous injury. Proximal suture line bleeding, particularly when posterior, can be difficult to control, especially if the proximal anastomosis is juxtarenal. Venous bleeding usually results from injury to the iliac or left renal veins during initial exposure. Often the distal aortic aneurysm or common iliac aneurysm is densely adherent to the associated iliac vein, making circumferential arterial dissection hazardous. In such cases, vascular clamps can usually be applied successfully without complete dissection of the posterior wall of the iliac artery or vascular control obtained with balloon occlusion catheters. A posterior left renal vein or a large lumbar vein may pose similar hazards during the proximal dissection. If undetected by preoperative CT scanning, such anomalies pose a high risk for venous injury. Diffuse bleeding after substantial intraoperative blood loss is usually due to exhausted coagulation factors and platelets, combined with hypothermia. Aggressive rewarming with platelet and coagulation factor replacement is required to overcome this complication.

Renal Failure

Although once common after infrarenal AAA repair, renal failure is now rare, due to adequate volume replacement and maintenance of normal cardiac output and renal blood flow. However, precautions are still required to reduce the risk of this complication. Because of the renal toxicity of IV contrast, it is prudent to delay AAA repair following arteriography or contrast-enhanced CT scanning to be certain that renal dysfunction has not been induced. A more likely cause of renal failure following infrarenal AAA repair is embolization of aortic atheromatous debris into the renal arteries during proximal aortic cross-clamping. Preoperative CT scanning may reveal pararenal atheromatous debris or thrombus, which should prompt temporary supraceliac cross-clamping until the infrarenal aorta is open. Because preoperative renal insufficiency is the best predictor of postoperative renal failure,[79,186] special precautions are appropriate in such patients. Some evidence supports a beneficial effect of IV mannitol when given before aortic cross-clamping (25 g).[186] Although some have advocated maintenance of higher urine volume using furosemide, the efficacy of this approach has not been proven and may hinder the assessment of fluid balance by artificially increasing urine output.

Gastrointestinal Complications

Some degree of bowel dysfunction occurs after any major abdominal procedure. However, the paralytic ileus that follows evisceration and dissection of the base of the mesentery during transperitoneal AAA repair often lasts longer than that occurring after other procedures. Consequently, one must use caution in reinstituting oral feeding postoperatively. Anorexia, periodic constipation, or diarrhea is commonly seen in the first few weeks following aneurysm surgery.

Sigmoid colon ischemia following AAA repair is a rare but devastating complication that occurs after approximately 1% of elective AAA repairs.[187,188] This may result from embolization into, or ligation of, the IMA or internal iliac arteries. Although the IMA is often chronically occluded, ligation too far from the aneurysm wall can obliterate important SMA collaterals. Fortunately, the abundance of collateral flow to the sigmoid colon usually prevents ischemia. Sigmoid ischemia is three to four times more likely following ruptured AAA repair, presumably due to the associated hypotension and shock added to the usual risk of this complication.[187–189] Careful inspection of the sigmoid colon following graft placement is important and may be facilitated by Doppler insonation of the bowel wall and mesentery. Preoperatively, patent IMAs should be carefully inspected for back-bleeding following the aortic reconstruction and ligated only when back-bleeding is pulsatile and colon viability is ensured. In questionable circumstances, IMA reimplantation or direct internal iliac revascularization is indicated.[190] Postoperatively, colon ischemia should be suspected in the presence of early diarrhea, usually containing blood; left lower quadrant abdominal pain; unexplained fever or leukocytosis; or excessive IV fluid or pressor requirement. This should prompt immediate flexible sigmoidoscopy or colonoscopy. In most cases, patchy, partial-thickness mucosal necrosis and sloughing are detected and often resolve with antibiotic therapy and bowel rest. However, in more severe cases of transmural infarction, early reexploration is indicated to avoid the high mortality rate associated with delayed treatment of this complication. Treatment requires sigmoid resection and colostomy, rarely combined with aortic graft excision followed by extra-anatomic bypass if substantial graft contamination has occurred.

Distal Embolization

Lower-extremity ischemia may occur after AAA repair, usually from embolization of aneurysmal debris that occurs during aneurysm mobilization or aortoiliac clamping. Usually such emboli are small (termed microemboli) and not amenable to surgical removal, and they result in transient, patchy areas of dusky skin or "blue toes." This can result in persistent pain or skin loss, occasionally necessitating amputation. Some have recommended treatment with low-molecular-weight dextran or even sympathectomy for such microembolic lesions, but their management is largely expectant. Occasionally, larger emboli or distal intimal flaps, particularly in diseased iliac arteries, may require operative intervention. For this reason, the legs should be carefully inspected intraoperatively for ischemia after AAA repair while the incision is still open, and arterial access can be easily obtained if necessary.

Paraplegia

Paraplegia due to spinal cord ischemia is rare following infrarenal AAA repair. It can result when important spinal artery collateral flow via the internal iliac arteries or an abnormally low origin of the accessory spinal artery (arterial magna radicularis or artery of Adamkiewicz) is obliterated or embolized during AAA repair.[191] Because the accessory spinal artery normally originates from the descending thoracic or upper abdominal aorta, this complication is much more common following thoracoabdominal aneurysm repair.

Impaired Sexual Function

Impotence or retrograde ejaculation may result after AAA repair due to injury of autonomic nerves during paraaortic dissection.[192] The incidence of this complication is difficult to determine due to the multiple causes of impotence in this age group and frequent underreporting. In the ADAM trial in US VA hospitals, 40% of men had impotence before AAA repair.[193] Contrary to most other reports that asked patients retrospectively if they had impotence before AAA repair, in the ADAM trial, less than 10% developed new impotence in the first year after repair. However, the proportion reporting new impotence increased over time such that by 4 years after AAA repair, more than 60% reported having

impotence, which underscores the multifactorial etiology of impotence in this age group. Careful preservation of nerves, particularly as they course along the left side of the infrarenal aorta, around the IMA, and cross the proximal left common iliac artery has been shown to substantially reduce this complication, which has reportedly occurred in up to 25% of patients.[194,195] Other possible causes of postoperative impotence include reduction in pelvic blood flow due to internal iliac occlusion or embolization. Sexual dysfunction is not confined to open AAA repair patients. A recent study by Pettersson et al. demonstrated that a group of patients when asked about their respective sexual function following EVAR reported increased postoperative impotence and ejaculatory function 1 year following AAA repair.[196]

Venous Thromboembolism

Pulmonary embolism and deep vein thrombosis are less common after AAA repair than after other abdominal operations, perhaps due to intraoperative anticoagulation. However, unrecognized deep vein thrombosis can occur in up to 18% of untreated patients.[197] Therefore perioperative prophylaxis with intermittent pneumatic compression stockings or subcutaneous heparin is appropriate.

FUNCTIONAL OUTCOME

Williamson and colleagues[198] reviewed their experience with open AAA repair with regard to functional outcome. They found that two-thirds of patients experienced complete recovery at an average time of 4 months, whereas one-third had not fully recovered at an average time of nearly 3 years. In addition, 18% said they would not undergo AAA repair again after knowing the recovery process, despite appearing to understand the implications of AAA rupture. Eleven percent were initially discharged to a skilled nursing facility, with an average stay of 3.7 months. This is similar to a 9% rate of discharge to a facility other than home, as reported in a review of national administrative data by Huber and colleagues.[199] Although all patients in Williamson's review were ambulatory preoperatively, at a mean of 25 months' follow-up, only 64% were fully ambulatory, whereas 22% required assistance and 14% were nonambulatory. Although it is difficult to determine the extent of the disability that is due to the AAA repair, this report highlights the high rate of disability after open AAA repair. More research into long-term functional outcomes and quality-of-life assessment is clearly necessary.

LONG-TERM SURVIVAL

As noted previously, the early (30-day) mortality after elective AAA repair in properly selected patients is less than or equal to 5%, whereas the early mortality after ruptured AAA repair averages 54% (not including patients who died from rupture before repair).[6,16] Five-year survival after successful AAA repair in modern series is approximately 70% compared with approximately 80% in the age- and gender-matched general population.[96,97,173,200–204] Ten-year survival after AAA repair is approximately 40%. Although survival is similar in men and women, women without AAA have longer survival than men. Therefore survival relative to gender-specific norms is lower in women after AAA repair than in men.[205] Survival after successful ruptured AAA repair versus successful elective repair was similar in one report[206] but reduced in others.[207,208] In a population-based analysis from Western Australia, survival after ruptured or elective AAA repair was similar for men but significantly reduced for women with ruptured AAA.[205] Overall, survival after AAA repair is reduced compared with an age- and sex-matched population because of greater associated comorbidity in patients with aneurysms.[88,201] Not surprisingly,

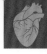

systemic complications of atherosclerosis cause most late deaths after AAA repair in this predominately elderly, male population. The cause of late deaths after AAA repair are cardiac disease (44%), cancer (15%), rupture of another aneurysm (11%), stroke (9%), and pulmonary disease (6%).[200,201,209] Combining cardiac causes, aneurysmal disease, and stroke indicates that vascular complications account for two-thirds of the late deaths following AAA repair.

When outcome is stratified according to these risk factors, the 5-year survival rate improves to 84% in patients without heart disease, which is substantially better than the 54% survival rate observed in patients with known heart disease.[200] Hypertension also reduces 5-year survival after AAA repair, from 84% to 59%.[200] In patients without hypertension or heart disease, late survival after AAA repair is identical to normal, age-matched controls.[201] Multivariate analysis indicates that uncorrected CAD is the most significant variable associated with late mortality after AAA repair, but that age, renal dysfunction, COPD, and peripheral occlusive disease also contribute.[96,97,173,210] One analysis of coronary artery bypass grafting performed in preparation for AAA repair indicates that it may improve long-term survival in patients younger than age 70 but that older patients do not benefit from this aggressive approach.[210] A recent prospective, multicentered study identified not only age, cardiac, carotid, and renal disease as independent predictors of late mortality following elective AAA repair but also aneurysm extent, as judged by size, suprarenal extension, and external iliac involvement.[202]

REFERENCES

1. Bobadilla JL, Kent KC. Screening for abdominal aortic aneurysms. *Adv Surg.* 2012;46:101–109.
2. McPhee JT, Hill JS, Eslami MH. The impact of gender on presentation, therapy, and mortality of abdominal aortic aneurysm in the United States, 2001-2004. *J Vasc Surg.* 2007;45(5):891–899.
3. Assar AN, Zarins CK. Ruptured abdominal aortic aneurysm: a surgical emergency with many clinical presentations. *Postgrad Med J.* 2009;85(1003):268–273.
4. Heller JA, Weinberg A, Arons R, et al. Two decades of abdominal aortic aneurysm repair: have we made any progress? *J Vasc Surg.* 2000;32(6):1091–1100.
5. Adam DJ, Mohan IV, Stuart WP, et al. Community and hospital outcome from ruptured abdominal aortic aneurysm within the catchment area of a regional vascular surgical service. *J Vasc Surg.* 1999;30(5):922–928.
6. Hallin A, Bergqvist D, Holmberg L. Literature review of surgical management of abdominal aortic aneurysm. *Eur J Vasc Endovasc Surg.* 2001;22(3):197–204.
7. Bown MJ, Sutton AJ, Bell PR, Sayers RD. A meta-analysis of 50 years of ruptured abdominal aortic aneurysm repair. *Br J Surg.* 2002;89(6):714–730.
8. Ernst CB. Abdominal aortic aneurysm. *N Engl J Med.* 1993;328(16):1167–1172.
9. Heikkinen M, Salenius JP, Auvinen O. Ruptured abdominal aortic aneurysm in a well-defined geographic area. *J Vasc Surg.* 2002;36(2):291–296.
10. Kantonen I, Lepäntalo M, Brommels M, Luther M, Salenius JP, Ylönen K. Mortality in ruptured abdominal aortic aneurysms. The Finnvasc Study Group. *Eur J Vasc Endovasc Surg.* 1999;17(3):208–212.
11. Bengtsson H, Bergqvist D. Ruptured abdominal aortic aneurysm: a population-based study. *J Vasc Surg.* 1993;18(1):74–80.
12. Pasch AR, Ricotta JJ, May AG, Green RM, DeWeese JE. Abdominal aortic aneurysm: the case for elective resection. *Circulation.* 1984;70(3 Pt 2):I1–I4.
13. Breckwoldt WL, Mackey WC, O'Donnell Jr TF. The economic implications of high-risk abdominal aortic aneurysms. *J Vasc Surg.* 1991;13(6):798–803. discussion 803–804.
14. Pearce WH, Slaughter MS, LeMaire S, et al. Aortic diameter as a function of age, gender, and body surface area. *Surgery.* 1993;114(4):691–697.
15. Johnston KW, Rutherford RB, Tilson MD, Shah DM, Hollier L, Stanley JC. Suggested standards for reporting on arterial aneurysms. Subcommittee on Reporting Standards for Arterial Aneurysms, Ad Hoc Committee on Reporting Standards, Society for Vascular Surgery and North American Chapter, International Society for Cardiovascular Surgery. *J Vasc Surg.* 1991;13(3):452–458.
16. Katz DA, Littenberg B, Cronenwett JL. Management of small abdominal aortic aneurysms. Early surgery vs watchful waiting. *JAMA.* 1992;268(19):2678–2686.
17. Brewster DC, Cronenwett JL, Hallett Jr JW, et al. Guidelines for the treatment of abdominal aortic aneurysms. Report of a subcommittee of the Joint Council of the American Association for Vascular Surgery and Society for Vascular Surgery. *J Vasc Surg.* 2003;37(5):1106–1117.
18. Brown LC, Powell JT. Risk factors for aneurysm rupture in patients kept under ultrasound surveillance. UK Small Aneurysm Trial Participants. *Ann Surg.* 1999;230(3):289–296. discussion 296–297.
19. Mortality results for randomised controlled trial of early elective surgery or ultrasonographic surveillance for small abdominal aortic aneurysms. The UK Small Aneurysm Trial Participants. *Lancet.* 1998;352(9141):1649–1655.
20. Lederle FA, Wilson SE, Johnson GR, et al. Immediate repair compared with surveillance of small abdominal aortic aneurysms. *N Engl J Med.* 2002;346(19):1437–1444.
21. Ouriel K, Clair DG, Kent KC, Zarins CK. Positive Impact of Endovascular Options for Treating Aneurysms Early (PIVOTAL) Investigators. Endovascular repair compared with surveillance for patients with small abdominal aortic aneurysms. *J Vasc Surg.* 2010;51(5):1081–1087.
22. Valentine RJ, Decaprio JD, Castillo JM, Modrall JG, Jackson MR, Clagett GP. Watchful waiting in cases of small abdominal aortic aneurysms—appropriate for all patients? *J Vasc Surg.* 2000;32(3):441–448. discussion 448–450.
23. Szilagyi DE, Smith RF, DeRusso FJ, Elliott JP, Sherrin FW. Contribution of abdominal aortic aneurysmectomy to prolongation of life. *Ann Surg.* 1966;164(4):678–699.
24. Foster JH, Bolasny BL, Gobbel Jr WG, Scott Jr HW. Comparative study of elective resection and expectant treatment of abdomianl aortic aneurysm. *Surg Gynecol Obstet.* 1969;129(1):1–9.
25. Darling RC, Messina CR, Brewster DC, Ottinger LW. Autopsy study of unoperated abdominal aortic aneurysms. The case for early resection. *Circulation.* 1977;56(3 Suppl):II161–II164.
26. Sterpetti AV, Cavallaro A, Cavallari N, et al. Factors influencing the rupture of abdominal aortic aneurysms. *Surg Gynecol Obstet.* 1991;173(3):175–178.
27. Lederle FA, Johnson GR, Wilson SE, et al. Rupture rate of large abdominal aortic aneurysms in patients refusing or unfit for elective repair. *JAMA.* 2002;287(22):2968–2972.
28. Tang W, Yao L, Roetker NS, et al. Lifetime risk and risk factors for abdominal aortic aneurysm in a 24-year prospective study: the ARIC study (Atherosclerosis Risk in Communities). *Arterioscler Thromb Vasc Biol.* 2016;36(12):2468–2477.
29. Sonesson B, Lanne T, Hansen F, Sandgren T. Infrarenal aortic diameter in the healthy person. *Eur J Vasc Surg.* 1994;8(1):89–95.
30. Ouriel K, Green RM, Donayre C, Shortell CK, Elliott J, DeWeese JA. An evaluation of new methods of expressing aortic aneurysm size: relationship to rupture. *J Vasc Surg.* 1992;15(1):12–18. discussion 19–20.
31. Sidloff DA, Saratzis A, Sweeting MJ, Holt PJ, Loftus IM, Thompson MM. Sex differences in mortality after abdominal aortic aneurysm repair in the UK. *Br J Surg.* 2017;104(12):1656–1664.
32. Malkawi AH, Hinchliffe RJ, Xu Y, et al. Patient-specific biomechanical profiling in abdominal aortic aneurysm development and rupture. *J Vasc Surg.* 2010;52(2):480–488.
33. McGloughlin TM, Doyle BJ. New approaches to abdominal aortic aneurysm rupture risk assessment: engineering insights with clinical gain. *Arterioscler Thromb Vasc Biol.* 2010;30(9):1687–1694.
34. Crawford JD, Chivukula VK, Haller S, et al. Aortic outflow occlusion predicts rupture of abdominal aortic aneurysm. *J Vasc Surg.* 2016;64(6):1623–1628.

35. Haller SJ, Crawford JD, Courchaine KM, et al. Intraluminal thrombus is associated with early rupture of abdominal aortic aneurysm. *J Vasc Surg.* 2018;67(4). 1051–1058-e1.

36. Darling 3rd RC, Brewster DC, Darling RC, et al. Are familial abdominal aortic aneurysms different? *J Vasc Surg.* 1989;10(1):39–43.

37. Verloes A, Sakalihasan N, Koulischer L, Limet R. Aneurysms of the abdominal aorta: familial and genetic aspects in three hundred thirteen pedigrees. *J Vasc Surg.* 1995;21(4):646–655.

38. Limet R, Sakalihassan N, Albert A. Determination of the expansion rate and incidence of rupture of abdominal aortic aneurysms. *J Vasc Surg.* 1991;14(4):540–548.

39. Cronenwett JL, Sargent SK, Wall MH, et al. Variables that affect the expansion rate and outcome of small abdominal aortic aneurysms. *J Vasc Surg.* 1990;11(2):260–268. discussion 268–269.

40. Hirose Y, Hamada S, Takamiya M. Predicting the growth of aortic aneurysms: a comparison of linear vs exponential models. *Angiology.* 1995;46(5):413–419.

41. Englund R, Hudson P, Hanel K, Stanton A. Expansion rates of small abdominal aortic aneurysms. *Aust N Z J Surg.* 1998;68(1):21–24.

42. Bengtsson H, Ekberg O, Aspelin P, Källerö S, Bergqvist D. Ultrasound screening of the abdominal aorta in patients with intermittent claudication. *Eur J Vasc Surg.* 1989;3(6):497–502.

43. Guirguis EM, Barber GG. The natural history of abdominal aortic aneurysms. *Am J Surg.* 1991;162(5):481–483.

44. Santilli SM, Littooy FN, Cambria RA, et al. Expansion rates and outcomes for the 3.0-cm to the 3.9-cm infrarenal abdominal aortic aneurysm. *J Vasc Surg.* 2002;35(4):666–671.

45. Vardulaki KA, Prevost TC, Walker NM, et al. Growth rates and risk of rupture of abdominal aortic aneurysms. *Br J Surg.* 1998;85(12):1674–1680.

46. Sterpetti AV, Schultz RD, Feldhaus RJ, Cheng SE, Peetz Jr DJ. Factors influencing enlargement rate of small abdominal aortic aneurysms. *J Surg Res.* 1987;43(3):211–219.

47. Chang JB, Stein TA, Liu JP, Dunn ME. Risk factors associated with rapid growth of small abdominal aortic aneurysms. *Surgery.* 1997;121(2): 117–122.

48. Brady AR, Thompson RW, Greenhalgh RM, Powell JT. Cardiovascular risk factors and abdominal aortic aneurysm expansion: Only smoking counts [abstract]. *Br J Surg.* 2003;90:492.

49. Lindholt JS, Heegaard NH, Vammen S, Fasting H, Henneberg EW, Heickendorff L. Smoking, but not lipids, lipoprotein(a) and antibodies against oxidised LDL, is correlated to the expansion of abdominal aortic aneurysms. *Eur J Vasc Endovasc Surg.* 2001;21(1):51–56.

50. MacSweeney ST, Ellis M, Worrell PC, Greenhalgh RM, Powell JT. Smoking and growth rate of small abdominal aortic aneurysms. *Lancet.* 1994;344(8923):651–652.

51. Brown PM, Zelt DT, Sobolev B. The risk of rupture in untreated aneurysms: the impact of size, gender, and expansion rate. *J Vasc Surg.* 2003;37(2):280–284.

52. Schewe CK, Schweikart HP, Hammel G, Spengel FA, Zöllner N, Zoller WG. Influence of selective management on the prognosis and the risk of rupture of abdominal aortic aneurysms. *Clin Investig.* 1994;72(8):585–591.

53. Bhak RH, Wininger M, Johnson GR, et al. Factors associated with small abdominal aortic aneurysm expansion rate. *JAMA Surg.* 2015;150(1): 44–50.

54. Wolf YG, Thomas WS, Brennan FJ, Goff WG, Sise MJ, Bernstein EF. Computed tomography scanning findings associated with rapid expansion of abdominal aortic aneurysms. *J Vasc Surg.* 1994;20(4):529–535. discussion 535–538.

55. Krupski WC, Bass A, Thurston DW, et al. Utility of computed tomography for surveillance of small abdominal aortic aneurysms. Preliminary report. *Arch Surg.* 1990;125(10):1345–1349. discussion 1349–1350.

56. Brophy CM, Tilson JE, Tilson MD. Propranolol stimulates the crosslinking of matrix components in skin from the aneurysm-prone blotchy mouse. *J Surg Res.* 1989;46(4):330–332.

57. Ricci MA, Slaiby JM, Gadowski GR, Hendley ED, Nichols P, Pilcher DB. Effects of hypertension and propranolol upon aneurysm expansion in the Anidjar/Dobrin aneurysm model. *Ann N Y Acad Sci.* 1996;800:89–96.

58. Simpson CF. Sotalol for the protection of turkeys from the development of B-aminopropionitrile-induced aortic ruptures. *Br J Pharmacol.* 1972;45(3):385–390.

59. Simpson CF, Boucek RJ. The B-aminopropionitrile-fed turkey: a model for detecting potential drug action on arterial tissue. *Cardiovasc Res.* 1983;17(1):26–32.

60. Simpson CF, Boucek RJ, Noble NL. Influence of d-, l-, and dl-propranolol, and practolol on beta-amino-propionitrile-induced aortic ruptures of turkeys. *Toxicol Appl Pharmacol.* 1976;38(1):169–175.

61. Leach SD, Toole AL, Stern H, DeNatale RW, Tilson MD. Effect of beta-adrenergic blockade on the growth rate of abdominal aortic aneurysms. *Arch Surg.* 1988;123(5):606–609.

62. Gadowski GR, Pilcher DB, Ricci MA. Abdominal aortic aneurysm expansion rate: effect of size and beta-adrenergic blockade. *J Vasc Surg.* 1994;19(4):727–731.

63. Propranolol Aneurysm Trial Investigators. Propranolol for small abdominal aortic aneurysms: results of a randomized trial. *J Vasc Surg.* 2002;35(1):72–79.

64. Wilmink AB, Hubbard CS, Day NE, Quick CR. Effect of propranolol on the expansion of abdominal aortic aneurysms: a randomized study. *Br J Surg.* 2000;87:499.

65. Takagi H, Matsui M, Umemoto TA. A meta-analysis of clinical studies of statins for prevention of abdominal aortic aneurysm expansion. *J Vasc Surg.* 2010;52(6):1675–1681.

66. Van Kuijk JP, Flu WJ, Witteveen OP, et al. The influence of statins on the expansion rate and rupture risk of abdominal aortic aneurysms. *J Cardiovasc Surg (Torino).* 2009;50(5):599–609.

67. Vammen S, Lindholt JS, Ostergaard L, et al. Randomized double-blind controlled trial of roxithromycin for prevention of abdominal aortic aneurysm expansion. *Br J Surg.* 2001;88(8):1066–1072.

68. Mosorin M, Juvonen J, Biancari F, et al. Use of doxycycline to decrease the growth rate of abdominal aortic aneurysms: a randomized, double-blind, placebo-controlled pilot study. *J Vasc Surg.* 2001;34(4):606–610.

69. Petersen E, Boman J, Persson K, et al. Chlamydia pneumoniae in human abdominal aortic aneurysms. *Eur J Vasc Endovasc Surg.* 1998;15(2):138–142.

70. Juvonen J, Juvonen T, Laurila A, et al. Demonstration of Chlamydia pneumoniae in the walls of abdominal aortic aneurysms. *J Vasc Surg.* 1997;25(3):499–505.

71. Vammen S, Lindholt JS, Andersen PL, Henneberg EW, Østergaard L. Antibodies against Chlamydia pneumoniae predict the need for elective surgical intervention on small abdominal aortic aneurysms. *Eur J Vasc Endovasc Surg.* 2001;22(2):165–168.

72. Curci JA, Petrinec D, Liao S, Golub LM, Thompson RW. Pharmacologic suppression of experimental abdominal aortic aneurysms: a comparison of doxycycline and four chemically modified tetracyclines. *J Vasc Surg.* 1998;28(6):1082–1093.

73. Curci JA, Mao D, Bohner DG, et al. Preoperative treatment with doxycycline reduces aortic wall expression and activation of matrix metalloproteinases in patients with abdominal aortic aneurysms. *J Vasc Surg.* 2000;31(2):325–342.

74. Abdul-Hussien H, Hanemaaijer R, Verheijen JH, van Bockel JH, Geelkerken RH, Lindeman JH. Doxycycline therapy for abdominal aneurysm: improved proteolytic balance through reduced neutrophil content. *J Vasc Surg.* 2009;49(3):741–749.

75. Dodd BR, Spence RA. Doxycycline inhibition of abdominal aortic aneurysm growth: a systematic review of the literature. *Curr Vasc Pharmacol.* 2011;9(4):471–478.

76. Steyerberg EW, Kievit J, de Mol Van Otterloo JC, van Bockel JH, Eijkemans MJ, Habbema JD. Perioperative mortality of elective abdominal aortic aneurysm surgery. A clinical prediction rule based on literature and individual patient data. *Arch Intern Med.* 1995;155(18):1998–2004.

77. Kazmers A, Perkins AJ, Jacobs LA. Outcomes after abdominal aortic aneurysm repair in those > or =80 years of age: recent Veterans Affairs experience. *Ann Vasc Surg.* 1998;12(2):106–112.

78. L'Italien GJ, Paul SD, Hendel RC, et al. Development and validation of a Bayesian model for perioperative cardiac risk assessment in a cohort of 1,081 vascular surgical candidates. *J Am Coll Cardiol.* 1996;27(4):779–786.

79. Johnston KW. Multicenter prospective study of nonruptured abdominal aortic aneurysm. Part II. Variables predicting morbidity and mortality. *J Vasc Surg.* 1989;9(3):437–447.

80. Brady AR, Fowkes FG, Greenhalgh RM, Powell JT, Ruckley CV, Thompson SG. Risk factors for postoperative death following elective surgical repair of abdominal aortic aneurysm: results from the UK Small Aneurysm Trial. On behalf of the UK Small Aneurysm Trial participants. *Br J Surg.* 2000;87(6):742–749.

81. Katz DJ, Stanley JC, Zelenock GB. Gender differences in abdominal aortic aneurysm prevalence, treatment, and outcome. *J Vasc Surg.* 1997;25(3):561–568.

82. Katz DA, Cronenwett JL. The cost-effectiveness of early surgery versus watchful waiting in the management of small abdominal aortic aneurysms. *J Vasc Surg.* 1994;19(6):980–990. discussion 990–991.

83. Iezzoni LI. Assessing quality using administrative data. *Ann Intern Med.* 1997;127(8 Pt 2):666–674.

84. Johnston KW, Scobie TK. Multicenter prospective study of nonruptured abdominal aortic aneurysms. I. Population and operative management. *J Vasc Surg.* 1988;7(1):69–81.

85. Beck AW, Goodney PP, Nolan BW, et al. Predicting 1-year mortality after elective abdominal aortic aneurysm repair. *J Vasc Surg.* 2009;49(4):838–843. discussion 843–844.

86. Eslami MH, Rybin DV, Doros G, Siracuse JJ, Farber A. External validation of Vascular Study Group of New England risk predictive model of mortality after elective abdominal aorta aneurysm repair in the Vascular Quality Initiative and comparison against established models. *J Vasc Surg.* 2018;67(1):143–150.

87. Lederle FA, Johnson GR, Wilson SE, et al. The aneurysm detection and management study screening program: validation cohort and final results. Aneurysm Detection and Management Veterans Affairs Cooperative Study Investigators. *Arch Intern Med.* 2000;160(10):1425–1430.

88. Newman AB, Arnold AM, Burke GL, O'Leary DH, Manolio TA. Cardiovascular disease and mortality in older adults with small abdominal aortic aneurysms detected by ultrasonography: the cardiovascular health study. *Ann Intern Med.* 2001;134(3):182–190.

89. Rodin MB, Daviglus ML, Wong GC, et al. Middle age cardiovascular risk factors and abdominal aortic aneurysm in older age. *Hypertension.* 2003;42(1):61–68.

90. Singh K, Bønaa KH, Jacobsen BK, Bjørk L, Solberg S. Prevalence of and risk factors for abdominal aortic aneurysms in a population-based study: The Tromso Study. *Am J Epidemiol.* 2001;154(3):236–244.

91. Törnwall ME, Virtamo J, Haukka JK, Albanes D, Huttunen JK. Life-style factors and risk for abdominal aortic aneurysm in a cohort of Finnish male smokers. *Epidemiology.* 2001;12(1):94–100.

92. Wilmink AB, Quick CR. Epidemiology and potential for prevention of abdominal aortic aneurysm. *Br J Surg.* 1998;85(2):155–162.

93. Johnston KW. Nonruptured abdominal aortic aneurysm: six-year follow-up results from the multicenter prospective Canadian aneurysm study. Canadian Society for Vascular Surgery Aneurysm Study Group. *J Vasc Surg.* 1994;20(2):163–170.

94. Batt M, Staccini P, Pittaluga P, Ferrari E, Hassen-Khodja R, Declemy S. Late survival after abdominal aortic aneurysm repair. *Eur J Vasc Endovasc Surg.* 1999;17(4):338–342.

95. Aune S, Amundsen SR, Evjensvold J, Trippestad A. Operative mortality and long-term relative survival of patients operated on for asymptomatic abdominal aortic aneurysm. *Eur J Vasc Endovasc Surg.* 1995;9(3):293–298.

96. Norman PE, Semmens JB, Lawrence-Brown MM. Long-term relative survival following surgery for abdominal aortic aneurysm: a review. *Cardiovasc Surg.* 2001;9(3):219–224.

97. Hertzer NR, Mascha EJ, Karafa MT, O'Hara PJ, Krajewski LP, Beven EG. Open infrarenal abdominal aortic aneurysm repair: the Cleveland Clinic experience from 1989 to 1998. *J Vasc Surg.* 2002;35(6):1145–1154.

98. Smoking, lung function and the prognosis of abdominal aortic aneurysm. The UK Small Aneurysm Trial Participants. *Eur J Vasc Endovasc Surg.* 2000;19(6):636–642.

99. Bastos Gonçalves F, Ultee KH, Hoeks SE, Stolker RJ, Verhagen HJ. Life expectancy and causes of death after repair of intact and ruptured abdominal aortic aneurysms. *J Vasc Surg.* 2016;63(3):610–616.

100. De Martino RR, Nolan BW, Goodney PP, et al. Outcomes of symptomatic abdominal aortic aneurysm repair. *J Vasc Surg.* 2010;52(1):5–12. e1.

101. Michaels JA. The management of small abdominal aortic aneurysms: a computer simulation using Monte Carlo methods. *Eur J Vasc Surg.* 1992;6(5):551–557.

102. Schermerhorn ML, Birkmeyer JD, Gould DA, Cronenwett JL. Cost-effectiveness of surgery for small abdominal aortic aneurysms on the basis of data from the United Kingdom Small Aneurysm Trial. *J Vasc Surg.* 2000;31(2):217–226.

103. United Kingdom Small Aneurysm Trial Participants, Powell JT, Brady AR, et al. Long-term outcomes of immediate repair compared with surveillance of small abdominal aortic aneurysms. *N Engl J Med.* 2002;346(19):1445–1452.

104. Suckow B, Schanzer AS, Hoel AW, et al. A national survey of disease-specific knowledge in patients with an abdominal aortic aneurysm. *J Vasc Surg.* 2016;63(5):1156–1162.

105. Goodney PP. *Preferences for Open versus Endovascular Repair for Aortic Abdominal Aneurysms - PROVE-AAA Trial.* White River Junction VA, VT: VA Office of Research and Development; 2017.

106. Eagle KA, Berger PB, Calkins H, et al. ACC/AHA guideline update for perioperative cardiovascular evaluation for noncardiac surgery—executive summary. A report of the American College of Cardiology/American Heart Association Task Force on Practice Guidelines (Committee to Update the 1996 Guidelines on Perioperative Cardiovascular Evaluation for Noncardiac Surgery). *Anesth Analg.* 2002;94(5):1052–1064.

107. Fagevik Olsén M, Hahn I, Nordgren S, Lönroth H, Lundholm K. Randomized controlled trial of prophylactic chest physiotherapy in major abdominal surgery. *Br J Surg.* 1997;84(11):1535–1538.

108. Hertzer NR, Young JR, Kramer JR, et al. Routine coronary angiography prior to elective aortic reconstruction: results of selective myocardial revascularization in patients with peripheral vascular disease. *Arch Surg.* 1979;114(11):1336–1344.

109. Eagle KA, Coley CM, Newell JB, et al. Combining clinical and thallium data optimizes preoperative assessment of cardiac risk before major vascular surgery. *Ann Intern Med.* 1989;110(11):859–866.

110. Creech Jr O. Endo-aneurysmorrhaphy and treatment of aortic aneurysm. *Ann Surg.* 1966;164(6):935–946.

111. Hollier LH, Reigel MM, Kazmier FJ, Pairolero PC, Cherry KJ, Hallett Jr JW. Conventional repair of abdominal aortic aneurysm in the high-risk patient: a plea for abandonment of nonresective treatment. *J Vasc Surg.* 1986;3(5):712–717.

112. Inahara T, Geary GL, Mukherjee D, Egan JM. The contrary position to the nonresective treatment for abdominal aortic aneurysm. *J Vasc Surg.* 1985;2(1):42–48.

113. Karmody AM, Leather RP, Goldman M, Corson JD, Shah DM. The current position of nonresective treatment for abdominal aortic aneurysm. *Surgery.* 1983;94(4):591–597.

114. Lynch K, Kohler T, Johansen K. Nonresective therapy for aortic aneurysm: results of a survey. *J Vasc Surg.* 1986;4(5):469–472.

115. Schwartz RA, Nichols WK, Silver D. Is thrombosis of the infrarenal abdominal aortic aneurysm an acceptable alternative? *J Vasc Surg.* 1986;3(3):448–455.

116. Shah DM, Chang BB, Paty PS, Kaufman JL, Koslow AR, Leather RP. Treatment of abdominal aortic aneurysm by exclusion and bypass: an analysis of outcome. *J Vasc Surg.* 1991;13(1):15–20. discussion 20–22.

117. Darling 3rd RC, Ozsvath K, Chang BB, et al. The incidence, natural history, and outcome of secondary intervention for persistent collateral flow in the excluded abdominal aortic aneurysm. *J Vasc Surg.* 1999;30(6):968–976.

118. Kline RG, D'Angelo AJ, Chen MH, Halpern VJ, Cohen JR. Laparoscopically assisted abdominal aortic aneurysm repair: first 20 cases. *J Vasc Surg.* 1998;27(1):81–87. discussion 88.

119. Lin JC, Kaul SA, Bhandari A, Peterson EL, Peabody JO, Menon M. Robotic-assisted aortic surgery with and without minilaparotomy for complicated occlusive disease and aneurysm. *J Vasc Surg.* 2012;55(1):16–22.

120. Wu T, Prema J, Zagaja G, Shalhav A, Bassiouny HS. Total laparorobotic repair of abdominal aortic aneurysm with sac exclusion obliteration and aortobifemoral bypass. *Ann Vasc Surg.* 2009;23(5):686 e11-6.

121. Parodi JC, Palmaz JC, Barone HD. Transfemoral intraluminal graft implantation for abdominal aortic aneurysms. *Ann Vasc Surg*. 1991;5(6):491–499.

122. Moore WS, Brewster DC, Bernhard VM. Aorto-uni-iliac endograft for complex aortoiliac aneurysms compared with tube/bifurcation endografts: results of the EVT/Guidant trials. *J Vasc Surg*. 2001;33(2 Suppl):S11–S20.

123. Matsumura JS, Brewster DC, Makaroun MS, Naftel DC. A multicenter controlled clinical trial of open versus endovascular treatment of abdominal aortic aneurysm. *J Vasc Surg*. 2003;37(2):262–271.

124. Zarins CK, White RA, Schwarten D, et al. AneuRx stent graft versus open surgical repair of abdominal aortic aneurysms: multicenter prospective clinical trial. *J Vasc Surg*. 1999;29(2):292–305. discussion 6–8.

125. Lee WA, Carter JW, Upchurch G, et al. Perioperative outcomes after open and endovascular repair of intact abdominal aortic aneurysms in the United States during 2001. *J Vasc Surg*. 2004;39(3):491–496.

126. Aquino RV, Jones MA, Zullo TG, Missig-Carroll N, Makaroun MS. Quality of life assessment in patients undergoing endovascular or conventional AAA repair. *J Endovasc Ther*. 2001;8(5):521–528.

127. Bernhard VM, Mitchell RS, Matsumura JS, et al. Ruptured abdominal aortic aneurysm after endovascular repair. *J Vasc Surg*. 2002;35(6):1155–1162.

128. Harris PL, Vallabhaneni SR, Desgranges P, Becquemin JP, van Marrewijk C, Laheij RJ. Incidence and risk factors of late rupture, conversion, and death after endovascular repair of infrarenal aortic aneurysms: the EUROSTAR experience. European Collaborators on Stent/graft Techniques for Aortic Aneurysm Repair. *J Vasc Surg*. 2000;32(4):739–749.

129. Holzenbein TJ, Kretschmer G, Thurnher S, et al. Midterm durability of abdominal aortic aneurysm endograft repair: a word of caution. *J Vasc Surg*. 2001;33(2 Suppl):S46–S54.

130. Schermerhorn ML, Finlayson SR, Fillinger MF, Buth J, van Marrewijk C, Cronenwett JL. Life expectancy after endovascular versus open abdominal aortic aneurysm repair: results of a decision analysis model on the basis of data from EUROSTAR. *J Vasc Surg*. 2002;36(6):1112–1120.

131. Prinssen M, Verhoeven EL, Buth J, et al. A randomized trial comparing conventional and endovascular repair of abdominal aortic aneurysms. *N Engl J Med*. 2004;351(16):1607–1618.

132. Blankensteijn JD, de Jong SE, Prinssen M, et al. Two-year outcomes after conventional or endovascular repair of abdominal aortic aneurysms. *N Engl J Med*. 2005;352(23):2398–2405.

133. Zarins CK, White RA, Fogarty TJ. Aneurysm rupture after endovascular repair using the AneuRx stent graft. *J Vasc Surg*. 2000;31(5):960–970.

134. Ohki T, Veith FJ, Shaw P, et al. Increasing incidence of midterm and long-term complications after endovascular graft repair of abdominal aortic aneurysms: a note of caution based on a 9-year experience. *Ann Surg*. 2001;234(3):323–334. discussion 34–35.

135. Suckow BD, Goodney PP, Columbo JA, et al. National trends in open surgical, endovascular, and branched-fenestrated endovascular aortic aneurysm repair in Medicare patients. *J Vasc Surg*. 2018;67(6):1690–1697. e1.

136. EVAR Trial Participants. Endovascular aneurysm repair versus open repair in patients with abdominal aortic aneurysm (EVAR trial 1): randomised controlled trial. *Lancet*. 2005;365(9478):2179–2186.

137. EVAR Trial Participants. Endovascular aneurysm repair and outcome in patients unfit for open repair of abdominal aortic aneurysm (EVAR trial 2): randomised controlled trial. *Lancet*. 2005;365(9478):2187–2192.

138. Rutherford RB. Randomized EVAR trials and advent of level I evidence: a paradigm shift in management of large abdominal aortic aneurysms? *Semin Vasc Surg*. 2006;19(2):69–74.

139. Lederle FA, Freischlag JA, Kyriakides TC, et al. Outcomes following endovascular vs open repair of abdominal aortic aneurysm: a randomized trial. *JAMA*. 2009;302(14):1535–1542.

140. Schermerhorn ML, Buck DB, O'Malley AJ, et al. Long-term outcomes of abdominal aortic aneurysm in the medicare population. *N Engl J Med*. 2015;373(4):328–338.

141. Kaiser AB, Clayson KR, Mulherin Jr JL, et al. Antibiotic prophylaxis in vascular surgery. *Ann Surg*. 1978;188(3):283–289.

142. Bender JS, Smith-Meek MA, Jones CE. Routine pulmonary artery catheterization does not reduce morbidity and mortality of elective vascular surgery: results of a prospective, randomized trial. *Ann Surg*. 1997;226(3):229–236. discussion 236–237.

143. Ziegler DW, Wright JG, Choban PS, Flancbaum L. A prospective randomized trial of preoperative "optimization" of cardiac function in patients undergoing elective peripheral vascular surgery. *Surgery*. 1997;122(3):584–592.

144. Birkmeyer JD, AuBuchon JP, Littenberg B, et al. Cost-effectiveness of preoperative autologous donation in coronary artery bypass grafting. *Ann Thorac Surg*. 1994;57(1):161–168. discussion 168–169.

145. Goodnough LT, Monk TG, Sicard G, et al. Intraoperative salvage in patients undergoing elective abdominal aortic aneurysm repair: an analysis of cost and benefit. *J Vasc Surg*. 1996;24(2):213–218.

146. Huber TS, Carlton LC, Irwin PB, et al. Intraoperative autologous transfusion during elective infrarenal aortic reconstruction. *J Surg Res*. 1997;67(1):14–20.

147. Ouriel K, Shortell CK, Green RM, DeWeese JA. Intraoperative autotransfusion in aortic surgery. *J Vasc Surg*. 1993;18(1):16–22.

148. Nelson AH, Fleisher LA, Rosenbaum SH. Relationship between postoperative anemia and cardiac morbidity in high-risk vascular patients in the intensive care unit. *Crit Care Med*. 1993;21(6):860–866.

149. Bush Jr HL, Hydo LJ, Fischer E, Fantini GA, Silane MF, Barie PS. Hypothermia during elective abdominal aortic aneurysm repair: the high price of avoidable morbidity. *J Vasc Surg*. 1995;21(3):392–400. discussion 400–402.

150. Frank SM, Fleisher LA, Breslow MJ, et al. Perioperative maintenance of normothermia reduces the incidence of morbid cardiac events. A randomized clinical trial. *JAMA*. 1997;277(14):1127–1134.

151. Ali ZA, Callaghan CJ, Lim E, et al. Remote ischemic preconditioning reduces myocardial and renal injury after elective abdominal aortic aneurysm repair: a randomized controlled trial. *Circulation*. 2007;116(11 Suppl):I98–105.

152. Mason RA, Newton GB, Cassel W, Maneksha F, Giron F. Combined epidural and general anesthesia in aortic surgery. *J Cardiovasc Surg (Torino)*. 1990;31(4):442–447.

153. Yeager MP, Glass DD, Neff RK, Brinck-Johnsen T. Epidural anesthesia and analgesia in high-risk surgical patients. *Anesthesiology*. 1987;66(6):729–736.

154. Baron JF, Bertrand M, Barré E, et al. Combined epidural and general anesthesia versus general anesthesia for abdominal aortic surgery. *Anesthesiology*. 1991;75(4):611–618.

155. Raggi R, Dardik H, Mauro AL. Continuous epidural anesthesia and postoperative epidural narcotics in vascular surgery. *Am J Surg*. 1987;154(2):192–197.

156. POISE Study Group, Devereaux PJ, Yang H, et al. Effects of extended-release metoprolol succinate in patients undergoing non-cardiac surgery (POISE trial): a randomised controlled trial. *Lancet*. 2008;371(9627):1839–1847.

157. Pasternack PF, Grossi EA, Baumann FG, et al. Beta blockade to decrease silent myocardial ischemia during peripheral vascular surgery. *Am J Surg*. 1989;158(2):113–116.

158. Mangano DT, Layug EL, Wallace A, Tateo I. Effect of atenolol on mortality and cardiovascular morbidity after noncardiac surgery. Multicenter Study of Perioperative Ischemia Research Group. *N Engl J Med*. 1996;335(23):1713–1720.

159. Wallace A, Layug B, Tateo I, et al. Prophylactic atenolol reduces postoperative myocardial ischemia. McSPI Research Group. *Anesthesiology*. 1998;88(1):7–17.

160. Deleted in review.

161. Deleted in review.

162. Goodney PP, Eldrup-Jorgensen J, Nolan BW, et al. A regional quality improvement effort to increase beta blocker administration before vascular surgery. *J Vasc Surg*. 2011;53(5):1316–1328. e1; discussion 1327–1328.

163. Gottlieb SS, McCarter RJ, Vogel RA. Effect of beta-blockade on mortality among high-risk and low-risk patients after myocardial infarction. *N Engl J Med*. 1998;339(8):489–497.

164. Cleland JG, McGowan J, Clark A, Freemantle N. The evidence for beta blockers in heart failure. *BMJ*. 1999;318(7187):824–825.

165. Chang BB, Paty PS, Shah DM, Leather RP, Kaufman JL, McClellan WR. The right retroperitoneal approach for abdominal aortic surgery. *Am J Surg*. 1989;158(2):156–158.

166. Sieunarine K, Lawrence-Brown MM, Goodman MA. Comparison of transperitoneal and retroperitoneal approaches for infrarenal aortic surgery: early and late results. *Cardiovasc Surg*. 1997;5(1):71–76.

167. Buck DB, Ultee KH, Zettervall SL, et al. Transperitoneal versus retroperitoneal approach for open abdominal aortic aneurysm repair in the targeted vascular National Surgical Quality Improvement Program. *J Vasc Surg*. 2016;64(3):585–591.

168. Samson RH, Lepore Jr MR, Showalter DP, et al. Long-term safety of left renal vein division and ligation to expedite complex abdominal aortic surgery. *J Vasc Surg*. 2009;50(3):500–504. discussion 504.

169. Mehta T, Wade RG, Clarke JM. Is it safe to ligate the left renal vein during open abdominal aortic aneurysm repair? *Ann Vasc Surg*. 2010;24(6):758–761.

170. Green RM, Ricotta JJ, Ouriel K, DeWeese JA. Results of supraceliac aortic clamping in the difficult elective resection of infrarenal abdominal aortic aneurysm. *J Vasc Surg*. 1989;9(1):124–134.

171. Breckwoldt WL, Mackey WC, Belkin M, O'Donnell Jr TF. The effect of suprarenal cross-clamping on abdominal aortic aneurysm repair. *Arch Surg*. 1992;127(5):520–524.

172. Nypaver TJ, Shepard AD, Reddy DJ, et al. Repair of pararenal abdominal aortic aneurysms. An analysis of operative management. *Arch Surg*. 1993;128(7):803–811. discussion 11-3.

173. Olsen PS, Schroeder T, Agerskov K, et al. Surgery for abdominal aortic aneurysms. A survey of 656 patients. *J Cardiovasc Surg (Torino)*. 1991;32(5):636–642.

174. Provan JL, Fialkov J, Ameli FM, St Louis EL. Is tube repair of aortic aneurysm followed by aneurysmal change in the common iliac arteries? *Can J Surg*. 1990;33(5):394–397.

175. Polterauer P, Prager M, Holzenbein T, et al. Dacron versus polytetrafluoroethylene for Y-aortic bifurcation grafts: a six-year prospective, randomized trial. *Surgery*. 1992;111(6):626–633.

176. Mabry CD, Thompson BW, Read RC. Activated clotting time (ACT) monitoring of intraoperative heparinization in peripheral vascular surgery. *Am J Surg*. 1979;138(6):894–900.

177. Ernst CB, Hagihara PF, Daugherty ME, Griffen Jr WO. Inferior mesenteric artery stump pressure: a reliable index for safe IMA ligation during abdominal aortic aneurysmectomy. *Ann Surg*. 1978;187(6): 641–646.

178. Thomas JH, Blake K, Pierce GE, et al. The clinical course of asymptomatic mesenteric arterial stenosis. *J Vasc Surg*. 1998;27(5):840–844.

179. Tollefson DF, Ernst CB. Natural history of atherosclerotic renal artery stenosis associated with aortic disease. *J Vasc Surg*. 1991;14(3):327–331.

180. Zierler RE, Bergelin RO, Davidson RC, et al. A prospective study of disease progression in patients with atherosclerotic renal artery stenosis. *Am J Hypertens*. 1996;9(11):1055–1061.

181. Dean RH, Benjamin ME, Hansen KJ. Surgical management of renovascular hypertension. *Curr Probl Surg*. 1997;34(3):209–308.

182. Cambria RP, Brewster DC, L'Italien G, et al. Simultaneous aortic and renal artery reconstruction: evolution of an eighteen-year experience. *J Vasc Surg*. 1995;21(6):916–924. discussion 25.

183. Benjamin ME, Hansen KJ, Craven TE, et al. Combined aortic and renal artery surgery. A contemporary experience. *Ann Surg*. 1996;223(5):555–565. discussion 65-7.

184. Williamson WK, Abou-Zamzam Jr AM, Moneta GL, et al. Prophylactic repair of renal artery stenosis is not justified in patients who require infrarenal aortic reconstruction. *J Vasc Surg*. 1998;28(1):14–20.

185. Nennhaus HP, Javid H. The distinct syndrome of spontaneous abdominal aortocaval fistula. *Am J Med*. 1968;44(3):464–473.

186. Haga M, Hoshina K, Shigematsu K, Watanabe T. A perioperative strategy for abdominal aortic aneurysm in patients with chronic renal insufficiency. *Surg Today*. 2016;46(9):1062–1067.

187. Jarvinen O, Laurikka J, Salenius JP, Lepantalo M. Mesenteric infarction after aortoiliac surgery on the basis of 1752 operations from the National Vascular Registry. *World J Surg*. 1999;23(3):243–247.

188. Bast TJ, van der Biezen JJ, Scherpenisse J, Eikelboom BC. Ischaemic disease of the colon and rectum after surgery for abdominal aortic aneurysm: a prospective study of the incidence and risk factors. *Eur J Vasc Surg*. 1990;4(3):253–257.

189. Welling RE, Roedersheimer LR, Arbaugh JJ, Cranley JJ. Ischemic colitis following repair of ruptured abdominal aortic aneurysm. *Arch Surg*. 1985;120(12):1368–1370.

190. Ernst CB. Prevention of intestinal ischemia following abdominal aortic reconstruction. *Surgery*. 1983;93(1 Pt 1):102–106.

191. Szilagyi DE, Hageman JH, Smith RF, Elliott JP. Spinal cord damage in surgery of the abdominal aorta. *Surgery*. 1978;83(1):38–56.

192. DePalma RG, Levine SB, Feldman S. Preservation of erectile function after aortoiliac reconstruction. *Arch Surg*. 1978;113(8):958–962.

193. Lederle FA, Johnson GR, Wilson SE, et al. Quality of life, impotence, and activity level in a randomized trial of immediate repair versus surveillance of small abdominal aortic aneurysm. *J Vasc Surg*. 2003;38(4):745–752.

194. Flanigan DP, Schuler JJ, Keifer T, et al. Elimination of iatrogenic impotence and improvement of sexual function after aortoiliac revascularization. *Arch Surg*. 1982;117(5):544–550.

195. Weinstein MH, Machleder HI. Sexual function after aorto-Iliac surgery. *Ann Surg*. 1975;181(6):787–790.

196. Pettersson M, Mattsson E, Bergbom I. Prospective follow-up of sexual function after elective repair of abdominal aortic aneurysms using open and endovascular techniques. *J Vasc Surg*. 2009;50(3): 492–499.

197. Olin JW, Graor RA, O'Hara P, Young JR. The incidence of deep venous thrombosis in patients undergoing abdominal aortic aneurysm resection. *J Vasc Surg*. 1993;18(6):1037–1041.

198. Williamson WK, Nicoloff AD, Taylor Jr LM, et al. Functional outcome after open repair of abdominal aortic aneurysm. *J Vasc Surg*. 2001;33(5):913–920.

199. Huber TS, Wang JG, Derrow AE, et al. Experience in the United States with intact abdominal aortic aneurysm repair. *J Vasc Surg*. 2001;33(2):304–310. discussion 10-11.

200. Crawford ES, Saleh SA, Babb 3rd JW, et al. Infrarenal abdominal aortic aneurysm: factors influencing survival after operation performed over a 25-year period. *Ann Surg*. 1981;193(6):699–709.

201. Hollier LH, Plate G, O'Brien PC, et al. Late survival after abdominal aortic aneurysm repair: influence of coronary artery disease. *J Vasc Surg*. 1984;1(2):290–299.

202. Koskas F, Kieffer E. Long-term survival after elective repair of infrarenal abdominal aortic aneurysm: results of a prospective multicentric study. Association for Academic Research in Vascular Surgery (AURC). *Ann Vasc Surg*. 1997;11(5):473–481.

203. Soreide O, Lillestol J, Christensen O, et al. Abdominal aortic aneurysms: survival analysis of four hundred thirty-four patients. *Surgery*. 1982;91(2):188–193.

204. Vohra R, Reid D, Groome J, et al. Long-term survival in patients undergoing resection of abdominal aortic aneurysm. *Ann Vasc Surg*. 1990;4(5):460–465.

205. Norman PE, Semmens JB, Lawrence-Brown MM, Holman CD. Long term relative survival after surgery for abdominal aortic aneurysm in western Australia: population based study. *BMJ*. 1998;317(7162): 852–856.

206. Stonebridge PA, Callam MJ, Bradbury AW, et al. Comparison of long-term survival after successful repair of ruptured and non-ruptured abdominal aortic aneurysm. *Br J Surg*. 1993;80(5):585–586.

207. Kazmers A, Perkins AJ, Jacobs LA. Aneurysm rupture is independently associated with increased late mortality in those surviving abdominal aortic aneurysm repair. *J Surg Res*. 2001;95(1):50–53.

208. Cho JS, Gloviczki P, Martelli E, et al. Long-term survival and late complications after repair of ruptured abdominal aortic aneurysms. *J Vasc Surg*. 1998;27(5):813–819. discussion 9-20.

209. Hertzer NR. Fatal myocardial infarction following abdominal aortic aneurysm resection. Three hundred forty-three patients followed 6-11 years postoperatively. *Ann Surg*. 1980;192(5):667–673.

210. Reigel MM, Hollier LH, Kazmier FJ, et al. Late survival in abdominal aortic aneurysm patients: the role of selective myocardial revascularization on the basis of clinical symptoms. *J Vasc Surg*. 1987;5(2):222–227.

613

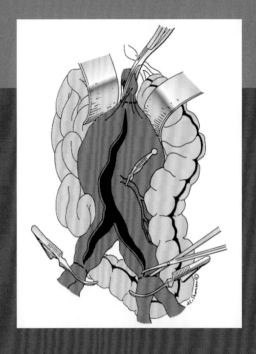

第38章
腹主动脉瘤的腔内修复术

　　虽然开放手术修复腹主动脉瘤取得了良好的疗效，但以微创的方法实现腹主动脉瘤修复始终还在不断探索。20世纪90年代，Parodi首次报道了主动脉瘤腔内修复术（endovascular aortic repair，EVAR）的应用。这种方法通过股动脉，置入腔内移植物，从而达到了瘤腔内隔绝动脉瘤的目的。作为里程碑式的事件，深深改变了当今腹主动脉瘤治疗的格局。历经几代腔内移植物的研发与测试，目前主动脉瘤腔内修复术已在临床上广泛应用。尽管手术适应证与开放手术相同，但主动脉瘤腔内修复术对患者的解剖条件却有着严格的要求，如何评估诸如瘤颈、直径、锚定区等解剖参数，如何选择适宜主动脉瘤腔内修复术的患者，将在本章内容中详细进行讨论。而作为治疗的核心，主动脉腔内支架移植物系统，也将被作为重点来详细阐述其结构组成、不同的性能特点等。尽管主动脉瘤腔内修复术减小了手术的创伤，但其特有的并发症和术后管理不容忽视。本章最后将详细分析内漏的产生原因、分类及治疗策略，以及其他一系列并发症防治的相关内容。

郭　伟

Endovascular Therapy for Abdominal Aortic Aneurysm

Alexander H. Shannon, Rishi A. Roy, and Gilbert R. Upchurch, Jr.

The surgical treatment of abdominal aortic aneurysms (AAAs) dates back centuries. Some of the initial approaches involved techniques similar, in some fashion, to modern endovascular techniques. In 1684, Moore reported on the use of large quantities of wire placed intraluminally into the aneurysm sac in order to induce thrombosis of AAA.[1] Later, electrical currents were passed through the wire to further promote thrombosis. A self-expanding endoluminally placed umbrella device was reported by Colt in the early 1900s to treat AAA.[2] In the mid-1900s, the use of endoluminally placed wire with the passage of electricity through it was revived and remained the procedure of choice until conventional operative therapy of AAA was introduced.[3] Operative repair of AAA evolved during the second half of the 20th century. Early techniques ranged from simple aortic ligation to aortic wrapping with cellophane.[4,5] Neither was successful. In 1951, the first replacement of an aortic aneurysm with an aortic homograft was described by Dubost.[6] However, homografts became aneurysmal over time and the procedure evolved to the use of prosthetic material to reconstruct the aorta.[7,8] This technique was later modified by Creech, who reported on endoaneurysmorrhaphy with intraluminal graft placement, leaving the aneurysm sac in situ[9]; this had become the mainstay of treatment until the mid-1990s.

Although excellent results have been obtained with conventional aneurysm repair, it remains a complex, challenging operation that initiates great physiologic stress for patients. The pursuit of a less invasive approach to AAA repair has subsequently evolved. Parodi and colleagues[10] reported the first use of endovascular aneurysm repair (EVAR). This approach allowed for the intraluminal exclusion of an aneurysm with the placement, through the femoral arteries, of an endograft. The hope was that this would decrease the morbidity and mortality of aneurysm repair and allow repairs to be performed in patients with significant comorbidities. The original endograft was constructed of a Dacron tube sutured to a Palmaz stent. Several generations of endografts have since been developed, tested, and put into general clinical use. With the evolution of aortic endografting, our knowledge about the pathophysiology of AAA has changed. Our understanding of the complexities of this mode of treatment is only just being realized and examined. This chapter reviews what is currently understood about endograft repairs of AAAs.

INDICATIONS

The indications for endovascular repair of an AAA remain the same as conventional repair with regard to the size of the aneurysm and its rate of growth. The classic teaching is that rupture rates for aneurysms depend on the size of the aneurysm. Rupture rates of 5% to 7% per year are estimated for aneurysms between 5 and 7 cm in diameter, and a greater than 20% rupture rate per year is estimated for larger aneurysms.[11] Surgical treatment for patients with these larger aneurysms significantly improves mortality compared with observation.[12] Although it is known that small aneurysms do have the potential to rupture, a recent meta-analysis looking at four randomized controlled trials (ADAM, UK small aneurysm trial, CAESAR, and PIVOTAL) demonstrated no advantage to early repair via open or endovascular surgery in men and women with asymptomatic AAA of diameter 4.0 to 5.5 cm. The authors recommend surveillance in this population.[13–15]

EVAR is a "less-invasive" technique than open surgery and offers several potential benefits over conventional AAA repair. It at most requires small femoral incisions instead of a large abdominal incision, which may decrease the incidence of postoperative pulmonary complications. The avoidance of extensive retroperitoneal dissection decreases the risk for perioperative bleeding. The period of aortic occlusion is minimal and accounts for the lower incidence of intraoperative hemodynamic and metabolic stress compared with patients undergoing open surgery.[16] Given these differences, endovascular aneurysm repair may be reasonable in patients who are "unfit" for conventional AAA surgery.[17] The durability of endovascular repair as a replacement for conventional surgery in relatively healthy patients has been proven by many clinical trials.[18]

ANATOMIC REQUIREMENTS

The exact anatomic requirements for placing an aortic endograft vary with device design. There are key aspects of each device and aortic anatomy to be aware of when assessing a patient as a potential candidate for endograft repair. Preprocedural imaging is paramount to properly assess the proximal and distal sites of fixation, as well as to assess the path the endograft will traverse before taking its postdeployment position.

Imaging

Successful endograft placement is completely dependent on adequate and accurate preoperative planning. One of the major elements distinguishing preoperative planning in open aneurysm repair from endovascular repair is the latter's increased dependency on imaging to provide information necessary for clinical decisions. Preprocedural imaging allows the surgeon to determine whether a patient is an acceptable candidate for endovascular aortic grafting and which device is best suited for a particular patient; this ultimately allows for determining the proper size of the endograft.

Historically, contrast aortography was used as a routine adjunct to axial imaging, as it was thought to allow for a more accurate determination of vessel length and angulation before CT reformatting was widely available. Preoperative angiography is now rarely employed and reserved for cases where an adjunctive therapeutic intervention (i.e., coil embolization) is necessary.[19] Recently, the advent of flat panel technology has allowed for the development of rotational angiography techniques that facilitate the construction of three-dimensional images found to be comparable to standard multidetector CTA. This technique has been termed C-arm cone-beam CT or FluoroCT. FluoroCT utilizes a modified C-arm with specialized software. This technique uses the spin rate of the C-arm around the gantry to acquire images. Most machines take between 6 and 8 seconds. To get good contrast imaging, it may require a large contrast bolus. This technology appears valuable in complicated aortic cases, such as fenestrated branched endovascular aneurysm repair, due to its ability to image graft to graft and graft to aorta apposition without the use of contrast.[20–22] However, concerns have developed regarding overall radiation doses delivered to patients and staff, due to pre-, intra-, and postoperative imaging and therefore FluoroCT is not routinely used.[23,24]

Spiral CT of the abdomen and pelvis is the mainstay of aortoiliac imaging. The imaging protocol is different from the standard protocol for most abdominal CT scans. Acquisition should use a 1:1.5 helical pitch and 3 to 5 mm collimation.[25] Slices of 1.5 mm are ideal for providing adequate information for stent graft planning. The two-dimensional (2-D) images, however, can often be misinterpreted. The axial images may "cut" vessels at an angle, particularly iliac arteries that have some degree of tortuosity—thus creating an ellipse as opposed to visualization of the true lumen diameter. Due to this problem, some physicians recommend three-dimensional (3-D) image processing as a better method to evaluate aortoiliac anatomy for endograft therapy.[26] Although it was common initially to perform an angiogram in addition to CT scan, recent evaluations suggest that high-quality 3-D CT scans alone may provide sufficient data for endovascular graft planning.[19,27] Currently, proprietary products for CT postprocessing provide the ability to evaluate the 3-D reconstruction of the aortoiliac system rapidly, rotate the images on the screen to obtain better vessel diameter measurements, and provide "virtual endograft" simulation.

Magnetic resonance angiography (MRA) can provide information similar to that of a CT scan. It, too, can provide thin-slice reconstructions and 3-D postprocessing. Its usefulness, however, is often limited by availability and physician expertise. MRA may provide a useful modality in patients in order to avoid the use of iodinated contrast agents. However, use of gadolinium-based contrast agents in MR is not without risk and may result in nephrogenic systemic fibrosis, and gadolinium deposition in bone and parts of the brain.[28]

Intravascular ultrasound (IVUS) is not routinely used in the preoperative evaluation of an endograft candidate. It is an invasive procedure, often performed at the time of angiography. Images produced by IVUS have a similar problem as viewing axial images on a 2-D CT scan. Unless the catheter remains centerline within the aorta, the images produced will be elliptical, which may also provide shorter than required length measurements. Its primary use is at the time of stent graft placement to assess graft position relative to the renal artery ostia; this can help to diminish the amount of contrast agent required.

Aortic Neck

The aortic neck is defined as the area of the aorta cephalad to the aneurysm in which the aortic endograft is placed (Fig. 38.1). This zone of the aorta is important for two reasons during aortic endografting. First, it is the site of proximal fixation that will prevent the device from migrating distally. Second, a circumferential seal must be obtained between the graft and the aorta in this area in order to prevent leakage of blood into the aneurysm sac. The exact length of aortic neck required is somewhat device dependent, but most commercially available devices require a 10- to 15-mm length of aortic neck below the level of the most caudal renal artery. Some investigational devices may allow for shorter

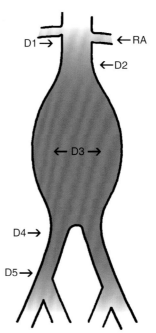

Fig. 38.1 Diagram Representing an Abdominal Aortic Aneurysm. D1 represents the diameter at the proximal aspect of the aortic neck, and D2 represents the diameter at the distal aspect of the aortic neck. The distance between D1 and D2, in general, must be 10 to 15 mm in order to adequately place an endograft. In addition, the difference between the diameter at D1 and D2 should not exceed 10%. D3 represents the aortic diameter. D4 and D5 represent the diameter within the common iliac artery where the distal fixation point of the aortic endograft occurs. The distance between D4 and D5 should also exceed 15 mm. RA is the left and, in this case, most caudal renal artery.

necks. One such device is the Medtronic Heli-FX EndoAnchor System, which is indicated for patients with aortic neck lengths <10 mm and >4 mm and <60-degree infrarenal angle. Prospective analysis of 1 year outcomes from 19 US and 3 EU sites demonstrated a rate of type Ia endoleak of 1.9%; however, these results come from a small-sample–size trial (n = 70).[29] The ANCHOR study demonstrated an overall rate of type Ia endoleak 9.9% in 202 patients who underwent EVAR for various indications.[30] Overall, EndoAnchors are useful in EVAR to prevent proximal site complications, and therefore has been given intent for use by the US Food and Drug Administration.

Additionally, several devices employ the use of a suprarenal, uncovered (or bare) stent to provide additional protection against graft migration. Suprarenal stent fixation may be useful, particularly in patients who have a shorter aortic neck, as it transfers protection against migration to a more normal segment of aorta. The suprarenal stent, however, does not provide any function with regard to creating a circumferential seal.

In addition to the length of the neck, other anatomic characteristics are important when determining whether patients are suitable candidates for endovascular aneurysm repair. These include aortic neck angulation, the shape of the neck, and the quality of the neck. Neck angulation refers to an alteration in the direction the aorta takes with regard to the centerline pathway. Acute angulation of the aortic neck can greatly affect the endograft's ability to obtain a proximal seal. Aortic neck angulation of greater than 60 degrees compared with the centerline is often considered prohibitive for endovascular aneurysm repair. There are devices undergoing preliminary trials that would allow for greater neck angulation, up to 90 degrees. The shape of the aortic neck also affects the ability of the graft to obtain a seal as well as fixation.

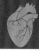

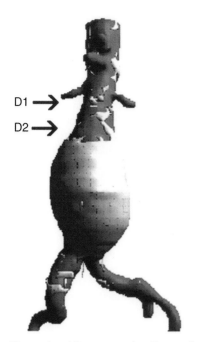

Fig. 38.2 Three-Dimensional Reconstruction From a Spiral CT Scan of an Abdominal Aortic Aneurysm. This is representative of a conical neck. The distance between D1 and D2 is 15 mm. The diameter at D1 is 23 mm and at D2 is 28 mm, representing a greater than 10% increase. The patient was not a suitable endograft candidate.

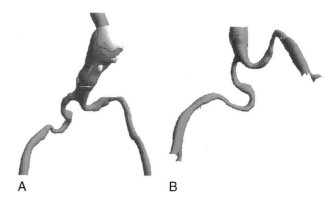

Fig. 38.3 Three-Dimensional Reconstruction From a Spiral CT Scan of an Abdominal Aortic Aneurysm. Note the tortuous iliac arteries (A). The degree of tortuosity may be underestimated in the direct anterior-posterior view, but on a more oblique angle (B) a more significant degree of tortuosity is visible.

A conical-shaped neck (Fig. 38.2) is generally thought to be unstable and predisposes to distal migration.[31] An increase in diameter from the top of the neck to the bottom of greater than 10% is often believed to be a contraindication to routine aortic endografting. The presence of circumferential thrombus or aortic calcification can also negatively affect an endograft's ability to obtain a proximal seal.

Iliac Arteries

The iliofemoral arterial system is important in endograft placement for two reasons. First, most endografts are placed through the common femoral artery and must traverse the iliofemoral system to reach the aorta. Iliac artery diameter and tortuosity can adversely affect the ease with which the endograft traverses this course. This topic is covered in more detail below. Certainly, the presence of significant atherosclerotic disease can cause arterial narrowing that inhibits the placement of the device. In addition, tortuosity of the iliac arteries can hinder placement of the grafts (Fig. 38.3). Second, the iliofemoral system is important because it is the site of the distal seal between the endograft and the iliac artery, preventing retrograde flow of blood into the aneurysm sac. Many of the features necessary for an adequate aortic neck are also necessary for the distal landing zone. The presence of thrombus, calcification, and tortuosity can significantly hinder the iliac limb seal. Ectatic or aneurysmal iliac arteries obviously affect the ability of the graft to seal against the iliac limb. Most available endograft systems require a femoral artery of 8 mm and common iliac artery diameter of 8 to 25 mm. Some endograft systems, such as Medtronic Endurant, require at least a 15-mm segment of iliac artery to be of adequate caliber and free of significant disease in order to obtain a distal seal, whereas others, such as Zenith from Cook Medical and Excluder from Gore, only require 10-mm distal landing zone.[32] If this is not present, adjunct interventions can be performed to assist in placing the device (i.e., iliac artery conduit placement or coil embolization of the internal iliac artery). Management of these complicated situations is discussed in more detail later.

ENDOGRAFT DESIGN

Endograft design can greatly affect the ability of the device to be placed in patients, particularly in patients with complex anatomy. Alterations in the characteristics of the grafts are what distinguish one manufacturer's device from another. Some of the key elements in endograft design are outlined as follows.

Delivery System

Standard endograft insertion involves placement of the device through an arteriotomy in the common femoral artery, from where the graft traverses the external iliac and common iliac arteries. The ability to deliver the endograft safely and effectively in this fashion is a prerequisite for effective repair. Three factors are important determinants of device delivery.[33]

Delivery System Size

With the placement of most endografts through the iliofemoral arterial system, any site along this pathway can represent a size limitation, the most common of which is the external iliac artery. Inadequate diameter or the presence of extensive calcifications can exclude standard endograft placement. It is intuitive that the size of the delivery system cannot be larger than the size of the iliac arteries that it traverses. Most sheaths are sized based on inner diameter, so knowledge of the outer diameter of the sheaths is therefore required for safe graft placement. Different manufacturer's devices have different size measurements for the delivery systems, and thus one device may be suitable for placement, whereas another is not. Most delivery systems easily traverse an iliofemoral segment of 7 to 8 mm in diameter (or a sheath that does not exceed 21 French [Fr] outer diameter), although several designs that provide a lower profile system are now available.[34,35] Lower profile delivery systems have allowed for the advent of totally percutaneous femoral artery access. A recent meta-analysis demonstrated no difference between percutaneous approach versus surgical cut-down for common femoral artery access including short-term mortality, aneurysm exclusion, wound infection, bleeding complications, and hematoma.[36]

Flexibility

Tortuosity, another anatomic variant, affects the ability to deliver adequately the endograft system. Tortuous iliac vessels can be "straightened" with the use of stiff guidewires, but this is not always possible or desirable. The ideal delivery system easily traverses these arteries on the basis of an intrinsic degree of flexibility. Again, different delivery systems have different abilities to track through tortuous iliac arteries, and thus some may be more successfully placed than others in this anatomic variant. Delivery systems composed of long, flexible, tapered tips pass more easily than those with short, stiff, blunt tips. In addition, other aspects of device construction, such as metallic struts that provide columnar strength, increase device rigidity and limit use in tortuous vessels.[33]

Deliverability

A number of features have been noted to affect the deliverability of endograft devices. As stated previously, long, flexible, tapered tips pass more easily than short, blunt, stiff ones. This allows for easier maneuverability through tortuous vessels, as well as past sites of narrowing. Larger-caliber devices are also more difficult to deliver, particularly in patients with smaller-diameter arteries.[33] Some delivery systems allow for the placement of the endograft system through alternate sheaths, whereas other systems necessitate the use of the manufacturer's own delivery system. This can greatly affect the placement of specific endografts in specific anatomic variants. A thorough understanding of the patient's arterial anatomy and the limitations of different endograft systems are important. The complexity of the delivery system also affects the ease with which it is placed. Some devices generally provide a simple maneuver to deploy the graft, whereas others have several complicated steps. However, there are some devices that allow for bareback device deployment without the use of sheath.

Endograft Features

The ideal endograft should be flexible enough to maneuver through tortuous and angulated vessels but also rigid enough to prevent kinking. It should have a low profile (having a small external diameter) that would allow it to be placed through as small of an arteriotomy as possible. Two general classifications of endografts exist: unibody and modular. A unibody device is a single-piece graft—including the main body and both limbs. Although this decreases the risk of endoleaks at the graft–graft interface, the unibody design often requires a larger delivery system and sizing can be more difficult. The modular system includes endografts that are composed of two to three pieces. Generally, there is a main body that may have one attached limb and one or two docking limbs. These devices can be introduced through smaller delivery systems and offer a greater degree of flexibility with regard to placement. With multiple sites of graft–graft interface, however, there is an increased risk of endoleak, as explained later.

Graft material is variable and can range from expanded polytetrafluorethylene to polyester. The graft material is typically supported by a metal framework, which is commonly stainless steel or its modified version, Elgiloy, or nitinol. The graft support can be placed inside the graft material (endoskeleton) or outside the graft (exoskeleton). Grafts can be fully supported, having stent material throughout, or only partially supported, with aspects of the device composed only of graft material and no metal. The graft skeleton provides several key elements to endograft makeup. First, it assists in graft fixation and in obtaining a seal. These stents provide some degree of radial force that helps to provide a seal, as well as providing a point of fixation. Most devices have hooks or barbs in the proximal aspect of the skeleton that help to anchor the graft onto the aortic wall and prevent migration. In addition, some devices employ metal framework that extends above the fabric and is used to engage the aorta in the pararenal or suprarenal location. The second function of the skeleton is to provide columnar strength, which may prevent graft migration. The skeleton can also prevent kinking and occlusion of limbs as they traverse the aortoiliac

anatomy. The lack of stents, however, may allow a graft to adapt more readily to morphological changes without dislocation of attachment sites. The interplay of the stent and fabric materials can lead to eventual erosion of the fabric.

Specific Grafts

Various endografts are currently commercially available or in clinical trials in the United States. A brief description of the currently commercially available endograft systems (in the United States) is outlined in Table 38.1 and depicted in Fig. 38.4.

GRAFT PLACEMENT AND POSTOPERATIVE MANAGEMENT

Once the patient is deemed an endograft candidate, the best graft has been chosen, and the device properly sized, the patient can undergo implantation. The majority of endografts are placed through the femoral arteries that have been operatively exposed. When choosing endograft placement through common femoral artery exposure, the majority of surgeons prefer the use of the transverse incision as it associated with a lower rate of wound complications (12.7% in transverse incision vs. 47.5% in vertical incisions).[37] Percutaneous access for EVAR has continued to grow in popularity. Suture-mediated closure devices facilitate this process, and using a "Preclose" technique has been described to allow closure of sheaths as large as 24-Fr.[38] Use of this procedure has been associated with 70% to 100% technical success, and immediate failures mandate surgical exploration of the femoral artery. Prospective analysis has demonstrated that use of a percutaneous approach may shorten operating times and reduce the rate of wound-related complications, without a significant increase in overall procedural cost.[38–40] The aorta is then cannulated with a guidewire and catheter. Small boluses of contrast agent are delivered to further define the anatomy and localize the renal arteries. With an angulated aorta, it is important to remember that the best view of the renal arteries and visualization of the fixation zone may not be in a direct anterior-posterior plane but at a more cranial-caudal angle. The device is then generally advanced over a stiff guidewire and correctly positioned to allow the most extensive coverage within the aortic neck without intruding on the orifice of the renal arteries. Each device has its own unique instruction for actual deployment. Once the main body and ipsilateral limb have been placed, the contralateral limb needs to be placed. The sequence of events for this varies depending on graft design—whether unibody or modular.

Recovery following EVAR is generally rapid and uncomplicated, and most patients are discharged home on the first or second postoperative day. Return to activities of daily living has been shown to be quicker following endovascular repair than open surgery. In addition, most patients report less postoperative pain. Aortic remodeling following EVAR, however, is a slow process that continues for several years. Anatomic changes in the native vessel, particularly at the proximal neck, can cause conformational changes in the implanted device which mandate close follow-up. In addition, late failures have been identified that have required reintervention.[41] Given these facts, routine surveillance following EVAR is universally recommended, although there are no standard regimens, and the requirements of a standard intensive regimen are debated. Nordon and colleagues performed a meta-analysis evaluating secondary intervention rates based on contemporary graft implants.[42] Their findings demonstrated that surveillance imaging alone initiated the secondary intervention in 1.4% to 9% of cases. Greater than 90% of EVAR cases, however, received no benefit from surveillance scans. Based on these findings, the group recommended that surveillance should be directed toward those patients identified

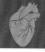

TABLE 38.1   Description of a Variety of Commercially Available Endografts

Company	Device	Initial FDA Approval Date	Deployment Type	Graft Material	Stent Material	Bifurcated Device Design	Main Body Sheath Size (OD)	Fixation
Cook (Bloomington, IN)	Zenith	May 2003	Self-expanding	Dacron	Stainless steel	Modular	21–26	Suprarenal
Cook (Bloomington, IN)	Zenith Fenestrated	April 2012	Self-expanding	Dacron	Stainless steel	Modular	20	Juxtarenal
Gore (Flagstaff, AZ)	Excluder	November 2002	Self-expanding	ePTFE	Nitinol	Modular	20–23	Infrarenal
Endologix (Irvine, CA)	Powerlink	October 2004	Self-expanding	High density ePTFE	Cobalt chromium alloy	Unibody	21	Anatomical (with either suprarenal or infrarenal proximal orientation)
Endologix (Irvine, CA)	AFX2	October 2015	Self-expanding	ePTFE	Cobalt chromium alloy	Modular	17	Anatomic (aortic bifurcation)
TriVascular (Santa Rosa, CA)	Ovation	November 2012	Self-expanding	PTFE	Nitinol	Tri-modular	15	Suprarenal
Lombard (Irvine, CA)	Aorfix	February 2015	Self-expanding	PTFE	Nitinol	Modular	22	Infrarenal, angulated neck
Cordis (San Francisco, CA)	INCRAFT	2014	Self-expanding	Polyester	Nitinol	Tri-modular	14	Suprarenal
Medtronic (Minneapolis, MN)	Endurant	May 2013	Self-expanding	Polyester	Electropolished nitinol	Modular	20	Suprarenal

ePTFE, Expanded polytetrafluoroethylene; *FDA,* US Food and Drug Administration; *PTFE,* polytetrafluoroethylene; *OD,* outer diameter.

as having a high-risk for postoperative complications. Identification of this group, however, is not obvious but may be necessary in patients with complicated aortic neck anatomy or in patients in whom the device was used outside of the indications for use (IFU).

Contrast-enhanced CT is the most widely used modality for follow-up after EVAR. It is widely available, has rapid data acquisition, reproducibility, and is uniform across institutions. The major concerns associated with its use are the use of contrast agent and the potential associated nephrotoxicity, radiation exposure, and cost. It is considered the gold standard for assessing aortic diameter with nearly a 100% sensitivity and specificity. The sensitivity and specificity rates for endoleak detection with CT are better than those with conventional angiography, at 92% and 90% for CT, versus 63% and 77% for angiography, respectively.[43–45] Triphasic CT (noncontrasted phase, arterial phase, and delayed phase) results in the greatest amount of information but at the cost of increased radiation exposure. Unenhanced CT imaging is useful for differentiation of endoleaks from calcifications from the metallic portion of a stent-graft, and can help detect small perigraft leaks compared with arterial-phase images. The use of arterial-phase alone has a lower diagnostic value compared to combined arterial and delayed-phase scanning.[46]

Repeated CT scanning exposes the patient to potential carcinogenic risks associated with ionizing radiation exposure. The estimated lifetime attributable risk of death from cancer following an abdominal CT scan in a patient greater than 50 years is 0.02%.[42,47] While this effect in itself is small, the cumulative effects over time with repeat imaging can be significant. Repetitive use of iodinated contrast can have a cumulative deleterious effect on renal function; especially in the elderly and those patients with preexisting renal impairment.[48] Given this, as well as the expense, the use of alternate modes of surveillance has been evaluated.

Magnetic resonance imaging (MRI) and MRA provide much of the same imaging information that can be acquired by CT scanning. Multiple format (T1, T2, gadolinium-enhanced) MR images can be viewed in 2-D and can be reformatted into 3-D volumes allowing dimensional measurements, assessment of luminal patency, device positioning, and the presence of an endoleak. Limitations of MRA/MRI include potential magnet-induced in vivo metallic heating or motion, which may prevent imaging in the immediate postimplant time period. In addition, postimplant artifacts, in particular with ferromagnetic metallic stents, will limit morphologic assessments. Furthermore, there is a risk of nephrogenic systemic fibrosis associated with gadolinium contrast use in patients with renal insufficiency.[49] Benefits of MR imaging are related to the lack of exposure to ionizing radiation and low nephrotoxicity of MR contrast medium. Disadvantages of MR are its lack of wide availability, longer procedure time than CT, patient claustrophobia, and contraindications for patients with cardiac pacemakers.

Color duplex ultrasonography (US) is a convenient, noninvasive, inexpensive portable means of postimplant surveillance. Its reliability as a useful surveillance tool, however, is still debated. Grayscale US is accurate for measurement of aortic aneurysm diameter. Endoleak detection by US requires color duplex. The reported specificity rates of color duplex US for endoleak detection are high (89% to 97%), but the sensitivity and diagnostic power of color duplex US for endoleak detection compared with CT is still debated.[50] The use of duplex US to detect an endoleak has a sensitivity of approximately 77%, with a specificity approaching 94%.[51] The addition of US contrast agents increases the sensitivity to 98%, with no significant change in the specificity.[51] The use of contrast agents is useful in identifying slow leaks that are not readily discernible on CT.[52,53] Detecting the flow direction of the endoleak is an advantage of US that is not easily discernable with CT.[54] The

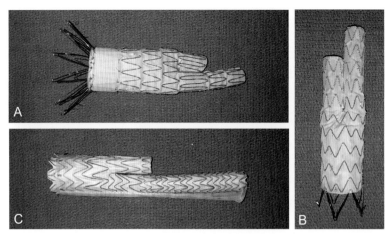

Fig. 38.4 Several Endograft Systems Illustrating Different Features. (A) The Zenith endograft represents a three-piece modular system with a main body and separate bilateral limbs. This graft design uses a bare suprarenal stent and internal stents at the sealing zones and is otherwise supported by a stainless steel Z-stent exoskeleton. (B) The Endurant stent graft system composed of nitinol exoskeleton. (C) The Excluder endograft, which represents a two-piece modular system. The graft is constructed from expanded polytetrafluoroethylene and is fully supported by a nitinol exoskeleton. ([A] Courtesy Cook, Inc., Bloomington, IN; [B] Courtesy Medtronic AVE, Santa Rosa, CA; [C] Courtesy WL Gore and Associates, Flagstaff, AZ.)

presence of a "to-and-fro" flow pattern is associated with spontaneous closure of the endoleak, while a monophasic or biphasic waveform is consistent with endoleak persistence.[54] Limitations of color duplex US include its operator dependence, variation based on patient physical size, and the need for optimal patient preparation. The substitution of duplex US imaging for CT, however, may result in long-term cost-savings.[55]

PROBLEMS WITH ENDOGRAFTING AND MANAGEMENT

Various problems can arise in the planning and placement of abdominal aortic endografts. Once the grafts are in place, several complications can arise over time that may require intervention to prevent the subsequent expansion and possible rupture of the previously excluded aneurysm. In the following section, several of the more common problems that occur following endograft placement are outlined.

Iliac Artery Disease

When iliac artery disease is present, whether it be aneurysmal disease, atherosclerotic disease, or severe tortuosity, the use of an iliac conduit can provide a safe route to deliver the endograft.[56] In the cases of iliac artery lumen narrowing resulting from atherosclerotic disease or increased vessel tortuosity, advancement of the device, despite the presence of resistance, can result in rupture of the iliac artery. Iliac artery rupture has been reported in 1% to 2% of cases.[57,58] To circumvent prohibitive iliac artery anatomy, an iliac conduit can be used. An iliac conduit involves suturing a prosthetic graft (generally 8 to 10 mm in diameter) to the mid–common iliac artery, even if it is aneurysmal. This can be done in an end-to-end or end-to-side fashion, although the latter often provides a greater lumen for passage of the device. The device is placed through the prosthetic graft, and the iliac limb of the endovascular graft traverses the common iliac artery and anastomosis and seals within the conduit. The distal end of the graft is tunneled along the natural course of the iliac artery and anastomosed to the femoral artery. The distal end of the common iliac artery is oversewn to allow retrograde flow through the external iliac artery to supply the

ipsilateral hypogastric artery. Alternatively, the hypogastric artery can be anastomosed directly to the conduit.

Iliac artery ectasia or aneurysms can present a problem in obtaining a distal seal. Enlarged common iliac arteries are present in up to 30% of patients presenting for endovascular aneurysm repair.[59-62] Newer endograft iliac limb options allow for ectatic iliac arteries up to a size in the range of 25 mm. As there are patients with ectatic or aneurysmal common iliac artery diameters beyond the IFU, distal seal may need to be obtained within the external iliac artery, which is often of normal caliber. If the distal seal occurs in the external iliac artery, the hypogastric artery is generally sacrificed using coil embolization. The presence of a hypogastric artery aneurysm would necessitate the same approach. Rarely, bilateral hypogastric artery embolization is required. Hypogastric artery embolization can occur before aneurysm repair or concurrently. If bilateral embolization is planned, it is generally performed in a staged fashion, although its occlusion is not always planned. Hypogastric artery embolization is not without risk, and side effects can occur in up to 50% of patients.[60] Buttock claudication is the predominant complaint after hypogastric artery occlusion. This occurs in 12% to 50% of the patients, but in most it generally resolves after several months.[59-64] Five percent to 25% of men complain of new-onset erectile dysfunction.[62,63] Buttock ischemia and bowel ischemia requiring resection are of theoretical concern, but they have not been described in any of the larger series. Patients requiring embolization in the more distal branches of the hypogastric artery (as might be done with the presence of an internal iliac artery aneurysm) and those in whom coil placement was not adequately controlled are at higher risk of developing pelvic symptoms.[64] Bilateral hypogastric artery embolization has not been associated with increased symptoms when compared with unilateral occlusion.[60,61,63] Coil embolization of the internal iliac artery is not necessary if it is not aneurysmal. In the face of common iliac artery aneurysms, Wyers and colleagues[65] have shown that if there is a 5-mm neck of iliac artery proximal to the hypogastric artery in addition to a 15-mm neck in the external iliac artery, coil embolization of the hypogastric artery is not necessary to obtain a distal seal. This may be possible in up to two-thirds of patients requiring coverage of the hypogastric artery.

Endoleaks

An endoleak is the persistence of blood flow outside the endograft, but in the aneurysm sac. Endoleaks are classified according to their etiology, and currently five types have been described (Table 38.2).[58,59] A type I endoleak (Fig. 38.5) arises from inadequate sealing at either the proximal aortic (allowing antegrade flow, Type IA) or distal iliac (allowing retrograde flow, type IB) attachment sites. Type II endoleaks (Fig. 38.6) arise from patent branch vessels off of the aortic sac that allow for retrograde flow into the aneurysm. Such branches may include a patent lumbar or inferior mesenteric artery. Type III endoleaks develop from defects in the fabric of the graft or at the junction zone between modular components. Type IV endoleaks develop secondary to diffuse "leaking" of blood between the interstices of the fabric or where the graft is sutured to a stent. Type V endoleaks describe a scenario in which the aneurysm sac remains pressurized and the aneurysm enlarges, but no demonstrable flow of blood into the sac can be visualized on current imaging modalities. These may be due to imaging that is not sophisticated enough to discern these leaks or due to intermittent episodes of leakage.[60] The pressure applied to the aneurysm sac causing it to continue to expand, in this situation, has been termed "endotension."[61,62] Controversy with regard to this concept exists, in particular with the ability of the thrombus to transmit pressure to the aneurysm wall. It is argued that these merely represent a type I, II, or III endoleak in

TABLE 38.2   Endoleak Classification

Endoleak	Cause	Blood Flow into Sac
Type I	Inadequate seal at aortic or iliac attachment sites	Antegrade or retrograde
Type II	Patent branches off aneurysm sac	Retrograde
Type III	Fabric defects or component junctions	Antegrade
Type IV	Leak at fabric interstices	Antegrade
Type V	Endotension	No clear leak

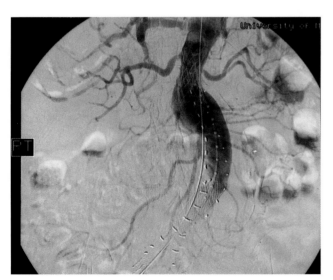

Fig. 38.5 Angiogram Demonstrating a Type I Endoleak. The contrast can be seen "leaking" around the proximal part of the graft and filling the aneurysm sac. The patient subsequently had a giant Palmaz stent placed in the aortic neck, and this ameliorated the endoleak.

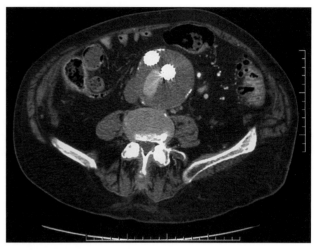

Fig. 38.6 CT Scan Representative of a Type II Endoleak. There is contrast within the aneurysm sac but outside of the limbs of the endograft. This aneurysm had continued expansion until the patient underwent embolization of the inferior mesenteric artery.

which the defect is large enough to allow blood to flow into the sac and transmit pressure to the sac, but the exit site is not present or too small to be detected.

Types I and III endoleaks are associated with significant risks of aneurysm enlargement and possible rupture, and these should be treated.[66,67] This may be accomplished with the placement of an extension cuff limb over the site of the leak. If the leak is a type I and the graft is juxtaposed to the inferior border of the renal arteries, a large balloon-expandable stent can be placed in the proximal aspect of the endograft. This provides increased radial force, causing better juxtaposition of the graft and aortic wall and thus ameliorating the leakage. If this is unsuccessful, open repair and graft explantation are generally indicated. Fabric tears are easily managed if the site of the leak is localized. In these situations, the tear can be covered with a cuff or extension. When it is more diffuse, the entire endograft can be relined with a second endograft, or the device can be removed and the aneurysm repaired in an open fashion.

Type II endoleaks are rarely associated with aneurysm rupture.[68] At least 10% to 15% of patients are identified with a type II endoleak during follow-up.[69–72] Warfarin treatment is not associated with an increased incidence of early or delayed postoperative endoleak, but type II endoleaks are less likely to undergo spontaneous resolution in these patients.[73] Type II endoleaks are generally observed unless they are associated with an increase in aneurysm size or are associated with aortic pulsatility on physical examination. In these situations, arteriography is the next step in order to identify the source of the endoleak. Superior mesenteric artery injection reveals retrograde inferior mesenteric artery flow as the source, whereas selective hypogastric artery injection demonstrates a lumbar artery filling the aneurysm. Super-selective arterial canalization can then be performed with embolization of the feeding vessels. Another approach is through direct aneurysm sac puncture.[74] With direct sac puncture, one can measure sac pressure and inject the sac directly with contrast agent to precisely identify the leak. The systolic sac pressure is related to the size of the leak, and the pulse amplitude is related to the resistance of the outflow vessels and sac compliance.[75] After localization of the leak, feeding vessels can be directly accessed and embolized.[76] In addition, the sac can be filled with substances such as coils, glue, or gel foam in order to further prevent flow. Differences in outcomes between these two different approaches has not been realized.[77]

Measurement of intrasac pressures may help determine if an endoleak is present at the time of the original surgery or if an endoleak has been adequately treated if it has been approached through direct sac puncture. In an ex vivo model of endoleaks, Parodi and colleagues[78] evaluated the pressure changes in the aortic sac with various types and sizes of endoleaks. In this model, sac pressures were significantly higher than systemic pressures in the presence of all endoleaks. This obviously places the aneurysm at significant risk for rupture. The presence of patent side branches significantly reduced the pressure within the sac, particularly the mean pressure and diastolic pressure. Clinically, persistent side branches augment the development of type II endoleaks and influence early sac behavior.[79,80] Gawenda and colleagues[81] evaluated the use of sac pressure monitoring and found it helpful in the detection and treatment of endoleaks. They noted, however, that intrasac pressure measurements did not correlate with AAA size change over ensuing follow-up. This may be an effective modality for monitoring aneurysms after endograft exclusion once less invasive methods of pressure measurement are developed.

Structural Failure

Material failure represents one of the most concerning problems for potential failure of endograft placement. This is a difficult event to identify, as patients are often asymptomatic and may not present with any acute changes in their endograft evaluation. Three modes of structural failure have been described in aortic endografting and involve fabric erosion, suture disruption, and metal fracture.[82]

The development of endoleaks secondary to graft erosion has been documented with some first-generation endograft devices (Fig. 38.7).[83,84] It has been speculated that the areas of graft erosion are secondary to friction between the stent material and the fabric, which

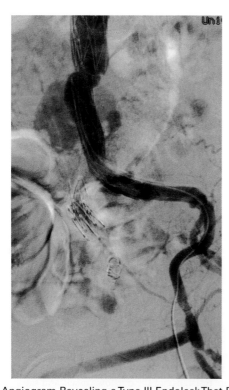

Fig. 38.7 Angiogram Revealing a Type III Endoleak That Developed at the Site of a Tear in the Graft Fabric. This was a "homemade" aorto-uniiliac graft that had been in place for approximately 5 years. The patient presented with new onset abdominal pain and had a CT scan that revealed an aneurysm sac that had significantly expanded in diameter. The tear was sealed by placement of a new endograft.

can be confounded by the pulsation of the aorta. Predicting the incidence of fabric fatigue is difficult, and although this does occur in grafts placed by conventional open aneurysm repair, it occurs much more rapidly and more commonly in the endograft systems.[85,86] In several device designs, the graft fabric is attached to the metal skeleton through the use of sutures. Disruption of these sutures is believed to explain graft failure in some instances.[87–89] The mechanism for suture failure is believed to be the same as for fabric erosion. Namely, motion of the stents with aortic pulsations causes friction and wear of the sutures with subsequent suture fracture.

The most common structural problem identified in aortic endograft systems has been metallic stent fractures.[86] Stent and hook fractures in the phase 1 trial of the Endovascular Technologie's graft resulted in suspension of the program and redesign of the metallic attachment system.[90] In a review of 686 patients who underwent endovascular aneurysm repair, Jacobs and colleagues[86] identified 60 patients who had material failure.[86] Forty-three (72%) of these failures were due to metallic stent fractures and occurred in various different endografts with different stent composition. The cause of metal failure has been attributed to stress fatigue and metal corrosion, particularly in nitinol stents.[91] Corrosion has not been seen in next-generation endografts and may reflect improved nitinol processing.[92–94] Tortuosity of the arterial system can also stress the stent graft system and lead to metal fracture.[95]

Fewer structural failures have been reported in second and third generation devices. Five-year outcomes from the Medtronic Endurant Stent graft system have been promising with good durability and minimal adverse events through 5 years.[96] The INNOVATION Trial looked at 4-year safety and effectiveness of INCRAFT AAA stent graft system by Cordis. Secondary reintervention rate at 1 year was 4.6%, and 97% of patients had no type I or III endoleaks or stent migration.[97] Similar results have been seen in the short term with the Endologix AFX2 and TriVascular Ovation abdominal stent grafts systems, although long-term results have yet to be reported.

Limb Thrombosis

Endograft limb thrombosis after endovascular repair of infrarenal AAA is a recognized complication in up to 11% of patients.[98–104] Various underlying factors have been purported to place patients at increased risk for limb thrombosis. One reported risk factor is the lack of device support. Although Carroccio and colleagues[99] reported on the results of 351 bifurcated grafts with no significant association between the use of unsupported devices and graft thrombosis, others have suggested there is a significant relationship. Baum and colleagues[105] specifically evaluated the rates of graft limb kinking and thrombosis between supported and unsupported abdominal aortic stent grafts. In total, 12% of the limbs in their series required an intervention for kinking. In the supported limbs, 5% required subsequent placement of arterial stents. Two percent required these for evidence of kinking at the time of the initial operation, whereas 3% required stenting in the postoperative period after the patients presented with limb thrombosis. In the unsupported grafts, there was an intervention rate of 44%. Approximately one-half of these had an additional stent placed at the time of the initial procedure, whereas the remainder had a subsequent stent placed in the postoperative follow-up period secondary to limb thrombosis or severe stenosis.

Another factor increasing the risk of limb thrombosis is oversizing of the iliac limb. Oversizing causes the graft material to have a significant amount of infolding, reducing the intraluminal diameter.[101] Along these lines, significant intraluminal vessel narrowing from underlying atherosclerotic disease or tortuosity can result in flow abnormalities and eventually cause graft limb thrombosis.[105] Extension of the graft limb into the external iliac artery has also been described as a risk factor for developing limb thrombosis.[99] It was believed that transition into the external iliac artery caused both a significant reduction in arterial diameter, as well as a kink in the graft due to acute angulation of the limb as it passed through the pelvis. Damage to the distal iliac or femoral artery, such as dissection during graft placement, can subsequently cause outflow obstruction and graft limb thrombosis.[98]

An additional factor is external compression of one or both limbs by calcific disease within the aorta. This compression results in luminal compromise with resultant thrombosis.

However, graft limb thrombosis does not appear to be associated with occlusion of the internal iliac artery. The internal iliac artery may be embolized intentionally if there is an aneurysm of the common iliac artery within 1 cm of the internal iliac, or unintentionally occluded due to trauma or coverage by an endograft. This may lead to a myriad of complications including colonic ischemia or disabling claudication, but does not appear to propagate aortic graft thrombus due to worsening outflow.[106]

Management of patients presenting with limb thrombosis depends on the severity of the patient's symptoms. In the series by Carroccio and colleagues,[99] nearly one-third of the patients presenting with symptoms had such mild symptoms that no intervention was required. Most patients in that study, however, underwent a femoral–femoral bypass to restore flow to the affected extremity. A more recent study by Oliveira and colleagues found that mural thrombus formation within the main body of the endograft did not appear to have an association with thromboembolic events over time, including limb thrombosis. Therefore they concluded a conservative approach of "watchful waiting" may be followed for known mural thrombus unless symptoms arise.[107] Few patients are successfully treated with thrombolysis or graft thrombectomy followed by endovascular repair of the underlying problem. In most series, patients with limb problems generally present early, within the first 6 months following endograft repair.[98,105,108–111] In fact, Sampram and colleagues[109] reported that no limb occlusions presented after 30 months of follow-up. In patients with possible limb compromise, IVUS is a useful tool to assess the luminal diameter and prompt index case intervention to possibly prevent limb thrombosis.

Migration

Distal stent-graft migration after abdominal aortic endografting has been reported to occur in 9% to 45% of patients.[72,112–115] Migration certainly has been identified as a risk for the development of a type I endoleak and delayed aneurysm rupture or late conversion to open repair.[116] The pathophysiology behind aortic endograft migration is complex, and various factors contribute to its occurrence.[117] A number of forces are at play within the aortic endograft, but blood flow acts as the main displacing force. As the tube of the aortic graft curves, there is a change in the velocity of the blood resulting in an increased displacement force. For many endografts, the forces providing protection against migration are friction forces of the graft against the aortic wall and the columnar strength of the graft. The friction forces depend on the apposition of the graft fabric and the aortic wall and obviously can be affected by the aortic wall composition (thrombus, calcifications), the size of the aorta, the radial force of the stent, and the nature of the graft fabric. It has been suggested that the presence of barbs or hooks in the proximal portion of the stent graft may provide additional protection.[118]

The infrarenal aortic neck length and its maximum diameter, shape, and angulation have all been implicated as causes of stent graft migration.[112,116,119,120] All of these work to decrease the friction between the stent graft and aortic wall. Albertini and colleagues[119] evaluated the

development of proximal perigraft endograft leak and device migration following endovascular aneurysm repair. Fifteen patients had graft migration, and 31 of 184 repairs developed a proximal endoleak. Neck angulation was the only factor found to be significant in the development of device migration, whereas neck angulation and neck diameter were the two factors important in developing a proximal perigraft endoleak.[119] Lee and colleagues,[121] however, were not able to identify any specific anatomical correlate and device migration. They did observe, however, that any device that migrated distally by more than 1 cm subsequently required an intervention.

Other hypotheses as to the cause of device migration have focused on the morphologic changes in the aneurysm and the aortic neck after EVAR. Specifically, aortic neck dilation, longitudinal sac shrinkage, and graft shortening have been described.[112,113,122,123] One of the more widely accepted hypotheses is aortic neck dilation following aortic endografting. After endovascular aneurysm repair, the aneurysm neck has been documented to dilate significantly, mostly in the first 2 years after graft placement.[124] In a review by Cao and colleagues,[115] 17 (15%) of 113 patients had an episode of device migration. The only two independent risk factors for device migration were neck dilation postoperatively and an AAA diameter of greater than 55 mm. Others have argued that neck dilation is not a significant event provided adequate graft oversizing was performed at initial endograft placement.[121] The amount to which the aortic neck dilated did not exceed the size of the original aortic endograft placed. Larger aneurysms have also been noted to have increased risks of developing type I endoleak, graft migration, and the subsequent need for open surgical conversion compared with larger aneurysms.[125]

OUTCOMES

Results of Aortic Endografting

Elective EVAR generally has a low mortality rate (1% to 3%) compared with open repair, and subsequent rates of aneurysm rupture after endovascular repair are reduced to 1% per year.[67,72,109,126] Endograft placement is not free of adverse events, however, and there is not an infrequent need for secondary interventions. Naslund and colleagues[127] reported technical complications in 26% of 34 endografts placed. Fairman and colleagues evaluated the occurrence of critical events during the deployment of their initial 75 endografts, and patients were divided into three groups corresponding to the time period in which the graft was placed.[110] Critical events were defined as unanticipated technical difficulties that occurred during the course of operation that threatened the success of the procedure. Difficulty in obtaining access occurred in nearly one quarter of all patients. Although it would be expected that the latter 25 patients should not have experienced as great a difficulty in obtaining access, these patients had increased complexity of their aortoiliac anatomy compared with endograft patients earlier in their experience. This group had a greater frequency of iliac artery balloon angioplasty, as well as the use of iliac artery conduits. Deployment difficulties existed and were composed mostly of graft foreshortening, necessitating the placement of additional distal covered extensions. Other deployment issues encountered included suprarenal graft displacement, infrarenal graft displacement, and device-related issues, such as iliac limb kinking or twisting. Malplacement of the graft did not correlate with anatomic complexity.

The need for subsequent secondary procedures has been evaluated by several large series of patients who had an abdominal aortic endograft placed.[102,109,128,129] The Eurostar registry reported the results of 1023 patients with a follow-up of 12 months or longer.[128] Overall,

186 (18%) patients required a secondary intervention. The majority of these interventions (76%) involved a transfemoral procedure, whereas the remaining patients required transabdominal (12%) or extra-anatomic (11%) surgery. The rates of freedom from intervention at 1, 3, and 4 years were 89%, 67%, and 62%, respectively. The transfemoral procedures performed most frequently were aortic or iliac limb extension for graft migration or endoleak. Late death was more frequent in those patients requiring a secondary intervention resulting in a 3-year cumulative survival of 85%, which is lower than the 90% rate ($P < .05$) observed in those that did not require reintervention. In addition, death was more frequently associated with those requiring a transabdominal procedure.

The Montefiore Medical Center and the Cleveland Clinic Foundation have published their single institution results on the durability of aortic endografting. Montefiore reported on 239 endografts placed over 9 years, with a technical success rate of 88.7%.[102] The 5-year survival rate in this group was only 37%. Secondary interventions were required in 10% of the patients, with more than half of the secondary procedures being performed for the presence of an endoleak. Sampram and colleagues[109] reported the results from the Cleveland Clinic Foundation on 703 patients undergoing endovascular aortic endografting with follow-up averaging 1 year. Survival in this group was 90% at 1 year and declined to 70% at 3 years. Overall, 128 secondary interventions were performed in 105 patients (15%). Freedom from intervention mirrored that of the Eurostar registry with freedom from intervention rates of 88%, 76%, and 65% at 1, 2, and 3 years, respectively. Mortality related to the secondary procedure was 8% but rose to 18% in those requiring a transabdominal procedure. Univariate analysis revealed that secondary procedures were more common in patients with larger major and minor sac axes, in patients who received a large aortic stent because of a proximal endoleak present at initial aneurysm repair, and in patients who received treatment later in the course of the review. This latter finding is thought to be secondary to the increased complexity of cases approached in an endovascular fashion.

The Cleveland Clinic Foundation review included the use of six different devices, which included two Zenith grafts—one that was part of the multicenter national trial and one group that was part of a sponsor-investigator investigational device exemption trial.[33] The overall freedom from risk of rupture was 98.7% at 2 years. The results of this review reveal that there are significant differences in outcomes between groups with different endovascular devices, in particular with regard to limb occlusion and rate of endoleak. Limb occlusion occurred most frequently with the Ancure device at a rate of 11% at 2 years. Endoleak of any kind was most common with the Excluder device at a rate of 64% at 1 year. Modular separations were the most frequent with the Zenith graft at 3.5%. Aneurysm sac shrinkage correlated inversely with the frequency of endoleaks, and aneurysm sac shrinkage was most common in the Zenith and Talent groups but least common in the Excluder group. There were no differences with regard to rate of secondary procedures, conversion to open repair, or migration. Sternbergh and colleagues[130] have reported similar findings. Outcomes were compared between the Zenith device and the AneuRx device, and it was determined that the Zenith graft was associated with fewer endoleaks and a higher rate and amount of aneurysm sac shrinkage. Bertges and associates[131] also reported similar findings in their evaluation. Regression of AAA size after endograft placement was more significant after placement of the Talent and Ancure endografts compared with the AneuRx or Excluder devices. During the first 2 years of follow-up the initial size of the AAA, the presence of an endoleak, and the type of graft used were significant predictors of sac shrinkage. After 2 years, however, only graft type was significant.

Ouriel and colleagues[125] have additionally concluded that the outcome after EVAR depends on the initial size of the aneurysm.

Comparison With Open Surgery

EVAR has been shown to be associated with lower postoperative morbidity, shorter length of hospital stay, and quicker return to normal function.[132] Direct comparison to open surgery, utilizing randomized prospective trials, however, has only recently been available for evaluation. There have been three randomized prospective trials evaluating the use of EVAR compared with open surgery. The EVAR 1 trial enrolled 1082 patients with AAA who were healthy enough to be suitable candidates for surgery.[132] They were randomized to either EVAR or open repair. Results from this trial demonstrated that the 30-day mortality rate was lower after EVAR (1.7%) compared to open surgery (4.7%, $P < .0001$). At 4-years follow-up, the aneurysm-related mortality rate in the EVAR group was half that in the open group ($P = .04$), but there was no difference in all cause-mortality (26% for the EVAR group and 29% for the open group). The Dutch Randomized Endovascular Aneurysm Management (DREAM) trial was a prospective, randomized trial that enrolled 351 patients. As in EVAR 1, the 30-day mortality rate was lower in patients who underwent endovascular repair compared with those that underwent open surgical reconstruction, but the 2-year outcomes were similar between the two groups. In addition, the results of the Open Versus Endovascular Repair (OVER) Veterans Affairs Cooperative Study Group results have been reported.[133] In this trial, 881 patients suitable for open or EVAR were randomized to one of the two surgical techniques. As with the other two trials, 30-day mortality was lower in the EVAR arm (0.5%) compared with the open surgery (3.0%, $P = .004$). This difference, however, resolved by 2-year follow-up time points (7.0% vs. 9.8%, respectively). Patients undergoing EVAR had shorter hospital stays, shorter operative durations, and required fewer blood transfusions, but they had increased exposure to fluoroscopy and contrast. Given its promising initial results, it is not surprising that EVAR has become increasingly popular over the past decade with both patients and providers.

One of the most controversial aspects of AAA repair, however, is when to perform EVAR and when to perform conventional open surgery. Open surgical repair of AAA has long been considered the gold standard, and there is evidence that this option provides good long-term durability.[134,135] Longer-term outcomes from both EVAR 1 and DREAM have been reported.[41,136] For EVAR 1,[41] the median follow-up was 6 years (5- to 10-year range), and at follow-up the overall aneurysm-related mortality was 1.0 deaths per 100 person-years in the EVAR group and 1.2 deaths per 100 person-years in the open repair group ($P = .73$). All-cause mortality was 7.2 deaths per 100 person-years (EVAR) and 7.1 deaths per 100 person-years (open surgery). Graft-related complication rates were higher in the EVAR group (12.6 per 100 person-years) compared to the open surgical arm (2.5 per 100 person-years, $P < .001$), and significantly more patients in the EVAR group required reintervention (5.1 per 100 person-years vs. 1.7 per 100 person-years, $P < .001$). In fact, new graft-related complications and reinterventions were reported for as long as 8 years following EVAR. For DREAM,[136] at a median follow-up of 6.4 years (5.1–8.2 years), cumulative survival rates were 69.9% for open repair and 68.9% for EVAR ($P = .97$). The cumulative rates of freedom from secondary interventions were 81.9% for the open repair group and 70.4% for EVAR ($P = .03$). Based on this data, it is clear that EVAR is not without its drawbacks. These factors may change as the technology improves and as we gain a better understanding of the long-term implications of placing an endovascular graft in the aorta.

While initial applications of EVAR were geared toward patients consider high risk for conventional surgery, this concept has come under some scrutiny after the results of the EVAR 2 trial.[137] In this trial, the outcomes of 404 patients with large AAAs (≥5.5 cm in diameter), who were considered to be physically ineligible for open repair were evaluated. Of this cohort, 197 patients were assigned to undergo endovascular repair, while 207 were assigned to have no intervention. The 30-day operative mortality rate for the EVAR group was 7.3%, while the overall rate of aneurysm rupture in the observation group was 12.4 per 100 person-years. While aneurysm-related mortality was lower in the endovascular-repair group, this did not provide any advantage when evaluating all-cause mortality, and during follow-up, EVAR required a considerable increase in expense. These results called into question the appropriateness of using EVAR in high-risk patients. The results, however, have been refuted by others demonstrating lower rates of perioperative mortality and better long-term survivals in these high-risk patients.[138] These improved outcomes are likely due to an aggressive, multidisciplinary approach to managing these patients' comorbidities.

OTHER CONSIDERATIONS

Endovascular Repair for Small Abdominal Aortic Aneurysms

Randomized prospective trials have demonstrated that there is no benefit to open repair of AAA for aneurysms that are less than 5.5 cm in diameter.[139,140] Operative mortality rates of 2.7% and 5.8% in these two trials raised the question of whether a procedure with lower operative mortality might provide benefit compared with observation in patients with smaller AAA. The Positive Impact of Endovascular Options for Treating Aneurysms Early (PIVOTAL) trial sought to evaluate whether endovascular repair of small AAA (4 to 5 cm) might provide a survival advantage compared with surveillance.[141] In this trial, 728 patients were randomly assigned to EVAR (N = 366) versus ultrasound surveillance (N = 362). Of the patients randomized to EVAR, 89% underwent repair, while of those assigned to surveillance 31% subsequently underwent repair during the course of the study (mean follow-up 20 ± 12 months, range 0 to 41 months). The unadjusted hazard ratio (95% confidence interval) for mortality after EVAR was 1.01 (0.49 to 2.07, P = .98), with 15 deaths (4.1%) occurring in each group. No survival advantage was demonstrated with EVAR. Similar findings were found in a recent meta-analysis looking at four randomized controlled trials (ADAM, UK small aneurysm trial, CAESAR, and PIVOTAL) demonstrated no advantage to early repair via open or endovascular surgery in men and women with asymptomatic AAA of diameter 4.0 to 5.5 cm. The authors recommend surveillance in this population.[14] It is important to note, however, women tend to rupture with smaller aortic diameters compared to men; however the diameter of the aneurysm at the time of rupture was 5.7 cm.[142]

Endovascular Treatment of Ruptured Abdominal Aortic Aneurysms

With the wide-spread application of EVAR for repair of AAA, its use in the repair of ruptured AAA has similarly expanded. Initially, there were several limitations to the application of this technology to treat the devastating problem of ruptured AAA: (1) unavailability of preoperative CT in patients with ruptured AAA; (2) unavailability of a dedicated operating room and ancillary staff equipped to perform emergent EVAR at all times; (3) unavailability of off-the-shelf stent grafts; and (4) the lack of data from multicenter randomized trials.[143] Many centers have developed protocols that allow the treatment teams to overcome these hurdles and provide emergent care for ruptured AAA with endovascular devices.[143–146] Gerassimidis and colleagues[144] reported on

the treatment of 69 patients with a ruptured AAA. Of these, 42 patients (63%) were suitable for EVAR. The in-hospital and 30-day mortality rates were 36% and 41%, respectively. Veith and colleagues[146] reported the worldwide experience with treating ruptured AAA with endovascular grafts. Data was collected from 49 centers, at which 1037 patients were treated with EVAR for ruptured AAA. Overall 30-day mortality was 21%, which was significantly lower than the 30-day mortality rate for the 763 patients undergoing open repair (36%, P < .001) for ruptured AAA at these same institutions during the same time period. Given these experiences, there is a trend toward even more centers instituting a program of EVAR for ruptured AAA. Certainly longer-term follow-up and larger series will be required to assess whether EVAR has ultimately affected outcomes from ruptured AAA.

Fenestrated and Branched Aortic Endografts

The most common reason for excluding patients from EVAR is the lack of a suitable proximal implantation site between the renal arteries and the aneurysm. Although commercially available devices provide a mechanism for supplementing fixation within the suprarenal aorta without detrimentally affecting renal function,[147] such a practice has not been advocated for the treatment of juxtarenal aneurysms. Despite evidence of short-term success with the treatment of short necks with devices intended to treat infrarenal aneurysms,[148] the risk of later failure remains high.[149] To overcome this fenestrated stent-graft technology was developed. The devices used currently are hybrids of original abdominal devices. The primary goal of treating an aneurysm with a fenestrated graft is to move the sealing and fixation region of the repair into healthy aorta with a parallel neck and without wall defects. A fenestration (hole in the graft) allows the stent graft to occupy this more proximal location while providing for transgraft flow to the renal arteries (or other significant branches) (Fig. 38.8). It is designed to incorporate the minimum number of visceral vessels required to achieve fixation and seal within healthy aorta. The fenestrations are constructed to match the ostial diameter of the visceral vessels and maximize the sealing zone. Several large series of fenestrated endograft deployments have been reported demonstrating the mid-term safety and efficacy of fenestrated stent grafting.[150–152] One of the largest series is reported by O'Neill and colleagues.[150] They outline a series of 119 patients with mean follow-up of 19 months. There was only one perioperative death, and survival at 12, 24, and 36 months was 92%, 83%, and 79%, respectively. The 30-day endoleak rate was 10%, and all endoleaks were type II in nature. Regression of the aneurysm sac was noted in 79% of the patients by 12 months. Complications related to the renal arteries was noted in 10 of the 231 stented renal arteries, and only one patient who did not have significant renal dysfunction preoperatively went on to require dialysis. Incorporation of the renal arteries raises questions about the effect of fenestrated stent-graft repair on long-term renal function.

Application of fenestrated technology has advanced to allow for the treatment of thoracoabdominal aortic aneurysms (TAAAs) in which the aneurysm involves the renal and visceral vessels. When treating TAAA with an endograft, however, the use of a simple fenestration is not adequate. Unlike fenestrated grafts where a hole in the graft suffices, in more complex aneurysms, such as TAAA, the branch arteries arise from the aneurysm. In this scenario blood flow has to be carried from the endograft, across the aneurysm and to the target vessel—without extravasation into the aneurysm (Fig. 38.9). There are two modes by which this can be assured. The first is the fenestrated branched stent graft[153] or reinforced fenestrated graft (see Fig. 38.8).[154] In this style, the addition of a covered bridging stent converts a fenestrated stent graft into a form of branched stent graft.[155] Sealing between

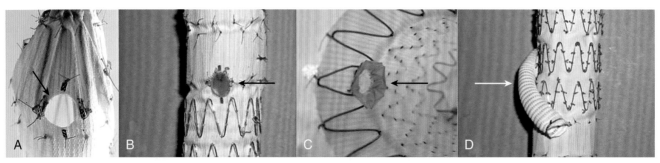

Fig. 38.8 Example of an endograft with (A) a fenestration *(arrow)* within the body of the endograft to accommodate a renal artery; (B) a reinforced fenestration *(arrow)* that allows for the placement of a (C) covered stent graft creating a form of a branched endograft for the treatment of a thoracoabdominal aortic aneurysm; and (D) a true directional branch *(arrow)* used to allow for continued flow to a visceral vessel when treating a thoracoabdominal aortic aneurysms.

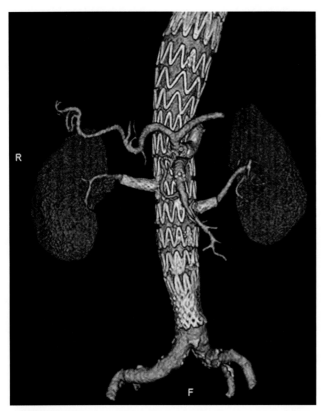

Fig. 38.9 Example of a thoracoabdominal aortic aneurysm that has been treated with a branched endograft that incorporates all of the visceral vessels.

the covered stent and the fenestration is tenuous because there is very limited overlap of material. A nitinol ring is added to the fenestration to reinforce the site of interaction between the covered stent and the fenestration. These are termed "reinforced" fenestrations. The second mode of branched graft design is the cuffed branched stent grafts[156] or directional branched stent grafts (see Fig. 38.8).[154] The cuff or branch creates an overlap zone between the stent graft and the branch artery. It provides a segment of overlap that can be used to provide better sealing and fixation than the thin joint between a reinforced fenestration and mating visceral stent graft. A longer overlap affords one the ability to use a self-expanding stent graft rather than a balloon-expandable stent graft. This may provide a means to better accommodate tortuosity and diameter discrepancies and may limit type I endoleaks and component separation from this region.

Investigators tend to pool results of both fenestrated branch grafts and cuffed branched grafts, with few series containing significant numbers of patients.[157–163] The largest single-center experience has been reported by the Cleveland Clinic. Greenberg et al.[161] performed a retrospective analysis on patients who underwent elective open surgical repair (N = 372) or endovascular repair (N = 352) of descending thoracic or TAAAs. The group of patients treated with endovascular repair was older and had more comorbid conditions than those undergoing open repair. Open repair, however, was more frequently applied to patients with type II or type III aneurysms and those that were associated with a chronic dissection. Despite the differences in patient age and comorbid conditions, mortality rates at 30 days (5.7% vs. 8.3%) and 12 months (15.6% vs. 15.9%) were not different between endovascular repair and surgical repair, nor was there a difference in the development of spinal cord ischemia (4% vs. 8%, respectively, P = .08). Bakoyiannis et al. performed a meta-analysis of all English-language literature published between 2000 and 2009 on endovascular procedures using fenestrated and/or branched technology.[163] The results of this analysis demonstrated that complex endografting can be performed with a technical success rate of 94% with a 30-day mortality of 7%. Typically, these procedures were performed in patients who were deemed high risk for conventional surgery. The 1-year mortality was 1.3%. The application of fenestrated and branched technology is very much in its infancy. As the technology progresses, we will be able to better discern who will best benefit from these procedures, and ultimately replace open surgery with this less invasive option.

SUMMARY

Abdominal aortic endografting provides a less invasive method of treating AAA. It provides a beneficial way of treating aneurysms in patients who are at high risk for conventional open surgical repair, and results of randomized trials suggests, at least in the short term, it provides clinical equipoise with conventional surgery. The durability of this procedure is still under evaluation. It is likely, however, that the application of endovascular technology will replace current open surgical options and ultimately the entire aortic tree will be treated with endovascular options.

REFERENCES

1. Criado FJ, Barnatan MF, Lingelbach JM, et al. Abdominal aortic aneurysm: overview of stent-graft devices. *J Am Coll Surg.* 2002;194(1 Suppl):S88.
2. Power D. Palliative treatment of aneurysms by wiring with Colt's apparatus. *Br J Surg.* 1927;9:27.

3. Blakemore A, King B. Electrothermic coagulation of aortic aneurysms. *JAMA*. 1938;111:1821.

4. Matas R. Ligation of the abdominal aorta: report of the ultimate result. 1 year, 5 months and 9 days after the ligation of the abdominal aorta for aneurysm of the bifurcation. *Ann Surg*. 1925;81:457.

5. Rea C. Surgical treatment of aneurysm of the abdominal aorta. *Minn Med*. 1948;31:153.

6. Dubost C, Allary M, Oeconomos N. Resection of an aneurysm of the abdominal aorta: resection of the continuity by a preserved arterial graft, with result after five months. *Arch Surg*. 1952;64:405.

7. Voorhees A, Jaretski A, Blakemore A. Use of tubes constructed from Vinyon "N" cloth in bridging arterial defects: a preliminary report. *Ann Surg*. 1952;135:322.

8. Edwards W, Tapp J. Chemically treated nylon tubes as arterial grafts. *Surgery*. 1955;38:61.

9. Creech O. Endo-aneurysmorrhaphy and treatment of aortic aneurysm. *Ann Surg*. 1966;164:935.

10. Parodi J, Palmaz J, Barone H. Transfemoral intraluminal graft implantation for abdominal aortic aneurysms. *Ann Vasc Surg*. 1991;5:491.

11. Ernst C. Abdominal aortic aneurysm. *N Engl J Med*. 1993;1993:1167.

12. Szilagyi D, Smith R, DeRusso F, et al. Contributions of abdominal aortic aneurysmectomy to prolongation of life. *Ann Surg*. 1966;164:678.

13. United Kingdom Small Aneurysm Trial Participants. Long-term outcomes of immediate repair compared with surveillance of small abdominal aortic aneurysms. *N Engl J Med*. 2002;346:1445.

14. Filardo G, Powell JT, Martinez MA, Ballard DJ. Surgery for small asymptomatic abdominal aortic aneurysms. *Cochrane Database Syst Rev*. 2015;(2):CD001835.

15. Cronenwett J, Johnston K. The United Kingdom Small Aneurysm Trial: implications for surgical treatment of abdominal aortic aneurysms. *J Vasc Surg*. 1999;29:191.

16. Baxendale B, Baker D, Hutchinson A, et al. Haemodynamic and metabolic response to endovascular repair of infra-renal aortic aneurysms. *Br J Anaesth*. 1996;77:581.

17. Laheij RJ, Van Marrewijk CJ. Endovascular stenting of abdominal aortic aneurysm in patients unfit for elective open surgery. Eurostar group. EUROpean collaborators registry on Stent-graft Techniques for abdominal aortic Aneurysm Repair. *Lancet*. 2000;356(9232):832.

18. Nordon IM, Thompson MM, Loftus IM. Are concerns about EVAR durability relevant with modern devices? *J Cardiovasc Surg (Torino)*. 2013;54(2):181–189.

19. Beebe H, Kritpracha B, Serres S, et al. Endograft planning without preoperative arteriography: a clinical feasibility study. *J Endovasc Ther*. 2000;7(8).

20. Eide K, Odegard A, Myhre H, et al. DynaCT during EVAR—a comparison with multidetector CT. *Eur J Endovasc Surg*. 2009;37:23.

21. Dijkstra ML, Eagleton MJ, Greenberg RK, et al. Intraoperative C-arm cone-beam computed tomography in fenestrated/branched aortic endografting. *J Vasc Surg*. 2011;53(3):583–590.

22. Nordon I, Hinchcliffe R, Malkawi A, et al. Validation of DynaCT in the morphological assessment of abdominal aortic aneurysm for endovascular repair. *J Endovasc Ther*. 2010;17:183.

23. Liu Y, Castro M, Lederlin M, et al. Edge-preserving denoising for intra-operative cone beam CT in endovascular aneurysm repair. *Comput Med Imaging Graph*. 2017;56:49–59.

24. Mohapatra A, Greenberg RK, Mastracci TM, et al. Radiation exposure to operating room personnel and patients during endovascular procedures. *J Vasc Surg*. 2013;58(3):702–709.

25. Beebe H, Kritpracha B. Imaging of abdominal aortic aneurysm: current status. *Ann Vasc Surg*. 2003;17:111.

26. Beebe H, Jackson T, Pigott J. Aortic aneurysm morphology for planning endovascular aortic grafts: limitations of conventional imaging methods. *J Endovasc Surg*. 1995;2:139.

27. Truijers M, Resch T, Van Den Berg JC, et al. Endovascular aneurysm repair: state-of-art imaging techniques for preoperative planning and surveillance. *J Cardiovasc Surg (Torino)*. 2009;50:423.

28. Fraum TJ, Ludwig DR, Bashir MR, Fowler KJ. Gadolinium-based contrast agents: a comprehensive risk assessment. *J Magn Reson Imaging*. 2017;46(2):338–353.

29. EVAR with Endoanchor Fixation for Short AAA Necks (<10 mm and >4 mm) Endurant II Stent Graft Systems. (October 2017). Retrieved from http://www.medtronic.com/us-en/healthcare-professionals/products/cardiovascular/aortic-stent-grafts/endurantii/endoanchor.html.

30. de Vries JP, Ouriel K, Mehta M, et al. Analysis of EndoAnchors for endovascular aneurysm repair by indications for use. *J Vasc Surg*. 2014;60(6):1460–1467.

31. Resch T, Ivancev K, Brunkwall J, et al. Distal migration of stent-grafts after endovascular repair of abdominal aortic aneurysms. *J Vasc Interv Radiol*. 1999;10(3):257–264.

32. England A, McWilliams R. Endovascular aortic aneurysm repair (EVAR). *Ulster Med J*. 2013;82(1):3–10.

33. Ouriel K. Endovascular repair of abdominal aortic aneurysms: the Cleveland Clinic experience with five different devices. *Semin Vasc Surg*. 2003;16(2):88–94.

34. de Donato G, Setacci F, Sirignano P, et al. Ultra-low profile Ovation device: is it the definitive solution for EVAR? *J Cardiovasc Surg (Torino)*. 2014;55(1):33–40.

35. Moulakakis KG, Dalainas I, Kakisis J, et al. Current knowledge on EVAR with the ultra-low profile Ovation Abdominal Stent-graft System. *J Cardiovasc Surg (Torino)*. 2012;53(4):427–432.

36. Gimzewska M, Jackson AI, Yeoh SE, Clarke M. Totally percutaneous versus surgical cut-down femoral artery access for elective bifurcated abdominal endovascular aneurysm repair. *Cochrane Database Syst Rev*. 2017;2:CD010185.

37. Swinnen J, Chao A, Tiwari A, et al. Vertical or transverse incisions for access to the femoral artery: a randomized control study. *Ann Vasc Surg*. 2010;24:336–341.

38. Lee W, Brown M, Nelson P, Huber T. Total percutaneous access for endovascular aortic aneurysm repair ("Preclose" technique). *J Vasc Surg*. 2007;45:1095–1101.

39. McDonnell C, Forlee M, Dowdall J, et al. Percutaneous endovascular abdominal aortic aneurysm repair leads to a reduction in wound complications. *Ir J Med Sci*. 2008;177:49–52.

40. Smith S, Timaran C, Valentine R, et al. Percutaneous access for endovascular abdominal aortic aneurysm repair: can selection criteria be expanded? *Ann Vasc Surg*. 2009;23:621–626.

41. The United Kingdom EVAR Trial Investigators. Endovascular versus open repair of abdominal aortic aneurysm. *N Engl J Med*. 2010;362:1863–1871.

42. Nordon I, Karthikesalingam R, Hinchliffe R, et al. Secondary interventions following endovascular aneurysm repair (EVAR) and the enduring value of graft surveillance. *Eur J Endovasc Surg*. 2010;39:547–554.

43. Armerding M, Rubin G, Beaulieu C, et al. Aortic aneurysmal disease: assessment of stent-graft treatment—CT versus conventional angiography. *Radiology*. 2000;215:138–146.

44. Rozenblit A, Marin M, Veith F, et al. Endovascular repair of abdominal aortic aneurysm: value of postoperative follow-up with helical CT. *Am J Roentgenol*. 1995;165:1473–1479.

45. Gorich J, Rlinger N, Sokirnaski R, et al. Leakages after endovascular repair of aortic aneurysms: classification based on findings at CT, angiography, and radiography. *Radiology*. 1999;213:767–772.

46. Buth J, Harris P, Marrewijk C. Causes and outcomes of open conversion and aneurysm rupture after endovascular abdominal aortic aneurysm repair: can type II endoleaks be dangerous? *J Am Coll Surg*. 2002;194:S98–S102.

47. Brenner D, Hall E. Computed tomography—an increasing source of radiation exposure. *N Engl J Med*. 2007;357:2277–2284.

48. Solomon R, DuMouchel W. Contrast media and nephropathy: findings from systematic analysis and food and drug administration reports of adverse effects. *Invest Radiol*. 2006;41:651–660.

49. Broome D, Giguis M, Baron P, et al. Gadodiamide-associated nephrogenic systemic fibrosis: why radiologists should be concerned. *Am J Roentgenol*. 2007;189:586–592.

50. Sun Z. Diagnostic value of color duplex ultrasonography in the follow-up of endovascular repair of abdominal aortic aneurysm. *J Vasc Interv Radiol*. 2006;17:759–764.

51. Mirza T, Karthikesalingam A, Jackson D, et al. Duplex ultrasound and contrast-enhanced ultrasound versus computed tomography for the detection of endoleak after EVAR: systematic review and bivariate meta-analysis. *Eur J Vasc Endovasc Surg*. 2010;39:418–428.

52. Napoli V, Bargellini I, Sardella S, et al. Abdominal aortic aneurysm: contrast-enhanced US for missed endoleaks after endoluminal repair. *Radiology*. 2004;233:217–225.

53. Henao E, Hodge M, Felkai D, et al. Contrast-enhanced duplex surveillance after endovascular abdominal aortic aneurysm repair: improved efficacy using a continuous infusion technique. *J Vasc Surg*. 2006;43:259–264.

54. Parent F, Meier G, Godziachvili V, et al. The incidence and natural history of type I and II endoleak: a 5-year follow-up assessment with 1 color duplex ultrasound scan. *J Vasc Surg*. 2002;35:474–481.

55. Beeman B, Doctor L, Doerr K, et al. Duplex ultrasound imaging alone is sufficient for midterm endovascular aneurysm repair surveillance: a cost analysis study and prospective comparison with computed tomography scan. *J Vasc Surg*. 2009;50:1019–1024.

56. Yao O, Faries P, Morrissey N, et al. Ancillary techniques to facilitate endovascular repair of aortic aneurysms. *J Vasc Surg*. 2001;34:69.

57. Zarins CK. The US AneuRx Clinical Trial: 6-year clinical update 2002. *J Vasc Surg*. 2003;37(4):904–908.

58. May J, White G, Waugh R, et al. Improved survival after endoluminal repair with second-generation prostheses compared with open repair in the treatment of abdominal aortic aneurysms: a 5-year concurrent comparison using life table method. *J Vasc Surg*. 2001;33:S21–S26.

59. Lee WA, O'Dorisio J, Wolf YG, et al. Outcome after unilateral hypogastric artery occlusion during endovascular aneurysm repair. *J Vasc Surg*. 2001;33(5):921–926.

60. Wolpert LM, Dittrich KP, Hallisey MJ, et al. Hypogastric artery embolization in endovascular abdominal aortic aneurysm repair. *J Vasc Surg*. 2001;33(6):1193–1198.

61. Criado FJ, Wilson EP, Velazquez OC, et al. Safety of coil embolization of the internal iliac artery in endovascular grafting of abdominal aortic aneurysms. *J Vasc Surg*. 2000;32(4):684–688.

62. Schoder M, Zaunbauer L, Holzenbein T, et al. Internal iliac artery embolization before endovascular repair of abdominal aortic aneurysms: frequency, efficacy, and clinical results. *AJR Am J Roentgenol*. 2001;177(3):599–605.

63. Mehta M, Veith F, Ohki T, et al. Unilateral and bilateral hypogastric artery interruption during aortoiliac aneurysm repair in 154 patients: a relatively innocuous procedure. *J Vasc Surg*. 2001;33:S27–S32.

64. Kritpracha B, Pigott JP, Price CI, et al. Distal internal iliac artery embolization: a procedure to avoid. *J Vasc Surg*. 2003;37(5):943–948.

65. Wyers MC, Schermerhorn ML, Fillinger MF, et al. Internal iliac occlusion without coil embolization during endovascular abdominal aortic aneurysm repair. *J Vasc Surg*. 2002;36(6):1138–1145.

66. Zarins CK, White RA, Hodgson KJ, et al. Endoleak as a predictor of outcome after endovascular aneurysm repair: AneuRx multicenter clinical trial. *J Vasc Surg*. 2000;32(1):90–107.

67. Holzenbein T, Kretschmer G, Thurnher S, et al. Midterm durability of abdominal aortic aneurysm endograft repair: a word of caution. *J Vasc Surg*. 2001;33:S46–S54.

68. Buth J, Harris PL, Van MC, Fransen G. The significance and management of different types of endoleaks. *Semin Vasc Surg*. 2003;16(2):95–102.

69. Chuter TA, Faruqi RM, Sawhney R, et al. Endoleak after endovascular repair of abdominal aortic aneurysm. *J Vasc Surg*. 2001;34(1):98–105.

70. Buth J, Laheji R. Early complications and endoleaks after endovascular abdominal aortic aneurysm repair: report of a multicenter study. *J Vasc Surg*. 2000;31:134–146.

71. Dattilo JB, Brewster DC, Fan CM, et al. Clinical failures of endovascular abdominal aortic aneurysm repair: incidence, causes, and management. *J Vasc Surg*. 2002;35(6):1137–1144.

72. Zarins C. The US AneuRx clinical trial: 6-year clinical update 2002. *J Vasc Surg*. 2003;37:904–908.

73. Fairman R, Carpenter J, Baum R, et al. Potential impact of therapeutic warfarin treatment on type II endoleaks and sac shrinkage rates on midterm follow-up examination. *J Vasc Surg*. 2002;35:679.

74. Baum RA, Carpenter JP, Cope C, et al. Aneurysm sac pressure measurements after endovascular repair of abdominal aortic aneurysms. *J Vasc Surg*. 2001;33(1):32–41.

75. Marty B, Sanchez LA, Ohki T, et al. Endoleak after endovascular graft repair of experimental aortic aneurysms: does coil embolization with

76. Baum R, Cope C, Fairman R, et al. Translumbar embolization of type 2 endoleaks after endovascular repair of abdominal aortic aneurysms. *J Vasc Interv Radiol*. 2001;12:111–116.

77. Stavropoulos S, Park J, Fairman R, Carpenter J. Type 2 endoleak embolization comparison: translumbar embolization versus modified transarterial embolization. *J Vasc Interv Radiol*. 2009;20:1299–1302.

78. Parodi J, Berguer R, Ferreira L, et al. Intra-aneurysmal pressure after incomplete endovascular exclusion. *J Vasc Surg*. 2001;33:909.

79. Back MR, Bowser AN, Johnson BL, et al. Patency of infrarenal aortic side branches determines early aneurysm sac behavior after endovascular repair. *Ann Vasc Surg*. 2003;17(1):27–34.

80. Fan CM, Rafferty EA, Geller SC, et al. Endovascular stent-graft in abdominal aortic aneurysms: the relationship between patent vessels that arise from the aneurysmal sac and early endoleak. *Radiology*. 2001;218(1):176–182.

81. Gawenda M, Heckenkamp J, Zaehringer M, Brunkwall J. Intra-aneurysm sac pressure—the holy grail of endoluminal grafting of AAA. *Eur J Vasc Endovasc Surg*. 2002;24(2):139–145.

82. Jacobs T, Teodorescu V, Morrissey N, et al. The endovascular repair of abdominal aortic aneurysm: an update analysis of structural failure modes of endovascular stent grafts. *Semin Vasc Surg*. 2003;16(2):103–112.

83. Stelter W, Umscheid T, Ziegler P. Three-year experience with modular stent-graft devices for endovascular AAA treatment. *J Endovasc Surg*. 1997;4(4):362–369.

84. Beebe HG. Lessons learned from aortic aneurysm stent graft failure; observations from several perspectives. *Semin Vasc Surg*. 2003;16(2):129–138.

85. Riepe G, Loos J, Imig H, et al. Long-term in vivo alterations of polyester vascular grafts in humans. *Endovasc Surg*. 1997;13:540.

86. Jacobs TS, Won J, Gravereaux EC, et al. Mechanical failure of prosthetic human implants: a 10-year experience with aortic stent graft devices. *J Vasc Surg*. 2003;37(1):16–26.

87. Alimi YS, Chakfe N, Rivoal E, et al. Rupture of an abdominal aortic aneurysm after endovascular graft placement and aneurysm size reduction. *J Vasc Surg*. 1998;28(1):178–183.

88. Riepe G, Heilberger P, Umscheid T, et al. Frame dislocation of body middle rings in endovascular stent tube grafts. *Eur J Vasc Endovasc Surg*. 1999;17(1):28–34.

89. Krajcer Z, Howell M, Dougherty K. Unusual case of AneuRx stent-graft failure two years after AAA exclusion. *J Endovasc Ther*. 2001;8(5):465–471.

90. Moore W, Rutherford R. Transfemoral endovascular repair of abdominal aortic aneurysm: results of the North American EVT phase I trial. *J Vasc Surg*. 1996;34:353.

91. Heintz C, Riepe G, Birken L, et al. Corroded nitinol wires in explanted aortic endografts: an important mechanism of failure? *J Endovasc Ther*. 2001;8(3):248–253.

92. Trepanier C, Tabrizian M, Yahia L, et al. Effect of modification of oxide layer on NiTi stent corrosion resistance. *J Biomed Mater Res (Appl Biomater)*. 1998;43:433.

93. Duerig T, Pelton A, Stockel D. An overview of nitinol medical applications. *Mater Sci Eng*. 1999;A273-275:149.

94. Starosvetsky E, Gotman I. Corrosion behavior of titanium nitride coated Ni-Ti shape memory surgical alloy. *Biomaterials*. 2001;22:1853.

95. Skibba AA, Evans JR, Greenfield DT, et al. Management of late main-body aortic endograft component uncoupling and type IIIa endoleak encountered with the Endologix Powerlink and AFX platforms. *J Vasc Surg*. 2015;62(4):868–875.

96. Singh MJ, Fairman R, Anain P, et al. Final results of the Endurant Stent Graft System in the United States regulatory trial. *J Vasc Surg*. 2016;64(1):55–62.

97. Pratesi G, Pratesi C, Chiesa R, et al. The INNOVATION Trial: four-year safety and effectiveness of the INCRAFT® AAA Stent-Graft System for endovascular repair. *J Cardiovasc Surg (Torino)*. 2017;58(5):650–657.

98. Fairman R, Baum R, Carpenter J, et al. Limb intervention in patients undergoing treatment with an unsupported bifurcated aortic endograft system: a review of the phase II EVT trial. *J Vasc Surg*. 2002;36:118–126.

angiographic "seal" lower intraaneurysmal pressure? *J Vasc Surg*. 1998;27(3):454–461.

99. Carroccio A, Faries P, Morrissey N, et al. Predicting iliac limb occlusion after bifurcated aortic stent grafting: anatomic and device-related causes. *J Vasc Surg*. 2002;36:679–684.

100. Baum R, Shetty S, Carpenter J, et al. Limb kinking in supported and unsupported abdominal aortic stent-grafts. *J Vasc Interv Radiol*. 2000;11:1165–1171.

101. Amesur NB, Zajko AB, Orons PD, Makaroun MS. Endovascular treatment of iliac limb stenoses or occlusions in 31 patients treated with the Ancure endograft. *J Vasc Interv Radiol*. 2000;11(4):421–428.

102. Ohki T, Veith FJ, Shaw P, et al. Increasing incidence of midterm and long-term complications after endovascular graft repair of abdominal aortic aneurysms: a note of caution based on a 9-year experience. *Ann Surg*. 2001;234(3):323–334.

103. Carpenter JP, Neschis DG, Fairman RM, et al. Failure of endovascular abdominal aortic aneurysm graft limbs. *J Vasc Surg*. 2001;33(2):296–302.

104. Cao P, De RP, Verzini F, Parlani G. Endoleak after endovascular aortic repair: classification, diagnosis and management following endovascular thoracic and abdominal aortic repair. *J Cardiovasc Surg (Torino)*. 2010;51(1):53–69.

105. Baum RA, Shetty SK, Carpenter JP, et al. Limb kinking in supported and unsupported abdominal aortic stent-grafts. *J Vasc Interv Radiol*. 2000;11(9):1165–1171.

106. Karch LA, Hodgson KJ, Mattos MA, et al. Adverse consequences of internal iliac artery occlusion during endovascular repair of abdominal aortic aneurysms. *J Vasc Surg*. 2000;32(4):676–683.

107. Oliveira NF, Bastos Gonçalves FM, Hoeks SE, et al. Clinical outcome and morphologic determinants of mural thrombus in abdominal aortic endografts. *J Vasc Surg*. 2015;61(6):1391–1398.

108. Carroccio A, Faries PL, Morrissey NJ, et al. Predicting iliac limb occlusions after bifurcated aortic stent grafting: anatomic and device-related causes. *J Vasc Surg*. 2002;36(4):679–684.

109. Sampram ES, Karafa MT, Mascha EJ, et al. Nature, frequency, and predictors of secondary procedures after endovascular repair of abdominal aortic aneurysm. *J Vasc Surg*. 2003;37(5):930–937.

110. Fairman RM, Velazquez O, Baum R, et al. Endovascular repair of aortic aneurysms: critical events and adjunctive procedures. *J Vasc Surg*. 2001;33(6):1226–1232.

111. Conners III M, Sternbergh III W, Carter G, et al. Secondary procedures after endovascular aortic aneurysm repair. *J Vasc Surg*. 2002;36:992.

112. Resch T, Ivancev K, Brunkwall J, et al. Distal migration of stent-grafts after endovascular repair of abdominal aortic aneurysms. *J Vasc Interv Radiol*. 1997;10:257–264.

113. Harris P, Vallabhaneni S, Desgranges P, et al. Incidence and risk factors of late rupture, conversion, and death after endovascular repair of infrarenal aortic aneurysms: the EUROSTAR experience. *J Vasc Surg*. 2000;32:739–749.

114. Albertini N, Kalliafas S, Travis S, et al. Anatomical risk factors for proximal perigraft endoleak and graft migration following endovascular repair of abdominal aortic aneurysms. *Eur J Endovasc Surg*. 2000;19:308–312.

115. Cao P, Verzini F, Zannetti S, et al. Device migration after endoluminal abdominal aortic aneurysm repair: analysis of 113 cases with a minimum follow-up period of 2 years. *J Vasc Surg*. 2002;35(2):229–235.

116. Cao P, Verzini F, Zannetti S, et al. Device migration after endoluminal abdominal aortic aneurysm repair: analysis of 113 cases with a minimum follow-up period of 2 years. *J Vasc Surg*. 2002;35:229–235.

117. Lawrence-Brown M, Semmens J, Hartley D, et al. How is durability related to patient selection and graft design with endoluminal grafting for abdominal aortic aneurysm? In: Greenhalgh R, ed. *Durability of Vascular and Endovascular Surgery*. London: WB Saunders; 1999:375–385.

118. Resch T, Malina M, Lindblad B, Ivancev K. The impact of stent-graft development on outcome of AAA repair—a 7-year experience. *Eur J Vasc Endovasc Surg*. 2001;22(1):57–61.

119. Albertini J, Kalliafas S, Travis S, et al. Anatomical risk factors for proximal perigraft endoleak and graft migration following endovascular repair of abdominal aortic aneurysms. *Eur J Vasc Endovasc Surg*. 2000;19(3):308–312.

120. Malina M, Lindblad B, Ivancev K, et al. Endovascular AAA exclusion: will stents with hooks and barbs prevent stent-graft migration? *J Endovasc Surg*. 1998;5(4):310–317.

121. Lee J, Lee J, Aziz I, et al. Stent-graft migration following endovascular repair of aneurysms with large proximal necks: anatomical risk factors and long-term sequalae. *J Endovasc Ther*. 2002;9:652–664.

122. White G, May J, Waugh R, et al. Shortening of endografts during deployment in endovascular AAA repair. *J Endovasc Ther*. 1999;6:4.

123. Prinssen M, Wever J, Mali W, et al. Concerns for the durability of the proximal abdominal aortic aneurysm endograft fixation from a 2-year and 3-year longitudinal tomography angiography study. *J Vasc Surg*. 2001;33:S64–S69.

124. Badran MF, Gould DA, Raza I, et al. Aneurysm neck diameter after endovascular repair of abdominal aortic aneurysms. *J Vasc Interv Radiol*. 2002;13(9 Pt 1):887–892.

125. Ouriel K, Srivastava SD, Sarac TP, et al. Disparate outcome after endovascular treatment of small versus large abdominal aortic aneurysm. *J Vasc Surg*. 2003;37(6):1206–1212.

126. Becker G, Kovacs M, Mathison M, et al. Risk stratification and outcomes of transluminal endografting for abdominal aortic aneurysm: 7-year experience and long-term follow-up. *J Vasc Interv Radiol*. 2003;12:1033–1046.

127. Naslund TC, Edwards Jr WH, Neuzil DF, et al. Technical complications of endovascular abdominal aortic aneurysm repair. *J Vasc Surg*. 1997;26(3):502–509.

128. Laheji R, Buth J, Harris P, et al. Need for secondary interventions after endovascular repair of abdominal aortic aneurysms. Intermediate-term follow-up results of a European collaborative registry (EUROSTAR). *Br J Surg*. 2000;87:1666.

129. May J, White G, Waugh R, et al. Life-table analysis and assisted success following endoluminal repair of abdominal aortic aneurysms: the role of supplementary endovascular intervention in improving outcome. *Eur J Vasc Endovasc Surg*. 2000;19:648.

130. Sternbergh III W, Conners M, Tonnessen B, et al. Aortic aneurysm sac shrinkage after endovascular repair is device-dependent: a comparison of Zenith and AneuRx endografts. *Ann Vasc Surg*. 2003;17:49.

131. Bertges D, Chow K, Wyers M, et al. Abdominal aortic aneurysm size regression after endovascular repair is endograft dependent. *J Vasc Surg*. 2003;37:716.

132. EVAR Trial Participants. Endovascular aneurysm repair versus open repair in patients with abdominal aortic aneurysm (EVAR trial 1): randomised controlled trial. *Lancet*. 2005;365:2179.

133. Lederle F, Freischlag J, Kyriakides T, et al. Outcomes following endovascular vs open repair of abdominal aortic aneurysm. A randomized trial. *JAMA*. 2009;302:1535–1542.

134. Hallet Jr J, Marshall D, Petterson T, et al. Graft-related complications after abdominal aortic aneurysm repair: reassurance from a 36-year population-based experience. *J Vasc Surg*. 1997;25:277–284.

135. Conrad M, Crawford R, Pedraza J, et al. Long-term durability of open abdominal aortic aneurysm repair. *J Vasc Surg*. 2007;46:669–675.

136. De Bruin J, Baas A, Buth J, et al. Long-term outcome of open or endovascular repair of abdominal aortic aneurysm. *N Engl J Med*. 2010;362:1881–1889.

137. The United Kingdom EVAR Trial Investigators. Endovascular repair of aortic aneurysm in patients physically ineligible for open repair. *N Engl J Med*. 2010;362(20):1872–1880.

138. Sobocinski J, Maurel B, Delsart P, et al. Should we modify our indications after the EVAR-2 trial conclusions? *Ann Vasc Surg*. 2011;25(5):590–597.

139. Lederle F, Wilson S, Johnson G, et al. Immediate repair compared with surveillance of small abdominal aneurysms. *N Engl J Med*. 2002;346:1437–1444.

140. Powell J, Brown L, Forbes J, et al. Final 12-year follow-up of surgery versus survillance in the UK small aneurysm trial. *Br J Surg*. 2007;94:702–708.

141. Ouriel K, Clair D, Kent C, Zarins C. Endovascular repair compared with surveillance for patients with small abdominal aortic aneurysms. *J Vasc Surg*. 2010;51:1081–1087.

142. Lo RC, Bensley RP, Hamdan AD, et al. Gender differences in abdominal aortic aneurysm presentation, repair, and mortality in the Vascular Study Group of New England. *J Vasc Surg*. 2013;57(5):1261–1268.

143. Mehta M, Taggert J, Darling III RC, et al. Establishing a protocol for endovascular treatment of ruptured abdominal aortic aneurysms: outcomes of a prospective analysis. *J Vasc Surg*. 2006;44(1):1–8.

144. Gerassimidis TS, Karkos CD, Karamanos DG, et al. Endovascular management of ruptured abdominal aortic aneurysms: an 8-year single-centre experience. *Cardiovasc Intervent Radiol.* 2009;32(2):241–249.

145. Starnes B, Quiroga E, Hutter C, et al. Management of ruptured abdominal aortic aneurysm in the endovascular era. *J Vasc Surg.* 2010;51:9–18.

146. Veith F, Lachat M, Mayer D, et al. Collected world and single center experience with endovascular treatment of ruptured abdominal aortic aneurysms. *Ann Vasc Surg.* 2009;250:818–824.

147. Greenberg RK, Chuter TA, Sternbergh III WC, Fearnot NE. Zenith AAA endovascular graft: intermediate-term results of the US multicenter trial. *J Vasc Surg.* 2004;39(6):1209–1218.

148. Greenberg R, Fairman R, Srivastava S, et al. Endovascular grafting in patients with short proximal necks: an analysis of short-term results. *Cardiovasc Surg.* 2000;8(5):350–354.

149. Waasdorp EJ, de Vries JP, Hobo R, et al. Aneurysm diameter and proximal aortic neck diameter influence clinical outcome of endovascular abdominal aortic repair: a 4-year EUROSTAR experience. *Ann Vasc Surg.* 2005;19(6):755–761.

150. O'Neill S, Greenberg RK, Haddad F, et al. A prospective analysis of fenestrated endovascular grafting: intermediate-term outcomes. *Eur J Vasc Endovasc Surg.* 2006;32(2):115–123.

151. Greenberg RK, Sternbergh III WC, Makaroun M, et al. Intermediate results of a United States multicenter trial of fenestrated endograft repair for juxtarenal abdominal aortic aneurysms. *J Vasc Surg.* 2009;50(4):730–737.

152. Greenberg RK, Haulon S, O'Neill S, et al. Primary endovascular repair of juxtarenal aneurysms with fenestrated endovascular grafting. *Eur J Vasc Endovasc Surg.* 2004;27(5):484–491.

153. Chuter TA. Fenestrated and branched stent-grafts for thoracoabdominal, pararenal and juxtarenal aortic aneurysm repair. *Semin Vasc Surg.* 2007;20(2):90–96.

154. Greenberg R. Aortic aneurysm, thoracoabdominal aneurysm, juxtarenal aneurysm, fenestrated endografts, branched endografts, and endovascular aneurysm repair. *Ann NY Acad Sci.* 2006;1085:187–196.

155. Anderson J, Adam D, Berce M, Hartley D. Repair of thoracoabdominal aortic aneurysms with fenestrated and branched endovascular stent grafts. *J Vasc Surg.* 2005;42:600–607.

156. Chuter TA. Fenestrated and branched stent-grafts for thoracoabdominal, pararenal and juxtarenal aortic aneurysm repair. *Semin Vasc Surg.* 2007;20(2):90–96.

157. Anderson JL, Adam DJ, Berce M, Hartley DE. Repair of thoracoabdominal aortic aneurysms with fenestrated and branched endovascular stent grafts. *J Vasc Surg.* 2005;42(4):600–607.

158. Chuter TA. Fenestrated and branched stent-grafts for thoracoabdominal, pararenal and juxtarenal aortic aneurysm repair. *Semin Vasc Surg.* 2007;20(2):90–96.

159. Chuter TA, Rapp JH, Hiramoto JS, et al. Endovascular treatment of thoracoabdominal aortic aneurysms. *J Vasc Surg.* 2008;47(1):6–16.

160. Roselli EE, Greenberg RK, Pfaff K, et al. Endovascular treatment of thoracoabdominal aortic aneurysms. *J Thorac Cardiovasc Surg.* 2007;133(6):1474–1482.

161. Greenberg R, Lu Q, Roselli E, et al. Contemporary analysis of descending thoracic and thoracoabdominal aneurysm repair. A comparison of endovascular and open techniques. *Circulation.* 2008;118(8):808–817.

162. Vourliotakis G, Bos WT, Beck AW, et al. Fenestrated stent-grafting after previous endovascular abdominal aortic aneurysm repair. *J Cardiovasc Surg (Torino).* 2010;51(3):383–389.

163. Bakoyiannis CN, Economopoulos KP, Georgopoulos S, et al. Fenestrated and branched endografts for the treatment of thoracoabdominal aortic aneurysms: a systematic review. *J Endovasc Ther.* 2010;17(2):201–209.

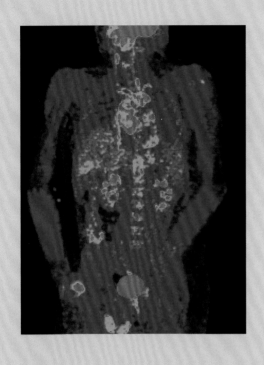

Vasculitis

血管炎

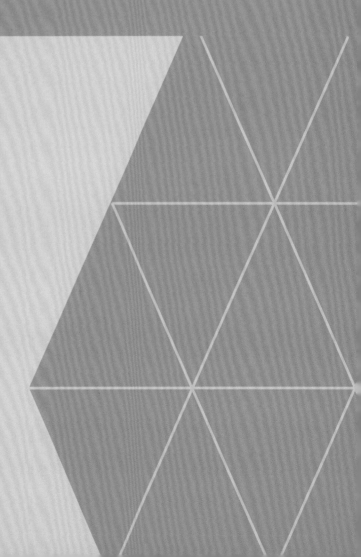

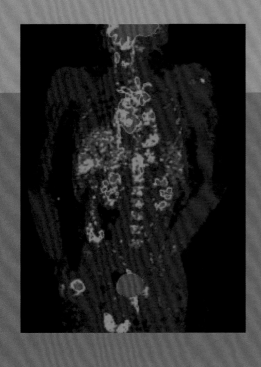

中文导读

第39章
血管炎概述

　　血管炎是一组临床表现与血管炎症性的病理结果相关的罕见疾病，其典型临床表现既可以为闭塞性疾病的缺血症状，也可存在类似于动脉瘤的退行性病变（专栏39.1）。这类疾病所涵盖的临床范围十分广泛，有多种临床和病理类型。然而，并非所有血管炎表型都是由真正的血管壁结构炎症反应引起。在某些病例中，血管炎的特点为出现发热、寒战、盗汗及不明原因的体重减轻等血管外表现。例如关节炎、葡萄膜炎和肺结节也属于血管炎的一部分，但临床表现并非血管闭塞所导致的缺血症状。血管炎的病理生理学在第10章和大血管血管炎的各个章节中进行了详细介绍，包括巨细胞动脉炎（giant cell arteritis，GCA）、大动脉炎（Takayasu arteritis，TAK）（第40章）、中小血管血管炎（第41章），以及黏膜皮肤淋巴结综合征（43章）。本章探讨的疾病是一类罕见病，每个病种都被认为是"孤儿"病，即那些在极少数人身上发生的疾病。与大多数罕见疾病一样，针对其所开展的高质量临床试验较少，大部分临床研究源于大型转诊中心的患者队列。得益于过去二十年诊治血管炎医疗中心之间国际合作的加强，几项重大随机对照临床试验对血管炎患者的诊治产生了具有里程碑意义的影响，包括抗中性粒细胞胞质抗体（antineutrophil cytoplasmic antibody，ANCA）相关的血管炎［嗜酸性肉芽肿性多血管炎（eosinophilic granulomatosis with polyangiitis，EGPA）、肉芽肿性多血管炎（granulomatosis with polyangiitis，GPA）和显微镜下多血管炎（microscopic polyangiitis，MPA）〕和GCA。此外，影像学和实验室检查的技术进步也为临床医师诊断和评估血管炎提供了极大的帮助，结果中提示存在多系统病变并伴有炎症标志物水平升高有助于血管炎的诊断。本章阐述了血管炎的主要类型，探讨了对可疑血管炎病例的诊断方法，并概述了各类血管炎的临床治疗和患者管理。由于此类血管疾病临床实践中所涉及的患者和病例具有临床范围广、病情复杂和极其罕见的特征，故本章还重点对如何区分炎症性和非炎症性疾病进行了探讨（表39.1）。最后，本章节简要综述了血管炎诊断和治疗的最新研究进展。

符伟国

Overview of Vasculitis

Peter A. Merkel

The vasculitides are a group of rare diseases linked by the pathological consequences of vascular inflammation, including bleeding, ischemia, and infarction of downstream organs (Box 39.1). However, the clinical spectrum of these diseases is wide ranging and includes a myriad of clinical and pathological findings. Not all disease phenotypes that occur in the vasculitides are due to true "vasculitis" (i.e., inflammation of vascular structures). Some damage in vasculitis is due to nonvascular inflammation. For example, arthritis, uveitis, and pulmonary nodules are parts of different vasculitides but are not due to interruption of vascular flow. The pathophysiology of vasculitis is covered in Chapter 10 and in individual chapters on large-vessel vasculitis, including giant cell arteritis (GCA) and Takayasu arteritis (TAK) (Chapter 40), medium- and small-vessel vasculitis (Chapter 41), and Kawasaki disease (Chapter 43).

The diseases outlined in this chapter are rare, and all are each considered "orphan" diseases, with fewer than 200,000 cases in the United States at any time. As with most rare diseases, few or no well-controlled clinical treatment trials have been performed for these disorders. Much of the clinical investigation stems from studies of patient cohorts at large referral centers. However, in the past two decades, increasing international cooperation among vasculitis centers has resulted in several important randomized controlled treatment trials that have had significant impacts on the care and management of patients with several forms of vasculitis, including antineutrophil cytoplasmic antibody (ANCA)-associated vasculitis (eosinophilic granulomatosis with polyangiitis [EGPA; Churg-Strauss], granulomatosis with polyangiitis [GPA], and microscopic polyangiitis [MPA]) and GCA. Similarly, advances in diagnostic imaging and laboratory testing have improved clinicians' ability to diagnose and evaluate patients with vasculitis.

This chapter reviews the major types of vasculitis, discusses evaluation of suspected cases of vasculitis, and outlines approaches to treatment and management of these disorders. There is a focus on differentiating *inflammatory* from *noninflammatory* disease as it relates to the types of patients physicians specializing in vascular medicine are likely to encounter in a consultative practice (Table 39.1). The newest advances in diagnosis and treatment are also reviewed briefly.

CLASSIFICATION OF VASCULITIS

The classification and nomenclature of vasculitis can be unnecessarily confusing. The most important first step in approaching these disorders is for clinicians to consider the possibility of "some sort of vasculitis" and, once clinical proof is found, to narrow down the specific type. Nevertheless, knowledge of the classification criteria is quite useful when considering treatment and clinical follow-up. Establishing a treatment plan for a case of vasculitis relies on both an understanding of the prognosis of a specific type and applying results of clinical trials that always include patients who meet specific classification criteria. For example, a patient with arthritis, purpura, and abdominal pain might well be treated with glucocorticoids alone if believed to have immunoglobulin A vasculitis (IgAV; Henoch-Schönlein) but would also receive an additional immunosuppressive drug (e.g., methotrexate, cyclophosphamide, or rituximab) if determined to have GPA. Similarly, the nature of follow-up visits, examinations, and subsequent evaluations is also heavily influenced by the specific type of vasculitis. For example, new-onset hemoptysis in a patient believed to be in remission after treatment for GCA would be concerning for infection or malignancy, whereas the same finding in a patient with GPA would usually prompt immediate reinstitution of high-dose glucocorticoids to treat potential alveolar hemorrhage while further evaluations, including for infection, are put in place.

Two major systems for sorting among the vasculitides exist: the American College of Rheumatology (ACR) classification system[1] and the Chapel Hill Consensus Conference definitions.[2] These systems were not meant to offer diagnostic criteria. The ACR system is used to establish vasculitis and differentiate one vasculitis from another. The Chapel Hill system is designed to standardize the definition of the diseases and was revised in 2012 with inclusion of new names for several entities to move away from eponyms and widely adopt more physiologically appropriate names. The main use of these systems has been for clinical trials and other types of clinical research. Nevertheless, these systems have been adapted for use by clinicians as helpful guides to practice but, when misapplied as diagnostic criteria, may lead to problems. Not all types of vasculitis are included in the ACR or Chapel Hill systems, and the ACR classification criteria are currently undergoing reevaluation and revision.[3]

The practice of differentiating among the inflammatory vasculitides by associated diagnostic antibodies is at this time limited to use of ANCAs. Specifically, many authors refer to *ANCA-associated vasculitis*, which includes GPA, MPA, renal-limited pauci-immune glomerulonephritis, and EGPA (Churg-Strauss). Although it is convenient to refer to these related diseases as "ANCA-associated" vasculitis, it is important to realize that patients may have any of these diseases and still test negative for the presence of ANCA.

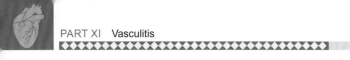

BOX 39.1　Classification of Vasculitis[a] by Predominant Size of Vessel Involvement

Large Vessel
Giant cell arteritis
Takayasu arteritis
Relapsing polychondritis
Cogan syndrome
Aortitis associated with spondyloarthropathies
Retroperitoneal fibrosis
Idiopathic aortitis

Medium Vessel
Polyarteritis nodosa
Kawasaki disease

Small Vessel
ANCA-associated vasculitis
　Granulomatosis with polyangiitis
　Microscopic polyangiitis
　Eosinophilic granulomatosis with polyangiitis (Churg-Strauss)
Cryoglobulinemic vasculitis
Anti–glomerular basement membrane disease
IgA vasculitis (Henoch-Schönlein)
Rheumatoid arthritis (rheumatoid vasculitis)
Sjögren syndrome
Systemic lupus erythematosus
Systemic sclerosis (scleroderma)
Drug-induced vasculitis

Variable Vessel
Behçet disease
Central nervous system vasculitis
Drug-induced vasculitis

[a]Most of these diseases can involve vessels of varying sizes but are listed here by the size of the most commonly affected arteries for convenience purposes. This is not an exhaustive list of vasculitides.

Perhaps the simplest method of sorting out the vasculitides, albeit also incomplete and not fully accurate, is to list them according to the size of artery involved (predominantly but not necessarily exclusively) (see Box 39.1). This results in considering *small-*, *medium-*, and *large-vessel vasculitides* and *variable-vessel vasculitis*. This system, although not applied for clinical trials or clinically for treatment purposes, is an easy one to use as a first approach to describing the diseases and their major manifestations and is used to outline the descriptions of the vasculitides in this chapter. However, when specific diseases and results of treatment trials are mentioned, the ACR and Chapel Hill Consensus systems are applied.

LARGE-VESSEL VASCULITIS

The large-vessel vasculitides are disorders in which the aorta and its main branches, including the subclavian, carotid, vertebral, renal, mesenteric, and iliac arteries, are affected (Fig. 39.1).[4] Because such vessels are so frequently involved in noninflammatory vascular diseases, and patients with these diseases are frequently encountered by specialists in vascular medicine, these disorders are particularly highlighted in this textbook. Also included are individual chapters on GCA and TAK (Chapter 40) and Kawasaki disease (Chapter 43). The vasculitides involving large arteries are briefly described in this section, but it is important to realize that many of them also involve smaller-sized vessels.

Giant Cell Arteritis

GCA, also commonly known as *temporal arteritis* and described in detail in Chapter 40, is the most common of the idiopathic vasculitides.[4,5] GCA affects men and women aged 50 and older but is especially prevalent after age 70. Many vascular and systemic manifestations are seen in this disease. Vascular disease occurs in the aorta and its branches, with predilection for the branches of the carotid arteries, especially the ophthalmic artery, with resulting headaches, jaw claudication, and visual impairment. Rapid-onset irreversible monocular blindness is the most feared complication, but stroke, limb ischemia, and aortic disease can occur, the latter much more common than generally appreciated, especially several years after the initial presentation. Common systemic manifestations include fever, anemia, proximal arthralgias (polymyalgia rheumatica), and fatigue. Diagnosis is often established by finding arteritis on temporal artery biopsy, but this is not required for a diagnosis. Elevated acute phase reactants are seen in 90% of cases. Treatment with high-dose glucocorticoids is highly effective but often results in significant drug-related morbidity. There is now good evidence from randomized controlled trials for the efficacy of methotrexate or tocilizumab (interleukin-6 [IL-6] receptor inhibitor) to treat GCA and act as "steroid-sparing" agents.[6–8]

Takayasu Arteritis

Takayasu arteritis, described in detail in Chapter 40, is a vasculitis that involves the aorta and all its major branches and the pulmonary arteries, including but not limited to, the brachiocephalic, carotid, vertebral, subclavian, renal, femoral, and coronary arteries. This disease often results in stenoses, occlusions, and ischemic damage to end organs and limbs.[4,9] Stroke, myocardial infarction, limb claudication, and severe renovascular hypertension are all complications well known to occur in this disease. It is mostly seen in women and usually first presents clinically in the second or third decade, but it can occur at older ages. Many patients have associated systemic symptoms of fever, arthralgias, and malaise. The disease has a waxing and waning course, and delay in diagnosis is common. Treatment involves glucocorticoids in almost all patients and often the addition of immunosuppressive medications. Surgical bypass procedures may be necessary in some cases.

Relapsing Polychondritis

Relapsing polychondritis is a rare connective tissue disease that predominantly affects the cartilaginous structures of the eyes, ears, nose, and subglottis/trachea but may also affect a wide variety of other organ systems and is associated with vasculitis, especially of large vessels.[11] The cardinal feature of polychondritis is auriculitis, inflammation of the outer ear, usually sparing the noncartilaginous lobe. Auriculitis, which is also a feature of GPA and EGPA but virtually of no other diseases, is readily treated with glucocorticoids and can result in disfigurement if allowed to go untreated. Other common manifestations include inflammatory eye disease that can lead to blindness, destruction of nasal cartilage leading to internal derangement and external disfigurement, sensorineural hearing loss and vertigo, arthritis, and subglottic inflammation with resulting stenosis, a life-threatening condition. Each of these features can also be seen in GPA, although auriculitis is rare in this disease, and relapsing polychondritis is not associated with parenchymal pulmonary manifestations.

The vasculitis seen in relapsing polychondritis can affect vessels of any size, but large-vessel vasculitis is the most common. Aortitis with associated aortic valvular dysfunction and accompanied by thoracic or abdominal aortic aneurysms is fairly common and can lead to heart failure,

TABLE 39.1 Manifestations of Vasculitis That Mimic Noninflammatory Cardiovascular Disease

Type of Vasculitis	Thoracic Aortic Disease	Abdominal Aortic Disease	Carotid/ Vertebral Arterial Disease	Stroke Due to Small- or Medium-Artery Disease	Upper- and Lower-Extremity Arterial Stenosis	Renal Arterial Disease	Coronary Artery Disease	Mesenteric Arteritis	Myocarditis	Pericarditis
GCA	++	+			+	+	Rare	Rare		
TAK	+++	++			+++	++	+	+	Rare	Rare
Other large-vessel diseases (RPC, CS, RPF, IA)	++	+	+	Rare	+	+	Rare	+	Rare	Rare
PAN				+	+	+	Rare	+++	+	+
Kawasaki disease	Rare		Rare	Rare			+++		++	+
GPA				Rare	+	Rare	Rare	+	Rare	+
MPA				Rare		Rare	Rare	+	Rare	+
EGPA				Rare			Rare	+	++	++
CV				Rare			Rare	Rare	+++	
IgAV								+++		
Small-vessel vasculitis of RA, SS, SLE, or SSc			Rare	+	Rare	+	+	++	+	+++
Behçet disease	+	++	Rare	Rare	+	Rare	Rare		+	
CNSV			++	++						

Rare, Reported but quite rare; +, well-described but relatively uncommonly seen; ++, moderately common manifestation; +++, common manifestation.
CNSV, Central nervous system vasculitis; *CS,* Cogan syndrome; *CV,* cryoglobulinemic vasculitis; *EGPA,* eosinophilic granulomatosis with polyangiitis; *GCA,* giant cell arteritis; *GPA,* granulomatosis with polyangiitis; *IA,* idiopathic aortitis; *IgAV,* IgA vasculitis (Henoch-Schönlein); *MPA,* microscopic polyangiitis; *PAN,* polyarteritis nodosa; *RA,* rheumatoid arthritis; *RPC,* relapsing polychondritis; *RPF,* retroperitoneal fibrosis; *SLE,* systemic lupus erythematosus; *SS,* Sjögren syndrome; *SSc,* systemic sclerosis (scleroderma); *TAK,* Takayasu arteritis.

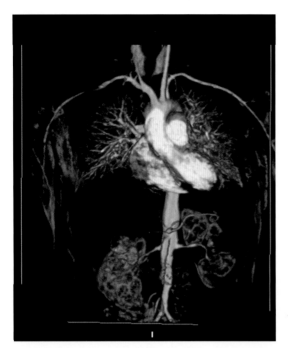

Fig. 39.1 Large-vessel vasculitis with stenotic lesions of abdominal aorta and left subclavian, left carotid, and bilateral renal arteries as imaged using three-dimensional dynamic gadolinium-enhanced magnetic resonance angiography.

aneurysmal rupture or dissection, and involvement of branch arteries. Small-vessel disease can affect nerves, eyes, kidneys, and other systems.

The histopathology of relapsing polychondritis includes destructive inflammation of various types of cartilage, necrotizing aortitis, vasculitis in small vessels (e.g., skin, glomeruli), and direct inflammatory infiltration of eye structures, heart valves, pericardium, skin, and other tissues.

Relapsing polychondritis has been associated with various other primary autoimmune diseases, such as inflammatory bowel disease, lupus, and others. The rarity of this syndrome has precluded comprehensive research that might help to both better differentiate cases from other conditions and learn more about the pathophysiology. Treatment almost always involves systemic glucocorticoids, and immunosuppressive agents are frequently prescribed for this often rapidly progressive disease.

Cogan Syndrome

Cogan syndrome is a rare disorder characterized by inflammatory eye and inner ear/vestibular disease that can also involve inflammatory vasculitis.[12] It is a disease of young adults, usually first affecting patients before age 40, although both children and older patients have also been affected.

The characteristic clinical manifestations of Cogan syndrome are interstitial keratitis, sensorineural hearing loss, and vestibulatory dysfunction. Although interstitial keratitis is the most common eye problem in Cogan syndrome, uveitis, scleritis, and many other types of ophthalmological inflammation can occur. The eye and ear damage is often permanent and can be quite debilitating. The combination of inflammatory eye disease and inner ear problems is required for a diagnosis of Cogan syndrome, but these findings can occur in other diseases as well, such as infections, malignancies, sarcoidosis, and various autoimmune diseases, including other vasculitides (e.g., GPA, relapsing polychondritis, Behçet disease). Other organ systems are less commonly involved.

Vasculitis occurs in up to 15% of patients with Cogan syndrome and is mostly large-vessel disease, with some medium-vessel manifestations reported. The large-vessel disease in Cogan syndrome is similar to that of TA and includes aortitis with aortic insufficiency, stenoses of the carotid, subclavian, and other aortic branch arteries, and even coronary artery disease (CAD). Treatment of Cogan syndrome includes both glucocorticoids and immunosuppressive drugs, appropriate rehabilitation (e.g., vestibular retraining), surgical correction of eye damage, and use of hearing aids or surgical correction of hearing loss.

Idiopathic Aortitis

Aortitis may be found in the absence of any other manifestations of a systemic inflammatory disease.[13-15] These cases often come to the attention of vascular medicine specialists when patients undergoing surgical repair of aortic aneurysms and dissections are found to have inflammation consistent with aortitis on pathological specimens. Autopsies and studies of large numbers of surgical specimens have demonstrated that noninfectious aortitis occurs in 4% to 15% of cases. Although, with detailed investigation, many of these patients are retrospectively found to have had evidence of GCA, TAK, relapsing polychondritis, GPA, or another definable vasculitis, it is common among these cases to find no evidence of more systemic inflammatory disease. The majority of cases of so-called idiopathic aortitis involve thoracic lesions, in contrast to the overall predominance of abdominal aortic lesions for noninflammatory disease.

It is possible that cases of isolated inflammatory aortic aneurysms will be increasingly identified earlier as magnetic resonance imaging (MRI) technology continues to improve and helps to demonstrate inflammation in the arterial wall. However, it can be difficult to differentiate inflammation due to true idiopathic aortitis and vasculitis from the vascular and periaortic inflammations seen in association with atherosclerotic disease. Currently, in the absence of pathological specimens or other evidence of a vasculitis, MRI alone is not diagnostic for inflammation. The emergence of positron emission tomography (PET) scanning for large-vessel disease may also help in the evaluation of such patients.[16]

The approach to treatment of idiopathic aortitis is unclear; many patients never develop other findings of vasculitis. However, new aneurysms and significant vascular disease do occur in some cases.[14] Comprehensive evaluation of evidence of systemic disease is necessary and should include a detailed physical examination, diagnostic imaging, laboratory studies, and other approaches outlined later in this chapter. Appropriate treatment should be given if inflammatory disease other than that seen in the surgical specimen is found, but not all patients require glucocorticoids, especially in the postoperative period. Furthermore, regular follow-up of such patients by a specialist knowledgeable about vasculitis is imperative because lesions may develop subtly and only years after the initial pathological diagnosis is made.

Miscellaneous Forms of Large-vessel Vasculitis

Although large-vessel vasculitis is rarely seen with other systemic inflammatory conditions, it is important to recognize these potential associations. Aortitis is rarely associated with long-standing seronegative spondyloarthropathies (ankylosing spondylitis, reactive arthritis, psoriatic arthritis, and inflammatory bowel disease) and can result in aortic insufficiency. Retroperitoneal fibrosis, a rare disease of proliferating fibroblasts usually causing ureteral obstruction and at times aortic stenosis and periaortitis, is also associated with true inflammatory aortitis. Rarely, IgG4-related disease can cause aortitis and is also frequently the etiology of retroperitoneal fibrosis.[17] There have been a few case reports of large-vessel vasculitis in patients with rheumatoid arthritis, systemic lupus erythematosus (SLE), and GPA.

MEDIUM-VESSEL VASCULITIS

Among the inflammatory vasculitides, the medium-vessel diseases have the greatest variety in clinical manifestations, which result from the broad range of vessel sizes actually involved in the process. As stated earlier, classifying the vasculitides by affected vessel size can be problematic but particularly so with the medium-vessel disorders.

Specialists in vascular medicine need to be aware of protean presentations of active medium-vessel disease and the lasting damage they can cause. As with large-vessel disease, these disorders can mimic noninflammatory cardiac, renal, cerebral, and other vascular disease. This fascinating set of diseases comprises the vasculitides for which the highest quality and quantity of clinical trial data are available to help guide therapy.

Polyarteritis Nodosa

Polyarteritis nodosa (PAN) is among the "purer" vasculitides in that most of its manifestations are due to true vascular inflammation.[18] With the identification of other types of vasculitis, the spectrum of what is now diagnosed as PAN has narrowed over the past 60 years. Although characterized as a medium-vessel disease, PAN may also involve small vessels such as those in the skin. PAN frequently involves inflammation leading to multiple small aneurysms that often appear angiographically as a "string of beads." Ischemia and infarction of kidneys, intestines, and skin are common in PAN, with arthralgias, myalgias, and fevers also frequently seen. Diagnosis is based on angiographic appearance (Fig. 39.2) or tissue pathology, often from surgical specimens such as a resected ischemic bowel segment.

After accurate diagnostic testing for hepatitis B virus (HBV) became widely available and implemented in clinical practice, it became apparent that many cases of PAN were caused by HBV infection. With the widespread use of highly effective vaccines to prevent HBV in many countries, the prevalence of PAN in these locations has fallen precipitously.

PAN is also associated with infection with hepatitis C virus but not as often as with HBV.[18,19] Importantly, there is a difference between hepatitis C–associated PAN and hepatitis C–associated cryoglobulinemic vasculitis (CV, see later section).

Cardiac manifestations of PAN are due to coronary arteritis or malignant hypertension (secondary to renal artery disease) and include myocardial ischemia, heart failure, and arrhythmias.

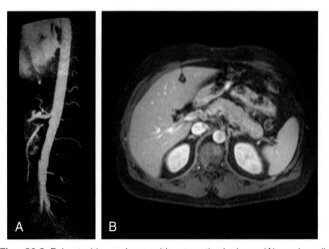

Fig. 39.2 Polyarteritis nodosa with stenotic lesions (A) and wall thickening and enhancement (B) of celiac and superior mesenteric arteries imaged using three-dimensional dynamic gadolinium-enhanced magnetic resonance angiography.

Treatment of PAN almost always involves high-dose glucocorticoids followed by a slow tapering of the dose. In more severe cases, an immunosuppressive agent is added. Hepatitis-associated PAN is now often treated with short courses of glucocorticoids and prolonged courses of antiviral agents. The rate of disease relapse in PAN is lower than that for many other types of vasculitis, and this relatively good prognosis is another important factor to take into consideration when deciding on a therapeutic regimen. Due to the rarity of the disease, controlled clinical trials for PAN are unlikely to occur; treatment is based on case series and expert opinion.

Kawasaki Disease

Kawasaki disease, a vasculitis of young children involving medium and small arteries, is a leading cause of acquired CAD in children.[35] The disease manifests as a systemic illness with high fevers, conjunctival injection, erythematous oropharyngeal lesions, erythematous rashes and skin desquamation, lymphadenopathy, and other signs and symptoms. Cardiac involvement is frequent in Kawasaki disease and can result in long-term morbidity. Myocarditis and pericarditis are common and can be serious, but coronary artery aneurysms are the most feared aspect of the disease. Both panarteritis and granulomas can be seen in the vessels, with subsequent scarring and aneurysm formation. Treatment includes aspirin and intravenous immunoglobulin; such regimens have been shown to markedly reduce the incidence of coronary complications. Kawasaki disease is described in detail in Chapter 43.

SMALL-VESSEL VASCULITIS

Granulomatosis with Polyangiitis

GPA, previously named Wegener granulomatosis,[20] is characterized by the triad of inflammation and destruction of tissue in the upper airway and sinuses (Fig. 39.3), lower airway (Fig. 39.4), and kidneys (Fig. 39.5), as well as the development of ANCAs.[21,22] More than 70% of patients with GPA are positive for ANCA at diagnosis, although some will develop the antibodies later in the course of their illness. Among patients with GPA and glomerulonephritis, more than 90% are positive for ANCA. Although the combination of these features is common in GPA, many patients present with only a subset of these findings. GPA also frequently involves many other organ systems. The upper airway lesions include destructive rhinitis, often leading to nasal bridge collapse and the "saddle nose" deformity, sinusitis, and subglottic inflammation that can lead to life-threatening tracheal stenosis. The most severe form of pulmonary disease in GPA is alveolar hemorrhage, and this is a common cause of early death. Other common pulmonary lesions include nodules, with or without cavitation, and tracheobronchitis. Additional common features of GPA include retroorbital pseudotumor with resulting proptosis, conductive and sensorineural hearing loss, mononeuritis multiplex, arthritis, and purpura. Peripheral vascular involvement with gangrene is seen in GPA and may be the presenting feature (Fig. 39.6).

Inflammatory cardiac disease is rare in GPA but can include myocarditis and pericarditis. Aortic or large-vessel involvement in GPA is extremely uncommon.

Venous thromboses, including both deep vein thromboses and pulmonary emboli, occur frequently in GPA and may be associated with active disease.[23,24] Although some of the pathology in GPA is indeed granulomatous with histiocytes, piecemeal necrosis, and occasional giant cells and eosinophils, other manifestations of inflammation are also seen in the disease. True vasculitis occurs and includes capillaritis. The renal disease of GPA is identical to other ANCA-positive diseases, and the pathology is that of rapidly progressive glomerulonephritis.

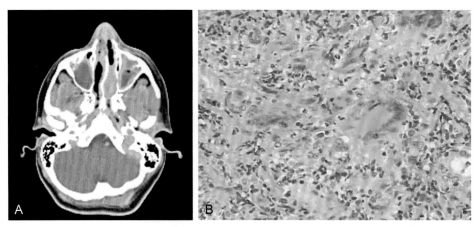

Fig. 39.3 Severe Sinusitis in a Patient With Granulomatosis With Polyangiitis. (A) Computed tomography scan during an acute flare of disease. (B) Hematoxylin and eosin stain of a sinus biopsy from this patient demonstrates characteristic inflammation, including a giant cell.

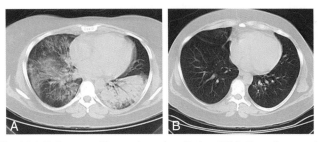

Fig. 39.4 Pulmonary Hemorrhage in a Patient With Granulomatosis With Polyangiitis as Seen on Chest Computed Tomography Scans. (A) During acute flare of disease. (B) Same patient after treatment with glucocorticoids and cyclophosphamide. Patient's dyspnea and plain radiographic changes mostly resolved within 2 weeks of starting glucocorticoids.

Untreated, GPA most often leads to death or serious damage.[25] Glucocorticoids are always used for treatment, but the prognosis of GPA changed considerably when a protocol using cyclophosphamide was introduced in the 1970s at the National Institutes of Health. The morbidity and mortality of GPA was markedly improved by cytotoxic therapy: 1-year mortality changed from more than 80% to less than 20%.[22,25,26] However, serious side effects are common with the use of cyclophosphamide, and the rate of recurrent disease in GPA after therapy is greater than 50%. In recent years, new treatment protocols have been tested in open and controlled trials that incorporate less toxic immunosuppressive drugs, including methotrexate and azathioprine.[27–29] Two multicenter randomized controlled trials have demonstrated that treatment with rituximab, a monoclonal antibody directed against the CD20 receptor on B cells, was equivalent to cyclophosphamide for induction of remission in ANCA-associated vasculitis (GPA and MPA).[30,31] In 2011 the US Food and Drug Administration approved rituximab for the treatment of GPA and MPA, and it has quickly become an established, and increasingly preferred, alternative to cyclophosphamide.

Microscopic Polyangiitis

With the publication of the Chapel Hill Consensus Conference classification system, recognition of MPA as a separate entity gained acceptance.[2,18] MPA is a mostly small- to medium-vessel ANCA-associated vasculitis with manifestations that strongly overlap with GPA. Its key features include glomerulonephritis, alveolar hemorrhage, skin lesions, and mononeuritis multiplex, but many other organ systems may also be involved. Unlike GPA, the pathology of MPA is nongranulomatous and does not involve the type of nonvascular disease seen in GPA or EGPA. The glomerulonephritis of MPA is identical to that seen in GPA.

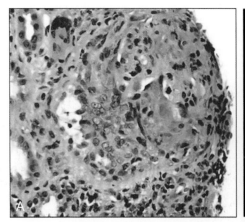
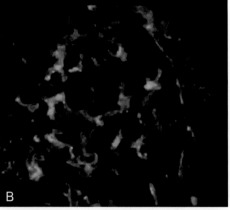

Fig. 39.5 Renal Biopsy in a Patient With Granulomatosis With Polyangiitis (GPA; Same Patient as in Fig. 39.4) With Rapidly Progressive Glomerulonephritis. (A) Hematoxylin and eosin stain demonstrates marked glomerular destruction as well as a multinucleated giant cell *(upper left)*. (B) Characteristic "pauci-immune" immunofluorescent staining seen in GPA and microscopic polyangiitis.

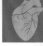

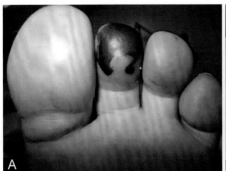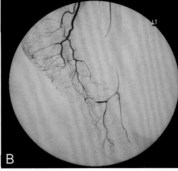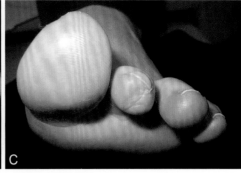

Fig. 39.6 Gangrenous Toe in a Patient With Granulomatosis With Polyangiitis. (A) Gangrenous left second toe pretreatment. (B) Conventional angiogram of left foot at time of gangrene seen in (A), demonstrating marked stenosis/occlusion of dorsal pedal artery and runoff. (C) Same toe months after initiation of glucocorticoids and cyclophosphamide. Only minimal tissue loss resulted, and toe is now well perfused.

Most patients with MPA are positive for ANCA, and the predominant ANCA antigen specificity is myeloperoxidase (MPO). Cardiac manifestations of MPA are uncommon, but peripheral artery disease (PAD) and gangrene are seen and may be confused with noninflammatory vascular disease. MPA should be differentiated from classic PAN. PAN is more of a medium-vessel disease and does not include glomerulonephritis or pulmonary capillaritis. MPA does not produce the microaneurysms seen in PAN. Treatment of MPA is essentially identical to that for GPA, although MPA is less likely to relapse than GPA.

Eosinophilic Granulomatosis with Polyangiitis (Churg-Strauss)

EGPA (Churg-Strauss) is a rare disease characterized by the triad of asthma, pulmonary infiltrates, and hypereosinophilia.[32,33] However, EGPA can involve almost all the clinical features seen in GPA, including the presence of ANCA in 30% to 40% of cases, almost always with specificity to MPO. As with GPA, much of the pathology seen in EGPA is due to inflammation that is not "vasculitis" per se but is every bit as damaging as vascular inflammation. Tissue eosinophilia, although seen in other types of vasculitis, is particularly common in EGPA and often striking. More than 90% of patients have asthma, often severe; the hypereosinophilia may be a marker of disease activity for some patients but is not always present. Pulmonary manifestations include dense infiltrates that rapidly clear with glucocorticoid therapy. In addition, neuropathies, especially mononeuritis multiplex and gastrointestinal ischemia, are common features and quite damaging. Diagnosis is based on the combination of clinical findings, hypereosinophilia, and pathology specimens that often show granulomatous and eosinophilic inflammation.

Cardiovascular manifestations of EGPA are fairly common and include myocarditis with resultant congestive heart failure and pericarditis. Angina is rare in EGPA. Cardiac involvement in EGPA may be rapid in onset and fatal.

Glucocorticoids are the mainstay of treatment for EGPA, but immunosuppressive agents are being used increasingly for more severe cases and to help wean patients from glucocorticoids. It is important to avoid overtreating the asthma component of the syndrome; asthma is not in itself a reason to start cytotoxic medications. In 2017, mepolizumab, a biological agent that binds to the IL-5 receptor, was approved by the US Food and Drug Administration for use in patients with EGPA based on the results of a randomized trial, the first drug ever approved for this type of vasculitis.[34]

IgA Vasculitis (Henoch-Schönlein)

IgAV (Henoch-Schönlein) is a small-vessel vasculitis that classically involves the clinical triad of inflammatory arthritis, ischemic abdominal pain, and purpura, although not all cases exhibit all three manifestations.[36] The most feared manifestation of IgAV is glomerulonephritis, which can lead to renal failure. Cardiac disease is not a feature of IgAV, but hypertension from renal insufficiency can be severe. The lesions in IgAV often involve leukocytoclasia and IgA deposition. An elevated serum IgA level is commonly seen in patients with IgAV.

IgAV is much more common among young children and is probably the most common type of vasculitis in this age group. Nevertheless, IgAV is also seen in adults. The disease is more often self-limited among children and more likely to lead to chronic renal insufficiency in adults. Relapse is common in all age groups. Treatment of IgAV varies from watchful waiting in some cases of pediatric IgAV, to high-dose glucocorticoids, to the addition of immunosuppressive agents. However, it is not clear whether immunosuppressive therapy substantially alters long-term outcomes for IgAV.

Cryoglobulinemic Vasculitis

CV occurs when cryoglobulins, any of various types of immunoglobins that precipitate from serum at temperatures less than body temperature, induce an immune complex–mediated inflammatory process in any organ.[37] Several types of cryoglobulins can occur, and cryoglobulinemia is subclassified based on the mix of IgG and IgM antibodies that make up the cryoglobulin portion of serum (the "cryocrit") and whether the excess cryoproteins are polyclonal or monoclonal.

CV was previously considered to be a quite rare phenomenon sometimes seen in chronic inflammatory diseases such as lupus or rheumatoid arthritis or associated with lymphoproliferative disorders. However, once the association between hepatitis C infection and type 2 mixed CV was established, it became apparent that coincident with the worldwide rise in hepatitis C infection, CV has been increasingly identified as a cause of vasculitis. The vast majority of cases of CV currently seen are associated with hepatitis C infection.

Major clinical manifestations of CV include cutaneous vasculitis (purpura), arthralgias, peripheral neuropathy, and nephropathy with associated renal insufficiency or nephrotic syndrome (or both). Cardiovascular manifestations of CV include Raynaud phenomenon, hypertension, and congestive heart failure. The hypertension in CV, which is often associated with renal disease, can be severe and lead to cardiac failure.

The histopathology of CV includes necrotizing vasculitis but may also involve Ig and complement deposition detected by immunofluorescence staining.

Treatment of CV is somewhat controversial. For patients with CV who are infected with hepatitis C virus, treatment with antiviral agents, even in the absence of significant liver disease, is crucial to provide, if possible. For acute disease exacerbations or when antiviral therapy is not efficacious or possible, treatment may include glucocorticoids, cytotoxic agents, and plasmapheresis. There is increasing evidence that rituximab (ant-CD20 B cell–depleting agent) is effective in treating CV. Although the introduction of direct-acting antiviral agents highly efficacious against hepatitis C virus can eradicate the virus within patients with viral-induced CV, and most such patients will no longer exhibit signs and symptoms of CV, some patients can still have active CV even in the absence of active viral infection.[38]

Vasculitis Secondary to Autoimmune/Connective Tissue Diseases

Vasculitis, especially of small arteries, can be seen in various systemic autoimmune diseases, including SLE, rheumatoid arthritis, Sjögren syndrome, and systemic sclerosis (scleroderma). In these diseases, vasculitis usually accompanies evidence of severe disease in other organs or long-standing disease (e.g., rheumatoid arthritis). Skin vasculitis is common, but mesenteric and CNS vasculitis are the most feared and dangerous vascular manifestations seen in these diseases.

Although coronary arteritis is rarely seen in these systemic autoimmune disorders, there is an increased recognition of early accelerated atherosclerotic CAD among patients with SLE, rheumatoid arthritis, and other chronic inflammatory diseases. The pathophysiology of this problem is under active investigation and parallels the increased attention vascular biologists are paying to the contribution of inflammation to atherosclerosis. When vasculitis occurs in SLE it is frequently severe and often necessitates treatment with high-dose glucocorticoids and cyclophosphamide. Vasculitis associated with rheumatoid arthritis, known as rheumatoid vasculitis, has become extremely rare due to the markedly improved treatments available for the linked arthritis.

VARIABLE-VESSEL VASCULITIS

Behçet Disease

Behçet disease is a systemic inflammatory disease with multiple mucocutaneous manifestations, especially including genital and oral ulcers and often severe sight-threatening inflammatory eye disease.[10] Arthritis, gastrointestinal disease (including mucosal lesions), epididymitis, and secondary amyloidosis can also occur. Although its prevalence is markedly increased in countries in the Eastern Mediterranean, Middle East, and East Asia, and in descendants of people from these regions, Behçet disease is found in populations worldwide.

Vasculitis occurs in up to one-third of patients with Behçet disease and is unique among the inflammatory vasculitides for the relatively common clinical involvement of venous disease. Both arterial and venous manifestations may occur in the same patients. Venous involvement includes superficial phlebitis, varices, and thromboses of deep veins, vena cava, cerebral sinuses, and other major veins.

The arterial lesions in Behçet disease are often in large vessels and frequently result in aneurysms, stenoses, or rupture. The most common sites of arteritis are the aorta and its branches and the pulmonary arteries; however, Behçet disease may also involve medium and small vessels.

Behçet disease can involve a wide range of different types of histopathologies, consistent with the protean disease manifestations. The oral and genital ulcers do not have specific pathognomonic features. Similarly, biopsy specimens of the gastrointestinal lesions cannot differentiate Behçet disease from inflammatory bowel disease. Although the vascular lesions can include large and small arteries as well as veins, these lesions are similar to those of other vasculitides.

Treatment of Behçet disease varies with the manifestation being addressed and may range from colchicine and topical glucocorticoids for aphthous ulcers to large doses of glucocorticoids for many problems including mucocutaneous, vascular, and eye lesions. The uveitis is treated with long-term immunosuppressive agents, including cyclosporine, azathioprine, chlorambucil, and cyclophosphamide. Inhibitors of tumor necrosis factor (TNF)-α are currently also used to treat this disorder. Many treatment protocols are based on expert opinion, but in recent years an increasing number of controlled clinical trials have been performed, especially involving mucocutaneous lesions or eye disease. Behçet disease can be a highly aggressive form of vasculitis that frequently results in significant morbidity and mortality.

Central Nervous System Vasculitis

Central nervous system vasculitis (CNSV), also known as primary angiitis of the central nervous system, is a quite rare necrotizing angiitis limited to the central nervous system.[39,40] CNSV is frequently associated with subacute nonfocal neurological deficits and chronic meningitis, although strokes and hemorrhage can also be seen.

Diagnosis of CNSV necessitates first suspecting this rare disease. Conventional angiography may be helpful in identifying other entities, such as aneurysms and emboli, but is often not diagnostic for vasculitis for several reasons (Fig. 39.7). First, in older patients the endothelial changes of atherosclerosis may mimic those of vasculitis. Second, vasospasm can be confused with stenosis from either atherosclerosis or inflammation. Finally, the resolution of conventional angiography is such that small arteries are not well visualized, and thus many cases of vasculitis may be missed by this technique. Leptomeningeal biopsies or larger tissue samples from affected brain areas are often necessary to demonstrate CNSV and provide the level of evidence required to institute therapy. The histopathology is that of vasculitis, but granulomas and giant cells are not always seen; there may be no inflammation in the vasospastic variant. Tests of cerebrospinal fluid are often normal in

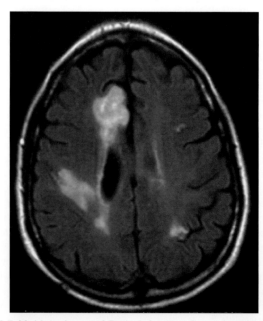

Fig. 39.7 Multiple Areas of Brain Infarction Secondary to Primary Angiitis of the Central Nervous System as Seen on Gadolinium-Enhanced Magnetic Resonance Angiography. The cerebral angiogram on this patient was unremarkable, but brain biopsy demonstrated small-vessel vasculitis.

patients with CNSV but are important in evaluating patients for other conditions, especially infection or malignancy.

Experts in vascular medicine need to be aware of CNSV because it can easily be mistaken for atherosclerotic disease with multiple infarcts. CNSV is extremely rare, but the approach to treatment is quite different from atherosclerotic disease.

Treatment recommendations are based solely on case series and an incomplete understanding of the pathophysiology. CNSV is treated with glucocorticoids, with other immunosuppressive agents often added.

It is imperative to differentiate CNSV from the increasingly recognized reversible cerebral vasoconstrictive syndrome (RCVS) previously referred to as *benign CNSV*[41]; RCVS is *not* a vasculitis. It is characterized by acute onset of severe headache ("thunderclap headaches") and a focal neurological event. RCVS is treated with vasodilators, including calcium channel blockers, and strict avoidance of smoking and vasoconstricting drugs and substances, such as caffeine, cocaine, sympathomimetics, and serotonin receptor agonists (e.g., sumatriptan).

Drug-Induced Vasculitis

Many drugs or other toxins have been implicated as causing inflammatory vasculitis involving vessels of all sizes, especially small arteries. A full list of drugs considered to be causative for vasculitis and details regarding the clinical syndromes of drug-induced vasculitis are available in recent reviews.[42,43] There is an interesting subset of patients with ANCA-associated vasculitis whose disease is caused by exposure to certain medications, especially hydralazine and propylthiouracil and related compounds.[44]

The clinical manifestations of drug-induced vasculitis range from skin-only disease to widespread life-threatening multisystemic disease. No clinical, laboratory, or pathological findings differentiate drug-induced from other types of vasculitis. Given that agents from most classes of drugs have been implicated in vasculitis, it is important that clinicians consider the possible contribution of not only every medication the patient was taking at the time of clinical presentation but also medications, supplements, and illegal drugs used in the previous year. The temporal association between drug exposure and disease, combined with the pattern of illness and evidence for or against a different vasculitic process, are helpful in establishing a diagnosis of drug-induced vasculitis.

Management of drug-induced vasculitis always includes discontinuation of the putative causative agent when possible but may also involve treatment with clinical observation alone, glucocorticoids, or immunosuppressive agents. Patients should be followed for an extended period, even after apparent disease resolution, to ensure the diagnosis of drug-induced vasculitis rather than waxing and waning idiopathic vasculitis.

A particularly interesting form of drug-induced vasculitis has only recently been described and is associated with immune checkpoint inhibitors.[45] These agents appear to cause a form of large-vessel vasculitis, as well as vasculitis of the nervous system. These observations are not surprising given that several other forms of immune-mediated diseases are seen among patients taking these drugs. A substantial challenge in treating such patients is that the use of the checkpoint inhibitors is usually quite imperative and good alternatives often do not yet exist.

EVALUATION AND DIAGNOSIS OF POSSIBLE VASCULITIS

When evaluating cases of potential vasculitis, the clinician's first challenge is to consider that one of these rare diseases is a possibility. Rather than quickly focusing on a specific type of vasculitis, it is best to consider first whether "some sort of" vasculitis is present and determine the specific type once more information becomes available. It is common that, when clinicians are evaluating patients for vasculitis, they are also conducting parallel evaluations for nonvasculitic diseases, an appropriate approach given the rarity of vasculitis and the urgency to diagnose and treat conditions that mimic vasculitis, such as infection.

Due to the protean potential manifestations of the vasculitides, clinicians must be comprehensive in their evaluation of patients for possible inflammatory vascular disease. By "looking everywhere" at all organ systems with complete history-taking, physical examinations, and selective laboratory and radiographic diagnostic tests, evidence is sought for both the presence of vasculitis and the size of vessel involved. Finding the "worst" manifestation of any new diagnosis or flare of disease is important, but the goal is to determine the diagnosis of a vasculitis and ensure all manifestations are documented. Treatment protocols will differ based on extent of disease, and later assessment of response depends on accurate baseline evaluation of all features of disease.

With the exception of tissue pathology, no single test is fully diagnostic for vasculitis. A comprehensive initial medical evaluation including medical history, physical examination, and routine laboratory studies can provide most of the information clinicians need to either dismiss the diagnosis of vasculitis or focus on more specific diagnostic testing. Finally, clinicians must reconsider a diagnosis of vasculitis or consider a coexisting problem when either the clinical course changes or treatment response is not characteristic for vasculitis.

Medical History

Medical history and physical examination remain key elements of evaluation for vasculitis. A comprehensive review of systems is essential, and the potential queries related to vasculitis are numerous. Examples of symptoms to inquire about include any visual changes or eye symptoms, changes in hearing, nasal discharge or epistaxis, sinusitis, headaches, any mental status change, any neurological symptom, stridor, wheezing, cough, hemoptysis, pleuritic chest pain, jaw or limb claudication, abdominal pain, any skin lesion, arthralgias, arthritis, myalgias, weakness, fevers, weight loss, and many other symptoms.

A full and accurate medication and drug use history is mandatory and should include any prescription drugs, over-the-counter products, illegal drugs, and alternative/herbal products taken within the *prior 6 to 12 months*, as well as accurate stop and start dates. If patients have been prescribed medications to address specific symptoms that may be vasculitic, documenting the response to these treatments may be important.

Physical Examination

A full physical examination is required whenever a patient is evaluated for potential vasculitis, and several examination findings should always prompt consideration of vasculitis in any patient. Blood pressure should be measured in both arms for discrepancies. Obtaining blood pressures in both arms and legs may be appropriate if upper- or lower-extremity stenoses are suspected. Hypertension may result from renal artery stenoses from vasculitis, and similar physiology occurs with some tight suprarenal aortic stenoses. A full examination of bilateral pulses should include radial, ulnar, brachial, carotid, femoral, popliteal, posterior tibial, and dorsalis pedis pulses. Bruits should be listened for over the aorta and the carotid, femoral, axillary, subclavian, and renal arteries. Presence of blood pressure discrepancies, absent pulses, or arterial bruits is each highly specific for major arterial disease but is not highly sensitive for major arterial lesions in large-vessel vasculitis.[46]

Careful examination of skin and mucosal surfaces can reveal many clues to vasculitis. Although palpable purpura is the classic vasculitis skin lesion, not all purpura is vasculitis, and not all skin vasculitis manifests as purpura. Macular lesions, both flat and raised, as well as bullae and nonerythematous lesions, can all occur in vasculitis. Livedo reticularis may be a clue to vasculitis or vasospasm. One should examine the patient for oral or genital aphthous ulcers. Extremity cyanosis and pallor may be seen and may be variable depending on the ambient temperature and limb positioning. Ulcerations and crusting should be sought in the nasopharynx. Nailfold capillary changes can be seen on bedside microscopic examination with an ophthalmoscope. Signs of capillary fragility, especially over sites of blood pressure cuff or tourniquet application, may be seen.

The rest of a full physical examination is also essential in evaluating for vasculitis. Lung examination may reveal any of the many abnormalities commonly seen in vasculitis, including rhonchi, pleural rubs, dullness due to effusions, and wheezing. Careful cardiac auscultation might reveal evidence of aortic regurgitation, as seen in aortitis or pericardial rubs. Gross inspection of the eyes may reveal signs of inflammation, and funduscopic examinations may show retinal pallor or other signs of ischemia. A full ophthalmological examination including slit lamp is necessary for any patient suspected of vasculitis with eye symptoms. A full joint examination may reveal even asymptomatic effusions. Detailed neurological examination is essential; subtle cranial and peripheral neuropathies often go unnoticed by both patients and physicians but are clues to severe disease.

Laboratory Studies

Acute Phase Reactants

Acute phase reactants, including the Westergren erythrocyte sedimentation rate (ESR), C-reactive protein (CRP), and others, are perhaps the most misunderstood and misused tests in the evaluation of vasculitis. ESR should never be considered a screening test for vasculitis, because acute phase reactants are neither highly sensitive nor specific diagnostically for any type of vasculitis. There is good evidence that a normal ESR can be found in active TAK, GCA, GPA, CNSV, drug-induced vasculitis, and other vasculitides. Although ESR is most helpful in evaluating patients for possible GCA, even in that disease, up to 10% of patients with documented GCA have normal sedimentation rates at the time of diagnosis. Furthermore, an elevated ESR can be seen in most of the disorders usually considered in the differential diagnosis of patients with possible vasculitis, notably infections and malignancies, thus emphasizing the lack of diagnostic usefulness of this test. Acute phase reactants are somewhat useful for monitoring disease activity and therefore in some cases may be supportive of a disease flare.

Renal Function Tests

Laboratory tests of renal function are an essential part of evaluating patients for possible vasculitis. A properly performed urinalysis is mandatory. Glomerulonephritis is a major feature of many small- and medium-vessel vasculitides and may manifest first as subtle findings on urinalysis, including proteinuria and hematuria. If the urine dipstick is abnormal, clinicians need to examine the urinary sediment. Clinicians must not count on hospital or reference laboratories to perform a manual urine sediment analysis, because urinary casts are often dissolved by the time laboratory personnel run the test. If clinicians are not comfortable examining the sediment themselves, they should consult a nephrologist or another provider expert in this key test. Creatinine elevations may reflect both acute renal disease and long-standing damage and scarring from prior flares of disease, and knowing a patient's baseline value is always important. Furthermore, the doses of many drugs used for patients with vasculitis are modified based on renal function; these include cyclophosphamide, methotrexate, cyclosporine, and nonsteroidal antiinflammatory drugs. Hematuria may also be a clue to

bladder toxicity from cyclophosphamide, including hemorrhagic cystitis and transitional cell carcinoma.

Complete Blood Cell Counts and White Blood Cell Differential Counts

No findings from a blood count and review of a blood smear are diagnostic for vasculitis, but the tests may provide clues to other diagnoses. Many, but certainly not all, patients with systemic vasculitis are anemic at initial presentation. Although eosinophilia is frequently present in EGPA, GPA, drug-induced disease, and other vasculitides, this finding is also neither sensitive nor specific enough for diagnosis. However, significant eosinophilia does help to narrow the potential diagnoses and may help in classifying patients with established vasculitis. In addition, it is not uncommon for patients with EGPA to have an increase in total eosinophil count before or during a flare of disease.

Antineutrophil Cytoplasmic Autoantibodies Testing

The discovery of ANCA and their association with GPA, MPA, EGPA, and renal-only pauci-immune glomerulonephritis was extremely important in the evolution of diagnostic testing for vasculitis.[47] ANCA testing, when performed properly, is highly specific for these syndromes and, in the correct clinical setting, may be the last piece of data necessary to establish a diagnosis, even in the absence of a tissue biopsy. In addition, the finding of a positive test for ANCA in a patient with already established vasculitis essentially narrows the diagnosis to one of four ANCA-associated diseases.

Currently, the methodology for conducting ANCA testing is not standardized, which leads to problems with reliability and interpretation of test results. At a minimum, a laboratory should perform both immunofluorescence testing to identify the cytoplasmic ("C") ANCA pattern or perinuclear ("P") pattern, as well as conduct enzyme-linked immunosorbent assay (ELISA) testing for antibodies to proteinase 3 (anti-PR3) and antibodies to MPO (anti-MPO). Antigen-specific ELISA tests are less prone to false-positive results (for the diagnosis of vasculitis) than the somewhat subjective immunofluorescence tests. Positive ANCA testing by the combined presence of C-pattern/anti-PR3 or P-pattern/anti-MPO is extremely specific for vasculitis, with other types of ANCA not helpful diagnostically.

Specificity of properly performed ANCA testing is better than 90% and may be closer to 99% in certain laboratories.[47,48] Sensitivity of ANCA testing varies with the type of disease and clinical manifestations. Although more than 90% of patients with GPA who have renal involvement are ANCA positive, this rate drops to approximately 70% for patients without renal disease. Most patients with MPA and renal-limited pauci-immune glomerulonephritis are ANCA positive, but the rate of ANCA positivity among patients with EGPA varies in the literature from 40% to 80%. Thus, although ANCA is highly specific for vasculitis when present, a negative test by no means excludes the diagnosis.

Other Immunology Tests

Tests for antinuclear antibodies (ANAs) and rheumatoid factor (RF) should be used only in selected cases. ANA is a useful screening test for SLE because 99% of patients with SLE have a positive ANA test, especially if they have vasculitis. However, a positive ANA is by no means specific for any autoimmune disease. In the absence of arthritis, a test for RF is rarely useful diagnostically because it can be seen in various infections and in type 2 cryoglobulinemia. In addition, the test often has false-positive results. Furthermore, it is not diagnostic in itself for rheumatoid arthritis but is almost always positive in patients with rheumatoid vasculitis.

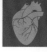

Testing for the presence of cryoglobulins is important. Their presence may not only help to make the diagnosis, but treatment may be different and include plasmapheresis or antiviral agents (or both) in cases of hepatitis C–associated disease. Testing for cryoglobulins is not simple and is frequently done incorrectly. The blood specimen must be kept at body temperature (37°C) from the moment it is drawn through transport to the laboratory, where it must be allowed to clot in a warm water bath or heated box. Once the clot forms at 37°C, further special processing is required. From a Bayesian perspective, it is not unreasonable to repeat testing for cryoglobulins when the likelihood of their presence is medium to high, especially if the patient is infected with hepatitis C virus.

Microbiological Testing

Cultures of blood, urine, and other specimens are often appropriate when evaluating patients with vasculitis. Furthermore, patients with established vasculitis are at considerably increased risk of infection when undergoing immunosuppressive therapy, necessitating a low threshold to test for infection in this population. Finally, it is important that some biopsy specimens, especially lung tissue, be sent for culture for both typical and atypical/opportunistic pathogens.

Diagnostic Vascular Imaging

Radiographic assessment of vascular structures has long been an important tool for diagnosing patients with vasculitis. This is especially true when medium and large vessels are involved, because they are much more likely to be visualized by the techniques available.[49] Although small- and even medium-sized arteries can often be seen on diagnostic biopsies or surgical specimens, large vessels are not usually amenable to tissue biopsy. Thus diagnostic imaging is crucial to assessment and management of patients with large-vessel vasculitis. The two great challenges inherent in interpretation of imaging of large vessels are (1) differentiating inflammatory disease from atherosclerotic disease and (2) trying to determine whether vascular lesions represent "active" disease. In recent years, interest in large-vessel vascular imaging has greatly increased as investigators and clinicians working in vasculitis strive to properly incorporate advances in various radiological modalities into practice. Imaging of organs and tissues other than arteries themselves is of obvious benefit for specific syndromes to help understand the extent of disease, facilitate choice of tissue biopsy, and rule out other pathology.

Specialists in vascular medicine need to be aware of the capabilities and limitations of various modalities for imaging the vascular system and differentiating atherosclerotic from inflammatory disease. Vascular imaging is much more commonly obtained to evaluate suspected atherosclerotic or structural disease, and thus it is vital that inflammatory disease is recognized, even when it is not expected. The increased recognition that atherosclerosis may have an inflammatory component and that vasculitis can result in some changes seen in atherosclerosis makes this differentiation even more challenging. Marked differences in treatment and prognosis for these different disorders make continued cooperative work by experts in cardiology, rheumatology, radiology, vascular surgery, and other specialties essential in evaluating patients and interpreting imaging data. The following sections summarize the progress to date in using various imaging modalities for evaluating vascular disease in the inflammatory vasculitides.

Conventional Angiography

Conventional angiography with intravascular injection of radiocontrast dye remains the "gold standard" for detecting stenoses and an-

eurysms in medium and large arteries and in diagnosing patients with vasculitis, especially TAK and PAN. It is important to ask radiologists to view the distal runoffs of arteries beyond the trunk; diagnostic and critical lesions more distally (e.g., axillary artery) may be missed by undue concentration on the proximal vessels. Additional advantages to conventional angiography include the ability to measure intraarterial blood pressure directly. Such pressure readings are especially important when caring for patients with subclavian or proximal aortic stenoses, where peripheral pressure readings may be inaccurate. Finally, conventional angiography is the only current imaging modality that assists catheter-based intervention, including angioplasty and stent placement.

There are several problems with and limitations to conventional angiography for evaluation of potential vasculitis. The direct toxicities of the contrast dye have the potential for hypersensitivity reactions, renal insufficiency, and volume overload. Catheters can potentially cause vascular injury. The resolution of conventional angiography is limited, and most small-vessel disease, such as in the brain or mesentery, is not well imaged by this technique. In addition, serial studies by conventional angiography, although sometimes necessary, are impractical, incur additive toxicity, and are thus not routinely performed to monitor patients. Finally, conventional angiography does not provide any information about the biological state of the arterial wall and therefore, except with serial images, cannot determine disease activity.

Magnetic Resonance Imaging

The use of MRI to help in the diagnosis and management of vasculitis continues to rapidly gain acceptance, although there are few properly done studies on the reliability of MRI for these purposes. MRI and magnetic resonance angiography (MRA) provide detailed information on luminal structures, arterial wall thickness and edema, tissue enhancement (by gadolinium contrast), and blood flow for large and some medium vessels. These structural measures have been proposed as useful in determining vasculitis disease activity. MRI and MRA can be performed repeatedly with little risk to the patient and can thus provide important serial data. The technology for magnetic resonance (MR) continues to improve, and it is anticipated that the reliability and breadth of information it provides in evaluating patients with vasculitis will continue to increase substantially in the next few years, especially for large-vessel pathology.

Several problems remain in the use of MR for diagnosing and following patients with vasculitis. First, not all vascular structures are easily imaged, and false-positive scans due to problems with imaging artifact (and possibly other reasons) do occur. Second, neither the protocols for data acquisition nor the methods of image interpretation are standardized, making comparison of research data and studies from different institutions or even different machines problematic. The specificity of MR as a disease activity measure remains controversial. Unlike conventional angiography, MR does not allow for pressure readings or catheter-based interventions. Finally, MR is currently not helpful for small- or even most medium-vessel disease, although resolution is improving.

Computed Tomography

Computed tomography (CT) is another promising imaging technique for large-vessel vasculitis. CT can demonstrate arterial calcification well and, with the newer machines and software, quite precise images are possible. Major drawbacks to CT include the associated toxicities of ionizing radiation and iodinated contrast dye. The best future use of CT may be in combination with other modalities, especially PET (see later discussion).

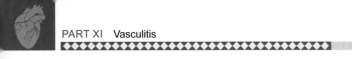

Ultrasound

Ultrasound has been used to evaluate vascular disease for many years, and well-developed literature is available on this technique. The non-invasive nature, widespread availability, and relatively low cost of ultrasound make it an attractive technique for vascular imaging. However, the work in ultrasound has mostly been on atherosclerotic disease and has focused on specific anatomical areas, including the carotid, vertebral, and ophthalmic arterial systems and the abdominal aorta.

Ultrasound is often the first vascular imaging test obtained for patients with suspected carotid or vertebral arterial disease or aortic aneurysms. Recognition by the examiner that the disease process may be something *other* than atherosclerosis is vital for proper early diagnosis. Greater awareness of the differences in foci of disease and in the size and appearances of lesions between atherosclerosis and vasculitis are important to emphasize.

Future use of ultrasound in evaluating inflammatory vascular disease depends on both (1) improved technology that better evaluates arterial wall structures and allows for examination of smaller-caliber vessels and (2) demonstration that ultrasound provides insight beyond that obtained from other modalities such as MR.

There is growing acceptance in some centers, especially in Europe, for the use of ultrasound of the temporal arteries as an initial diagnostic screening test for GCA, and some investigators feel this modality can often replace temporal artery biopsy. This remains an exceptionally controversial topic, with strong disagreements within the vasculitis research community about the methodology used to test ultrasound in this setting and the diagnostic specificity of routine ultrasonography for the diagnosis of GCA.

Positron Emission Tomography

PET is an intriguing imaging modality for vascular disease. Because it relies on uptake of an isotope, it may be able to provide a biological link to disease activity. Case series on the use of PET in evaluating aortitis provide evidence that it may help to detect and diagnose aortitis that is not otherwise apparent. However, the rate of so-called false-positive tests is not clear, and data from PET studies must be carefully considered within the clinical context. The utility of serial PET studies evaluating disease activity and guiding treatment for large-vessel vasculitis is an area of active investigation. Although the work on PET for large-vessel vasculitis is still in the early stages, and the lack of standardization, paucity of direct comparisons with MRI, and high cost are all important issues to consider, it is likely that some form of PET, MR, or a related technology will become more central to evaluating patients with large-vessel vasculitis.[16]

Tissue Biopsy

Given the need to often exclude infection, malignancy, or other processes, as well as the need for immunosuppressive medications for vasculitis, biopsy evidence is often crucial, and empirical therapy is strongly discouraged. With the exception of some cases of large-vessel vasculitis and some situations in patients with ANCA-positive disease, tissue biopsy is usually necessary to establish a firm diagnosis of vasculitis.

A temporal artery biopsy is almost always appropriate when GCA is a consideration, even if there are no cranial symptoms. A positive biopsy is such strong evidence for GCA that, although a negative temporal artery biopsy does not exclude the diagnosis, a second contralateral biopsy is sometimes advised if the initial specimen is nondiagnostic.

For large-vessel diseases other than GCA, a vessel biopsy is almost never obtained because a medium- to full-thickness biopsy of the aorta or its main branches has obvious morbidity. However, obtaining surgical specimens during bypass procedures or biopsies under highly controlled situations such as during aortic valve or graft surgery should be considered when a diagnosis of large-vessel disease has not yet been established or when disease activity status is unclear.

For the other vasculitides, it is usually preferred to obtain a biopsy from the most accessible tissue. Skin biopsies are simple, have low risk of morbidity, and can be instrumental in diagnosis. Too often, purpuric lesions are assumed to be vasculitis, and biopsies not performed. In addition, skin biopsies can be examined for evidence of embolic, thrombotic, or infectious diseases.

In the proper setting, biopsies of kidneys or lungs involve moderate risks but can be of high yield, whereas biopsies of other tissues (e.g., sinus mucosa, nerve, myocardium) are lower risk but also have lower diagnostic yields. Biopsies of other organs, such as intestine and liver, offer low yields and higher risks but may be appropriate, especially during a surgical procedure, in certain circumstances.

TREATMENT OF VASCULITIS

The goals of treatment for inflammatory vasculitis are to stop the active inflammation and prevent permanent damage. Unlike many other systemic inflammatory diseases, true clinical remission is not only possible in many cases of vasculitis but should be the goal of treatment. Thus protocols are increasingly being referred to as involving either "remission induction" or "remission maintenance" treatments. The mainstays of therapy for vasculitis remain glucocorticoids and various immunosuppressive drugs. Treatment protocols are tailored to the specific type of vasculitis and the extent of disease. Clinical trial data are increasingly available to guide treatment for GPA, MPA, Kawasaki disease, and GCA, whereas other diseases rely on either case series for guidance or extrapolated data from studies in related, but not identical, vasculitides. Box 39.2 outlines the treatments used for patients with inflammatory vasculitis.

BOX 39.2   Treatments for Inflammatory Vasculitis

Commonly Used Medications/Treatments

Aspirin
Glucocorticoids
Cyclophosphamide
Azathioprine
Methotrexate
Mycophenolate mofetil
Cyclosporine and tacrolimus (FK506)
Antiviral agents
Plasmapheresis
Intravenous immunoglobulin

Newer and/or Experimental Agents

Rituximab (anti-CD20)
Inhibitors of tumor necrosis factor-α
Tociluzumab (anti–IL-6)
Mepolizumab (anti–IL-5)
Abatacept (CTLA4-Ig)
Other experimental biologics

Surgical/Invasive Treatments

Balloon angioplasty
Intravascular stents ($\pm$ drug-eluting coating)
Vascular bypass or replacement grafts
Reconstructive surgery

Ensuring long-term follow-up of patients with inflammatory vasculitis is extremely important. Relapse of vasculitis, even after complete remission, is quite common in many forms, including both large- and small-vessel diseases. Relapse may occur weeks to years from the time of clinical remission and manifest with different clinical findings than those seen on initial presentation. For example, aortic aneurysms may be seen in patients with GCA years after the patient was believed to be in "remission." Other manifestations may also occur, even in the absence of clinical symptoms, and are more likely missed when patients are believed to be "cured" of their vasculitis. For example, inadequate surveillance may allow renal insufficiency in patients with ANCA-associated vasculitis to go undetected until end-stage renal failure has occurred.

Medical Therapies for Vasculitis

Medical management of patients with vasculitis should only be directed by physicians familiar with both the use of chronic immunosuppressive agents and the clinical presentation and management of vasculitis. The acute and chronic toxicities of these drugs should not be underestimated and can result in significant morbidity. Treatment protocols are beyond the scope of this chapter, but the most commonly used medications for vasculitis are briefly outlined. Many different agents have been used for vasculitis (see Box 39.2).

Glucocorticoids are used for almost all patients with almost all types of vasculitis during the acute presentation or during flares. They have a rapid onset of action, and high doses often stabilize patients even with severe manifestations such as alveolar hemorrhage or glomerulonephritis. The toxicities of glucocorticoids, especially with prolonged use, are serious and common and include weight gain, osteoporosis, osteonecrosis, glucose intolerance, Cushingoid habitus, adrenal suppression, hypertension, mood disturbances, frank psychosis, cataracts, glaucoma, and many others.

Other immunosuppressive drugs are often used in conjunction with glucocorticoids, either to provide more effective therapy and induce a remission or to act as "steroid-sparing" drugs, allowing for safe tapering of the glucocorticoids.

Cyclophosphamide is widely considered the most effective agent for inducing and maintaining remission in multiple types of vasculitis.[22] The introduction of cyclophosphamide-based therapy changed the prognosis of many of these diseases. Although cyclophosphamide is extremely effective, its multiple toxicities are severe and include cytopenias, especially neutropenia with associated infections, gonadal failure, teratogenicity, hemorrhagic cystitis, transitional cell carcinoma of the bladder, myelodysplasia, mucositis, hair loss, and others. Controversy exists about the best route of administration for cyclophosphamide, orally or intravenously.

Multiple alternative agents have been tested and proposed to limit use of cyclophosphamide. Methotrexate, taken orally or intramuscularly weekly, has demonstrated efficacy as both a remission-induction agent and remission-maintenance agent for GPA and is used for both purposes for multiple vasculitides.[50] The toxicities of methotrexate include cytopenias, gastrointestinal upset, oral ulcers, teratogenicity, and hepatic disease. Azathioprine is another commonly used agent for remission maintenance in vasculitis.[27] Azathioprine can cause cytopenias, infections, nausea, mucositis, hair loss, pancreatitis, and other problems but, like methotrexate, is usually well tolerated even for extended periods. Mycophenolate mofetil is also used for vasculitis. Cyclosporine has long been used in Behçet disease and occasionally in other vasculitides.

Rituximab has been demonstrated in two randomized controlled trials to have similar efficacy to cyclophosphamide for induction of remission in ANCA-associated vasculitis (GPA and MPA). The risks of rituximab include allergic reactions and potential for infections. Repeated courses of rituximab have now become a standard method of maintaining remission in ANCA-associated vasculitis, and this approach is the subject of several recent and current clinical trials.[51,52]

Plasmapheresis (plasma exchange) has a central role in treating anti–glomerular basement membrane antibody–associated disease (Goodpasture syndrome). Plasmapheresis was regularly used at some centers to treat both alveolar hemorrhage and severe glomerulonephritis in ANCA-associated vasculitis. However, the results of the PEXIVAS trial have called into question the utility of this treatment for GPA and MPA.[53] Plasmapheresis is frequently used to treat acute manifestations of CV and occasionally other vasculitides. Intravenous Ig is a mainstay of therapy for Kawasaki disease and has been advocated for several other types of vasculitis, often as a second or third line regimen, and based mostly on small case series.

Many biological agents ("biologics") have been, and continue to be, studied as treatment for vasculitides (see Box 39.2).[29] This rapidly expanding group of agents that inhibit specific targets within the immune system is having a remarkable impact on the care of patients with a wide variety of autoimmune and systemic inflammatory diseases. The studies of rituximab for GPA and MPA demonstrated efficacy of the agent, and it has become the standard of care in many situations.[30,31] Mepolizumab, a biological agent directed against IL-5, has been proven efficacious for patients with EGPA.[34] In contrast, despite initial enthusiasm from open-label studies, randomized trials studying the use of inhibitors of TNF-α did not demonstrate efficacy of this class of drug for treatment of either GPA[54] or GCA.[55] However, two randomized trials have demonstrated the efficacy of tocilizumab (IL-6 inhibition) benefit for the treatment of GCA.[7,8] These missed experiences highlight the need for properly conducted randomized clinical trials in vasculitis. Studies testing the efficacy of several other biologics for various forms of vasculitis are either currently in process or in the planning stages.

Surgical or Procedural Interventions for Vasculitis

In addition to medical therapies, interventional and surgical treatments for vasculitis remain options for certain types of problems, especially in larger vessels after damage has become permanent. Angioplasty and stent placement have been performed for patients with TAK and other diseases when severe arterial stenoses occur in large vessels. Results of these interventions are mixed, with restenosis a commonly reported problem. Whether or not drug-eluting stents offer advantages for the vasculitides remains to be demonstrated.

Surgical bypass or grafts of stenotic vessels, including the aorta and coronary, subclavian, carotid, and renal arteries, are an option for patients with large-vessel vasculitides. Several questions are unanswered regarding the proper timing of such surgery in the presence of "active" disease or when patients are on chronic glucocorticoids. Reconstructive surgery also plays a role in the care of patients with vasculitis, especially in patients with GPA who suffer deforming damage from nasal collapse or other upper airway and retroorbital disease.

Miscellaneous Issues in the Treatment of Vasculitis
Pneumocystis Jiroveci Pneumonia Prophylaxis
It is now standard practice to prescribe trimethoprim-sulfamethoxazole or another agent for prophylaxis against *P. jiroveci* (formerly *carinii*) pneumonia for patients on medium to high doses of glucocorticoids in combination with another immunosuppressive agent.

Gonadal Function and Pregnancy-Related Problems
Treatment of vasculitis often involves drugs that adversely affect patients' gonadal function or are problematic during pregnancy, or

both.[56] Cyclophosphamide can cause both male and female sterility and is a highly teratogenic agent. Methotrexate is teratogenic and an abortifacient drug. Glucocorticoids cause significant maternal and some fetal problems. Several of the other treatments in Box 39.2 are either directly contraindicated during pregnancy, or their safety during pregnancy has not been established.

It is imperative that patients in their reproductive years be counseled at the time of diagnosis and regularly thereafter regarding issues of fertility, pregnancy, and contraception. Full discussion of these issues often leads to careful planning that may involve freezing sperm, empirical ovarian-preserving medication protocols, and reevaluation of contraceptive choices.

Prevention of Osteoporosis

Because patients with inflammatory vasculitis are often treated with repeated courses of high-dose glucocorticoids, it is essential that treating physicians give consideration to preservation of bone mass and assessments of osteoporosis. Most patients need to be given calcium and vitamin D supplementation, and many patients may be candidates for bisphosphonates or other treatments for prophylaxis or treatment of glucocorticoid-induced osteoporosis. A baseline bone density scan is often useful for risk stratification.

Accelerated Atherosclerosis

There is mounting evidence and concern that patients with inflammatory vasculitis are at increased risk of accelerated atherosclerosis and CAD, as is seen in patients with other chronic inflammatory diseases such as rheumatoid arthritis and SLE.[57,58] The etiology of the atherosclerosis is likely multifactorial but includes glucocorticoid use, lipid disorders associated with disease and treatment regimens, and other treatment-related problems, such as nephrotic syndrome and diabetes mellitus. However, the impact of chronic inflammation itself may be the most important factor in the development of atherosclerosis. Ongoing research is directed at the interaction between inflammation and atherogenesis. Whether or not chronic therapy with statins or other agents that act via lipid or inflammatory pathways is appropriate has yet to be proven in clinical studies.

REFERENCES

1. Bloch DA, Michel BA, Hunder GG, et al. The American College of Rheumatology 1990 criteria for the classification of vasculitis. Patients and methods. *Arthritis Rheum.* 1990;33:1068–1073.
2. Jennette JC, Falk RJ, Bacon PA, et al. 2012 revised International Chapel Hill Consensus Conference Nomenclature of Vasculitides. *Arthritis Rheum.* 2013;65(1):1–11.
3. Watts RA, Suppiah R, Merkel PA, et al. Systemic vasculitis—is it time to reclassify? *Rheumatology (Oxford).* 2011;50:643–645.
4. Kissin GY, Merkel PA. Large-vessel vasculitis. In: Coffman JD, Eberhardt RT, eds. *Peripheral Arterial Disease: Diagnosis and Treatment.* Totawa, NJ: Humana Press; 2002:319.
5. Weyand CM, Goronzy JJ. Giant-cell arteritis and polymyalgia rheumatica. *Ann Intern Med.* 2003;139:505–515.
6. Mahr AD, Jover JA, Spiera RF, et al. Adjunctive methotrexate for treatment of giant cell arteritis: an individual patient data meta-analysis. *Arthritis Rheum.* 2007;56(8):2789–2797.
7. Villiger PM, Adler S, Kuchen S, et al. Tocilizumab for induction and maintenance of remission in giant cell arteritis: a phase 2, randomised, double-blind, placebo-controlled trial. *Lancet.* 2016;387(10031):1921–1927.
8. Stone JH, Tuckwell K, Dimonaco S, et al. Trial of tocilizumab in giant-cell arteritis. *N Engl J Med.* 2017;377(4):317–328.
9. Kerr GS, Hallahan CW, Giordano J, et al. Takayasu arteritis. *Ann Intern Med.* 1994;120:919–929.
10. Sakane T, Takeno M, Suzuki N, et al. Behcet's disease. *N Engl J Med.* 1999;341:1284–1291.
11. Sridharan ST. Relapsing polychondritis. In: Hoffman GS, Weyand CM, eds. *Inflammatory Diseases of Blood Vessels.* New York: Marcel Dekker; 2001:675.
12. St Clair EW, McCallum RM. Cogan's syndrome. *Curr Opin Rheumatol.* 1999;11:47–52.
13. Liang KP, Chowdhary VR, Michet CJ, et al. Noninfectious ascending aortitis: a case series of 64 patients. *J Rheumatol.* 2009;36:2290–2297.
14. Merkel PA. Noninfectious ascending aortitis: staying ahead of the curve. *J Rheumatol.* 2009;36:2137–2140.
15. Rojo-Leyva F, Ratliff NB, Cosgrove 3rd DM, et al. Study of 52 patients with idiopathic aortitis from a cohort of 1,204 surgical cases. *Arthritis Rheum.* 2000;43:901–907.
16. Quinn KA, Ahlman MA, Malayeri AA, et al. Comparison of magnetic resonance angiography and 18F-fluorodeoxyglucose positron emission tomography in large-vessel vasculitis. *Ann Rheum Dis.* 2018;77(8):1165–1171.
17. Stone JH, Khosroshahi A, Deshpande V, Stone JR. IgG4-related systemic disease accounts for a significant proportion of thoracic lymphoplasmacytic aortitis cases. *Arthritis Care Res (Hoboken).* 2010;62(3):316–322.
18. Guillevin L. Polyarteritis nodosa and microscopic polyangiitis. In: Ball GV, Bridges L, eds. *Vasculitis.* New York: Oxford University Press; 2002:300.
19. Guillevin L, Lhote F, Cohen P, et al. Polyarteritis nodosa related to hepatitis B virus. A prospective study with long-term observation of 41 patients. *Medicine (Baltimore).* 1995;74:238–253.
20. Falk RJ, Gross WL, Guillevin L, et al. Granulomatosis with polyangiitis (Wegener's): an alternative name for Wegener's granulomatosis. *Arthritis Rheum.* 2011;63(4):863–864.
21. Hoffman GS, Gross WL. Wegener's granulomatosis: clinical aspects. In: Hoffman GS, Weyand CM, eds. *Inflammatory Diseases of Blood Vessels.* New York: Marcel Dekker; 2001:381.
22. Hoffman GS, Kerr GS, Leavitt RY, et al. Wegener's granulomatosis: an analysis of 158 patients. *Ann Intern Med.* 1992;116:488–498.
23. Allenbach Y, Seror R, Pagnoux C, et al. High frequency of venous thromboembolic events in Churg-Strauss syndrome, Wegener's granulomatosis and microscopic polyangiitis but not polyarteritis nodosa: a systematic retrospective study on 1130 patients. *Ann Rheum Dis.* 2009;68:564–567.
24. Merkel PA, Lo GH, Holbrook JT, et al. Brief communication: high incidence of venous thrombotic events among patients with Wegener granulomatosis: the Wegener's Clinical Occurrence of Thrombosis (WeCLOT) Study. *Ann Intern Med.* 2005;142:620–626.
25. Walton EW. Giant-cell granuloma of the respiratory tract (Wegener's granulomatosis). *BMJ.* 1958;2:265–270.
26. Reinhold-Keller E, Beuge N, Latza U, et al. An interdisciplinary approach to the care of patients with Wegener's granulomatosis: long-term outcome in 155 patients. *Arthritis Rheum.* 2000;43:1021–1032.
27. Jayne D, Rasmussen N, Andrassy K, et al. A randomized trial of maintenance therapy for vasculitis associated with antineutrophil cytoplasmic autoantibodies. *N Engl J Med.* 2003;349:36–44.
28. Langford CA. Treatment of ANCA-associated vasculitis. *N Engl J Med.* 2003;349:3–4.
29. Langford CA, Sneller MC. Biologic therapies in the vasculitides. *Curr Opin Rheumatol.* 2003;15:3–10.
30. Jones RB, Tervaert JW, Hauser T, et al. Rituximab versus cyclophosphamide in ANCA-associated renal vasculitis. *N Engl J Med.* 2010;363:211–220.
31. Stone JH, Merkel PA, Spiera R, et al. Rituximab versus cyclophosphamide for ANCA-associated vasculitis. *N Engl J Med.* 2010;363:221–232.
32. Guillevin L, Lhote F, Cohen P. Churg-Strauss syndrome: clinical aspects. In: Hoffman GS, Weyand CM, eds. *Inflammatory Diseases of Blood Vessels.* New York: Marcel Dekker; 2001:399.
33. Guillevin L, Cohen P, Gayraud M, et al. Churg-Strauss syndrome. Clinical study and long-term follow-up of 96 patients. *Medicine (Baltimore).* 1999;78:26–37.

34. Wechsler ME, Akuthota P, Jayne D, et al. Mepolizumab or placebo for eosinophilic granulomatosis with polyangiitis. *N Engl J Med.* 2017;376(20):1921–1932.

35. Barron KS. Kawasaki disease: etiology, pathogenesis, and treatment. *Cleve Clin J Med.* 2002;69(Suppl 2):SII69–SII78.

36. Saulsbury FT. Henoch-Schonlein purpura. *Curr Opin Rheumatol.* 2001;13:35–40.

37. Cacoub P, Costedoat-Chalumeau N, Lidove O, et al. Cryoglobulinemia vasculitis. *Curr Opin Rheumatol.* 2002;14:29–35.

38. Ghosn M, Palmer MB, Najem CE, et al. New-onset hepatitis C virus-associated glomerulonephritis following sustained virologic response with direct-acting antiviral therapy. *Clin Nephrol.* 2017;87(5):261–266 [2017].

39. Calabrese LH, Duna GF, Lie JT. Vasculitis in the central nervous system. *Arthritis Rheum.* 1997;40:1189–1201.

40. Hajj-Ali RA, Singhal AB, Benseler S, et al. Primary angiitis of the CNS. *Lancet Neurol.* 2011;10:561–572.

41. Calabrese LH, Dodick DW, Schwedt TJ, et al. Narrative review: reversible cerebral vasoconstriction syndromes. *Ann Intern Med.* 2007;146:34–44.

42. Merkel PA. Drug-induced vasculitis. *Rheum Dis Clin North Am.* 2001;27:849–862.

43. Merkel PA. Drug-induced vasculitis. In: Hoffman GS, Weyand CM, eds. *Inflammatory Diseases of Blood Vessels.* New York: Marcel Dekker; 2001:727.

44. Choi HK, Merkel PA, Walker AM, et al. Drug-associated antineutrophil cytoplasmic antibody-positive vasculitis: prevalence among patients with high titers of antimyeloperoxidase antibodies. *Arthritis Rheum.* 2000;43:405–413.

45. Daxini A, Cronin K, Sreih AG. Vasculitis associated with immune checkpoint inhibitors—a systematic review. *Clin Rheumatol.* 2018;37(9):2579–2584.

46. Grayson PC, Tomasson G, Cuthbertson D, et al. Association of vascular physical examination findings and arteriographic lesions in large vessel vasculitis. *J Rheumatol.* 2012;39:303–309.

47. Niles JL. Antineutrophil cytoplasmic antibodies in the classification of vasculitis. *Annu Rev Med.* 1996;47:303–313.

48. Merkel PA, Polisson RP, Chang Y, et al. Prevalence of antineutrophil cytoplasmic antibodies in a large inception cohort of patients with connective tissue disease. *Ann Intern Med.* 1997;126:866–873.

49. Kissin EY, Merkel PA. Diagnostic imaging in Takayasu arteritis. *Curr Opin Rheumatol.* 2004;16:31–37.

50. Langford CA, Sneller MC, Hoffman GS. Methotrexate use in systemic vasculitis. *Rheum Dis Clin North Am.* 1997;23:841–853.

51. Guillevin L, Pagnoux C, Karras A, et al. Rituximab versus azathioprine for maintenance in ANCA-associated vasculitis. *N Engl J Med.* 2014;371(19):1771–1780.

52. Gopaluni S, Smith RM, Lewin M, et al. Rituximab versus azathioprine as therapy for maintenance of remission for anti-neutrophil cytoplasm antibody-associated vasculitis (RITAZAREM): study protocol for a randomized controlled trial. *Trials.* 2017;18(1):112.

53. Walsh M, Merkel PA, Peh CA, et al. Plasma exchange and glucocorticoid dosing in the treatment of anti-neutrophil cytoplasm antibody associated vasculitis (PEXIVAS): protocol for a randomized controlled trial. *Trials.* 2013;14:73.

54. WGET Research Group. Etanercept plus standard therapy for Wegener's granulomatosis. *N Engl J Med.* 2005;352:351–361.

55. Hoffman GS, Cid MC, Rendt-Zagar KE, et al. Infliximab for maintenance of glucocorticosteroid-induced remission of giant cell arteritis: a randomized trial. *Ann Intern Med.* 2007;146:621–630.

56. Langford CA, Kerr GS. Pregnancy in vasculitis. *Curr Opin Rheumatol.* 2002;14:36–41.

57. Hahn BH. Systemic lupus erythematosus and accelerated atherosclerosis. *N Engl J Med.* 2003;349:2379–2380.

58. Argyropoulou OD, Protogerou AD, Sfikakis PP. Accelerated atheromatosis and arteriosclerosis in primary systemic vasculitides: current evidence and future perspectives. *Curr Opin Rheumatol.* 2018;30(1):36–43.

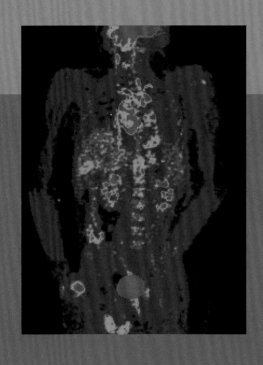

中文导读

第40章
大血管血管炎

　　本章重点介绍大动脉炎的两种主要形式，大动脉炎（takayasu arteritis，TAK）和巨细胞动脉炎（giant cell arteritis，GCA），详细阐述大动脉炎是由主动脉和（或）其主要大动脉分支的炎症病变引起。临床表现包括肢体缺血、中风、视力丧失、心脏病、高血压和主动脉瘤。影像学检查可以发现上肢和主动脉弓上动脉血管狭窄或闭塞形态上变化特征。治疗上主要是根据病情进展，控制和稳定动脉炎症反应，再行相关血管缺血干预治疗。本章还介绍了大动脉炎与其他动脉炎病变或全身性风湿病［如白塞综合征、柯根综合征、免疫球蛋白G4（IgG4）相关疾病、复发性多软骨炎或脊柱关节炎］的鉴别。该类血管疾病尽管不常见，但由于病因不明，临床表现无特异性，早期诊断及治疗困难，常常出现临床症状和并发症后才引起注意，值得关注和重视。

赵纪春

Large Vessel Vasculitis

Peter A. Merkel and Maria C. Cid

Large vessel vasculitis refers to a group of diseases involving inflammation of the aorta and/or its major large artery branches not caused by infection, radiation, or trauma. These diseases may come to the attention of vascular medicine specialists through any one of the multiple clinical manifestations of disease the disorders cause, including claudication, limb ischemia, stroke, visual loss, cardiac disease, hypertension, and aortic aneurysms. Large vessel vasculitis may also be suspected after arterial changes are found incidentally through imaging studies. This chapter focuses on the two main forms of large vessel vasculitis, Takayasu arteritis (TAK) and giant cell arteritis (GCA), as well as isolated aortitis. Large vessel vasculitis can also rarely be seen in other forms of vasculitis or systemic rheumatic disease such as Behçet disease, Cogan syndrome, immunoglobulin G4 (IgG4)-related disease, relapsing polychondritis, or spondyloarthropathy.

TAKAYASU ARTERITIS

TAK is a rare chronic inflammatory large vessel form of vasculitis that affects the aorta and its primary branches. Chronic vascular inflammation leads to vessel stenosis and, less commonly, aneurysm formation. The presentation and progression may be insidious, but the disease can lead to organ- and life-threatening complications and all clinicians specializing in vascular medicine should be familiar with the clinical manifestations of TAK.

Epidemiology

TAK is a rare disorder that has variable incidence and prevalence depending on the country where it has been studied. In the United States, incidence estimates from Olmstead County, Minnesota, are 2.6 cases/million/year, whereas in Sweden they are 1.2 cases/million/year.[1,2] Autopsy studies in Japan document a high prevalence, with evidence of TAK found in 1 of every 3000 individuals.[3] Similar postmortem studies have not been performed elsewhere to provide comparative data. Approximately 90% of patients with TAK are female. The peak incidence of TAK is in the third decade of life. However, the distinction between TAK and GCA with large artery involvement can be difficult, and the diagnosis a patient, who presents after age 50 years, receives may vary by geographic location and specialty.

Pathogenesis

The etiopathogenesis of TAK is unknown. Differences in disease prevalence and characteristics among different racial and ethnic cohorts suggest a genetic predisposition for TAK, and recent data are finding some allelic associations that have provided intriguing leads to pathogenic pathways of disease susceptibility.[4-6] There has long been speculation that, because of the increased prevalence of *Mycobacterium tuberculosis* (TB) infection in countries with a high prevalence of TAK

(e.g., India, Korea, Mexico), mycobacterial infection may play a role in the etiology TAK. However, this theory has not been consistently upheld and a causal link has not been established.[7,8] Interestingly, the current treatment approaches to TAK include medications that could promote reactivation of mycobacterial infection.

Clinical Manifestations

Systemic symptoms and signs occur in less than half of all patients and include fever, weight loss, malaise, and generalized arthralgias and myalgias. Patients more often present with signs and/or symptoms of tissue ischemia, never having had more diffuse constitutional symptoms. The most common symptom of TAK is upper-extremity claudication, occurring in more than 60% of patients and reflecting disease predilection for aortic arch vessels (~90% of cases) (Figs. 40.1–40.3).[9] The most frequent clinical findings include blood pressure asymmetry in paired extremities and bruits found most often over the carotid, subclavian, and aortic vessels.[10] Aneurysms most often affect the aortic root and lead to stretching of the atrioventricular annulus and producing valvular regurgitation (~20% of patients) that often eventually requires surgical intervention. Hypertension occurs in at least 40% of patients in US cohorts and is even more common in Japanese and Indian cohorts (80%). Hypertension is most frequently due to renal artery stenosis, but it may also result from suprarenal aortic stenosis (Figs. 40.4–40.6).[9,11] However, the diagnosis of hypertension can easily be missed in patients with disease involving both upper extremities where peripheral cuff measurements in either arm will be an inaccurate reflection of central aortic pressure. Hypertension with vascular bruits or claudication, especially in younger patients, should lead to a suspicion of TAK and to further evaluation of all four extremity pulses and blood pressures for asymmetry. Vascular imaging of the entire aorta and primary branch vessels should then confirm anatomical abnormalities compatible with the diagnosis and delineate the extent of disease and types of lesions.

Coronary artery disease in TAK may be the result of either coronary arteritis, obstruction of the coronary arteries at their take off from an inflamed aorta, or coronary artery aneurysms. Young women with TAK who present to medical attention with chest pain are often not immediately evaluated for possible angina due to lack of understanding and knowledge about TAK on the part of the evaluating physician; such delays in care can be fatal. Angina should be considered not a rare event in patients with TAK who present with chest pain. However, aortitis without coronary artery involvement can also be a TAK-related cause of chest pain, as can aortic dissection.

The most common morbidity in TAK results primarily from extremity claudication leading to discomfort and reduced functional capacity that may affect the patient's ability to work. Less common but regularly seen and highly problematic are cardiac, renal, and central nervous system manifestations that include myocardial infarction,

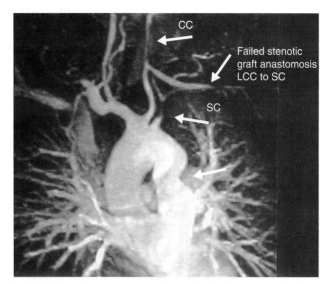

Fig. 40.1 Magnetic resonance angiography illustrating stenotic lesions involving aorta, left common carotid *(LCC)*, and left subclavian *(SC)* arteries.

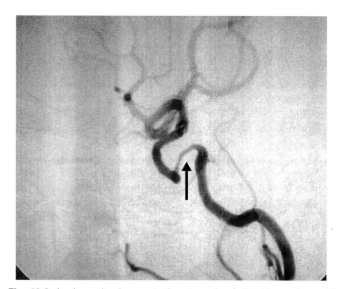

Fig. 40.3 Angiography demonstrating stenosis of distal internal carotid artery *(arrow)*.

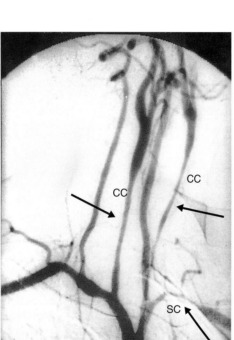

Fig. 40.2 Angiography demonstrating stenoses of left subclavian *(SC)* and bilateral common carotid *(CC)* arteries.

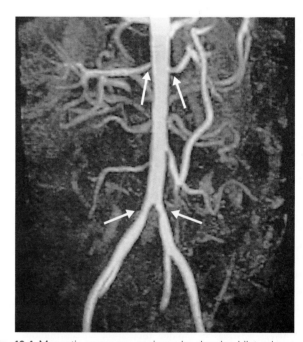

Fig. 40.4 Magnetic resonance angiography showing bilateral common iliac and renal arterial stenoses *(arrows)*.

renal artery hypertension, heart failure, and stroke. Undetected and/ or untreated hypertension is a significant cofactor in these disease sequelae. Causes of death include stroke, congestive heart failure, sudden death of uncertain cause, unrecognized or inadequately treated hypertension, and infection secondary to effects of immunosuppressive medications.[12,13]

Differential Diagnosis

A thorough and careful investigation is necessary to distinguish TAK from its mimics (Box 40.1). Congenital and acquired disorders of tissue matrix may present with aortic root dilation, valvular insuffi-

ciency, and aneurysms in other sites; however, the findings are not generally associated with large vessel stenoses, the hallmark of TAK. In many cases, there are also genetic studies and extravascular features that help to identify the syndromic disorders (e.g., Marfan, Loeys-Dietz, Ehlers-Danlos syndromes). Exceptions better known for matrix abnormalities usually leading to stenoses are fibromuscular dysplasia and Grange syndrome.[14] The most common disease process that needs to be differentiated from TAK is atherosclerosis, which can result in all of the arterial lesions seen in TAK. Although lesions of TAK generally have a different appearance than atherosclerotic lesions, there is a major unmet need to develop imaging or other approaches to improve the identification of each type of arterial pathology. Furthermore, inflammatory disease and atherosclerosis may coexist, especially as patients age.

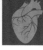

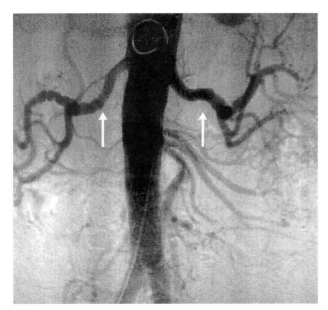

Fig. 40.5 Angiography demonstrating bilateral renal artery lesions mimicking fibromuscular dysplasia *(arrows)*.

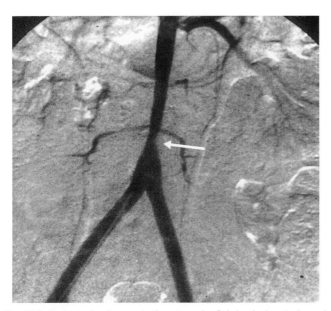

Fig. 40.6 Angiography demonstrating stenosis of abdominal aorta *(arrow)*.

Although other autoimmune disorders can be associated with large vessel vasculitis, they are most often distinguished by their other associated disease manifestations and age preferences. Aortitis restricted to the aortic arch has emerged as one of numerous examples of single-organ vasculitis.[15] Distinguishing it from TAK requires complete evaluation of the large vessel anatomy and careful follow-up over years to be certain that it is not the first sign of TAK. It is important to distinguish isolated aortitis from TAK because, after surgical intervention, further therapy may not always be required.[16–18]

A significant and often underappreciated clinical variation exists between the clinical presentations of TAK and GCA. A comparative cohort study of TAK and GCA identified numerous shared features of disease, much of this coming to light with the advent and increased use of noninvasive vascular imaging studies.[19] TAK and GCA may be indistinguishable in patients who present in middle age (45 to 55 years

BOX 40.1 Differential Diagnosis of Takayasu Arteritis

Autoimmune Disease
Behçet disease
Cogan syndrome
Kawasaki disease
Relapsing polychondritis
Sarcoidosis
Spondyloarthropathy
Immunoglobulin G4–related disease with aortitis
Idiopathic single-organ vasculitis restricted to the aortic arch

Collagen Vascular Disease (Congenital or Acquired)
Ehlers-Danlos syndrome
Fibromuscular dysplasia
Grange syndrome
Loeys-Dietz syndrome
Marfan syndrome
Idiopathic aortic dissection/aneurysm

Infectious
Tuberculosis
Syphilis
Coxiella burnetii
Salmonella typhimurium
Staphylococcus aureus

Other
Atherosclerotic vascular disease
Aortic aneurysm associated with congenital bicuspid aortic valve

When vasculitis is a complication of these diseases, it most often takes the form of small vessel disease.

of age) with large artery stenoses and less often aneurysms, especially of the aortic root. This overlap in clinical manifestations of TAK and GCA has led some to propose using a similar set of outcome measures when studying these diseases.[20,21] However, the different epidemiology between TAK and GCA, some differences in large arterial involvement, and the differences in genetic associations and response to targeted therapies found to date provide compelling evidence that these two diseases may be part of a clinical spectrum of vasculitis but have different etiologies or pathogenic mechanisms.[4–6,22–25]

Infectious causes of large vessel aneurysms should always be considered irrespective of age or sex. Stenosis of large vessels is unusual in the setting of infection, where aneurysms dominate.

Diagnosis

Serological tests do not exist to identify TAK. Rarely, the diagnosis is first considered after a surgical procedure provides biopsy findings that are compatible with the diagnosis. Most often the diagnosis is based on clinical findings in the presence of compatible vascular imaging abnormalities.[26,27] A delay in establishing a diagnosis is common; not infrequently, several years pass between an initial clinical symptom, such as upper limb claudication or even pulselessness, and diagnosis. Catheter-directed angiography allows for luminal imaging and pressure measurements and provides opportunities for intervention (e.g., angioplasty), but it provides little direct information about the vessel wall. Computed tomography (CT) or magnetic resonance imaging and angiography (MRI/MRA) are now the much-preferred imaging modality for establishing a diagnosis of TAK and provide more information regarding vessel wall thickening and edema, but the clinical implications of these findings, although suggestive of active vascular disease, do not always correlate with disease activity or progression.[28] Studies examining the use of positron emission tomography (PET) imaging combined with either CT or MRA and are underway to determine whether more useful information may be derived about the vessel lumen and wall (Fig. 40.7). The presence or absence of increased tagged glucose uptake within large vessels may have improved sensitivity and specificity for identifying active disease in TAK.[29-32]

Although systemic signs and symptoms or elevated acute phase reactants, including erythrocyte sedimentation rate (ESR) and C-reactive protein (CRP), may be suggestive of active disease, they are inadequately sensitive in patients who have only vascular symptoms or findings. Sequential angiographic evaluations have revealed progression of disease, based on the presence of new vascular abnormalities, in more than 50% of patients with normal ESRs.[11] In addition, histopathological proof of vascular inflammation has been documented in 44% of surgical specimens from patients with TAK who underwent bypass surgery at a time when their disease was believed to be quiescent. Thus among the major challenges in caring for patients with TAK is determining whether active disease is present.

Treatment

Essential to effective treatment is accurate determination of disease activity, a goal that may not always be possible. Often the development of new arterial lesions in TAK is a completely asymptomatic process until a critical stenosis occurs. In addition, because the time of progression of lesions is highly variable and often slow, collateral vessels often form around the site of stenoses. It is common for a patient with TAK to be declared to have active disease only when a new arterial lesion has been found on serial imaging. Thus the challenge is to determine when patients with TAK have active disease meriting treatment, as well as whether treatment is effective in halting progression of disease and/or preventing new disease activity. Compared with many other forms of systemic inflammatory disease, including some other forms of vasculitis, the current ability of physicians to determine disease state activity in TAK and predict outcome is poor. Nonetheless, an approach to

treatment has been established and continues to develop as new treatments are tested in this complex disease.

Due to a chronic and relapsing pattern of disease in TAK, most patients are treated with chronic or repeated courses of immunosuppressive therapy, often for many years. Studies that have incorporated sequential angiography have demonstrated that the majority of patients continue to develop new lesions in new vascular territories, even if they appear clinically to be in remission.[9,11,13,19] Because clinical symptoms and serological tests are often unreliable in monitoring disease activity, serial imaging studies are routinely used for assessment of disease progression.

Therapy with glucocorticoids induces improvement in nearly all patients and initial disease remission in approximately 50%, but in 96% of patients, relapses occur during the course of tapering medication (with a mean of 2.8 relapses per patient in one study).[11,19] Therapy with other immunosuppressive agents may aid in achieving lower glucocorticoid requirements in such individuals or those with glucocorticoid-responsive and relapsing disease.

Many different nonglucocorticoid immunosuppressive agents have been proposed to treat TAK with evidence of efficacy stemming only from case series.[33] Further complicating the comparison of studies of these agents is that the definitions used to assess the drugs' efficacy were highly variable.[34] Among the agents purported to be of possible benefit in the treatment of TAK include more traditional antirheumatic agents, often orally administered, including azathioprine, leflunomide, methotrexate, and mycophenolate mofetil. Cyclophosphamide, an alkylating agent with more substantial potential toxicities than the previously mentioned agents, is generally reserved for use in severe cases of TAK. There has been keen interest in the use of targeted biologic agents to treatment TAK. Tumor necrosis factor (TNF)-α inhibitors have been shown in multiple case series to seemingly provide benefit for some patients with TAK and allow for less use of glucocorticoids. Other biological agents of interest in the treatment of TAK include anti–interleukin-6 (IL-6) agents, ustekinumab (anti–IL-12/23), and rituximab (anti-CD20).

There have been only two randomized controlled trials conducted in TAK. The first trial, conducted by the Vasculitis Clinical Research Consortium in North America, tested the efficacy of abatacept (CTLA4-Ig) as adjunctive therapy to glucocorticoids and found

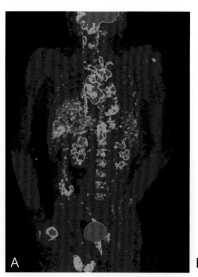
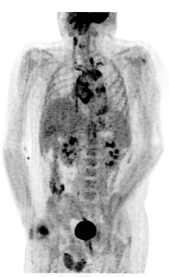
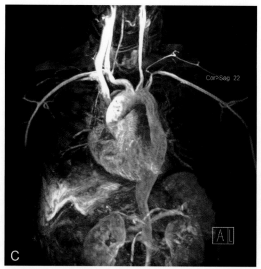

Fig. 40.7 FDG-PET-CT from a 24-Year-Old Man With Takayasu Arteritis Demonstrating PET Activity Throughout the Thoracic Aorta and Arch Vessels, Left Subclavian Stenosis, and a Diffusely Ectatic Thoracic Aorta. (A) and (B) are from maximum intensity projection reconstructions (A with color filter applied) with a corresponding magnetic resonance angiography of the chest (C). (Images courtesy Peter C. Grayson, MD, MSc.)

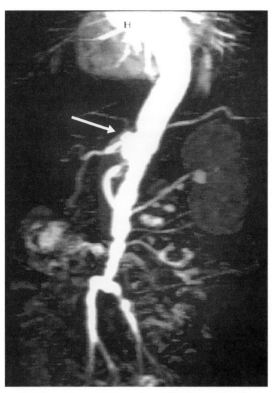

Fig. 40.8 Angiography demonstrating diffuse ectasia of abdominal aorta and bilateral common iliac arteries, significant stenosis of left iliac artery, and dilation of origin of celiac artery *(arrow)*.

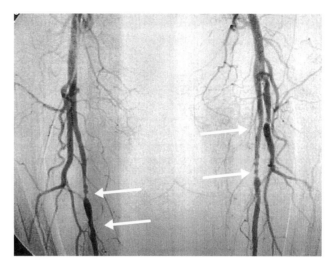

Fig. 40.9 Angiography demonstrating multiple stenoses of superficial femoral arteries *(arrows)*.

no difference between treatment groups.[35] The second trial was conducted in Japan and tested tocilizumab (anti–IL-6) and glucocorticoids versus glucocorticoids alone; this trial had equivocal results, but there were some outcomes indicating possible efficacy of the test drug.[36] Additional randomized trials are critical to help demonstrate efficacy and safety of new or existing therapies for TAK.

Hypertension is a major source of morbidity and mortality in TAK. Delay in the diagnosis of hypertension is common because of the high frequency of subclavian and innominate artery involvement, which may result in markedly inaccurate and reduced measurement of blood pressure in the affected upper extremity; bilateral disease is common, making use of either upper limb inappropriate for clinical care and necessitating the use of lower extremity blood pressure measurements only. However, stenotic lesions also may be present in lower-extremity vessels, leaving some patients without any extremity capable of providing cuff blood pressure measurements that reliably represent those within the aortic root (Figs. 40.8 and 40.9). This emphasizes the need for complete vascular imaging of the entire aorta and its primary branches at the time of diagnosis and during extended follow-up. If stenoses of extremity vessels and/or the abdominal aorta preclude accurate determination of central aortic pressure by using an extremity blood pressure cuff, invasive angiography should be considered to obtain direct central aortic pressure measurements and gradient determinations. Effective blood pressure management is crucial and can be complex in TAK. Even with reliable peripheral recordings, determining and attaining a target pressure range without causing compromised perfusion in the setting of arterial stenotic lesions affecting major organs (e.g., cerebral or coronary stenoses) can be challenging. For this reason, careful monitoring is essential when treatment for blood pressure control is necessary. In addition, medical management must take into consideration renal artery stenosis if present.

Arterial stenoses may affect any organ system. Intervention to correct lesions should be considered in the setting of severely impaired daily function or evidence of significant organ ischemia. Multiple studies demonstrate impressive initial patency rates of 80% to 100% with percutaneous angioplasty.[37–39] However, the rates of vascular restenosis vary widely, from 20% to 71% of cases followed up to 45 months post procedure. The utility of drug-eluting stents in TAK is not clear.

Bypass procedures also may be complicated by vessel restenosis, but rates of sustained patency are higher than with angioplasty (65% to 88%; mean follow-up period 44 to 60 months).[39,40] When interventions are planned, it is preferred that they occur in the setting of disease remission[41] and it may be appropriate to consider prescribing a short course of glucocorticoids before and after any vascular procedure or surgery. When feasible, tissue should be obtained from the origin or insertion of grafts, because histopathological examination can provide critical information in assessing disease activity and later assist in medical management.

A multidisciplinary approach to the care of TAK patients is essential for optimizing patient outcomes. The team should include a rheumatologist, a radiologist expert in vascular imaging, and experts in cardiovascular medicine and surgery.

GIANT CELL ARTERITIS

Giant cell (temporal) arteritis is a chronic inflammatory arteritis that preferentially involves large and medium-sized arteries and affects persons older than 50 years of age. Although autopsy and imaging studies have shown that the aorta and its major tributaries are frequently involved, most of the major clinical manifestations and complications of the disease arise from involvement of the carotid artery branches and include headaches, visual loss, and stroke.[42–44] Aneurysms due to aortitis, as well as extremity arterial occlusions and claudication, can also be seen in GCA, especially in late disease.[45–47] Histopathological diagnosis is usually determined from examination of a biopsy of the superficial temporal artery (Figs. 40.10 and 40.11).

Some 50% of patients with GCA develop *polymyalgia rheumatica* (PMR), an inflammatory disease involving proximal joints and periarticular structures. PMR is clinically characterized by aching and stiffness in the neck, shoulders, or pelvic girdle. PMR can also exist as a distinct entity with no evidence of vascular involvement.[45]

This section of the chapter presents the epidemiology, pathophysiology, clinical manifestations, and treatment options for GCA, with

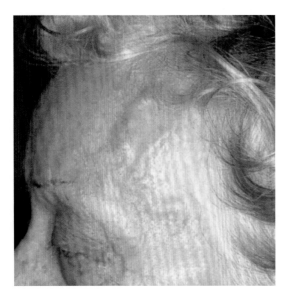

Fig. 40.10 Enlarged, hardened, and pulseless temporal and frontal arteries in a patient with giant cell arteritis.

particular reference to manifestations likely encountered by vascular medicine specialists.

Epidemiology

GCA characteristically occurs in people older than 50 years of age, and its frequency increases with age.[48–50] Maximal incidence of GCA occurs in persons between 75 and 85, and it is twice as frequent in women as men. Although there is a markedly increased incidence of GCA among whites in northern Europe and in populations with similar ethnic background,[46,51] the disease can occur in all populations. GCA is not an uncommon disease. Studies conducted in northern Europe and North America disclose an annual incidence of 19 to 32 cases per 100,000 people older than 50[46,47] and a rate of 49 per 100,000 for individuals in their 80s.[46–51] In Mediterranean countries, the annual incidence is lower, approximately 6 to 10 cases per 100,000.[51] Isolated PMR is even more frequent, with an average annual incidence of 52 to 59 per 100,000 among people older than age 50.[43,45]

Pathology

GCA involves large and medium arteries, and the cranial branches of the carotid and vertebral arteries are the most typically involved. The artery wall is infiltrated by T lymphocytes and macrophages, frequently forming a granulomatous reaction with the presence of multinucleated giant cells (see Fig. 40.11).[48,49] B lymphocytes are less abundant and occasionally form ectopic lymphoid follicles.[50] Scattered polymorphonuclear leukocytes can be occasionally identified.

Inflammatory infiltrates usually reach the artery through the adventitial layer and subsequently expand to involve the entire vessel thickness. Inflammatory lesions are typically segmental, and the extent of inflammatory infiltrates is highly variable among patients, even in different sections of the same specimen.[48,52] The internal elastic lamina is usually disrupted, and giant cells often accumulate in its vicinity but are not required for the diagnosis. In well-developed lesions, the lumen is occluded by intimal hyperplasia. Small arteries and arterioles in the vicinity of the superficial temporal artery are almost invariably involved.[53] In some specimens, inflammation of the vasa vasorum and small vessels surrounding the temporal artery is the only apparent abnormality. The diagnostic specificity of this finding is lower,[54] and, in this setting, other forms of small and medium vessel vasculitis or other systemic diseases must be excluded.[54] Autopsy studies have demonstrated that inflammatory infiltrates are often detected in the aorta and its major tributaries.[55]

Histopathological findings in PMR include chronic synovitis and bursitis of proximal joints.[56,57] Synovitis is usually mild, and inflammatory infiltrates contain CD4 T lymphocytes and macrophages, with scarce granulocytes. Muscle biopsies do not disclose specific abnormalities.

Pathogenesis
Genetic Predisposition

The predominance of GCA and PMR among whites, especially those of northern European origin, strongly suggests a genetic component in the pathogenesis of GCA and PMR. A large-scale genome-wide association study recently confirmed the association of GCA with class II HLA-DRB1*04 alleles, previously reported in candidate polymorphism studies.[24] Outside the HLA region, association of GCA with variants in the plasminogen *(PLG)* and prolyl hydroxylase 4 *(P4HA2)* genes achieved genome-wide significance.[23] Additional variants in genes

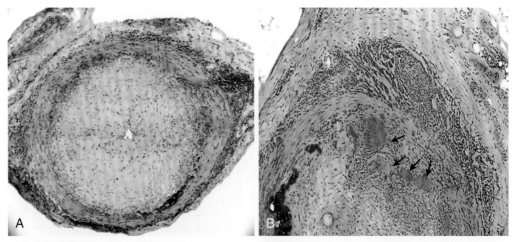

Fig. 40.11 Classic Fully Developed Lesions in Temporal Artery Biopsy Specimens from Patients With Giant Cell Arteritis. (A) Inflammatory infiltrates involving entire arterial wall and predominating at adventitial layer and intima media junction, where a granulomatous reaction around internal elastic lamina can be appreciated. Note prominent intimal hyperplasia virtually occluding lumen. (B) Enlargement of another specimen. Thin arrows indicate multinucleated giant cells.

involved in immune and inflammatory responses have been associated with increased risk of GCA, including protein tyrosine phosphatase nonreceptor type 22 (PTPN22),[58] vascular endothelial growth factor (VEGF),[59] endothelial nitric oxide synthase (eNOS),[59] IL-6, and IL-17, among others.[59,60]

Possible Triggering Agents

Several observations suggest that GCA may be triggered by an environmental agent yet to be defined. Cyclic fluctuations in the incidence of GCA occurring every 6 or 7 years have been reported.[61] In addition, the characteristic granulomatous reaction with multinucleated giant cells has also prompted a search for an infectious agent that may cause a delayed-type hypersensitivity reaction. However, attempts to identify specific pathogens, including Chlamydia pneumoniae, parvovirus B19, or varicella-zoster virus, have led to conflicting results and the search for an infectious trigger continues.[62]

Immunopathogenic Mechanisms

It has been postulated that inflammatory lesions in GCA develop as a consequence of an antigen-specific immune response against antigens present in the vessel wall. Activated dendritic cells have been detected in inflammatory lesions of GCA,[63,64] where they are thought to serve as antigen-presenting cells and provide costimulatory signals for CD4 T cell activation. Innate immune system activation through Toll-like receptors (TLRs) seems to be relevant in the activation of dendritic cells.[63] Immunopathological studies have demonstrated that inflammatory infiltrates in GCA mainly consist of activated T lymphocytes, particularly of the CD4 subset, and macrophages.[49] Expansion of CD4 T lymphocyte clones derived from different areas of temporal artery biopsy specimens has shown that some of them share identical sequences at the third complementary determining region of the T cell receptor,[64] suggesting a specific immune recognition of a disease-relevant antigen. Inhibitory immune checkpoint function would be reduced in GCA, favoring lymphocyte activation during antigen presentation.[65] Activated CD4 T lymphocytes undergo T helper 1 (Th1) differentiation, with vigorous production of interferon (IFN)-γ, a key cytokine in macrophage activation and granuloma formation.[66] IL-17 is also produced in GCA lesions, providing evidence for the participation of Th17-mediated responses in the pathophysiology of GCA.[67] The role of T cells is further supported by epigenetic studies showing marked hypomethylation of genes related to T cell activation in GCA lesions.[68]

Mechanisms of Vascular Injury

Multiple processes have been implicated in the vascular injury seen in GCA. Activated macrophages produce oxygen radicals and proteolytic enzymes that participate in disruption of the vessel wall and tissue destruction.[69,70] Increased levels of lipid peroxidation products, aldose reductase, inducible nitric oxide synthase (iNOS), and functionally active matrix metalloproteases MMP-2 and MMP-9 have been demonstrated in GCA.[69,70]

Systemic Inflammatory Response

Activated macrophages produce proinflammatory cytokines IL-1, TNF-α, and IL-6, which are major inducers of the systemic inflammatory response (fever, weight loss, anemia, and hepatic synthesis of acute phase proteins) often prominent in patients with GCA. Expression of these cytokines in the arterial tissue of patients, as well as circulating levels of TNF-α and IL-6, correlate with the intensity of the systemic inflammatory reaction.[71] As discussed later, these cytokines are able to activate proinflammatory cascades such as chemokine release, adhesion molecule expression, and angiogenesis.[72,73]

Vascular Response to Inflammation

Vessel wall components, particularly endothelial cells and smooth muscle cells (SMCs), actively react to cytokines and growth factors released by infiltrating leukocytes, become pro-inflammatory, and promote amplification and perpetuation of the inflammatory process.[72-75] Inflammation-induced angiogenesis is remarkable in GCA lesions and preferentially occurs at the adventitial layer and within inflammatory infiltrates, particularly in granulomatous areas at the intima media junction.[72,73]

Neovessels may have a protective role at distal sites where providing new blood supply may prevent organ ischemia.[73,76] In addition, neovessels provide a population of endothelial cells that may exert a variety of proinflammatory activities.[72,77] Vascular response to inflammation may eventually lead to vessel occlusion, with subsequent ischemia of the tissues supplied by involved vessels. In GCA, vessel occlusion results mostly from intimal hyperplasia driven by proliferation and matrix production by myointimal cells; platelet-derived growth factor (PDGF) and endothelin-1 appear to be crucial cytokines in this process.[74,78]

Clinical Manifestations

Patients with GCA may present with a wide variety of clinical features, summarized in Table 40.1. Disease-related manifestations may appear rapidly or develop insidiously. A delay of weeks or even months

TABLE 40.1 Clinical Findings in a Series of 250 Patients with Giant Cell Arteritis	
General Features	
Age (mean, range)	75 (50–94)
Sex (female/male)	178/72
Weight loss	61%
Fever	47%
Cranial Symptoms	**86%**
Headache	77%
Temporal artery abnormality (swollen, tender, weak/absent pulse)	74%
Jaw claudication	44%
Scalp tenderness	39%
Facial pain	18%
Earache	18%
Odynophagia	12%
Ocular pain	8%
Tongue pain	5%
Carotidynia	5%
Toothache	5%
Trismus	1%
Ophthalmic Events	**22%**
Blindness (permanent)	14%
Amaurosis fugax	10%
Transient diplopia	4%
Cerebrovascular Accident	**2%**
Symptomatic Large Vessel Involvement (claudication and/or bruit)	**5%**
Polymyalgia Rheumatica (PMR)	**48%**

Modified from Cid MC, Hernandez-Rodriquez J, Grau JM. Vascular manifestations in giant-cell arteritis. In: Asherson RA, Cervera R, ed. *Vascular Manifestations of Systemic Autoimmune Diseases*. London: CRC Press; 2001.

between the onset of clinical symptoms and diagnosis is common, particularly in patients with predominantly systemic complaints in whom more prevalent diseases (e.g., infections, malignancies) are usually suspected. Ischemic complications tend to accumulate in some patients and are frequently early events during the course of the disease.[79,80]

Some data suggest that an initial presentation of GCA that includes signs and symptoms of systemic inflammation (elevated acute phase reactants, fever, anemia, weight loss) is associated with a specific pattern of clinical illness. For unclear reasons, patients with a strong systemic inflammatory response are at lower risk of ischemic events but are more refractory to therapy[76,80,81] than are patients with a seemingly weaker initial inflammatory response. Similarly, as with cranial ischemic complications, symptomatic stenosis of large vessels has been shown to be negatively associated with prominent inflammatory markers at the time of diagnosis.[82]

Systemic Manifestations

Patients with GCA or PMR frequently experience malaise, anorexia, weight loss, and depression.[42–44] Nearly 50% of patients with GCA have fever, and in some patients, fever or constitutional symptoms are the most prominent findings. Approximately 10% of patients present with fever of unknown origin with subtle or no cranial manifestations.[83]

Clinical Manifestations of Cranial Arterial Involvement

Headache is one of the most common and classic symptoms and occurs in 60% to 98% of cases of GCA.[42–44] Intensity and location of headache are highly variable, but it frequently predominates at the temporal areas. Scalp tenderness is also common. Approximately 40% of patients experience jaw claudication when eating, a symptom highly specific for GCA but occasionally seen in other vascular diseases (e.g., necrotizing vasculitis, systemic amyloidosis). Other manifestations, such as facial swelling, tongue ischemia, or edema, are less frequently seen (see Table 40.1).[42–44,86] Patients may also present with a variety of unusual pains in the craniofacial area, including ocular pain, earache, toothache, odynophagia, odontalgia, and carotidynia. When certain of these symptoms predominate, a substantial delay in diagnosis is common.

Visual impairment is the most feared complication of GCA and occurs in approximately 15% of cases.[42–44,82,83] Blindness is most commonly due to anterior ischemic optic neuropathy derived from inflammatory involvement of posterior ciliary arteries supplying the optic nerve.[42–44] Less frequently, central retinal artery occlusion, retrobulbar neuritis, or cortical blindness can occur. Visual loss can be bilateral or unilateral, complete or partial. It usually appears suddenly but is often preceded by transient visual loss (*amaurosis fugax*), diplopia, or, occasionally, blue vision.

Less common ischemic complications include stroke due to involvement of carotid or vertebral tributaries, and scalp or tongue necrosis. Strokes, when they do occur, are more frequent in territories supplied by the vertebral arteries (Fig. 40.12). Additional ischemic manifestations include hearing loss and vestibular dysfunction.[84]

Cardiac, Aortic, and Peripheral Vascular Manifestations

Aortitis and inflammatory involvement of the main branches of the aorta are more common in GCA than previously considered (Fig. 40.13). In a small autopsy series, aortic inflammation was observed in 12 out of 13 patients with GCA.[55] Imaging techniques are now used to indirectly measure aortic inflammation in living individuals.[85–88] Evidence of probable aortic involvement can be detected by PET, computed tomographic angiography (CTA), or MRA in 50% to 65% of patients at the time of diagnosis (see Fig. 40.13).[88–91] Aortic involvement is asymptomatic unless aortic dissection or dilation occurs (Fig. 40.14). Systematic screening of 54 patients revealed that aortic dilatation occurs in 22.5% of patients after a median follow-up of 5.6 years and in 33% after a median follow-up of 8.7 years.[89,90] Interestingly, unlike noninflammatory aortic disease, there is a markedly increased ratio of thoracic to abdominal aortic aneurysms in patients with GCA, and the risk of thoracic disease may be 17-fold higher among patients with a history of GCA.[91,92]

GCA may also involve aortic branches (see Fig. 40.13). PET, CTA, or MRA studies show that subclavian arteries may be involved in 70% of patients, axillary arteries in 40%, iliac arteries in 37%, and femoral arteries in 37%.[88–91] Studies using color duplex ultrasonography have disclosed abnormalities in these territories in approximately one-third of patients.[93] Distal lower-limb arteries (e.g., femoropopliteal, tibial, peroneal) may also be affected.[94] Although in most instances, extremity involvement is asymptomatic, some patients develop claudication and even critical ischemia when significant vascular stenoses occur.

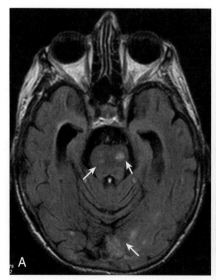
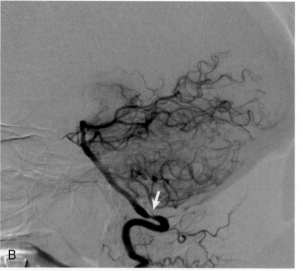

Fig. 40.12 Neurological Complications in Giant Cell Arteritis (GCA). (A) Magnetic resonance imaging discloses multiple ischemic lesions in the vertebral territory in patient with GCA presenting with subacute dementia and ataxia *(arrows)*. (B) Stenosis in left vertebral artery in patient with GCA presenting with recurrent transient ischemic attacks *(arrow)*.

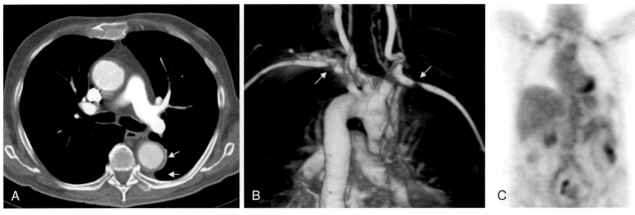

Fig. 40.13 Large Artery Involvement in Giant Cell Arteritis (GCA). (A) Concentric thickening with contrast enhancement of thoracic descending aorta in patient with newly diagnosed GCA (computed tomographic angiography) *(arrows)*. (B) Bilateral subclavian stenosis in patient with newly diagnosed GCA and subclavian bruits (magnetic resonance angiogram) *(arrows)*. (C) Subclavian, axillary, aortic, and iliac arteries fluorodeoxyglucose-18 (^{18}F-FDG) uptake in patient with active GCA (positron emission tomography scan).

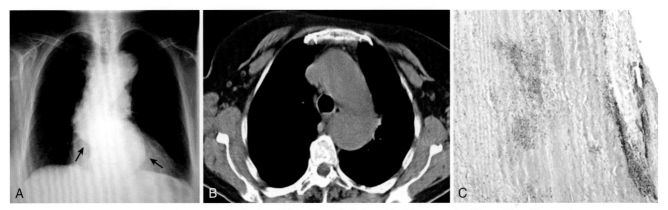

Fig. 40.14 Aortic Aneurysm in Patient With Giant Cell Arteritis Discovered 5 Years After Diagnosis. (A) Plain chest radiography indicating aortic dilatation *(arrows)*. (B) Computed tomography confirming aortic aneurysm. (C) Histology from surgical aortic specimen showing remaining scattered inflammatory infiltrates.

Large vessel occlusions may be late manifestations of GCA, occurring years after initial diagnosis. When they become clinically significant, they often are misdiagnosed as secondary to atherosclerotic disease. For this reason, the frequency of clinically relevant peripheral artery disease in GCA is not well known.

Patients with GCA should be followed indefinitely for complications of large vessel disease, even when there is no evidence of other active disease. In patients with GCA, aortic valvular disease, aortic aneurysms or dissections, and peripheral vascular occlusions should all be considered possibly related to vasculitis. New vascular bruits or cardiac murmurs, asymmetry in blood pressure readings, weak or absent peripheral pulses, and limb claudication or ischemia are all warning signs easily inquired about and examined for in physicians' offices.

Myocardial or mesenteric infarction due to GCA is seen infrequently.[95,96] Because GCA occurs in older people, some cases of inflammatory coronary or mesenteric arteritis may be misdiagnosed as due to atherosclerotic disease. However, even among patients with GCA, atherosclerosis is a much more common cause of cardiac or mesenteric ischemia than vasculitis. With increased interest in the role of inflammation in coronary artery disease and new tools to study the disease process, investigators are now better able to study the contributions, if any, of inflammatory arteritis to coronary artery disease among patients with GCA and other vasculitides.

Polymyalgia Rheumatica

Approximately 50% of patients with GCA present with symptoms of PMR, a syndrome clinically defined by the presence of aching and stiffness in the neck, shoulders, or pelvic girdle. Pain is exacerbated with movement. Morning stiffness is a prominent finding and may last for many hours. Proximal muscles are usually tender, but true weakness or myopathy is not seen. Ultrasonography, MRI, and PET studies indicate that the underlying abnormalities are synovitis and bursitis of proximal joints.[45,97]

PMR can appear simultaneously with cranial symptoms or may precede development of GCA symptoms by months or even years. Some patients without PMR develop PMR symptoms during GCA relapses, and PMR may sometimes be the only clinical manifestation of GCA.[98]

PMR can exist as an isolated entity without any evidence of vascular inflammation. The demography of patients with isolated PMR is similar to that reported for GCA. Genetic risk has been less extensively investigated, and in some studies the risk alleles for PMR are similar to GCA. However, studies exhibit more variability, possibly indicating heterogeneity within patients diagnosed with PMR, because diagnosis is primarily based on clinical judgement. Temporal artery biopsies disclosing GCA can be demonstrated in approximately 10% to 20% of patients with apparently isolated PMR.[45,99] This frequency is lower when cranial symptoms are ruled out by a detailed inquiry and when abnormalities at careful physical examination of the temporal arteries are excluded. Imaging may also reveal large vessel involvement in some patients.[100] It is important that patients with PMR be followed with the same rigor as patients with GCA and evaluated for any clue suggesting vascular involvement.

Patients with GCA may develop peripheral synovitis; knees, wrists, and metacarpophalangeal joints are most frequently involved.[45,99] Peripheral manifestations usually occur in patients with PMR but may also occasionally appear in patients without proximal symptoms of PMR. Other associated manifestations include tenosynovitis, carpal tunnel syndrome, and distal swelling with pitting edema.[45,92] Some patients develop a clinical picture indistinguishable from seronegative rheumatoid arthritis.[80]

Incidentally Discovered Giant Cell Arteritis

Occasionally, GCA may be unexpectedly diagnosed when vascular surgical specimens reveal arteritis with or without giant cells. In these patients, retrospective investigation may reveal prior signs or symptoms attributable to GCA.[17] In this setting, a positive temporal artery biopsy may confirm the diagnosis of GCA. Similarly, imaging with PET, CTA, or MRA performed after surgery recovery may reveal persistent abnormalities suggesting areas of inflammation in the remaining aorta or in aortic primary or secondary branches and blood tests of acute phase reactants may be elevated, supporting a decision to institute pharmacological treatment in addition to surgery.

Physical Examination

Physical examination is extremely important, not only for initial evaluation of patients with possible GCA but also for following patients after the diagnosis has been established. Blood pressure measurements should be taken in both arms at each visit (and periodically in both legs). Asymmetry of pressures may indicate aortic, subclavian, or other peripheral artery involvement. A careful comprehensive examination of all pulses is key to evaluating GCA. The temporal arteries may be swollen, hard, or pulseless in GCA, although they may appear fully normal even in arteries later found to have active arteritis. At times, just a slight asymmetry, decrease, or irregularity in the pulse can be detected in temporal or other cranial arteries. Auscultation for bruits should be performed over carotid, subclavian, axillary, renal, iliac, and other arteries and the aorta. The scalp should be examined for tenderness. Ophthalmological examination, including funduscopy, visual field assessment, and acuity testing, should be performed for evidence of optic ischemia or other abnormalities of GCA. Evidence of synovitis or enthesitis should be sought. A comprehensive examination is important to help evaluate patients for disorders with overlapping features of GCA.

Laboratory Findings

With few exceptions, both GCA and PMR are characterized by a strong acute phase reaction. The ESR is usually markedly elevated, frequently around 100 mm/h (Westergren method). Plasma concentrations of acute phase proteins such as CRP, haptoglobin, and fibrinogen are also elevated. Protein electrophoresis shows an increase in α_2-globulins.[42-44] Thrombocytosis and chronic disease–type anemia are common, and some patients have abnormal liver function tests, particularly increased levels of alkaline phosphatase.[42-44] Hyperbilirubinemia with visible jaundice is rare but may also occur. Symptomatic anemia may occasionally be the first clinical manifestation of GCA. Nonspecific immunological abnormalities, such as decreased numbers of circulating CD8 lymphocytes and elevated levels of soluble IL-2 receptors, are common in GCA and PMR.[42-44,51,86]

Several lymphocyte, monocyte, or endothelial cell activation products can be detected at increased concentrations in plasma from patients with GCA and PMR. These include cytokines such as IL-6,[81,101] TNF-α,[81] B cell–activating factor (BAFF),[102] soluble adhesion molecules such as ICAM-1,[103] S-100 proteins,[104] and von Willebrand factor (vWF) antigen, among others.[42-44] The role these or other cytokines or cellular markers may play in the diagnosis and management of GCA is an area of active investigation.

Diagnosis

Diagnosis of GCA is arrived at by a combination of clinical history, physical examination findings, laboratory studies, and imaging or arterial biopsy results. No one feature or finding is fully diagnostic on its own because even "positive" temporal artery biopsies can occasionally be seen in other types of arteritis and other disorders can also result in similar systemic features, headaches, or visual changes.[105,106] Nonetheless, a positive temporal artery biopsy is an extremely strong finding and is almost always diagnostic.[107] Similarly, no feature or finding is absolutely required to make the diagnosis. For example, the ESR may be normal in up to 10% of patients with GCA at presentation, but certain symptoms and findings should prompt a high suspicion of GCA. It is the initial consideration of GCA that is crucial for initiating the diagnostic process that often leads to empirical treatment even before a diagnosis is fully established.

In parallel with an evaluation of GCA itself, physicians will usually need to consider alternative diagnoses such as brain lesions, infections, or malignancies and conduct appropriate evaluations for these disorders. Even if GCA is established by history and biopsy, other inflammatory vasculitides, such as granulomatosis with polyangiitis or polyarteritis nodosa, must at least be considered and screened for, because they can rarely present with temporal artery involvement.[53,105] Finally, although there are differences between patients with GCA and TAK in terms of the frequency of specific clinical manifestations, distribution of lesions, response to therapy, use of nonglucocorticoid immunosuppressive agents, and outcomes, there are many similar features.[87] Thus all patients with either diagnosis should be screened for manifestations of the other.

In evaluating and treating patients with GCA, the best management often includes collaboration among rheumatologists, ophthalmologists, neurologists, and vascular medicine specialists.

Temporal Artery Biopsy

Histopathological examination of a temporal artery biopsy often provides the definitive diagnosis of GCA.[48,107] The area to be excised is carefully selected, guided by symptoms and physical examination findings. At least a 2-cm fragment should be removed and multiple sections examined histologically. When the initial biopsy is negative for evidence of GCA, excision of the contralateral artery is not routinely recommended but may increase diagnostic sensitivity in selected cases. Temporal artery biopsy is highly sensitive for the diagnosis of GCA.[107] Occasionally, the temporal artery may be involved in the context of other systemic vasculitides or other disorders such as systemic amyloidosis.[48,105] When systemic necrotizing vasculitis involves the temporal artery or its tributaries, it may present with cranial symptoms and complications similar to GCA.

Although the diagnostic yield of a temporal artery biopsy (if performed and examined appropriately) is high, a normal temporal artery biopsy does not necessarily exclude GCA, owing to the segmental distribution of inflammatory infiltrates or involvement of other arteries, and imaging can be essential in these cases. Given the frequent existence of overlapping features among vasculitides, criteria sets have been established to classify patients with vasculitis into specific categories. The most commonly used classification criteria are those of the American College of Rheumatology[108]; the criteria for GCA are outlined in

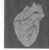

BOX 40.2 American College of Rheumatology Criteria for Classification of Giant Cell (Temporal) Arteritis

1. Age at disease onset ≥50 years
2. New onset of headache or new type of localized pain in the head
3. Temporal artery tenderness or decreased pulsation
4. Erythrocyte sedimentation rate ≥50 mm/h (Westergren)
5. Temporal artery biopsy showing vasculitis with a predominance of mononuclear cells or granulomatous inflammation, usually with multinucleated giant cells

A patient is considered to have giant cell arteritis if at least three of the above criteria are present. Presence of any three or more criteria yields a sensitivity of 93.5% and a specificity of 91.2%.

From Hunder GG, Bloch DA, Michel BA, et al. The American College of Rheumatology 1990 criteria for the classification of giant cell arteritis. *Arthritis Rheum.* 1990;33(8):1122–1128.

Box 40.2. Although not intended for use diagnostically, these criteria are useful when evaluating patients. In addition, they are adopted for use as inclusion criteria for most research studies of GCA. However, to ensure that patients with nonvasculitic conditions are not mistakenly labeled as having GCA, caution must be exercised when applying these criteria. Moreover, these criteria do not allow inclusion of patients with predominantly large vessel involvement. Classification criteria for this and other vasculitides are currently under reconsideration.[109]

Diagnostic Imaging

A variety of imaging modalities are in use or under investigation for the diagnosis and long-term management of GCA.[110,111] These modalities currently include ultrasound, MRA, PET, or PET-CT, and CTA (Figs. 40.13, 40.14, and 40.15). Furthermore, as these imaging techniques continue to be used extensively for evaluation of patients with fever of unknown origin, presumed cancer, or atherosclerotic disease, additional patients who actually have inflammatory vascular disease are likely to be encountered and diagnosed. Thus vascular medicine

specialists, vascular surgeons, and vascular radiologists need to consider GCA when reviewing such imaging studies.

Color duplex ultrasonography and high-resolution MRI of the cranial arteries may be particularly useful in diagnosing GCA. The ultrasonographic finding of a dark hypoechoic halo surrounding the lumen, or MRI evidence of thickening and contrast enhancement of the artery wall, has remarkable specificity.[110] By exploring several artery branches in both sides, ultrasonography may have higher diagnostic sensitivity than temporal artery biopsy, but specificity remains lower.[112] Although much controversy remains about these newer diagnostic studies, they are increasingly considered as potential surrogates when biopsy is not feasible or when other arteries such as the occipital or axillary arteries are involved.[93] MRI/MRA and CT/CTA are increasingly used imaging modalities for screening and evaluating large vessel disease in GCA.[110,111] MRA or CTA can detect arterial wall thickening and contrast enhancement of the artery wall, indicating inflammation as well as abnormal vascular remodeling resulting in dilatation or stenoses. MRA is a relatively low-risk method to screen and monitor patients for large vessel disease in GCA and is increasingly part of the standard management for such patients.

Fluorodeoxyglucose-18 (^{18}F-FDG) PET is another modality for evaluating patients with suspected GCA. PET scans may demonstrate FDG uptake in the aorta and its branches in patients with GCA and also in some patients thought to have just PMR.[100] Furthermore, FDG uptake in the abdominal aorta and arteries of the lower limbs also can be seen in severe atherosclerosis, so specificity is lower in these locations.[113] Its diagnostic sensitivity and specificity have to be tested in larger studies, but ^{18}F-FDG PET may have a role in evaluation of vascular inflammation in patients with atypical symptoms, in patients with fever of unknown origin, and when assessing vascular involvement in patients with apparently isolated PMR. The combination of PET with CT imaging may also have a role in evaluating these patients because it takes advantage of the properties of both techniques.

Imaging may have an important role in the assessment of disease activity and response to therapies during the course of the disease, as well as in detecting vascular damage (dilatation or stenoses). Vascular thickening by CTA or MRA and FDG uptake improve with treatment,

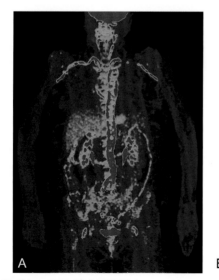
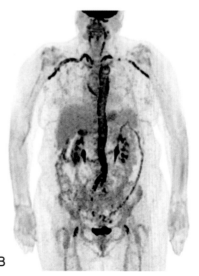

A   B

Fig. 40.15 (A) and (B) FDG-PET-CT from a 68-year-old woman with biopsy-proven giant cell arteritis who underwent FDG-PET-CT at time of diagnosis that showed diffuse FDG uptake throughout the aorta and branch vessels consistent with active vasculitis (A with color filter applied). (Images courtesy Peter C. Grayson, MD, MSc.)

but persistent/recurrent abnormalities may be observed in some patients.[31,114,115] Increased FDG uptake during treatment may predict subsequent relapses.[31] Correlation between imaging findings and clinically active disease is not always clear, and more research is needed before imaging may be routinely used as an outcome measure.

Conventional contrast angiography may confirm involvement of large vessels in patients with bruits or limb claudication, but it is no longer used for screening purposes or serial examination due to its invasive nature. Advantages of catheter-based angiography dictating its current use include the ability to measure blood pressure at various locations to evaluate the functional effect of stenoses and as a prelude for intervention with angioplasty or stent placement.

Diagnosis of Polymyalgia Rheumatica

Diagnosis of PMR relies at present on clinical criteria; imaging modalities may provide supportive evidence.[116,117] MRI, PET, and ultrasound are able to detect subdeltoid or trochanteric bursitis, biceps tenosynovitis, or glenohumeral or hip synovitis, the sources of many polymyalgic symptoms.[45,100,117] An American College of Rheumatology/European League Against Rheumatic Disease classification algorithm[116] has been proposed (Table 40.2). PMR diagnosis requires evaluation to exclude other disorders, particularly rheumatoid arthritis, but also

TABLE 40.2 Polymyalgia Rheumatica Classification Criteria Scoring Algorithm

Criteria	Points Without Ultrasound (0–6)	Points With Ultrasound (0–8)[a]
Morning stiffness >45 minutes	2	2
Hip pain or limited range of motion	1	1
Normal RF or ACPA	2	2
Absence of other joint movement	1	1
At least one shoulder with subdeltoid bursitis and/or biceps tenosynovitis and/or glenohumeral synovitis (either posterior or axillary) and At least one hip with synovitis and/or trochanteric bursitis	NA	1
Both shoulders with subdeltoid bursitis, biceps tenosynovitis, or glenohumeral synovitis	NA	1

[a]Optional ultrasound criteria.
Required criteria: age ≥50 years, bilateral shoulder aching, and abnormal C-reactive protein and/or erythrocyte sedimentation rate. A score of 4 or more is categorized as polymyalgia rheumatica in the algorithm without ultrasound, and a score of 5 or more is categorized as polymyalgia rheumatica in the algorithm with ultrasound.
ACPA, Anticitrullinated protein antibody; NA, not applicable; RF, rheumatoid factor.
From Dasgupta B, Cimmino MA, Maradit-Kremers H, et al. International Polymyalgia Rheumatica Classification Criteria Work Group. European League Against Rheumatism/American College of Rheumatology classification criteria for polymyalgia rheumatica. Ann Rheum Dis. 2012;71:484–492.

inflammatory myopathies, other vasculitides, and infections that occasionally present with similar symptoms.[116]

Treatment and Management

Glucocorticoid therapy is the initial treatment of choice for GCA and, in most cases, induces a dramatic amelioration of disease manifestations within a few days. The most widely recommended initial dose is 40 to 60 mg/day of prednisone (or equivalent glucocorticoid).[118] Presence of transient ocular manifestations (e.g., amaurosis fugax, diplopia, blurred vision) should be considered a medical emergency. Treatment should be started immediately in this setting, even before histological confirmation of GCA is obtained. Glucocorticoid treatment for several days, and even weeks, does not clear the inflammatory infiltrates and therefore should not hinder histopathological diagnosis.[119] When visual loss occurs, glucocorticoid pulses of 1 g/day of methylprednisolone (or equivalent glucocorticoid) for 3 days is frequently recommended, although it has not been clearly demonstrated that this dose regimen is more effective than the standard oral treatment to prevent irreversible visual loss. Treatment within the first 12 to 24 hours appears to be the major determinant of visual recovery, which can be expected in only 4% to 12% of cases.[120,121] In case of ischemic symptoms, it is reasonable to recommend antiplatelet drugs, but their efficacy is not proven.[118] Some patients with visual symptoms experience further visual loss during the first 1 to 2 weeks of glucocorticoid treatment. Visual loss beyond this point or during controlled relapses is rare.

The starting dose of prednisone (or equivalent) is maintained for 2 to 4 weeks. The daily dose is then tapered progressively by approximately 5 to 10 mg/week with close surveillance. Usually a target dose of 15 to 20 mg/day is achieved within 2 to 3 months and ≤5 mg/day after 1 year. Although most patients do well with a daily maintenance dose of 7.5 to 10 mg, some patients require higher doses. Tapering is guided primarily by clinical evaluation. The ESR is a useful parameter for following patients with GCA, but therapeutic decisions must not rely solely on ESR values. The usual initial dose of prednisone for patients with isolated PMR is 10 to 20 mg/day.[122] Guidelines for reduction are similar to those recommended for GCA. Total duration of therapy may vary, but most patients require treatment for approximately 2 to 3 years. Reduction in dose below the maintenance doses must be made gradually to avoid relapses, which are common during the first 2 years after diagnosis.[123] Approximately 40% to 60% of patients require low-dose glucocorticoid therapy for longer periods of time, some perhaps indefinitely.[124]

In the majority of patients, the ESR normalizes quickly after initiation of glucocorticoid therapy. However, other inflammatory markers (e.g., IL-6, CRP, haptoglobin, vWF antigen) may persist slightly elevated in patients who appear to be in clinical remission, possibly indicating persistent low-level inflammatory activity.[125] Long-term consequences of persistent subclinical activity are unknown. Persistent slight elevation of inflammatory markers should not lead to an increase in glucocorticoid dose in the setting of clinical remission, particularly in the absence if imaging abnormalities.

Complications of glucocorticoid therapy are quite common among patients with GCA and PMR.[123,124] These include osteoporosis, weight gain, mood and sleep disturbances, glucose intolerance, congestive heart failure, cataracts, glaucoma, hypertension, and other problems. GCA affects elderly patients, a population particularly susceptible to serious complications of glucocorticoid therapy. Physicians treating GCA should anticipate such complications, screen for them, and, when feasible, prescribe prophylactic treatments such as calcium, vitamin D, and bisphosphonates to prevent osteoporosis.[118]

Other immunosuppressive drugs may be considered as "steroid-sparing agents" to reduce the cumulative toxicity of glucocorticoid therapy.

Methotrexate, was evaluated in three randomized placebo-controlled double-blind studies.[126–128] An individual patient-level meta-analysis of these trials demonstrated modest but significant benefits of methotrexate, including prevention of relapses and reduction of glucocorticoid use.[129] Although small case series reported beneficial effects of TNF blockers for GCA, TNF-α blockade with infliximab was not superior to placebo in maintaining glucocorticoid-induced remission in an international randomized double-masked placebo-controlled trial.[130] Recently IL-6 receptor blockade with tocilizumab was demonstrated to have efficacy in maintaining glucocorticoid-induced remission and sparing glucocorticoids in phase 2 and 3 randomized controlled trials,[115,131] both in newly diagnosed and relapsing patients. Tocilizumab has been approved in several countries for the treatment of GCA and is usually administered at 162 mg subcutaneously every 1 to 2 weeks. Interfering with CD28-mediated T cell activation with abatacept has been tested in a small randomized controlled trial resulting in a decrease in relapse rate, but efficacy needs to be confirmed in larger trials.[132] Other biological agents targeting cytokines (i.e., IL-1 or IL-12/23p40) or therapies targeting signaling pathways (JAK inhibitors) are currently being tested and more safety and efficacy data are needed. Patients with both GCA and PMR require long-term follow-up care, often for many years if not for their lifetime, following apparent disease remission. Disease relapse is common, and the long-term problems of large vessel disease are now being fully appreciated. Finally, it is imperative that patients and their family members be educated and reminded about the warning symptoms of GCA, which necessitate urgent medical evaluation.

ISOLATED IDIOPATHIC AORTITIS

Isolated aortitis is an inflammatory disease of unknown etiology restricted to the aorta and periaortic tissues and currently included in the category of single organ vasculitis.[133] The thoracic aorta is more frequently involved. When the abdominal aorta is involved, it may be in the form of aortitis, chronic periaortitis (potentially associated with retroperitoneal fibrosis), or inflammatory aortic aneurysm. It is unclear whether these disorders belong to a spectrum of diseases or are different conditions.

Clinical Manifestations

Isolated aortitis can be found incidentally after histopathological examination of aortic tissue removed during aneurysm surgical repair. Awareness of this condition comes from retrospective analysis of surgical or autopsy series of aortic specimens demonstrating noninfectious aortitis in 1% to 15% of cases.[15,17,134] Less than 50% of the patients had associated clinical or imaging data suggesting a systemic vasculitis such as GCA or TAK or other chronic inflammatory conditions known to be occasionally associated with aortitis. These data highlight the clinical impression that idiopathic aortitis is frequently asymptomatic unless complicated by aneurysm formation. Isolated aortitis can be incidentally detected by imaging (CTA, MRA, or PET scan) performed to evaluate patients for many other medical issues. Elevation of acute phase reactants, ESR or CRP, are inconsistently detected.

Differential Diagnosis

It is important to keep in mind that the most frequent causes of aortitis are systemic large vessel vasculitis (GCA or TAK) and that these diseases may be ruled out by accurate clinical evaluation, imaging, or temporal artery biopsy when applicable. Imaging of the entire aorta and its primary branches is extremely useful to detect involvement of other arterial segments which may suggest a systemic large vessel vasculitis rather than isolated aortitis. Similarly, the absence of additional large arterial abnormalities is useful in ruling out other forms of vasculitis. If aortitis is detected after surgery, imaging should be delayed for several weeks as surgery-related inflammation or repair may result in imaging abnormalities. Infectious aortitis should be ruled out other chronic inflammatory conditions that occasionally may be associated with aortitis.

Treatment

Patients with isolated aortitis that is fully surgically excised, who have no clinical symptoms or elevation of acute phase reactants and no apparent involvement of additional artery segments by extensive imaging, may not need additional treatment. In cases with remaining inflammation, glucocorticoids with or without other immunosuppressive agents may be added following the schedules recommended for large vessel vasculitis. However, such empiric treatment may interfere with healing from the surgery and this may influence when therapy is started.

It is important to recognize that follow-up studies of incidentally discovered aortitis have shown that untreated patients may develop new vascular abnormalities over time. However, most studies are retrospective and it is unknown how extensively systemic vasculitis was excluded at the time of diagnosis. The experiences to date indicate that regardless of whether patients with seemingly isolated aortitis are treated, it is essential that such patients are followed regularly and that careful clinical evaluation and periodic imaging may guide management during follow-up.

ACKNOWLEDGMENT

The authors acknowledge Dr. Kathleen Maksimowicz-McKinnon and Dr. Gary S. Hoffman for their contributions to parts of this chapter in an earlier edition of this textbook.

REFERENCES

1. Hall S, Barr W, Lie JT, et al. Takayasu arteritis: a study of 32 North American patients. *Medicine (Baltimore)*. 1985;64:89–99.
2. Waern AU, Anderson P, Hemmingsson A. Takayasu's arteritis: a hospital-region based study on occurrence, treatment, and prognosis. *Angiology*. 1983;34:311–320.
3. Nasu T. Takayasu's truncoarteritis in Japan: a statistical observation of 76 autopsy cases. *Pathol Microbiol (Basel)*. 1975;43:140–146.
4. Renauer PA, Saruhan-Direskeneli G, Coit P, et al. Identification of susceptibility loci in IL6, RPS9/LILRB3, and an intergenic locus on chromosome 21q22 in Takayasu arteritis in a genome-wide association study. *Arthritis Rheumatol*. 2015;67(5):1361–1368.
5. Saruhan-Direskeneli G, Hughes T, Aksu K, et al. Identification of multiple genetic susceptibility loci in Takayasu arteritis. *Am J Hum Genet*. 2013;93(2):298–305.
6. Terao C, Yoshifuji H, Kimura A, et al. Two susceptibility loci to Takayasu arteritis reveal a synergistic role of the IL12B and HLA-B regions in a Japanese population. *Am J Hum Genet*. 2013;93(2):289–297.
7. Chauhan SK, Tripathy NK, Sinha N, et al. Cellular and humoral immune responses to mycobacterial heat shock protein-65 and its human homologue in Takayasu's arteritis. *Clin Exp Immunol*. 2004;138:547–553.
8. Chauhan SK, Tripathy NK, Nityanand S. Antigenic targets and pathogenicity of anti-aortic endothelial cell antibodies in Takayasu's arteritis. *Arthritis Rheum*. 2006;54:2326–2333.
9. Numano F. Takayasu's arteritis: clinical aspects. In: Hoffman GS, Weyand CM, eds. *Inflammatory Diseases of Blood Vessels*. New York: Marcel Dekker; 2002:455.
10. Hotchi M. Pathologic studies on Takayasu arteritis. *Heart Vessels*. 1992;7(Suppl 1):11–17.
11. Kerr G, Hallahan C, Giordano J, et al. Takayasu arteritis. *Ann Intern Med*. 1994;120:919–929.

12. Lupi-Herrara E, Sánchez-Torrez G, Marchushamer J, et al. Takayasu arteritis: clinical study of 107 cases. *Am Heart J.* 1977;93:94–103.

13. Numano F, Kobayashi Y. Takayasu arteritis—beyond pulselessness. *Intern Med.* 1999;38:226–232.

14. Grange DK, Balfour IC, Chen SC, et al. Familial syndrome of progressive arterial occlusive disease consistent with fibromuscular dysplasia, hypertension, congenital cardiac defects, bone fragility, brachysyndactyly, and learning disabilities. *Am J Med Genet.* 1998;75:469–480.

15. Merkel PA. Noninfectious ascending aortitis: staying ahead of the curve. *J Rheumatol.* 2009;36(10):2137–2140.

16. Hoffman GS. Large-vessel vasculitis: unresolved issues. *Arthritis Rheum.* 2003;48:2406–2414.

17. Rojo-Leyva F, Ratliff N, Cosgrove 3rd DM, Hoffman GS. Study of 52 patients with idiopathic aortitis from a cohort of 1,204 surgical cases. *Arthritis Rheum.* 2000;43:901–907.

18. Hernández-Rodriguez J, Molloy ES, Hoffman GS. Single organ vasculitis. *Curr Opin Rheumatol.* 2008;20:40–46.

19. Maksimowicz-McKinnon K, Clark TM, Hoffman GS. Takayasu arteritis and giant cell arteritis: a spectrum within the same disease? *Medicine (Baltimore).* 2009;88:221–226.

20. Aydin SZ, Direskeneli H, Merkel PA. International Delphi on Disease Activity Assessment in Large-vessel Vasculitis. Assessment of disease activity in large-vessel vasculitis: results of an international Delphi exercise. *J Rheumatol.* 2017;44(12):1928–1932.

21. Sreih AG, Alibaz-Oner F, Kermani TA, et al. Development of a core set of outcome measures for large-vessel vasculitis: report from OMERACT 2016. *J Rheumatol.* 2017;44(12):1933–1937.

22. Cid MC, Prieto-González S, Arguis P, et al. The spectrum of vascular involvement in giant-cell arteritis: clinical consequences of detrimental vascular remodelling at different sites. *APMIS Suppl.* 2009;127:10–20.

23. Carmona FD, Vaglio A, Mackie SL, et al. A genome-wide association study identifies risk alleles in plasminogen and P4HA2 associated with giant cell arteritis. *Am J Hum Genet.* 2017;100(1):64–74.

24. Carmona FD, Mackie SL, Martín JE, et al. A large-scale genetic analysis reveals a strong contribution of the HLA class II region to giant cell arteritis susceptibility. *Am J Hum Genet.* 2015;96(4):565–580.

25. Carmona FD, Coit P, Saruhan-Direskeneli G, et al. Analysis of the common genetic component of large-vessel vasculitides through a meta-immunochip strategy. *Sci Rep.* 2017;7:43953.

26. Arnaud L, Haroche J, Limal N, et al. Takayasu arteritis in France: a single-center, retrospective study of 82 cases comparing white, North African, and black patients. *Medicine (Baltimore).* 2010;89:1–17.

27. Bicakcigil M, Aksu K, Ozbalkan Z, et al. Takayasu's arteritis in Turkey-clinical and angiographic features of 248 patients. *Clin Exp Rheumatol.* 2009;27(Suppl 52):S59–S64.

28. Tso E, Flamm SD, White RD, et al. Takayasu arteritis. Utility and limitations of magnetic resonance imaging in diagnosis and treatment. *Arthritis Rheum.* 2002;46:1634–1642.

29. Webb M, Chambers A, Al-Nahhas A, et al. The role of 18-FDG PET in characterizing disease activity in Takayasu arteritis. *Eur J Nucl Med Mol Imaging.* 2004;31:627–634.

30. Walter MA, Melzer RA, Schindler C, et al. The value of F-18 FDG-PET in the diagnosis of large-vessel vasculitis and the assessment of activity and extent of disease. *Eur J Nucl Med Mol Imaging.* 2005;32:674–681.

31. Grayson PC, Alehashemi S, Bagheri AA, et al. 18 F-fluorodeoxyglucose-positron emission tomography as an imaging biomarker in a prospective, longitudinal cohort of patients with large vessel vasculitis. *Arthritis Rheumatol.* 2018;70(3):439–449.

32. Quinn KA, Ahlman MA, Malayeri AA, et al. Comparison of magnetic resonance angiography and 18F-fluorodeoxyglucose positron emission tomography in large-vessel vasculitis. *Ann Rheum Dis.* 2018;77(8):1165–1171.

33. Barra L, Yang G, Pagnoux C. Canadian Vasculitis Network (CanVasc). Non-glucocorticoid drugs for the treatment of Takayasu's arteritis: a systematic review and meta-analysis. *Autoimmun Rev.* 2018;17(7):683–693.

34. Direskeneli H, Aydin SZ, Kermani TA, et al. Development of outcome measures for large-vessel vasculitis for use in clinical trials: opportunities, challenges, and research agenda. *J Rheumatol.* 2011;38(7):1471–1479.

35. Langford CA, Cuthbertson D, Ytterberg SR, et al. A randomized, double-blind trial of abatacept (CTLA-4Ig) for the treatment of Takayasu arteritis. *Arthritis Rheumatol.* 2017;69(4):846–853.

36. Nakaoka Y, Isobe M, Takei S, et al. Efficacy and safety of tocilizumab in patients with refractory Takayasu arteritis: results from a randomised, double-blind, placebo-controlled, phase 3 trial in Japan (the TAKT study). *Ann Rheum Dis.* 2018;77(3):348–354.

37. Sharma BK, Jain S, Bali HK, et al. A follow-up study of balloon angioplasty and de-novo stenting in Takayasu arteritis. *Int J Cardiol.* 2000;75:S147–S152.

38. Tyagi S, Gambhir DS, Kaul UA, et al. A decade of subclavian angioplasty: aortoarteritis versus atherosclerosis. *Indian Heart J.* 1996;48:667–671.

39. Bali HK, Bhargava M, Jain AK, Sharma BK. De novo stenting of descending thoracic aorta in Takayasu arteritis: intermediate-term follow-up results. *J Invasive Cardiol.* 2000;12:612–617.

40. Liang P, Tan-Ong M, Hoffman GS. Takayasu's arteritis: vascular interventions and outcomes. *J Rheumatol.* 2004;31:102–106.

41. Pajari R, Hekali P, Harjola PT. Treatment of Takayasu's arteritis: an analysis of 29 operated patients. *Thorac Cardiovasc Surg.* 1986;34:176–181.

42. Hoffman GS. Giant cell arteritis. *Ann Intern Med.* 2016;165(9):ITC65–ITC80.

43. Buttgereit F, Dejaco C, Matteson EL, Dasgupta B. Polymyalgia rheumatica and giant cell arteritis: a systematic review. *JAMA.* 2016;315(22):2442–2458.

44. Salvarani C, Pipitone N, Versari A, Hunder GG. Clinical features of polymyalgia rheumatica and giant cell arteritis. *Nat Rev Rheumatol.* 2012;8(9):509–521.

45. Matteson EL, Dejaco C. Polymyalgia rheumatica. *Ann Intern Med.* 2017;166(9):ITC65–ITC80.

46. Hunder GG. Epidemiology of giant-cell arteritis. *Cleve Clin J Med.* 2002;69(Suppl 2):SII79–SII82.

47. Baldursson O, Steinsson K, Bjornsson J. Giant cell arteritis in Iceland. An epidemiologic and histopathologic analysis. *Arthritis Rheum.* 1994;37:1007–1012.

48. Lie J. Histopathologic specificity of systemic vasculitis. *Rheum Dis Clin North Am.* 1995;21:883–909.

49. Cid MC, Campo E, Ercilla G, et al. Immunohistochemical analysis of lymphoid and macrophage cell subsets and their immunologic activation markers in temporal arteritis. Influence of corticosteroid treatment. *Arthritis Rheum.* 1989;32:884–893.

50. Graver JC, Sandovici M, Diepstra A, et al. Artery tertiary lymphoid organs in giant cell arteritis are not exclusively located in the media of temporal arteries. *Ann Rheum Dis.* 2018;77(3):e16.

51. Gonzalez-Gay MA, Vazquez-Rodriguez TR, Lopez-Diaz MJ, et al. Epidemiology of giant cell arteritis and polymyalgia rheumatica. *Arthritis Rheum.* 2009;61:1454–1461.

52. Hernández-Rodríguez J, Murgia G, Villar I, et al. Description and validation of histological patterns and proposal of a dynamic model of inflammatory infiltration in giant-cell arteritis. *Medicine (Baltimore).* 2016;95(8):e2368.

53. Esteban MJ, Font C, Hernandez-Rodriguez J, et al. Small-vessel vasculitis surrounding a spared temporal artery: clinical and pathological findings in a series of twenty-eight patients. *Arthritis Rheum.* 2001;44:1387–1395.

54. Le Pendu C, Meignin V, Gonzalez-Chiappe S, et al. Poor predictive value of isolated adventitial and periadventitial infiltrates in temporal artery biopsies for diagnosis of giant cell arteritis. *J Rheumatol.* 2017;44(7):1039–1043.

55. Ostberg G. Temporal arteritis in a large necropsy series. *Ann Rheum Dis.* 1971;30:224–235.

56. Meliconi R, Pulsatelli L, Uguccioni M, et al. Leukocyte infiltration in synovial tissue from the shoulder of patients with polymyalgia rheumatica. Quantitative analysis and influence of corticosteroid treatment. *Arthritis Rheum.* 1996;39:1199–1207.

57. Meliconi R, Pulsatelli L, Melchiorri C, et al. Synovial expression of cell adhesion molecules in polymyalgia rheumatica. *Clin Exp Immunol.* 1997;107:494–500.

58. Serrano A, Márquez A, Mackie SL, et al. Identification of the PTPN22 functional variant R620W as susceptibility genetic factor for giant cell arteritis. *Ann Rheum Dis.* 2013;72:1882–1886.

59. Enjuanes A, Benavente Y, Hernández-Rodríguez J, et al. Association of NOS2 and potential effect of VEGF, IL6, CCL2, and IL1RN polymorphisms and haplotypes on susceptibility to giant cell arteritis. A simultaneous study of 130 potentially functional SNPs in 14 candidate genes. *Rheumatology (Oxford)*. 2012;51:841–851.

60. Márquez A, Hernández-Rodríguez J, Cid MC, et al. Influence of the IL17A locus in giant cell arteritis susceptibility. *Ann Rheum Dis*. 2014;73(9):1742–1745.

61. Chandran AK, Udayakumar PD, Crowson CS, et al. The incidence of giant cell arteritis in Olmsted County, Minnesota, over a 60-year period 1950-2009. *Scand J Rheumatol*. 2015;44(3):215–218.

62. Rhee RL, Grayson PC, Merkel PA, Tomasson G. Infections and the risk of incident giant cell arteritis: a population-based, case-control study. *Ann Rheum Dis*. 2017;76(6):1031–1035.

63. Ma-Krupa W, Jeon MS, Spoerl S, et al. Activation of arterial wall dendritic cells and breakdown of self-tolerance in giant cell arteritis. *J Exp Med*. 2004;199(2):173–183.

64. Weyand CM, Schönberger J, Oppitz U, et al. Distinct vascular lesions in giant cell arteritis share identical T cell clonotypes. *J Exp Med*. 1994;179(3):951–960.

65. Zhang H, Watanabe R, Berry GJ, et al. Immunoinhibitory checkpoint deficiency in medium and large vessel vasculitis. *Proc Natl Acad Sci U S A*. 2017;114(6):E970–E979.

66. Deng J, Younge BR, Olshen RA, et al. Th17 and Th1 T-cell responses in giant cell arteritis. *Circulation*. 2010;121:906–915.

67. Espígol-Frigolé G, Corbera-Bellalta M, Planas-Rigol E, et al. Increased IL-17A expression in temporal artery lesions is a predictor of sustained response to glucocorticoid treatment in patients with giant-cell arteritis. *Ann Rheum Dis*. 2013;72(9):1481–1487.

68. Coit P, De Lott LB, Nan B, et al. DNA methylation analysis of the temporal artery microenvironment in giant cell arteritis. *Ann Rheum Dis*. 2016;75(6):1196–1202.

69. Rittner HL, Kaiser M, Brack A, et al. Tissue-destructive macrophages in giant cell arteritis. *Circ Res*. 1999;84:1050–1058.

70. Segarra M, Garcia-Martinez A, Sanchez M, et al. Gelatinase expression and proteolytic activity in giant-cell arteritis. *Ann Rheum Dis*. 2007;66:1429–1435.

71. Hernandez-Rodriguez J, Segarra M, Vilardell C, et al. Tissue production of pro-inflammatory cytokines (IL-1beta, TNF-alpha and IL-6) correlates with the intensity of the systemic inflammatory response and with corticosteroid requirements in giant-cell arteritis. *Rheumatology (Oxford)*. 2004;43:294–301.

72. Cid MC, Cebrian M, Font C, et al. Cell adhesion molecules in the development of inflammatory infiltrates in giant cell arteritis: inflammation-induced angiogenesis as the preferential site of leukocyte-endothelial cell interactions. *Arthritis Rheum*. 2000;43:184–194.

73. Cid MC, Hernandez-Rodriguez J, Esteban MJ, et al. Tissue and serum angiogenic activity is associated with low prevalence of ischemic complications in patients with giant-cell arteritis. *Circulation*. 2002;106:1664–1671.

74. Lozano E, Segarra M, García-Martínez A, et al. Imatinib mesylate inhibits in vitro and ex vivo biological responses related to vascular occlusion in giant cell arteritis. *Ann Rheum Dis*. 2008;67(11):1581–1588.

75. Corbera-Bellalta M, Planas-Rigol E, Lozano E, et al. Blocking interferon γ reduces expression of chemokines CXCL9, CXCL10 and CXCL11 and decreases macrophage infiltration in ex vivo cultured arteries from patients with giant cell arteritis. *Ann Rheum Dis*. 2016;75(6):1177–1186.

76. Hernandez-Rodriguez J, Segarra M, Vilardell C, et al. Elevated production of interleukin-6 is associated with a lower incidence of disease-related ischemic events in patients with giant-cell arteritis: angiogenic activity of interleukin-6 as a potential protective mechanism. *Circulation*. 2003;107:2428–2434.

77. Wen Z, Shen Y, Berry G, et al. The microvascular niche instructs T cells in large vessel vasculitis via the VEGF-Jagged1-Notch pathway. *Sci Transl Med*. 2017;9(399). pii: eaal3322.

78. Planas-Rigol E, Terrades-Garcia N, Corbera-Bellalta M, et al. Endothelin-1 promotes vascular smooth muscle cell migration across the artery wall: a mechanism contributing to vascular remodelling and intimal hyperplasia in giant-cell arteritis. *Ann Rheum Dis*. 2017;76:1624–1634.

79. Font CC, Cid MC, Coll-Vinent B, et al. Clinical features in patients with permanent visual loss due to biopsy–proven giant cell arteritis. *Br J Rheumatol*. 1997;36:251–254.

80. Cid MC, Font C, Oristrell J, et al. Association between strong inflammatory response and low risk of developing visual loss and other cranial ischemic complications in giant cell (temporal) arteritis. *Arthritis Rheum*. 1998;41:26–32.

81. Hernández-Rodríguez J, García-Martínez A, Casademont J, et al. A strong initial systemic inflammatory response is associated with higher corticosteroid requirements and longer duration of therapy in patients with giant-cell arteritis. *Arthritis Rheum*. 2002;47(1):29–35.

82. Nuenninghoff DM, Hunder GG, Christianson TJ, et al. Incidence and predictors of large-artery complication (aortic aneurysm, aortic dissection, and/or large-artery stenosis) in patients with giant cell arteritis: a population-based study over 50 years. *Arthritis Rheum*. 2003;48:3522–3531.

83. Huston KA, Hunder GG, Lie JT, et al. Temporal arteritis: a 25-year epidemiologic, clinical, and pathologic study. *Ann Intern Med*. 1978;88:162–167.

84. Amor-Dorado JC, Llorca J, Garcia-Porrua C, et al. Audiovestibular manifestations in giant cell arteritis: a prospective study. *Medicine (Baltimore)*. 2003;82:13–26.

85. Blockmans D, de Ceuninck L, Vanderschueren S, et al. Repetitive 18F-fluorodeoxyglucose positron emission tomography in giant cell arteritis: a prospective study of 35 patients. *Arthritis Rheum*. 2006;55:131–137.

86. Prieto-González S, Arguis P, García-Martínez A, et al. Large vessel involvement in biopsy-proven giant cell arteritis: prospective study in 40 newly diagnosed patients using CT angiography. *Ann Rheum Dis*. 2012;71(7):1170–1176.

87. Grayson PC, Maksimowicz-McKinnon K, Clark TM, et al. Distribution of arterial lesions in Takayasu's arteritis and giant cell arteritis. *Ann Rheum Dis*. 2012;71(8):1329–1334.

88. Prieto-González S, Depetris M, García-Martínez A, et al. Positron emission tomography assessment of large vessel inflammation in patients with newly diagnosed, biopsy-proven giant cell arteritis: a prospective, case-control study. *Ann Rheum Dis*. 2014;73:1388–1392.

89. Garcia-Martinez A, Hernandez-Rodriguez J, Arguis P, et al. Development of aortic aneurysm/dilatation during the followup of patients with giant cell arteritis: a cross-sectional screening of fifty-four prospectively followed patients. *Arthritis Rheum*. 2008;59:422–430.

90. García-Martínez A, Arguis P, Prieto-González S, et al. Prospective long term follow-up of a cohort of patients with giant cell arteritis screened for aortic structural damage (aneurysm or dilatation). *Ann Rheum Dis*. 2014;73(10):1826–1832.

91. Evans JM, O'Fallon WM, Hunder GG. Increased incidence of aortic aneurysm and dissection in giant cell (temporal) arteritis. A population-based study. *Ann Intern Med*. 1995;122(7):502–507.

92. Kermani TA, Warrington KJ, Crowson CS, et al. Large-vessel involvement in giant cell arteritis: a population-based cohort study of the incidence-trends and prognosis. *Ann Rheum Dis*. 2013;72(12):1989–1994.

93. Schmidt WA, Seifert A, Gromnica-Ihle E, et al. Ultrasound of proximal upper extremity arteries to increase the diagnostic yield in large-vessel giant cell arteritis. *Rheumatology (Oxford)*. 2008;47:96–101.

94. Assie C, Janvresse A, Plissonnier D. Long-term follow-up of upper and lower extremity vasculitis related to giant cell arteritis: a series of 36 patients. *Medicine (Baltimore)*. 2011;90:40–51.

95. Scola CJ, Li C, Upchurch KS. Mesenteric involvement in giant cell arteritis. An underrecognized complication? Analysis of a case series with clinico anatomic correlation. *Medicine (Baltimore)*. 2008;87:45–51.

96. Udayakumar PD, Chandran AK, Crowson CS, et al. Cardiovascular risk and acute coronary syndrome in giant cell arteritis: a population-based retrospective cohort study. *Arthritis Care Res (Hoboken)*. 2015;67(3):396–402.

97. Camellino D, Cimmino MA. Imaging of polymyalgia rheumatica: indications on its pathogenesis, diagnosis and prognosis. *Rheumatology (Oxford)*. 2012;51(1):77–86.

98. Hernandez-Rodriguez J, Font C, Garcia-Martinez A, et al. Development of ischemic complications in patients with giant cell arteritis presenting with apparently isolated polymyalgia rheumatica: study of a series of 100 patients. *Medicine (Baltimore)*. 2007;86:233–241.

99. Chuang TY, Hunder GG, Ilstrup DM, Kurland LT. Polymyalgia rheumatica: a 10-year epidemiologic and clinical study. *Ann Intern Med*. 1982;97(5):672–680.

100. Blockmans D, De Ceuninck L, Vanderschueren S, et al. Repetitive 18-fluorodeoxyglucose positron emission tomography in isolated polymyalgia rheumatica: a prospective study in 35 patients. *Rheumatology (Oxford)*. 2007;46(4):672–677.

101. Roche NE, Fulbright JW, Wagner AD, et al. Correlation of interleukin-6 production and disease activity in polymyalgia rheumatica and giant cell arteritis. *Arthritis Rheum*. 1993;36:1286–1294.

102. van der Geest KS, Abdulahad WH, Rutgers A, et al. Serum markers associated with disease activity in giant cell arteritis and polymyalgia rheumatica. *Rheumatology (Oxford)*. 2015;54(8):1397–1402.

103. Coll-Vinent B, Vilardell C, Font C, et al. Circulating soluble adhesion molecules in patients with giant cell arteritis. Correlation between soluble intercellular adhesion molecule-1 (sICAM-1) concentrations and disease activity. *Ann Rheum Dis*. 1999;58:189–192.

104. Springer JM, Monach P, Cuthbertson D, et al. Serum S100 proteins as a marker of disease activity in large vessel vasculitis. *J Clin Rheumatol*. 2018;24(7):393–395.

105. Genereau T, Lortholary O, Pottier MA, et al. Temporal artery biopsy: a diagnostic tool for systemic necrotizing vasculitis. *French Vasculitis Study Group Arthritis Rheum*. 1999;42:2674–2681.

106. Duran E, Merkel PA, Sweet S, et al. ANCA-associated small vessel vasculitis presenting with ischemic optic neuropathy. *Neurology*. 2004;62(1):152–153.

107. Vilaseca J, Gonzalez A, Cid MC, et al. Clinical usefulness of temporal artery biopsy. *Ann Rheum Dis*. 1987;46:282–285.

108. Hunder GG, Bloch DA, Michel BA, et al. The American College of Rheumatology 1990 criteria for the classification of giant cell arteritis. *Arthritis Rheum*. 1990;33:1122–1128.

109. Basu N, Watts R, Bajema I, et al. EULAR points to consider in the development of classification and diagnostic criteria in systemic vasculitis. *Ann Rheum Dis*. 2010;69:1744–1750.

110. Blockmans D, Bley T, Schmidt W. Imaging for large-vessel vasculitis. *Curr Opin Rheumatol*. 2009;21(1):19–28.

111. Prieto-González S, Espígol-Frigolé G, García-Martínez A, et al. The expanding role of imaging in systemic vasculitis. *Rheum Dis Clin North Am*. 2016;42:733–751.

112. Luqmani R, Lee E, Singh S, et al. The role of ultrasound compared to biopsy of temporal arteries in the diagnosis and treatment of giant cell arteritis (TABUL): a diagnostic accuracy and cost-effectiveness study. *Health Technol Assess*. 2016;20(90):1–238.

113. Yun M, Jang S, Cucchiara A, et al. 18F FDG uptake in the large arteries: a correlation study with the atherogenic risk factors. *Semin Nucl Med*. 2002;32(1):70–76.

114. Prieto-González S, García-Martínez A, Tavera-Bahillo I, et al. Effect of glucocorticoid treatment on computed tomography angiography detected large-vessel inflammation in giant-cell arteritis. A prospective, longitudinal study. *Medicine (Baltimore)*. 2015;94(5):e486.

115. Reichenbach S, Adler S, Bonel H, et al. Magnetic resonance angiography in giant cell arteritis: results of a randomized controlled trial of tocilizumab in giant cell arteritis. *Rheumatology (Oxford)*. 2018;57(6):982–986.

116. Dasgupta B, Cimmino MA, Maradit-Kremers H, et al. European League Against Rheumatism/American College of Rheumatology classification criteria for polymyalgia rheumatica. *Ann Rheum Dis*. 2012;71:484–492.

117. Cantini F, Salvarani C, Olivieri I, et al. Shoulder ultrasonography in the diagnosis of polymyalgia rheumatica: a case-control study. *J Rheumatol*. 2001;28:1049–1055.

118. Mukhtyar C, Guillevin L, Cid MC, et al. EULAR recommendations for the management of large vessel vasculitis. *Ann Rheum Dis*. 2009;68(3): 318–323.

119. Achkar AA, Lie JT, Hunder GG, et al. How does previous corticosteroid treatment affect the biopsy findings in giant cell (temporal) arteritis? *Ann Intern Med*. 1994;120:987–992.

120. Foroozan R, Deramo VA, Buono LM, et al. Recovery of visual function in patients with biopsy-proven giant cell arteritis. *Ophthalmology*. 2003;110:539–542.

121. Gonzalez-Gay MA, Blanco R, Rodriguez-Valverde V, et al. Permanent visual loss and cerebrovascular accidents in giant cell arteritis: predictors and response to treatment. *Arthritis Rheum*. 1998;41:1497–1504.

122. Dejaco C, Singh YP, Perel P, et al. 2015 Recommendations for the management of polymyalgia rheumatica: a European League Against Rheumatism/American College of Rheumatology collaborative initiative. *Ann Rheum Dis*. 2015;74(10):1799–1807.

123. Alba MA, García-Martínez A, Prieto-González S, et al. Relapses in patients with giant cell arteritis: prevalence, characteristics, and associated clinical findings in a longitudinally followed cohort of 106 patients. *Medicine (Baltimore)*. 2014;93(5):194–201.

124. Proven A, Gabriel SE, Orces C, et al. Glucocorticoid therapy in giant cell arteritis: duration and adverse outcomes. *Arthritis Rheum*. 2003;49:703–708.

125. Weyand CM, Fulbright JW, Hunder GG, et al. Treatment of giant cell arteritis: interleukin-6 as a biologic marker of disease activity. *Arthritis Rheum*. 2000;43:1041–1048.

126. Jover JA, Hernandez-Garcia C, Morado IC, et al. Combined treatment of giant-cell arteritis with methotrexate and prednisone. a randomized, double-blind, placebo-controlled trial. *Ann Intern Med*. 2001;134: 106–114.

127. Spiera RF, Mitnick HJ, Kupersmith M, et al. A prospective, double-blind, randomized, placebo controlled trial of methotrexate in the treatment of giant cell arteritis (GCA). *Clin Exp Rheumatol*. 2001;19:495–501.

128. Hoffman GS, Cid MC, Hellmann DB, et al. A multicenter, randomized, double-blind, placebo-controlled trial of adjuvant methotrexate treatment for giant cell arteritis. *Arthritis Rheum*. 2002;46(5):1309–1318.

129. Mahr AD, Jover JA, Spiera RF, et al. Adjunctive methotrexate for treatment of giant cell arteritis: an individual patient data meta-analysis. *Arthritis Rheum*. 2007;56:2789–2797.

130. Hoffman GS, Cid MC, Rendt-Zagar KE, et al. Infliximab for maintenance of glucocorticosteroid-induced remission of giant cell arteritis: a randomized trial. *Ann Intern Med*. 2007;146(9):621–630.

131. Stone JH, Tuckwell K, Dimonaco S, et al. Trial of tocilizumab in giant-cell arteritis. *N Engl J Med*. 2017;377(4):317–328.

132. Langford CA, Cuthbertson D, Ytterberg SR, et al. A randomized, double-blind trial of abatacept (CTLA-4Ig) for the treatment of giant cell arteritis. *Arthritis Rheumatol*. 2017;69(4):837–845.

133. Jennette JC, Falk RJ, Bacon PA, et al. 2012 revised International Chapel Hill Consensus Conference Nomenclature of Vasculitides. *Arthritis Rheum*. 2013;65:1–11.

134. Liang KP, Chowdhary VR, Michet CJ, et al. Noninfectious ascending aortitis: a case series of 64 patients. *J Rheumatol*. 2009;36(10):2290–2297.

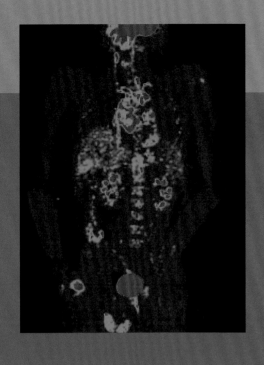

中文导读

第41章
中小血管血管炎

　　本章主要介绍了中小动脉血管疾病，主要包括结节性多动脉炎、皮肤小血管炎、抗中性粒细胞细胞质抗体相关血管炎、免疫球蛋白A血管炎。尽管这些血管疾病临床上较少见，但遇到这些患者时常常诊断和治疗较为棘手，患者非常痛苦，在国内书籍里少有介绍。本章较详细介绍了国际上对这几种血管疾病的最新研究结果，包括流行病学、病因、组织病理学、临床表现、诊断和鉴别诊断、治疗和预后，值得相关专业临床医师研究、学习和作为参考书查阅。

赵纪春

Medium and Small Vessel Vasculitis

Matthew J. Koster, Kenneth J. Warrington, and Tanaz A. Kermani

MEDIUM VESSEL VASCULITIS

Polyarteritis Nodosa

Polyarteritis nodosa (PAN) is a medium vessel vasculitis affecting the main visceral arteries and their branches.[1] The 2012 International Chapel Hill Consensus Conference (CHCC) defines PAN as a necrotizing arteritis of medium and small arteries without glomerulonephritis or vasculitis in arterioles, capillaries, or venules, and not associated with antineutrophil cytoplasmic antibodies (ANCA).[1] The association of PAN with hepatitis B virus (HBV) has been well documented.[2,3] PAN is generally a systemic vasculitis that can affect multiple organs such as the skin, nerves, kidneys, and gastrointestinal (GI) tract. A localized form of PAN involving the skin is cutaneous PAN (c-PAN).[4-7] Other "single-organ" isolated forms, where necrotizing vasculitis is found on surgical specimens of resected abdominal or reproductive organs, are also occasionally encountered.[8-10]

Epidemiology

PAN is a rare disease with an estimated annual incidence of 0.9 to 9.7 per million.[11,12] Prevalence estimates range from 9 to 31 per million, based on studies from Europe.[13,14] In a study from a hyperendemic area for HBV, an incidence of 7.7 per 100,000 was reported,[15] but a more recent study found that HBV-associated PAN may be declining.[16] In a cohort of 341 cases of PAN, HBV-associated PAN accounted for 17.4% of all cases of PAN in patients diagnosed between 1990 and 2002 compared to earlier decades, when prevalence of HBV among patients with PAN was as high as 52%.[16] There appears to be a slight male predominance in PAN.[13]

Etiology

Based on recent developments, it has been proposed that necrotizing vasculitis represents a broad range of diseases with different etiopathogeneses.[17] While most cases of PAN are idiopathic, the association of HBV with PAN has been well documented.[2,3] Hepatitis C virus (HCV)-associated PAN has also been reported, but is infrequent.[18] The availability of ANCA testing has allowed us to distinguish PAN from other forms of systemic necrotizing vasculitis like microscopic polyangiitis (MPA), which can cause similar clinical manifestations.[1,19,20] Medications like minocycline can rarely cause both c-PAN and systemic PAN.[21] Recently, loss of function mutations in the cat eye syndrome chromosome region, candidate 1 (*CECR1*) gene, which encodes for adenosine deaminase 2, has been associated with an autoinflammatory condition characterized by early onset vasculopathy with clinical and histopathologic features of PAN, as well as hemorrhagic and ischemic strokes.[22-24]

Pathogenesis and Histopathology

In the case of HBV-associated PAN, circulating immune complexes or direct injury of the vessel wall from viral replication have been implicated.[3,25-27] In contrast, the pathogenesis of the idiopathic or primary form of PAN is not well understood. Immunohistochemistry of the affected biopsy tissue reveals macrophages and T cells in the inflammatory infiltrates, suggesting PAN is a T-cell mediated disease.[28,29] Elevated circulating soluble adhesion molecules have also been reported and activation of endothelial cells is also thought to play a role in disease pathogenesis.[28-30]

PAN is segmental and predominates at vessel branching points.[31] Fibrinoid, transmural necrosis of the vessel wall with a mixed inflammatory infiltrate consisting of macrophages, lymphocytes, neutrophils, and eosinophils is observed.[31] Temporal variability of lesions with both active necrotizing lesions and healed or fibrotic lesions representing different stages of the inflammatory process can be seen concurrently in the same specimen.[28,30,31] Thrombosis can lead to vascular occlusion, while severe vessel wall injury may result in the formation of microaneurysms.[28,30-32]

Clinical Manifestations

Constitutional symptoms including fever, weight loss, myalgias, and arthralgias are frequently observed.[33] In a large series of 348 patients with PAN, the most frequently affected organs were nerves, genitourinary system, and the skin.[33] Mononeuritis multiplex or sensorimotor peripheral neuropathy can occur in up to 74% of patients with PAN.[33] Renal manifestations may include new onset hypertension, proteinuria, and hematuria while testicular tenderness or orchitis has been reported in about 17% patients.[33] PAN does not cause glomerulonephritis; therefore, the presence of an active urine sediment and dysmorphic red blood cells in the urine should prompt evaluation for small vessel vasculitis, mainly ANCA-associated vasculitis.[1] The most frequent cutaneous manifestations are purpura followed by subcutaneous nodules and livedo reticularis (Fig. 41.1).[33] In severe cases, digital ischemia from peripheral arterial occlusions or ischemic ulcerations can also occur. GI manifestations may occur in 38%, with the most frequent manifestation being abdominal pain.[33] However, mesenteric ischemia, hemorrhage, bowel perforation, cholecystitis, appendicitis, and pancreatitis have all been described, and may require surgical intervention.[33-35] Cardiac involvement with cardiomyopathy and pericarditis have been reported in 5% to 8% of patients with PAN.[33] Pulmonary manifestations including lung infiltrates and pleural effusions are rare, being noted in only about 3% of patients.[33] Indeed, the presence of pulmonary abnormalities in a patient with suspected vasculitis should prompt careful evaluation for ANCA-associated vasculitis. Although rare, PAN may cause ocular manifestations, including retinal vasculitis.[33]

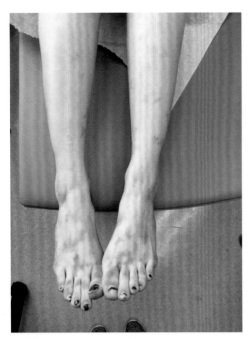

Fig. 41.1 Livedo reticularis in patient with polyarteritis nodosa.

Hepatitis B–associated PAN vs. idiopathic PAN. The clinical features of HBV-associated PAN are overall similar to those of idiopathic PAN. However, in a series of 348 patients, 225 with idiopathic PAN and 123 with HBV-associated PAN, there were some differences.[33] Patients with HBV-associated PAN had more frequent peripheral neuropathy and mononeuritis multiplex (88% and 85%, respectively, compared to 68% and 64% with idiopathic PAN).[33] Other manifestations that differed included the presence of a high frequency of recent onset hypertension, orchitis/testicular pain, abdominal pain, and severe organ manifestations including GI manifestations requiring surgery and cardiomyopathy in patients with HBV-associated PAN.[33] In contrast, patients with idiopathic PAN had more cutaneous manifestations (58% vs. 35% with HBV-associated PAN).[33]

Cutaneous PAN vs. systemic PAN. Patients with c-PAN generally present with tender subcutaneous nodules and/or other skin manifestations of vasculitis, but in the absence of other organ manifestations. Few studies have compared the clinical features and outcomes of c-PAN with systemic PAN.[4,6,36,37] As opposed to systemic PAN, c-PAN appears to affect women more frequently than men.[4,6,7,36,37] HBV infection is infrequent in patients with c-PAN, and most cases are idiopathic or drug-induced.[4,6,7,36,37] While patients with c-PAN may have constitutional symptoms, arthralgias, and, in some cases a mild peripheral neuropathy, progression to systemic PAN is almost never observed.[4,6,7,36] Additionally, the peripheral neuropathy in c-PAN is often localized to the same area as the skin lesions.[7] While c-PAN does not typically cause organ failure, it follows a chronic, relapsing course which can be associated with disease and treatment-related morbidity.[4,36,37]

Single-organ vasculitis versus systemic PAN. Isolated necrotizing vasculitis noted on histopathology of abdominal or reproductive organs in the absence of systemic manifestations of PAN, so called "single-organ vasculitis" (SOV), has also been described.[8–10] There have been studies comparing isolated testicular, gallbladder, and GI vasculitis to systemic PAN.[8,10,36] In the case of isolated testicular or gallbladder vasculitis, constitutional symptoms and elevated markers of inflammation were infrequent compared to those with systemic PAN.[8,10] Surgical resection is thought to be curative in SOV and generally patients are not treated with immunosuppressive therapy.[38] However, it is important to evaluate patients with SOV carefully to ensure this is not an organ manifestation of systemic PAN.[38] In a recent series evaluating isolated GI vasculitis compared to systemic PAN, 67% of patients with GI vasculitis were treated with systemic glucocorticoids (compared to 94% with systemic PAN) and additional immunosuppressive therapy was used in 37% of patients with GI vasculitis compared to 67% with systemic PAN.[36] While patients with isolated GI vasculitis did not have relapses or progression to systemic PAN, a higher mortality was observed, particularly in the first year with 61% survival compared to 93% survival for systemic PAN.[36]

Diagnosis

The 1990 American College of Rheumatology (ACR) classification criteria for PAN are listed in Table 41.1.[39] However, these criteria predate the discovery of ANCA and are therefore of limited utility in clinical practice.[39] There are ongoing collaborative efforts between the ACR and European League Against Rheumatism (EULAR) for the development of diagnostic and classification criteria for several forms of systemic vasculitis including PAN.[40] In a study evaluating 949 patients with systemic vasculitis (262 with PAN), positive predictors for PAN were presence of hepatitis B viral antigen, arteriographic abnormalities (arteriogram showing aneurysms or occlusions of the visceral arteries not due to arteriosclerosis, fibromuscular dysplasia, or other noninflammatory causes), and mononeuropathy or polyneuropathy while factors that made PAN less likely were presence of ANCA, glomerulonephritis, asthma, ear/nose/throat signs, or cryoglobulinemia.[20]

Laboratory testing in patients with PAN often shows findings of systemic inflammation with elevated sedimentation rate, C-reactive protein, anemia, and leukocytosis. Testing should include evaluation of renal parameters (serum creatinine, urinalysis), liver function testing, chronic hepatitis serologies (HBV and hepatitis C), muscle enzymes, and markers of other forms of systemic vasculitis including ANCA, antinuclear antibody (ANA), cryoglobulins, complement C3, complement C4, and rheumatoid factor (RF). Testing for human immunodeficiency virus (HIV) should be considered in the appropriate clinical context. Other diagnostic testing may include nerve conduction studies and electromyography in cases of suspected neurologic involvement. As there is no diagnostic laboratory marker for PAN, imaging or tissue diagnosis in the form of a biopsy is often essential in the diagnostic evaluation. While computed tomography (CT) of the abdomen can be useful in detecting organ infarcts (Fig. 41.2A), hemorrhage, bowel wall thickening or ischemia, these findings are fairly nonspecific and therefore visceral angiography is often needed. Characteristic findings on conventional angiography such as multiple aneurysms (fusiform, sacular, or microaneurysm) of the celiac, mesenteric, and renal artery branches can be diagnostic for PAN (see Fig. 41.2B and C).[41] Biopsies from affected areas of involvement including skin, muscle, or nerve can allow the histopathologic confirmation of vasculitis. Surgical specimens from patients with visceral involvement (e.g., small intestine, gallbladder) may also provide the diagnosis. Diagnostic confirmation is important, given the medications used for treatment are associated with significant adverse effects.

Treatment and Prognosis

Treatment of PAN should be tailored according to underlying cause (if known), disease severity, and organs that are affected. Patients with idiopathic systemic PAN are generally treated with high-dose glucocorticoids (pulse and/or oral) and cyclophosphamide for induction of remission.[42] Cyclophosphamide is usually given orally at a dose of 1.5 to 2 mg/kg/day or by monthly intravenous infusion (600 to 750 mg/m^2).[42] The dose should be carefully adjusted depending on response

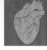

TABLE 41.1   1990 American College of Rheumatology Classification Criteria

Disease	Criterion	Definition
Polyarteritis nodosa[a]	1. Weight loss > 4 kg	Loss of 4 kg or more of body weight since illness began, not due to dieting or other factors
	2. Livedo reticularis	Mottled reticular pattern over the skin or portions of the extremities or torso
	3. Testicular pain or tenderness	Pain or tenderness of the testicles, not due to infection, trauma, or other causes
	4. Myalgias, weakness, or leg tenderness	Diffuse myalgias (excluding shoulder and hip girdle) or weakness of muscles or tenderness of leg muscles
	5. Mononeuropathy or polyneuropathy	Development of mononeuropathy, multiple mononeuropathies, or polyneuropathy
	6. Diastolic BP > 90 mm Hg	Development of hypertension with diastolic BP > 90 mm Hg
	7. Elevated BUN or creatinine	Elevation of BUN > 40 mg/dL or creatinine > 1.5 mg/dL, not due to dehydration or obstruction
	8. Hepatitis B virus	Presence of hepatitis B surface antigen or antibody in serum
	9. Arteriographic abnormality	Arteriogram showing aneurysms or occlusions of the visceral arteries, not due to arteriosclerosis, fibromuscular dysplasia, or other noninflammatory causes
	10. Biopsy of small or medium-sized artery containing PMN	Histologic changes showing the presence of granulocytes or granulocytes and mononuclear leukocytes in the artery wall
Granulomatosis with polyangiitis (GPA), (formerly Wegener granulomatosis)[b]	1. Nasal or oral inflammation	Development of painful or painless oral ulcers, or purulent or bloody nasal discharge
	2. Abnormal chest radiograph	Chest radiograph showing the presence of nodules, fixed infiltrates, or cavities
	3. Urinary sediment	Microscopic hematuria (> 5 red blood cells per high power field) or red cell casts in urine sediment
	4. Granulomatous inflammation on biopsy	Histologic changes showing granulomatous inflammation within the wall of an artery or in the perivascular or extravascular area (artery or arteriole)
Eosinophilic granulomatosis with polyangiitis (EGPA), (formerly Churg-Strauss syndrome)[c]	1. Asthma	History of wheezing or diffuse pitched rales on expiration
	2. Eosinophilia > 10%	Eosinophilia > 10% on white blood cell count differential
	3. Mononeuropathy or polyneuropathy	Development of mononeuropathy, multiple mononeuropathies, or polyneuropathy (i.e., glove/stocking distribution) attributable to a systemic vasculitis
	4. Pulmonary infiltrates, nonfixed	Migratory or transient pulmonary infiltrates (not including fixed infiltrates) on radiographs attributable to a systemic vasculitis
	5. Paranasal sinus abnormality	History of acute or chronic paranasal sinus pain or tenderness or radiographic opacification of the paranasal sinuses
	6. Extravascular eosinophils	Biopsy including artery, arteriole, or venule, showing accumulations of eosinophils in extravascular areas

[a]For classification purposes, a patient shall be said to have polyarteritis nodosa if at least 3 of the 10 criteria are present. The presence of any 3 or more criteria yields a sensitivity of 82.2% and a specificity of 86.6%.

[b]For purposes of classification, a patient shall be said to have Wegener granulomatosis if at least 2 of these 4 criteria are present. The presence of any 2 or more criteria yields a sensitivity of 88.2% and a specificity of 92.0%

[c]For purposes of classification, a patient shall be said to have EGPA if at least 4 of the 6 criteria are positive. The presence of any 4 or more of the 6 criteria yields a sensitivity of 85% and a specificity of 99.7%.

BP, Blood pressure; *BUN,* blood urea nitrogen; *PMN,* polymorphonuclear cell.

From Lightfoot Jr RW, Michel BA, Bloch DA, et al. The American College of Rheumatology 1990 criteria for the classification of polyarteritis nodosa. *Arthritis Rheum.* 1990;33(8):1088–1093; Leavitt RY, Fauci AS, Bloch DA, et al. The American College of Rheumatology 1990 criteria for the classification of Wegener granulomatosis. *Arthritis Rheum.* 1990;33(8):1101–1107; Masi AT, Hunder GG, Lie JT, et al. The American College of Rheumatology 1990 criteria for the classification of Churg-Strauss syndrome (allergic granulomatosis and angiitis). *Arthritis Rheum.* 1990;33(8):1094–1100.

to therapy, renal function, and hematologic parameters. Treatment with cyclophosphamide is typically continued for at least 6 months, after which it is replaced with a remission maintenance agent such as methotrexate or azathioprine, for total treatment duration of 12 to 18 months. One study showed superiority of treatment with 12 cycles of intravenous pulse cyclophosphamide compared to 6 months of treatment.[43] Although benefit was seen early in the disease course, this was not sustained and at 10 years, there was no difference in survival or disease outcomes between the two groups.[43] In less severe cases of PAN, glucocorticoid monotherapy at a dose of 1 mg/kg/day for 4 weeks followed by a gradual taper over months may be reasonable with the addition of adjunctive immunosuppressive therapy if needed in relapsing cases.[44]

For HBV-related PAN, recommendations for treatment are use of a short course of glucocorticoids (2 weeks) along with antiviral agents to treat the underlying HBV infection, and plasma exchange to remove circulating immune complexes.[42,45] Treatment should be aimed at achieving seroconversion and stopping viral replication which, generally, results in remission of the disease and prevents long-term hepatic complications.[16] Prolonged glucocorticoid therapy and cyclophosphamide should be avoided in order to allow immunological clearance of HBV-infected hepatocytes.

The treatment of c-PAN also depends on disease severity. Mild cases may respond to nonsteroidal antiinflammatory medications, colchicine, or dapsone, while refractory disease often requires additional immunosuppressive therapy.[4,6,7,36,37] In the case of isolated SOV that is detected incidentally at surgery, resection is thought to be curative.[8–10,46]

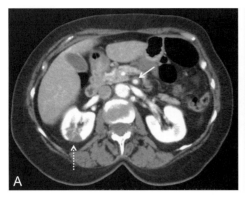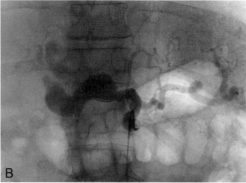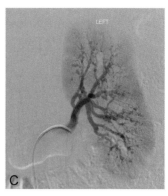

Fig. 41.2 Angiographic findings in patients with polyarteritis nodosa may demonstrate (A) thickening of visceral arteries (*arrow*, superior mesenteric artery) and abdominal organ infarcts *(dotted arrow, left renal)* (computed tomography angiography [axial view]). Conventional angiography may reveal large saccular aneurysms (B, common and right hepatic artery) or multiple microaneurysms (C, left renal artery branches).

The presence of renal, GI, cardiac, or central nervous system involvement in systemic necrotizing vasculitis portends a poorer prognosis with increased risk of mortality.[33,47] The "Five-Factor Score," which includes creatinine of > 1.58 mg/dL, proteinuria > 1 g/24 h, cardiac symptoms, central nervous system, or GI involvement, can be used to estimate disease severity and outcomes in patients with systemic necrotizing vasculitis.[47] A higher "Five-Factor Score" has been associated with increased mortality—11% in patients with a score of 0 compared to 46% in those with a score of > 2.[47] Death in the first year was usually associated with poorly controlled vasculitis.[33,48] In one study, patients with HBV-associated PAN had fewer relapses but more severe disease and increased mortality (34%) compared to non–HBV-associated PAN (20% mortality).[33] In a French cohort study, GI manifestations were the most frequent cause of death in patients with HBV-associated PAN.[48]

SMALL VESSEL VASCULITIS

The 2012 CHCC divided primary small vessel vasculitis into two broad categories: (1) immune complex–mediated vasculitis (antiglomerular basement membrane disease, idiopathic cryoglobulinemic vasculitis [CV], IgA vasculitis [previously Henoch-Schönlein purpura {HSP}], and hypocomplementemic vasculitis), and (2) ANCA-associated vasculitis (granulomatosis with polyangiitis [GPA; previously Wegener's], MPA, and eosinophilic granulomatosis with polyangiitis [EGPA; previously Churg-Strauss]) (Table 41.2).[1] Additionally, while there are numerous secondary causes of medium and small vessel vasculitis, they proposed separate categories for "Vasculitis associated with systemic disease" (e.g., systemic lupus erythematosus, Sjögren's, rheumatoid arthritis) and "Vasculitis associated with probable etiology" (e.g., CV associated with hepatitis C, drug-associated vasculitis, hepatitis B-associated PAN) to account for these.[1]

TABLE 41.2 Definitions Adopted by the 2012 International Chapel Hill Consensus Conference on the Nomenclature of Vasculitides

Disease	Definition
Polyarteritis nodosa	Necrotizing arteritis of medium or small arteries without glomerulonephritis or vasculitis in arterioles, capillaries, or venules, and not associated with antineutrophil cytoplasmic antibodies (ANCAs).
ANCA-associated vasculitis (AAV)	Necrotizing vasculitis, with few or no immune deposits, predominantly affecting small vessels (i.e., capillaries, venules, arterioles, and small arteries), associated with myeloperoxidase (MPO) ANCA or proteinase 3 (PR3) ANCA. Not all patients have ANCA. Add a prefix indicating ANCA reactivity (e.g., MPO-ANCA, PR3-ANCA, ANCA-negative).
Granulomatosis with polyangiitis (GPA)	Necrotizing granulomatous inflammation usually involving the upper and lower respiratory tract, and necrotizing vasculitis affecting predominantly small to medium vessels (e.g., capillaries, venules, arterioles, arteries, and veins). Necrotizing glomerulonephritis is common.
Microscopic polyangiitis (MPA)	Necrotizing vasculitis, with few or no immune deposits, predominantly affecting small vessels (i.e., capillaries, venules, or arterioles). Necrotizing arteritis involving small and medium arteries may be present. Necrotizing glomerulonephritis is very common. Pulmonary capillaritis often occurs. Granulomatous inflammation is absent.
Eosinophilic granulomatosis with polyangiitis (EGPA)	Eosinophil-rich and necrotizing granulomatous inflammation often involving the respiratory tract, and necrotizing vasculitis predominantly affecting small to medium vessels, and associated with asthma and eosinophilia. ANCA is more frequent when glomerulonephritis is present.
IgA vasculitis (IgAV, formerly Henoch-Schönlein purpura)	Vasculitis, with IgA1-dominant immune deposits, affecting small vessels (predominantly capillaries, venules, or arterioles). Often involves skin and gastrointestinal tract, and frequently causes arthritis. Glomerulonephritis indistinguishable from IgA nephropathy may occur.
Cryoglobulinemic vasculitis	Vasculitis with cryoglobulin-immune deposits affecting small vessels (predominantly capillaries, venules, or arterioles) and associated with serum cryoglobulins. Skin, glomeruli, and peripheral nerves are often involved.

Modified from Jennette JC, Falk RJ, Bacon PA, et al. 2012 revised International Chapel Hill Consensus Conference Nomenclature of Vasculitides. *Arthritis Rheum*. 2013;65:1–11.

Cutaneous Small Vessel Vasculitis

It is helpful to consider the CHCC nomenclature when evaluating a patient with cutaneous small vessel vasculitis, which typically presents as palpable purpura. Palpable purpura has a broad differential and may be a manifestation of systemic vasculitis; it may be isolated to the skin (so-called "SOV") or related to multiple other causes including autoimmune diseases, medications, and infections (Box 41.1).[49–52] A systematic approach to the evaluation of these cutaneous lesions is important for several reasons. First, the skin finding can be a manifestation of a systemic process that is affecting other internal organs. Second, appropriate history and consideration of the differential diagnosis allow for appropriate diagnostic testing. Finally, treatment choice is dependent on disease severity and potential triggering factors. For example, in the case of drug-associated cutaneous vasculitis, withdrawal of the offending agent would be sufficient and would obviate the need for any immunosuppressive therapy. The term "leukocytoclastic vasculitis" (LCV) refers to a histopathologic pattern of injury in small vessel vasculitides and is not by itself a distinct form of vasculitis.[53]

Epidemiology

In population-based studies, the estimated annual incidence of cutaneous vasculitis is between 15.4 to 45 per million.[49,54,55] All of these studies included both isolated cutaneous as well as systemic vasculitides that cause cutaneous manifestations, including IgA vasculitis (formerly HSP).[49,54,55] In a population-based study from Olmsted County, MN, USA, the incidence of idiopathic cutaneous small vessel vasculitis was 16 cases per million.[49]

Etiology

The differential diagnosis of palpable purpura is extensive (see Box 41.1). The proportion of cases attributed to different etiologies varies. In a population-based study, the majority of the cases (76%) of cutaneous small vessel vasculitis were idiopathic.[49] Medications may account for up to 20% of cases of cutaneous vasculitis, also termed "hypersensitivity" vasculitis or angiitis. However, in a population-based cohort, only 3% of cases were attributed to medications.[49–52] Approximately 5% to 25% of cases can be from autoimmune conditions like connective tissue diseases or systemic vasculitis like IgA vasculitis, while 22% have been attributed to infections and approximately 8% to malignancies.[49–52]

Histopathology

Biopsy of a purpuric lesion due to vasculitis typically shows findings of LCV.[56] LCV is characterized by a predominantly polymorphonuclear neutrophilic infiltrate primarily affecting the superficial postcapillary venules with fibrinoid deposits in and around the vessel wall, endothelial swelling, and extravasation of red blood cells.[56] Findings on immunofluorescence staining of skin tissue are affected by the age of the lesion biopsied. Ideally, biopsy for immunofluorescence should be performed from a lesion taken within 8 to 24 hours after appearance.[56] The pattern and component of staining on immunofluorescence is particularly helpful in conditions such as IgA vasculitis, which can account for up to 30% of cases of cutaneous vasculitis.[49,56]

Clinical Manifestations

Palpable purpuric lesions are typically characterized by recurrent crops of purpura, primarily involving the dependent areas such as the lower extremities and buttocks, occasionally with findings such as necrosis, ulceration, or bullae (Fig. 41.3).[56] The skin lesions may also appear in areas of pressure or friction, and may be painful, pruritic, or associated with burning.[56] In the case of isolated cutaneous vasculitis, other associated symptoms are absent or very mild (constitutional, arthralgias). The presence of organ manifestations outside the skin (e.g., neurologic, GI, arthritis) should raise concern for systemic vasculitis or other causes such as infections or systemic autoimmune diseases. Patients with associated conditions such as systemic lupus erythematosus, Sjögren syndrome, and rheumatoid arthritis usually have an established diagnosis of a rheumatic disease preceding the presentation of vasculitis. In the study from Olmsted County, systemic involvement

---

BOX 41.1 Differential Diagnosis of Cutaneous Vasculitis

Medications
Antiinflammatories
Antimicrobials—including minocycline which can induce antineutrophil cytoplasmic antibodies
Antitumor necrosis factor
Antiepileptics
Hydralazine (can induce antineutrophil cytoplasmic antibodies)
Propylthiouracil (can induce antineutrophil cytoplasmic antibodies)

Infections
Bacterial
  Endocarditis
  Neisseria
  Pseudomonas
  Staphylococcus aureus
  Streptococcus pyogenes
  Rickettsia
Viral
  Hepatitis B
  Hepatitis C
  Human immunodeficiency virus
Fungal
  Aspergillus

Primary Forms of Vasculitis
Pauci-immune
  Eosinophilic granulomatosis with polyangiitis
  Granulomatosis with polyangiitis
  Microscopic polyangiitis
Immune complex mediated
  Cryoglobulinemic vasculitis
  Immunoglobulin A vasculitis (previously Henoch-Schönlein purpura)
  Urticarial vasculitis

Other Autoimmune Diseases
Antiphospholipid antibody syndrome
Inflammatory bowel disease
Rheumatoid arthritis
Sjögren syndrome
Systemic lupus erythematosus

Malignancies

Illicit Drugs
Cocaine; including levamisole adulterated cocaine

Idiopathic

Common causes in each category are listed.

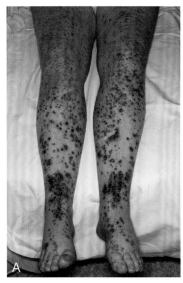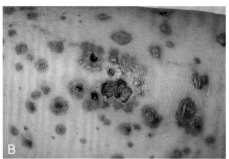

Fig. 41.3 Cutaneous vasculitis can manifest as palpable purpura (A) or ulceration (B).

was present in 46% of cases of cutaneous vasculitis with renal manifestations accounting for 44% of those cases.[49] Other systemic organ involvement in order of decreasing frequency included musculoskeletal (36%), GI (31%), constitutional (31%), ear/nose/throat (8%), pulmonary (5%), and neurologic (3%).[49]

Diagnosis

While histopathology is necessary to confirm the diagnosis of cutaneous vasculitis, a careful history and examination is of paramount importance in the evaluation of palpable purpura. In particular, emphasis should be placed on the time course, preceding triggers (e.g., medications, infections), and presence of manifestations that suggest a systemic process. Laboratory testing should at least include complete blood count, liver function panel, assessment of renal function, and urinalysis.[52] In acute cases without any other concerning clinical features and with normal laboratory evaluation, monitoring alone may be reasonable. In chronic cases, recurrent cases, or in patients where history suggests other organ involvement or a systemic condition, additional serologic testing for infections and autoantibodies can help clarify the diagnosis (Box 41.2). The testing should be individualized based on the clinical symptoms and degree of suspicion. The diagnosis of cutaneous vasculitis should be confirmed by histopathology with biopsy sent for evaluation by hematoxylin and eosin staining, and also by immunofluorescence, especially given that IgA vasculitis is a common cause among autoimmune diseases that can cause palpable purpura (up to 30% cases).[49,52,56] Imaging studies and other organ-specific testing may be indicated in cases where systemic vasculitis is suspected.

Treatment and Prognosis

It is important to identify any potential triggers of palpable purpura as treatment is directed toward the underlying cause. If it is associated with a medication, withdrawal of the offending agent would be appropriate. In the case of infections, systemic autoimmune diseases, or cancer, treatment of the underlying condition is important. Frequently, cutaneous vasculitis is idiopathic and isolated to the skin. In such cases, leg elevation and symptomatic measures like antiinflammatories or antihistamines may be beneficial.[51,52,56] Other options for idiopathic isolated cutaneous vasculitis include glucocorticoids, colchicine, dapsone, or immunosuppressive therapy, but

> ### BOX 41.2 Recommended Laboratory Testing for Evaluation of Cutaneous Vasculitis
>
> Recommended in all patients:
>   Complete blood count with differential
>   Hepatic function panel
>   Creatinine
>   Urinalysis with microscopy
>   Urine protein-creatinine ratio
>   Markers of inflammation (erythrocyte sedimentation rate and C-reactive protein)
> Recommended based on clinical suspicion, in patients with evidence of multi-system involvement, or in chronic recurrent cases:
> Infections
>   Viral: Hepatitis B, Hepatitis C, Human immunodeficiency virus
>   Bacterial: Blood cultures, Antistreptolysin O (ASO), Deoxyribonuclease (DNase), echocardiogram
> Connective tissue disease related
>   Antinuclear antibody (ANA), double-stranded DNA (dsDNA), SSA, SSB, anti-Smith, anti-ribonuclear protein (RNP), C3, C4, rheumatoid factor.
> Rheumatoid arthritis related
>   Rheumatoid factor, cyclic citrullinated peptide (CCP), C3, C4
> Cryoglobulinemic vasculitis (should also include appropriate evaluation for other causes of cryoglobulinemia)
>   C3, C4, rheumatoid factor, cryoglobulin, serum protein electrophoresis, immunofixation
> Antineutrophil cytoplasmic antibody associated vasculitis
>   Antineutrophil cytoplasmic antibody (ANCA) including:
>   perinuclear (p) ANCA via immunofluorescence
>   cytoplasmic (c) ANCA via immunofluorescence
>   Myeloperoxidase (MPO) antibody
>   Proteinase-3 (PR3) antibody

the data on treatment is primarily anecdotal.[51,52,56] Recurrences may be frequent.[49] In one study, overall survival in patients with cutaneous vasculitis, even when isolated to the skin, was lower than expected for the general population, but the reason for this finding is unclear.[49]

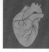

PAUCI-IMMUNE SMALL VESSEL VASCULITIS

Antineutrophil Cytoplasmic Antibodies-Associated Vasculitis

Nomenclature

ANCA are autoantibodies that react against proteins that are primarily found in cytoplasmic granules of neutrophils. Indirect immunofluorescence (IIF) of neutrophils has identified two main positive staining patterns, c-ANCA (cytoplasmic) and p-ANCA (perinuclear). The c-ANCA pattern is usually due to antibodies targeting the neutrophil protein proteinase-3 (PR3, PR3-ANCA) and the p-ANCA pattern due to antibodies directed against myeloperoxidase (MPO, MPO-ANCA).[57] The ANCA-associated vasculitides (AAV) are a group of diseases characterized by a necrotizing vasculitis with few or no immune deposits, predominantly affecting small vessels and associated with MPO-ANCA or PR3-ANCA.[1] The three main subsets of systemic AAV include GPA (formerly Wegener granulomatosis), EGPA (formerly Churg-Strauss syndrome), and MPA.

Epidemiology

The annual incidences of GPA and MPA are each estimated to be 6 to 12 per million population and the incidence of EGPA is 0.5 to 2 per million.[11,58] While the combined incidence of AAV is roughly similar across different populations, geographical and ethnic variations have been observed. For instance, GPA is more prevalent among populations in Australasia, the United Kingdom, and Norway, whereas MPA is more common in China, Japan, and Kuwait.[59] Incidence appears to increase with age with a peak mean age of onset between 50 and 65 years of age.[60,61] The gender distribution is overall similar among AAV, though a slight male predominance has been seen in some cohorts.

Genetics

AAV are not directly inherited genetic disorders, but genetic alterations conferring susceptibility have been identified through international genome-wide association studies (GWAS) leading to alteration of the innate and adaptive immune response. Genetic variants in the major histocompatibility complex (MHC) system highlight a genetic contribution to the immunopathogenesis of AAV. The most reproducible and significant contribution that increases risk of AAV has been observed at the *HLA-DPB1* gene.[62–64] In addition, polymorphisms near *SEMA6A*, a gene coding for semaphorin6A, which is involved in angiogenesis through regulation of endothelial cell survival and growth, has also reached genome-wide significance in patients with GPA.[64] More recent studies have identified that distinct genetic associations may be more closely linked to ANCA specificity (i.e., PR3 vs. MPO) rather than the clinical disease spectrum (GPA vs. MPA). Anti-PR3 ANCA was strongly associated with *HLA-DP*, proteinase 3 *(PRTN3)*, and *SERPINA1*, whereas anti-MPO ANCA was associated with *HLA-DQ*.[63] *SERPINA1* encodes for alpha-1 anti-trypsin, which inhibits PR3 activity. The observed null mutation leading to alpha-1 anti-trypsin deficiency is thought to result in decreased regulation of PR3 activity, which consequently leads to ongoing tissue inflammation and generation of ANCA.[65]

Etiology

The exact cause of AAV remains unidentified. In addition to genetic risk, several nongenetic environmental factors may contribute to an increased likelihood of AAV. Chronic nasal carriage of *Staphylococcus aureus* has been observed at high rates in patients with GPA and is associated with increased relapse risk; however, a direct pathogenic contribution has yet to be confirmed.[66] Inhalation of silica dust has demonstrated an increased risk in several case-control studies and is

most strongly supported by the two-fold increase in incidence in AAV directly following the Kobe, Japan earthquake.[67] Several medications have been identified as causal agents of drug-induced AAV, with the most common offending drugs being propylthiouracil, hydralazine, D-penicillamine, minocycline, sulfasalazine, tumor necrosis factor-alpha (TNF-α) inhibitors, and levamisole-contaminated cocaine.[68]

Pathogenesis

The etiologic mechanism(s) for developing AAV remain incompletely understood, but ANCA are considered to have a pathogenic role. The generation of ANCA is likely multifactorial in nature, but a current area of focus in their generation is the contribution of neutrophil extracellular traps (NETs). NETs are web-like structures that consist of decondensed fibers of chromatin and cytosolic antimicrobial proteins, including MPO and PR3.[69] Their function is to trap, kill, and remove microbial pathogens. However, if dysregulated, NETs can contribute to the pathogenesis of immune-related disease.[70] Indeed, transfer of MPO and PR3 from neutrophils undergoing NETosis to antigen-presenting cells with resultant production of anti-MPO ANCA and the generation of vasculitis have been observed in animal models.[71] In addition, studies of sera from human subjects with MPA have demonstrated in vitro evidence that MPO-ANCA can stimulate NETs.[72] The involvement of NETS in patients with AAV is further observed through increased levels of NETs and NET-associated proteins, both in circulation[73,74] and in lesioned tissue.[75]

The combined findings from multiple animal models and human studies have led to a proposed sequence of events that result in the observed vascular damage in AAV. Neutrophils are pre-activated through a process known as "priming," which is facilitated by pro-inflammatory mediators in response to a danger signal/stimulus.[76] The primed neutrophils can express PR3 or MPO on their surface or release these proteins into the local environment.[77] Circulating ANCA can bind to either MPO or PR3, resulting in full activation of the primed neutrophils.[78] This activation can result in neutrophil adhesion to the vascular endothelium[79] and release of factors that activate neutrophil chemoattractant complement component 5a (C5a).[80] Recruited neutrophils can be further primed and activated by C5a, increasing the inflammatory signal through an amplification loop.[81] The activated neutrophils can traffic through the vascular wall and release reactive oxygen species and toxic granules, leading to injury and necrosis of vessel wall and the adjacent extravascular tissue.[82,83] Moreover, neutrophils guide other immune cells, particularly T lymphocytes, which also appear to play a significant role in vascular injury.[84]

Clinical Features

AAV and its subsets are multi-system diseases that have a variety of disease presentations ranging from mild, limited disease to life-threatening organ destruction. While there is notable overlap between these subsets, the main characteristics and differences between GPA, MPA, and EGPA are summarized in Table 41.3.

The upper respiratory tract is a common site of pathology in AAV. While it can occur in MPA, it is more common in GPA and EGPA.[85] The frequently observed features include epistaxis, nasal crusting, nasal polyposis, and chronic refractory sinusitis. Nasal sores and ulceration can range from mild to severe in nature (Fig. 41.4). In general, sinus lesions are less severe and less destructive in MPA and EGPA when compared to GPA. Osteocartilaginous inflammation can lead to septal erosion/perforation, bony destruction, and saddle nose deformity (Fig. 41.5).[86] Serous otitis media is the most common type of otologic involvement.[85] Development of this finding in patients over the age of 50 years should raise the suspicion for AAV, particularly if associated with conductive hearing loss.

TABLE 41.3 Main Clinical Characteristics of ANCA-Associated Vasculitis

Characteristic (Key Features)	Granulomatosis With Polyangiitis	Microscopic Polyangiitis	Eosinophilic Granulomatosis With Polyangiitis
Ear, nose, throat	60%–95% (sinusitis can be destructive, septal perforation, saddle nose deformity, otitis media)	<15%	30%–60% (allergic rhinitis, polyposis, nondestructive sinusitis)
Pulmonary parenchymal abnormalities	50%–80% (nodules, cavitary lesions)	20%–40% (interstitial lung disease)	20%–30% (ground glass opacities)
Alveolar hemorrhage	10%–20%	20%–50%	<5%
Asthma	No	No	Yes
Cardiac	30%–40%	Rare	60%–90%
Glomerulonephritis	60%–80%	60%–80%	10%–20%
Mononeuritis multiplex	20%–40%	30%–40%	60%–75%
Eye	35%–55% (scleritis, episcleritis, orbital pseudotumor)	<10%	<10%
Leukocytoclastic vasculitis	30%–40%	30%–60%	50%–60%
Granulomatous inflammation	Yes	No	Yes
Eosinophilia	No	No	Yes
ANCA positive	80%–90% (primarily c-ANCA/PR3)	80%–90% (primarily p-ANCA/MPO)	30%–50% (primarily p-ANCA/MPO)

ANCA, Antineutrophil cytoplasmic antibodies; *MPO,* myeloperoxidase.

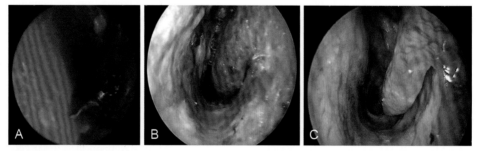

Fig. 41.4 Nasal endoscopic views of severe inferior turbinate ulceration prior to (A), 6 weeks after (B) and 3 months following (C) induction with high-dose prednisone and rituximab.

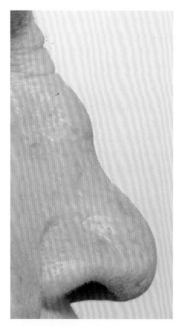

Fig. 41.5 Saddle nose deformity in patient with granulomatosis with polyangiitis.

Laryngotracheal involvement can range from mild vocal hoarseness to life-threatening tracheal obstruction. Subglottic stenosis can occur in approximately 20% of patients,[85] leading to respiratory dysfunction and difficulty with intubation if pulmonary compromise develops. Involvement of the lower respiratory tract with pulmonary capillaritis resulting in alveolar hemorrhage can be seen in all subsets of AAV, whereas granulomatous lung nodules and cavitary lesions are associated with GPA and EGPA, but not MPA. In a patient with small vessel vasculitis, the presence of asthma, particularly if present in the context of eosinophilia, is strongly suggestive of EGPA.

Renal disease is frequent in MPA and GPA (60% to 80%) but is less common in EGPA.[87] Hematuria with dysmorphic red blood cells, red blood cell casts, proteinuria, or rising creatinine may indicate glomerular abnormalities. In some patients, AAV may be renal-limited, without evidence of other systemic findings. In both limited and systemic forms, the hallmark findings on renal biopsy include pauci-immune (i.e., without immune complex deposition) necrotizing crescentic glomerulonephritis.

Among patients with AAV, cardiac involvement is most commonly seen in patients with EGPA (60% to 90%), followed by GPA (30% to 40%) and much less likely in MPA. If present, cardiac involvement is a major contributor to disease-related death in EGPA.[88] The two main mechanisms attributed to cardiac dysfunction in EGPA

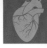

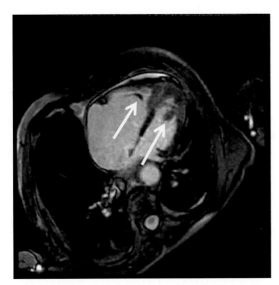

Fig. 41.6 Two-chamber view cardiac magnetic resonance imaging with delayed myocardial enhancement demonstrating right and left ventricular apical mural thrombi (arrows) and pericardial enhancement in patient with eosinophilic granulomatosis with polyangiitis.

are eosinophilic infiltration of the cardiac layers and vasculitis-associated ischemia. Ventricular and supraventricular arrhythmias can be seen but resultant sudden cardiac death is rare. Coronary arteritis has been reported but is exceptional. Pericarditis and pericardial effusion are detected in 25% to 40%, infrequently accompanied by tamponade.[89,90] Eosinophilic myocarditis is common (60%) and considered a severe manifestation, as it can lead to cardiomyopathy and heart failure and carries a poor prognosis.[88] Endomyocardial inflammation in EGPA can occur in three main stages: acute inflammation/necrosis, fibrin deposition ± thrombus formation, and fibrosis.[91] Ventricular thrombi (Fig. 41.6) can occur in either the right or left chambers and, if biopsied, show dense lymphoplasmacytic infiltrate with > 10% eosinophils. Absence of patient-reported cardiac symptoms and lack of abnormalities on electrocardiogram does not exclude the presence of cardiac involvement and systematic testing of EGPA patients with echocardiography and/or cardiac magnetic resonance imaging (MRI) is often needed to identify cardiac pathology.[90]

Additional features that can raise suspicion of AAV include, but are not limited to, inflammatory pathology of the eye (scleritis, episcleritis, retro-orbital pseudotumor), skin (purpuric LCV), nervous system (peripheral sensory neuropathy, mononeuritis multiplex, cranial nerve abnormalities, pachymeningitis), and GI tract (bowel wall edema, viscus perforation, mesenteric vasculitis).[92] A subset of patients may present with inflammatory arthritis and ANCA testing should be considered in patients with clinical features of inflammatory arthritis in which RF, anti-citrullinated protein antibodies (ACPA), and antinuclear antigen (ANA) are negative.[93]

Due to the multiple organ systems that can be involved, a comprehensive physical examination is requisite when evaluating patients for AAV. At a minimum, cranial nerve assessment, visual scleral inspection, speculum examination of the ears and nose, pulmonary auscultation, peripheral sensory and motor nerve evaluation, and skin examination should be performed in all patients. Formal consultation with otorhinolaryngology, ophthalmology, and/or pulmonology may be required for advanced examination procedures to confirm or exclude each specialty's respective organ involvement.

Laboratory Findings

Routine laboratory parameters are nonspecific but can primarily demonstrate an inflammatory state with findings of a normocytic anemia, thrombocytosis, leukocytosis, and increased inflammatory markers (erythrocyte sedimentation rate and/or C-reactive protein). A complete blood count with differential is particularly helpful, as the presence of eosinophilia (> 1500 cells/microliter or > 10% leukocyte count) should prompt suspicion for EGPA. Creatinine with estimated glomerular filtration rate and urinalysis with microscopy should be evaluated in all patients to assess for renal abnormalities. If proteinuria is present, quantification should be pursued via 24-hour protein measurement.

All patients suspected of AAV should have ANCA testing. IIF testing (i.e., c-ANCA, p-ANCA) is generally combined with ELISA (MPO-ANCA, PR3-ANCA) assays to provide optimal sensitivity and specificity. A reasonable approach is to evaluate first with IIF and, if positive, reflex to ELISA; however, the sequence of testing may vary, depending on local laboratory practice.[94] Overall, 80% to 90% of patients with GPA and MPA will have positive ANCA, whereas only approximately 30% to 50% in EGPA are ANCA positive.[89] In patients with positive ANCA testing, c-ANCA/PR3 is most frequently seen in patients with GPA (80%), whereas p-ANCA/MPO is more common among ANCA-positive MPA (90%) and EGPA (70% to 80%).

While in the appropriate clinical context, positive ANCA testing has a high positive predictive value for AAV, ANCA (p-ANCA or atypical-ANCA) have also been reported in several other inflammatory conditions including, but not limited to, systemic lupus erythematosus (25%), Sjögren syndrome (20%), ulcerative colitis (40%), and primary sclerosing cholangitis (80%).[95,96] In addition, ANCA can also be seen in patients with infections like tuberculosis (40%), endocarditis (8% to 18%), and HIV (up to 80%). Positive p-ANCA/MPO can also be observed in patients taking certain medications including propylthiouracil, hydralazine, minocycline, D-penicillamine, and allopurinol.[97] In such cases, circulating antibody is not necessarily pathologic; however, drug-induced vasculitis from these agents has been noted to occur. Additional laboratory studies to rule out other etiologies with similar systemic findings should be considered (see Box 41.2).

Diagnosis

At current, there are no diagnostic criteria or validated diagnostic algorithms for AAV; however, an international collaboration to develop these tools is ongoing.[40] As such, the diagnosis of patients with AAV can be challenging and relies on the presence of clinical features, laboratory parameters, radiographic findings, and biopsy.

A positive tissue biopsy is strongly supportive of the diagnosis of AAV and has been recommended by expert consensus guidelines.[98] However, the diagnostic yield of sites with active disease varies based on the organ system targeted. Renal biopsies in patients with declining renal function, hematuria, or worsening proteinuria have the highest diagnostic yield (85% to 90%), classically demonstrating evidence of pauci-immune glomerulonephritis.[99] Lung biopsies, if pursued, should be done with open or thoracoscopic approach because transbronchial biopsies obtain sufficient tissue for diagnosis in only 10% to 15% of cases.[100,101] Lung findings strongly suggestive of AAV include pulmonary capillaritis (MPA, GPA, EGPA) and necrotizing granulomatosis (GPA), the latter of which is eosinophil-rich in EGPA. Sinus biopsies, though less invasive, are often nonspecific, demonstrating only chronic inflammatory changes without overt granulomas or vasculitis.[102]

Because of the complexity of diagnosing patients with AAV in a timely manner in order to initiate treatment, evaluation of patients with concern for AAV should be undertaken at centers with expertise

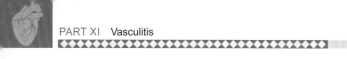

in both diagnosing and managing these conditions. A multispecialty approach is often required with coordination between rheumatology, pulmonary medicine, nephrology, otorhinolaryngology, and pathology.

Prognosis and Treatment

If left untreated, the prognosis of severe systemic AAV is dismal, with a mortality reaching 90% at 2 years, usually due to pulmonary complications or renal failure.[92] The introduction of immunosuppressive therapy has led to marked improvement in long-term outcomes with 10-year survival now reaching 75%. Relapse is common, with 20% to 40% of patients experiencing one or more relapses during the course of disease and occurs more commonly in patients with PR3-ANCA, lung disease, and upper respiratory tract abnormalities.[103]

All patients with evidence of AAV require treatment. Mild and limited forms with non–life-threatening manifestations of AAV may be treated with low to moderate doses of glucocorticoids and conventional immunosuppressive agents such as mycophenolate mofetil, azathioprine, or methotrexate. In contrast, the treatment of severe AAV involves more intensive management with two main stages of treatment: induction to remission followed by maintenance of remission.

Induction to remission. Remission induction is initiated with high-dose glucocorticoids (1 mg/kg/day oral prednisone, sometimes preceded by intravenous methylprednisolone 1000 mg daily for 3 days) followed by taper, in combination with cyclophosphamide or rituximab. Cyclophosphamide can be given as either monthly intravenous boluses (750 mg/m^2) or daily oral tablets (target 2 mg/kg/day). Patients receiving daily oral administration have a lower relapse rate (20%) compared to intravenous bolus (40%),[104] but have higher total cumulative cyclophosphamide exposure which has been linked to infertility, bladder cancer, skin cancer, and lymphoma risk.

The benefit of rituximab, a chimeric monoclonal antibody directed against the cell surface protein CD20 on B cells, was confirmed in two landmark clinical trials showing noninferiority of a single cycle of rituximab (375 mg/m^2, weekly for 4 weeks) to 6 months of cyclophosphamide in the induction to remission for GPA and MPA.[105,106] Although short-term adverse events of cyclophosphamide and rituximab were similar in these studies, the concern for long-term complications of cyclophosphamide has led many providers to consider rituximab as a first-line option in patients with AAV. It should be noted that patients with EGPA were not included in these studies. Although preliminary efficacy has been observed, the overall benefit of rituximab in EGPA is less well known and limited to retrospective studies and case series.[107,108] Ongoing clinical trials are evaluating the benefit of rituximab in EGPA (Clinicaltrials.gov Identifier NCT02807103).

Mepolizumab, a monoclonal antibody directed against interleukin (IL)-5, is the first medication in a randomized, controlled trial to show definitive benefit in relapsing or refractory EGPA. Patients receiving mepolizumab (300 mg, subcutaneous, monthly) had a higher percentage of remission at week 48 compared to placebo (32% vs. 3%).[109] These findings have led mepolizumab to become the first-ever FDA approved medication for EGPA.

The addition of plasma exchange to induction regimens has been utilized in AAV patients with severe renal manifestations and alveolar hemorrhage with variable short- and long-term benefit.[110,111] While current consensus guidelines suggest plasma exchange should be considered in rapidly progressive glomerulonephritis and can be considered in diffuse alveolar hemorrhage,[98] an ongoing randomized clinical trial (PEXIVAS) evaluating use of plasma exchanges in such scenarios is expected to provide further guidance.[112]

The use of high-dose glucocorticoids in the induction to remission phase can cause significant adverse events and morbidity, and the requirement of such use is being challenged. In a phase 2 trial, the addition of a new oral complement 5a-receptor blocking agent, CCX168 (Avacopan), to the standard induction regimen (cyclophosphamide or rituximab) for patients with GPA and MPA has demonstrated the capacity to dramatically reduce and potentially eliminate the need for glucocorticoids during induction.[113] A phase 3 trial further evaluating the safety and efficacy of CCX168 in induction and maintenance of remission is underway (Clinicaltrials.gov Identifier NCT02994927).

Maintenance of remission. Following induction, patients who have achieved remission on cyclophosphamide are transitioned to a less toxic immunosuppressant. The most commonly used medication is azathioprine (2 mg/kg/day), which has shown benefit over mycophenolate mofetil.[114] Methotrexate (0.3 mg/kg/week, up to maximum dose of 25 mg weekly) has similar efficacy to azathioprine, but must be avoided in patients with moderate-severe renal insufficiency.[115] Following induction therapy with rituximab, this same agent can be used intermittently for maintenance of remission but the dose, timing, and frequency lack consensus. Some experts have suggested re-treatment only at the sign of clinical relapse, return of depleted CD19/CD20 B cells, and/or reappearance or rise in ANCA titer, while others suggest scheduled interval maintenance infusions.[116,117] Ongoing clinical trials evaluating dosing based on ANCA titers and CD19/CD20 counts versus fixed-schedule dosing of rituximab will provide further guidance once completed (Clinicaltrials.gov Identifiers NCT01731561, NCT02433522, NCT01697267). Regardless of the immunosuppressive agent chosen, maintenance therapy should be continued for at least 24 months after remission is achieved before consideration of de-escalating or discontinuing therapy.[98] In patients with life-threatening organ manifestations at disease onset or with recurrent relapses, ongoing treatment may be required.

IMMUNE COMPLEX MEDIATED SMALL VESSEL VASCULITIS

Immunoglobulin-A Vasculitis

Epidemiology

Immunoglobulin-A vasculitis (IgAV), previously known as HSP, is an immune complex–mediated vasculitis affecting small blood vessels. IgAV can affect individuals of any age but is primarily observed in children and adolescents with an annual incidence ranging from 10 to 20 per 100,000 among those < 17 years of age[118–120] and a peak incidence between 4 and 6 years of age (70 per 100,000).[119] The annual incidence among adults is less well-defined but is estimated at 0.5 to 5 cases per 100,000 population.[121] A slight male predominance (male-to-female ratios of 1.1 to 1.8:1) have been described.[118,122] The etiology of IgAV is unknown; however, evidence of detected seasonal variations has led to the hypothesis of a potential infectious trigger. Indeed, approximately half of patients affected describe a recent upper respiratory infection prior to symptom onset,[123] and GI infections preceding diagnosis have also been reported.

Pathogenesis

Immunoglobulin A (IgA) exists in both secretory and circulating forms, and is present in two isotypes, IgA1 and IgA2. IgA1 is the predominant IgA subclass in the circulation (90%), while IgA2 is less frequent (10%).[124] IgAV is characterized by IgA1-autoantibody deposition in the vasculature, but the antigen to which IgA1 binds remains unknown. The etiopathogenesis of IgAV remains under investigation but a multi-hit hypothesis has been proposed.[125] In this model, it is suggested that (1) genetic and/or environmental stimuli increase levels of circulating IgA1 antiendothelial cell antibodies (AECA); (2) IgA1-AECA undergo enhanced binding to endothelial cells in the presence of circulating TNF-α; (3) endothelial cells then produce IL-8, resulting in neutrophil migration; (4) IgA1-activated neutrophils release chemoattractants resulting in a neutrophil attracting/activating feedback loop; and (5) activation of neutrophils results in multiple pro-inflammatory sequelae including phagocytosis, reactive oxygen species generation, inflammatory cytokine/chemokine secretion, and antibody-mediated cellular cytotoxicity, which culminate in vascular damage.[125]

Clinical Features

The main clinical tetrad of IgA vasculitis is palpable purpura, arthritis, GI, and renal involvement. Cutaneous findings are present in all patients at some point of the disease course and account for the presenting feature in approximately 75% of patients.[122,126]

The skin findings (Fig. 41.7) typically appear as clusters of lesions but can coalesce and become more confluent. Varying stages of cutaneous involvement can be observed with initial inflammatory lesions presenting as urticarial, macular, erythematous changes that progress into palpable purpuric lesions and then into post-inflammatory hyperpigmented macules/plaques. Hemorrhagic vesiculobullous findings can be seen in up to 35% of patients.[127] Skin lesions tend to be symmetrically distributed and predominantly in the lower extremities and buttocks, but can also progress proximally, infrequently rising higher than the umbilicus. Less commonly, lesions can be seen on the trunk and upper extremities.[128] Reactive subcutaneous edema is common in affected limbs.

Renal involvement in IgA vasculitis is detected in 20% to 54% of pediatric cases[122,129,130] and can manifest as hematuria (micro- or macroscopic) and/or proteinuria (sub-nephrotic or nephrotic). The majority of renal abnormalities are identified at, or within, 4 weeks of diagnosis in 85% of cases with an additional 12% being seen between 1 and 6 months after disease onset.[131] Adults tend to have more frequent and more severe renal disease at diagnosis, with a higher proportion presenting with nephrotic syndrome and elevated creatinine.[132] Other nonrenal genitourinary manifestations include scrotal pain and/or swelling. Such findings are more common in pediatric and adolescent cases (occurring in up to 22% of males), can be unilateral or bilateral, and rarely may be the initial presenting symptom.[133]

Arthralgia is present in up to 40% to 70% of patients and the most commonly involved areas include the knees and ankles.[122,132] Inflammatory arthritis can occur and lead to significant discomfort during the course of disease but is typically self-limiting and nondestructive.

GI involvement is observed in 40% to 50% of cases and typically follows onset of rash.[127] However, GI symptoms may rarely precede cutaneous manifestations in 10% to 20%. Abdominal pain is acute, diffuse, and colicky in 60% to 70% of patients[134] and thought to be due to submucosal bleeding and/or bowel wall edema. Intussusception can occur in pediatric cases but is rare in adults.[122,135] Melena, hematemesis, or hematochezia can occur in 15% to 26% of patients.[132,136]

Involvement of the peripheral and central nervous systems, as well as pulmonary and ocular manifestations have been reported in rare cases but are considered highly atypical and the presence of such findings should prompt thorough evaluation for other forms of small vessel vasculitis.

Diagnosis

The diagnosis of IgAV remains primarily based on clinical manifestations. Classification criteria for IgAV have primarily focused on pediatric populations and have not been validated prospectively in adults.[137] While several classification criteria exist, the EULAR/PRINTOS/PRES criteria have the highest sensitivity (100%) and specificity (87%) (Table 41.4).[138] Because of clinical overlap, exclusion of other forms of small vessel vasculitis is recommended (see Box 41.2). Serum IgA levels may be elevated, but are nonspecific and should not be relied upon to confirm or refute the diagnosis of IgAV.[139,140] Infective endocarditis has rarely been associated with precipitating IgAV and should be considered in patients with clinical features of endocarditis such as fever or new/worsening valvular murmur.

In pediatric cases, the clinical tetrad of nonthrombocytopenic palpable purpura, arthritis, renal involvement, and GI symptoms is pathognomonic. Biopsy of the skin is not absolutely necessary for diagnosis. However, it is helpful for confirmation, particularly in atypical presentations and in adult patients in which other small vessel vasculitides are seen at higher frequencies than in pediatric populations.

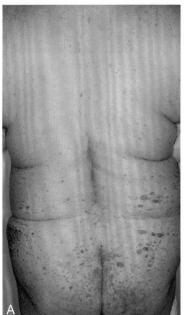
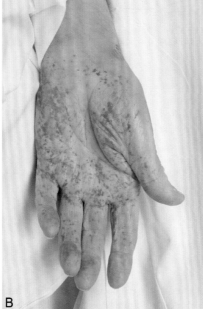
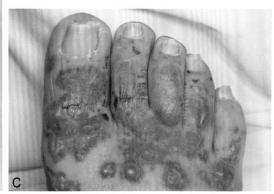

Fig. 41.7 Cutaneous findings of IgA vasculitis include lower extremity predominant palpable purpura that can progress cephalad to the buttocks and trunk (A) and less frequently the upper extremity and hands (B). Vesiculobullous lesions are uncommon but can occur (C).

TABLE 41.4   EULAR/PRINTO/PRES Classification Criteria for Childhood IgA Vasculitis

Criterion	Definition
Purpura (mandatory criterion) plus ≥ 1 of the following	Purpura (commonly palpable and in crops) or petechiae, with lower limb predominance,[a] not related to thrombocytopenia
1. Abdominal pain	Diffuse abdominal colicky pain with acute onset assessed by history and physical examination. May include intussusception and gastrointestinal bleeding
2. Histopathology	Typically leukocytoclastic vasculitis with predominant IgA deposit or proliferative glomerulonephritis with predominant IgA deposit
3. Arthritis or arthralgias	Arthritis of acute onset defined as joint swelling or joint pain with limitation on motion Arthralgia of acute onset defined as joint pain without joint swelling or limitation on motion
4. Renal involvement	Proteinuria > 0.3 g/24 h or > 30 mmol/mg of urine albumin/creatinine ratio on a spot morning sample; and/or Hematuria or red blood cell casts: > 5 red blood cells/high power field or red blood cells casts in the urinary sediment or ≥ 2 + on dipstick

[a]For purpura with atypical distribution, a demonstration of an IgA deposit in a biopsy is required.

If mandatory criterion + ≥ 1 additional criterion present sensitivity 100%, specificity 87%.

EULAR, European League Against Rheumatism; *PRES,* Paediatric Rheumatology European Society, *PRINTO,* Paediatric Rheumatology International Trials Organisation.

Modified from Ozen S, Pistorio A, Iusan SM, et al. EULAR/PRINTO/PRES criteria for Henoch-Schonlein purpura, childhood polyarteritis nodosa, childhood Wegener granulomatosis and childhood Takayasu arteritis: Ankara 2008. Part II: Final classification criteria. *Ann Rheum Dis.* 2010;69(5):798–806.

Biopsies typically demonstrate evidence of LCV. Performance of direct immunofluorescence on skin samples is essential to confirm isolated IgA deposition, which would be confirmatory for this disease. When choosing location of biopsy, lesions that are less than 24 hours old should be sampled to minimize false-negative results.

Renal biopsy is not routinely required unless severe renal disease is present or if there is diagnostic uncertainty. In such cases, biopsy may be helpful to distinguish between IgAV and other autoimmune causes of renal compromise including ANCA-associated vasculitis or SLE. The renal histopathologic findings of IgAV are indistinguishable from IgA nephropathy and the severity can range from mild isolated mesangial proliferation to markedly severe crescentic glomerulonephritis.[1] Similar to skin biopsies, immunofluorescence is requisite and demonstrates IgA deposition in the renal mesangium.

For patients with mild abdominal pain without findings of enteritis or mucosal bleeding, abdominal imaging is not required, but if obtained may show bowel wall edema or mural thickening (Fig. 41.8A). Pediatric patients with severe abdominal pain should undergo evaluation with ultrasound (preferred) or CT to exclude intussusception or obstruction. Spontaneous visceral perforation can occur but is rare. In patients with GI hemorrhage, endoscopy may demonstrate mucosal erythema, petechiae, or ulceration in the stomach or duodenum (see Fig. 41.8B). In such cases, biopsies of these lesions often demonstrate nonspecific inflammation with staining of IgA in the capillaries.[141]

Prognosis and Treatment

The main indicator of long-term morbidity is the presence of renal disease. Persistent proteinuria and mild hematuria can be observed in approximately 12% of patients.[139] Progression to chronic renal failure can occur in 1.8% to 15.7% of children[128,142] and in 10% to 30% of adults.[127,128] Females and patients aged > 50 years at diagnosis tend to have poorer long-term renal outcomes.[127,131] Baseline renal failure, macroscopic hematuria, and proteinuria > 1 g/L have also been associated with higher risk of end-stage renal disease.[127,128] Among patients in whom renal biopsy has been performed, the presence of crescents involving ≥ 50% of glomeruli is strongly predictive of development of chronic kidney or end-stage renal disease.[143]

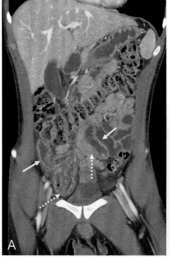
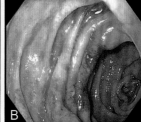

Fig. 41.8 (A) Abdominal computed tomography (coronal view) demonstrating bowel wall thickening *(dotted arrows)* and contrast enhancement *(solid arrows)* demonstrating intestinal inflammation in patient with IgA vasculitis. (B) Upper endoscopy with duodenal mucosal hyperemia in which biopsy showed evidence of IgA deposition in capillaries.

Relapses of IgAV are common and occur in 12% to 52% of patients.[139,144] Among those that relapse, recurrence of skin lesions is the predominant (88%–100%) manifestation, whereas reemergence of GI symptoms can occur in 27% to 85%.[134,145] The presence of severe abdominal pain at diagnosis increases the likelihood of such relapses.[134] However, provided GI manifestations do not present with severe hemorrhage requiring surgical intervention, late-stage residual complications of the GI tract are rarely encountered.

In the majority of cases, IgAV is self-limited with complete recovery occurring in 90% of cases.[146] Discomfort from skin lesions and arthralgia is treated symptomatically with mild analgesics. Nonsteroidal antiinflammatory medications can be utilized provided severe renal or GI manifestations are not concomitantly present. Limited observational studies have shown dapsone,[147] colchicine,[148] and montelukast[149] to have

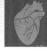

variable success for treatment of chronic purpuric skin lesions, but have little impact on joint, renal, and GI symptoms. Significant controversy surrounds the use of glucocorticoids in IgAV. Patients with crescentic glomerulonephritis due to IgAV may benefit from early pulse intravenous methylprednisolone,[150] but there are no randomized controlled trials demonstrating that high-dose oral glucocorticoid therapy has any substantial long-term benefit in patients with renal involvement.

On the other hand, glucocorticoids appear to have short-term benefit on the severity and duration of abdominal pain, often significantly reducing or eliminating abdominal pain within 24 to 48 hours.[151,152] In patients with abdominal pain severe enough to limit oral intake or to require hospitalization, it is reasonable to consider prednisone 1 mg/kg/day (or equivalent) with a taper over 4 to 8 weeks. Bowel wall edema may impair absorption and if present intravenous forms of methylprednisolone may be required in those not tolerating oral intake or for patients failing to respond to oral prednisone within 2 to 3 days.

The efficacy of additional immunosuppressive therapy is unclear. Cyclophosphamide has demonstrated no significant benefit in a prospective trial of adults with severe IgAV.[153] There is limited evidence suggesting that azathioprine[154,155] or mycophenolate mofetil[156] may be effective in IgAV, mostly in patients with renal involvement. Plasmapheresis has been used in severe cases with variable results, but is not routinely recommended.[157,158] Rituximab, a chimeric anti-CD20 monoclonal antibody, has shown preliminary signals of efficacy in several reported cases of relapsing, refractory, or glucocorticoid-dependent IgAV.[159,160] However, further studies of B-cell depleting agents are needed prior to recommending routine use.

Cryoglobulinemic Vasculitis

CV is a systemic small vessel vasculitis that frequently affects the skin, nerves, and kidneys (glomerulonephritis).[161] CV is defined by vasculitis with cryoglobulin-immune deposits affecting small vessels (predominantly capillaries, venules, or arterioles) and associated with cryoglobulins in the serum.[1] Cryoglobulins are circulating immunoglobulins (Ig) that precipitate when serum is cooled below core body temperature and resolubilize on rewarming.[161] As in the case of palpable purpura, there are many causes of cryoglobulinemia including hematologic conditions, autoimmune diseases, HCV, other infections including HBV, HIV, and idiopathic (so-called "essential") cryoglobulinemia.[1,161] While a significant proportion of patients with the above conditions may have cryoglobulinemia (presence of detectable cryoglobulins in serum), the diagnosis of CV is based on manifestations of vasculitis. In the sections below, the findings of cryoglobulinemia which may be asymptomatic are distinguished from CV when reviewing the different studies. Advances in treatment of HCV, including curative therapy, have led to significant improvements in treatment of HCV-associated CV while the use of rituximab appears efficacious for many different forms of CV.[162–170]

Epidemiology and Etiology

The incidence of CV is unknown. Among patients infected with HCV, cryoglobulins are detected in up to 52% with only a minority developing CV.[165,171,172] Other studies have evaluated cryoglobulinemia in other conditions with prevalence estimates of 17% in HIV (up to 42% in subjects co-infected with HCV),[173] 25% of patients with SLE,[174] and 12% of subjects with Sjögren syndrome (12%).[175]

Conversely, when looking at a large group of patients with cryoglobulinemia, the common causes were infections (75% including HCV, HBV, HIV), autoimmune diseases (21%), idiopathic or "essential" (11%), and hematologic (7%).[176] In a GWAS comparing patients with HCV-associated CV to HCV patients without CV, polymorphisms

in major histocompatibility class II and NOTCH4 genes were associated with CV.[177]

Pathogenesis and Histopathology

Cryoglobulins are Ig generated by the clonal expansion of B cells related to lymphoproliferative disorders or persistent immune stimulation due to infections or autoimmune diseases.[178,179] The Brouet classification is frequently used to classify cryoglobulins as follows[178]:

- Type I—Monoclonal Ig, typically IgM or IgG. This form is most frequently associated with hematologic conditions including monoclonal gammopathies, Waldenstrom macroglobulinemia, or multiple myeloma.[178,179]
- Type II—Monoclonal IgM with RF activity (i.e., ability to bind the Fc portion of IgG) and polyclonal IgG
- Type III—Polyclonal IgM and IgG.

Types II and III are also referred to as "mixed" cryoglobulins and can be seen in chronic infections, autoimmune diseases, and rarely, lymphoproliferative malignancies.[178,179]

The circulating cryoglobulins can induce tissue injury by precipitation in the microcirculation and immune complex formation with inflammation of blood vessels.[179] Vascular occlusion is more frequent with type I cryoglobulins and hyperviscosity.[179] Increased levels of circulating cytokines such as IL-1, IL-6, TNF-α, and chemokine (C–X–C motif) ligand (CXCL)10, CXCL11, and chemokine (C–C motif) ligand (CCL)2 have been found in patients with HCV-associated cryoglobulinemia, but the role in the pathogenesis of CV is unclear.[180,181] A deficiency of regulatory T cells was reported in patients with HCV and cryoglobulinemia, suggesting a possible role of T regulatory cells in the autoimmune conditions related to HCV.[182]

Biopsies of affected tissue often show mixed inflammatory infiltrates involving the small blood vessels. Fibrinoid necrosis can occur. Skin biopsies generally show findings of LCV. High levels of type I monoclonal cryoglobulins often also result in occlusive vasculopathy with intraluminal aggregates of cryoglobulins in the small blood vessels of the dermis as well as the capillaries of the subcutaneous fat lobules in the absence of inflammation. Direct immunofluorescence reveals deposits of IgM, IgG, and/or C3.[53,179]

Renal biopsy shows membranoproliferative glomerulonephritis in the vast majority of cases (92%), characterized by mesangial hypercellularity, capillary wall remodeling, and focal to diffuse endocapillary leukocyte infiltration.[164] Intraluminal thrombi may be observed, especially in cases of CV-associated renal involvement in primary Sjögren syndrome. Other glomerular lesions including mesangial proliferative glomerulonephritis or crescentic extra-capillary proliferation are less frequently observed.[164] Granular deposits of IgG, IgM, and C3 are often observed in the glomerular capillary wall and less frequently in the mesangium.[164] Neuropathy is characterized by perineural and endoneural vasculitis with axonal degeneration and demyelination, again with occasional deposits of Ig and/or complement.[179]

Clinical Manifestations

The triad of purpura, arthralgia, and fatigue has been reported in 80% of patients at disease onset.[a] Constitutional symptoms like fatigue (80% to 90%) and fever may be reported. Arthralgia without frank arthritis is observed in 20% to 70%.[a] The skin is the most frequently affected organ, accounting for 53% to 96% of cases.[a] The most common cutaneous manifestation is palpable purpura, although Raynaud-like phenomenon, distal acrocyanosis, livedo, ischemic digits, skin ulcerations,

---

[a]References 161, 164, 176, 179, 183, 184

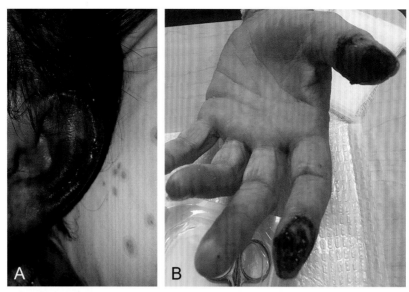

Fig. 41.9 Acrocyanosis of the ear with ischemia and hemorrhagic bullae in a patient with cryoglobulinemic vasculitis (A) and digital ischemia with dry gangrene of the left thumb and index fingers in a patient with cryoglobulinemic vasculitis (B).

and necrosis may also occur (Fig. 41.9).[a] Neurologic involvement appears to be the next most common clinical manifestation, occurring in 11% to 74% of individuals.[a] The most common neurologic manifestation is sensorimotor polyneuropathy.[a] Renal involvement is observed in approximately 20% to 40% of patients.[a] Other rare but serious organ manifestations may include GI tract involvement, pulmonary involvement, central nervous system manifestations, and myocardial disease.[161,179] There is significant clinical heterogeneity in CV, and different disease "subsets" have variable clinical manifestations. These are briefly discussed below.

Type I cryoglobulinemia vs. mixed (type II and type III) cryoglobulinemia. In a study evaluating 33 patients with type I cryoglobulinemia compared to 57 patients with mixed cryoglobulinemia, cutaneous manifestations (53% vs. 30% for type I) and peripheral neuropathy (26% vs. 6% for type I) were more frequently observed in patients with mixed cryoglobulinemia.[176]

Hepatitis C–associated CV vs. other CV. When evaluating HCV-associated cryoglobulinemia, no significant clinical differences were noted compared to those who were HCV negative in one study.[176] However, a cohort study of 306 patients with non–HCV-associated CV (64 with type I and 242 with type II) demonstrated that compared to 165 patients with HCV-associated CV, cutaneous manifestations like necrosis and ulcerations were significantly more frequent in non–HCV-associated CV (14% to 28%) compared to HCV-associated CV (1% to 4%).[161] Peripheral neuropathy, on the other hand, was more frequently observed with HCV-associated CV (74%) compared to patients with CV without HCV (44% to 52%)[161]. Frequency of renal involvement was similar between the two groups.[161]

Renal manifestations of CV compared to those without renal involvement. In a large series of 230 patients with noninfectious mixed CV, patients with renal involvement (80 patients) were less likely to have skin manifestations (OR 0.26, 95% CI 0.10–0.64) or peripheral neuropathy (OR 0.32, 95% CI 0.15–0.68), but more likely to have type II cryoglobulinemia (OR 24.5, 95% CI 2.87–209.08).[164]

Non-HCV infectious CV. Other infections have also rarely been associated with cryoglobulinemia. In a series of 342 patients with CV, 18 cases (5%) were related to infections other than HCV.[185]

The infections included HBV (4 cases); ear, nose, and throat infections (3 cases); and one case each of Epstein-Barr virus (EBV), parvovirus B19, HIV, *Streptococcus* endocarditis, *Staphylococcus aureus* skin infection, *Staphylococcus aureus* joint infection, leprosy, candidiasis, ascariasis, Leishmaniasis.[185] The most common clinical manifestations were purpuric lesions (78%), arthralgia (28%), glomerulonephritis (28%), and peripheral neuropathy (22%).[185] The cryoglobulinemia was type II in 67% and type III in 33%.[176] Based on their review of 27 other cases of CV from the literature, 22% of cases of non–HCV-associated CV were in cases of HBV, 18% from endocarditis infection, 13% from Leishmaniasis, and 11% due to other pyogenic infections.[185] Other viral infections included cytomegalovirus (7%), EBV (5%), HIV (5%), and hepatitis A (2%).[185]

Diagnosis

There are no diagnostic criteria for CV. Classification criteria using a combination of symptoms and serologic abnormalities have been proposed.[186] While the criteria appear to have good sensitivity of about 90%, the specificity was only about 66% when trying to distinguish CV from other forms of small vessel vasculitis.[186]

The diagnosis of CV is based on clinical symptoms, laboratory evaluation, and histopathology. Laboratory testing in the evaluation of patients with suspected CV should include complete blood count, measures of renal function (creatinine, urinalysis, urine protein-creatinine ratio), liver function testing, complement C3, complement C4, RF, and cryoglobulins. Additionally, evaluation for causes of cryoglobulinemia should include testing for infections like HBV, HCV, and HIV, and testing for hematologic conditions including serum protein electrophoresis with immunofixation, and autoimmune testing including lupus (ANA, dsDNA, SSA, SSB, Sm, RNP) and Sjögren's (ANA, SSA, SSB) should be pursued (see Box 41.2). Laboratory abnormalities often include presence of RF and low complement C4, which may indirectly signal the presence of cryoglobulins.[161,179] Other diagnostic testing may include electromyography in cases of suspected neurologic involvement. This more typically shows a polyneuropathy than findings of mononeuritis multiplex.[161,179] Finally, biopsy of the affected areas including skin, kidney, or nerve can allow the histopathologic confirmation of vasculitis.

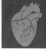

Treatment and Prognosis

The general principles that guide the treatment of CV are (1) to evaluate and address the underlying cause of cryoglobulinemia, (2) assess areas of involvement, and (3) assess severity of the organ involvement.[179] Immunomodulatory therapy may include glucocorticoids, rituximab, cyclophosphamide, and/or plasma exchange. In cases of CV associated with a viral or other infection, treatment of the underlying infectious etiology would need to be addressed, while in the case of a hematologic etiology, treatment of the underlying disorder would also be needed.[165,187]

Initial treatment includes glucocorticoids with gradual taper. In severe cases, pulse methylprednisolone 1 g intravenously once daily for 3 days followed by oral prednisone at 1 mg/kg/day orally may be needed. In life-threatening or organ-threatening cases, plasmapheresis to remove the circulating immune complexes can be helpful but has to be followed by cytotoxic therapy with cyclophosphamide or rituximab to reduce the production of cryoglobulins.[179] While data specific to CV is lacking, extrapolating from treatment of other forms of necrotizing vasculitis, cyclophosphamide (oral daily dosing or intravenously monthly) has been used to treat severe manifestations from CV.[162,164] However, recent retrospective and prospective studies have demonstrated the efficacy of rituximab for both noninfectious CV and HCV-associated CV.[165–167] In an open label study of patients with HCV-associated CV who failed antiviral therapy, rituximab 375 mg/m² of body surface area once a week for 3 weeks was efficacious and did not cause any exacerbation of HCV viremia or liver abnormalities.[167] The study by De Vita et al., which also included patients with HCV, compared rituximab 1 g administered twice 2 weeks apart to conventional treatment (azathioprine or cyclophosphamide) and showed similar efficacy with overall decrease in disease activity.[166] In a large study of 145 patients with noninfectious mixed CV, use of rituximab was associated with a decreased risk of relapse.[162–164] In another study of 242 cases of noninfectious mixed CV, treatment with rituximab and glucocorticoids was superior to treatment with glucocorticoids alone or to treatment with glucocorticoids in conjunction with alkylating medications; however, the rituximab-treated patients had an increased risk of severe infections.[162] Caution must be used for cases of HBV-associated CV, given the association of rituximab treatment with reactivation of HBV.

In the case of HCV-associated CV, treatment of the underlying infection is an essential component of the treatment plan.[165] Recently, non–interferon-based antiviral medications that directly target specific viral functions have become available for the treatment of patients with HCV. These newer antiviral therapies may eliminate the need for immunosuppressive therapy in some cases of HCV-associated CV.[168–170] Treatment guidelines have been published for HCV-related extrahepatic disorders including CV.[188] Treatment of HCV-associated CV requires collaboration with a gastroenterologist or liver specialist. For type I cryoglobulinemia, efficacy of treatment with alkylating agents, rituximab, thalidomide, lenalidomide, and bortezomib have all been reported.[187] Again, treatment should be decided in collaboration with the hematology experts.

Increased mortality has been reported in patients with HCV-associated CV with severe organ manifestations such as GI manifestations, central nervous system disease, or pulmonary hemorrhage.[189] Likewise, in the case of noninfectious mixed CV, age > 65 years, GI manifestations, pulmonary disease, or renal failure are associated with increased mortality.[185] The most common causes of mortality in patients with CV are infections or poorly controlled vasculitis.[162,164,183,185,190] Patients with CV are also at increased risk of lymphoproliferative malignancies and should be monitored closely.[162,164,183,191]

REFERENCES

1. Jennette JC, Falk RJ, Bacon PA, et al. 2012 revised International Chapel Hill Consensus Conference Nomenclature of Vasculitides. *Arthritis Rheum.* 2013;65:1–11.
2. Trepo C, Thivolet J. Hepatitis associated antigen and periarteritis nodosa (PAN). *Vox Sang.* 1970;19:410–411.
3. Trepo CG, Zucherman AJ, Bird RC, Prince AM. The role of circulating hepatitis B antigen/antibody immune complexes in the pathogenesis of vascular and hepatic manifestations in polyarteritis nodosa. *J Clin Pathol.* 1974;27:863–868.
4. Daoud MS, Hutton KP, Gibson LE. Cutaneous periarteritis nodosa: a clinicopathological study of 79 cases. *Br J Dermatol.* 1997;136:706–713.
5. Morgan AJ, Schwartz RA. Cutaneous polyarteritis nodosa: a comprehensive review. *Int J Dermatol.* 2010;49:750–756.
6. Chen KR. Cutaneous polyarteritis nodosa: a clinical and histopathological study of 20 cases. *J Dermatol.* 1989;16:429–442.
7. Furukawa F. Cutaneous polyarteritis nodosa: an update. *Ann Vasc Dis.* 2012;5:282–288.
8. Hernandez-Rodriguez J, Tan CD, Koening CL, et al. Testicular vasculitis: findings differentiating isolated disease from systemic disease in 72 patients. *Medicine (Baltimore).* 2012;91:75–85.
9. Hernandez-Rodriguez J, Tan CD, Rodriguez ER, Hoffman GS. Gynecologic vasculitis: an analysis of 163 patients. *Medicine (Baltimore).* 2009;88:169–181.
10. Hernandez-Rodriguez J, Tan CD, Rodriguez ER, Hoffman GS. Single-organ gallbladder vasculitis: characterization and distinction from systemic vasculitis involving the gallbladder. An analysis of 61 patients. *Medicine (Baltimore).* 2014;93:405–413.
11. Mohammad AJ, Jacobsson LT, Westman KW, et al. Incidence and survival rates in Wegener's granulomatosis, microscopic polyangiitis, Churg-Strauss syndrome and polyarteritis nodosa. *Rheumatology (Oxford).* 2009;48:1560–1565.
12. Watts RA, Gonzalez-Gay MA, Lane SE, et al. Geoepidemiology of systemic vasculitis: comparison of the incidence in two regions of Europe. *Ann Rheum Dis.* 2001;60:170–172.
13. Lane SE, Watts R, Scott DG. Epidemiology of systemic vasculitis. *Curr Rheumatol Rep.* 2005;7:270–275.
14. Mohammad AJ, Jacobsson LT, Mahr AD, et al. Prevalence of Wegener's granulomatosis, microscopic polyangiitis, polyarteritis nodosa and Churg-Strauss syndrome within a defined population in southern Sweden. *Rheumatology (Oxford).* 2007;46:1329–1337.
15. McMahon BJ, Heyward WL, Templin DW, et al. Hepatitis B-associated polyarteritis nodosa in Alaskan Eskimos: clinical and epidemiologic features and long-term follow-up. *Hepatology.* 1989;9:97–101.
16. Guillevin L, Mahr A, Callard P, et al. Hepatitis B virus-associated polyarteritis nodosa: clinical characteristics, outcome, and impact of treatment in 115 patients. *Medicine (Baltimore).* 2005;84:313–322.
17. Ozen S. The changing face of polyarteritis nodosa and necrotizing vasculitis. *Nat Rev Rheumatol.* 2017;13:381–386.
18. Saadoun D, Terrier B, Semoun O, et al. Hepatitis C virus-associated polyarteritis nodosa. *Arthritis Care Res (Hoboken).* 2011;63:427–435.
19. Watts R, Lane S, Hanslik T, et al. Development and validation of a consensus methodology for the classification of the ANCA-associated vasculitides and polyarteritis nodosa for epidemiological studies. *Ann Rheum Dis.* 2007;66:222–227.
20. Henegar C, Pagnoux C, Puechal X, et al. A paradigm of diagnostic criteria for polyarteritis nodosa: analysis of a series of 949 patients with vasculitides. *Arthritis Rheum.* 2008;58:1528–1538.
21. Kermani TA, Ham EK, Camilleri MJ, Warrington KJ. Polyarteritis nodosa-like vasculitis in association with minocycline use: a single-center case series. *Semin Arthritis Rheum.* 2012;42:213–221.
22. Navon Elkan P, Pierce SB, Segel R, et al. Mutant adenosine deaminase 2 in a polyarteritis nodosa vasculopathy. *N Engl J Med.* 2014;370:921–931.
23. Zhou Q, Yang D, Ombrello AK, et al. Early-onset stroke and vasculopathy associated with mutations in ADA2. *N Engl J Med.* 2014;370:911–920.
24. Caorsi R, Penco F, Grossi A, et al. ADA2 deficiency (DADA2) as an unrecognised cause of early onset polyarteritis nodosa and stroke: a multicentre national study. *Ann Rheum Dis.* 2017;76:1648–1656.

25. Gower RG, Sausker WF, Kohler PF, et al. Small vessel vasculitis caused by hepatitis B virus immune complexes. Small vessel vasculitis and HBsAG. *J Allergy Clin Immunol.* 1978;62:222–228.

26. Guillevin L, Ronco P, Verroust P. Circulating immune complexes in systemic necrotizing vasculitis of the polyarteritis nodosa group. Comparison of HBV-related polyarteritis nodosa and Churg Strauss Angiitis. *J Autoimmun.* 1990;3:789–792.

27. Michalak T. Immune complexes of hepatitis B surface antigen in the pathogenesis of periarteritis nodosa. A study of seven necropsy cases. *Am J Pathol.* 1978;90:619–632.

28. Cid MC, Grau JM, Casademont J, et al. Immunohistochemical characterization of inflammatory cells and immunologic activation markers in muscle and nerve biopsy specimens from patients with systemic polyarteritis nodosa. *Arthritis Rheum.* 1994;37:1055–1061.

29. Panegyres PK, Faull RJ, Russ GR, et al. Endothelial cell activation in vasculitis of peripheral nerve and skeletal muscle. *J Neurol Neurosurg Psychiatry.* 1992;55:4–7.

30. Coll-Vinent B, Grau JM, Lopez-Soto A, et al. Circulating soluble adhesion molecules in patients with classical polyarteritis nodosa. *Br J Rheumatol.* 1997;36:1178–1183.

31. Lie JT. Systemic and isolated vasculitis. A rational approach to classification and pathologic diagnosis. *Pathol Annu.* 1989;24(Pt 1): 25–114.

32. Bonsib SM. Polyarteritis nodosa. *Semin Diagn Pathol.* 2001;18:14–23.

33. Pagnoux C, Seror R, Henegar C, et al. Clinical features and outcomes in 348 patients with polyarteritis nodosa: a systematic retrospective study of patients diagnosed between 1963 and 2005 and entered into the French Vasculitis Study Group Database. *Arthritis Rheum.* 2010;62:616–626.

34. Levine SM, Hellmann DB, Stone JH. Gastrointestinal involvement in polyarteritis nodosa (1986-2000): presentation and outcomes in 24 patients. *Am J Med.* 2002;112:386–391.

35. Pagnoux C, Mahr A, Cohen P, Guillevin L. Presentation and outcome of gastrointestinal involvement in systemic necrotizing vasculitides: analysis of 62 patients with polyarteritis nodosa, microscopic polyangiitis, Wegener granulomatosis, Churg-Strauss syndrome, or rheumatoid arthritis-associated vasculitis. *Medicine (Baltimore).* 2005;84:115–128.

36. Alibaz-Oner F, Koster MJ, Crowson CS, et al. Clinical spectrum of medium-sized vessel vasculitis. *Arthritis Care Res (Hoboken).* 2017;69:884–891.

37. Kint N, De Haes P, Blockmans D. Comparison between classical polyarteritis nodosa and single organ vasculitis of medium-sized vessels: a retrospective study of 25 patients and review of the literature. *Acta Clin Belg.* 2016;71:26–31.

38. Hernandez-Rodriguez J, Molloy ES, Hoffman GS. Single-organ vasculitis. *Curr Opin Rheumatol.* 2008;20:40–46.

39. Lightfoot Jr RW, Michel BA, Bloch DA, et al. The American College of Rheumatology 1990 criteria for the classification of polyarteritis nodosa. *Arthritis Rheum.* 1990;33:1088–1093.

40. Craven A, Robson J, Ponte C, et al. ACR/EULAR-endorsed study to develop Diagnostic and Classification Criteria for Vasculitis (DCVAS). *Clin Exp Nephrol.* 2013;17:619–621.

41. Miller DL. Angiography in polyarteritis nodosa. *AJR Am J Roentgenol.* 2000;175:1747–1748.

42. Mukhtyar C, Guillevin L, Cid MC, et al. EULAR recommendations for the management of primary small and medium vessel vasculitis. *Ann Rheum Dis.* 2009;68:310–317.

43. Samson M, Puechal X, Mouthon L, et al. Microscopic polyangiitis and non-HBV polyarteritis nodosa with poor-prognosis factors: 10-year results of the prospective CHUSPAN trial. *Clin Exp Rheumatol.* 2017;35(Suppl 103):176–184.

44. Samson M, Puechal X, Devilliers H, et al. Long-term follow-up of a randomized trial on 118 patients with polyarteritis nodosa or microscopic polyangiitis without poor-prognosis factors. *Autoimmun Rev.* 2014;13:197–205.

45. Guillevin L, Mahr A, Cohen P, et al. Short-term corticosteroids then lamivudine and plasma exchanges to treat hepatitis B virus-related polyarteritis nodosa. *Arthritis Rheum.* 2004;51:482–487.

46. Hernandez-Rodriguez J, Hoffman GS. Updating single-organ vasculitis. *Curr Opin Rheumatol.* 2012;24:38–45.

47. Guillevin L, Lhote F, Gayraud M, et al. Prognostic factors in polyarteritis nodosa and Churg-Strauss syndrome. A prospective study in 342 patients. *Medicine (Baltimore).* 1996;75:17–28.

48. Bourgarit A, Le Toumelin P, Pagnoux C, et al. Deaths occurring during the first year after treatment onset for polyarteritis nodosa, microscopic polyangiitis, and Churg-Strauss syndrome: a retrospective analysis of causes and factors predictive of mortality based on 595 patients. *Medicine (Baltimore).* 2005;84:323–330.

49. Arora A, Wetter DA, Gonzalez-Santiago TM, et al. Incidence of leukocytoclastic vasculitis, 1996 to 2010: a population-based study in Olmsted County, Minnesota. *Mayo Clin Proc.* 2014;89:1515–1524.

50. Carlson JA, Cavaliere LF, Grant-Kels JM. Cutaneous vasculitis: diagnosis and management. *Clin Dermatol.* 2006;24:414–429.

51. Chen KR, Carlson JA. Clinical approach to cutaneous vasculitis. *Am J Clin Dermatol.* 2008;9:71–92.

52. Goeser MR, Laniosz V, Wetter DA. A practical approach to the diagnosis, evaluation, and management of cutaneous small-vessel vasculitis. *Am J Clin Dermatol.* 2014;15:299–306.

53. Sunderkotter CH, Zelger B, Chen KR, et al. Nomenclature of cutaneous vasculitis: dermatologic addendum to the 2012 Revised International Chapel Hill Consensus Conference Nomenclature of Vasculitides. *Arthritis Rheumatol.* 2018;70:171–184.

54. Garcia-Porrua C, Gonzalez-Gay MA. Comparative clinical and epidemiological study of hypersensitivity vasculitis versus Henoch-Schonlein purpura in adults. *Semin Arthritis Rheum.* 1999;28:404–412.

55. Watts RA, Jolliffe VA, Grattan CE, et al. Cutaneous vasculitis in a defined population-clinical and epidemiological associations. *J Rheumatol.* 1998;25:920–924.

56. Russell JP, Gibson LE. Primary cutaneous small vessel vasculitis: approach to diagnosis and treatment. *Int J Dermatol.* 2006;45:3–13.

57. Falk RJ, Jennette JC. Anti-neutrophil cytoplasmic autoantibodies with specificity for myeloperoxidase in patients with systemic vasculitis and idiopathic necrotizing and crescentic glomerulonephritis. *N Engl J Med.* 1988;318:1651–1657.

58. Watts RA, Lane SE, Scott DG, et al. Epidemiology of vasculitis in Europe. *Ann Rheum Dis.* 2001;60:1156–1157.

59. Watts RA, Mahr A, Mohammad AJ, et al. Classification, epidemiology and clinical subgrouping of antineutrophil cytoplasmic antibody (ANCA)-associated vasculitis. *Nephrol Dial Transplant.* 2015;30(Suppl 1):i14–i22.

60. Gonzalez-Gay MA, Garcia-Porrua C, Guerrero J, et al. The epidemiology of the primary systemic vasculitides in northwest Spain: implications of the Chapel Hill Consensus Conference definitions. *Arthritis Rheum.* 2003;49:388–393.

61. Berti A, Cornec D, Crowson CS, et al. The epidemiology of antineutrophil cytoplasmic autoantibody-associated vasculitis in Olmsted County, Minnesota: a twenty-year US population-based study. *Arthritis Rheumatol.* 2017;69:2338–2350.

62. Jagiello P, Gencik M, Arning L, et al. New genomic region for Wegener's granulomatosis as revealed by an extended association screen with 202 apoptosis-related genes. *Hum Genet.* 2004;114:468–477.

63. Lyons PA, Rayner TF, Trivedi S, et al. Genetically distinct subsets within ANCA-associated vasculitis. *N Engl J Med.* 2012;367:214–223.

64. Xie G, Roshandel D, Sherva R, et al. Association of granulomatosis with polyangiitis (Wegener's) with HLA-DPB1*04 and SEMA6A gene variants: evidence from genome-wide analysis. *Arthritis Rheum.* 2013;65:2457–2468.

65. Merkel PA, Xie G, Monach PA, et al. Identification of functional and expression polymorphisms associated with risk for antineutrophil cytoplasmic autoantibody-associated vasculitis. *Arthritis Rheumatol.* 2017;69:1054–1066.

66. Popa ER, Tervaert JW. The relation between Staphylococcus aureus and Wegener's granulomatosis: current knowledge and future directions. *Intern Med.* 2003;42:771–780.

67. Takeuchi Y, Saito A, Ojima Y, et al. The influence of the Great East Japan earthquake on microscopic polyangiitis: a retrospective observational study. *PLoS One.* 2017;12:e0177482.

68. Gao Y, Zhao MH. Review article: drug-induced anti-neutrophil cytoplasmic antibody-associated vasculitis. *Nephrology (Carlton).* 2009;14:33–41.

69. Brinkmann V, Reichard U, Goosmann C, et al. Neutrophil extracellular traps kill bacteria. *Science*. 2004;303:1532–1535.

70. Papayannopoulos V. Neutrophil extracellular traps in immunity and disease. *Nat Rev Immunol*. 2018;18:134–147.

71. Sangaletti S, Tripodo C, Chiodoni C, et al. Neutrophil extracellular traps mediate transfer of cytoplasmic neutrophil antigens to myeloid dendritic cells toward ANCA induction and associated autoimmunity. *Blood*. 2012;120:3007–3018.

72. Nakazawa D, Shida H, Tomaru U, et al. Enhanced formation and disordered regulation of NETs in myeloperoxidase-ANCA-associated microscopic polyangiitis. *J Am Soc Nephrol*. 2014;25:990–997.

73. Soderberg D, Kurz T, Motamedi A, et al. Increased levels of neutrophil extracellular trap remnants in the circulation of patients with small vessel vasculitis, but an inverse correlation to anti-neutrophil cytoplasmic antibodies during remission. *Rheumatology (Oxford)*. 2015;54:2085–2094.

74. Surmiak M, Hubalewska-Mazgaj M, Wawrzycka-Adamczyk K, et al. Neutrophil-related and serum biomarkers in granulomatosis with polyangiitis support extracellular traps mechanism of the disease. *Clin Exp Rheumatol*. 2016;34:S98–104.

75. Abreu-Velez AM, Smith Jr JG, Howard MS. Presence of neutrophil extracellular traps and antineutrophil cytoplasmic antibodies associated with vasculitides. *N Am J Med Sci*. 2009;1:309–313.

76. Reumaux D, Hordijk PL, Duthilleul P, Roos D. Priming by tumor necrosis factor-alpha of human neutrophil NADPH-oxidase activity induced by anti-proteinase-3 or anti-myeloperoxidase antibodies. *J Leukoc Biol*. 2006;80:1424–1433.

77. Falk RJ, Terrell RS, Charles LA, Jennette JC. Anti-neutrophil cytoplasmic autoantibodies induce neutrophils to degranulate and produce oxygen radicals in vitro. *Proc Natl Acad Sci U S A*. 1990;87:4115–4119.

78. Porges AJ, Redecha PB, Kimberly WT, et al. Anti-neutrophil cytoplasmic antibodies engage and activate human neutrophils via Fc gamma RIIa. *J Immunol*. 1994;153:1271–1280.

79. Radford DJ, Luu NT, Hewins P, et al. Antineutrophil cytoplasmic antibodies stabilize adhesion and promote migration of flowing neutrophils on endothelial cells. *Arthritis Rheum*. 2001;44:2851–2861.

80. Xiao H, Dairaghi DJ, Powers JP, et al. C5a receptor (CD88) blockade protects against MPO-ANCA GN. *J Am Soc Nephrol*. 2014;25:225–231.

81. Schreiber A, Xiao H, Jennette JC, et al. C5a receptor mediates neutrophil activation and ANCA-induced glomerulonephritis. *J Am Soc Nephrol*. 2009;20:289–298.

82. Ewert BH, Jennette JC, Falk RJ. Anti-myeloperoxidase antibodies stimulate neutrophils to damage human endothelial cells. *Kidney Int*. 1992;41:375–383.

83. Lu X, Garfield A, Rainger GE, et al. Mediation of endothelial cell damage by serine proteases, but not superoxide, released from antineutrophil cytoplasmic antibody-stimulated neutrophils. *Arthritis Rheum*. 2006;54:1619–1628.

84. Al-Hussain T, Hussein MH, Conca W, et al. Pathophysiology of ANCA-associated vasculitis. *Adv Anat Pathol*. 2017;24:226–234.

85. Gubbels SP, Barkhuizen A, Hwang PH. Head and neck manifestations of Wegener's granulomatosis. *Otolaryngol Clin North Am*. 2003;36:685–705.

86. D'Anza B, Langford CA, Sindwani R. Sinonasal imaging findings in granulomatosis with polyangiitis (Wegener granulomatosis): a systematic review. *Am J Rhinol Allergy*. 2017;31:16–21.

87. Franssen C, Gans R, Kallenberg C, et al. Disease spectrum of patients with antineutrophil cytoplasmic autoantibodies of defined specificity: distinct differences between patients with anti-proteinase 3 and anti-myeloperoxidase autoantibodies. *J Intern Med*. 1998;244:209–216.

88. Neumann T, Manger B, Schmid M, et al. Cardiac involvement in Churg-Strauss syndrome: impact of endomyocarditis. *Medicine (Baltimore)*. 2009;88:236–243.

89. Guillevin L, Cohen P, Gayraud M, et al. Churg-Strauss syndrome. Clinical study and long-term follow-up of 96 patients. *Medicine (Baltimore)*. 1999;78:26–37.

90. Dennert RM, van Paassen P, Schalla S, et al. Cardiac involvement in Churg-Strauss syndrome. *Arthritis Rheum*. 2010;62:627–634.

91. Lanham JG, Cooke S, Davies J, Hughes GR. Endomyocardial complications of the Churg-Strauss syndrome. *Postgrad Med J*. 1985;61:341–344.

92. Hoffman GS, Kerr GS, Leavitt RY, et al. Wegener granulomatosis: an analysis of 158 patients. *Ann Intern Med*. 1992;116:488–498.

93. Draibe J, Salama AD. Association of ANCA associated vasculitis and rheumatoid arthritis: a lesser recognized overlap syndrome. *Springerplus*. 2015;4:50.

94. Stone JH, Talor M, Stebbing J, et al. Test characteristics of immunofluorescence and ELISA tests in 856 consecutive patients with possible ANCA-associated conditions. *Arthritis Care Res*. 2000;13:424–434.

95. Blockmans D, Stevens E, Marien G, Bobbaers H. Clinical spectrum associated with positive ANCA titres in 94 consecutive patients: is there a relation with PR-3 negative c-ANCA and hypergammaglobulinaemia? *Ann Rheum Dis*. 1998;57:141–145.

96. Weiner M, Segelmark M. The clinical presentation and therapy of diseases related to anti-neutrophil cytoplasmic antibodies (ANCA). *Autoimmun Rev*. 2016;15:978–982.

97. Choi HK, Merkel PA, Walker AM, Niles JL. Drug-associated antineutrophil cytoplasmic antibody-positive vasculitis: prevalence among patients with high titers of antimyeloperoxidase antibodies. *Arthritis Rheum*. 2000;43:405–413.

98. Yates M, Watts RA, Bajema IM, et al. EULAR/ERA-EDTA recommendations for the management of ANCA-associated vasculitis. *Ann Rheum Dis*. 2016;75:1583–1594.

99. Aasarod K, Bostad L, Hammerstrom J, et al. Renal histopathology and clinical course in 94 patients with Wegener's granulomatosis. *Nephrol Dial Transplant*. 2001;16:953–960.

100. Travis WD, Hoffman GS, Leavitt RY, et al. Surgical pathology of the lung in Wegener's granulomatosis. Review of 87 open lung biopsies from 67 patients. *Am J Surg Pathol*. 1991;15:315–333.

101. Schnabel A, Holl-Ulrich K, Dalhoff K, et al. Efficacy of transbronchial biopsy in pulmonary vaculitides. *Eur Respir J*. 1997;10:2738–2743.

102. Devaney KO, Travis WD, Hoffman G, et al. Interpretation of head and neck biopsies in Wegener's granulomatosis. A pathologic study of 126 biopsies in 70 patients. *Am J Surg Pathol*. 1990;14:555–564.

103. Hogan SL, Falk RJ, Chin H, et al. Predictors of relapse and treatment resistance in antineutrophil cytoplasmic antibody-associated small-vessel vasculitis. *Ann Intern Med*. 2005;143:621–631.

104. Harper L, Morgan MD, Walsh M, et al. Pulse versus daily oral cyclophosphamide for induction of remission in ANCA-associated vasculitis: long-term follow-up. *Ann Rheum Dis*. 2012;71:955–960.

105. Jones RB, Tervaert JW, Hauser T, et al. Rituximab versus cyclophosphamide in ANCA-associated renal vasculitis. *N Engl J Med*. 2010;363:211–220.

106. Stone JH, Merkel PA, Spiera R, et al. Rituximab versus cyclophosphamide for ANCA-associated vasculitis. *N Engl J Med*. 2010;363:221–232.

107. Mohammad AJ, Hot A, Arndt F, et al. Rituximab for the treatment of eosinophilic granulomatosis with polyangiitis (Churg-Strauss). *Ann Rheum Dis*. 2016;75:396–401.

108. Thiel J, Troilo A, Salzer U, et al. Rituximab as induction therapy in eosinophilic granulomatosis with polyangiitis refractory to conventional immunosuppressive treatment: a 36-month follow-up analysis. *J Allergy Clin Immunol Pract*. 2017;5:1556–1563.

109. Wechsler ME, Akuthota P, Jayne D, et al. Mepolizumab or placebo for eosinophilic granulomatosis with polyangiitis. *N Engl J Med*. 2017;376:1921–1932.

110. Walsh M, Catapano F, Szpirt W, et al. Plasma exchange for renal vasculitis and idiopathic rapidly progressive glomerulonephritis: a meta-analysis. *Am J Kidney Dis*. 2011;57:566–574.

111. Cartin-Ceba R, Diaz-Caballero L, Al-Qadi MO, et al. Diffuse alveolar hemorrhage secondary to antineutrophil cytoplasmic antibody-associated vasculitis: predictors of respiratory failure and clinical outcomes. *Arthritis Rheumatol*. 2016;68:1467–1476.

112. Walsh M, Merkel PA, Peh CA, et al. Plasma exchange and glucocorticoid dosing in the treatment of anti-neutrophil cytoplasm antibody associated vasculitis (PEXIVAS): protocol for a randomized controlled trial. *Trials*. 2013;14:73.

113. Jayne DRW, Bruchfeld AN, Harper L, et al. Randomized trial of C5a receptor inhibitor avacopan in ANCA-associated vasculitis. *J Am Soc Nephrol*. 2017;28:2756–2767.

114. Hiemstra TF, Walsh M, Mahr A, et al. Mycophenolate mofetil vs azathioprine for remission maintenance in antineutrophil cytoplasmic antibody-associated vasculitis: a randomized controlled trial. *JAMA*. 2010;304:2381–2388.

115. Pagnoux C, Mahr A, Hamidou MA, et al. Azathioprine or methotrexate maintenance for ANCA-associated vasculitis. *N Engl J Med*. 2008;359:2790–2803.

116. Cartin-Ceba R, Golbin JM, Keogh KA, et al. Rituximab for remission induction and maintenance in refractory granulomatosis with polyangiitis (Wegener's): ten-year experience at a single center. *Arthritis Rheum*. 2012;64:3770–3778.

117. Smith RM, Jones RB, Guerry MJ, et al. Rituximab for remission maintenance in relapsing antineutrophil cytoplasmic antibody-associated vasculitis. *Arthritis Rheum*. 2012;64:3760–3769.

118. Yang YH, Hung CF, Hsu CR, et al. A nationwide survey on epidemiological characteristics of childhood Henoch-Schonlein purpura in Taiwan. *Rheumatology (Oxford)*. 2005;44:618–622.

119. Gardner-Medwin JM, Dolezalova P, Cummins C, Southwood TR. Incidence of Henoch-Schonlein purpura, Kawasaki disease, and rare vasculitides in children of different ethnic origins. *Lancet*. 2002;360:1197–1202.

120. Dolezalova P, Telekesova P, Nemcova D, Hoza J. Incidence of vasculitis in children in the Czech Republic: 2-year prospective epidemiology survey. *J Rheumatol*. 2004;31:2295–2299.

121. Hocevar A, Rotar Z, Ostrovrsnik J, et al. Incidence of IgA vasculitis in the adult Slovenian population. *Br J Dermatol*. 2014;171:524–527.

122. Trapani S, Micheli A, Grisolia F, et al. Henoch Schonlein purpura in childhood: epidemiological and clinical analysis of 150 cases over a 5-year period and review of literature. *Semin Arthritis Rheum*. 2005;35:143–153.

123. Saulsbury FT. Epidemiology of Henoch-Schonlein purpura. *Cleve Clin J Med*. 2002;69(Suppl 2):SII87–9.

124. Crago SS, Kutteh WH, Moro I, et al. Distribution of IgA1-, IgA2-, and J chain-containing cells in human tissues. *J Immunol*. 1984;132:16–18.

125. Heineke MH, Ballering AV, Jamin A, et al. New insights in the pathogenesis of immunoglobulin A vasculitis (Henoch-Schonlein purpura). *Autoimmun Rev*. 2017;16:1246–1253.

126. Jauhola O, Ronkainen J, Koskimies O, et al. Clinical course of extrarenal symptoms in Henoch-Schonlein purpura: a 6-month prospective study. *Arch Dis Child*. 2010;95:871–876.

127. Pillebout E, Thervet E, Hill G, et al. Henoch-Schonlein purpura in adults: outcome and prognostic factors. *J Am Soc Nephrol*. 2002;13:1271–1278.

128. Kang Y, Park JS, Ha YJ, et al. Differences in clinical manifestations and outcomes between adult and child patients with Henoch-Schonlein purpura. *J Korean Med Sci*. 2014;29:198–203.

129. Stewart M, Savage JM, Bell B, McCord B. Long term renal prognosis of Henoch-Schonlein purpura in an unselected childhood population. *Eur J Pediatr*. 1988;147:113–115.

130. Chang WL, Yang YH, Wang LC, et al. Renal manifestations in Henoch-Schonlein purpura: a 10-year clinical study. *Pediatr Nephrol*. 2005;20:1269–1272.

131. Narchi H. Risk of long term renal impairment and duration of follow up recommended for Henoch-Schonlein purpura with normal or minimal urinary findings: a systematic review. *Arch Dis Child*. 2005;90:916–920.

132. Uppal SS, Hussain MA, Al-Raqum HA, et al. Henoch-Schonlein's purpura in adults versus children/adolescents: a comparative study. *Clin Exp Rheumatol*. 2006;24:S26–S30.

133. Ha TS, Lee JS. Scrotal involvement in childhood Henoch-Schonlein purpura. *Acta Paediatr*. 2007;96:552–555.

134. Calvo-Rio V, Hernandez JL, Ortiz-Sanjuan F, et al. Relapses in patients with Henoch-Schonlein purpura: analysis of 417 patients from a single center. *Medicine (Baltimore)*. 2016;95:e4217.

135. Chang WL, Yang YH, Lin YT, Chiang BL. Gastrointestinal manifestations in Henoch-Schonlein purpura: a review of 261 patients. *Acta Paediatr*. 2004;93:1427–1431.

136. Hong S, Ahn SM, Lim DH, et al. Late-onset IgA vasculitis in adult patients exhibits distinct clinical characteristics and outcomes. *Clin Exp Rheumatol*. 2016;34:S77–S83.

137. Mills JA, Michel BA, Bloch DA, et al. The American College of Rheumatology 1990 criteria for the classification of Henoch-Schonlein purpura. *Arthritis Rheum*. 1990;33:1114–1121.

138. Ozen S, Pistorio A, Iusan SM, et al. EULAR/PRINTO/PRES criteria for Henoch-Schonlein purpura, childhood polyarteritis nodosa, childhood Wegener granulomatosis and childhood Takayasu arteritis: Ankara 2008. Part II: Final classification criteria. *Ann Rheum Dis*. 2010;69:798–806.

139. Calvino MC, Llorca J, Garcia-Porrua C, et al. Henoch-Schonlein purpura in children from northwestern Spain: a 20-year epidemiologic and clinical study. *Medicine (Baltimore)*. 2001;80:279–290.

140. Davin JC, Ten Berge IJ, Weening JJ. What is the difference between IgA nephropathy and Henoch-Schonlein purpura nephritis? *Kidney Int*. 2001;59:823–834.

141. Kato S, Shibuya H, Naganuma H, Nakagawa H. Gastrointestinal endoscopy in Henoch-Schonlein purpura. *Eur J Pediatr*. 1992;151:482–484.

142. Goldstein AR, White RH, Akuse R, Chantler C. Long-term follow-up of childhood Henoch-Schonlein nephritis. *Lancet*. 1992;339:280–282.

143. Counahan R, Winterborn MH, White RH, et al. Prognosis of Henoch-Schonlein nephritis in children. *Br Med J*. 1977;2:11–14.

144. Rigante D, Candelli M, Federico G, et al. Predictive factors of renal involvement or relapsing disease in children with Henoch-Schonlein purpura. *Rheumatol Int*. 2005;25:45–48.

145. Prais D, Amir J, Nussinovitch M. Recurrent Henoch-Schonlein purpura in children. *J Clin Rheumatol*. 2007;13:25–28.

146. Blanco R, Martinez-Taboada VM, Rodriguez-Valverde V, et al. Henoch-Schonlein purpura in adulthood and childhood: two different expressions of the same syndrome. *Arthritis Rheum*. 1997;40:859–864.

147. Bech AP, Reichert LJ, Cohen Tervaert JW. Dapsone for the treatment of chronic IgA vasculitis (Henoch-Schonlein). *Neth J Med*. 2013;71:220–221.

148. Padeh S, Passwell JH. Successful treatment of chronic Henoch-Schonlein purpura with colchicine and aspirin. *Isr Med Assoc J*. 2000;2:482–483.

149. Wu SH, Liao PY, Chen XQ, et al. Add-on therapy with montelukast in the treatment of Henoch-Schonlein purpura. *Pediatr Int*. 2014;56:315–322.

150. Niaudet P, Habib R. Methylprednisolone pulse therapy in the treatment of severe forms of Schonlein-Henoch purpura nephritis. *Pediatr Nephrol*. 1998;12:238–243.

151. Szer IS. Gastrointestinal and renal involvement in vasculitis: management strategies in Henoch-Schonlein purpura. *Cleve Clin J Med*. 1999;66:312–317.

152. Weiss PF, Feinstein JA, Luan X, et al. Effects of corticosteroid on Henoch-Schonlein purpura: a systematic review. *Pediatrics*. 2007;120:1079–1087.

153. Pillebout E, Alberti C, Guillevin L, et al. Addition of cyclophosphamide to steroids provides no benefit compared with steroids alone in treating adult patients with severe Henoch Schonlein Purpura. *Kidney Int*. 2010;78:495–502.

154. Shin JI, Park JM, Shin YH, et al. Can azathioprine and steroids alter the progression of severe Henoch-Schonlein nephritis in children? *Pediatr Nephrol*. 2005;20:1087–1092.

155. Fotis L, Tuttle PVt, Baszis KW, et al. Azathioprine therapy for steroid-resistant Henoch-Schonlein purpura: a report of 6 cases. *Pediatr Rheumatol Online J*. 2016;14:37.

156. Ren P, Han F, Chen L, et al. The combination of mycophenolate mofetil with corticosteroids induces remission of Henoch-Schonlein purpura nephritis. *Am J Nephrol*. 2012;36:271–277.

157. Shah R, Ramakrishnan M, Vollmar A, et al. Henoch-Schonlein purpura presenting as severe gastrointestinal and renal involvement with mixed outcomes in an adult patient. *Cureus*. 2017;9:e1088.

158. Shenoy M, Ognjanovic MV, Coulthard MG. Treating severe Henoch-Schonlein and IgA nephritis with plasmapheresis alone. *Pediatr Nephrol*. 2007;22:1167–1171.

159. Pillebout E, Rocha F, Fardet L, et al. Successful outcome using rituximab as the only immunomodulation in Henoch-Schonlein purpura: case report. *Nephrol Dial Transplant*. 2011;26:2044–2046.

160. Ishiguro H, Hashimoto T, Akata M, et al. Rituximab treatment for adult purpura nephritis with nephrotic syndrome. *Intern Med*. 2013;52:1079–1083.

161. Cacoub P, Comarmond C, Domont F, et al. Cryoglobulinemia vasculitis. *Am J Med*. 2015;128:950–955.
162. Terrier B, Krastinova E, Marie I, et al. Management of noninfectious mixed cryoglobulinemia vasculitis: data from 242 cases included in the CryoVas survey. *Blood*. 2012;119:5996–6004.
163. Terrier B, Marie I, Launay D, et al. Predictors of early relapse in patients with non-infectious mixed cryoglobulinemia vasculitis: results from the French nationwide CryoVas survey. *Autoimmun Rev*. 2014;13:630–634.
164. Zaidan M, Terrier B, Pozdzik A, et al. Spectrum and prognosis of noninfectious renal mixed cryoglobulinemic GN. *J Am Soc Nephrol*. 2016;27:1213–1224.
165. Dammacco F, Sansonno D. Therapy for hepatitis C virus-related cryoglobulinemic vasculitis. *N Engl J Med*. 2013;369:1035–1045.
166. De Vita S, Quartuccio L, Isola M, et al. A randomized controlled trial of rituximab for the treatment of severe cryoglobulinemic vasculitis. *Arthritis Rheum*. 2012;64:843–853.
167. Sneller MC, Hu Z, Langford CA. A randomized controlled trial of rituximab following failure of antiviral therapy for hepatitis C virus-associated cryoglobulinemic vasculitis. *Arthritis Rheum*. 2012;64:835–842.
168. Gragnani L, Visentini M, Fognani E, et al. Prospective study of guideline-tailored therapy with direct-acting antivirals for hepatitis C virus-associated mixed cryoglobulinemia. *Hepatology*. 2016;64:1473–1482.
169. Saadoun D, Pol S, Ferfar Y, et al. Efficacy and safety of sofosbuvir plus daclatasvir for treatment of HCV-associated cryoglobulinemia vasculitis. *Gastroenterology*. 2017;153:49–52. e5.
170. Saadoun D, Resche Rigon M, Thibault V, et al. Peg-IFNalpha/ribavirin/protease inhibitor combination in hepatitis C virus associated mixed cryoglobulinemia vasculitis: results at week 24. *Ann Rheum Dis*. 2014;73:831–837.
171. Ramos-Casals M, Munoz S, Medina F, et al. Systemic autoimmune diseases in patients with hepatitis C virus infection: characterization of 1020 cases (The HISPAMEC Registry). *J Rheumatol*. 2009;36:1442–1448.
172. Vigano M, Lampertico P, Rumi MG, et al. Natural history and clinical impact of cryoglobulins in chronic hepatitis C: 10-year prospective study of 343 patients. *Gastroenterology*. 2007;133:835–842.
173. Bonnet F, Pineau JJ, Taupin JL, et al. Prevalence of cryoglobulinemia and serological markers of autoimmunity in human immunodeficiency virus infected individuals: a cross-sectional study of 97 patients. *J Rheumatol*. 2003;30:2005–2010.
174. Garcia-Carrasco M, Ramos-Casals M, Cervera R, et al. Cryoglobulinemia in systemic lupus erythematosus: prevalence and clinical characteristics in a series of 122 patients. *Semin Arthritis Rheum*. 2001;30:366–373.
175. Ramos-Casals M, Brito-Zeron P, Solans R, et al. Systemic involvement in primary Sjogren's syndrome evaluated by the EULAR-SS disease activity index: analysis of 921 Spanish patients (GEAS-SS Registry). *Rheumatology (Oxford)*. 2014;53:321–331.
176. Trejo O, Ramos-Casals M, Garcia-Carrasco M, et al. Cryoglobulinemia: study of etiologic factors and clinical and immunologic features in 443 patients from a single center. *Medicine (Baltimore)*. 2001;80:252–262.
177. Zignego AL, Wojcik GL, Cacoub P, et al. Genome-wide association study of hepatitis C virus- and cryoglobulin-related vasculitis. *Genes Immun*. 2014;15:500–505.
178. Brouet JC, Clauvel JP, Danon F, et al. Biologic and clinical significance of cryoglobulins. A report of 86 cases. *Am J Med*. 1974;57:775–788.
179. Ramos-Casals M, Stone JH, Cid MC, Bosch X. The cryoglobulinaemias. *Lancet*. 2012;379:348–360.
180. Antonelli A, Fallahi P, Ferrari SM, et al. Chemokine (CXC motif) ligand 9 serum levels in mixed cryoglobulinaemia are associated with circulating levels of IFN-gamma and TNF-alpha. *Clin Exp Rheumatol*. 2012;30:864–870.
181. Antonelli A, Fallahi P, Ferrari SM, et al. High circulating chemokines (C-X-C motif) ligand 9, and (C-X-C motif) ligand 11, in hepatitis C-associated cryoglobulinemia. *Int J Immunopathol Pharmacol*. 2013;26:49–57.
182. Boyer O, Saadoun D, Abriol J, et al. CD4+CD25+ regulatory T-cell deficiency in patients with hepatitis C-mixed cryoglobulinemia vasculitis. *Blood*. 2004;103:3428–3430.
183. Ferri C, Sebastiani M, Giuggioli D, et al. Mixed cryoglobulinemia: demographic, clinical, and serologic features and survival in 231 patients. *Semin Arthritis Rheum*. 2004;33:355–374.
184. Terrier B, Carrat F, Krastinova E, et al. Prognostic factors of survival in patients with non-infectious mixed cryoglobulinaemia vasculitis: data from 242 cases included in the CryoVas survey. *Ann Rheum Dis*. 2013;72:374–380.
185. Terrier B, Marie I, Lacraz A, et al. Non HCV-related infectious cryoglobulinemia vasculitis: results from the French nationwide CryoVas survey and systematic review of the literature. *J Autoimmun*. 2015;65:74–81.
186. Quartuccio L, Isola M, Corazza L, et al. Validation of the classification criteria for cryoglobulinaemic vasculitis. *Rheumatology (Oxford)*. 2014;53:2209–2213.
187. Terrier B, Karras A, Kahn JE, et al. The spectrum of type I cryoglobulinemia vasculitis: new insights based on 64 cases. *Medicine (Baltimore)*. 2013;92:61–68.
188. Zignego AL, Ramos-Casals M, Ferri C, et al. International therapeutic guidelines for patients with HCV-related extrahepatic disorders. A multidisciplinary expert statement. *Autoimmun Rev*. 2017;16:523–541.
189. Retamozo S, Diaz-Lagares C, Bosch X, et al. Life-threatening cryoglobulinemic patients with hepatitis C: clinical description and outcome of 279 patients. *Medicine (Baltimore)*. 2013;92:273–284.
190. Landau DA, Scerra S, Sene D, et al. Causes and predictive factors of mortality in a cohort of patients with hepatitis C virus-related cryoglobulinemic vasculitis treated with antiviral therapy. *J Rheumatol*. 2010;37:615–621.
191. Saadoun D, Sellam J, Ghillani-Dalbin P, et al. Increased risks of lymphoma and death among patients with non-hepatitis C virus-related mixed cryoglobulinemia. *Arch Intern Med*. 2006;166:2101–2108.

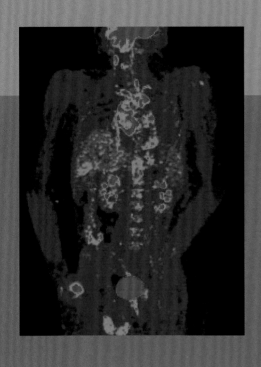

第42章
血栓闭塞性脉管炎

血栓闭塞性脉管炎（thromboangiitis obliterans，TAO），又称Buerger病，是一类主要累及肢体动静脉和神经的节段性、非动脉粥样硬化性炎症疾病。该病好发于青年男性，偶见女性患者。血栓闭塞性脉管炎的主要病理特点为炎症反复刺激血管壁导致血栓形成，但具体机制尚不清楚。目前认为，血栓闭塞性脉管炎发病的主要危险因素为吸烟，且与免疫功能异常、内皮功能不全、感染等相关，并表现出了一定的遗传倾向。血栓闭塞性脉管炎的常见临床表现为因动脉闭塞导致的间歇性跛行与肢体活动耐力降低、雷诺现象、感觉异常及特征性的浅静脉血栓性静脉炎等。临床上应注意将血栓闭塞性脉管炎与系统性红斑狼疮、类风湿关节炎和其他血管炎等结缔组织病相鉴别。

现主要根据患者病史对血栓闭塞性脉管炎做出临床诊断，治疗上应根据患者具体病情采取以戒烟和应用血管活性药物为主，必要时辅以血管重建手术的个体化综合治疗方案。

吴学君

Thromboangiitis Obliterans (Buerger Disease)

Gregory Piazza and Jeffrey W. Olin

Thromboangiitis obliterans (TAO) describes a segmental, nonatherosclerotic inflammatory disorder that primarily involves the small and medium arteries, veins, and nerves of the extremities.[1] Although TAO was initially thought to be a disease confined exclusively to men, epidemiologic studies demonstrate a growing population of women with the disorder. Also known as Buerger disease, TAO has an extremely strong pathophysiological relationship with tobacco use, usually in the form of heavy cigarette smoking.

In 1879, von Winiwarter provided the first description of a patient with TAO. He presented the case of a 57-year-old man who had reported pain in his feet for 12 years. Histopathological examination of an amputation specimen from this patient demonstrated intimal proliferation, luminal thrombosis, and fibrosis. von Winiwarter hypothesized that the observed endarteritis and endophlebitis were distinct from atherosclerosis. In his landmark paper 29 years later, Leo Buerger published a detailed report of the pathological findings of 11 amputated limbs from patients with the disease. Buerger coined the term "thromboangiitis obliterans" to describe the characteristic observations of endarteritis and endophlebitis typical of the disease. Like von Winiwarter, Buerger made a point to distinguish the clinical and pathological findings of TAO from those of atherosclerosis.

In 1928, Allen and Brown described the clinical and pathological characteristics of 200 cases of TAO seen at the Mayo Clinic from 1922 to 1926.[2] All patients were heavy smokers, and the pathological findings were virtually identical to those described in Buerger's original paper.

EPIDEMIOLOGY

Although it is observed worldwide, TAO is more prevalent in the Middle East and Far East than in North America and Western Europe. Prior to the late 1960s, overdiagnosis of TAO was frequent. Of 205 cases originally diagnosed as TAO at Mount Sinai Hospital from 1933 to 1963, only 33 were later believed to be compatible with the diagnosis, 28 were considered questionable, and 144 were determined to be incorrect.[3]

The reported number of new patients diagnosed with TAO in the United States and Europe has declined largely due to the adoption of stricter diagnostic criteria and a reduction in tobacco use. The overall incidence of TAO is higher in regions of the world where the consumption of tobacco is greater. At the Mayo Clinic, over a 40-year period, the prevalence rate of patients with the diagnosis of TAO has decreased from 104 per 100,000 patient registrations in 1947 to 13 per 100,000 patient registrations in 1986.[4] The prevalence rate of TAO in patients with peripheral artery disease varies across Europe and Asia: 1% to 3% in Switzerland, 0.5% to 5% in West Germany, 1.2% to 5.6% in France, 4% in Belgium, 0.5% in Italy, 0.25% in the United Kingdom,

3.3% in Poland, 6.7% in East Germany, 11.5% in Czechoslovakia, 39% in Yugoslavia, 80% in Israel (among Ashkenazy Jews), 45% to 53% in India, and 16% to 66% in Japan and Korea.[5] In Asia, a greater proportion of patients with limb ischemia has been attributed to TAO than in the United States and Europe.

The overall incidence of TAO also appears to be declining in South Asia and Japan. In particular, the ratio of new patients with TAO to new patients with atherosclerotic peripheral artery disease has declined precipitously. In particular areas of Southeast Asia, including India, TAO has been associated with lower socioeconomic class and smoking unrefined homemade tobacco cigarettes called bidi.

Although it has been considered a disease of young men, TAO also occurs in women. The mean age at onset of TAO is estimated to be 38 years.[6] The reported incidence was less than 2% in the majority of published case series before 1970. Subsequent studies have demonstrated a much higher prevalence of TAO among women, ranging from 11% to 23%.[1] The increasing prevalence of TAO among women has been attributed to rising consumption of tobacco products.

ETIOLOGY AND PATHOGENESIS

TAO is a vasculitis characterized by a highly cellular inflammatory thrombus with relative sparing of the vessel wall. The precise etiology of TAO remains unknown. TAO is distinct from other vasculitides because levels of acute-phase reactants such as erythrocyte sedimentation rate and C-reactive protein and commonly measured autoantibodies are typically normal. However, it has been suggested that abnormalities in immunoreactivity and other factors may contribute to the inflammatory process.

Tobacco

Exposure to tobacco is critical to the initiation, maintenance, and progression of TAO. Although smoking tobacco is by far the most frequent precipitating factor, TAO may also develop as a result of chewing tobacco, snuff, or marijuana use. The association between heavy tobacco use and TAO is so strong that it is typically considered to be a *sine qua non* for the diagnosis. The mean Brinkman index score (number of cigarettes smoked per day multiplied by the number of years of smoking) is 780.[6] It has been hypothesized that some patients develop an immunological reaction to a constituent of tobacco that triggers small vessel occlusive disease. Because only a small proportion of smokers worldwide eventually develop TAO, other factors are believed to contribute to disease pathogenesis.

In South Asia, a large proportion of patients diagnosed with TAO belong to the lowest socioeconomic class and smoke bidi, a hand-rolled herbal cigarette made from dried betel leaves and tobacco. Bidi smoking is believed to account for the higher incidence of TAO in the Indian population.

In addition to its role in disease initiation, tobacco use is a critical factor in disease progression and continued symptoms associated with TAO. While second-hand or passive smoking has not been associated with the onset of TAO, it may play an important role in continuation of the disease process.

Genetic Predisposition

Several studies have suggested that there may be a genetic predisposition to develop TAO. Although there appears to be an association between certain human lymphocyte antigen (HLA) haplotypes and the development of TAO, no consistent pattern has been identified across patient populations. Lack of consistency in HLA haplotype predominance among various populations with TAO is likely due to genetic diversity and methodological differences in each of the studies.

In a study comparing 21 TAO patients with healthy age-, gender-, and race-matched controls, the frequency of mutations associated with arterial vasospasm (stromelysin-1 5A/6A, eNOS T-786C) was evaluated.[7] 5A/6A stromelysin-1 homozygosity was present in 7 of 21 (33%) TAO cases compared with 5 of 21 (24%) controls (risk ratio 1.4; 95% confidence interval [CI] 0.5 to 3.7), and eNOS T-786C homozygosity was present in 3 of 21 (14%) TAO cases compared with 1 of 21 (5%) controls (risk ratio 3.0; 95% CI 0.3 to 26.6). In another study, endothelial nitric oxide synthase (eNOS) 894 G→T and endothelin-1 (ET-1) 8000 T→C polymorphisms were assessed to determine whether either played a role in the development of TAO.[8] Investigators found that the T allele of the eNOS 894 G→T polymorphism was protective against TAO.

Hypercoagulable States

The role of hypercoagulable states in the pathogenesis of TAO remains unclear because studies have failed to demonstrate a consistent pattern of association. Increased levels of anticardiolipin antibodies have been reported in patients with TAO.

Immunologic Mechanisms

Abnormalities in immunoreactivity are believed to play a critical role in the inflammatory process that characterizes TAO. Cellular and humoral immune responses to native human collagen Type I and Type III are increased in patients with TAO compared with those with atherosclerosis or in healthy male controls. Circulating immune complexes found in peripheral arteries of patients with TAO provide further evidence for an immunologic basis for this disease.

While the architecture of blood vessel walls is well preserved regardless of the stage of disease, cell infiltration is observed involving the thrombus and intima. Among infiltrating cells, CD3(+) T cells greatly outnumber CD20(+) B cells, and CD68(+) macrophages or S-100(+) dendritic cells are detected in higher number in the intima during acute and subacute phases. Deposits of immunoglobulins G, A, and M (IgG, IgA, IgM) and complement factors 3d and 4c are noted along the internal elastic lamina. These observations indicate that TAO represents an endarteritis that is characterized by both T-cell (cellular) and B-cell (humoral) mediated immunity in association with activation of antigen-presenting cells in the intima.

In patients with a definite diagnosis of TAO as determined by clinical criteria, linear arrangement of macrophages, B-lymphocytes, and T-lymphocytes along vascular elastic fibers has been found to be a predictable and specific inflammatory response to the internal elastic lamina of affected vessels. This finding indicates that elastic fibers are an important immunogen in the pathogenesis of the disease.

A study of 11 TAO patients detected autoantibodies directed against G-protein coupled receptors in 82%.[9] The majority of these autoantibodies were directed against loop1 of the α1-adrenergic receptor, the endothelin-A receptor, the angiotensin-1 epitope 1 or 2, and the protease-activated receptor (PAR) loop1/2.

Endothelial Dysfunction

Abnormalities of endothelial function also appear to contribute to the pathogenesis of TAO. Although various autoantibodies commonly observed in vasculitides are typically absent, elevations in antiendothelial cell antibody titers have been documented in patients with active TAO. In the future, measurement of antiendothelial cell antibody titers among other biomarkers may serve as a useful tool in following disease activity.

Patients with TAO also demonstrate impairment of endothelium-dependent vasodilation in the peripheral vasculature. The increase in forearm blood flow response to intraarterial acetylcholine infusion is diminished in patients with TAO. In contrast, there is no significant difference in the increase in forearm blood flow response to sodium nitroprusside infusion and reactive hyperemia between the TAO patients and healthy controls.

In a study of 13 young male TAO patients and age-matched healthy smokers ($n = 11$) and nonsmokers ($n = 12$), TAO patients had lower numbers of endothelial progenitor cells (EPCs) and EPC colonies than both nonsmokers and smokers.[10] These results suggest that TAO patients may have an intrinsic decrease in EPCs resulting in endothelial dysfunction that is not completely due to smoking.

Infection

Nearly two-thirds of patients with TAO have severe periodontal disease. Moderate periodontitis, severe periodontitis, and edentulism has been observed in 31%, 56%, and 13% of TAO patients, respectively.[6] Polymerase chain reaction analysis demonstrated DNA fragments from anaerobic bacteria, in particular *Treponema denticola*, in both arterial lesions and oral cavities of patients with TAO but not in arterial samples from health control subjects.

PATHOLOGY

Pathologically, TAO is distinguished by inflammatory thrombus that affects small- and medium-sized arteries and veins. The histopathology of the involved blood vessels varies according to the stage at which the tissue sample is obtained. TAO involves three phases: acute, subacute, and chronic (Fig. 42.1). The histopathology is most likely to be diagnostic of TAO in samples obtained during the acute phase of the disease. As the disease progresses from the subacute to chronic phases, the histopathology of TAO becomes virtually indistinguishable from other obstructive vascular diseases that result in fibrosis of the blood vessels in their end-stage. Because the histological appearance can vary from patient to patient and depends upon the stage of the disease, a pathological diagnosis of TAO may be challenging in some cases. Furthermore, the pathological diagnosis may be inconclusive if only amputated specimens or occluded arteries and veins are examined. Subacute and chronic phase lesions have far fewer characteristic features and therefore are rarely diagnostic for TAO.

Acute Phase

The acute phase of TAO comprises an occlusive, highly cellular, inflammatory thrombus. Polymorphonuclear neutrophils, microabscesses, and multinucleated giant cells are often present around the periphery of the thrombus (Fig. 42.2). The presence of multinucleated giant cells is characteristic of, but not specific for, TAO.

Inflammatory thrombus is observed with greatest frequency in biopsies of areas demonstrating acute superficial thrombophlebitis taken from patients with TAO. While it is unclear whether the vascular

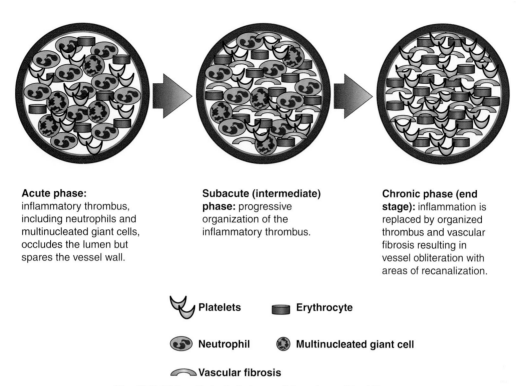

Acute phase: inflammatory thrombus, including neutrophils and multinucleated giant cells, occludes the lumen but spares the vessel wall.

Subacute (intermediate) phase: progressive organization of the inflammatory thrombus.

Chronic phase (end stage): inflammation is replaced by organized thrombus and vascular fibrosis resulting in vessel obliteration with areas of recanalization.

Platelets   Erythrocyte

Neutrophil   Multinucleated giant cell

Vascular fibrosis

Fig. 42.1 Histopathological stages of thromboangiitis obliterans.

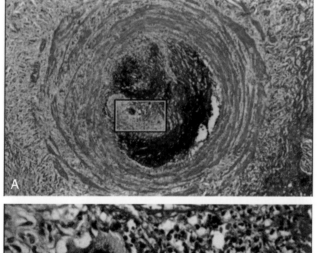

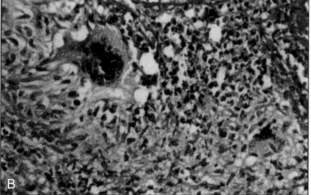

Fig. 42.2 Typical acute histological lesion in a vein obtained from a patient with thromboangiitis obliterans (A). Close-up of the boxed area in A, demonstrating a microabscess in the thrombus and two multinucleated giant cells (hematoxylin and eosin, ×64 [A], ×400 [B]). (From Lie JT. Thromboangiitis obliterans (Buerger disease) revisited. *Pathol Annu.* 1988;23[Pt 2]:257–291.)

lesions of TAO are primarily thrombotic or inflammatory, the pattern of intense inflammatory cell infiltration and cellular proliferation observed in the acute phase of the disease is particularly distinctive. Acute phlebitis without thrombosis, acute phlebitis with thrombosis, and acute phlebitis with thrombus containing microabscesses and giant cells may coexist in different segments of the same affected vein if it is biopsied at an early stage.

Subacute (Intermediate) Phase

During the subacute or intermediate phase, progressive organization of the inflammatory thrombus takes place in affected arteries and veins. While some degree of inflammatory infiltrate remains within the thrombus, the vessel wall is generally spared. Partial recanalization of the vessel and disappearance of microabscesses may also be observed in the subacute phase.

Chronic (End-Stage) Phase

The chronic phase is characterized by organized thrombus with areas of extensive recanalization, prominent vascularization of the media, and adventitial and perivascular fibrosis. Because they represent the end products of vascular injury and occlusive thrombosis, chronic phase arterial lesions are the least distinctive of the three morphological stages of TAO. However, focal residual inflammation within the organized thrombus may suggest TAO in an end-stage lesion. Chronic phase lesions in TAO frequently mimic atherosclerotic vascular disease. In some patients, especially those over 40 years of age, both TAO and atherosclerotic vascular disease may coexist and thereby create further diagnostic uncertainty.

Additional Histologic Features

In all three phases of TAO, the normal architecture of the vessel wall adjacent to the occlusive thrombus, including the internal elastic lamina, remains intact. This observation distinguishes TAO from atherosclerotic vascular disease and from other systemic vasculitides in which there is typically disruption of the internal elastic lamina and the media. "Skip" areas in which normal vessel segments are observed between diseased ones are common in TAO. In addition, the intensity of the periadventitial inflammatory reaction can be quite variable in different segments of the same vessel.

Corkscrew collateral vessels, typically seen in areas of arterial occlusion in patients with TAO, may originate from the vasa nervorum rather than the vasa vasorum.[11]

Immunohistochemical Features

Studies focusing on immunohistochemistry have provided a limited understanding of the role of the cytoskeleton and other cellular elements in TAO. Soon after the inflammatory thrombus has occluded the vessel lumen, spindle cells migrate from the media through fenestrations in the internal elastic lamina into the intima to populate the periphery of the thrombus. These spindle cells express vimentin and alpha-1-actin and originate from smooth muscle cells of the media. Capillaries appear along the margins of the thrombus. Endothelial cells express factor VIII-related antigen and *Ulex europaeus* agglutinin.

As the thrombus organizes during later stages of the disease, the spindle cells differentiate into fibroblasts and lose their positive staining for alpha-1-actin. Demonstration of the internal elastic lamina by collagen type IV markers confirms that the lamina remains intact in TAO and that smooth muscle cells migrate from the media to the intima via fenestrations. Newly formed capillaries within the thrombus are noted.

Immunohistochemically, the process of thrombus organization in TAO is virtually identical to that of ordinary thrombus with the exception of the characteristic inflammatory component. However, infiltration of smooth muscle cells from the media results in a more hypercellular thrombus and rapid organization.

CLINICAL PRESENTATION

The typical patient with TAO is a young man or woman with a heavy tobacco smoking history who presents with the onset of ischemic symptoms of the extremities before age 45 years. However, patients should be questioned about chewing tobacco, snuff, and marijuana use, especially if they deny smoking and present with a history compatible with TAO. Ischemic symptoms typically result from stenosis or occlusion of the distal small arteries and veins. However, TAO frequently progresses proximally and involves multiple limbs. TAO may involve the femoral arteries, iliac arteries, and the abdominal aorta and its visceral branches in 25%, 8%, and 6%, respectively.[6] Large artery involvement rarely occurs in the absence of small vessel occlusive disease. The most common symptoms result from arterial occlusive disease, secondary vasospasm, and superficial thrombophlebitis (Table 42.1).

Arterial Occlusive Disease

Arterial occlusive disease resulting from TAO most often presents as intermittent claudication of the feet, legs, hands, or arms. Foot or arch claudication may be a presenting symptom and is frequently attributed to an orthopedic problem resulting in diagnostic delay. As lower extremity disease progresses proximally, patients with TAO may report classical calf claudication.

Symptoms and signs of critical limb ischemia, including rest pain, ulcerations, and digital gangrene, occur with advanced arterial occlusive disease. At the time of presentation, 76% of patients have ischemic ulcerations (Figs. 42.3A and 42.4). With early recognition of the symptoms and signs of TAO, many patients can be identified and treated before critical limb ischemia develops.

TABLE 42.1	Frequency of Common Presenting Symptoms and Signs in Patients with Thromboangiitis Obliterans	
Clinical Finding	**Frequency, %**
Rest pain	81
Ischemic ulcerations	76
Sensory findings	69
Intermittent claudication	63
Abnormal Allen test	63
Raynaud phenomenon	44
Thrombophlebitis	38

From Olin JW, Young JR, Graor RA, et al. The changing clinical spectrum of thromboangiitis obliterans (Buerger's disease). *Circulation.* 1990;82(5 Suppl):IV3–IV8.

While only one limb may be affected clinically, arterial occlusive disease always involves two or more extremities on angiographic evaluation.

Raynaud Phenomenon

A common complaint in TAO, cold sensitivity may represent one of the earliest manifestations of the disease. Indeed, presentations of TAO appear to be more common in the winter. Cold sensitivity likely results from ischemia or markedly increased muscle sympathetic nerve activity which has been demonstrated in patients with TAO compared with control subjects. Raynaud phenomenon is present in greater than 40% of patients with TAO and may be asymmetrical. The extremities, particularly the digits, may be characterized by either rubor or cyanosis. This discoloration has been termed "Buerger's color."

Superficial Thrombophlebitis

Although it may also be observed in Behçet disease, superficial thrombophlebitis differentiates TAO from other vasculitides and atherosclerotic vascular disease (see Fig. 42.3B). Superficial thrombophlebitis occurs in approximately 40% of patients with TAO. Superficial thrombophlebitis may predate the onset of ischemic symptoms caused by arterial occlusive disease and may parallel disease activity. Some patients may describe a migratory pattern of tender nodules that follow a venous distribution.

Neurological Findings

Sensory abnormalities are common in TAO and are observed in up to 70% of patients. Sensory findings are most likely due to ischemic neuropathy, which is a late finding in the course of TAO. Sensory findings may also be due to primary involvement of the nerves themselves since earlier studies have suggested that the inflammatory cell infiltrate may surround the nerves.

Unusual Presentations

TAO is typically a disease of the distal extremities. However, TAO has been reported to involve unusual vascular beds, including the great vessels and pulmonary, proximal extremity, mesenteric, cerebral, coronary, renal, pelvic, and ophthalmic arteries. TAO in atypical vascular beds is characterized by similar pathological findings as found in the extremities. Of note, reports of TAO in unusual locations should be interpreted with caution because the diagnosis of TAO in such cases may not meet the criteria outlined in this chapter.

TAO of large elastic arteries such as the pulmonary arteries and iliac arteries has been rarely documented. Visceral involvement may present as abdominal pain, nausea, vomiting, diarrhea, melena, hematochezia,

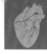

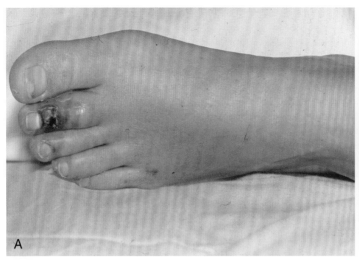
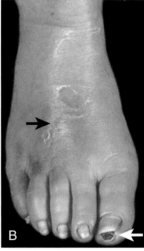

Fig. 42.3 Ischemic ulceration on the second toe in a young woman with thromboangiitis obliterans (A). Superficial thrombophlebitis on the dorsum of the right foot *(arrow)* in a patient with thromboangiitis obliterans (B). Note the ischemic ulceration on the distal right great toe. (From Olin JW, Lie JT. Current management of hypertension and vascular disease. In Cooke JP, Frohlich ED, eds. *Thromboangiitis Obliterans [Buerger's Disease]*. St. Louis: Mosby-Yearbook; 1992:65.)

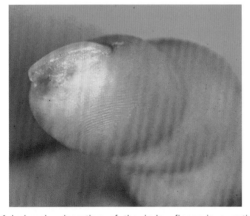

Fig. 42.4 Ischemic ulceration of the index finger in a patient with thromboangiitis obliterans.

weight loss, and anorexia and result in mesenteric ischemia or infarction. Cerebrovascular involvement may manifest as transient ischemic attack, ischemic stroke, and psychotic disorders.

Coronary artery involvement may present as myocardial ischemia or infarction. TAO affecting the intrarenal arterial branches has been reported. Rarely, TAO may involve the pelvic vessels, including the pudendal arteries and veins, resulting in erectile dysfunction. TAO involving the temporal and ophthalmic arteries may mimic giant cell arteritis.

Involvement of saphenous vein bypass grafts in patients with TAO is a truly rare occurrence.

DIFFERENTIAL DIAGNOSIS

A clinical diagnosis of TAO requires the exclusion of disorders that may mimic the disease (Box 42.1). The most important disorders to exclude are atherosclerotic vascular disease, thromboembolic disease, and autoimmune diseases such as scleroderma or CREST syndrome. In most cases, the combination of serological testing, echocardiography, and arteriography can exclude these disorders and help establish the diagnosis of TAO.

The diagnosis of scleroderma or limited scleroderma (formally called the CREST syndrome) is typically suggested by the clinical

> ### BOX 42.1 Disorders That May Mimic Thromboangiitis Obliterans
>
> - Atherosclerotic vascular disease
> - Thromboembolic disease
> - Endocarditis
> - Rheumatologic disorders
>   - Scleroderma
>   - CREST syndrome
>   - Systemic lupus erythematosus
>   - Rheumatoid arthritis
>   - Mixed connective tissue diseases
>   - Other vasculitides
> - Hypercoagulable states
>   - Antiphospholipid antibody syndrome
> - Syndromes of repetitive mechanical trauma
>   - Hypothenar hammer syndrome
>   - Vibration-related vascular injury
> - Thoracic outlet syndrome
> - Popliteal entrapment syndrome
> - Cystic adventitial disease
> - Drug
>   - Ergotamine abuse
>   - Cocaine abuse
>   - Amphetamine abuse

presentation, including skin findings. Nailfold capillaroscopy may be performed and is usually quite distinctive in patients with scleroderma or CREST syndrome. However, characteristic findings of capillary loop drop-out may also be observed in some patients with TAO. The detection of serological markers such as anti–ACL-70 or anti-centromere antibodies provides further evidence for these disorders.

Clinicians should evaluate patients for features of other autoimmune diseases such as systemic lupus erythematosus, rheumatoid arthritis, and other vasculitides. Serological markers are often helpful in excluding such disorders. Patients with antiphospholipid antibody syndrome pose a particular diagnostic challenge because they may present with both arterial and venous thrombotic events. Antiphospholipid antibody syndrome is suggested by detection of lupus-type anticoagulants or the presence of elevated titers of anticardiolipin antibodies, anti-β2 glycoprotein-1 antibodies, anti-phosphotidylserine antibodies, or anti-prothrombin (PT) antibodies. Of note, lupus anticoagulant and anticardiolipin antibodies may be detected in some patients with TAO but may also indicate an unrelated thrombophilia.[1] Pathological examination can clearly differentiate between the two disorders because antiphospholipid antibody syndrome is characterized by the presence of bland thrombosis whereas TAO results in an inflammatory thrombus.

TAO is differentiated from other vasculitides because it results in distal extremity ischemia while patients with Takayasu arteritis or giant cell arteritis present with more proximal arterial involvement. The arteriographic features of TAO are also quite distinctive from those observed in Takayasu arteritis or giant cell arteritis. In addition, vasculitides such as Takayasu arteritis and giant cell arteritis are typically associated with elevations in inflammatory markers, including erythrocyte sedimentation rate and C-reactive protein.

Clinicians evaluating patients with suspected TAO should inquire about possible ergotamine, amphetamine, or cocaine use in addition to disorders of repetitive mechanical trauma such as vibration-induced vascular injury and hypothenar hammer syndrome. Serum ergotamine levels can be obtained to exclude vascular injury caused by this drug. Because it can mimic TAO, all patients should be questioned about cocaine abuse. A particularly virulent form of TAO may occur in patients who smoke marijuana (cannabis arteritis). In some countries, it is common to mix marijuana with tobacco and smoke it like a cigarette. A complete toxicology screen is recommended in patients who present with a history and physical compatible with TAO, especially if they deny tobacco use.

DIAGNOSIS

TAO is a clinical diagnosis that requires a compatible history in combination with supportive physical examination findings and vascular abnormalities on imaging studies (Fig. 42.5).

Physical Examination

The physical examination of a patient with suspected TAO should include a detailed vascular evaluation with palpation of peripheral pulses, auscultation for arterial bruits, and measurement of ankle:brachial indices, toe pressures and finger pressures (when the upper extremity is involved). Extremities should be carefully inspected for superficial thrombophlebitis which may present as tender superficial venous nodules and cords. The hands and feet should be examined for findings of digital ischemia. Neurological examination may document peripheral nerve involvement in the form of sensory deficits.

Although nonspecific, an abnormal Allen test in a young smoker with digital ischemia is strongly suggestive of TAO because it provides evidence for disease in the arteries distal to the wrist (Fig. 42.6). Documentation of an abnormal Allen test is helpful because the distal nature of TAO and involvement of both upper and lower extremities distinguishes it from atherosclerotic vascular disease. With the exception of chronic kidney disease patients with diabetes or those who have undergone renal transplantation, atherosclerosis does not involve the hand and rarely occurs distal to the subclavian artery.

Diagnostic Criteria

Several diagnostic criteria have been proposed for the evaluation of patients with suspected TAO. The most commonly used criteria are those of Shionoya and Olin (Table 42.2). An increasing number of individuals who fulfill clinical criteria for TAO have risk factors for atherosclerotic vascular disease such as hypertension and hyperlipidemia. A subset of these patients may subsequently develop concomitant atherosclerotic vascular disease after the original diagnosis of TAO. Accordingly, if patients meet criteria of distal extremity involvement, tobacco use, and exclusion of a proximal source of emboli, atherosclerosis, and thrombophilia, hyperlipidemia or hypertension should not exclude the diagnosis of TAO.

Laboratory Evaluation

Although there are no specific blood tests to aid in the diagnosis, laboratory evaluation in patients with suspected TAO is useful for excluding alternative diagnoses. Initial laboratory studies should include a complete blood count, chemistry panel, liver function tests, fasting blood glucose, urinalysis, inflammatory markers such as erythrocyte sedimentation rate and C-reactive protein, cold agglutinins, and cryoglobulins. In addition, serological markers of autoimmune disease,

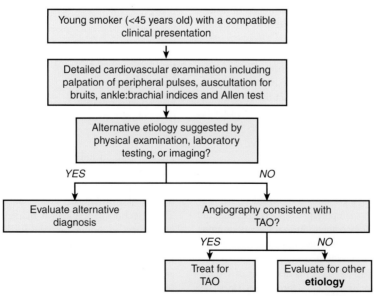

Fig. 42.5 A diagnostic algorithm for patients with suspected thromboangiitis obliterans *(TAO)*.

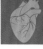

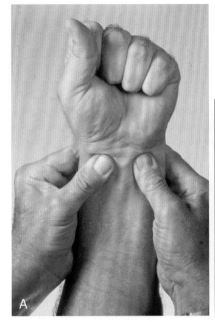

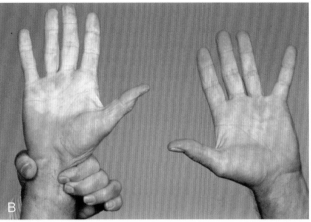

Fig. 42.6 Allen test with occlusion of the radial and ulnar pulse by manual compression (A). When compression of the ulnar pulse is released while continuing to compress the radial artery, the hand does not fill with blood (B). The pallor of the right hand when compared with the left hand is consistent with distal arterial occlusive disease of the ulnar artery (right portion of the image). (From Olin JW, Lie JT. Current management of hypertension and vascular disease. In Cooke JP, Frohlich ED, eds. *Thromboangiitis Obliterans [Buerger's Disease]*. St. Louis: Mosby-Yearbook; 1992:65.)

TABLE 42.2 Common Criteria for the Diagnosis of Thromboangiitis Obliterans

Shionoya's Criteria[a]	Olin's Criteria[b]
Onset before age 50	Onset before age 45
Smoking history	Current (or recent past) tobacco use
Infrapopliteal arterial occlusions	Distal extremity ischemia (claudication, rest pain, ischemic ulcers, gangrene) documented with noninvasive testing
Upper limb involvement or phlebitis migrans	Laboratory tests to exclude autoimmune diseases, hypercoagulable states, and diabetes mellitus
Absence of atherosclerotic risk factors other than smoking	Exclude a proximal source of emboli with echocardiography and arteriography
	Demonstrate consistent arteriographic findings in the involved and clinically noninvolved limbs

A biopsy is rarely needed to make the diagnosis unless the patient presents with unusual characteristics such as large artery involvement or age greater than 45.

[a]Shionoya S. Diagnostic criteria of Buerger's disease. *Int J Cardiol.* 1998;66(Suppl 1):S243–S245.
[b] Olin JW. Thromboangiitis obliterans. *N Engl J Med.* 2000;343:864–869.

including antinuclear antibody, rheumatoid factor, anticentromere antibody, and anti–SCL-70 antibody, should be obtained and are typically negative in patients with TAO. An evaluation for hypercoagulable states is frequently performed. Of note, antiphospholipid and anticardiolipin antibodies are detected in some patients with TAO but may also indicate an isolated thrombophilia.

Imaging

Imaging in patients with suspected TAO is not only utilized to establish the diagnosis but also to exclude alternative etiologies for the presentation that may require a radically different therapeutic approach. For example, echocardiography is frequently indicated to exclude a cardiac source of embolism resulting in acute arterial occlusion. Likewise, catheter-based angiography provides evidence for TAO but also excludes proximal sources of artery-to-artery embolism.

Noninvasive vascular laboratory studies such as segmental arterial pressure measurements with pulse volume recordings demonstrating distal abnormalities in the absence of proximal disease suggest a diagnosis of TAO. Digital plethysmography, finger and toe pressures, and transcutaneous oxygen measurement may be useful in documenting distal small vessel disease in the absence of more proximal upper or lower extremity abnormalities in patients with TAO. Arterial duplex scanning can also be used to exclude proximal atherosclerotic lesions and identify distal arterial occlusive disease. Corkscrew collaterals, a finding frequently observed in patients with TAO, may also be visualized on arterial duplex scanning. Abdominal aortic ultrasonography may be used to exclude abdominal aortic aneurysm or atherosclerosis as a source of distal embolization to the lower extremities.

Computed tomographic angiography (CTA), magnetic resonance angiography (MRA), or catheter-based angiography may be performed to exclude a proximal arterial source of embolism and to define the anatomy and severity of distal arterial occlusive disease. Although advances in CTA and MRA have shown promise for imaging distal vessels, the majority of patients will require catheter-based angiography to provide the spatial resolution necessary to detect small-artery pathology, especially of the hands and feet. In patients with ischemic ulcerations and in whom secondary infection is a concern, MR may be useful in determining the presence of osteomyelitis.

Catheter-based angiography plays a critical role in establishing the diagnosis of TAO and excluding proximal arterial pathology that may result in distal arterial occlusive disease. While there are no pathognomonic angiographic findings in TAO, angiography helps to establish the diagnosis when taken in context with a compatible clinical presentation. The classic angiographic picture of TAO consists of arterial occlusive disease confined to the distal circulation, most often infrapopliteal and infrabrachial, with proximal arteries free of atheroma, aneurysms, and other sources of emboli (Fig. 42.7). There are often areas of disease interspersed with normal appearing vessels (skip areas). In the absence of diabetes, isolated arterial occlusive disease distal to the popliteal artery virtually never occurs in atherosclerosis. Commonly, angiographic abnormalities are observed in the digital arteries of the fingers and toes, the palmar and plantar arteries of the hands and feet, and the radial, ulnar, anterior tibial, posterior tibial, and peroneal arteries.

Distal small-to-medium artery involvement, segmental occlusions, and corkscrew-shaped collaterals around areas of occlusions are characteristic angiographic findings in TAO (Fig. 42.8). Corkscrew collaterals are not specific for TAO and may be observed with any disease process that results in small vessel occlusive disease. In particular, arterial occlusive disease due to scleroderma or limited scleroderma (CREST syndrome) can closely mimic the angiographic appearance of TAO. Findings of arterial wall irregularity, vascular calcification, and proximal artery involvement should call a diagnosis of TAO into question.

Role for Biopsy

Tissue biopsy is rarely required for the diagnosis of TAO unless the clinical presentation involves an unusual vascular territory or a patient older than 45 to 50 years at the onset of symptoms. Biopsy is most likely to be diagnostic when obtained from a vein with superficial thrombophlebitis during the acute phase of the disease. A highly inflammatory

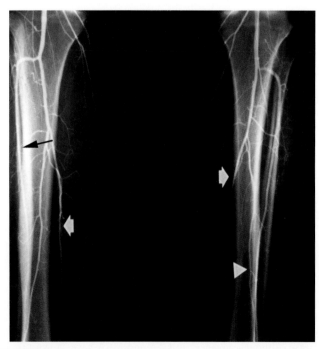

Fig. 42.7 Catheter-based angiogram demonstrating severe infrapopliteal arterial occlusive disease in a patient with thromboangiitis obliterans. In the right leg, the anterior tibial artery is occluded *(red arrow)*. The posterior tibial artery tapers and then occludes in the mid-to-distal calf *(white arrow)*. In the left leg, the posterior tibial artery *(white arrow)* occludes several centimeters after its origin. The peroneal artery *(arrowhead)* tapers in the mid-to-distal calf.

thrombus, relative sparing of the blood vessel wall, and preservation of the internal elastic lamina in arterial biopsies are characteristic histological findings in TAO.

PROGNOSIS

The prognosis for patients with TAO greatly depends on their ability to discontinue tobacco use. Continued smoking strongly correlates with the risk of limb amputation. Quality of life is substantially diminished in patients with TAO. TAO-related limb amputation is strongly correlated with unemployment.

MANAGEMENT

While various options exist for the management of TAO, discontinuation of tobacco use is the definitive and most effective therapy for the disease (Box 42.2). The efficacy of alternative therapies in TAO is profoundly limited in the setting of ongoing tobacco exposure.

Tobacco Cessation

The cornerstone of therapy for TAO is total discontinuation of any tobacco use (Box 42.3). Complete tobacco cessation is critical because even a few cigarettes a day may drive disease progression and culminate in amputation.[1] Patients should be counseled to abstain from using smokeless tobacco as well as smoking marijuana, as both have been associated with TAO. Patient education on the role of tobacco exposure in the initiation, maintenance, and progression of TAO is of paramount importance. Adjunctive measures to assist in discontinuation of tobacco use such as pharmacotherapy and smoking cessation groups should be made available to all patients with TAO. However, nicotine replace therapy should be avoided in patients with TAO because it may contribute to disease activity. Agents such as bupropion and varenicline may be preferred as smoking cessation aids in patients with TAO. Although it remains unclear whether passive smoke exposure can cause TAO, patients with active disease should be advised to avoid second-hand smoke as much as possible.

Patients with TAO have a similar degree of tobacco dependence as those with atherosclerotic cardiovascular disease. Patients with TAO may have a higher frequency of tobacco cessation than those with atherosclerotic vascular disease. Patients with TAO should be reassured that if they are able to discontinue tobacco use, the disease will become quiescent and the risk of amputation will greatly diminish provided critical limb ischemia is not present. If significant arterial occlusive disease has developed, symptoms of intermittent claudication and secondary vasospasm (Raynaud phenomenon) may continue but should not progress. Vasodilators may help reduce the symptomatic burden in such patients.

Vasodilators

The use of vasodilators in patients with TAO is largely palliative. The most extensive clinical experience with vasodilators in TAO comes from trials evaluating the intravenous prostacyclin analogue iloprost. A Cochrane Database Systematic Review suggested that intravenous iloprost was more effective than aspirin for treatment of rest pain and healing ischemic ulcers in patients with TAO.[12] In contrast, oral iloprost was not more effective than placebo. Transcutaneous oxygen ($TcPO_2$) and carbon dioxide ($TcPCO_2$) monitoring and laser Doppler flow measurement have shown promise for measuring the efficacy of intravenous iloprost in patients with TAO.[13]

Phosphodiesterase inhibitors with vasodilator properties have the potential to play a role in the management of TAO but require evaluation in prospective trials. Although not specifically described in patients

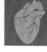

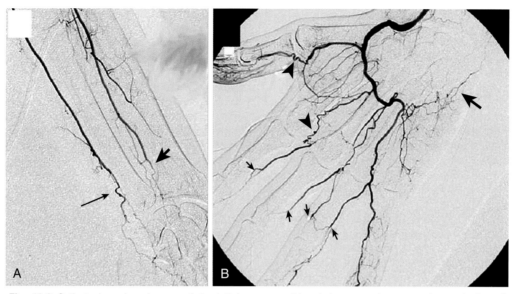

Fig. 42.8 Catheter-based angiogram of the left forearm and hand demonstrating a tapering occlusion of the left radial artery *(arrowhead)* and ulnar artery *(arrow)* at the wrist (A). All proximal arteries were normal. The right hand of the same patient demonstrated an occluded ulnar artery at the wrist *(large arrow;* B). A patent radial artery fills the deep palmar arch. Multiple segmental digital artery occlusions are present *(small arrows).* Numerous "corkscrew collaterals" *(arrowheads),* which represent collateralization around occluded segments, are visualized. (From Olin JW, Shih A. *Thromboangiitis obliterans [Buerger's disease]. Curr Opin Rheumatol.* 2006;18:18–24.)

BOX 42.2 Therapeutic Options for the Management of Thromboangiitis Obliterans

- Tobacco cessation
- Vasodilators
  - Prostacyclin analogues
  - Alpha-adrenergic receptor antagonists
  - Calcium channel antagonists
  - Phosphodiesterase inhibitors (cilostazol, sildenafil, tadalafil)
  - Transdermal nitrates
- Peripheral periarterial sympathectomy
- Regional sympathetic blockade
- Spinal cord stimulation
- Intermittent pneumatic compression
- Therapeutic angiogenesis
- Endovascular therapy
  - Intraarterial fibrinolysis
  - Angioplasty/stenting
  - Radiofrequency ablation
- Surgical Revascularization
  - Arterial bypass surgery
  - Omental transfer
  - Amputation
- Local Wound Care
  - Debridement
  - Vacuum-assisted wound closure

BOX 42.3 Pearls for Tobacco Cessation in Patients with Thromboangiitis Obliterans

- Educate patients on the critical role of tobacco in the initiation, maintenance, and progression of thromboangiitis obliterans
- Counsel patients and members of their households about the role of secondhand smoke exposure in perpetuating the disease process
- Ask the patient at every office visit if they have been successful in tobacco cessation. This approach lets the patient know that tobacco cessation is the single most important step in treating this disease.
- Explain to patients the limited efficacy of alternative therapies for thromboangiitis obliterans in the absence of complete and continued tobacco cessation
- Measure urinary nicotine, cotinine, and cannabis in patients who continue to have signs and symptoms consistent with active disease despite claims of tobacco cessation
- Offer adjunctive therapies such as pharmacotherapy and smoking cessation groups to aid with discontinuation of tobacco use
- Prescribe bupropion and varenicline as the preferred pharmacological adjuncts to assist in tobacco cessation because nicotine replacement therapy may contribute to ongoing disease activity

---

with TAO, cilostazol has been reported to aid in the healing of ischemic ulcerations in patients who were not eligible for revascularization.[14,15] Although it is also helpful in the treatment of claudication due to atherosclerotic peripheral vascular disease, the clinical experience with cilostazol for this indication in patients with TAO is limited. Sildenafil and tadalafil may represent another option in this drug class for patients with TAO but requires investigation.

Other vasodilators such as alpha-adrenergic receptor antagonists, calcium channel antagonists, and transdermal nitrates may be helpful in patients who experience vasospasm but have not been studied in prospective clinical trials.

Periarterial Sympathectomy and Sympathetic Blockade

Peripheral periarterial sympathectomy may be considered for patients with refractory pain and digital ischemia due to TAO but remains controversial. Sympathectomy has anecdotally been reported to occasionally assist the healing of ischemic ulcerations. In a single case report, intravenous regional sympathetic blockade (Bier block) with guanethidine and lidocaine increased finger blood flow and resulted in complete disappearance of fingertip ischemic ulcerations and rest pain in a patient with advanced TAO.[16]

Spinal Cord Stimulation

Epidural spinal cord stimulation has been evaluated in a limited number of patients to decrease ischemic pain and avoid amputation when revascularization is not feasible and other therapeutic interventions have not been effective.[17] In a retrospective study, 29 patients were evaluated to determine the effect of epidural spinal cord stimulation in the treatment of TAO.[18] The regional perfusion index (the ratio between the foot and chest transcutaneous oxygen pressure) at baseline was 0.27 ± 0.25. Three months after spinal cord stimulation implantation, the regional perfusion index increased to 0.41 ± 0.22. During the 1- and 3-year follow-up period, a sustained improvement in the microcirculation was recorded. The most pronounced improvement in the regional perfusion index values was observed in the subgroup of 13 patients with trophic lesions. In this group, the regional perfusion index increased significantly from 0.17 ± 0.21 to 0.4 ± 0.18 ($P < .02$) after a mean follow-up of 5.7 years. Limb survival rate was 93.1%.

Intermittent Pneumatic Compression

Intermittent pneumatic compression of the foot and calves has been used to augment perfusion to the lower extremities in patients with severe claudication or critical limb ischemia who are not candidates for revascularization because of advanced distal arterial occlusive disease, including those with TAO.

Therapeutic Angiogenesis and Cell-Based Therapy

Limited options for patients with severe distal arterial occlusive disease and critical limb ischemia due to TAO has driven a growing interest in therapeutic angiogenesis. In a study of 6 patients with TAO and critical limb ischemia, direct intramuscular injection of naked plasmid DNA-encoding vascular endothelial growth factor (VEGF) resulted in complete healing of ischemic ulcerations that were nonhealing for more than 1 month in three of five limbs.[19] Nocturnal rest pain was relieved in the remaining two patients. Evidence of improved perfusion to the distal ischemic limb included an increase of more than 0.1 in the ankle:brachial index in three limbs, improved flow shown by MR imaging in all seven limbs studied, and newly formed collateral vessels demonstrated on serial catheter-based angiography in all seven limbs studied. Two patients with advanced distal extremity gangrene ultimately required below-knee amputation despite the evidence of improved perfusion. Based on these preliminary observations, therapeutic angiogenesis with VEGF gene transfer may provide benefit to patients with TAO who have not developed frank gangrene but are unresponsive to medical or surgical treatment.

Several subsequent studies have evaluated autologous bone marrow mononuclear cell implantation for patients with critical limb ischemia due to TAO.[20–23] Although short-term results with autologous bone marrow mononuclear cell implantation have been promising, long-term safety and efficacy remain to be demonstrated.[24] Autologous whole bone marrow stem cell transplantation may represent another promising avenue for therapeutic angiogenesis in patients with TAO.[25,26]

Revascularization Strategies

Endovascular Therapy

Endovascular therapy for arterial revascularization in patients with TAO remains controversial. Selective intraarterial infusion of fibrinolytic therapy has been reported as an adjunctive treatment in patients with TAO. However, the efficacy of intraarterial fibrinolysis for TAO may not be as high as initially reported. From a pathological standpoint, the highly inflammatory thrombus observed in TAO is quickly invaded by fibroblasts and subsequently organized, making it quite resistant to fibrinolysis. In patients facing amputation and in whom no other alternatives for revascularization exist, a short trial of intraarterial fibrinolysis may be reasonable to avoid amputation in the absence of contraindications.

Other percutaneous techniques, including angioplasty and stent placement, have a very limited role in treatment of TAO because of the distal and small-vessel nature of the disease. Intravascular ultrasound (IVUS) may assist in identification of lesions in TAO patients that may have favorable outcomes with percutaneous revascularization.[27] Percutaneous approaches for limb salvage in TAO patients are associated with a higher rate of reintervention (62.8% vs. 27.7%, $P < .001$) and lower primary (19% in the femoropopliteal segment and 14.4% in the tibioperoneal segment vs. 60.4%, $P = .008$ and $P < .001$, respectively) and secondary patency rates (33.9% in the femoropopliteal segment and 21.3% in the tibioperoneal segment vs. 68.8%, $P = .04$ and $P = .002$, respectively) at 3 years compared with surgical revascularization.[28] However, amputation-free survival in percutaneous revascularization patients was similar to that of the surgical bypass patients at 1 year (92.9% vs. 93.2%, $P = .81$) and 3 years (87.8% vs. 90.6%, $P = .66$). Percutaneous intervention may be a valid strategy for limb salvage in TAO patients in whom surgical revascularization is not an option.

In a study of 30 patients with unilateral TAO, endovascular radiofrequency ablation was associated with decreased pain score and an increase in the ankle:brachial index compared with the baseline and immediate post-procedure measurement.[29] Based on these findings, further investigation of endovascular radiotherapy for TAO is warranted.

Surgical Revascularization

Surgical revascularization is usually not possible in patients with TAO because of the distal and diffuse nature of the disease with extremely poor run-off. In addition, there is rarely a suitable distal target vessel for bypass. Short- and long-term patency rates are poor. Superficial thrombophlebitis of the lower extremities frequently limits the number and quality of venous conduits available for bypass surgery. However, surgical bypass using autologous vein may be considered in select patients with severe ischemia, suitable distal target vessels, and good quality venous conduits. In a retrospective study of 101 patients with TAO who were followed for a mean of 10.6 years, outcomes after surgical bypass were often suboptimal with primary patency rates of 41%, 32%, and 30% and secondary patency rates of 54%, 47%, and 39% at 1, 5, and 10 years, respectively.[30] Graft patency rates are nearly 50% lower in TAO patients who continue to smoke after surgical revascularization. For reasons mentioned above, lower extremity bypass surgery in patients with TAO is rarely carried out in the United States.

While long-term patency of surgical bypass grafts is limited, short-term patency may be sufficient to allow healing of ischemic ulcerations due to TAO and preservation of the at-risk limb. Despite these low patency rates, limb salvage rates exceed 90%. Accordingly, every effort should be taken to achieve limb salvage in patients with TAO who are often young with many years of potential productivity ahead of them.

Another surgical option for patients with TAO consists of omental transfer. Despite promising data from a limited number of centers, omental transfer has not been widely adopted. The reason may be the lack of published data from centers outside of India where the technique has been pioneered.

Unfortunately, for a subset of patients with TAO, amputation is necessary to treat refractory rest pain or to prevent progression of local infection, including osteomyelitis. The amputation rate is substantially reduced among patients who discontinue tobacco use compared with those who do not. In general, the increased risk of amputation in former smokers is eliminated by eight years following tobacco cessation.

Local Wound Care

For patients with areas of frank or threatened ischemic ulceration due to TAO, local wound care is of paramount importance. Consultation with wound care specialists can provide recommendations for dressings and other local interventions to aid wound healing. In addition, wound care specialists can educate patients about daily care and warning signs of progression or infection. In patients with more advanced ischemic ulcerations or gangrene, local debridement and appropriate antibiotic therapy may be required. Vacuum-assisted wound closure may be promising in patients with TAO and ischemic ulcerations, but requires further investigation.[31]

Supportive Care

Supportive care in patients with TAO and ischemic rest pain or ulcerations is identical to that for patients with critical limb ischemia due to any other arterial occlusive disease. A reverse Trendelenburg position should be used in patients who have severe ischemic rest pain. Adequate analgesia, with narcotics if required, should be used to manage periods of severe ischemic pain. Maintenance of central and peripheral warmth is crucial to reduce cold-induced vasospasm. Meticulous skin care of the hands and feet is important to prevent new ulcerations.

Unproven Therapies

Other alternative therapies that remain unproven in the treatment of patients with TAO include antiplatelet agents, anticoagulants, and hyperbaric oxygen therapy. Although they may be prescribed on an individual basis, the role of antiplatelet agents such as aspirin and clopidogrel has not been established in TAO. Likewise, therapeutic anticoagulation has never been shown to be effective in treatment of TAO.

Despite this, some clinicians have anecdotally used anticoagulation in an effort to delay amputation and improve collateral flow in severe critical limb ischemia. A short 30- to 45-day course of anticoagulation may also be used in patients with severe symptoms due to superficial thrombophlebitis.[32,33] Pentoxifylline increases red blood cell membrane flexibility and has been used with limited benefit in patients with claudication due to atherosclerotic peripheral vascular disease of the lower extremities. Its role, if any, in TAO remains to be defined. Hyperbaric oxygen therapy has shown promise in the healing of cutaneous wounds due to a variety of disorders but has not been evaluated in the treatment of patients with TAO. Although they have pleomorphic effects, including the modulation of inflammatory pathways, which may benefit patients with TAO, the role of statins and selective cannabinoid receptor antagonists in management of this disorder is unclear.

Overall Therapeutic Algorithm

An overall therapeutic algorithm for patients with TAO emphasizes tobacco cessation and then addresses symptoms based on the extent of arterial and venous occlusive disease (Fig. 42.9).

FUTURE PERSPECTIVES

Although the pathophysiology of TAO is not completely understood, the role of tobacco use in disease initiation and activity is indisputable. Continued population- and individual-based efforts to decrease tobacco use will not only lower the frequency of TAO but also other smoking-related illnesses such as lung cancer, chronic obstructive pulmonary disease, venous thromboembolism, and atherosclerotic cardiovascular disease. For patients who are unable to discontinue tobacco use or for those patients who require palliative therapy to help them get through an episode of critical limb ischemia, more effective therapeutic alternatives, such as vasodilators, would be beneficial. The use of gene therapy or cell-based therapy may hold the greatest promise in this regard. Further prospective randomized trials are warranted to determine if, in fact, therapeutic angiogenesis is a useful treatment strategy for patients with TAO. However, it is difficult to complete

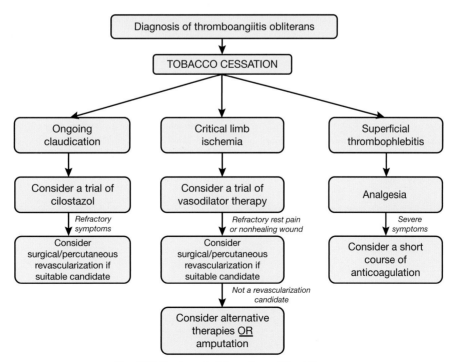

Fig. 42.9 Treatment of thromboangiitis obliterans.

these studies because achieving an adequate sample size to answer the question at hand has proven to be difficult. Since TAO is a vasculitis characterized by inflammatory thrombus, an improved understanding of the mechanisms of inflammation in this disease as well as medications that modulate vascular inflammation may result in more effective therapy for this disorder.

REFERENCES

1. Piazza G, Creager MA. Thromboangiitis obliterans. *Circulation*. 2010;121:1858–1861.
2. Allen EV, Brown GE. Thrombo-angiitis obliterans: a clinical study of 200 cases. *Ann Intern Med*. 1928;1:535–549.
3. Herman BE. Buerger's syndrome. *Angiology*. 1975;26:713–716.
4. Lie JT. The rise and fall and resurgence of thromboangiitis obliterans (Buerger's disease). *Acta Pathol Jpn*. 1989;39:153–158.
5. Cachovan M. Epidemiologie und geographisches verteilungsmuster der thromboangiitis obliterans. In: Heidrich J, ed. *Thromboangiitis obliterans morbus Winiwarter-Buerger*. Stuttgart, New York: George Thieme; 1988:31–36.
6. Igari K, Inoue Y, Iwai T. The epidemiologic and clinical findings of patients with Buerger disease. *Ann Vasc Surg*. 2016;30:263–269.
7. Glueck CJ, Haque M, Winarska M, et al. Stromelysin-1 5A/6A and eNOS T-786C polymorphisms, MTHFR C677T and A1298C mutations, and cigarette-cannabis smoking: a pilot, hypothesis-generating study of gene-environment pathophysiological associations with Buerger's disease. *Clin Appl Thromb Hemost*. 2006;12:427–439.
8. Adiguzel Y, Yilmaz E, Akar N. Effect of eNOS and ET-1 polymorphisms in thromboangiitis obliterans. *Clin Appl Thromb Hemost*. 2010;16:103–106.
9. Klein-Weigel PF, Bimmler M, Hempel P, et al. G-protein coupled receptor auto-antibodies in thromboangiitis obliterans (Buerger's disease) and their removal by immunoadsorption. *Vasa*. 2014;43:347–352.
10. Park HS, Cho KH, Kim KL, et al. Reduced circulating endothelial progenitor cells in thromboangiitis obliterans (Buerger's disease). *Vasc Med*. 2013;18:331–339.
11. Bas A, Dikici AS, Gulsen F, et al. Corkscrew collateral vessels in Buerger disease: vasa vasorum or vasa nervorum. *J Vasc Interv Radiol*. 2016;27:735–739.
12. Cacione DG, Macedo CR, Baptista-Silva JC. Pharmacological treatment for Buerger's disease. *Cochrane Database Syst Rev*. 2016;3:CD011033.
13. Melillo E, Grigoratos C, Sanctis FD, et al. Noninvasive transcutaneous monitoring in long-term follow-up of patients with thromboangiitis obliterans treated with intravenous iloprost. *Angiology*. 2015;66:531–538.
14. Dean SM, Vaccaro PS. Successful pharmacologic treatment of lower extremity ulcerations in 5 patients with chronic critical limb ischemia. *J Am Board Fam Pract*. 2002;15:55–62.
15. Dean SM, Satiani B. Three cases of digital ischemia successfully treated with cilostazol. *Vasc Med*. 2001;6:245–248.
16. Paraskevas KI, Trigka AA, Samara M. Successful intravenous regional sympathetic blockade (Bier's block) with guanethidine and lidocaine in a patient with advanced Buerger's disease (thromboangiitis obliterans)--a case report. *Angiology*. 2005;56:493–496.
17. Boari B, Salmi R, Manfredini R. Buerger's disease: spinal cord stimulation may represent a useful tool for delaying amputation in young patients. *Eur J Intern Med*. 2007;18:259.
18. Donas KP, Schulte S, Ktenidis K, Horsch S. The role of epidural spinal cord stimulation in the treatment of Buerger's disease. *J Vasc Surg*. 2005;41:830–836.
19. Isner JM, Baumgartner I, Rauh G, et al. Treatment of thromboangiitis obliterans (Buerger's disease) by intramuscular gene transfer of vascular endothelial growth factor: preliminary clinical results. *J Vasc Surg*. 1998;28:964–973. discussion 973-965.
20. Saito Y, Sasaki K, Katsuda Y, et al. Effect of autologous bone-marrow cell transplantation on ischemic ulcer in patients with Buerger's disease. *Circ J*. 2007;71:1187–1192.
21. Saito S, Nishikawa K, Obata H, Goto F. Autologous bone marrow transplantation and hyperbaric oxygen therapy for patients with thromboangiitis obliterans. *Angiology*. 2007;58:429–434.
22. Matoba S, Tatsumi T, Murohara T, et al. Long-term clinical outcome after intramuscular implantation of bone marrow mononuclear cells (therapeutic angiogenesis by cell transplantation [TACT] trial) in patients with chronic limb ischemia. *Am Heart J*. 2008;156:1010–1018.
23. Durdu S, Akar AR, Arat M, et al. Autologous bone-marrow mononuclear cell implantation for patients with Rutherford grade II-III thromboangiitis obliterans. *J Vasc Surg*. 2006;44:732–739.
24. Miyamoto K, Nishigami K, Nagaya N, et al. Unblinded pilot study of autologous transplantation of bone marrow mononuclear cells in patients with thromboangiitis obliterans. *Circulation*. 2006;114:2679–2684.
25. Kim SW, Han H, Chae GT, et al. Successful stem cell therapy using umbilical cord blood-derived multipotent stem cells for Buerger's disease and ischemic limb disease animal model. *Stem Cells*. 2006;24:1620–1626.
26. Kim DI, Kim MJ, Joh JH, et al. Angiogenesis facilitated by autologous whole bone marrow stem cell transplantation for Buerger's disease. *Stem Cells*. 2006;24:1194–1200.
27. Kawarada O, Kume T, Ayabe S, et al. Endovascular therapy outcomes and intravascular ultrasound findings in thromboangiitis obliterans (Buerger's disease). *J Endovasc Ther*. 2017;24:504–515.
28. Ye K, Shi H, Qin J, et al. Outcomes of endovascular recanalization versus autogenous venous bypass for thromboangiitis obliterans patients with critical limb ischemia due to tibioperoneal arterial occlusion. *J Vasc Surg*. 2017;66. 1133–1142 e1131.
29. Tang J, Gan S, Zheng M, et al. Efficacy of endovascular radiofrequency ablation for thromboangiitis obliterans (Buerger's disease). *Ann Vasc Surg*. 2017;42:78–83.
30. Ohta T, Ishioashi H, Hosaka M, Sugimoto I. Clinical and social consequences of Buerger disease. *J Vasc Surg*. 2004;39:176–180.
31. Canter HI, Isci E, Erk Y. Vacuum-assisted wound closure for the management of a foot ulcer due to Buerger's disease. *J Plast Reconstr Aesthet Surg*. 2009;62:250–253.
32. Geerts WH, Bergqvist D, Pineo GF, et al. Prevention of venous thromboembolism: American College of Chest Physicians Evidence-Based Clinical Practice Guidelines (8th edition). *Chest*. 2008;133:381S–453S.
33. Decousus H, Prandoni P, Mismetti P, et al. Fondaparinux for the treatment of superficial-vein thrombosis in the legs. *N Engl J Med*. 2010;363:1222–1232.

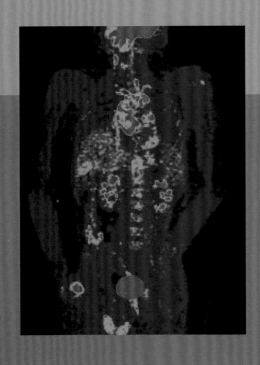

第43章
川崎病

　　川崎病（Kawasaki disease，KD）是一种病因不明的急性、系统性、自限性血管炎，可见于全人群，主要见于婴幼儿，致病机制不明。川崎病的血管病理改变包括坏死性动脉炎期、亚急性慢性血管炎期和管腔肌纤维母细胞增生期3个阶段。其中，冠状动脉扩张与冠状动脉瘤形成主要发生于坏死性动脉炎期，而管腔肌纤维母细胞增生期表现以附壁血栓形成为主。

　　川崎病的主要临床表现包括心律失常、腹泻、呕吐、咳嗽、流涕、非渗出性结膜炎、口腔黏膜炎症、皮疹、颈部淋巴结肿大、手足部位肿胀、手掌脚底发红等，实验室检查可见红细胞沉降率加快、C反应蛋白水平升高、低蛋白血症、脑脊液单核细胞增多等。川崎病急性期的主要治疗方案为通过阿司匹林、丙种球蛋白、皮质醇等药物减少全身炎症反应，尽量减少冠状动脉瘤的发生。由于该病为自限性疾病，急性期后大多数患者可以痊愈，但已产生冠状动脉瘤的患者需接受密切随访并预防冠状动脉血栓形成。

吴学君

Kawasaki Disease

Kevin G. Friedman and Jane W. Newburger

Kawasaki disease (KD), initially described by Dr. Tomisaku Kawasaki in 1967,[1] is an acute systemic vasculitis of uncertain etiology that predominantly affects infants and young children. The disease has been described worldwide and occurs in all populations. The acute illness is self-limited and is characterized by a nonexudative conjunctivitis, inflammation of the oral mucosa, rash, cervical adenopathy, and findings in the extremities, including swollen hands and feet as well as red palms and soles (Box 43.1). Coronary artery dilation or aneurysms affect up to 25% of those who are not treated with intravenous gamma globulin (IVIG) early in the course of the disease.[2] Angina, myocardial infarction (MI), and death may ensue——during the acute phase[3] or months to years later[4]——in patients who develop aneurysms.

EPIDEMIOLOGY

Despite its description in diverse areas of the world, the incidence of KD differs according to race and ethnicity, with the highest rates in Asia. Indeed, in the most recent Japanese nationwide survey performed in calendar years 2011 and 2012, the incidence rate was approximately 250 per 100,000 children younger than 5 years of age.[5] The incidence of KD has continued to increase in Japan, either because of a greater number of cases or increased awareness and diagnosis of patients with incomplete criteria. Genetic factors have long been recognized to play an important role in susceptibility to KD. Children of Japanese ancestry have a relative risk 10 to 15 times higher than that of Caucasian children, whether they live in Japan or the United States. Furthermore, siblings have a relative risk 6 to 10 times greater than that of children without a family history. The parents of Japanese children with KD are twice as likely than expected in the general population to have had the disease themselves in childhood.[6] Lack of a mandatory national reporting system in the United States hinders epidemiological analysis, but administrative data from hospital discharge indicates that more than 4000 US hospitalizations per year are due to KD.[7] In the United States, the incidence is approximately 21 cases per 100,000 children, higher among Asians and Pacific Islanders (30 per 100,000), followed by non-Hispanic African Americans (17 per 100,000), Hispanics (16 per 100,000) and Caucasians (12 per 100,000).[7] The incidence rate in the United States has been stable. Outbreaks are more likely in the late winter and early spring, suggesting an infectious etiology, but a steady background activity of cases is noted throughout the remainder of the year. Males outnumber females, generally in a ratio of 1.4:1. Although KD is most common in children younger than age 5, the illness is being more commonly recognized in older children and adolescents.[8,9]

ETIOLOGY AND PATHOGENESIS

The search for an etiological agent has been wide-ranging over the course of the past four decades, but to date the cause of KD is unknown.

An infectious cause or trigger in genetically susceptible individuals is the most widely accepted theory. Although KD is not spread by person-to-person transmission, features suggesting an infectious etiology include its self-limited and typically nonrecurring course; peak incidence in young children; clinical features including fever, rash, and conjunctivitis; the increase in incidence in winter and early spring; and the past occurrence of nationwide epidemics in Japan. Some researchers hold that KD is caused by a single agent,[10] but others believe the marked immune response typical in KD can be triggered by a variety of different agents.[11] Reports of selective expansion of $V_\beta2$ and $V_\beta8$ T-cell receptor families have implicated specific superantigens, including TSST-1-secreting strains of *Staphylococcus aureus* and streptococcal pyrogenic exotoxin B- and C-producing streptococci.[12] The only animal model of KD, which uses *Lactobacillus casei* to induce coronary arteritis in mice, implicates a toxin-mediated etiology.[13] By contrast, studies by Rowley et al. suggest a possible typical antigen-driven response to infection with a novel ribonucleic acid virus that enters through the upper respiratory tract.[14-18] Other studies propose an idiosyncratic immune response, influenced by host genetics, that is triggered by an environmental exposure carried by winds.[19,20] This theory is suggested by links between the seasonality of KD to tropospheric wind patterns. The importance of genetic factors in susceptibility is supported by the influence of race and family history on its incidence. In addition, an increasing literature has explored the association of genetic polymorphisms to susceptibility to the disease and to the development of aneurysms.[21-27]

KD is accompanied by significant derangements in the immunoregulatory system that lead to coronary inflammation and coronary artery abnormalities (dilation, aneurysm formation, and giant aneurysms) in some patients. Profound immune activation is evidenced by the release of proinflammatory cytokines and growth factors, endothelial cell (EC) activation, and infiltration of the coronary arterial wall——first by neutrophils and then by $CD68^+$ monocytes and macrophages; $CD8^+$, $CD3^+$, and $CD20^+$ lymphocytes; and IgA plasma cells.[28-32] Release of matrix metalloproteinases (MMPs) may further disrupt arterial wall integrity, leading to aneurysms of the coronary arteries and occasionally of other extraparenchymal medium-sized muscular arteries.[33] KD patients with coronary artery lesions have higher levels of MMPs and higher ratios of MMPs to tissue inhibitors of metalloproteinases (TIMPs) than those without coronary abnormalities,[34] suggesting that these circulating proteins may play an active role in the remodeling of coronary arteries. Data suggesting an important role for MMPs in the pathogenesis of aneurysms also come from recent research on genetic risk factors, showing that MMP-3 rs3025058 (–/T) and haplotypes containing MMP-3 rs3025058 (–/T) and MMP-12 rs2276109 (A/G) were associated with a higher risk of aneurysm formation.[35] In addition to MMP haplotypes, increased susceptibility to KD has been related to genetic variations in the transforming growth factor (TGF)-β pathway,[31] CC chemokine receptor 5 (CCR5) and/or its ligand CCL3L1,[36] and

BOX 43.1　Principal Clinical Findings in Kawasaki Disease

Fever persisting at least 5 days or more without other source in association with at least four principal features:

1. Oral changes that may include erythema or cracking of the lips, strawberry tongue, erythema of the oral mucosa
2. Bilateral nonexudative conjunctival injection
3. Polymorphous rash, generally truncal involvement, nonvesicular
4. Changes of extremities——may include erythema and edema of the hands or feet, desquamation of fingers and toes 1–3 weeks after onset of illness
5. Cervical lymphadenopathy, often unilateral, with at least 1 node ≥1.5 cm
   Patients with fever and fewer than four criteria can be diagnosed with the presence of coronary artery disease by two-dimensional echocardiography or coronary angiography.

Modified from American Heart Association Scientific Statement. Diagnosis, treatment, and long-term management of Kawasaki disease. *Circulation.* 2004;110:2751.

ITPKC (a negative regulator of T cell activation),[37] among others. In a genome-wide association study, investigators recently identified a single functional network containing LNX1, CAMK2D, ZFHX3, CSMD1, and TCP1, believed to be relevant to inflammation and apoptosis.[38] Functional genomics may eventually lead to the development of new diagnostic tests and therapies for KD.

PATHOLOGY

Because mortality in this disease is uncommon (ranging from 0% to 0.17% in the United States), published studies on the histopathology of early KD are limited.[39,40] The original pathological description of KD by Fujiwara and Hamashima was based on autopsy findings of children dying in the acute and subacute phases of KD before IVIG treatment became available.[39] More recent work has described the pathologic mechanisms of coronary artery aneurysm development in greater detail.[41,42] Three linked processes are responsible for KD vasculopathy: necrotizing arteritis, subacute chronic vasculitis, and luminal myofibroblastic proliferation. Necrotizing arteritis begins in the acute phase, is complete after about 2 weeks of illness, and is characterized by neutrophilic infiltration of arterial walls initiated at the endothelial surface. This process can result in progressive necrosis of the endothelium as well as the media and adventitia, and the formation of large saccular coronary artery aneurysms; in the most severe cases, this process leaves only a residual rim of adventitia in the affected segment. These lesions are responsible for the rare but catastrophic cases of coronary artery rupture. The second process is subacute chronic vasculitis, which begins within the initial 2 weeks of illness and can persist for months to years. It is characterized by the infiltration of vessel walls by lymphocytes, plasma cells, and eosinophils, starting at the adventitia and progressing inward toward the endothelium. The third process, luminal myofibroblastic proliferation, occurs in close concert with subacute chronic vasculitis and involves smooth muscle–derived myofibroblasts and their associated matrix products laying down a concentric mass within the vessel wall. The activated myofibroblasts can persist for months or years after KD and lead to progressive coronary obstruction. This partially explains why coronary artery stenosis in KD is often progressive over years and even decades. Large fusiform aneurysms with a preserved medial layer frequently narrow due to luminal myofibroblastic proliferation with or without associated thrombus. Giant saccular aneurysms, in which only the adventitial layer is preserved, typically develop stenosis due to the repetitive layering of thrombi. In both types

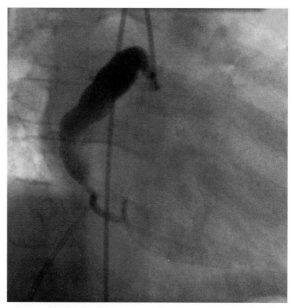

Fig. 43.1 Isolated giant aneurysm of the left anterior descending coronary artery in a 7-year-old boy who received multiple doses of intravenous gamma globulin and plasmapheresis for persistent fever.

of aneurysms, markedly abnormal flow conditions are present with low wall sheer, wall stress, and stasis in combination with the activation of platelets, clotting factors, and the endothelium; all of these promote thrombosis.[2]

The outcome of coronary aneurysms over time largely depends on their size in the acute phase.[43–45] Mildly dilated coronary arteries typically remodel to a normal internal luminal diameter. However, large aneurysms that have lost their intimal and medial layers cannot remodel to normal. Thrombus can develop in coronary aneurysms, particularly giant aneurysms, and may be completely occlusive but may also organize, recanalize, and calcify (Fig. 43.1). Arteries with partially preserved media can develop thrombosis or progressive stenosis from luminal myofibroblastic proliferation.

Myocarditis is found in the majority of patients and is the earliest cause of death.[39,46] Small histopathological series have demonstrated myocardial edema and a variable cellular inflammatory infiltrate with neutrophils, monocytes, macrophages, and/or eosinophils.[47] After the first 10 days, death is most often caused by MI due to thrombosis. Mortality peaks between 15 and 45 days after the onset of fever, when patients are in a hypercoagulable state, with thrombocytosis and disrupted vascular endothelium.[2] Beyond the first 1 to 2 years after onset of the illness, mortality declines significantly, but MI may occur many years later because of progressive coronary artery stenosis.[43,44]

CLINICAL PRESENTATION

Because no laboratory test or pathognomonic feature is available for KD, the diagnosis must be made on clinical grounds. First described by Kawasaki on the basis of his observations in Japanese children,[48] the classic criteria have continued to serve as the diagnostic standard adopted by the American Heart Association (AHA; see Box 43.1).[2] They include fever for 5 days or more and at least four of the five following findings: (1) a nonexudative bilateral conjunctivitis; (2) oral changes with erythematous or dry cracked lips, strawberry tongue, or pharyngitis; (3) a nonvesicular rash, often involving the trunk, perineum, and extremities; (4) erythema of the palmar and plantar surfaces, edema of the hands or feet, or periungual desquamation 2 weeks after illness onset; and (5) anterior cervical lymphadenopathy of 1.5 cm or greater, usually unilateral. Alternatively, the diagnosis can be made with fewer than four of five criteria in the presence of coronary artery abnormalities. Not all criteria have to be present simultaneously to make the diagnosis; indeed, it is common for some findings to resolve as others appear, making serial evaluation of the child essential.

The classic epidemiological case definition is not fulfilled in almost one-third of children who develop coronary artery aneurysms.[49] To capture these incomplete cases, the 2017 AHA recommendations include an algorithm for the evaluation and treatment of suspected KD in children with at least 5 days of fever and only two or three clinical criteria.[2] Furthermore, infants younger than 6 months of age present a particular challenge because they often have incomplete criteria yet are at greater risk for the development of coronary artery abnormalities.[43,50] The diagnosis should be considered and echocardiography performed in young infants who have had a fever for at least 7 days without a documented source and who have high systemic inflammatory markers.[2]

Other supportive signs are present in many children with KD (Box 43.2). When it is perineal in location, the rash often desquamates

---

BOX 43.2   Other Significant Clinical and Laboratory Findings in Kawasaki Disease

Cardiovascular
On auscultation, gallop rhythm or distant heart sounds; ECG changes (arrhythmias, abnormal Q waves, prolonged PR and/or QT intervals; occasionally low-voltage or ST-T wave changes); chest x-ray abnormalities (cardiomegaly); echocardiographic changes (pericardial effusion, coronary aneurysms, or decreased contractility); mitral and/or aortic valvular insufficiency; rarely, aneurysms of peripheral arteries (e.g., axillary), angina pectoris, or MI

Gastrointestinal
Diarrhea, vomiting, abdominal pain, hydrops of gallbladder, paralytic ileus, mild jaundice, and mild increase of serum transaminase levels

Blood
Increased ESR, leukocytosis with left shift, positive CRP, hypoalbuminemia, and mild anemia in acute phase of illness (thrombocytosis in subacute phase)

Urine
Sterile pyuria of urethral origin and occasional proteinuria

Skin
Perineal rash and desquamation in subacute phase and transverse furrows of fingernails (Beau lines) during convalescence

Respiratory
Cough, rhinorrhea, and pulmonary infiltrate

Joints
Arthralgia and arthritis

Neurological
Mononuclear pleocytosis in cerebrospinal fluid, striking irritability, and (rarely) facial palsy

CRP, C-reactive protein; *ECG,* electrocardiogram; *ESR,* erythrocyte sedimentation rate; *MI,* myocardial infarction.
Modified from American Heart Association Scientific Statement. Diagnosis, treatment, and long-term management of Kawasaki disease. *Circulation.* 2004;110:2751.

---

by the end of the first week of illness. Anterior uveitis can be identified by slit-lamp examination in 83% of patients early in the course.[51] Arthralgia and arthritis of large and small joints may be severe enough that children refuse to walk or perform tasks with their hands, but the arthritis is virtually never chronic. Abdominal signs including vomiting, diarrhea, or hydrops of the gallbladder are common.

Laboratory values in the acute phase are consistent with systemic inflammation. Acute-phase reactants, including erythrocyte sedimentation rate (ESR) and C-reactive protein (CRP), are markedly increased. The white blood cell (WBC) count is elevated with a leftward shift, and a normochromic, normocytic anemia is noted within the first week of illness. Thrombocytosis is usually present by the second week of the disease, often peaking at counts greater than 1,000,000 mm^3 in association with hypercoagulability. These parameters often persist over the first month of the illness and gradually decline. Hepatocellular inflammation is accompanied by increases in γ-glutamyl transferase. Sterile pyuria and pleocytosis of cerebrospinal fluid,[52] both with mononuclear cells, are found frequently. Laboratory measures of systemic inflammation usually return to normal by 6 to 8 weeks after illness onset.

CARDIAC MANIFESTATIONS

Coronary Artery Abnormalities

Coronary artery aneurysms are the most serious long-term complication of KD. Long-term outcomes are related to the extent of dilation of the coronary arteries in the first month of illness. Coronary artery abnormalities occur in 15% to 25% of patients who are not treated in the acute phase of the disease with high-dose IVIG.[2] Coronary abnormalities may be observed by echocardiography as early as 1 week from fever onset, with further aneurysmal enlargement over the ensuing 3 to 4 weeks and occasionally beyond this time.[43] Given the difficulty in reaching diagnostic confirmation of the illness using the classic criteria, identification of those at higher risk for coronary disease and for whom early treatment could reduce extent of involvement has led investigators to focus on predictive factors for coronary artery abnormalities. Late diagnosis with resultant delayed IVIG treatment beyond 10 days of illness is the most important modifiable risk factor.[34,43] Infants younger than age 6 months are at the highest risk for developing aneurysms even when they are treated within the first 10 days of illness.[50,53] The youngest infants frequently present with incomplete or atypical features, further increasing their risk of aneurysms by delaying diagnosis and IVIG treatment. Older children are also at higher risk for coronary aneurysms, in part because care providers do not consider KD as high in the differential diagnosis of the older child with fever.[54,55] Many studies have highlighted the association of coronary aneurysms with persistent and recrudescent fever (IVIG resistance).[56–59] Greater derangement of laboratory measures of the acute-phase response, reflecting more severe vasculitis, are also predictive and include lower hematocrit or hemoglobin (Hb), lower serum albumin, lower serum sodium, higher alanine aminotransferase, higher CRP and ESR, lower baseline serum IgG as well as elevations in interleukin (IL)-6, IL-8, and other biomarkers.[60] In addition, genetic polymorphisms (e.g., MMP haplotypes,[29] polymorphisms of vascular endothelial growth factor [VEGF] and its receptors[27]) affect host susceptibility to aneurysms.

Myocarditis

Approximately 10% of KD patients present with shock in the acute phase due to decreased myocardial systolic function and/or peripheral vasodilation with associated capillary leak.[61,62] In acute KD, myocarditis is a frequent finding at autopsy and by biopsy.[39,63] Gallium-67 citrate

scans[64] and technetium-99 m-labeled WBC scans[65] have also identified inflammatory myocardial changes in 50% to 70% of patients.
Congestive heart failure (CHF) in the acute phase of the illness is generally the result of myocarditis and improves rapidly with IVIG treatment, in many cases within 24 hours from initiation of treatment.[66]
Later implications of these early changes are speculative, but several
investigators have evaluated pathology and clinical function late after
KD. Myocardial biopsies in patients with long-term follow-up have
shown fibrosis, abnormal branching, and hypertrophy of myocytes
unrelated to duration from illness onset.[67] The clinical significance of
these findings is uncertain. Noninvasive studies of myocardial function in childhood through early adulthood show normal left ventricular (LV) function among patients who were unaffected by coronary
aneurysms. To our knowledge, however, there are no systematically
collected and unbiased studies of myocardial function in middle-aged
patients with a history of KD.

Valve Regurgitation

Mitral and aortic regurgitation have been associated with KD in both
early and chronic phases of the disease. In the acute stage, one in four
children has mitral regurgitation of mild to moderate severity detected
by two-dimensional (2D) echocardiography, which resolves in most
children by the convalescent phase.[68] The frequency of aortic regurgitation has been reported to be as high as 5% in Japanese children[69] but
only 1% in a recent North American population with KD,[68] and there
are rare reports of late-onset aortic regurgitation necessitating valve replacement.[70,71] The cause of aortic insufficiency is not known; however,
it has been reported that the aortic root enlarges from baseline and
remains dilated during the first year after illness onset,[68,72] raising the
possibility that coaptation of the leaflets is disturbed.

Other Cardiac Findings

Rarely, patients in the acute or subacute phase of KD can develop tamponade due to a pericardial effusion, although effusions greater than
1 mm occur in fewer than 5% of patients.[68,73] Rupture of a giant aneurysm into the pericardial space is an even rarer cause of pericardial
tamponade.[74–76]

CARDIAC TESTING

Electrocardiographic (ECG) findings are nonspecific and include sinus
tachycardia, prolonged PR interval, and diffuse ST-T wave changes. In
children with coronary artery aneurysms, ECG abnormalities are useful in detecting myocardial ischemia and infarction.

Using 2D echocardiography, visualization of the proximal coronary
arteries in young children is almost always possible, and measurements
correlate closely with angiographic measurements. In addition to measurements of the proximal left main, anterior descending, circumflex,
proximal, and middle right and posterior descending branches, assessments of ventricular function, pericardial fluid, and mitral and aortic regurgitation should be obtained. Coronary artery dilation may be
present as early as the first week of illness. In addition, findings on
echocardiography are used to determine the need for IVIG treatment
in children with suspected KD on the basis of fever and incomplete
criteria.[2] Echocardiography should be undertaken at the time of diagnosis or, in children with suspected incomplete KD, when the diagnosis is entertained.[2,77] In those with no coronary artery abnormalities,
serial studies are obtained within 1 to 2 weeks and 4 to 6 weeks after treatment to assess for the presence of aneurysm development.
Echocardiography should be performed more frequently in the child
with coronary dilation at baseline, persistent fever, or other factors
raising the likelihood of development of coronary aneurysms. Finally,

children with giant aneurysms (z-score ≥ 10 or absolute dimension ≥ 8
mm) are at highest risk for the development of coronary thrombosis in
the first months after illness onset. For this reason, echocardiography
should be performed once or twice a week until approximately 6 weeks
after illness onset or until the coronary arteries stop enlarging and systemic inflammation has subsided.

Classification systems for coronary artery aneurysms in terms of
size differ in Japan and the United States. The most recent criteria
from the Japanese Circulation Society (JCS) Joint Working Group
classify aneurysms as small if <4 mm, medium if 4 to 8 mm, and giant
if ≥ 8 mm; in children >5 years of age, small if <1.5 times the adjacent
segment, medium if 1.5 to 4 times, and giant if >4 times. However,
these criteria do not account for variation in body size, nor do they
differentiate between coronary artery segments. Because the use of
absolute dimension may underestimate coronary artery aneurysm
severity, particularly in infants and smaller children, coronary artery
z-scores have been proposed as a potentially superior method of coronary artery aneurysm classification.[44,78–80] The 2017 AHA guidelines
use body surface area (BSA)-adjusted coronary artery z-scores to define aneurysms as follows: small aneurysm has z-score ranging from
≥ 2.5 to <5, medium aneurysm has z-score ≥ 5 to <10 and absolute
dimension <8 mm, and large or giant aneurysm have a z-score of ≥ 10
or absolute dimension ≥ 8 mm.[2]

Echocardiography in the acute phase of KD is also useful for assessing LV dysfunction. Among patients without coronary aneurysms,
systolic function rapidly improves following IVIG administration.[66,68]
Diastolic function, specifically relaxation, is impaired in acute KD.
Patients with coronary aneurysms may continue to have long-term diastolic dysfunction even when systolic function is preserved.[81]

Although echocardiography has high sensitivity and specificity for
the detection of dilation in the proximal coronary arteries, it is less
useful for detection of coronary stenoses and aneurysms in the distal
coronary vasculature. The quality of coronary imaging by echocardiography also diminishes as children grow larger, limiting its utility
in long-term follow-up of the patient with KD. Therefore imaging of
the coronary arteries by ultrafast computed tomographic angiography
(CTA) and magnetic resonance angiography (MRA) is used to obtain
high-resolution images.[82–86] The quality of coronary artery imaging is
superior with CTA, and radiation dosage in the most state-of-the-art
systems is much lower than it was in the past. MRA has the advantages
of not requiring ionizing radiation, and, in the child who is too young
to exercise on a treadmill or bicycle, can be used with dobutamine or
adenosine stress to delineate reversible ischemia.

Children with aneurysms should undergo periodic stress testing
with assessment of myocardial perfusion or function. Most methods
of stress testing used in adult cardiology have been reported in small
series of children with KD.[87–92] Because the sensitivity and specificity
of tests to provoke myocardial ischemia have been exhaustively studied in adults with coronary artery disease, adult guidelines should be
followed to choose the best test based upon specific characteristics of
the patients.[2] Additional factors in the choice of modality for testing
include institutional expertise with particular techniques as well as
the age and ability of the child to cooperate with exercise. To avoid
false-positive test results, stress testing should be performed only in
children with a history of coronary artery aneurysms.

Coronary angiography has traditionally been the gold standard
for the diagnostic assessment of coronary abnormalities. With rapid
technical improvement in noninvasive imaging modalities and concerns about the use of ionizing radiation in children, invasive studies are now generally reserved for children with aneurysms in whom
noninvasive testing is insufficient to guide treatment or in whom revascularization is needed.[2] Aneurysms are described as *localized* or

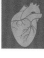

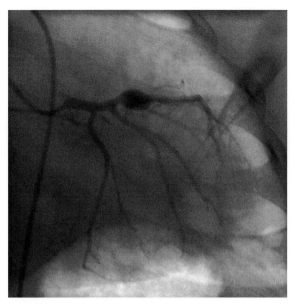

Fig. 43.2 Ectatic giant aneurysm of the right coronary artery (maximum diameter 11 mm) from the same patient as in Fig. 43.1.

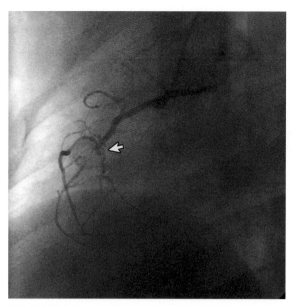

Fig. 43.3 Calcified thrombotic right coronary artery giant aneurysm in a 10-year-old boy diagnosed with Kawasaki disease at 1 year of age. The lesion is stenotic proximally *(arrow)* with recanalized distal vessels.

extensive, the former being further subclassified as *fusiform* or *saccular* (see Fig. 43.1). Extensive aneurysms, those that involve more than one segment, are *ectatic* (dilated uniformly, Fig. 43.2, or *segmented*, with multiple dilated segments joined by normal or stenotic segments). Aneurysms may also involve other medium- to large-sized extraparenchymal arteries, so-called peripheral artery aneurysms, particularly involving the subclavian, axillary, femoral, iliac, renal, and mesenteric arteries. Occasionally aneurysms of the aorta may occur. However, aneurysms outside the coronary arterial system rarely occur in the absence of giant coronary aneurysms.

CLINICAL COURSE

Persistent Coronary Aneurysms

After expanding in diameter over the first 4 to 6 weeks of illness, coronary aneurysms in KD tend to regress over time. Their regression to a normal internal luminal diameter occurs in about 55% to 70% of patients within 1 to 2 years of illness.[43,93] Substantial regression in aneurysmal diameter after 2 years is unlikely. The strongest predictor of regression is the initial size of the aneurysm, with smaller coronary aneurysms being more likely to improve.[43,44,94] Giant aneurysms are unlikely to regress.[95] In regressed aneurysms, intravascular ultrasound examination reveals myointimal thickening, which is most severe in patients whose coronary diameters were initially the largest.[96,97] Furthermore, coronary and peripheral vascular reactivity may be impaired in patients with either persistent or regressed aneurysms.[81]

Among patients with persistent coronary aneurysms, the prevalence of arterial stenosis increases linearly with time owing to myointimal proliferation at the entrance or exit of the aneurysm. Giant aneurysms are at highest risk; stenoses commonly occur at the distal end of these lesions (Fig. 43.3) and, together with sluggish blood flow in the grossly dilated arterial segment, predispose to thrombosis and infarction. Relative to smaller aneurysms, giant aneurysms are more frequently associated with late stenosis and sudden death from infarction.[43,44,98] A recent Japanese study using maximal coronary dimensions during initial illness reported a 20-year prevalence of stenotic lesions of 84% for those with z-scores ≥10, 29% for those with z-scores

≥5 and <10, and 0% for those with z-scores <5.[44] In the largest reported series of patients with giant aneurysms (median observation 19 years), survival rates at 10, 20, and 30 years after disease onset were 95%, 88%, and 88%, and cumulative rates of coronary intervention at 5, 15, and 25 years were 28%, 43%, and 59%, respectively.[95] In addition to stenoses, coronary arteries that have been affected by aneurysm formation may become increasingly tortuous and calcified, and they are prone to thrombotic occlusion. Rupture of an aneurysm is a rare event that occurs in the first months after illness onset in children whose aneurysms are expanding rapidly.

The principal cause of death in KD is MI, resulting from thrombotic occlusion and/or stenosis. MI in children can be clinically silent or present with atypical symptoms.[99] The highest risk for infarction occurs in patients with giant aneurysms, where sluggish flow, sometimes combined with stenosis at the aneurysm exit, increases the risk of thrombosis. The risk of MI is highest in the first year following diagnosis and seems to decrease after 2 years, although risk of myocardial ischemia is lifelong. Indeed, a history of KD may first become apparent when MI occurs in an adult with coronary aneurysms.[100] In San Diego county, 5% of patients under the age of 40 years with acute coronary syndrome had events resulting from earlier KD.[101] Fatalities due to MI are more likely with occlusion of the left main coronary artery or proximal segments of the right and anterior descending coronaries. Thrombosis of the right coronary artery is more likely to be silent and to recanalize. Patients with prior MI are at risk for further ischemic events, although the risk can be decreased with effective revascularization. Not surprisingly, ejection fraction is a significant predictor of long-term survival after MI, with poor 30-year survival when ejection fraction is 45% or less.[102]

Regressed Coronary Aneurysms

Regression of aneurysms appears to result from myofibroblastic proliferation,[41,42,103,104] suggesting that even patients with coronary aneurysms that have remodeled to a normal internal luminal diameter have lifelong abnormalities of coronary structure and function. In a study of patients with KD receiving isosorbide dinitrate at catheterization, those segments with regressed aneurysms as well as regions with persistent

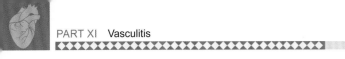

aneurysms had diminished reactivity relative to coronary arteries that had never been dilated or to coronary arteries of control patients.[105]

No Detectable Lesions

Autopsy studies of incidental deaths are limited. In one series, five children who died of incidental causes following KD underwent postmortem examination.[39] Microscopic examination of the coronary arteries revealed intimal thickening and fibrosis indistinguishable from that of atherosclerosis, but correlation with clinical status was not possible. On positron emission tomography (PET), Kawasaki patients who never had aneurysms had lower myocardial reserve and higher total coronary resistance without regional perfusion abnormalities compared with controls, suggesting an abnormal coronary microcirculation.[106] Testing of coronary endothelial function by infusing acetylcholine in the epicardial coronary arteries of Kawasaki patients and comparison patients has yielded conflicting results,[107,108] as have studies on peripheral arterial stiffness and brachial reactivity.[109–111]

The preponderance of evidence, however, suggests that individuals who had KD with always normal coronary arteries have an outlook similar to that of the normal population.[112] In the absence of a history of coronary aneurysms, KD has not been associated with an increase in standardized mortality ratio in adulthood.[112] Moreover, coronary artery calcium scores by CTA are normal in adults with a history of KD who never had coronary aneurysms, in contrast to findings in the aneurysm population.[113] Undue emphasis on coronary and myocardial sequelae in KD patients without detectable coronary dilation in any phase of illness can have the adverse effect of creating a "cardiac nondisease."[114] These considerations led to the 2017 AHA recommendation that patients in whom coronary artery dimensions were always normal do not need long-term cardiac follow-up.

TREATMENT

Therapy in the acute phase of the illness is aimed at reducing the systemic inflammatory response, minimizing the occurrence of coronary artery aneurysms, and preventing acute coronary thrombosis in those who develop aneurysms. Late management focuses on the prevention of myocardial ischemia and infarction among patients with persistent aneurysms and the reduction in risk factors for later atherosclerotic coronary artery disease (CAD) in all patients.

Antiinflammatory Therapy During Acute Kawasaki Disease

Aspirin

Aspirin has been a mainstay of therapy for KD, both for its antiinflammatory and antithrombotic effects. Meta-analysis has shown that low-dose or high-dose aspirin regimens in conjunction with IVIG lead to a similar incidence of coronary abnormalities at 30 and 60 days from the onset of illness.[115] The 2017 AHA guidelines recommend the administration of moderate (30 to 50 mg/kg/day) to high-dose (80 to 100 mg/kg/day) ASA divided into four daily doses until the patient is afebrile and then reducing the dosage to antiplatelet-dose aspirin (81 mg once daily; Box 43.3) to reduce the likelihood of Reye syndrome or gastrointestinal bleeding. In patients with aneurysms, low-dose aspirin therapy is continued, sometimes in combination with anticoagulants or other antiplatelet agents.

Intravenous Gamma Globulin

IVIG was first administered to children with KD in 1984[116]; it has been shown reduce the likelihood of coronary aneurysms and the inflammatory response in the acute phase. Many subsequent studies have confirmed the efficacy of high-dose IVIG and identified optimal

> ### BOX 43.3 Accepted Therapy for Acute Kawasaki Disease
>
> Intravenous gamma globulin (IVIG) 2 g/kg as a single infusion over 8–12 hours
> *and*
> High- (80–100 mg/kg/day) or moderate- (30–50 mg/kg/day) dose aspirin divided equally four times daily until patient has been afebrile for at least 48 hours
> *followed by*
> Aspirin 3–5 mg/kg in a single daily dose; discontinued at 6–8 weeks if echocardiogram is normal

dosing as a single administration of 2 g/kg given over 8 to 12 hours (see Box 43.3).[116–118] Children who are acutely ill with KD should be given IVIG no later than the 10th day of illness and ideally within the first 7 days.[118,119] Meta-analyses of IVIG treatment compared with placebo have shown a conclusive decrease in coronary artery abnormalities among IVIG-treated patients, reducing the prevalence of aneurysms approximately fivefold to <5%.[120,121] The mechanism of action of IVIG remains unknown. Patients with fever beyond 10 days of illness should also receive IVIG, as should those with aneurysm formation and evidence of persistent inflammation.[119] Approximately 15% of children have persistent or recrudescent fever after IVIG treatment (so-called IVIG resistance).[2] Although not tested in a randomized trial, retreatment with IVIG 2 g/kg or an alternative antiinflammatory agent (see later) is often administered if recurrent or recrudescent fever is present more than 36 hours after completion of an initial course of IVIG.[122] Of note, patients with a non-O blood type who receive multiple doses of IVIG in the context of ongoing inflammation are at increased risk for hemolytic anemia and should be appropriately monitored.[123]

Corticosteroids

Corticosteroids are widely used in the treatment of other vasculitides but their use in KD has long been controversial. Corticosteroids were used as the initial therapy prior to the first report of IVIG efficacy, and early studies showed no ill effects and possible benefit.[124–128] More recently, the RAISE (Randomized Controlled Trial to Assess Immunoglobulin Plus Steroid Efficacy for KD) study group conducted a multicenter, prospective, randomized, open-label, blinded end-points trial to assess the efficacy of IVIG (2 g/kg) plus intravenous prednisolone (2 mg/kg/day) for 5 days followed by an oral steroid taper over weeks in Japanese patients who were at high risk for coronary aneurysms based on clinical scoring criteria (Kobayashi score).[129] The steroid group had a lower incidence of coronary artery abnormalities and treatment resistance, lower coronary artery z-scores, and more rapid resolution of fever as well as decline in CRP levels. A recent meta-analysis that included this trial, using different regimens of steroids and different prediction scores, found that a combination of corticosteroid with standard-dose IVIG as primary treatment in high-risk patients reduced the rate of coronary artery abnormalities.[130] Unfortunately the Japanese scoring systems for IVIG resistance and aneurysms have low sensitivity in North American populations; therefore further work is needed to develop predictive scores of high-risk patients outside of Japan and to test the efficacy of the RAISE steroid protocol in this population.[131,132]

Corticosteroids are often used as rescue therapy in the patient with IVIG-resistant KD, with most reports comprising case series.[133–135] Kobayashi et al. reported on a retrospective cohort of 359 consecutive IVIG-resistant patients and found lower rates of coronary anomalies and a lower rate of persistent or recrudescent fever in those treated

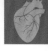

with steroids plus IVIG for rescue therapy compared with those who received only IVIG or only steroids for rescue therapy.[136]

Additional Therapies

Limited data are available concerning efficacy of other therapies that can be used in the IVIG-resistant patient. Plasmapheresis has been reported to lower the incidence of coronary disease,[137] but it is technically complex, requiring placement of large-bore catheters and the commitment of the local blood bank to assist in the exchange. Infliximab, a chimeric monoclonal antibody to tumor necrosis factor (TNF)-α, has been used as rescue therapy in IVIG-resistant patients.[138,139] A two-center retrospective study suggested that infliximab as rescue therapy shortens fever duration; however, at least in a low-risk population, it has marginal to no effect on the prevalence or size of aneurysms.[140] A small, open label, single-arm pilot trial in Japan studied cyclosporine treatment in 28 children with IVIG resistance.[141] After receiving an oral dose of 4 to 6 mg/kg/day, 78% of patients responded. Recently there has been anecdotal evidence of efficacy using anakinra, a recombinant nonglycosylated form of the human IL-1 receptor antagonist, for the treatment of IVIG-resistant KD.[142,143] Finally, in the most refractory cases of KD, where coronary aneurysms are progressively enlarging despite all other medical therapies, treatment with cytotoxic agents including cyclophosphamide has been reported.[144]

Antithrombotic Therapy

The combination of active vasculitis with endothelial damage, thrombocytosis, and hypercoagulable state creates the clinical milieu for coronary artery thrombosis. Peak occurrence for such events is 15 to 45 days from onset of illness.[2] The AHA 2017 guidelines recommend aspirin 3 to 5 mg/kg/day for 6 to 8 weeks for all patients. If the echocardiogram is normal at that time, aspirin is discontinued. If there is persistent dilation or aneurysms, aspirin is continued until regression to a normal internal luminal diameter is seen. For patients with moderate-sized aneurysms, some clinicians use combination antiplatelet therapy consisting of aspirin together with an inhibitor of adenosine diphosphate (ADP)–induced platelet aggregation (e.g., a thienopyridine).[2]

Finally, patients with large or giant aneurysms have the greatest risk for coronary thrombosis and are conventionally treated with a combination of anticoagulation and aspirin.[145] Although there has never been a randomized trial of antithrombotic treatment in KD, one series has shown that patients with giant aneurysms have a lower risk of MI if treated with aspirin and warfarin than with aspirin alone.[146] Low-molecular-weight heparin (LMWH) is used in young infants and in the first few weeks of KD, when regulation of the international normalized ratio (INR) is particularly challenging. LMWH may also be used over the longer term in those for whom warfarin management is difficult. Newer oral direct thrombin inhibitors and factor Xa inhibitors have not yet been approved for use in the pediatric population but hold promise for the future treatment of KD patients requiring anticoagulation. Women of childbearing age who have giant coronary aneurysms and are contemplating pregnancy should be counseled about the effects of warfarin and, once pregnant, should be treated in accordance with a protocol similar to that used for the pregnant woman with a mechanical prosthetic valve.[147]

Acute Coronary Thrombosis

In patients presenting with ST-elevation myocardial infarction (STEMI), timely restoration of coronary blood flow is critical to preserving myocardial function. The most effective intervention in adults with STEMI is cardiac catheterization for revascularization (i.e., percutaneous coronary intervention [PCI]). Although this is a standard procedure in adults, PCI in children may be limited by timely recognition of MI (particularly in young children), available technical expertise, and patient size. In patients who are likely have a large thrombotic burden, use of fibrinolytic therapy in conjunction with PCI may be considered.[148] In small children or those having events in remote places without capability of PCI in children, or for those with asymptomatic nonocclusive thrombus in the acute phase, thrombolytic therapy alone is used. No prospective randomized study has been undertaken to assess the preferred thrombolytic medication in KD because adequate power is precluded by the limited number of affected patients. Therapy should be instituted as soon as possible. After reperfusion of the affected vessel, anticoagulation is started with the combination of intravenous unfractionated heparin (UFH) and aspirin. This regimen is converted to warfarin or LMWH in place of intravenous UFH for chronic therapy.

CORONARY REVASCULARIZATION FOR LATE STENOSIS

The criteria for coronary revascularization in KD are based on the consensus of experts, experience in adult patients with atherosclerotic CAD, and small retrospective reviews of experience in KD.[149-154]

Coronary Artery Bypass Surgery

The decision to undertake coronary artery bypass graft (CABG) surgery is generally based on a combination of factors, including evidence of reversible ischemia on stress-imaging tests, viable myocardium in the region of distribution of the affected vessel, and absence of evidence for severe disease distal to the site of the planned graft.[152,153] Initial reports of bypass grafting in KD involved the use of saphenous veins; but early failures, particularly among younger children, led to the introduction of internal mammary artery grafts. In the current era, systemic arterial grafts (e.g., internal mammary, radial) are preferred because they increase in length and diameter with somatic growth.[149-153] Even young children have undergone successful surgical revascularization, but freedom from reintervention is longer when bypass is performed at an older age. A Japanese survey of national experience with CABG showed 15-year patency rate of 91% for those >12 years of age and 64 % for those below age 12. Of 244 patients who were included in this survey, there were 15 deaths (1 operative death, 12 late deaths, and 2 noncardiac deaths).[150] Of the total, 14 patients required repeat CABG operations, and another 17 required PCI for graft stenoses.

Percutaneous Coronary Intervention

Experience with PCI in children affected by KD is even more limited than that with CABG, but techniques for interventional catheterization procedures used in these patients are similar to those utilized in adults. Based on recommendations of the Research Committee of the Japanese Ministry of Health, Labor, and Welfare, patients with the following criteria should be considered for PCI: ischemic symptoms, presence of reversible ischemia on stress testing, or at least 75% stenosis of the left anterior descending (LAD) coronary artery.[155,156] These recommendations suggest that CABG is superior to PCI in the setting of severe LV dysfunction or in the presence of multiple ostial or long-segment coronary artery stenoses. Although early success rates for percutaneous transluminal coronary angiography, rotational ablation, and stent placement are all high, restenosis is common.[155,156] Furthermore, neoaneurysm formation is a risk of percutaneous dilation related to use of the high inflation pressures necessary to dilate the heavily calcified arteries found in KD patients.[157] For this reason, after a few years have passed since disease onset, rotational ablation and stent placement are generally preferred to percutaneous transluminal coronary angioplasty.

Because pediatric cardiologists have limited experience with interventional coronary artery techniques, percutaneous intervention should be performed by adult invasive cardiologists with support from pediatric teams when children are small.

Randomized clinical trials of CABG versus PCI have not been conducted; sample size and power would be limited by the infrequency with which revascularization is required, even in Japanese children. Using survey data comparing outcomes in patients whose first intervention was either PCI or CABG, rates of mortality and MI were similar. However, repeat revascularization therapies were administered more often to children whose first intervention was percutaneous.[156]

Cardiac transplantation is reserved for patients with end-stage ischemic cardiomyopathy who can no longer be helped by coronary revascularization.

PREVENTIVE CARDIOLOGY

Data are conflicting about whether atherosclerotic changes are more prevalent in coronary aneurysms, with some autopsy studies reporting histopathological findings of atherosclerosis[158] and others finding no evidence of atherosclerosis within aneurysmal segments.[41,42] Intravascular ultrasound studies have shown increased myointimal thickness in the coronary arteries of those with a history of aneurysms[96,97] and evidence of premature atherosclerosis in the carotid arteries at 6 to 20 years after illness onset.[158] High-sensitivity CRP levels are greater in KD patients with a history of aneurysms than among those who never developed aneurysms or in normal children.[159,160]

All patients with a history of KD should be counseled about risk factors for atherosclerotic cardiovascular disease, including the importance of a heart-healthy diet, exercise, avoidance of smoking, and, for parents, the importance of maintaining a smoke-free home.[161] In the AHA recommendations, the threshold for pharmacological treatment of hypertension and hyperlipidemia is lower for children with current and regressed coronary aneurysms.[2] Exercise recommendations for participation in competitive sports are tailored to the severity of coronary disease, but all patients with a history of KD should avoid a sedentary lifestyle.[2,162]

SUMMARY

KD is an acute vasculitis of uncertain etiology in children. Despite appropriate IVIG and ASA treatment within the first 10 days of illness, approximately 4% of patients still develop coronary artery aneurysms. Many coronary aneurysms remodel to a normal luminal diameter by myofibroblastic proliferation, but larger aneurysms may persist and can be associated with progressive stenosis, leading to ischemia and MI. Patients with coronary aneurysms are followed with regular stress testing to guide the need for invasive testing and catheter or surgical interventions. Individuals with KD without detected coronary aneurysms appear to have a later risk for atherosclerotic cardiovascular disease similar to that of the general population. As the oldest individuals with a history of KD who have had systematic surveillance are only now in middle age, the long-term natural history of KD will continue to be delineated.

REFERENCES

1. Kawasaki T. Acute febrile mucocutaneous syndrome with lymphoid involvement with specific desquamation of the fingers and toes in children (Japanese). *Jpn J Allergy*. 1967;116(3):178–222.

2. McCrindle BW, Rowley AH, Newburger JW, et al. Diagnosis, treatment, and long-term management of Kawasaki disease. A statement for health professionals from the Committee on Rheumatic Fever, Endocarditis and Kawasaki Disease, Council on Cardiovascular Disease in the Young, American Heart Association. *Circulation*. 2017;137(1):2747–2771.

3. Hayasaka S, Nakamura Y, Yashiro M, et al. Analyses of fatal cases of Kawasaki disease in Japan using vital statistical data over 27 years. *J Epidemiol*. 2003;13(5):246–250.

4. Tsuda E, Matsuo M, Naito H, et al. Clinical features in adults with coronary arterial lesions caused by presumed Kawasaki disease. *Cardiol Young*. 2007;17(1):84–89.

5. Makino N, Nakumara Y, Yashiro M, et al. Descriptive epidemiology of Kawasaki disease in Japan, 2011-2012: from the results of the 22nd nationwide survey. *J Epidemiol*. 2015;25(3):239–245.

6. Uehara R, Yashiro M, Nakamura Y, et al. Kawasaki disease in parents and children. *Acta Paediatr*. 2003;92(6):694–697.

7. Holman RC, Curns AT, Belay ED, et al. Kawasaki syndrome hospitalizations in the United States, 1997 and 2000. *Pediatrics*. 2003;112(3 Pt 1):495–501.

8. Stockheim JA, Innocentini N, Shulman ST. Kawasaki disease in older children and adolescents. *J Pediatr*. 2000;137(2):250–252.

9. Burns JC, Mason WH, Glode MP, et al. Clinical and epidemiologic characteristics of patients referred for evaluation of possible Kawasaki disease. *J Pediatr*. 1991;118(5):680–686.

10. Rowley AH, Shulman ST. Recent advances in the understanding and management of Kawasaki disease. *Curr Infect Dis Rep*. 2010;12(2):96–102.

11. Burns JC, Glode MP. Kawasaki syndrome. *Lancet*. 2004;364(9433):533–544.

12. Leung DYM. Superantigens related to Kawasaki syndrome. *Springer Semin Immunopathol*. 1996;17(4):385–396.

13. Yeung RS. Lessons learned from an animal model of Kawasaki disease. *Clin Exp Rheumatol*. 2007;25(1 Suppl 44):S69–S71.

14. Rowley AH. Kawasaki disease: novel insights into etiology and genetic susceptibility. *Annu Rev Med*. 2011;62:69–77.

15. Rowley AH, Baker SC, Shulman ST, et al. Cytoplasmic inclusion bodies are detected by synthetic antibody in ciliated bronchial epithelium during acute Kawasaki disease. *J Infect Dis*. 2005;192(10):1757–1766.

16. Rowley AH, Baker SC, Shulman ST, et al. RNA-containing cytoplasmic inclusion bodies in ciliated bronchial epithelium months to years after acute Kawasaki disease. *PLoS ONE*. 2008;3(2):e1582.

17. Rowley AH, Baker SC, Shulman ST, et al. Ultrastructural, immunofluorescence, and RNA evidence support the hypothesis of a "new" virus associated with Kawasaki disease. *J Infect Dis*. 2011;203(7):1021–1030.

18. Rowley AH, Shulman ST, Spike BT, et al. Oligoclonal IgA response in the vascular wall in acute Kawasaki disease. *J Immunol*. 2001;166(2):1334–1343.

19. Rodó X, Curcoll R, Robinson M, et al. Tropospheric winds from northeastern China carry the etiologic agent of Kawasaki disease from its source to Japan. *Prox Natl Acad Sci USA*. 2014;111(22):7952–7957.

20. Rodó X, Ballester J, Cayan D, et al. Association of Kawasaki disease with tropospheric wind patterns. *Sci Rep*. 2011;1:152.

21. Onouchi Y. Genetics of Kawasaki disease: what we know and don't know. *Circ J*. 2012;76:1581–1586.

22. Khor CC, Davila S, Shimizu C, et al. Genome-wide linkage and association mapping identify susceptibility alleles in ABCC4 for Kawasaki disease. *J Med Genet*. 2011;48:467–472.

23. Onouchi Y, Ozaki K, Buns JC, et al. Common variants in CASP3 confer susceptibility to Kawasaki disease. *Hum Mol Genet*. 2010;19:2898–2906.

24. Onouchi Y, Ozaki K, Burns JC, et al. A genome-wide association study identifies three new risk loci for Kawasaki disease. *Nat Genet*. 2012;44:517–521.

25. Ouchi K, Suzuki Y, Shirakawa T, Kishi F. Polymorphism of SLC11A1 (formerly NRAMP1) gene confers susceptibility to Kawasaki disease. *J Infect Dis*. 2003;187:326–329.

26. Tomasdottir H, Hjartarson H, Ricksten A, et al. Tumor necrosis factor gene polymorphism is associated with enhanced systemic inflammatory response and increased cardiopulmonary morbidity after cardiac surgery. *Anesth Analg*. 2003;97:944–949.

27. Kariyazono H, Ohno T, Khajoee V, et al. Association of vascular endothelial growth factor (VEGF) and VEGF receptor gene polymorphisms with coronary artery lesions of Kawasaki disease. *Pediatr Res.* 2004;56:953–959.

28. Yasukawa K, Terai M, Shulman ST, et al. Systemic production of vascular endothelial growth factor and FMS-like tyrosine kinase-1 receptor in acute Kawasaki disease. *Circulation.* 2002;105(6):766–769.

29. Asano T, Ogawa S. Expression of monocyte chemoattractant protein-1 in Kawasaki disease: the anti-inflammatory effect of gamma globulin therapy. *Scand J Immunol.* 2000;51(1):98–103.

30. Ohno T, Yuge T, Kariyazono H, et al. Serum hepatocyte growth factor combined with vascular endothelial growth factor as a predictive indicator for the occurrence of coronary artery lesions in Kawasaki disease. *Eur J Pediatr.* 2002;161(2):105–111.

31. Nomura Y, Masuda K, Maeno N, et al. Serum levels of interleukin-18 are elevated in the subacute phase of Kawasaki syndrome. *Int Arch Allergy Immunol.* 2004;135(2):161–165.

32. Takahashi K, Oharaseki T, Naoe S, et al. Neutrophilic involvement in the damage to coronary arteries in acute stage of Kawasaki disease. *Pediatr Int.* 2005;47(3):305–310.

33. Takeshita S, Tokutomi T, Kawase H, et al. Elevated serum levels of matrix metalloproteinase-9 (MMP-9) in Kawasaki disease. *Clin Exp Immunol.* 2001;125(2):340–344.

34. Gavin PJ, Crawford SE, Shulman ST, et al. Systemic arterial expression of matrix metalloproteinases 2 and 9 in acute Kawasaki disease. *Arterioscler Thromb Vasc Biol.* 2003;23(4):576–581.

35. Shimizu C, Matsubara T, Onouchi Y, et al. Matrix metalloproteinase haplotypes associated with coronary artery aneurysm formation in patients with Kawasaki disease. *J Hum Genet.* 2010;55(12):779–784.

36. Mamtani M, Matsubara T, Shimizu C, et al. Association of CCR2-CCR5 haplotypes and CCL3L1 copy number with Kawasaki disease, coronary artery lesions, and IVIG responses in Japanese children. *PLoS ONE.* 2010;5(7):e11458.

37. Onouchi Y, Gunji T, Burns JC, et al. ITPKC functional polymorphism associated with Kawasaki disease susceptibility and formation of coronary artery aneurysms. *Nat Genet.* 2008;40(1):35–42.

38. Burgner D, Davila S, Breunis WB, et al. A genome-wide association study identifies novel and functionally related susceptibility loci for Kawasaki disease. *PLoS Genet.* 2009;5(1):e1000319.

39. Fujiwara H, Hamashima Y. Pathology of the heart in Kawasaki disease. *Pediatrics.* 1978;61(1):100–107.

40. Naoe S, Takahasha M, Masuda H, et al. Kawasaki disease with particular emphasis on arterial lesions. *Acta Pathol Jpn.* 1991;41(1):785–797.

41. Orenstein JM, Shulman ST, Fox LM, et al. Three linked vasculopathic processes characterize Kawasaki disease: a light and transmission electron microscopic study. *PLoS One.* 2012;7(6):e38998.

42. Rowley AH, Orenstein JM. Clinical implications of a new model of Kawasaki disease arteriopathy. *Pediatr Cardiol.* 2013;34(5):1290–1291.

43. Friedman KG, Gauvreau K, Hamaoka-Okamoto A, et al. Coronary artery aneurysms in Kawasaki disease: risk factors for progressive disease and adverse cardiac events in US population. *J Am Heart Assoc.* 2016;5(9):15.

44. Tsuda E, Tsujii N, Hayama Y. Cardiac events and maximum diameter of coronary artery aneurysms in Kawasaki disease. *J Pediatr.* 2017;188:70–74.

45. Friedman KG, Newburger JW. Coronary artery stenosis in Kawasaki disease: size matters. *J Pediatr.* 2018;194:8–10.

46. Ino T, Akimoto K, Nishimoto K, et al. Myocarditis in Kawasaki disease. *Am Heart J.* 1989;117(6):1400–1401.

47. Yutani G, Go S, Kamiya T, et al. Cardiac biopsy of Kawasaki disease. *Arch Pathol Lab Med.* 1981;105(9):470–473.

48. Kawasaki T, Kosaki F, Okawa S, et al. A new infantile acute febrile mucocutaneous lymph node syndrome (MLNS) prevailing in Japan. *Pediatrics.* 1974;54(3):271–276.

49. Yellen ES, Gauvreau K, Takahashi M, et al. Performance of 2004 American Heart Association recommendations for treatment of Kawasaki disease. *Pediatrics.* 2010;125(2):e234–e241.

50. Salgado A, Ashouri N, Berry EK, et al. High risk of coronary artery aneurysms in infants younger than 6 months of age with Kawasaki disease. *J Pediatr.* 2017;185:112–116.

51. Burns JC, Joffe L, Sargent RA, et al. Anterior uveitis associated with Kawasaki syndrome. *Pediatr Infect Dis.* 1985;4(3):258–261.

52. Dengler LD, Capparelli EV, Bastian JF, et al. Cerebrospinal fluid profile in patients with acute Kawasaki disease. *J Ped Inf Dis.* 1998;17(6):478–481.

53. Minich LL, Sleeper LA, Atz AM, et al. Delayed diagnosis of Kawasaki disease: what are the risk factors? *Pediatrics.* 2007;120(6):e1434–e1440.

54. Muta H, Ishii M, Sakaue T, et al. Older age is a risk factor for the development of cardiovascular sequelae in Kawasaki disease. *Pediatrics.* 2004;114(3):751–754.

55. Song D, Yeo Y, Ha K, et al. Risk factors for Kawasaki disease-associated coronary abnormalities differ depending on age. *Eur J Pediatr.* 2009;168(11):1315–1321.

56. Kim T, Choi W, Woo CW, et al. Predictive risk factors for coronary artery abnormalities in Kawasaki disease. *Eur J Pediatr.* 2007;166(5):421–425.

57. Beiser AS, Takahashi M, Baker AL, et al. A predictive instrument for coronary artery aneurysms in Kawasaki disease. *Am J Cardiol.* 1998;81(9):1116–1120.

58. Sabharwal T, Manlhiot C, Benseler SM, et al. Comparison of factors associated with coronary artery dilation only versus coronary artery aneurysms in patients with Kawasaki disease. *Am J Cardiol.* 2009;104(12):1743–1747.

59. McCrindle BW, Li JS, Minich LL, et al. Coronary artery involvement in children with Kawasaki disease: risk factors from analysis of serial normalized measurements. *Circulation.* 2007;116(2):174–179.

60. Burns JC, Franco A. The immunomodulatory effects of immunoglobulin therapy in Kawasaki disease. *Expert Rev Clinc Immunol.* 2015;11(7):819–825.

61. Dominguez SR, Friedman K, Seewald R, et al. Kawasaki disease in a pediatric intensive care unit: a case-control study. *Pediatrics.* 2008;122(4):e786–e790.

62. Dionne A, Dadah N. Myocarditis and Kawasaki disease. *Intensive Care Med.* 2012;38(5):872–878.

63. Yutani C, Okano K, Kamiya T, et al. Histopathological study on right endomyocardial biopsy of Kawasaki disease. *Br Heart J.* 1980;43(5):589–592.

64. Matsuura H, Ishikita T, Yamamoto S, et al. Gallium-67 myocardial imaging for the detection of myocarditis. *Br Heart J.* 1987;58(4):385–392.

65. Kao CH, Hsieh KS, Wang YL, et al. Tc-99m HMPAO labeled WBC scan for the detection of myocarditis in different phases of Kawasaki disease. *Clin Nucl Med.* 1992;17(3):185–190.

66. Moran AM, Newburger JW, Sanders SP, et al. Abnormal myocardial mechanics in Kawasaki disease: rapid response to gamma-globulin. *Am Heart J.* 2000;139(2 Pt 1):217–223.

67. Tanaka N, Naoe S, Masuda H, et al. Pathological study of sequelae of Kawasaki disease (MCLS). With special reference to the heart and coronary arterial lesions. *Acta Pathol Jpn.* 1986;36(10):1513–1527.

68. Printz BF, Sleeper LA, Newburger JW, et al. Noncoronary cardiac abnormalities are associated with coronary artery dilation and with laboratory inflammatory markers in acute Kawasaki disease. *J Am Coll Cardiol.* 2010;57(1):86–92.

69. Nakano H, Nojima K, Saito A, et al. High incidence of aortic regurgitation following Kawasaki disease. *J Pediatr.* 1985;107(1):59–63.

70. Gidding SS. Late onset valvular dysfunction in Kawasaki disease. *Prog Clin Biol Res.* 1987;250:305–309.

71. Gidding SS, Shulman ST, Ilbawi M, et al. Mucocutaneous lymph node syndrome (Kawasaki disease): delayed aortic and mitral insufficiency secondary to active valvulitis. *J Am Coll Cardiol.* 1986;7(4):894–897.

72. Ravekes WJ, Colan SD, Gauvreau K, et al. Aortic root dilation in Kawasaki disease. *Am J Cardiol.* 2001;87(7):919–922.

73. Ozdogu H, Boga C. Fatal cardiac tamponade in a patient with Kawasaki disease. *Heart Lung.* 2005;34(4):257–259.

74. Kuppuswamy M, Gukop P, Sutherland G, et al. Kawasaki disease presenting as cardiac tamponade with ruptured giant aneurysm of the right coronary artery. *Interact Cardiovasc Thorac Surg.* 2010;10(2):317–318.

75. Imai Y, Sunagawa K, Ayusawa M, et al. A fatal case of ruptured giant coronary artery aneurysm. *Eur J Pediatr.* 2005;165(2):1–4.

76. Maresi E, Passantino R, Midulla R, et al. Sudden infant death caused by a ruptured coronary aneurysm during acute phase of atypical Kawasaki disease. *Hum Pathol.* 2001;32(12):1407–1409.

77. Council on Cardiovascular Disease in the Young Committee on Rheumatic Fever Endocarditis and Kawasaki Disease American Heart Association. Diagnostic guidelines for Kawasaki disease. *Circulation*. 2001;103(2):335–336.

78. de Zorzi A, Colan SD, Gauvreau K, et al. Coronary artery dimensions may be misclassified as normal in Kawasaki disease. *J Pediatr*. 1998;133(2):254–258.

79. Manhliot C, Millar K, Golding F, McCrindle BW. Improved classification of coronary artery abnormalities based only on coronary artery z-scores after Kawasaki disease. *Pediatr Cardiol*. 2010;31(2):242–249.

80. Ronai C, Hamaoka-Okamoto A, Baker AL, et al. Coronary artery aneurysm measurement and z-score variability in Kawasaki disease. *J Am Soc Echocardiogr*. 2016;29(2):150–157.

81. Tierney ES, Newburger JW, Graham D, et al. Diastolic function in children with Kawasaki Disease. *Int J Cardiol*. 2009;148(3):309–312.

82. Greil GF, Stuber M, Botnar RM, et al. Coronary magnetic resonance angiography in adolescents and young adults with Kawasaki disease. *Circulation*. 2002;105(8):908–911.

83. Danias PG, Stuber M, Botnar RM, et al. Coronary MR angiography: clinical applications and potential for imaging coronary artery disease. *Magn Reson Imaging Clin N Am*. 2003;11(1):81–99.

84. Mavrogeni S, Papadopoulos G, Douskou M, et al. Magnetic resonance angiography is equivalent to x-ray coronary angiography for the evaluation of coronary arteries in Kawasaki disease. *J Am Coll Cardiol*. 2004;43(4):649–652.

85. Sohn S, Kim HS, Lee SW. Multidetector row computed tomography for follow-up of patients with coronary artery aneurysms due to Kawasaki disease. *Pediatr Cardiol*. 2004;25(1):35–39.

86. Dietz SM, Tacke CE, Kuipers IM, et al. Cardiovascular imaging in children and adults following Kawasaki disease. *Insights Imaging*. 2015;6(6):697–705.

87. Jan SL, Hwang B, Fu YC, et al. Comparison of 201Tl SPET and treadmill exercise testing in patients with Kawasaki disease. *Nucl Med Commun*. 2000;21:431–435.

88. Pahl E, Sehgal R, Chrystof D, et al. Feasibility of exercise stress echocardiography for the follow-up of children with coronary involvement secondary to Kawasaki disease. *Circulation*. 1995;91:122–128.

89. Noto N, Kamiyama H, Karasawa H, et al. Long-term prognostic impact of dobutamine stress echocardiography in patients with Kawasaki disease and coronary artery lesions: a 15-year follow-up study. *J Am Coll Cardiol*. 2014;63(4):337–344.

90. Noto N, Ayusawa M, Karasawa K, et al. Dobutamine stress echocardiography for detection of coronary artery stenosis in children with Kawasaki disease. *J Am Coll Cardiol*. 1996;27:1251–1256.

91. Kimball TR, Witt SA, Daniels SR. Dobutamine stress echocardiography in the assessment of suspected myocardial ischemia in children and young adults. *Am J Cardiol*. 1997;79:380–384.

92. Fukuda T, Ishibashi M, Ykoyama T, et al. Myocardial ischemia in Kawasaki disease: evaluation with dipyridamole stress technetium 99m tetrofosmin scintigraphy. *J Nucl Cardiol*. 2002;9(6):632–637.

93. Kato H, Sugimura T, Akagi T, et al. Long-term consequences of Kawasaki disease. A 10- to 21-year follow-up study of 594 patients. *Circulation*. 1996;94(6):1379–1385.

94. Kamiya T, Suzuki A, Ono Y, et al. Angiographic follow-up study of coronary artery lesion in the cases with a history of Kawasaki disease - with a focus on the follow-up more than ten years after the onset of the disease. In: Kato H, ed. *Kawasaki disease. Proceedings of the 5th International Kawasaki Disease Symposium, Fukuoka, Japan, May 22-25, 1995*. The Netherlands: Elsevier Science B.V; 1995:569–573.

95. Suda K, Iemura M, Nishiono H, et al. Long-term prognosis of patients with Kawasaki disease complicated by giant coronary aneurysms: a single-institution experience. *Circulation*. 2011;123(17):1836–1842.

96. Tsuda E, Kamiya T, Kimura K, et al. Coronary artery dilatation exceeding 4.0 mm during acute Kawasaki disease predicts a high probability of subsequent late intima-medial thickening. *Pediatr Cardiol*. 2002;23(1):9–14.

97. Iemura M, Ishii M, Sugimura T, et al. Long term consequences of regressed coronary aneurysms after Kawasaki disease: vascular wall morphology and function. *Heart*. 2000;83(3):307–311.

98. Tsuda E, Kamiya T, Ono Y, et al. Incidence of stenotic lesions predicted by acute phase changes in coronary arterial diameter during Kawasaki disease. *Pediatr Cardiol*. 2005;26(1):73–79.

99. Kato H, Ichinose E, Kawasaki T. Myocardial infarction in Kawasaki disease: clinical analyses in 195 cases. *J Pediatr*. 1986;108(6):923–927.

100. Rizk SR, El Said G, Daniels LB, et al. Acute myocardial ischemia in adults secondary to missed Kawasaki disease in childhood. *Am J Cardiol*. 2015;201:429–437.

101. Gordon JB, Kahn AM, Burns JC. When children with Kawasaki disease grow up: myocardial and vascular complications in adulthood. *J Am Coll Cardiol*. 2009;54(21):1911–1920.

102. Tsuda E, Hirata T, Matsuo O, et al. The 30-year outcome for patients after myocardial infarction due to coronary artery lesions caused by Kawasaki disease. *Pediatr Cardiol*. 2010;32(2):176–182.

103. Sugimura T, Kato H, Inoue O, et al. Intravascular ultrasound of coronary arteries in children. Assessment of the wall morphology and the lumen after Kawasaki disease. *Circulation*. 1994;89(1):258–265.

104. Sasaguri Y, Kato H. Regression of aneurysms in Kawasaki disease: a pathological study? *J Pediatr*. 1982;100(2):225–231.

105. Sugimura T. Coronary artery distensibility in Kawasaki disease—evaluation by intracoronary infusion of isosorbide dinitrate in long-term follow-up. *Kurume Med J*. 1991;38(4):317–325.

106. Muzik O, Paridon SM, Singh TP, et al. Quantification of myocardial blood flow and flow reserve in children with a history of Kawasaki disease and normal coronary arteries using positron emission tomography. *J Am Coll Cardiol*. 1996;28(3):757–762.

107. Mitani Y, Okuda Y, Shimpo H, et al. Impaired endothelial function in epicardial coronary arteries after Kawasaki disease. *Circulation*. 1997;96:454–461.

108. Yamakawa R, Ishii M, Sugimura T, et al. Coronary endothelial dysfunction after Kawasaki disease: evaluation by intracoronary injection of acetylcholine. *J Am Coll Cardiol*. 1998;31(5):1074–1080.

109. Cheung YF, Wong SJ, Ho MH. Relationship between carotid intima-media thickness and arterial stiffness in children after Kawasaki disease. *Arch Dis Child*. 2007;92(1):43–47.

110. Deng YB, Li TL, Xiang HJ, et al. Impaired endothelial function in the brachial artery after Kawasaki disease and the effects of intravenous administration of vitamin C. *Pediatr Infect Dis J*. 2003;22(1):34–39.

111. McCrindle BW, McIntyre S, Kim C, et al. Are patients after Kawasaki disease at increased risk for accelerated atherosclerosis? *J Pediatr*. 2007;151(3):244–248.

112. Nakumara Y, Aso E, Yashiro M, et al. Mortality among Japanese with history Kawasaki disease: results at the end of 2009. *J Epidemiol*. 2013;23(6):429–434.

113. Kahn AM, Budoff MJ, Daniels LB, et al. Usefulness of calcium scoring as a screening examination in patients with a history of Kawasaki disease. *Am J Cardiol*. 2017;119(7):687–696.

114. Gersony WM. The adult after Kawasaki disease: the risks for late coronary events. *J Am Coll Cardiol*. 2009;54(21):1921–1923.

115. Durongpisitkul K, Gururaj VJ, Park JM, et al. The prevention of coronary artery aneurysm in Kawasaki disease: a meta-analysis on the efficacy of aspirin and immunoglobulin treatment. *Pediatrics*. 1995;96(6):1057–1061.

116. Furusho K, Kamiya T, Nakano H, et al. High-dose intravenous gammaglobulin for Kawasaki disease. *Lancet*. 1984;2(8411): 1055–1058.

117. Red book: report of the committee on infectious disease. kawasaki disease. ed 26. In: Pickering LK, ed. Elk Grove Village, IL: American Academy of Pediatrics; 2003:394.

118. Tse SM, Silverman ED, McCrindle BW, et al. Early treatment with intravenous immunoglobulin in patients with Kawasaki disease. *J Pediatr*. 2002;140(4):450–455.

119. Marasini M, Pongiglione G, Gazzolo D, et al. Late intravenous gamma globulin treatment in infants and children with Kawasaki disease and coronary artery abnormalities. *Am J Cardiol*. 1991;68(8):796–797.

120. Oates-Whitehead RM, Baumer JH, Haines L, et al. Intravenous immunoglobulin for the treatment of Kawasaki disease in children. *Cochrane Database Syst Rev*. 2003;(4):CD004000.

121. Mori M, Miyamae T, Imagawa T, et al. Meta-analysis of the results of intravenous gamma globulin treatment of coronary artery lesions in Kawasaki disease. *Mod Rheumatol.* 2004;14:361–366.

122. Lo MS, Newburger JW. Role of intravenous immunoglobulin in treatment of Kawasaki disease. *Int J Rheum Dis.* 2017;21(1):64–69.

123. Luban NL, Wong EC, Lobo RH, et al. Intravenous immunoglobulin related hemolysis in patients treated for Kawasaki disease. *Transfusion.* 2015;55(Suppl 2):S90–S94.

124. Newburger JW, Sleeper LA, McCrindle BW, et al. Randomized trial of pulsed corticosteroid therapy for primary treatment of Kawasaki disease. *N Engl J Med.* 2007;356(7):663–675.

125. Sundel RP, Baker AL, Fulton DR, et al. Corticosteroids in the initial treatment of Kawasaki disease: report of a randomized trial. *J Pediatr.* 2003;142(6):611–616.

126. Okada Y, Shinohara M, Kobayashi T, et al. Effect of corticosteroids in addition to intravenous gamma globulin therapy on serum cytokine levels in the acute phase of Kawasaki disease in children. *J Pediatr.* 2003;143(3):363–367.

127. Shinohara M, Sone K, Tomomasa T, et al. Corticosteroids in the treatment of the acute phase of Kawasaki disease. *J Pediatr.* 1999;135(4):465–469.

128. Nonaka Z, Maekawa K, Okabe T, et al. Randomized controlled study of intravenous prednisolone and gamma globulin treatment in 100 cases with Kawasaki disease. In: *Proceedings of the Fifth International Symposium on Kawasaki Disease*; 1995.

129. Kobayashi T, Saji T, Otani T, et al. Efficacy of immunoglobulin plus prednisolone for prevention of coronary artery abnormalities in severe Kawasaki disease (RAISE study): a randomized, open-label, blinded-endpoints trial. *Lancet.* 2012;379(9826):1613–1620.

130. Wardle AJ, Connolly GM, Seager MJ, Tulloh RM. Corticosteroids for the treatment of Kawasaki disease in children. *Cochrane Database Syst Rev.* 2017;1:CD011188.

131. Sleeper LA, Minich LL, McCrindle BM, et al. Evaluation of Kawasaki disease risk-scoring systems for intravenous immunoglobulin resistance. *J Pediatr.* 2011;158:831–835.

132. Son MBF, Gauvreau K, Kim S, et al. Predicting coronary artery aneurysms in Kawasaki disease at a North American center: an assessment of baseline z-scores. *J Am Heart Assoc.* 2017;6:e005378.

133. Dale RC, Saleem MA, Daw S, et al. Treatment of severe complicated Kawasaki disease with oral prednisolone and aspirin. *J Pediatr.* 2000;137(5):723–726.

134. Wallace CA, French JW, Kahn SJ, et al. Initial intravenous gammaglobulin treatment failure in Kawasaki disease. *Pediatrics.* 2000;105(6):E78.

135. Hashino K, Ishii M, Iemura M, et al. Re-treatment for immune globulin-resistant Kawasaki disease: a comparative study of additional immune globulin and steroid pulse therapy. *Pediatr Int.* 2001;43(3):211–217.

136. Kobayashi T, Kobayashi T, Morikawa A, et al. Efficacy of intravenous immunoglobulin combined with prednisolone following resistance to initial intravenous treatment of acute Kawasaki disease. *J Pediatr.* 2013;163:521–526.

137. Imagawa T, Mori M, Miyamae T, et al. Plasma exchange for refractory Kawasaki disease. *Eur J Pediatr.* 2004;163(4–5):263–264.

138. Weiss JE, Eberhard BA, Chowdhury D, et al. Infliximab as a novel therapy for refractory Kawasaki disease. *J Rheumatol.* 2004;31(4):808–810.

139. Burns JC, Best BM, Mejias A, et al. Infliximab treatment of intravenous immunoglobulin-resistant Kawasaki disease. *J Pediatr.* 2008;153(6):833–838.

140. Son MB, Gauvreau K, Burns JC, et al. Infliximab for intravenous immunoglobulin resistance in Kawasaki disease: a retrospective study. *J Pediatr.* 2011;158(4):644–649.

141. Suzuki H, Terai M, Hamada H, et al. Cyclosporin A treatment for Kawasaki disease refractory to initial and additional intravenous immunoglobulin. *Pediatr Infect Dis J.* 2011;30:871–876.

142. Shafferman A, Birmingham JD, Cron RQ. High dose anakinra for treatment of severe neonatal Kawasaki disease: a case report. *Pediatr Rheumatol Online J.* 2014;12:26.

143. Suzuki H, Terai M, Hamada H, et al. A child with severe relapsing Kawasaki disease rescued by IL-1 receptor blockade and extracorporeal membrane oxygenation. *Ann Rheum Dis.* 2012;71:2059–2061.

144. Saneeymehri S, Baker K, So TY. Overview of pharmacological options for pediatric patients with refractory Kawasaki disease. *J Pediatr Pharmacol Ther.* 2015;20(30):163–177.

145. Manlhiot C, Brandao LR, Somji Z, et al. Long-term anticoagulation in Kawasaki disease: initial use of low molecular weight heparin is a viable option for patients with severe coronary artery abnormalities. *Pediatr Cardiol.* 2010;31(6):834–842.

146. Sugahara Y, Ishii M, Muta H, et al. Warfarin therapy for giant aneurysm prevents myocardial infarction in Kawasaki disease. *Pediatr Cardiol.* 2008;29(2):398–401.

147. Tsuda E, Ishihara Y, Kawamata K, et al. Pregnancy and delivery in patients with coronary artery lesions caused by Kawasaki disease. *Heart.* 2005;91(11):1481–1482.

148. Harada M, Akimoto K, Ogawa S, et al. National Japanese survey of thrombolytic therapy selection for coronary aneurysm: intracoronary thrombolysis or intravenous coronary thrombolysis in Kawasaki disease. *Pediatr Int.* 2013;55(6):690–695.

149. Tsuda E, Kitamura S, Kimura K, et al. Long-term patency of internal thoracic artery grafts for coronary artery stenosis due to Kawasaki disease: comparison of early with recent results in small children. *Am Heart J.* 2007;153(6):995–1000.

150. Tsuda E, Kitamura S. National survey of coronary artery bypass grafting for coronary stenosis caused by Kawasaki disease in Japan. *Circulation.* 2004;110(11 Suppl 1):II61–II66.

151. Kitamura S, Tsuda E, Kobayashi J, et al. Twenty-five-year outcome of pediatric coronary artery bypass surgery for Kawasaki disease. *Circulation.* 2009;120(1):60–68.

152. Akagi T. Interventions in Kawasaki disease. *Pediatr Cardiol.* 2005;26(2):206–212.

153. Subcommittee of Cardiovascular Sequelae. Subcommittee of Surgical Treatment, Kawasaki Disease Research Committee: guidelines for treatment and management of cardiovascular in Kawasaki disease. *Heart Vessels.* 1987;3(1):50–54.

154. Ishii M, Ueno T, Akagi T, et al. Guidelines for catheter intervention in coronary artery lesion in Kawasaki disease. *Pediatr Int.* 2001;43(5):558–562.

155. Ishii M, Ueno T, Ikeda H, et al. Sequential follow-up results of catheter intervention for coronary artery lesions after Kawasaki disease: quantitative coronary artery angiography and intravascular ultrasound imaging study. *Circulation.* 2002;105(25):3004–3010.

156. Muta H, Ishii M. Percutaneous coronary intervention versus coronary artery bypass grafting for stenotic lesions after Kawasaki disease. *J Pediatr.* 2010;157(1):120–126.

157. Takahashi K, Oharaseki T, Naoe S. Pathological study of postcoronary arteritis in adolescents and young adults: with reference to the relationship between sequelae of Kawasaki disease and atherosclerosis. *Pediatr Cardiol.* 2001;22(2):138–142.

158. Noto N, Okada T, Yamasuge M, et al. Noninvasive assessment of the early progression of atherosclerosis in adolescents with Kawasaki disease and coronary artery lesions. *Pediatrics.* 2001;107(5):1095–1099.

159. Cheung YF, Ho MH, Tam SC, et al. Increased high sensitivity C reactive protein concentrations and increased arterial stiffness in children with a history of Kawasaki disease. *Heart.* 2004;90(11):1281–1285.

160. Mitani Y, Sawada H, Hayakawa H, et al. Elevated levels of high-sensitivity c-reactive protein and serum amyloid-A late after Kawasaki disease. Association between inflammation and late coronary sequelae in Kawasaki disease. *Circulation.* 2005;111(1):38–43.

161. Kavey RE, Allada V, Daniels SR, et al. Cardiovascular risk reduction in high-risk pediatric patients: a scientific statement from the American Heart Association Expert Panel on Population and Prevention Science; the Councils on Cardiovascular Disease in the Young, Epidemiology and Prevention, Nutrition, Physical Activity and Metabolism, High Blood Pressure Research, Cardiovascular Nursing, and the Kidney in Heart Disease; and the Interdisciplinary Working Group on Quality of Care and Outcomes Research. *Circulation.* 2006;114(24):2710–2738.

162. Graham TP Jr, Driscoll DJ, Gersony WM, et al. Task Force 2: congenital heart disease. *J Am Coll Cardiol.* 2005;45(8):1326–1333.

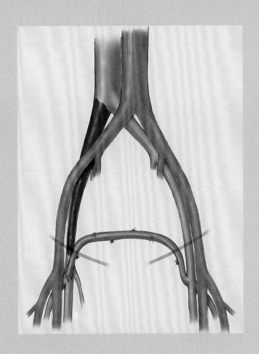

PART **XII**

第十二部分

Acute Limb Ischemia

急性肢体缺血

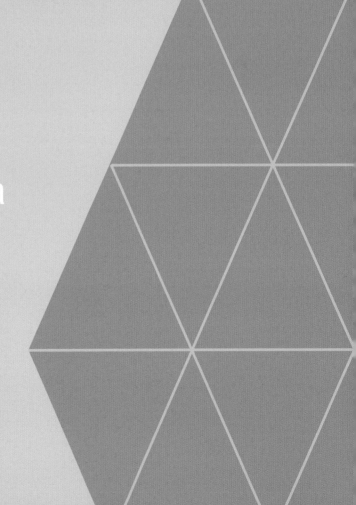

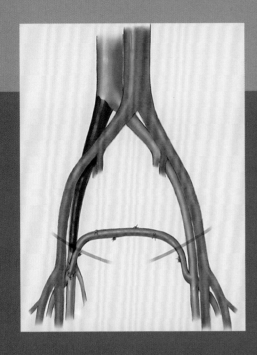

第44章
急性动脉闭塞

　　急性动脉闭塞（acute arterial occlusion，AAO）是指供应肢体或脏器的动脉非创伤性急性闭塞，脏器组织突然失去血供而导致一系列急性缺血症状。急性动脉闭塞若发生在下肢，几小时内即可造成不可逆性组织损伤，因此，急性动脉闭塞为临床急症，快速识别和急诊干预对保肢和挽救生命十分关键。需要指出的是，在临床工作中，急性动脉闭塞多指急性肢体缺血（acute limb ischemia，ALI）。由Piotr Sobieszczyk所撰写的ALI一章，虽然篇幅不大，但作者深入浅出地从ALI的流行病学、病因学、病理生理学、影像学检查和临床诊断到现代治疗方法进行了详细阐述，尤其是ALI所致筋膜室综合征的病理生理学改变和最终带来的严重后果，内容不仅细致入微，而且很自然过渡到此类患者"生命高于肢体"的原则性治疗策略。治疗方面，着重强调了经导管接触溶栓（catheter-directed thrombolysis，CDT）、机械血栓清除装置（angiojet）、真空抽栓装置（indigo system）、超声辅助溶栓装置（EKOS endowave）等腔内治疗在ALI快速恢复血流所起到的重要作用，但对于一些病情复杂患者，诸如动脉切开取栓、血管重建和杂交手术等外科手段仍不可或缺，辅助治疗方法在ALI再灌注损伤处理方面也有详尽描述。ALI是一种临床急症，本章节无论对年轻医师还是有临床经验的医师，都具有极高的临床治疗指导价值和教学价值。

翟水亭

Acute Arterial Occlusion

Piotr Sobieszczyk

Nontraumatic, acute occlusion of arterial supply to a limb or organ presents with a constellation of symptoms specific to the tissue suddenly deprived of arterial perfusion. Irrespective of the arterial segment involved, this syndrome represents a vascular emergency. Irreversible organ injury may occur within seconds in the case of acute embolic occlusion of a middle cerebral artery or take hours when arterial supply of a lower limb is involved. In everyday clinical practice, *acute arterial occlusion* is synonymous with *acute limb ischemia*. Rapid recognition and treatment are required to prevent limb loss and life-threatening morbidity. *Acute limb ischemia* is thus defined as a sudden limb-threatening decrease in arterial perfusion of less than 14 days' duration. It can occur as a result of embolic occlusion or in situ arterial thrombosis. Over the last several decades, the etiology of acute limb ischemia has varied with changing prevalence of causative conditions. The management of the syndrome has evolved, but the diagnostic skills required to recognize this clinical entity remain unchanged.

EPIDEMIOLOGY OF ACUTE LIMB ISCHEMIA

Acute limb ischemia is a rare vascular event and its incidence eludes exact quantification. It has been influenced by the ever-changing medical landscape. Increasing numbers of patients treated with antiplatelet and antithrombotic therapies, effective therapy for atrial fibrillation, and advances in treatment of valvular and ischemic heart disease have had an impact on the incidence of acute limb ischemia by decreasing the number of embolic events. This may be counterbalanced by increasing numbers of patients undergoing elective surgical and endovascular revascularization therapies, which carry a low but measurable risk of graft or stent thrombosis. An estimate in the 1990s proposed that a vascular center serving a community of 500,000 may expect an annual incidence of 75 patients with acute limb ischemia of the lower extremity.[1] Other studies report similar data, estimating the incidence of acute lower limb ischemia between 13 and 17 cases per 100,000 people per year with mortality as high as 18%, even in the modern era.[2,3] Contemporary studies report amputation rates as high as 13% in patients presenting with acute limb ischemia of the lower extremity.[4] Retrospective analysis suggests that 1-year amputation-free survival in patients with acute limb ischemia who present to the emergency department at a tertiary care facility is 71%, with 8% of survivors suffering from permanent motor deficit in the involved limb.[5]

Acute limb ischemia affects men and women equally. It is infrequent in patients with established peripheral artery disease (PAD), except in those who have undergone surgical or endovascular revascularization and developed acute thrombosis of the conduit, graft, or stent. Patients with symptomatic PAD who do not have atrial fibrillation develop acute limb ischemia at an annual rate of 1.3%. The majority (69%) of these events are due to graft or stent thrombosis, while in situ thrombosis is responsible for 27% of acute ischemic episodes.[6] Acute limb ischemia is typically a disease of middle aged and older populations, but can affect younger patients when unusual clinical events such as paradoxical embolism, intracardiac masses, and endocarditis or hypercoagulable syndromes affect the arterial circulation.

Acute, nontraumatic ischemia of the upper extremity is even more uncommon. It is less likely to result in limb loss and thus its importance has been overshadowed by lower extremity ischemic syndromes. Few published series have been reported and there are no randomized trials evaluating this clinical syndrome and its treatment; a recent review identified only 23 retrospective studies of acute upper extremity ischemia.[7] While the overall limb salvage rates exceed 90%,[7] the consequences of functional impairment in the upper extremity can be equally devastating to the patient.[8] On average, acute arm ischemia accounts for 16.6% of cases of acute ischemia of the extremities and, by extrapolation, occurs with an incidence of 1.2 to 3.5 cases per 100,000 per year.[9] However, these estimates are based primarily on surgical series which usually include only patients who underwent surgical treatment. Surveys of all patients presenting with acute arm ischemia estimate an incidence of 1.13 per 100,000 per year.[10] In the absence of more meticulous population studies, the true incidence can only be estimated. Patients with upper extremity ischemia tend to be older than those with lower extremity ischemia, with mean ages of 74 and 70, respectively.[11]

Amputation-free survival is influenced by many modifiable and nonmodifiable factors.[12] Among the former, delay in diagnosis stands out as a major factor. Non-Caucasian race, older age, malignancy, congestive heart failure, and low body weight decrease, while systemic atherosclerosis increases the likelihood of amputation-free survival.[12,13] Among patients older than 75 years, overall 30-day mortality rates approach 42%.[14] Survival and functional recovery among patients with acute limb ischemia are directly related to the underlying comorbidities and delay in diagnosis and treatment.

ETIOLOGY OF ACUTE LIMB ISCHEMIA

Acute Upper Extremity Ischemia

The most common sites of arterial occlusion in the upper extremity are the brachial and axillary arteries, representing 85% of cases of embolic occlusion.[7,9] Subclavian artery occlusion is thought to be

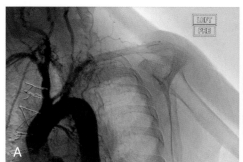 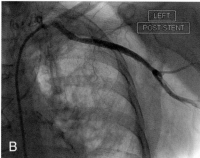 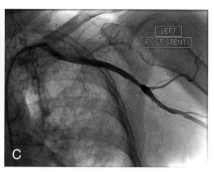

Fig. 44.1 In Situ Thrombosis of Subclavian Artery in a Patient Presenting With an Inferior ST-Segment Elevation Myocardial Infarction and Symptoms of Acute Left Arm and Hand Ischemia. Panel (A) depicts occlusion of the subclavian artery with angiographic changes suggestive of in situ thrombosis. After balloon angioplasty and stenting of the subclavian artery, the thrombotic component of the lesion is seen trapped in the filter embolic protection device positioned in the axillary artery (B). Panel (C) shows a patent vessel after filter retrieval.

the most frequent site of occlusion in uncommon cases of in situ thrombosis (Fig. 44.1).

Iatrogenic Causes

In the past, acute ischemia of the arm was primarily caused by cardiac catheterization performed via brachial artery access (Fig. 44.2). In a series from the 1980s reporting on 37 cases of acute arm ischemia treated surgically over a period of 5 years, 56% of the cases were caused by this iatrogenic complication, 24% were related to embolic events, while the remainder was due to stab wounds.[15] Since brachial artery catheterization fell out of favor, causes of upper extremity ischemia have changed. In a later series of 65 patients with acute arm ischemia treated surgically in a span of 8 years, a cardioembolic source was identified in 41% of patients, 17% of events were attributed to arterial source of embolism, and 28% of cases were related to iatrogenic occlusion, mainly a result of cardiac catheterization.[16] The resurgence of interest in radial artery access for coronary procedures is unlikely to result in a rise in frequency of upper extremity ischemia. Occlusion of the radial artery, seen in up to 5% of procedures, is unlikely to compromise perfusion of the hand in a patient with proper preprocedural assessment of a patent palmar arch.

Embolism

Embolic occlusion is the most frequent cause of acute arm ischemia accounting for 74% to 100% of cases in several reported series.[9,10,16–18] Of these, 72% are thought to be cardioembolic in source, 12% originate from

the proximal vessel, and the remainder are of unknown origin.[9] Atrial fibrillation and left ventricular thrombus in patients with ventricular dysfunction are the most frequent causes of cardiac emboli. Other rare causes of embolization are atrial myxoma[19–21] and paradoxical embolism[22] via a patent foramen ovale. Proximal arteries of the arm can be a source of arterial embolism. Artery-to-artery embolization may cause occlusion of a large or medium caliber artery, but more commonly presents with digital embolization. Atherosclerotic stenosis of the subclavian artery is a rare cause of embolism, but can result in acute hand or arm ischemia.[23–25] The rare primary subclavian artery aneurysm, or one caused by external compression in thoracic outlet syndrome, can result in thromboembolic occlusion of upper extremity arteries.[24,26–28] Aortic arch atheroma has also been implicated as the source of acute arm ischemia.[18,29] Other rare arterial sources of embolic events are malignant emboli or paradoxical embolism through intracardiac shunting (Fig. 44.3).[30,31]

Thrombosis

Atherosclerotic disease is much less frequent in the upper extremity compared to the lower limb. Consequently, in situ thrombosis is uncommon and has been estimated to account for 5% of ischemic cases in population studies and 5% to 35% of cases in surgical series.[10,17,18,32] Many of the proximal arterial lesions responsible for distal embolization can cause in situ thrombosis. Arteritis, radiation injury, and hypercoagulable syndromes have been reported as rare causes of in situ arterial thrombosis of the upper extremity.[24,26,33,34]

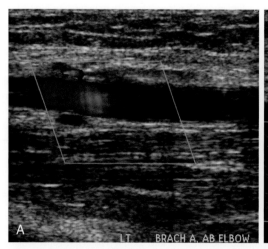 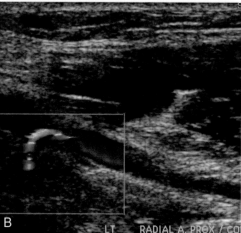

Fig. 44.2 Acute Hand Ischemia After Coronary Angiography via Left Brachial Artery Access. (A) Ultrasound examinations depict occlusion of the left brachial artery. (B) The radial artery reconstitutes via collaterals.

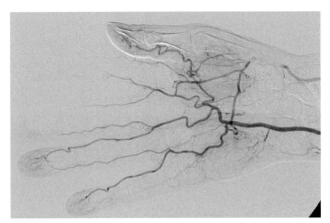

Fig. 44.3 Embolic occlusion of the right radial artery and ischemia of the index and middle fingers in a patient with a patent foramen ovale.

Acute Ischemia of the Lower Extremity

The distinction between embolism and in situ thrombosis should not detract from the need to establish a rapid diagnosis and to institute immediate therapy. Nevertheless, embolic etiology is more commonly associated with rapid onset of symptoms, history of cardiac disease, and absence of prior history of PAD. The contralateral limb is likely to have a normal exam without stigmata of systemic atherosclerosis. Some of the causes of acute limb ischemia are listed in Table 44.1.

In Situ Thrombosis

In situ thrombosis rather than embolism was responsible for 85% of the acute limb ischemia cases enrolled in the Thrombolysis or Peripheral Arterial Surgery (TOPAS) trial. The rate of embolic cases has been decreasing over the last few decades. In a Greek study evaluating the causes of acute limb ischemia at a referral center between 2000 and 2004, 40% of cases were caused by embolic events, in situ thrombosis was responsible for 50% of cases, and the remaining 10% were due to trauma, iatrogenic injury, vasculitis, or aortic dissection.[35] As many as 78% of the embolic events were of cardiac origin; the source of 9% of embolic events could not be determined. Among cases of in situ thrombosis, 30% involved native arteries and 70% involved thrombosis of vessels after an intervention (65% represented graft thrombosis and 5% iliac or infrainguinal stent thrombosis). Surgical graft thrombosis represented 30% of all cases of acute limb ischemia. Patients with surgical grafts can develop graft thrombosis and symptoms of acute limb ischemia due to graft degeneration or mechanical problems such as anastomotic stenosis or retained valves. Graft compression or kink can also cause thrombosis. With the advent of stent grafting for aortoiliac aneurysmal disease, acute stent graft thrombosis has been added as a cause of acute limb ischemia (Fig. 44.4).

In situ thrombosis of a popliteal artery aneurysm usually presents with acute limb ischemia. A review of nearly 900 patients presenting with acute limb ischemia secondary to a thrombosed popliteal aneurysm reported amputation rates of 14%. In this study, catheter-directed thrombolysis prior to surgery did not lower the likelihood of amputation, but it significantly improved the long-term patency of the graft, presumably by maximizing patency of the tibial vessel.[36] The decision to perform catheter-directed thrombolysis must depend on the clinical situation and urgency of revascularization. In a Swedish Vascular Registry, amputation rates for acute thrombosis of the popliteal aneurysm were 17% in patients presenting with acute ischemia and only 1.8% for asymptomatic, electively repaired aneurysms.[37]

Embolism

Acute limb ischemia is often caused by an embolic event, commonly from a cardiac source. The embolus most frequently lodges in the aortoiliac bifurcation, femoral bifurcation, or popliteal trifurcation. Over the last several decades, the etiology of cardioembolic events has evolved. Embolic events caused by rheumatic mitral stenosis with left atrial enlargement have become a rare occurrence because the prevalence of rheumatic valve disease has decreased substantially. Age-related atrial fibrillation and left ventricular dysfunction with apical thrombus formation are the most common causes of cardioembolic events (Fig. 44.5). Less common causes include endocarditis, intracardiac myxoma, or paradoxical embolism due to a patent foramen ovale allowing transit of venous thrombus into the arterial circulation. Acute embolic occlusion related to aortic aneurysmal disease and intramural thrombus is a rare event.

Iatrogenic Causes

Iatrogenic acute limb ischemia can be caused by arterial access in the common femoral artery and injury of the vessel at the access site, be it by deployment of a vascular closure device or direct injury to the common femoral or iliac artery. Similarly, catheter associated thrombosis and embolism of the popliteal artery can occur.

Other Causes

Intense vasospasm, such as can be caused by ergotism[38,39] or cocaine ingestion,[40] have been reported to cause acute limb ischemia. Aortic dissection can result in occlusion of the distal aorta and iliac vessels when the true lumen is compressed by a pressurized false lumen. Iliofemoral deep vein thrombosis with massive swelling of the thigh can compromise arterial inflow to the leg. The syndrome of phlegmasia

TABLE 44.1	Causes of Acute Limb Ischemia	
Embolism	**In Situ Thrombosis**	**Other Causes**
Cardiac source of embolism	*Atherosclerotic peripheral artery disease*	Trauma
Atrial fibrillation	*Iatrogenic*	Vasospasm
Left ventricular thrombus	Catheter-associated in situ thrombosis	Ergotism
Cardiac myxoma	*Stent and graft thrombosis*	Cocaine use
Valvular heart disease	Restenosis	Phlegmasia cerulea dolens
Infectious endocarditis	Intimal hyperplasia	
Prosthetic valve thrombosis	Stent or stent-graft underexpansion	
Rheumatic valve disease	Mechanical	
Paradoxical embolism via patent foramen ovale	*Arterial aneurysm*	
Artery-to-artery source	Popliteal aneurysm thrombosis	
Arterial aneurysm	*Hypercoagulable states*	
Atherosclerotic plaque	Antiphospholipid antibody syndrome	
Iatrogenic	Advanced malignancy	
Catheter-associated embolism	Hyperviscosity syndromes	
Vascular closure device malfunction	*Low flow states*	
Other	Cardiogenic shock and preexisting PAD	
Tumor embolism	Vasopressor-induced vasospasm	
Amniotic fluid	*Arterial dissection*	
Fat embolism	Access site artery dissection	
Air	Aortic dissection	

PAD, Peripheral artery disease.

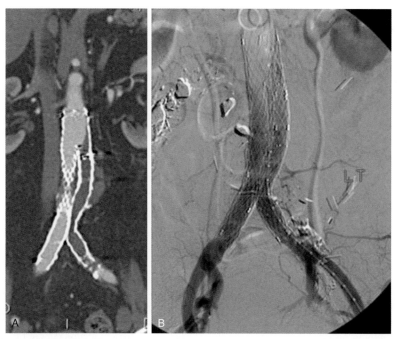

Fig. 44.4 Acute limb ischemia due to collapse of the right iliac endograft limb (A) treated with ultrasound-accelerated thrombolysis (B).

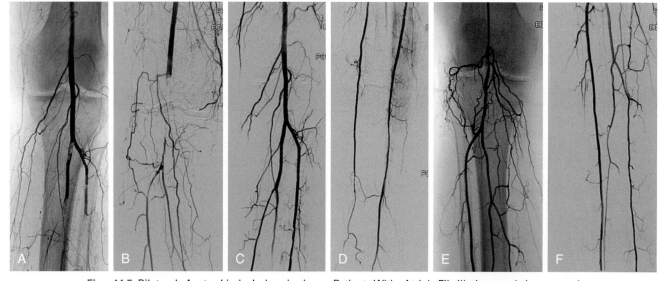

Fig. 44.5 Bilateral Acute Limb Ischemia in a Patient With Atrial Fibrillation and Interrupted Anticoagulation. The left anterior tibial artery and tibioperoneal trunk are occluded (A) as is the right popliteal artery (B). Mechanical thrombectomy and catheter suction embolectomy restored flow in the left (C and D) and right calf (E and F).

cerulea dolens requires urgent catheter-directed thrombolysis to restore venous outflow and, thus, arterial inflow to the limb.

PATHOPHYSIOLOGY OF ACUTE LIMB ISCHEMIA

Most emboli lodge in points of arterial branching: aortic, iliac, femoral, or popliteal bifurcations in the leg and brachial bifurcation in the arm. In situ thrombosis most commonly affects the femoral or popliteal artery, particularly in the setting of an existing arterial bypass, ruptured atherosclerotic plaque, or low output state. Sudden cessation of arterial flow to the extremity triggers a series of complex pathophysiological processes. Malperfused tissues shift from aerobic to anaerobic

metabolism. The shift in lactate to pyruvate ratio further increases lactate production, increases the concentration of hydrogen ions, and induces acidosis. Progressive ischemia results in cell dysfunction and eventual cell death. Muscle hypoxia depletes the intracellular adenosine triphosphate (ATP) stores, and the consequent dysfunction of the sodium-potassium ATPase and the calcium/sodium pumps causes leakage of intracellular calcium into the myocytes.[41] Intracellular free calcium levels rise and interact with actin, myosin, and proteases, leading to necrosis of muscle fibers. As the cellular membranes and microvascular integrity fail, intracellular potassium, phosphate, creatinine kinase, and myoglobin leak into the systemic circulation. Reperfusion further amplifies these cellular changes.

Nerve and muscle tissue are quite susceptible to ischemic injury, so presence or absence of neuromotor deficit is thus of paramount importance in assessing the severity of acute limb ischemia. Irreversible muscle damage begins after 3 hours of ischemia and is nearly complete after 6 hours.[42] In addition to myocyte injury, progressive microvascular damage follows skeletal muscle injury. The more severe the cellular damage, the greater the microvascular changes. In the setting of muscle necrosis, microvascular flow stops within a few hours. Traditionally a window of 6 hours has been assumed before irreversible functional injury occurs. This time window may be longer in a "preconditioned" limb with collateral pathways.

Ischemic insult sets the stage for reperfusion injury, a process triggered by restoration of perfusion and mediated by a complex cascade of cytokines, reactive oxygen species, and neutrophils. Reactive oxygen species (e.g., superoxide anion, hydrogen peroxide, hydroxyl radicals, peroxynitrite) are produced by activated neutrophils and xanthine oxidase, an enzyme located on microvascular endothelial cells of skeletal muscle and activated during ischemic conditions.[43] Under normal conditions, xanthine dehydrogenase uses nicotinamide adenine dinucleotide to oxidize hypoxanthine to xanthine. Xanthine dehydrogenase is converted to xanthine oxidase after 2 hours of ischemia.[44] During ischemia, ATP is degraded to hypoxanthine, but xanthine oxidase requires oxygen to convert hypoxanthine to xanthine. Thus hypoxanthine accumulates during ischemia. When oxygen is reintroduced during reperfusion, xanthine dehydrogenase isoform becomes active again. Conversion of massive amounts of hypoxanthine generates reactive oxygen species.[45]

The essential substrate for production of these radicals, molecular oxygen, is provided by reperfusion. Xanthine oxidase-derived oxidants mediate the increased vascular permeability in postischemic muscle. The importance of elemental oxygen and the role of oxygen radicals in reperfusion injury is underscored by studies showing that reperfusion initially with deoxygenated autologous blood prevents increase in permeability after ischemia. Changing the perfusate to oxygenated blood during reperfusion mimicked the microvascular injury response seen after normoxic reperfusion.[46] Similarly, gradual reintroduction of oxygen early in reperfusion decreases postischemic injury.[46] Additional supplementation with free radical scavengers and reduced oxygen delivery further reduces injury of postischemic necrosis.[47]

Activated neutrophils are the principal agents responsible for local and systemic damage caused by reperfusion. Leukocytes play an equally important role in reperfusion injury. Activated neutrophils accumulate in the reperfusing muscle and produce reactive oxygen metabolites, release cytotoxic enzymes, and occlude microcirculation pathways.[48] Leukocyte depletion has been shown to reduce the ischemia-reperfusion injury. Reperfusion with oxygenated blood depleted of leukocytes by the use of filters completely prevents development of vascular permeability in canine skeletal muscle.[49,50] Interestingly, inducing neutropenia before ischemia in rats restores transmembrane potential and contractile function in postischemic rat muscle.[51,52]

Skeletal muscle ischemia and reperfusion triggers a number of additional inflammatory cascades that include complement activation, increased expression of adhesion molecules, cytokine release, eicosanoid synthesis, free radical formation, cytoskeletal alterations, adenine nucleotide depletion, alterations in calcium and phospholipid metabolism, leukocyte activation, and endothelial dysfunction.[53] Interleukin (IL)-1β and tumor necrosis factor α (TNF-α) are detected soon after reperfusion and induce adhesion molecules on the surface of endothelial cells, increase capillary leak, and stimulate production of IL-6 and IL-8, which further increase endothelial permeability, destroy endothelial integrity, and activate leukocytes.[54–58]

The clinical impact of these cellular responses to reperfusion results in tissue swelling, a catastrophic event in the closed spaces of the forearm, thigh, calf, and buttock. Elevated compartment pressures within fascial boundaries cause *compartment syndrome*, defined as elevated compartment pressures that reduce the perfusion gradient and capillary blood flow below the metabolic requirement, resulting in further ischemia and necrosis. Release of myoglobin can result in renal injury. Increased endothelial permeability can lead to acute lung injury, a process attenuated in animal models by chemically induced neutropenia, suggesting that activation and transmigration of neutrophils and loss of endothelial integrity are critical in acute lung injury caused by reperfusion of ischemic skeletal muscle.[59] Thus non-cardiogenic pulmonary edema can develop after reperfusion of lower limbs, a process that can be prevented by granulocyte depletion.[59,60]

The reperfusion syndrome consists of two components. The local response to reperfusion triggers tissue swelling, while the systemic response can result in multiorgan failure and death. It is the latter that mitigates intervention in advanced and irreversible limb ischemia. The degree of inflammatory response following reperfusion is variable. There is little inflammatory response when muscle necrosis is uniform. The degree of ischemic damage, however, will vary depending on the proximity of the tissue to the occlusion and the efficiency of the collateral supply. The magnitude of the inflammatory response will be determined by the extent of the ischemic, but not completely necrotic, zone. Thus, reperfusion of large muscle groups with advanced ischemic injury and tissue necrosis will result in the release of large amounts of toxic inflammatory mediators into the systemic circulation. This detrimental effect of reperfusion favors amputation in patients with irreversible ischemic injury.

DIAGNOSIS OF ACUTE LIMB ISCHEMIA

The diagnosis of acute limb ischemia may be elusive, especially in patients who present with sensory and motor deficits that direct attention toward neurological evaluation. Modern audits of emergency room triage, diagnosis, and treatment of patients with acute limb ischemia continue to identify significant delays in treatment not normally accepted for other cardiovascular emergencies.[5,61] The current guidelines stress rapid evaluation and revascularization of a threatened limb within 6 hours of symptom onset.[62]

Clinical signs and symptoms of acute limb ischemia manifest as a spectrum of findings directly related to the severity of ischemia and duration or arterial malperfusion. Diagnosis of acute limb ischemia is made on the basis of physical examination. Confirmatory imaging with computed tomographic angiography (CTA) or magnetic resonance angiography (MRA) introduces a potentially costly delay in therapeutic intervention. Bedside duplex ultrasonography can be rapidly performed and can add information about the level of occlusion and arterial access strategy for endovascular procedure. A careful physical exam including Doppler evaluation of arterial and venous signals is usually sufficient for obtaining this information. A comprehensive physical exam can determine the level of arterial occlusion and obviate the need for additional imaging.

The classic symptoms and physical exam findings of an acutely ischemic limb are commonly known as the six P's: *pulselessness, pallor, pain, poikilothermia, paralysis,* and *paresthesia.* Pain is the most common symptom and progresses with ischemia. Pallor is an early finding in an ischemic extremity and is caused by complete emptying and vasospasm of the arteries (Fig. 44.6). Subsequent stagnation of microvascular circulation will cause mottling of the skin which initially blanches with pressure. As ischemia continues, paresthesia develops and numbness replaces pain, often falsely reassuring both patient and physician. In the final stages of ischemic injury, paralysis sets in and the skin mottling is fixed and nonblanching. Loss of motor function and marble-like appearance of the skin herald irreversible ischemic injury.

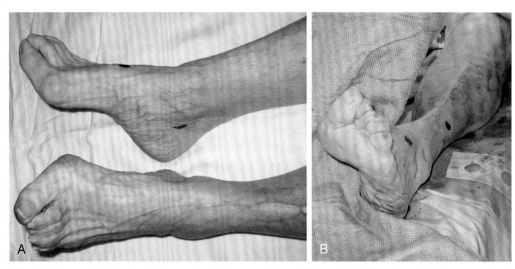

Fig. 44.6 Acute Limb Ischemia Due to Left Common Femoral Artery Embolism. Panel (A) shows marked pallor of the left foot which resolves after surgical embolectomy (B). (Image courtesy Dr. Edwin Gravereaux.)

A careful physical exam can determine the level of occlusion by detecting a temperature gradient along the limb and a deficit in pulses either on palpation or by arterial Doppler exam. The cutaneous changes of pallor and temperature change are detected one level below the occluded arterial segment. Physical exam must also include a search for potential sources of acute limb ischemia. Recognition of atrial fibrillation, cardiac murmur of valvular disease, or symptoms of congestive heart failure may implicate a cardioembolic cause of the event. Systemic symptoms of fevers, night sweats, and chills may hint at endocarditis as the etiology of cardiac embolism. Stigmata of PAD in the contralateral limb or signs of prior surgical revascularization point toward an in situ arterial thrombosis, whereas chest pain, hypertension, and asymmetry in arterial pulses of the upper extremity may require additional imaging to exclude an aortic dissection.

More importantly, it is the physical exam which allows classification of the severity of ischemia, urgency of revascularization, and prognosis after revascularization (Table 44.2).[63] The following clinical classes are also useful for determining the best intervention strategies. In general, Rutherford class I represents a viable and nonthreatened limb, akin to patients with chronic and noncritical ischemia. Rutherford class II symptoms describe a directly threatened limb. A class IIa limb is characterized by intact sensory and motor exam despite an absent arterial Doppler signal in the foot. This limb is marginally threatened. Class IIb includes patients with an immediately threatened limb characterized by sensory loss, mild motor function impairment, and absent Doppler arterial signals. This limb can be salvaged if treated immediately.

Irreversible limb ischemia falls into Rutherford class III with permanent nerve damage, profound sensory loss and motor paralysis, and absent arterial and venous Doppler signals. Revascularization of such a limb is harmful; amputation is required.

The presence of preexisting arterial occlusive disease may "precondition" the limb by fostering development of collaterals that lessen the severity of tissue malperfusion when acute occlusion occurs. Thus, patients with thrombosis in situ in an atherosclerotic vessel and those with graft failure may tolerate acute ischemia better than patients with no underlying arterial disease who develop acute limb ischemia due to a cardioembolic or an iatrogenic event. Several clinical characteristics may allow differentiation between an embolic event and in situ thrombosis. Patients with the former report a more abrupt onset of pain with clearer demarcation of ischemic temperature change and skin mottling. These patients usually present with symptoms and signs in Rutherford class IIb and III. Patients with in situ arterial thrombosis usually have signs of established PAD and report a more vague onset of symptoms. The physical exam findings are less striking with a less distinct demarcation of ischemic changes and more cyanosis than pallor. These patients often fall in the Rutherford class I and IIa categories.

TREATMENT OF ACUTE LIMB ISCHEMIA

Prompt recognition of acute limb ischemia and rapid restoration of arterial perfusion are cornerstones of therapy. The decision of whether

TABLE 44.2 Rutherford Classification of Acute Limb Ischemia

Rutherford Class	Prognosis	Sensory Exam	Motor Exam	Arterial Doppler Signal	Venous Doppler Signal	Skin Exam
Class I: Viable, not threatened	Threatened	Normal sensory exam	Normal	Audible	Audible	Normal capillary return
Class IIa: Marginally threatened	Salvageable with prompt therapy	Minimal sensory loss	Normal	Often audible	Audible	Decreased capillary return
Class IIb: Immediately threatened	Salvageable if treated immediately	Mild sensory loss and rest pain	Mildly to moderately abnormal	Usually inaudible	Audible	Pallor
Class III: Irreversible	Irreversible tissue and nerve damage	Profound sensory loss	Paralysis and rigor	Inaudible	Inaudible	No capillary return, skin marbling

Modified from Rutherford RB, Baker JD, Ernst C, et al. Recommended standards for reports dealing with lower extremity ischemia: revised version. *J Vasc Surg.* 1997;26(3):517–538

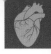

revascularization or primary amputation should be undertaken depends largely on the viability of the affected limb. In patients with a salvageable limb, selection of the type of revascularization therapy is equally important. The two major factors affecting morbidity and mortality among patients with acute limb ischemia are the burden of medical co-morbidities and the delay in recognition and treatment of the ischemic limb. Other factors associated with reduced amputation-free survival rates are increased age, race, diabetes, and absence of prompt initiation of anticoagulation.[64]

Surgical intervention has been traditionally associated with high perioperative mortality rates. In a compilation of 3000 patients treated surgically for acute limb ischemia in 30 centers between 1963 and 1978, 30-day mortality rates were as high as 25%.[65] Despite rapid advances in surgical and anesthesia techniques, Jivegard reported a 20% mortality rate a decade later.[13] Even in the 1990s, 30-day mortality after surgical intervention among selected patients enrolled in several trials— TOPAS, Surgery versus Thrombolysis for Ischemia of the Lower Extremity (STILE), and the Rochester randomized trials—ranged from 5% to 18%.[12,66,67] A modern series describing patients with Rutherford class IIa and IIb treated between 2005 and 2011 reported a 5-year mortality rate of 54% and amputation rate of 28%, reflecting the burden of medical co-morbidities and an aging population.[68]

The high burden of cardiopulmonary disease and high surgical mortality in the population affected by acute limb ischemia provided an impetus for the development of less invasive endovascular strategies. Evidence from randomized trials suggests equipoise between endovascular and surgical therapies in selected patients, particularly those with class I and IIa symptoms. The cause of limb ischemia, location of the occlusion, Rutherford class, as well as patient characteristics, play a crucial role in selection of the appropriate revascularization strategy. The Rochester, STILE, and TOPAS trials form a framework for selection of patients for endovascular therapies.[12,66,67] These trials demonstrated that patients with underlying PAD or graft thrombosis and with Rutherford class I and IIa, thrombolytic-based endovascular therapies do indeed have better outcomes. Patients with cardioembolic events usually present with Rutherford class IIb symptoms and may be better served by prompt surgical embolectomy.[4]

In modern practice, a rigid division between open surgical and endovascular treatment is artificial and these two treatment modalities should be viewed as complementary.[69] Although many patients can be treated with an entirely endovascular approach and others require traditional surgical embolectomy, large numbers of patients are treated with hybrid approaches. Indeed, routine use of perioperative angiography suggests a high rate of residual thrombus necessitating additional combined surgical and endovascular intervention in up to 90% of complex cases.[70] The Michigan Cardiovascular Consortium Vascular Intervention Collaborative reported that in over 1400 patients with Rutherford class IIa and IIb ischemia treated between 2012 and 2015, endovascular therapy alone was used in 55% of patients, 13% of patients underwent open surgical intervention, and 32% were treated with a hybrid approach.[71] Endovascular therapy has increasingly become the first line therapy for acute limb ischemia.[72] The 30-day amputation rates have been reported to be as low as 4% with the use of endovascular therapy.[71]

In addition to revascularization therapies, the sequelae of acute limb ischemia include the ischemia-reperfusion injury, which may range from mild injury without functional or systemic consequences, to systemic inflammatory response and multiorgan failure. Treatment of these metabolic consequences of acute limb ischemia is essential to patients' survival.

Initial Medical Management

Regardless of the revascularization strategy selected, the basic principles of initial therapy are the same: fluid resuscitation, analgesia, and administration of antithrombin and antiplatelet therapy. After decades of clinical experience, heparin therapy has been shown to decrease ischemic injury, reduce thrombus propagation, and improve survival.[4,73-75] Some studies dispute the benefit of perioperative anticoagulation even in patients with a cardiac source of emboli, but the overwhelming amount of data supports perioperative anticoagulation with heparin.[76] Unfractionated heparin should be administered at high doses with a goal of rapidly achieving a therapeutic level of anticoagulation and rise in partial thromboplastin time (PTT) by a factor of 2 to 2.5 above baseline. Patients with heparin-induced thrombocytopenia should be treated with intravenous direct thrombin inhibitors such as lepirudin or argatroban. Bivalirudin, another direct thrombin inhibitor commonly used in coronary and endovascular interventions, has a relatively short half-life and is more familiar to most vascular specialists. The decision regarding long-term anticoagulation must be made based on the etiology of the ischemic event, outcome of revascularization, and the balance between bleeding and thrombotic risk.

Correction of laboratory abnormalities and stabilization of underlying acute medical conditions are imperative for achieving the best clinical outcomes. Certain laboratory characteristics predict the ultimate therapeutic success. Patients presenting with elevated creatinine kinase and neutrophil count had a 50% risk of amputation as compared to a 5% risk among those with normal enzyme and neutrophil levels.[77] This finding underscores the poor clinical outcomes in patients with advanced ischemic injury of skeletal muscle. In patients who present with irreversible tissue loss, alkalinization of urine may be required to prevent renal injury from myoglobinuria. In some cases, the cause of acute limb ischemia is itself immediately life threatening, such as myocardial infarction complicated by left ventricular thrombus and cardiogenic shock, aortic dissection, or infective endocarditis with hemodynamic compromise due to valvular incompetence. In such cases, the principle of "life over limb" should guide best therapeutic strategy.

Endovascular Therapy of Acute Limb Ischemia

The basic principle behind endovascular therapy is to restore arterial flow either by thrombus lysis or unmasking and treating an underlying lesion, thus eliminating the need for surgery or reducing the extent of the surgical procedure.

Endovascular therapy for acute limb ischemia became possible when Tillet and Garner discovered the fibrinolytic properties of hemolytic streptococcus in 1933.[78] It was not long after the first use of intravenous streptokinase in healthy volunteers by Tillet in 1955 that Cliffton reported on the therapeutic use of streptokinase to dissolve pathologic thrombi in arteries and veins in 1957.[79,80] Catheter-based delivery of intraarterial streptokinase was pioneered by Charles Dotter in 1974.[81] Berridge subsequently confirmed that catheter delivery of fibrinolytic agents directly into the affected artery was superior to intravenously-administered thrombolytic agents and improved limb salvage rates (80% vs 45%) and lowered hemorrhagic complications.[82]

Modern thrombolytic agents work by enhancing the intrinsic fibrinolytic process through activation of plasminogen and its conversion into plasmin, which degrades fibrin (Table 44.3). The conversion of plasminogen into plasmin requires hydrolysis of a lysine-arginine bond, a step catalyzed by the tissue-type plasminogen activator, the model for today's recombinant plasminogen activators. Technical success of catheter-directed thrombolysis is defined as restoration of antegrade flow and complete or near complete resolution of thrombus. Clinical success is defined as relief of acute ischemic symptoms or reduction of the level of the subsequent surgical intervention or amputation.[83] Enzymatic dissolution of thrombus may be more complete compared to surgical embolectomy, particularly in the distal arterial beds and in cases of distal embolization. Endovascular therapies

TABLE 44.3 Properties of Thrombolytic Agents Used in Treatment of Acute Limb Ischemia

Thrombolytic Agent	Properties	Half-Life	Dosing	Major Bleeding Complications	Fibrin Affinity	Fibrin Specificity
Urokinase	Direct plasminogen activator: cleavage of plasminogen converts it into active plasmin	7–20 min	240,000 IU/h for 4 h, then 120,000 IU/h	5.6–12.5%	Low	Low
Alteplase (rtPA)	Recombinant tissue plasminogen activator. Fibrin-mediated conversion of plasminogen to active plasmin	3–6 min	0.5–1 mg/h, maximum dose 40 mg	6.1–6.8%	High	High
Reteplase (r-PA)	Superior thrombus penetration	14–18 min	0.25–1 U/h, maximum dose 20 Units in 24 h	6.1–6.8%	Low	Moderate
Tenecteplase (TNK-rt-tPA)	Increased fibrin affinity and longer half-life	20–24 min	0.25–1.0 mg/h Low dose regimen: 0.125 mg/h	5.4–13.3% 2.9%	Low	Very High

evolved and became more effective as cumulative experience grew in the 1980s and 1990s. Development of multi-hole infusion catheters and recognition of the importance of traversing the thrombotic occlusion with the infusion catheter, and infusion of the drug into the clot rather than above the occlusion, have markedly increased the efficacy of these procedures.

Three randomized trials performed in the 1990s compared endovascular therapy to surgical intervention in patients with acute limb ischemia. The Rochester trial randomized 114 patients with limb-threatening ischemia from embolic and thrombotic occlusion of native vessels or grafts to treatment with intraarterial delivery of urokinase or surgery.[67] Catheter-directed thrombolysis resulted in resolution of thrombus in 70% of patients. After 1 year, amputation rates were identical in both arms at 18%, while mortality was significantly higher in the surgical arm: 16% versus 42% with the majority of deaths in the surgical arm related to cardiopulmonary complications. Thrombolytic therapy was also associated with lower cost.

The larger STILE trial enrolled 393 patients with native vessel or graft thrombosis of less than 6 months duration who were randomized to surgical intervention or thrombolytic therapy.[66] The trial was handicapped by inclusion of patients with chronic ischemic symptoms unlikely to respond to thrombolysis. Indeed, 70% of patients in the thrombolytic arm had symptoms of a chronic nature. Technical failure accounted for a large fraction of clinical failures in the fibrinolytic arms. Failure to traverse the occlusive lesion was noted in 28% of patients. In patients who underwent successful catheter placement, patency was restored in 81% of bypass grafts and 69% of native arteries (P = NS). The ability to cross the lesion with a wire was predictive of therapeutic success, a key finding which has guided endovascular therapy for acute limb ischemia ever since.

In the fibrinolytic arm, patients received either recombinant tissue plasminogen activator (tPA) at a dose of 0.05 mg/kg per hour for up to 12 hours or urokinase for up to 36 hours. The dose of tPA used in this trial was much larger than usual doses of 1 mg/h used in clinical practice today. The trial was terminated early after a combined end point of death, major amputation, and recurrent ischemia occurred in 61.7% and 36.1% of patients in the lytic and surgical arms, respectively (P < .001). The 30-day mortality rates were 4.0% in the thrombolysis arm and 4.9% in the surgical arm (P = NS) with amputation rates of 5.2% and 6.3% respectively (P = NS). The difference in major morbidity of 21% in the thrombolysis arm and 16% in the surgical group stemmed primarily from the hemorrhagic and vascular access complications and recurrent ischemia observed in the former group.

Patients in the thrombolysis arm had a reduction in the extent of surgical revascularization.

A post hoc analysis stratified patients according to the duration of symptoms: among patients with symptoms less than 14 days in duration, thrombolytic therapy was associated with a trend toward a lower rate of major amputation compared to surgical intervention (5.7% vs. 17.9%, P = .06). Among patients with a longer duration of symptoms, 5.3% of those in the thrombolytic arm and 2.1% in the surgical arm underwent amputation (P = NS). Among patients with symptoms for 14 days, the rates of death and amputation at 6 months were 15.3% in the fibrinolytic arm and 37.5% in the surgical arm (P = .01). This study firmly established that thrombolytic therapy was not effective in most cases of chronic limb ischemia.

The TOPAS trial, the third trial comparing surgical intervention to catheter-directed thrombolysis, enrolled only patients with symptoms of less than 14 days' duration.[12] Thrombotic events were the predominant etiology of acute limb ischemia, responsible for 85% of the cases, and occurred more frequently in arterial grafts than native arteries. In addition, only 19% of the grafts consisted of autologous vein conduits, a departure from modern practice. The first dose-finding phase of the trial randomized 213 patients to initial infusion of variable doses of urokinase, followed by prolonged low-dose infusion. Complete thrombolysis was achieved in 71% of patients without a statistically significant difference in 12-month limb salvage or mortality rates in the surgical and urokinase arms. Patients treated with urokinase had a prohibitively high rate of intracranial hemorrhage (2.1%), particularly associated with the use of higher urokinase dose. In the second phase of the trial, 542 patients were randomized to surgical intervention or treatment with the safest dose of urokinase infusion. Recanalization occurred in 79.7% of patients and complete thrombolysis in 67.9% of patients. After 1 year, amputation-free survival in the thrombolytic and surgical arms was nearly identical (65% vs. 69.9%, P = NS), but came at a cost of higher rates of intracranial hemorrhage of 1.6% in the thrombolytic arm. Intracranial hemorrhage was associated with concomitant infusion of therapeutic doses of unfractionated heparin and occurred in as many as 4.8% of patients receiving doses aimed at full systemic anticoagulation, compared to 0.5% of patients who received subtherapeutic doses of heparin.

Major bleeding complications were higher in the thrombolytic arm compared to the surgical group (12.5% vs.5.5%, P = .005). At the time of discharge, death occurred in 5.9% of surgical patients and 8.8% of urokinase-treated patients (P = NS). Thrombolytic therapy with urokinase was associated with a higher rate of bleeding complications, but effectively reduced the need for surgical interventions without compromising amputation-free survival in patients with primarily thrombotic rather than embolic etiology of acute limb ischemia.

A Cochrane review of five trials of catheter-directed thrombolysis included 1283 patients and reported that there was no significant difference between the two strategies when limb salvage or mortality were compared at 30 days or 1 year. Patients undergoing catheter-directed thrombolysis were more likely to suffer bleeding complications (8.8% vs. 3.3%, 95% CI:1.7–4.6) and stroke (1.3% vs. 0%, 95% CI: 1.57–26.22).[84] A "real world" experience with catheter-directed thrombolysis was reported in the National Audit of Thrombolysis for Acute Limb Ischemia (NATALI) registry of 1133 patients treated with thrombolytic drugs between 1990 and 1999. This study showed amputation-free survival of 75%, with amputation and death rates each at 12% in the first 30 days with a 7.8% rate of major hemorrhage. It is not clear whether registries of such type included patients in whom thrombolytic therapy was selected due to high perioperative mortality risk.[85]

Modern outcomes in Rutherford IIa and IIb patients treated with arterial thrombolysis suggest that as many as 50% of these patients will avoid amputation or reintervention 5 years after the index event. Amputation-free survival is still only 42% at 5 years.[86] The long-term results of catheter-directed thrombolysis are better in patients who develop acute limb ischemia due to embolism, compared to those who suffer graft or stent thrombosis.

Multivariable analysis identified several factors predicting success of thrombolytic therapy.[87] Ability to traverse the thrombus and position a thrombolytic-infusing catheter directly in the thrombus favored successful fibrinolysis. Similarly, a native artery or prosthetic graft was more responsive to thrombolysis, whereas patients with diabetes were less likely to have successful treatment.

The success of thrombolytic therapy has led to an intense search for the optimal agent and dosing regimen in an ongoing effort to provide maximal thrombolysis effect with minimal bleeding complications. The largest experience in arterial thrombolysis comes from streptokinase, urokinase, and recombinant tPA. Urokinase has been shown to achieve more rapid thrombolysis and fewer bleeding complications when compared to streptokinase.[88] Streptokinase use has been therefore abandoned owing to its immunogenic effects, platelet-activating effects, and higher bleeding rates compared to later generation agents. Urokinase was withdrawn from production in 1999 after concerns about contamination in the production process. Since that time, recombinant tPA agents have become the dominant fibrinolytic used in clinical practice. Three agents are available in this class: alteplase, reteplase, and tenecteplase.

Alteplase and tenecteplase have a higher affinity for activation of fibrin-bound plasminogen compared to urokinase and reteplase, which are less fibrin specific. Reduced fibrin binding of reteplase could allow greater availability of the unbound drug for thrombus penetration and faster lysis compared to tPA. Alteplase is commonly used for catheter-directed thrombolysis. Catheter-directed thrombolysis using recombinant tPA has been shown to be superior to streptokinase, achieving better angiographic results and superior 30-day limb salvage rates.[82] When compared with urokinase, alteplase was found to have superior efficacy in thrombus resolution, but a price of higher incidence of access-site hematoma.[89] In the STILE trial, however, there were no differences between urokinase and alteplase. A review of multiple studies evaluating alteplase concluded that the risk of bleeding was directly related to the duration of infusion and the overall dose, but did not differ from complications encountered with urokinase.[90] Reteplase, a third generation tPA derivative, has a longer half-life of 13 to 16 minutes and has been successfully tested in a small number of patients with acute limb ischemia.[91,92] Proliferation of adjunctive

endovascular treatments has made direct comparisons between various lytic agents increasingly difficult, but there is no convincing evidence that one thrombolytic is superior to another in terms of efficacy and safety.

Adjuvant therapy with glycoprotein IIb/IIIa inhibitor abciximab was piloted in a small trial of thrombolysis with reteplase. Study results suggested that combined therapy allowed shorter thrombolytic infusion without an increase in bleeding complications.[93] Efficacy of combining infusion of fibrinolytic and glycoprotein IIb/IIIa inhibitors was further evaluated in the randomized RELAX trial (Reteplase Monotherapy and Reteplase/abciximab Combination Therapy in Acute Peripheral Arterial Occlusive Disease). In this study, 74 patients with acute occlusion received variable doses of reteplase alone or reteplase and abciximab infusion.[94] At 90 days, the composite end point in patients treated with the tPA dose of 1 mg/h did not differ whether they received concomitant placebo or abciximab. Interestingly, no instances of intracranial hemorrhage were observed in either arm. In selected patients, direct intraarterial infusion of abciximab mixed with tPA has also been described to facilitate thrombus resolution and reduce resource utilization without increasing the risk of bleeding.[95] The use of these adjuvant agents has not been accepted as standard therapy. Unfractionated heparin, on the other hand, is routinely infused through the catheter's side arm to achieve a PTT of 40 to 50. Subgroup analysis of the STILE trial suggested that heparin administration during alteplase infusion was associated with reduction in the composite end points of death, amputation, major morbidity, and recurrent ischemia. More importantly, adjunctive infusion of heparin in either urokinase or alteplase arms was not associated with increased bleeding.[63] Infusion of heparin through the side arm also lowers the risk of catheter thrombosis.[96] Thus, low-dose heparin of 400 to 600 U/h should be administered, while some recommend a lower dose of 100 U/h.

Risk of hemorrhagic complications increases with duration of therapy. It has been estimated that the risk of major complications associated with thrombolytic therapy increases with the duration of the infusion from 4% at 8 hours to 34% at 40 hours.[97] The optimal duration of thrombolytic infusion is not well defined. There has been a gradual decrease in the duration of therapy from 48-hour infusions in the early trials, to 6- to 18-hour infusions used currently in the era of adjunctive techniques. Monitoring of fibrinogen levels during thrombolytic infusion has long been advocated. Fibrinogen levels are checked serially during infusion and a level below 100 to 150 mg/dL indicates significant dysfibrinogenemia and requires lowering the drug dose or stopping the infusion altogether. Lower fibrinogen correlated with bleeding in the STILE trial, but it is not clear whether the fibrinogen level is a reliable predictor of bleeding complications.

Some of the drawbacks of catheter-directed thrombolysis are the prolonged infusion times, high costs of fibrinolytic agents, need for repeat angiographic imaging, and monitoring of patients in the intensive care units. Delays in restoring vessel patency made this therapy unsuitable for patients who require immediate revascularization, so surgical intervention has been recommended for patients with Rutherford class IIb symptoms. The drive to overcome these shortcomings, reduce the dose of thrombolytics required to achieve clinical success, and lower hemorrhagic complications has led to the development of several adjunctive techniques and devices designed to achieve more rapid reperfusion of the threatened limb.[98–100] Mechanical thrombectomy, pulse-spray thrombectomy, and ultrasound-accelerated thrombolysis are examples of these techniques. In modern practice, endovascular procedures for acute limb ischemia combine catheter-directed thrombolysis with mechanical thrombectomy, pulse-spray thrombectomy, catheter-suction embolectomy, ultrasound-assisted thrombolysis, distal embolic protection devices, and angioplasty and stenting. Despite the variety of adjunctive therapies, certain basic principles apply to endovascular thrombolysis. The entire occluded segment must be crossed and an infusion catheter with multiple sideholes must be positioned across the thrombus to directly infuse the thrombolytic drug into the thrombus. Recombinant tPA is the most commonly used thrombolytic agent, infused at a rate of 0.5 to 1 mg/h for a minimum of 12 hours.

Mechanical Thrombectomy Devices

The AngioJet rheolytic thrombectomy catheter (Boston Scientific, Marlborough, MA) is the most commonly used mechanical thrombectomy catheter. This small-caliber catheter uses a system of forced saline jets at its tip to fragment the thrombus, while the vacuum created proximal to the jets by the Venturi effect aids in aspiration of the fragmented debris. A simple modification allows substitution of thrombolytic agents for saline, which can be sprayed into the thrombus without concomitant aspiration. Some 20 to 30 minutes after such "pulse-spray" treatment, the thrombus laced with fibrinolytic agents is fragmented and aspirated in standard thrombectomy mode, reducing the thrombotic burden and restoring arterial flow.[101] Mechanical thrombectomy can be performed without the pulse-spray technique to restore flow in patients intolerant of thrombolytics. In early trials, thrombectomy with the AngioJet catheter in acute limb ischemia of native arteries and bypass grafts reestablished arterial flow in 90% of patients, with clinical improvement seen in 82% of patients, and distal embolization of thrombus occurring in only 2% of patients.[102] Catheter-directed thrombolysis is routinely used with this adjuvant therapy, but the dose and duration of fibrinolytic therapy is reduced.[103]

Rheolytic thrombectomy was evaluated in a small multicenter registry of patients, mostly with Rutherford class IIa and IIb symptoms, who were treated with catheter-directed infusion before or after rheolytic thrombectomy. After adjunctive angioplasty and stenting or elective surgery was performed in 80% of these patients, amputation rates were 7.1% and mortality 4.0% at 30 days.[104] Experience with rheolytic thrombectomy suggests that it is particularly effective in cases of in situ thrombosis irrespective of the conduit type (Fig. 44.7).[103] The thrombectomy devices fail to remove organized and adherent thrombi and are best used to treat acute thrombi. The overall technical success rates with AngioJet range from 56% to 95%, with distal embolization rates of 9.5%, and amputation-free survival rates reaching 75% at 2 years. The device can be also used without concomitant thrombolytics, with limb salvage rates reported to be as high as 95%.[103,105–107] The largest experience of AngioJet in acute limb ischemia comes from the PEARL Registry which enrolled 283 patients, predominantly with Rutherford class IIa and IIb ischemia. In 52% of procedures, technical and clinical success was achieved without the need for adjunctive thrombolytic infusion.[108]

Several other devices have been used for percutaneous mechanical thrombectomy. The Trellis device consists of a catheter with multiple infusion holes bordered by proximal and distal balloons, which when inflated localizes the thrombolytic agent to the thrombosed segment and potentially limits the systemic effect of these agents. A battery-powered sinusoidal wire rotates around the catheter, effectively mixing the thrombus and thrombolytic agents. Before the balloons are deflated, the debris contained between the balloons is aspirated. The use of this device, more common in venous thrombosis, has been described in a handful of patients with arterial occlusions, but its use was associated with an 11.5% rate of distal embolization.[109] The Rotarex device (Straub Medical AG, Wangs, Switzerland) is available in Europe and has been tested to be safe and effective in peripheral arterial thromboembolic disease.[110] This over-the-wire catheter is designed for thrombus removal in peripheral vessels. A spiral at the catheter's tip rotates at 40,000 rpm, and fragments and aspirates particles at 180 mL/min. The catheter is advanced into the thrombus and gently withdrawn during aspiration. The strength of suction can be adjusted to avoid collapse and injury of the vessel around the catheter. The Hydrolyser catheter (Cordis, Warren, NJ) was originally designed for management of dialysis access thrombosis. This 6F, 0.018″ guidewire-compatible catheter uses the Venturi effect to create a vacuum when powered by a standard contrast injector filled with saline. It has been reported to be effective in treatment of graft thrombosis, and in vitro evaluations have been associated with a lower distal embolization rate compared to the Angiojet.[111] The technical success rates of 88% in grafts and 73% in native arteries have been reported with amputation rates of 11% reported.

All thrombectomy devices require frequent use of thrombolysis. None of these devices have been studied rigorously, but they firmly belong in the arsenal of adjunctive devices accelerating reperfusion and decreasing the amount of thrombolytic used. Reduction in procedural time and thrombolytic dose is likely counterbalanced by more traumatic effect compared to pharmacotherapy alone. The thrombolytic agent also affects patency of the side branches and collateral vessels that are too small to be treated with these devices.

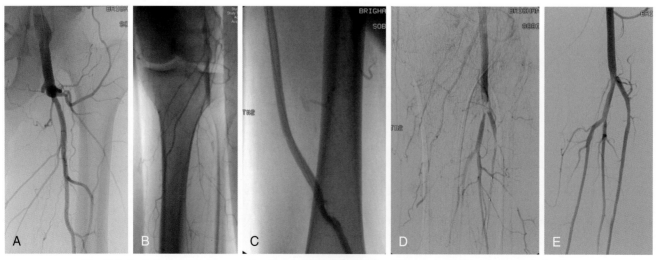

Fig. 44.7 Acute limb ischemia caused by thrombosis of the left femoral bypass graft (A) and distal embolization to the popliteal artery (B). Pulse-spray thrombectomy restored patency of the graft (C) and reduced thrombotic burden in the popliteal artery (D) allowing catheter-directed thrombolysis to restore patency (E).

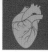

Suction Embolectomy

Percutaneous aspiration thrombectomy may be particularly effective for popliteal and tibial vessels (Figs. 44.8 and 44.9). A large lumen catheter (6F to 8F) connected to a 60 mL syringe is advanced into the proximal aspect of the occlusion, vacuum is attached by aspirating the syringe, and the thrombus is aspirated into the catheter and removed from the artery.[112,113] A combination of catheter-suction embolectomy and thrombolysis can result in success rates of up to 90% with limb salvage of 86% in 4-year follow-up.[114] The vacuum-assisted thrombectomy catheter, such as the Indigo System (Penumbra, Inc.), combines aspiration and fragmentation of the thrombus without the need for upfront thrombolytic use. This system consists of a tapered catheter which does not collapse during suction, a separator wire at its tip designed to break up the thrombus and keep the catheter from occluding, and an automated suction pump attached to the catheter. This system has been shown to be quite effective in arterial thrombus removal.[115]

Ultrasound Assisted Thrombolysis

Ultrasound emitting catheters have been used to assist and accelerate thrombolysis. Administration of high energy ultrasound can mechanically fragment a thrombus[116,117] while low energy ultrasound accelerates enzymatic thrombus lysis by dissociating fibrin strands, exposing more fibrin binding sites, and increasing thrombus permeability and penetration by thrombolytics.[118,119] These effects have the potential for accelerating reperfusion and reducing hemorrhagic complications of thrombolytic therapy.

Four small studies investigated ultrasound-assisted thrombolysis for acute limb ischemia. The EKOS EndoWave low energy system (Ekos Corp, Bothell, WA) was tested in 25 patients with acute lower extremity arterial occlusion. Complete thrombus resolution was noted in 88% of patients after mean therapy time of only 16.9 ± 10.9 hours.[120] Another study compared ultrasound accelerated thrombolysis with mechanical thrombectomy using the Rotarex device (Straub, Wangs, Switzerland) in 20 patients with acute femoro-popliteal graft occlusion.[121] Motarjeme

used ultrasound accelerated thrombolysis to treat 24 subacute arterial occlusions, with a technical success rate of 100% and complete thrombus lysis in 96% of cases after a mean treatment period of 16.4 hours (range 3 to 25 hours).[122] The mean duration of thrombolytic infusion in the ultrasound arm was 15 hours, with a technical success rate of 90%. Another prospective study of 21 patients treated with ultrasound-accelerated thrombolysis showed that complete lysis was achieved in 20 patients without hemorrhagic complications and 30-day vessel or graft patency of 81%.[123] The Dutch DUET study compared the efficacy of standard catheter-directed thrombolysis and ultrasound-assisted thrombolysis in a randomized trial of acute and chronic thrombosis of native and bypassed infrainguinal vessels with Rutherford class I and IIa symptoms.[124] Effective thrombolysis was faster in patients treated with the ultrasound-assisted catheter (17.7 vs. 29 hours) and the thrombolytic drug dose was significantly reduced.

Gradual dissolution of the thrombus may provoke embolization of smaller fragments into the distal circulation. This complication can occur in up to 19% of procedures and is manifested by sudden worsening of pain or loss of distal pulses.[125] This complication requires a temporary increase in the thrombolytic dose and, if symptoms do not improve in the course of the next 1 to 2 hours, repeat angiography may be warranted.

In modern practice, the distinction between surgical and endovascular techniques is often blurred and patients with acute ischemic symptoms are often treated with catheter-directed thrombolysis followed by either endovascular, combined, or open procedures.[126] For example, as reviewed above, in the Michigan Cardiovascular Consortium Vascular Intervention Collaborative study of 1480 patients with acute limb ischemia of the lower extremity, 32% of patients underwent a hybrid procedure combining both endovascular and surgical techniques.[71]

Surgical Therapy of Acute Limb Ischemia

Modern surgical therapy for acute limb ischemia was introduced in 1963 in a landmark study by Fogarty.[127] Prior to the development of the Fogarty catheter, the emboli were retrieved by direct exposure of

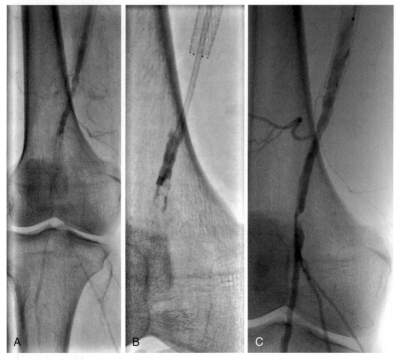

Fig. 44.8 Acute Limb Ischemia Due to Restenosis and Thrombosis of the Superficial Femoral Artery. Embolic occlusion noted distal to the stent (A) is engaged with a catheter under suction (B) and retrieved unmasking additional atherosclerotic disease (C).

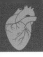

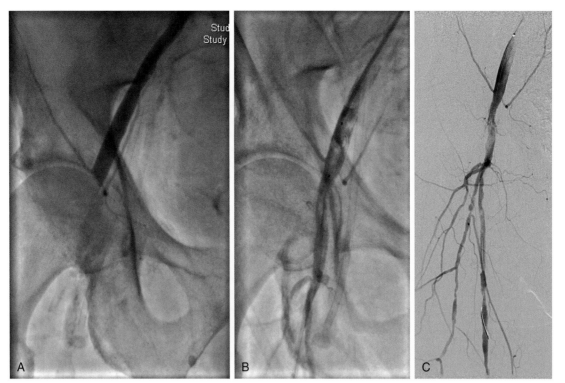

Fig. 44.9 Acute Limb Ischemia After Manual Compression of the Right Common Femoral Artery Access Site. Panel (A) depicts thrombotic occlusion of the right common femoral artery. In (B), the thrombus is trapped in a filter embolic protection device and withdrawn from the artery toward a sheath. Arterial flow is restored immediately after percutaneous thrombus removal with evidence of calcified atherosclerotic disease in the common femoral artery (C).

the occluded artery and its exploration with rigid instruments and suction devices. These methods were not only largely ineffective, but also damaging to the artery.[128,129] Fogarty's technique allowed arterial exposure away from the occluded segment with much lower risk of arterial injury. Physical exam guides the site of surgical exposure; absence of a palpable popliteal pulse requires femoral artery exposure regardless of the presence of femoral pulse. This approach allows embolectomy of the iliac, superficial femoral, profunda, and popliteal arteries. Physical exam supporting infrapopliteal occlusion will guide popliteal artery exposure and allow cannulation of individual tibial vessels. In cases of upper extremity acute limb ischemia, the brachial artery is the preferred exposure site. Appropriately sized balloon-tipped embolectomy catheters are advanced into the occluded artery, inflated distally, and pulled back, thus removing the thrombus (Fig. 44.10). Appropriate technique is essential to avoid arterial dissection and excessive endothelial injury.

When embolectomy does not reconstitute pedal perfusion, intraoperative angiography is performed to determine whether adjunctive surgical or endovascular intervention is required to treat residual distal thrombus. Direct exploration of the tibial vessels at the ankle is associated with high rates of re-thrombosis, so intraoperative fibrinolytic therapy may be a more effective therapy. Intraoperative angiography should be performed to confirm complete embolectomy. Residual thrombus can be seen in as many as 30% of embolectomy procedures.[130,131] Similarly, Doppler exam should accompany completion angiography to document restoration of arterial perfusion, although arterial spasm may attenuate the detected signals. Arterial rupture, perforation, intimal injury, and distal embolization can complicate embolectomy and underscore the importance of performing the completion angiography.

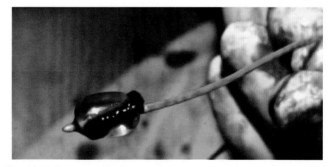

Fig. 44.10 Fogarty embolectomy balloon with thrombus removed from the popliteal artery. (Image courtesy Dr. Edwin Gravereaux.)

In cases of acute limb ischemia caused by embolism, embolectomy is usually sufficient; removal of the intravascular debris from a healthy vessel restores perfusion without the need for additional intervention. In patients with acute ischemia due to thrombosis, the underlying atherosclerotic disease must be addressed either by a surgical bypass or hybrid endovascular approach with angioplasty or stent placement. Indeed, as the population presenting with acute limb ischemia has shifted toward the elderly patients with preexisting PAD and in situ thrombosis, Fogarty embolectomy has ceased to be a standalone technique. Instead, modern surgical therapy for acute limb ischemia incorporates complex vascular reconstruction, embolectomy, angiography, and hybrid endovascular techniques.[130]

Treatment of Upper Extremity Ischemia

Most of the reported series regarding management of upper extremity ischemia come from surgical experience and, therefore, carry an inherent bias by underreporting the outcomes of conservative management. The development of simple and well-tolerated embolectomy techniques has increased the frequency of surgical interventions for upper extremity ischemia.

Before surgical embolectomy techniques gained popularity, conservative management included warming, pharmacologic vasodilation, and anticoagulation, with sympathectomy reserved for intractable pain. Baird reported a series of 95 patients treated before the advent of the Fogarty balloon. Among the 78 patients treated conservatively, 68% did not suffer any residual effect, 24% suffered from residual weakness or claudication, and 8% required amputation or had complete loss of function in the extremity. These results and the superior collateral circulation of the upper extremity led to recommendations for conservative treatment, a practice largely abandoned today in favor of surgical embolectomy. Subsequent reports showed that as many as 50% of patients treated conservatively were left with significant functional impairment, strengthening the argument for more aggressive intervention.[132]

Prior to the development of balloon embolectomy, surgical interventions involved arteriotomies at multiple sites and removal of the clot by "milking out" the arm or use of corkscrew wires and forceps. The introduction of the Fogarty balloon catheter enabled removal of a thrombus under local anesthesia through a single brachial arteriotomy in the antecubital fossa. Modern surgical techniques result in amputation-free and symptom-free outcomes in 80% to 90% of patients.[133,134] A more recent series of 251 patients treated with surgical embolectomy over a period of two decades reported amputation rates of 2% and mortality rates of 5.6% from cardiac and cerebrovascular complications, despite the fact that general anesthesia was used in only 3% of procedures.[135] The high perioperative mortality and 40% subsequent mortality underscores the severity of coexisting medical conditions in patients with acute arterial occlusions.

Catheter-directed thrombolysis has not been widely used in the treatment of acute arm ischemia. Upper limb salvage rates are much higher than in lower limb arterial occlusion and the risk of bleeding associated with thrombolytic therapy may thus be more justified in lower extremity interventions. Nevertheless, initial reports of catheter-directed thrombolysis have been successful. Coulon described a series of 13 patients with acute occlusion of the axillary and brachial arteries largely due to atrial fibrillation. Catheter-directed thrombolysis resulted in complete thrombus resolution in 8 patients, full recovery in 11, and no limb loss.[136] Others have reported similar results in small groups of patients.[137,138] Thrombolytic therapy may be particularly useful in cases of digital vessel thrombosis. Today, upper extremity ischemia is still more likely to be treated surgically than with endovascular techniques.[7]

Compartment Syndrome

Compartment syndrome follows intracranial hemorrhage as the most feared complication of revascularization procedures in patients with acute limb ischemia. Postreperfusion compartment syndrome most frequently occurs in patients with surgically treated Rutherford class IIb and III symptoms, but can also occur in patients with less severe ischemia undergoing endovascular therapies. Ischemic reperfusion injury can occur even after only an hour of ischemia.[139] Mortality from this syndrome ranged from 7.5% to 41% in the 1960s and 1970s and remains high today.[140] The likelihood of developing compartment syndrome is directly related to the duration of ischemia; the longer the ischemic period, the higher the likelihood of reperfusion syndrome and a worse clinical outcome. Reperfusion within 12 hours of ischemia onset has been associated with mortality and limb salvage rates of 12% and 93%, respectively. Reperfusion after more than 12 hours

of ischemia carries a much worse prognosis; mortality rates can be as high as 31% and limb salvage rates 78%.[141] High serum creatine kinase, positive volume status in the first 48 hours after revascularization, inadequate intraoperative backflow from arteries distal to the occlusion, and severity of ischemia at presentation also predict the likelihood of developing compartment syndrome.[142]

Compartment syndrome is caused by tissue swelling following restoration of blood flow and reperfusion injury.[143] The tissue injury initiated during the ischemic period is continued by reperfusion with oxygenated blood, with introduction of oxygen free radicals and inflammatory cells. Free radicals peroxidate the lipid component of cell membranes, thus enhancing capillary permeability and muscle edema.[139,144] Compartment syndrome occurs when high pressure in a confined fascial space reduces capillary perfusion below a level needed to maintain tissue viability.[145] The resulting pressure decreases venous drainage from swollen muscle groups encased in firm fascial layers. The pressure in the limb compartment increases to further decrease venous and capillary flow and eventually overcomes arterial pressure and stops arterial perfusion. Unless rapidly decompressed, the compartment pressures will result in irreversible neuromuscular damage.

The clinical signs and symptoms of the syndrome include rapidly progressive pain out of proportion to the clinical situation. Clinical exam is characterized by pain on passive stretch of the muscle in the affected compartment, parasthesias of the muscles in the compartment, and hypoaesthesia in the distribution of the nerve traversing the affected compartment. The limb exam is notable for a pale and painful swollen calf, thigh, or forearm. Distal pulses may become undetectable if the pressure becomes severe enough, but their presence does not exclude the syndrome.[146] Timely recognition of this complication is crucial, as compartment pressure exceeding 30 mm Hg for 6 to 8 hours leads to irreversible limb injury and limb loss. Some reports indicate that untreated compartment syndrome results in muscle necrosis within 3 hours.[147] The diagnosis of the syndrome is established by physical exam, though compartment pressure measurement can help in confirming the diagnosis in some cases. The compartment pressure criteria used to guide the decision for urgent fasciotomy vary from 30 mm Hg, 45 mm Hg, or any pressure exceeding the diastolic arterial pressure by 10 to 30 mm Hg.[148–152]

Once recognized, urgent fasciotomy of the three compartments in the thigh or four compartments in the calf (anterior, lateral, deep posterior, and superficial posterior) is recommended. Delay in therapy results in limb loss, rhabdomyolysis, tissue necrosis, renal failure, and death.[153,154] Even after successful fasciotomy, amputation rates can be as high as 11% to 21%.[155,156] Among patients undergoing fasciotomy for reperfusion injury, even successful limb salvage leaves 36% of the limbs with some degree of dysfunction.[156]

The frequency of fasciotomies after revascularization has been reported to be as high as 16% to 22%, though many of these procedures are performed prophylactically to prevent compartment syndrome.[157,158] Patients undergoing thrombolysis usually have less severe ischemia and the reperfusion is more gradual. Consequently, compartment syndrome in patients treated with endovascular therapies occurs in 2% of procedures. Some increase in compartment pressure is routinely seen after revascularization of an ischemic limb, but the pressure rarely reaches levels high enough to cause a clinical syndrome.[159,160] Experimental evidence suggests that prophylactic fasciotomies performed at the time of reperfusion reduce the amount of muscle injury compared to fasciotomies performed several hours later. Some authors recommend prophylactic fasciotomies in cases when ischemia exceeds 6 hours, the patients are young, reperfusion is incomplete, and tissue swelling develops immediately on or even before reperfusion.[146,157,161]

Adjunctive Medical Therapy

In addition to the underlying medical comorbidities, reperfusion injury is the principal cause of mortality and morbidity after revascularization. To reduce ischemic reperfusion injury, gradual reperfusion with modified reperfusate has been evaluated in experimental animal models. Hypothermia and low initial flow rates have been shown to decrease the severity of reperfusion injury in animal skeletal muscle.[162] Controlled reperfusion consists of a 30 minute infusion of crystalloid reperfusion solution mixed with oxygenated blood directly into the revascularized artery and muscle bed.[163] Controlled reperfusion does not eliminate reperfusion injury but may significantly attenuate it with a decrease in tissue edema and preservation of muscle viability and contraction force.[164,165] Other strategies have been proposed over the years, but none have penetrated into clinical practice. Administration of free radical scavengers and antiinflammatory agents has been shown to mitigate the deleterious effects of reperfusion.[47] Controlled reperfusion with blood mixed in with crystalloid to obtain an alkalotic, hypocalcemic, and substrate-rich perfusate has been shown to successfully reduce the degree of reperfusion injury.[163,166-168] Patients undergoing controlled reperfusion have been shown to have a superior functional recovery and lower rate of amputation.[169]

Iloprost, a synthetic analogue of prostacyclin, has been investigated as adjunctive therapy to reduce limb-related complications by improving microcirculation.[170] In a randomized study of 300 patients with acute limb ischemia, patients treated with intraarterial and intravenous infusion of iloprost had a statistically significant lower 90-day mortality compared to patients in the placebo arm. There was, however, no difference in the rate of amputation. None of these investigational therapies have reached the mainstream of modern clinical practice.

Efforts to attenuate the systemic inflammation associated with reperfusion have also focused on modulating the molecular mediators of end-organ injury. These early studies have been limited to animal models. T-cell sequestration agents have been shown to decrease systemic inflammation and to reduce transcription of injury-associated target genes in multiple end-organs.[171] Inhibition of cytokines involved in the early stages of the inflammatory cascade has been shown to reduce the expression of downstream mediators of inflammation such as TNF-α, IL-6, and MMP-9. This modulation could preserve vascular homeostasis and integrity, and facilitate perfusion of the ischemic limb.[172] Caffeine infusion has been shown to mitigate lung injury after reperfusion for acute limb ischemia.[173]

Long-term antiplatelet and antithrombotic therapy in survivors of acute limb ischemia should be guided by the cause of arterial occlusion and revascularization strategy. Systemic antithrombotic therapy may be appropriate in patients with a cardioembolic source of arterial embolism. Patients who suffered acute limb ischemia due to stent or graft failure may require the addition of an antithrombotic agent to their antiplatelet therapy. While there are no randomized controlled trials to guide optimal pharmacotherapy after an episode of acute limb ischemia, there is an increasing body of evidence regarding primary prevention of acute limb ischemia in patients with PAD.

Vorapaxar, an oral thrombin receptor antagonist, has been shown to reduce the incidence of acute limb ischemia. In the randomized, placebo-controlled Trial to Assess the Effects of Vorapaxar in Preventing Heart Attack and Stroke in Patients With Atherosclerosis (TRA2 P-TIMI50 study), addition of this thrombin receptor antagonist to the antiplatelet therapy in patients with symptomatic PAD reduced the incidence of acute limb ischemia by 41%.[6] The benefit was similar in patients with surgical grafts, endovascular stents, and those without prior interventions. Increased risk of bleeding associated with vorapaxar therapy has hindered its acceptance in clinical practice. The Prevention of Cardiovascular Events in Patients With Prior Heart Attack Using Ticagrelor Compared to Placebo on a Background of

Aspirin (PEGASUS-TIMI 54) study suggested that addition of ticagrelor to low-dose aspirin therapy can reduce the incidence of acute limb ischemia in high-risk patients. This randomized controlled trial included 1143 patients with a history of both myocardial infarction and PAD. The treatment arm in this trial received ticagrelor, a potent and reversible antiplatelet agent inhibiting the P2Y$_{12}$ subtype of the platelet adenosine diphosphate (ADP) receptor. After a follow-up of 3 years, patients treated with aspirin and ticagrelor had a 51% lower rate of acute limb ischemia and revascularization for ischemia compared to patients treated with aspirin alone.[174]

The clinical benefit of adding the antithrombotic agent rivaroxaban to low-dose aspirin in patients with PAD or carotid artery disease was investigated in the Cardiovascular Outcomes for People using Anticoagulation Strategies (COMPASS) trial.[175] Patients were randomized to one of three treatments groups: low-dose (100 mg) aspirin alone, low-dose aspirin and rivaroxaban (2.5 mg twice daily), or rivaroxaban (5 mg twice daily) without aspirin. After a median follow up of 21 months, the risk of developing acute limb ischemia was 44% lower in the low-dose rivaroxaban plus aspirin group and 43% lower in the rivaroxaban alone group compared to the aspirin alone group. Unlike the combination of rivaroxaban and aspirin, rivaroxaban monotherapy did not reduce the rate of major adverse cardiovascular events compared to aspirin monotherapy. Thus the combination of low-dose rivaroxaban and aspirin appears to reduce the risk of major adverse cardiovascular events and acute limb ischemia in patients with CAD or PAD.[176]

REFERENCES

1. Earnshaw JJ. Demography and etiology of acute leg ischemia. *Semin Vasc Surg.* 2001;14:86–92.
2. Davies B, Braithwaite BD, Birch PA, et al. Acute leg ischaemia in Gloucestershire. *Br J Surg.* 1997;84:504–508.
3. Bergqvist D, Troeng T, Elfstrom J, et al. Auditing surgical outcome: ten years with the Swedish Vascular Registry--Swedvasc. The Steering Committee of Swedvasc. *Eur J Surg Suppl.* 1998;(581):3–8.
4. Eliason JL, Wainess RM, Proctor MC, et al. A national and single institutional experience in the contemporary treatment of acute lower extremity ischemia. *Ann Surg.* 2003;238:382–389. discussion 9-90.
5. Langenskiold M, Smidfelt K, Karlsson A, et al. Weak links in the early chain of care of acute lower limb ischaemia in terms of recognition and emergency management. *Eur J Vasc Endovasc Surg.* 2017;54: 235–240.
6. Bonaca MP, Gutierrez JA, Creager MA, et al. Acute limb ischemia and outcomes with vorapaxar in patients with peripheral artery disease: results from the trial to assess the effects of vorapaxar in preventing heart attack and stroke in patients with atherosclerosis-thrombolysis in myocardial infarction 50 (TRA2 degrees P-TIMI 50). *Circulation.* 2016;133:997–1005.
7. Wong VW, Major MR, Higgins JP. Nonoperative management of acute upper limb ischemia. *Hand (N Y).* 2016;11:131–143.
8. Williams N, Bell PR. Acute ischaemia of the upper limb. *Br J Hosp Med.* 1993;50:579–582.
9. Eyers P, Earnshaw JJ. Acute non-traumatic arm ischaemia. *Br J Surg.* 1998;85:1340–1346.
10. Dryjski M, Swedenborg J. Acute ischemia of the extremities in a metropolitan area during one year. *J Cardiovasc Surg (Torino).* 1984;25:518–522.
11. Stonebridge PA, Clason AE, Duncan AJ, et al. Acute ischaemia of the upper limb compared with acute lower limb ischaemia; a 5-year review. *Br J Surg.* 1989;76:515–516.
12. Ouriel K, Veith FJ, Sasahara AA. A comparison of recombinant urokinase with vascular surgery as initial treatment for acute arterial occlusion of the legs. Thrombolysis or Peripheral Arterial Surgery (TOPAS) Investigators. *N Engl J Med.* 1998;338:1105–1111.

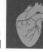

13. Jivegard L, Holm J, Schersten T. Acute limb ischemia due to arterial embolism or thrombosis: influence of limb ischemia versus pre-existing cardiac disease on postoperative mortality rate. *J Cardiovasc Surg (Torino)*. 1988;29:32–36.

14. Braithwaite BD, Davies B, Birch PA, et al. Management of acute leg ischaemia in the elderly. *Br J Surg*. 1998;85:217–220.

15. Lambert M, Ball C, Hancock B. Management of acute brachial artery occlusion due to trauma or emboli. *Br J Surg*. 1983;70:639–640.

16. Katz SG, Kohl RD. Direct revascularization for the treatment of forearm and hand ischemia. *Am J Surg*. 1993;165:312–316.

17. Wirsing P, Andriopoulos A, Botticher R. Arterial embolectomies in the upper extremity after acute occlusion. Report on 79 cases. *J Cardiovasc Surg (Torino)*. 1983;24:40–42.

18. James EC, Khuri NT, Fedde CW, et al. Upper limb ischemia resulting from arterial thromboembolism. *Am J Surg*. 1979;137:739–744.

19. Darling RC, Austen WG, Linton RR. Arterial embolism. *Surg Gynecol Obstet*. 1967;124:106–114.

20. Kaar G, Broe PJ, Bouchier-Hayes DJ. Upper limb emboli. A review of 55 patients managed surgically. *J Cardiovasc Surg (Torino)*. 1989;30:165–168.

21. Yamashita M, Eguchi K, Ogawa M, et al. A case of left atrial myxoma whose initial symptom was finger ischemic symptom. *Int Heart J*. 2018;59:233–236.

22. Gazzaniga AB, Dalen JE. Paradoxical embolism: its pathophysiology and clinical recognition. *Ann Surg*. 1970;171:137–142.

23. Bryan AJ, Hicks E, Lewis MH. Unilateral digital ischaemia secondary to embolisation from subclavian atheroma. *Ann R Coll Surg Engl*. 1989;71:140–142.

24. Rapp JH, Reilly LM, Goldstone J, et al. Ischemia of the upper extremity: significance of proximal arterial disease. *Am J Surg*. 1986;152:122–126.

25. Keen RR, McCarthy WJ, Shireman PK, et al. Surgical management of atheroembolization. *J Vasc Surg*. 1995;21:773–780. discussion 780-781.

26. Ricotta JJ, Scudder PA, McAndrew JA, et al. Management of acute ischemia of the upper extremity. *Am J Surg*. 1983;145:661–666.

27. Banis Jr JC, Rich N, Whelan Jr TJ. Ischemia of the upper extremity due to noncardiac emboli. *Am J Surg*. 1977;134:131–139.

28. Nehler MR, Taylor Jr LM, Moneta GL, Porter JM. Upper extremity ischemia from subclavian artery aneurysm caused by bony abnormalities of the thoracic outlet. *Arch Surg*. 1997;132:527–532.

29. Sachatello CR, Ernst CB, Griffen Jr WO. The acutely ischemic upper extremity: selective management. *Surgery*. 1974;76:1002–1009.

30. Prioleau PG, Katzenstein AL. Major peripheral arterial occlusion due to malignant tumor embolism: histologic recognition and surgical management. *Cancer*. 1978;42:2009–2014.

31. Lorentzen JE, Roder OC, Hansen HJ. Peripheral arterial embolism. A follow-up of 130 consecutive patients submitted to embolectomy. *Acta Chir Scand Suppl*. 1980;502:111–116.

32. Jivegard LE, Arfvidsson B, Holm J, Schersten T. Selective conservative and routine early operative treatment in acute limb ischaemia. *Br J Surg*. 1987;74:798–801.

33. Vohra R, Lieberman DP. Arterial emboli to the arm. *J R Coll Surg Edinb*. 1991;36:83–85.

34. Quraishy MS, Cawthorn SJ, Giddings AE. Critical ischaemia of the upper limb. *J R Soc Med*. 1992;85:269–273.

35. Klonaris C, Georgopoulos S, Katsargyris A, et al. Changing patterns in the etiology of acute lower limb ischemia. *Int Angiol*. 2007;26:49–52.

36. Kropman RH, Schrijver AM, Kelder JC, et al. Clinical outcome of acute leg ischaemia due to thrombosed popliteal artery aneurysm: systematic review of 895 cases. *Eur J Vasc Endovasc Surg*. 2010;39:452–457.

37. Ravn H, Bergqvist D, Bjorck M. Nationwide study of the outcome of popliteal artery aneurysms treated surgically. *Br J Surg*. 2007;94:970–977.

38. Marine L, Castro P, Enriquez A, et al. Four-limb acute ischemia induced by ergotamine in an AIDS patient treated with protease inhibitors. *Circulation*. 2011;124:1395–1397.

39. Zavaleta EG, Fernandez BB, Grove MK, Kaye MD. St. Anthony's fire (ergotamine induced leg ischemia)--a case report and review of the literature. *Angiology*. 2001;52:349–356.

40. Mirzayan R, Hanks SE, Weaver FA. Cocaine-induced thrombosis of common iliac and popliteal arteries. *Ann Vasc Surg*. 1998;12:476–481.

41. Knochel JP. Mechanisms of rhabdomyolysis. *Curr Opin Rheumatol*. 1993;5:725–731.

42. Blaisdell FW. The pathophysiology of skeletal muscle ischemia and the reperfusion syndrome: a review. *Cardiovasc Surg*. 2002;10:620–630.

43. Gillani S, Cao J, Suzuki T, Hak DJ. The effect of ischemia reperfusion injury on skeletal muscle. *Injury*. 2012;43(6):670–675.

44. Rubin BB, Romaschin A, Walker PM, et al. Mechanisms of postischemic injury in skeletal muscle: intervention strategies. *J Appl Physiol (1985)*. 1996;80:369–387.

45. Collard CD, Gelman S. Pathophysiology, clinical manifestations, and prevention of ischemia-reperfusion injury. *Anesthesiology*. 2001;94:1133–1138.

46. Korthuis RJ, Smith JK, Carden DL. Hypoxic reperfusion attenuates postischemic microvascular injury. *Am J Physiol*. 1989;256:H315–H319.

47. Walker PM, Lindsay TF, Labbe R, et al. Salvage of skeletal muscle with free radical scavengers. *J Vasc Surg*. 1987;5:68–75.

48. Jerome SN, Akimitsu T, Korthuis RJ. Leukocyte adhesion, edema, and development of postischemic capillary no-reflow. *Am J Physiol*. 1994;267:H1329–H1336.

49. Korthuis RJ, Grisham MB, Granger DN. Leukocyte depletion attenuates vascular injury in postischemic skeletal muscle. *Am J Physiol*. 1988;254:H823–H827.

50. Carden DL, Smith JK, Korthuis RJ. Neutrophil-mediated microvascular dysfunction in postischemic canine skeletal muscle. Role of granulocyte adherence. *Circ Res*. 1990;66:1436–1444.

51. Walden DL, McCutchan HJ, Enquist EG, et al. Neutrophils accumulate and contribute to skeletal muscle dysfunction after ischemia-reperfusion. *Am J Physiol*. 1990;259:H1809–H1812.

52. Yokota J, Minei JP, Fantini GA, Shires GT. Role of leukocytes in reperfusion injury of skeletal muscle after partial ischemia. *Am J Physiol*. 1989;257:H1068–H1075.

53. Rubin BB, Romaschin A, Walker PM, et al. Mechanisms of postischemic injury in skeletal muscle: intervention strategies. *J Appl Physiol*. 1996;80:369–387.

54. Welbourn R, Goldman G, O'Riordain M, et al. Role for tumor necrosis factor as mediator of lung injury following lower torso ischemia. *J Appl Physiol*. 1991;70:2645–2649.

55. Yassin MM, Harkin DW, Barros D'Sa AA, et al. Lower limb ischemia-reperfusion injury triggers a systemic inflammatory response and multiple organ dysfunction. *World J Surg*. 2002;26:115–121.

56. Ascer E, Mohan C, Gennaro M, Cupo S. Interleukin-1 and thromboxane release after skeletal muscle ischemia and reperfusion. *Ann Vasc Surg*. 1992;6:69–73.

57. Hashimoto M, Shingu M, Ezaki I, et al. Production of soluble ICAM-1 from human endothelial cells induced by IL-1 beta and TNF-alpha. *Inflammation*. 1994;18:163–173.

58. Sato N, Goto T, Haranaka K, et al. Actions of tumor necrosis factor on cultured vascular endothelial cells: morphologic modulation, growth inhibition, and cytotoxicity. *J Natl Cancer Inst*. 1986;76:1113–1121.

59. Klausner JM, Anner H, Paterson IS, et al. Lower torso ischemia-induced lung injury is leukocyte dependent. *Ann Surg*. 1988;208:761–767.

60. Welbourn CR, Goldman G, Paterson IS, et al. Pathophysiology of ischaemia reperfusion injury: central role of the neutrophil. *Br J Surg*. 1991;78:651–655.

61. Normahani P, Standfield NJ, Jaffer U. Sources of delay in the acute limb ischemia patient pathway. *Ann Vasc Surg*. 2017;38:279–285.

62. Gerhard-Herman MD, Gornik HL, Barrett C, et al. 2016 AHA/ACC guideline on the management of patients with lower extremity peripheral artery disease: executive summary: a report of the American College of Cardiology/American Heart Association Task Force on Clinical Practice Guidelines. *Circulation*. 2017;135:e686–e725.

63. Rutherford RB, Baker JD, Ernst C, et al. Recommended standards for reports dealing with lower extremity ischemia: revised version. *J Vasc Surg*. 1997;26:517–538.

64. Henke PK. Contemporary management of acute limb ischemia: factors associated with amputation and in-hospital mortality. *Semin Vasc Surg*. 2009;22:34–40.

65. Blaisdell FW, Steele M, Allen RE. Management of acute lower extremity arterial ischemia due to embolism and thrombosis. *Surgery*. 1978;84:822–834.

66. Results of a prospective randomized trial evaluating surgery versus thrombolysis for ischemia of the lower extremity. The STILE trial. *Ann Surg.* 1994;220:251–266. discussion 266-268.

67. Ouriel K, Shortell CK, DeWeese JA, et al. A comparison of thrombolytic therapy with operative revascularization in the initial treatment of acute peripheral arterial ischemia. *J Vasc Surg.* 1994;19:1021–1030.

68. Genovese EA, Chaer RA, Taha AG, et al. Risk factors for long-term mortality and amputation after open and endovascular treatment of acute limb ischemia. *Ann Vasc Surg.* 2016;30:82–92.

69. Wang JC, Kim AH, Kashyap VS. Open surgical or endovascular revascularization for acute limb ischemia. *J Vasc Surg.* 2016;63:270–278.

70. Zaraca F, Stringari C, Ebner JA, Ebner H. Routine versus selective use of intraoperative angiography during thromboembolectomy for acute lower limb ischemia: analysis of outcomes. *Ann Vasc Surg.* 2010;24:621–627.

71. Davis FM, Albright J, Gallagher KA, et al. Early outcomes following endovascular, open surgical, and hybrid revascularization for lower extremity acute limb ischemia. *Ann Vasc Surg.* 2018;51:106–112.

72. Baril DT, Ghosh K, Rosen AB. Trends in the incidence, treatment, and outcomes of acute lower extremity ischemia in the United States Medicare population. *J Vasc Surg.* 2014;60:669–677. e2.

73. Tawes Jr RL, Harris EJ, Brown WH, et al. Arterial thromboembolism. A 20-year perspective. *Arch Surg.* 1985;120:595–599.

74. Hobson 2nd RW, Neville R, Watanabe B, et al. Role of heparin in reducing skeletal muscle infarction in ischemia-reperfusion. *Microcirc Endothelium Lymphatics.* 1989;5:259–276.

75. Wright JG, Kerr JC, Valeri CR, Hobson 2nd RW. Heparin decreases ischemia-reperfusion injury in isolated canine gracilis model. *Arch Surg.* 1988;123:470–472.

76. Jivegard L, Holm J, Bergqvist D, et al. Acute lower limb ischemia: failure of anticoagulant treatment to improve one-month results of arterial thromboembolectomy. A prospective randomized multi-center study. *Surgery.* 1991;109:610–616.

77. Currie IS, Wakelin SJ, Lee AJ, Chalmers RT. Plasma creatine kinase indicates major amputation or limb preservation in acute lower limb ischemia. *J Vasc Surg.* 2007;45:733–739.

78. Tillet WS, Garner RL. The fibrinolytic activity of hemolytic streptococci. *J Exp Med.* 1933;58:485–502.

79. Tillett WS, Johnson AJ, McCarty WR. The intravenous infusion of the streptococcal fibrinolytic principle (streptokinase) into patients. *J Clin Invest.* 1955;34:169–185.

80. Clifton EE. The use of plasmin in humans. *Ann NY Acad Sci.* 1957;68:209–229.

81. Dotter CT, Rosch J, Seaman AJ. Selective clot lysis with low-dose streptokinase. *Radiology.* 1974;111:31–37.

82. Berridge DC, Gregson RH, Hopkinson BR, Makin GS. Randomized trial of intraarterial recombinant tissue plasminogen activator, intravenous recombinant tissue plasminogen activator and intraarterial streptokinase in peripheral arterial thrombolysis. *Br J Surg.* 1991;78:988–995.

83. Karnabatidis D, Spiliopoulos S, Tsetis D, Siablis D. Quality improvement guidelines for percutaneous catheter-directed intraarterial thrombolysis and mechanical thrombectomy for acute lower-limb ischemia. *Cardiovasc Intervent Radiol.* 2011;34(6):1123–1136.

84. Berridge DC, Kessel D, Robertson I. Surgery versus thrombolysis for acute limb ischaemia: initial management. *Cochrane Database Syst Rev.* 2002;3:CD002784.

85. Earnshaw JJ, Whitman B, Foy C. National Audit of Thrombolysis for Acute Leg Ischemia (NATALI): clinical factors associated with early outcome. *J Vasc Surg.* 2004;39:1018–1025.

86. Grip O, Wanhainen A, Acosta S, Bjorck M. Long-term outcome after thrombolysis for acute lower limb ischaemia. *Eur J Vasc Endovasc Surg.* 2017;53:853–861.

87. Ouriel K, Shortell CK, Azodo MV, et al. Acute peripheral arterial occlusion: predictors of success in catheter-directed thrombolytic therapy. *Radiology.* 1994;193:561–566.

88. Olin JW, Graor RA. Thrombolytic therapy in the treatment of peripheral arterial occlusions. *Ann Emerg Med.* 1988;17:1210–1215.

89. Schweizer J, Altmann E, Stosslein F, et al. Comparison of tissue plasminogen activator and urokinase in the local infiltration thrombolysis of peripheral arterial occlusions. *Eur J Radiol.* 1996;22:129–132.

90. Semba CP, Murphy TP, Bakal CW, et al. Thrombolytic therapy with use of alteplase (rtPA) in peripheral arterial occlusive disease: review of the clinical literature. *The Advisory Panel J Vasc Interv Radiol.* 2000;11:149–161.

91. Hanover TM, Kalbaugh CA, Gray BH, et al. Safety and efficacy of reteplase for the treatment of acute arterial occlusion: complexity of underlying lesion predicts outcome. *Ann Vasc Surg.* 2005;19:817–822.

92. Laird JR, Dangas G, Jaff M, et al. Intra-arterial reteplase for the treatment of acute limb ischemia. *J Invasive Cardiol.* 1999;11:757–762.

93. Drescher P, Crain MR, Rilling WS. Initial experience with the combination of reteplase and abciximab for thrombolytic therapy in peripheral arterial occlusive disease: a pilot study. *J Vasc Interv Radiol.* 2002;13:37–43.

94. Ouriel K, Castaneda F, McNamara T, et al. Reteplase monotherapy and reteplase/abciximab combination therapy in peripheral arterial occlusive disease: results from the RELAX trial. *J Vasc Interv Radiol.* 2004;15:229–238.

95. Salzler GG, Graham A, Connolly PH, et al. Safety and effectiveness of adjunctive intraarterial abciximab in the management of acute limb ischemia. *Ann Vasc Surg.* 2016;30:66–71.

96. McNamara TO, Fischer JR. Thrombolysis of peripheral arterial and graft occlusions: improved results using high-dose urokinase. *AJR Am J Roentgenol.* 1985;144:769–775.

97. Sullivan KL, Gardiner Jr GA, Shapiro MJ, et al. Acceleration of thrombolysis with a high-dose transthrombus bolus technique. *Radiology.* 1989;173:805–808.

98. Ritchie JL, Hansen DD, Vracko R, Auth DC. Mechanical thrombolysis: a new rotational catheter approach for acute thrombi. *Circulation.* 1986;73:1006–1012.

99. Drasler WJ, Jenson ML, Wilson GJ, et al. Rheolytic catheter for percutaneous removal of thrombus. *Radiology.* 1992;182:263–267.

100. Schmitz-Rode T, Gunther RW, Muller-Leisse C. US-assisted aspiration thrombectomy: in vitro investigations. *Radiology.* 1991;178:677–679.

101. Allie DE, Hebert CJ, Lirtzman MD, et al. Novel simultaneous combination chemical thrombolysis/rheolytic thrombectomy therapy for acute critical limb ischemia: the power-pulse spray technique. *Catheter Cardiovasc Interv.* 2004;63:512–522.

102. Mathie AG, Bell SD, Saibil EA. Mechanical thromboembolectomy in acute embolic peripheral arterial occlusions with use of the AngioJet Rapid Thrombectomy System. *J Vasc Interv Radiol.* 1999;10:583–590.

103. Kasirajan K, Gray B, Beavers FP, et al. Rheolytic thrombectomy in the management of acute and subacute limb-threatening ischemia. *J Vasc Interv Radiol.* 2001;12:413–421.

104. Ansel GM, George BS, Botti CF, et al. Rheolytic thrombectomy in the management of limb ischemia: 30-day results from a multicenter registry. *J Endovasc Ther.* 2002;9:395–402.

105. Wagner HJ, Muller-Hulsbeck S, Pitton MB, et al. Rapid thrombectomy with a hydrodynamic catheter: results from a prospective, multicenter trial. *Radiology.* 1997;205:675–681.

106. Silva JA, Ramee SR, Collins TJ, et al. Rheolytic thrombectomy in the treatment of acute limb-threatening ischemia: immediate results and six-month follow-up of the multicenter AngioJet registry. *Possis Peripheral AngioJet Study AngioJet Investigators Cathet Cardiovasc Diagn.* 1998;45:386–393.

107. Muller-Hulsbeck S, Kalinowski M, Heller M, Wagner HJ. Rheolytic hydrodynamic thrombectomy for percutaneous treatment of acutely occluded infra-aortic native arteries and bypass grafts: midterm follow-up results. *Invest Radiol.* 2000;35:131–140.

108. Leung DA, Blitz LR, Nelson T, et al. Rheolytic pharmacomechanical thrombectomy for the management of acute limb ischemia: results from the PEARL Registry. *J Endovasc Ther.* 2015;22:546–557.

109. Sarac TP, Hilleman D, Arko FR, et al. Clinical and economic evaluation of the trellis thrombectomy device for arterial occlusions: preliminary analysis. *J Vasc Surg.* 2004;39:556–559.

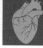

110. Stanek F, Ouhrabkova R, Prochazka D. Mechanical thrombectomy using the Rotarex catheter--safe and effective method in the treatment of peripheral arterial thromboembolic occlusions. *Vasa*. 2010;39:334–340.

111. Bucker A, Schmitz-Rode T, Vorwerk D, Gunther RW. Comparative in vitro study of two percutaneous hydrodynamic thrombectomy systems. *J Vasc Interv Radiol*. 1996;7:445–449.

112. Wagner HJ, Starck EE. Acute embolic occlusions of the infrainguinal arteries: percutaneous aspiration embolectomy in 102 patients. *Radiology*. 1992;182:403–407.

113. Zehnder T, Birrer M, Do DD, et al. Percutaneous catheter thrombus aspiration for acute or subacute arterial occlusion of the legs: how much thrombolysis is needed? *Eur J Vasc Endovasc Surg*. 2000;20:41–46.

114. Wagner HJ, Starck EE, Reuter P. Long-term results of percutaneous aspiration embolectomy. *Cardiovasc Intervent Radiol*. 1994;17: 241–246.

115. Baumann F, Sharpe 3rd E, Pena C, et al. Technical results of vacuum-assisted thrombectomy for arterial clot removal in patients with acute limb ischemia. *J Vasc Interv Radiol*. 2016;27:330–335.

116. Siegel RJ, Fishbein MC, Forrester J, et al. Ultrasonic plaque ablation. A new method for recanalization of partially or totally occluded arteries. *Circulation*. 1988;78:1443–1448.

117. Steffen W, Fishbein MC, Luo H, et al. High intensity, low frequency catheter-delivered ultrasound dissolution of occlusive coronary artery thrombi: an in vitro and in vivo study. *J Am Coll Cardiol*. 1994;24:1571–1579.

118. Braaten JV, Goss RA, Francis CW. Ultrasound reversibly disaggregates fibrin fibers. *Thromb Haemost*. 1997;78:1063–1068.

119. Francis CW, Blinc A, Lee S, Cox C. Ultrasound accelerates transport of recombinant tissue plasminogen activator into clots. *Ultrasound Med Biol*. 1995;21:419–424.

120. Wissgott C, Richter A, Kamusella P, Steinkamp HJ. Treatment of critical limb ischemia using ultrasound-enhanced thrombolysis (PARES Trial): final results. *J Endovasc Ther*. 2007;14:438–443.

121. Wissgott C, Kamusella P, Richter A, et al. Treatment of acute femoropopliteal bypass graft occlusion: comparison of mechanical rotational thrombectomy with ultrasound-enhanced lysis. *Rofo*. 2008;180:547–552.

122. Motarjeme A. Ultrasound-enhanced thrombolysis. *J Endovasc Ther*. 2007;14:251–256.

123. Schrijver AM, Reijnen MM, van Oostayen JA, et al. Initial results of catheter-directed ultrasound-accelerated thrombolysis for thromboembolic obstructions of the aortofemoral arteries: a feasibility study. *Cardiovasc Intervent Radiol*. 2012;35(2):279–285.

124. Schrijver AM, van Leersum M, Fioole B, et al. Dutch randomized trial comparing standard catheter-directed thrombolysis and ultrasound-accelerated thrombolysis for arterial thromboembolic infrainguinal disease (DUET). *J Endovasc Ther*. 2015;22:87–95.

125. Schernthaner MB, Samuels S, Biegler P, et al. Ultrasound-accelerated versus standard catheter-directed thrombolysis in 102 patients with acute and subacute limb ischemia. *J Vasc Interv Radiol*. 2014;25:1149–1156. quiz 1157.

126. Kashyap VS, Gilani R, Bena JF, et al. Endovascular therapy for acute limb ischemia. *J Vasc Surg*. 2011;53:340–346.

127. Fogarty TJ, Cranley JJ, Krause RJ, et al. A method for extraction of arterial emboli and thrombi. *Surg Gynecol Obstet*. 1963;116:241–244.

128. Dale WA. Endovascular suction catheters for thrombectomy and embolectomy. *J Thorac Cardiovasc Surg*. 1962;44:557–558.

129. Green RM, DeWeese JA, Rob CG. Arterial embolectomy before and after the Fogarty catheter. *Surgery*. 1975;77:24–33.

130. Hill SL, Donato AT. The simple Fogarty embolectomy: an operation of the past? *Am Surg*. 1994;60:907–911.

131. Plecha FR, Pories WJ. Intraoperative angiography in the immediate assessment of arterial reconstruction. *Arch Surg*. 1972;105:902–907.

132. Galbraith K, Collin J, Morris PJ, Wood RF. Recent experience with arterial embolism of the limbs in a vascular unit. *Ann R Coll Surg Engl*. 1985;67:30–33.

133. Davies MG, O'Malley K, Feeley M, et al. Upper limb embolus: a timely diagnosis. *Ann Vasc Surg*. 1991;5:85–87.

134. Pentti J, Salenius JP, Kuukasjarvi P, Tarkka M. Outcome of surgical treatment in acute upper limb ischaemia. *Ann Chir Gynaecol*. 1995;84:25–28.

135. Hernandez-Richter T, Angele MK, Helmberger T, et al. Acute ischemia of the upper extremity: long-term results following thrombembolectomy with the Fogarty catheter. *Langenbecks Arch Surg*. 2001;386:261–266.

136. Coulon M, Goffette P, Dondelinger RF. Local thrombolytic infusion in arterial ischemia of the upper limb: mid-term results. *Cardiovasc Intervent Radiol*. 1994;17:81–86.

137. Michaels JA, Torrie EP, Galland RB. The treatment of upper limb vascular occlusions using intraarterial thrombolysis. *Eur J Vasc Surg*. 1993;7:744–746.

138. Widlus DM, Venbrux AC, Benenati JF, et al. Fibrinolytic therapy for upper-extremity arterial occlusions. *Radiology*. 1990;175:393–399.

139. Beyersdorf F. Protection of the ischemic skeletal muscle. *Thorac Cardiovasc Surg*. 1991;39:19–28.

140. Dormandy J, Heeck L, Vig S. Acute limb ischemia. *Semin Vasc Surg*. 1999;12:148–153.

141. Abbott WM, Maloney RD, McCabe CC, et al. Arterial embolism: a 44 year perspective. *Am J Surg*. 1982;143:460–464.

142. Orrapin S, Orrapin S, Arwon S, Rerkasem K. Predictive factors for post-ischemic compartment syndrome in non-traumatic acute limb ischemia in a lower extremity. *Annals of Vascular Diseases*. 2017;10:378–385.

143. Perry MO. Compartment syndromes and reperfusion injury. *Surg Clin North Am*. 1988;68:853–864.

144. McCord JM. Oxygen-derived free radicals in postischemic tissue injury. *N Engl J Med*. 1985;312:159–163.

145. Mubarak SJ, Hargens AR. Acute compartment syndromes. *Surg Clin North Am*. 1983;63:539–565.

146. Hyde GL, Peck D, Powell DC. Compartment syndromes. Early diagnosis and a bedside operation. *Am Surg*. 1983;49:563–568.

147. Vaillancourt C, Shrier I, Vandal A, et al. Acute compartment syndrome: how long before muscle necrosis occurs? *CJEM*. 2004;6:147–154.

148. Mubarak SJ, Owen CA, Hargens AR, et al. Acute compartment syndromes: diagnosis and treatment with the aid of the wick catheter. *J Bone Joint Surg Am*. 1978;60:1091–1095.

149. Rorabeck CH. The treatment of compartment syndromes of the leg. *J Bone Joint Surg Br*. 1984;66:93–97.

150. Matsen 3rd FA, Winquist RA, Krugmire Jr RB. Diagnosis and management of compartmental syndromes. *J Bone Joint Surg Am*. 1980;62:286–291.

151. Whitesides TE, Haney TC, Morimoto K, Harada H. Tissue pressure measurements as a determinant for the need of fasciotomy. *Clin Orthop Relat Res*. 1975;43–51.

152. Frink M, Hildebrand F, Krettek C, et al. Compartment syndrome of the lower leg and foot. *Clin Orthop Relat Res*. 2010;468:940–950.

153. Rush DS, Frame SB, Bell RM, et al. Does open fasciotomy contribute to morbidity and mortality after acute lower extremity ischemia and revascularization? *J Vasc Surg*. 1989;10:343–350.

154. Jensen SL, Sandermann J. Compartment syndrome and fasciotomy in vascular surgery. A review of 57 cases. *Eur J Vasc Endovasc Surg*. 1997;13:48–53.

155. Finkelstein JA, Hunter GA, Hu RW. Lower limb compartment syndrome: course after delayed fasciotomy. *J Trauma*. 1996;40:342–344.

156. Heemskerk J, Kitslaar P. Acute compartment syndrome of the lower leg: retrospective study on prevalence, technique, and outcome of fasciotomies. *World J Surg*. 2003;27:744–747.

157. Papalambros EL, Panayiotopoulos YP, Bastounis E, et al. Prophylactic fasciotomy of the legs following acute arterial occlusion procedures. *Int Angiol*. 1989;8:120–124.

158. Allenberg JR, Meybier H. The compartment syndrome from the vascular surgery viewpoint. *Chirurgie*. 1988;59:722–727.

159. Qvarfordt P, Christenson JT, Eklof B, Ohlin P. Intramuscular pressure after revascularization of the popliteal artery in severe ischaemia. *Br J Surg*. 1983;70:539–541.

160. Melberg PE, Styf J, Biber B, et al. Muscular compartment pressure following reconstructive arterial surgery of the lower limbs. *Acta Chir Scand*. 1984;150:129–133.

161. Patman RD. Compartmental syndromes in peripheral vascular surgery. *Clin Orthop Relat Res*. 1975;103–110.

162. Wright JG, Belkin M, Hobson 2nd RW. Hypothermia and controlled reperfusion: two non-pharmacologic methods which diminish ischemia-reperfusion injury in skeletal muscle. *Microcirc Endothelium Lymphatics.* 1989;5:315–334.

163. Beyersdorf F, Schlensak C. Controlled reperfusion after acute and persistent limb ischemia. *Semin Vasc Surg.* 2009;22:52–57.

164. Dick F, Li J, Giraud MN, et al. Basic control of reperfusion effectively protects against reperfusion injury in a realistic rodent model of acute limb ischemia. *Circulation.* 2008;118:1920–1928.

165. Anderson RJ, Cambria R, Kerr J, Hobson 2nd RW. Sustained benefit of temporary limited reperfusion in skeletal muscle following ischemia. *J Surg Res.* 1990;49:271–275.

166. Defraigne JO, Pincemail J, Laroche C, et al. Successful controlled limb reperfusion after severe prolonged ischemia. *J Vasc Surg.* 1997;26:346–350.

167. Walker PM, Romaschin AD, Davis S, Piovesan J. Lower limb ischemia: phase 1 results of salvage perfusion. *J Surg Res.* 1999;84:193–198.

168. Mowlavi A, Neumeister MW, Wilhelmi BJ, et al. Local hypothermia during early reperfusion protects skeletal muscle from ischemia-reperfusion injury. *Plast Reconstr Surg.* 2003;111:242–250.

169. Wilhelm MP, Schlensak C, Hoh A, et al. Controlled reperfusion using a simplified perfusion system preserves function after acute and persistent limb ischemia: a preliminary study. *J Vasc Surg.* 2005;42:690–694.

170. de Donato G, Gussoni G, de Donato G, et al. The ILAILL study: iloprost as adjuvant to surgery for acute ischemia of lower limbs: a randomized, placebo-controlled, double-blind study by the Italian Society for Vascular and Endovascular Surgery. *Ann Surg.* 2006;244:185–193.

171. Foster AD, Vicente D, Sexton JJ, et al. Administration of FTY720 during tourniquet-induced limb ischemia reperfusion injury attenuates systemic inflammation. *Mediators Inflamm.* 2017;2017:4594035.

172. Liu Y, Zhou C, Jiang J, et al. Blockade of HMGB1 preserves vascular homeostasis and improves blood perfusion in rats of acute limb ischemia/reperfusion. *Microvasc Res.* 2017;112:37–40.

173. Chou WC, Kao MC, Yue CT, et al. Caffeine mitigates lung inflammation induced by ischemia-reperfusion of lower limbs in rats. *Mediators Inflamm.* 2015;2015:361638.

174. Bonaca MP, Bhatt DL, Storey RF, et al. Ticagrelor for prevention of ischemic events after myocardial infarction in patients with peripheral artery disease. *J Am Coll Cardiol.* 2016;67:2719–2728.

175. Anand SS, Bosch J, Eikelboom JW, et al. Rivaroxaban with or without aspirin in patients with stable peripheral or carotid artery disease: an international, randomised, double-blind, placebo-controlled trial. *Lancet.* 2018;391:219–229.

176. Anand SS, Caron F, Eikelboom JW, et al. Major adverse limb events and mortality in patients with peripheral artery disease: the COMPASS Trial. *J Am Coll Cardiol.* 2018;71:2306–2315.

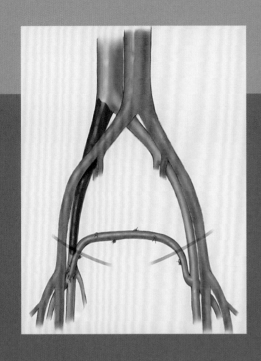

第45章
动脉粥样硬化栓塞

　　动脉粥样性栓塞又称动脉粥样硬化栓塞、胆固醇结晶栓塞等，是一种少见但严重的多系统功能不全。本章将从该病的发病、症状、治疗等方面系统介绍相关知识。

　　动脉粥样硬化斑块自发或在外力作用下破裂后，胆固醇结晶等内容物会进入血液循环并栓塞远端小动脉，造成脑、眼、肾等终末器官及肢体末梢的缺氧及组织损害。其中，最常受累的部位为肾与皮肤。该病的主要危险因素包括动脉粥样硬化、经动脉介入治疗史、高龄等。由于动脉粥样性栓塞可累及多个器官，其症状多样，难以准确诊断。典型体征包括蓝趾、网状青斑、视网膜Hollenhorst斑。短暂性脑缺血发作、一过性黑矇、急/慢性肾功能不全等为该病常见的临床表现。目前尚无有效的可确诊动脉粥样性栓塞的实验室检查，实践中主要依据患者病史及临床表现给出该病的临床诊断。对动脉粥样性栓塞而言，预防才是最有效的治疗。一旦发病，伤口护理、止痛、器官替代治疗等支持手段为主要治疗方法，但也应根据具体情况决定是否取栓。该病的预后主要取决于患者基础状况及器官受累程度。编者认为，由于介入诊疗技术已在我国得到了相当的发展与推广，有必要提高对该病的警惕性，以预防为主，防微杜渐，让先进技术更好地服务患者。

罗明尧

Atheroembolism

Roger F.J. Shepherd

Atheroembolism is a rare but serious disorder with significant morbidity from stroke, renal failure, and limb loss. This systemic disorder affects multiple organs and carries a high mortality rate. Atheroembolism can be a single event or recurrent. It can occur spontaneously or following an invasive vascular procedure. It can originate from atherosclerotic or aneurysmal disease and involve single or multiple sites. There is no specific laboratory test that can reliably distinguish cholesterol embolization from other disorders. A definitive diagnosis can only be made with biopsy of involved tissue and histological examination. A high index of clinical suspicion is necessary because atheroembolism may mimic a number of other disorders, leading to potential misdiagnosis. The focus of this chapter will be review of pathophysiology, precipitating factors, clinical syndromes, and management of atheroembolic disease. Prognosis is determined by the extent of systemic involvement and risk of recurrent episodes. As in many vascular disorders, prevention is the best treatment.

Atheroembolism occurs when tiny fragments of an atherosclerotic plaque (in particular, cholesterol crystals) break off from a proximal artery and travel distally in the circulation, ending up in small arteries downstream from the origin. The consequence of this event is microvascular obstruction with tissue ischemia. The abdominal aorta is the most common origin for atheroembolism to the abdominal organs and lower extremities, but any artery with atheromatous disease may be a potential embolic source. End-organ targets include the brain, eye, heart, kidney, gastrointestinal tract, fingers, toes, and skin. The kidneys and skin are the two most common targets in many cases.[1] In the setting of an elderly patient with atherosclerosis, who develops sudden onset of pain and ischemia of the distal extremities and unexplained renal failure after an invasive angiographic procedure, atheroembolism should be high on the list of likely diagnoses.[2]

It is important to differentiate between two types of arterial embolization: thromboemboli and atheroemboli. Atheroembolism is a much different disease and can be more difficult to diagnose and manage. Thromboembolism occurs when a section of thrombus breaks off from a proximal site, such as the heart, and occludes downstream vessels. Thromboembolism can be diagnosed by computed tomography, magnetic resonance, or invasive imaging, as it causes obstruction of large proximal vessels. By contrast, an atheroembolic event is a shower of tiny particles originating from atherosclerotic plaque, causing very distal end organ embolization and tissue ischemia. This chapter will only deal with atheroembolism. Thromboembolism causing acute limb/organ ischemia is reviewed in Chapter 44.

Atheroembolism can present in a number of distinct clinical syndromes (Box 45.1). The *blue toe syndrome* occurs when arteries to the distal parts of the feet and toes become obstructed by atheromatous embolization, causing toe ischemia (Fig. 45.1). *Livedo reticularis* (localized mottling of the skin) occurs when the atheroembolism involves small cutaneous vessels (Figs. 45.2 and 45.3). When present, this can be an important diagnostic indicator of atheroembolism. *Acute and chronic kidney failure* can result from aortic or renal artery atheroembolism. Atheroemboli can also travel to the mesenteric arteries, causing *intestinal necrosis*, or to the splenic, hepatic, or pancreatic arteries, causing *localized infarction*. *Transient ischemic episodes and stroke* may result from atheromatous disease of the aortic arch, internal carotid, or vertebral arteries. Atheroembolism to the retinal arteries may present with temporary horizontal monocular visual loss called *amaurosis fugax*. Funduscopic examination may identify a bright reflection from a cholesterol crystal in a retinal artery known as a *Hollenhorst plaque*.[3] The unifying cause of all atheroembolic syndromes is the presence of atheromatous disease in a proximal artery and ischemic damage to a distal organ or extremity when these fragments embolize and lodge in distal vessels.

A number of terms for this syndrome are used interchangeably in the literature, including *cholesterol crystal embolization*, *atheromatous embolization*, and *atheroembolism*. Vascular medicine covers a great deal of internal medicine, and atheroembolism should be in the differential diagnosis of many diseases including vasculitis, infective endocarditis, malignancy, hematological diseases, atypical infections, Raynaud syndrome, and acute and chronic renal failure. Atheroembolism has been called "the great masquerader" because it may resemble many other conditions.[4] Diagnosis of atheroembolism is usually made on the basis of clinical suspicion, by history and examination, but most importantly by an astute clinician who considers this entity when presented with unusual vascular diseases.

PATHOBIOLOGY

Atheroembolism originates from atherosclerotic plaque. The pathobiology of atherosclerosis is reviewed in detail in Chapter 6.

ETIOLOGY

Atheroembolism may occur spontaneously or be precipitated by angiographic or surgical procedures (iatrogenic). Earlier reports indicated spontaneous episodes of atheroembolism were more common.[5,6] Today with increased numbers of vascular procedures, iatrogenic catheter-induced atheroembolism outnumbers spontaneous cases. Currently, over three-fourths of atheroembolic renal disease is procedure-related, occurring during or after an angiographic or endovascular procedure (Figs. 45.4 through 45.6).[7,8]

Spontaneous Atheroembolism
Who Is at Risk?

Spontaneous atheroembolism occurs in older patients with advanced atherosclerosis. In Fine's review of 221 cases of atheroembolism in the

BOX 45.1 Clinical Syndromes and Manifestations of Atheroembolism

Skin
Livedo reticularis
Petechiae
Purpura
Splinter hemorrhages
Fissures and nodules
Ulceration and skin necrosis

Extremities
Blue toe syndrome
Digital gangrene
Trash foot
Genital skin necrosis
Scrotal and penile necrosis

Renal
Acute and chronic renal failure
Progressive renal failure
Proteinuria
Renal infarction
Worsening or uncontrolled hypertension

Gastrointestinal
Abdominal pain
Nausea/vomiting
Gastrointestinal hemorrhage
Bowel perforation/infarction
Pancreatitis
Cholecystitis
Splenic infarcts
Abnormal liver transaminases

Central Nervous System
Amaurosis fugax
Hollenhorst plaque
Transient ischemic attack/stroke
Spinal cord infarction

Cardiac
Myocardial infarction

General Symptoms
Myalgias
Fever
Malaise
Weight loss
Anorexia

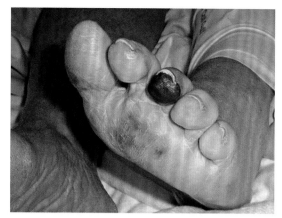

Fig. 45.1 Classic Blue Toe Syndrome. Note impending infarction of affected third toe, with livedo reticularis of the plantar surface.

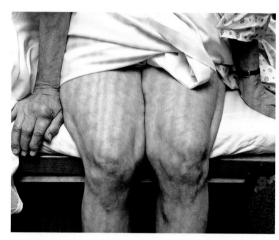

Fig. 45.2 Patient With Previously Undiagnosed Abdominal Aortic Aneurysm Presenting With Atheroembolism to Lower Extremities. Note typical lacy reticular skin pattern of both thighs.

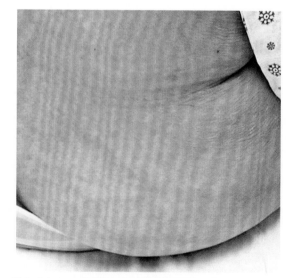

Fig. 45.3 Atheroembolism to Buttock and Flank. Same patient as in Fig. 45.2, with renal failure and livedo reticularis as presenting symptoms of previously unknown abdominal aortic aneurysm.

English literature, he noted a predominance of patients with underlying atherosclerotic disease including cardiac, carotid, and kidney disease. In particular, many had significant preexisting chronic kidney disease (CKD) evidenced by elevated serum creatinine (Cr) (CKD stage 3 or 4). There was also a high incidence of aortic aneurysms, present in 25% of these patients.[5] Many patients with atheroembolic events present with multisystem manifestations. Common presentations of spontaneous atheroembolism included blue toe syndrome, livedo reticularis, and progressive renal failure. Stroke/transient ischemic events due to carotid atherosclerosis is one of the best examples of a spontaneous

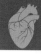

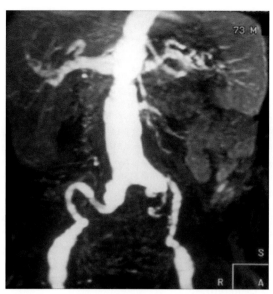

Fig. 45.4 Abdominal Magnetic Resonance Image Showing Diffuse Atherosclerosis of Aorta, With "Arteriomegaly." This disease has a high risk of atheroembolism.

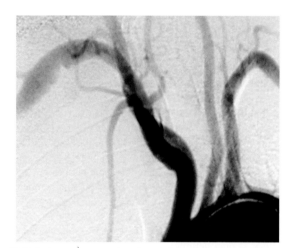

Fig. 45.5 Arch aortogram showing right subclavian aneurysm with ulcerated atheromatous disease in nonsmoking young woman with thoracic outlet syndrome, presenting with atheroemboli to fingers.

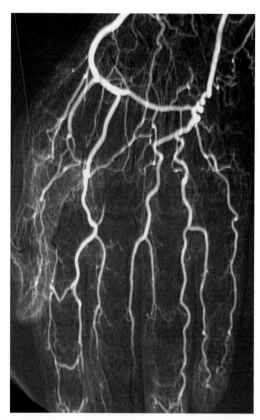

Fig. 45.6 Upper-Extremity Angiogram in Patient With Hypothenar Hammer Syndrome, Multiple Digital Artery Occlusions Resulting in Critical Ischemia of Fingers. Note abnormal ulnar artery tortuosity secondary to local trauma to hand.

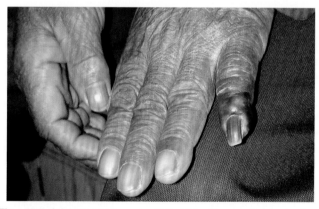

Fig. 45.7 Atheroembolism to Left Fifth Finger. Origin is from subclavian atheromatous plaque.

atheroembolic episode. The mechanism of blue toe syndrome has been likened to a brain transient ischemic attack (TIA), but affecting a lower extremity.[9] Today, many cases of unexplained progressive renal failure may be due to unsuspected atheroembolism.

In most series, males are more affected by atheroembolism than females, with mean ages ranging from 63 to 69 years.[1,5,10] Skin lesions and renal failure are often the two most common manifestations.[1,5] Skin lesions may be the initial clinical sign of atheroembolization (see Fig. 45.3), of which blue toes and livedo reticularis make up 88% of cutaneous findings.[1] African Americans are less likely to be diagnosed with atheroembolism, perhaps because the faint cutaneous pattern of livedo is more difficult to see in skin that is more deeply pigmented (Fig. 45.7).[11]

How Common Is Spontaneous Atheroembolism?

Autopsy studies from the 1940s found an atheroembolic incidence of 3.4% (9 of 267 patients with aortic atherosclerosis).[12] A larger and more recent autopsy study involving 2126 elderly patients over a period of

7 years found only 16 cases of spontaneous atheroembolism (incidence <0.1%), despite the high prevalence of severe aortoiliac atheromatous disease and aortic aneurysms.[13] Another autopsy study of 372 patients found spontaneous cholesterol embolization occurred in only seven individuals; all were over age 60, and all but one were male, for an incidence of 1.9%. Lesions of different ages were noted, suggesting recurrent episodes to the kidneys and spleen.[10] A review of autopsy data at Johns Hopkins from 1973 to 1995 found 0.7% had histological features of atheroembolism.[14]

The actual incidence of spontaneous atheroembolism is difficult to determine; symptoms may be vague, and clinical features can be subtle or not recognized.[15]

Procedure-Related Atheroembolism
Cardiovascular Surgery

Atheroembolism can occur as a complication of any invasive cardiac or vascular procedure or operation. Atheroembolism has been reported following abdominal aortic aneurysm (AAA) repair, aortoiliac bypass, and aortic and renal arteriography. Atheromatous debris can be dislodged during left heart catheterization, external cardiac massage, blunt abdominal trauma, coronary artery bypass surgery, and many endovascular procedures.[2,16]

The advent of aortography in the 1930s transformed the ability to make accurate vascular diagnosis and expanded treatment options, but brought with it the risk of atheroembolism, especially in patients with atheromatous or aneurysmal disease. A 30% incidence of atheroembolism after abdominal aortography was reported in patients who subsequently died within 6 months of the procedure. The organs most commonly affected were the kidneys and spleen.[17]

In the 1950s, Thurlbeck and Castleman first reported atheroembolism associated with vascular surgery and attributed this to operative manipulations that included arterial incisions, cannulation, and clamping of major arteries. Postmortem examination of those who died following AAA repair found cholesterol embolization to the kidneys in as many as 77% of patients.[18] In a more recent large retrospective series of 1011 patients undergoing angiographic procedures prior to aortic or infrainguinal vascular surgery, 2.9% (29 patients) were identified with atheroembolism. The majority of iatrogenic cases were attributed to aortography as opposed to surgery. The primary sources of embolism in these patients were the abdominal aorta, iliac arteries, and femoropopliteal arteries.[19]

Massive atheroembolism following aortoiliac stent placement for treatment of aortic aneurysmal disease has been reported but is uncommon.[20,21] A study using Doppler ultrasound to identify microembolism found a significantly higher degree of peripheral embolization during endovascular aneurysm repair, compared to conventional surgical aneurysm repair.[22]

Atheroembolism can also occur after coronary artery bypass grafting (CABG) and valve surgery. Fatal myocardial infarction (MI) due to atheroembolism has been reported during coronary artery bypass operations.[23] Procedures that provoke atheroembolism include aortic cannulation, initiation of cardiopulmonary bypass (CPB), and anastomosis of bypass grafts to the ascending aorta during cardiac surgery. Atheroemboli may originate from the aortic root at the origin of vein grafts or from ruptured plaque in a coronary artery. In one series of 29 patients who died after cardiac surgery, atheroembolism was the causative factor in 22% of all deaths. In this series, atheroembolism to the coronary circulation caused cardiac failure; to the brain caused massive stroke; and to the gastrointestinal tract caused abdominal pain and bleeding.[14] Fortunately this is rare. Of 4095 CABG procedures, atheroembolism was found in only nine patients, for an incidence of 0.22%.[23] Those undergoing reoperation were found to have a higher incidence of 2.3%.[23]

Atherosclerosis involving the ascending aorta is a major risk factor for stroke during cardiac surgery. A large autopsy study of 221 patients found severe atherosclerosis of the ascending aorta in patients who died from atheroembolism after cardiac procedures. Atheroembolism occurred in 46 of 123 patients with severe ascending aortic disease, but only 2 of 98 (2%) without ascending aortic disease. The incidence of atheroembolism was three times as high after CABG than valve surgery (26.1% vs. 8.9%).[24] Older patients with more advanced atheromatous disease of the ascending aorta were at the highest risk. Atheroemboli traveled to the brain in 16%, the spleen in 11%, kidney in 10%, and pancreas in 7%. Two-thirds of patients had multiple sites of atheroembolism.[24] A 12% stroke risk during CPB was noted in one recent study

if aortic arch atheromas were seen with intraoperative transesophageal echocardiography (TEE).[25]

Transcranial Doppler (TCD) has documented that the greatest number of microembolic events was found during aortic clamping and initiation of bypass.[26] A study where an intraaortic filter was deployed and left in place until the patient was weaned from bypass found that 62% of filters contained atheroma in addition to platelet and fibrin strands.[27]

Off-pump CABG may reduce cerebral damage due to microembolism.[28] A study comparing effects of CABG with and without CPB assessed retinal microembolization by fluorescein angiography and fundus photography. Doppler high-intensity transient signals (HITS) was used to assess emboli to the brain. Five of nine pump patients had retinal microvascular damage, but none was evident in the off-pump patients. Doppler HITS were 20 times more frequent in the CPB patients.[28] Off-pump coronary artery bypass may have less risk of atheroembolism by avoiding arterial cannulation and the abrasive effect of CPB on the arterial wall.[24,28]

Cardiac Catheterization

Cholesterol embolization after left heart catheterization is rare but can be devastating when it occurs. Coronary angiography is the most common invasive procedure associated with atheroembolism.[8] Clinically detectable cholesterol embolization occurring after cardiac catheterization has resulted in stroke, renal failure, mesenteric ischemia, and lower-extremity tissue loss with gangrene. In some situations, it has a high fatality rate.[29-33]

A retrospective British study by Drost et al. reported 7 cases out of a total of 4587 cardiac catheterization procedures. Most had extensive atherosclerosis and suffered multisystem atheroembolization, with a retinal embolism in one patient, renal failure in five patients, and three requiring toe amputations. Six of the seven had extensive atherosclerosis. Four of these patients died within 4.5 months of this procedure.[29]

In a large prospective Japanese study, Fukumoto et al. prospectively reviewed 1786 consecutive patients undergoing left heart catheterization in a multicenter study. Diagnostic criteria for atheroembolism included livedo reticularis, blue toe syndrome, digital gangrene, or renal dysfunction. They found an incidence of 1.4 % (25 patients), of which cutaneous findings and renal failure were the two most common clinical findings. If only definite cases were counted, the incidence was lower at 0.75%. Prognosis is poor in some patients, with an in-hospital mortality rate of 16%.[34]

Saklayen et al. prospectively evaluated 267 patients undergoing coronary angiography at a Veterans Administration (VA) medical center. A rise in Cr of 0.5 mg/dL or more at 3 weeks after the procedure was the main indicator of atheroembolism. They found an incidence of atheroembolic renal dysfunction of 1.9% (5/263 of patients undergoing coronary angiography).[31] Frock identified 17 patients with atheroembolic renal disease out of 14,998 angiographic procedures, an incidence of 0.1%.[35] In a prospective study of 1579 patients, Johnson et al. also found the incidence of cholesterol embolization to be very low—a single patient in 1579 coronary angiograms (0.06%).[36]

Passage of a catheter into the aorta for any endovascular procedure may not only loosen atheromatous plaque but can also scrape off aortic debris into the coronary guiding catheters. During contrast injection, this debris could be injected into the coronary or cerebral artery. In a study of 1000 consecutive coronary interventions, the amount of atheromatous material entering a guiding catheter from passage up the aorta was assessed by allowing blood to passively exit the back of the catheter into a sterile towel. Depending on the catheter shape, aortic debris was recovered in 24% to 65% of interventional cases. Surprisingly, the finding of aortic debris did not correlate with clinically apparent neurological, coronary, or renal ischemic events. Allowing adequate back-bleeding of guiding catheters before injecting contrast was suggested to decrease the risk of atheroembolism found in the guiding catheter from scraping the wall of the aorta during placement.[37]

Today, with more advanced surgical techniques and greater awareness of atheroembolic risk, the incidence of atheroembolism during vascular and cardiac catheterization procedures is less common. The promise of distal protection devices to decrease the risk of atheroembolism during a procedure is still being assessed. Atheromatous debris can be recovered from the majority of angioplasty procedures. Development of more flexible catheters and lower-profile devices, along with improved operator technique, should allow for lower incidence of atheroembolic events in the future.[38]

Karalis et al. addressed the risk of atheroembolism in patients undergoing catheterization when they have a so-called shaggy aorta. In this study, 70 patients were identified with aortic debris found on echocardiography, and 10 had a procedure-related embolic episode. A radial approach may be a better option in these patients.[39] Spinal cord atheroembolism is a very rare complication of angiography.[13,40,41] Spinal cord infarction likely occurs secondary to embolic occlusion of small spinal cord arteries.

Intraaortic balloon pumps. Intraaortic balloon pumps have especially high potential for embolization when placed in an aorta with atherosclerotic debris. In one study, 5 of 10 patients (50%) had an embolic event related to placement of an intraaortic balloon pump.[39] If aortic debris is mobile, risk of embolization is especially high.

Anticoagulation/Thrombolysis Issues

A number of large studies have shown no increased risk of atheroembolism in patients treated with warfarin. Blackshear et al. addressed concerns of warfarin anticoagulation in patients with atrial fibrillation and documented aortic plaque. The SPAF III (Stroke Prevention in Atrial Fibrillation) trial looked at patients with atrial fibrillation and aortic plaque documented by TEE and found that patients assigned to warfarin therapy had an annual cholesterol embolization rate of 0.7 per patient-year, which was lower than those randomized to warfarin plus aspirin. The authors conclude that "elderly patients with AF and aortic plaque can receive adjusted-dose warfarin with a relatively low risk of cholesterol embolism."[42] The French Study of Aortic Plaques in Stroke found no difference in recurrent brain infarction in patients receiving warfarin compared to those on aspirin.[43]

Many cardiovascular patients are on anticoagulation and in most case reports of atheroembolism, causation from anticoagulation is difficult to prove. Delayed recognition of an acute event or recurrent showers in patients with shaggy aortas may account for the temporal association of atheroembolism with an oral anticoagulant.[44] Elderly patients are more likely to have advanced atherosclerosis and other chronic disorders such as atrial fibrillation requiring long-term anticoagulation. Often these patients had undergone other procedures including angiography, which is more likely an explanation for atheroembolic events.

A sensible conclusion is to continue anticoagulation when compelling conditions exist, such as atrial fibrillation and thromboembolism, but consider stopping it if there is a lesser indication.[38]

Atheroembolism has also been reported to occur after thrombolytic therapy for MI.[45–48] In some of these case reports, atheroembolism occurred in the absence of any invasive procedure, therefore implicating thrombolysis as a possible culprit. The mechanism of atheroembolism is thought to be dissolution of thrombus overlying atheromatous plaque, exposing ulcerated plaque that can embolize distally to the arterial circulation. Large trials of thrombolysis for acute myocardial infarction (AMI), including GISSI 2 and GUSTO, did not cite atheroembolism as

a complication of thrombolytic therapy, so concern of atheroembolization should not be a reason to withhold thrombolysis.[49]

Blankenship et al. prospectively followed 60 patients with AMI who later underwent CABG. Half of these patients received thrombolytic therapy and half did not. It was concluded the prevalence of cholesterol embolization was not higher in those who received thrombolytic therapy.[50]

ATHEROEMBOLIC SYNDROMES

Livedo Reticularis and Skin Atheroembolism

Skin findings are the earliest, and at times the only, clinical finding of atheroembolism. Livedo reticularis is the most common manifestation of skin involvement, noted in 49% of patients.[51,52] The incidence of cutaneous manifestations of atheroembolism ranges from 35% to 96%.[1,53,54] Livedo reticularis has been labeled an underutilized clue to the diagnosis of atheroembolism. It should be considered an important and common indicator of atheroembolism elsewhere—in particular, to the kidneys or mesenteric organs.[51,55] For example, the suspicion of renal atheroembolism is markedly strengthened by the finding of livedo reticularis affecting the trunk or abdomen.

Livedo reticularis has a classic appearance as a reddish-blue lacy or netlike color pattern of the skin (Fig. 45.8). It is noted when the cutaneous venous plexus becomes visible owing to desaturated venous blood. In the presence of atheroembolism, small arteries are obstructed, reducing flow into the venous plexus and resulting in stasis of deoxygenated blood.[56] Characteristics of livedo reticularis include blanching with local pressure. It is more prominent when the patient is upright and may not be apparent if the patient is examined in the supine position.[51] Atheroembolism is less frequently diagnosed in nonwhite individuals because darker skin may disguise visible manifestations.[11] Livedo reticularis is most commonly seen on the feet and legs, but thighs, buttocks, lower back, abdomen, and upper extremities can also be affected, depending on the source of the atheroembolism.[1]

Less common cutaneous findings in atheroembolism include splinter hemorrhages, petechiae, purpura, and erythematous nodules. Cholesterol embolism to the skin has been called a *pseudovasculitic syndrome*.[57] Livedo reticularis due to atheroembolism has been mistaken for small-vessel vasculitis in 16% of patients.[58] The diagnosis of atheroembolism can be confirmed by skin biopsy, and is positive in 92% of cases.[53,58]

In young women, livedo reticularis may be a common normal finding due to cold-induced vasospasm of skin vessels, and classically disappears with warming. It can also be seen in a number of diseases including collagen vascular disorders, vasculitides such as systemic

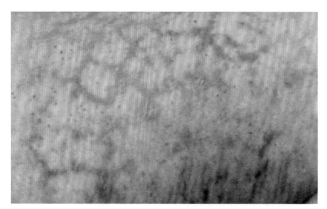

Fig. 45.8 Unusual nonblanching livedo reticularis of thigh in patient with suspected livedo vasculitis.

lupus erythematosus (SLE) and polyarteritis nodosa, antiphospholipid antibody syndrome, disseminated intravascular coagulation (DIC), infective endocarditis, cryoglobulinemia, and hyperviscosity disorders.[38]

Atheroembolic Renal Disease

About half of all reported cases of atheroembolism involve the kidney.[8] The kidney receives a major percentage of the cardiac output and is the most common site for atheroembolism, followed by skin and gastrointestinal tract.[1,59] In clinical practice, it has been estimated that up to 10% of all cases of acute renal failure may be due to atheroembolism.[60]

Atheroembolic renal disease is defined as a syndrome of renal failure secondary to obstruction of small kidney arteries, arterioles, and glomerular capillaries by cholesterol crystal atheroembolism dislodged from the aorta or proximal renal arteries.[61] Renal atheroembolism may occur spontaneously in patients who have advanced atheromatous disease of the abdominal aorta, but more frequently it occurs as a complication of an angiographic or endovascular procedure. As noted earlier, passage of a catheter or guidewire through the aorta or renal arteries may dislodge atheromatous plaque fragments that travel to the kidneys, where they occlude small vessels. Today, approximately three-fourths of renal atheroembolization cases are iatrogenic secondary to invasive procedures, in particular angiography. Coronary angiography is the most common angiographic procedure.[7,8]

The exact incidence of spontaneous atheroembolic renal disease is difficult to determine because most studies are retrospective. However, approximately 20% of atheroembolic episodes to the kidneys are thought to be unprovoked spontaneous episodes.[61] In addition, many atheroembolic episodes are subclinical, difficult to diagnose, and may be missed unless specifically looked for.

In renal biopsy studies, the prevalence of renal atheroembolism in all patients and age groups is quite low, ranging from 0.31% to 2.4%.[8,10] Moolenaar and Lamers reviewed the Netherlands' experience of 842 cases of cholesterol crystal embolization in the Dutch National Pathology Information System and found an incidence of 6.0 cases per million population. Among autopsy reports, they also found a low incidence of 0.31%.[59] In other renal biopsy series, Greenberg et al. found 24/500 had atheroembolic findings.[62] In another large series of 755 renal biopsies, atheroemboli were discovered in 8 patients (1.1%).[63] Selection bias may account for the low prevalence; these patients were selected for biopsy because of unexplained recent worsening of renal function.

Atheroembolism to the kidneys can also occur during any vascular surgical procedure, in particular AAA resection, renal revascularization, and aortoiliac or aortofemoral bypass. In those who died after aortic surgery or an angiographic procedure, the finding of atheroembolism at autopsy ranged from 12% to 77%.[8] Atheromatous emboli to the kidney was documented in 77% of patients following surgical repair of AAAs.[2]

Atheroembolism to the kidneys also occurs as a complication of endovascular procedures; Modi and Rao reports 85% of patients presenting with atheroembolic renal disease underwent an invasive vascular procedure within the prior 3 months (abdominal aorta, coronary, or carotid angiography).[61]

Another study by Kawarada et al. used intrarenal duplex ultrasound to detect microembolic signals during renal artery interventions. They found emboli occurred in all 13 patients undergoing renal artery stent implantation, in particular post dilation of the stent.[64]

Underappreciation of this frequent occurrence is because clinicians attribute acute renal failure after a procedure to another cause such as contrast-induced nephropathy.

A prospective study at a VA medical center looked at renal failure after cardiac catheterization. Atheroembolism was suspected on the basis of a 0.5 mg/dL or more rise in Cr 3 weeks after a coronary angiogram. Although the incidence of renal impairment was low in this group, two of the five died of renal failure. Of note, none of the five had skin signs of livedo reticularis, and the diagnosis of atheroembolism would have been missed on examination.[31]

Atheroembolism to the kidneys is underrecognized as a cause of acute and chronic renal disease. In one review of 259 patients who underwent renal biopsy for acute renal failure, cholesterol emboli were found in 6.9% of cases. Of note, 15 of 18 of these patients were clinically unsuspected to have atheroembolism as a cause of renal failure. Another study found 7.5% of patients with acute renal failure had documented atheroembolism on renal biopsy.[65]

In one review, Mayo and Swartz estimated that 4% of all inpatient nephrology consults were due to atheroembolism. This may be a conservative estimate because older patients with multiple risk factors accounted for a higher proportion of in-hospital nephrology consults. Of those consults seen with acute renal failure, 5% to 10% were felt to be due to atheroembolic renal disease.[60]

Atheromatous emboli and cholesterol crystals tend to lodge in arcuate and interlobar arteries, which are 150 to 200 microns in diameter.[8,61] Cholesterol crystal emboli not only cause mechanical vessel obstruction but also set up an endothelial inflammatory reaction that some have labeled *microcrystalline angiitis*.[8] This is characterized by polymorphonuclear leukocyte and eosinophil infiltration around the vessel, and subsequently mononuclear cells with giant cell formation in the perivascular tissues. Endothelial distortion, intimal proliferation, perivascular fibrosis, and sometimes extraluminalization of crystals can be seen.[63] With thrombus formation, there is further microvascular occlusion of renal vessels. Over 2 to 4 weeks, there is a progressive gradual decline in renal function following an acute atheroembolic episode. Renal infarction or necrosis is rare because the process is patchy and does not obstruct the larger feeding arteries to the kidney.

Atheroembolic renal disease presents as acute or subacute renal dysfunction in older patients, rarely younger than age 50, usually affecting those with preexisting renal insufficiency.[5,35,66] Patients with atheroembolism have multiple risk factors including smoking, diabetes, hypertension, and hyperlipidemia. A review of 52 cases of atheroembolic renal failure at the Massachusetts General Hospital from 1981 to 1990 found these patients were more likely to have significant hypertension and coronary and peripheral artery disease (PAD).[67]

The clinical course may be variable. In contrast-induced nephropathy, renal failure occurs immediately after dye infusion, with a peak in creatinine within several days and resolving in less than 2 weeks.[8] Unlike contrast-induced nephropathy, atheroembolic renal failure may slowly worsen over a period of weeks to months, likely because of recurrent spontaneous showers of emboli. The kidney responds to ischemic damage with inflammatory changes that lead to glomerular sclerosis, tubular atrophy, and interstitial fibrosis.[38,61] Sometimes, features of focal segmental necrotizing glomerulonephritis and crescentic glomerulonephritis are seen in renal biopsy specimens.[61,62,68]

Atheroembolism to kidneys may also be subclinical. Subacute presentation is more common with progressive renal failure over several weeks. In one report, the average time interval between an angiographic procedure and diagnosis of atheroembolic renal disease was 5 weeks.[35] Renal function declined over 3 to 8 weeks.[67]

A chronic form of renal failure may be mild and can be clinically silent. Clinical manifestations may present acutely, with onset within 1 week, or be subacute with delayed onset of renal impairment 2 to 6 weeks after an inciting procedure. A step-and-plateau drop in renal function has been described, perhaps owing to intermittent recurrent showers of cholesterol crystals over a period of time. One- to two-thirds of patients with atheroembolic renal disease will need dialysis.

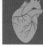

Lye et al. reviewed the English literature in 1993, noting that 40% of patients required dialysis.[6] Only 20% to 30% will recover sufficient renal function to stop dialysis.[6,8,69]

Clinical features are often absent but may include flank pain and gross hematuria due to renal infarction. Abdominal pain, nausea, vomiting, and blood loss can result from embolization to the gastrointestinal tract. In approximately half of these patients, there may be livedo reticularis or purple toe discoloration due to cholesterol embolization to the skin. Fever, malaise, and weight loss may be accompanying systemic symptoms.[61]

Severe or resistant hypertension has been noted in up to half of patients with atheroembolic renal disease.[6,15] Hypertension may result from activation of the renin angiotensin system, or be volume mediated secondary to inability of the kidney to excrete excess fluid. Malignant hypertension can occur with atheromatous embolization to the kidneys.[70]

Laboratory Testing

Laboratory testing generally shows nonspecific findings in patients with suspected atheroembolism. Although elevated creatinine, proteinuria, and eosinophilia have been reported in up to 80% of patients in the acute stage, these findings are found inconsistently.[15,71] Anemia, leukocytosis, thrombocytopenia, and elevated inflammatory markers including erythrocyte sedimentation rate and C-reactive protein (CRP) are occasionally noted.[1]

The finding of eosinophils in the urine is considered to be a very important diagnostic feature of renal atheroembolism. In a report by Wilson et al., urine eosinophils were found in 8 of 24 patients who had biopsy-proven atheroembolic disease. In six of the eight patients, more than 5% of urinary white cells were eosinophils.[72] Hansel's stain may increase the identification of urinary eosinophils. Urinary eosinophils, however, can be seen in other kidney disorders such as acute interstitial nephritis and other allergic disorders. Urinalysis may show hyaline or granular casts. Proteinuria may be present but is rarely severe enough to cause nephrotic syndrome.[73] Urine sediment is usually inactive and unremarkable.[73,74]

Blood tests may show eosinophilia ranging from 14% to 80%, but this is not a consistent finding.[8,67] Eosinophilia is thought to be due to inflammatory changes in the kidney with immune activation. Kasinath et al. reviewed the literature and observed that 29 of 36 reports noted eosinophilia in association with renal atheroembolism. In this patient series, they found eosinophil counts ranging from 540 to 2000 cells/mm^3.[71] Modi and Rao found that 60% of patients had eosinophilia,[61] and Lye et al. reported an incidence of 71%.[6] Eosinophilia may be transient and seen only in the acute phase. Despite not always being present, an eosinophil count greater than 500 cells per µL may contribute to the diagnosis of atheroembolism.[7]

The definitive diagnosis of atheroembolic kidney disease is confirmed histologically by the demonstration of cholesterol crystals in arcuate and interlobular arteries of the kidney. The sensitivity of a single renal biopsy may be only 75%, owing to the patchy distribution of atheroembolism; however, with two biopsies, 94% of patients are positive.[61]

Renal biopsies are not done in every patient with renal insufficiency, but a high degree of suspicion of atheroembolism in the appropriate setting (e.g., after an invasive vascular procedure) is necessary to make the correct diagnosis. It is important to be aware of many potential causes of renal failure in vascular patients, including contrast nephropathy, volume depletion from diuretics, renal artery or vein thrombosis, renal artery stenosis, nephrotoxic agents (e.g., antiinflammatory agents, angiotensin inhibitors), drug-induced interstitial nephritis, and glomerulonephritis (Box 45.2). Atheroembolic renal disease can also mimic vasculitis. In many cases, renal failure after an angiographic

---

BOX 45.2 Differential Diagnosis of Renal Failure in Vascular Patients

Contrast-Induced Nephropathy
Acute tubular necrosis: rapid rise in creatinine, peaks in 3 days and back to baseline in 2 weeks

Atheroembolic Renal Disease
Slow progressive or stepwise decline in renal function over 3–8 weeks. Increased likelihood of end-stage renal disease.

Ischemic Renal Failure
Renal artery stenosis, often severe hypertension

Small-Vessel Vasculitis
Active urine sediment, autoimmune markers (ANA or ANCA)

Drug-Induced Interstitial Nephritis
Drug fever, rash, eosinophilia

Thrombotic Thrombocytopenic Purpura
Smear for schistocytes

Bacterial Endocarditis
Transesophageal echocardiography

ANA, Antinuclear antibody; *ANCA*, antineutrophil cytoplasmic autoantibody.

---

procedure is incorrectly attributed to contrast-induced acute tubular necrosis. Clinical differentiation between the two is important.

Prognosis and Treatment

The prognosis for atheroembolic renal disease is generally poor.[1] Some 30% to 40% of patients with recurrent atheroembolic events have irreversible end-stage kidney failure requiring long-term hemodialysis.[6,75,76] Dialysis dependency is also an indicator of poor prognosis. In one study, those who progressed to end-stage renal failure had a mortality rate of 75% over a 107-month period, compared to 17% in those who recovered renal function.[35] Scolari et al. reported poor outcomes for 354 subjects followed for 2 years, of whom 116 required dialysis and 102 died. These patients were elderly with advanced cardiovascular disease and comorbidities including heart failure and renal disease.[7,77] Another series also reported an overall mortality rate of 58% over 15 months. Most of these patients died of cardiac failure.[1] The overall outcome and prognosis is influenced by severity of atheroembolism and presence of preexisting kidney and cardiovascular comorbidities.

Treatment of renal atheroembolism is preventative (to avoid further episodes of atheroembolism) and supportive.[8] General measures include avoidance of nephrotoxic agents, including angiographic contrast and antiinflammatory drugs. Hypertension and congestive heart failure (CHF) should be managed with appropriate medications such as vasodilators and diuretics. Aggressive management of hypertension may decrease proteinuria.[74] Dialysis may be needed for uremia, volume excess, and electrolyte imbalances.

Belenfant et al. showed positive outcomes with aggressive supportive care in 67 patients admitted to a renal intensive care unit (ICU) for management of acute renal failure in the setting of multisystem cholesterol embolization.[75] Clinical features included pulmonary edema, gastrointestinal ischemia, cutaneous ischemia, and retinal embolism. Treatment consisted of anticoagulation withdrawal, avoidance of invasive procedures, management of CHF with angiotensin-converting enzyme (ACE) inhibitors, and loop diuretics. Ultrafiltration or hemodialysis was used when needed for renal support. Enteral or parenteral nutrition supplementation was provided when needed. Some patients were treated empirically with steroids. Improved outcomes in multiorgan cholesterol embolism were reported, although the in-hospital mortality rate was 16%. Of the 56 patients who survived initial hospitalization and were ultimately discharged, there was a 77% 1-year and 52% 4-year survival; 32% remained on maintenance hemodialysis for irreversible renal failure.[75]

Pharmacological treatment for renal atheroembolism is empirical because there are no prospective clinical trials, and no definitive treatment has been established. Cholesterol crystals act like foreign bodies setting up an inflammatory reaction with a cascade of systemic mediators of inflammation. Steroids may reduce the inflammatory reaction and may have a favorable response.[78]

Statins have been used empirically to treat cholesterol crystal embolism. Simvastatin (40 mg daily) was associated with improved renal function in some patients with renal biopsy–documented atheroembolism.[79]

Prevention is the best management, in particular avoiding additional invasive angiographic procedures in high-risk patients with extensive atheromatous disease of the aorta. If procedures are necessary, distal embolic protection devices may improve outcomes for arterial interventions.[80]

Gastrointestinal Tract Atheroembolism

The gastrointestinal tract is one of the common sites for aortic atheroembolism and ranks as the third most frequently affected organ system after skin and renal involvement.[59] Cholesterol embolization should be in the differential diagnosis of all patients with atherosclerosis presenting with gastrointestinal symptoms after a vascular interventional procedure. Symptoms may be nonspecific and difficult to diagnose but include abdominal pain, fever, and diarrhea. Gastrointestinal bleeding due to mucosal infarcts and ulceration caused by bowel ischemia may occur.[53,81,82] In severe cases, intestinal infarction may require urgent surgery for necrotic bowel or bowel perforation. The colon is most commonly involved. Multiple emboli over time may result in stricture formation, bowel obstruction, or polypoid lesions.[83–85] Rarely, atheroembolism to the gut can mimic colon cancer.[86] Sometimes symptoms may be misdiagnosed for months until a catastrophic event such as small-bowel perforation with peritonitis or bleeding occurs.[87] The liver, gallbladder, and pancreas are also uncommon sites for atheroembolism, but there are case reports of acute pancreatitis and acute acalculous cholecystitis from aortic atheroembolism.[88–93] The stomach is rarely involved. An endoscopic biopsy should include submucosa to detect cholesterol clefts in small arterioles.[59] Most patients with atheroembolism to the gastrointestinal tract have advanced atherosclerosis, and atheroembolism affects multiple organs.[82] When atheroembolism involves the gastrointestinal tract, cholesterol embolization can also be seen as livedo reticularis or associated blue toe syndrome.[87] At least half of these cases are precipitated by an angiographic procedure and have a high mortality rate.[81]

Lower Extremities and Blue Toe Syndrome

In 1961, Feder and Auerbach were the first to describe blue toe syndrome in six patients who presented with painful purple toes and noted findings of dark-tinged discoloration of the plantar surfaces of the toes. They reported the toes were painful and tender to touch, and that the blue discoloration of the skin blanched with local pressure, which differentiated this entity from localized hematoma or purpura. These patients were older, with ages ranging from 53 to 69, and had atherosclerotic cardiovascular diseases including diabetes, stroke, or CHF. Most of these patients had intact peripheral pulses. Feder and Auerbach

associated these skin changes with initiation of warfarin anticoagulation but recognized these features were not due to warfarin-induced skin necrosis.[94]

In 1976, Karmody et al. established the term *blue toe syndrome*, recognizing that the sudden onset of pain and cyanosis was the result of a microembolic event to the digital arteries. Angiography in a number of these patients localized the source of emboli to the femoral, popliteal, or aortoiliac arteries.[9]

The typical patient with blue toe syndrome presents with sudden onset of painful cyanotic skin lesions that may involve one or many toes. Cyanosis results from decreased arterial inflow along with impaired venous outflow, leading to stasis of desaturated blood. Initially, the cyanosis blanches with pressure, but with worsening ischemia and tissue damage, the blue discoloration may become nonblanchable. The affected toe is dark blue in color, painful due to ischemia, and exquisitely tender to touch. Digital ischemia can progress to cause skin necrosis, ulceration, and gangrene. Livedo reticularis of the foot may also be present, involving the base of the affected toe, forefoot, plantar surface, or heel (Figs. 45.9 through 45.13). Myalgias due to muscle atheroembolism may occur, with clinical features of local muscle tenderness and sometimes with actual myonecrosis.[95]

Clinical examination should be the initial step to determine the source of atheroembolism. In 78% of patients, peripheral pulses including pedal pulses are intact.[1] Although distal pulses are palpable in the classic case of blue toe syndrome, occlusive arterial disease is present in up to half of patients, based on ankle-brachial indices (ABIs) less than 0.9.[96] Careful pulse examination with auscultation for bruits may suggest proximal arterial disease. A widened expansile common femoral or popliteal pulse may suggest an aneurysm. Palpation of the abdomen

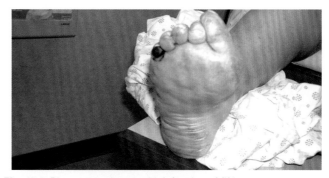

Fig. 45.9 Blue toe syndrome with infarction of fifth toe.

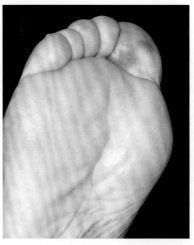

Fig. 45.10 Atheroembolic mottling of the big toe.

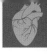

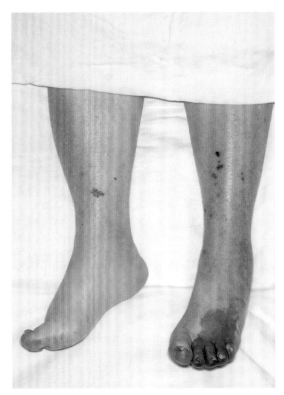

Fig. 45.11 Severe episode of atheroembolism to forefoot.

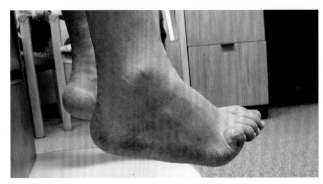

Fig. 45.13 Livedo reticularis from atheroembolism involving lateral aspect of foot and heel.

may reveal an aortic aneurysm. The location of livedo reticularis, such as the foot, thigh, or abdomen, suggests a more proximal site.

Lower-extremity atheromatous emboli can originate from focal or diffuse atherosclerosis, from stenotic or aneurysmal disease, and from disease above or below the inguinal ligament.[96] If both lower extremities are involved, this suggests the origin of the atheroembolism is proximal to the aortic bifurcation. In unilateral blue toe syndrome, the culprit site is likely at or distal to the iliac artery. Common sites of atherosclerosis are the common or external iliac artery (EIA), the superficial femoral artery (SFA) at the adductor hiatus (due to stenotic disease), and the popliteal artery (arising from a local aneurysm). The aortoiliac segment is the most common origin for atheroembolism, accounting for two-thirds of cases.[96–100] One-third of cases are found to arise from the femoropopliteal arteries.[96]

When no embolic source is readily identifiable, imaging of the thoracic aorta is important and may reveal a coral reef or mobile plaque as the source of distal atheroemboli. Coral reef plaque is a calcified discrete mass in the posterior wall of the suprarenal aorta that is prone to distal embolization.[101,102] They can be treated by surgical thromboendarterectomy or bypass.[103,104] Endovascular stent placement has also been successful in patients symptomatic with claudication from aortic lumen compromise by a coral reef.[105] Sometimes a solitary embolic source cannot be isolated, owing to the diffuse nature of atherosclerosis. For example, in one study, arteriograms showed diffuse disease at both aortoiliac and femoropopliteal levels in 40% of patients, making it difficult to discern the likely source of atheroembolism.[96]

Only a few years ago, angiography was the gold standard to search for a culprit lesion, but now with advances in noninvasive imaging, computed tomographic angiography (CTA), magnetic resonance angiography (MRA), duplex ultrasound, and TEE are all first-line well-established methods to image the aorta.[100,106]

Blue toes due to atheroembolism should be differentiated from other skin and systemic disorders (Fig. 45.14). Blue toes can also be caused by benign cold-induced reversible vasospasm, similar to Raynaud phenomenon of the fingers (see Chapter 46). Other vascular diseases that can present with a blue toe include pernio (see Chapter 49), thromboangiitis obliterans (TAO) (Buerger disease) (see Chapter 42), and digital artery thrombosis. Paraproteinemia (e.g., myeloma) or myeloproliferative disorders (e.g., polycythemia vera, essential thrombocytosis) may cause small-vessel thrombosis. Cryofibrinogenemia results from complexes of fibrinogen, fibrin, and proteins that precipitate with cold. Secondary forms are associated with cancers, rheumatological diseases, and infections. Cryoglobulinemia results from immunoglobulins (Igs) that precipitate in the cold. There are three types: type 1 cryoglobulinemia occurs in association with lymphoproliferative disease (e.g., chronic lymphocytic lymphoma); types 2 and 3 may be

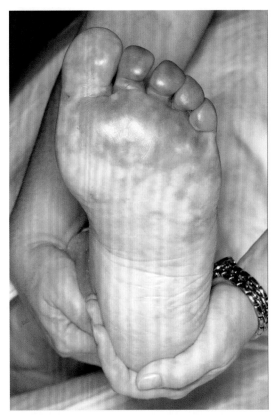

Fig. 45.12 Plantar surface of same patient as in Fig. 45.11, showing purple toes and severe atheroembolism to forefoot.

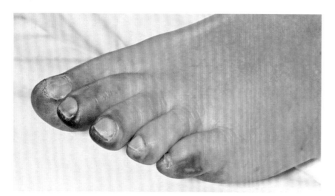

Fig. 45.14 Blue toes from unknown cause.

associated with viral hepatitis infections. Hirschmann and Raugi define the blue toe syndrome as a "blue or violaceous discoloration of one or more toes in the absence of trauma (fracture or strain), cold-induced injury (pernio or frostbite), or disorders that produce systemic cyanosis (methemoglobinemia or hypoxia)."[56]

The short- and long-term outcome after an atheroembolic episode is variable depending on the extent of atheroembolism and resulting tissue damage. For many patients, the prognosis for atheroembolism is poor, sometimes requiring limb amputation. Improvement may occur but may take several weeks for pain to slowly subside, and longer for skin color changes to improve. In more severe cases, the affected toe(s) may progress to necrosis with black gangrene. If carefully managed, the gangrene may stay dry and demarcate from healthy tissue, allowing future autoamputation of the distal or entire toe. Wet gangrene may lead to infection and may require surgical amputation. A toe amputation may heal satisfactorily at a demarcation line if large-vessel arterial perfusion is intact.

Although some individuals recover after a single episode of atheroembolism, a recurrent episode can cause further irreparable damage resulting in extensive tissue damage and necrosis. Spontaneous embolic episodes tend to be recurrent. With very extensive atheroembolism, skin necrosis may occur, affecting much of the foot; this has been referred to as *trash foot* (Fig. 45.15).[19] This is potentially limb threatening and is associated with a high mortality rate, owing to coexistent multisystem disease. In one study where trash foot occurred in 19 of 29 patients (7 bilateral) following abdominal aorta or lower-extremity revascularization, 8 patients underwent major amputations, and 5 underwent minor amputations.[19] The risk of major amputation after extensive atheroembolism varies from 10% to 27%, depending on

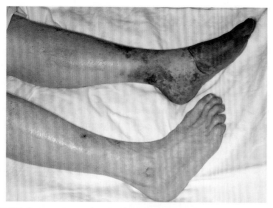

Fig. 45.15 Postangiographic atheroembolism to foot, resulting in critical irreversible foot ischemia requiring below-knee amputation.

the reported series.[9,96,107] Mortality is also significant in multisystem atheroembolism, as in one study where 31% of patients died during a follow-up period of 15 months.[108]

Operative Management

Once lower-extremity atheroembolism occurs, management principles are to prevent recurrent embolic episodes and provide local care for the affected extremity. General treatment measures are discussed later under the section on treatment.

Surgical or endovascular intervention has been advocated because of the high likelihood of recurrent atheroembolic events leading to worsening irreversible tissue ischemia with risk of limb amputation.[9,107] Embolic recurrence may be as high as 50% to 80%, with a 40% to 60% risk of tissue loss.[96,97] The goal of surgical intervention is to remove or exclude the source of embolization and prevent recurrent episodes leading to organ and extremity loss. Treatment choice is determined by location and severity of disease. The optimal surgical intervention depends on the individual patient. Arterial bypass, endarterectomy, and angioplasty with stent placement have been reported to be effective in selected patients by preventing recurrent embolization.[97,109]

A retrospective study at Washington University Medical Center found 62 patients with renal or cutaneous manifestations of atheroembolism. Angiography was done in almost all patients. The aorta and iliac arteries (80%) were felt to be the most common source of atheroembolism, followed by femoral (13%), popliteal (3%), and subclavian (3%) arteries. Bypass grafting procedures were performed on 42 patients to exclude the native diseased artery. Other patients underwent a combination of endarterectomy and bypass grafts. Limb salvage was accomplished in 98%, although 31% had minor amputations. No further episodes of atheroembolism occurred over a mean follow-up period of 20 months.[98]

Keen et al. reviewed their experience of surgical management of atheroembolism in 100 patients with lower-extremity, visceral, and upper-extremity atheroembolism who were followed for 12 years.[99] Aortoiliac occlusive disease was present in 47 patients, and aortic aneurysm was present in 20 patients (average size, 3.5 cm). Operations to exclude the embolic source included aortic bypass or aortoiliac endarterectomy, femoral and popliteal endarterectomy, or bypass graft. Several patients underwent extra-anatomical reconstruction. Despite surgery, 6 of 97 had recurrent events, and 9 required major leg amputations with 10 toe amputations.[99]

Friedman and Krishnasastry reviewed a small group of high-risk surgical patients presenting with rest pain, ulceration, or gangrene due to atheroemboli to both lower extremities. These patients, who were not candidates for direct aortic reconstruction because of preexisting medical comorbidities, underwent ligation of the EIA with axillary-bifemoral bypass. Initial limb salvage was accomplished in all, with no limb loss over the next 52 months.[110] Kaufman et al. also reported a small group of high-risk patients in whom limb salvage and healing of foot ulcers was accomplished in the majority with an axillobifemoral bypass with exclusion of the external iliacs.[111]

Hollier et al. reviewed 88 patients with shaggy aorta syndrome who suffered atheromatous embolization (Fig. 45.16). Surgical correction was performed in 27 patients, including endarterectomy, external iliac ligation, and graft replacement. The best outcome (lowest morbidity and mortality) for those with lower-extremity atheroembolism was with ligation of the distal EIA and extra-anatomical bypass.[112] The author noted that surgery was not always successful in preventing visceral infarction or renal failure.[112]

Primary angioplasty for iliac or superficial femoral lesions can also be successful for focal high-grade stenotic lesions of the iliac or SFA.[109,113] Although there may be concern of provoking further

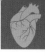

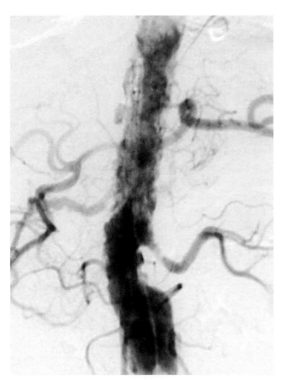

Fig. 45.16 Aortogram demonstrating diffuse atheromatous disease, so-called shaggy aorta, with high atheroembolic potential.

embolization, some studies show good results. In one series of 10 patients treated with primary angioplasty, none had embolization at the time of the procedure, and 8 of the 10 had no recurrent atheroembolic episodes. The patients in this series were more likely to have single focal high-grade stenotic lesions of an iliac or SFA amenable to angioplasty, as opposed to more diffuse proximal atherosclerotic plaque.[107,109]

A self-expanding stent has been used to treat atheroembolism arising from an isolated segment of the iliac artery.[97] For more complex plaques, a covered stent has been successfully deployed and offers the advantage of excluding the diseased segment by trapping the atheroma and thrombus under the covered stent.[11,97] In one case report of three patients with iliac artery disease treated with a self-expanding stent covered with Dacron, no recurrences of microembolism were noted after 16 months, and the toe lesions healed.[97]

Aortic stent grafting is now commonly used in the management of AAAs. In a retrospective study of 19 patients with symptomatic lower-extremity atheroembolism presenting with ischemic ulcers or toe gangrene and an abdominal aneurysm, an aortic stent graft was deployed to exclude an AAA. At 1-year follow-up, eight of nine patients had resolution of ischemic toe symptoms.[101] The authors note that although stent graft repair of AAA may prevent future embolization, it is important to not miss coexisting thoracic aortic disease.

Arterial filters have also been employed in the SFA, carotid, renal, and many other vessels. As filter development continues to advance, this may become an adjunctive procedure in the future.[114]

Upper-Extremity Atheroembolism

Atheroembolism is uncommon in the upper extremity.[98] Atherosclerosis may involve the aortic arch and branch vessels. The subclavian artery is a common site for atherosclerosis. Unequal upper-extremity blood pressures should raise suspicion of disease at or proximal to the sub-

clavian artery level. Most individuals with subclavian atherosclerotic disease are asymptomatic, but this can be a source of atheroembolism to the arm and the fingers (Fig. 45.17).

Ascending Aorta/Arch Atheroma and Stroke

With the advent of TEE, aortic arch plaque has been identified as an important potential source of cerebral embolic stroke.[115,116] Case-controlled prospective studies have shown a clear association between atherosclerotic disease of the ascending aorta/aortic arch and risk of ischemic stroke.[117] Autopsy studies found ulcerated plaque in the aortic arch to be present in 26% of 239 patients with cerebrovascular disease (both stroke and brain hemorrhage), but only 5% of patients with neurological diagnoses.[117,118] Another large study using TEE to detect aortic atheroma compared 215 consecutive patients with first stroke or TIA to 202 control subjects. This technique confirmed that atheroma in the ascending aorta and arch were a significant risk factor for stroke.[119]

Characterization of aortic plaque morphology (hypoechoic plaque, ulceration, calcification, sessile or mobile thrombus) is important in prediction of stroke.[120] In particular, the thickness of plaque in the ascending aorta and arch correlates with risk of stroke. When patients with acute stroke were compared to consecutive controls, 28% had plaques of 4 mm or more in thickness in those with unexplained stroke, compared to 8% of 172 patients who had a known or suspected cause of brain infarct.[117] In the French Study of Aortic Plaques in Stroke, TEE was done to quantify aortic arch atheromatous disease in 331 patients aged 60 or older admitted to hospital with an acute ischemic stroke. The incidence of recurrent brain infarction was 11.9% per 100 person-years in those with aortic plaque thickness greater than 4 mm, compared to 2.8% for those with minimal plaque (<1 mm). The presence of atherosclerotic arch plaque thickness of 4 mm or greater was found to be an independent predictor of recurrent brain infarction and cardiovascular events.[43] Even moderate atheromatous disease (defined as intimal thickness of the ascending aorta and arch of >2 mm) is a significant risk factor for stroke after cardiac surgery.[121]

Mobile Atheroma

The presence of mobile components denotes the highest risk for stroke.[25,99,122–128] In a study of 118 elderly patients undergoing CPB and studied with intraoperative TEE, 3 of 12 patients (25%) with a mobile aortic arch atheroma had suffered a perioperative stroke, compared to 2 of 118 (2%) patients without a mobile atheroma.[123] A mobile mass overlying an atheromatous plaque is likely adherent thrombus and therefore is more likely to respond to anticoagulation than the underlying plaque itself.

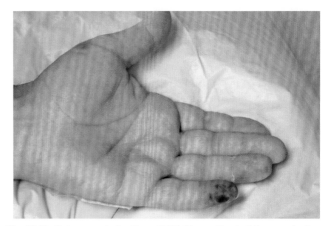

Fig. 45.17 Cutaneous Infarction of Fifth Finger Due to Atheroembolism. Note subtle ischemic mottling of other fingers.

Whether to use anticoagulation for mobile thrombus in the aorta, however, remains controversial. Warfarin anticoagulation has been advocated for the management of mobile aortic atheroma. A study by Dressler et al. documented effectiveness of warfarin compared to no anticoagulation in preventing recurrent embolic events in those with symptomatic thoracic aorta mobile atheroma.[129] They reviewed 31 patients with mobile aortic atheroma who presented with a systemic embolic event. At follow-up, those patients not receiving warfarin had a much higher incidence of vascular events (45% vs. 5%). Recurrent strokes occurred in 38% of patients. There were no strokes in those on warfarin. Of note, those with small mobile atheroma were not treated with warfarin, and recurrent strokes occurred in 37% of these patients.[129] Warfarin was noted to be more effective than antiplatelet medications in another study of patients with severe ascending aortic atheromatous disease.[127] Further randomized controlled trials would be needed to address anticoagulation versus antiplatelet therapy for this important issue.

Stroke due to atheroembolism can also occur during carotid surgery. Microemboli occur during carotid endarterectomy and can be detected by TCD ultrasound. Ackerstaff et al. found a positive correlation with the occurrence of microembolism during carotid endarterectomy and perioperative TIA and stroke. Magnetic resonance imaging also documented new ischemic brain lesions in these patients.[130] Carotid sinus massage may reproduce not only syncope in patients with carotid sinus hypersensitivity, but also cause inadvertent atheroembolic stroke in patients with carotid atherosclerosis.[131]

Atheroembolic stroke should be suspected in the proper clinical setting. In some patients, TEE has identified unsuspected mobile aortic arch thrombus on atherosclerotic plaque.[116] Brain imaging characteristically shows multiple small ischemic lesions. Brain pathology has also documented multiple cholesterol emboli.[132] Lacunar infarcts are generally thought to be due to small brain infarcts from hypertension. However, some lacunar infarcts may be due to cholesterol emboli.[133]

GENERAL TREATMENT MEASURES FOR ATHEROEMBOLIC DISEASE PREVENTION

Preventative

Preventative interventions should be considered in patients at risk for atheroembolism.[134–139] Angiography is the most common iatrogenic cause of atheroembolism, responsible for up to 80% of cases, so safer angiographic techniques and newer technologies may decrease the incidence of catheter-induced atheroembolism.[8] For example, a "no-touch technique" has been advocated to reduce potential for intimal disruption during renal artery stenting. A second guide is placed within the guide catheter to minimize contact between the guide catheter and aorta.[135] Arterial filters have also been successfully employed in the superficial artery.[114] Distal protection devices are available for renal and cerebral angioplasty. Cerebral protection devices may reduce stroke during carotid artery stenting, but device-related complications can occur.[134,139]

Reduction of atherosclerotic burden and plaque stabilization is a major focus for preventing recurrent atheroembolism. Measures directed at stabilizing atherosclerotic plaque and potentially reducing the risk of atheroembolism include lifestyle modifications such as cessation of cigarette smoking and avoidance of all tobacco products, and pharmacological therapy including statin medications and antiplatelet agents. Many large trials have confirmed the benefits of statin agents in secondary prevention of cardiovascular events.[140] Unfortunately, there are no large randomized trials of statin or antiplatelet medica-

tions in atheroembolism, but there are a number of observational case reports. Tunick et al. looked at the rate of cholesterol embolism in 519 patients with complex aortic plaque seen during TEE in a retrospective study in which atheroembolism occurred in 21% of patients. Although the treatment arms were not randomized, the multivariate analysis showed a benefit for statin medication with an absolute risk reduction of 17%. No protective effect was found for warfarin or antiplatelet drugs.[141] Antiplatelet agents, however, are a mainstay in the prevention of cardiovascular disease and may be effective in preventing recurrent atheroembolism.[142] Commonly used oral antiplatelet agents include aspirin (75 to 325 mg/day), dipyridamole plus aspirin, and clopidogrel 75 mg daily. Iloprost therapy has been used for cholesterol emboli syndrome.[143] Anecdotal treatment of blue toe syndrome has included nifedipine and pentoxifylline.[144] With fixed microvascular disease, there is no clear benefit of vasodilator therapy in the majority of patients with atheroembolism. Although anticoagulation may be of benefit for mobile thrombus overlying atheromatous plaque, it is not routinely used in asymptomatic patients with nonmobile atheroma.[145]

Supportive Therapies

Although there is no cure for atheroembolism, supportive care is a mainstay of treatment. Wound care may be needed for management of lower-extremity skin necrosis, using surgical wound debridement and application of topical agents and dressings. Limited amputation of toes or forefoot is necessary in some patients, and limb amputations may be necessary for patients with irreversible ischemia with gangrene. Antibiotics may be necessary for infection. A fluffy, soft vascular boot can protect the ischemic foot from trauma. Pneumatic arterial pumps can improve arterial perfusion in some patients.

Effective pain control is very important; ischemic pain can be severe and persist for weeks after lower-extremity atheroembolism. The degree of pain from blue toe syndrome may seem to be out of proportion to the extent of tissue involvement but reflects microvascular necrosis. Besides narcotic and neurotransmitter inhibitor agents, several other modalities have been used for pain associated with lower-extremity ischemia.[146]

Other treatment options may include hyperbaric oxygen or pneumatic leg compression to improve distal perfusion in selected cases of extremity atheroembolism.[147]

Finally, organ failure must be treated. Kidney disease must be monitored, with correction of electrolyte abnormalities, volume excess, and uremia. Renal replacement therapy with dialysis may be temporary or permanent. However, Ishiyama et al. found that low-density lipoprotein apheresis (LDL-A) reduced incidence of maintenance dialysis compared to a control group (8% vs. 33%) in 49 patients with cholesterol crystal embolism caused after a vascular procedure.[148]

CONCLUSIONS

Atheroembolism is a rare but serious disorder that can occur spontaneously or be a complication of invasive cardiac and vascular procedures. Angiography is the most common iatrogenic cause, responsible for up to 80% of cases.[8] Atheroembolic skin changes may mimic many other disorders but, if present with or without other syndrome manifestations, should raise clinical suspicion.

A presumptive diagnosis is often based on clinical features. The diagnosis requires a high index of suspicion in an appropriate clinical setting as in a patient with known atherosclerotic disease or aortic aneurysm who develops unexplained renal failure, and cutaneous signs of atheroembolization after an invasive angiographic procedure.

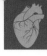

A definitive diagnosis requires histological confirmation of cholesterol crystals in a biopsy of muscle, skin, or affected organ. There is no single definitive laboratory test except biopsy of involved tissue to confirm the diagnosis of atheroembolic disease.

It is important to determine the most likely embolic source. When atheroembolism involves the lower extremities, atherosclerotic or aneurysmal disease of the aortoiliac segment accounts for two-thirds of cases.

Atheroembolism can be recurrent, and in those patients, there is a 40% to 60% risk of tissue loss with recurrent episodes. These patients often have a poor prognosis due to irreversible renal failure and increased mortality from diffuse atherosclerosis. Surgical or endovascular intervention may be indicated to exclude the embolic source and prevent recurrent episodes. A covered stent or extra-anatomical bypass may be an option in high-risk patients.

Management of mobile atheroma is controversial, but warfarin seems to be effective in preventing symptomatic thromboembolism in some patients. Anticoagulation is not routine therapy in patients with diffuse atherosclerosis. Anticoagulation, if indicated for another condition such as atrial fibrillation, should not be withheld in patients with atherosclerosis. Although older anecdotal reports suggest warfarin anticoagulation may be associated with increased risk of atheroembolism, causal relationship has not been documented. The correct therapeutic strategy for atheroemboli are treatments to prevent atherosclerosis and atherosclerotic events.

REFERENCES

1. Jucgla A, Moreso F, Muniesa C, et al. Cholesterol embolism: still an unrecognized entity with a high mortality rate. *J Am Acad Dermatol.* 2006;55(5):786–793.
2. Kiechle FL, McLaughlin JH, Yang SS, Bernstein J. Atheromatous embolization. *Am J Emerg Med.* 1983;1(3):299–301.
3. Hollenhorst RW. Significance of bright plaques in the retinal arterioles. *Trans Am Ophthalmol Soc.* 1961;59:252–273.
4. Lie JT. Cholesterol atheromatous embolism. The great masquerader revisited. *Pathol Annu.* 1992;27(Pt 2):17–50.
5. Fine MJ, Kapoor W, Falanga V. Cholesterol crystal embolization: a review of 221 cases in the English literature. *Angiology.* 1987;38(10):769–784.
6. Lye WC, Cheah JS, Sinniah R. Renal cholesterol embolic disease. Case report and review of the literature. *Am J Nephrol.* 1993;13(6):489–493.
7. Scolari F, Ravani P, Gaggi R, et al. The challenge of diagnosing atheroembolic renal disease: clinical features and prognostic factors. *Circulation.* 2007;116(3):298–304.
8. Scolari F, Ravani P. Atheroembolic renal disease. *Lancet.* 2010;375(9726):1650–1660.
9. Karmody AM, Powers SR, Monaco VJ, Leather RP. "Blue toe" syndrome. An indication for limb salvage surgery. *Arch Surg.* 1976;111(11):1263–1268.
10. Cross SS. How common is cholesterol embolism? *J Clin Pathol.* 1991;44(10):859–861.
11. Saklayen MG. Atheroembolic renal disease: preferential occurrence in whites only. *Am J Nephrol.* 1989;9(1):87–88.
12. Flory C. Arterial occlusions produced by emboli from eroded aortic atheromatous plaques. *Am J Pathol.* 1945;21:549–565.
13. Kealy WF. Atheroembolism. *J Clin Pathol.* 1978;31(10):984–989.
14. Doty JR, Wilentz RE, Salazar JD, et al. Atheroembolism in cardiac surgery. *Ann Thorac Surg.* 2003;75(4):1221–1226.
15. Rosman HS, Davis TP, Reddy D, Goldstein S. Cholesterol embolization: clinical findings and implications. *J Am Coll Cardiol.* 1990;15(6):1296–1299.
16. Hertzer NR. Peripheral atheromatous embolization following blunt abdominal trauma. *Surgery.* 1977;82(2):244–247.
17. Ramirez G, O'Neill Jr WM, Lambert R, Bloomer HA. Cholesterol embolization: a complication of angiography. *Arch Internal Med.* 1978;138(9):1430–1432.
18. Thurlbeck WM, Castleman B. Atheromatous emboli to the kidneys after aortic surgery. *N Engl J Med.* 1957;257(10):442–447.
19. Sharma PV, Babu SC, Shah PM, Nassoura ZE. Changing patterns of atheroembolism. *Cardiovasc Surg.* 1996;4(5):573–579.
20. Lindholt JS, Sandermann J, Bruun-Petersen J, et al. Fatal late multiple emboli after endovascular treatment of abdominal aortic aneurysm. *Case Report Int Angiol.* 1998;17(4):241–243.
21. Zempo N, Sakano H, Ikenaga S, et al. Fatal diffuse atheromatous embolization following endovascular grafting for an abdominal aortic aneurysm: report of a case. *Surg Today.* 2001;31(3):269–273.
22. Thompson MM, Smith J, Naylor AR, et al. Microembolization during endovascular and conventional aneurysm repair. *J Vasc Surg.* 1997;25(1):179–186.
23. Keon WJ, Heggtveit HA, Leduc J. Perioperative myocardial infarction caused by atheroembolism. *J Thorac Cardiovasc Surg.* 1982;84(6):849–855.
24. Blauth CI, Cosgrove DM, Webb BW, et al. Atheroembolism from the ascending aorta. An emerging problem in cardiac surgery. *J Thorac Cardiovasc Surg.* 1992;103(6):1104–1111. discussion 1111-2.
25. Tunick PA, Krinsky GA, Lee VS, Kronzon I. Diagnostic imaging of thoracic aortic atherosclerosis. *AJR Am J Roentgenol.* 2000;174(4):1119–1125.
26. Baker AJ, Naser B, Benaroia M, Mazer CD. Cerebral microemboli during coronary artery bypass using different cardioplegia techniques. *Ann Thorac Surg.* 1995;59(5):1187–1191.
27. Harringer W. Capture of particulate emboli during cardiac procedures in which aortic cross-clamp is used. International Council of Emboli Management Study Group. *Ann Thorac Surg.* 2000;70(3):1119–1123.
28. Ascione R, Ghosh A, Reeves BC, et al. Retinal and cerebral microembolization during coronary artery bypass surgery: a randomized, controlled trial. *Circulation.* 2005;112(25):3833–3838.
29. Drost H, Buis B, Haan D, Hillers JA. Cholesterol embolism as a complication of left heart catheterisation. Report of seven cases. *Br Heart J.* 1984;52(3):339–342.
30. Colt HG, Begg RJ, Saporito JJ, et al. Cholesterol emboli after cardiac catheterization. Eight cases and a review of the literature. *Medicine.* 1988;67(6):389–400.
31. Saklayen MG, Gupta S, Suryaprasad A, Azmeh W. Incidence of atheroembolic renal failure after coronary angiography. A prospective study. *Angiology.* 1997;48(7):609–613.
32. Gaines PA, Cumberland DC, Kennedy A, et al. Cholesterol embolisation: a lethal complication of vascular catheterisation. *Lancet.* 1988;1(8578):168–170.
33. Gjesdal K, Orning OM, Smith E. Fatal atheromatous emboli to the kidneys after left-heart catheterisation. *Lancet.* 1977;2(8034):405.
34. Fukumoto Y, Tsutsui H, Tsuchihashi M, et al. Cholesterol Embolism Study I. The incidence and risk factors of cholesterol embolization syndrome, a complication of cardiac catheterization: a prospective study. *J Am Coll Cardiol.* 2003;42(2):211–216.
35. Frock J, Bierman M, Hammeke M, Reyes A. Atheroembolic renal disease: experience with 22 patients. *Nebr Med J.* 1994;79(9):317–321.
36. Johnson LW, Esente P, Giambartolomei A, et al. Peripheral vascular complications of coronary angioplasty by the femoral and brachial techniques. *Cathet Cardiovasc Diagn.* 1994;31(3):165–172.
37. Keeley EC, Grines CL. Scraping of aortic debris by coronary guiding catheters: a prospective evaluation of 1,000 cases. *J Am Coll Cardiol.* 1998;32(7):1861–1865.
38. Liew YP, Bartholomew JR. Atheromatous embolization. *Vasc Med.* 2005;10(4):309–326.
39. Karalis DG, Quinn V, Victor MF, et al. Risk of catheter-related emboli in patients with atherosclerotic debris in the thoracic aorta. *Am Heart J.* 1996;131(6):1149–1155.
40. Blankenship JC, Mickel S. Spinal cord infarction resulting from cardiac catheterization. *Am J Med.* 1989;87(2):239–240.
41. Harrington D, Amplatz K. Cholesterol embolization and spinal infarction following aortic catheterization. *Am J Roentgenol Radium Ther Nucl Med.* 1972;115(1):171–174.
42. Blackshear JL, Zabalgoitia M, Pennock G, et al. Warfarin safety and efficacy in patients with thoracic aortic plaque and atrial fibrillation.

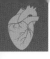

SPAF TEE Investigators. Stroke Prevention and Atrial Fibrillation. Transesophageal Echocardiography. *Am J Cardiol.* 1999;83(3):453–455.

43. Amarenco P, Cohen A, et al. French Study of Aortic Plaques in Stroke Group. Atherosclerotic disease of the aortic arch as a risk factor for recurrent ischemic stroke. *N Engl J Med.* 1996;334(19):1216–1221.

44. Bols A, Nevelsteen A, Verhaeghe R. Atheromatous embolization precipitated by oral anticoagulants. *Int Angiol.* 1994;13(3):271–274.

45. Boudes P. Cholesterol emboli and streptokinase therapy. *JAMA.* 1988;259(8):1180.

46. Gupta BK, Spinowitz BS, Charytan C, Wahl SJ. Cholesterol crystal embolization-associated renal failure after therapy with recombinant tissue-type plasminogen activator. *Am J Kidney Dis.* 1993;21(6):659–662.

47. Wong FK, Chan SK, Ing TS, Li CS. Acute renal failure after streptokinase therapy in a patient with acute myocardial infarction. *Am J Kidney Dis.* 1995;26(3):508–510.

48. Arora RR, Magun AM, Grossman M, Katz J. Cholesterol embolization syndrome after intravenous tissue plasminogen activator for acute myocardial infarction. *Am Heart J.* 1993;126(1):225–228.

49. GUSTO Investigators. An international randomized trial comparing four thrombolytic strategies for acute myocardial infarction. *N Engl J Med.* 1993;329(10):673–682.

50. Blankenship JC, Butler M, Garbes A. Prospective assessment of cholesterol embolization in patients with acute myocardial infarction treated with thrombolytic vs. conservative therapy. *Chest.* 1995;107(3):662–668.

51. Chaudhary K, Wall BM, Rasberry RD. Livedo reticularis: an underutilized diagnostic clue in cholesterol embolization syndrome. *Am J Med Sci.* 2001;321(5):348–351.

52. Faraggiana T, Muda AO. Atheromatous embolism. *Contrib Nephrol.* 1996;119:67–73.

53. Ben-Horin S, Bardan E, Barshack I, et al. Cholesterol crystal embolization to the digestive system: characterization of a common, yet overlooked presentation of atheroembolism. *Am J Gastroenterol.* 2003;98(7):1471–1479.

54. Scolari F, Tardanico R, Zani R, et al. Cholesterol crystal embolism: a recognizable cause of renal disease. *Am J Kidney Dis.* 2000;36(6):1089–1109.

55. Chesney TM. Atheromatous embolization to the skin. *Am J Dermatopathol.* 1982;4(3):271–273.

56. Hirschmann JV, Raugi GJ. Blue (or purple) toe syndrome. *J Am Acad Dermatol.* 2009;60(1):1–20. quiz 21-2.

57. Cappiello RA, Espinoza LR, Adelman H, et al. Cholesterol embolism: a pseudovasculitic syndrome. *Semin Arthritis Rheum.* 1989;18(4):240–246.

58. Falanga V, Fine MJ, Kapoor WN. The cutaneous manifestations of cholesterol crystal embolization. *Arch Dermatol.* 1986;122(10):1194–1198.

59. Moolenaar W, Lamers CB. Cholesterol crystal embolization in the Netherlands. *Arch Intern Med.* 1996;156(6):653–657.

60. Mayo RR, Swartz RD. Redefining the incidence of clinically detectable atheroembolism. *Am J Med.* 1996;100(5):524–529.

61. Modi KS, Rao VK. Atheroembolic renal disease. *J Am Soc Nephrol.* 2001;12(8):1781–1787.

62. Greenberg A, Bastacky SI, Iqbal A, et al. Focal segmental glomerulosclerosis associated with nephrotic syndrome in cholesterol atheroembolism: clinicopathological correlations. *Am J Kidney Dis.* 1997;29(3):334–344.

63. Jones DB, Iannaccone PM. Atheromatous emboli in renal biopsies. An ultrastructural study. *Am J Pathol.* 1975;78(2):261–276.

64. Kawarada O, Yokoi Y, Takemoto K. The characteristics of dissemination of embolic materials during renal artery stenting. *Catheter Cardiovasc Interv.* 2007;70(6):784–788.

65. Haas M, Spargo BH, Wit EJ, Meehan SM. Etiologies and outcome of acute renal insufficiency in older adults: a renal biopsy study of 259 cases. *Am J Kidney Dis.* 2000;35(3):433–447.

66. Hara S, Asada Y, Fujimoto S, et al. Atheroembolic renal disease: clinical findings of 11 cases. *J Atheroscler Thromb.* 2002;9(6):288–291.

67. Thadhani RI, Camargo Jr CA, Xavier RJ, et al. Atheroembolic renal failure after invasive procedures. Natural history based on 52 histologically proven cases. *Medicine.* 1995;74(6):350–358.

68. Goldman M, Thoua Y, Dhaene M, Toussaint C. Necrotising glomerulonephritis associated with cholesterol microemboli. *Br Med J (Clin Res Ed).* 1985;290(6463):205–206.

69. Theriault J, Agharazzi M, Dumont M, et al. Atheroembolic renal failure requiring dialysis: potential for renal recovery? A review of 43 cases. *Nephron.* 2003;94(1):c11–c18.

70. Dalakos TG, Streeten DH, Jones D, Obeid A. "Malignant" hypertension resulting from atheromatous embolization predominantly of one kidney. *Am J Med.* 1974;57(1):135–138.

71. Kasinath BS, Corwin HL, Bidani AK, et al. Eosinophilia in the diagnosis of atheroembolic renal disease. *Am J Nephrol.* 1987;7(3):173–177.

72. Wilson DM, Salazer TL, Farkouh ME. Eosinophiluria in atheroembolic renal disease. *Am J Med.* 1991;91(2):186–189.

73. Haqqie SS, Urizar RE, Singh J. Nephrotic-range proteinuria in renal atheroembolic disease: report of four cases. *Am J Kidney Dis.* 1996;28(4):493–501.

74. Williams HH, Wall BM, Cooke CR. Reversible nephrotic range proteinuria and renal failure in atheroembolic renal disease. *Am J Med Sci.* 1990;299(1):58–61.

75. Belenfant X, Meyrier A, Jacquot C. Supportive treatment improves survival in multivisceral cholesterol crystal embolism. *Am J Kidney Dis.* 1999;33(5):840–850.

76. Herzog AL, Wanner C. Case report: atheroembolic renal disease in a 72-year-old patient through coronary intervention after myocardial infarction. *Hemodial Int.* 2008;12(4):406–411.

77. Scolari F, Ravani P, Pola A, et al. Predictors of renal and patient outcomes in atheroembolic renal disease: a prospective study. *J Am Soc Nephrol.* 2003;14(6):1584–1590.

78. Graziani G, Santostasi S, Angelini C, Badalamenti S. Corticosteroids in cholesterol emboli syndrome. *Nephron.* 2001;87(4):371–373.

79. Woolfson RG, Lachmann H. Improvement in renal cholesterol emboli syndrome after simvastatin. *Lancet.* 1998;351(9112):1331–1332.

80. Dubel GJ, Murphy TP. Distal embolic protection for renal arterial interventions. *Cardiovasc Intervent Radiol.* 2008;31(1):14–22.

81. Moolenaar W, Lamers CB. Gastrointestinal blood loss due to cholesterol crystal embolization. *J Clin Gastroenterol.* 1995;21(3):220–223.

82. Paraf F, Jacquot C, Bloch F, et al. Cholesterol crystal embolization demonstrated on GI biopsy. *Am J Gastroenterol.* 2001;96(12):3301–3304.

83. Blundell JW. Small bowel stricture secondary to multiple cholesterol emboli. *Histopathology.* 1988;13(4):459–462.

84. Mulliken JB, Bartlett MK. Small bowel obstruction secondary to atheromatous embolism. A case report and review of the literature. *Ann Surg.* 1971;174(1):145–150.

85. Gramlich TL, Hunter SB. Focal polypoid ischemia of the colon: atheroemboli presenting as a colonic polyp. *Arch Pathol Lab Med.* 1994;118(3):308–309.

86. Chan T, Levine MS, Park Y. Cholesterol embolization as a cause of cecal infarct mimicking carcinoma. *AJR Am J Roentgenol.* 1988;150(6):1315–1316.

87. Fujiyama A, Mori Y, Yamamoto S, et al. Multiple spontaneous small bowel perforations due to systemic cholesterol atheromatous embolism. *Intern Med.* 1999;38(7):580–584.

88. Funabiki K, Masuoka H, Shimizu H, et al. Cholesterol crystal embolization (CCE) after cardiac catheterization: a case report and a review of 36 cases in the Japanese literature. *Jpn Heart J.* 2003;44(5):767–774.

89. Orvar K, Johlin FC. Atheromatous embolization resulting in acute pancreatitis after cardiac catheterization and angiographic studies. *Arch Intern Med.* 1994;154(15):1755–1761.

90. Moolenaar W, Kreuning J, Eulderink F, Lamers CB. Ischemic colitis and acalculous necrotizing cholecystitis as rare manifestations of cholesterol emboli in the same patient. *Am J Gastroenterol.* 1989;84(11):1421–1422.

91. Moolenaar W, Lamers CB. Cholesterol crystal embolization and the digestive system. *Scand J Gastroenterol Suppl.* 1991;188:69–72.

92. Harvey RL, Doberneck RC, Black 3rd WC. Infarction of the stomach following atheromatous embolization. Report of a case and literature review. *Gastroenterology.* 1972;62(3):469–472.

93. Bourdages R, Prentice RS, Beck IT, et al. Atheromatous embolization to the stomach: an unusual cause of gastrointestinal bleeding. *Am J Dig Dis.* 1976;21(10):889–894.

94. Feder W, Auerbach R. "Purple toes": an uncommon sequela of oral coumarin drug therapy. *Ann Intern Med.* 1961;55:911–917.

95. Donohue KG, Saap L, Falanga V. Cholesterol crystal embolization: an atherosclerotic disease with frequent and varied cutaneous manifestations. *J Eur Acad Dermatol Venereol*. 2003;17(5):504–511.

96. Wingo JP, Nix ML, Greenfield LJ, Barnes RW. The blue toe syndrome: hemodynamics and therapeutic correlates of outcome. *J Vasc Surg*. 1986;3(3):475–480.

97. Kumins NH, Owens EL, Oglevie SB, et al. Early experience using the Wallgraft in the management of distal microembolism from common iliac artery pathology. *Ann Vasc Surg*. 2002;16(2):181–186.

98. Baumann DS, McGraw D, Rubin BG, et al. An institutional experience with arterial atheroembolism. *Ann Vasc Surg*. 1994;8(3):258–265.

99. Keen RR, McCarthy WJ, Shireman PK, et al. Surgical management of atheroembolization. *J Vasc Surg*. 1995;21(5):773–780. discussion 780-1.

100. Applebaum RM, Kronzon I. Evaluation and management of cholesterol embolization and the blue toe syndrome. *Curr Opin Cardiol*. 1996;11(5):533–542.

101. Rosenberg GD, Killewich LA. Blue toe syndrome from a "coral reef" aorta. *Ann Vasc Surg*. 1995;9(6):561–564.

102. Schlieper G, Grotemeyer D, Aretz A, et al. Analysis of calcifications in patients with coral reef aorta. *Ann Vasc Surg*. 2010;24(3):408–414.

103. Schulte KM, Reiher L, Grabitz L, Sandmann W. Coral reef aorta: a long-term study of 21 patients. *Ann Vasc Surg*. 2000;14(6):626–633.

104. Teebken OE, Pichlmaier MA, Kühn C, Haverich A. Severe obstructive calcifications affecting the descending and suprarenal abdominal aorta without coexisting peripheral atherosclerotic disease–coral reef aorta. *Vasa*. 2006;35(3):206–208.

105. Holfeld J, Gottardi R, Zimpfer D, et al. Treatment of symptomatic coral reef aorta by endovascular stent-graft placement. *Ann Thorac Surg*. 2008;85(5):1817–1819.

106. Spittell PC, Seward JB, Hallett Jr JW. Mobile thrombi in the abdominal aorta in cases of lower extremity embolic arterial occlusion: value of extended transthoracic echocardiography. *Am Heart J*. 2000;139(2 Pt 1):241–244.

107. Matchett WJ, McFarland DR, Eidt JF, Moursi MM. Blue toe syndrome: treatment with intra-arterial stents and review of therapies. *J Vasc Interv Radiol*. 2000;11(5):585–592.

108. Carroccio A, Olin JW, Ellozy SH, et al. The role of aortic stent grafting in the treatment of atheromatous embolization syndrome: results after a mean of 15 months follow-up. *J Vasc Surg*. 2004;40(3):424–429.

109. Kumpe DA, Zwerdlinger S, Griffin DJ. Blue digit syndrome: treatment with percutaneous transluminal angioplasty. *Radiology*. 1988;166(1 Pt 1):37–44.

110. Friedman SG, Krishnasastry KV. External iliac ligation and axillary-bifemoral bypass for blue toe syndrome. *Surgery*. 1994;115(1):27–30.

111. Kaufman JL, Saifi J, Chang BB, et al. The role of extraanatomic exclusion bypass in the treatment of disseminated atheroembolism syndrome. *Ann Vasc Surg*. 1990;4(3):260–263.

112. Hollier LH, Kazmier FJ, Ochsner J, et al. "Shaggy" aorta syndrome with atheromatous embolization to visceral vessels. *Ann Vasc Surg*. 1991;5(5):439–444.

113. Brewer ML, Kinnison ML, Perler BA, White Jr RI. Blue toe syndrome: treatment with anticoagulants and delayed percutaneous transluminal angioplasty. *Radiology*. 1988;166(1 Pt 1):31–36.

114. Van Thielen J, Hendriks JMH, Hertoghs M, et al. Filters placed in the superficial femoral arteries for limb salvage in a high-surgical-risk patient with atheroembolism: results at 2 years. *J Endovasc Ther*. 2010;17(3):399–401.

115. Bernard Y. Value of transoesophageal echocardiography for the diagnosis of embolic lesions from the thoracic aorta. *J Neuroradiol*. 2005;32(4):266–272.

116. Laperche T, Laurian C, Roudaut R, Steg PG. Mobile thromboses of the aortic arch without aortic debris. A transesophageal echocardiographic finding associated with unexplained arterial embolism. The Filiale Echocardiographie de la Société Française de Cardiologie. *Circulation*. 1997;96(1):288–294.

117. Amarenco P, Cohen A, Tzourio C, et al. Atherosclerotic disease of the aortic arch and the risk of ischemic stroke. *N Engl J Med*. 1994;331(22):1474–1479.

118. Amarenco P, Duyckaerts C, Tzourio C, et al. The prevalence of ulcerated plaques in the aortic arch in patients with stroke. *N Engl J Med*. 1992;326(4):221–225.

119. Jones EF, Kalman JM, Calafiore P, et al. Proximal aortic atheroma. An independent risk factor for cerebral ischemia. *Stroke*. 1995;26(2):218–224.

120. Cohen A, Tzourio C, Bertrand B, et al. Aortic plaque morphology and vascular events: a follow-up study in patients with ischemic stroke. FAPS Investigators. French Study of Aortic Plaques in Stroke. *Circulation*. 1997;96(11):3838–3841.

121. Djaiani G, Fedorko L, Borger M, et al. Mild to moderate atheromatous disease of the thoracic aorta and new ischemic brain lesions after conventional coronary artery bypass graft surgery. *Stroke*. 2004;35(9):e356–e358.

122. Di Tullio MR, Homma S, Jin Z, Sacco RL. Aortic atherosclerosis, hypercoagulability, and stroke the APRIS (Aortic Plaque and Risk of Ischemic Stroke) study. *J Am Coll Cardiol*. 2008;52(10):855–861.

123. Katz ES, Tunick PA, Rusinek H, et al. Protruding aortic atheromas predict stroke in elderly patients undergoing cardiopulmonary bypass: experience with intraoperative transesophageal echocardiography. *J Am Coll Cardiol*. 1992;20(1):70–77.

124. Karalis DG, Chandrasekaran K, Victor MF, et al. Recognition and embolic potential of intraaortic atherosclerotic debris. *J Am Coll Cardiol*. 1991;17(1):73–78.

125. Tunick PA, Kronzon I. Protruding atherosclerotic plaque in the aortic arch of patients with systemic embolization: a new finding seen by transesophageal echocardiography. *Am Heart J*. 1990;120(3):658–660.

126. Tunick PA, Perez JL, Kronzon I. Protruding atheromas in the thoracic aorta and systemic embolization. *Ann Intern Med*. 1991;115(6):423–427.

127. Ferrari E, Vidal R, Chevallier T, Baudouy M. Atherosclerosis of the thoracic aorta and aortic debris as a marker of poor prognosis: benefit of oral anticoagulants. *J Am Coll Cardiol*. 1999;33(5):1317–1322.

128. Naghavi M, Libby P, Falk E, et al. From vulnerable plaque to vulnerable patient: a call for new definitions and risk assessment strategies. Part I. *Circulation*. 2003;108(14):1664–1672.

129. Dressler FA, Craig WR, Castello R, Labovitz AJ. Mobile aortic atheroma and systemic emboli: efficacy of anticoagulation and influence of plaque morphology on recurrent stroke. *J Am Coll Cardiol*. 1998;31(1):134–138.

130. Ackerstaff RG, Jansen C, Moll FL, et al. The significance of microemboli detection by means of transcranial Doppler ultrasonography monitoring in carotid endarterectomy. *J Vasc Surg*. 1995;21(6):963–969.

131. Beal MF, Park TS, Fisher CM. Cerebral atheromatous embolism following carotid sinus pressure. *Arch Neurol*. 1981;38(5):310–312.

132. Ezzeddine MA, Primavera JM, Rosand J, et al. Clinical characteristics of pathologically proved cholesterol emboli to the brain. *Neurology*. 2000;54(8):1681–1683.

133. Laloux P, Brucher JM. Lacunar infarctions due to cholesterol emboli. *Stroke*. 1991;22(11):1440–1444.

134. Cremonesi A, Manetti R, Setacci F, et al. Protected carotid stenting: clinical advantages and complications of embolic protection devices in 442 consecutive patients. *Stroke*. 2003;34(8):1936–1941.

135. Feldman RL, Wargovich TJ, Bittl JA. No-touch technique for reducing aortic wall trauma during renal artery stenting. *Catheter Cardiovasc Interv*. 1999;46(2):245–248.

136. Henry M, Henry I, Klonaris C. et al. Renal angioplasty and stenting under protection: the way for the future? *Catheter Cardiovasc Interv*. 2003;60(3):299–312.

137. Henry M, Henry I, Klonaris C, et al. Benefits of cerebral protection during carotid stenting with the PercuSurge GuardWire system: midterm results. *J Endovasc Ther*. 2002;9(1):1–13.

138. Kawarada O, Yokoi Y, Takemoto K, Morioka N. Double-wire technique in balloon-protected carotid artery stenting. *J Interv Cardiol*. 2007;20(1):55–62.

139. Kastrup A, Gröschel K, Krapf H, et al. Early outcome of carotid angioplasty and stenting with and without cerebral protection devices: a systematic review of the literature. *Stroke*. 2003;34(3):813–819.

140. Blanco-Colio LM, Tuñón J, Martín-Ventura JL, Egido J. Anti-inflammatory and immunomodulatory effects of statins. *Kidney Int*. 2003;63(1):12–23.

141. Tunick PA, Nayar AC, Goodkin GM, et al. Effect of treatment on the incidence of stroke and other emboli in 519 patients with severe thoracic aortic plaque. *Am J Cardiol*. 2002;90(12):1320–1325.

142. Ling G, Ovbiagele B. Oral antiplatelet therapy in the secondary prevention of atherothrombotic events. *Am J Cardiovasc Drugs*. 2009;9(3):197–209.

143. Elinav E, Chajek-Shaul T, Stern M. Improvement in cholesterol emboli syndrome after iloprost therapy. *BMJ*. 2002;324(7332): 268–269.

144. Carr Jr ME, Sanders K, Todd WM. Pain relief and clinical improvement temporally related to the use of pentoxifylline in a patient with documented cholesterol emboli--a case report. *Angiology*. 1994;45(1):65–69.

145. Jennings WC, Corder CN, Jarolim DR, et al. Atheromatous embolism: varied clinical presentation and prognosis. *South Med J*. 1989;82(7):849–852.

146. Ghilardi G, Massaro F, Gobatti D, et al. Temporary spinal cord stimulation for peripheral cholesterol embolism. *J Cardiovasc Surg (Torino)*. 2002;43(2):255–258.

147. Vella A, Carlson LA, Blier B, et al. Circulator boot therapy alters the natural history of ischemic limb ulceration.[Erratum appears in *Vasc Med*. 2000;5(2):128]. *Vasc Med*. 2000;5(1):21-5.

148. Ishiyama K, Sato T, Taguma Y. Low-density lipoprotein apheresis ameliorates renal prognosis of cholesterol crystal embolism. *Ther Apher Dial*. 2015;19(4):355–360.

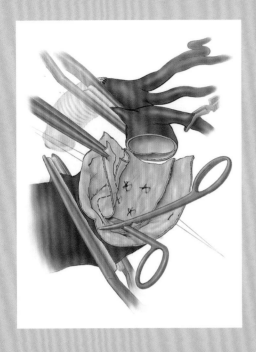

PART **XIII**

第十三部分

Vasospasm and Other
Related Vascular
Diseases

血管痉挛及其他相关
血管疾病

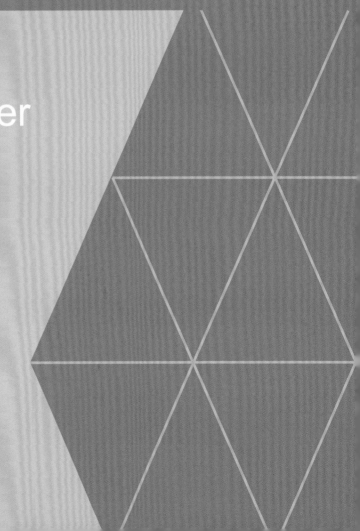

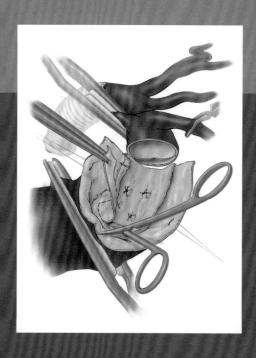

第46章
雷诺现象

雷诺现象是指手指在寒冷、情绪变化等刺激因素作用下因手指动脉收缩导致的发作性缺血改变，典型者包括苍白、发绀和发红三个阶段。第一阶段，指端末梢血管痉挛导致手指缺血苍白，同时微动脉、毛细血管及小静脉扩张；第二阶段，静脉血流入使手指发绀，手指在前两个阶段可伴有发冷、麻木、感觉异常等症状；第三阶段，在去除刺激因素后，痉挛的血管舒张并显著增加手指血流量，手指发红、复温并逐渐恢复正常，此阶段常伴有抽搐样疼痛。两次发作期间手指通常无异常表现。雷诺现象可分为原发性和继发性两大类。原发性雷诺现象更常见，继发性雷诺现象则常与系统性结缔组织病、动脉闭塞性疾病、周围神经病、药物作用等相关。雷诺现象的主要诊断依据为患者病史，但也可用节段性压力测量、冷刺激试验、超声检查等无创性血管检查进行临床评估。继发性雷诺现象的治疗以治疗原发病为基础，而治疗原发性雷诺现象时则应根据疾病的严重程度为患者选择戒烟、保暖等保守治疗手段，或利用钙通道阻滞剂、交感神经系统抑制剂等药物进行扩血管治疗，或行交感神经切除术、肉毒素注射等。临床上应根据患者具体情况，结合各专业意见制订诊疗计划，以实现患者获益最大化。

罗明尧

Raynaud Phenomenon

Stanislav Henkin and Mark A. Creager

In its simplest form, local syncope is a condition perfectly compatible with health. Persons who are attacked with it are ordinarily females. Under the least stimulus, sometimes without appreciable cause, one or many fingers become pale and cold all at once; in many cases, it is the same finger that is always first attacked; the others become dead successively and in the same order. It is the phenomenon known as "dead finger." The attack is indolent, the duration varies from a few minutes to many hours. The determining cause is often the impression of cold; but that which is only commonly produced under the influence of the most severe cold, appears in the subjects of whom I speak on the occasion of the least lowering of temperatures; sometimes even a simple mental emotion is enough … the skin of the affected parts assumes a dead white or sometimes a yellow colour; it appears completely exsanguine. The cutaneous sensibility becomes blunted, then annihilated; the fingers become like foreign bodies to the subject … the slight importance of this local abolition of the circulation is probably due to the fact that it is so transient … the attack is followed by a period of reaction, which is often very painful, and which gives place to a sensation quite analogous to that of being numbed by cold … and in the more pronounced cases, which the patients compared to tingling from cold, or to the stinging of nettles…Finally, a patch of deep red is formed on the extremities of the fingers. This patch gives place to the normal pink colour, and then the skin is found to have entirely returned to the primitive condition.

—Maurice Raynaud[1]

Episodic vasospastic ischemia of the digits was first described by Maurice Raynaud in the quotation above (Fig. 46.1).[1] Raynaud phenomenon comprises sequential development of digital blanching, cyanosis, and rubor following cold exposure and subsequent rewarming (Fig. 46.2).[2] Emotional stress also precipitates Raynaud phenomenon. The color changes are usually well demarcated and primarily confined to fingers or toes. Blanching, or pallor, occurs during the ischemic phase of the phenomenon and is secondary to digital vasospasm. During ischemia, arterioles, capillaries, and venules dilate. Cyanosis results from the deoxygenated blood in these vessels. Cold, numbness, or paresthesias of the digits often accompany the phases of pallor and cyanosis. With rewarming, digital vasospasm resolves, and blood flow dramatically increases into the dilated arterioles and capillaries. This "reactive hyperemia" imparts a bright red color to the digits. In addition to rubor and warmth, patients often experience a throbbing sensation during the hyperemic phase. Thereafter, the color of the digits

gradually returns to normal. Although the triphasic color response is typical of Raynaud phenomenon, some patients may develop only pallor and cyanosis. Others may experience only cyanosis.

The classification of Raynaud phenomenon is broadly separated into two categories: (1) the idiopathic variety, termed *primary Raynaud phenomenon*, and (2) the secondary variety, associated with other disease states or known causes of vasospasm (Box 46.1). Secondary causes of Raynaud phenomenon include collagen vascular diseases, arterial occlusive disease, thoracic outlet syndrome, several neurological disorders, blood dyscrasias, trauma, and several drugs or toxins.

OVERVIEW OF PRIMARY RAYNAUD PHENOMENON

Primary Raynaud phenomenon, or idiopathic episodic digital vasospasm, is the most common diagnosis of patients who present with Raynaud phenomenon.[2] The diagnosis is based on criteria originally established by Allen and Brown,[3] including (1) intermittent attacks of ischemic discoloration of the extremities, (2) absence of organic arterial occlusions, (3) bilateral distribution, (4) trophic changes—when present, limited to the skin and never consisting of gross gangrene, (5) absence of any symptoms or signs of systemic disease that might account for the occurrence of Raynaud phenomenon, and (6) symptom duration for 2 years or longer. Recent international expert consensus criteria for the diagnosis of Raynaud phenomenon[4] includes (1) sensitivity to cold; *AND* (2) biphasic color change during vasospastic episode; *AND* (3) additional 3 out of 7 criteria such as triggers besides cold (i.e., emotional stressor), involvement of both hands, presence of numbness and/or paresthesias, triphasic color change, well-demarcated border between affected and unaffected skin, patient photographs with findings consistent with Raynaud phenomenon, and presence of symptoms at other body sites (nose, ears, feet). The diagnosis is more secure with normal nailfold capillaroscopy, no history of connective tissue disease and a negative physical examination for signs of secondary causes, negative or low titer antinuclear antibodies (ANA) (1:40 by indirect immunofluorescence), and normal erythrocyte sedimentation rate (ESR) or C-reactive protein (CRP).

Primary Raynaud phenomenon is common and may affect up to 8% of the general population in the United States;[5] women are significantly more affected than men. Onset usually occurs before the fourth decade of life, with higher prevalence in cooler climates. Raynaud phenomenon is also known to occur in children, more often in girls than boys, and prevalence increases in age.[6] There is a significant familial aggregation of primary Raynaud phenomenon, as approximately 26%

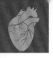

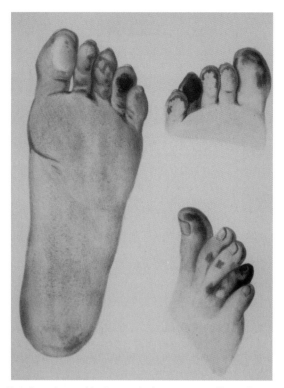

Fig. 46.1 A patient with Raynaud phenomenon. (From Raynaud M. *Local asphyxia and symmetrical gangrene of the extremities.* London: New Sydenham Society; 1862. Courtesy Boston Medical Library in the Francis A. Countway Library of Medicine.)

to 41% of patients may know of one or more relatives who have the phenomenon, suggesting a genetic predisposition.[7,8]

In the vast majority of patients, the fingers are the initial sites of involvement. At first, blanching or cyanosis may involve only one or two fingers (Fig. 46.3). Later, color changes may develop in additional fingers, and symptoms occur bilaterally. In about 40% of patients, Raynaud phenomenon involves the toes as well as the fingers. Isolated Raynaud phenomenon of the toes occurs in only 1% to 2% of patients. Rarely, the ear lobes, tip of the nose, or tongue are affected.

Episodes of Raynaud phenomenon are usually precipitated by exposure to a cool environment or by direct exposure of the extremities to low temperatures. Some patients may experience Raynaud phenomenon during either cold exposure or emotional stress; infrequently, emotional stress may be the only precipitating factor. Duration, frequency, and severity of Raynaud phenomenon increase during cold months.

Multiple studies have correlated Raynaud phenomenon with vasospastic disorders, including migraine headaches,[9] variant angina,[10,11] and vasospasm in the kidney,[12] retina,[13] and pulmonary vessels.[14] However, differences in the responses of pharmacological intervention make the hypothesis of a common mechanism less appealing. For example, metoprolol and propranolol have been successfully used to prevent migraines headaches,[15] but are not beneficial in variant angina and may precipitate Raynaud phenomenon.[16] Ergot alkaloids are effective for treating migraine headaches but can cause coronary and digital vasospasm.[17,18] Finally, there is contradicting evidence regarding genetic predisposition; one report describes a family with three generations of systemic arterial vasospastic disease involving Raynaud phenomenon, variant angina, and migraine headaches.[19] Additionally, up to 50% of patients report a first-degree relative with Raynaud when

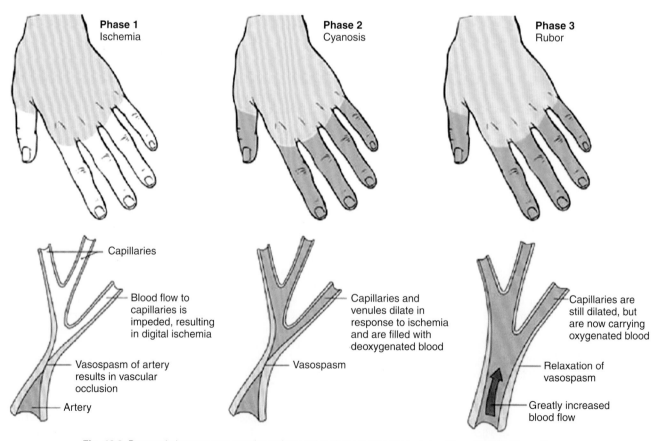

Fig. 46.2 Raynaud phenomenon may have three color phases: blanching, cyanosis, and rubor. (From Creager MA. Raynaud's phenomenon. *Med Illus.* 1983;2:84.)

BOX 46.1 Secondary Causes of Raynaud Phenomenon

Collagen Vascular Diseases
Systemic sclerosis (scleroderma)
Systemic lupus erythematosus (SLE)
Rheumatoid arthritis
Dermatomyositis and polymyositis
Mixed connective tissue disease (MCTD)
Sjögren syndrome
Necrotizing vasculitis

Arterial Occlusive Disease
Atherosclerosis of the extremities
Thromboangiitis obliterans (TAO) (Buerger disease)
Thromboembolism

Neurological Disorders
Carpal tunnel syndrome
Complex regional pain syndrome
Stroke
Intervertebral disk disease
Syringomyelia
Poliomyelitis

Thoracic Outlet Syndrome

Trauma
Exposure to vibrating tools ("vibration white finger")

Electric shock injury
Thermal injury
Percussive injury
Hypothenar hammer syndrome

Drugs and Toxins
Ergot alkaloids
Methysergide
Vinblastine
Bleomycin
Gemcitabine
β-Adrenoceptor antagonists
Vinyl chloride

Blood Dyscrasias
Hyperviscosity syndrome
Cold agglutinin disease
Cryoglobulinemia
Cryofibrinogenemia

Myeloproliferative Disease

Miscellaneous Causes
Hypothyroidism
Arteriovenous fistula (AVF)
Pulmonary hypertension

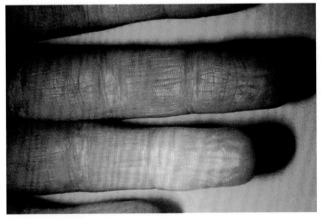

Fig. 46.3 Raynaud phenomenon presenting as blanching of one finger.

asked by survey.[7] However, a study exploring an association between known polymorphisms of vasoactive mediator genes and Raynaud phenomenon found no significant association.[8]

Physical examination of patients with primary Raynaud phenomenon is often entirely normal. Sometimes the fingers and toes are cool and may perspire excessively. The pulse examination is normal; radial, ulnar, and pedal pulses should be easily palpable. Trophic changes such as sclerodactyly (thickening and tightening of the digital subcutaneous tissue) occur in less than 10% of patients. The physical examination is most important to exclude secondary causes of Raynaud phenomenon.

Of all the forms of Raynaud phenomenon, primary Raynaud phenomenon has the most benign prognosis. In a historical group of patients identified by Gifford and Hines[20] followed for a period of 1 to 32 years (average 12 years), 16% reported worsening of their symptoms, and 38%, 36%, and 10%, respectively, reported no change,

improvement, or disappearance of symptoms. Sclerodactyly or trophic changes of the digits occurred in approximately 3% of patients during follow-up, and less than 1% of patients lost part of a digit. In some patients, scleroderma may develop after Raynaud phenomenon has been present as the only symptom for many years. Pavlov-Dolijanovic et al.[21] reported that of patients with primary Raynaud phenomenon diagnosed around age 40, in whom ANA anticentromere antibody and anti-topoisomerase I antibodies were measured and nailfold capillaroscopy was available, 32% of patients developed scleroderma over the next 2.3 ± 1.9 years of follow-up. Scleroderma pattern on nailfold capillaroscopy was the most sensitive marker of scleroderma development, while absence of anti-topoisomerase I antibodies was the most specific. In a prospective study of 784 patients with diagnosis of primary Raynaud's, ~13% developed scleroderma during the follow-up period of ~4 years; for patients with normal nailfold capillaroscopy and negative scleroderma antibodies, only 1.8% developed scleroderma.[22]

PATHOPHYSIOLOGY

The precise cause of Raynaud phenomenon has not been clearly identified. It is quite likely that a variety of physiological and pathological conditions may contribute to or cause digital vasospasm (Box 46.2 and Fig. 46.4).[2]

Normally, regulation of peripheral blood flow depends on several factors that include intrinsic vascular tone, sympathetic nervous system activity, hemorrheological properties such as blood viscosity, and various circulating hormonal substances. In contrast to other regional circulations that are supplied by both vasoconstrictor and vasodilator sympathetic fibers, the cutaneous vessels of the hands and feet are innervated only by sympathetic adrenergic vasoconstrictor fibers. In these vascular beds, neurogenic vasodilation occurs by *withdrawal* of a sympathetic stimulus. Cooling evokes reflex sympathetic-mediated vasoconstriction in the hands and feet via neurons originating in cutaneous receptors. Environmental cooling or cooling of specific

BOX 46.2   Possible Pathophysiological Mechanisms of Raynaud Phenomenon

Vasoconstrictive Stimuli

Digital vascular hyperreactivity ("local fault")

Increased sympathetic nervous system activity

β-Adrenoceptor blockade (unopposed α-adrenergic activity)

Circulating vasoactive hormones

Angiotensin II (Ang II)

Serotonin

Thromboxane

Endothelin-1 (ET-1)

Exogenous administration of vasoconstrictor agents

Ergot alkaloids

Sympathomimetic drugs

Decreased Intravascular Pressure

Low systemic blood pressure

Arterial occlusive disorder (e.g., atherosclerosis, thromboangiitis obliterans [TAO])

Digital arterial occlusions (e.g., scleroderma)

Hyperviscosity

body parts, such as the head, neck, or trunk, also causes a reduction in digital blood flow. Local digital cooling also induces vasoconstriction, independent of increased sympathetic tone.[23] Thus, digital vasoconstriction may be a physiological response to local cooling or to reflex activation of the sympathetic nervous system by environmental cold exposure or emotional stress.

Raynaud phenomenon is not a normal physiological response but rather an episode of digital artery vasospasm causing decrease of blood flow to the digits. The term *vasospasm* must be distinguished from *vasoconstriction*. *Vasoconstriction* may be defined as the expected reduction in vessel lumen size as a result of endogenous neural, hormonal, or metabolic factors that cause smooth muscle contraction. *Vasospasm* implies an excessive vasoconstrictor response to stimuli that would normally cause modest smooth muscle contraction, but that instead has resulted in obliteration of the vascular lumen. Patency of the digital artery depends on a favorable balance between the contractile forces of the muscular wall of the digital artery and its intraluminal pressure. Thus, a situation in which there is excessive vasoconstrictive force or decreased intravascular pressure upsets this balance and results in vasospasm. It is with these rather simple concepts that several theories have been proposed to explain the episodic digital vasospasm that defines Raynaud phenomenon.

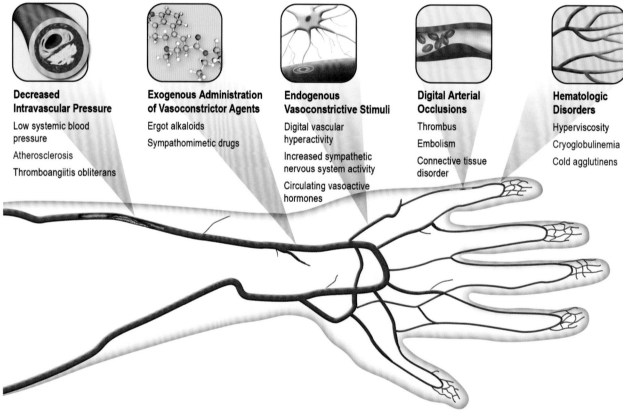

Fig. 46.4 Pathophysiology of Digital Vasospasm. Digital vasospasm may be due to vasoconstrictive stimuli, decreased intravascular pressure, or both. Mechanisms that contribute to exercise vasoconstriction include local vascular hypersensitivity to vasoactive stimuli (e.g., increased α-adrenoceptor sensitivity), sympathetic efferent activity, and local or circulating vasoactive hormones such as angiotensin II, endothelin-1, serotonin, or thromboxane A₂. Low blood pressure, even in a healthy young person, may predispose to Raynaud phenomenon when the person encounters vasoconstrictive stimuli. Pathological conditions that may decrease intravascular pressure include arterial occlusion in proximal arteries (e.g., atherosclerosis), digital vascular occlusion (e.g., scleroderma), or hyperviscosity.

Increased Vasoconstrictive Stimuli

Several theories implicate excessive vasoconstrictive stimuli as a cause of Raynaud phenomenon. Postulated causes include local vascular hyperreactivity, increased sympathetic nervous system activity, elevated levels of vasoconstrictor hormones (e.g., angiotensin II [Ang II], serotonin, thromboxane A_2 [TxA_2]), and exogenously administered agents such as ergot alkaloids and sympathomimetic drugs.

Local Vascular Hyperreactivity

The observation that episodic digital vasospasm occurs during cold exposure has led several investigators to consider the possibility that Raynaud phenomenon occurs as a result of a local vascular hyperreactivity. In 1929, Sir Thomas Lewis observed that following exposure of the finger to cold, vasospasm could be produced even after nerve blockade or sympathectomy.[24] These experiments were repeated and confirmed 60 years later.[25] Therefore the vasospastic response of the Raynaud phenomenon may occur in the absence of efferent digital nerves. The possibility of local vascular hyperreactivity was examined by Jamieson et al.[26] They compared the magnitude of reflex vasoconstriction in each hand following application of ice to the neck while one hand was kept at 26°C and the other at 36°C. At 36°C, the reflex vasoconstrictor response was comparable in normal subjects and patients with primary Raynaud phenomenon. In the hand cooled to 26°C, however, reflex vasoconstriction was exaggerated in patients with Raynaud phenomenon. This response led these investigators to hypothesize that digital adrenoceptors were sensitized by cold exposure. Coffman and Cohen reported that systemic cooling also causes an exaggerated reduction in digital blood flow in individuals with Raynaud phenomenon compared to those without.[27]

A series of studies by Vanhoutte et al.[28] have supported the hypothesis that cooling potentiates the vascular response to sympathetic nerve activation. Vasoconstriction, in response to exogenous norepinephrine, also is increased by cooling. Augmentation of adrenergic-mediated vasoconstriction by cooling occurs despite generalized depression of contractile machinery and diminished release of norepinephrine from sympathetic nerve endings in the vessel wall. The most likely hypothesis is that cold causes changes at the level of the adrenoceptor, such as an increase in the affinity for norepinephrine or greater efficacy of the agonist/receptor complex. Vanhoutte et al.[28] have reported that α_2 adrenoceptors are more sensitive than α_1 adrenoceptors to temperature change. Whereas cooling slightly depresses α_1 adrenergic-mediated vasoconstriction, it markedly augments α_2 adrenergic-mediated responses. Conversely, warming augments α_1-adrenergic vasoconstriction and depresses α_2-adrenergic vasoconstriction.[29]

These experimental observations may have important implications regarding the pathophysiology of Raynaud phenomenon. Flavahan et al.[30] examined the distribution of α_1 and α_2 adrenoceptors in arterial tissue from amputated limbs of patients who did not have vascular disease. They reported that α_2 adrenoceptors were more prominent in digital arteries. Chotani et al.[31] found that human dermal arterioles selectively expressed α_{2C} adrenoceptors. Jeyaraj et al.[32] observed that cooling redistributed α_{2C} adrenoceptors from the Golgi to the plasma membrane in human embryonic kidney cells. It is therefore an intriguing observation by Keenan and Porter that the density of α_2 adrenoceptors is increased in platelets from patients with Raynaud disease.[33]

In support of these findings, Coffman and Cohen reported that α_2 adrenoceptors were more important than α_1 adrenoceptors in mediating sympathetic nerve-induced vasoconstriction in the fingers.[34] They administered the α_1-antagonist prazosin and the α_2-antagonist yohimbine to normal individuals during reflex sympathetic vasoconstriction caused by body cooling. Whereas prazosin caused no significant change in finger blood flow or finger vascular resistance, yohimbine significantly increased finger blood flow and decreased finger vascular resistance. This study confirmed that postjunctional α_2 adrenoceptors are present in human digits and play a more important role than α_1-adrenoceptors in sympathetic digital vasoconstriction.

Thereafter, Coffman and Cohen demonstrated that compared to normal subjects, patients with Raynaud phenomenon were hypersensitive to the vasoconstrictor effects of clonidine, an α_2-adrenoceptor agonist, but not to phenylephrine, an α_1-adrenoceptor agonist,[35] a finding confirmed by several other studies.[36,37] Even with combined systemic and local cooling, selective inhibition of only α_2-adrenoceptors significantly reduced the number of vasospastic episodes in individuals with Raynaud phenomenon.[38] In contrast, Cooke et al.[39] found that both α_1- and α_2-adrenoceptor antagonists induced digital vasodilation in patients with acute Raynaud phenomenon, yet did not inhibit digital vasoconstriction caused by local digital cooling. Overall, these studies suggest that episodic digital vasospasm may be secondary to a predominance of postjunctional α_2 adrenoceptors in digits of patients with either primary or secondary Raynaud phenomenon.[40]

Increased Sympathetic Nervous System Activity

Although appealing as a potential mechanism for digital vasospasm, the concept of exaggerated reflex sympathetic vasoconstrictor responses to cold environment has not been convincingly demonstrated. Increased concentrations of epinephrine and norepinephrine in peripheral venous blood at the wrist were found to be higher in patients with primary Raynaud phenomenon than in normal subjects by one investigator,[41] but others found normal local levels of norepinephrine in brachial arterial and venous blood samples.[42] The latter group of investigators reported that the reflex vasoconstrictor response of the hand to a cold stimulus in affected patients is similar to that in a control group, and there were comparable vasoconstrictor responses to the intraarterial infusion of tyramine, a drug that causes vasoconstriction by releasing norepinephrine from sympathetic nerve terminals. Central thermoregulatory control of skin temperature has also been reported to be comparable in normal individuals and patients with primary Raynaud phenomenon.[43] Finally, microelectrode recordings of skin sympathetic nerve activity do not demonstrate an abnormality in patients with primary Raynaud phenomenon; there was no hypersensitivity of the vessels to strong sympathetic stimuli or abnormal increase in sympathetic outflow.[44]

β-Adrenergic Blockade

Raynaud phenomenon is observed frequently in individuals treated with β-adrenoceptor antagonists, with an estimated prevalence of ~15% in a meta-analysis.[45] It may be inferred from this observation that β-adrenergic vasodilation normally attenuates digital vasoconstrictor tone. Cohen and Coffman[46] examined the effect of isoproterenol and propranolol on fingertip blood flow after vasoconstriction had been induced by a brachial artery infusion of norepinephrine or angiotensin, or reflexively by environmental cooling. Intraarterial isoproterenol administration increased fingertip blood flow during infusions of norepinephrine and angiotensin, but not during reflex sympathetic vasoconstriction. Conversely, propranolol served to potentiate vasoconstriction caused by intraarterial norepinephrine, but not that caused by reflex sympathetic vasoconstriction. These investigators concluded that a β-adrenergic vasodilator mechanism may be active in human digits but does not modulate sympathetic vasoconstriction. There is no evidence to support the contention that decreased sensitivity or number of β adrenoceptors contribute to the pathophysiology of Raynaud phenomenon in the absence of pharmacological blockade of β adrenoceptors.

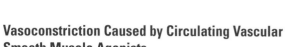

Vasoconstriction Caused by Circulating Vascular Smooth Muscle Agonists

Various neurotransmitters, hormones, and platelet release byproducts are capable of constricting vascular smooth muscle and causing digital vasoconstriction. These include Ang II, serotonin, TxA$_2$, and endothelin-1 (ET-1). It would be difficult to attribute all causes of Raynaud phenomenon to excessive levels of these vasoconstrictor agents, but in some secondary causes of Raynaud phenomenon, any one of them might contribute to vasoconstriction.

Serotonin (5-hydroxytryptamine [5-HT]) is a neurotransmitter that is synthesized and released by selective neurons and enterochromaffin cells. Serotonin can cause vasoconstriction by directly activating serotoninergic receptors on the smooth muscle cells (SMCs). Vasoconstriction may also be caused by direct activation of α adrenoceptors on SMCs or indirectly by facilitating release of norepinephrine from adrenergic nerve terminals. Although some evidence implicates a role for serotonin in the pathophysiology of Raynaud phenomenon, as patients may experience improvement of symptoms with serotonin reuptake inhibitors,[47] the contribution of serotonin to digital vasospasm remains speculative.

The possibility that vasoconstrictors released during platelet aggregation may be pertinent to the pathophysiology of Raynaud phenomenon has been further evaluated by studies that have either measured levels of TxA$_2$ or administered a thromboxane synthetase inhibitor.[48,49] Coffman and Rasmussen compared the thromboxane synthetase inhibitor, dazoxiben, to placebo in patients with either primary or secondary Raynaud phenomenon.[48] Dazoxiben did not affect total fingertip blood flow or fingertip capillary blood flow, whether measured in a warm (28.3°C) or cool (20°C) environment. With chronic treatment, there was a small decrease in frequency of vasospastic episodes in patients with primary Raynaud phenomenon. To date, however, there is insufficient evidence to support a role for TxA$_2$ in digital vasospasm.

Plasma concentration of the potent vasoconstrictor Ang II is rarely elevated in patients with Raynaud phenomenon.[50] This hormone is therefore unlikely to contribute to the pathophysiology of digital vasospasm in most patients.

ET-1 is an endothelium-derived, powerful, and prolonged-acting vasoconstrictor agent suggested to play a part in the pathogenesis of Raynaud phenomenon. It rises in response to a cold pressor test and constricts cutaneous blood vessels. Studies measuring ET-1 in primary or secondary Raynaud phenomenon have been conflicting.[51,52] Controlled clinical trials of ET-1 receptor antagonism in the treatment of primary Raynaud phenomenon have achieved little success, although ET-1 antagonists may play a role in reducing the risk of new ulcer formation in secondary Raynaud's due to scleroderma.[53-55] It is therefore doubtful that ET-1 plays a role in primary Raynaud phenomenon.

Decreased Intravascular Pressure

Patency of a blood vessel requires balance between arterial wall tension (favoring closure of the vessel) and intravascular distending pressure. Landis measured intravascular pressure in patients with Raynaud phenomenon by introducing a micropipette into a large digital capillary.[56] During cyanosis, capillary pressure fell to approximately 5 mm Hg, and flow ceased. These findings suggested that the site of closure was proximal to the capillaries at the arterial level. Interestingly, Thulesius reported that brachial artery blood pressure in patients with primary Raynaud phenomenon was significantly lower than that in a normal control population.[57] Cohen and Coffman also found that blood pressure was lower in patients with primary Raynaud phenomenon compared with normal subjects.[58] In addition to lower brachial blood pressure, systolic blood pressure (SBP) measured at the proximal and distal digital arteries averaged 18 mm Hg less than that in normal digits.

A low digital artery pressure may occur in various disorders associated with Raynaud phenomenon, such as large-vessel arterial occlusive disease secondary to atherosclerosis, embolism, or thoracic outlet syndrome. When extrinsic vasoconstrictor force is applied, these vessels may collapse and cause digital ischemia. Distal vascular occlusions secondary to thromboangiitis obliterans (TAO), vasculitis, or vibration injury may also reduce digital arterial pressure distal to the diseased vascular segment.

Hyperviscosity may reduce blood flow velocity in digital vessels, leading to a decrease in intravascular pressure. Indeed, Raynaud phenomenon occurs in patients with hyperviscosity due to polycythemia vera or Waldenström macroglobulinemia. In patients with Raynaud phenomenon secondary to disorders such as cryoglobulinemia and cold agglutinin disease, hyperviscosity caused by cooling may contribute to digital vasospasm. Indeed, cooling has been shown to abolish hand blood flow in patients with cold agglutinins, possibly because the vessels become occluded by agglutinated red cells.[59] Data invoking hyperviscosity as a cause of primary Raynaud phenomenon in patients who do not have an established blood dyscrasia, however, are less compelling.[60,61]

SECONDARY CAUSES OF RAYNAUD PHENOMENON

The secondary causes of Raynaud phenomenon include collagen vascular diseases, arterial occlusive disorders, thoracic outlet syndrome, several neurological disorders, blood dyscrasias, trauma, and several drugs or toxins (see Box 46.1).

Collagen Vascular Diseases

Systemic Sclerosis (Scleroderma)

Raynaud phenomenon occurs in 80% to 90% of patients with systemic sclerosis; it may be the presenting symptom in up to a third of patients. In some patients, scleroderma may develop after Raynaud phenomenon has been present as the only symptom for many years. The frequency and severity of Raynaud phenomenon in patients with systemic sclerosis is often worse than that observed in patients with primary Raynaud phenomenon, due at least in part to the presence of endothelial dysfunction, which manifests as reduced activity of vasodilators and increased activity of inflammatory, thrombotic, and vasoconstrictor factors.[62] The incidence of digital ulceration and gangrene is increased, possibly leading to amputation. Quality of life of patients with Raynaud phenomenon secondary to systemic sclerosis is significantly worse than those with primary phenomenon.[63]

Diagnosis of systemic sclerosis is suggested by the appearance of typical sclerotic skin changes. These include tightness, thickening, and nonpitting induration involving the extremities, face, neck, or trunk. When present in the digits, these abnormalities produce changes in the contour of the fingers and toes, referred to as sclerodactyly. Other manifestations of systemic sclerosis include pitting scars of the tips of the digits, normal skin pigmentation, and telangiectasia. Visceral manifestations include pulmonary fibrosis, esophageal dysmotility, and colonic sacculation. The kidney and heart may also be involved. As the disease progresses, skin and subcutaneous tissue of the fingers become stiffer, joints become immobile, and contractures develop. A variant of systemic sclerosis is the CREST syndrome, a form of limited scleroderma that includes calcinosis, Raynaud phenomenon, esophageal dysmotility, sclerodactyly, and telangiectasia in the absence of internal organ involvement.

Several serological studies are consistent with the diagnosis of scleroderma. ESR and CRP may be elevated, and ANAs are present in the majority of individuals with this disorder. Patients may have antibodies to nucleolar antigens, nuclear ribonucleoprotein (RNP), and to the centromeric region of metaphase chromosomes. In patients with systemic sclerosis and Raynaud phenomenon, capillary microscopy often demonstrates enlarged and deformed capillary loops surrounded by relatively avascular areas, particularly in the nailfolds.[64] Angiography frequently demonstrates digital vascular obstruction.

Systemic Lupus Erythematosus

Raynaud phenomenon occurs in approximately 10% to 35% of patients with systemic lupus erythematosus (SLE). Persistent digital vasospasm, often due to proliferative endarteritis of the small digital vessels, also occurs and may result in gangrene. Diagnosis of SLE is based on the presence of at least 4 of the following 17 criteria, including at least 1 of 11 clinical criteria *and* at least 1 of 6 immunologic criteria; **or** biopsy-proven nephritis compatible with SLE *and* presence of ANA or anti-double-stranded DNA (anti-dsDNA).[65]

Clinical criteria:
1. Malar rash or photosensitive rash or acute cutaneous lupus
2. Discoid rash
3. Oral ulcers
4. Nonscarring alopecia
5. Synovitis involving ≥2 joints
6. Serositis, including pleuritis or pericarditis
7. Renal manifestation (i.e., urine protein/creatinine ratio >500 mg/24 hours; or red blood cell casts)
8. Neurological disorders, such as seizures and psychosis
9. Hemolytic anemia
10. Leukopenia or lymphopenia
11. Thrombocytopenia

Immunologic criteria:
1. Abnormal ANA titer
2. Abnormal anti-dsDNA titer
3. Presence of anti-Sm antibody
4. Positive antiphospholipid antibody
5. Low complement levels
6. Positive direct Coombs test without hemolytic anemia[65]

Compared to prior diagnostic criteria developed by American College of Rheumatology in 1997,[66] more recent criteria have higher sensitivity (97% vs. 83%) but lower specificity (84% vs. 96%).[65]

Rheumatoid Arthritis

Raynaud phenomenon also occurs in more than 20% of patients with rheumatoid arthritis.[67] These patients may have vasculitis of medium-sized vessels, as well as proliferative endarteritis of small vessels. Crops of small brown spots may be observed in the nail beds and digital pulp. Digital blood flow is often reduced in patients with rheumatoid arthritis, and angiography frequently reveals occlusions of one or more digital arteries. The diagnosis is suggested in patients who have at least one joint with synovitis, with the synovitis not explained by another disease, and who score 6/10 points or more on the following consensus diagnostic criteria:[68]
1. Involvement of 2 to 10 large joints (1 point)
2. 1 to 3 small joints (2 points)
3. 4 to 10 small joints (3 points)
4. More than 10 joints (5 points)
5. Low-positive rheumatoid factor (RF) or low-positive anticitrullinated protein/peptide (ACPA) (2 points)
6. High-positive RF or high-positive ACPA (3 points)
7. Abnormal CRP or abnormal ESR (1 point)
8. Duration of symptoms 6 weeks or more (1 point)

Dermatomyositis and Polymyositis

Thirty percent of patients with dermatomyositis and polymyositis have associated Raynaud phenomenon. Muscular manifestations include weakness of the proximal girdle muscles, particularly those involving the lower extremities. Patients may also experience aching in the buttocks, thighs, and calves. Some patients complain of dysphagia or dyspnea. Myocarditis develops in approximately one third of these individuals. The dermatological abnormalities in dermatomyositis include localized or diffuse erythema, a maculopapular rash, and eczematoid dermatitis. A purplish (heliotrope) rash may develop on the upper eyelids, face, chest, limbs, or around the nail beds. Laboratory diagnosis of dermatomyositis and polymyositis is based on elevated serum levels of the skeletal muscle enzymes, including creatine kinase, aldolase, serum glutamic oxaloacetic transaminase, and lactic acid dehydrogenase. There may be myoglobinuria, and ESR is often elevated. Electromyogram reveals evidence of a myopathy.

Primary Sjögren Syndrome

Sjögren syndrome is an autoimmune disease that mainly affects exocrine glands and leads to dryness of the eyes and mouth, but it can have extraglandular manifestations. Raynaud phenomenon has been reported in 13% of patients and may precede the sicca symptomatology in up to 50% of patients.[69] Presence of anticentromere antibody increases the likelihood of associated Raynaud phenomenon, possibly because of an association with an increase in fibrous tissues.[70] The clinical course is usually milder than in patients with systemic sclerosis. Diagnosis is made with a score of ≥4 points of 5 weighed criteria in an individual who presents with oral or ocular dryness:[71]
1. Labial gland with focal lymphocytic sialadenitis (3 points)
2. Positive anti-SSa/Ro antibody (3 points)
3. Ocular Staining Score ≥5 (1 point)
4. Schirmer test ≤5 mm in 5 minutes (1 point)
5. Unstimulated saliva flow rate ≤0.1 mL per minute (1 point)

Mixed Connective Tissue Disease

Mixed connective tissue disease (MCTD) is a disorder with overlapping clinical features of SLE, scleroderma, and myositis, and presence of a distinctive antibody against U1-RNP. Raynaud phenomenon is the main symptom in MCTD, and trophic abnormalities of the fingers are frequently observed.[72] Elevated anti–U1-RNP antibody titers and an abnormal capillaroscopic pattern are specific for the condition.[73]

Arterial Occlusive Disease

Occlusive disease of arteries proximal to the digital vessels is often associated with Raynaud phenomenon. Proximal arterial occlusive disease may decrease intravascular pressure and upset the balance between tension in the arterial wall and intravascular distending pressure. This may make the vessel more prone to vasospasm when subjected to sympathetic nervous system stimuli.

Atherosclerosis of the extremities tends to occur most frequently in males older than 50 years of age and females older than 60. When Raynaud phenomenon occurs in these individuals, it tends to be unilateral and related to the affected extremity. Usually only one or two digits are involved. The diagnosis is suggested by clinical history and physical examination. Symptoms of claudication or findings that would suggest atherosclerosis elsewhere, such as in the coronary or cerebral vasculature, often indicate the underlying disorder. Physical findings are noteworthy for decreased or absent pulses in the involved extremity. These abnormalities can be confirmed by noninvasive vascular testing. Severe ischemia may manifest as persistent digital pallor or cyanosis and must be distinguished from the episodic digital vasospasm of Raynaud phenomenon. Digital ischemic ulcers may develop in these individuals.

TAO [Buerger disease]) is an inflammatory occlusive vascular disorder involving small- and medium-sized arteries and veins, often accompanied by Raynaud phenomenon (see Chapter 42). In addition to Raynaud phenomenon, clinical features of TAO include claudication of the affected extremity and migratory superficial vein thrombosis in a young male. Smoking cessation is a mainstay of treatment.

Thoracic Outlet Syndrome

Compression of the neurovascular bundle as it courses through the neck and shoulder can result in a symptom complex that includes Raynaud phenomenon as well as shoulder and arm pain, weakness, paresthesias, and claudication of the affected upper extremity (see Chapter 63). Raynaud phenomenon may result from the decreased intravascular pressure caused by extrinsic compression of the subclavian artery. Most common causes include trauma or presence of a cervical rib. Whether compression of the brachial plexus alters sympathetic nervous system activity is unknown.

Neurological Disorders

Various neurological conditions, particularly those causing disuse of the limb, may be associated with disorders of circulatory vasomotion. These include stroke, syringomyelia, intervertebral disk disease, spinal cord tumors, and poliomyelitis. The affected limb, including the hand or foot in addition to the digits, may be cool and cyanotic. In contrast to the episodic nature of Raynaud phenomenon, these changes tend to be persistent.

Raynaud phenomenon has been reported in approximately 16% of patients with carpal tunnel syndrome.[74] This entrapment neuropathy is due to compression of the median nerve as it passes through the carpal tunnel. It may result from pregnancy, localized tenosynovitis, trauma, hypothyroidism, amyloidosis, or activities associated with repeated motion of the wrist. Patients usually experience paresthesias or weakness in the distribution of the median nerve. The diagnosis is suggested when symptoms are reproduced by tapping the volar surface of the wrist (Tinel sign) or by maintaining flexion of the wrist (Phalen maneuver). Nerve conduction tests usually demonstrate abnormalities of the median nerve at the wrist. Supportive treatment includes splints and antiinflammatory drugs. Individuals with concurrent carpal tunnel and Raynaud phenomenon respond less well to corticosteroid injections than those with only carpal tunnel syndrome.[75] With severe persistent symptoms, surgical release of the carpal ligament may be beneficial.

Complex regional pain syndrome, previously known as *reflex sympathetic dystrophy* or *causalgia*, is another neurological disorder associated with cyanotic extremities and involves pain, swelling, and sensitivity to hand or touch, with accompanying vasomotor instability.

Blood Dyscrasias

Hyperviscosity syndromes, cold-precipitable plasma proteins, abnormalities of red cell agglutination, and certain myeloproliferative disorders are associated with Raynaud phenomenon, as well as with persistent digital ischemia.

Patients with cold agglutinins occasionally develop Raynaud phenomenon. It is generally thought that Raynaud phenomenon develops when proteins precipitate on red blood cells and agglutinate within the digital vessel during exposure to cold. Prolonged exposure may cause thrombosis and subsequent digital gangrene. Cold agglutinin disease usually involves immunoglobulin (Ig)M antibodies that are reactive with I antigen of the red blood cell, which consequently activates the complement cascade.[76] The antibody titer is high at 4°C and low at 37°C. These antibodies also may cause cold-induced hemolysis. Agglutination usually does not occur in temperatures above 32°C. Cold agglutinins may arise spontaneously or occur in patients with mycoplasma pneumonia, infectious mononucleosis, or lymphoproliferative

disorders. Cold agglutinin disease may be short lived in patients with infectious causes but is often persistent in patients with lymphoproliferative disease.

Cryoglobulins are a group of proteins that precipitate in cold serum and may cause Raynaud phenomenon.[77] Cryoglobulins are associated with monoclonal and polyclonal gammopathies in disorders such as Waldenström macroglobulinemia, SLE, and rheumatoid arthritis. Cryoglobulinemia has been categorized into three subtypes. Type I cryoglobulins include monoclonal immunoglobulins of a single class, usually associated with lymphoproliferative disorders such as multiple myeloma. Type II encompasses mixed cryoglobulins containing monoclonal IgM or RF and polyclonal IgG. This may occur in patients with Waldenström macroglobulinemia or chronic active hepatitis. In patients with Waldenström macroglobulinemia, about 10% of macroglobulins are cryoglobulins. Type III cryoglobulinemia includes polyclonal IgM and IgG immunoglobulins, as may occur in SLE. Approximately 80% of patients with lupus have cold-insoluble precipitates. In these patients, there is a significantly higher level of cryoprecipitating IgM class RFs than in other patients. Most patients with mixed cryoglobulinemia have a chronic hepatitis C infection.

Cryofibrinogenemia is a rare condition that may be associated with digital vasospasm.[78] The plasma, but not the serum, of patients with cryofibrinogenemia forms a gelatinous precipitate at 4°C. Disorders associated with cryofibrinogenemia include disseminated intravascular coagulation, collagen vascular diseases, thromboembolism, and diabetes mellitus.

Trauma

Various traumatic injuries are associated with Raynaud phenomenon and have been designated *traumatic vasospastic diseases*. Causes of traumatic vasospastic disease include electric shock injury, thermal injuries such as frostbite, and mechanical percussive injury associated with piano playing and typing. The most common traumatic cause of Raynaud phenomenon is repeated exposure to vibrating tools. This has occasionally been referred to as *vibration white finger syndrome*. It has been reported in lumberjacks and other users of chainsaws, stonecutters who use air hammers, operators of pneumatic hand grinders and impact wrenches in the engine manufacturing industry, and road drillers. Prevalence of Raynaud phenomenon induced by vibration ranges from 33% to 71% among members of populations at risk and increases with exposure time.[79,80] A recent meta-analysis has found that those exposed to hand-arm vibration have up to seven times the risk of developing Raynaud compared to the nonexposed group.[81] It has been suggested that the combination of vibration and cold exposure in many of these workers is responsible for development of Raynaud phenomenon.[82] Pathophysiological changes may involve both the vascular and neurological systems in these individuals and may contribute to digital vasospasm. Intimal thickening of peripheral arteries has been reported in animals exposed to repeated vibration,[83] but pathological changes of the blood vessels have not consistently been demonstrated.[84] Medial muscular hypertrophy and subintimal fibrosis have been found in biopsy specimens of digital arteries of patients in one study, but not in others.[85] Nailbed capillaroscopy has shown a reduction in the number of capillaries. Arteriograms of these patients have shown arterial occlusion of the distal radial and ulnar arteries and frequently of the palmar arch.

Neurophysiological abnormalities have not been consistently demonstrated in patients with Raynaud phenomenon secondary to vibration. Although some have found a high instance of abnormal electromyograms,[86] others have found that episodes of Raynaud phenomena occur independently of electromyographic abnormalities.[87] Peripheral nerve conduction velocities are often abnormal in vibrating tool operators, and pathological changes have also been reported in the nerves of patients with vibration white finger, including axonal degeneration, demyelination, and collagenization of perineurium and endoperineurium. Thus, the precise pathophysiology of Raynaud phenomenon in patients repeatedly exposed to vibratory stimuli is unclear. Some have suggested that overexcitation of the Pacinian corpuscles causes reflex efferent sympathetic nerve activity. Others have suggested that following vibration, cutaneous vessels become more reactive to sympathetic stimuli.

Another trauma-induced cause of Raynaud phenomenon is the hypothenar hammer syndrome. Patients develop an ulnar artery thrombosis after hammering with the palms of their hands or practicing karate.

Drugs and Toxins

Various drugs have been implicated in producing Raynaud phenomenon or digital vasospasm (see Box 46.1). Although some of these drugs act by directly causing vasoconstriction, the mechanism whereby others cause Raynaud phenomenon is not known.

Ergot derivatives, such as bromocriptine mesylate or methysergide, cause vasospasm, primarily by stimulating α adrenoceptors, but also have affinity for serotonin, dopamine, and norepinephrine receptors. Vasospasm usually occurs when excessive doses of these drugs have been administered. Spasm may affect digital vessels as well as the coronary, carotid, femoral, and splanchnic vessels. The tricyclic antidepressant imipramine and the amphetamines also have been reported to cause arterial spasm.

Raynaud phenomenon has also been associated with use of at least four chemotherapeutic agents: cisplatin, vinblastine, gemcitabine, and bleomycin. Although it is unknown how these compounds cause Raynaud phenomenon, one hypothesis is that chemotherapeutic agents cause endothelial dysfunction that may persist after cessation of chemotherapy.[88] Vinblastine can induce peripheral neuropathy and perhaps interfere with the autonomic reflexes. Gemcitabine therapy has been associated with Raynaud phenomenon and digital ischemia due to endothelial damage secondary to inflammatory changes, and from thrombotic microangiopathy.[89] There seems to be a dose-dependent relationship.[16]

Industrial exposure to vinyl chloride polymerization processes may cause endothelial dysfunction and significantly higher likelihood of developing Raynaud phenomenon compared to nonexposed individuals, with prevalence of up to 30%.[90]

β-Adrenoceptor blocking drugs may cause Raynaud phenomenon. Although the mechanism of action is unknown, possibilities include unopposed stimulation of vascular α adrenoceptors or reflex sympathetic vasoconstriction initiated by the central cardiovascular depressant effect of β-adrenergic blockade. It remains controversial whether cardioselective β-adrenoceptor blocking drugs cause Raynaud phenomenon less frequently than nonselective drugs, and whether there is less digital vasospasm with drugs that also have α-adrenoceptor blocking properties or intrinsic sympathomimetic activity. One placebo-controlled study examined both cardioselective and nonselective β-adrenoceptor blockers in patients who already had Raynaud phenomenon.[91] Compared with placebo, neither metoprolol nor propranolol decreased fingertip blood flow, despite exposure to a cool environment, a finding confirmed in another study.[92] Furthermore, chronic treatment did not increase the number of vasospastic attacks in patients receiving either drug compared with placebo. A recent meta-analysis found a significant difference in incidence of Raynaud phenomenon in those using β-adrenoceptor blocking drugs compared to controls (7% vs. 4.6%), although this was mostly driven by patients on either atenolol or propranolol.[93] One might conclude from these observations that β-adrenoceptor blocking drugs may cause Raynaud phenomenon in some individuals, but these drugs do not seem to adversely affect frequency of vasospastic attacks, nor do they decrease finger blood flow in patients with Raynaud phenomenon.

Miscellaneous Causes

Hypothyroidism may be associated with Raynaud phenomenon.[94] In these cases, thyroid replacement alleviates the episodes of digital vasospasm. Although the mechanism is unknown, peripheral vasoconstriction may occur in hypothyroid patients to conserve heat. Alternatively, edematous thickening of the vascular wall could predispose to vessel closure during normal sympathetic stimuli.

Patients with arteriovenous fistula (AVF) may develop Raynaud phenomenon; it is particularly prevalent in patients undergoing hemodialysis.[95] This may be secondary to decreased blood flow and blood pressure in the digits of the limb with the fistula.

Pulmonary hypertension and Raynaud phenomenon may occur in the same patients. Some of these may have a connective tissue disorder such as scleroderma.[96] Ten percent of women with pulmonary arterial hypertension (PAH) have Raynaud phenomenon.[97] This prevalence is not significantly different from that occurring in the general population, so it is not clear whether the association of PAH and Raynaud phenomenon is coincidence or related to a common neurohumoral or immunological mechanism.

Paraneoplastic Raynaud phenomenon is a rare complication of a number of different malignancies (e.g., carcinomas, sarcomas, lymphomas, leukemias), at times accompanied by paraneoplastic dermatomyositis and characterized by capillaroscopic findings similar to scleroderma.[98-100]

DIAGNOSTIC TESTS

Noninvasive vascular tests may be employed to evaluate patients with Raynaud phenomenon (see Chapter 12). The effect on finger systolic pressure of local cooling with ischemia is an objective test for Raynaud phenomenon, but this is too cumbersome a test for routine use because it involves measuring digital systolic pressure with cooling plus 5 minutes of ischemia at four different temperatures (Fig. 46.5). Patients with Raynaud phenomenon have a greater reduction or loss of finger systolic pressure with cooling compared with normal subjects, who show a gradual decrease.

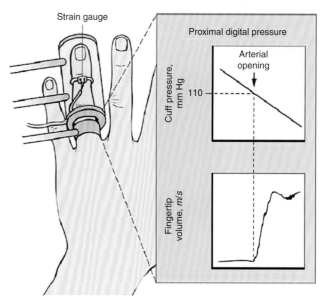

Fig. 46.5 Measurement of proximal finger systolic blood pressure using strain gauge to detect increase in fingertip volume as proximal cuff is slowly deflated from suprasystolic pressure. Fingertip pulsations and volume increase are not detected until cuff pressure deflates to 110 mm Hg, the point of digital artery opening.

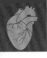

The pulse volume waveform may distinguish patients with Raynaud phenomenon who have digital ischemia secondary to vascular occlusive lesions (Fig. 46.6). During local digital warming, the vessels dilate. The pulse waveform is usually normal during warming in patients with Raynaud phenomenon if obstructive lesions are not present, and may be abnormal if atherosclerosis, TAO, or other fixed obstructive digital vascular pathology impairs digital blood flow.

Various serological studies such as for collagen vascular disorders or blood dyscrasias are useful to screen for secondary causes of Raynaud phenomenon. These tests include inflammatory markers (ESR and/or CRP), serum protein electrophoresis, and assays for ANA, RF, cryoglobulins, and cold agglutinins. Indications for these and other serological studies are usually suggested by the history and physical examination.

Nailfold capillary microscopy may be used to detect the deformed capillary loops and avascular areas typical of collagen vascular disorders (Fig. 46.7).[64] Roentgenography of the cervical spine is used to detect cervical ribs as a screen for thoracic outlet syndrome.

Angiography is rarely indicated, since Raynaud phenomenon is a diagnosis based primarily on history and physical examination. Angiography may be indicated, however, in patients with persistent digital ischemia secondary to atherosclerosis, TAO, or emboli from a subclavian artery aneurysm, in order to plan revascularization procedures (Fig. 46.8).

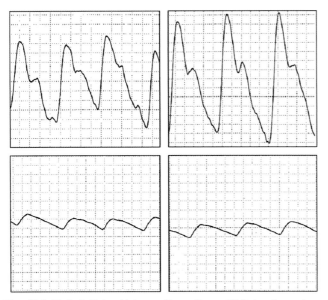

Fig. 46.6 Digital Pulse Volume Recordings. Digital pulse volume waveforms were recorded during cooling (*left;* 24°C) and rewarming (*right;* 44°C). In healthy subject *(top),* pulse volume amplitude increased during warming. In patient with digital ischemia secondary to vascular occlusion, pulse volume amplitude is diminished during both cooling and rewarming *(bottom).*

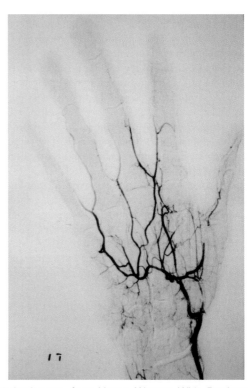

Fig. 46.8 Angiogram from Young Woman With Persistent Digital Ischemia. Multiple areas demonstrate digital vascular occlusion. Blood vessel biopsy was performed to make the diagnosis of necrotizing vasculitis.

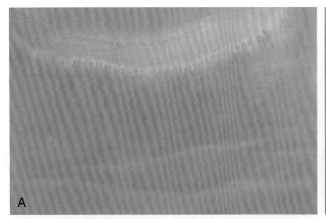
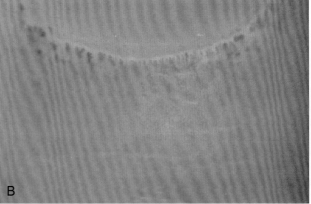

Fig. 46.7 Nailfold capillary microscopy is performed using magnifying glass, ophthalmoscope, or compound microscope (magnification, ×10) to view clean nailfold covered with immersion oil. (A) Normally, superficial capillaries are regularly spaced hairpin loops. (B) Results of this test are abnormal in patients with connective tissue disorders. Avascular areas and enlarged and deformed capillary loops are present in nailfold of this patient with scleroderma. Disorganized nailfold capillaries associated with avascular areas and hemorrhage are present in patients with dermatomyositis and polymyositis (magnification, ×10). (Courtesy H. Maricq, MD.)

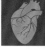

TREATMENT

Treatment programs must be individualized and designed according to the underlying cause of Raynaud phenomenon and severity of symptoms. Therapy directed specifically at the symptoms of Raynaud phenomenon can be categorized as (1) conservative measures, (2) pharmacological intervention, and (3) surgical sympathectomy (Box 46.3). In individuals with well-defined secondary causes of Raynaud phenomenon, treatment should also be directed specifically at the underlying cause. For example, if a patient has been taking a vasoactive medication, such as an ergot alkaloid, or has been treated with a β-adrenergic blocking drug for hypertension, removal of the offending agent may reduce or eliminate the Raynaud phenomenon. Similarly, specific treatment may be directed at other secondary causes such as arterial occlusive disorders, connective tissue diseases, and blood dyscrasias. The following discussion focuses on treatment designed to palliate Raynaud phenomenon.

BOX 46.3 Treatment of Raynaud Phenomenon

Conservative Measures
Warm clothing
Avoidance of cold exposure
Abstinence from nicotine
Remove offending drug (if present)
Behavioral therapy

Pharmacological Interventions
Calcium Channel Blockers
Nifedipine
Diltiazem
Felodipine
Isradipine
Amlodipine

Sympathetic Nervous System Inhibitors
Prazosin
Doxazosin
Terazosin

Organic Nitrates
Topical nitrates

Phosphodiesterase Type-5 Inhibitors
Sildenafil
Tadalafil

Classes of Drugs with Uncertain Efficacy
Selective serotonin reuptake inhibitors
Vasodilator prostaglandins
Thromboxane inhibitors
Angiotensin-converting enzyme inhibitors
Angiotensin receptor antagonists
Endothelin receptor antagonists

Sympathectomy
Stellate ganglionectomy
Lumbar sympathectomy
Digital sympathectomy

Botulinum Toxin Injection

Conservative Measures

Patients with primary Raynaud phenomenon often benefit from education and reassurance. An explanation describing the frequency of the disease in the general population, its precipitating factors, and its benign prognosis is reassuring and allays fears of amputation. Patients should avoid unnecessary cold exposure and should wear loose, warm clothing; electrically heated gloves and socks may be helpful. In addition to adequate hand and foot protection, the trunk and head should be kept warm to avoid reflex vasoconstriction. Moving to a warmer climate is rarely feasible; furthermore, vasospasm may be induced after a move by even small changes in environmental temperature. Patients should use a moisturizing cream on their digits to prevent drying and cracking. Cigarette smoking should be avoided, since nicotine causes cutaneous vasoconstriction. Behavioral therapy has been proposed as a means of ameliorating the symptoms of Raynaud phenomenon. Results have been conflicting; however, each study used a different biofeedback technique, making comparison between studies difficult.[101] In one controlled study that compared temperature biofeedback with nifedipine for treatment of primary Raynaud phenomenon, biofeedback was not better than control treatment, and inferior to the drug.[102] Thus, although behavioral therapy may be effective in some individuals, there are insufficient data to support its routine use for patients with Raynaud phenomenon. Other forms of complementary therapy including acupuncture, herbal agents, and laser therapy are not helpful.[103]

Pharmacological Intervention

The most commonly used and most effective drug class for treatment of Raynaud phenomenon is calcium channel blockers. Other agents that have been used include sympathetic nervous system inhibitors, serotonin antagonists and selective serotonin reuptake inhibitors (SSRIs), angiotensin-converting enzyme inhibitors (ACEIs), angiotensin II receptor blockers (ARBs), endothelin antagonists, and direct-acting smooth muscle relaxants such as nitrates, phosphodiesterase type 5 (PDE5) inhibitors, and vasodilator prostaglandins (PGs).[2]

Calcium Channel Blockers

Calcium entry blockers are the most effective drugs for treating Raynaud phenomenon. Most of the evidence accumulated to date involves nifedipine, which interferes with vascular smooth muscle contraction by antagonizing calcium influx. This drug decreases digital vascular resistance in patients with Raynaud phenomenon during environmental cold exposure and increases digital SBP and digital skin temperature during local cold exposure.[104,105] Recent Cochrane reviews have suggested that dihydropyridine calcium channel blockers decreased the frequency, severity, pain, and disability due to Raynaud phenomenon.[106,107] Patients with secondary Raynaud phenomenon may show improvement, although less so than those with primary Raynaud phenomenon.[106] Extended-action preparations should be used, starting with lower doses and increasing to higher doses if necessary.[2,106] Side effects include hypotension, lightheadedness, indigestion, and peripheral edema, which may result in discontinuation in up to 15% of patients.[106] Verapamil is not effective in patients with Raynaud phenomenon.[108]

Sympathetic Nervous System Inhibitors

The vasoconstrictor response to cold exposure or emotional stress is mediated via the sympathetic nervous system, and sympathetic nervous system inhibitors have been used to treat Raynaud phenomenon. Prazosin hydrochloride is an α_1-adrenoceptor blocker. Since postsynaptic α_1 adrenoceptors are found on digital vessels, clinical improvement following administration of this drug might be anticipated.

Several studies have shown reduction in the number and duration of attacks with prazosin in patients with both primary and secondary Raynaud phenomenon.[109] Tachyphylaxis may occur with prazosin, often necessitating dosage increments up to 10 mg three times daily. Side effects of prazosin include hypotension, particularly after the first few doses, leading to lightheadedness or syncope. In addition, patients may develop headache, drowsiness, or fatigue. Long-acting α_1-adrenoceptor blockers, such as doxazosin and terazosin, although less extensively studied than prazosin, seem to also be effective for Raynaud phenomenon.[110]

Selective Serotonin Reuptake Inhibitors

One small study found that fluoxetine, an SSRI, reduced the number and severity of vasospastic attacks in 53 patients with primary or secondary Raynaud phenomenon compared with nifedipine; more clinical trial data are needed.[47] Erythromelalgia has been reported as a complication of SSRI therapy for Raynaud phenomenon.[111]

Renin-Angiotensin System Inhibitors

Angiotensin II is unlikely to mediate digital vasospasm in most patients with Raynaud phenomenon.[112] If elevation of this hormone is due to other pathological conditions, it could conceivably contribute to digital vasospasm in patients already predisposed to Raynaud phenomenon. The results, however, have been mixed, with limited evidence to support the efficacy of angiotensin converting enzyme inhibitors.[113] The angiotensin receptor antagonist, losartan, has been reported to decrease the frequency and severity of vasospastic attacks in patients with both primary and secondary Raynaud phenomenon, with fewer side effects when compared to nifedipine.[114] More studies of this class of drug are necessary.

Endothelin Receptor Antagonists

ET-1, a strong vasoconstrictor, is implicated in the pathogenesis of secondary Raynaud phenomenon in patients with scleroderma, but not in primary Raynaud phenomenon.[2] Bosentan, an endothelin receptor antagonist, has been successfully used to treat refractory secondary Raynaud phenomenon and digital ulcers in several clinical trials of patients with scleroderma.[115,116] Other studies, however, have shown less promise. In a large multicenter double-blind, placebo-controlled trial of 24 weeks of therapy in 188 patients with systemic sclerosis, bosentan reduced occurrence of new digital ulcers but had no effect on ulcer healing; other secondary endpoints such as pain and disability were negative.[54] In a separate small placebo-controlled trial of patients with secondary Raynaud phenomenon, bosentan did not lessen frequency, duration, pain, or severity of attacks.[53] Studies with other preparations, including macitentan and ambrisentan, have been disappointing.[117,118]

Phosphodiesterase Type 5 Inhibitors

The PDE5 inhibitors prevent breakdown of cyclic guanosine monophosphate, causing relaxation of vascular smooth muscle cells and vasodilation. Accumulating evidence supports use of these agents in patients with Raynaud phenomenon.[119-123] A meta-analysis of randomized controlled trials with PDE5 inhibitors showed significant improvement in symptoms due to secondary Raynaud phenomenon and significant decrease in number and duration of attacks.[123]

Direct Vascular Smooth Muscle Relaxants

The problem with most vasodilators is that they cause a general reduction in vascular resistance and may actually divert blood flow from the affected digits. As a result, patients often experience adverse side effects, including hypotension, without deriving significant benefit for Raynaud phenomenon.

Organic nitrate preparations including nitropaste are often used in patients with Raynaud phenomenon. Topical glyceryl trinitrate may be considered for treatment of patients with Raynaud phenomenon, but is limited in utility because of headache.[124] A meta-analysis of 7 placebo-controlled trials of a heterogeneous group of topical nitrate preparation showed improvement of symptoms with nitrates, especially in individuals with secondary Raynaud phenomenon.[125]

Prostaglandins inhibit platelet aggregation and are vasodilators. Intravenous formulations have shown benefit, while results with oral preparations have been disappointing. Intravenous iloprost has been shown to reduce the frequency, duration, and severity of attacks and to promote wound healing in secondary Raynaud phenomenon.[126] When compared to nifedipine, patients derive similar benefits albeit with more side effects.[127] Although intravenous epoprostenol increases fingertip skin temperature and laser Doppler flow, these effects are sustained for less than 1 week.[128] Side effects of iloprost depend on dosage and include headaches, flushing, nausea, vomiting, and jaw pain. Oral prostacyclin preparations, unfortunately, have not proven of value in the treatment of Raynaud phenomenon.[129]

Statins

HMG-CoA reductase inhibitors ("statins") exhibit pleiotropic effects on endothelial function and therefore might be anticipated to retard the vascular pathology of Raynaud phenomenon. Multiple studies have shown benefits in patients with secondary Raynaud phenomenon due to scleroderma by decreasing severity of attacks and formation of new digital ulcers, as well as improving healing of ulcers.[130-133]

Sympathectomy

The success rate of sympathectomy for episodic digital vasospasm of the upper extremity is not as good as might be anticipated. Raynaud phenomenon recurs in the majority of patients.[2] Successful relief of digital ischemia can be achieved in both primary and secondary Raynaud phenomenon, although this effect may be short-lasting.[134,135]

Digital sympathectomy, also referred to as *adventitial stripping*, has been advocated by some surgeons for treatment of digital ischemia, particularly that of secondary severe Raynaud phenomenon.[136] This technique may improve digital blood flow and allow healing of digital ulcerations.

Botulinum Injection

Botulinum toxin type A is a neurotoxin that results in flaccid muscle paralysis. Injection of botulinum toxin into the perineurovascular tissue of the wrist or the distal palm, or along the digits, has been reported to relieve recalcitrant Raynaud phenomenon in several case series, but no controlled clinical trial has been reported.[137,138]

REFERENCES

1. Raynaud M. *L'Asphyxie Locale et de la Gangrene Semmetrique des Extremities*. London: New Sydenham Soc; 1862.
2. Wigley FM, Flavahan NA. Raynaud's phenomenon. *N Engl J Med*. 2016;375(6):556–565.
3. Allen E, Brown G. Raynaud's disease: a critical review of minimal requisites for diagnosis. *Am J Med Sci*. 1932;183.
4. Maverakis E, Patel F, Kronenberg DG, et al. International consensus criteria for the diagnosis of Raynaud's phenomenon. *J Autoimmun*. 2014;48–49:60–65.
5. Garner R, Kumari R, Lanyon P, et al. Prevalence, risk factors and associations of primary Raynaud's phenomenon: systematic review and meta-analysis of observational studies. *BMJ Open*. 2015;5(3):e006389.
6. Jones GT, Herrick AL, Woodham SE, et al. Occurrence of Raynaud's phenomenon in children ages 12-15 years: prevalence and association with other common symptoms. *Arthritis Rheum*. 2003;48(12):3518–3521.

7. Freedman RR, Mayes MD. Familial aggregation of primary Raynaud's disease. *Arthritis Rheum*. 1996;39(7):1189–1191.

8. Smyth A, Hughes A, Bruce I, Bell A. A case-control study of candidate vasoactive mediator genes in primary Raynaud's phenomenon. *Rheumatology*. 1999;38(11):1094–1098.

9. Cakir N, Pamuk ON, Dönmez S, et al. Prevalence of Raynaud's phenomenon in healthy Turkish medical students and hospital personnel. *Rheumatol Int*. 2008;29(2):185–188.

10. O'Keeffe ST, Tsapatsaris NP, Beetham WP. Increased prevalence of migraine and chest pain in patients with primary Raynaud disease. *Ann Intern Med*. 1992;116(12 Pt 1):985–989.

11. Miller D, Waters D, Warnica W, Al E. Is variant angina the coronary manifestation of a generalized vasospastic disorder? *N Engl J Med*. 1981;304:763–766.

12. Cannon P, Hassar M, Case D, Al E. The relationship of hypertension and renal failure in scleroderma (progressive systemic sclerosis) to structural and functional abnormalities of the renal cortical circulation. *Medicine (Baltimore)*. 1974;53:1–46.

13. Salmenson BD, Reisman J, Sinclair SH, Burge D. Macular capillary hemodynamic changes associated with Raynaud's phenomenon. *Ophthalmology*. 1992;99(6):914–919.

14. Vergnon JM, Barthélémy JC, Riffat J, et al. Raynaud's phenomenon of the lung. A reality both in primary and secondary Raynaud syndrome. *Chest*. 1992;101(5):1312–1317.

15. Silberstein SD, Holland S, Freitag F, et al. Evidence-based guideline update: pharmacologic treatment for episodic migraine prevention in adults: report of the Quality Standards Subcommittee of the American Academy of Neurology and the American Headache Society. *Neurology*. 2012;78(17):1337–1345.

16. Khouri C, Blaise S, Carpentier P, et al. Drug-induced Raynaud's phenomenon: beyond β-adrenoceptor blockers. *Br J Clin Pharmacol*. 2016;82(1):6–16.

17. Curry Jr RC, Pepine CJ, Sabom MB, et al. Effects of ergonovine in patients with and without coronary artery disease. *Circulation*. 1977;56(5):803–809.

18. Schroeder J, Bolen J, Quint R, Al E. Provocation of coronary spasm with ergonovine maleate. New test with results in 57 patients undergoing coronary arteriography. *Am J Cardiol*. 1977;40:487–491.

19. Krumholz HM, Goldberger AL. Systemic arterial vasospastic syndrome: familial occurrence with variant angina. *Am J Med*. 1992;92(3):334–335.

20. Gifford Jr R, Hines Jr E. Raynaud's disease among women and girls. *Circulation*. 1957;16:1012–1021.

21. Pavlov-Dolijanovic SR, Damjanov NS, Vujasinovic Stupar NZ, et al. The value of pattern capillary changes and antibodies to predict the development of systemic sclerosis in patients with primary Raynaud's phenomenon. *Rheumatol Int*. 2013;33(12):2967–2973.

22. Koenig M, Joyal F, Fritzler MJ, et al. Autoantibodies and microvascular damage are independent predictive factors for the progression of Raynaud's phenomenon to systemic sclerosis: a twenty-year prospective study of 586 patients, with validation of proposed criteria for early systemic sclerosis. *Arthritis Rheum*. 2008;58(12):3902–3912.

23. Honda M, Suzuki M, Nakayama K, Ishikawa T. Role of alpha2C-adrenoceptors in the reduction of skin blood flow induced by local cooling in mice. *Br J Pharmacol*. 2007;152(1):91–100.

24. Lewis T. Experiments relating to the peripheral mechanism involved in spasmodic arrest of the circulation in the fingers, a variety of Raynaud's disease. *Heart*. 1929;15:7–101.

25. Freedman RR, Mayes MD, Sabharwal SC. Induction of vasospastic attacks despite digital nerve block in Raynaud's disease and phenomenon. *Circulation*. 1989;80(4):859–862.

26. Jamieson G, Ludbrook J, Wilson A. Cold hypersensitivity in Raynaud's phenomenon. *Circulation*. 1971;44:254–264.

27. Coffman J, Cohen A. Total and capillary fingertip blood flow in Raynaud's phenomenon. *N Engl J Med*. 1971;285:259–263.

28. Vanhoutte PM, Cooke JP, Lindblad LE, et al. Modulation of postjunctional alpha-adrenergic responsiveness by local changes in temperature. *Clin Sci (Lond)*. 1985;68(Suppl 1):121s–123s.

29. Cooke JP, Shepherd JT, Vanhoutte PM. The effect of warming on adrenergic neurotransmission in canine cutaneous vein. *Circ Res*. 1984;54(5):547–553.

30. Flavahan NA, Cooke JP, Shepherd JT, Vanhoutte PM. Human postjunctional alpha-1 and alpha-2 adrenoceptors: differential distribution in arteries of the limbs. *J Pharmacol Exp Ther*. 1987;241(2):361–365.

31. Chotani MA, Mitra S, Su BY, et al. Regulation of alpha(2)-adrenoceptors in human vascular smooth muscle cells. *Am J Physiol Heart Circ Physiol*. 2004;286(1):H59–H67.

32. Jeyaraj SC, Chotani MA, Mitra S, et al. Cooling evokes redistribution of alpha2C-adrenoceptors from Golgi to plasma membrane in transfected human embryonic kidney 293 cells. *Mol Pharmacol*. 2001;60(6):1195–1200.

33. Keenan EJ, Porter JM. Alpha-adrenergic receptors in platelets from patients with Raynaud's syndrome. *Surgery*. 1983;94(2):204–209.

34. Coffman JD, Cohen RA. Role of alpha-adrenoceptor subtypes mediating sympathetic vasoconstriction in human digits. *Eur J Clin Invest*. 1988;18(3):309–313.

35. Coffman J, Cohen R. A alpha2-adrenergic and 5-HT2 receptor hypersensitivity in Raynaud's phenomenon. *J Vasc Med Biol*. 1990;2:100–106.

36. Freedman RR, Sabharal SC, Desai N, et al. Increased alpha-adrenergic responsiveness in idiopathic Raynaud's disease. *Arthritis Rheum*. 1989;32(1):61–65.

37. Freedman RR, Moten M, Migály P, Mayes M. Cold-induced potentiation of alpha 2-adrenergic vasoconstriction in primary Raynaud's disease. *Arthritis Rheum*. 1993;36(5):685–690.

38. Freedman RR, Baer RP, Mayes MD. Blockade of vasospastic attacks by alpha 2-adrenergic but not alpha 1-adrenergic antagonists in idiopathic Raynaud's disease. *Circulation*. 1995;92(6):1448–1451.

39. Cooke JP, Creager SJ, Scales KM, et al. Role of digital artery adrenoceptors in Raynaud's disease. *Vasc Med*. 1997;2(1):1–7.

40. Flavahan NA, Flavahan S, Liu Q, et al. Increased alpha2-adrenergic constriction of isolated arterioles in diffuse scleroderma. *Arthritis Rheum*. 2000;43(8):1886–1890.

41. Peacock J. Peripheral venous blood concentrations of epinephrine and norepinephrine in primary Raynaud's disease. *Circ Res*. 1959;7:821–827.

42. Kontos H, Wasserman A. Effect of reserpine in Raynaud's phenomenon. *Circulation*. 1969;39:259–266.

43. Downey JA, LeRoy EC, Miller JM, Darling RC. Thermoregulation and Raynaud's phenomenon. *Clin Sci*. 1971;40(3):211–219.

44. Fagius J, Blumberg H. Sympathetic outflow to the hand in patients with Raynaud's phenomenon. *Cardiovasc Res*. 1985;19(5):249–253.

45. Mohokum M, Hartmann P, Schlattmann P. The association of Raynaud syndrome with β-blockers: a meta-analysis. *Angiology*. 2012;63(7):535–540.

46. Cohen RA, Coffman JD. Beta-adrenergic vasodilator mechanism in the finger. *Circ Res*. 1981;49(5):1196–1201.

47. Coleiro B, Marshall SE, Denton CP, et al. Treatment of Raynaud's phenomenon with the selective serotonin reuptake inhibitor fluoxetine. *Rheumatology (Oxford)*. 2001;40(9):1038–1043.

48. Coffman JD, Rasmussen HM. Effect of thromboxane synthetase inhibition in Raynaud's phenomenon. *Clin Pharmacol Ther*. 1984;36(3):369–373.

49. Polidoro L, Barnabei R, Giorgini P, et al. Platelet activation in patients with the Raynaud phenomenon. *Intern Med J*. 2012;42(5):531–535.

50. Coppo M, Boddi M, Poggesi L, et al. Exaggerated local hand sympathetic but not renin-angiotensin system activation in patients with primary Raynaud's phenomenon. *Microvasc Res*. 2006;71(2):128–134.

51. Smyth AE, Bell AL, Bruce IN, et al. Digital vascular responses and serum endothelin-1 concentrations in primary and secondary Raynaud's phenomenon. *Ann Rheum Dis*. 2000;59(11):870–874.

52. Rychlik-Golema W, Mastej K, Adamiec R. The role of endothelin-1 and selected cytokines in the pathogenesis of Raynaud's phenomenon associated with systemic connective tissue diseases. *Int Angiol*. 2006;25(2):221–227.

53. Nguyen VA, Eisendle K, Gruber I, et al. Effect of the dual endothelin receptor antagonist bosentan on Raynaud's phenomenon secondary to systemic sclerosis: a double-blind prospective, randomized, placebo-controlled pilot study. *Rheumatology (Oxford)*. 2010;49(3):583–587.

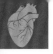

54. Matucci-Cerinic M, Denton CP, Furst DE, et al. Bosentan treatment of digital ulcers related to systemic sclerosis: results from the RAPIDS-2 randomised, double-blind, placebo-controlled trial. *Ann Rheum Dis*. 2011;70(1):32–38.

55. Cutolo M, Ruaro B, Pizzorni C, et al. Longterm treatment with endothelin receptor antagonist bosentan and iloprost improves fingertip blood perfusion in systemic sclerosis. *J Rheumatol*. 2014;41(5):881–886.

56. Landis E. Micro-injection studies of capillary blood pressure in Raynaud's disease. *Heart*. 1930;15:247.

57. Thulesius O. Methods for the evaluation of peripheral vascular function in the upper extremities. *Acta Chir Scand Suppl*. 1976;465:53–54.

58. Cohen R, Coffman J. Reduced fingertip arterial pressure in Raynaud's disease. *J Vasc Med Biol*. 1989;1:21.

59. Hillestad LK. The peripheral circulation during exposure to cold in normals and in patients with the syndrome of high-titre cold haemagglutination. I. The vascular response to cold exposure in normal subjects. *Acta Med Scand*. 1959;164:203–229.

60. Jahnsen T, Nielsen SL, Skovborg F. Blood viscosity and local response to cold in primary Raynaud's phenomenon. *Lancet*. 1977;2(8046):1001–1002.

61. Lacombe C, Mouthon JM, Bucherer C, et al. Raynaud's phenomenon and blood viscosity. *J Mal Vasc*. 1992;17(Suppl B):132–135.

62. Flavahan NA. A vascular mechanistic approach to understanding Raynaud phenomenon. *Nat Rev Rheumatol*. 2015;11(3):146–158.

63. Hughes M, Snapir A, Wilkinson J, et al. Prediction and impact of attacks of Raynaud's phenomenon, as judged by patient perception. *Rheumatology (Oxford)*. 2015;54(8):1443–1447.

64. Maricq HR, LeRoy EC, D'Angelo WA, et al. Diagnostic potential of in vivo capillary microscopy in scleroderma and related disorders. *Arthritis Rheum*. 1980;23(2):183–189.

65. Petri M, Orbai A-M, Alarcón GS, et al. Derivation and validation of the Systemic Lupus International Collaborating Clinics classification criteria for systemic lupus erythematosus. *Arthritis Rheum*. 2012;64(8):2677–2686.

66. Hochberg MC. Updating the American College of Rheumatology revised criteria for the classification of systemic lupus erythematosus. *Arthritis Rheum*. 1997;40(9):1725.

67. Pope JE, Al-Bishri J, Al-Azem H, Ouimet JM. The temporal relationship of Raynaud's phenomenon and features of connective tissue disease in rheumatoid arthritis. *J Rheumatol*. 2008;35(12):2329–2333.

68. Aletaha D, Neogi T, Silman AJ, et al. 2010 Rheumatoid arthritis classification criteria: an American College of Rheumatology/European League Against Rheumatism collaborative initiative. *Arthritis Rheum*. 2010;62(9):2569–2581.

69. García-Carrasco M, Sisó A, Ramos-Casals M, et al. Raynaud's phenomenon in primary Sjögren's syndrome. Prevalence and clinical characteristics in a series of 320 patients. *J Rheumatol*. 2002;29(4):726–730.

70. Nakamura H, Kawakami A, Hayashi T, et al. Anti-centromere antibody-seropositive Sjögren's syndrome differs from conventional subgroup in clinical and pathological study. *BMC Musculoskelet Disord*. 2010;11:140.

71. Shiboski CH, Shiboski SC, Seror R, et al. 2016 American College of Rheumatology/European League Against Rheumatism classification criteria for primary Sjögren's syndrome: a consensus and data-driven methodology involving three international patient cohorts. *Ann Rheum Dis*. 2017;76(1):9–16.

72. Sen S, Sinhamahapatra P, Choudhury S, et al. Cutaneous manifestations of mixed connective tissue disease: study from a tertiary care hospital in eastern India. *Indian J Dermatol*. 2014;59(1):35–40.

73. Hoffman RW, Maldonado ME. Immune pathogenesis of mixed connective tissue disease: a short analytical review. *Clin Immunol*. 2008;128(1):8–17.

74. Hartmann P, Mohokum M, Schlattmann P. The association of Raynaud's syndrome with carpal tunnel syndrome: a meta-analysis. *Rheumatol Int*. 2012;32(3):569–574.

75. Roh YH, Noh JH, Gong HS, Baek GH. Comparative study on the effectiveness of a corticosteroid injection for carpal tunnel syndrome in patients with and without Raynaud's phenomenon. *Bone Joint J*. 2017;99-B(12):1637–1642.

76. Swiecicki P, Hegerova T, Gertz M. Cold agglutinin disease. *Blood*. 2013;122:1114–1121.

77. Trejo O, Ramos-Casals M, García-Carrasco M, et al. Cryoglobulinemia: study of etiologic factors and clinical and immunologic features in 443 patients from a single center. *Medicine*. 2001;80(4):252–262.

78. Soyfoo MS, Goubella A, Cogan E, et al. Clinical significance of Cryofibrinogenemia: possible pathophysiological link with Raynaud's phenomenon. *J Rheumatol*. 2012;39(1):119–124.

79. Letz R, Cherniack MG, Gerr F, et al. A cross sectional epidemiological survey of shipyard workers exposed to hand-arm vibration. *Br J Ind Med*. 1992;49(1):53–62.

80. Mirbod SM, Yoshida H, Nagata C, et al. Hand-arm vibration syndrome and its prevalence in the present status of private forestry enterprises in Japan. *Int Arch Occup Environ Health*. 1992;64(2):93–99.

81. Nilsson T, Wahlström J, Burström L. Hand-arm vibration and the risk of vascular and neurological diseases—a systematic review and meta-analysis. *PLoS One*. 2017;12(7):e0180795.

82. Su AT, Darus A, Bulgiba A, et al. The clinical features of hand-arm vibration syndrome in a warm environment—a review of the literature. *J Occup Health*. 2012;54(5):349–360.

83. Inaba R, Furuno T, Okada A. Effects of low- and high-frequency local vibration on the occurrence of intimal thickening of the peripheral arteries of rats. *Scand J Work Environ Health*. 1988;14(5):312–316.

84. Okada A, Inaba R, Furuno T. Occurrence of intimal thickening of the peripheral arteries in response to local vibration. *Br J Ind Med*. 1987;44(7):470–475.

85. Sakakibara H, Yamada S. Vibration syndrome and autonomic nervous system. *Cent Eur J Public Health*. 1995;3(Suppl):11–14.

86. Murata K, Araki S, Okajima F, et al. Effects of occupational use of vibrating tools in the autonomic, central and peripheral nervous system. *Int Arch Occup Environ Health*. 1997;70(2):94–100.

87. Hisanaga H. Studies of peripheral nerve conduction velocities in vibrating tool operators. *Sangyo Igaku*. 1982;24(3):284–293.

88. Glendenning JL, Barbachano Y, Norman AR, et al. Long-term neurologic and peripheral vascular toxicity after chemotherapy treatment of testicular cancer. *Cancer*. 2010;116(10):2322–2331.

89. Kuhar CG, Mesti T, Zakotnik B. Digital ischemic events related to gemcitabine: report of two cases and a systematic review. *Radiol Oncol*. 2010;44(4):257–261.

90. Fontana L, Marion M-J, Ughetto S, Catilina P. Glutathione S-transferase M1 and GST T1 genetic polymorphisms and Raynaud's phenomenon in French vinyl chloride monomer-exposed workers. *J Hum Genet*. 2006;51(10):879–886.

91. Coffman JD, Rasmussen HM. Effects of beta-adrenoreceptor-blocking drugs in patients with Raynaud's phenomenon. *Circulation*. 1985;72(3):466–470.

92. Franssen C, Wollersheim H, de Haan A, Thien T. The influence of different beta-blocking drugs on the peripheral circulation in Raynaud's phenomenon and in hypertension. *J Clin Pharmacol*. 1992;32(7):652–659.

93. Khouri C, Jouve T, Blaise S, et al. Peripheral vasoconstriction induced by β-adrenoceptor blockers: a systematic review and a network meta-analysis. *Br J Clin Pharmacol*. 2016;82(2):549–560.

94. Nielsen SL, Parving HH, Hansen JE. Myxoedema and Raynaud's phenomenon. *Acta Endocrinol (Copenh)*. 1982;101(1):32–34.

95. Nielsen SL, Løkkegaard H. Cold hypersensitivity and finger systolic blood pressure in hemodialysis patients. *Scand J Urol Nephrol*. 1981;15(3):319–322.

96. Preston IR, Hill NS. Evaluation and management of pulmonary hypertension in systemic sclerosis. *Curr Opin Rheumatol*. 2003;15(6):761–765.

97. Rich S, Dantzker DR, Ayres SM, et al. Primary pulmonary hypertension. A national prospective study. *Ann Intern Med*. 1987;107(2):216–223.

98. Madabhavi I, Revannasiddaiah S, Rastogi M, Gupta MK. Paraneoplastic Raynaud's phenomenon manifesting before the diagnosis of lung cancer. *BMJ Case Rep*. 2012;2012:PMC3391388.

99. Schildmann EK, Davies AN. Paraneoplastic Raynaud's phenomenon—good palliation after a multidisciplinary approach. *J Pain Symptom Manage*. 2010;39(4):779–783.

100. Lambova S, Müller-Ladner U. Capillaroscopic pattern in paraneoplastic Raynaud's phenomenon. *Rheumatol Int*. 2013;33(6):1597–1599.

101. Karavidas MK, Tsai P-S, Yucha C, et al. Thermal biofeedback for primary Raynaud's phenomenon: a review of the literature. *Appl Psychophysiol Biofeedback*. 2006;31(3):203–216.

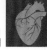

102. Comparison of sustained-release nifedipine and temperature biofeedback for treatment of primary Raynaud phenomenon. Results from a randomized clinical trial with 1-year follow-up. *Arch Intern Med.* 2000;160(8):1101–1108.

103. Malenfant D, Catton M, Pope JE. The efficacy of complementary and alternative medicine in the treatment of Raynaud's phenomenon: a literature review and meta-analysis. *Rheumatology (Oxford).* 2009;48(7):791–795.

104. Creager MA, Pariser KM, Winston EM, et al. Nifedipine-induced fingertip vasodilation in patients with Raynaud's phenomenon. *Am Heart J.* 1984;108(2):370–373.

105. Nilsson H, Jonason T, Leppert J, Ringqvist I. The effect of the calcium-entry blocker nifedipine on cold-induced digital vasospasm. A double-blind crossover study versus placebo. *Acta Med Scand.* 1987;221(1):53–60.

106. Rirash F, Tingey PC, Harding SE, et al. Calcium channel blockers for primary and secondary Raynaud's phenomenon. *Cochrane Database Syst Rev.* 2017;12:CD000467.

107. Ennis H, Hughes M, Anderson ME, et al. Calcium channel blockers for primary Raynaud's phenomenon. *Cochrane Database Syst Rev.* 2016;2:CD002069.

108. Kinney EL, Nicholas GG, Gallo J, et al. The treatment of severe Raynaud's phenomenon with verapamil. *J Clin Pharmacol.* 1982;22(1):74–76.

109. Pope J, Fenlon D, Thompson A, et al. Prazosin for Raynaud's phenomenon in progressive systemic sclerosis. *Cochrane Database Syst Rev.* 2000;2:CD000956.

110. Landry GJ. Current medical and surgical management of Raynaud's syndrome. *J Vasc Surg.* 2013;57(6):1710–1716.

111. Rey J, Cretel E, Jean R, et al. Serotonin reuptake inhibitors, Raynaud's phenomenon and erythromelalgia. *Rheumatology (Oxford).* 2003;42(4):601–602.

112. Challenor VF. Angiotensin converting enzyme inhibitors in Raynaud's phenomenon. *Drugs.* 1994;48(6):864–867.

113. Stewart M, Morling JR. Oral vasodilators for primary Raynaud's phenomenon. *Cochrane Database Syst Rev.* 2012;7:CD006687.

114. Dziadzio M, Denton CP, Smith R, et al. Losartan therapy for Raynaud's phenomenon and scleroderma: clinical and biochemical findings in a fifteen-week, randomized, parallel-group, controlled trial. *Arthritis Rheum.* 1999;42(12):2646–2655.

115. Tsifetaki N, Botzoris V, Alamanos Y, et al. Bosentan for digital ulcers in patients with systemic sclerosis: a prospective 3-year followup study. *J Rheumatol.* 2009;36(7):1550–1552.

116. Parisi S, Bruzzone M, Centanaro Di Vittorio C, et al. Efficacy of bosentan in the treatment of Raynaud's phenomenon in patients with systemic sclerosis never treated with prostanoids. *Reumatismo.* 2014;65(6):286–291.

117. Khanna D, Denton CP, Merkel PA, et al. Effect of macitentan on the development of new ischemic digital ulcers in patients with systemic sclerosis: DUAL-1 and DUAL-2 randomized clinical trials. *JAMA.* 2016;315(18):1975–1988.

118. Bose N, Bena J, Chatterjee S. Evaluation of the effect of ambrisentan on digital microvascular flow in patients with systemic sclerosis using laser Doppler perfusion imaging: a 12-week randomized double-blind placebo controlled trial. *Arthritis Res Ther.* 2015;17:44.

119. Fries R, Shariat K, von Wilmowsky H, Böhm M. Sildenafil in the treatment of Raynaud's phenomenon resistant to vasodilatory therapy. *Circulation.* 2005;112(19):2980–2985.

120. Shenoy PD, Kumar S, Jha LK, et al. Efficacy of tadalafil in secondary Raynaud's phenomenon resistant to vasodilator therapy: a double-blind randomized cross-over trial. *Rheumatology (Oxford).* 2010;49(12):2420–2428.

121. Herrick AL, van den Hoogen F, Gabrielli A, et al. Modified-release sildenafil reduces Raynaud's phenomenon attack frequency in limited cutaneous systemic sclerosis. *Arthritis Rheum.* 2011;63(3):775–782.

122. Andrigueti FV, Ebbing PCC, Arismendi MI, Kayser C. Evaluation of the effect of sildenafil on the microvascular blood flow in patients with systemic sclerosis: a randomised, double-blind, placebo-controlled study. *Clin Exp Rheumatol.* 2017;35(4, Suppl 106):151–158.

123. Roustit M, Blaise S, Allanore Y, et al. Phosphodiesterase-5 inhibitors for the treatment of secondary Raynaud's phenomenon: systematic review and meta-analysis of randomised trials. *Ann Rheum Dis.* 2013;72(10):1696–1699.

124. Teh LS, Manning J, Moore T, et al. Sustained-release transdermal glyceryl trinitrate patches as a treatment for primary and secondary Raynaud's phenomenon. *Br J Rheumatol.* 1995;34(7):636–641.

125. Curtiss P, Schwager Z, Cobos G, et al. A systematic review and meta-analysis of the effects of topical nitrates in the treatment of primary and secondary Raynaud's phenomenon. *J Am Acad Dermatol.* 2018;78(6):1110–1118. e3.

126. Pope J, Fenlon D, Thompson A, et al. Iloprost and cisaprost for Raynaud's phenomenon in progressive systemic sclerosis. *Cochrane Database Syst Rev.* 2000;2:CD000953.

127. Scorza R, Caronni M, Mascagni B, et al. Effects of long-term cyclic iloprost therapy in systemic sclerosis with Raynaud's phenomenon. A randomized, controlled study. *Clin Exp Rheumatol.* 2001;19(5):503–508.

128. Kingma K, Wollersheim H, Thien T. Double-blind, placebo-controlled study of intravenous prostacyclin on hemodynamics in severe Raynaud's phenomenon: the acute vasodilatory effect is not sustained. *J Cardiovasc Pharmacol.* 1995;26(3):388–393.

129. Wigley FM, Korn JH, Csuka ME, et al. Oral iloprost treatment in patients with Raynaud's phenomenon secondary to systemic sclerosis: a multicenter, placebo-controlled, double-blind study. *Arthritis Rheum.* 1998;41(4):670–677.

130. Furukawa S, Yasuda S, Amengual O, et al. Protective effect of pravastatin on vascular endothelium in patients with systemic sclerosis: a pilot study. *Ann Rheum Dis.* 2006;65(8):1118–1120.

131. Kuwana M, Kaburaki J, Okazaki Y, et al. Increase in circulating endothelial precursors by atorvastatin in patients with systemic sclerosis. *Arthritis Rheum.* 2006;54(6):1946–1951.

132. Abou-Raya A, Abou-Raya S, Helmii M. Statins: potentially useful in therapy of systemic sclerosis-related Raynaud's phenomenon and digital ulcers. *J Rheumatol.* 2008;35(9):1801–1808.

133. Ladak K, Pope JE. A review of the effects of statins in systemic sclerosis. *Semin Arthritis Rheum.* 2016;45(6):698–705.

134. Hashmonai M, Cameron AEP, Licht PB, et al. Thoracic sympathectomy: a review of current indications. *Surg Endosc.* 2016;30(4):1255–1269.

135. Coveliers HME, Hoexum F, Nederhoed JH, et al. Thoracic sympathectomy for digital ischemia: a summary of evidence. *J Vasc Surg.* 2011;54(1):273–277.

136. Balogh B, Mayer W, Vesely M, et al. Adventitial stripping of the radial and ulnar arteries in Raynaud's disease. *J Hand Surg Am.* 2002;27(6):1073–1080.

137. Mannava S, Plate JF, Stone AV, et al. Recent advances for the management of Raynaud phenomenon using botulinum neurotoxin A. *J Hand Surg Am.* 2011;36(10):1708–1710.

138. Neumeister MW. Botulinum toxin type A in the treatment of Raynaud's phenomenon. *J Hand Surg Am.* 2010;35(12):2085–2092.

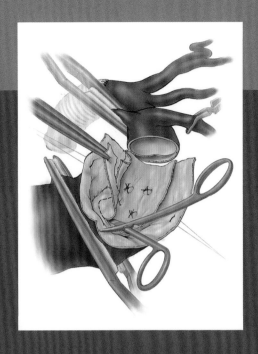

中文导读

第47章
肢端发绀

本章主要介绍肢端发绀的流行病学、病因、病理生理学、临床表现、诊断及其治疗。肢端发绀是一种罕见的功能性血管痉挛性疾病，好发于女性，常见发病年龄为 20~30 岁，其特征是持续的淡蓝色变色，变色呈对称分布，通常无疼痛或组织损伤，可有轻微的手指肿胀及局部多汗，主要发生于四肢，寒冷暴露或情绪压力可能会加剧肢端发绀。肢端发绀分为原发性肢端发绀和继发性肢端发绀，原发性肢端发绀病因不明，通常预后良好，极少使用药物治疗；继发性肢端发绀潜在病因通常为结缔组织病或其他系统性疾病，预后较差，取决于其相关疾病的严重程度。此外，肢端发绀还须与其他肢端综合征和血管活性相关疾病区分开来，如冻疮、肢端萎缩、红斑性肢痛症、雷诺现象和网状青斑等。

李　鑫

Acrocyanosis

Robert T. Eberhardt

The term *acrocyanosis* is derived from the Greek words *akron* (meaning "extremity") and *kyanos* (meaning "blue"). As a medical condition, acrocyanosis is an uncommon functional vasospastic disorder characterized by persistent bluish discoloration, primarily of the hands and feet. However, the term acrocyanosis is often used to describe diverse conditions and lacks a uniform definition. The original description of acrocyanosis is credited to Crocq in 1896, thus the eponym *Crocq disease*.[1] Classically, acrocyanosis affects young females with asthenic habitus residing in regions with cooler climates. In contrast to Raynaud syndrome, the bluish discoloration of acrocyanosis is relatively persistent rather than episodic and is not associated with discomfort or triphasic color changes.[1] Similar to Raynaud syndrome, acrocyanosis may be exacerbated by cold exposure or emotional stress. *Primary acrocyanosis* is not associated with an identifiable cause (i.e., idiopathic) and is usually a benign disorder with a good prognosis; skin ulceration and tissue loss are extremely rare. Primary acrocyanosis typically responds well to behavioral measures, such as avoidance of exposure to cold, and pharmacological therapy is rarely necessary. *Secondary acrocyanosis* occurs in association with another underlying disorder, such as a connective tissue disease or other systemic disorder. Treatment and prognosis of secondary acrocyanosis depends on the underlying condition.[1] It often conveys a worse prognosis than primary disease, that is based upon the specific associated disorder and its severity. Acrocyanosis must be differentiated from other so-called acrosyndromes and vasoactive related disorders, such as pernio, acrorygosis, erythromelalgia, Raynaud syndrome, and livedo reticularis. In addition, an acrocyanotic appearance may be seen in conjunction with any disease that causes central cyanosis or markedly decreases blood flow to the distal extremity.

EPIDEMIOLOGY

There is limited information available on many of the epidemiological aspects of primary acrocyanosis, including its precise incidence and prevalence. Specific factors that contribute to its development remain incompletely defined. Acrocyanosis is associated more frequently with a low body mass index, outdoor occupations, and areas with cooler climates.[2] Despite early reports suggesting similar gender predilection, most studies suggest that primary acrocyanosis affects women more frequently than men, with a female-to-male ratio of up to 6 to 8:1.[1] It occurs more commonly in younger adults, typically in the second and third decades of life.[1] In addition, occurrence of acrocyanosis seems to decrease with increasing age, with few cases seen in women after menopause, suggesting hormonal influences.[3] It has been suggested that as many as 10% of patients have a family history of acrocyanosis in one of the first-degree relatives, suggesting a genetic basis.[2]

The epidemiology of secondary acrocyanosis is related to the underlying disorder. It is seen frequently in patients with anorexia nervosa, affecting up to 20% of women with this disorder.[4]

ETIOLOGY

Primary acrocyanosis is not associated with an identifiable cause. Secondary acrocyanosis occurs in association with connective tissue disorders, some hematological conditions, anorexia nervosa, neurovascular disorders, drugs, toxins, infections, heritable metabolic diseases, and certain malignancies (Box 47.1).[5] An acrocyanotic appearance also occurs in conjunction with any disease that causes central cyanosis or markedly decreases blood flow to the extremities.

PATHOPHYSIOLOGY

Acrocyanosis may be caused by different pathophysiologic mechanisms that lead to similar clinical manifestations. Several mechanisms for primary acrocyanosis have been proposed, but the precise mechanism remains elusive. Potential pathophysiological disturbances include abnormal arteriolar tone, alteration of microvascular responsiveness with capillary and venular dilation, arteriovenous subpapillary plexus shunting, and abnormal autonomic nervous system activity (Box 47.2).

The essential abnormality in primary acrocyanosis seems to be peripheral cutaneous vasoconstriction due to increased tone of the arterioles, associated with secondary vasodilation of capillaries and subpapillary venous plexi.[1] Arteriolar vasoconstriction produces the cyanotic discoloration, and compensatory venular dilation in the postcapillary sphincter. Persistent vasoconstriction at the precapillary sphincter creates a local hypoxic environment that may cause increased release of vasodilatory mediators, such as adenosine, in the capillary beds.[6] This in turn leads to dilation of postcapillary venules and possible arteriovenous subpapillary plexus shunting. The difference in the vessel tone may create a countercurrent exchange system in an attempt to retain heat, and this leads to local sweating. Potential mediators that may contribute to the pathogenesis of acrocyanosis include serotonin, adrenaline, noradrenaline, and endothelin (ET)-1. Levels of these mediators have been shown to be increased in acrocyanosis.[1,3]

The exact cause of the disordered arteriolar tone in acrocyanosis is unknown. Most evidence points to local sensitivity of the arterioles to cold and an exaggerated local sympathetic nerve response. Earlier studies had suggested a key role of exaggerated digital arteriolar vasoconstrictive response to cold stimuli,[7] whereas subsequent studies have also implicated excessive local sympathetic nervous system

BOX 47.1   Causes of Acrocyanosis

Primary or Idiopathic Acrocyanosis

Secondary Acrocyanosis
Connective Tissue Disorders
Scleroderma
Systemic lupus erythematosus (SLE)
Rheumatoid arthritis
Mixed connective tissue disease
Antiphospholipid antibody syndrome

Hematological Disorders
Cryoglobulins
Cold agglutinins
Lymphoproliferative disorders

Infections
Mycoplasma pneumonia
Mononucleosis
Hepatitis C

Medications and Toxins
Tricyclic antidepressants, interferon alpha (IFN-α), amphotericin B deoxycholate
Blasticidin S
Arsenic, butyl nitrate

Anorexia Nervosa

Heritable Disorders
Ethylmalonic aciduria
Mitochondrial disease
Fucosidosis
Fabry disease

Neurovascular Disorders
Spinal cord injury
Complex regional pain syndrome
Postural orthostatic tachycardia syndrome

Malignancy
Lymphoma

Cardiopulmonary Disease
Pulmonary hypertension (PH)
Cyanotic heart disease
Respiratory failure

Arterial Occlusive Disease
Atheromatous embolism
Disseminated intravascular coagulation (DIC)
Heparin-induced thrombocytopenia (HIT)
Septic embolism

BOX 47.2   Proposed Pathophysiological Mechanisms of Primary Acrocyanosis

Abnormal arteriolar tone
Alteration in microvascular reactivity
Abnormal autonomic nervous system balance
- Local or systemic sympathetic nervous system overactivity
- Diminished parasympathetic activity
Increased blood viscosity
Persistently elevated vasoconstrictive mediators

CLINICAL PRESENTATION

Primary acrocyanosis has typically been described in thin young women who are not physically active. The principal manifestation is persistent bluish discoloration of the hands and feet. The distribution of the discoloration is symmetrical.[1] It may also involve forearms, ears, lips, nose, or nipples, but less often. It is the discoloration that often is of concern and prompts patients to seek medical care. In addition, patients may also describe a sensation of coolness of the affected areas, but typically will not have pain or tissue injury. There may be mild swelling of the digits and local hyperhidrosis. Although the discoloration is persistent, emotional stress and cold exposure can intensify the acrocyanotic appearance, and warmth can diminish it. The discoloration and coolness are worse in cold weather, but typically persist even during the warmer weather of the summer months.

Examination reveals symmetric bluish discoloration of the hands and feet, which are cool and yet still often moist (Fig. 47.1). The color has also been described as bluish-pink or orange-like tinged with red, and differing hues may be seen at various times. A brownish-yellow color on the dorsum of hands and feet has been described and attributed to exposure to the warmth of the sun because it is most obvious in summer. Pressure on the discolored skin causes pallor, and color returns slowly from the periphery in an irregular manner. Fingers may appear puffy with shiny skin due to local edema, but trophic skin changes or ulceration do not typically occur with primary disease. However, trophic skin findings may be seen in a variant known as remitting necrotizing acrocyanosis.

In patients with primary disease, there are few other abnormal physical findings. Arterial pulses are normal, suggesting there is no

activity.[1] Other observations have suggested a key role of the central autonomic nervous system including increased sympathetic and decreased parasympathetic activity.[8] Other mechanisms hypothesized include increased blood viscosity, decreased distal blood flow at low temperatures, and persistently elevated levels of vasoconstrictive mediators such as ET-1, but convincing supporting evidence for these is not readily available.[1]

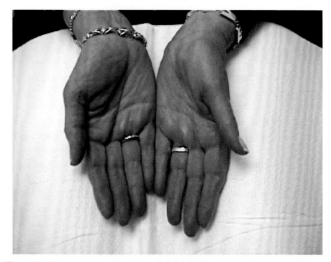

Fig. 47.1 Primary acrocyanosis involving the hands.

large-vessel arterial obstruction. Elevation of a cyanotic limb above heart level produces pallor, suggesting venous obstruction is not present. Patients with secondary acrocyanosis often have clinical features of the underlying condition, and these occasionally are the presenting manifestation. Episodes of digital pallor or rubor do not occur, although patients may have both acrocyanosis and Raynaud phenomenon. This is especially true in patients with scleroderma or systemic lupus erythematosus as an underlying cause.

DIAGNOSIS

Primary acrocyanosis is diagnosed clinically based on a careful history and physical examination. Laboratory or imaging studies typically are not necessary.[9] Cyanosis is symmetrical in distribution and should be present at the time of examination, owing to its persistent nature. In addition, there is usually no localized pain, trophic skin changes, or ulcerations. Peripheral pulse examination is normal, excluding significant peripheral artery occlusive disease. Pulse oximetry reveals normal oxygen saturation.

Secondary acrocyanosis is suggested by asymmetrical distribution of the discoloration, presence of pain, or trophic skin changes of the fingers or toes. Hypoxemia or absent pulses suggest central cyanosis or arterial obstructive disease, respectively. Selected laboratory tests are necessary to confirm the diagnosis of secondary acrocyanosis. Arterial blood gas assessment is appropriate to evaluate for hypoxemia. Antinuclear antibodies may suggest an underlying connective tissue disorder. If the history and physical examination are suggestive, directed testing for cryoglobulins, antiphospholipid antibodies, cold agglutinins, or antibodies to Epstein-Barr virus should be performed.

Capillaroscopy may be performed at the nail folds or mucous membrane to assess capillary morphology, distribution, and blood flow in acrocyanosis.[1] Nailfold capillaroscopy is often abnormal but nonspecific. Features on capillaroscopy include abnormal capillary morphology, pericapillary edema, and even hemorrhage. Such findings on capillaroscopy are not diagnostic and may be associated with secondary disease. Mean capillary density is decreased in patients with acrocyanosis compared with normal subjects, but not to the extent seen in patients with Raynaud phenomenon due to scleroderma.[10] Other capillary abnormalities include tortuous and dilated capillary loops. The presence of megacapillaries and areas of sparse or absent capillaries suggest underlying scleroderma or mixed connective tissue, whereas bushy capillaries may suggest systemic lupus erythematosus. Additional test findings such as decreased oscillations over the radial artery and decreased digital vessel sounds when assessed by Doppler have been described in acrocyanosis but are nonspecific.[11]

HISTOPATHOLOGY

Cutaneous biopsy is usually unnecessary for the diagnosis of acrocyanosis. The findings are nonspecific and may include mild thickening of the medial coat of arterioles and dilation of papillary and subpapillary capillaries. Other features include mild perivascular infiltration, local dermal edema and fibrosis, and possible formation of new blood vessels.[1] An increase in the number and size of arteriovenous anastomoses has also been shown in acrocyanosis.

DIFFERENTIAL DIAGNOSIS

Primary acrocyanosis should be distinguished from other cold-related or vasospastic conditions such as Raynaud syndrome, pernio, and livedo reticularis.[9] This determination is based upon general appearance, distribution, and persistence of the cyanosis. Then the finding

of acrocyanosis requires consideration of other local or systemic features that suggest an underlying secondary disorder (see Box 47.1).[5] Distinguishing findings of secondary causes of acrocyanosis include asymmetric distribution and the cyanotic discoloration, associated pain, and tissue injury.

Other disorders in the differential diagnosis include systemic hypoxemia, as well as abnormal hemoglobin variants. Systemic hypoxemia with increased deoxyhemoglobin is a common cause of an acrocyanotic appearance. The presence of central cyanosis with arterial hypoxemia should prompt a search for underlying cardiopulmonary disease. Cyanosis may also result from an alteration in hemoglobin with accumulation of methemoglobin and sulfahemoglobin.[12] This may be seen with exposure to oxidizing agents such as aniline, benzocaine, dapsone, phenazopyridine, nitrates, and naphthalene. In addition, several medications and toxins are associated with acrocyanosis, including tricyclic antidepressants, interferon-α, interferon-β, amphotericin B, arsenic, and butyl nitrite.[13,14] Therefore it is important to consider medications or toxic substances as a potential cause of cyanosis.

Hematologic conditions such as cold agglutinins and cryoglobulinemia may cause acrocyanosis.[15,16] Cold agglutinins may be associated with infectious mononucleosis and *Mycoplasma* pneumonia, while cryoglobulinemia may be associated with hepatitis C infection and several other diseases.[16] Acrocyanosis also has been reported in conditions and malignancies both with and without cold agglutinins, such as lymphoproliferative disorders including Hodgkin lymphoma and chronic lymphocytic leukemia.[17,18]

Acrocyanosis has been well described in anorexia nervosa and starvation.[4] It is reported in 20% to 40% of persons with anorexia nervosa and tends to occur in severely ill and malnourished patients. Typically, these patients have pallor of the face and trunk, decreased distal blood flow, and impaired vasodilation to a heat stimulus.

Numerous connective tissue disorders may manifest acrocyanosis, but other signs of these diseases are usually present. Patients with scleroderma and systemic lupus erythematosus may have both acrocyanosis and episodic attacks of Raynaud phenomenon.[17,19] Antinuclear antibodies may be abnormal and help to identify those with connective tissue disorders. Acrocyanosis has been reported in nearly one third of patients with antiphospholipid antibodies and may be seen in conjunction with other cutaneous manifestations such as dermatographism, urticaria, livedo reticularis, cutaneous nodules, purpura, and digital ulceration.[20]

Acrocyanosis also occurs in several associated neurological disorders that have suspected neurovascular instability. An acrocyanotic appearance may be seen following spinal cord injuries or with complex regional pain syndrome.[21] This latter disorder often occurs following trauma and is typified by pain and autonomic dysregulation. Acrocyanosis and lower-extremity edema have also been described in postural orthostatic tachycardia syndrome and have been ascribed to venous pooling.[22]

Acrocyanosis secondary to inherited metabolic disorders is more likely to present during childhood or adolescence. These disorders are suspected when other characteristic associated manifestations are present. Infants with ethylmalonic aciduria have petechiae, diarrhea, pyramidal signs, and mental retardation. Children with mitochondrial disease may have hair abnormalities, pigmentation disorders, and hypertrichosis.

Acrocyanosis may also be present in patients with microemboli, microthrombi, or atheromatous embolism. Patients with atheromatous emboli are typically older with other signs of atherosclerosis, and they have other cutaneous signs such as petechiae, livedo reticularis, and painful skin lesions on the toes (so-called blue toe syndrome). Microthrombi and/or microemboli may occur in acutely ill patients with disseminated intravascular coagulation (DIC), heparin-induced thrombocytopenia (HIT), or septic embolism due to endocarditis.

TREATMENT

Primary acrocyanosis is a benign condition that usually requires only conservative measures; there is no standard or effective curative medical or surgical treatment (Box 47.3). Treatments often focus on cosmetic appearance and occasionally symptom relief. Some patients are so affected that they avoid social contact.[9] Reassurance and behavioral measures, such as avoidance of exposure to cold and use of protective clothing with moisture wicking properties, often improve the discoloration and associated manifestations such as hyperhidrosis.[23] In addition, psychophysiological measures such as biofeedback training, conditioning of reflexes, and hypnosis may give partial relief.

Pharmacological intervention is rarely necessary. Various drugs have been advocated, although few controlled studies have been performed. A variety of vasodilator agents have been tried, such as calcium channel blockers and adrenergic blocking agents (rauwolfia, guanethidine, reserpine, and α-blockers), but have not shown consistent benefit. Other agents such as nicotinic acid derivatives, cyclandelate, topical minoxidil, and rutin compounds have also been suggested to provide some improvement to a variable extent.[1] Bromocriptine has been reported to relieve acrocyanosis within a few days, but may induce Raynaud phenomenon in about one-third of patients.[24] Sympathectomy or disrupting the fibers of the sympathetic nervous system to the affected area usually will alleviate acrocyanosis, but is reserved for severe cases and is rarely appropriate for primary disease.[1]

Treatment of secondary acrocyanosis depends on the underlying condition, as the treatment may alleviate or resolve the acrocyanosis.

PROGNOSIS

Although there is no curative treatment, the prognosis of primary acrocyanosis is excellent. It is not associated with increased risk of death, amputation, or other complications. Apart from the discoloration and potential associated concern, patients with primary acrocyanosis usually have no other signs or symptoms such as pain, skin ulcerations, or tissue loss. Patients can expect to lead normal lives

with minor behavioral modifications. In contrast, the prognosis of secondary acrocyanosis varies widely depending upon the underlying condition.

REFERENCES

1. Kurklinsky AK, Miller VM, Rooke TW. Acrocyanosis: the Flying Dutchman. *Vasc Med.* 2011;16:288–301.
2. Carpentier PH. Definition and epidemiology of vascular acrosyndromes. *Rev Prat.* 1998;48:1641–1646.
3. Creager MA, Loscalzo J. Vascular disease of the extremity. In: Jameson JL, Fauci AS, Kasper DL, et al., eds. *Harrison's Principles of Internal Medicine.* 20th ed. New York: McGraw-Hill; 2018.
4. Strumia R. Eating disorders and the skin. *Clin Dermatol.* 2013;31:80–85.
5. Brown PJ, Zirwas MJ, English JC. The purple digit an algorithmic approach to diagnosis. *Am J Clin Dermatol.* 2010;11:103–116.
6. Bollinger A. Function of the precapillary vessels in peripheral vascular disease. *J Cardiovasc Pharmacol.* 1985;7:S147–S151.
7. Lottenbach K. Vascular response to cold in acrocyanosis. *Helvetia Medica Acta.* 1967;33:437–444.
8. Yilmaz S, Yokuşoğlu M, Çinar M, et al. Autonomic functions in acrocyanosis assessed by heart rate variability. *Eur J Rheumatol.* 2014;1:18–20.
9. Heidrich H. Functional vascular diseases: Raynaud's syndrome, acrocyanosis and erythromelalgia. *Vasa.* 2010;39:33–41.
10. Monticone G, Colonna L, Palmeri G, et al. Quantitative nailfold capillary microscopy findings in patients with acrocyanosis compared with patients having systemic sclerosis and normal subjects. *J Am Acad Dermatol.* 2000;42:787–790.
11. Davis E. Oscillometry of radial artery in acrocyanosis and cold sensitivity. *J Mal Vasc.* 1992;17:214–217.
12. Lata K, Janardhanan R. Methemoglobinemia: a diagnosis not to be missed. *Am J Med.* 2015;128:e45–e46.
13. Masuda H, Mori M, Araki N, Kuwabara S. Bilateral foot acrocyanosis in an interferon-β-treated MS patient. *Intern Med.* 2016;55:319.
14. Zhang X, Jin J, Cai C, et al. Amphotericin B liposome-induced acrocyanosis and elevated serum creatinine. *Indian J Pharmacol.* 2016;48:321–323.
15. Gregory GP, Farrell A, Brown S. Cold agglutinin disease complicated by acrocyanosis and necrosis. *Ann Hematol.* 2017;96:509–510.
16. Mosdósi B, Nyul Z, Nagy A, et al. Severe acrocyanosis precipitated by cold agglutinin secondary to infection with mycoplasma pneumoniae in a pediatric patient. *Croat Med J.* 2017;58:424–430.
17. El Habr C, Sammour R, El-Murr T, et al. Acrocyanosis and necrotic purpura: a manifestation of multiple myeloma and type I cryoglobulinemia. *Int J Dermatol.* 2015;54:946–950.
18. Lesesve JF. Acrocyanosis revealing chronic lymphocytic leukemia. *Clin Case Rep.* 2016;4:404–405.
19. Richter JG, Sander O, Schneider M, et al. Diagnostic algorithm for Raynaud's phenomenon and vascular skin lesions in systemic lupus erythematosus. *Lupus.* 2010;19:1087–1095.
20. Diógenes MJ, Diógenes PC, de Morais Carneiro RM, et al. Cutaneous manifestations associated with antiphospholipid antibodies. *Int J Dermatol.* 2004;43:632–637.
21. Glazer E, Pacanowski JP, Leon LR. Asymptomatic lower extremity acrocyanosis: report of two cases and review of the literature. *Vascular.* 2011;19:105–110.
22. Steward JM, Gewitz MH, Weldon A, et al. Patterns of orthostatic intolerance: the orthostatic tachycardia syndrome and adolescent chronic fatigue. *J Pediatr.* 1999;135:218–221.
23. Planchon B, Becker E, Carpentier PH, et al. Acrocyanosis: changing concepts and nosological limitations. *J Mal Vasc.* 2001;26:5–15.
24. Morrish DW, Crockford PM. Acrocyanosis treated with bromocriptine. *Lancet.* 1976;2:851.

BOX 47.3 **Treatment of Primary Acrocyanosis**

Reassurance
Behavioral measures:
  Avoidance of exposure to cold
  Use of protective clothing
Psychophysiological measures:
  Biofeedback training
  Conditioning of reflexes
  Hypnosis
Pharmacological interventions:
  Calcium channel blockers
  Nicotinic acid derivatives
  Adrenergic blocking agents
  Cyclandelate
  Topical minoxidil
  Bromocriptine
Sympathectomy

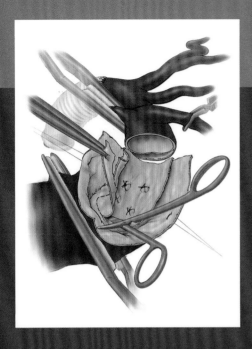

第48章
红斑性肢痛症

　　红斑性肢痛症是一种罕见的四肢疾病，早在150年前，医学文献中就有过描述，1878年，Mitchell将其命名为红斑性肢痛症。其表现为间歇性的四肢皮肤发红、发热、疼痛。虽然红斑性肢痛症在命名、诊断标准、临床严重程度评分及发病机制等方面均存在争议，但现有的研究正在逐渐揭露其神秘的面纱。红斑性肢痛症可以发生在任何年龄段，以白人和女性为主，常因环境温度上升导致受累及的肢端部分温度升高，进而诱发症状。诊断主要通过病史分析明确。红斑性肢痛症的病因可以分为原发性及继发性，未明确病因及遗传病因划为原发性病因；继发性病因与骨髓增生性疾病、血液疾病、药物、传染病、食物摄入（蘑菇）、肿瘤、结缔组织病、生理状况（妊娠）和神经病等有关，其中与骨髓增生性疾病关系最密切。病理生理学上也存在血管性、神经性及遗传性等学说。红斑性肢痛症对生活质量有明显的负面影响，但治疗非常困难，目前并没有确切的治疗药物及方法。主要处理措施就是避免诱发因素和缓解疼痛，如局部药物治疗（如利多卡因贴片、肉毒素局部注射等）和全身药物治疗（如阿司匹林、β受体阻滞剂）等，药物干预可能有益，非药物治疗的效果也不同，疼痛康复是严重者及疼痛相关患者的有效治疗方法。

陈海生

Erythromelalgia

Julio C. Sartori-Valinotti, Mark D.P. Davis, and Thom W. Rooke

DEFINITION AND HISTORICAL PERSPECTIVE

Erythromelalgia is a rare condition of the extremities characterized by the triad of redness, warmth, and pain. The symptom complex of intermittent acral warmth, pain, and erythema that defines erythromelalgia has been well documented in the medical literature for more than 150 years. Graves[1] described cases of "hot and painful legs" in 1834. The term *erythromelalgia* was coined in 1878 by Mitchell[2] from *erythros* (red), *melos* (extremity), and *algos* (pain); some have since referred to it as *Mitchell disease*. As we discover more about the link between a vasculopathy and neuropathy in this syndrome, it seems that Mitchell was prophetically accurate when he entitled the original manuscript "On a Rare Vasomotor Neurosis of the Extremities." Smith and Allen[3] emphasized another essential component of this syndrome when they renamed it *erythermalgia* in 1938 to denote the heat *(thermé)* in the affected extremity during periods of redness. Although many authors agree that *erythermalgia* is perhaps more accurate, *erythromelalgia* is the term most commonly used, and it is the term used in this chapter.

Although poorly characterized initially,[4-6] there have been considerable advances in the characterization of this clinical syndrome, with large case series[7-10] published. Although the condition is mysterious, it is not as mysterious as was once believed.[9,10] Much of our current understanding of erythromelalgia derives from the larger case series reported.[7-9,11,12]

NOMENCLATURE

Considerable confusion exists regarding the nomenclature of erythromelalgia.[13] Many terms have been used, and some authors have proposed that these terms should refer to different forms of erythromelalgia, as detailed later. However, these synonyms are not widely used, and most authors currently use the term *erythromelalgia* as originally used by Silas Weir Mitchell (1829–1914). Related names used by some include *Weir-Mitchell disease*, *Mitchell disease*, and *acromelalgia*. Michiels et al.[14] proposed that the term *erythromelalgia* be restricted to cases due to myeloproliferative disorders responsive to aspirin therapy. They used the term *erythermalgia* to describe idiopathic conditions or conditions due to other diseases that are unresponsive to aspirin therapy. An unwieldy term, *erythermomelalgia*, accounts for the four cardinal symptoms and signs of the condition, but it is not in general use.[15] *Erythralgia* has been used.[6,16] *Erythroprosopalgia*, derived from *prosopon* (face), is used in the German literature to describe facial erythromelalgia.[6,14,16]

CRITERIA FOR DIAGNOSIS

No objective criteria exist for the diagnosis of erythromelalgia, making it difficult to interpret some of the cases reported in the literature.[13]

The diagnosis is most often clinically based, dependent on the medical history and physical findings, because no objective diagnostic or laboratory tests are available[14] and because the physical findings of erythromelalgia may be absent owing to the frequently intermittent nature of the condition.[8]

Different diagnostic criteria have been suggested by different authors. Weir Mitchell[2,8] applied the three inclusion criteria used in the original description of the syndrome: red, hot, and painful extremities. Brown[17] added three additional criteria in 1932: induction and exacerbation of symptoms by warming, relief by cooling, and unresponsiveness to therapy. The criteria were described as follows: (1) during attacks (bilateral or symmetrical burning pain in hands and feet), affected parts are flushed, congested, and warm; (2) attacks are initiated or aggravated by standing, exercising, or exposing the extremity to temperatures warmer than 34°C; (3) symptoms are relieved by elevation of the extremity or exposure of the extremity to cold; and (4) the condition is refractory to treatment. Thompson et al.[18] suggested the following five criteria: (1) burning extremity pain, (2) pain aggravated by warming, (3) pain relieved by cooling, (4) erythema of the affected skin, and (5) increased temperature of the affected skin. These five criteria have been used in several publications.[9,13,19]

Lazareth et al.[20] used three major and two of four minor criteria to satisfy the diagnosis. Major criteria were paroxysmal pain, burning pain, and redness of affected skin. Minor criteria were typical precipitating factors (heat exposure, effort), typical relieving factors (cold, rest), elevated skin temperature in affected skin, and response of symptoms to acetylsalicylic acid. Drenth et al.[21-24] distinguished three types of red, congested, and painful conditions of the extremities that must be distinguished for effective treatment according to their cause: (1) erythromelalgia in thrombocythemia, (2) primary erythromelalgia, and (3) secondary erythromelalgia.

Littleford et al.[25] used a classification of type 1 erythromelalgia (the typical form) and type 2 erythromelalgia (the abortive form), in which the burning nature of the pain is absent and symptomatic relief is not always provided by cooling or elevation of the limb. Mørk and Kvernebo[13] made the following distinctions: (1) *Syndrome* is used when initial and gradual symptoms localized to the feet and legs appear in childhood or adolescence and when there is a family history of erythromelalgia; *phenomenon* is used for all other cases. (2) Erythromelalgia is *primary* when it is idiopathic. It is *secondary* when symptoms are caused by a primary disease such as a hemorrheological, metabolic, connective tissue, musculoskeletal, or infectious disease; are induced by drugs; or are part of a paraneoplastic phenomenon. (3) *Acute* is used when symptoms reach maximal strength within 1 month after onset of symptoms. (4) *Borderline erythromelalgia*, *erythromelalgia*, and *severe erythromelalgia* may be useful.[13]

CLINICAL CONTROVERSIES

Several controversies persist concerning erythromelalgia: nomenclature, diagnostic criteria, scoring systems for clinical severity, and pathogenesis. Classification of erythromelalgia into primary and secondary types may be controversial when comorbid conditions are mislabeled as underlying diseases that cause erythromelalgia. Classification of incomplete forms of erythromelalgia is also controversial; for example, some patients report that their feet are blue when symptoms are present. The problem with all definitions is that each criterion depends on clinical subjective judgment. The diagnosis of erythromelalgia is based on history because there are no objective physical findings. This may lead to an erroneous diagnosis.

CLINICAL PRESENTATION

The essential elements of this clinical syndrome, as described by its name, are intermittent (occasionally continuous) redness of an acral area (i.e., extremities, head and neck area) associated with heat and pain. Common terms used to describe the pain include "piercing," "burning," and "discomfort."[8] The pain and burning sensation can be extremely severe. Patients report that they make major adjustments to their lifestyles to avoid precipitating an event. During an episode, they try to cool their feet in many ways, sometimes resorting to extraordinary measures to alleviate the pain, such as putting their feet in ice or walking barefoot in snow.

Erythromelalgia involves the feet in most circumstances (Fig. 48.1A and B); a minority of these patients have similar symptoms involving the hands.[8] Occasionally, only the hands are involved. Erythromelalgia may extend proximally to the knees in the lower extremities (see Fig. 48.1C) and to the elbows in the upper extremities. Involvement of the extremities is generally symmetrical. Rarely, erythromelalgia involves the ears and face. In the largest reported series (168 patients), symptoms predominantly involved feet (148 patients, 88.1%) and hands (43 patients, 25.6%).[8]

In the majority of patients, symptoms are intermittent; episodes, precipitated by specific triggers, can last from minutes to hours. In a minority of patients, erythromelalgia symptoms are continuous, although they may wax and wane. Patients with continuous symptoms usually report that their symptoms started intermittently and then became more frequent and prolonged until they were continuous.

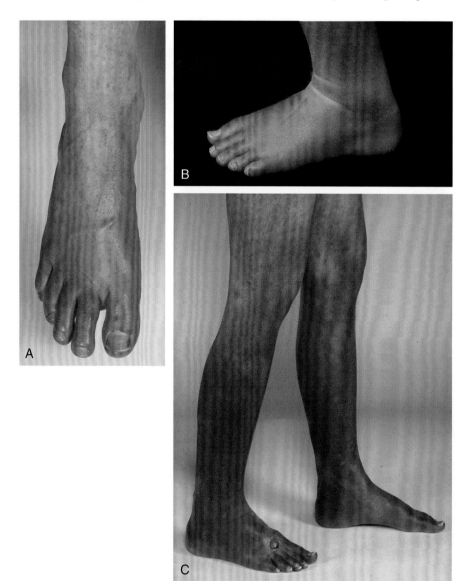

Fig. 48.1 Erythromelalgia (red, hot, acral areas) involving lower extremities may affect toes only, distal forefoot (A), or entire foot (B) or may extend up the leg, even beyond the knee (C). It is usually bilateral (C).

In the series of 168 patients,[8] symptoms were intermittent in 163 patients (97%) and continuous in 5 (3%).

The specific precipitant for erythromelalgia varies from person to person, but the most frequent precipitant is an increase in temperature of the affected acral area. This may be caused by an increase in ambient temperature, and patients may experience increases in severity and frequency of attacks during the summer. Erythromelalgia affecting the feet is often precipitated by an increase in local temperature from aerobic exercise. Symptoms can also be precipitated or intensified by lowering the affected part. Common aggravating factors include warm rooms, floors, or water; placing the extremity near heating appliances; sleeping under bedcovers; and wearing shoes and gloves. Walking, exercise, sitting, dependency of the extremities, and application of skin pressure may intensify symptoms. Some patients relate that episodes of erythromelalgia occur spontaneously without clear precipitating factors.

Aspirin may dramatically relieve symptoms in a subset of patients with underlying myeloproliferative disease, but otherwise aspirin is rarely effective. Other agents that have been reported to relieve symptoms are presented later in the section on treatment. Many patients report that plunging their feet into ice water during an episode relieves their symptoms. Patients frequently report that the affected extremities must be exposed to cold surfaces or air-conditioned rooms or be immersed in buckets of cool or ice water to relieve their symptoms. A decrease in local temperature may decrease the severity of erythromelalgia or even abort an episode. Some patients sleep with their extremities outside the bedcovers, and some engage in unusual behaviors such as sleeping with their feet out a window, putting their feet in a refrigerator, walking barefoot in the snow, or storing shoes in a freezer. Kvernebo[9] described a patient who, for almost 25 years day and night, lived with a bucket of ice water at her side, immersing her feet intermittently for 15 to 30 minutes an hour. Thus, in what superficially appears to be the antithesis of Raynaud phenomenon, patients seek relief by cooling the affected extremity.

Symptoms of erythromelalgia are intermittent, and the clinical examination is often normal. If the patient is examined during an episode of erythromelalgia, the affected extremity is tender, erythematous, and objectively hot. In up to two-thirds of patients, affected extremities are discolored (blue/cyanotic, red, or mottled) and cool or cold to the touch, with varying degrees of discomfort between episodes. Raynaud phenomenon is not uncommon between episodes. The syndrome of erythromelalgia is frequently worsened when patients try to relieve their symptoms. For example, patients soak their feet in water and ice, which can lead to immersion irritant contact dermatitis or even frostbite. Allergic contact dermatitis due to substances that have been applied to the affected feet can occur. Other common vascular problems in the lower extremities such as edema, venous insufficiency, and lymphedema can be worsened by erythromelalgia. Patients may have high requirements for pain medications and become addicted to or dependent on narcotic analgesics. Psychiatric problems such as depression and obsessive-compulsive behaviors to avoid episodes of erythromelalgia can occur. The syndrome can be socially disabling if patients avoid exercising, walking, participating in sports, or leaving their homes, which leads to a sense of disablement, isolation, and loneliness. The syndrome frequently affects performance in the workplace (especially with manual work or jobs that entail standing) and at home.

Erythromelalgia predominantly affects individuals who are white and of any age. In the largest published series,[8] all 168 patients were white, the female-to-male ratio was approximately 3:1, and the mean age was 55.8 years (range, 5 to 91 years). Symptoms had been present since childhood in seven patients (4.2%), and six patients (3.6%) had a first-degree relative with erythromelalgia.

Erythromelalgia can also occur in the pediatric age group. In the largest pediatric series reported—32 patients (girls, 22 [69%]) seen at the Mayo Clinic[26]—mean age was 14.1 years (range, 5 to 18 years) and the diagnosis was delayed; mean time to diagnosis was 5.2 years. Seven patients (22%) had a first-degree relative with erythromelalgia; four were from the same family. Physical activity was limited in 21 patients (66%), and school attendance was affected in 11 patients (34%). Hypertension was not a feature of these patients. In contrast, Drenth et al.[27] described nine children in whom erythromelalgia was transient (seven girls and two boys; mean age, 11.6 years); in seven, hypertension was directly related to the symptoms, and treatment of the hypertension with intravenous (IV) sodium nitroprusside relieved symptoms.

DIAGNOSIS

Making the diagnosis is often a problem because objective findings may not be present during the physical examination, so the diagnosis may rest on history alone. However, because the differential diagnosis includes many possibilities, it is best to have evidence to support the diagnosis. The following may help:

1. Examine and assess the patient both during an episode and between episodes. Ask the patient to engage in an activity, such as climbing stairs that will precipitate an episode.
2. If it is not possible to examine a patient during an episode, ask the patient to obtain a photograph of the affected areas during an episode.

CLASSIFICATION

Most authors agree on the fundamentals of the diagnosis of erythromelalgia, but there are many described criteria for diagnosis and many subclassifications of erythromelalgia. Use of these subclassifications may depend on whether one is a "lumper" or "splitter."[22] The most popular classification of erythromelalgia is into primary and secondary forms.

Primary Erythromelalgia

Primary erythromelalgia is defined by patients in whom no identifiable cause is found. This group includes the hereditary forms.

Secondary Erythromelalgia

Potential causes of secondary erythromelalgia are presented in Box 48.1. Erythromelalgia has been reported in association with myeloproliferative diseases, blood disorders, drugs, infectious diseases, food ingestion (mushrooms), neoplasms, connective tissue disease, physiological conditions (pregnancy), and neuropathies. The relationship of many underlying disorders to erythromelalgia is sometimes unclear, and the disorder may be a coincidental comorbidity rather than an underlying disease.

Among the reported series, the association with myeloproliferative disease seems most constant.[8] Evidence of underlying myeloproliferative disease should be sought at diagnosis and subsequently. Erythromelalgia can herald the onset of underlying myeloproliferative disease. In one series, erythromelalgia was the presenting symptom of essential thrombocythemia in 26 of 40 patients (65%)[28]; in another series, erythromelalgia was the presenting symptom in 11 of 268 patients with thrombocythemia (4%).[29]

INCIDENCE

In a population-based study from Olmsted County, Minnesota, the overall age- and sex-adjusted incidence rate (95% confidence interval [95% CI]) was calculated to be 1.3 (0.8 to 1.7) per 100,000 persons per year. The incidence of primary and secondary erythromelalgia

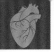

was 1.1 (0.7 to 1.5) and 0.2 (0.02 to 0.4) per 100,000 persons per year, respectively.[30] The incidence was noted to have increased over the past 3 decades. This incidence was approximately five times higher than that reported from Norway, where the incidence was calculated to be 2.5 to 3.3 per 1 million inhabitants per year in the Norwegian population, with a corresponding annual prevalence of 18 to 20 per 1 million.[9] Cases of borderline erythromelalgia were not included in these figures.[10]

PATHOPHYSIOLOGY

The pathophysiology of erythromelalgia is not clearly understood. Part of the difficulty in understanding this disorder has been the heterogeneity of the affected population.[31] The underlying pathological mechanisms most likely involve a complex dysregulation of cutaneous blood flow that ultimately results in microvascular ischemia. Determining the nature of this dysfunction has also been challenging because control of cutaneous blood flow depends on an intricate interplay of systemic and local signals and is not completely understood.[31] A small-fiber neuropathy likely contributes to this dysregulation.[32,33]

Erythromelalgia: A Vasculopathy?

Thermoregulatory control of human skin blood flow is vital to maintenance of normal body temperatures during challenges to thermal homeostasis. Sympathetic neural control of skin blood flow includes the noradrenergic vasoconstrictor system and a sympathetic active vasodilator system, the latter being responsible for 80% to 90% of the substantial cutaneous vasodilation that occurs with whole-body heat stress. With body heating, the magnitude of skin vasodilation is striking; skin blood flow can reach 6 to 8 L/min during hyperthermia.[34]

Erythromelalgia is a cutaneous microvascular disorder. The pathophysiology appears to relate to disorders of local or reflex thermoregulatory control of skin circulation.[34] Two paradoxical observations concerning blood flow during an episode of erythromelalgia have been made. During symptoms, there is increased blood flow. Sandroni et al.,[33] Mørk et al.[10] and Kvernebo[9] confirmed that the observed erythema and warmth are associated with increased blood flow. Using laser Doppler, Sandroni et al. measured blood flow during symptoms and demonstrated increased perfusion during attacks. However, paradoxically, this increased blood flow is accompanied by local hypoxia. Although there is increased perfusion during attacks, the values for transcutaneous oxygen tension are critically low, low, or unchanged—in other words, during symptoms, transcutaneous oximetry values decrease or do not change.[9,10,32,33] To explain this paradox, Mørk et al.[35] theorized and demonstrated that the increased blood flow is probably due to shunting through arteriovenous anastomoses, which results in hypoperfusion of the more superficial nutritive capillaries. If available blood is shunted away from normal skin capillaries, the skin will be hypoxic. Mørk et al. demonstrated that despite increased overall blood flow to the skin, the induction of erythromelalgia symptoms is accompanied by decreased perfusion of the superficial vascular plexus, as evidenced by a decreased density of skin capillaries. Thus their hypothesis is that dilation of arteriovenous anastomoses is directly responsible for shunting nutritive blood flow away from the superficial vascular plexus. Furthermore, Mørk et al. postulated that erythromelalgia is not a disease but rather a physiological response to stimuli such as infection, trauma, or tumor, and symptoms are caused by tissue hypoxia induced by maldistribution of microvascular blood flow in the skin, with increased thermoregulatory flow and inadequate perfusion.

Sandroni et al.[33] theorized that the effects of diminished perfusion could be exacerbated by increased metabolic demands in response to hyperthermia, ultimately resulting in hypoxic tissue damage and pain.

Pain relief by cooling could be explained by a resultant decrease in the metabolic rate and a corresponding decrease in the need for oxygen.

Littleford et al.[25] described an underlying vasoconstrictor tendency in patients with erythromelalgia that may be related to functional or structural changes in skin microvessels and noted that basal skin erythrocyte flux and skin temperature were lower in patients with a history of erythromelalgia than in controls. As noted earlier, Raynaud phenomenon has been described in patients with erythromelalgia.[36] Acrocyanosis has also been described.[36] Davis et al.[32] have also noted that at baseline the skin is cool and occasionally cyanotic between episodes in two-thirds of patients.

Erythromelalgia: A Neuropathy?

Several lines of evidence suggest that a neuropathy is associated with erythromelalgia, because the disorder has been described in association with many types of neuropathy. Both large- and small-fiber neuropathies are observed in a large proportion of patients with erythromelalgia (see Box 48.1).[32,33,37]

Among 57 patients with erythromelalgia who were evaluated with use of an autonomic reflex screen, results for 49 (86%) were abnormal, indicating a small-fiber neuropathy. The most common abnormalities were sudomotor abnormalities (i.e., absent or reduced sweat production).[32] In an earlier series, findings were similar for 17 of 27 patients (63%); whether the observed neuropathy led to erythromelalgia, or vice versa, is unclear.[33,38] In support of this, thermoregulatory sweat testing results were abnormal in 28 (88%) of 32 patients, and quantitative sudomotor axon reflex test results were abnormal in 22 patients (69%); abnormalities noted on thermoregulatory sweat testing varied from local hypohidrosis or anhidrosis to global anhidrosis.[37]

Conversely, in a series of 321 cases of disorders of autonomic neuropathy, the majority had erythromelalgia.[39] Ørstavik et al.[40] used erythromelalgia as a model to study chronic pain and found changes in the conductive properties of C fibers in patients with erythromelalgia that were indicative of a small-fiber neuropathy. In addition, an active contribution of mechanoinsensitive fibers to chronic pain was postulated. Uno and Parker[41] reported that the density of both acetylcholinesterase-positive and catecholamine-containing nerve terminals in the periarterial and sweat gland plexuses was much less in the skin of the erythermalgic foot than in the unaffected skin of the same patient and much less than in the foot skin of a healthy person.

Layzer[42] wrote that it seems plausible to regard erythromelalgia as a problem of polymodal C fiber receptors in sensitized skin. The threshold of C fibers to activation by heat would decrease to between 32°C and 36°C; activated C fibers would cause vasodilation by axon reflexes, resulting in redness, heat, and swelling. With cooling, the threshold for the nociceptors would increase.

Kazemi et al.[43] reported that 72.7% of the patients studied had abnormal sympathetic reflexes, which may result from an abnormality of the sympathetic nerves. Littleford et al.[44] also noted findings suggesting that patients with erythromelalgia have diminished sympathetic vasoconstrictor responses to both cold challenge of the contralateral arm and inspiratory gasp; an interplay between neural and vasoactive agents was postulated.

Inherited Erythromelalgia

There is a subset of erythromelalgia that is inherited. In the largest reported series, the proportion of cases that are inherited was approximately 5%.[8] Inheritance in familial autosomal dominant (29 persons were affected in five generations) and X-linked dominant fashions have been reported. Clinical onset in familial cases usually occurs in childhood, most frequently prior to the age of 5 or 6, but occasionally is seen up to 10 or 12 years of age and, in rare families, at even older ages.

Gain-of-Function Mutations in Sensory Nerves and Consequent Nerve Hyperexcitability

In the inherited forms of erythromelalgia, there have been developments in understanding the disease. It currently appears that mutations in particular sodium channels in the nociceptors of sensory nerves lead to firing of nerves with little provocation; in other words, sensory nerves are hyperexcitable. In 2001, Drenth et al. investigated DNA from five families with hereditary erythromelalgia using linkage analysis and located the gene responsible to chromosome 2q31-32.[45] Based on this work, Yang et al. subsequently reported that mutations in the gene SCN9A on this chromosome caused primary erythromelalgia.[46] Cummins et al. showed that functionally this gene encoded the Nav1.7 sodium channel; mutations in this gene lead to altered channel function in nerves.[47] These mutations are preferentially expressed by the dorsal root ganglion and sympathetic ganglion neuron. In 2005, Michiels et al. reported that a mutation in this gene occurred in all five affected members of a Flemish family and in none of five unaffected members.[48] Han et al. described a patient with onset of erythromelalgia in the second decade and suggested that mutations that lead to lesser changes in sodium channel activation are associated with lesser neuron excitability and later onset of clinical signs.[49]

The implications of these findings are significant because these mutated sodium channels could be a therapeutic target, and more widely, other pain syndromes also involve altered sodium channel function.[50] In an editorial in 2005, Waxman and Dib-Hajj stated, "Erythromelalgia is the first human disorder in which it has been possible to associate an ion channel mutation with chronic neuropathic pain … erythromelalgia may emerge as a model disease that holds more general lessons about the molecular neurobiology of chronic pain."[51] Erythromelalgia can therefore be regarded as a painful channelopathy.[52]

Most recently a new mutation within the Nav1.7-encoding gene SCN9A, c.2477T>A (p. F826Y), has been shown to cosegregate with the disease phenotype. It seems that this mutation renders dorsal root ganglion neurons hyperexcitable, partially explaining the etiopathogenesis of this disorder (28990532). Not surprisingly, patients with Nav1.7, 1.8, or 1.9 mutation exhibit differential sensitivity to intradermal lidocaine, to suprathreshold heat, and mechanical pain stimuli.[53]

As previously stated, targeting of Nav1.7 may become a therapeutic option for patients who harbor the mutation, but studies thus far have been rather disappointing. For example, the analgesic benefit of single oral dose of a compound called PF-05089771 was modest.[54]

Homozygous recessive and heterozygous missense mutations in the transient receptor potential vanilloid 3 (TRPV3) have been implicated in the development of erythromelalgia in patients with Olmsted syndrome (bilateral palmoplantar keratoderma and periorificial keratotic plaques).[55,56]

It is important to bear in mind that these findings have been described in the inherited form of erythromelalgia thus far and not the more common noninherited forms. In addition, SCN9A mutation is not always present in inherited erythromelalgia. Drenth et al. identified this mutation in only 1 of 15 patients with a family history of the disease.[57]

Erythromelalgia Associated With a Myeloproliferative Disease

Erythromelalgia in the setting of thrombocythemia or myeloproliferative diseases seems to be a separate entity, although it presents similarly to other forms of erythromelalgia. Recognition of the associated myeloproliferative disease is vital because in these specific types of erythromelalgia, aspirin provides immediate and long-lived relief from symptoms. Thrombin, platelet function, and genetics have been considered in studies of erythromelalgia. van Genderen et al.[58] noted that thrombocythemia-associated erythromelalgia may develop despite treatment with oral anticoagulants or heparin, suggesting that generation of thrombin is not a prerequisite for development of erythromelalgia. Disordered platelet function affecting the microvasculature has been implicated in thrombocythemia-related erythromelalgia.[59]

Pathophysiological Controversies

Several questions about erythromelalgia remain. Does a neuropathy cause the vasculopathy, or does the vasculopathy cause a neuropathy?[32] What causes the neuropathy if it is not caused by the vasculopathy? In the inherited form, mutations in the sodium channel lead to hyperexcitability of sensory nerves. Similar mutations have not been described in the sporadic form, which accounts for 95% of cases. What is the pathophysiology in these forms? How does dysfunction of the precapillary sphincter affect this disease? Schechner[31] pointed out that it is unknown whether shunting of blood through arteriovenous anastomoses alone can induce hypoxia severe enough to induce pain, particularly in areas that contain few arteriovenous anastomoses. Potentially inadequate compensatory dilation, or even inappropriate constriction of the precapillary sphincter, may compound the effects of the relative hypoperfusion. What factors are responsible for vascular dysfunction? Both autonomic neuropathy[33] and endothelial injury[60] have been observed in patients with erythromelalgia, but it is not known whether this damage to critical vasoregulatory components is primary or secondary to chronic hypoxia.

DIFFERENTIAL DIAGNOSIS

Any condition causing extremity pain could be mistaken for erythromelalgia. In particular, unwarranted diagnosis of erythromelalgia can result from any clinical situation that includes burning sensations in the limbs. However, the syndrome of erythromelalgia is specific for red, hot extremities. The following conditions are included in the differential diagnosis:

- Neuropathies: peripheral neuropathy, small-fiber neuropathy, reflex sympathetic dystrophy (complex regional pain syndrome)
- Vascular: large-vessel disease, small-vessel disease, postural orthostatic tachycardia syndrome (which causes "evanescent hyperemia"), Raynaud phenomenon, Raynaud disease, arterial insufficiency, venous insufficiency (which can produce sensations of warm feet, often at bedtime, with edema and an increase in local heat)
- Metabolic: painful crises associated with Fabry disease (a hereditary sphingolipidosis transmitted on chromosome X that occurs predominantly in men, often starting early in childhood with a burning sensation in the limbs)
- Skin: dermatitis, immersion foot
- Infectious: erysipelas
- Bone: osteomyelitis
- Exogenous: acrodynia (a rare disease caused by excessive mercury intake and confirmed by high mercury levels in the urine, in which the main sign is vasomotor impairment in the limbs, and the red hands and feet have an intense, paroxysmal, burn-type pain)

INVESTIGATIONS

To investigate the possibility of erythromelalgia, the clinician should take the following steps:

1. Get a detailed history, and perform a physical examination with respect to each element of the history outlined earlier.
2. If signs of erythromelalgia are not present during the examination, ask the patient to photograph the affected area when symptoms are apparent.

3. Evaluate the results of a complete blood cell (CBC) count, including total and differential leukocyte counts.
4. Investigate the possibility of underlying disease, as indicated by the patient's age, history, and physical examination.
5. Consider further investigations as outlined in Box 48.2, especially for small-fiber neuropathy and large-fiber neuropathy, and for noninvasive vascular studies during symptoms and between symptoms (as detailed by Davis et al.[32]) to better define the pathophysiology. Results of these tests are useful to confirm the diagnosis and help to guide therapy.
6. In the inherited form, molecular genetic testing for mutations in *SCN9A* is available on a clinical basis.

Biopsy Findings

Reports of skin biopsies for erythromelalgia are scant. In the series reported by Davis et al.,[8] only 12 of the 168 patients with primary erythromelalgia had a biopsy, and the biopsy specimens showed no specific abnormalities. Three cases of primary erythromelalgia were reported by Drenth et al.,[60] and similarly, the biopsy specimens showed nonspecific changes.

The histopathological changes in cases of erythromelalgia related to thrombocythemia showed arteriolar inflammation, fibromuscular intimal proliferation, and thrombotic occlusions.[61] Croue et al.[62] noted similar changes in a case of erythromelalgia related to essential thrombocythemia. Biopsies from a few patients with drug-induced erythromelalgia have been described. Biopsies from a patient with verapamil-induced erythromelalgia showed mild perivascular mononuclear infiltrate and moderate perivascular edema.[63]

BOX 48.2 Investigation Protocol for Patients Presenting with Erythromelalgia

Clinical
History
Physical examination

Peripheral Vascular Laboratory
Studies of the following parameters in affected extremities, with and without symptoms:
Color change
Skin temperature and core temperature
Blood flow (laser Doppler flowmetry)
Oxygen saturation (transcutaneous oximetry)
Ankle-brachial indices (ABIs)

Neurological Evaluation
Electromyography
Autonomic nerve studies:
Quantitative sudomotor axon reflex test (QSART)
Heart rate response to deep breathing and Valsalva ratio (cardiovagal functioning)
Adrenergic function testing
Thermoregulatory sweat testing
Consultation with neurologist specializing in autonomic nerve studies if results of the above tests are abnormal

Modified from Davis MD, Sandroni P, Rooke TW, Low PA. Erythromelalgia: vasculopathy, neuropathy, or both? A prospective study of vascular and neurophysiologic studies in erythromelalgia. *Arch Dermatol.* 2003;139:1337–1343.

Thickening of blood vessel walls with intramural and perivascular mucin deposition has been reported in a patient with erythromelalgia secondary to primary myelofibrosis.[64] Similarly, thickening of arterioles with intramural mucin deposition, marked perivascular mucin deposition, and acute perivascular inflammation was noted in a patient with polycythemia vera.[65] These studies suggest that mucin deposition may be a unique histopathologic finding in erythromelalgia secondary to myeloproliferative disease.

Contrary to other painful conditions of the lower extremities, erythromelalgia patients have normal epidermal nerve fiber density on skin biopsy. However, although the number of fibers is not decreased, functionality is impaired as evidenced by abnormal sweat test results, pain thresholds, and blood pressure or heart rate control.[66]

NATURAL HISTORY AND PROGNOSIS

Information concerning the prognosis of this condition is limited.[8,11] In a study of the natural history of erythromelalgia in which 168 patients were studied, with a mean follow-up of 8.7 years (range, 1.3 to 20 years), Kaplan-Meier survival curves showed a significant decrease in survival compared with expected survival among people matched for age and sex from the US general population ($P < .001$).[8] Of 94 patients questioned about their symptoms, 30 (31.9%) reported that their symptoms had worsened, 25 (26.6%) had not changed, 29 (30.9%) had improved, and 10 (10.6%) had completely resolved.

At the time of the most recent follow-up, 45 of the 168 patients (26.8%) had died. Causes of death included myeloproliferative disease, cardiovascular disease, and cancer. Importantly, three patients with severe symptoms had committed suicide. In a series of patients with pediatric erythromelalgia, one patient had committed suicide.[26]

Kalgaard et al.[11] reported that approximately two-thirds of 87 patients studied had primary cases and approximately three-quarters had some form of chronic condition. Over time in the patients with erythromelalgia, the condition gradually became worse. In patients with primary or secondary acute erythromelalgia, the condition improved, and in patients with primary or secondary chronic erythromelalgia, the condition remained stable.

Thus overall, it can be concluded from these studies that the course of the disease is unpredictable; some patients become worse, some have a stable course, and some get better or even have full resolution of erythromelalgia with time. It is notable that some patients experienced cure.[8]

Quality of Life

Erythromelalgia has a markedly negative effect on quality of life. One study has directly measured quality-of-life parameters.[8] The Medical Outcomes Study 36-Item Short Form Health Survey was used, and the results of this questionnaire were compared with scores obtained from a cohort from the US general population. The questionnaire is a standard survey that measures health-related quality-of-life outcomes and measures each of eight health concepts (or domains) on a five-point Likert scale: physical functioning, role limitations due to physical disease, bodily pain, general health, vitality (energy and fatigue), social functioning, role limitations due to emotional problems, and mental health (psychological stress and psychological well-being). Scores for all but one of the health domains were significantly less in the study population than in the US general population. The lowest scores were in the physical functioning domain.

MANAGEMENT

Management of erythromelalgia is difficult. There are no randomized controlled studies of treatments for erythromelalgia, and no single treatment is effective in all cases. The literature is replete with case reports and small case series describing a response to one treatment or another. When a larger group of erythromelalgia patients was surveyed, the majority reported that no treatment was very effective. Various treatments used in the management of erythromelalgia have been reviewed.[67]

One algorithmic approach to the management of erythromelalgia is as follows:

1. General measures:
   a. Patient education regarding the condition
   b. Avoidance of factors that precipitate events
   c. Judicious use of factors to relieve pain during symptoms
   d. Patient support groups such as the Erythromelalgia Association
2. Topical medications:
   a. Lidocaine patches[68,69]
   b. Amitriptyline/ketamine[70]
   c. Midodrine[71]
   d. Botulinum toxin (local injection)[72]
3. Systemic medications (see later discussion)
4. Pain rehabilitation program[73]

Aspirin[3,74] has been reported to abolish erythromelalgia, especially in initial reports of the syndrome. It has become increasingly evident that aspirin may be effective in erythromelalgia due to myeloproliferative disease, but it is rarely effective in other forms of erythromelalgia.[8,75]

Increasingly, drugs acting on the nervous system are reported to be useful in inducing remission of disease or in controlling symptoms. These include selective serotonin reuptake inhibitors (SSRIs) such as venlafaxine and sertraline,[76,77] tricyclic antidepressants such as amitriptyline,[78] and anticonvulsants such as gabapentin.[79] IV lidocaine followed by oral mexiletine[80] induced remission in a patient with long-standing erythromelalgia. Mexiletine normalizes aberrant gating properties of the L858F gain-of-function mutation in Nav1.7.[81]

Benzodiazepines such as clonazepam are effective occasionally.[82] Sympathectomy and sympathetic nerve blocks have been reported to both relieve and exacerbate erythromelalgia.[16,83] Stereotactic thalamotomy,[84] ankle nerve crushing and neurectomy,[85] spinal cord stimulation[86] and lumbar sympathetic pulsed radiofrequency[87] have been reported to be helpful. Patient-controlled epidural analgesia and interferon α-2b provided relief of erythromelalgia symptoms in a patient with polycythemia vera.[88] Drugs acting on the vascular system (vasoactive drugs) may be effective. β-Blockers such as propranolol[89] and labetalol[27] have been reported to be successful in single cases. Calcium antagonists have been reported to both relieve and exacerbate erythromelalgia.[8,75] Various doses of magnesium have been reported to relieve symptoms.[90] Sodium nitroprusside infusions may be helpful in children with erythromelalgia,[91] but one adult experienced worsening of the disease with this medication.[75] Prostaglandin E_1 (PGE_1), a potent vasodilator and platelet inhibitor administered intravenously, has successfully induced remission.[9,25] Iloprost, a synthetic prostacyclin analog, improved patients' symptoms more than placebo did.[92] Use of ergot alkaloids, such as methysergide maleate, has been described in isolated case reports.[93] Low-molecular-weight heparin (LMWH) has been reported to exacerbate erythromelalgia.[94]

Control of pain is an extremely important factor in erythromelalgia. Anesthetics have been used, including topical lidocaine (lidocaine patch),[68] a combination of topical amitriptyline and ketamine,[70] and epidural infusion of narcotic analgesic medications such as bupivacaine, sometimes in combination with other narcotic drugs.[95] Narcotic analgesic drugs may be administered by various routes—oral, IV, intramuscular (IM), epidural, or intrathecal, alone or in combination with other drugs.

Pizotyline, a benzocycloheptathiophene derivative used primarily for migraine prophylaxis, has been used for erythromelalgia.[27]

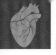

A retrospective cohort of 31 patients showed that a window of corticosteroid responsiveness may exist in patients with a traumatic, surgical, or infectious precipitant before permanent and irreversible nociceptive remodeling ensues.[96] Antihistamines such as cyproheptadine[96] have been reported to help, but many patients find them unhelpful. A single case report documented successful treatment with high-dose IV immunoglobulin.[97]

A combination of pharmacological interventions may be of benefit. Nonmedicinal therapies such as acupuncture, biofeedback, hypnosis, and magnets have been variably effective.[75,98]

Pain rehabilitation is a useful method for managing pain-related impairment in physical and emotional functioning in patients with severe forms of erythromelalgia.[73]

REFERENCES

1. Graves RJ. *Clinical lectures on the practice of medicine*. Dublin: Fannin; 1834.
2. Mitchell SW. On a rare vaso-motor neurosis of the extremities and on the maladies with which it may be confounded. *Am J Med Sci*. 1878;76:17.
3. Smith LA, Allen EV. Erythermalgia (erythromelalgia) of the extremities: a syndrome characterized by redness, heat, and pain. *Am Heart J*. 1938;16:175.
4. Housley E. What is erythromelalgia and how should it be treated? *BMJ*. 1986;293:117.
5. Lewis T. Clinical observations and experiments relating to burning pain in extremities and to so-called "erythromelalgia" in particular. *Clin Sci*. 1933;1:175.
6. Snapper I, Kahn AI. *Bedside Medicine*. ed 2. London: William Heinemann Medical Books; 1967:106.
7. Babb RR, Alarcon-Segovia D, Fairbairn 2nd JF. Erythermalgia. Review of 51 Cases. *Circulation*. 1964;29:136–141.
8. Davis MD, O'Fallon WM, Rogers 3rd RS, Rooke TW. Natural history of erythromelalgia: presentation and outcome in 168 patients. *Arch Dermatol*. 2000;136(3):330–336.
9. Kvernebo K. Erythromelalgia: a condition caused by microvascular arteriovenous shunting. *VASA J Vasc Dis Suppl*. 1998;51:1.
10. Mørk C, Kalgaard OM, Kvernebo K. Erythromelalgia: a clinical study of 102 cases (abstract). *Australas J Dermatol*. 1997;38(Suppl 2):50.
11. Kalgaard OM, Seem E, Kvernebo K. Erythromelalgia: a clinical study of 87 cases. *J Intern Med*. 1997;242(3):191–197.
12. Levesque H. Classification of erythermalgia. *J Mal Vasc*. 1996;21(2):80–83.
13. Mørk C, Kvernebo K. Erythromelalgia—a mysterious condition? *Arch Dermatol*. 2000;136(3):406–409.
14. Michiels JJ, Drenth JP, Van Genderen PJ. Classification and diagnosis of erythromelalgia and erythermalgia. *Int J Dermatol*. 1995;34(2):97–100.
15. Zoppi M, Zamponi A, Pagni E, Buoncristiano U. A way to understand erythromelalgia. *J Auton Nerv Syst*. 1985;13(1):85–89.
16. Regli F. Facial neuralgia and vascular facial pain. *Praxis*. 1969;58(7):210–215.
17. Brown GE. Erythromelalgia and other disturbances of the extremities accompanied by vasodilatation and burning. *Am J Med Sci*. 1932;183:468.
18. Thompson GH, Hahn G, Rang M. Erythromelalgia. *Clin Orthop Relat Res*. 1979;(144):249–254.
19. Mørk C, Asker CL, Salerud EG, Kvernebo K. Microvascular arteriovenous shunting is a probable pathogenetic mechanism in erythromelalgia. *J Invest Dermatol*. 2000;114(4):643–646.
20. Lazareth I, Fiessinger JN, Priollet P. Erythermalgia, rare acrosyndrome. 13 cases. *Presse Med*. 1988;17(42):2235–2239.
21. Drenth JP, Michiels JJ. Erythromelalgia and erythermalgia: diagnostic differentiation. *Int J Dermatol*. 1994;33(6):393–397.
22. Drenth JP, Michiels JJ. Erythromelalgia versus primary and secondary erythermalgia. *Angiology*. 1994;45(4):329–331.
23. Drenth JP, Michiels JJ, van Joost T. Primary and secondary erythermalgia. *Ned Tijdschr Geneeskd*. 1994;138(45):2231–2234.
24. Drenth JP, van Genderen PJ, Michiels JJ. Thrombocythemic erythromelalgia, primary erythermalgia, and secondary erythermalgia: three distinct clinicopathologic entities. *Angiology*. 1994;45(6):451–453.
25. Littleford RC, Khan F, Belch JJ. Skin perfusion in patients with erythromelalgia. *Eur J Clin Invest*. 1999;29(7):588–593.
26. Cook-Norris RH, Tollefson MM, Cruz-Inigo AE, et al. Pediatric erythromelalgia: a retrospective review of 32 cases evaluated at Mayo Clinic over a 37-year period. *J Am Acad Dermatol*. 2012;66(3):416–423.
27. Drenth JP, Michiels JJ, Ozsoylu S. Acute secondary erythermalgia and hypertension in children. Erythermalgia Multidisciplinary Study Group. *Eur J Pediatr*. 1995;154(11):882–885.
28. Michiels JJ, ten Kate FJ. Erythromelalgia in thrombocythemia of various myeloproliferative disorders. *Am J Hematol*. 1992;39(2):131–136.
29. McCarthy L, Eichelberger L, Skipworth E, Danielson C. Erythromelalgia due to essential thrombocythemia. *Transfusion*. 2002;42(10):1245.
30. Reed KB, Davis MD. Incidence of erythromelalgia: a population-based study in Olmsted County. *Minnesota J Eur Acad Dermatol Venereol*. 2009;23(1):13–15.
31. Schechner J. Red skin re-read. *J Invest Dermatol*. 2002;119(4):781–782.
32. Davis MD, Sandroni P, Rooke TW, Low PA. Erythromelalgia: vasculopathy, neuropathy, or both? A prospective study of vascular and neurophysiologic studies in erythromelalgia. *Arch Dermatol*. 2003;139(10):1337–1343.
33. Sandroni P, Davis MD, Harper CM, et al. Neurophysiologic and vascular studies in erythromelalgia: a retrospective analysis. *J Clin Neuromuscul Dis*. 1999;1(2):57–63.
34. Charkoudian N. Skin blood flow in adult human thermoregulation: how it works, when it does not, and why. *Mayo Clin Proc*. 2003;78(5):603–612.
35. Mørk C, Kvernebo K, Asker CL, Salerud EG. Reduced skin capillary density during attacks of erythromelalgia implies arteriovenous shunting as pathogenetic mechanism. *J Invest Dermatol*. 2002;119(4):949–953.
36. Lazareth I, Priollet P. Coexistence of Raynaud's syndrome and erythromelalgia. *Lancet*. 1990;335(8700):1286.
37. Davis MD, Genebriera J, Sandroni P, Fealey RD. Thermoregulatory sweat testing in patients with erythromelalgia. *Arch Dermatol*. 2006;142(12):1583–1588.
38. Davis MD, Rooke TW, Sandroni P. Mechanisms other than shunting are likely contributing to the pathophysiology of erythromelalgia. *J Invest Dermatol*. 2000;115(6):1166–1167.
39. Liu Y. A study of erythromelalgia in relation to the autonomic nervous system. Report of 321 cases of functional disorders of the autonomic nervous system. *Zhonghua Shen Jing Jing Shen Ke Za Zhi*. 1990;23(1):47–48. 64.
40. Ørstavik K, Weidner C, Schmidt R, et al. Pathological C-fibres in patients with a chronic painful condition. *Brain*. 2003;126(Pt 3):567–578.
41. Uno H, Parker F. Autonomic innervation of the skin in primary erythermalgia. *Arch Dermatol*. 1983;119(1):65–71.
42. Layzer RB. Hot feet: erythromelalgia and related disorders. *J Child Neurol*. 2001;16(3):199–202.
43. Kazemi B, Shooshtari SM, Nasab MR, et al. Sympathetic skin response (SSR) in erythromelalgia. *Electromyogr Clin Neurophysiol*. 2003;43(3):165–168.
44. Littleford RC, Khan F, Belch JJ. Impaired skin vasomotor reflexes in patients with erythromelalgia. *Clin Sci (Lond)*. 1999;96(5):507–512.
45. Drenth JP, Finley WH, Breedveld GJ, et al. The primary erythermalgia-susceptibility gene is located on chromosome 2q31-32. *Am J Hum Genet*. 2001;68(5):1277–1282.
46. Yang Y, Wang Y, Li S, et al. Mutations in SCN9A, encoding a sodium channel alpha subunit, in patients with primary erythermalgia. *J Med Genet*. 2004;41(3):171–174.
47. Cummins TR, Dib-Hajj SD, Waxman SG. Electrophysiological properties of mutant Nav1.7 sodium channels in a painful inherited neuropathy. *J Neurosci*. 2004;24(38):8232–8236.
48. Michiels JJ, te Morsche RH, Jansen JB, Drenth JP. Autosomal dominant erythermalgia associated with a novel mutation in the voltage-gated sodium channel alpha subunit Nav1.7. *Arch Neurol*. 2005;62(10):1587–1590.
49. Han C, Dib-Hajj SD, Lin Z, et al. Early- and late-onset inherited erythromelalgia: genotype-phenotype correlation. *Brain*. 2009;132(Pt 7):1711–1722.
50. Estacion M, Waxman SG, Dib-Hajj SD. Effects of ranolazine on wild-type and mutant hNav1.7 channels and on DRG neuron excitability. *Mol Pain*. 2010;6:35.

51. Waxman SG, Dib-Hajj S. Erythermalgia: molecular basis for an inherited pain syndrome. *Trends Mol Med*. 2005;11(12):555–562.

52. Bennett DL, Woods CG. Painful and painless channelopathies. *Lancet Neurol*. 2014;13(6):587–599.

53. Helås T, Sagafos D, Kleggetveit IP, et al. Pain thresholds, supra-threshold pain and lidocaine sensitivity in patients with erythromelalgia, including the I848Tmutation in NaV 1.7. *Eur J Pain*. 2017;21(8):1316–1325.

54. Alexandrou AJ, Brown AR, Chapman ML, et al. Subtype-selective small molecule inhibitors reveal a fundamental role for Nav1.7 in nociceptor electrogenesis, axonal conduction and presynaptic release. *PLoS One*. 2016;11(4):e0152405.

55. Duchatelet S, Guibbal L, de Veer S, et al. Olmsted syndrome with erythromelalgia caused by recessive transient receptor potential vanilloid 3 mutations. *Br J Dermatol*. 2014;171(3):675–678.

56. Duchatelet S, Pruvost S, de Veer S, et al. A new TRPV3 missense mutation in a patient with Olmsted syndrome and erythromelalgia. *JAMA Dermatol*. 2014;150(3):303–306.

57. Drenth JP, Te Morsche RH, Mansour S, Mortimer PS. Primary erythermalgia as a sodium channelopathy: screening for SCN9A mutations: exclusion of a causal role of SCN10A and SCN11A. *Arch Dermatol*. 2008;144(3):320–324.

58. van Genderen PJ, Lucas IS, van Strik R, et al. Erythromelalgia in essential thrombocythemia is characterized by platelet activation and endothelial cell damage but not by thrombin generation. *Thromb Haemost*. 1996;76(3):333–338.

59. Kurzrock R, Cohen PR. Erythromelalgia: review of clinical characteristics and pathophysiology. *Am J Med*. 1991;91(4):416–422.

60. Drenth JP, Vuzevski V, Van Joost T, et al. Cutaneous pathology in primary erythermalgia. *Am J Dermatopathol*. 1996;18(1):30–34.

61. Michiels JJ, ten Kate FW, Vuzevski VD, Abels J. Histopathology of erythromelalgia in thrombocythaemia. *Histopathology*. 1984;8(4):669–678.

62. Croue A, Gardembas-Pain M, Verret JL, et al. Histopathologic lesions in erythromelalgia during essential thrombocythemia. *Ann Pathol*. 1993;13(2):128–130.

63. Drenth JP, Michiels JJ, Van Joost T, Vuzevski VD. Verapamil-induced secondary erythermalgia. *Br J Dermatol*. 1992;127(3):292–294.

64. Blake T, Mortimore R, De Ambrosis K. A case of secondary erythromelalgia with perivascular and intramural mucin. *Australas J Dermatol*. 2016;57(1):e26–e28.

65. Bakkour W, Motta L, Stewart E. A case of secondary erythromelalgia with unusual histological findings. *Am J Dermatopathol*. 2013;35(4):489–490.

66. Mantyh WG, Dyck PJ, Dyck PJ, et al. Epidermal nerve fiber quantification in patients with erythromelalgia. *JAMA Dermatol*. 2016. [Epub ahead of print].

67. Davis MD, Rooke T. Erythromelalgia. *Curr Treat Options Cardiovasc Med*. 2002;4(3):207–222.

68. Davis MD, Sandroni P. Lidocaine patch for pain of erythromelalgia. *Arch Dermatol*. 2002;138(1):17–19.

69. Davis MD, Sandroni P. Lidocaine patch for pain of erythromelalgia: follow-up of 34 patients. *Arch Dermatol*. 2005;141(10):1320–1321.

70. Sandroni P, Davis MD. Combination gel of 1% amitriptyline and 0.5% ketamine to treat refractory erythromelalgia pain: a new treatment option? *Arch Dermatol*. 2006;142(3):283–286.

71. Davis MD, Morr CS, Warndahl RA, Sandroni P. Topically applied midodrine, 0.2%, an alpha1-agonist, for the treatment of erythromelalgia. *JAMA Dermatol*. 2015;151(9):1025–1026.

72. da Costa AF, Meireles J, Festas MJ, et al. Therapeutic success with local botulinum toxin in erythromelalgia. *Pain Physician*. 2014;17(5):E658–E660.

73. Durosaro O, Davis MD, Hooten WM, Kerkvliet JL. Intervention for erythromelalgia, a chronic pain syndrome: comprehensive pain rehabilitation center. *Mayo Clinic Arch Dermatol*. 2008;144(12):1578–1583.

74. Naldi L, Brevi A, Cavalieri d'Oro L, et al. Painful distal erythema and thrombocytosis. Erythromelalgia secondary to thrombocytosis. *Arch Dermatol*. 1993;129(1):105–106, 109.

75. Cohen JS. Erythromelalgia: new theories and new therapies. *J Am Acad Dermatol*. 2000;43(5 Pt 1):841–847.

76. Moiin A, Yashar SS, Sanchez JE, Yashar B. Treatment of erythromelalgia with a serotonin–noradrenaline reuptake inhibitor. *Br J Dermatol*. 2002;146(2):336–337.

77. Rudikoff D, Jaffe IA. Erythromelalgia: response to serotonin reuptake inhibitors. *J Am Acad Dermatol*. 1997;37(2 Pt 1):281–283.

78. Herskovitz S, Loh F, Berger AR, Kucherov M. Erythromelalgia: association with hereditary sensory neuropathy and response to amitriptyline. *Neurology*. 1993;43(3 Pt 1):621–622.

79. McGraw T, Kosek P. Erythromelalgia pain managed with gabapentin. *Anesthesiology*. 1997;86(4):988–990.

80. Kuhnert SM, Phillips WJ, Davis MD. Lidocaine and mexiletine therapy for erythromelalgia. *Arch Dermatol*. 1999;135(12):1447–1449.

81. Cregg R, Cox JJ, Bennett DL, et al. Mexiletine as a treatment for primary erythromelalgia: normalization of biophysical properties of mutant L858F NaV 1.7 sodium channels. *Br J Pharmacol*. 2014;171(19):4455–4463.

82. Kraus A. Erythromelalgia in a patient with systemic lupus erythematosus treated with clonazepam. *J Rheumatol*. 1990;17(1):120.

83. Seishima M, Kanoh H, Izumi T, et al. A refractory case of secondary erythermalgia successfully treated with lumbar sympathetic ganglion block. *Br J Dermatol*. 2000;143(4):868–872.

84. Kandel EI. Stereotactic surgery of erythromelalgia. *Stereotact Funct Neurosurg*. 1990;54-55:96–100.

85. Sadighi PJ, Arbid EJ. Neurectomy for palliation of primary erythermalgia. *Ann Vasc Surg*. 1995;9(2):197–198.

86. Graziotti PJ, Goucke CR. Control of intractable pain in erythromelalgia by using spinal cord stimulation. *J Pain Symptom Manage*. 1993;8(7):502–504.

87. Lee JY, Sim WS, Kang RA, et al. Lumbar sympathetic pulsed radiofrequency treatment for primary erythromelalgia: a case report. *Pediatr Dermatol*. 2017;34(1):e47–e50.

88. Li X, Li Y, Qu Y, Lu L. Secondary erythromelalgia successfully treated with patient-controlled epidural analgesia and interferon alpha-2b: a case report and review of the literature. *Exp Ther Med*. 2016;11(5):1823–1826.

89. Bada JL. Treatment of erythromelalgia with propranolol. *Lancet*. 1977;2(8034):412.

90. Cohen JS. High-dose oral magnesium treatment of chronic, intractable erythromelalgia. *Ann Pharmacother*. 2002;36(2):255–260.

91. Stone JD, Rivey MP, Allington DR. Nitroprusside treatment of erythromelalgia in an adolescent female. *Ann Pharmacother*. 1997;31(5):590–592.

92. Kalgaard OM, Mørk C, Kvernebo K. Prostacyclin reduces symptoms and sympathetic dysfunction in erythromelalgia in a double-blind randomized pilot study. *Acta Derm Venereol*. 2003;83(6):442–444.

93. Vendrell J, Nubiola A, Goday A, et al. Erythromelalgia associated with acute diabetic neuropathy: an unusual condition. *Diabetes Res*. 1988;7(3):149–151.

94. Conri CL, Azoulai P, Constans J, et al. Erythromelalgia and low molecular weight heparin. *Therapie*. 1994;49(6):518–519.

95. Stricker LJ, Green CR. Resolution of refractory symptoms of secondary erythermalgia with intermittent epidural bupivacaine. *Reg Anesth Pain Med*. 2001;26(5):488–490.

96. Pagani-Estévez GL, Sandroni P, Davis MD, Watson JC. Erythromelalgia: identification of a corticosteroid-responsive subset. *J Am Acad Dermatol*. 2017;76(3):506–511. e1.

97. Kuroda T, Sugimoto A, Ishigaki S, et al. A case of primary erythromelalgia successfully treated with high-dose intravenous immunoglobulin therapy. *Brain Nerve*. 2014;66(2):185–189.

98. Chakravarty K, Pharoah PD, Scott DG, Barker S. Erythromelalgia—the role of hypnotherapy. *Postgrad Med J*. 1992;68(795):44–46.

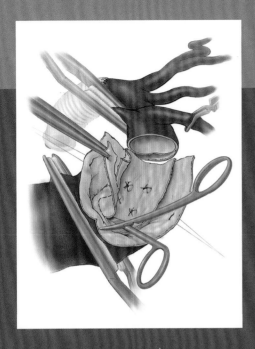

第49章
冻 疮

冻疮是一种由寒冷引起的局部炎症性疾病，主要表现为未受保护的肢端区域的皮肤损伤，通常出现在手指和脚趾的近节指骨背侧。1894年，由Corlett首次描述冻疮的临床特征，他将其称为冻疮性皮炎。冻疮在年轻女性中较常见，但在所有年龄段及性别都有报道，主要出现在潮湿、寒冷气候的地区。但随着生活、工作环境的供暖改善，这种疾病逐渐减少。冻疮的病理基础是机体对冷刺激的第一反应，实际是真皮和皮下组织的血管收缩。通过关闭远端毛细血管床和减少四肢肢端部分的血液供应以维持中心体温，可以最大限度地减少热量损失。病理继发于小动脉收缩、小静脉松弛和与寒冷相关的血液黏度增加，血流从浅表血管流出的停滞和分流，这些变化的结果是表面组织缺氧和缺血。

冻疮病变通常发生于脚趾的肢端区域和近端的背侧指骨，但也可能涉及鼻子、耳朵和大腿。询问病史和体格检查是正确诊断冻疮的主要手段，因寒冷发作，天气转暖后症状减轻，提示冻疮诊断。冻疮发生的主要诱因是冷暴露，预防是关键，需保证居住及工作环境的温暖，着装也要充分保暖。二氢吡啶类钙通道阻滞剂被认为对治疗冻疮有效果，建议可局部涂抹硝苯地平乳膏，其他药物如硝酸甘油、己酮可可碱、羟氯喹可能有效，交感神经切除术可增强活动性病变的解决并改善主观感受，但不能防止复发。

陈海生

Pernio (Chilblains)

Jeffrey W. Olin

Pernio, commonly known as *chilblains*, is a cold-induced localized inflammatory condition presenting as skin lesions predominantly on unprotected acral areas. Typically there is swelling of the dorsa of the proximal phalanges of fingers and toes (Fig. 49.1). *Pernio* is a Latin term meaning "frostbite." *Chilblains* is an Anglo-Saxon term used in older literature and means "cold sore." The tissue and vascular damage is less severe in pernio than in frostbite, in which the skin is actually frozen. The numerous names that were used to describe this syndrome created much confusion and misunderstanding of this entity (Box 49.1).[1] In the mid-1800s, there were attempts to better classify the disease[2] and in 1894, Corlett was the first to describe the clinical characteristics of pernio, which he called *dermatitis hiemalis*.

EPIDEMIOLOGY

The first epidemiological study to explicate the prevalence of chilblains and its impact on productivity in servicewomen was carried out in 1942 by the US Medical Department of the War Office.[3] The study concluded that at least 50% of questionnaire participants had chilblains by age 40 during World War II (1939-1943). Although pernio is most common in young women, it has also been reported in all ages and both sexes.[4-8] The number of reported cases of pernio is higher during times of wet near-freezing weather, and less common in dry freezing weather or in a bitterly cold climate.[9] Pernio is most commonly encountered in the northern and western parts of the United States; isolated cases have been reported in warmer climates in times of cooler damp weather.[5,10,11]

As shown in a cross-sectional study conducted by the US Army, the yearly rate of cold weather injuries declined from 38.2/100,000 in 1985 to 0.2/100,000 in 1999.[12] This and other observations from clinical practice suggest that the disease is becoming less common with higher standards of home and workplace heating and greater use of appropriate clothing during the cold winter months.

PATHOPHYSIOLOGY

The first response to cold exposure is vasoconstriction in the dermis and subcutaneous tissue. Heat loss is minimized by shutting down distal capillary beds and diminishing blood supply to the acral portions of the extremities to maintain central body temperature. Stasis and shunting of blood flow away from the superficial vessels occurs secondary to arteriolar constriction, venular relaxation, and cold-associated increased blood viscosity. The result of these changes is superficial tissue anoxia and ischemia.[9,13-15] The arteriolar vasoconstriction described in pernio has been demonstrated in pathological and radiographic studies.[5] Female predominance may be related to increased responsiveness of their cutaneous circulation to cold. Indeed, there is a higher frequency of vasomotor instability, cold hands and feet, and Raynaud phenomenon in women.[6,8,15-17]

Humidity has an important role in the pathophysiology of pernio because it enhances air conductivity, promoting heat loss from the skin.[6,8] Most individuals tolerate exposure to nonfreezing damp cold, but others may experience pernio, Raynaud phenomenon, acrocyanosis, or cold urticaria.[6,17] The clinical manifestations of cold injuries are related to duration, severity, and dampness of cold exposure as well as the individual's underlying predisposition to cold injury and the stage at which medical attention was sought. The exposed skin of affected subjects remains cool longer and warms slower than that of controls, further highlighting the importance of individual susceptibility for development of pernio after cold exposure.[5,6,18] The increased incidence of pernio among relatives of affected patients suggests the possibility of genetic or familial predisposition.[3,19-23] Several other conditions have been proposed to promote vulnerability to the disease (Box 49.2).[7]

Why one patient exposed to cold develops Raynaud phenomenon and another pernio is unclear. Raynaud phenomenon and pernio frequently coexist in the same patient, so these diseases may be part of a continuum, with Raynaud phenomenon representing acute and readily reversible vasospasm, and pernio representing more prolonged vasospasm with more chronic changes.[6,18]

A number of conditions have been associated with pernio. Weston and Morelli reported the presence of cryoproteins in four of eight children presenting with pernio.[10,15,24-26] Since cryoproteins and cold agglutinins may be detected transiently after viral infections, they hypothesized that exposure to cold wet weather during the brief cryoproteinemia may lead to exaggerated tissue injury manifesting as pernio. In a large series reported from the Mayo Clinic, 11 of 20 patients (55%) tested for cold agglutinins were positive.[8] Pernio has been described both in women with large amounts of leg fat and in women with inadequate fat pads, as seen in anorexia nervosa.[6] The possibility that pernio may be a manifestation of a pre-leukemic state, namely the chronic myelomonocytic type, or a presenting feature of lymphoblastic leukemia has been suggested in several reports.[4,25,27]

Viguier and colleagues reported observations over 38 months in a cohort of 33 patients with severe chilblains, defined as duration of lesions greater than 1 month.[28] Two-thirds of the patients had clinical and/or laboratory features supporting a diagnosis of connective tissue disorders: 12 patients had systemic lupus erythematosus (SLE) and 10 patients presented with at least one of the American College of Rheumatology revised criteria for SLE at the time of the diagnosis of pernio. In the latter group, all patients except one had positive antinuclear antibody (ANA) titers. These observations led the authors to conclude that when the lesions persist beyond the cold season, perniotic

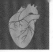

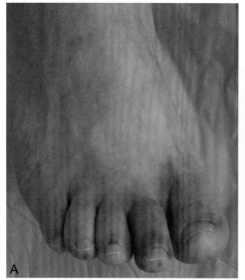
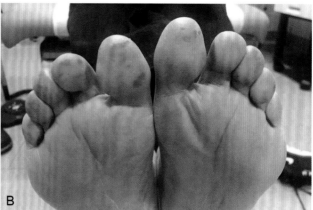

Fig. 49.1 Typical changes of pernio on dorsal portion (A) and pads of toes (B). Distribution around nail beds (A) and swollen toes with brownish yellow and red lesions (B) are characteristic of pernio. At this stage, affected extremities often itch and burn.

BOX 49.1   Different Names Used in the Literature to Describe Pernio or Pernio-Like Conditions

Pernio
Chilblains
Nodular vasculitis
Erythrocyanosis
Erythrocyanose sur malléolair
Erythema induratum
Lupus pernio
Kibes
Perniosis
Dermatitis hiemalis
Frostschaden
Erythrocyanosis frigida
Erythrocyanosis crurum puellaris
Bazin disease
L'engelune
Cold panniculitis

BOX 49.2   Categories of Diseases Associated with Pernio

Defective Cutaneous Vasomotor Reactivity
Raynaud phenomenon
Acrocyanosis
Complex regional pain syndrome (reflex sympathetic dystrophy [RSD])
Anterior poliomyelitis
Syringomyelia
Livedo reticularis
Erythromelalgia

Underlying Chronic Limb Ischemia
Peripheral artery disease (PAD)

Hyperviscosity Syndrome
Dysproteinemia (cryoproteins)

Abnormal Fat Distribution
Obesity with excess leg fat
Inadequate fat pads (anorexia nervosa)

Other
Leukemia
Systemic lupus erythematosus (SLE)

---

lesions may be a clue to underlying SLE. Therefore, targeted laboratory investigations to search for conditions listed in Box 49.2, as well as long-term follow-up, are recommended for patients who present with pernio.[7,29]

HISTOPATHOLOGY

Although not routinely required to establish the diagnosis, biopsies are occasionally sought by healthcare providers unfamiliar with the disease.[30–32] The histopathological features of perniotic lesions may vary depending upon the chronological stage of the disease and presence or absence of superimposed secondary pathology such as infection or ulceration.[31–33] The characteristic histopathological features of pernio are usually seen in the dermis and subcutaneous tissue, but are not pathognomonic. These consist of edema of the papillodermis, vasculitis

characterized by perivascular infiltration of the arterioles and venules of the dermis and subcutaneous fat by mononuclear and lymphocytic cells, thickening and edema of blood vessel walls, fat necrosis, and chronic inflammatory reaction with giant cell formation.[6] Not all these changes are necessarily present, and fat necrosis and giant cell formation are frequently absent. The most consistent feature is perivascular lymphocytic or mononuclear infiltrates.[31]

Repeated episodes of vasospasm or prolonged vasospasm may cause tissue anoxia, thus causing the identical histopathological picture that occurs in pernio.[1,15] The histological pattern of pernio lesions may mimic cutaneous vasculitis but typically lacks fibrinoid deposition, inflammatory

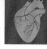

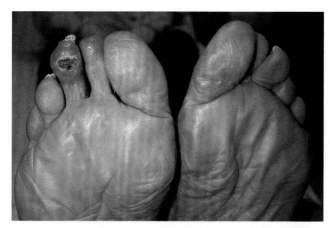

Fig. 49.2 Advanced Stage of Pernio. Toes are cyanotic, and there is a shallow ulcer on right third toe. This stage of pernio is often quite painful and may be mistaken for atheromatous embolization in the elderly patient.

cells in the vessel wall, and thrombosis, typical of true vasculitis.[4,5,30,32–34] Blood vessels in long-standing pernio resemble those of any chronic occlusive vascular disease. The occlusion and fibrosis present are due to long-standing injury; this histopathological appearance may be seen in many other types of vascular disease. When this occurs, the seasonal variation disappears and the patient may have ischemic lesions year round.

Review of published case series and case reports support the notion that pernio may display different and loosely related histological features.[33] Cribier and associates retrospectively compared the biopsies of hand lesions from 17 patients with chilblains to those of 10 patients with proven SLE and associated pernio-like hand lesions.[30] The study included only acute lesions (<1 month duration) occurring during the cold period of the year. The most characteristic finding in chilblains (47% of cases) was the association of edema and reticular dermis infiltrate that showed a periecrine reinforcement: dermal edema (70% of chilblains lesions vs. 20% of SLE lesions), superficial (papillary) and deep (reticular) infiltrate (82% vs. 80%), and deep periecrine reinforcement (76% vs. 0%). The infiltrate was composed primarily of T cells, which were predominantly CD3+. Remarkably, 29% of the chilblain lesions in this group showed evidence of microthrombi (compared to 10% in the lupus group), usually a feature seen in vasculitis, and 6% had conspicuous vacuolation (compared to 60% in the lupus group).

In another study, Viguier et al. prospectively studied 33 patients with severe prolonged chilblains (i.e., lesions persisted >1 month) and attempted to differentiate the histopathological characteristics of lesions of "idiopathic" pernio from those of pernio-like lesions in patients with connective tissue diseases or lupus pernio.[28] Skin punch biopsies were performed on 5 of 11 patients of the "idiopathic" pernio group, and these showed deep dermal, perisudoral lymphocytic infiltrate (100%), dermal edema (75%), keratinocyte necrosis (62.5%), and keratinocyte vacuolization (50%). In comparison, biopsies from 7 of the 12 patients with the diagnosis of SLE (LE chilblain) demonstrated perisudoral cellular infiltrate in only two patients (vs. 8/8 in the "idiopathic" chilblains group; P = .007). Biopsy is rarely needed to make the diagnosis of pernio, but a biopsy may be helpful in differentiating atheromatous embolization from pernio in an ischemic-looking lesion (Fig. 49.2).

CLINICAL FEATURES

Pernio most commonly affects females in adolescence and early adulthood, but may occur at any age and in either sex. The lesions typically affect the acral areas of the toes and the dorsa of the proximal

phalanges but may involve the nose, ears, and thighs (Fig. 49.3).[1–3,8,28,35–39] Generally, the most common location of the lesions are on the toes. Hands and fingers appear more commonly affected in milkers and gardeners, the buttocks have been involved in women driving tractors in winter, and involvement of the lateral thighs have been described in women who wear thin pants and ride horses or motorcycles in winter.[17,35,40–43] There was a report of perniotic lesions on the hips of young girls wearing tight-fitting jeans with a low waistband.[44] Facial lesions have been described in infants and rarely in adults.[28,43,44]

Typically the initial presentation is one of *acute pernio*, where the lesions appear during the cold months and disappear when the weather warms up. This may recur for several years and follows a similar seasonal pattern.[6] Lesions vary in shape, number, and size and usually are associated with functional symptoms such as itching, burning, or pain. They can be described as brownish, yellow, or cyanotic on a base of doughy subcutaneous swelling or erythema (see Figs. 49.1 and 49.3). They may be cool to the touch or cooler than surrounding skin. Acute lesions may be self-limited and resolve within a few days to a few weeks (especially in children) unless cold exposure persists, the lesions become infected, or the skin is broken by iatrogenic causes such as self-treatment with severe heat or vigorous massage.[39,45] Otherwise, ulceration is not common in acute pernio, and when it happens, the lesions are usually shallow with a hemorrhagic base (see Figs. 49.2 and 49.3B).[6]

Chronic pernio ensues if repeated and prolonged exposure to cold persists throughout the acute phase and/or the patient goes through several seasons of acute pernio. The lesions of chronic pernio are similar to those seen in acute pernio but, if they occur over many seasons, may be associated with scarring, atrophy, permanent discoloration, and possibly ulceration (see Fig. 49.2). Initially, pernio may start late in the fall or early winter and resolve in early spring. If left untreated, the lesions of pernio may start earlier in the cold season and resolve later, until eventually all seasonal variation is lost.

Pernio tends to be more severe in adults and may, if left untreated, eventually cause macrovascular occlusive disease.[5,6] Children, on the other hand, tend to have recurrent acute pernio over several seasons.[39] Although most children outgrow the disease, middle-aged individuals presenting with pernio may occasionally recall a history of acute pernio during childhood. Several different forms of pernio have been described.

Milker pernio usually affects the hands and could be debilitating and force the affected individual to quit milking (Fig. 49.4).[42] *Kibe* is defined as a chapped or inflamed area on the skin, especially on the heel, resulting from exposure to cold or an ulcerated chilblain.[46] This has been described in overweight women who ride horses and wear tight pants, in women who ride motorcycles and wear thin pants, and in men who cross cold rivers with their thighs inadequately clothed.[17,43] Lesions tend to localize on the outer thighs and often cause severe pain and disability. The pain may last up to a week and usually resolves once the lesions heal.[17] A similar form has been described in women who drive tractors in winter, who tend to have lesions on the buttocks.

Lupus pernio applies to papular lesions involving the extremities and is associated with SLE.[47] Whether this is a subtype of pernio or a pernio-like lupus manifestation remains controversial. Some authors suggested that most lupus pernio patients have lesions on the hands, but this anatomical localization was not a differentiating factor between idiopathic pernio and lupus pernio according to others.[6,28,29] Features that suggest pernio secondary to SLE include onset of pernio during the third decade, female sex, African origin, and presence of pernio long after the cold weather has abated.

Erythrocyanosis affects adolescent girls and young women and typically involves the lower extremities. Some have classified this as the "nodular chronic form" of pernio; lesions take on a swollen, dusky red appearance.[6]

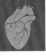

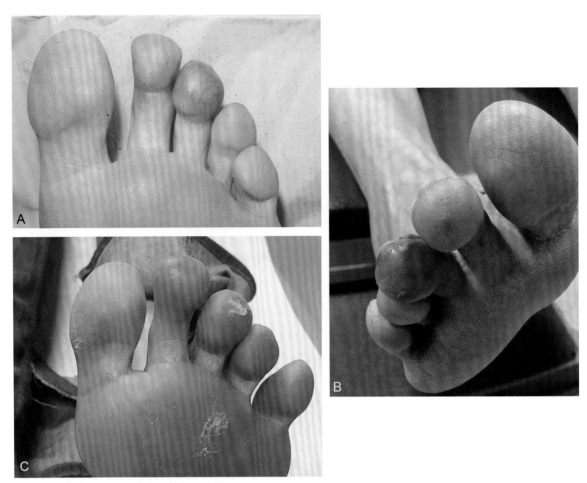

Fig. 49.3 Characteristic bulbous swelling brownish red appearance of left (A) and right (B) third toe. Flaking (C), itching, burning, and pain are common.

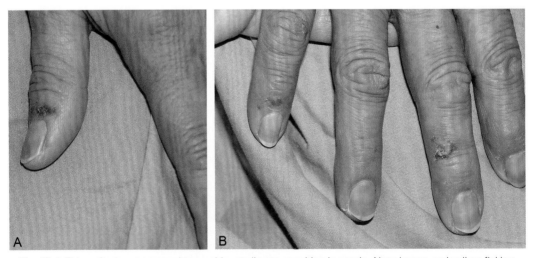

Fig. 49.4 This patient was exposed to a cold wet climate, resulting in pernio. Note brown and yellow flaking lesion on thumb (A) and healing lesions on index and ring fingers (B).

DIAGNOSIS

Pernio usually is not difficult to diagnose. A comprehensive history and complete physical exam are the primary means by which the diagnosis of pernio can be correctly established. Chronological correlation between nonfreezing cold and onset of typical lesions that improve with onset of warm weather should strongly suggest the diagnosis.

Within hours of exposure to damp cold, and commonly at the onset of winter, the patient develops violet or yellow blisters, brown plaques, or shallow ulcers on the toes, which often burn, itch, or become painful (see Figs. 49.1 and 49.3). These lesions typically disappear when the weather warms up at the beginning of spring. However, in some chronic cases in which the lesions do not disappear in warm weather, or in which the lesions cause severe pigmentation and disfiguration of the lower part of the leg, the diagnosis may be more difficult.

The main obstacle to establishing the diagnosis of pernio is unfamiliarity of the healthcare provider with the disease. Since many of the dermatological manifestations associated with pernio overlap with other serious diseases, it is not uncommon for pernio patients to be subjected to unnecessary investigations and suffer needless delay in proper treatment.[4,45,48] Characteristically, peripheral pulses and peripheral blood pressure measurements are normal unless the patient has underlying peripheral artery disease (PAD) or the pernio has been of such long duration that chronic occlusive vascular disease has developed.[5] Pulse volume recordings (PVR) and segmental blood pressures may be abnormal in patients with pernio if there is vasospasm (the study will normalize with warming of the extremity) or fixed vascular disease has occurred due to long-standing pernio. Because the diagnosis of pernio is a clinical diagnosis, sophisticated laboratory tests are often not needed, but it is important to rule out other entities that can mimic pernio. The following tests may be obtained: complete blood cell count (CBC) with differential, ANA titer, rheumatoid factor (RF), comprehensive metabolic panel, cryoglobulin, cryofibrinogen, cold agglutinin, and serum viscosity measurements.[7] Arteriography and skin biopsy are not warranted to establish the diagnosis of pernio, except in the occasional case where a clear history could not be obtained or a concomitant vascular pathology (e.g., atheromatous embolization) is suspected.[49]

The differential diagnosis of pernio includes a variety of diseases. Atheromatous emboli (blue toe syndrome) is the most challenging diagnostic entity to differentiate from pernio because similar lesions may be present in each disorder (see Chapter 45). When the history of cold exposure is uncertain and in patients with established or suspected atherosclerosis, imaging studies often are warranted to demonstrate atheroma in the aorta or iliac vessels. A biopsy of these lesions showing characteristic cholesterol clefts establishes the diagnosis of atheromatous emboli.[49] The next group of diseases that may be confused with pernio include those with chronic recurrent erythematous, nodular, and ulcerative lesions: erythema induratum, nodular vasculitis, erythema nodosum, and cold panniculitis. Erythema induratum (Bazin disease) is often but not always a cutaneous form of tuberculosis that affects adolescent girls and is manifested by nodular ulcerating lesions of the calves.[50] Nontuberculous forms of recurrent painful nodules are called *nodular vasculitis*.[50] Women over the age of 30 years are usually affected, and no apparent cause is known. Although the nodules of nodular vasculitis are extremely painful, they rarely ulcerate. Erythema nodosum may be differentiated from pernio in that it may be associated with fever, arthralgias, malaise, and an underlying disease. The lesions are painful and generally do not ulcerate. Cold panniculitis is another important entity characterized by painful nodules that appear on the skin after cold exposure and can be reproduced by application of an ice cube. The histology of these lesions reveals fat necrosis.[51] The palpable purpuric lesion sometimes present in pernio must be differentiated from other types of vasculitis, especially leukocytoclastic vasculitis. Lack of the systemic manifestations and laboratory abnormalities that occur in leukocytoclastic vasculitis and the relation of the lesions to cold exposure in pernio serve to separate these two conditions. Rarely, a skin biopsy may be needed to make a definitive diagnosis.

TREATMENT

Since the primary trigger for development of pernio is cold exposure, prevention is the mainstay of management. Working in a damp cold basement or living in a poorly heated apartment may necessitate change of profession or moving to a properly heated residence. Patients do not always volunteer information about the climate of their residence and workplace, so the physician may need to ask specifically about the quality of heating systems and the degree of humidity present. The patient should be instructed on methods of proper dress. Adequate body insulation with gloves, stockings, footwear, and headwear may be needed. As is the case in the treatment of Raynaud phenomenon, the entire body must be kept warm. A dihydropyridine calcium channel blocker, such as nifedipine, may be quite effective in patients with pernio. In a double-blind placebo-controlled randomized crossover pilot study, Dowd et al. reported that treatment with 20 mg of short-acting nifedipine three times daily, when given shortly after the appearance of lesions, led to resolution of the lesions within 7 to 10 days, compared to 20 to 28 days with placebo. In addition, the pain disappeared within 5 days in the treated group, compared to 20 to 25 days in the group receiving placebo.[20] In a double-blind placebo-controlled randomized trial, Rustin et al. have shown that nifedipine given at a daily dose of 20 to 60 mg was shown to reduce severity of symptoms, shorten their duration, enhance resolution of existing lesions, and prevent development of new lesions.[52] However, a recent study in 32 patients with chronic pernio randomized to nifedipine controlled release, 30 mg twice daily compared to placebo showed no significant difference between the two groups.[53] Despite this one negative trial, either nifedipine or amlodipine frequently is prescribed by the author to facilitate healing of the lesions and prevent their recurrence. Often pernio occurs in trim young women with low blood pressures. Thus, administration of an oral agent such as nifedipine may cause symptomatic hypotension. In these circumstances, I recommend the use of topical nifedipine, 5% in non-ionic cream, applied to the feet or toes twice a day. A compounding pharmacy will need to make this formulation. Other agents such as topical nitroglycerin, oral pentoxifylline, and hydroxychloroquine have been used with variable degrees of success.[54-56]

In one study, 4 of 5 patients treated with hydroxychloroquine demonstrated improvement.[56] However, it should be noted that all four of the patients showing improvement had an underlying connective tissue disease (Sjögren syndrome [1], SLE [2], or a family history of connective tissue disease [1]).

Despite speculation that it may enhance resolution of active lesions and provide subjective improvement, sympathectomy does not prevent recurrence of new lesions and has little effect if any on pigmentation and thickness at the sites of perniotic lesions. Conflicting reports exist about use of other treatment modalities such as topical or systemic corticosteroids, calcium, vitamin D, and intramuscular (IM) vitamin K. Given the controversy and lack of prospective studies, routine use of these agents is not recommended.

REFERENCES

1. McGovern T, Wright IS, Kruger E. Pernio: a vascular disease. *Am Heart J.* 1941;22:583.
2. Bazin E. *Lecons theoriques et cliniques sur la scrofule.* 2nd ed. Paris; 1861.
3. Winner A, Cooper-Willis E. Chilblains in service women. *Lancet.* 1946;1:663.
4. Goette DK. Chilblains (perniosis). *J Am Acad Dermatol.* 1990;23:257–262.
5. Jacob JR, Weisman MH, Rosenblatt SI, Bookstein JJ. Chronic pernio. A historical perspective of cold-induced vascular disease. *Arch Intern Med.* 1986;146:1589–1592.
6. Olin JW, Arrabi W. Vascular diseases related to extremes in environmental temperature. In: Young JR, Olin JW, Bartholomew JR, eds. *Peripheral Vascular Disease.* 2nd ed. St. Louis: Mosby-Year Book; 1996:611–613.
7. Takci Z, Vahaboglu G, Eksioglu H. Epidemiological patterns of perniosis, and its association with systemic disorder. *Clin Exp Dermatol.* 2012;37:844–849.

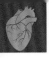
8. Cappel JA, Wetter DA. Clinical characteristics, etiologic associations, laboratory findings, treatment, and proposal of diagnostic criteria of pernio (chilblains) in a series of 104 patients at Mayo Clinic, 2000 to 2011. *Mayo Clin Proc.* 2014;89:207–215.

9. Purdue GF, Hunt JL. Cold Injury: a collective review. *J Burn Care Rehabil.* 1986;7:417–421.

10. Weston WL, Morelli JG. Childhood pernio and cryoproteins. *Pediatr Dermatol.* 2000;17:97–99.

11. Chan Y, Tang W, Lam WY, et al. A cluster of chilblains in Hong Kong. *Hong Kong Med J.* 2008;14:185–191.

12. DeGroot DW, Castellani JW, Williams JO, Amoroso PJ. Epidemiology of U.S. Army cold weather injuries, 1980-1999. *Aviat Space Environ Med.* 2003;74:564–570.

13. Kulka JP. Vasomotor microcirculatory insufficiency: observations on nonfreezing cold injury of the mouse ear. *Angiology.* 1961;12:491–506.

14. Ozmen M, Kurtoglu V, Can G, et al. The capillaroscopic findings in idiopathic pernio: is it a microvascular disease? *Mod Rheumatol.* 2013;23:897–903.

15. Shahi V, Wetter DA, Cappel JA, et al. Vasospasm is a consistent finding in pernio (chilblains) and a possible clue to pathogenesis. *Dermatology.* 2015;231:274–279.

16. Goodfield M. Cold-induced skin disorders. *Practitioner.* 1989;233:1616–1620.

17. Price RD, Murdoch DR. Perniosis (chilblains) of the thigh: report of five cases, including four following river crossings. *High Alt Med Biol.* 2001;2:535–538.

18. Lewis ST. Observations on some normal and injurious effects of cold upon the skin and underlying tissues: chilblains and allied conditions. *Br Med J.* 1941;2:837.

19. Gunther C, Berndt N, Wolf C, Lee-Kirsch MA. Familial chilblain lupus due to a novel mutation in the exonuclease III domain of 3' repair exonuclease 1 (TREX1). *JAMA Dermatol.* 2015;151:426–431.

20. Dowd PM, Rustin MH, Lanigan S. Nifedipine in the treatment of chilblains. *Br Med J (Clin Res Ed).* 1986;293:923–924.

21. Konig N, Fiehn C, Wolf C, et al. Familial chilblain lupus due to a gain-of-function mutation in STING. *Ann Rheum Dis.* 2017;76:468–472.

22. Souwer IH, Smaal D, Bor JH, et al. Phenotypic familial aggregation in chronic chilblains. *Fam Pract.* 2016;33:461–465.

23. Spiteri MA, Matthey F, Gordon T, et al. Lupus pernio: a clinico-radiological study of thirty-five cases. *Br J Dermatol.* 1985;112:315–322.

24. Lutz V, Cribier B, Lipsker D. Chilblains and antiphospholipid antibodies: report of four cases and review of the literature. *Br J Dermatol.* 2010;163:645–646.

25. Nazzaro G, Genovese G, Marzano AV. Idiopathic chilblains in myelomonocytic leukemia: not a simple association. *Int J Dermatol.* 2018;57(5):596–598.

26. Yang X, Perez OA, English III JC. Adult perniosis and cryoglobulinemia: a retrospective study and review of the literature. *J Am Acad Dermatol.* 2010;62:e21–e22.

27. Park KK, Tayebi B, Uihlein L, et al. Pernio as the presenting sign of blast crisis in acute lymphoblastic leukemia. *Pediatr Dermatol.* 2018;35(1):e74–e75.

28. Viguier M, Pinquier L, Cavelier-Balloy B, et al. Clinical and histopathologic features and immunologic variables in patients with severe chilblains. A study of the relationship to lupus erythematosus. *Medicine (Baltimore).* 2001;80:180–188.

29. Stagaki E, Mountford WK, Lackland DT, Judson MA. The treatment of lupus pernio: results of 116 treatment courses in 54 patients. *Chest.* 2009;135:468–476.

30. Cribier B, Djeridi N, Peltre B, Grosshans E. A histologic and immunohistochemical study of chilblains. *J Am Acad Dermatol.* 2001;45:924–929.

31. Herman EW, Kezis JS, Silvers DN. A distinctive variant of pernio. Clinical and histopathologic study of nine cases. *Arch Dermatol.* 1981;117:26–28.

32. Wall LM, Smith NP. Perniosis: a histopathological review. *Clin Exp Dermatol.* 1981;6:263–271.

33. Boada A, Bielsa I, Fernandez-Figueras MT, Ferrandiz C. Perniosis: clinical and histopathological analysis. *Am J Dermatopathol.* 2010;32:19–23.

34. Page EH, Shear NH. Temperature-dependent skin disorders. *J Am Acad Dermatol.* 1988;18:1003–1019.

35. Corlett WT. Cold as an etiological factor in diseases of the skin. In: *Eleventh International Medical Congress.* Rome; 1894:153.

36. McCleskey PE, Winter KJ, Devillez RL. Tender papules on the hands. Idiopathic chilblains (perniosis). *Arch Dermatol.* 2006;142:1501–1506.

37. Parra SL, Wisco OJ. What is your diagnosis? Perniosis (Chilblain). *Cutis.* 2009;84:15, 27–29.

38. Prakash S, Weisman MH. Idiopathic chilblains. *Am J Med.* 2009;122:1152–1155.

39. Simon TD, Soep JB, Hollister JR. Pernio in pediatrics. *Pediatrics.* 2005;116:e472–e475.

40. Beacham BE, Cooper PH, Buchanan CS, Weary PE. Equestrian cold panniculitis in women. *Arch Dermatol.* 1980;116:1025–1027.

41. De Silva BD, McLaren K, Doherty VR. Equestrian perniosis associated with cold agglutinins: a novel finding. *Clin Exp Dermatol.* 2000;25:285–288.

42. Duffill MB. Milkers' chilblains. *N Z Med J.* 1993;106:101–103.

43. Winter kibes in horsey women. *Lancet.* 1980;2:1345.

44. Weismann K, Larsen FG. Pernio of the hips in young girls wearing tight-fitting jeans with a low waistband. *Acta Derm Venereol.* 2006;86:558–559.

45. Gardinal-Galera I, Pajot C, Paul C, Mazereeuw-Hautier J. Childhood chilblains is an uncommon and invalidant disease. *Arch Dis Child.* 2010;95:567–568.

46. *The American Heritage® Dictionary for the English Language.* 4th ed; 2000.

47. Millard LG, Rowell NR. Chilblain lupus erythematosus (Hutchinson). A clinical and laboratory study of 17 patients. *Br J Dermatol.* 1978;98:497–506.

48. Giusti R, Tunnessen Jr WW. Picture of the month. Chilblains (pernio). *Arch Pediatr Adolesc Med.* 1997;151:1055–1056.

49. Olin JW, Bartholomew JR. Atheromatous embolization syndrome. In: Cronenwett JL, Johnston KW, eds. *Rutherford's Vascular Surgery.* 8th ed. Philadelphia: W.B. Saunders; 2010:2555–2570.

50. Montgomery H, O'Leary PA, Barker NW. Nodular vascular disease of the legs. *JAMA.* 1945;128:335.

51. Solomon LM, Beerman H. Cold panniculitis. *Arch Dermatol.* 1961;88:897.

52. Rustin MH, Newton JA, Smith NP, Dowd PM. The treatment of chilblains with nifedipine: the results of a pilot study, a double-blind placebo-controlled randomized study and a long-term open trial. *Br J Dermatol.* 1989;120:267–275.

53. Souwer IH, Bor JH, Smits P, Lagro-Janssen AL. Nifedipine vs placebo for treatment of chronic chilblains: a randomized controlled trial. *Ann Fam Med.* 2016;14:453–459.

54. Al-Sudany NK. Treatment of primary perniosis with oral pentoxifylline (a double-blind placebo-controlled randomized therapeutic trial). *Dermatol Ther.* 2016;29:263–268.

55. Verma P. Topical nitroglycerine in perniosis/chilblains. *Skinmed.* 2015;13:176–177.

56. Yang X, Perez OA, English III JC. Successful treatment of perniosis with hydroxychloroquine. *J Drugs Dermatol.* 2010;9:1242–1246.

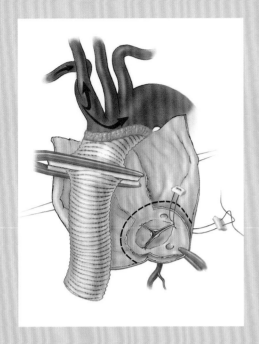

PART XIV

第十四部分

Venous Thromboem-
bolic Disease

静脉血栓栓塞性疾病

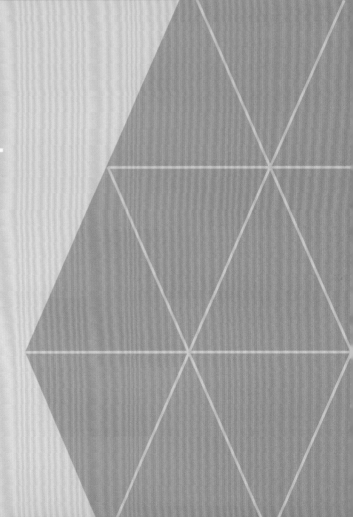

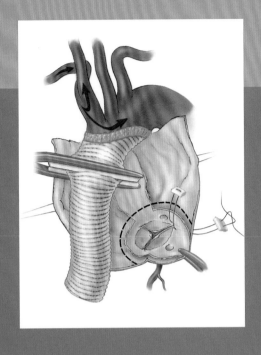

第50章
静脉血栓栓塞性疾病的
流行病学

　　静脉血栓栓塞作为仅次于冠心病和脑卒中的第三大心血管疾病，主要包括深静脉血栓形成及肺栓塞，其并发症的发生显著降低患者生活质量，严重威胁患者生命，也极大提高了医疗成本。全面深入地了解静脉血栓栓塞的流行病学有助于疾病的预防、分类与管理。静脉血栓栓塞的总体发病率并没有随着时间推移而出现显著变化，但影像诊断技术的进步及新兴诊断设备的应用提高了静脉血栓栓塞的诊断效率，因而显著增加了因静脉血栓栓塞住院的患者数量，也增加了肺栓塞在疾病总体中的占比。在静脉血栓栓塞的危险因素中，住院、人口老龄化及肥胖对疾病的影响已得到了证实，而研究新兴危险因素如较高的身高、慢性肾疾病和不同的人种等对于预防疾病和减轻医疗负担也具有重要意义。静脉血栓栓塞可根据其危险因素进行分类，但在分类和临床治疗时需要综合考虑危险因素的多样性及其叠加效应以达到有效的疾病预防、治疗及防止复发。

周为民

Epidemiology of Venous Thromboembolic Disease

Marc Carrier and Mary Cushman

INCIDENCE AND CLINICAL RELEVANCE OF VENOUS THROMBOEMBOLISM

Venous thromboembolism (VTE), consisting of deep vein thrombosis (DVT) and pulmonary embolism (PE), is the third leading cardiovascular disease after coronary heart disease and stroke. The age-standardized incidence rate is 1 to 2 per 1000 people per year. There is no surveillance for VTE, so the precise incidence and prevalence are not clear; three data sources present disparate results as recently reviewed.[1] Estimates from the United States Centers for Disease Control suggest there are 300,000 to 600,000 cases annually in the United States. In contrast, another study suggested 465,715 DVT, 296,000 PE, and 370,000 VTE deaths annually in six European countries with a population size together that is similar to the United States. The American Heart Association estimated that there were 676,000 DVT cases in the United States in 2014.

Estimation of lifetime risk is another way to consider the impact of VTE on the population. A report from an observational cohort of blacks and whites in the United States estimated that the lifetime risk of VTE after age 45 was 8.1% overall and 11.5% in blacks. Reflecting the association of common risk factors for VTE, lifetime risk was 10.9% in those with obesity and 17% to 18% in those with sickle cell anemia/trait or factor V Leiden (the most common genetic thrombophilia).[2] The risk of VTE differs by race-ethnicity, being lower in populations of Asian descent and perhaps higher in those of African descent, compared to Caucasians.[3]

VTE is a chronic disease that is associated with increased short- and long-term complications. In the short term, recurrent VTE and major bleeding predominate, while in the long term post-thrombotic syndrome (PTS), recurrent VTE and chronic thromboembolic pulmonary hypertension (CTEPH) cause morbidity and mortality. The case fatality rate for both recurrent VTE and major bleeding is approximately 11% during the first three months of anticoagulation therapy. PTS is a long-term complication in up to 25% to 50% of patients with DVT, and CTEPH complicates the course of approximately 1% of patients with PE.[4,5] Hence, VTE is an important cause of disability-adjusted life years lost and poses significant healthcare costs.[6,7] To reduce incidence and complications of VTE a better understanding of its incidence and associated risk factors is required.

SECULAR TRENDS IN INCIDENCE OF VENOUS THROMBOEMBOLISM

In North America, the overall incidence of VTE seems to have remained relatively unchanged over time. A large US population-based study reported an age- and sex-adjusted incidence of a first episode of VTE of 10.2 (95% CI: 10.2 to 10.3) per 10,000 person-years and demonstrated that the incidence did not change over a 30-year period (1991 to 2010).[8] A Canadian study also reported a stable age- and sex-adjusted incidence of VTE of 13.8 (95% CI: 13.7 to 14.0) per 10,000 person-years between 2004 and 2012.[9] Finally, a study from the Netherlands reported a stable overall age-adjusted incidence rate of first episode of VTE over a 10-year period from 2003 to 2012.[7] Interestingly, although the incidence rate of overall VTE remained stable over time, a number of studies have reported a decrease in the incidence of DVT but an increase in the incidence of PE. A French study comparing the 2013 incidence rate of VTE to that of 1998 using age- and sex-adjusted standardized incidence ratios (SIRs) reported a lower incidence for isolated DVT (without PE) in 2013 (SIR 0.53 [95% CI: 0.47 to 0.60]) but an increase in the incidence of isolated PE (without DVT) (SIR 1.29 [95% CI: 1.10 to 1.52]).[10] Other studies in the United States and the Netherlands also reported a decrease in the incidence of first (distal or proximal) DVT but an increase in the incidence of PE.[7,11] These observations are consistent with findings from the large population-based Norwegian Tromsø study that reported that the age-adjusted incidence of PE increased from 4.5 (95% CI: 2.3 to 6.7) per 10,000 person-years in 1996 to 11.3 (95% CI: 8.2 to 14.4) in 2010, whereas the incidence of isolated DVT in the same timeframe decreased from 11.2 (95% CI: 7.7 to 14.6) to 8.8 (95% CI: 6.1 to 11.5).[12] In contrast, as shown in Fig. 50.1, the 2018 statistical update of the American Heart Association reported a tripling of PE hospitalization and an approximate 50% increase in DVT hospitalization over the last two decades in the United States.[1] There are many potential reasons for this reported increase in DVT hospitalization. One explanation could relate to increased detection due to improvements in the sensitivity of imaging tests, such as using full-length leg ultrasonography, which may detect small distal DVTs that would not have been diagnosed with a diagnostic algorithm using proximal ultrasonography alone. However, the differences in findings from these studies with varied designs remain unexplained.

The reason for the increase in the overall incidence rate of PE over time remains unclear. The introduction of computed tomographic pulmonary angiography (CTPA) and its recent increasing availability in hospital emergency rooms is an important factor to consider. Detection of incidental PE, discussed below, might contribute. Advances in technology, more specifically the implementation of multiple-detector CTPA in clinical practice, has led to improvement in the sensitivity of PE diagnosis by allowing better resolution of the 2 to 3 mm diameter subsegmental pulmonary arteries. A large study from the US reported

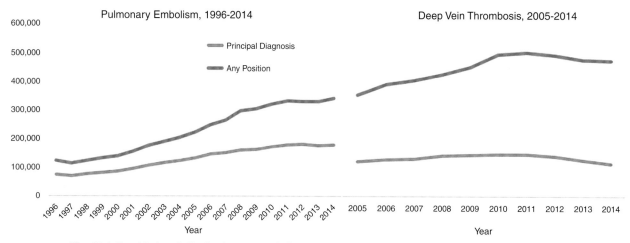

Fig. 50.1 Trend in hospitalized pulmonary embolism and deep vein thrombosis in the United States. Data is based on appearance of diagnosis codes in the principal position (*blue;* reason for the hospital stay) or any position *(orange)* in the list of discharge diagnosis codes. (From Benjamin EJ, Virani SS, Callaway CW, et al. Heart disease and stroke statistics-2018 update: a report from the American Heart Association. *Circulation.* 2018;137:e67–e492.)

that the increased use of multiple-detector CTPA for the diagnosis of PE seems to have led to a significant increase in the overall incidence of PE diagnosis.[13] Other factors besides improved sensitivity of CTPA may also be contributing, including improvements in effectiveness of PE diagnosis (using diagnostic algorithms including pre-test probability assessment), increased clinical awareness of healthcare providers to the diagnosis, a true increase in the incidence, or overdiagnosis. One study reported a decreasing age-adjusted, in-hospital case fatality rate from 12.1% to 7.8% between 1998 and 2006 without any significant change in overall mortality, suggesting that at least some of the increased PE diagnoses are less severe (or overdiagnosed).[13] Similar findings were reported in an Italian study assessing hospitalization for patients with acute PE. In this study, the incidence of PE increased from 4.0 to 6.2 per 10,000 person-years in women and from 3.5 to 4.6 in men between 2002 and 2012. The case-fatality rate decreased over the same time frame from 15.6% to 10.2% in women and 17.6% to 10.2% in men.[14]

The reported increased incidence of PE diagnosis since the introduction of multiple-detector CTPA may be correlated with an increase in the diagnosis of PE localized in the subsegmental pulmonary arteries without involvement in larger-order vessels (i.e., subsegmental PE, SSPE). A systematic review and meta-analysis of the literature reported that the rate of SSPE diagnosis among patients that underwent single-detector CTPA was 4.7% as compared to 9.4% for those that underwent multiple-detector CTPA.[15] Thus the rate of SSPE diagnosis seems to be increasing with the number of detectors used for PE diagnosis. These rates have been reported to range from 7% to 15% in patients undergoing 4- to 64-detector CTPA, respectively.

In summary, although not all reports agree, the overall incidence of VTE seems to have remained relatively unchanged over time, with lower-limb DVT decreasing and PE increasing in recent years. The rise in PE is likely, in part, a manifestation of the greater sensitivity of diagnostic tests for PE in smaller caliber vessels (e.g., subsegmental pulmonary arteries). The clinical importance of these isolated SSPE is not clear[15] and further studies are required to guide clinical management.

RISK FACTORS FOR VENOUS THROMBOEMBOLISM

Established Risk Factors

The incidence of VTE is dependent on the prevalence of its associated risk factors. A list including known important independent risk factors for VTE is depicted in Table 50.1. Most of these risk factors are transient (e.g., hospitalization) or modifiable (e.g., obesity). It is important

TABLE 50.1 Independent Risk Factors for Venous Thromboembolism	
Risk Factor	**Relative Risk**
Established	
Age, per decade	2
Body mass index >30 kg/m²	2
Body mass index >40 kg/m²	3
Major surgery	20
Hospitalization for acute medical illness	5
Immobilization	2
Nursing home confinement	5
Trauma/fracture	5
Active cancer	15
Neurologic disease with leg paresis	6
Pregnancy or postpartum	4
Oral contraceptives	2–3
Postmenopausal oral hormones	2
Hereditary thrombophilia	2–12
Emerging	
Elevated factor VIII or von Willebrand factor	4
Elevated D-dimer	4
Height (per 10 cm)	1.5
Chronic kidney disease	2
Venous insufficiency	2
Sickle cell trait	1.6
African American ethnicity vs. Caucasian (in United States)	1.8

to consider that the impact of combinations of risk factors tends to be at least additive and often multiplicative, such that the more factors present, the higher the risk. A well-known example is the combination of oral contraceptive pills (relative risk 2 to 3) and factor V Leiden (relative risk 4 to 7), which lead to a relative risk of 34 for VTE.

Hospitalization (due to acute medical illness or major surgery) is the most important risk factor, with about 40% of all VTE occurring after

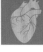

hospital stay. The risk of VTE in hospitalized medically ill patients may be stratified further based on a combination of additional risk factors (e.g., age, obesity, previous VTE, or other co-morbid conditions). Risk assessment models for predicting VTE have been derived for this high-risk population, however the models are not fully validated so may not be generalizable to all settings.[16] Among surgical patients, who tend to have higher risk than medical patients, the incidence of postoperative VTE is greater in older patients (≥ 65 years old) and following certain types of procedures (e.g., major orthopedic surgery, abdominal, or pelvic surgery).[17] The total number of high-risk surgeries has been increasing over time. For example, hip and knee arthroplasties have doubled in the Netherlands between 1995 and 2010.[7] Given this increase in the prevalence of high-risk procedures and the fact that about 40% of all VTE occur during or shortly after hospitalization, there is a strong and unmet potential to prevent events and reduce the burden of disease.

Secular trends in two risk factors in particular are also important to consider in relation to VTE incidence in recent decades: the aging population and the obesity epidemic. Age is a critical determinant of this disease. The incidence of VTE ranges from 1 in 10,000 annually in young people, to 1 to 3 per 1000 in middle age, and nearly 1% per year in the very old; essentially the incidence doubles with every decade of age. As such, with the graying of the population, we could anticipate an increase in incidence over time. The second key factor is obesity, which is associated with a two- to threefold increased risk of VTE. Between 1990 and 2000, the obesity prevalence in the United States rose from 10% to 25%. We can calculate based on the change in population over this time that this factor alone would lead to 32,500 more cases of VTE annually in the United States. If the obesity rate had remained unchanged there would have been 21,000 events attributable to obesity in 2000 rather than an estimated 52,500 cases. Further, obesity seems to be more closely associated with PE than DVT,[18] so might relate to increases in PE diagnosis discussed above.

It can also be expected that the prevalence of cancer will increase in the upcoming years.[19] Active cancer accounts for approximately 20% of all incident VTE, and VTE is the second leading cause of death in this patient population. The risk of VTE is higher for patients with certain tumor types (e.g., brain, stomach, pancreas) and those with metastatic disease.

Emerging Risk Factors

As shown in Table 50.1, emerging risk factors for VTE include taller height, chronic kidney disease (CKD), sickle cell trait, elevated factor VIII/von Willebrand factor, elevated D-dimer, and African American ethnicity. While these factors are important risk factors, the clinical role of considering these risk factors is uncertain since they have rarely been incorporated into prediction scores for VTE. However, these risk factors are generally persistent risk factors, so consideration and understanding is important, especially for researchers.

Of these risk factors, D-dimer is probably the most widely used clinically, being present in risk prediction scores for cancer-related VTE[20] and recurrent VTE among patients with unprovoked first VTE.[21] While higher D-dimer is also strongly associated with risk of a first VTE in the future in healthy people[22] at this time there is no role for testing for predicting first VTE. There are also strong associations of coagulation factor VIII levels with first and recurrent VTE risk.[23]

Several studies investigated taller height or longer legs in relation to VTE risk with a hypothesis that venous return is impaired in taller people. More definitive data on height as a VTE risk factor was published by Roetker and colleagues who reported that a genetic risk score for taller height increased the risk of VTE, providing solid evidence of a causal relationship between height and VTE risk.[24] This association may be due to impaired venous return with taller height.

CKD has a global prevalence of 11% to 13%,[25] and increases the risk of VTE about twofold, although it is not yet clear whether stage 0 CKD or

isolated albuminuria is related to risk.[26,27] Most of the association of CKD with VTE can be explained by a higher factor VIII level in the presence of CKD,[28] suggesting the mechanism might involve a procoagulant state or endothelial dysfunction in CKD as the link. This suggests that interventions to reduce procoagulation in CKD patients might be worthy of study.

About 8% of African Americans are carriers of the sickle cell trait, the heterozygous form of sickle cell disease. Several studies have now documented that sickle cell trait increases VTE risk, especially PE, which is a more fatal disease.[29] This finding may play a role in the known disparity in VTE affecting African Americans compared to whites in the United States, a disparity that is also partly explained by obesity.[3]

Overall, the prevalence of a majority of VTE risk factors is increasing over time and improvements in preventative strategies should hold promise for avoiding a concurrent increase in the incidence of VTE and its complications.

CLASSIFICATION OF VENOUS THROMBOEMBOLISM

The diagnostic classification of VTE is critical to consider as it leads directly to information on prognosis and on treatment duration. In general, VTE is either provoked by an acquired risk factor or unprovoked.[30] Acquired risk factors can be transient (e.g., major surgery) or persistent (e.g., metastatic carcinoma). VTE may be divided into unprovoked (~50% of cases), provoked with transient risk factors (~25% of cases), or provoked by persistent risk factors (~25% of cases).

Transient risk factors usually resolve after the VTE event (e.g., major surgery, trauma, etc.) and can be divided into major and minor risk factors. Patients with major and minor transient risk factors in the 2 to 3 months prior to VTE diagnosis, typically have a 50% lower recurrence risk than those with unprovoked VTE (Box 50.1). Patients with VTE provoked by a major transient risk factor (e.g., major surgery) are usually at very low risk of recurrent VTE after stopping treatment

---

BOX 50.1 Classification of Venous Thromboembolism (VTE)

VTE Provoked by a Transient Risk Factor

Major risk factors (up to 3 months prior to VTE)
- Surgery with general anesthesia for greater than 30 minutes
- Confined to bed ("bathroom privileges") for ≥3 days with acute illness
- Cast immobilization
- Cesarean section

Minor risk factors (up to 2 months prior to VTE)
- Surgery with general anesthesia for less than 30 minutes
- Admission to hospital for less than 3 days with an acute illness
- Estrogen therapy
- Pregnancy or puerperium
- Confined to bed out of hospital for less than 3 days with acute illness
- Leg injury associated with reduced mobility for at least 3 days

VTE Provoked by a Persistent Risk Factor
- Active cancer (ongoing treatment or metastatic/progressive disease)
- Neurologic disease with leg paresis

Unprovoked VTE
- Not in either of the above classifications

Modified from Kearon C, Ageno W, Cannegieter SC, et al. Categorization of patients as having provoked or unprovoked venous thromboembolism: guidance from the SSC of ISTH. *J Thromb Haemost.* 2016;14(7):1480–1483.

and short-term anticoagulation (3 months) is usually recommended. Patients with VTE provoked by persistent risk factors (e.g., metastatic cancer) are at high risk of recurrent VTE and extended treatment duration is often warranted to minimize the risk of recurrence. Transient risk factors may also fluctuate over time (e.g., inflammatory bowel disease) making it difficult to categorize and prognosticate the expected VTE recurrence rate. Patients with transient risk factors that fluctuate over time have a higher risk of recurrent VTE than those with truly transient risk factors, but lower than those with persistent risk factors. Guidelines recommend that clinicians tailor anticoagulation duration based of the risk benefit ratio and patient preference.[30]

Unprovoked VTE is not associated with any identifiable acquired risk factors (either transient or permanent) and can be considered a chronic disease in many patients. The term "unprovoked" is preferred over the previously used term "idiopathic" which suggests that there is no identifiable reason for the VTE. Patients may have non-acquired risk factors (e.g., hereditary thrombophilia) which do not qualify the VTE as provoked and may influence the underlying risk of recurrent VTE after stopping anticoagulation. Patients with unprovoked VTE have an intermediate risk of recurrent VTE after stopping therapy and need risk stratification and determination of patient preferences to help clinicians decide on length of anticoagulation. Essentially all of these patients are candidates for long-term anticoagulation, and consultation with a clinician experienced in VTE care is advisable.

INCIDENTAL VENOUS THROMBOEMBOLISM

The most common setting for incidental VTE is in cancer patients.[31] Approximately 50% of all VTE diagnosed in cancer patients are incidentally detected without any clinical suspicion of a symptomatic event. The prevalence of incidental VTE varies widely (from 1% to 15%) depending on tumor type and stage and type of diagnostic test used. Most incidental VTE are PE diagnosed on staging multi-detector CT. Approximately 60% of all incidental PEs involve the main or lobar pulmonary arteries and they are bilateral in about 30% of cases.[31] Small studies have suggested that incidental PE may present with a lower thrombotic burden when compared to symptomatic events.[32] However, these studies might have underestimated the actual embolic burden.

Data on the prevalence of incidental DVT of the extremities is scarce. The reported prevalence is variable from < 1% to 7%.[31] These estimates likely underestimate the actual prevalence of asymptomatic DVT in high-risk patients as imaging of the leg veins is not routinely performed. A recent prospective study reported that 9% of cancer patients initiating chemotherapy had asymptomatic DVT detected when screening lower extremity ultrasonography was performed.[33]

To consider treatment options for incidental VTE, prognosis must be considered. The prognosis seems to be similar for patients with incidental and symptomatic VTE.[34] A prospective cohort study reported rates of recurrent VTE of 11% among cancer patients with incidental VTE and 18% in those with symptomatic VTE.[35] The overall survival was 71% in both groups. Therefore, current clinical practice guidelines recommend treating incidental VTE using the same approach as symptomatic VTE.[36]

CONCLUSION

An understanding of the epidemiology and trends over time in VTE and its risk factors is important in considering diagnosis and management of this often-chronic disease. Correct diagnosis and classification are critical to designing treatment plans for patients since many patients are treated with long-term anticoagulants after a single event. Established and emerging risk factors discussed above should be

considered by clinicians when they educate their patients. For example, occurrence of VTE in an obese patient should be accompanied by weight loss counseling. Proper interpretation of imaging findings has important clinical implications, for example in consideration of SSPE or incidental PE. The changing landscape of an individual's risk with aging and over time has implications for prevention as well.

REFERENCES

1. Benjamin EJ, Virani SS, Callaway CW, et al. Heart disease and stroke statistics—2018 update: a report from the American Heart Association. *Circulation*. 2018;137(12):e67–e492.
2. Bell EJ, Lutsey PL, Basu S, et al. Lifetime risk of venous thromboembolism in two cohort studies. *Am J Med*. 2016;129(3):339. e19-26.
3. Zakai NA, McClure LA, Judd SE, et al. Racial and regional differences in venous thromboembolism in the United States in 3 cohorts. *Circulation*. 2014;129(14):1502–1509.
4. Ten Cate-Hoek AJ. Prevention and treatment of the post-thrombotic syndrome. *Res Pract Thromb Haemost*. 2018;2(2):209–219.
5. Ende-Verhaar YM, Cannegieter SC, Vonk Noordegraaf A, et al. Incidence of chronic thromboembolic pulmonary hypertension after acute pulmonary embolism: a contemporary view of the published literature. *Eur Respir J*. 2017;49(2).
6. Raskob GE, Angchaisuksiri P, Blanco AN, et al. Thrombosis: a major contributor to global disease burden. *Arterioscler Thromb Vasc Biol*. 2014;34(11):2363–2371.
7. Scheres LJJ, Lijfering WM, Cannegieter SC. Current and future burden of venous thrombosis: not simply predictable. *Res Pract Thromb Haemost*. 2018;2(2):199–208.
8. Heit JA, Ashrani A, Crusan DJ, et al. Reasons for the persistent incidence of venous thromboembolism. *Thromb Haemost*. 2017;117(2):390–400.
9. Alotaibi GS, Wu C, Senthilselvan A, McMurtry MS. Secular trends in incidence and mortality of acute venous thromboembolism: the AB-VTE population-based study. *Am J Med*. 2016;129(8):879. e19-25.
10. Delluc A, Tromeur C, Le Ven F, et al. Current incidence of venous thromboembolism and comparison with 1998: a community-based study in Western France. *Thromb Haemost*. 2016;116(5):967–974.
11. Huang W, Goldberg RJ, Anderson FA, et al. Secular trends in occurrence of acute venous thromboembolism: the Worcester VTE study (1985-2009). *Am J Med*. 2014;127(9):829–839. e5.
12. Arshad N, Isaksen T, Hansen JB, Braekkan SK. Time trends in incidence rates of venous thromboembolism in a large cohort recruited from the general population. *Eur J Epidemiol*. 2017;32(4):299–305.
13. Wiener RS, Schwartz LM, Woloshin S. Time trends in pulmonary embolism in the United States: evidence of overdiagnosis. *Arch Intern Med*. 2011;171(9):831–837.
14. Dentali F, Ageno W, Pomero F, et al. Time trends and case fatality rate of in-hospital treated pulmonary embolism during 11 years of observation in Northwestern Italy. *Thromb Haemost*. 2016;115(2):399–405.
15. Carrier M, Righini M, Wells PS, et al. Subsegmental pulmonary embolism diagnosed by computed tomography: incidence and clinical implications. A systematic review and meta-analysis of the management outcome studies. *J Thromb Haemost*. 2010;8(8):1716–1722.
16. Rothberg MB. Venous thromboembolism prophylaxis for medical patients: who needs it? *JAMA Intern Med*. 2014;174(10):1585–1586.
17. Heit JA, Spencer FA, White RH. The epidemiology of venous thromboembolism. *J Thromb Thrombolysis*. 2016;41(1):3–14.
18. Cushman M, O'Meara ES, Heckbert SR, et al. Body size measures, hemostatic and inflammatory markers and risk of venous thrombosis: the Longitudinal Investigation of Thromboembolism Etiology. *Thromb Res*. 2016;144:127–132.
19. Torre LA, Bray F, Siegel RL, et al. Global cancer statistics, 2012. *CA Cancer J Clin*. 2015;65(2):87–108.
20. Pabinger I, van Es N, Heinze G, et al. A clinical prediction model for cancer-associated venous thromboembolism: a development and validation study in two independent prospective cohorts. *Lancet Haematol*. 2018;5(7):e289–e298.

21. Tosetto A, Iorio A, Marcucci M, et al. Predicting disease recurrence in patients with previous unprovoked venous thromboembolism: a proposed prediction score (DASH). *J Thromb Haemost*. 2012;10(6):1019–1025.

22. Folsom AR, Alonso A, George KM, et al. Prospective study of plasma D-dimer and incident venous thromboembolism: the Atherosclerosis Risk in Communities (ARIC) Study. *Thromb Res*. 2015;136(4): 781–785.

23. Timp JF, Lijfering WM, Flinterman LE, et al. Predictive value of factor VIII levels for recurrent venous thrombosis: results from the MEGA follow-up study. *J Thromb Haemost*. 2015;13(10):1823–1832.

24. Roetker NS, Armasu SM, Pankow JS, et al. Taller height as a risk factor for venous thromboembolism: a Mendelian randomization meta-analysis. *J Thromb Haemost*. 2017;15(7):1334–1343.

25. Hill NR, Fatoba ST, Oke JL, et al. Global prevalence of chronic kidney disease - a systematic review and meta-analysis. *PLoS One*. 2016;11(7):e0158765.

26. Mahmoodi BK, Gansevoort RT, Naess IA, et al. Association of mild to moderate chronic kidney disease with venous thromboembolism: pooled analysis of five prospective general population cohorts. *Circulation*. 2012;126(16):1964–1971.

27. Cheung KL, Zakai NA, Folsom AR, et al. Measures of kidney disease and the risk of venous thromboembolism in the REGARDS (Reasons for Geographic and Racial Differences in Stroke) Study. *Am J Kidney Dis*. 2017;70(2):182–190.

28. Cheung KL, Zakai NA, Callas PW, et al. Mechanisms and mitigating factors for venous thromboembolism in chronic kidney disease: the REGARDS Study. *J Thromb Haemost*. 2018;16(9):1743–1752.

29. Folsom AR, Tang W, Roetker NS, et al. Prospective study of sickle cell trait and venous thromboembolism incidence. *J Thromb Haemost*. 2015;13(1):2–9.

30. Kearon C, Ageno W, Cannegieter SC, et al. Categorization of patients as having provoked or unprovoked venous thromboembolism: guidance from the SSC of ISTH. *J Thromb Haemost*. 2016;14(7):1480–1483.

31. Di Nisio M, Carrier M. Incidental venous thromboembolism: is anticoagulation indicated? *Hematology Am Soc Hematol Educ Program*. 2017;2017(1):121–127.

32. den Exter PL, Kroft LJ, van der Hulle T, et al. Embolic burden of incidental pulmonary embolism diagnosed on routinely performed contrast-enhanced computed tomography imaging in cancer patients. *J Thromb Haemost*. 2013;11(8):1620–1622.

33. Khorana AA, Francis CW, Kuderer NM, et al. Dalteparin thromboprophylaxis in cancer patients at high risk for venous thromboembolism: a randomized trial. *Thromb Res*. 2017;151:89–95.

34. den Exter PL, Hooijer J, Dekkers OM, Huisman MV. Risk of recurrent venous thromboembolism and mortality in patients with cancer incidentally diagnosed with pulmonary embolism: a comparison with symptomatic patients. *J Clin Oncol*. 2011;29(17):2405–2409.

35. Font C, Farrus B, Vidal L, et al. Incidental versus symptomatic venous thrombosis in cancer: a prospective observational study of 340 consecutive patients. *Ann Oncol*. 2011;22(9):2101–2106.

36. Lyman GH, Bohlke K, Khorana AA, et al. Venous thromboembolism prophylaxis and treatment in patients with cancer: American Society of Clinical Oncology clinical practice guideline update 2014. *J Clin Oncol*. 2015;33(6):654–656.

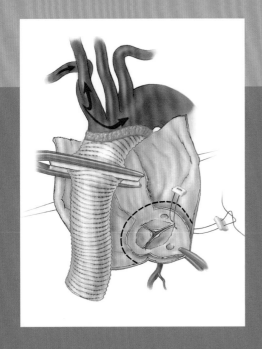

第51章
静脉血栓栓塞性疾病的
临床评估

　　静脉血栓栓塞是一种常见的心血管疾病，通常表现为深静脉血栓形成（deep vein thrombosis，DVT）或肺栓塞（pulmonary embolism，PE）。血栓栓塞事件是世界上仅次于冠心病和脑卒中的第三大心血管疾病；60岁后患该疾病的风险显著增加。既往学者总结了可能导致血栓栓塞事件发生的3大因素，包括血液高凝状态、血管内皮完整性被破坏及血流停滞，至今仍被认可。除此之外，血管壁炎症反应目前也被认为是驱使血栓栓塞事件发生发展的关键因素。深静脉血栓形成是血栓栓塞事件患者常见的临床表现之一，深静脉血栓形成患者就诊时通常以下肢肿胀为主要表现。肺栓塞患者常见的临床表现包括突发性呼吸困难和胸痛。血栓栓塞事件患者的诊断和风险评估可从3个方面进行，包括风险评分、实验室检查及影像学检查。Wells风险评估表是目前深静脉血栓形成和肺栓塞患者最常用的临床风险分层工具；D-二聚体是评估疑似血栓栓塞事件患者最常用的检测指标；双功能多普勒超声及肺栓塞患者肺动脉CT血管造影是确诊深静脉血栓形成类疾病首选的影像学检查方式；除此之外，还包括心电图、胸部X线等辅助检查手段。综合多种诊断技术对血栓栓塞事件患者进行评估可获得更好的诊断效能。总的来说，需综合考量血栓栓塞事件患者的既往史、家族史、风险评分及影像学指标以达到诊断和区分不同风险层患者的目的，为患者个性化治疗方案的制定提供重要理论基础。

戴向晨

Clinical Evaluation of Venous Thromboembolism

Brett J. Carroll and Gregory Piazza

Venous thromboembolism (VTE), most often presenting as deep vein thrombosis (DVT) or pulmonary embolism (PE), is a frequently encountered cardiovascular disorder. After myocardial infarction and stroke, VTE is the third most common cardiovascular disease with an estimated 10 million cases per year globally.[1] VTE is prevalent across all ages; however, the incidence increases significantly after the age of 60, with an 8% lifetime risk in those older than 45 years.[2,3] Lower extremity DVT is the source of the majority of PEs. Approximately 70% of patients with symptomatic PE will have a concomitant DVT on imaging study.[4,5] PE is estimated to be present in about one-third of patients with symptomatic DVT.[6]

CLINICAL PRESENTATION

Risk Factors

Risk factors for VTE can be both inherited and acquired (Box 51.1). The Virchow triad of hypercoagulability, endothelial injury, and venous stasis holds true for more than 150 years after its initial description. More recently, inflammation has been identified as a key mechanistic driver in the development of VTE.[7] Among one of the strongest risk factors for VTE is a history of prior VTE. There is a high risk of recurrence in patients with both provoked and unprovoked prior VTE: up to 50% over 10 years in those with a prior unprovoked event and up to 25% over 10 years in those with a prior provoked event.[8] An individual patient's risk factors should be considered when assessing likelihood of VTE as a possible cause of their clinical presentation.

Clinical Manifestation

In a large registry of patients presenting with DVT, the most common complaint was swelling of the extremity, present in 82% of outpatients and 59% of inpatients.[9] Patients with lower extremity DVT also often complain of a cramping or pulling sensation in the calf that may be exacerbated by ambulation. Extremity discomfort was reported in 70% of outpatients, but only 37% of inpatients. Though much less prevalent, DVT can also occur in the upper extremities, most frequently in the setting of an indwelling catheter or pacemaker, or in the presence of venous outflow obstruction. Symptoms are similar with swelling and discomfort in the affected arm. Symptoms of an associated PE are also reported in patients presenting with a DVT.

The physical exam is often notable for swelling and tenderness, but warmth and erythema can also be present. The presentation is most often unilateral, although it can present bilaterally in those that are hypercoagulable or have the rare instance of inferior vena cava (IVC) thrombosis. A palpable cord or prominent superficial venous collaterals may also be present. Signs and symptoms tend to be more common in those patients diagnosed as an outpatient compared to those hospitalized at the time of diagnosis, with over 10% of inpatients

having no signs or symptoms and compared to only 2% of outpatients.[9] In rare, severe cases, patients may exhibit signs of impaired perfusion due to venous obstruction secondary to massive DVT resulting in diminished arterial flow. Phlegmasia alba dolens is the early stage of decreased perfusion as the leg will appear white. This may progress further to become phlegmasia cerulea dolens—frank venous gangrene of the limb.[10]

The two most common presenting symptoms of PE are sudden onset dyspnea and chest pain, which is commonly described as pleuritic in nature.[11,12] Other presenting symptoms include cough with or without hemoptysis, dizziness, or syncope, or upper abdominal pain. One-quarter to half of patients will also complain of symptoms of a concomitant DVT.[4,5,11,12] Small PEs can also be asymptomatic and found incidentally on imaging performed for an alternative reason. The prognostic implications of these small asymptomatic PEs remain a matter of debate.

Presenting signs of PE include tachycardia, tachypnea, respiratory distress, diaphoresis, and clinical evidence of DVT.[11,12] Rales, decreased breath sounds, an accentuated pulmonic component of the second heart sound, right ventricular (RV) heave, and jugular venous distension can also be seen.[12] In patients with suspicion for PE, signs of DVT increase the pre-test probability. In the most severe cases, patients can present with hypotension, shock, active cardiac arrest, or respiratory failure. Overall, clinical signs and symptoms in isolation have poor specificity, thus further evaluation of risk factors and clinical risk stratification is required.[11,13]

The signs and symptoms of DVT and PE are associated with a broad differential diagnoses, thus limiting the use of assessment of clinical presentation alone when making the diagnosis (Boxes 51.2 and 51.3).

DIAGNOSIS

Risk Scores

Multiple risk scores have been developed to aid in the diagnostic evaluation of VTE given the broad range of possible alternative diagnoses. These risk scores assist in the assessment of the pre-test probability and are utilized as a guide for the appropriateness of further evaluation with laboratory testing and imaging for DVT and PE. A generally accepted bedside score for evaluation of the likelihood of DVT, the Wells DVT risk score incorporates risk factors, signs, and symptoms for DVT (Table 51.1).[14] Similar scores for PE are also available and have been validated for use with D-dimer testing (<1%) when appropriate (see Table 51.1).[15–18]

Clinical decision scores are valuable tools in the urgent care and emergency department setting but appear to be less helpful in the primary care setting. In a study of 1,293 patients in primary care clinics, 12% of those with a low probability score were found to have a

BOX 51.1   Risk Factors for Venous Thromboembolism (VTE)

Acquired
- Prior personal history of VTE
- Advanced age (>60 years old)
- Malignancy
- Estrogen therapy
- Pregnancy/postpartum
- Obesity
- Antiphospholipid antibodies
- Chronic inflammatory diseases (e.g., rheumatologic disease, inflammatory bowel disease)
- Chronic medical conditions (e.g., heart failure, chronic kidney disease, chronic obstructive pulmonary disease, infection, atherosclerosis)
- Venous obstructive processes (e.g., May-Thurner syndrome, thoracic outlet syndrome, tumor compression)
- Indwelling central venous catheter or pacemaker
- Recent hospitalization for medical or surgical issue (within 90 days)
- Recent trauma or surgery (within 90 days)
- Heparin-induced thrombocytopenia

Inherited
- Family history of VTE
- Factor V Leiden
- Prothrombin gene mutation
- Antithrombin deficiency
- Protein C deficiency
- Protein S deficiency

BOX 51.2   Alternative Diagnoses to Deep Vein Thrombosis

- Superficial vein thrombosis
- Phlebitis without thrombosis
- Venous insufficiency without acute thrombosis
- Varicose veins
- Post-thrombotic syndrome
- Muscle or soft tissue injury
- Ruptured Baker cyst
- Hematoma
- Cellulitis
- Lymphedema
- Lymphangitis
- Peripheral edema secondary to:
  - congestive heart failure
  - liver failure
  - renal failure
  - nephrotic syndrome

BOX 51.3   Alternative Diagnoses to Pulmonary Embolism

- Acute coronary syndrome
- Aortic dissection
- Chronic obstructive pulmonary disease exacerbation
- Pneumonia
- Acute bronchitis
- Decompensated heart failure
- Pulmonary hypertension
- Intrathoracic malignancy
- Pneumothorax
- Pleuritis
- Pericardial disease
- Musculoskeletal pain
- Hepatobiliary or splenic pathology
- Anxiety

Laboratory Tests

D-dimer is a nonspecific marker of endogenous fibrinolysis and is elevated in VTE, as well as other systemic illnesses and conditions (Box 51.4). D-dimer is most useful in the evaluation of outpatients or emergency department patients with suspected VTE, as these patients are less likely to have an alternative cause for an elevated D-dimer than inpatients. Enzyme-linked immunofluorescent assays (ELISA) are the most sensitive testing method. A systematic review of D-dimer studies in patients with suspected acute DVT demonstrated that the quantitative D-dimer by ELISA had negative likelihood ratios similar to those for negative venous duplex ultrasonography.[24] In evaluation of D-dimer in a high-volume emergency department for patients with suspected PE, a normal D-dimer had a sensitivity of 96.4% and a negative predictive value of 99.6%.[25] Though D-dimer can be checked in isolation, it is best used when in conjunction with clinical risk or likelihood scores.[26] D-dimer values increase with age, thus further limiting specificity in older patients. One meta-analysis compared the specificity of conventional cutoff values (<500 ng/mL) with age-adjusted values (age [years] × 10 ng/mL for patients over 50) and demonstrated higher specificity when an age-adjusted value was utilized.[27]

For patients suspected of having a PE, complete blood count and serum chemistries should be ordered. Arterial blood gases may demonstrate hypoxemia, increased alveolar to arterial gradient, and a respiratory alkalosis secondary to hypocapnia, but also may be normal. Because of their potential to mislead a clinician into missing the diagnosis, arterial blood gas measurement is not recommended in the routine evaluation of patients with suspected PE. Brain-type natriuretic peptide (BNP) and cardiac troponin are also frequently evaluated in patients with symptoms of a PE; however, they are of limited specificity and sensitivity for the diagnosis of PE.

Diagnostic Imaging Studies

Duplex ultrasonography for DVT and computed tomographic (CT) angiography of the pulmonary arteries for PE are the preferred imaging modalities to confirm a diagnosis. Duplex ultrasonography of the affected limb is the initial imaging testing in the evaluation of suspected upper and lower extremity DVT (see Chapter 12). Ultrasound offers accurate imaging with no exposure of radiation or iodinated contrast to the patient. Sensitivity and specificity for the evaluation of proximal lower extremity DVT are greater than 95%.[28] Duplex venous ultrasound combines vein compression with B-mode imaging and pulsed Doppler spectrum analysis, with and without color. Inability to fully

DVT.[19] The Wells score for DVT is also less predictive in patients that are older, have more comorbidities, and are hospitalized.[20–22] Clinical decision rules help to organize the clinical assessment, though perform similarly when compared to clinical gestalt in a meta-analysis.[23] The risk scores are of improved predictive value when utilized in conjunction with evaluation of D-dimer levels.

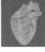

TABLE 51.1 Generally Accepted Clinical Risk Scores

Risk Score	Original Points	Simplified/Modified Points
Wells Rule for DVT		
Active cancer	+1	+1
Paralysis, paresis, or recent lower extremity cast	+1	+1
Recent immobilization >3 days or major surgery within 4 weeks	+1	+1
Localized tenderness of deep venous system	+1	+1
Swelling of entire leg	+1	+1
Calf swelling >3 cm compared to asymptomatic side	+1	+1
Unilateral pitting edema	+1	+1
Collateral superficial veins	+1	+1
Alternative diagnosis at least as likely as DVT	−2	−2
Prior DVT	−	+1
Classification of score	Low probability ≤0 Moderate probability 1–2 High probability ≥3	Unlikely <1 Likely ≥2
Wells Rule for PE		
Clinical signs and symptoms of DVT	+3	+1
Heart rate >100 beats/min	+1.5	+1
Previous DVT or PE	+1.5	+1
Immobilization or surgery within past 4 weeks	+1.5	+1
Active cancer	+1	+1
Hemoptysis	+1	+1
Alternative diagnosis is less likely than PE	+3	+1
Classification of score	Unlikely ≤4 Likely >4	Unlikely ≤1 Likely >1
Revised Geneva Score for PE		
Heart rate ≥95 beats/min	+5	+2
Heart rate 75–94 beats/min	+3	+1
Pain or lower limb deep venous palpation or unilateral edema	+4	+1
Unilateral lower extremity pain	+3	+1
Previous DVT or PE	+3	+1
Active cancer	+2	+1
Hemoptysis	+2	+1
Surgery or fracture within the past 4 weeks	+2	+1
Age >65 years	+1	+1
Classification of scores	Low probability <3 Intermediate probability 4–10 High probability ≥11	Non-high probability ≤2 High probability >3

DVT, Deep vein thrombosis; *PE*, pulmonary embolism.
Modified from Di Nisio M, van Es N, Buller HR. Deep vein thrombosis and pulmonary embolism. *Lancet*. 2016;388:3060–3073. Reprinted with permission from Elsevier.

compress a vein is diagnostic of DVT (Fig. 51.1A and B). Evaluation of the pelvic veins and upper extremity veins proximal to the clavicle is limited; however, pulsed Doppler of the proximal upper and lower extremity veins can also assess venous velocities (see Fig. 51.1C and D). Blunted peak velocities, especially if different than the contralateral extremity, are suggestive of more proximal obstruction. Calf veins can also be more difficult to assess due to their size. If only the proximal veins are assessed on initial imaging, an isolated calf vein can be missed, and follow-up ultrasound in 1 week is required to assure there has not been extension of a distal DVT. Prior studies demonstrate presence of new proximal DVT in 2% of patients on these follow-up ultrasounds.[29,30] Whole-leg compression ultrasonography can generally be

completed within 15 minutes with good interobserver agreement and few inconclusive results.[31–33]

Ultrasound can be utilized in the majority of cases of suspected DVT. In rare instances, additional imaging with CT venography or magnetic resonance (MR) venography is required. CT venography has been utilized in conjunction with CT pulmonary angiography; however, it exposes the patient to increased radiation and studies suggest it may be less accurate than ultrasound evaluation of the lower extremity veins.[34] The most valuable role for CT and MR venography is the contrast-enhanced evaluation of the proximal veins, including subclavian in the upper extremities, and the iliac and IVC in the pelvis (Fig. 51.2). Ultrasonography can also be limited in the evaluation

BOX 51.4 Alternative Causes for an Elevated D-Dimer

- Cancer
- Pregnancy
- Post-operative state
- Infection
- Liver disease
- Renal disease
- Trauma
- Aortic dissection
- Myocardial infarction
- Stroke
- Disseminated intravascular coagulation

of recurrent DVT as 50% of patients will have persistent abnormalities on ultrasound one year after the initial event.[5] Direct comparison with the initial ultrasound can be helpful to determine whether there is a recurrent DVT (including distribution of the thrombus and residual diameter of the thrombus within the vein); however, interobserver agreement is only moderate and additional imaging may be required.[35] MR venography is also useful in the evaluation of the change in thrombus volume over time and is a reproducible technique to distinguish acute from chronic DVT.[36,37] CT and MR venography also allows for the evaluation of concomitant anatomy that may be important in a patient's presentation (e.g., May-Thurner syndrome, discussed later). CT and MR venography may also be helpful when a mass invading or compressing the veins is suspected. Though rarely performed, invasive contrast venography can still be used if other imaging remains inconclusive.

Chest CT pulmonary angiogram is the first-choice imaging modality for the assessment of PE as it offers excellent sensitivity and specificity when incorporated into diagnostic algorithms, evaluates other potential causes of a patient's symptoms, is widely available, and can be obtained quickly (Fig. 51.3; see Chapter 14). Advances in multi-detector array CT technology with up to 320-slice imaging has improved temporal and spatial resolution. The frequency of non-diagnostic studies has decreased with these technological advancements.[38] A systematic review of CT evaluation of PE demonstrated a negative predictive value of 99.1% for PE and 99.4% for PE-attributed mortality, which was at least as accurate as the traditional gold standard of invasive pulmonary angiography.[39] An initial limitation of CT scan was the evaluation of the smaller arterial tree including segmental and subsegmental pulmonary arteries; however, with advancement in technology, multi-detector array CT detects twice as many subsegmental PEs than single-array detectors.[40] CT is not only diagnostic but also offers an assessment of RV enlargement, which can be utilized in risk stratification, discussed later.

Alternative imaging options include ventilation perfusion (V/Q) scan, and less frequently, invasive pulmonary angiography or MR angiography. V/Q scans are generally reserved for patients with severe chronic kidney disease, anaphylaxis to intravenous iodinated contrast, or pregnancy. V/Q scans are generally reported as normal, low-probability, intermediate-probability, or high-probability for PE. V/Q scans can be helpful if a patient has a low clinical risk (including normal D-dimer) and a normal or low-probability V/Q scan with a follow-up incidence of PE of < 3%.[41,42] A high-probability scan in the setting of a moderate to high clinical suspicion is sufficient to make a diagnosis. However, in patients with intermediate clinical risk and an indeterminate-probability scan, further definitive imaging is required. A normal perfusion scan essentially rules out the diagnosis of PE.

Invasive catheter-based pulmonary angiography had been the traditional gold standard prior to the emergence of CT. It is now rarely performed, and thus, the diagnostic accuracy is variable and dependent on the operator's experience. Its use is now mostly limited to patients that are undergoing catheter-directed therapy. MR pulmonary angiography is also infrequently used, but is an option in a patient with indeterminate V/Q scan who cannot undergo CT angiography. The test can take more than 30 minutes and is also dependent on a center's experience with such testing. In one study, the sensitivity of MR pulmonary angiography was low at 78%, but with a specificity of 99%.[43]

Complementary Imaging
Electrocardiography

An ECG should be checked in all patients with clinical suspicion for PE as there may be clues to suggest an alternative cause of the patient's presentation (e.g., MI or pericarditis) and may also demonstrate findings to suggest PE. Evidence of RV strain may be present, including T wave inversions in the anterior precordium or a complete or incomplete right bundle branch block. The pattern of an S wave in lead I and a Q wave and T wave inversion in lead III (S1Q3T3) has been classically described in PE and is a sign of acute cor pulmonale; however, it has poor sensitivity and specificity with one study finding an equal prevalence in patients with confirmed PE and those with suspected PE but negative confirmatory testing.[44] The most frequently seen findings on ECG are sinus tachycardia and non-specific T wave changes; however, when evidence of RV strain is present on ECG it can assist in risk stratification (discussed later). PE may also be accompanied by atrial fibrillation.

Chest X-ray

Similar to ECG, chest x-ray can serve an important role in the initial diagnostic evaluation of patients with symptoms suggestive of a PE to detect alternative diagnoses like pneumonia. A normal or near-normal chest x-ray in a patient with dyspnea or hypoxemia may be suggestive of PE. The classically described findings such as a peripheral wedge-shaped opacity (Hampton hump), focal oligemia (Westermark sign), or an enlarged right descending pulmonary artery (Palla sign) are rare and mostly of historical interest.

Echocardiography

Echocardiography plays an important role in risk assessment for patients with confirmed PE, but is not sensitive enough for diagnosis. Transthoracic echocardiography can rarely demonstrate thrombus within the proximal pulmonary arteries. Only occasionally is a thrombus in-transit in the right atrium or right ventricle visualized (Fig. 51.4). A classic finding of RV hypokinesis with sparing of the apex (McConnell sign) may suggest PE, but is insensitive for the diagnosis of PE (sensitivity of 77%).[45] In a study of 511 consecutive patients with echocardiography after PE, 71% had no significant abnormality consistent with PE.[46] A recent meta-analysis demonstrated that evidence of right heart strain had a sensitivity of 53% and specificity of 83% for the presence of PE, suggesting that it is inadequate to rule out a PE, but may be helpful in ruling in a PE.[47] Transesophageal echocardiography has been used to diagnose proximal PE at the bedside when first-line imaging techniques are unavailable in a timely fashion or simply not feasible. The presence of DVT on a lower extremity ultrasound may be helpful to suggest PE in patients with elevated clinical suspicion for PE; however, absence of DVT is insufficient to rule out a PE as DVT may be absent in over 50% of patients with a PE.[48]

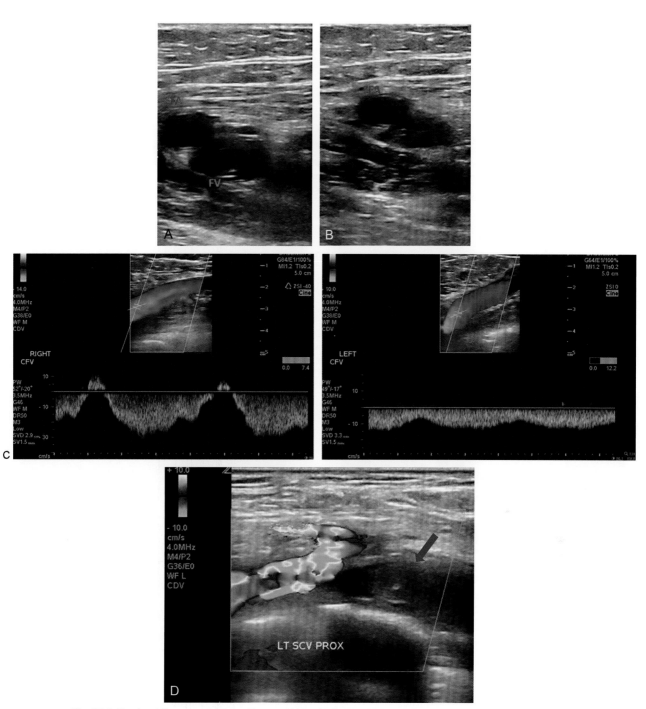

Fig. 51.1 Duplex Ultrasound of the Femoral Vein *(FV)*. (A) Initial image without compression. (B) Same location after compression demonstrates minimal change in the diameter of the femoral artery (as expected); however, the femoral vein also does not compress confirming the presence of a deep vein thrombosis. There is slightly increased echogenicity present within the lumen of the femoral vein which is suggestive of thrombus. (C) Pulsed-wave Doppler of the right and left common femoral vein demonstrating reduced pulsatility on the left suggestive of a possible proximal obstruction. (D) Color duplex ultrasound of the left subclavian vein *(SCV)*. Because of the subclavicular location of the subclavian vein, compression cannot be used to evaluate for thrombus; however, color duplex can assist and demonstrate lack of flow in a segment of the vein *(red arrow)*. *SFA,* Superficial femoral artery.

Integrated Approach to Diagnosis

An integrated approach to the diagnosis of VTE which includes assessment of the clinical presentation in addition to D-dimer and diagnostic imaging offers improved diagnostic utility than either alone. The modified Wells score was evaluated in a randomized trial with or without D-dimer testing in 1,096 patients with suspected DVT. DVT was found in 3-month follow-up in only 0.4% of patients unlikely to have a DVT by risk score and a normal D-dimer, where the rate of DVT was 1.4% in those with utilization of the risk score only.[30] When comparing the original Wells score, simplified Wells score, original revised Geneva

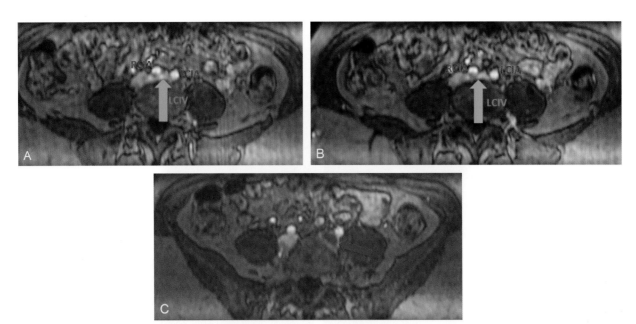

Fig. 51.2 Magnetic Resonance Venography (MRV) Demonstrating May-Thurner Syndrome. (A and B) MRV axial images of the left common iliac vein (LCIV) is being compressed by the right common iliac artery (RCIA) (blue arrow). (C) There is thrombus in the LCIV distal to the compressed portion of the vein (red arrow).

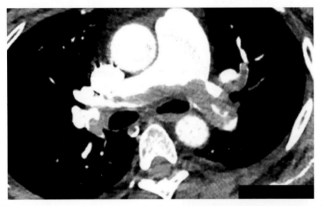

Fig. 51.3 Computed Tomography Pulmonary Angiography. Computed tomography pulmonary angiography axial image demonstrating a saddle pulmonary embolism with extension of the thrombus into the left and right main pulmonary arteries.

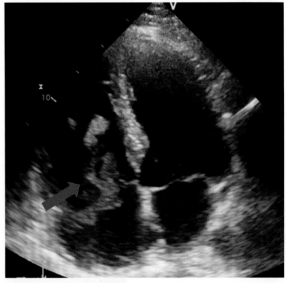

Fig. 51.4 Transthoracic Echocardiography Demonstrating Clot-in-Transit. Sixty-five-year-old man presented with subacute dyspnea on exertion over 7 days. Transthoracic echocardiography was performed to evaluate for left ventricular systolic dysfunction as initial ECG demonstrated findings consistent with possible myocardial ischemia. Images demonstrated a large thrombus (red arrow) in the right atrium traversing the tricuspid valve into the right ventricle.

score, and the modified revised Geneva score in 807 patients with suspected first acute PE, all were similar with 1 failure in follow-up when a low clinical score and a normal D-dimer was present.[18]

The PE Rule Out Criteria (PERC) was designed to identify patients that are at sufficiently low risk and do not warrant D-dimer or imaging evaluation. If a patient has a low probability initial clinical risk score and fulfill all 8 PERC criteria, no further testing is needed. The PERC rule includes age <50 years, heart rate <100 beats per minute, oxygen saturation ≥95%, no hemoptysis, no estrogen use, no prior DVT or PE, no unilateral leg swelling, and no surgery or trauma requiring hospitalization within the last 4 weeks.[49] In a large multicenter trial of patients with suspected PE in the emergency room, there was a false-negative rate of 1% in patients with a low probability clinical score and a negative PERC.[49]

An overall approach to the evaluation of a patient with suspected DVT or PE is summarized in Fig. 51.5. D-dimer should not be checked if it is likely to be elevated for another reason. Notably, in patients who are at high risk for DVT or PE by clinical risk assessment, D-dimer should not be checked as it is not sufficiently sensitive to rule out the

diagnosis in such patients. Further, in patients with very high clinical probability and are either very ill or there is an expected delay in imaging, treatment should be started empirically with anticoagulation if no contraindication is present.

DIAGNOSIS IN PREGNANCY

Pregnancy and the postpartum period are associated with elevated risk of VTE due to hypercoagulability from increased resistance to activated protein C, increased fibrinogen, and decreased protein S,

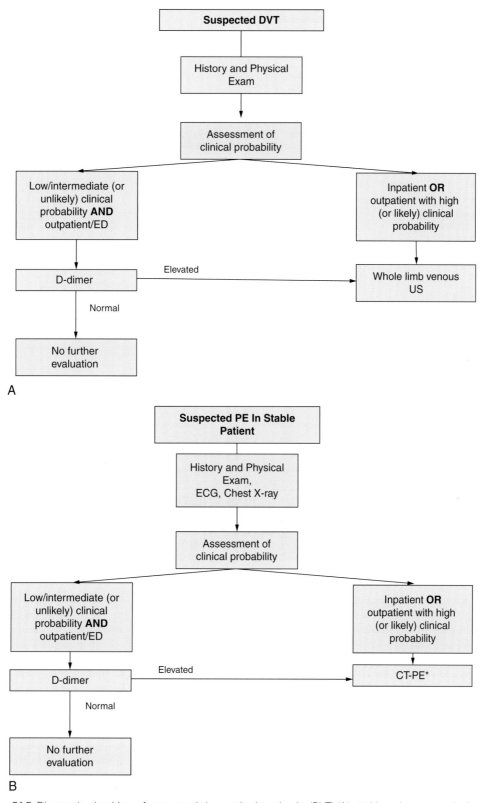

Fig. 51.5 Diagnostic algorithm of suspected deep vein thrombosis *(DVT)* (A), stable pulmonary embolism *(PE)* (B), and unstable PE (C). *In patients at very high clinical probability or expected delay in imaging, anticoagulation can be considered prior to confirmed diagnosis if no contraindication. V/Q scan is alternative diagnostic option in patients with contraindication to computed tomography *(CT). ED*, Emergency department; *IV*, intravenous; *RV*, right ventricular; *US*, ultrasound.

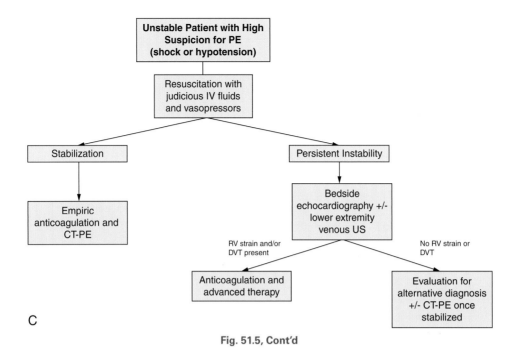

Fig. 51.5, Cont'd

along with greater venous capacitance, venous outflow obstruction, and a tendency toward decreased mobility. Diagnosis is more difficult in pregnancy as D-dimer can be elevated in the absence of VTE. Guidelines differ on the appropriate use of D-dimer in pregnancy with some advocating its use and others recommending against it.[50,51] There are ongoing trials evaluating diagnostic algorithms for PE in pregnancy (NCT00771303 and NTR5913), both of which include D-dimer in pregnant women with low clinical risk.[52]

Lower extremity edema is common in pregnancy and often is due to an alternative process other than DVT. When present in pregnancy, DVTs are more commonly left-sided due to compression of the left iliac vein by a gravid uterus. A clinical risk score was devised specifically for assessment of DVT in pregnancy which includes symptoms in the left leg, calf circumference of ≥2 cm, and presentation during first trimester (LEFt prediction rule).[53] When evaluated in 157 pregnant women with suspected DVT, 11 were found to have a DVT. None of the 46 women with a score of 0 were found to have a DVT on imaging. The rule can be incorporated into assessment with D-dimer and imaging when appropriate. The Wells score has not been validated in pregnancy. Ultrasound can be performed when there is elevated suspicion for DVT and does not pose a risk to the fetus.

Assessment of PE is complicated by potential radiation exposure to the fetus with V/Q scan or CT pulmonary angiography. The European Society of Cardiology guidelines recommend bilateral lower extremity ultrasound as the first line test.[51] If DVT is found, PE-specific diagnostic testing will not change management unless the patient has concerning clinical features and there is consideration of advanced treatments in addition to anticoagulation. A negative ultrasound does not rule out PE, however, and further definitive testing may be required. V/Q scans expose the fetus to a higher amount of radiation than CT; however, both V/Q scans and CT pulmonary angiography are below the danger threshold to the fetus. Though V/Q scans are associated with higher radiation overall, they may be preferred over CT as it avoids a radiation dose delivered to the breasts in young female patients. Additionally, because of changes during pregnancy including hemodilution and

a hyperdynamic state, CT results in pregnant women are more frequently inconclusive compared to those that are not pregnant and have similar diagnostic accuracy as V/Q scans in the pregnant population.[54] Overall, the benefit of confirming the diagnosis of PE is generally greater than the risk of radiation exposure to the patient and fetus and imaging should not be avoided if the clinical pre-test probability warrants such testing.

RISK STRATIFICATION

All patients without contraindications should receive anticoagulation for the management of DVT and PE. Risk stratification, particularly for PE, is essential to aid in assessment of prognosis and decision-making regarding appropriateness of advanced therapy.

Risk Stratification for Deep Vein Thrombosis

Risk stratification of DVT is primarily based on clinical assessment. Beyond the risk of PE and recurrent DVT, DVT can lead to the long-term complication of post-thrombotic syndrome in as many as 50% of patients with a DVT who are treated with anticoagulation (see Chapter 54).[55] A recent randomized-control trial of 692 patients evaluated pharmacomechanical catheter-directed thrombolysis for acute proximal DVT and found no difference in the prevalence of post-thrombotic syndrome in those that received an intervention plus anticoagulation compared to those that received anticoagulation alone at 24 months. There was a lower rate of moderate to severe post-thrombotic syndrome in the intervention arm (18% vs. 24%, P = .04), however.[56] Catheter-directed therapy should not be routinely performed for patients with DVT. Clinical circumstances may warrant consideration for catheter-directed intervention in some patients who exhibit significant swelling or persistent symptoms despite anticoagulation in the setting of acute iliofemoral DVT and are at low risk for bleeding.

Phlegmasia cerulea dolens is a rare but potentially life- or limb-threatening presentation of DVT due to significant venous outflow obstruction leading to impaired arterial perfusion. Patients can present with a spectrum from phlegmasia alba dolens, where the leg is

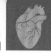

swollen and appears pale due to decreased arterial flow to phlegmasia cerulea dolens, frank venous gangrene. With more severe presentations, the leg will be swollen, cyanotic, with a violaceous discoloration and persistent severe pain.[10] Risk factors for phlegmasia cerulea dolens include malignancy, antiphospholipid antibody, and heparin-induced thrombocytopenia. Early recognition is important as advanced therapy with catheter-directed thrombolysis or venous thrombectomy in addition to anticoagulation is often required to rapidly improve limb perfusion (see Chapter 52).

Risk Stratification for Pulmonary Embolism

Risk stratification for PE is a vital aspect of the clinical evaluation as it guides consideration for therapy in addition to anticoagulation. Because of the risks associated with advanced therapy (e.g., bleeding with fibrinolysis), risk stratification is essential in limiting exposure to such treatments to those patients that are most likely to benefit (see Chapter 52). Primary in the initial assessment is the patient's hemodynamic status. If a patient is hypotensive or displays findings of cardiogenic shock, advanced therapy is warranted when no contraindications are present given the high rate of mortality in this subset of patients.[57] Decision-making is more complex in those patients with hemodynamic stability. Comprehensive risk stratification incorporates both the patient's history and physical exam findings, comorbidities, along with complementary data from laboratory and imaging testing. Much of the risk differentiation occurs by assessment of RV strain, as RV dysfunction is the primary pathophysiologic mechanism that can lead to hemodynamic collapse and persistent symptoms.[58]

The most frequently utilized clinical risk assessment tool is the PE Severity Index (PESI) and simplified PESI (sPESI) (Tables 51.2 to 51.5).[59,60] The PESI score includes 11 clinical parameters that can be cumbersome to calculate, thus the sPESI score is more frequently utilized with six easy-to-score features. The ability to predict 30-day mortality was similar between the two scoring systems (C statistic 0.75 for both).[60]

PE can cause abrupt increases in RV afterload due to direct vascular obstruction and pulmonary vasoconstriction secondary to hypoxemia and release of mediators of arterial vasoconstrictors. The increase in RV afterload leads to RV dilation and hypokinesis along with increased RV wall tension. These changes induce RV ischemia with worsening of RV dilation and bowing of the interventricular septum into the LV, decreasing systemic preload and potentiating RV ischemia and RV failure. In the most profound presentations, this cycle can result in circulatory collapse. Evidence of RV dysfunction by both imaging and

TABLE 51.3 Pulmonary Embolism Severity Index Risk Classification and 30-Day Mortality

Score	Class	Risk	30-Day Mortality (%)
<66	I	Low	0–1.6
66–85	II		1.7–3.5
86–105	III	High	3.2–7.1
106–125	IV		4.0–11.4
>125	V		10.0–24.5

TABLE 51.4 Simplified Pulmonary Embolism Severity Index Score

Clinical Feature	Points
Age >80 years	1
History of cancer	1
Chronic cardiopulmonary disease	1
Pulse ≥110 beats/min	1
Systolic blood pressure <100 mm Hg	1
Arterial oxygenation saturation <90%	1

TABLE 51.5 Simplified Pulmonary Embolism Severity Index Risk Classification and 30-Day Mortality

Score	Risk	30-Day Mortality (%)
0	Low	1.0–1.1
≥1	High	8.9–10.9

cardiac biomarkers has been demonstrated in numerous studies to be independently associated with poor clinical outcome.

Detection of an increased RV-to-left ventricular (LV) diameter ratio (abnormal >0.9) can be accomplished using the same axial CT data used to diagnose the PE and corresponds with increased PE-related mortality (Fig. 51.6). In a recent meta-analysis, the RV-to-LV diameter ratio was the most predictive CT finding for all-cause mortality (OR 2.5, 95% CI 1.8 to 2.5; $P < .0001$) and PE-related mortality (OR 5.0, 95% CI 2.7 to 9.2; $P < .0001$).[61] An increased RV-to-LV diameter ratio is less predictive in patients that are hemodynamically stable (all-cause mortality, OR 1.85, 95% CI 1.15 to 2.98, $P = .08$). Interventricular septal flattening (bowing) or contrast reflux into the IVC are associated with increased mortality.[61] Thrombus burden has also been associated with PE-related mortality, but not all-cause mortality. Central location of thrombus is not associated with all-cause or PE-related mortality, indicative of the effect of the thrombus on RV function rather than the thrombus load itself as being the primary driver of morbidity.[61,62]

Echocardiography offers a greater breadth of assessment of RV size and function with a variety of potential parameters compared to CT. Most commonly evaluated is the RV diameter and RV-to-LV diameter ratio, overall RV function, tricuspid regurgitation, pulmonary hypertension, and bowing of the interventricular septum suggestive of volume or pressure overload.[63–65] A study of 411 normotensive patients with PE evaluated numerous parameters on transthoracic echocardiography and demonstrated only an abnormal tricuspid annular plane systolic excursion (TAPSE) to be predictive of a complicated clinical course in multivariable analysis (HR 27.9, 95% CI 6.2 to 124.6; $P < .001$).[64]

TABLE 51.2 Pulmonary Embolism Severity Index Score

Clinical Feature	Points
Age	No. of years
Male gender	10
History of cancer	30
Heart failure	10
Chronic lung disease	10
Pulse ≥110 beats/min	20
Systolic blood pressure <100 mm Hg	30
Respiratory rate ≥30 breaths/min	20
Temperature <36°C	20
Altered mental status	60
Arterial oxygen saturation <90%	20

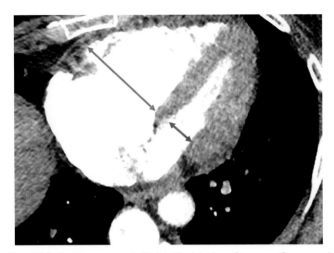

Fig. 51.6 Assessment of Right Ventricular Size on Computed Tomography. Right ventricular– *(blue arrows)* to–left ventricular *(red arrows)* diameter ratio measured as 2.7 on axial images of a computed tomographic pulmonary angiogram in a patient presenting with a large pulmonary embolism.

AHA	ESC*	(+) RV Strain on CT or Echo	(+) Elevated cardiac biomarkers	Shock or hypotension
Massive	High-risk	+	+†	+
Submassive‡	Intermediate-high-risk	+	+	-
	Intermediate-low-risk†	+ or -	+ or -	-
Low-Risk	Low-risk	-	-	-

*ESC guidelines also utilize clinical risk stratification with PESI or simplified PESI score. PESI class I-II or sPESI score of 0 with negative RV strain are considered low-risk. PESI class ≥III or sPESI ≥I are considered at least intermediate low-risk regardless of presence of RV strain. †Cardiac biomarkers are not required in patients with shock or hypotension, though if checked are likely to be positive. ‡Submassive: RV strain on imaging and/or biomarkers. Intermediate-low: RV strain on imaging or biomarkers.

Fig. 51.7 Risk stratification of pulmonary embolism by the American Heart Association *(AHA)* and the European Society of Cardiology *(ESC)*. *RV*, Right ventricular. (Data from Konstantinides SV, Torbiki A, Agnelli G, et al. ESC Guidelines on the diagnosis and management of acute pulmonary embolism. *Eur Heart J.* 2014;35:3033–3080.)

More complex evaluation of the RV by echocardiography including speckle-tracking, 3-dimensional assessment, and Tei index have also been associated with poor clinical outcomes, but can be time consuming.[66,67]

As noted earlier, cardiac ischemia plays a role in the pathophysiology of PE, and congruent with that understanding is the association of elevated troponin and adverse outcomes. Though no optimal cut-off value for risk stratification has been identified, there is a clear association with short-term mortality, PE-attributable mortality, and adverse outcomes.[68] BNP has similarly been associated with adverse outcomes in patients with PE.[69] Cardiac biomarkers are recommended by the European Society of Cardiology (ESC) for detection and differentiation of intermediate-low- and intermediate-high-risk patients.[51]

Other findings associated with adverse outcome include thrombus in the RV and the presence of a coexisting DVT; however, neither are frequently incorporated into risk assessment tools or guidelines.[70,71]

Many patients presenting with signs or symptoms of a PE have ECG evidence of RV strain; however, the ECG is not incorporated into most risk assessment tools.[72–75]

Similar to the diagnosis of PE, an integrated approach to risk assessment is also recommended. Evaluation of RV dysfunction by imaging or cardiac biomarkers in isolation is of limited positive predictive value for early mortality after an acute PE (<10%); however, they do demonstrate very good negative predictive value (>93%) and are most useful in determining those patients at low risk.[51] There are numerous other clinical risk scores that incorporate a variety of clinical and RV strain parameters, and when evaluated in a recent meta-analysis, most have high sensitivity (88% to 97%), though with relatively poor specificity (<49%) to predict adverse outcomes.[76]

The various clinical and complementary risk assessment tools have been incorporated into guidelines (Fig. 51.7).[51,77,78] Evaluation of the patient's hemodynamic status (hypotension ≤90 mm Hg for >15 minutes, need for vasopressor, or evidence of shock) is paramount on initial assessment, as those patients are considered to have massive or high-risk PE. If a patient is stable, further risk stratification with imaging and cardiac biomarkers is recommended (Fig. 51.8).

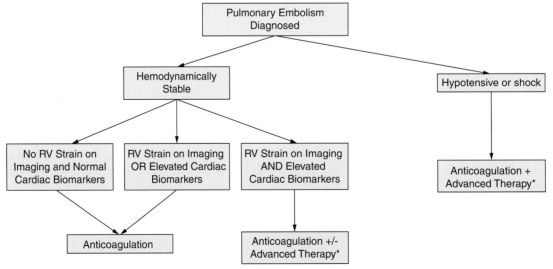

Fig. 51.8 Initial Risk Stratification and Treatment Consideration Algorithm for Pulmonary Embolism. *Systemic intravenous fibrinolysis, catheter-directed fibrinolysis/embolectomy, pulmonary embolectomy, inferior vena cava filter depending on patient comorbidities and bleeding risk profile.

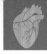

ADJUNCTIVE CLINICAL EVALUATION FOR ETIOLOGY OF VENOUS THROMBOEMBOLISM

In patients presenting with VTE, it is important that appropriate evaluation of the underlying etiology of the VTE be performed. Assessment for provoking factors is essential in the determination of duration of anticoagulation given the high risk of recurrence in those with unprovoked VTE when treated with a limited course of anticoagulation.[8] Thrombophilia testing should not be routinely performed. Though thrombophilias are a risk factor for initial VTE, there is a limited association with recurrent VTE, and testing should not generally be utilized in the determination of duration of anticoagulation.[79,80] There are specific cases where testing may be considered such as in patients with first-degree relatives who are women of child-bearing age, given the elevated risk of concomitant thrombophilia and oral contraceptive use, or in those with clinical suspicion for antiphospholipid antibodies as these results may affect choice of anticoagulant and duration of anticoagulation.

All patients should have sex- and age-appropriate cancer screening soon after their diagnosis of VTE (e.g., colonoscopy, Pap smear, mammography, prostate cancer screening). Given the high frequency of concomitant malignancy in VTE, more advanced evaluation for occult malignancy with CT chest and/or CT abdomen/pelvis after an unprovoked VTE has been evaluated. Though malignancy was discovered with a slightly greater frequency, there does not appear to be a clinical benefit of a more aggressive screening approach.[81,82]

Evaluation for possible anatomic causes of venous obstruction should be considered when suspected by the particular clinical presentation. May-Thurner syndrome classically describes the external compression of the left iliac vein by the overlying right common iliac artery, although right-sided and bilateral forms have also been described (see Fig. 51.2).[83] Dedicated evaluation for May-Thurner syndrome can be considered in patients that present with rapid onset left lower extremity swelling and pain due to a proximal DVT (i.e., common femoral vein DVT on ultrasound). Patients are more frequently female and may have a prior history of left lower extremity swelling, varicose veins, or proximal left-sided superficial venous collaterals which are suggestive of a proximal venous obstruction. Ultrasound may be of limited value in the assessment of pelvic venous anatomy as body habitus and bowel gas can make acquisition of high-quality images difficult. Surrogate markers of obstruction with dampened venous waveforms isolated to the left proximal veins may suggest a proximal obstruction; however, waveforms cannot be obtained when a proximal clot is present. Further imaging with CTV or MRV can be considered to better delineate pelvic venous anatomy. In patients that are appropriate candidates for catheter-based therapy, direct venography with pressure measurements can be performed to evaluate for the presence and severity of obstruction, as venous stent placement may be warranted (see Chapter 63).

Thoracic outlet syndrome (also known as Paget-Schroetter syndrome or "effort" thrombosis) should be considered in patients with isolated upper extremity DVT without other risk factors (e.g., pacemaker or venous catheter). Patients classically have a history of vigorous and repetitive exertion of the upper extremities, most frequently at or above the shoulders.[84] The repetitive activity can lead to scarring and stenosis of the subclavian vein in the region of the thoracic outlet. Patients may have a prior history of unilateral arm swelling, development of superficial venous collaterals, or symptoms of thoracic outlet nerve compression with paresthesia of the fingers. There may be findings suggestive of proximal stenosis on ultrasound, but most frequently, CTV or MRV is required to better evaluate the venous anatomy. If present, consideration for catheter-directed fibrinolysis with subsequent decompressive surgical therapy is warranted (Fig. 51.9) (see Chapter 63).[85,86]

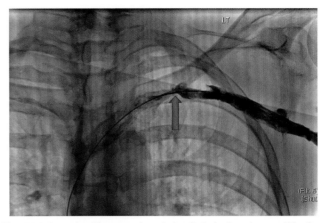

Fig. 51.9 Invasive Venography of the Subclavian Artery. Fifty-five-year-old man presented with left upper extremity swelling and was found to have a left subclavian deep vein thrombosis on ultrasound. He was taken to the cardiac catheterization lab for invasive venography, given suspicion for thoracic outlet syndrome. He was found to have stenosis of the left subclavian vein at the thoracic outlet *(red arrow).*

REFERENCES

1. Raskob GE, Angchaisuksiri P, Blanco AN, et al. Thrombosis: a major contributor to the global disease burden. *J Thromb Haemost.* 2014;12(10):1580–1590.
2. Silverstein MD, Heit JA, Mohr DN, et al. Trends in the incidence of deep vein thrombosis and pulmonary embolism. *Arch Intern Med.* 1998;158:585–593.
3. Bell EJ, Lutsey PL, Basu S, et al. Lifetime risk of venous thromboembolism in two cohort studies. *Am J Med.* 2016;129(3):e319–e326.
4. Heit JA. Epidemiology of venous thromboembolism. *Nat Rev Cardiol.* 2015;12(8):464–474.
5. Kearon C. Natural history of venous thromboembolism. *Circulation.* 2003;107(23):22–30.
6. Stein PD, Matta F, Musani MH, et al. Silent pulmonary embolism in patients with deep venous thrombosis: a systematic review. *Am J Med.* 2010;123(5):426–431.
7. Piazza G, Ridker PM. Is venous thromboembolism a chronic inflammatory disease? *Clin Chem.* 2015;61(2):313–316.
8. Prandoni P, Noventa F, Ghirarduzzi A, et al. The risk of recurrent venous thromboembolism after discontinuing anticoagulation in patients with acute proximal deep vein thrombosis or pulmonary embolism. A prospective cohort study in 1,626 patients. *Haematologica.* 2007;92(2):199–205.
9. Goldhaber SZ, Tapson VF. A prospective registry of 5,451 patients with ultrasound-confirmed deep vein thrombosis. *Am J Card.* 2004;93: 259–262.
10. Mumoli N, Invernizzi C, Luschi R, et al. Phlegmasia cerulea dolens. *Circulation.* 2012;125(8):1056–1057.
11. Pollack CV, Schreiber D, Goldhaber SZ, et al. Clinical characteristics, management, and outcomes of patients diagnosed with acute pulmonary embolism in the emergency department: initial report of EMPEROR (Multicenter Emergency Medicine Pulmonary Embolism in the Real World Registry). *J Am Coll Cardiol.* 2011;57(6):700–706.
12. Stein PD, Beemath A, Matta F, et al. Clinical characteristics of patients with acute pulmonary embolism: data from PIOPED II. *Am J Med.* 2007;120(10):871–879.
13. Sandler DA, Duncan JS, Ward P, et al. Diagnosis of deep-vein thrombosis: comparison of clinical evaluation, ultrasound, plethysmography, and venoscan with x-ray venogram. *Lancet.* 1984;2(8405):716–719.
14. Wells PS, Anderson DR, Bormanis J, et al. Value of assessment of pretest probability of deep-vein thrombosis in clinical management. *Lancet.* 1997;350(9094):1795–1798.

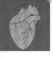

15. Gibson NS, Sohne M, Kruip MJ, et al. Further validation and simplification of the Wells clinical decision rule in pulmonary embolism. *Thromb Haemost.* 2008;99(1):229–234.

16. Le Gal G, Righini M, Roy PM, et al. Prediction of pulmonary embolism in the emergency department: the revised Geneva score. *Ann Intern Med.* 2006;144:165–171.

17. Klok FA, Mos IC, Nijkeuter M, et al. Simplification of the revised Geneva score for assessing clinical probability of pulmonary embolism. *Arc Intern Med.* 2008;168(19):2131–2136.

18. Douma RA, Mos IC, Erkens PM, et al. Performance of 4 clinical decision rules in the diagnostic management of acute pulmonary embolism. *Ann Intern Med.* 2011;154:709–718.

19. Oudega R, Hoes AW, Moons KG. The Wells rule does not adequately rule out deep venous thrombosis in primary care patients. *Ann Intern Med.* 2005;143:100–107.

20. Goodacre S, Sutton AJ, Sampson FC. Meta-analysis: the value of clinical assessment in the diagnosis of deep venous thrombosis. *Ann of Intern Med.* 2005;143:129–139.

21. Schouten HJ, Geersing GJ, Oudega R, et al. Accuracy of the Wells clinical prediction rule for pulmonary embolism in older ambulatory adults. *J Am Geriatr Soc.* 2014;62(11):2136–2141.

22. Silveira PC, Ip IK, Goldhaber SZ, et al. Performance of Wells score for deep vein thrombosis in the inpatient setting. *JAMA Intern Med.* 2015;175(7):1112–1117.

23. Lucassen W, Geersing GJ, Erkens PM, et al. Clinical decision rules for excluding pulmonary embolism: a meta-analysis. *Ann of Intern Med.* 2011;155:448–460.

24. Stein PD, Hull RD, Patel KC, et al. D-dimer for the exclusion of acute venous thrombosis and pulmonary embolism. *Ann Intern Med.* 2004;140:589–602.

25. Dunn KL, Wolf JP, Dorfman DM, et al. Normal d-dimer levels in emergency department patients suspected of acute pulmonary embolism. *J Am Coll Cardiol.* 2002;40(8):1475–1478.

26. Wells PS, Owen C, Doucette S, et al. Does this patient have deep vein thrombosis? *JAMA.* 2006;295:199–207.

27. Schouten HJ, Geersing GJ, Koek HL, et al. Diagnostic accuracy of conventional or age adjusted d-dimer cut-off values in older patients with suspected venous thromboembolism: systematic review and meta-analysis. *BMJ.* 2013;346:f2492.

28. Habscheid W, Hohmann M, Wilhelm T, et al. Real-time ultrasound in the diagnosis of acute deep venous thrombosis of the lower extremity. *Angiology.* 1990;41(8):599–608.

29. Birdwell BG, Raskob GE, Whitsett TL, et al. The clinical validity of normal compression ultrasonography in outpatients suspected of having deep venous thrombosis. *Ann of Intern Med.* 1998;128:1–7.

30. Wells PS, Anderson DR, Rodger M, et al. Evaluation of d-dimer in the diagnosis of suspected deep-vein thrombosis. *N Eng J Med.* 2003;349:1227–1235.

31. Elias A, Mallard L, Elias M, et al. A single complete ultrasound investigation of the venous network for the diagnostic management of patients with a clinically suspected first episode of deep venous thrombosis of the lower limbs. *Thromb Haemost.* 2003;89:221–227.

32. Schellong SM, Schwarz T, Halbritter K, et al. Complete compression ultrasonography of the leg veins as a single test for the diagnosis of deep vein thrombosis. *J Thromb Haem.* 2003;89:228–234.

33. Schwarz T, Schmidt B, Schmidt B, et al. *Clin App Thromb Hemos.* 2002;8(1):45–49.

34. Duwe KM, Shiau M, Budorick NE, et al. Evaluation of the lower extremity veins in patients with suspected pulmonary embolism: a retrospective comparison of helical CT venography and sonography. *Am J Roent.* 2000;175:1525–1531.

35. Linkins LA, Stretton R, Probyn L, et al. Interobserver agreement on ultrasound measurements of residual vein diameter, thrombus echogenicity and doppler venous flow in patients with previous venous thrombosis. *Thromb Res.* 2006;117(3):241–247.

36. Tan M, Mol GC, van Rooden CJ, et al. Magnetic resonance direct thrombus imaging differentiates acute recurrent ipsilateral deep vein thrombosis from residual thrombosis. *Blood.* 2014;124(4):623–627.

37. Westerbeek RE, Van Rooden CJ, Tan M, et al. Magnetic resonance direct thrombus imaging of the evolution of acute deep vein thrombosis of the leg. *J Thromb Haemost.* 2008;6(7):1087–1092.

38. Hunsaker AR, Lu MT, Goldhaber SZ, et al. Imaging in acute pulmonary embolism with special clinical scenarios. *Circ Cardiovasc Imaging.* 2010;3(4):491–500.

39. Quiroz R, Kucher N, Zou KH, et al. Clinical validity of a negative computed tomography scan in patients with suspected pulmonary embolism. *JAMA.* 2005;293:2012–2017.

40. Carrier M, Righini M, Wells PS, et al. Subsegmental pulmonary embolism diagnosed by computed tomography: Incidence and clinical implications. A systematic review and meta-analysis of the management outcome studies. *J Thromb Haemost.* 2010;8(8):1716–1722.

41. Kruip MJ, van der Heul C, Prins MH, et al. Diagnostic strategies for excluding pulmonary embolism in clinical outcome studies. *Ann Intern Med.* 2003;138:941–951.

42. The PIOPED Investigators. Value of the ventilation/perfusion scan in acute pulmonary embolism: results of the prospective investigation of pulmonary embolism diagnosis (PIOPED). *JAMA.* 1990;263:2753–2759.

43. Stein PD, Chenevert TL, Fowler SE, et al. Gadolinium-enhanced magnetic resonance angiography for pulmonary embolism. *Ann Intern Med.* 2010;152:434–443.

44. Rodger M, Makropoulos D, Turek M, et al. Diagnostic value of the electrocardiogram in suspected pulmonary embolism. *Am J Cardiol.* 2000;86:807–809.

45. McConnell MV, Solomon SD, Rayan ME, et al. Regional right ventricular dysfunction detected by echocardiography in acute pulmonary embolism. *Am J Cardiol.* 1996;78:469–473.

46. Kurnicka K, Lichodziejewska B, Goliszek S, et al. Echocardiographic pattern of acute pulmonary embolism: analysis of 511 consecutive patients. *J Am Soc Echocardiogr.* 2016;29(9):907–913.

47. Fields JM, Davis J, Girson L, et al. Transthoracic echocardiography for diagnosing pulmonary embolism: a systematic review and meta-analysis. *J Am Soc Echocardiogr.* 2017;30(7):714–723.

48. Turkstra F, Kuijer PM, van Beek EJ, et al. Diagnostic utility of ultrasonography of leg veins in patients suspected of having pulmonary embolism. *Annals of Internal Medicine.* 1997;126:775–781.

49. Kline JA, Courtney DM, Kabrhel C, et al. Prospective multicenter evaluation of the pulmonary embolism rule-out criteria. *J Thromb Haemost.* 2008;6(5):772–780.

50. Leung AN, Bull TM, Jaeschke R, et al. An official American Thoracic Society/Society of Thoracic Radiology clinical practice guideline: evaluation of suspected pulmonary embolism in pregnancy. *Am J Respir Crit Care Med.* 2011;184(10):1200–1208.

51. Konstantinides SV, Torbicki A, Agnelli G, et al. 2014 ESC guidelines on the diagnosis and management of acute pulmonary embolism. *Eur Heart J.* 2014;35(43):3033–3069.

52. Tromeur C, van der Pol LM, Klok FA, et al. Pitfalls in the diagnostic management of pulmonary embolism in pregnancy. *Thromb Res.* 2017;151:S86–S91.

53. Righini M, Jobic C, Boehlen F, et al. Predicting deep venous thrombosis in pregnancy: external validation of the left clinical prediction rule. *Haematologica.* 2013;98(4):545–548.

54. Cahill AG, Stout MJ, Macones GA, et al. Diagnosing pulmonary embolism in pregnancy using computed-tomographic angiography or ventilation–perfusion. *Obst Gynec.* 2009;114:124–129.

55. Ashrani AA, Heit JA. Incidence and cost burden of post-thrombotic syndrome. *J Thromb Thrombolysis.* 2009;28(4):465–476.

56. Vedantham S, Goldhaber SZ, Julian JA, et al. Pharmacomechanical catheter-directed thrombolysis for deep-vein thrombosis. *N Engl J Med.* 2017;377(23):2240–2252.

57. Casazza F, Becattini C, Bongarzoni A, et al. Clinical features and short term outcomes of patients with acute pulmonary embolism. The Italian Pulmonary Embolism Registry (IPER). *Thromb Res.* 2012;130(6):847–852.

58. Piazza G, Goldhaber SZ. Management of submassive pulmonary embolism. *Circulation.* 2010;122(11):1124–1129.

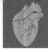

59. Aujesky D, Obrosky S, Stone RA, et al. Derivation and validation of a prognostic model for pulmonary embolism. *Am J Respir Crit Care Med.* 2005;172:1041–1046.

60. Jimenez D, Aujesky D, Moores L, et al. Simplification of the pulmonary embolism severity index for prognostication in patients with acute symptomatic pulmonary embolism. *Arch Intern Med.* 2010;170(15): 1383–1389.

61. Meinel FG, Nance Jr JW, Schoepf UJ, et al. Predictive value of computed tomography in acute pulmonary embolism: systematic review and meta-analysis. *Am J Med.* 2015;128:747–759.

62. Gouin B, Blondon M, Jimenez D, et al. Clinical prognosis of nonmassive central and noncentral pulmonary embolism: a registry-based cohort study. *Chest.* 2017;151(4):829–837.

63. Kucher N, Rossi E, De Rosa M, et al. Prognostic role of echocardiography among patients with acute pulmonary embolism and a systolic arterial pressure of 90 mm hg or higher. *Arch Int Med.* 2005;165:1777–1781.

64. Pruszczyk P, Goliszek S, Lichodziejewska B, et al. Prognostic value of echocardiography in normotensive patients with acute pulmonary embolism. *JACC Cardiovasc Imag.* 2014;7(6):553–560.

65. Khemasuwan D, Yingchoncharoen T, Tunsupon P, et al. Right ventricular echocardiographic parameters are associated with mortality after acute pulmonary embolism. *J Am Soc Echocardiogr.* 2015;28(3):355–362.

66. Vitarelli A, Barilla F, Capotosto L, et al. Right ventricular function in acute pulmonary embolism: a combined assessment by three-dimensional and speckle-tracking echocardiography. *J Am Soc Echocardiogr.* 2014;27(3):329–338.

67. Dahhan T, Siddiqui I, Tapson VF, et al. Clinical and echocardiographic predictors of mortality in acute pulmonary embolism. *Cardiovasc Ultrasound.* 2016;14(1):44.

68. Becattini C, Vedovati MC, Agnelli G. Prognostic value of troponins in acute pulmonary embolism: a meta-analysis. *Circulation.* 2007;116(4):427–433.

69. Klok FA, Mos IC, Huisman MV. Brain-type natriuretic peptide levels in the prediction of adverse outcome in patients with pulmonary embolism: a systematic review and meta-analysis. *Am J Respir Crit Care Med.* 2008;178(4):425–430.

70. Torbicki A, Galié N, Covezzoli A, et al. Right heart thrombi in pulmonary embolism. *J Am Coll Cardiol.* 2003;41(12):2245–2251.

71. Jimenez D, Aujesky D, Diaz G, et al. Prognostic significance of deep vein thrombosis in patients presenting with acute symptomatic pulmonary embolism. *Am J Respir Crit Care Med.* 2010;181(9):983–991.

72. Shopp JD, Stewart LK, Emmett TW, et al. Findings from 12-lead electrocardiography that predict circulatory shock from pulmonary embolism: systematic review and meta-analysis. *Acad Emerg Med.* 2015;22(10):1127–1137.

73. Daniel KR, Courtney DM, Kline JA. Assessment of cardiac stress from massive pulmonary embolism with 12-lead ECG. *Chest.* 2001;120:474–481.

74. Keller K, Beule J, Balzer JO, et al. Right bundle branch block and SIQIII-type patterns for risk stratification in acute pulmonary embolism. *J Electrocardiol.* 2016;49(4):512–518.

75. Kukla P, McIntyre WF, Fijorek K, et al. Use of ischemic ECG patterns for risk stratification in intermediate-risk patients with acute PE. *Am J Emerg Med.* 2014;32(10):1248–1252.

76. Kohn CG, Mearns ES, Parker MW, et al. Prognostic accuracy of clinical prediction rules for early post-pulmonary embolism all-cause mortality: a bivariate meta-analysis. *Chest.* 2015;147(4):1043–1062.

77. Jaff MR, McMurtry MS, Archer SL, et al. Management of massive and submassive pulmonary embolism, iliofemoral deep vein thrombosis, and chronic thromboembolic pulmonary hypertension: a scientific statement from the American Heart Association. *Circulation.* 2011;123(16):1788–1830.

78. Kearon C, Akl EA, Ornelas J, et al. Antithrombotic therapy for VTE disease: CHEST guideline and expert panel report. *Chest.* 2016;149(2):315–352.

79. Christiansen SC, Cannegieter SC, Koster T, et al. Thrombophilia, clinical factors, and recurrent venous thrombotic events. *JAMA.* 2005;293(19):2352–2361.

80. Connors JM. Thrombophilia testing and venous thrombosis. *N Engl J Med.* 2017;377(12):1177–1187.

81. Carrier M, Lazo-Langner A, Shivakumar S, et al. Screening for occult cancer in unprovoked venous thromboembolism. *N Engl J Med.* 2015;373(8):697–704.

82. Van Doormaal FF, Terpstra W, Van Der Griend R, et al. Is extensive screening for cancer in idiopathic venous thromboembolism warranted? *J Thromb Haemost.* 2011;9(1):79–84.

83. Moudgill N, Hager E, Gonsalves C, et al. May-Thurner Syndrome: case report and review of the literature involving modern endovascular therapy. *Vascular.* 2009;17(6):330–335.

84. Sanders RJ, Hammond SL, Rao NM. Diagnosis of thoracic outlet syndrome. *J Vasc Surg.* 2007;46(3):601–604.

85. Urschel HC, Razzuk MA. Paget-Schroetter syndrome: what is the best management? *Ann Thorac Surg.* 2000;69:1663–1669.

86. Molina JE, Hunter DW, Dietz CA. Paget-Schroetter syndrome treated with thrombolytics and immediate surgery. *J Vasc Surg.* 2007;45(2):328–334.

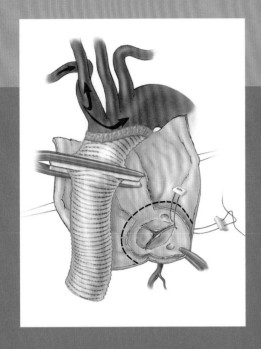

第52章
静脉血栓栓塞性疾病的管理

　　血栓栓塞事件的管理需要综合考虑临床治疗、经济效益和社会心理学等方面因素。同时，还需要关注血栓栓塞事件相关不良并发症的发生。通过全面考量这些因素，可为患者制定个性化治疗方案及二级预防措施提供充足的证据支持。抗凝治疗是血栓栓塞事件患者基础治疗手段，临床常用的抗凝药物分为胃肠外抗凝药及直接口服抗凝药（direct oral anticoagulants，DOACs）。DOACs目前已经成为血栓栓塞事件患者主要的抗凝治疗药物；然而，肾功能不全患者禁忌及较高的DOACs相关出血事件发生率使得DOACs的使用具有一定局限性。对于血栓栓塞事件患者最佳抗凝时间仍有争议，但大多数临床医师认为延长抗凝治疗时间可为患者带来更大收益。血栓栓塞事件的高级治疗方式包括溶栓（经静脉全身溶栓或经导管定向溶栓）、手术取栓和下腔静脉滤器置入。对于血栓栓塞事件相关不良并发症的管理目前仍有争议，但多数临床医师建议进行长期抗凝治疗。由于部分血栓栓塞事件患者及其家属会因疾病的发生而过度焦虑，因此，与患者及其家属建立良好的沟通将有助于患者的心理健康。血栓栓塞事件患者最佳的管理方式是一级预防，然而在现实生活中却难以实现。单一药物的使用或外科手术治疗无法解决血栓栓塞事件的复发及并发症的发生。因此，需要依据患者情况制定个性化治疗方案及二级预防措施，使患者长期受益。

戴向晨

Management of Venous Thromboembolism

Samuel Z. Goldhaber and Gregory Piazza

Optimal management of venous thromboembolism (VTE) hinges upon understanding the medical, economic, and psychosocial consequences of pulmonary embolism (PE) and deep vein thrombosis (DVT). In an international registry of 23,858 patients with acute PE over 13 years, the mean length of hospital stay decreased 32% and the risk of all-cause 30-day mortality decreased from 6.6% to 4.9%. The risk-adjusted 30-day PE-related mortality decreased from 3.3% to 1.8%.[1] Of special concern, however, is that the annual VTE event rate is increasing.[2] The adverse effects of concomitant DVT on prognosis of PE,[3] the association of VTE with atherosclerosis,[4] and the late effects of VTE—postthrombotic syndrome (PTS)[5] and chronic thromboembolic pulmonary hypertension (CTEPH)[6]—factor into the construction of a comprehensive program for immediate treatment and secondary prevention. The best management, though not always feasible, is primary prevention of VTE.

The Nationwide Inpatient Sample data show that US hospital admissions for PE increased from 23 per 100,000 in 1993 to 65 per 100,000 in 2012. The percent of massive PE admissions decreased from 5.3% to 4.4%, even though the absolute number of admissions for massive PE increased from 1.5 to 2.8 per 100,000. The median length of hospital stay for PE was halved from 8 days to 4 days. However, adjusted hospital charges increased from $16,475 in 1993 to $25,728 in 2012. All-cause hospital mortality for PE decreased from 7.1% to 3.2%.[7] Patients residing in zip codes with lower socioeconomic status had increased in-hospital mortality rates compared with patients residing in higher socioeconomic status zip codes.[8] In a Dutch study that encompassed 1.4 million inhabitants, higher neighborhood socioeconomic status was associated with a lower incidence of VTE.[9]

In an Australian study of patients hospitalized with PE, the post-discharge mortality of 8.5% per patient-year was 2.5-fold higher than that of an age- and sex-matched general population. Patients with known cardiovascular disease at baseline had a 2.2-fold greater all-cause mortality than those without cardiovascular disease; 40% of the post-discharge deaths were attributed to cardiovascular causes.[10]

The Framingham Heart Study reported VTE incidence from 1995 to 2014. The age-adjusted incidence rate was 20.3/10,000; 40% of events were PE, and 60% were DVT. Increasing age and obesity were associated with VTE.[11]

Management of VTE should strive to be cost-effective. In the US, treatment of an acute VTE has an incremental direct medical cost of about $12,000 to $15,000 among first-year survivors. Subsequent complications increase cumulative costs to $18,000 to $23,000 per incident case. Annual incident VTE events cost the U.S. healthcare system $7 to $10 billion per year for 375,000 to 475,000 newly diagnosed, medically treated cases.[12]

The psychosocial impact of VTE should also be recognized. Among patients 13 to 33 years of age, the diagnosis of VTE is associated with a poorer mental health prognosis compared with non-VTE patients. In a Danish study, 20% received prescriptions for psychotropic medications such as antidepressants, anxiolytics, or sedatives.[13] Global public awareness is lower for PE (54%) and DVT (44%) than for myocardial infarction (88%) and stroke (85%). For those stricken with VTE, they are less likely to present themselves for medical evaluation if they are not aware of the existence of VTE and its symptoms and signs (Box 52.1).[14]

PATHOPHYSIOLOGY AND RISK FACTORS FOR VENOUS THROMBOEMBOLISM

Deep Vein Thrombosis

Most venous thrombosis originates in the pelvic or deep leg veins. The clot initially is in the center of the vein. Over the ensuing days to weeks, most venous thrombi develop some fibrosis and become tethered to the vein wall. For reasons that remain uncertain, some thrombi dislodge from the vein wall and embolize to the lungs. Others never adhere to the vein wall securely and embolize to the lungs.

Certain conditions seem to cause increased adherence to the vein wall, thus lessening the chance of developing PE. The best-known example is factor V Leiden, which predisposes to VTE. The "factor V Leiden paradox" is the term used to describe this observation. These patients have more DVT than expected but less PE than would be predicted. Other apparent risk factors that share this good prognostic finding include oral contraceptive use, pregnancy, minor leg injuries, and obesity. In contrast, conditions that appear to predispose to embolization of leg DVT and result in acute PE include chronic obstructive lung disease, pneumonia, and sickle cell disease.[15]

Unresolved DVT leads to increased ambulatory venous pressure, which in turn impairs venous return, reduces calf muscle perfusion, increases tissue permeability at the microvasculature, and leads to chronic venous hypertension. The two principal mechanisms are persistent venous obstruction and valvular reflux (Fig. 52.1). Inflammation delays thrombus resolution, resulting in chronic thrombosis in the vein wall and further promoting valvular reflux. Activated inflammatory cells and platelets interact at the interface of the thrombus and vein wall.[16]

Because of inflammation in the venous thrombus, with its associated white blood cells and activated platelets, VTE is no longer classified as a "red clot" disease. Thrombi due to PE and DVT are filled with polymorphonuclear leukocytes and activated platelets, which release procoagulant microparticles and proinflammatory mediators. Neutrophil extracellular traps (NETs) consist of DNA extruded from white blood cells. These NETs are prothrombotic and procoagulant. NETs provide the scaffold that binds erythrocytes and that promotes further platelet aggregation.[17]

- In-hospital PE mortality has declined by about 50% over the past decade.
- Median length of hospital stay for PE has halved during the past decade.
- Annual incident VTE events cost the US healthcare system $7–$10 billion.
- VTE occurs more often in communities with lower socioeconomic status.
- Global public awareness of PE and DVT is lower than of myocardial infarction and stroke.

DVT, Deep vein thrombosis; PE, pulmonary embolism; VTE, venous thromboembolism.

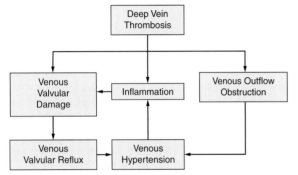

Fig. 52.1 Pathophysiology of symptoms in deep venous thrombosis.

Pulmonary Embolism

The right ventricle plays a central role in the pathophysiology of PE (Fig. 52.2A). Increased pulmonary vascular resistance leads to right ventricular overload, which in turn can cause right ventricular dilatation and hypokinesis. Increased right ventricular systolic pressure causes deviation of the interventricular septum toward the left ventricle. In severe cases, right ventricular cardiac output decreases (see Fig. 52.2B). Although the left ventricle remains intrinsically normal, left ventricular filling can be impaired, leading to decreased left ventricular cardiac output, with consequent decrease of systemic arterial pressure. Increased right ventricular myocardial wall tension impedes oxygen supply to the right ventricle, resulting in decreased coronary arterial perfusion, especially to the right coronary artery. The result is right ventricular ischemia and microinfarction of the right ventricle.

Right ventricular myocardial stretch leads to elevation of brain natriuretic peptide (BNP) levels. Right ventricular microinfarction leads to elevation of cardiac biomarkers such as troponin[18] and heart-type fatty acid-binding protein.[19]

Impaired gas exchange occurs because of: (1) increased alveolar dead space due to vascular obstruction, (2) hypoxemia from alveolar hypoventilation and right-to-left shunting, (3) impaired carbon monoxide transfer caused by loss of gas exchange surface, (4) alveolar hyperventilation caused by reflex stimulation of irritant receptors, (5) increased airway resistance due to bronchoconstriction, and (6) decreased pulmonary compliance due to lung edema, lung hemorrhage, and loss of surfactant.

The "Post-PE Syndrome" is characterized by suboptimal cardiac function, abnormal pulmonary gas exchange in combination with chronic dyspnea, exercise intolerance, chronic functional limitations, and decreased quality of life.[20] The pathophysiology is thought most likely due to impaired endogenous fibrinolysis coupled with abnormal thrombus remodeling.

Root Causes of Venous Thromboembolism

Optimal strategies for VTE management can be facilitated by identifying root causes of PE and DVT. Virchow's triad of stasis, hypercoagulability, and endothelial injury has served as the foundation of our understanding of VTE pathophysiology. However, contemporary concepts prioritize inflammation as possibly the most important root cause of VTE.[21]

VTE is now considered part of a pan-vascular syndrome of thrombosis-related illnesses that include myocardial infarction,[22] stroke, and peripheral artery disease.[23] Classic cardiovascular risk factors for coronary artery disease serve as risk factors associated with VTE, including obesity, hypertension, diabetes mellitus, smoking, and hypercholesterolemia, as well as low HDL cholesterol levels.[24] A more recent study only showed an association between VTE and cigarette smoking.[25] Other inflammatory illnesses associated with VTE include psoriasis[26] and sepsis.[27]

In a registry of 991 acute VTE patients, independent predictors of all-cause mortality included age, active cancer, diabetes mellitus, sedentary lifestyle, and polypharmacy.[28] In a meta-analysis of seven PE cohorts with 7868 participants, the presence of concomitant DVT almost doubled the 30-day mortality rate compared to PE patients without DVT (6.2% versus 3.8%, respectively).[29] Another adverse prognostic factor is the "weekend effect," with a risk-adjusted 17% increased PE mortality rate compared with weekdays.[30]

Thrombophilia

The two most common inherited thrombophilias are factor V Leiden and the prothrombin gene mutation. A single point mutation in the factor V gene, designated factor V Leiden, causes resistance to the endogenous anticoagulant, activated protein C. A single point mutation in the prothrombin gene increases the levels of prothrombin and doubles the risk of VTE. Clinical characteristics suggesting an inherited thrombophilia include thrombosis at a young age in association with unprovoked VTE or weak provoking factors, a strong family history of VTE, recurrent VTE especially at a young age, or VTE in unusual sites, such as splanchnic or cerebral veins.[31]

Thrombophilia can impact women's contraceptive therapy, fertility, and pregnancy. Use of estrogen-containing contraceptive pills can triple the risk of VTE and, in the presence of thrombophilia such as factor V Leiden, can increase the VTE risk by at least 30-fold. Thrombophilia may manifest as difficulty with conception, recurrent pregnancy loss, or both. Thrombophilia also increases the risk of pregnancy-related complications such as preeclampsia and placental abruption.[32]

The antiphospholipid syndrome is an acquired prothrombotic disorder that can affect both the venous and arterial circulations. The deep leg veins and the cerebral arterial circulation are the most common sites of thromboses. Catastrophic antiphospholipid syndrome is characterized by thrombi in multiple small vascular beds. It can cause multisystem organ failure. The syndrome is also associated with obstetrical complications such as otherwise unexplained miscarriages and premature birth before the 34th week of gestation, often in the setting of eclampsia or severe preeclampsia.[33]

ANTICOAGULATION

Parenteral Anticoagulants: Unfractionated Heparin, Low-Molecular-Weight Heparins, Fondaparinux, and Direct Thrombin Inhibitors

Anticoagulation comprises the foundation of therapy for VTE. There are three fundamental anticoagulation strategies for treatment of acute PE or DVT: (1) parenteral monotherapy, (2) parenteral anticoagulation either overlapping or abruptly switching to oral anticoagulation, and

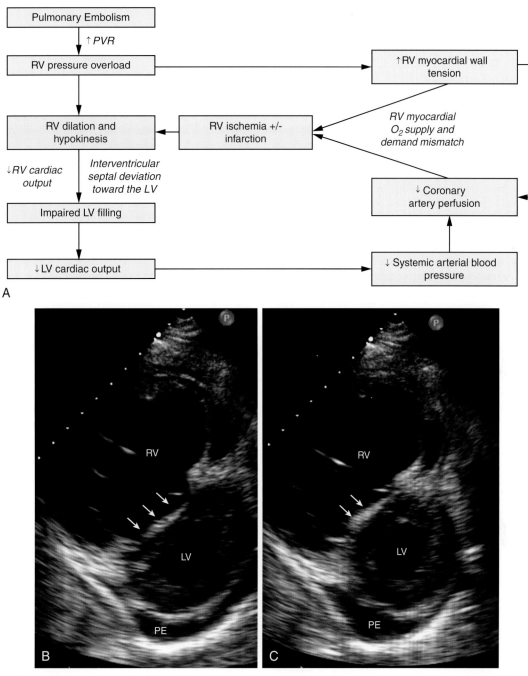

Fig. 52.2 (A) Central role of the right ventricle in the pathophysiology of pulmonary embolism. (B) and (C) Parasternal short-axis views of the right ventricle *(RV)* and left ventricle *(LV)* in diastole (B) and systole (C). There is diastolic and systolic bowing of the interventricular septum *(arrows)* into the LV, due to RV volume and pressure overload, respectively. The RV is dilated and hypokinetic, with little change in the RV area from diastole to systole, indicated poor cardiac output. There is a small pericardial effusion *(PE)*.

(3) oral anticoagulation alone, without parenteral therapy. At times, ill patients with acute VTE are initiated on continuous intravenous unfractionated heparin (UFH), followed by a switch to low-molecular-weight heparin (LMWH) as they become more clinically stable, followed by initiation of oral anticoagulation.

Unfractionated Heparin

UFH is a partially purified, highly sulfated glycosaminoglycan that is most often obtained from pig intestinal mucosa. Heparin binds to the protein, antithrombin, and changes the conformation of antithrombin so that its activity is markedly accelerated. Antithrombin, in turn, inhibits coagulation factors XII, XI, X, IX, and II (thrombin) and thus prevents additional thrombus formation. Although heparin itself does not dissolve thrombus, endogenous fibrinolytic mechanisms often lyse some of the clot that has already formed.

Inflammation contributes critically to the development of thrombosis, principally through disruption of endothelial functions, local leukocyte recruitment, and promotion of a pro-coagulant milieu. Heparin has a biological basis as a modulator of inflammation. Heparin inhibits the activation and function of neutrophils. It interacts with the vascular endothelium to prevent expression of inflammatory mediators which initiate activation of the innate immune system. Heparin also inhibits proliferation of the vascular smooth muscle cell. The anti-inflammatory effect of LMWH is at least as strong as that of UFH.[34]

Low-Molecular-Weight Heparins

UFH has an average molecular weight of about 15,000 Da, whereas LMWH has an average molecular weight of about 5000 Da. LMWH is manufactured by depolymerizing UFH using chemical or enzymatic processes. LMWH potently inhibits activated clotting factor X. It has greater bioavailability with a more predictable dose response and longer half-life than UFH. LMWH is dosed by weight in patients with normal renal function. However, because it is metabolized by the kidneys, dose reductions are required in patients with impaired renal function. Whether LMWH should be titrated using anti-Xa levels, particularly in special populations such as obese or pregnant patients, remains uncertain. When used for low-dose primary VTE prophylaxis, the typical regimen for enoxaparin is 40 mg once daily. LMWH in full dose as monotherapy is the guideline-recommended treatment for cancer patients with VTE.

Heparin-induced thrombocytopenia (HIT) and thrombosis-associated HIT occur less often with LMWH than with UFH. One hospital reduced the hospital burden of HIT by switching from UFH to LMWH.[35]

Fondaparinux

Fondaparinux is a synthetically manufactured pentasaccharide that binds to and potentiates the effect of antithrombin III in blocking activated clotting factor X. It has a long half-life, approximately 17 hours. It is metabolized by the kidney and must be downward dose-adjusted in patients with renal dysfunction. Fondaparinux has no reliable reversal agent (Box 52.2). It is often used off-label in patients with suspected or proven HIT.[36]

Direct Thrombin Inhibitors

Bivalirudin, metabolized by the kidney, and argatroban, metabolized by the liver, are the two direct thrombin inhibitors available in the United States. Argatroban is FDA approved for treatment of HIT-associated thrombosis. Bivalirudin is FDA approved for use during percutaneous coronary intervention in patients with acute or previous HIT and in patients with HIT-associated thrombosis.[37] Overall, bivalirudin is frequently used off-label for anticoagulation of any patient with suspected or proven HIT.

Oral Anticoagulation With Warfarin and Other Vitamin K Antagonists

Warfarin is the most widely used vitamin K antagonist. It prevents gamma-carboxylation of clotting factors II, VII, IX, and X. Attaining its full effect requires 5 to 7 days, and therefore, most patients are initially "bridged" with UFH, LMWH, or fondaparinux. Warfarin is usually dosed to achieve a target International Normalized Ratio (INR) between 2.0 and 3.0. Three large randomized trials of pharmacogenetic-guided versus routine clinical dosing of vitamin K antagonists showed

either no usefulness with the pharmacogenetic approach[38,39] or, at best, marginal utility.[40] The pharmacogenetic approach was also expensive and inconvenient for patients and practitioners.

In a meta-analysis of individual patient data, self-monitoring and self-management of warfarin were found to be safe options suitable for patients of all ages. In 11 trials with data for 6417 participants and 12,800 person-years of follow-up, there was a 49% reduction in thromboembolic events in the self-monitoring group. However, the 12% reduction in major hemorrhagic events with self-monitoring did not achieve statistical significance.[41]

Warfarin remains a potentially dangerous drug that can be difficult to dose and regulate, even by experienced clinicians. In a study of emergency hospitalizations for adverse drug events in older Americans, warfarin was the most frequent drug causing adverse events (33%) followed by insulin (14%), oral antiplatelet agents (13%), and oral hypoglycemic agents (11%).[42] In Denmark, increased antithrombotic drug use, especially vitamin K antagonists, was associated with a higher risk of subdural hematoma. The highest odds of subdural hematoma occurred with the combination of a vitamin K antagonist and an antiplatelet drug.[43] Almost half of intracranial hemorrhages in warfarin-treated patients occur with INRs in the desired target range of 2.0 to 3.0.

In addition to hemorrhage, warfarin is associated with an increase in coronary and peripheral vascular calcification.[44] This is due to inhibition of the enzyme matrix gamma-carboxyglutamate Gla Protein (MGP).[45] In women undergoing routine mammography, breast arterial calcification may correlate with calcification of peripheral arteries.[46] The clinical ramifications of warfarin-associated vascular calcification remain undefined.

Warfarin's anticoagulant effect can be most effectively reversed with 4-factor prothrombin complex concentrates, administered in conjunction with intravenous vitamin K. In a systematic review and meta-analysis, prothrombin complex concentrates compared with fresh frozen plasma reversed warfarin with a significant reduction in all-cause mortality, more rapid INR reduction, and less volume overload, without an increased risk of thromboembolic events.[47]

Efficacy and Safety of Direct Oral Anticoagulants (Non–vitamin K Oral Anticoagulants) for Treatment of Venous Thromboembolism

Direct oral anticoagulants (DOACs) have become the predominant anticoagulants to manage VTE. Six randomized controlled pivotal trials recruited more than 27,000 patients and led to approval of dabigatran, rivaroxaban, apixaban, and edoxaban for the treatment of PE and DVT. There are about 200,000 patients who have been studied with DOACs versus warfarin in observational cohort studies. Thus far, there is no contradiction between results from the randomized trials compared with the observational clinical practice trials.[48] In general, DOACs should be avoided in patients with a creatinine clearance less than 30 mL/min because this was an exclusion criterion in the randomized controlled pivotal VTE trials.[49]

The DOACs have noninferior efficacy but superior safety compared to warfarin for VTE treatment. When meta-analyzing the six pivotal acute VTE trials of DOACs versus warfarin, DOACs show a nonsignificant 10% reduction in recurrent VTE or VTE-related death. Regarding specific VTE subgroups, patients 75 years of age or older had a significant 44% reduction in recurrent VTE, and patients with cancer had a significant 43% reduction in recurrent VTE. In these same trials, DOACs exhibit a highly significant 39% reduction in major bleeding compared to warfarin. There was a 64% reduction in fatal bleeding and a 63% reduction in intracranial bleeding.[50]

BOX 52.2   Parenteral Anticoagulants for Acute Venous Thromboembolism

- Intravenous unfractionated heparin: 80 U/kg loading dose; 18 U/kg/h
- Subcutaneous enoxaparin: 1 mg/kg twice daily—with normal renal function
- Subcutaneous fondaparinux: 7.5 mg once daily for weight 50–100 kg; 10 mg for weight >100 kg; 5 mg for weight <50 kg—with normal renal function

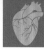

Dabigatran

Dabigatran is an oral direct thrombin inhibitor that is about 80% metabolized by the kidneys. Its half-life is about 12 to 17 hours. Dabigatran should be taken on a full stomach to minimize the possibility of gastrointestinal upset. It should not be administered if the creatinine clearance is less than 30 mL per minute.

For anticoagulation of acute VTE, the FDA has approved dabigatran in a dose of 150 mg twice daily, after a 5-day course of UFH, LMWH, or fondaparinux. This approval is based upon two pivotal randomized controlled trials, RE-COVER and RE-COVER II, comparing dabigatran to warfarin.[51,52] The pooled analysis of these two trials, comprising 5107 subjects, showed that dabigatran was noninferior to warfarin for preventing recurrent VTE and that dabigatran reduced the rate of any bleeding by 30% compared with warfarin.

Among dabigatran-treated elderly patients, as renal function worsened, recurrent VTE/VTE-related death decreased, from 3.1% with normal renal function to 1.9% for mild renal impairment, and to 0.0% with moderate renal impairment. This is probably because plasma dabigatran levels increased with worsening renal function. For warfarin-treated patients, the recurrent VTE rates were 2.6%, 1.6%, and 4.1%, respectively. Major bleeding increased with increasing renal impairment and with increasing age, with no apparent difference between dabigatran and warfarin patients.[53]

When analyzing the subset of patients who presented with symptomatic PE (with or without DVT) as the index event, dabigatran was noninferior to warfarin with respect to efficacy. Regarding major bleeding events in symptomatic PE patients, there was a significant 40% reduction in major bleeding with dabigatran compared with warfarin.[54]

Two pivotal extension studies were undertaken with dabigatran in patients who had completed at least 3 months of anticoagulation for VTE. The active control study, RE-MEDY, tested dabigatran against warfarin for 6 to 36 months in 2866 patients. In RE-MEDY, dabigatran was noninferior to warfarin with respect to efficacy and showed a significant 46% reduction in major or clinically relevant bleeding. The placebo control study, RE-SONATE, tested dabigatran against placebo for 6 months in 1353 patients. In RE-SONATE, there was a significant 92% reduction in recurrent VTE in the dabigatran group and a 3-fold increase in major or clinically relevant bleeding compared with placebo.[55]

When the efficacy of dabigatran versus warfarin in acute VTE patients with thrombophilia was studied, results were pooled from RE-COVER, RE-COVER II, and RE-MEDY. The efficacy and safety of dabigatran were not significantly affected by the presence of thrombophilia or the antiphospholipid antibody syndrome.[56]

Dabigatran administered for 6 months is currently being tested after a 72-hour course of parenteral heparin anticoagulation for acute submassive PE in a European study called PEITHO-2.[57] The target enrollment is 700 patients.

Rivaroxaban

Rivaroxaban is an oral direct anti-Xa anticoagulant that is about 35% metabolized by the kidneys. Its half-life is about 5 to 9 hours. To maximize its half-life, rivaroxaban should be taken on a full stomach. The loading dose is 15 mg twice daily for 3 weeks. The maintenance dose with normal renal function is 20 mg once daily with the dinner meal. Rivaroxaban should not be administered if the creatinine clearance is less than 30 mL per minute.

In a pivotal randomized trial, EINSTEIN-DVT, of 3449 acute DVT patients allocated to rivaroxaban or to warfarin, rivaroxaban was noninferior to warfarin with respect to efficacy and safety. DVT patients, regardless of their participation in EINSTEIN-DVT, who had completed at least 6 months of anticoagulation, were eligible to participate

in the EINSTEIN-Extension trial. These latter patients were randomized to rivaroxaban 20 mg daily versus placebo and were treated for 1 year. The rivaroxaban patients had an 82% reduction in recurrent VTE compared with placebo-treated patients. There was no significant difference in major bleeding complications between rivaroxaban and placebo, 0.7% versus 0.0%, respectively.[58]

In a "real world" observational study of rivaroxaban versus standard anticoagulation of acute DVT patients, XALIA, the rivaroxaban-treated patients had a lower risk profile at baseline than those treated with standard anticoagulation. Propensity score-adjusted results showed that rivaroxaban was a safe and effective alternative to standard anticoagulation in a broad range of patients.[59]

In another large, observational study of 13,609 rivaroxaban patients compared with 32,244 warfarin patients being treated for VTE, rivaroxaban patients had a 19% reduction in recurrent VTE and 21% reduction in major bleeding compared with warfarin patients. Rivaroxaban patients had a 60% reduction in intracranial hemorrhage and a 28% reduction in gastrointestinal bleeding compared with warfarin patients.[60]

Apixaban

Apixaban is a direct oral anti-Xa anticoagulant that is about 25% metabolized by the kidneys. Its half-life is about 12 hours. The loading dose is 10 mg twice daily for 1 week. The maintenance dose is 5 mg twice daily. Apixaban should not be administered if the creatinine clearance is less than 25 ml per minute.

The pivotal AMPLIFY Trial enrolled 5395 acute VTE patients. They were randomized to apixaban versus warfarin for a 6-month treatment course. Apixaban was noninferior to warfarin with respect to efficacy and resulted in a 69% reduction in major bleeding compared with warfarin.[61]

A 12-month extension study was undertaken in acute VTE patients who had completed 6 to 12 months of anticoagulation. Two doses of apixaban, 2.5 mg twice daily and 5 mg twice daily, were compared against placebo. The primary efficacy outcome was recurrent VTE or death from any cause. There was a highly significant 64% reduction in the primary efficacy outcome for apixaban 5 mg twice daily versus placebo and 67% reduction in the primary efficacy endpoint for apixaban 2.5 mg twice daily versus placebo. The rates of major bleeding were 0.5% in the placebo group, 0.2% in the 2.5 mg twice daily apixaban group, and 0.1% in the 5 mg twice daily apixaban group.[62]

In a substudy of AMPLIFY, the clinical presentation of bleeding events and the clinical course of bleeding events were analyzed. Of the major bleeds, there was a more severe clinical presentation in the warfarin patients (45%) compared with the apixaban patients (28%). The clinical course of major bleeds was similar.[63]

Edoxaban

Edoxaban is a direct oral anti-Xa anticoagulant that is about 50% metabolized by the kidneys. Its half-life is about 10 to 14 hours. Edoxaban can be administered with or without food. It should not be administered to patients with a creatinine clearance less than 30 mL per minute.

Edoxaban is the only DOAC that incorporated an option for reduced dosing in a pivotal VTE trial, Hokusai-VTE, leading to FDA approval.[64] Hokusai-VTE is also the largest ever randomized DOAC versus warfarin VTE trial (N = 8240: 4921 with DVT and 3319 with PE). All patients required 5 days of UFH or LMWH prior to being randomized to edoxaban versus warfarin. The standard dose of edoxaban was 60 mg once daily. However, patients with a creatinine clearance of 30 to 50 mL per minute, or a body weight of 60 kg or less, or those receiving concomitant potent P-glycoprotein inhibitors, were placed on a reduced dose of 30 mg once daily. Edoxaban or warfarin was administered for 3 to 12 months.

Edoxaban was noninferior compared to warfarin with respect to overall efficacy. However, a subgroup of 938 of the PE patients had right ventricular dysfunction, defined as an elevated NT-pro-BNP level at baseline. In a prespecified analysis of this subgroup of PE patients with right ventricular dysfunction, there was a significant 48% reduction in recurrent VTE: 3.3% with edoxaban compared with 6.2% with warfarin.[65]

In the overall trial, edoxaban was superior to warfarin with respect to safety. There was a significant 19% reduction in major or clinically relevant nonmajor bleeding.

Further analyses were carried out in high-risk VTE patients identified by older age, multiple comorbidities, and polypharmacy. There was a nonsignificant trend toward fewer episodes of recurrent VTE in edoxaban-treated high-risk patients. The relative safety of edoxaban compared to warfarin was maintained.[66]

Selecting the Optimal Oral Anticoagulant

Selection of the optimal oral anticoagulant incorporates the clinical presentation, comorbidities, patient preferences, and recognition of any obstacles to medication adherence (Box 52.3). In our practices, we select warfarin for patients who have had difficulty with medication adherence. INR monitoring keeps them in close contact with healthcare providers and ensures rapid feedback to the patient if there is no INR evidence of a warfarin effect. We also use warfarin for patients who require an intensive anticoagulation regimen, often due to clinical failure of anticoagulation with standard intensity anticoagulation. Warfarin allows us to modulate and titrate the intensity of anticoagulation.

We select dabigatran for patients with average or increased body weight who have normal renal function. Dabigatran appears suitable for patients with anatomically extensive VTE. We remind these patients to take dabigatran with a large breakfast and large dinner. Dabigatran has the most robust trial data for extended duration therapy, with one trial comparing it to warfarin and another comparing it to placebo. It is also the DOAC with which we have the longest market experience.

Rivaroxaban has a short half-life. After the 3-week loading dose is complete, it is administered once daily with the dinner meal. It seems particularly well suited for patients with anatomically mild or moderate VTE. There are excellent trial data to justify its use for extended duration, especially in patients with provoked VTE.

Apixaban is dosed twice daily and is primarily metabolized by the liver. It appears particularly suitable for frail patients at high risk of bleeding. The extended duration data with 2.5 mg twice daily dosing make it especially appealing because of its low major bleeding complication rate.

Edoxaban has a niche of being superior to warfarin in patients with large PE that elevates the biomarker, pro-BNP. It has no restrictions on the time of day it is administered and can be taken with or without food. Edoxaban is convenient because it is a once daily medication and

is the only DOAC which incorporated a lower dose into the pivotal clinical trial for patients with moderately severe chronic kidney disease or for low body weight. Another important niche is that edoxaban has the best data of any DOAC to support its use in patients with cancer and VTE.

Specialty Society Guidelines for Management of Venous Thromboembolism With Oral Anticoagulants

The 2016 update of the American College of Chest Physicians Guidelines recommends DOACs in preference to warfarin for the initial and long-term treatment of VTE in patients without cancer. This guideline is based on the lower bleeding rate with DOACs compared to warfarin in VTE trials and the greater convenience of DOACs for patients and healthcare providers.[67]

Fundamental Approach to Managing Major Bleeding due to DOACs
General Considerations

DOACs cause less major bleeding than warfarin and have about a 50% lower intracranial hemorrhage rate than warfarin. The DOACs are also much more convenient to administer because they are prescribed in fixed doses, without the need for any routine laboratory coagulation testing. Furthermore, unlike warfarin, there are no restrictions on eating vitamin K-rich green leafy vegetables.

To minimize bleeding risks with DOACs, downward off-label dose adjustment can be considered in the setting of moderate renal dysfunction, even though this was not an option in the protocol design for the pivotal acute VTE trials of dabigatran, rivaroxaban, or apixaban. If feasible, avoid concomitant use of antiplatelet agents. Commonly used coagulation tests such as prothrombin time or thrombin time can provide qualitative information on DOACs that may be clinically useful (Box 52.4).[68] The approach we take is to measure the thrombin time to assess the presence and effect of dabigatran and to measure anti-Xa levels to gauge the effects of rivaroxaban, apixaban, and edoxaban.

There is considerable concern about how best to manage major bleeding complications due to DOACs. The populations at greatest risk for major bleeding are elderly patients, those with moderate or severe renal disease, and those who are prescribed concomitant antiplatelet therapy.

Anticoagulant-related bleeding should first be stratified according to severity and location. Because of short half-lives, DOAC-related mild bleeding can often be controlled by temporarily withholding the anticoagulant. Aside from "tincture of time," consider other general

---

BOX 52.3   Direct Oral Anticoagulants for Acute Venous Thromboembolism

- Dabigatran 150 mg twice daily with a large breakfast and dinner—after 5 days of parenteral anticoagulation
- Rivaroxaban 15 mg twice daily for 3 weeks, then 20 mg once daily with the dinner meal
- Apixaban 10 mg twice daily for 1 week, then 5 mg twice daily
- Edoxaban 60 mg once daily (reduced to 30 mg once daily with low body weight or severe chronic kidney disease)—after 5 days of parenteral anticoagulation

---

BOX 52.4   Assessment of Patients Prescribed Anticoagulants Who Present with Bleeding

Is a Vitamin K Antagonist Effect Present?
- Drug: warfarin
- Test: international normalized ratio (INR)

Is a Direct Thrombin Inhibitor Effect Present?
- Drug: dabigatran
- Test: dilute thrombin time (TT)

Is a Direct Xa Inhibitor Effect Present?
- Drug: unfractionated heparin, low-molecular-weight heparin, fondaparinux, rivaroxaban, apixaban, edoxaban
- Test: anti-Xa assay

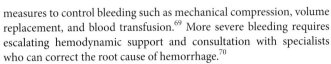

measures to control bleeding such as mechanical compression, volume replacement, and blood transfusion.[69] More severe bleeding requires escalating hemodynamic support and consultation with specialists who can correct the root cause of hemorrhage.[70]

Major therapeutic agents to reverse bleeding complications include the following: (1) coagulation factor replacement with prothrombin complex concentrates, (2) prohemostatic agents such as recombinant activated factor VII or activated prothrombin complex concentrate, which is commercially available as factor eight inhibitor bypassing activity (FEIBA), and (3) antidotes such as idarucizumab, andexanet, and ciraparantag.[71]

Steps to follow when confronted with bleeding due to DOACs include the following: (1) review the overall clinical situation, (2) remove the DOAC, if possible, with gastric lavage or hemodialysis (dabigatran), (3) repair the bleeding problem, which might require gastrointestinal endoscopy or surgery, and (4) administer reversal agents.[72]

After the major bleeding problem has been controlled, it is important to resume anticoagulation as soon as possible. Failure to resume anticoagulation in patients who have bled leads to a decrease in survival and an increase in ischemic events such as stroke and myocardial infarction, without any reduction in subsequent major hemorrhagic events.[73]

Current Trends in Clinical Practice

At Brigham and Women's Hospital, we have found that DOACs are often downward dose-adjusted even when standard dosing is recommended by the package insert.[74] As a quality improvement initiative, we are expanding our Anticoagulation Management Service from a warfarin/LMWH Service to include DOACs.[75]

Reversal Agents

Major bleeding from DOACs that cannot be controlled with conventional measures warrants management with specific reversal agents (Fig. 52.3). In addition, certain patients taking DOACs may require urgent or emergency surgery or invasive procedures that cannot safely be postponed until the DOACs are metabolized, even with their relatively short half-lives.[76] Definite indications for reversal agents include life-threatening bleeding or bleeding into a closed space or critical organ such as intracranial, intraspinal, or pericardial bleeding.[77]

Idarucizumab

This humanized monoclonal antibody fragment binds dabigatran with an affinity about 350 times greater than the affinity of dabigatran for thrombin. Idarucizumab is available as a ready-to-use solution

in a package containing two 50 mL glass vials, each with 2.5 g of idarucizumab at a concentration of 50 mg/mL. No reconstitution is necessary, thus facilitating rapid administration. Vials must be refrigerated and have a shelf life of 24 months. The total dose is 5 g administered intravenously as two consecutive 2.5-g infusions, no more than 15 minutes apart.[78]

The pivotal trial of idarucizumab for dabigatran reversal enrolled 503 patients: 301 with uncontrolled bleeding, including 46% with gastrointestinal bleeding and 33% with intracranial hemorrhage, and 202 who needed to undergo an urgent procedure or operation. In all patients, the dilute thrombin time normalized within minutes of the idarucizumab infusion. Thrombotic events at 90 days occurred in 6.3% of the cohort with uncontrolled bleeding and in 7.4% requiring an urgent procedure. The 90-day mortality rates were 19% in both groups.[79]

Andexanet

This recombinant modified Xa decoy molecule was designed as a universal reversal agent for bleeding from all DOACs that are anti-Xa agents. DOACs are more strongly attracted to the inert andexanet decoy molecule than to the real clotting factor, Xa. Theoretically, andexanet might also reverse UFH and LMWH and possibly fondaparinux due to these anticoagulants' anti-Xa activity. Serine, the active site of factor Xa, was substituted with alanine, rendering the molecule unable to cleave and activate prothrombin. The Gla domain of factor Xa was removed to prevent its assembly into the prothrombinase complex, thus removing any anticoagulant effects.[73]

Andexanet was tested in a trial that initially enrolled 67 patients with acute major bleeding within 18 hours after administration of an anti-Xa DOAC. All patients received a bolus of andexanet followed by a 2-hour infusion. The mean age was 77 years. Most bleeding was gastrointestinal or intracranial. After completion of the infusion, anti-factor Xa activity decreased by about 90%.[80]

Ciraparantag

This small synthetic new molecule binds to heparin, LMWH, and the DOACs, but it has no effect on warfarin or argatroban. The mechanism of action is not well described but involves noncovalent hydrogen bonding and charge-charge interactions. Edoxaban 60 mg was administered to each of 80 male normal volunteers. Then a single intravenous dose of 100 mg to 300 mg of ciraparantag was infused. Full reversal of anticoagulation occurred within 10 minutes and was sustained for at least 24 hours. Fibrin diameter within clots was restored to normal within 30 minutes.[81]

RECURRENT VENOUS THROMBOEMBOLISM AND OPTIMAL DURATION OF ANTICOAGULATION

One of the most contentious areas of VTE management is figuring out the optimal duration of anticoagulation for patients with PE and DVT. The classic dogma has been disrupted and is no longer operational. This outdated approach dichotomized VTE events into "provoked" or "unprovoked" categories. Provoked VTE was considered far less likely to recur after a short course of anticoagulation than unprovoked VTE, which was identified as having a high risk of recurrence after cessation of anticoagulation. Even the classic model acknowledged that over a 10-year period after cessation of anticoagulation, the recurrence rate of provoked VTE was as high as 20%. By contemporary standards, this "low" rate of recurrence is high and would be considered unacceptable for stroke or myocardial infarction. However, the major bleeding complication rate for warfarin is about 2% per year. Therefore, after 10 years of anticoagulation, the major bleeding complication rate could

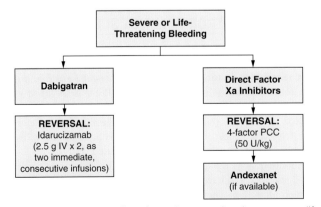

Fig. 52.3 Management of anticoagulant-associated severe or life-threatening bleeding in patients prescribed direct oral anticoagulants.

be as high as the VTE recurrence rate for provoked VTE. However, this calculation of risks versus benefits of extended-duration anticoagulation for provoked VTE has now changed because DOACs have much lower bleeding complication rates than warfarin.

Another issue is that accurate classification of provoked versus unprovoked VTE events can be difficult or impossible. The International Society of Thrombosis and Haemostasis attempted to create four categories in a cumbersome and not-well-validated approach: (1) VTE provoked by a major transient risk factor during the 3 months before the VTE, (2) VTE provoked by a "minor (yet important) transient risk factor during the 2 months prior to the VTE," (3) VTE provoked by a persistent risk factor such as cancer or "ongoing non-malignant condition associated with a least a 2-fold risk of recurrent VTE after stopping anticoagulant therapy (such as inflammatory bowel disease)," or (4) unprovoked VTE.[82]

With unprovoked VTE, the recurrence rate after cessation of anticoagulation is reported to be between 30% and 50% over the ensuing 10 years.[83] The risk of recurrence is highest during the first year.[84] One risk factor for recurrent PE is residual PE on lung scan imaging 6 months after initiation of oral anticoagulation.[85] The Vienna Prediction Model helps assess the likelihood of recurrent VTE in patients with an initial unprovoked VTE. The most important factors for predicting recurrence were male gender, PE (rather than DVT), and the degree of elevation of the D-dimer level at the time that VTE was diagnosed.[86] Residual pulmonary vascular obstruction, as assessed with lung scanning at 6 months after a first PE, is an independent predictor of recurrent VTE.[87]

Two anticoagulant management approaches to prevent recurrent VTE in patients with an initial unprovoked VTE have been tested and have been invalidated. The first strategy was used in a multicentered French study, PADIS-PE, of patients with idiopathic PE. Patients were randomized to 6 months versus 24 months of anticoagulation. The hypothesis was that a "legacy effect" would prevent recurrent PE in patients after 24 months of anticoagulation. However, the benefit of prolonged anticoagulation was not maintained after warfarin was discontinued.[88]

The second failed strategy to predict recurrence in patients with a first unprovoked VTE is anticoagulation for 3 to 7 months followed by temporary cessation of anticoagulation and D-dimer testing. The theory was that a normal D-dimer indicated that recurrent VTE would be very unlikely. In fact, the recurrence rate in patients with normal D-dimer levels was unacceptably high: 6.7% per patient-year.[89]

Our assessment is that most VTE is chronic and susceptible to recurrence, and that, in many instances, inflammation explains the recurrent nature of VTE.[90] We question the utility of trying to differentiate between provoked and unprovoked VTE to determine the optimal duration of anticoagulation.

Role of Aspirin

With inflammation, platelet activation, and platelet aggregation playing a causal role in many patients with VTE, it is appealing to consider extended duration low-dose aspirin for prevention of recurrent VTE. Aspirin is low cost and requires no special monitoring.

Aspirin also reduces the long-term incidence of some adenocarcinomas. In a meta-analysis of five large trials totaling 17,285 patients of low-dose aspirin to prevent vascular events in the UK, aspirin reduced the risk of fatal adenocarcinomas by 35%, probably by preventing distant metastasis.[91] In 34 trials of 69,224 participants randomized to aspirin versus placebo to prevent vascular events, there was a 15% reduction in cancer deaths. In six trials of low-dose aspirin for primary prevention of vascular events, reduction in nonvascular deaths accounted for most of the deaths that were prevented.[92]

> **BOX 52.5   Provoked Minor Risk Factors that Predispose to Recurrent Venous Thromboembolism after Discontinuing Anticoagulation**
>
> - Inflammatory bowel disease
> - Congestive heart failure
> - Obesity
> - Immobilization
> - Long-haul air travel
> - Estrogen/pregnancy

Low-dose aspirin versus placebo was studied in two randomized trials to prevent recurrent VTE in patients who had completed an initial course of anticoagulation for idiopathic PE or DVT.[93,94] These trials were then meta-analyzed according to a prespecified plan. Among 1224 patients, aspirin reduced recurrent VTE by 32% compared with placebo.[95]

Need for Extended-Duration Anticoagulation in Provoked Venous Thromboembolism

Most disruptive to the dogma of 3 to 6 months of anticoagulation for provoked VTE and extended duration anticoagulation restricted to unprovoked VTE are results from the EINSTEIN CHOICE trial[96]; 59% of the 3365 patients in this trial had provoked VTE. EINSTEIN CHOICE tested the hypothesis that patients with provoked VTE would benefit from extended duration anticoagulation. All patients recruited to this trial had completed 6 to 12 months of anticoagulation prior to enrollment. They were randomized to rivaroxaban 20 mg daily versus rivaroxaban 10 mg daily versus aspirin 100 mg daily. The rate of recurrent VTE was higher in unprovoked VTE patients compared to provoked VTE patients who were allocated aspirin: 5.6% versus 3.6%, respectively. However, there was a 70% reduction in recurrent VTE in the provoked VTE patients as well as in the unprovoked VTE patients randomized to receive either of the two doses of rivaroxaban compared with low-dose aspirin.

Provoked minor persisting risk factors predisposing to recurrence included: inflammatory bowel disease, lower limb paresis or paralysis, congestive heart failure, obesity, family history of VTE, and hereditary thrombophilia. Provoked minor transient risk factors predisposing to recurrence included: immobilization, long-haul travel, estrogen/pregnancy, and leg injury with impaired mobility (Box 52.5).[97]

ADVANCED MANAGEMENT OF VENOUS THROMBOEMBOLISM: WHEN ANTICOAGULATION ALONE MAY NOT OR WILL NOT SUFFICE

PE has a wide spectrum of clinical severity and mortality risk. The principal factors that determine disease severity are clinical stability, right ventricular dysfunction, and right ventricular microinfarction. The Pulmonary Embolism Severity Index (PESI) is the most extensively validated clinical prediction rule. The simplified version of PESI predicts a 30-day mortality risk of 1.0% in the absence of age greater than 80 years, cancer, chronic heart failure or pulmonary disease, tachycardia, hypotension, or oxygen desaturation.[98]

About 70% of PE patients are low risk. They have mild symptoms and signs of PE and have no evidence of right ventricular dysfunction or microinfarction. Their prognosis is excellent with anticoagulation alone. A meta-analysis of 1675 patients in 13 studies suggests that properly selected low-risk acute PE patients can be treated at home effectively and safely.[99] This strategy is being tested rigorously in a single-arm trial of 1050 patients using a standardized rivaroxaban protocol. The trial is called Home Treatment of PE (HoT-PE).[100]

Patients with preserved systemic arterial pressure and right ventricular dysfunction (diagnosed on echocardiography or chest CT) or right ventricular microinfarction (diagnosed by an elevated troponin level) have submassive, intermediate risk PE. These patients' risk can be further subdivided. "Intermediate High Risk" patients have both right ventricular dysfunction and right ventricular microinfarction. "Intermediate Low Risk" patients have either right ventricular dysfunction or right ventricular microinfarction, but not both. In our experience, the prognosis depends far more on right ventricular function rather than right ventricular microinfarction.

Most intermediate low-risk patients are hospitalized and observed, without the need for advanced therapy. Whether to administer advanced therapy to intermediate high-risk patients remains controversial. At Brigham and Women's Hospital, we usually recommend advanced therapy rather than watchful waiting. We have observed some patients in this category receive anticoagulation alone and then, with little warning, deteriorate with worsening hypoxia, respiratory distress, and hypotension. When this occurs, it is often in the middle of the night.

Massive (high-risk) PE is characterized by systemic arterial hypotension with poor perfusion of vital organs, leading to multisystem organ failure (Fig. 52.4). These patients often warrant emergent thrombolysis or surgical pulmonary embolectomy.

Interventional options for advanced management of VTE are rapidly expanding.[101] The three major categories of advanced therapy are thrombolysis (systemic or catheter-directed), surgical embolectomy (occasionally with extracorporeal membrane oxygenation [ECMO]), and vena caval filter insertion (Box 52.6).

Multidisciplinary Pulmonary Embolism Response Teams (PERTs) are being formed at most hospitals to assess patients with submassive and massive PE. These teams facilitate communication among hospital staff with expertise in vascular medicine, interventional cardiology and radiology, cardiac surgery, pulmonary vascular disease, hematology, and multimodality cardiovascular imaging. The PERT provides a consensus recommendation to the patient, family, and primary team, thus

> ## BOX 52.6 Advanced Venous Thromboembolism Management Options
>
> - FDA-approved "full-dose" alteplase (TPA): 100 mg as a continuous infusion (without heparin) over 2 hours
> - Off-label "half-dose" TPA: 50 mg—first 10 mg as a bolus over 1 minute, then 40 mg as a continuous infusion over 2 hours (with heparin 10 U/kg/h, not to exceed 1,000 U/h)
> - Ultrasound-facilitated catheter-directed thrombolysis—with 24 mg TPA
> - Inferior vena caval filter insertion
> - Surgical embolectomy
> - Extracorporeal membrane oxygenation

facilitating communication and minimizing the likelihood of contradictory messaging. PERTs offer immediate multidisciplinary cognitive and technical expertise. These teams foster cohesiveness and increase awareness of advanced therapies for submassive and massive PE.[102]

In the first 30 months of PERT at Massachusetts General Hospital, 143 submassive and 80 massive PE patients were evaluated; 11% received systemic or catheter-directed thrombolysis. The all-cause 30-day mortality rate was 12%.[103] The PERT at Beth Israel Deaconess Medical Center evaluated 72 PE patients in the first 14 months of operation; 11% received systemic thrombolysis; 18% received catheter-directed thrombolysis; 3% received ECMO; and 15% underwent inferior vena caval (IVC) filter insertion.[104] While PERTs show great potential, high-quality prospective data are required to demonstrate that PERTs help to standardize PE care, improve outcomes, and optimize cost-effectiveness.[105]

Systemic Thrombolysis Administered Through a Peripheral Vein

Thrombolysis reduces right ventricular dilatation and dysfunction by dissolving some of the thrombus obstructing the pulmonary arteries. The reduction in right ventricular pressure overload prevents continued release of serotonin which, in turn, reduces pulmonary hypertension. Dissolution of thrombus in situ in the pelvic and deep leg veins

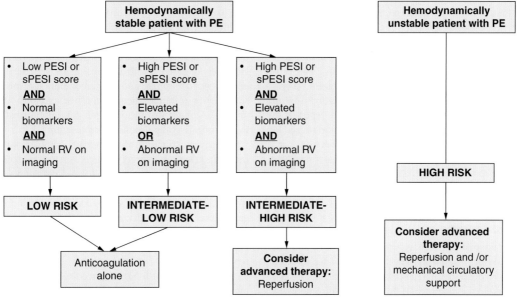

Fig. 52.4 An overall algorithm for management of pulmonary embolism based on risk stratification. *PE,* Pulmonary embolism; *PESI,* Pulmonary Embolism Severity Index; *RV,* right ventricle.

should remove much of the source of clot that could otherwise cause recurrent PE. A long-held theory, never proven, is that thrombolysis might also improve pulmonary capillary blood flow and, therefore, reduce the risk of developing CTEPH.

Full-Dose Thrombolysis

The FDA has approved full-dose alteplase (TPA) as a continuous infusion of 100 mg over 2 hours to treat massive PE without concomitant heparin. The time window for administration is up to 2 weeks after the onset of symptoms. Immediately after completion of the alteplase infusion, a partial thromboplastin time (PTT) is obtained. If the PTT is less than 80 seconds, and it almost always is, UFH is started as a continuous infusion without a bolus, with a target PTT between 60 and 80 seconds. If the PTT is greater than 80 seconds, hold heparin and repeat the PTT 4 hours later. Intracranial hemorrhage occurs in 2% to 3% of patients.

A meta-analysis was undertaken of submassive PE patients randomized in trials to thrombolysis plus heparin versus heparin alone. Thrombolysis resulted in a 47% reduction in all-cause mortality, a 60% reduction in recurrent PE, a 2.7-fold increase in major bleeding, and a 4.6-fold increase in intracranial hemorrhage.[106]

PEITHO was the largest full-dose systemic thrombolysis trial ever undertaken; 1006 patients with submassive PE were randomized to full-dose tenecteplase plus heparin versus heparin alone. At 7 days, there was a 56% reduction in death or cardiovascular collapse in the tenecteplase group. There was a 2% rate of hemorrhagic stroke in the tenecteplase patients compared with a 0.2% rate in the heparin-alone patients.[107] After a median follow-up of 38 months, about one-third of the PEITHO patients reported some persistent functional limitation, usually chronic shortness of breath. These symptoms are characteristic of the Post-PE Syndrome. Thrombolysis did not affect long-term mortality rates and did not reduce residual dyspnea or right ventricular dysfunction compared with anticoagulation alone.[108] Nor did it prevent development of CTEPH. PEITHO shows that PE is a chronic illness with long-term adverse consequences.[109] Though early death and cardiovascular collapse can be averted with full-dose systemic thrombolysis, the price is steep—a hemorrhagic stroke rate of 2%.

Reduced-Dose Systemic Thrombolysis

The "MOPETT" Trial randomized submassive PE patients to heparin plus "half-dose TPA," 50 mg administered over 2 hours, versus heparin plus placebo. The first 10 mg was given as an intravenous push within 1 minute, followed by 40 mg as a continuous infusion over 2 hours. During the alteplase infusion, the maintenance dose of UFH was reduced to 10U/kg/h, not to exceed 1000 U/hour. There were no major bleeding complications with reduced-dose thrombolysis. The estimated pulmonary artery systolic pressure by echocardiogram was reduced more in the TPA group than in the heparin alone group: 16 mm Hg versus 10 mm Hg, respectively.[110] Similar results were reported in a Chinese study of massive and submassive PE patients randomized to half-dose TPA (50 mg) versus full-dose TPA (100 mg). There was similar efficacy in the two TPA dosing regimens, with less major bleeding in the 50 mg/2 h group compared with the 100 mg/2 h group. Five studies of half-dose versus full-dose TPA thrombolysis for PE were meta-analyzed with similar results.[111]

Catheter-Directed Therapy

The high rate of intracranial hemorrhage with systemic thrombolysis has increased enthusiasm for pharmacomechanical catheter-directed reperfusion with lower doses of TPA. Efficacy with catheter-directed thrombolysis appears to be comparable to systemic thrombolysis. However, the lower doses of thrombolytic agent that are used likely lower the rate of major bleeding complications compared with systemic

thrombolysis. Multiple endovascular devices are available for interventional treatment of PE. The largest device is the AngioVac, with a 26-French access for inflow and a 16- to 20-French access for outflow. It requires a perfusion team. It is used as an alternative to open surgical embolectomy for massive PE. The AngioJet, which has lost popularity, utilizes rheolytic thrombectomy with the option of thrombolytic or saline spray. It frequently causes hypotension, bradycardia, and hemolysis. Most popular is the EkoSonic endovascular system, which utilizes ultrasound-assisted catheter-directed thrombolysis with a 24-mg dose of TPA. It is the only device with FDA approval for acute PE.[112]

Ultrasound-Facilitated Catheter-Directed Thrombolysis

With ultrasound-facilitated thrombolysis, ultrasound disaggregates fibrin strands, increases clot permeability, and disperses infused fibrinolytic drug into the clot through acoustic microstreaming effects. A thrombolytic agent is delivered via the outer infusion catheter, which contains an inner ultrasonic core wire that delivers high frequency, low-power ultrasound waves into the adjacent thrombus. This technology has the added benefit of causing the fibrin strands to thin and loosen, allowing for greater exposure of intrathrombus TPA binding sites as well as possibly increasing thrombus permeability, which can result in greater penetration of the drug. The outer EKOS catheter delivers the lytic drug, while the noncavitational ultrasound energy from the inner core wire gently drives the drug deeper into the clot. This, in turn, limits the amount of drug that escapes into the systemic circulation.[113]

The pivotal trial in the USA was SEATTLE II: a prospective single-arm, multicenter trial of the EkoSonic system for acute massive and submassive PE with 24 mg of TPA. This strategy decreased right ventricular dilatation, reduced pulmonary hypertension, and decreased anatomic thrombus burden, without intracranial hemorrhage in the 150 patients who were enrolled.[114] In a substudy, multiple venous access attempts were associated with major bleeding.[115] Another substudy showed that there was a similar improvement in right ventricular function among elderly patients compared with younger patients.[116] TPA doses as low as 8 mg with infusion durations as short as 2 hours are currently being tested.

Surgical Pulmonary Embolectomy

In the 1990s, surgical pulmonary embolectomy was abandoned and almost discarded as a credible operation and management strategy. The harshest critics were cardiac surgeons, especially those in senior positions. They berated their usually junior colleagues for operating on massive PE patients. The senior surgeons said that massive PE patients who survived were not sufficiently ill to have warranted surgery. However, for patients who died postoperatively, the operation itself was characterized as futile, and the junior staff surgeon was chastised for squandering resources, being impulsive, and for not knowing when to say "no." At many institutions, there was an informal, unspoken moratorium on surgical pulmonary embolectomy.[117]

The near-extinction of pulmonary embolectomy came about because the criteria for surgery, which were not evidence based, required that patients be hypotensive despite maximum doses of two vasopressor agents. Therefore, most patients undergoing pulmonary embolectomy were in cardiogenic shock and had already developed multisystem organ failure. The mortality, not surprisingly, hovered around 50%, and younger surgeons rarely had the appetite for undertaking the risk of operating because of the potential damage to their budding careers and reputations.[117]

Management of PE has advanced so that we now know the warning signs of impending cardiogenic shock, particularly moderate or severe right ventricular dysfunction. Multidisciplinary PERTs can now refer patients for a spectrum of advanced therapies, including surgical

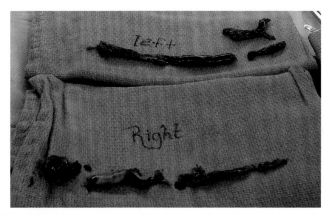

Fig. 52.5 Pulmonary embolism removed during open surgical embolectomy in a patient who developed acute onset dyspnea, hypoxemia, and systemic arterial hypotension after total hip arthroplasty.

pulmonary embolectomy. The rebirth of pulmonary embolectomy started with the case series by Aklog et al., in which 29 patients underwent embolectomy in a 2-year period, with 89% 30-day survival. All patients received permanent vena caval filters perioperatively. The report focused on lessons learned from the 11% who did not survive: (1) do not operate on a patient in cardiac arrest if a spontaneous heart rate cannot be restored preoperatively, (2) do not operate on an octogenarian if there are relative contraindications such as failed thrombolysis, (3) do not wait until an ill patient becomes critically ill.[118] This case series from Brigham and Women's Hospital was subsequently expanded to 115 patients undergoing surgical pulmonary embolectomy and reported an overall operative mortality rate of 6.6%.[119] In a series of 44 patients from Emory, 80% had submassive PE, and embolectomy was accomplished with only one in-hospital death.[120]

Surgical pulmonary embolectomy is an excellent option for patients with high-risk submassive PE or with massive PE who have a contraindication to thrombolysis (Fig. 52.5). Some patients will need cardiac surgery because of PE with clot-in-transit or paradoxical embolism to a crucial arterial site such as the aorta. During cardiopulmonary bypass, the activated clotting time is targeted to at least 480 seconds. The operation is usually done without aortic cross-clamping. Blind exploration of the pulmonary arteries should be avoided.[121]

Extracorporeal Membrane Oxygenation

With veno-arterial extracorporeal membrane oxygenation (VA ECMO), blood is extracted from a venous inflow cannula in the vena cava and returned to the arterial system via an outflow cannula, thus bypassing the heart and lungs. VA ECMO is not dependent on the patient's cardiac output and, therefore, can be used for patients in cardiogenic shock. Blood flow through the circuit is driven by an external pump, which can generate up to 8 to 10 L/min of flow.[122]

In a review of ECMO to manage massive PE, 66 cases of patient survival were identified. The mean duration of ECMO was 5 days. Half had ECMO as a bridge to surgical pulmonary embolectomy. One-quarter had ECMO and anticoagulation, without any additional therapy. The other one-quarter of patients had ECMO with systemic thrombolysis.[123]

Inferior Vena Caval Filter Insertion

The use of IVC filters increased about 25-fold from 1980 to 2000 in the United States, from approximately 2000 insertions to 50,000 insertions annually. Retrievable IVC filters were approved in the US in 2003 and, by 2006, accounted for about half of all filter insertions.

From 1993 to 2010, annual rates of IVC filter insertion in the United States increased from about 28,000 to 130,000. However, an inflection point was identified in 2010, correlating with the year the FDA issued an advisory to try to remove retrievable filters whenever medically justified and to ensure close follow-up of patients undergoing IVC filter insertion. By 2014, the annual IVC filter insertion rate fell to 96,000 per year.[124]

Generally accepted recommendations for IVC filter insertion include: (1) major bleeding on full-dose anticoagulation, (2) major contraindication to full-dose anticoagulation, and (3) new onset acute PE (especially recurrent PE) despite well-documented full-dose anticoagulation for an existing PE or DVT. However, the most common reason for IVC filter insertion currently is for patients at risk for PE who have suffered neither PE nor DVT.[125]

In a review of Medicare hospitalizations of PE patients, about 15% receive IVC filters. Insertion rates vary widely by region and are highest in the South Atlantic region and lowest in the Mountain region. Mortality associated with PE hospitalization appears to be declining, regardless of IVC filter insertion.[126]

The most recent large randomized trial, PREPIC2, enrolled 399 patients in 17 French centers. Patients were allocated retrievable IVC filter placement plus anticoagulation versus anticoagulation alone. At the 3-month endpoint, there was no reduction in recurrent VTE in the IVC filter group.[127] The fundamental flaw in this trial is that all patients were eligible to receive full-dose anticoagulation. Therefore, the trial does not reflect clinical practice, and the trial does not study the primary population of interest.

A review of the US Nationwide Inpatient Sample showed that among 21,095 unstable patients with PE, vena caval filters were associated with a reduced in-hospital all-cause case fatality rate.[128] In the RIETE registry, 371 VTE patients underwent filter insertion because of a significant bleeding risk. The risk-adjusted PE-related mortality was lower for filter insertion than no insertion patients, 1.7% versus 4.9%, respectively.[129]

A systemic review and meta-analysis of vena caval filter trials identified 11 studies with 4204 patients. Patients receiving IVC filters had a 50% lower risk for subsequent PE, a 70% increased risk for subsequent DVT, a 49% nonsignificant lower PE-related mortality rate, and no change in all-cause mortality. For every 100 patients receiving vena caval filters, these data suggest there would be 5 fewer subsequent PEs, two excess DVTs, and no change in all-cause mortality.[130]

The most recent innovation in IVC filters is the Angel Catheter (Bio2 Medical, San Antonio, TX) which combines an IVC filter with a central venous catheter. It can be placed at the bedside with ultrasound guidance to identify the femoral vein, and there is no need for fluoroscopy. The catheter was tested in a single-arm study of 163 critically ill trauma patients. No patient developed clinically significant PE, but 7% developed new or worsening proximal DVT during the first 7 days. There were no catheter-related bloodstream infections. Overall, the device prevented clinically significant and fatal PE in this critically ill major trauma population.[131]

STRATEGIES FOR MANAGING ACUTE VENOUS THROMBOEMBOLISM

Pulmonary Embolism

Most PE patients can be treated with anticoagulants alone and do not require advanced therapy such as thrombolysis or embolectomy or IVC filter placement. There are many choices for anticoagulant therapy, such as parenteral bridging or abruptly switching to oral medication versus entirely oral anticoagulation for some VTE patients who are completely stable. Selecting an appropriate anticoagulant regimen is as much an art as a science.

All patients with submassive and massive PE should be evaluated for possible advanced therapy. Patients who have elevated troponin levels indicating right ventricular microinfarction will mostly remain clinically stable if right ventricular function remains normal. In contrast, patients with moderate or severe right ventricular dysfunction are at risk of rapid hemodynamic deterioration and should be considered for advanced therapy while they are clinically stable. The alternative approach is to heparinize, observe, and resort to advanced therapy only if the patient begins to show signs of hemodynamic instability.

It is easy to identify the patient with massive PE. These patients are acutely ill, and their survival is threatened. Choosing which advanced therapies they will receive depends upon the clinical expertise at the specific institution or that institution's tertiary hospital to which such patients are emergently transferred.

Deep Venous Thrombosis and Minimizing Postthrombotic Syndrome

PTS is a potentially debilitating complication of DVT resulting in chronic pain, persistent edema, and, in advanced cases, venous ulceration (Fig. 52.6). The American Heart Association Scientific Statement on PTS is a comprehensive compendium of contemporary approaches to its diagnosis and treatment.[132] In acute DVT patients randomized to graduated compression stockings versus placebo stockings for 2 years of stocking therapy, there was no reduction in the incidence of PTS in the real compression stocking group compared with the placebo stocking group: 14% versus 13%, respectively.[133] In a trial of ultrasound-assisted versus conventional catheter-directed thrombolysis for acute iliofemoral DVT, there was no reduction in PTS in the ultrasound-assisted catheter group.[134]

A Norwegian Trial randomized 209 first-time iliofemoral DVT patients to catheter-directed thrombolysis versus standard anticoagulant treatment. The co-primary endpoints were frequency of PTS at 24 months and iliofemoral patency at 6 months. Both endpoints favored catheter-directed thrombolysis. PTS frequency at 2 years was 41% versus 56%, respectively. Iliofemoral patency at 6 months was 66% versus 47%, respectively.[135] Catheter-directed thrombolysis was also cost-effective.[136]

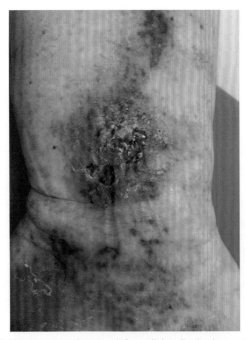

Fig. 52.6 Venous ulceration over left medial malleolus in a patient with recurrent deep vein thrombosis of the left lower extremity.

The most comprehensive study of pharmacomechanical catheter-directed thrombolysis for DVT to prevent PTS is the National Heart, Lung, and Blood Institute–sponsored ATTRACT Trial, in which 692 patients with femoral or iliofemoral DVT were randomized to pharmacomechanical therapy with catheter-directed thrombolysis plus anticoagulation versus anticoagulation alone. The primary endpoint was development of PTS 24 months after enrollment in the trial. The study showed that pharmacomechanical catheter-directed thrombolysis did not lower the risk of PTS compared with anticoagulation alone. However, the catheter-directed thrombolysis group had a higher rate of major bleeding complications.[137]

Cancer and Venous Thrombosis

LMWH as monotherapy is the standard anticoagulation regimen for cancer patients with VTE. In a landmark trial, the CLOT Trial, dalteparin as monotherapy halved the recurrent VTE rate compared with warfarin.[138] In a subsequent trial with LMWH monotherapy using tinzaparin, the bleeding rate was about 40% lower with tinzaparin than with warfarin.[139] In our experience, most cancer patients with VTE tire or become unacceptably bruised after about 6 months of self-injection with LMWH as monotherapy. We have routinely switched them off-label to a DOAC.

The Hokusai VTE Cancer trial randomized 1050 patients with cancer who had symptomatic or incidental VTE to either edoxaban or full therapeutic-dose dalteparin as monotherapy. Recurrent VTE occurred in 7.9% of the edoxaban patients versus 11.3% receiving dalteparin (risk difference −3.4%; 95% CI, −7.0 to 0.2). Major bleeding occurred in 6.9% of edoxaban patients versus 4.0% receiving dalteparin (risk difference 2.9%; 95% CI, 0.1 to 5.6). Most of the excess bleeding was gastrointestinal.[140] The trial met its primary endpoint: noninferiority of edoxaban compared with dalteparin when combining recurrent VTE and major bleeding endpoints. These results allow providers and cancer patients to make more informed decisions about anticoagulation strategy. Guideline committees are starting to endorse DOACs as an alternative to LMWH monotherapy.

Heparin-Induced Thrombocytopenia

VTE and arterial thrombosis can be caused by HIT. Diagnosis of HIT is critical because management differs for HIT patients with VTE compared with patients who have VTE without HIT. The most important immediate intervention in patients with suspected or confirmed HIT is the prompt cessation of UFH or LMWH.[141] Keep in mind that catheters may be heparin coated and that heparin flushes may be administered without specific orders to do so.[37] In the United States, the direct thrombin inhibitor, bivalirudin, is the most commonly prescribed anticoagulant for HIT patients. Off-label use of fondaparinux to treat HIT has gained popularity due to its convenience and high success rate in this population.[36] A preliminary report using DOACs to manage HIT appears promising.[142]

Isolated Calf Deep Vein Thrombosis

Optimal management of isolated calf DVT has generated controversy for several generations. We anticoagulate patients with symptomatic calf DVT for at least 3 months, unless their bleeding risk is prohibitive. In a retrospective cohort study of 280 isolated calf DVT patients who were symptomatic and who were anticoagulated for 4 to 6 weeks, 42 (15%) developed recurrent VTE within 42 months of follow-up. Half of the recurrent events were either proximal leg DVT or PE.[143] The rates of recurrence in this cohort are sufficiently high that most clinicians would recommend longer-term or indefinite-duration anticoagulation.[144] The link between inflammation and VTE, even isolated calf DVT, may be among the most plausible explanations for such a high recurrence rate after anticoagulation is discontinued.[90]

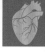

THE MULTITUDE OF CHALLENGES IN MANAGING VENOUS THROMBOSIS

It would be a mistake to think that management of VTE is mostly about choosing which anticoagulants should be prescribed and which advanced therapies, if any, should be considered. The allure of VTE management is the opportunity to empathize with the patient and family and to have them reveal and discuss their fears and concerns.

What might seem like a straightforward acute popliteal DVT that can be managed entirely with outpatient oral anticoagulation is, for most patients, a major life event. The most pressing question is: "Why did this happen to me?" The answer is often that the etiology tends to be multifactorial. For example, a viral infection during the winter season might have triggered an inflammatory response at a time when the patient felt too tired to exercise and had gained weight after the Holiday Season and New Year celebrations. However, sometimes we have no reasonable explanation, which is especially frustrating for the patient, family, and healthcare provider.

The next question the patient probably has is: "How long do I need to be anticoagulated and, when I stop anticoagulation, what is the chance I'll suffer a recurrence?" This is a difficult question without any easy answers. You can share with the patient the results of the EINSTEIN CHOICE trial and the growing consensus that VTE is often due to chronic, perhaps sporadic, inflammation.

The patient will want to know the implications for other family members. This is tricky because a negative workup for thrombophilia does not exclude a strong hereditary tie. Certainly, obtaining a careful and extensive family history is useful.

We have found that many of these issues can be discussed meaningfully, and with empathy from peers, in patient support groups. We run both live and online support groups under the sponsorship of a nonprofit organization, the North American Thrombosis Forum (www.NATFonline.org). Our live support group has been held one evening per month at Brigham and Women's Hospital for more than 25 years.

Our messaging about VTE is positive and encouraging. The in-hospital death rate from PE is decreasing rapidly. Our understanding of the etiology of VTE is becoming more comprehensive. We have more anticoagulants in our toolbox than ever before. The DOACs have fewer bleeding complications and are far more convenient to administer than warfarin. As for advanced therapy, we are learning to utilize lower doses of thrombolytic agents, which will improve safety. And we manage submassive and massive PE as a multidisciplinary team. Patients can be reassured that in most cases, the prognosis and outlook are encouraging.

A LOOK INTO THE FUTURE

The in-hospital death rate for acute PE is decreasing rapidly. But the best approach to VTE management will be primary prevention, so that PE and DVT become much less frequent. Addressing modifiable cardiovascular risk factors such as cigarette smoking, hypertension, hyperlipidemia, obesity, and sedentary lifestyle might help decrease VTE incidence as well as the incidence of myocardial infarction and stroke.

With respect to primary VTE prevention, we have made great strides by routinely prescribing prophylactic UFH and LMWH in hospitalized patients. Nevertheless, about 75% of VTE events occur out-of-hospital, many within the first month of hospital discharge.[145] To address the unmet need to prevent VTE early after hospital discharge, a new DOAC, betrixaban, was tested in a large randomized trial against enoxaparin.[146] Betrixaban is an anti-Xa anticoagulant. It has a longer half-life, 19 to 25 hours, than the other DOACs. Betrixaban also has less renal excretion than the other DOACs, only

7% to 17%. The vulnerable period following hospitalization is responsible for hundreds of thousands of VTE events annually in the United States alone. The pivotal APEX trial randomized (double-blind, double-dummy) hospitalized medically ill patients to an average of 10 days of enoxaparin 40 mg once daily versus betrixaban 80 mg tablets once daily for 35 to 42 days. Compared with enoxaparin, the betrixaban group had a 24% reduction in overall VTE and a 46% reduction in symptomatic VTE.[146] Betrixaban also cut the stroke rate by 56%[147] and reduced VTE-related rehospitalization by 56% compared with enoxaparin.[147] In 2017, the FDA approved betrixaban for prevention of VTE during hospitalization for medical illness and for the first month after hospital discharge. The MARINER trial utilized rivaroxaban and prevented VTE among hospitalized medically ill patients after discharge.[148]

REFERENCES

1. Jimenez D, de Miguel-Diez J, Guijarro R, et al. Trends in the management and outcomes of acute pulmonary embolism: analysis from the RIETE registry. *J Am Coll Cardiol.* 2016;67(2):162–170.
2. Huang W, Goldberg RJ, Anderson FA, et al. Secular trends in occurrence of acute venous thromboembolism: the Worcester VTE study (1985-2009). *Am J Med.* 2014;127(9):829–839. e825.
3. Prandoni P, Lensing AWA, Prins MH, et al. Does the presence of clinical symptoms of pulmonary embolism affect the outcome of patients with deep vein thrombosis? *Thromb Res.* 2017;157:134–135.
4. Prandoni P, Bilora F, Marchiori A, et al. An association between atherosclerosis and venous thrombosis. *N Engl J Med.* 2003;348(15):1435–1441.
5. Winter MP, Schernthaner GH, Lang IM. Chronic complications of venous thromboembolism. *J Thromb Haemost.* 2017;15(8):1531–1540.
6. Simonneau G, Torbicki A, Dorfmuller P, et al. The pathophysiology of chronic thromboembolic pulmonary hypertension. *Eur Respir Rev.* 2017;26(143).
7. Smith SB, Geske JB, Kathuria P, et al. Analysis of national trends in admissions for pulmonary embolism. *Chest.* 2016;150(1):35–45.
8. Agarwal S, Menon V, Jaber WA. Residential zip code influences outcomes following hospitalization for acute pulmonary embolism in the United States. *Vasc Med.* 2015;20(5):439–446.
9. Kort D, van Rein N, van der Meer FJM, et al. Relationship between neighborhood socioeconomic status and venous thromboembolism: results from a population-based study. *J Thromb Haemost.* 2017;15(12):2352–2360.
10. Ng AC, Chung T, Yong AS, et al. Long-term cardiovascular and noncardiovascular mortality of 1023 patients with confirmed acute pulmonary embolism. *Circ Cardiovasc Qual Outcomes.* 2011;4(1):122–128.
11. Puurunen MK, Gona PN, Larson MG, et al. Epidemiology of venous thromboembolism in the Framingham heart study. *Thromb Res.* 2016;145:27–33.
12. Grosse SD, Nelson RE, Nyarko KA, et al. The economic burden of incident venous thromboembolism in the United States: a review of estimated attributable healthcare costs. *Thromb Res.* 2016;137:3–10.
13. Hojen AA, Dreyer PS, Lane DA, et al. Adolescents' and young adults' lived experiences following venous thromboembolism: "It will always lie in wait". *Nurs Res.* 2016;65(6):455–464.
14. Wendelboe AM, Raskob GE. Global burden of thrombosis: epidemiologic aspects. *Circ Res.* 2016;118(9):1340–1347.
15. van Langevelde K, Flinterman LE, van Hylckama Vlieg A, et al. Broadening the factor V Leiden paradox: pulmonary embolism and deep-vein thrombosis as 2 sides of the spectrum. *Blood.* 2012;120(5):933–946.
16. Rabinovich A, Kahn SR. The postthrombotic syndrome: current evidence and future challenges. *J Thromb Haemost.* 2017;15(2):230–241.
17. Savchenko AS, Martinod K, Seidman MA, et al. Neutrophil extracellular traps form predominantly during the organizing stage of human venous thromboembolism development. *J Thromb Haemost.* 2014;12(6):860–870.

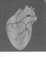

18. Bajaj A, Saleeb M, Rathor P, et al. Prognostic value of troponins in acute nonmassive pulmonary embolism: a meta-analysis. *Heart Lung.* 2015;44(4):327–334.

19. Bajaj A, Rathor P, Sehgal V, et al. Risk stratification in acute pulmonary embolism with heart-type fatty acid-binding protein: a meta-analysis. *J Crit Care.* 2015;30(5):1151–1157. 1151 e.

20. Sista AK, Klok FA. Late outcomes of pulmonary embolism: the post-PE syndrome. *Thromb Res.* 2018;164:157–162.

21. Riva N, Donadini MP, Ageno W. Epidemiology and pathophysiology of venous thromboembolism: similarities with atherothrombosis and the role of inflammation. *Thromb Haemost.* 2015;113(6):1176–1183.

22. Rinde LB, Lind C, Smabrekke B, et al. Impact of incident myocardial infarction on the risk of venous thromboembolism: the Tromsø Study. *J Thromb Haemost.* 2016;14(6):1183–1191.

23. Becattini C, Vedovati MC, Ageno W, et al. Incidence of arterial cardiovascular events after venous thromboembolism: a systematic review and a meta-analysis. *J Thromb Haemost.* 2010;8(5):891–897.

24. Ageno W, Becattini C, Brighton T, et al. Cardiovascular risk factors and venous thromboembolism: a meta-analysis. *Circulation.* 2008;117(1):93–102.

25. Mahmoodi BK, Cushman M, Anne Naess I, et al. Association of traditional cardiovascular risk factors with venous thromboembolism: an individual participant data meta-analysis of prospective studies. *Circulation.* 2017;135(1):7–16.

26. Chung WS, Lin CL. Increased risks of venous thromboembolism in patients with psoriasis. A nationwide cohort study. *Thromb Haemost.* 2017;117(8):1637–1643.

27. Kaplan D, Casper TC, Elliott CG, et al. VTE incidence and risk factors in patients with severe sepsis and septic shock. *Chest.* 2015;148(5):1224–1230.

28. Faller N, Limacher A, Mean M, et al. Predictors and causes of long-term mortality in elderly patients with acute venous thromboembolism: a prospective cohort study. *Am J Med.* 2017;130(2):198–206.

29. Becattini C, Cohen AT, Agnelli G, et al. Risk stratification of patients with acute symptomatic pulmonary embolism based on presence or absence of lower extremity DVT: systematic review and meta-analysis. *Chest.* 2016;149(1):192–200.

30. Nanchal R, Kumar G, Taneja A, et al. Pulmonary embolism: the weekend effect. *Chest.* 2012;142(3):690–696.

31. Connors JM. Thrombophilia testing and venous thrombosis. *N Engl J Med.* 2017;377(12):1177–1187.

32. Piazza G. Thrombophilia testing, recurrent thrombosis, and women's health. *Circulation.* 2014;130(3):283–287.

33. Giannakopoulos B, Krilis SA. The pathogenesis of the antiphospholipid syndrome. *N Engl J Med.* 2013;368(11):1033–1044.

34. Poterucha TJ, Libby P, Goldhaber SZ. More than an anticoagulant: do heparins have direct anti-inflammatory effects? *Thromb Haemost.* 2017;117(3):437–444.

35. McGowan KE, Makari J, Diamantouros A, et al. Reducing the hospital burden of heparin-induced thrombocytopenia: impact of an avoid-heparin program. *Blood.* 2016;127(16):1954–1959.

36. Kang M, Alahmadi M, Sawh S, et al. Fondaparinux for the treatment of suspected heparin-induced thrombocytopenia: a propensity score-matched study. *Blood.* 2015;125(6):924–929.

37. Salter BS, Weiner MM, Trinh MA, et al. Heparin-induced thrombocytopenia: a comprehensive clinical review. *J Am Coll Cardiol.* 2016;67(21):2519–2532.

38. Kimmel SE, French B, Kasner SE, et al. A pharmacogenetic versus a clinical algorithm for warfarin dosing. *N Engl J Med.* 2013;369(24):2283–2293.

39. Verhoef TI, Ragia G, de Boer A, et al. A randomized trial of genotype-guided dosing of acenocoumarol and phenprocoumon. *N Engl J Med.* 2013;369(24):2304–2312.

40. Pirmohamed M, Burnside G, Eriksson N, et al. A randomized trial of genotype-guided dosing of warfarin. *N Engl J Med.* 2013;369(24):2294–2303.

41. Heneghan C, Ward A, Perera R, et al. Self-monitoring of oral anticoagulation: systematic review and meta-analysis of individual patient data. *Lancet.* 2012;379(9813):322–334.

42. Budnitz DS, Lovegrove MC, Shehab N, et al. Emergency hospitalizations for adverse drug events in older Americans. *N Engl J Med.* 2011;365(21):2002–2012.

43. Gaist D, Garcia Rodriguez LA, Hellfritzsch M, et al. Association of antithrombotic drug use with subdural hematoma risk. *JAMA.* 2017;317(8):836–846.

44. Poterucha TJ, Goldhaber SZ. Warfarin and vascular calcification. *Am J Med.* 2016;129(6):631–634. 635 e.

45. Schurgers LJ, Cranenburg EC, Vermeer C. Matrix Gla-protein: the calcification inhibitor in need of vitamin K. *Thromb Haemost.* 2008;100(4):593–603.

46. Tantisattamo E, Han KH, O'Neill WC. Increased vascular calcification in patients receiving warfarin. *Arterioscler Thromb Vasc Biol.* 2015;35(1):237–242.

47. Chai-Adisaksopha C, Hillis C, Siegal DM, et al. Prothrombin complex concentrates versus fresh frozen plasma for warfarin reversal. A systematic review and meta-analysis. *Thromb Haemost.* 2016;116(5):879–890.

48. Schulman S, Singer D, Ageno W, et al. NOACs for treatment of venous thromboembolism in clinical practice. *Thromb Haemost.* 2017;117(7):1317–1325.

49. Fanikos J, Burnett AE, Mahan CE, et al. Renal function and direct oral anticoagulant treatment for venous thromboembolism. *Am J Med.* 2017;130(10):1137–1143.

50. van Es N, Coppens M, Schulman S, et al. Direct oral anticoagulants compared with vitamin K antagonists for acute venous thromboembolism: evidence from phase 3 trials. *Blood.* 2014;124(12):1968–1975.

51. Schulman S, Kearon C, Kakkar AK, et al. Dabigatran versus warfarin in the treatment of acute venous thromboembolism. *N Engl J Med.* 2009;361(24):2342–2352.

52. Schulman S, Kakkar AK, Goldhaber SZ, et al. Treatment of acute venous thromboembolism with dabigatran or warfarin and pooled analysis. *Circulation.* 2014;129(7):764–772.

53. Goldhaber SZ, Schulman S, Eriksson H, et al. Dabigatran versus warfarin for acute venous thromboembolism in elderly or impaired renal function patients: pooled analysis of RE-COVER and RE-COVER II. *Thromb Haemost.* 2017;117(11):2045–2052.

54. Goldhaber SZ, Schellong S, Kakkar A, et al. Treatment of acute pulmonary embolism with dabigatran versus warfarin. A pooled analysis of data from RE-COVER and RE-COVER II. *Thromb Haemost.* 2016;116(4):714–721.

55. Schulman S, Kearon C, Kakkar AK, et al. Extended use of dabigatran, warfarin, or placebo in venous thromboembolism. *N Engl J Med.* 2013;368(8):709–718.

56. Goldhaber SZ, Eriksson H, Kakkar A, et al. Efficacy of dabigatran versus warfarin in patients with acute venous thromboembolism in the presence of thrombophilia: findings from RE-COVER(R), RE-COVER II, and RE-MEDY. *Vasc Med.* 2016;21(6):506–514.

57. Klok FA, Ageno W, Barco S, et al. Dabigatran after short heparin anticoagulation for acute intermediate-risk pulmonary embolism: rationale and design of the single-arm PEITHO-2 study. *Thromb Haemost.* 2017;117(12):2425–2434.

58. EINSTEIN Investigators, Bauersachs R, Berkowitz SD, et al. Oral rivaroxaban for symptomatic venous thromboembolism. *N Engl J Med.* 2010;363(26):2499–2510.

59. Ageno W, Mantovani LG, Haas S, et al. Safety and effectiveness of oral rivaroxaban versus standard anticoagulation for the treatment of symptomatic deep-vein thrombosis (XALIA): an international, prospective, non-interventional study. *Lancet Haematol.* 2016;3(1):e12–e21.

60. Coleman CI, Bunz TJ, Turpie AGG. Effectiveness and safety of rivaroxaban versus warfarin for treatment and prevention of recurrence of venous thromboembolism. *Thromb Haemost.* 2017;117(10):1841–1847.

61. Agnelli G, Buller HR, Cohen A, et al. Oral apixaban for the treatment of acute venous thromboembolism. *N Engl J Med.* 2013;369(9):799–808.

62. Agnelli G, Buller HR, Cohen A, et al. Apixaban for extended treatment of venous thromboembolism. *N Engl J Med.* 2013;368(8):699–708.

63. Bleker SM, Cohen AT, Buller HR, et al. Clinical presentation and course of bleeding events in patients with venous thromboembolism, treated with apixaban or enoxaparin and warfarin. Results from the AMPLIFY trial. *Thromb Haemost.* 2016;116(6):1159–1164.

64. Büller HR, Décousus H, Grosso MA, et al. Edoxaban versus warfarin for the treatment of symptomatic venous thromboembolism. *N Engl J Med.* 2013;369(15):1406–1415.

65. Brekelmans MP, Ageno W, Beenen LF, et al. Recurrent venous thromboembolism in patients with pulmonary embolism and right ventricular dysfunction: a post-hoc analysis of the Hokusai-VTE study. *Lancet Haematol.* 2016;3(9):e437–e445.

66. Vanassche T, Verhamme P, Wells PS, et al. Impact of age, comorbidity, and polypharmacy on the efficacy and safety of edoxaban for the treatment of venous thromboembolism: an analysis of the randomized, double-blind Hokusai-VTE trial. *Thromb Res.* 2017;162:7–14.

67. Kearon C, Akl EA, Ornelas J, et al. Antithrombotic therapy for VTE disease: chest guideline and expert panel report. *Chest.* 2016;149(2):315–352.

68. Ruff CT, Giugliano RP, Antman EM. Management of bleeding with non-vitamin K antagonist oral anticoagulants in the era of specific reversal agents. *Circulation.* 2016;134(3):248–261.

69. Niessner A, Tamargo J, Morais J, et al. Reversal strategies for non-vitamin K antagonist oral anticoagulants: a critical appraisal of available evidence and recommendations for clinical management—a joint position paper of the European Society of Cardiology Working Group on Cardiovascular Pharmacotherapy and European Society of Cardiology Working Group on Thrombosis. *Eur Heart J.* 2017;38(22):1710–1716.

70. Weitz JI, Pollack Jr CV. Practical management of bleeding in patients receiving non-vitamin K antagonist oral anticoagulants. *Thromb Haemost.* 2015;114(6):1113–1126.

71. Siegal DM, Crowther MA. Acute management of bleeding in patients on novel oral anticoagulants. *Eur Heart J.* 2013;34(7):489–498b.

72. Kovacs RJ, Flaker GC, Saxonhouse SJ, et al. Practical management of anticoagulation in patients with atrial fibrillation. *J Am Coll Cardiol.* 2015;65(13):1340–1360.

73. Milling Jr TJ, Kaatz S. Preclinical and clinical data for factor Xa and "universal" reversal agents. *Am J Med.* 2016;129(11S):S80–S88.

74. Barra ME, Fanikos J, Connors JM, et al. Evaluation of dose-reduced direct oral anticoagulant therapy. *Am J Med.* 2016;129(11):1198–1204.

75. Sylvester KW, Ting C, Lewin A, et al. Expanding anticoagulation management services to include direct oral anticoagulants. *J Thromb Thrombolysis.* 2018;45(2):274–280.

76. Weitz JI, Harenberg J. New developments in anticoagulants: past, present and future. *Thromb Haemost.* 2017;117(7):1283–1288.

77. Ageno W, Buller HR, Falanga A, et al. Managing reversal of direct oral anticoagulants in emergency situations. Anticoagulation Education Task Force White Paper. *Thromb Haemost.* 2016;116(6):1003–1010.

78. Eikelboom JW, Quinlan DJ, van Ryn J, et al. Idarucizumab: the antidote for reversal of dabigatran. *Circulation.* 2015;132(25):2412–2422.

79. Pollack Jr CV, Reilly PA, van Ryn J, et al. Idarucizumab for dabigatran reversal - full cohort analysis. *N Engl J Med.* 2017;377(5):431–441.

80. Connolly SJ, Milling Jr TJ, Eikelboom JW, et al. Andexanet alfa for acute major bleeding associated with factor Xa inhibitors. *N Engl J Med.* 2016;375(12):1131–1141.

81. Ansell JE, Bakhru SH, Laulicht BE, et al. Single-dose ciraparantag safely and completely reverses anticoagulant effects of edoxaban. *Thromb Haemost.* 2017;117(2):238–245.

82. Kearon C, Ageno W, Cannegieter SC, et al. Categorization of patients as having provoked or unprovoked venous thromboembolism: guidance from the SSC of ISTH. *J Thromb Haemost.* 2016;14(7):1480–1483.

83. Kyrle PA, Kammer M, Eischer L, et al. The long-term recurrence risk of patients with unprovoked venous thromboembolism: an observational cohort study. *J Thromb Haemost.* 2016;14(12):2402–2409.

84. Arshad N, Bjori E, Hindberg K, et al. Recurrence and mortality after first venous thromboembolism in a large population-based cohort. *J Thromb Haemost.* 2017;15(2):295–303.

85. Wan T, Rodger M, Zeng W, et al. Residual pulmonary embolism as a predictor for recurrence after a first unprovoked episode: results from the reverse cohort study. *Thromb Res.* 2018;162:104–109.

86. Eichinger S, Heinze G, Jandeck LM, et al. Risk assessment of recurrence in patients with unprovoked deep vein thrombosis or pulmonary embolism: the Vienna prediction model. *Circulation.* 2010;121(14):1630–1636.

87. Pesavento R, Filippi L, Palla A, et al. Impact of residual pulmonary obstruction on the long-term outcome of patients with pulmonary embolism. *Eur Respir J.* 2017;49(5).

88. Couturaud F, Sanchez O, Pernod G, et al. Six months vs extended oral anticoagulation after a first episode of pulmonary embolism: the PADIS-PE randomized clinical trial. *JAMA.* 2015;314(1):31–40.

89. Kearon C, Spencer FA, O'Keeffe D, et al. D-dimer testing to select patients with a first unprovoked venous thromboembolism who can stop anticoagulant therapy: a cohort study. *Ann Intern Med.* 2015;162(1):27–34.

90. Piazza G. Beyond Virchow's Triad: does cardiovascular inflammation explain the recurrent nature of venous thromboembolism? *Vasc Med.* 2015;20(2):102–104.

91. Rothwell PM, Wilson M, Price JF, et al. Effect of daily aspirin on risk of cancer metastasis: a study of incident cancers during randomised controlled trials. *Lancet.* 2012;379(9826):1591–1601.

92. Rothwell PM, Price JF, Fowkes FG, et al. Short-term effects of daily aspirin on cancer incidence, mortality, and non-vascular death: analysis of the time course of risks and benefits in 51 randomised controlled trials. *Lancet.* 2012;379(9826):1602–1612.

93. Becattini C, Agnelli G, Schenone A, et al. Aspirin for preventing the recurrence of venous thromboembolism. *N Engl J Med.* 2012;366(21):1959–1967.

94. Brighton TA, Eikelboom JW, Mann K, et al. Low-dose aspirin for preventing recurrent venous thromboembolism. *N Engl J Med.* 2012;367(21):1979–1987.

95. Simes J, Becattini C, Agnelli G, et al. Aspirin for the prevention of recurrent venous thromboembolism: the INSPIRE collaboration. *Circulation.* 2014;130(13):1062–1071.

96. Weitz JI, Lensing AWA, Prins MH, et al. Rivaroxaban or aspirin for extended treatment of venous thromboembolism. *N Engl J Med.* 2017;376(13):1211–1222.

97. Prins MH, Lensing AWA, Prandoni P, et al. Risk of recurrent venous thromboembolism according to baseline risk factor profiles. *Blood Adv.* 2018;2:788–796.

98. Konstantinides SV, Warntges S. Acute phase treatment of venous thromboembolism: advanced therapy. Systemic fibrinolysis and pharmacomechanical therapy. *Thromb Haemost.* 2015;113(6):1202–1209.

99. Zondag W, Kooiman J, Klok FA, et al. Outpatient versus inpatient treatment in patients with pulmonary embolism: a meta-analysis. *Eur Respir J.* 2013;42(1):134–144.

100. Barco S, Lankeit M, Binder H, et al. Home treatment of patients with low-risk pulmonary embolism with the oral factor Xa inhibitor rivaroxaban. Rationale and design of the HoT-PE trial. *Thromb Haemost.* 2016;116(1):191–197.

101. Jaber WA, Fong PP, Weisz G, et al. Acute pulmonary embolism: with an emphasis on an interventional approach. *J Am Coll Cardiol.* 2016;67(8):991–1002.

102. Dudzinski DM, Piazza G. Multidisciplinary pulmonary embolism response teams. *Circulation.* 2016;133(1):98–103.

103. Kabrhel C, Rosovsky R, Channick R, et al. A multidisciplinary pulmonary embolism response team: initial 30-month experience with a novel approach to delivery of care to patients with submassive and massive pulmonary embolism. *Chest.* 2016;150(2):384–393.

104. Carroll BJ, Pemberton H, Bauer KA, et al. Initiation of a multidisciplinary, rapid response team to massive and submassive pulmonary embolism. *Am J Cardiol.* 2017;120(8):1393–1398.

105. Giri JS, Piazza G. A midterm report card for pulmonary embolism response teams. *Vasc Med.* 2018;23(1):72–74.

106. Chatterjee S, Chakraborty A, Weinberg I, et al. Thrombolysis for pulmonary embolism and risk of all-cause mortality, major bleeding, and intracranial hemorrhage: a meta-analysis. *JAMA.* 2014;311(23):2414–2421.

107. Meyer G, Vicaut E, Danays T, et al. Fibrinolysis for patients with intermediate-risk pulmonary embolism. *N Engl J Med.* 2014;370(15):1402–1411.

108. Konstantinides SV, Vicaut E, Danays T, et al. Impact of thrombolytic therapy on the long-term outcome of intermediate-risk pulmonary embolism. *J Am Coll Cardiol.* 2017;69(12):1536–1544.

109. Goldhaber SZ. PEITHO long-term outcomes study: data disrupt dogma. *J Am Coll Cardiol.* 2017;69(12):1545–1548.

110. Sharifi M, Bay C, Skrocki L, et al. Moderate pulmonary embolism treated with thrombolysis (from the "MOPETT" trial). *Am J Cardiol.* 2013;111(2):273–277.

111. Zhang Z, Zhai ZG, Liang LR, et al. Lower dosage of recombinant tissue-type plasminogen activator (rt-PA) in the treatment of acute pulmonary embolism: a systematic review and meta-analysis. *Thromb Res.* 2014;133(3):357–363.

112. Dudzinski DM, Giri J, Rosenfield K. Interventional treatment of pulmonary embolism. *Circ Cardiovasc Interv.* 2017;10(2):116. e004345.

113. Garcia MJ. Endovascular management of acute pulmonary embolism using the ultrasound-enhanced EkoSonic system. *Semin Intervent Radiol.* 2015;32(4):384–387.

114. Piazza G, Hohlfelder B, Jaff MR, et al. A prospective, single-arm, multicenter trial of ultrasound-facilitated, catheter-directed, low-dose fibrinolysis for acute massive and submassive pulmonary embolism: the SEATTLE II study. *JACC Cardiovasc Interv.* 2015;8(10):1382–1392.

115. Sadiq I, Goldhaber SZ, Liu PY, et al. Risk factors for major bleeding in the SEATTLE II trial. *Vasc Med.* 2017;22(1):44–50.

116. Carroll BJ, Goldhaber SZ, Liu PY, et al. Ultrasound-facilitated, catheter-directed, low-dose fibrinolysis in elderly patients with pulmonary embolism: a SEATTLE II sub-analysis. *Vasc Med.* 2017;22(4):324–330.

117. Goldhaber SZ. Surgical pulmonary embolectomy: the resurrection of an almost discarded operation. *Tex Heart Inst J.* 2013;40(1):5–8.

118. Aklog L, Williams CS, Byrne JG, et al. Acute pulmonary embolectomy: a contemporary approach. *Circulation.* 2002;105(12):1416–1419.

119. Neely RC, Byrne JG, Gosev I, et al. Surgical embolectomy for acute massive and submassive pulmonary embolism in a series of 115 patients. *Ann Thorac Surg.* 2015;100(4):1245–1251. discussion 1251 1242.

120. Keeling WB, Leshnower BG, Lasajanak Y, et al. Midterm benefits of surgical pulmonary embolectomy for acute pulmonary embolus on right ventricular function. *J Thorac Cardiovasc Surg.* 2016;152(3):872–878.

121. Poterucha TJ, Bergmark B, Aranki S, et al. Surgical pulmonary embolectomy. *Circulation.* 2015;132(12):1146–1151.

122. Lawler PR, Silver DA, Scirica BM, et al. Extracorporeal membrane oxygenation in adults with cardiogenic shock. *Circulation.* 2015;131(7):676–680.

123. Yusuff HO, Zochios V, Vuylsteke A. Extracorporeal membrane oxygenation in acute massive pulmonary embolism: a systematic review. *Perfusion.* 2015;30(8):611–616.

124. Ahmed O, Patel K, Patel MV, et al. Declining national annual IVC filter utilization: an analysis on the impact of societal and governmental communications. *Chest.* 2017;151(6):1402–1404.

125. Goldhaber SZ. Requiem for liberalizing indications for vena caval filters? *Circulation.* 2016;133(21):1992–1994.

126. Bikdeli B, Wang Y, Minges KE, et al. Vena caval filter utilization and outcomes in pulmonary embolism: Medicare hospitalizations from 1999 to 2010. *J Am Coll Cardiol.* 2016;67(9):1027–1035.

127. Mismetti P, Laporte S, Pellerin O, et al. Effect of a retrievable inferior vena cava filter plus anticoagulation vs anticoagulation alone on risk of recurrent pulmonary embolism: a randomized clinical trial. *JAMA.* 2015;313(16):1627–1635.

128. Stein PD, Matta F. Vena cava filters in unstable elderly patients with acute pulmonary embolism. *Am J Med.* 2014;127(3):222–225.

129. Muriel A, Jimenez D, Aujesky D, et al. Survival effects of inferior vena cava filter in patients with acute symptomatic venous thromboembolism and a significant bleeding risk. *J Am Coll Cardiol.* 2014;63(16):1675–1683.

130. Bikdeli B, Chatterjee S, Desai NR, et al. Inferior vena cava filters to prevent pulmonary embolism: systematic review and meta-analysis. *J Am Coll Cardiol.* 2017;70(13):1587–1597.

131. Tapson VF, Hazelton JP, Myers J, et al. Evaluation of a device combining an inferior vena cava filter and a central venous catheter for preventing pulmonary embolism among critically ill trauma patients. *J Vasc Interv Radiol.* 2017;28(9):1248–1254.

132. Kahn SR, Comerota AJ, Cushman M, et al. The postthrombotic syndrome: evidence-based prevention, diagnosis, and treatment strategies: a scientific statement from the American Heart Association. *Circulation.* 2014;130(18):1636–1661.

133. Kahn SR, Shapiro S, Wells PS, et al. Compression stockings to prevent post-thrombotic syndrome: a randomised placebo-controlled trial. *Lancet.* 2014;383(9920):880–888.

134. Engelberger RP, Stuck A, Spirk D, et al. Ultrasound-assisted versus conventional catheter-directed thrombolysis for acute iliofemoral deep vein thrombosis: 1-year follow-up data of a randomized-controlled trial. *J Thromb Haemost.* 2017;15(7):1351–1360.

135. Enden T, Haig Y, Klow NE, et al. Long-term outcome after additional catheter-directed thrombolysis versus standard treatment for acute iliofemoral deep vein thrombosis (the CaVenT study): a randomised controlled trial. *Lancet.* 2012;379(9810):31–38.

136. Enden T, Resch S, White C, et al. Cost-effectiveness of additional catheter-directed thrombolysis for deep vein thrombosis. *J Thromb Haemost.* 2013;11(6):1032–1042.

137. Vedantham S, Goldhaber SZ, Julian JA, et al. Pharmacomechanical catheter-directed thrombolysis for deep-vein thrombosis. *N Engl J Med.* 2017;377(23):2240–2252.

138. Lee AY, Levine MN, Baker RI, et al. Low-molecular-weight heparin versus a coumarin for the prevention of recurrent venous thromboembolism in patients with cancer. *N Engl J Med.* 2003;349(2):146–153.

139. Lee AYY, Kamphuisen PW, Meyer G, et al. Tinzaparin vs warfarin for treatment of acute venous thromboembolism in patients with active cancer: a randomized clinical trial. *JAMA.* 2015;314(7):677–686.

140. Raskob GE, van Es N, Verhamme P, et al. Edoxaban for the treatment of cancer-associated venous thromboembolism. *N Engl J Med.* 2018;378:615–624.

141. Greinacher A. Clinical practice. Heparin-induced thrombocytopenia. *N Engl J Med.* 2015;373(3):252–261.

142. Warkentin TE, Pai M, Linkins LA. Direct oral anticoagulants for treatment of hit: update of Hamilton experience and literature review. *Blood.* 2017;130(9):1104–1113.

143. Donadini MP, Dentali F, Pegoraro S, et al. Long-term recurrence of venous thromboembolism after short-term treatment of symptomatic isolated distal deep vein thrombosis: a cohort study. *Vasc Med.* 2017;22(6):518–524.

144. Barnes GD. Preventing recurrence from distal deep vein thrombosis: still searching for answers. *Vasc Med.* 2017;22(6):525–526.

145. Amin AN, Varker H, Princic N, et al. Duration of venous thromboembolism risk across a continuum in medically ill hospitalized patients. *J Hosp Med.* 2012;7(3):231–238.

146. Cohen AT, Harrington RA, Goldhaber SZ, et al. Extended thromboprophylaxis with betrixaban in acutely ill medical patients. *N Engl J Med.* 2016;375(6):534–544.

147. Gibson CM, Chi G, Halaby R, et al. Extended-duration betrixaban reduces the risk of stroke versus standard-dose enoxaparin among hospitalized medically ill patients: an APEX trial substudy (acute medically ill venous thromboembolism prevention with extended duration betrixaban). *Circulation.* 2017;135(7):648–655.

148. Spyropoulos AC, Ageno W, Albers GW, et al. Rivaroxaban for thromboprophylaxis after hospitalization for medical illness. *N Engl J Med.* 2018;379(12):1118–1127.

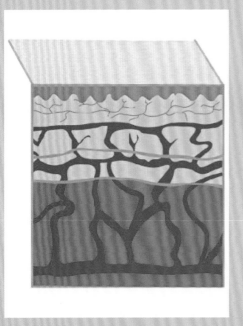

PART XV

第十五部分

Chronic Venous Disorders

慢性静脉疾病

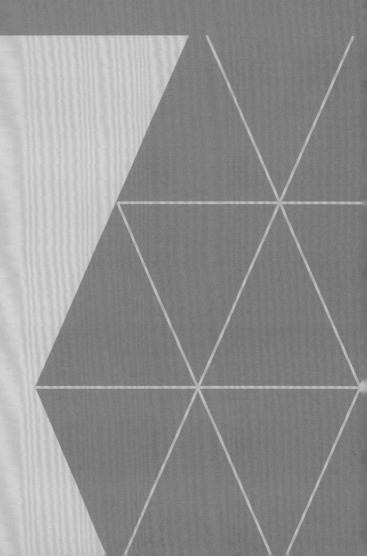

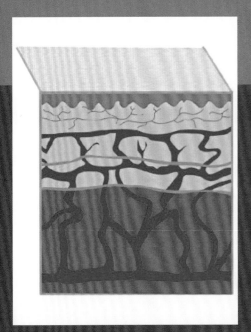

中文导读

第53章
静脉曲张

　　下肢浅静脉曲张（varicose veins，VVs）是血管外科的常见病，主要是下肢浅表静脉出现扩张，表现为团块状或者蚯蚓状的静脉团，严重时可能出现肢体水肿、曲张静脉破裂出血、色素沉着、湿疹或静脉性溃疡，影响患者的工作与生活。其发病机制目前认为有：①静脉壁薄弱和瓣膜缺陷，静脉壁相对薄弱，静脉压增大造成血管扩张，瓣窦处的扩张导致原有的静脉瓣膜无法紧密闭合，发生瓣膜功能相对不全，血液倒流；②瓣膜发育不良或缺失，不能有效防止血液倒流；③静脉内压力持久升高，对瓣膜产生一定的压力，瓣膜逐渐松弛、脱垂，最终关闭不全。发生病变的主要血管为大隐静脉或小隐静脉，该疾病在欧美国家的发病率为20%～40%，而在我国约为10%，对于下肢浅静脉曲张，保守治疗的方法有使用医用弹力袜、抬高患肢、药物治疗等，传统的手术治疗方法是曲张静脉的高位结扎和抽剥、缝扎术，若合并交通静脉或深静脉病变，可以行交通静脉结扎等多种手术。近10年来，随着微创手术技术的发展，下肢浅静脉曲张的治疗也出现了许多新的方法，包括泡沫硬化剂注射法（foam sclero therapy）、腔内激光治疗（endovenous laser therapy）、射频消融（radiofrequency ablation）、腔内微波治疗（endovenous microwave therapy）等，这些治疗方法可以在减少手术并发症的基础上取得相同甚至更好的疗效，并逐渐成为目前主流的下肢浅静脉曲张治疗方法。

李晓强

53

Varicose Veins

Aditya Sharma and Suman Wasan

EPIDEMIOLOGY

Varicose veins (VVs) are tortuous, dilated, bulging, superficial veins typically measuring 3 mm or larger.[1-3] They are the most common manifestation of chronic venous insufficiency (CVI) and affect up to 25% of women and 15% of men.[2,4] In the Framingham Study, which includes men and women between the ages of 30 and 62 from the town of Framingham, Massachusetts, the annual incidence of VVs is 2.6% among women and 1.9% among men.[5] Risk factors include female gender, advancing age, family history, pregnancy, prolonged standing, obesity, vascular malformations, and hormone therapy.[2,6] Varicose veins are more common in patients of European ancestry compared to Blacks or Asians.[5] Approximately 4% of the women presenting with VVs have pelvic vein reflux as the underlying etiology.[7] Pregnancy and deep venous reflux are also associated with VV recurrence after treatment.[6] Other patterns of venous pathology include reticular veins, which are smaller, 1- to 3- mm diameter, flat, blue-green colored, less tortuous veins.[2] Telangiectasias, or spider veins, are 1 mm or less, and blue, black, purple, or reddish in appearance.[2] A cross-sectional study of a random sample of 1,566 subjects 18 to 64 years of age from the general population in Scotland found that telangiectasias and reticular veins were each present in approximately 80% of men and 85% of women.[8]

The chronic nature of VVs has a major impact on healthcare resources. It is estimated that venous ulcers cause the loss of approximately 2 million working days annually, generating a cost of more than $3 billion per year in the United States alone.[5] Moreover, beyond the purely economic impact of VVs, chronic venous disease is associated with reduced quality of life, with particularly negative impact on pain, physical function, and mobility measures.[5] The same is true for patients who develop venous ulcers, with effect on quality of life directly related to severity of disease.[5]

ANATOMY

Broadly, the veins of the lower extremity are divided into three systems confluent in a single network, which ultimately drains into the external iliac vein. This venous network includes the superficial veins, deep venous system, and their mutual connections, as well as the perforators (Fig. 53.1). The *deep compartment* includes the deep venous system and it is bordered by the fascia muscularis. The *superficial compartment* is externally bordered by the dermis.[9] The tissue situated under the dermis is called the *tela subcutanea* (subcutaneous tissue) and contains the saphenous vein. Within the superficial compartment,

a narrow anatomical space called the *saphenous compartment* can be identified by ultrasound evaluation. Externally bordered by the saphenous fascia, this compartment covers the proper venae saphenae and their beginnings. The term *perforating veins* or *perforators* is reserved only for those veins that penetrate the fascia muscularis to connect the superficial system to the deep venous system. Conversely, communicating veins connect veins of the same venous system.

The *great saphenous vein* (GSV) is the longest vein in the human body. It starts at the medial side of the foot and courses proximally along the medial side of the calf as the marginal medial vein together with the saphenous nerve.[9] The main tributaries are the posterior accessory GSV and the anterior accessory GSV. The vein continues alone on the medial side of the thigh and crosses through the saphenous hiatus into the common femoral vein. The normal caliber of the GSV is 3 to 4 mm, and it has 10 to 20 valves.[9] The GSV is bifid in about 20% of legs, but two venous trunks of the GSV in the same compartment, constituting a true duplication, occurs in only 1% of cases. The *small saphenous vein* (SSV) is the second largest vein of the lower limb. It begins on the lateral side of the foot dorsum and runs along the lateral margin of the foot as the lateral marginal vein. It penetrates the popliteal fascia into the popliteal vein. In one-third of cases, blood flows via various communicating veins to the system of the great saphenous. In one-tenth of cases, it flows via the gastrocnemii veins and perforating veins into the deep venous system. The SSV is usually 3 mm wide and contains 7 to 13 valves. It is accompanied by the small saphenous artery, which must not be confused with the vein during sclerotherapy injection.[9]

Some of the perforating veins are consistently located. The *thigh perforators* include the medial thigh (formerly Hunter perforator), anterior thigh, lateral thigh, and posterior thigh perforating veins, and the pudendal perforating vein. The *knee perforators* include the medial knee (formerly Boyd perforator), suprapatellar, lateral knee, infrapatellar, and popliteal fossa perforating veins. The *leg perforators* include the paratibial, posterior tibial (formerly Cockett perforating vein), anterior leg, lateral leg, and posterior leg (medial and lateral gastrocnemius, intergemellar, para-Achillean) perforating veins. Other groups include the gluteal, ankle, and foot perforating veins. The perforator system does play a key role in calf muscle pump function (Fig. 53.2A).

A system of subcutaneous veins spreads on the lateral aspect of the thigh and leg as a developmental remnant of the embryonic lateral marginal vein, which fades out and is replaced with the system of the saphenous veins and may be abnormally developed in patients with Klippel-Trénaunay or Parkes-Weber syndromes. In relation to the surface, there are three levels of venous plexuses: dermal, hypodermal,

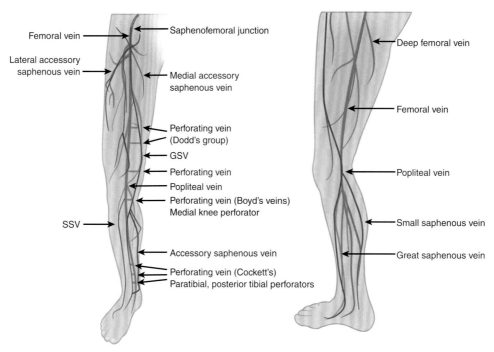

Fig. 53.1 Lower-extremity venous anatomy schematics. *GSV,* Great saphenous vein; *SSV,* small saphenous vein.

and deep. The dermal veins involve the superficial subpapillary venous plexus and the deep dermal venous plexus (Fig. 53.3).[9]

PATHOGENESIS

Varicose veins are caused by weakness in the vein wall, and according to their underlying etiology can be divided into primary or secondary. *Primary VVs* result from idiopathic structural or functional defects in the venous system. *Secondary VVs* result from underlying venous obstruction, most commonly deep vein thrombosis (DVT) or underlying deep venous insufficiency (see Fig. 53.2B and C).[2] Primary valvular incompetence is more frequent. Approximately 8 in 10 individuals with VVs have primary valvular incompetence. Secondary valvular reflux is usually due to trauma or thrombosis. Congenital anomalies only occur in about 2% of cases.[5] Secondary chronic venous disease progresses faster than primary.

A key factor in the development of VVs is venous hypertension. Venous pressure is directly proportional to the weight of the column of blood from the right atrium to the foot and is reduced by pressures generated by muscle contractions. When standing, venous pressure is as high as 90 mm Hg. It temporarily increases with muscle pumping, but then rapidly decreases as the functioning venous valves guide blood flow toward the heart. A well-functioning calf muscle pumping mechanism decreases the venous pressure to less than 30 mm Hg.[5] The constant insult of increased venous pressure degenerates in stretching, splitting, tearing, thinning, and adhesion of valves, causing inflammation.[5] Adjuvant factors for development of excessive venous hypertension include failure of the calf muscle pump and obesity. Ultimately, prolonged venous hypertension leads to venous valvular incompetence or reflux and venous dilation.[2] Venous defects increase venous hypertension and cause weakened venous walls, abnormal distention of the surrounding connective tissue, and separation of valve cusps.

Elevated venous pressure may also generate edema. Prominent swelling is not a usual feature of VVs, but episodic ankle edema is common.[10] A small percentage of patients develop complications including dermatitis, superficial thrombophlebitis, or bleeding. Thrombophlebitis may occur spontaneously or result from an injury. Skin changes in chronic

venous disease are proportionately related to the severity of venous hypertension. Up to 100% of patients with postexercise venous pressures of more than 90 mm Hg develop venous ulcers.[5] Patients with CVI and deep vein incompetence are at greatly increased risk of developing ulcers.[11] Conversely, frequent dorsiflexion of the ankle and an effective calf muscle pump are protective factors (see Fig. 53.2A). Poor prognostic factors favoring progression include the combination of reflux and obstruction, ipsilateral recurrent DVT, and multisegmental involvement.[12]

Inflammatory changes also contribute to the genesis of VVs. Blood returning from feet that have been passively dependent for 40 to 60 minutes is depleted of leukocytes, suggesting that leukocytes accumulate and locally participate in the inflammatory cascade.[5] Circulating leukocytes and vascular endothelial cells (ECs) express several types of adhesion molecules. Integrin binding promotes firm adhesion of leukocytes, the starting point for their migration out of the vasculature and degranulation. The activated leucocytes shed L-selectin into the plasma and express members of the integrin family.[5] This is the backbone of the microvascular leukocyte-trapping hypothesis. Local inflammation associated with intercellular adhesion molecule (ICAM)-1 expression increases monocyte and macrophage adhesion. The valve damage is augmented by disturbed excessive collagen type 1 synthesis, which increases venous rigidity.[5] Finally, matrix metalloproteinases (MMPs) and serine proteinases favor the accumulation of extracellular matrix (ECM) material in VVs.[5,13]

CLINICAL MANIFESTATIONS

Clinical manifestations of VV range from cosmetic problems to severe symptoms, including ulceration. Chronic venous insufficiency can be classified by clinical presentation, etiology, anatomy, and pathophysiology (CEAP Classification) (see Chapter 54).[10,14] Clinically, however, the patterns may be classified as *complicated* and *uncomplicated varices.* Uncomplicated VVs may need only cosmetic treatment or reassurance. Patients with complicated VVs may develop heaviness, fatigue, local pain, spontaneous bleeding, and superficial thrombophlebitis. Varicose veins may cause edema, pain, and skin changes such as stasis dermatitis and ulceration. Venous ulcerations can take more than

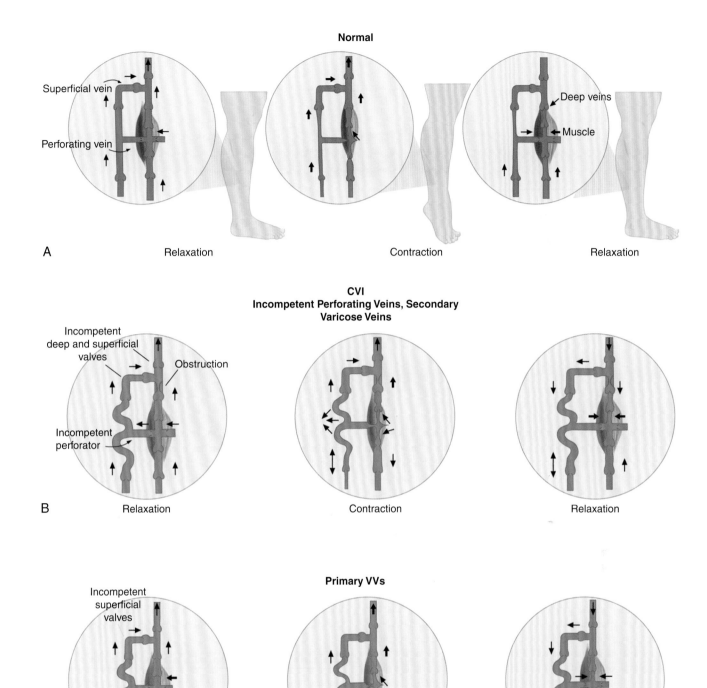

Fig. 53.2 Calf "Muscle Pump" and Varicose Veins *(VVs)*. (A) Normal calf muscle pump physiology during relaxation and contraction. (B) Deep vein obstruction heralds perforator vein incompetence and associated secondary VV. (C) Conversely, deep venous system and perforator system are independent of primary VV. *CVI,* Chronic venous insufficiency. (Modified from Sumner DS. Venous dynamics–varicosities. *Clin Obstet Gynecol.* 1981;24:743–760.)

9 months to heal, with one study reporting that 66% of ulcers last longer than 5 years.[2] All these symptoms impair activities of daily living.[2]

Multiple questionnaires and instruments measure the effect of venous disease on quality of life. Most are subjective and completed by the patient. The Chronic Venous Insufficiency Questionnaire (CIVIQ) was validated in a sample of 2,001 patients and measures the psychological, social, physical, and pain domains. A revised version of the instrument, the CIVIQ 2, equally weighted the categories across 20 questions to provide a global score. This measure is used to follow quality-of-life (QOL) improvement after therapy for chronic venous insufficiency,

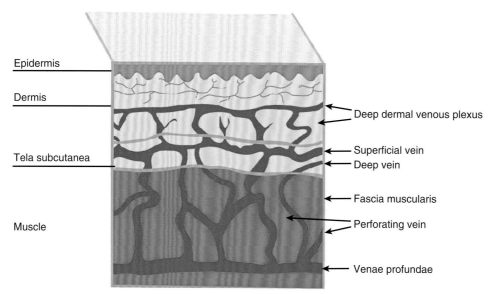

Fig. 53.3 Venous drainage of the lower limb. (Modified from Kachlik D, Pechacek V, Baca V, Musil V. The superficial venous system of the lower extremity: new nomenclature. *Phlebology*. 2010; 25:113–123.)

Labels in figure:
Epidermis
Dermis
Tela subcutanea
Muscle
Deep dermal venous plexus
Superficial vein
Deep vein
Fascia muscularis
Perforating vein
Venae profundae

including VVs. The Aberdeen Varicose Vein Questionnaire (AVVQ) includes 13 questions on physical symptoms and social issues, including pain, ankle edema, ulcers, compression therapy use, and the effect of VVs on daily activities. The disease-specific index is graded from 0 to 100 (extreme venous symptoms).[15] This measure has also been validated for patient follow-up after intervention.[16] The Venous Insufficiency Epidemiological and Economic Study (VEINES) instrument consists of 35 items in two categories to generate two summary scores. It includes the VEINES-QOL, with 25 QOL questions, and the VEINES-Sym, with 10 symptom questions.[16] The focus of this measure is on physical symptoms of venous disease, in particular postthrombotic syndrome. It has been validated in patients with DVT. In 2004, Kahn et al. compared the VEINES and the 36-item Short-Form Health Survey (SF-36) with CEAP classification in 1,531 patients from four countries to examine the effect of patient-related QOL reporting on interpreting outcomes in venous studies. Higher CEAP class was directly associated with and predictive of the VEINES-QOL.[16] The Charing Cross Venous Ulceration Questionnaire (CXVUQ) was developed for patients with venous ulcers, and its performance is not impaired by the treatment option selected.[16] Finally, the Venous Severity Score (VSS) system was derived from the CEAP classification and has three elements: the venous disability score (VDS), venous segmental disease score (VSDS), and venous clinical severity score (VCSS). The VCSS has been recently revised and includes multiple parameters: pain, VVs, inflammation, edema, skin induration, pigmentation, ulcers (size, number, duration), and compression therapy.[17] The Venous Clinical Severity Score is useful for following changes with treatment.[16,17]

PHYSICAL EXAMINATION

Initial inspection of the leg may reveal edema, prominent VVs, cyanosis, plethora, hyperpigmentation, lipodermatosclerosis, or ulcerations. On inspection, VVs may be observed as tortuous, dilated, bulging, superficial veins measuring 3 mm or larger; the patient is ideally examined in the standing position to allow venous reflux.[2] *Lipodermatosclerosis* is a consequence of localized chronic inflammation and fibrosis of the skin and subcutaneous tissue of the lower part of the leg.[1] The skin changes will often occur at the "gaiter area" above the medial malleolus. *Atrophie blanche* is a localized circular, whitish, avascular, atrophic

skin area surrounded by capillaries and sometimes hyperpigmentation, consistent with severe chronic venous insufficiency. Similarly, a *phlebectasic crown* (fan-shaped small intradermal veins on medial or lateral aspects of the foot) may herald severe venous insufficiency.

Trendelenburg and Perthes tests may be used during the exam to differentiate superficial from deep venous insufficiency (also see Chapter 54). In the Trendelenburg test, the leg is elevated and a tourniquet applied above the knee. This obstructs the superficial veins, which will promptly fill after standing if the patient has deep vein incompetence (secondary VVs). If after standing, the vein requires more than 20 seconds to refill, but prompt filling follows tourniquet removal, the exam is consistent with primary VVs. In the Perthes test, the leg is elevated and the tourniquet placed at the midthigh or proximal calf. When the patient stands and walks, the VVs will refill owing to incompetent perforators (Figs. 53.4 and 53.5).[1] These maneuvers may be complemented with Brodie Trendelenburg percussion: a finger is placed over the distal area of a VV while the proximal segment of the vein is percussed. A transmitted impulse at the lower end suggests incompetence.

IMAGING AND PHYSIOLOGICAL TESTING

Duplex ultrasonography is useful in the evaluation of VVs (also see Chapter 12). The test is performed with the patient standing or in reverse Trendelenburg position, and is used to detect acute or chronic thrombosis, postthrombotic changes, obstructive flow, and incompetence in the deep veins. Reflux, demonstrated by reversal of flow, is pathological whenever longer than 0.5 seconds.[1] Duplex ultrasonography is not reliable for assessment of the iliac and caval veins, but it is sensitive for evaluation of saphenous vein reflux and useful for identification of incompetent perforator veins.

Impedance plethysmography, strain gauge plethysmography, and air plethysmography may be used to detect venous obstruction and reflux in large veins above the knee. Photoplethysmography, most commonly used with and without a tourniquet, is a screening test that can be employed to evaluate deep and superficial venous insufficiency. A venous refilling time less than 20 seconds *without* a tourniquet that normalizes to over 20 seconds *with* a tourniquet is compatible with GSV incompetence.[1] Kurstjens et al. assessed air plethysmography for chronic deep venous obstruction and compared it to duplex

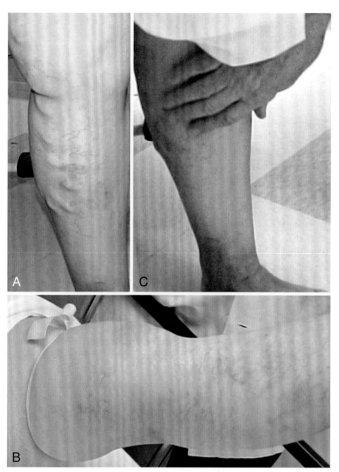

Fig. 53.4 Physical Examination of Varicose Veins (VVs). (A) Medial great saphenous vein VVs are observed on a right leg. (B) Limb is elevated and tourniquet positioned above knee. (C) With tourniquet applied and patient standing, VVs are not evident. This is suggestive of primary venous incompetence.

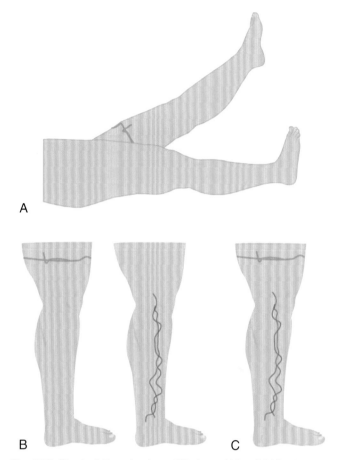

Fig. 53.5 Physical Examination of Varicose Veins (VVs). (A) Leg is elevated so VVs are drained. (B) Return of VVs only after tourniquet is removed. (C) Findings suggestive of incompetent perforator veins, consistent with secondary varicosities.

ultrasound and magnetic resonance venogram. It showed very poor correlation with sensitivity of 34% and negative predictive value of 29.6% indicating minimal clinical benefit.[18] However, air plethysmography may account for the presence of collateral channels. The 2013 appropriate use criteria on venous ultrasound by multiple vascular societies suggested that plethysmography with provocative maneuvers are appropriate for assessing signs and symptoms of venous insufficiency, including varicose veins, venous ulcer, and chronic skin changes related to venous disease; however, it was not recommended for acute deep venous thrombosis.[19]

Venography may provide information regarding pelvic vein obstruction in patients with postthrombotic disease.[1] Ascending venography is performed with the patient at 45 degrees, non–weight-bearing, with legs down as contrast is infused. Contrast filling the superficial vein denotes incompetence. Ascending venography is useful to determine vein obstruction, collateralization, and recanalization. Descending venography is more useful to diagnose venous insufficiency. In this scenario, the contrast is injected into the common femoral vein above the saphenofemoral junction. The patient is initially in supine position, and after the contrast dye injection, the table is tilted feet downward. Contrast leakage to the knee or distally is abnormal.[1] Venography is usually indicated in the setting of endovenous intervention but is difficult in the setting of a swollen leg. There is limited experience with magnetic resonance venography (MRV) or computed tomography (CT) to evaluate venous insufficiency and VVs. Their use

is clinically limited for usual causes of VV; however, they may assist in diagnosing and treating unusual anatomic causes of varicose veins such as persistent sciatic vein incompetence, Klippel-Trénaunay syndrome, congenital venous malformation, round ligament varicosity, and portosystemic collateral-related varicose vein.[20]

MANAGEMENT

Treatment Suitability

Varicose vein treatment may be divided into conservative and invasive modalities. Conservative treatment for VVs and subsequent CVI include lifestyle modifications, compression therapy, and pharmacotherapy. All patients are appropriate for conservative measures. The use of more invasive techniques depends on the size of the vein and the presence of complications. Most commonly, ablation of an incompetent or varicose great saphenous vein is performed first to decompress more distal varicosities; however, most patients require additional treatments for adequate therapeutic and cosmetic results. Thermal ablation of the GSV using endovenous laser therapy (EVLT) or radiofrequency ablation (RFA) is the most frequently employed technique; GSVs with diameters of 3 to 12 mm are candidates for RFA; EVLT is an option for those larger than 3 mm. A less invasive technique, foam sclerotherapy of the GSV, may also be performed in veins smaller than 1 cm, but has been used to treat larger veins as well.[21] When the GSV is larger than 12 mm in diameter, surgery is an option.[22] Tortuosity of the vessel is also relevant. For RFA and EVLT, the straight segment of the GSV should extend 15 to 20 cm immediately distal to the saphenofemoral junction.[21]

In a study of 577 patients with GSV reflux, 55% were suitable for RFA or EVLT, and 57% were suitable for foam sclerotherapy. Stressing the need for careful patient selection, only 41% of the limbs were suitable for all the procedures.[21] In one study evaluating patients with recurrent VVs, less than 40% had limbs suitable for RFA or EVLT, while foam sclerotherapy was an option in 58% of the cases.[21] Owing to the risk of skin burns, superficial tributary veins are not suitable for catheter-based thermal ablation. Optimal therapeutic results may be achieved with an approach of combined modalities.[21] Recently, newer nonthermal tumescentless techniques are gaining momentum.[23]

Conservative Management

Diet and Lifestyle Changes

Prolonged standing or sitting may exacerbate signs and symptoms of VVs. The patient should elevate the legs above the level of the heart as much as possible, lose excess weight, and exercise to minimize swelling and improve calf muscle function.[24] Furthermore, moderate-intensity lower-limb exercise training improves microvascular endothelial vasodilator function in postsurgical VV patients.[25]

Compression

External compression is the cornerstone of therapy for VVs. Compression therapy, including graduated elastic compression stockings and short-stretch bandages, is effective in reducing lower-extremity pain and swelling and preventing progression of VVs and CVI to venous ulceration.[24] Among patients with venous ulcerations, improved healing is achieved with multicomponent compression systems. Compression garments should be individualized for maximal patient compliance.[24,26]

Pharmacotherapy

Low-dose diuretics are often prescribed for patients with significant edema due to VVs, but they are minimally effective in reducing the symptoms of pain and discomfort.[24] Patients with stasis dermatitis may be treated with a short course of topical corticosteroids to reduce inflammation. Antibiotics with gram-positive coverage are prescribed to treat cellulitis or infected ulcerations. Antibiotic coverage should be expanded to include gram-negative and anaerobic organisms in diabetic patients.[24] Because of the increasing problem of bacterial resistance to antibiotics, current guidelines recommend that antibacterial preparations should only be used in cases of clinical infection and not for bacterial colonization. At present, there is no evidence to support routine use of systemic antibiotics to promote healing in venous leg ulcers.[27]

Phlebotonics

These are venoactive medications which are often utilized for treatment of CVI symptoms. These are natural such as horse chestnut seed extract (aescin), flavonoids such as rutosides, diosmin, and hesperidin; the micronized purified flavonoid fraction (MPFF), and other plant extracts such as French maritime pine bark extract, grape seed extract, and Centella asiatica as well as synthetic products such as calcium dobesilate, naftazone, aminaftone, chromocarbe, and benzarone.[5] A Cochrane review of 110 publications found that there was improvement in edema with diosmin, MPFF, rutosides, and hesperidin. Calcium dobesilate reduced cramps. Diosmin and hesperidin improved skin changes.[28] These drugs are effective in CVI regardless of presence or absence of VV.

Short-term studies have shown the efficacy of horse chestnut seed (Aesculus hippocastanum) extract in reducing edema, ankle and calf circumference, and symptoms of VVs with insufficiency. The horse chestnut is native to southeast Europe, with aescin the active ingredient.[24,29]

This extract has antiinflammatory and vasoconstrictive properties that may exert a positive influence on venous tone and increase the flow velocity of venous blood.[29] It can be administered orally as a 20- or 50-mg dose. In a meta-analysis by Suter et al., a treated population of 219 adults with CVI stage I/II showed improvement; eight patients reported gastrointestinal upset.[29] In 2012, a Cochrane review identified 17 randomized controlled trials with either placebo-controlled or compression stockings or other therapies. Leg swelling, edema, pruritis, leg volume, and circumference were significantly reduced. However, most of the reduction was seen in studies compared to placebo rather than compression stockings.[30]

MPFF consists of 90% diosmin and 10% flavonoids. MPFF protects the microcirculation from raised ambulatory venous pressure. It decreases the interaction between leucocytes and ECs by inhibiting expression of endothelial ICAM-1 and vascular cell adhesion molecule (VCAM).[31] A meta-analysis of randomized prospective studies using MPFF that included 723 patients with venous ulcers suggested improved healing at 6 months among those who used MPFF compared with conventional therapy alone.[31] In the RELIEF study, 5,052 patients with CVI (class C0 to C4 with or without reflux) received MPFF for 6 months. MPFF showed reduction in venous symptoms of pain, heaviness, swelling, and cramps regardless of presence or absence of reflux.[32]

Calcium dobesilate was studied in a double-blinded RCT and noted significant reduction in venous symptoms including edema independent of the concomitant usage of compression stockings. However, a more recent RCT involving 351 patients showed no significant volume change in general; a difference was seen, though, in the most pathological leg at the end of follow-up.[33] Aziz et al. reviewed 15 RCTs involving 1,643 participants receiving rutosides and showed improvements in symptoms of chronic venous insufficiency such as pain (SMD –1.07; 95% confidence interval (CI) –1.44 to –0.70), heavy legs (odds ratio [OR] 0.50; 95% CI 0.28 to 0.91), and cramps (SMD –1.07; 95% CI –1.45 to –0.69).[34] French maritime pine bark extract and grape leaf extract have very limited data, with registry data noting possible benefit in reducing edema and pain.[24,35,36]

In 2016, a Cochrane review on venous insufficiency evaluated 53 randomized controlled trials utilizing phlebotonics involving 6,013 participants. Ten of those studies included use of diosmin and hidrosmine; 28 used rutosides; 9 used dobesilate; 2 each used Centella asiatica, aminaftone, and French maritime pine bark extract; and 1 used grape seed extract.[28] Overall, it was noted that there may be benefits with reduction in edema and other venous symptoms with lack of benefit in ulcer healing.[28] Although herbal products may be beneficial short term, their efficacy and safety have not been proven long term, and these preparations with varying amounts of active and inactive ingredients are not regulated by the US Food and Drug Administration (FDA).

Pentoxifylline

In a double-blinded placebo controlled trial, pentoxifylline use showed complete healing of venous ulcers in 64% of patients receiving pentoxifylline compared to 53% of the patients receiving placebo.[37] Other trials showed ulcer healing faster too, with 800 mg three times a day dosing; however, the higher dose may be associated with gastrointestinal upset.[38,39] In 2011, clinical practice guidelines of the Society for Vascular Surgery and the American Venous Forum recommended venoactive drugs (diosmin, hesperidin, rutosides, sulodexide, micronized purified flavonoid fraction, or horse chestnut seed extract [aescin]) for patients with pain and swelling due to chronic venous disease as a class 2B recommendation.[40,41] Pentoxifylline or MPFF are suggested to accelerate venous ulcer healing with compression therapy as a class 2B recommendation. The European Society for Vascular Surgery guidelines recommend venotonic drugs for swelling and pain from chronic venous disease as class IIa B recommendation.[40] Pentoxifylline is not useful in VV without active ulcers (see Chapter 54).

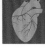

Invasive Therapy

For large VVs, invasive therapy is divided into endovenous procedures, including chemical and thermal ablation, nonthermal ablation, and surgical procedures (Table 53.1).

Chemical Sclerotherapy

Liquid sclerosants have been a treatment for VVs for almost a century. The introduction of endovenous foam sclerotherapy (EFS) in 1944, with standardization of the method by Cabrera in the early 1990s, improved the nonsurgical obliteration of VVs. EFS is especially effective when administered using ultrasound guidance.[24]

Procedure. A chemical sclerosant (e.g., polidocanol, sodium morrhuate, sodium tetradecyl sulfate) is combined with carbon dioxide/oxygen (CO_2/O_2) or room air to produce foam (concentration 1% to 3%; volume 6 to 10 mL) using the two-syringe, or Tessari, method (Fig. 53.6).[42] Because it is more soluble in blood and water than the nitrogen in room air, CO_2/O_2 may reduce the risk of microbubble embolization. The Tessari method generates foam by pumping the contents of two disposable syringes, one containing the liquid sclerosant and the other containing air, backward and forward through a two-way stopcock.[42] Ultrasound is performed to localize the most superficially accessible segment of the varicosity or GSV proper into which a catheter can be easily inserted. The foam is prepared immediately before the procedure and injected into the GSV or its tributaries under ultrasound guidance.[42] The leg is elevated 45 degrees during injection, and the foam is massaged distally to fill the tributaries. Subsequently, a compression garment is applied to the treated leg.[42,43]

The foam displaces the blood in the vein, resulting in local inflammation, sclerosis, and obliteration of the VV over 1 to 2 weeks.[42,44] The effectiveness of foam sclerotherapy lies in the utilization of detergent sclerosants that work by denaturation of proteins. By forming a lipid bilayer, the endothelial surface is disrupted in the absence of essential proteins, which produces a delayed cell death.[43]

A systematic review of EFS by van den Bos et al. that selected 64 studies and assessed 12,320 limbs followed for an average of 32 months determined an overall obliteration rate of 82.1% at 3 months (95% CI, 72.5 to 88.9), 80.9% at 1 year (95% CI, 71.8 to 87.6), and 73.5% at 5 years (95% CI, 62.8 to 82.1) (see Table 53.1).[45] Contrary to catheter thermal-based techniques, increasing age does not impact sclerotherapy suitability.[21] Endovenous foam sclerotherapy is also effective in treating venous stasis ulcers and congenital vascular malformations.[2] In a study by Barrett et al. that analyzed a total of 100 randomly chosen legs with VVs treated with ultrasound-guided EFS, patient satisfaction was rated highly, with a 90% improvement in QOL 2 years after treatment with EFS (see Table 53.1).[2] In the van den Bos review, after adjusting for follow-up, EFS and RFA were as effective as surgical stripping.[45] In the absence of large comparative randomized clinical trials between multiple techniques, the minimally invasive techniques appear to be at least as effective as surgery in the treatment of lower-extremity VVs. EFS is often used in conjunction with thermal ablation for sclerosis of tributary VVs.

TABLE 53.1   Comparison of Varicose Vein Treatment Outcomes

Treatment	PERCENT OBLITERATION (95% CI)			Complications
	1 Year	**3 Years**	**5 Years**	
Saphenofemoral ligation and stripping	79.7% (71.8–85.8)	77.8% (70.0–84.0)	83% (72–90)	Hematomas (<30%) Paresthesias (4%–25%) Wound infection (2%–15%) DVT (<2%)
EVLT	93.3% (91.1–95.0)	94.5% (87.2–97.7)	88% (82–92)	Pain (50%) Ecchymosis (40%) Hematoma (24%) Phlebitis (12%) Paresthesias (10%) DVT (7%) Hyperpigmentation (<4%)
RFA	87.7% (83.1–91.2)	84.2% (75.5–90.4)	79.9% (59.9–91.5)	Bruising (50%) Paresthesias (3%–20%) DVT (16%) Hematoma (<7%) Burns (2%–7%) Infection (<2%)
EFS	80.9% (71.8–87.6)	77.4% (68.7–84.3)	34% (26–44)	Pain (common) Hyperpigmentation (common) Phlebitis (5%) DVT (<1%) TIA (<1%) Skin necrosis (rare)

CI, Confidence interval; *DVT*, deep vein thrombosis; *EFS*, endovenous foam sclerotherapy; *EVLT*, endovenous laser therapy; *RFA*, radiofrequency ablation; *TIA*, transient ischemic attack.

Modified from Nael R, Rathbun S. Treatment of varicose veins. *Curr Treat Options Cardiovasc Med.* 2009; 11:91–103; van den Bos R, Arends L, Kockaert M, et al. Endovenous therapies of lower extremity varicosities: a meta-analysis. *J Vasc Surg.* 2009; 49:230–239; Hamann SAS, Giang J, De Maeseneer MGR, et al. Editor's choice – five year results of great saphenous vein treatment: a meta-analysis. *Eur J Vasc Endovasc Surg.* 2017;54(6):760–770.

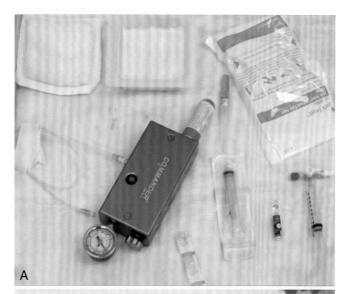

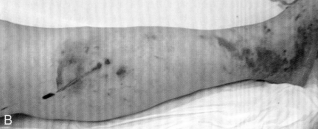

Fig. 53.6 Tray prepared for sclerotherapy (A), and leg marked for access (B).

In a study of 1,931 treatment sessions that included 852 patients treated with ultrasound-guided EFS, the risk of deep venous occlusion was lower when treating veins less than 5 mm in diameter, and when restricting the volume of foam injected to less than 10 mL.[46] The most common complications include mild to moderate pain and hyperpigmentation (up to 30%).[2,46a] Hyperpigmentation typically resolves within 6 to 12 months.[2] Less common adverse events include superficial thrombophlebitis, DVT and pulmonary embolism (PE), trapped coagulum, hematoma, skin necrosis, transient neurological events (migraines, visual disturbance), and pulmonary symptoms (cough). Trapped coagulum resulting in superficial thrombophlebitis occurs in less than 5% of treated veins. Deep vein thrombosis results from propagation of foam into the deep venous system and typically involves the popliteal and calf veins. The incidence of DVT/PE is less than 1%.[2,14] Transient neurological events may occur with the use of large amounts of foam in patients with a patent foramen ovale. To date, there have been three reported cases of major posttreatment neurological events (transient ischemic attack [TIA] and cerebrovascular accident) suspected to be associated with EFS. A systematic search reported 12 cases of imaging-confirmed cerebrovascular accidents and 9 cases of transient ischemic attacks in literature.[47] Research postulates the increased risk of release of endothelin 1 as the cause of visual symptoms, migraines, and cerebral symptoms.[48] Myocardial infarction has also been rarely reported in the presence of patent foramen ovale.[49] In a meta-analysis evaluating 5-year outcomes, sclerotherapy had lower anatomical success compared to high ligation stripping (HLS), EVLT and EVLT with high ligation, i.e., 34% (95% CI 26 to 44) versus 83% (95% CI 72 to 90) and 88% (95% CI 82 to 92), and 88% (95% CI 17 to 100) respectively; $P \le .001$.[50] Recurrent reflux rates were higher for foam sclerotherapy compared to HLS and EVLT (29% vs. 12% vs. 12%). Rathbun et al. published a more comprehensive meta-analysis in 2012 regarding efficacy

and safety of EFS including 104 studies which showed similar vein occlusion rates to EVLT, but not as effective to HLS. Nineteen percent of the studies were RCTs, 79% were observational studies.[51] The current SVS and AVF guidelines recommend foam sclerotherapy for telangiectasia, reticular veins, and varicose veins (class 1B).[40] The ESVS does not recommend sclerotherapy as the first choice of treatment for chronic venous disease. Foam sclerotherapy is recommended for recurrent varicose veins and in elderly and frail patients with ulcers (class IIa B). Foam sclerotherapy is recommended as the second choice of treatment of varicose veins and for advanced disease in saphenous vein incompetence, not eligible for surgery or endovenous ablation (class IA). Liquid sclerotherapy can be considered for telangiectasias and reticular veins (class IIa B).[40,41]

Polidocanol endovenous foam (PEM) (1%, Varithena [polidocanol injectable foam], unlike physician-compounded foam (PCF), is made with a low concentration of nitrogen ($<0.8\%$) plus carbon dioxide and oxygen and is dispensed from a proprietary canister device.[52] This combination provides more consistent bubble size, better cohesiveness, and longer contact with the endothelium. PCF has reports of adverse events such as stroke and other neurological events; however, use of carbon dioxide can result in fewer such events. Additional PCF sclerotherapy has many variables such as volume, concentrations, and type of sclerosant used; method of preparation; and number of needles and cannulas used.[52] Also, as noted earlier, failure rate is high using PCF sclerotherapy. PEM reduces likelihood of gas embolism–related adverse events and provides more stability and cohesive properties in the foam. It is also FDA approved for GSV incompetence. In the VANISH-2 trial, 0.5% and 1% PEM was compared to placebo for GSV incompetence.[53] On 8-week follow-up, there was significant improvement in symptoms; however, on 1-year follow-up, 87.9% patients had required additional PEM. Sixty percent had adverse events compared to 39% in placebo group; however, 95% of adverse events were mild with no reports of neurological events or pulmonary embolism. In 2017, two additional trials showed similar risk and improved symptoms with most common side effect being thrombophlebitis.[54,55] PEM has been studied in over 1,300 patients with improvement in symptoms but GSV closure rates are lower than other established techniques. DVT rates may be higher than thermal ablation, but are usually distal, often not requiring treatment with anticoagulant therapy. PEM may be useful in situations where other therapies are difficult to use or unlikely to benefit such as neovascularized or scarred veins in the setting of thickened skin or lipodermatosclerosis.[23]

Mechanochemical endovenous ablation: Mechanochemical endovenous ablation (MOCA) performs venous closure by mechanical abrasion of the endothelium and ablation by sclerosant therapy. It uses the ClariVein device, which contains a rotating wire within the infusion catheter. When the catheter is withdrawn, the wire disrupts the endothelium and the sclerosant is injected in to the vein leading to venous closure. Bishawi et al. performed a trial using MOCA for GSV incompetence treatment in 126 patients and reported a 94% closure rate at 6 months with improvement in symptom scores.[56] Adverse events seen were thrombophlebitis (10%), ecchymosis (9%), and hematoma (1%). Bootun et al. performed RCT of 119 patients with GSV incompetence to MOCA or RFA. At 1-month follow-up, MOCA and RFA had 83% and 92% complete closure respectively.[57] Its use in SSV and below the knee GSV alone is very limited. In a 2017 systemic review of MOCA using ClariVein, 1,521 veins (1,267 great and 254 small saphenous veins) reported 92% and 91% occlusion rates at 6 and 12 months respectively.[58] Occlusion rates at 2 and 3 years were 91% and 87% respectively with a nonsignificant number of major complications. It is approved by FDA for large VVs.

Cyanoacrylate: The VenaSeal closure system (VCSC) delivers cyanoacrylate (CAC), a glue, through a specific delivery system. It does not require use of tumescence anesthesia, eliminating the risk of nerve injury and pain related to conventional thermal endovenous therapy and the patient can return to regular activities soon after the procedure without the need to wear compression stockings. Morrison et al. treated 70 patients with GSV reflux using CAC with 1-year closure rate of 93%. The VeClose study, a RCT comparing CAC (N = 108) to RFA (N = 112) for incompetent GSV closure reported that CAC was noninferior to RFA.[59] At 3 months, complete closure was 99% and 96% with CAC and RFA respectively. Ecchymosis was less in the CAC group; however, pain, adverse events, and quality of life scores such as VCSS and AVVQ were similar with both groups. Adverse events were very few between the two groups. The WAVES study, a postmarket evaluation study, reported outcomes for great, small, and accessory saphenous veins in 50 subjects treated in a single session.[60] Compression stockings were not used postprocedure. There was 100% closure of all treated veins noted in 1-month follow-up with venous ultrasound. The mean time to return to work and normal activities was 0.2 ± 1.1 and 2.4 ± 4.1 days respectively. Thrombophlebitis was seen in 20% of subjects on initial evaluation postprocedure but only 2% had it at 1-month follow up. VCSS score 1.8 ± 1.4 ($p < .001$) and AVVQ score 8.9 ± 6.6 ($p < .001$) had improved from presentation. It is also FDA approved.[5]

Endovenous Laser Therapy

EVLT was introduced in 1999 for obliteration of the GSV and its tributaries. The direct action of the laser on the vein wall and heating of the venous blood results in damage to the vein wall and, over weeks to months, obliteration of the varicosity.[24] The pattern of injury is eccentrically distributed, with maximum injury occurring along the path of laser contact. Temperatures during EVLT may reach 1,000° C at the fiber tip and 300° C in the firing zone. There is also steam generated during the photothermolytic process, but this accounts for only 2% of applied energy dose.[61] The occlusion and complication rate after EVLT are proportional to the total energy (joules) per centimeter of vein (J/cm). The laser energy can be applied in continuous or pulsed mode, the continuous mode being more effective.

Procedure. Endovenous laser therapy is performed using tumescent anesthesia. Preprocedure, the leg is marked to outline the veins to be treated (Fig. 53.7). A 5-mL syringe with a 25-gauge needle may be used to subcutaneously infiltrate 2 mL of tumescent anesthetic solution (420 mL of normal saline, 60 mL of 1% lidocaine with epinephrine, and 20 mL of sodium bicarbonate) over the access site. This solution is delivered manually or with an infusion pump under ultrasound guidance, aiming to surround the vein segment to be treated.[24,62] A laser-tipped catheter is inserted into the GSV at the level of the knee and advanced just distal to the saphenofemoral junction with ultrasound guidance (Fig. 53.8). The laser is continuously pulled distally in the GSV as continuous energy is applied to the vein.

The systematic review by van den Bos et al. (see Table 53.1) reported an overall obliteration rate of 92.9% at 3 months (95% CI, 90.2 to 94.8), 93.3% at 1 year (95% CI, 91.1 to 95.0), and 95.4% at 5 years (95% CI, 79.7 to 99.1).[45] Several studies have reported that EVLT is more effective than, if not at least as effective as, venous stripping and other endovenous procedures in terms of obliteration and recurrence rates.[2] Post EVLT recurrence of reflux in the treated vein occurs secondary to new incompetent perforators in the thigh and calf, and new saphenofemoral junction incompetence accounted for the progression of new vein disease.[21] In a study of 3,000 treated limbs by Ravi et al., overall patient satisfaction, as assessed by symptom relief and absence of VVs after ablation, was 86%.[63] There are no absolute contraindications for EVLT.[40] Relative contraindications include uncorrectable coagulopathy, liver dysfunction limiting local anesthetic use, immobility, pregnancy, and breastfeeding.[40] Higher energy results in increased occlusion rates but

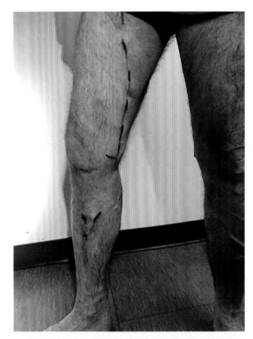

Fig. 53.7 Photo depicting marking of varicose vein to be treated.

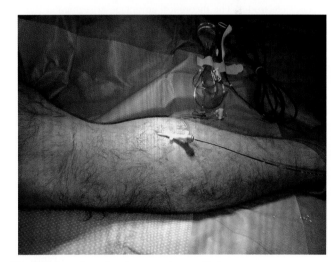

Fig. 53.8 Insertion of endovenous laser catheter.

is associated with higher complication rates, including paresthesia and thermal injuries. Other complications include pain, edema, erythema, ecchymosis, hematoma, vesiculation, hypo- or hyperpigmentation, superficial thrombophlebitis, and DVT.[2,64] In a meta-analysis of 29 studies, Luebke and Brunkwall described more than a 50% incidence of ecchymosis in 12 of the studies where this complication was reported.[46a] In the same meta-analysis, the incidence of paresthesias was 1.7%. Moderate pain along the treated vein and superficial thrombophlebitis occurs in up to 50% and 12% of the limbs, respectively.[65] In the same meta-analysis, seven studies with a total of 9,317 patients reported only 27 cases of incident DVT (0.3%). In other studies, the incidence of DVT has been reported to be as much as 7%.[2,46a] Pulmonary embolism has not been a reported complication with EVLT.[46a] Because EVLT is usually performed in the outpatient setting, it may be more cost-effective than surgical treatment for VVs.[2] In another meta-analysis comparing EVLT to HLS including 23 studies with 2,245 limbs (1,128 treated with EVLT and 1,117 treated with high ligation and stripping), no difference was seen in technical success between EVLT and HLS in up to 2-year follow-up, and duplex detected and clinical recurrence rate were similar between them in the same time period. Adverse events such as bleeding and hematoma (1.28% versus 4.83%), wound infection (0.33% versus 1.91%), and paresthesia (6.73% versus 11.27%) were fewer with EVLT.[66] A 5-year follow-up study evaluating 130 legs undergoing EVLT vs. HLS for GSV incompetence showed more recurrent varicose veins in EVLT group (31% vs. 7%; *P* < .01) likely caused by neoreflux in incompetent tributaries.[67] Clinically visible recurrences originating from the SFJ region were seen more in EVLT (33% vs. 17%; *P* < .04). In both treatment groups, venous symptoms, CEAP class, and visualized changes improved significantly. In contrast, in a Cochrane review, three RCTs compared EVLT with HLS including 311 participants (185 in EVLT and 126 in HLS).[68] Recurrence of reflux at 1 year was less frequent in the EVLT group than in the HLS group (OR 0.24; 95% CI 0.07 to 0.77). Clinical evidence of recurrence (i.e., presence of new visible varicose veins) at 1 year was similar (OR 0.54; 95% CI 0.17 to 1.75). No difference was seen in disease-specific QOL evaluations. Sural nerve injury, wound infection, and deep venous thrombosis (one in each group) were the complications reported.[68]

Radiofrequency Ablation

Radiofrequency ablation, introduced in the United States in 1999, results in obliteration of the GSV and its tributaries by delivering controlled heat using radiofrequency energy passed through an endovenous electrode.[2] The theoretical advantage of segmental RFA is greater consistency in the vein treatment and increased speed of ablation; each 7-cm segment can be treated in 20 seconds.[69]

Procedure. Radiofrequency ablation is performed under general or local anesthesia. Tumescent anesthesia is required, and a dilute mixture of lidocaine in normal saline may be used (50 mL of 1% lidocaine with 1:200,000 epinephrine in 500 mL 0.9% saline for unilateral procedures, or in 1,000 mL 0.9% saline for bilateral procedures). The volumes of tumescence are commonly between 75 and 100 mL per 10 cm of vein.[69] Ultrasound is used for catheter placement and guidance during the procedure. The GSV is cannulated at the knee, and the catheter is advanced to the saphenofemoral junction.

Radiofrequency ablation's mechanism of action is based on resistive (or ohmic) heating caused by current. The heat generated in the vein wall (not in the catheter tip) is then dissipated and causes controlled collagen contraction or total thermocoagulation of the vein. The outcome is controlled tissue destruction that ultimately seals the lumen with minimal thrombus or coagulum.[70] The thermal effect is proportional to the temperature and treatment time. For instance, with a temperature of 85°C to 90°C and a pullback speed of 3 to 4 cm/min, the thermal effect is sufficient to cause collagen contraction and occlude the lumen.[70]

A compression garment is applied for several days after the procedure. Recovery time is 3 to 5 days. Complications include paresthesia, hematoma, skin burns, infection, bruising, and thrombophlebitis/thromboembolism. Transient paresthesia is reported in up to 15%, hematoma in 5%, skin burns in 2.1%, superficial thrombophlebitis in 2.1%, DVT in 16%, and nonfatal PE in 1% of 286 treated limbs.[2] Venous size of less than 2 mm or more than 15 mm, previous superficial thrombophlebitis with residual obstruction, and GSV tortuosity are relative contraindications for RFA.[40]

In a systematic review of more than 12,000 limbs of patients who received stripping, foam sclerotherapy, or thermal ablation, the overall occlusion rate for RFA was 88.8% at 3 months (95% CI, 83.6 to 92.5), 87.7% at 1 year (95% CI, 83.1 to 91.2), and 79.9% at 5 years (95% CI, 59.5 to 91.5).[45] Symptomatic improvement was reported in 85% to 94% of limbs with anatomical success and 70% to 80% of limbs with anatomical failures.[2] In a meta-analysis by Luebke and Brunkwall, the

QOL at 72 hours and 1 week was significantly better with RFA than with surgery.[46a]

Ultrasound examination is recommended within 72 hours to 1 week after the procedure to evaluate for DVT. Although no studies exist validating efficacy and safety of VTE prevention, patients with high thromboembolic risk can be considered for medical thromboprophylaxis after the procedure.[2] Radiofrequency ablation requires less hospitalization and recovery time than surgical procedures. In a study of 458 patients treated with RFA followed at 3 months and 1 year, the main predictors of long-term occlusion were pullback speed (OR 3.7; 95% CI, 1.1 to 12.4) and CEAP classification (OR 3.1; 95% CI, 1.7 to 5.6).[71] Murad et al. performed a meta-analysis and identified four RCTs and three observational studies comparing RFA to HLS for symptomatic varicose veins with maximum follow-up for 3 years.[72] The RFA group had a faster return to work (1.15 vs. 3.89 days; *P* = .02), to normal activities (7 vs. 14 days; *P* < .05), lower pain scores, better QOL, and similar rates for recurrent varicosities (RR, 0.94; 95% CI, 0.25 to 3.46). Another meta-analysis comparing RCTs of RFA vs. HLS identified similar primary failure rate (pooled RR of 1.2 [95% CI, 0.5 to 2.8]) and similar recurrence rate (pooled RR of 0.9 [95% CI, 0.6 to 1.4]).[73] When comparing RFA vs. EVLT, four RCTs were also identified in the same meta-analysis with a pooled RR of 1.5 (95% CI, 0.7 to 3.4) for primary failure which was not statistically significant. Both EVLT and RFA had 70% lower rates of wound infection (NNT of 80) and 50% to 60% lower rates of hematoma (NNT of 4 to 10) with a 3- to 5-day earlier return to work and normal activities compared to HLS.[73]

Surgical Procedures

Surgical interventions were traditionally the alternative treatment for VVs when conservative management had been unsuccessful. These are now rarely performed. Surgical treatments of VVs include saphenous vein stripping, ligation of the saphenofemoral junction, and ambulatory phlebectomy.[2] The hemodynamic effectiveness of surgical procedures is supported by air plethysmography studies. In a study of 2,120 limbs by Park et al., hemodynamic parameters including venous volume, venous filling index, residual volume function, and ejection fraction were significantly improved after surgery.[74]

Saphenous Vein Stripping. First reported in 1844, this procedure is performed in patients with incompetent GSVs or SSVs, reflux through the saphenofemoral or saphenopopliteal junctions, or superficial thrombophlebitis identified by duplex ultrasound.[1] Additional chemical sclerotherapy is often needed for residual tributary VVs.[75]

Saphenous vein stripping is performed under general anesthesia and involves making an incision in the groin, along with ligation of the GSV and its major branches. A stiff but flexible wire is inserted into the free end of the GSV and advanced along its length and out through a second incision at the upper calf. The vein is then tied to the wire in the groin and retrieved through the second incision at the upper calf, stripping the entire GSV. The incisions are then closed and compression bandages applied.[2]

Of note, venous stripping from ankle to groin is not always necessary. Ligation of the vein at the saphenofemoral junction in conjunction with removal of the thigh portion of the vein can also reduce venous reflux. Venous stripping may be performed in conjunction with ligation of the saphenofemoral junction, phlebectomy, or chemical sclerotherapy. Saphenous vein stripping has a higher initial cost due to hospitalization and results in more time lost from work compared with endovenous procedures.[2] Recovery time varies from 2 to 3 weeks. The procedure is contraindicated in patients with a history of DVT, Klippel-Trénaunay syndrome, or the presence of severe peripheral artery disease (PAD) or neuropathy, which may impede wound healing and increase the risk of infection.

In a large systematic review, there was persistent GSV and SSV obliteration of 80.4% (95% CI, 72.3 to 86.5) at 3 months, 79.7% (95% CI, 71.8 to 85.8) at 1 year, and 75.7% (95% CI, 67.9 to 82.1) at 5 years after saphenous vein stripping.[2,45] In a study of 245 extremities in 210 patients operated on for either GSV or SSV incompetence, there was a recurrence rate of 30%, as determined by ultrasound examination 14 years after the procedure, with only 6.9% having clinically significant recurrence of their VVs.[13] A multicenter study evaluated predictors of persistence or redevelopment of reflux in 1,638 limbs. After adjustment for follow-up, independent predictors were found to be groin mapping by ultrasound (OR, 0.28; 95% CI, 0.20 to 0.40), less than 3-cm groin incisions at or below groin crease (OR, 0.50; 95% CI, 0.32 to 0.78), prior parity (OR, 2.69; 95% CI, 1.45 to 4.97), body mass index (BMI) over 29 (OR, 1.65; 95% CI, 1.12 to 2.43), less than 3-cm suprainguinal incisions (OR, 3.71; 95% CI, 1.70 to 5.88), stripping to the ankle (OR, 2.43; 95% CI, 1.71 to 3.46), and interim pregnancy (OR, 4.74; 95% CI, 2.47 to 9.12).[76] Perforating vein incompetence and postthrombotic deep vein incompetence are also relevant considerations for postoperative VV recurrence.[77] The exact causes of VV recurrence are speculative, but may include neovascularization, presence of superficial and deep venous insufficiency, presence of incompetent perforator veins, or surgical failure.[6,10]

Although saphenous vein stripping improves the QOL for patients with symptomatic VVs, in a multicenter retrospective analysis of 376 limbs of 296 patients treated for primary VVs due to GSV insufficiency, the patient satisfaction rate decreased from 86% at 1 year to 74% at 5 years.[6] Complications of venous stripping include pain, bleeding (24%), infection (2% to 15%), nerve injury (25%), superficial thrombophlebitis, and venous thromboembolism (<2%).[78]

Ligation of the Saphenofemoral Junction. Ligation of the saphenofemoral junction can be performed in patients with saphenofemoral reflux. However, owing to the high VV recurrence rate, it is typically performed in conjunction with venous stripping, phlebectomy, or EFS.[2]

Ligation is performed under local anesthesia through an incision made parallel to the inguinal ligament at the site of the saphenofemoral junction. Saphenous vein tributaries are identified and ligated until reaching the saphenofemoral junction. The GSV is then ligated at its junction with the common femoral vein. The incision is then closed, and compression garments are applied.[2] Ligation has been used with endovenous ablation techniques to improve efficacy and safety. In one study of 210 legs in 182 patients with primary saphenofemoral junction incompetence, the recurrence rate for saphenofemoral junction ligation was 5.4% at 1 year and 35.5% at 4 years. The relative risk of recurrence after ligation of the saphenofemoral junction alone is 2.4 times greater than that of venous stripping.[79] However, the percentage of patients with symptomatic recurrence of their varicosities is low. In a study with long-term follow-up of 10 years of 245 extremities in 210 patients operated on for either GSV or SSV incompetence, only 7% of the limbs had recurrence (>3 mm diameter), with neovascularization as the main cause.[80] Complications of saphenofemoral ligation include pain, bleeding, and hematoma (<30%); infection (2% to 15%); nerve injury (4% to 25%); thrombophlebitis; and DVT/PE (<2%).[78] Contraindications are similar to saphenous vein stripping.

Stab or Transilluminated Phlebectomy. Transilluminated phlebectomy (TIPP) was proposed in 2000 as a more reliable and less invasive outpatient alternative to saphenous vein stripping.[2] The use of TIPP is associated with fewer incisions compared with conventional stab phlebectomy, but with a potentially higher cost, longer operating time, and greater complication rate.

For incision phlebectomy, small incisions are made along the GSV and its tributaries, which are retrieved with the use of a phlebectomy hook and subsequently avulsed.[2] Transilluminated phlebectomy is performed with a fiberoptic light channel inserted into the GSV. A mixture of saline and local anesthetic is infused into the subcutaneous tissue to produce tumescence and transilluminate the vein. With an endoscopic dissector provided with a rotating blade and suction channel, the GSV and its tributaries are resected and aspirated.[78] Contraindications are similar to those for saphenous vein stripping.

A randomized prospective trial on 188 limbs comparing stab phlebectomy with TIPP reported a significant difference in the number of incisions for phlebectomy between the two groups (29 ± 1.28 vs. 5 ± 0.17; $P < .001$). However, there was a higher recurrence rate at 52 weeks with TIPP (21.2% vs. 6.2%), with no significant difference in complication rates.[81] Complications include pain, hyperpigmentation (<2%), cellulitis (<3%), hematoma (5% to 12%), and nerve injury (up to 25%). The rate of calf hematoma is higher for TIPP than for stab phlebectomy (25% vs. 2.5%). Phlebectomy is useful for larger truncal veins, in which higher venous flow limits the use of endovenous procedures, and in younger patients with thicker vein walls.[2] This procedure is often performed in conjunction with traditional surgical ligation of the saphenofemoral junction.[2] Both stab phlebectomy and TIPP prolong the return to work and resumption of activities of daily living. However, most patients recover fully by 6 weeks postsurgery.[82]

Microphlebectomy. Dr. Robert Muller, a Swiss dermatologist from Neuchâtel, Switzerland, rediscovered this technique in 1956.[83] Ambulatory phlebectomy is a minimally invasive technique that can be performed in an office-based practice. This technique may be suitable for GSV, SSV, and pudendal veins in the groin, but more commonly is used to treat reticular varices in the popliteal fold or lateral part of the thigh.[83]

The VVs are carefully identified with a marking pen while the patient is standing. After tumescent anesthesia, with the patient in Trendelenburg position, cutaneous incisions are made with a #11 scalpel blade or 18-gauge needle, vertically oriented along the thigh and lower leg following the skin lines at the knee or the ankle.[83] The distance between the incisions is determined by experience, anatomy, and history of phlebitis. The vein is then dissected with the phlebectomy hook and mosquito forceps. Incompetent perforators can be dissected and eliminated with gentle traction or torsion, but this is more difficult. Venous ligation is not necessary, since hemostasis may be achieved with local compression during and after surgery. No skin closure is needed with small incisions of 1 to 3 mm. Postoperative bandaging is essential.[84] Dressings are removed after 24 or 48 hours. Ongoing compression therapy with elastic bandages or compression stockings is recommended for up to 3 weeks. Complementary chemical sclerotherapy may be used several weeks after the initial procedure.

Complications are minor and benign and usually resolve spontaneously. Periprocedurally, patients should avoid early sun exposure because hyperpigmentation may result at the puncture or incision sites.[83] Complications include edema, bleeding, hematoma formation, scarring, trauma-induced telangiectatic matting, neotelangiectasia, occasional nerve injury with sensory disturbances, and blisters due to wound dressings.[84] Very rarely, skin necrosis due to the high pH caused by adding excess bicarbonate to the anesthetic solution may occur. Deep venous thrombosis has not been reported.[84] Contraindications to ambulatory phlebectomy include reflux at the saphenofemoral or saphenopopliteal junctions. These junctions may be treated by thermal ablation.[83] Small studies and case series have reported a high rate of success with this procedure.

CHIVA Cure

This is a relatively new outpatient method described by Franceschi in 1988. "Cure Conservatrice et Hémodynamique de l'Insuffisance

Veineuse en Ambulatoire" (CHIVA), or "Ambulatory Conservative Hemodynamic Management of Varicose Veins," aims for preservation of the superficial venous system and its cutaneous and subcutaneous drainage. The CHIVA method consists of breaking up the hydrostatic pressure column by disconnecting venous shunts. This is achieved by using venous ligatures guided by hemodynamic and duplex ultrasonographic data derived from the deep and superficial venous system.[85] A variation of the CHIVA technique may be done using sclerotherapy.[86] Recurrence at 5 years of follow-up were 44.3% cured, 24.6% improved, and 31.1% failure in a study by Pares et al.[85] There were no occurrences of DVT, pulmonary thromboembolism, saphenous vein neuralgia, or deaths. Potential complications include bruises (47.5%), wound infection (2.5%), and phlebitis (1.3%).[85] Although the technique was invented in 1988, it is not yet widely available in the United States. The practice guidelines of the American Venous Forum and the Society for Vascular Surgery do not currently endorse widespread use of the CHIVA technique.[40]

MANAGEMENT OF INCOMPETENT PERFORATOR VEINS

Poor deep venous function caused by venous reflux, obstruction, or calf muscle pump failure will ultimately lead to an increase in ambulatory venous pressure and recurrence of VV through incompetent perforators, resulting in chronic venous insufficiency. Incompetent perforator veins in patients with venous ulcerations were previously treated with ligation using the open Linton procedure, and now occasionally with subfascial endoscopic perforator surgery (SEPS).[2] More commonly, endovenous thermal ablation or sclerotherapy is the treatment of choice for patients with venous ulcers who have failed conservative compression therapy and require ablation of incompetent perforator veins. The current SVS and AVF guidelines do suggest treatment of so-called pathological perforating veins, defined as those with outward flow of 500-ms duration, diameter of 3.5 mm, and located beneath a healed or open venous ulcer.[40]

Surgical Treatments of Incompetent Perforator Veins

Patients who undergo ligation of perforator veins typically have severe resistant CVI complicated by venous ulcerations. The Linton procedure was introduced in the 1950s for treating perforator veins and has largely been replaced by SEPS. About 45% of incompetent perforator veins are located in an area 10 to 15 cm above the medial malleolus, the typical Cockett 2/3 area, but the anatomy of the subfascial compartments makes only 32% of Cockett 2, 4% of Cockett 3, and 40% of Cockett 4 perforators available in the superficial posterior compartment for interruption via a SEPS procedure.[87,88]

Linton or Subfascial Endoscopic Perforator Surgery Procedure

The Linton procedure involves making a long incision across the calf including the diseased tissue, forming a skin/soft tissue/fascial flap, and ligating the perforator veins under direct visualization.[2] SEPS can be performed in the ambulatory care setting, with less time away from work required. The SEPS procedure involves making two incisions below the knee and inserting ports into the subfascial space.[2] The subfascial plane is kept open with infusion of CO_2 for visualization of the structures. The perforator veins are identified and ligated.

As noted, the Linton procedure has largely been replaced by SEPS because of higher complication rates, including wound infections (40% to 50%), nerve injury (11%), and DVT (4%). Complications associated with SEPS are less frequent and include wound infection (5% to 7%), nerve injury (6%), superficial thrombophlebitis (3%), and cellulitis (2.5%).[21,24,81] Presence of peripheral artery disease, which carries the

risk of poor wound healing, is a relative contraindication to these procedures. Similarly, performance of these procedures in patients with deep vein occlusion is associated with poor outcomes.[89]

Lower-extremity activity is limited for 5 to 7 days.[2] SEPS may be performed in conjunction with other surgical and endovenous procedures that ablate an incompetent GSV.

Sclerotherapy

Ultrasound-guided sclerotherapy uses a relatively small catheter to gain access to the incompetent perforator or its tributary. Masuda et al. treated 80 limbs in 68 patients by sclerotherapy using liquid sodium morrhuate. The initial incompetent perforator closure rate was 90%, but fell to 70% at a mean follow-up of 20 months.[87] After treatment, the VCSS was improved from a median of 8 to 2. Skin necrosis is a reported adverse effect. Kiguchi et al. treated 73 perforator veins in 62 patients with UGFS with 52% ulcer healing at 30-month mean follow-up.[90] Male gender and warfarin use was noted as negative predictors for perforator vein thrombosis. For ulcer healing, large ulcers were negative predictors and perforator thrombosis were positive predictors. Calf vein thrombosis was seen in 3% of patients. Another study reported ulcer recurrence rate of 28% at 5 years.[91]

Endovenous Thermal Ablation

Endovenous thermal ablation (EVTA) of incompetent perforator veins can be carried out with a small incision or puncture site in the calf. However, because this entry site is usually made in compromised skin directly over the perforator, there may be risk of infection or exacerbation of the wound. In a meta-analysis of 1,573 incompetent perforator veins treated by RFA, the occlusion rate varied from 64% to 99% during a short follow-up.[87] A study published after the meta-analysis prospectively evaluated 482 limbs of which 534 perforators of 303 limbs underwent EVLT. High occlusion rates were noted on follow-up with only 7.6% of perforator veins needing reintervention.[92] Another study of 171 perforating veins reported 94% of perforators remained occluded after 3 months with 96% of patients having symptoms resolution. DVT was seen in one case.[93] In a study of 37 patients who underwent Doppler ultrasound surveillance 5 years after incompetent perforator ablation, of 125 incompetent perforators analyzed, 101 were closed (81%).[94] Studies have shown that patients with active venous ulcers healed within 4 weeks to 4 months after undergoing RFA of incompetent superficial and perforating veins especially when compression therapy was continued.[87,95–97] EVLT has been studied also. Hissink et al. treated 58 perforators with EVLT, five of which had ulcers. Four of five ulcers healed within 6 weeks of intervention.[98] Studies have shown EVLA provides faster ulcer healing and less recurrence compared to compression alone.[95]

The current approach to perforator vein ablation suggests that there is no advantage over GSV ablation alone in patients with CEAP class 2 or 3, or mild-moderate venous symptoms. Perforator interventions should be considered in patients with severe venous symptoms such as active ulcers not healing with conventional therapy or those with recurrent ulcers associated with incompetent perforators.

Small saphenous veins: Although SSVs constitute up to 15% of VVs, often most trials and data specifically analyze GSV. In 2016, Boersma et al. published a meta-analysis and systematic review on treatment outcomes for SSV insufficiency. In this analysis, pooled anatomical success was assessed and was reported as 58.0% (95% CI, 40.9% to 75.0%) for surgery (798 SSVs), 98.5% (95% CI, 97.7% to 99.2%) for EVLT (2950 SSVs), 97.1% (95% CI, 94.3% to 99.9%) for RFA (386 SSVs), 63.6% (95% CI, 47.1% to 80.1%) for ultrasound guided EFS (494 SSVs), and 94% in one study for MOCA. EVTA was superior to EFS and surgery for SSV in general.[99]

MANAGEMENT OF TELANGIECTASIA/RETICULAR VEINS

Surface Transcutaneous Laser Therapy

Surface transcutaneous laser therapy has been used for treating telangiectasias and reticular veins since the 1970s. Laser obliterates the vein by heating the hemoglobin (Hb) within the vessel and injuring the endothelium. New advances in laser technology have allowed delivery of sufficient energy to achieve pan-endothelial necrosis without affecting structures in the epidermal layer. High-intensity pulsed light therapy was developed in 1990 for treating small VVs. It differs from laser by emitting a spectrum of light, rather than a wavelength, to obliterate the vein.

Procedure

Patients undergo skin cooling with water-cooled chambers applied to the skin, cooling coupling gel, air-blowing cooling devices, or refrigerated cooling sprays before and after the procedure to provide comfort during the procedure and minimize postprocedure adverse effects. The amount of precooling depends on the patient's skin type and size of varicosities; those with higher amounts of melanin in their skin require longer precooling. The amount of postcooling depends on the size of the vessels to be treated, with smaller vessels requiring longer postcooling.

The laser is applied to the surface of the skin and targets a wavelength of light to the Hb within the vessel, resulting in heating and obliteration of the vessel. Small (<1 mm) superficial vessels with higher oxygenated Hb content are treated with shorter wavelengths (580 to 1,064 nm), shorter pulse durations (15 to 30 ms), higher fluences (350 to 600 J/cm^2), and smaller spot sizes (<2 mm).[69] Larger, deeper vessels with lower oxygenated Hb content are treated with longer wavelengths (800 to 1,064 nm), longer pulse durations (30 to 50 ms), moderate fluences (100 to 350 J/cm^2), and larger spot sizes (2 to 8 mm).[2] Pulsed light therapy delivers a high-intensity spectrum of light to the vessel, resulting in its obliteration. Pulsed light therapy generally is used for longer vessels. Typically, one to three laser treatments are scheduled at 6- to 12-week intervals.[2]

Reports of effectiveness are based on case series reporting small numbers of patients. In a study of 40 female patients 24 to 58 years old, the leg veins were treated with synchronized micropulses from a long-pulsed 1,064-nm Nd:YAG laser, 6-mm diameter spot size, and 130 and 140 J/cm.[4] After one to three laser treatment sessions, there was a 50% to 75% disappearance of veins in approximately 60% of the limbs at 4 weeks, and in more than 80% of the limbs at 12 weeks. The patient subjective satisfaction index, measuring cosmetics, increased from 42.5% at 6 months to 75% at 12 months. Objective improvement in cosmetic appearance, measured with computer-assessed medical photography, increased from 57% at 6 months to 82.5% at 12 months.[100]

Postprocedure pain is a common side effect of laser and light therapy. Other complications include edema, erythema, bruising, vesiculation, hypo/hyperpigmentation, transient hemosiderin staining, telangiectatic matting, and scarring. This procedure is contraindicated during pregnancy and in those with tanned or dark skin, history of photosensitivity disorder, or keloidal scarring. Patients are advised to avoid tanning before the procedure to avoid absorption of shorter wavelengths from the laser by sun-induced melanin, resulting in blistering and hyperpigmentation.[5] Sunscreen is advised after treatment with laser.

Laser and light therapies are more expensive than liquid sclerotherapy, owing to the cost of equipment. VeinGogh and Veinwave are FDA-exempt devices employing percutaneous radiofrequency ablation for telangiectasias. There is a paucity of published data on their efficacy and safety, mostly anecdotal cases promoted by the manufacturers.

Chemical Sclerotherapy

Sclerotherapy for treating telangiectasias and reticular veins is generally performed using liquid sclerosant (glycerin, hypertonic saline, polidocanol, and sodium tetradecyl sulfate) rather than foam, although foam can also be used in lower volumes. To decrease telangiectatic matting and postsclerosis hyperpigmentation, a reduced amount of foam per injection (0.5 mL) and per treatment session is recommended for telangiectasias and reticular veins. *Telangiectatic matting* describes a network of tiny vessels less than 0.2 mm in diameter that may appear after sclerotherapy treatment.[101] In a large retrospective analysis of 2,120 patients, the overall incidence of telangiectatic matting was 16%.[101]

FOLLOW-UP AND PROGNOSIS

A relevant disclosure before treating the patient with VVs is that current methodologies continue to require long-term follow-up and retreatment. The possibility of recurrence at 5 years is 5% to 30%, depending on the treatment administered and ongoing risk factors. Obesity, multiple pregnancies, incompetent perforators, and saphenofemoral junction incompetence are some of the often-mentioned risk factors for recurrence. Regular compression stocking use will minimize the signs and symptoms associated with recurrent VVs and progression of chronic venous insufficiency. However, patients will commonly return for repeated treatments over their lifetime.[76,77]

Quality Assurance and Patient Reported Outcomes

With the increased requirement for documentation of medical necessity for venous disorders treatment, including treatment of varicose veins, central registries have been developed. Most notable are the American College of Phlebology PRO registry and the American Venous Forum VQI Varicose vein registry. These registries collect both patient- and physician-reported outcomes post vein treatment and are designed to interact with the electronic health record. Further, the International Accreditation Commission has established minimal standards for vein center accreditation that includes documentation of vein treatment outcomes. Capture of patient reported outcomes continues to be a focus of CMS and third-party coverage for treatment of chronic venous disease.

REFERENCES

1. Gloviczki P, Comerota AJ, Dalsing MC, et al. The care of patients with varicose veins and associated chronic venous diseases: clinical practice guidelines of the Society for Vascular Surgery and the American Venous Forum. *J Vasc Surg.* 2011;53(5 Suppl):2S–48S.
2. Nael R, Rathbun S. Treatment of varicose veins. *Curr Treat Options Cardiovasc Med.* 2009;11(2):91–103.
3. Rumwell C, McPharlin M. *Vascular Technology.* ed 4. Pasadena, CA: Davies; 2009.
4. Callam MJ. Epidemiology of varicose veins. *Br J Surg.* 1994;81(2):167–173.
5. Bergan JJ, Schmid-Schonbein GW, Smith PD, et al. Chronic venous disease. *N Engl J Med.* 2006;355(5):488–498.
6. Miyazaki K, Nishibe T, Sata F, et al. Long-term results of treatments for varicose veins due to greater saphenous vein insufficiency. *Int Angiol.* 2005;24(3):282–286.
7. Marsh P, Holdstock J, Harrison C, et al. Pelvic vein reflux in female patients with varicose veins: comparison of incidence between a specialist private vein clinic and the vascular department of a National Health Service District General Hospital. *Phlebology.* 2009;24(3):108–113.

8. Evans CJ, Fowkes FG, Ruckley CV, Lee AJ. Prevalence of varicose veins and chronic venous insufficiency in men and women in the general population: Edinburgh Vein Study. *J Epidemiol Community Health*. 1999;53(3):149–153.

9. Kachlik D, Pechacek V, Baca V, Musil V. The superficial venous system of the lower extremity: new nomenclature. *Phlebology*. 2010;25(3):113–123.

10. Raju S, Neglen P. Clinical practice. Chronic venous insufficiency and varicose veins. *N Engl J Med*. 2009;360(22):2319–2327.

11. Robertson L, Lee AJ, Gallagher K, et al. Risk factors for chronic ulceration in patients with varicose veins: a case control study. *J Vasc Surg*. 2009;49(6):1490–1498.

12. Labropoulos N, Gasparis AP, Pefanis D, et al. Secondary chronic venous disease progresses faster than primary. *J Vasc Surg*. 2009;49(3):704–710.

13. Raffetto JD, Khalil RA. Matrix metalloproteinases in venous tissue remodeling and varicose vein formation. *Curr Vasc Pharmacol*. 2008;6(3):158–172.

14. Rutherford RB, Padberg Jr FT, Comerota AJ, et al. Venous severity scoring: an adjunct to venous outcome assessment. *J Vasc Surg*. 2000;31(6):1307–1312.

15. Ward A, Abisi S, Braithwaite BD. An online patient completed Aberdeen Varicose Vein Questionnaire can help to guide primary care referrals. *Eur J Vasc Endovasc Surg*. 2013;45:178–182.

16. Vasquez MA, Munschauer CE. Venous Clinical Severity Score and quality-of-life assessment tools: application to vein practice. *Phlebology*. 2008;23(6):259–275.

17. Vasquez MA, Rabe E, McLafferty RB, et al. Revision of the venous clinical severity score: venous outcomes consensus statement: special communication of the American Venous Forum Ad Hoc Outcomes Working Group. *J Vasc Surg*. 2010;52(5):1387–1396.

18. Kurstjens RL, de Wolf MA, Alsadah SA, et al. The value of hemodynamic measurements by air plethysmography in diagnosing venous obstruction of the lower limb. *J Vasc Surg Venous Lymphat Disord*. 2016;4(3):313–319.

19. Gornik HL, Gerhard-Herman MD, Misra S, et al. ACCF/ACR/AIUM/ASE/IAC/SCAI/SCVS/SIR/SVM/SVS/SVU 2013 appropriate use criteria for peripheral vascular ultrasound and physiological testing part II: testing for venous disease and evaluation of hemodialysis access: a report of the American College of Cardiology Foundation Appropriate Use Criteria Task Force. *J Am College Cardiol*. 2013;62(7):649–665.

20. Jung SC, Lee W, Chung JW, et al. Unusual causes of varicose veins in the lower extremities: CT venographic and Doppler US findings. *Radiographics*. 2009;29(2):525–536.

21. Goode SD, Kuhan G, Altaf N, et al. Suitability of varicose veins for endovenous treatments. *Cardiovasc Intervent Radiol*. 2009;32(5):988–991.

22. Luebke T, Gawenda M, Heckenkamp J, Brunkwall J. Meta-analysis of endovenous radiofrequency obliteration of the great saphenous vein in primary varicosis. *J Endovasc Ther*. 2008;15(2):213–223.

23. Kolluri R. Interventions for varicose veins: beyond ablation. *Curr Treat Options Cardiovasc Med*. 2016;18(7):43.

24. Rathbun SW, Kirkpatrick AC. Treatment of chronic venous insufficiency. *Curr Treat Options Cardiovasc Med*. 2007;9(2):115–126.

25. Klonizakis M, Tew G, Michaels J, Saxton J. Exercise training improves cutaneous microvascular endothelial function in post-surgical varicose vein patients. *Microvasc Res*. 2009;78(1):67–70.

26. Milic DJ, Zivic SS, Bogdanovic DC, et al. The influence of different sub-bandage pressure values on venous leg ulcers healing when treated with compression therapy. *J Vasc Surg*. 2010;51(3):655–661.

27. O'Meara S, Al-Kurdi D, Ologun Y, et al. Antibiotics and antiseptics for venous leg ulcers. *Cochrane Database Syst Rev*. 2014;(1):CD003557.

28. Martinez-Zapata MJ, Vernooij RW, Uriona Tuma SM, et al. Phlebotonics for venous insufficiency. *Cochrane Database Syst Rev*. 2016;4:CD003229.

29. Suter A, Bommer S, Rechner J. Treatment of patients with venous insufficiency with fresh plant horse chestnut seed extract: a review of 5 clinical studies. *Adv Ther*. 2006;23(1):179–190.

30. Pittler MH, Ernst E. Horse chestnut seed extract for chronic venous insufficiency. *Cochrane Database Syst Rev*. 2012;11:CD003230.

31. Coleridge-Smith P, Lok C, Ramelet AA. Venous leg ulcer: a meta-analysis of adjunctive therapy with micronized purified flavonoid fraction. *Eur J Vasc Endovasc Surg*. 2005;30(2):198–208.

32. Jantet G. Chronic venous insufficiency: worldwide results of the RELIEF study. Reflux assEssment and quaLity of lIfe improvEment with micronized Flavonoids. *Angiology*. 2002;53(3):245–256.

33. Rabe E, Ballarini S, Lehr L. A randomized, double-blind, placebo-controlled, clinical study on the efficacy and safety of calcium dobesilate in the treatment of chronic venous insufficiency. *Phlebology*. 2016;31(4):264–274.

34. Aziz Z, Tang WL, Chong NJ, Tho LY. A systematic review of the efficacy and tolerability of hydroxyethylrutosides for improvement of the signs and symptoms of chronic venous insufficiency. *J Clin Pharm Ther*. 2015;40(2):177–185.

35. Belcaro G, Dugall M, Luzzi R, et al. Management of varicose veins and chronic venous insufficiency in a comparative registry with nine venoactive products in comparison with stockings. *Int J Angiol*. 2017;26(3):170–178.

36. Belcaro G. A clinical comparison of pycnogenol, antistax, and stocking in chronic venous insufficiency. *Int J Angiol*. 2015;24(4):268–274.

37. Dale JJ, Ruckley CV, Harper DR, et al. Randomised, double blind placebo controlled trial of pentoxifylline in the treatment of venous leg ulcers. *BMJ*. 1999;319(7214):875–878.

38. Falanga V, Fujitani RM, Diaz C, et al. Systemic treatment of venous leg ulcers with high doses of pentoxifylline: efficacy in a randomized, placebo-controlled trial. *Wound Repair Regen*. 1999;7(4):208–213.

39. Nelson EA, Prescott RJ, Harper DR, et al. A factorial, randomized trial of pentoxifylline or placebo, four-layer or single-layer compression, and knitted viscose or hydrocolloid dressings for venous ulcers. *J Vasc Surg*. 2007;45(1):134–141.

40. Gloviczki P, Comerota AJ, Dalsing MC, et al. The care of patients with varicose veins and associated chronic venous diseases: clinical practice guidelines of the Society for Vascular Surgery and the American Venous Forum. *J Vasc Surg*. 2011;53(5 Suppl):2s–48s.

41. Wittens C, Davies AH, Baekgaard N, et al. Editor's choice - management of chronic venous disease: clinical practice guidelines of the European Society for Vascular Surgery (ESVS). *Eur J Vasc Endovasc Surg*. 2015;49(6):678–737.

42. Breu FX, Guggenbichler S. European consensus meeting on foam sclerotherapy, April 4-6, 2003, Tegernsee, Germany. *Dermatol Surg*. 2004;30(5):709–717. discussion 17.

43. Bergan J, Cheng V. Foam sclerotherapy for the treatment of varicose veins. *Vascular*. 2007;15(5):269–272.

44. Belcaro G, Cesarone MR, Di Renzo A, et al. Foam-sclerotherapy, surgery, sclerotherapy, and combined treatment for varicose veins: a 10-year, prospective, randomized, controlled, trial (VEDICO trial). *Angiology*. 2003;54(3):307–315.

45. van den Bos R, Arends L, Kockaert M, et al. Endovenous therapies of lower extremity varicosities: a meta-analysis. *J Vasc Surg*. 2009;49(1):230–239.

46. Myers KA, Jolley D. Factors affecting the risk of deep venous occlusion after ultrasound-guided sclerotherapy for varicose veins. *Eur J Vasc Endovasc Surg*. 2008;36(5):602–605.

46a. Luebke T, Brunkwall J. Systematic review and meta-analysis of endovenous radiofrequency obliteration, endovenous laser therapy, and foam sclerotherapy for primary varicosis. *J Cardiovasc Surg (Torino)*. 2008;49(2):213–233.

47. Sarvananthan T, Shepherd AC, Willenberg T, Davies AH. Neurological complications of sclerotherapy for varicose veins. *J Vasc Surg*. 2012;55(1):243–251.

48. Frullini A, Felice F, Burchielli S, Di Stefano R. High production of endothelin after foam sclerotherapy: a new pathogenetic hypothesis for neurological and visual disturbances after sclerotherapy. *Phlebology*. 2011;26(5):203–208.

49. Stephens R, Dunn S. Non-ST-elevation myocardial infarction following foam ultrasound-guided sclerotherapy. *Phlebology*. 2014;29(7):488–490.

50. Hamann SAS, Giang J, De Maeseneer MGR, et al. Editor's choice - five year results of great saphenous vein treatment: a meta-analysis. *Eur J Vasc Endovasc Surg*. 2017;54(6):760–770.

51. Rathbun S, Norris A, Stoner J. Efficacy and safety of endovenous foam sclerotherapy: meta-analysis for treatment of venous disorders. *Phlebology*. 2012;27(3):105–117.

52. Carugo D, Ankrett DN, Zhao X, et al. Benefits of polidocanol endovenous microfoam (Varithena(R)) compared with physician-compounded foams. *Phlebology*. 2016;31(4):283–295.

53. Todd 3rd KL, Wright DI. Durability of treatment effect with polidocanol endovenous microfoam on varicose vein symptoms and appearance (VANISH-2). *J Vasc Surg Venous Lymphat Disord*. 2015;3(3):258–264.e1.

54. Vasquez M, Gasparis AP. A multicenter, randomized, placebo-controlled trial of endovenous thermal ablation with or without polidocanol endovenous microfoam treatment in patients with great saphenous vein incompetence and visible varicosities. *Phlebology*. 2017;32(4):272–281.

55. Gibson K, Kabnick LA. A multicenter, randomized, placebo-controlled study to evaluate the efficacy and safety of Varithena(R) (polidocanol endovenous microfoam 1%) for symptomatic, visible varicose veins with saphenofemoral junction incompetence. *Phlebology*. 2017;32(3):185–193.

56. Bishawi M, Bernstein R, Boter M, et al. Mechanochemical ablation in patients with chronic venous disease: a prospective multicenter report. *Phlebology*. 2014;29(6):397–400.

57. Bootun R, Lane TR, Dharmarajah B, et al. Intra-procedural pain score in a randomised controlled trial comparing mechanochemical ablation to radiofrequency ablation: the Multicentre Venefit versus ClariVein(R) for varicose veins trial. *Phlebology*. 2016;31(1):61–65.

58. Witte ME, Zeebregts CJ, de Borst GJ, et al. Mechanochemical endovenous ablation of saphenous veins using the ClariVein: a systematic review. *Phlebology*. 2017;32(10):649–657.

59. Morrison N, Gibson K, McEnroe S, et al. Randomized trial comparing cyanoacrylate embolization and radiofrequency ablation for incompetent great saphenous veins (VeClose). *J Vasc Surg*. 2015;61(4):985–994.

60. Gibson K, Ferris B. Cyanoacrylate closure of incompetent great, small and accessory saphenous veins without the use of post-procedure compression: initial outcomes of a post-market evaluation of the VenaSeal System (the WAVES Study). *Vascular*. 2017;25(2):149–156.

61. Fan CM, Rox-Anderson R. Endovenous laser ablation: mechanism of action. *Phlebology*. 2008;23(5):206–213.

62. Perkowski P, Ravi R, Gowda RC, et al. Endovenous laser ablation of the saphenous vein for treatment of venous insufficiency and varicose veins: early results from a large single-center experience. *J Endovasc Ther*. 2004;11(2):132–138.

63. Ravi R, Trayler EA, Barrett DA, Diethrich EB. Endovenous thermal ablation of superficial venous insufficiency of the lower extremity: single-center experience with 3000 limbs treated in a 7-year period. *J Endovasc Ther*. 2009;16(4):500–505.

64. Nwaejike N, Srodon PD, Kyriakides C. 5-years of endovenous laser ablation (EVLA) for the treatment of varicose veins--a prospective study. *Int J Surg*. 2009;7(4):347–349.

65. Pannier F, Rabe E. Endovenous laser therapy and radiofrequency ablation of saphenous varicose veins. *J Cardiovasc Surg (Torino)*. 2006;47(1):3–8.

66. Pan Y, Zhao J, Mei J, et al. Comparison of endovenous laser ablation and high ligation and stripping for varicose vein treatment: a meta-analysis. *Phlebology*. 2014;29(2):109–119.

67. Gauw SA, Lawson JA, van Vlijmen-van Keulen CJ, et al. Five-year follow-up of a randomized, controlled trial comparing saphenofemoral ligation and stripping of the great saphenous vein with endovenous laser ablation (980 nm) using local tumescent anesthesia. *J Vasc Surg*. 2016;63(2):420–428.

68. Paravastu SC, Horne M, Dodd PD. Endovenous ablation therapy (laser or radiofrequency) or foam sclerotherapy versus conventional surgical repair for short saphenous varicose veins. *Cochrane Database Syst Rev*. 2016;11:CD010878.

69. Gohel MS, Davies AH. Radiofrequency ablation for uncomplicated varicose veins. *Phlebology*. 2009;24(Suppl 1):42–49.

70. Roth SM. Endovenous radiofrequency ablation of superficial and perforator veins. *Surg Clin North Am*. 2007;87(5):1267–1284. xii.

71. Boon R, Akkersdijk GJ, Nio D. Percutaneus treatment of varicose veins with bipolar radiofrequency ablation. *Eur J Radiol*. 2010;75(1):43–47.

72. Murad MH, Coto-Yglesias F, Zumaeta-Garcia M, et al. A systematic review and meta-analysis of the treatments of varicose veins. *J Vasc Surg*. 2011;53(5 Suppl):49S–65S.

73. Siribumrungwong B, Noorit P, Wilasrusmee C, et al. A systematic review and meta-analysis of randomised controlled trials comparing endovenous ablation and surgical intervention in patients with varicose vein. *Eur J Vasc Endovasc Surg*. 2012;44(2):214–223.

74. Park UJ, Yun WS, Lee KB, et al. Analysis of the postoperative hemodynamic changes in varicose vein surgery using air plethysmography. *J Vasc Surg*. 2010;51(3):634–638.

75. Nishibe T, Kondo Y, Dardik A, et al. Fate of varicose veins after great saphenous vein stripping alone. *Int Angiol*. 2009;28(4):311–314.

76. Fischer R, Chandler JG, Stenger D, et al. Patient characteristics and physician-determined variables affecting saphenofemoral reflux recurrence after ligation and stripping of the great saphenous vein. *J Vasc Surg*. 2006;43(1):81–87.

77. Allegra C, Antignani PL, Carlizza A. Recurrent varicose veins following surgical treatment: our experience with five years follow-up. *Eur J Vasc Endovasc Surg*. 2007;33(6):751–756.

78. Beale RJ, Gough MJ. Treatment options for primary varicose veins--a review. *Eur J Vasc Endovasc Surg*. 2005;30(1):83–95.

79. Winterborn RJ, Foy C, Heather BP, Earnshaw JJ. Randomised trial of flush saphenofemoral ligation for primary great saphenous varicose veins. *Eur J Vasc Endovasc Surg*. 2008;36(4):477–484.

80. Hartmann K, Klode J, Pfister R, et al. Recurrent varicose veins: sonography-based re-examination of 210 patients 14 years after ligation and saphenous vein stripping. *VASA Zeitschrift fur Gefasskrankheiten*. 2006;35(1):21–26.

81. Aremu MA, Mahendran B, Butcher W, et al. Prospective randomized controlled trial: conventional versus powered phlebectomy. *J Vasc Surg*. 2004;39(1):88–94.

82. Chetter IC, Mylankal KJ, Hughes H, Fitridge R. Randomized clinical trial comparing multiple stab incision phlebectomy and transilluminated powered phlebectomy for varicose veins. *Br J Surg*. 2006;93(2):169–174.

83. Ramelet AA. Phlebectomy. Technique, indications and complications. *Int Angiol*. 2002;21(2 Suppl 1):46–51.

84. Weiss RA, Dover JS. Leg vein management: sclerotherapy, ambulatory phlebectomy, and laser surgery. *Semin Cutan Med Surg*. 2002;21(1):76–103.

85. Pares JO, Juan J, Tellez R, et al. Varicose vein surgery: stripping versus the CHIVA method: a randomized controlled trial. *Ann Surg*. 2010;251(4):624–631.

86. Bernardini E, Piccioli R, De Rango P, et al. Echo-sclerosis hemodynamic conservative: a new technique for varicose vein treatment. *Ann Vasc Surg*. 2007;21(4):535–543.

87. O'Donnell TF. The role of perforators in chronic venous insufficiency. *Phlebology*. 2010;25(1):3–10.

88. O'Donnell Jr TF, Passman MA, Marston WA, et al. Management of venous leg ulcers: clinical practice guidelines of the Society for Vascular Surgery (R) and the American Venous Forum. *J Vasc Surg*. 2014;60(2 Suppl):3S–59S.

89. Gloviczki P, Bergan JJ, Rhodes JM, et al. Mid-term results of endoscopic perforator vein interruption for chronic venous insufficiency: lessons learned from the North American Subfascial Endoscopic Perforator Surgery Registry. The North American Study Group. *J Vasc Surg*. 1999;29(3):489–502.

90. Kiguchi MM, Hager ES, Winger DG, et al. Factors that influence perforator thrombosis and predict healing with perforator sclerotherapy for venous ulceration without axial reflux. *J Vasc Surg*. 2014;59(5):1368–1376.

91. Kulkarni SR, Slim FJ, Emerson LG, et al. Effect of foam sclerotherapy on healing and long-term recurrence in chronic venous leg ulcers. *Phlebology*. 2013;28(3):140–146.

92. Corcos L, Pontello D, DE Anna D, et al. Endovenous 808-nm diode laser occlusion of perforating veins and varicose collaterals: a prospective study of 482 limbs. *Dermatol Surg*. 2011;37(10):1486–1498.

93. Chehab M, Dixit P, Antypas E, et al. Endovenous laser ablation of perforating veins: feasibility, safety, and occlusion rate using a 1,470-nm laser and bare-tip fiber. *J Vasc Interv Radiol*. 2015;26(6):871–877.

94. Bacon JL, Dinneen AJ, Marsh P, et al. Five-year results of incompetent perforator vein closure using TRans-Luminal Occlusion of Perforator. *Phlebology*. 2009;24(2):74–78.

95. Harlander-Locke M, Lawrence P, Jimenez JC, et al. Combined treatment with compression therapy and ablation of incompetent superficial and perforating veins reduces ulcer recurrence in patients with CEAP 5 venous disease. *J Vasc Surg*. 2012;55(2):446–450.

96. Harlander-Locke M, Lawrence PF, Alktaifi A, et al. The impact of ablation of incompetent superficial and perforator veins on ulcer healing rates. *J Vasc Surg*. 2012;55(2):458–464.

97. Alden PB, Lips EM, Zimmerman KP, et al. Chronic venous ulcer: minimally invasive treatment of superficial axial and perforator vein reflux speeds healing and reduces recurrence. *Ann Vasc Surg*. 2013;27(1):75–83.

98. Hissink RJ, Bruins RM, Erkens R, et al. Innovative treatments in chronic venous insufficiency: endovenous laser ablation of perforating veins: a prospective short-term analysis of 58 cases. *Eur J Vasc Endovasc Surg*. 2010;40(3):403–406.

99. Boersma D, Kornmann VN, van Eekeren RR, et al. Treatment modalities for small saphenous vein insufficiency: systematic review and meta-analysis. *J Endovasc Ther*. 2016;23(1):199–211.

100. Trelles MA, Allones I, Martin-Vázquez MJ, et al. Long pulse Nd:YAG laser for treatment of leg veins in 40 patients with assessments at 6 and 12 months. *Lasers Surg Med*. 2004;35(1):68–76.

101. Davis LT, Duffy DM. Determination of incidence and risk factors for postsclerotherapy telangiectatic matting of the lower extremity: a retrospective analysis. *J Dermatol Surg Oncol*. 1990;16(4):327–330.

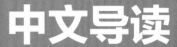

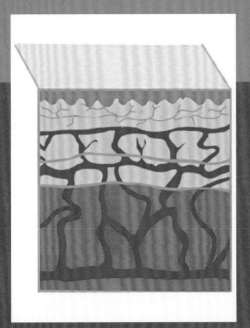

第54章
慢性静脉功能不全

慢性静脉功能不全是血管外科临床最常见的疾病，人群患病率高达25%左右。由于对其病理生理学理解的不断进展，初级预防已得到了更多的重视。患者对疾病的耐受程度不同，大部分就诊时常症状明显，甚至已经出现足踝部皮肤溃疡。合并盆腔静脉高压及髂静脉闭塞者的诊治更困难。多普勒超声仍是最普及的无创检查方式，CT静脉造影检查（CT venography，CTV）及血管内超声为病情复杂患者提供了更精准的影像依据。此类疾病早期症状轻微，药物及压力治疗更容易为患者接受，尤其是相关药物进展及合理的压力治疗值得临床关注，症状严重时常需进一步干预。既往创伤较大的外科修复瓣膜功能的手术越来越少应用，因为效果不确切及复发率较高，外科手术仅建议在不合适腔内治疗时或某些特殊情况下采用。随着影像检查及微创技术的进展与普及，如何精准修复或改善局部异常静脉血流动力学已经成为临床治疗的研究热点。超声引导下的静脉消融治疗在浅静脉瓣膜病变治疗中得到了广泛应用，穿支病变也得到了有效关注与治疗。静脉支架是目前治疗髂静脉阻塞性病变的主要方式，尽管静脉支架对这些疾病的治疗效果明显，但在血栓导致的深静脉病变中仍需更多的数据支持与研究，通畅率更高的腔内静脉支架系统与干预模式是未来研究的方向。

李震

Chronic Venous Insufficiency

Arjun Jayaraj and Peter Gloviczki

Chronic venous insufficiency (CVI) refers to clinical conditions of varying severity, from varicose veins at one end of the spectrum to venous ulceration. Advanced chronic venous disease (CVD) has a more severe clinical presentation than simple varicose veins, reticular veins, or telangiectasia but may be part of the clinical syndrome of CVI that typically presents with swelling, skin changes, and/or leg ulcers. The prevalence of varicose veins has been estimated to be 25% to 33% of the general population.[1,2] The progression of isolated varicose veins to CVI is rare and noted to be approximately 2% per year.[3] The prevalence of skin changes and ulceration is thought to be approximately 2% to 5% of the general population, whereas the prevalence of venous ulcers alone is approximately 1%.[4-6] Although the direct costs associated with the treatment of CVI have historically been estimated to be 1 billion dollars/year, the actual number is likely much higher.[7,8] There are additional indirect costs due to impairment of quality of life (QOL) and consequent societal impact. The management of simple varicose veins are considered in Chapter 53.

The CEAP (Clinical, Etiologic, Anatomic, and Pathophysiologic) classification groups chronic venous disorders on the basis of clinical presentation, etiology, anatomy, and pathophysiology and is denoted in the basic and full forms. This classification, considered in Box 54.1, was first described in 1995 and revised in 2004.[9-11] Although C1 clinical presentation is considered a chronic disorder, patients with C2 to C6 clinical presentation have CVD and the term CVI applies to those patients who have a clinical presentation of C3 to C6. The group of CVI patients with a history of deep vein thrombosis are described as having postthrombotic syndrome (PTS).

ANATOMY

The veins in the lower extremity can broadly be grouped into three categories: superficial, perforator, and deep. Superficial veins are those that run superficial to the muscle fascia and include the great saphenous, small saphenous, and accessory veins (Fig. 54.1). There exist multiple connections between these veins. Deep veins run deep to the muscle fascia and are axial veins that parallel the course of the arteries. Perforating veins are those that connect the superficial system to the deep veins in the process traversing the fascia (see Fig. 54.1). The veins that connect the superficial veins among themselves and which stay above the fascia are termed connecting veins. The great saphenous vein (GSV) starts at the medial end of the dorsal venous arch, runs anterior to the medial malleolus, rising up the medial leg and thigh, and empties into the common femoral vein (CFV) after piercing the fascia approximately 4 cm lateral and inferior to the pubic tubercle.[12] The small saphenous vein (SSV) starts at the lateral end of the dorsal venous arch, courses behind the lateral malleolus, and ascends along the lateral leg before emptying into the popliteal vein approximately

60% of the time.[12,13] The outflow is into the femoral, profunda femoral, or internal iliac veins, and the GSV the reminder of the time. The two saphenous veins can be connected by a communicating vein, the intersaphenous vein (Giacomini vein). The deep veins originate in the foot as the continuation of the dorsalis pedis vein (anterior tibial) and from the plantar aspect as the continuation of the deep venous plantar arch in the form of the lateral and medial plantar veins and then the posterior tibial veins. Continuation in the leg and the thigh is through accompaniment of corresponding arteries. There is often duplication of the deep veins, especially in the calf where the posterior tibial, anterior tibial, and peroneal veins accompany the corresponding artery as venae comitantes.[12] The incidence of duplication of the femoral vein, popliteal vein, common femoral, or the iliac veins is much lower. The profunda femoris vein communicates directly with the popliteal vein in 38% of limbs and communicates via a tributary in a further 48% of limbs.[12] The direct perforator veins can be divided into those of the foot, ankle, calf, and thigh. The foot perforators are grouped into medial, lateral, dorsal, and plantar, but unlike the perforating veins elsewhere the flow is from the deep veins into the superficial veins. The calf has three main group of perforating veins, including medial (paratibial and posterior tibial), lateral, and anterior perforating veins. Although the upper, middle, and lower posterior tibial perforators connect the posterior accessory GSV to the posterior tibial veins, the paratibial perforators connect the GSV to the posterior tibial veins. Four to five paraperoneal perforators typically exist along the lateral calf. In the thigh, the femoral canal perforators connect the GSV with the femoral or cranial popliteal vein approximately 10 to 15 cm proximal to the knee.

The veins in the lower extremities serve the dual purpose of being a conduit to conduct blood back to the heart and also as a reservoir. They are aided in these functions by two aspects unique to the venous system—the presence of unidirectional bicuspid valves in the veins and the calf pump. There is variation in the number and location of valves in the superficial, perforator, and deep venous systems. The GSV typically has at least six valves, with varicosity decreasing this number.[14,15] The most constant valve is usually the one within 2 to 3 cm of the saphenofemoral junction, present in more than 94% of the population.[14] The mean number valves in the SSV is quite variable, 1.8 to 13.[13,16,17] The perforator veins have valves that normally allow blood flow from superficial to the deep systems. The deep system has a valve pattern that decreases in number with cranial progression. The inferior vena cava (IVC) does not have any valves, and the common iliac vein (CIV) valve is seen in only 1.2%.[18] Valves are present in the external iliac vein (EIV; right more often than left) in 27% of veins and in the internal iliac in 10%.[18] The CFV above the SFJ usually has a valve, and there are approximately five valves between the SFJ and the knee joint.[19] The deep veins of the calf typically have valves every 2 cm.[19,20] The mean distance between valves in the GSV has been estimated to be 3.8 ±

BOX 54.1   The CEAP Classification (Basic)

1. Clinical classification

C0	No visible or palpable signs of venous disease
C1	Telangiectases or reticular veins
C2	Varicose veins
C3	Edema
C4a	Pigmentation and/or eczema
C4b	Lipodermatosclerosis and/or atrophie blanche
C5	Healed venous ulcer
C6	Active venous ulcer
S	Symptoms including ache, pain, tightness, skin irritation, heaviness, and muscle cramps, as well as other complaints attributable to venous dysfunction
A	Asymptomatic

2. Etiologic classification

Ec	Congenital
Ep	Primary
Es	Secondary (postthrombotic)
En	No venous etiology identified

3. Anatomic classification

As	Superficial veins
Ap	Perforator veins
Ad	Deep veins
An	No venous location identified

4. Pathophysiologic classification

Pr	Reflux
Po	Obstruction
Pr,o	Reflux and obstruction
Pn	No venous pathophysiology identifiable

Modified from Eklöf B, Rutherford RB, Bergan JJ, et al. Revision of the CEAP classification for chronic venous disorders: consensus statement. *J Vasc Surg.* 2004;40:1248–1252, used with permission.

0.4 cm and in the femoral vein was 4.6 ± 0.3 cm.[21] This study found that the valve cusps were at a minimum angle of 60% to one another and that the angle between the valves correlated with the distance between the valves. However, no relation was noted between the diameter of the normal vein and the angle between the valves.[21] Four stages of valve function have been defined—opening, equilibrium, closing, and closed.[22] Although it was originally believed that valve closure was related to the reversal of flow, contemporary thinking is that it is due to the vortex generated by the part of the flow that goes into the valve sinus. This vortex, while keeping the valve leaflets away from the vein wall, forces the closure of the valve by virtue of pressure exerted once the flow through the valve itself slows.[23]

The calf pump or peripheral heart is akin to a peripheral pump whose role is to store and subsequently "pump" blood back into the central circulation through muscle contraction that occurs with lower extremity activity. This pump is composed of venous sinusoids that constitute the reservoir of the pump embedded in skeletal muscle which provided the contractile effect. These sinusoids lie within the gastrocnemius and soleus muscles, with those in the latter being more developed. The inflow for the sinusoids is the superficial veins, reticular veins, and from the muscle itself via muscular veins and postcapillary venules. The outflow for the soleal sinusoids is constituted by the posterior tibial and peroneal veins via indirect perforators, while that for the gastrocnemius sinusoids is the popliteal vein via the gastrocnemius veins. Although thigh and foot pumps also exist, they play a

secondary role to the calf pump.[24] Valves exist in the network of veins that constitute the inflow and outflow but are absent in the sinusoids themselves. The presence of proximal deep venous obstruction or reflux from incompetent valves can lead to calf pump dysfunction and manifestation of CVI.

ETIOLOGY

The CEAP classification defines etiology in chronic venous disorders as being congenital, primary, or secondary. Congenital etiology primarily involves venous and arteriovenous (AV) malformations and, to a very limited extent, iliac vein compression because some cases of such compression occur at embryological fusion sites. Congenital absence or anomalies of veins or venous valves and persistent embryonic veins also belong to this group. Primary etiology refers to degenerative changes in the vein wall and valves leading to reflux and varicosity. Most patients with nonthrombotic iliac vein lesions have primary etiology. Secondary refers to an acquired origin could be due to a variety of causes, including postthrombotic changes, extrinsic compression of the deep veins from fibrosis or tumor, and iatrogenic from placement of IVC filters. Of these the postthrombotic changes are the predominant secondary etiology. Although Bauer noted that most of the advanced cases of CVI were due to primary etiology,[25] more recent data from increasing use of duplex ultrasound (DUS) and intravascular ultrasound (IVUS) support PTS as the most common etiology for CVI.[26]

PATHOPHYSIOLOGY

The primary driver for CVI is reflux involving the superficial and/or deep veins, obstruction involving the deep veins, or a combination of the same. The common pathway that leads to clinical manifestations is venous hypertension.

Venous reflux can arise as discussed previously by failure of valves either from primary or secondary etiology. In the superficial veins, such reflux can arise by primary degeneration of the vein valve leaflets, dilation of the vein wall, or secondary etiology, including superficial thrombophlebitis, trauma, or hormonal effects. Primary etiology has been found to be responsible for 11% to 75% of deep venous reflux (DVR).[27–30] Primary DVR arises due to stretching/elongation of the valve cusps or dilation of the affected venous segment.[27] A developmental etiology has also been recognized due to symptoms predating the age of actual presentation, often as early as teenage years.[31] Trauma has also been presented as a cause. Degeneration of the fibroelastic tissue of the valve that gradually develops over time is deemed the most plausible cause in a majority of patients.[31] Secondary DVR usually results from DVT. With regard to progression of DVR, it has been postulated that an initial incompetent valve high in the femoral vein creates an excess stress on the valve below and leads to it becoming incompetent. For clinical manifestations, the reflux must involve multiple venous segments in the thigh and calf (axial reflux) as opposed to segmental reflux. A functioning, competent popliteal valve has been considered a barrier to development of severe symptoms, even in the presence of reflux involving the entire femoral vein because it protects the calf pump from the deleterious effect of reflux.[32,33] This is particularly true for patients with venous ulcer (C6 disease) in whom Danielsson et al. noted axial distribution of reflux in a majority of patients (79%). In their series, no patient had isolated DVR below the knee with primary etiology as the predominant cause.[34] However, the role of the competent popliteal valve is still debated. More recent work by Neglen et al. has shown the popliteal valve not to be an important determinant of venous hemodynamics or clinical severity by itself. The authors note that reflux in additional segments must also be considered.[35] Secondary DVR

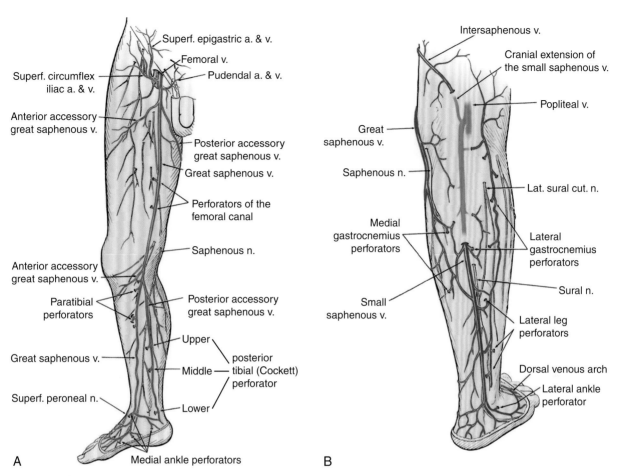

Fig. 54.1 (A) Medial superficial and perforating veins of the lower limb. (B) Posterior superficial and perforating veins of the leg. (Used with permission of Mayo Foundation for Medical Education and Research.)

resulting from DVT often involves not only the thrombosed segment but also the adjacent segment(s). As Caps et al. have pointed out, permanent valvular damage can occur even in the absence of thrombosis of the deep venous segment. Although the precise mechanism has not been identified, release of inflammatory mediators and localized vein dilation have been proposed as potential contributing factors.[36] The most frequent pathophysiology in secondary DVR is direct damage to the vein valve cusps by the thrombus. Dysfunction of the valves of the deep veins has been shown to increase the rate of progression of venous disease with a higher rate of ulcer formation. Failure of the valves can also occur in the perforator system with resultant blood flow from deep to the superficial system. The resultant impact on the latter is dilation and secondary failure of the vein valves. Reflux may also occur in the venous tributaries without concomitant reflux in the superficial/deep or perforator system, leading to localized symptoms. Clinical severity increases with an increase in DVR (higher CEAP clinical class correlates with worsening axial reflux).[37] This has been supported by other studies.[38,39] The prevalence of both superficial and deep reflux is very common in patients with venous ulceration. In 264 patients with venous ulceration the anatomic distribution of reflux was noted as follows: deep reflux (71%), superficial reflux (57%), and perforator reflux (17%).[40] This relative distribution varies according to the practice setting. In one series, up to 80% had superficial reflux alone or in combination with perforator and/or deep insufficiency.[41] Occurrence of reflux in more than one venous compartment is extremely common, occurring in up to two-thirds of patients with healed or active ulceration.[40,41] Isolated perforator insufficiency is extremely rare as a basis

of venous leg ulcers because most are associated with reflux in other territories.[38]

Obstruction of the deep veins leads to limitation of limb blood outflow leading to development of elevated venous pressure in addition to calf pump dysfunction. The etiology of such obstruction can be primary due to extrinsic compression (e.g., nonocclusive iliac vein lesions, such as May-Thurner syndrome [MTS]) or secondary due to extrinsic compression (retroperitoneal fibrosis, pelvic masses or tumors) or intrinsic, such as PTS. With increasing use of IVUS the increasing incidence of PTS in causing venous obstruction has come to the fore. Also important is the presence of combined venous obstruction and reflux. Coexistence of deep venous obstruction with DVR reinforces the pathology with earlier occurrence of symptoms than would be the case if obstruction did not exist. Most postthrombotic reflux is associated with obstruction.[42] Furthermore, the prevalence of having combined reflux and obstruction significantly increases in patients with skin changes constituting CEAP clinical class 4, 5, and 6 disease when compared with those without skin damage.[41] In one study of patients with venous leg ulcers, only 1% was found to be due to obstruction alone without reflux.[43]

Although calf pump dysfunction can occur due to primary causes such as muscular or neuromuscular disorders, it is more commonly due to severe reflux or obstruction. The overwhelming of the calf pump renders it less efficient in the process, leading to venous hypertension and sequelae thereof. Calf pump dysfunction appears to be a noteworthy mechanism responsible for development of more advanced stages of clinical disease, including venous ulcers.[44,45]

The final pathway for reflux, obstruction, and/or calf pump dysfunction to exert its impact is through venous hypertension. The hemodynamic changes resulting from changes in the macrovenous milieu reflect on to the microcirculation, leading to a constellation of findings collectively termed venous microangiopathy.[46] Activation of inflammatory pathways and dysfunction of microvenous valves can also contribute to the development of such microangiopathy (elongation, dilation and tortuosity of capillary beds, endothelial damage, and thickening of basement membrane).[47–49] Although the precise mechanism is not known for the development of venous microangiopathy, white blood cell and growth factor trapping, in addition to fibrin cuff formation, have been hypothesized as potential mechanisms.[46]

DIAGNOSIS

The history should focus on establishing the etiology—congenital versus primary versus secondary or a combination thereof—by focusing on personal or family history of venous thromboembolic episodes (VTEs) or thrombophilia, medication history (hormone replacement therapy, oral contraceptive pills, or use of testosterone), obstetric history, and smoking. Risk factors for CVI include age, positive family history, and obesity.[50] Examination should always be performed with the patient in the standing position in a warm room with good light and should establish the size, location, and distribution of varicose veins and also focus on other signs of venous disease such as edema (partially pitting or nonpitting), skin changes (induration, pigmentation, lipodermatosclerosis, atrophie blanche, eczema, dermatitis, skin discoloration, increased skin temperature), and ulceration (healed or active). Inspection and palpation are essential parts of the examination, and auscultation (bruit) is particularly helpful in those with vascular malformation and AV fistula.[51] Varicose dilations or venous aneurysms, palpable cord in the vein, tenderness, thrill, bruit, or pulsatility should be recorded. Ankle mobility should also be examined because patients with advanced venous disease frequently have decreased mobility in the ankle joints. Sensory and motor functions of the limb and foot are assessed to help differentiate from diabetic neuropathy or any underlying neurologic problem. An abdominal mass or lymphadenopathy can provide a clue to venous compression and outflow obstruction. Corona phlebectatica (ankle flare or malleolar flare) is a fan-shaped pattern of small intradermal veins located around the ankle or the dorsum of the foot.[11] This is considered to be an early sign of advanced venous disease. Inspection of the abdominal wall and perineal and inguinal region should be routinely performed. Perineal, vulvar, or groin varicosities can be seen in iliac vein obstruction or internal iliac vein or gonadal vein incompetence causing pelvic congestion syndrome (PCS). Scrotal varicosity may be a sign of gonadal vein incompetence, left renal vein compression between the superior mesenteric artery and the aorta (Nutcracker syndrome), or occasionally even IVC lesions or renal carcinoma. Skin lesions, other than those listed previously, such as capillary malformations, tumors, onychomycosis, or excoriations, should be noted. An aneurysmal saphenous vein can be misdiagnosed as a femoral hernia or vice versa. The presence of a longer limb, lateral varicosity noted soon after birth, and associated capillary malformations are tip-offs for congenital venous-lymphatic malformation (Klippel-Trénaunay syndrome).[52] A complete pulse examination is performed to exclude underlying peripheral artery disease. The physical examination can be complemented by a handheld Doppler ultrasound examination, although the latter does not replace evaluation of the venous circulation with color duplex scanning. The aim of the clinical evaluation is not only to determine the presenting signs and symptoms and the type of venous disease (primary, secondary, congenital) but also to exclude other etiologies (peripheral artery disease, rheumatoid disease,

infection, tumor, or allergies). The physician should also establish the degree of disability caused by the venous disease and its impact on the patient's QOL. The American Venous Forum recommends using the revised Venous Clinical Severity Score (VCSS)[53] to grade and document the presenting symptoms of patients with CVD (Table 54.1).

Clinical Features

Patients with CVI can present with a variety of symptoms and signs. Such manifestations can overlap for PTS and nonthrombotic iliac vein lesions including MTS. In fact, MTS can be identified in 18% to 49% of patients presenting with left lower limb DVT.[54] MTS can affect any age group. It is more commonly seen in women and usually involves the left side. Another aspect previously noted is the worsened clinical manifestation in patients with combined deep venous obstruction and reflux. Patients may present with one or more of the following—limb swelling; pain; venous claudication (pelvic, thigh, or hip pain that develops after exercise); venous varicosities; hyperpigmentation; skin and subcutaneous inflammatory changes (eczema, lipodermatosclerosis, induration, and venous ulcerations). One review noted swelling followed by venous claudication as the most common symptoms at presentation in patients undergoing intervention for nonmalignant obstruction of the iliocaval system.[55] This study also observed the incidence of active ulcers as approximately 19%.[55]

Limb Swelling

DVR and obstruction can both cause limb swelling, although swelling from reflux is usually less severe and more intermittent than that caused by obstruction. Such limb swelling in the presence of skin damage can lead to recurrent bouts of cellulitis, which is not uncommon in patients presenting with massive limb edema. Patients presenting with limb swelling that is more diffuse than just overlying varicose veins should undergo careful interrogation for deep venous obstruction/reflux.[56,57]

Pain

Patients with CVI can experience pain that is focal in nature involving the thigh, calf, or shin, or be more diffuse involving the entire extremity. Such pain can be of varying quality—achiness, heaviness, shooting, or bursting. Relief from such pain is usually by measures which reduce limb venous pressure, including elevation and ambulation. It is also possible for CVI patients with deep venous obstruction to experience venous claudication, pain that arises with exercise. Arterial pathology can be ruled out in such patients with pulse exam and exercise ankle-brachial index. Hyperesthesia can also be the presenting symptom at times. Atypical pain that occurs when a patient is recumbent and relieved with ambulation is also seen. Another condition is venous hypertension syndrome where patients complain of severe pain in an otherwise normal-appearing limb and is seen in approximately 10% of patients. Iliac vein obstruction usually presents with pain out of proportion to signs.

Skin Changes

Hyperpigmentation and lipodermatosclerosis include skin manifestations in patients presenting with CVI. They represent the final end points of venous hypertension that leads to skin damage. Obstructive venous pathology or combined obstruction/reflux is generally more responsible for this as opposed to isolated DVR. Reflux leading to such skin changes can occur with substantial reflux that requires either axial DVR or a refluxing large-caliber saphenous vein (usually >10 mm). The prevalence of having combined reflux and obstruction significantly increases in patients with skin changes constituting CEAP clinical class 4, 5, and 6 disease when compared with those with a lack of substantial skin damage.[41] In patients with venous leg ulcers, only 1% was found to be due to obstruction alone without reflux.[43]

TABLE 54.1 Revised Venous Clinical Severity Score

Pain	None: 0	Mild: 1	Moderate: 2	Severe: 3
Or other discomfort (i.e., aching, heaviness, fatigue, soreness, burning); presumes venous origin		Occasional pain or other discomfort (i.e., not restricting regular daily activity)	Daily pain or other discomfort (i.e., interfering with but not preventing regular daily activities)	Daily pain or discomfort (i.e., limits most regular daily activities)
Varicose Veins	**None: 0**	**Mild: 1**	**Moderate: 2**	**Severe: 3**
"Varicose" veins must be ≥3 mm in diameter in the standing position to qualify		Few: scattered (i.e., isolated branch varicosities or clusters); also includes corona phlebectatica (ankle flare)	Confined to calf or thigh	Involves calf and thigh
Venous Edema	**None: 0**	**Mild: 1**	**Moderate: 2**	**Severe: 3**
Presumes venous origin		Limited to foot and ankle area	Extends above ankle but below knee	Extends to knee and above
Skin Pigmentation	**None: 0**	**Mild: 1**	**Moderate: 2**	**Severe: 3**
Presumes venous origin; does not include focal pigmentation over varicose veins or pigmentation due to other chronic diseases (i.e., vasculitis purpura)	None or focal	Limited to perimalleolar area	Diffuse over lower third of calf	Wider distribution above lower third of calf
Inflammation	**None: 0**	**Mild: 1**	**Moderate: 2**	**Severe: 3**
More than just recent pigmentation (i.e., erythema, cellulitis, venous eczema, dermatitis)		Limited to perimalleolar area	Diffuse over lower third of calf	Wider distribution above lower third of calf
Induration	**None: 0**	**Mild: 1**	**Moderate: 2**	**Severe: 3**
Presumes venous origin of secondary skin and subcutaneous changes (i.e., chronic edema with fibrosis, hypodermitis); includes white atrophy and lipodermatosclerosis		Limited to perimalleolar area	Diffuse over lower third of calf	Wider distribution above lower third of calf
No. of Active Ulcers	**0**	**1**	**2**	**≥3**
Active ulcer duration (longest active)	N/A	<3 months	>3 months but <1 year	Not healed for >1 year
Active ulcer size (largest active)	N/A	Diameter <2 cm	Diameter 2–6 cm	Diameter >6 cm
Use of Compression Therapy	**None: 0**	**Occasional: 1**	**Frequent: 2**	**Always: 3**
	Not used	Intermittent use of stockings	Wears stockings most days	Full compliance: stockings

Modified from Vasquez MA, Rabe E, McLafferty RB, et al. Revision of the venous clinical severity score: venous outcomes consensus statement: special communication of the American Venous Forum Ad Hoc Outcomes Working Group. *J Vasc Surg.* 2010;52:1387–1396, used with permission.

Restless Legs

Patients with CVI can also have restless legs at night waking them from sleep or causing them to remain awake at night. These can also be a manifestation of CVI, especially obstructive deep venous lesions. Relief of the obstruction leads to respite from the symptom or even complete resolution.

Lymphedema Versus Venous Swelling

Limb swelling due to CVI can mimic that from lymphedema, and such patients can present with humping of dorsum of foot, squaring of toes, and inability to pinch the skin off the second toe (Stemmer sign). Secondary lymphedema from overloading of the lymphatic system from venous obstruction/reflux is more common than previously thought and responds to correction of relevant venous pathology including obstruction. It is essential to evaluate patients presenting with lymphedema for possible venous obstruction/reflux.

Pelvic Congestion Syndrome

PCS denotes a collection of symptoms and signs in women arising from incompetence of the pelvic veins and accounts for up to 20% of outpatient gynecological consultations. Patients with PCS can present with pain (pelvic, lower abdominal, lower back, hip, and/or dyspareunia), urinary frequency, dysmenorrhea, and/or varicose veins of the vulva, perineum, buttocks, and lower extremity, in addition to ovarian point tenderness.

Diagnostic Studies

A variety of studies are used to screen and confirm diagnosis in patients with CVI.

Duplex Ultrasound

Venous DUS is the most commonly used tool given its noninvasive nature and cost effectiveness. DUS can be used to evaluate the superficial, deep, and perforator systems, and ascertain pathology: reflux versus obstruction versus combination. A 5-MHz linear array pulsed wave Doppler transducer is used most frequently for the deeper veins, with the higher-frequency probe (up to 18 MHz) for detailed assessment of the superficial veins. Evaluation of reflux should be performed with the patient in the upright position, with the leg rotated outward, heel on the ground, and weight taken on the opposite limb.[33] The veins below the knee can also be assessed in the sitting position. Using the supine position for reflux gives both false-positive and false-negative results.[38] All deep veins of the leg are evaluated followed by the superficial veins, including the GSV, SSV, accessory saphenous veins, and perforating veins, for a complete examination. The four components that are essential in a complete duplex scanning examination for CVI are visibility, compressibility, venous flow, and augmentation. Asymmetry in flow velocity, lack of respiratory variations in venous flow, and waveform patterns at rest and during flow augmentation in the CFVs indicate proximal obstruction. Reflux in the superficial system is elicited by increased intraabdominal pressure using a Valsalva maneuver followed by manual compression of the calf/foot.[58,59] Reflux in the deep veins of the lower extremity is typically evaluated in the standing position[60] using the cuff deflation technique put forth by van Bemmelen et al.[59] Based on studies by Masuda et al. and Araki et al. the standing cuff deflation technique appears to be a superior method when compared with other techniques, including the Valsalva maneuver.[61,62] Four stages of the venous valve cycle—opening, equilibrium, closing, and closed phases—have been described.[22] The ability of the valve to maintain the closed phase determines occurrence of reflux. Although metrics such as valve closure time/reflux time (VCT/RT) have been postulated and used to grade reflux, these represent more qualitative than quantitative indices. The latter include peak reflux velocity (PRV) and time-averaged flow (TAF), which have demonstrated good correlation with both hemodynamic parameters and clinical severity in multiple studies.[35,63] The most common criteria used for defining reflux is derived from data published by multiple groups,[59,64,65] including Labropoulos et al., and have since been incorporated into the clinical practice guidelines of the Society for Vascular Surgery and the American Venous Forum.[66,67] Per the guidelines, DVR is defined as reflux lasting for 500 ms or more in the deep veins below the knee and the deep femoral vein (DFV) and lasting for 1000 ms or more in the femoral and popliteal veins. For the superficial truncal veins in the lower extremity, reflux is pathologic if it lasts longer than 500 ms. The perforator veins are noted to have pathologic reflux if they have a diameter >3.5 mm and outward flow of >500 ms, located beneath a healed or open venous ulcer. Duplex scanning also ascertains location and extent of the obstructive pathology, besides providing inflow and outflow data. Normal luminal diameter cutoffs used for the CFV, EIV, and CIV are 12, 14, and 16 mm, respectively (Table 54.2). The corresponding areas used for the three segments are 125, 150, and 200 mm^2, respectively. Luminal diameter/areas less than these cutoffs in the symptomatic patient require further investigation in the form of IVUS.

Air Plethysmography

Air plethysmography (APG) is a noninvasive technique of evaluating lower extremity reflux, obstruction, and calf pump function using calf volumetric changes (Fig. 54.2). Other forms of plethysmography have fallen out of favor due to a variety of shortcomings. APG is performed using the technique described by Christopoulos et al. where a tubular bag is placed around the leg of the patient in the supine position.[68] The leg is subsequently elevated to 45 degrees, emptying the veins and allowing the calibration of the device. The patient then stands up quickly, holding onto a frame with the body weight on the contralateral limb. The increase in the calf volume that results is known as the functional venous volume (VV), and the time taken to achieve 90% of this volume is known as the venous filling time (VFT). The venous filling index (VFI), which is a comprehensive measure of reflux, is computed by

dividing 90% of VV by VFT.[68] The subject is then asked to take one tiptoe and with weight on both legs and return to the baseline position. Contraction of the calf muscles during this action ejects venous blood with resultant reduction in calf volume. The volume forced out is the ejection volume (EV), and (EV/VV) × 100 is the ejection fraction. The subject is then asked to perform 10 tiptoes and return to baseline. The calf volume at the end of the 10 tiptoes is the residual volume (RV).[68] The residual volume fraction (RVF) is represented by (RV/VV) × 100. EV, EF, RV, and RVF all represent calf pump metrics. A recent study has suggested a body weight transfer maneuver (subject rocks forward shifting most of his or her weight onto the leading foot and then back again onto the rear foot) as being better than the tiptoe maneuver in evaluating calf pump function given a 40% relative increase in EF.[69] Venous obstruction is evaluated by the venous occlusion method, in which patients are placed in a supine position with the leg elevated to empty the veins. A 14-cm thigh tourniquet is placed close to the groin and inflated to 80 mm Hg with resultant increase in the VV (beyond the original value previously noted). Following attainment of a steady state (arterial inflow equals venous outflow), the thigh tourniquet is deflated rapidly leading to a rapid decrease in calf volume. The amount of venous blood that leaves the leg in the first second is calculated (V1). Outflow fraction (OF) is computed as (V1/VV) × 100. Repetition of the process with digital occlusion of the long saphenous and small saphenous veins at the level of the knee gives the OF with superficial occlusion.[70] Venous outflow resistance (VOR) is another metric that can be used to determine outflow obstruction and is computed by simultaneous recording of the volume and pressure outflow curves. The resistance is estimated by dividing the pressure on the curve by the flow. OF and VOR are plethysmographically calculated measures of outflow obstruction.[70] Kurstjens et al. compared OF, ejection fraction, and RVF as a quantitative metric of outflow obstruction with DUS and magnetic resonance venography (MRV). They found poor correlation between OF, EF, and RVF and presence of deep venous obstruction.[71] The same group in a separate study using receiver operator curves demonstrated that venous occlusion APG could not be used to identify obstruction proximal to the femoral venous confluence or those who would benefit from femoroiliocaval stenting.[72] Lattimer et al. have put forth venous drainage index (VDI) as a metric for quantitative assessment of venous obstruction based on the inverse relation between the rate of reduction of calf volume on leg elevation with the degree of proximal venous obstruction.[73] Further study is required to elucidate the usefulness of this metric.

Peripheral Venous Pressure

Ambulatory venous pressure (AMVP), dorsal foot venous pressure (DFVP) with and without hyperemia, hand-foot pressure differential, and deep venous pressure (femoral/common femoral venous) are some of the metrics that have been used as diagnose venous hypertension. The normal supine peripheral venous pressure is 11 mm Hg or less. AMVP is measured by cannulation of the dorsal foot vein connected to a transducer with pressure noted at baseline and after 15 toe stands.[68] The accuracy with which the AMVP reflects the deep venous pressure has been questioned. Neglen and Raju in a study that had patients with only superficial reflux at baseline without any deep venous obstruction or reflux noted that AMVP is not always accurate in detecting changes in pressure in the tibial and popliteal veins. They also observed that deep venous pressure might be increased or decreased while the AMVP is normal.[74] Kurstjens et al. observed that the pressure in the CFV and not the DFVP was what was able to identify significant venous outflow obstruction.[75] The group also noted during a treadmill study on PTS patients that CFV pressure increased significantly with ambulation in patients with iliofemoral PTS compared with the unaffected control

TABLE 54.2 Optimal Diameters and Luminal Areas for the Femoroiliocaval Segment		
Vein	Luminal Area (mm^2)	Diameter (mm)
CFV	125	12
EIV	150	14
CIV	200	16

CFV, Common femoral vein; *CIV*, common iliac vein; *EIV*, external iliac vein.

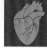

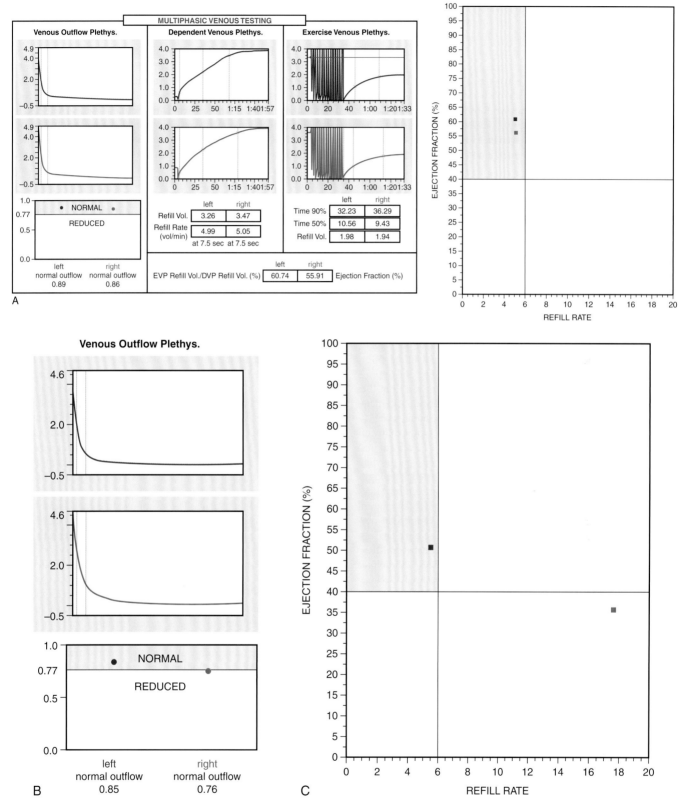

Fig. 54.2 (A–C) Plethysmography images.

limb. The authors came to the conclusion that change in CFV pressure after walking yielded the best discrimination between affected and normal limbs (area under the receiver operated characteristic curve of 0.94 [95% confidence interval [CI], 0.85 to 1.00], compared with 0.57 [95% CI, 0.37 to 0.76] in the dorsal foot vein, *P* < .001).[76]

These observations are reflective of the possibility that CFV pressure is a better index of venous hypertension than the DFVP and that the pressure changes in the superficial system are not reflective of the deep system. Another metric that has been considered for obstruction is the pressure difference between the femoral vein and the vena cava.

In this regard a resting pressure differential of 5 mm Hg or greater, or a lower pressure at rest but increasing to 10 mm Hg (or twofold) after exercise (10 dorsiflexions of the ankle or 20 isometric contractions of the calf muscle) are considered evidence for significant obstruction. Neglen and Raju noted the arm-foot pressure differential combined with pressure elevation with reactive hyperemia to be a reliable test for detecting and grading global chronic obstruction (normal arm-foot pressure differential <4 mm Hg; normal foot venous pressure elevation to reactive hyperemia <6 mm Hg).[77] However, caution should be exercised when using such indices given that when compared with the "gold standard," IVUS, all the aforementioned pressure metrics have concordance of less than 60%.

Cross-sectional Imaging

Studies such as computed tomographic venography (CTV), magnetic resonance (MR) time-of-flight imaging, and MRV help to recognize venous obstruction in addition to identifying etiology of same (obstructing mass, tumor, fibrosis etc.). Such cross-sectional imaging also provides information about venous anatomy, collateral circulation, and nature of obstruction—stenosis or occlusion. Although such imaging has advantages over on-table venography in being less invasive and providing more information about the femoroiliocaval lesions, validation of such imaging against the gold standard IVUS is not yet available. For the CTV, as Arnoldussen et al. have noted, the biggest challenge is sufficient and homogeneous opacification of all the lower extremity veins.[78] Using weight-based dosing of contrast and appropriate rate of injection with delay (110-second delay to scan from the symphysis to the diaphragm) helps to overcome this issue. Alternate protocols have been suggested by Szapiro et al. and Chung et al.[79,80] Several studies have demonstrated the feasibility and reproducibility of MRV using a variety of different imaging protocols.[81–83] Such studies had demonstrated that MR imaging (MRI) of the veins can provide accurate visualization of the venous anatomy and associated pathology. In a study comparing obstruction and collateralization seen on MRV with variables of venous occlusion plethysmography in PTS, Blomgren et al. scored and analyzed 28 patients (33 legs) and found that obstruction of the IVC correlated with an overall increase of collaterals ($P < .001$). The authors found only modest correlation between MRV scores and venous occlusion plethysmography variables.[84] Rudolphi et al. evaluated whether sonographically (DUS) measured vascular hemodynamic parameters were reproducible using MRI basing their study on the finding that the ratio of venous to arterial volume flow in the common femoral vessels, the venous-arterial flow index (VAFI), is increased in patients with varicose veins and/or CVD.[85] The authors noted the existence of a significant correlation between VAFI's measured using sonography and MRI.[85] Although both CTV and MRV can give a precise assessment of nature and etiology of compressive pathology and can aid in operative planning, they are not without drawbacks. Although there is radiation exposure and risk of contrast nephropathy from CTV, the MRV's drawbacks include time required, potential for claustrophobia, and risk of nephrogenic systemic sclerosis in patients with impaired renal dysfunction. Like peripheral venous pressure, cross-sectional imaging modalities have also not been validated against IVUS or against standard clinical scoring systems such as VCSS, Villalta-Prandoni, or the CEAP score. This represents an area requiring further work.

Venogram

Historically, venography, both ascending and descending, were the mainstay of work-up of patients presenting with symptoms of CVI. Ascending venography (AV) is done by cannulation of the dorsal vein of the foot to assess the lower extremity venous outflow and a transfemoral approach to assess the femoroiliocaval system. AV helps to define sites of obstruction, delineates collateral venous circulation, and identifies patterns of preferential flow. Descending venography is performed by placement of an end hole catheter at the level of the upper border of the femoral head and performing the venogram with the patient in a semi-upright (60-degree tilt with feet down) position to evaluate reflux. This allows for evaluation of reflux in the saphenous and deep system and subsequent grading.[86] The current role of descending phlebography in assessing reflux is deemed only of historical importance, with duplex technology having currently supplanted it.[87,88] For ascending venography, it is important to note that because compression can be in the coronal or sagittal plane, multiplanar views are required to recognize compressive lesions. A recent prospective study evaluated the diagnostic efficacy of IVUS with multiplanar venography for iliofemoral vein obstruction and found that, although venography identified stenotic lesions in 51 of 100 subjects, IVUS identified lesions in 81 of 100 subjects.[89] Gagne et al. noted that compared with IVUS, the diameter reduction was on average 11% less for venography ($P < .001$). IVUS identified significant lesions not detected with three-view venography in 26.3% of patients. There was a change in the treatment plan in 57 patients on the basis of the IVUS findings.[89] In a follow-up analysis of the same study, the authors found that for PTS patients, IVUS measurement of area stenosis was most predictive (area under the curve, 0.70; $P = .004$) of clinical improvement as opposed to venographic measurements of baseline stenosis and stenotic change which were not predictive of later improvement.[90] For patients with nonthrombotic iliac vein lesions, IVUS diameter rather than area measurements of baseline stenosis was a more significant predictive of clinical success.[90] However, this study did not include C3 (edema) patients, so how such metrics will hold up in this group is not known. In another study, Murphy et al. compared IVUS and venogram (154 patients) in their ability to identify: location of iliocaval confluence; location/degree of maximal CFV, EIV, and CIV stenosis; and location of distal landing zone.[91] Existence of a lesion was missed by venography in 25% ($n = 40$) of patients. The location of maximal disease (CIV, EIV, CFV) identified by venography was correct in only 52 (33%). There was significant variation in maximum degree of stenosis, with a mean difference of 28.8% between venogram and IVUS ($P < .001$). Venogram underestimated the degree of stenosis in 68.8% of patients.[91]

Intravascular Ultrasound

The gold standard for diagnosis of obstructive femoroiliocaval lesions is IVUS. Accurate diagnosis, disease characterization, and intraoperative treatment guidance (determining proximal and distal landing zones, stent sizing, confirming stent apposition and treatment adequacy) all require IVUS. In addition, it plays a critical role in follow-up of patients presenting with recurrent symptoms. The device typically consists of an 8.2-Fr, 10-MHz transducer (Volcano, San Diego, CA). Planimetric evaluation of the luminal areas of the CFV, EIV and CIV are made; 125, 150, and 200 mm^2 are used as normal luminal area cutoffs corresponding to 12, 14, and 16 mm as normal luminal diameters in the CFV, EIV and CIV, respectively (see Table 54.2). Any decrease in a symptomatic patient is considered abnormal, meriting angioplasty and stenting with stent sizing dictated by such findings. The aforementioned luminal diameters/areas were derived by using iliofemoral outflow calibers using duplex in healthy volunteers and IVUS data from 345 CVD limbs.[92] Raju et al. postulated that values at the right tail end of the curve should approach normal vein caliber values according to distribution theory. In addition, concordance was sought using alternate metrics, including the Poiseuille equation and Young scaling rule.[92] Patients who undergo femoroiliocaval stenting for obstructive pathology can redevelop symptoms suggestive of stent malfunction.

Such patients should undergo IVUS interrogation of the stented areas and treatment pursued depending on findings—angioplasty alone or with stent extension.

Laboratory Evaluation

Selective patients, based on their history, with recurrent DVT, thrombosis at a young age, or thrombosis in an unusual site, should undergo screening for thrombophilia.[93] Laboratory examination is also needed in patients with long-standing recalcitrant venous ulcers, because a small percentage of these patients could have an underlying secondary etiology, including neoplasia or chronic inflammation.[94] Patients who undergo general anesthesia for treatment of CVI should undergo appropriate testing to assess suitability for such procedures.

TREATMENT

Severity of Venous Disease

The aforementioned diagnostic evaluation should provide adequate information to quantify and classify the severity of venous disease, using CEAP clinical class and VCSS.[11,53] The revised VCSS instrument helps determine disease severity at baseline in addition to quantifying improvement/deterioration at follow-up. In the basic CEAP classification only the highest score is used to denote the clinical class and only the main anatomic groups (s, p, d) are noted.

The revised format of the classification[11] includes two elements in addition to the C-E-A-P findings: the date of the examination and the diagnostic level of the evaluation:
Level 1: History, physical, Doppler examination (handheld)
Level 2: Noninvasive—duplex scan, plethysmography
Level 3: Invasive—venography, venous pressure, IVUS, CTV, MRV

Recording the date and method used to confirm the clinical impression can be added in parentheses after the CEAP recording. The main purpose of using the CEAP classification in patients with varicose veins is to distinguish primary venous disease causing simple varicose veins from secondary, postthrombotic venous insufficiency.[95]

Evaluation and treatment of the two conditions are distinctly different. Complete CEAP classification and QOL evaluation is recommended before and after treatment to help to assess the patient's perception of the burden of the disease for research purposes. A general QOL instrument such as the SF-36 and one of the disease-specific QOL instruments (e.g., VEINES, CIVIQ 2, Aberdeen, Charing Cross) should both be used.[96–99]

Treatment of Chronic Venous Insufficiency

Treatment of CVI requires a multimodality approach and has role for both medical and interventional therapy. A concise flowchart for surgical/interventional treatment decision-making is presented in Fig. 54.3.

Drug Treatment

Multiple phlebotonic drugs have been available and used for treatment of symptoms of CVD, and they have also been used to decrease ankle swelling and accelerate ulcer healing. Many compounds have been tried with varying success, but the most promising drugs include gamma-benzopyrones (flavonoids) such as rutoside, diosmin, and hesperidin, the micronized purified flavonoid fraction (MPFF), saponins such as the horse chestnut seed extract (aescin), pentoxifylline, and other plant extracts such as French maritime pine bark extract and synthetic products include calcium dobesilate, naftazone, aminophtone, and chromocarb.[100]

A precise mechanism of action of most of these drugs is unknown and they are postulated to improve venous tone and capillary permeability. Flavonoids appear to affect leukocytes and the endothelium by modifying the degree of inflammation and reducing edema.[101] Two different Cochrane reviews found that flavonoids[102] and aescin[103] appeared to have an effect on edema and on restless leg syndrome but these meta-analyses concluded that there is insufficient evidence to support the global use of phlebotonics in the treatment of CVD.

Recent randomized controlled trials (RCTs) for pentoxifylline have showed some benefit in venous ulcer healing although all three trials failed to show any statistically significant benefit.[104–106]

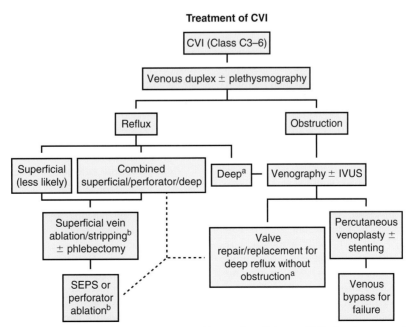

Fig. 54.3 Evaluation and Management of Chronic Venous Insufficiency *(CVI)*. Good compression therapy, although not listed, is a must in any treatment protocol. [a]Essential to rule out occult underlying obstruction. [b]Dotted lines: in select cases only. *IVUS,* Intravascular ultrasound; *SEPS,* Subfascial Endoscopic Perforator Surgery.

The venous guidelines of the American College of Chest Physicians (ACCP) suggest use of oral pentoxifylline (400 mg three times daily) in patients with venous ulcers in addition to local care, compression garment, or intermittent compression pump (ICP) (grade 2B).[107] A meta-analysis of five RCTs that included 723 patients with venous ulcers found that at 6 months the chance of healing ulcer was 32% better in patients treated with adjunctive MPFF than in those managed by conventional therapy alone (relative risk reduction, 32%; 95% CI, 3% to 70%).[108] For patients with persistent venous ulcers, flavonoids in the form of MPFF given orally or sulodexide administered intramuscularly and then orally are suggested in the guidelines of the ACCP (grade 2B).[107]

Compression Therapy

Compression therapy remains the standard of care for patients with advanced CVD and venous ulcers (class C3 to C6). Compression is recommended to decrease ambulatory venous hypertension in patients with CVD, in addition to lifestyle modifications that include weight loss, exercise, and elevation of the legs whenever possible. Ambulatory compression techniques and devices include elastic compression stockings, paste gauze boots (Unna boot), multilayer elastic wraps, dressings, and elastic and nonelastic bandages and nonelastic garments. Pneumatic compression devices (e.g., ICP), applied primarily at night, are also used in patients with refractory edema and venous ulcers.[109] The rationale of compression treatment is to compensate for the increased ambulatory venous hypertension. Pressures to compress the superficial veins in supine patients range from 20 to 25 mm Hg, whereas in the upright position, pressures approximately 35 to 40 mm Hg have been shown to narrow the superficial veins, and pressures higher than 60 mm Hg are needed to occlude them.[110]

Compression therapy improves calf muscle pump function and decreases reflux in vein segments in patients with CVI.[111,112] Although graded compression is effective as the primary treatment to aid healing of venous ulceration and as adjuvant therapy to interventions to prevent recurrence of venous ulcers, compliance is important.[113] In this study, ulcer healing was 97% in compliant patients and 55% in noncompliant patients ($P < .0001$); recurrence was 16% in compliant patients and 100% in noncompliant patients.[113]

Systematic reviews on compression treatment for venous ulcers concluded that compression treatment improves the healing of ulcers compared with no compression and that high compression is more effective than low compression.[114–116] A recent meta-analysis examined data of 692 ulcer patients in eight RCTs and found that ulcer healing was faster with an average of 3 weeks with stockings than with bandages ($P = .0002$) with significantly less pain ($P < .0001$).[117] There is no evidence that hydrocolloid or other dressing beneath compression is more effective than compression alone.[118] The ESCHAR trial randomized 500 patients with leg ulcers to either compression treatment alone or compression in combination with superficial venous surgery.[119,120] Compression consisted of multilayer compression bandaging followed by class 2 (medium compression, 18 to 24 mm Hg) below-knee stockings. Compression treatment alone was as effective as compression with surgery for ulcer healing (65% vs. 65%; hazard ratio, 0.84 [95% CI, 0.77 to 1.24]), but 12-month ulcer recurrence rates were reduced in the compression with surgery group versus those with compression alone (12% vs. 28%; hazard ratio, −2.76 [95% CI, −1.78 to −4.27]). This difference in ulcer recurrence rates persisted between the two groups at 4 years.[121] Unfortunately, this trial did not have a surgery-only arm, because evidence suggests that saphenous vein disconnection improves venous function and heals venous ulcers even without compression bandaging if the deep veins are normal.[122]

Surgical Treatment

Treatment of Superficial Vein Incompetence

Superficial reflux treatment is the primary treatment modality in patient with CVI. Treatment of superficial reflux leads to decrease in ulcer recurrence as proved in the ESCHAR trial.[119,120] We refer the readers to Chapter 53 for details on technique and results of surgical treatment of superficial venous incompetence.

High ligation, division, and stripping. Surgical stripping of the GSV and/or SSV is performed selectively now with the advent of endovenous ablation techniques. Patients who could benefit from open vein stripping include those with a very superficial primary or accessory saphenous vein, large tortuous or aneurysmal saphenous veins, and partially recanalized veins which cannot be cannulated using the ablation probe or injected using ultrasound guidance. Preservation of GSV using CHIVA[123] or ASVAL[124] techniques have limited data for CVI patients and are used selectively in few centers.

Phlebectomy. Ambulatory phlebectomy or powered phlebectomy can be used to eliminate large venous tributaries.[125,126] These are important adjuncts to treatment of superficial and/or perforator incompetence and can be safely performed even in patients with CVI.

Treatment of Perforator Vein Incompetence

An association between incompetent perforating veins and venous ulcers was established more than a century ago by Gay,[127] and surgical perforator interruption was recommended to treat venous ulcers by multiple authors in the past.[128–131] The importance of incompetent perforators in CVI is supported by the observation that most skin changes and ulcers are seen in the gaiter area, where large incompetent medial perforating veins are located. A correlation between number and size of duplex-based incompetent perforating veins and severity of CVI has been demonstrated.[39] Still, the contribution of perforator incompetence to CVI changes is debated.

Perforator interruption is reserved for patients with advanced CVI and documented perforator reflux on duplex (suing established criteria as outlined previously) after superficial reflux has been successfully corrected or in those with no or limited superficial reflux. In many cases, superficial reflux correction would lead to resolution of perforator vein incompetence,[119,132] although one study showed conflicting results.[133] Contraindications to perforator interruption include moderate to severe arterial occlusive disease, infected ulcer, or medically unfit or nonambulatory patient. Relative contraindications include diabetes, renal/liver failure, morbid obesity, autoimmune disorders, recent DVT, and severe lymphedema. Popliteal or proximal deep venous obstruction is also a relative contraindication. A brief description of anatomy of perforator veins is described in the preceding section and illustrated in Fig. 54.1, and details can be found in the article by Mozes et al.[134] All identified incompetent perforators are marked on the skin with a nonerasable marker during preoperative duplex.

Open perforator interruption. Linton's original open subfascial ligation[128] was abandoned because of wound complication rates of up to 24%.[135,136] Many modifications were proposed to this technique, and currently the only potential role for open perforator ligation is in the lateral fascial compartment due to limited space in this compartment. Open perforator ligation using duplex guidance and small incisions may limit the extent of surgery. An RCT observed a significantly higher rate of wound complications after open perforator ligation, using a modified Linton procedure, than after endoscopic perforator ligation (53% vs. 0%; $P < .001$).[137]

Subfascial endoscopic perforator surgery (SEPS). Hauer's[138] technique of SEPS, introduced in 1985, uses a single port and is practiced mostly in Europe. O'Donnell[139] was the first to use laparoscopic instrumentation with a two-port technique, and the Mayo Clinic team[140] and Conrad[141] improved the technique and added carbon dioxide insufflation to the procedure. Between 1992 and 2008, SEPS became the technique of choice for perforator ablation, primarily because of the reduced rate of wound complications.[137,142] SEPS is performed under general or epidural anesthesia. Either the single or double endoscopic port techniques can be used for dissection and division of medial calf perforators. Most authors use balloon dissection and carbon dioxide insufflation with a pressure of 30 mm Hg and a pneumatic thigh tourniquet, inflated to 300 mm Hg, to avoid any bleeding in the surgical field.[143] Division of the fascia of the deep posterior compartment with a paratibial fasciotomy is required to identify all important medial perforating veins. Occlusion of the perforators can be done with endoscopic clips, although most surgeons use an ultrasonic harmonic scalpel for division and transection of the perforators. The wounds are closed, the tourniquet is deflated, and the extremity is wrapped with an elastic bandage. The operation is an outpatient procedure, and patients are encouraged to ambulate 3 hours after the operation.

The North American SEPS registry[144] reported on results of SEPS performed in 17 US centers on 155 limbs, 85% with class C5 and C6 disease. Ulcer healing at 1 year was 88%, with the median time to ulcer healing of 54 days. Ulcer recurrence was 16% at 1 year and 28% at 2 years. In this registry, there were 27 patients with class C6 disease who underwent SEPS alone; 78% of the ulcers healed and the ulcer healing rate was significantly lower (79%) at 2 years than it was in those who had SEPS and superficial ablation (95%) ($P < .05$). However, the ulcer recurrence rate (35%) in the SEPS-only group at 2 years was not significantly worse than that in patients who underwent SEPS and superficial ablation alone (25%). In a systematic review, Tenbrook et al.[145] reported results of the SEPS procedure performed with or without superficial ablation on 1140 limbs in one RCT and 19 case series. Ulcers in 88% of limbs healed and recurred in 13%, at a mean time of 21 months. Risk factors for nonhealing and recurrence included postoperative incompetent perforating veins, pathophysiologic obstruction, previous DVT, and ulcer diameter greater than 2 cm. The authors concluded that surgical treatment including SEPS, with or without saphenous ablation, is recommended for patients with venous ulcers, but RCTs are needed to discern the contributions of compression therapy, superficial venous surgery, and SEPS in patients with advanced CVI. A recent meta-analysis of SEPS by Luebke and Brunkwall[146] reviewed data of studies published between 1985 and 2008 and concluded that SEPS, used as part of a treatment regimen for severe CVI, benefits most patients in the short term regarding ulcer healing and the prevention of ulcer recurrence but further prospective RCTs are needed to define the long-term benefits of SEPS.

Treatment of Deep Vein Incompetence

The first open venous valve reconstruction was reported by Kistner in 1968.[147,148] Since then, many techniques have been developed and modified to treat deep venous insufficiency. Deep valve reconstruction is reserved for advanced CVI patients who have failed other treatment strategies, including compression therapy. Preoperative assessment includes venography in all patients, primarily to rule out underlying proximal venous obstruction causing secondary valvular reflux, but also to grade the severity of reflux as described previously. No specific strategies exist to quantify reflux at a single valve station. Pathological appearance of valves would vary depending on the underlying cause for incompetence, with both primary and secondary (postthrombotic) deep vein reflux contributing to about half the cases.[149] In primary valve reflux patients, valves grossly have normal texture, with a widened commissure. On the other hand, postthrombotic valves have a fibrosis of the vein wall and valve cusp thickening, trabeculation, and, sometimes, complete destruction of the valve structure. In cases with extensive damage to valve structure, valvuloplasty is not an option and reconstruction is usually carried out using valve or vein transposition. Exposure and preparation of valves is similar for both repair and transfer techniques. An arm is prepped out, to provide access to the axillary/brachial vein in case vein transfer is needed. Usually only one valve is repaired, the first femoral vein valve, despite reflux at multiple stations in the femoral vein. DFV valve is also repaired, in case it is incompetent. Meticulous dissection is carried out to identify the valve attachment lines, which may require subadventitial dissection in some postthrombotic cases. Intact valve lines signify a preserved valve apparatus that can be repaired in most cases, in contrast to absence or disruption of valve attachment lines, when repair is not possible.[149] A strip test is used to confirm valve incompetence.

Valvuloplasty. Can be performed from within (internal, as originally described by Kistner) or from outside (external). The goal for both approaches is to appose the commissure and achieve valve tightening. Obvious advantage of internal valvuloplasty is repair under direct vision, although opening the vein increases the risk of surgical trauma to the vein and valve apparatus. To overcome this disadvantage of external valvuloplasty, we have used angioscopic external valvuloplasty technique, where an angioscope is introduced from a tributary proximal to the repaired valve and helps with visualization during suture placement.[150]

Valve transfer. Can be achieved using two methods—either transfer of a segment of vein with a competent valve and use as interposition graft (usually axillary/brachial vein segment from the arm) or transposition of the incompetent vein onto a competent vein segment (usually femoral vein is transposed to the adjacent GSV or DFV).

Vein transposition. Requires an adjacent patent competent vein, which is not always true in many cases where the GSV has already been ablated/stripped and the DFV is also incompetent. In addition, long-term competence is a concern due to increased chance of reflux with dilatation, as a result of increased flow.[151] Axillary vein transfer is technically demanding, with 40% incidence of incompetent axillary valves in situ and carries additional morbidity of a second incision.

Other less commonly used techniques include prosthetic sleeve reconstruction, de novo valve reconstruction, cryopreserved allograft, and artificial venous valves. None of these techniques have been widely adopted and all previous attempts at artificial or cryopreserved valves were met with failure. A new "neovalve" technique described by Lugli et al.[152] holds promise, but their excellent results at least in the short term have not been duplicated at other centers yet.

Perioperative complications are rare with minimal or no mortality in these cases. The incidence of DVT has been reported to be between 0% and 11%, with higher rates in postthrombotic patients.[27,30] Long-term outcomes of deep vein incompetence have reported 60% to 80% ulcer healing,[149] with better outcomes in primary disease and better outcomes with valvuloplasty compared with valve transfer techniques.[27]

Prevention of postthrombotic superficial/deep vein incompetence could be a key point of intervention in view of limited success with valve reconstruction once the valves are damaged in these patients. It has been shown that duration of venous occlusion clearly affects the likelihood of secondary reflux.[153] Multilevel disease and recurrent thrombosis are the two most predictive factors for future CVI.[154] Early spontaneous lysis may lead to preserved valve function and fewer symptoms.[155] The role of thrombus lysis to prevent venous reflux and postthrombotic syndrome is discussed in Chapter 52. Data suggest that venous obstruction is more important than valvular incompetence. In a study of 504 patients who underwent iliac vein stenting, stenting was sufficient to control symptoms in the majority of patients with combined outflow obstruction and DVR without need to correct underlying reflux.[26]

Treatment of Deep Vein Obstruction

Open surgical reconstructions have been challenging due to multiple factors affecting graft patency,[156] including inadequate graft material, low venous flow, and the frequent thrombophilia in these patients. Endovascular stenting is currently the first-line therapy with excellent mid-term and some long-term results in chronic symptomatic venous stenosis and short occlusions,[157] but stenting is not possible or successful in all patients with long, femoroiliocaval venous occlusions.[158]

Femorofemoral crossover bypass. This can be performed for unilateral iliofemoral obstruction with suprapubic transposition of the GSV (Palma-Dale procedure) (Fig. 54.4). Contralateral GSV is tunneled subcutaneously to the groin incision of the affected limb. End-to-side anastomosis is performed between the saphenous vein and ipsilateral CFV. This anastomosis can be spatulated onto the ipsilateral GSV if the femoral or DFVs are diseased and the GSV is the predominant outflow in the affected leg. An externally supported 10- to 12-mm diameter PTFE graft is used if the GSV is inadequate, less than 5 mm in diameter, or of poor quality. An AV fistula is performed between the conduit and superficial femoral artery in selective cases and is marked with a silastic sheath for easy identification at a later time.

Femoroiliac or iliocaval bypass. The iliac vein is exposed via a flank incision and the femoral vein through a standard groin incision. In cases with CIV occlusion, infrahepatic cava is used as outflow, exposed through a midline incision. These "short" bypasses have a hemodynamic advantage due to the length and high flow. We prefer an externally supported 10- to 14-mm PTFE graft for these bypasses.

Femorocaval or complex bypass. Long bypasses from the femoral vein to the IVC have poor results due to the hemodynamics of flow across the femoral vein. Most of these patients also have extensive postphlebitic changes in the femoral and distal veins, making these procedures technically challenging and prone to failure due to poor inflow. Patients with bilateral disease or those with obstruction of suprarenal or suprahepatic IVC who have failed endovascular intervention are evaluated for a complex reconstruction using either a bifurcated graft or tube graft with contralateral jump graft.

Saphenopopliteal bypass. This is popularly known as the May-Husni procedure and is indicated for femoral or proximal popliteal vein obstruction. The GSV, which most commonly is the major outflow from the leg via collaterals in these patients, is exposed above the knee joint and a direct anastomosis is performed between the GSV and popliteal vein (end to side). Alternatively, a free vein conduit or prosthetic can be used in case the ipsilateral GSV is not suitable.

In a recent report on open surgical reconstruction for chronic iliofemoral occlusion, 50 patients underwent 52 open reconstructive procedures for CVI over a 25-year period[159]; 29 patients underwent a femorofemoral crossover bypass and 17 underwent a short bypass (femoroiliac or iliocaval). Early graft occlusion occurred in 17%, requiring reoperation and discharge patency was 96%. There was no mortality or pulmonary embolism. Five-year primary and secondary patency for Palma vein grafts was 70% and 78%, for femoroiliac and ilioinfrahepatic IVC bypasses it was 63% and 86%, and for femoroinfrahepatic IVC bypasses it was 31% and 57%, respectively. MTS with associated chronic thrombosis, use of prosthetic grafts, and endoscopic vein harvesting were noted to be adversely related to long-term graft patency. More than 60% of the patients had no venous claudication and no or minimal swelling. In multiple large series, the Palma procedure has shown good to excellent patency rates of 70% to 85% on mid- to long-term follow-up.[160]

Endovenous Treatment
Treatment of Superficial Vein Incompetence

Endovenous treatment of superficial vein incompetence using radiofrequency ablation (RFA) or laser (endovenous laser treatment [EVLT]) ablation or foam sclerotherapy has made significant advancement over the past decade and has replaced open surgical treatment in most centers. We again refer the readers to Chapter 53 for details on technique and results of endovenous treatment of superficial venous incompetence.

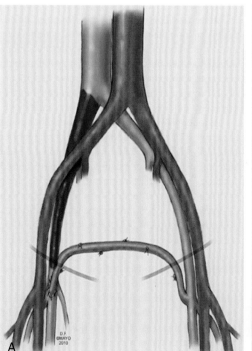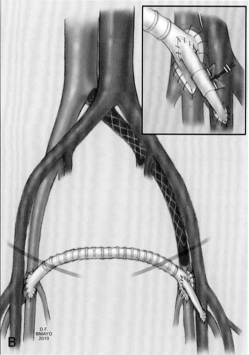

Fig. 54.4 Schematic presentation of femorofemoral crossover venous bypass with either the contralateral great saphenous vein (A) or prosthetic graft (B). An arteriovenous fistula is shown in inset with the marking silastic sheath. (Used with permission of Mayo Foundation for Medical Education and Research.)

Treatment of Perforator Incompetence

The emergence of ultrasonographically guided thermal ablations and sclerotherapy in recent years has transformed the techniques of perforator ablation.[142,161–163] Advantages of percutaneous ablation of perforators (PAPs) include the low risk of a minimally invasive procedure that is easily repeatable and can be performed under local anesthesia in an office setting.[164] PAPs is performed under ultrasound guidance, with direct needle puncture of the perforating vein, performed under local anesthesia, with the patient in the reverse Trendelenburg position to allow for full venous distention. The tip of the needle should be at or just below the fascia in the vein to minimize deep vessel and nerve injury. After confirmation of probe position, local anesthesia is used to infiltrate the surrounding tissues before treatment, and the patient is then placed in the Trendelenburg position.

Radiofrequency ablation. RFA of the perforating veins can be accomplished using a new intravascular ablation device (Closure RFS Stylet, VNUS Medical Technologies, San Jose, California); intraluminal placement of the RF stylet is confirmed by ultrasonography and also by measuring impedance: values between 150 and 350 ohms indicate the intravascular location of the tip of the probe. Treatment is performed with a target temperature of 85°C. All four quadrants of the vein wall are treated for 1 minute each. The catheter is then withdrawn 1 to 2 mm, and a second treatment is performed. The treatment is finished with applying compression to the region of the treated perforating vein.

Perforator endovenous laser treatment. Performed with a 16-gauge angiocatheter (for 600-micrometer laser fiber) or a 21-gauge micro puncture needle (for a 400-micrometer laser fiber) can be used.[165] Intraluminal placement of the access catheter is confirmed by ultrasonography and by aspiration of blood, at or just below the fascial level. Various methods of energy application are used and perforating veins are treated at three locations, each segment receiving between 60 and 120 joules in one to two treatments.[163,165] The rest of the procedure is similar to RFA.

Sclerotherapy. Is done with a 25-, 27-, or 30-gauge needle. A wire may be placed into the deep system for better control of the access. Ultrasonographically guided sclerotherapy can be performed using different agents, and care should be taken to avoid injection of the agent into the accompanying artery. 0.5 to 1 mL of the sclerosant is injected with the leg elevated to avoid flow into the deep system and compression is applied over the treated perforators.[165]

Outcomes in PAPs are largely unknown and most publications have a small number of patients with short follow-up, frequently treated for mild disease (class C2 to C3). Most data provided are on safety and surrogate end points such as perforating vein occlusions but less so on clinical and functional end points. A systematic review of five cohort studies and seven unpublished case series found a mean occlusion rate of 80% and a mean follow-up of less than 2 months.[142] Ultrasonographically guided sclerotherapy is gaining rapid acceptance because perforating veins can be accessed easily with a small needle without much pain to the patient. After ultrasonographically guided sclerotherapy using morrhuate sodium in 80 limbs with predominantly perforator incompetence, significant improvement in VCSS was noted, and ulcers rapidly healed in 86.5%, with a mean time to heal of 36 days.[162] The ulcer recurrence rate was 32% at a mean of 20 months despite low compliance (15%) with compression hose. New and recurrent perforators were identified in 33% of limbs, and ulcer recurrence was statistically associated with perforator recurrence and presence of PTS.

Treatment of Deep Vein Incompetence

Endovascular treatment of deep vein incompetence using stents mounted with native or artificial valves have been frought with failure, and new designs in development are still in infancy, awaiting good clinical data.[166]

Treatment of Deep Vein Obstruction

Deep vein obstruction, either postthrombotic or nonthrombotic, has recently been shown to be a significant contributor to CVD. Due to lack of adequate tests to quantify the exact role of deep vein obstruction, experts currently recommend the routine use of IVUS for detailing venous assessment.[157] In one study, more than one-fourth of patients were shown to have greater than 50% stenosis based on IVUS, whereas venogram failed to reveal any obstruction.[167]

Endovenous stenting. This is performed under local or general anesthesia in an endovascular suite. Access is achieved under ultrasound guidance, either via femoral or jugular vein. After venography and IVUS (as needed), the obstructed segments are crossed using a hydrophilic wire. Predilatation is performed with high-pressure balloons and the risk of rupture is low to none, and chronic occlusive lesions usually require serial dilation to a final diameter of 12 to 18 mm. Self-expanding stents are used in the entire diseased segment with stent sizes tailored according to the segments involved.[92] Wallstent (Boston Scientific, Marlborough, MA) is the typically used stent given extensive experience with the same, with the Gianturco Z stent (Cook Medical, Bloomington, IN) used across the iliocaval confluence to overcome the choke point effect (Fig. 54.5).[168] Newer nitinol stents are currently in trials in the United States. Extension of a stent across the inguinal ligament is less of a concern in the venous segment.[169] Chronic occlusive changes in the iliocaval segment can be stented in a similar manner post recanalization.[158,170,171] An indwelling IVC filter in such cases can either be removed or crushed and stented across.[170,172] Coverage of the renal veins has not been of concern in our experience and of some others.[173]

Hybrid reconstruction. In patients with CFV obstruction and proximal disease, vascular access could be impossible. Endovenous recanalization and stent placement is combined with femoral vein endophlebectomy and patch angioplasty in these cases. Balloon angioplasty and stenting is performed prior to or at completion of the patch angioplasty. Jugular vein access is obtained for retrograde recanalization as an alternative to or in combination with femoral access. The stent is extended proximally to the

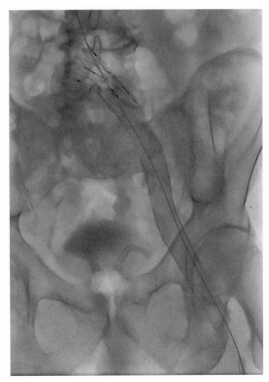

Fig. 54.5 Femoroiliocaval stenting performed using a combination of Wallstent-Gianturco stent for obstructive iliac pathology.

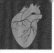

healthy vein and across the inguinal ligament distally. With recent experience, we extend the distal end of the stent into the venous patch.

Technical success for endovascular iliac vein recanalization is reported to be 87% to 100% in multiple series.[174] IVC occlusion does decrease the ability to cross the occluded segment and technical success in these cases was reported to be 66% in one series.[173] Mid-long–term secondary patency is very good in successful cases, ranging from 75% at 48 months to 93% at 36 months.[174] Patients with nonthrombotic

obstruction fare much better than those with thrombotic occlusion.[175] Cumulative rate of improvement of pain and swelling at 5 years after treatment of venous outflow obstruction was 78% and 55%, respectively, and reflux parameters did not deteriorate after stenting in one large study.[26] In a study from Mayo Clinic, we also observed marked improvement in hemodynamics, venous function, and symptoms after successful treatment of venous outflow obstruction with stenting (Fig. 54.6).[176] We noted improvement in both venous outflow (OF) and

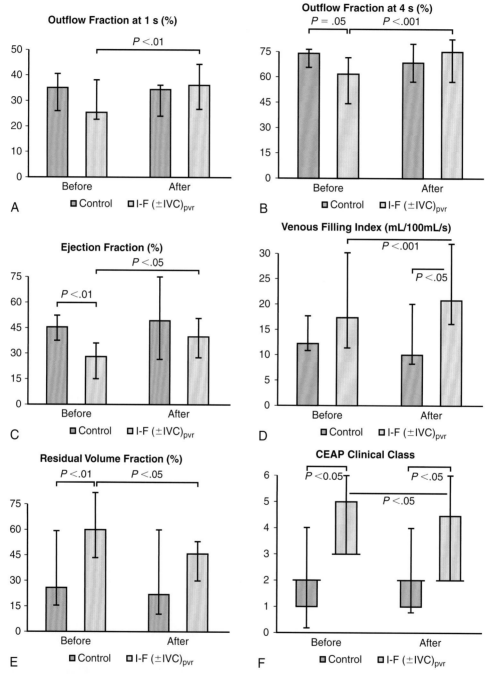

Fig. 54.6 (A–F) The effects of successful treatment of venous outflow obstruction using venous stents. Venous hemodynamics, including venous outflow (outflow fraction at 1 and 4 seconds; A, B), calf muscle pump function (ejection fraction; C), amount of venous reflux (venous filling index; D) and venous hypertension (residual volume fraction; E), and the CEAP clinical class (F) in 23 limbs with chronic iliofemoral (I-F) inferior vena cava (IVC) thrombosis (DVT) and 9 control limbs, before (30 days) and after (median, 8.4; interquartile range, 3–11.8 months) successful I-F (IVC) venous stenting. Data are median and interquartile range. (From Delis KT, Bjarnason H, Wennberg PW, et al. Successful iliac vein and inferior vena cava stenting ameliorates venous claudication and improves venous outflow, calf muscle pump function, and clinical status in post-thrombotic syndrome. *Ann Surg.* 2007;24:130–139.)

calf muscle pump function (EF) ($P < .05$) and the RVF had decreased ($P < .05$), at the expense of venous reflux, which increased (increase of median VFI, by 24%; $P < .05$) in our study. Stenting improved the CEAP class status of the patients ($P < .05$). Incapacitating venous claudication noted in 62.5% of patients before stenting was eliminated in all after stenting ($P < .05$). This study concluded that successful treatment of venous outflow obstruction in patients with CVI ameliorates venous claudication, normalizes outflow, and enhances calf muscle pump function, compounded by a significant clinical improvement of CVD. The significant increase in the amount of venous reflux of the stented limbs indicated that elastic or inelastic compression support of the successfully stented limbs would be pivotal in preventing disease progression.[176] The study also supports the notion that venous obstruction is likely more important than venous valvular incompetence.

Assessment of Treatment Outcome

Clinical outcome studies evaluate the results of procedures on patient-focused outcomes, including symptom improvement, recurrence of varicosity, healing or recurrence of skin ulcers, improvement in the chronic, progressive symptoms of CVD, improved QOL, and cosmetic improvement.[177] These can be assessed using multiple carriers, including QOL measures for symptom relief and CEAP classification in combination with revised VCSS for disease severity outcomes (reader is referred to previous section on "Severity of Venous Disease" for details) The Recurrent Varicose Veins After Surgery (REVAS) classification,[178] a descriptive evaluation of recurrent and residual varicosities based on the physician's assessment, can be used for cosmetic outcome, although it has some limitations. Surrogate outcome measures are commonly used in reporting outcomes of treatment, although caution should be used. Surrogate outcomes may include patency of the ablated saphenous or perforating vein, patency of a venous bypass or stent, or hemodynamic results after interventions.

CONCLUSIONS

Although treatment of CVI has evolved significantly over the past decade, as a result of better understanding of the pathophysiology, more awareness among both patients and care providers and the advent of endovascular techniques and technology, there is still significant room for improvement. It is mandatory that both primary care and specialists not only provide the best evidence-based treatment in care of these patients but also primary prevention given the paramount importance of the latter. Endovenous ablation therapy has replaced both open treatment of superficial reflux and open treatment of perforator incompetence. Endovenous stenting is currently the first line of treatment for deep venous obstruction, and open surgical reconstruction is indicated only in patients who fail or are not candidates for minimally invasive treatment. Further research is needed in development of more effective treatment of deep vein incompetence, although the role of venous stenting in these cases is rapidly evolving. Noninvasive treatment modalities are also lacking in this field.

REFERENCES

1. Fowkes FG, Lee AJ, Evans CJ, et al. Lifestyle risk factors for lower limb venous reflux in the general population: Edinburgh Vein Study. *Int J Epidemiol.* 2001;30(4):846–852.
2. Bradbury A, Evans CJ, Allan P, et al. The relationship between lower limb symptoms and superficial and deep venous reflux on duplex ultrasonography: The Edinburgh Vein Study. *J Vasc Surg.* 2000;32(5):921–931.
3. Neglen P, Eklöf B, et al. Prevention and treatment of venous ulcers in primary chronic venous insufficiency. *J Vasc Surg.* 2010;52(5 Suppl):15S–20S.
4. Krijnen RM, de Boer EM, Bruynzeel DP. Epidemiology of venous disorders in the general and occupational populations. *Epidemiol Rev.* 1997;19(2):294–309.
5. Callam MJ, Ruckley CV, Harper DR, Dale JJ. Chronic ulceration of the leg: extent of the problem and provision of care. *Br Med J (Clin Res Ed).* 1985;290(6485):1855–1856.
6. Fowkes FG, Evans CJ, Lee AJ. Prevalence and risk factors of chronic venous insufficiency. *Angiology.* 2001;52(Suppl 1):S5–15.
7. Olin JW, Beusterien KM, Childs MB, et al. Medical costs of treating venous stasis ulcers: evidence from a retrospective cohort study. *Vasc Med.* 1999;4(1):1–7.
8. Heit JA, Rooke TW, Silverstein MD, et al. Trends in the incidence of venous stasis syndrome and venous ulcer: a 25-year population-based study. *J Vasc Surg.* 2001;33(5):1022–1027.
9. Porter JM, Moneta GL. Reporting standards in venous disease: an update. International Consensus Committee on Chronic Venous Disease. *J Vasc Surg.* 1995;21(4):635–645.
10. Beebe HG, Bergan JJ, Bergqvist D, et al. Classification and grading of chronic venous disease in the lower limbs. A consensus statement. *Eur J Vasc Endovasc Surg.* 1996;12(4):487–491. discussion 91-2.
11. Eklof B, Rutherford RB, Bergan JJ, et al. Revision of the CEAP classification for chronic venous disorders: consensus statement. *J Vasc Surg.* 2004;40(6):1248–1252.
12. Browse N, Burnand K, Thomas M. *Diseases of the Veins: Pathology, Diagnosis, and Treatment.* London: Edward Arnold; 1988.
13. Schweighofer G, Muhlberger D, Brenner E. The anatomy of the small saphenous vein: fascial and neural relations, saphenofemoral junction, and valves. *J Vasc Surg.* 2010;51(4):982–989.
14. Pang AS. Location of valves and competence of the great saphenous vein above the knee. *Ann Acad Med Singapore.* 1991;20(2):248–250.
15. Cotton LT. Varicose veins. Gross anatomy and development. *Br J Surg.* 1961;48:589–598.
16. Kosinski C. Observations on the superficial venous system of the lower extremity. *J Anat.* 1926;60(Pt 2):131–142.
17. Gray H. *Gray's Anatomy of the Human Body.* Bartleby.com; 2000.
18. LePage PA, Villavicencio JL, Gomez ER, et al. The valvular anatomy of the iliac venous system and its clinical implications. *J Vasc Surg.* 1991;14(5):678–683.
19. Negus D. The surgical anatomy of the veins of the lower limb. In: Dodd H, Cockett FB, eds. *The Pathology and Surgery of the Veins of the Lower Limb.* Edinburgh: Churchill Livingstone; 1976:18–49.
20. Basmajian JV. The distribution of valves in the femoral, external iliac, and common iliac veins and their relationship to varicose veins. *Surg Gynecol Obstet.* 1952;95(5):537–542.
21. Lurie F, Kistner RL. The relative position of paired valves at venous junctions suggests their role in modulating three-dimensional flow pattern in veins. *Eur J Vasc Endovasc Surg.* 2012;44(3):337–340.
22. Lurie F, Kistner RL, Eklöf B, Kessler D. Mechanism of venous valve closure and role of the valve in circulation: a new concept. *J Vasc Surg.* 2003;38(5):955–961.
23. Lurie F, Kistner RL, Eklöf B. The mechanism of venous valve closure in normal physiologic conditions. *J Vasc Surg.* 2002;35(4):713–717.
24. Ludbrook J. The musculovenous pumps of the human lower limb. *Am Heart J.* 1966;71(5):635–641.
25. Bauer G. The etiology of leg ulcers and their treatment by resection of the popliteal vein. *J Inter Chir.* 1948;8:937–967.
26. Raju S, Darcey R, Neglen P. Unexpected major role for venous stenting in deep reflux disease. *J Vasc Surg.* 2010;51(2):401–408. discussion 8.
27. Masuda EM, Kistner RL. Long-term results of venous valve reconstruction: a four- to twenty-one-year follow-up. *J Vasc Surg.* 1994;19(3):391–403.
28. Cheatle TR, Perrin M. Venous valve repair: early results in fifty-two cases. *J Vasc Surg.* 1994;19(3):404–413.
29. Raju S. Venous insufficiency of the lower limb and stasis ulceration. Changing concepts and management. *Ann Surg.* 1983;197(6):688–697.
30. Raju S, Fredericks R. Valve reconstruction procedures for nonobstructive venous insufficiency: rationale, techniques, and results in 107 procedures with two- to eight-year follow-up. *J Vasc Surg.* 1988;7(2):301–310.

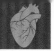

31. Kistner RL. Primary venous valve incompetence of the leg. *Am J Surg.* 1980;140(2):218–224.

32. Brittenden J, Bradbury AW, Allan PL, et al. Popliteal vein reflux reduces the healing of chronic venous ulcer. *Br J Surg.* 1998;85(1):60–62.

33. Rosfors S, Lamke LO, Nordstrom E, Bygdeman S. Severity and location of venous valvular insufficiency: the importance of distal valve function. *Acta Chir Scand.* 1990;156(10):689–694.

34. Danielsson G, Arfvidsson B, Eklöf B, et al. Reflux from thigh to calf, the major pathology in chronic venous ulcer disease: surgery indicated in the majority of patients. *Vasc Endovasc Surg.* 2004;38(3):209–219.

35. Neglen P, Egger 3rd JF, Olivier J, Raju S. Hemodynamic and clinical impact of ultrasound-derived venous reflux parameters. *J Vasc Surg.* 2004;40(2):303–310.

36. Caps MT, Manzo RA, Bergelin RO, et al. Venous valvular reflux in veins not involved at the time of acute deep vein thrombosis. *J Vasc Surg.* 1995;22(5):524–531.

37. Welch HJ, Young CM, Semegran AB, et al. Duplex assessment of venous reflux and chronic venous insufficiency: the significance of deep venous reflux. *J Vasc Surg.* 1996;24(5):755–762.

38. Neglen P, Raju S. A rational approach to detection of significant reflux with duplex Doppler scanning and air plethysmography. *J Vasc Surg.* 1993;17(3):590–595.

39. Labropoulos N, Delis K, Nicolaides AN, et al. The role of the distribution and anatomic extent of reflux in the development of signs and symptoms in chronic venous insufficiency. *J Vasc Surg.* 1996;23(3):504–510.

40. Marston WA, Carlin RE, Passman MA, et al. Healing rates and cost efficacy of outpatient compression treatment for leg ulcers associated with venous insufficiency. *J Vasc Surg.* 1999;30(3):491–498.

41. Labropoulos N, Patel PJ, Tiongson JE, et al. Patterns of venous reflux and obstruction in patients with skin damage due to chronic venous disease. *Vasc Endovasc Surg.* 2007;41(1):33–40.

42. Johnson BF, Manzo RA, Bergelin RO, Strandness Jr DE. Relationship between changes in the deep venous system and the development of the postthrombotic syndrome after an acute episode of lower limb deep vein thrombosis: a one- to six-year follow-up. *J Vasc Surg.* 1995;21(2):307–312. discussion 13.

43. Labropoulos N, Volteas N, Leon M, et al. The role of venous outflow obstruction in patients with chronic venous dysfunction. *Arch Surg.* 1997;132(1):46–51.

44. Araki CT, Back TL, Padberg FT, et al. The significance of calf muscle pump function in venous ulceration. *J Vasc Surg.* 1994;20(6):872–877. discussion 8-9.

45. Christopoulos D, Nicolaides AN, Cook A, et al. Pathogenesis of venous ulceration in relation to the calf muscle pump function. *Surgery.* 1989;106(5):829–835.

46. Abdel-Naby D, Duran WN, Lal BK, et al. Pathogenesis of varicose veins and cellular pathophysiology of chronic venous insufficiency. In: Gloviczki P, ed. *Handbook of Venous and Lymphatic Disorders.* 4th ed. Boca Raton: CRC Press; 2017.

47. Vincent JR, Jones GT, Hill GB, van Rij AM. Failure of microvenous valves in small superficial veins is a key to the skin changes of venous insufficiency. *J Vasc Surg.* 2011;54(6 Suppl):62S-9S. e1-3.

48. Pappas PJ, DeFouw DO, Venezio LM, et al. Morphometric assessment of the dermal microcirculation in patients with chronic venous insufficiency. *J Vasc Surg.* 1997;26(5):784–795.

49. Wenner A, Leu HJ, Brunner U. Ultrastructural changes of capillaries in chronic venous insufficiency. *Exp Cell Biol.* 1980;48:1–14.

50. Rabe E, Pannier F. Epidemiology of chronic venous disorders. In: Gloviczki P, ed. *Hanbook of Venous and Lymphatic Disorders.* 4th ed. Boca Raton: CRC Press; 2017:121–127.

51. Onida S, Lane TRA, Davies AH. Clinical presentation and assessment of patients with venous disease. In: Gloviczki P, ed. *Handbook of Venous and Lymphatic Disorders.* 4th ed. Boca Raton: CRC Press; 2017:361–377.

52. Gloviczki P, Driscoll DJ. Klippel-Trenaunay syndrome: current management. *Phlebology.* 2007;22(6):291–298.

53. Vasquez MA, Rabe E, McLafferty RB, et al. Revision of the venous clinical severity score: venous outcomes consensus statement: special communication of the American Venous Forum Ad Hoc Outcomes Working Group. *J Vasc Surg.* 2010;52(5):1387–1396.

54. Bruins B, Masterson M, Drachtman RA, Michaels LA. Deep venous thrombosis in adolescents due to anatomic causes. *Pediatr Blood Cancer.* 2008;51(1):125–128.

55. Garg N, Gloviczki P, Karimi KM, et al. Factors affecting outcome of open and hybrid reconstructions for nonmalignant obstruction of iliofemoral veins and inferior vena cava. *J Vasc Surg.* 2011;53(2):383–393.

56. Raju S, Ward M. Utility of iliac vein stenting in elderly population older than 80 years. *J Vasc Surg Venous Lymphat Disord.* 2015;3(1):58–63.

57. Raju S, Tackett Jr P, Neglen P. Spontaneous onset of bacterial cellulitis in lower limbs with chronic obstructive venous disease. *Eur J Vasc Endovasc Surg.* 2008;36(5):606–610.

58. Labropoulos N, Leon M, Nicolaides AN, et al. Venous reflux in patients with previous deep venous thrombosis: correlation with ulceration and other symptoms. *J Vasc Surg.* 1994;20(1):20–26.

59. van Bemmelen PS, Bedford G, Beach K, Strandness DE. Quantitative segmental evaluation of venous valvular reflux with duplex ultrasound scanning. *J Vasc Surg.* 1989;10(4):425–431.

60. Szendro G, Nicolaides AN, Zukowski AJ, et al. Duplex scanning in the assessment of deep venous incompetence. *J Vasc Surg.* 1986;4(3):237–242.

61. Masuda EM, Kistner RL, Eklof B. Prospective study of duplex scanning for venous reflux: comparison of Valsalva and pneumatic cuff techniques in the reverse Trendelenburg and standing positions. *J Vasc Surg.* 1994;20(5):711–720.

62. Araki CT, Back TL, Padberg Jr. FT, et al. Refinements in the ultrasonic detection of popliteal vein reflux. *J Vasc Surg.* 1993;18(5):742–748.

63. Marston WA, Brabham VW, Mendes R, et al. The importance of deep venous reflux velocity as a determinant of outcome in patients with combined superficial and deep venous reflux treated with endovenous saphenous ablation. *J Vasc Surg.* 2008;48(2):400–405. discussion 5-6.

64. Sarin S, Sommerville K, Farrah J, et al. Duplex ultrasonography for assessment of venous valvular function of the lower limb. *Br J Surg.* 1994;81(11):1591–1595.

65. Masuda EM, Kistner RL. Prospective comparison of duplex scanning and descending venography in the assessment of venous insufficiency. *Am J Surg.* 1992;164(3):254–259.

66. Labropoulos N, Giannoukas AD, Delis K, et al. Where does venous reflux start? *J Vasc Surg.* 1997;26(5):736–742.

67. Gloviczki P, Comerota AJ, Dalsing MC, et al. The care of patients with varicose veins and associated chronic venous diseases: clinical practice guidelines of the Society for Vascular Surgery and the American Venous Forum. *J Vasc Surg.* 2011;53(5 Suppl):2S–48S.

68. Christopoulos DG, Nicolaides AN, Szendro G, et al. Air-plethysmography and the effect of elastic compression on venous hemodynamics of the leg. *J Vasc Surg.* 1987;5(1):148–159.

69. Lattimer CR, Franceschi C, Kalodiki E. Optimizing calf muscle pump function. *Phlebology.* 2018;33(5):353–360.

70. Nicolaides A, Clark H, Labropoulos N, et al. Quantitation of reflux and outflow obstruction in patients with CVD and correlation with clinical severity. *Int Angiol.* 2014;33(3):275–281.

71. Kurstjens RL, de Wolf MA, Alsadah SA, et al. The value of hemodynamic measurements by air plethysmography in diagnosing venous obstruction of the lower limb. *J Vasc Surg Venous Lymphat Disord.* 2016;4(3):313–319.

72. Kurstjens RL, Catarinella FS, Lam YL, et al. The inability of venous occlusion air plethysmography to identify patients who will benefit from stenting of deep venous obstruction. *Phlebology.* 2018;33(7):483–491.

73. Lattimer CR, Doucet S, Geroulakos G, Kalodiki E. Validation of the novel venous drainage index with stepwise increases in thigh compression pressure in the quantification of venous obstruction. *J Vasc Surg Venous Lymphat Disord.* 2017;5(1):88–95.

74. Neglen P, Raju S. Ambulatory venous pressure revisited. *J Vasc Surg.* 2000;31(6):1206–1213.

75. Kurstjens R, de Wolf M, de Graaf R, Wittens C. Hemodynamic changes in iliofemoral disease. *Phlebology.* 2014;29(1 suppl):90–96.

76. Kurstjens RL, de Wolf MA, Konijn HW, et al. Intravenous pressure changes in patients with postthrombotic deep venous obstruction: results using a treadmill stress test. *J Thromb Haemost.* 2016;14(6):1163–1170.

77. Neglen P, Raju S. Detection of outflow obstruction in chronic venous insufficiency. *J Vasc Surg.* 1993;17(3):583–589.

78. Arnoldussen CW, de Graaf R, Wittens CH, de Haan MW. Value of magnetic resonance venography and computed tomographic venography in lower extremity chronic venous disease. *Phlebology*. 2013;28(Suppl 1):169–175.

79. Szapiro D, Ghaye B, Willems V, et al. Evaluation of CT time-density curves of lower-limb veins. *Invest Radiol*. 2001;36(3):164–169.

80. Chung JW, Yoon CJ, Jung SI, et al. Acute iliofemoral deep vein thrombosis: evaluation of underlying anatomic abnormalities by spiral CT venography. *J Vasc Interv Radiol*. 2004;15(3):249–256.

81. Asciutto G, Mumme A, Marpe B, et al. MR venography in the detection of pelvic venous congestion. *Eur J Vasc Endovasc Surg*. 2008;36(4):491–496.

82. Fraser DG, Moody AR, Morgan PS, Martel A. Iliac compression syndrome and recanalization of femoropopliteal and iliac venous thrombosis: a prospective study with magnetic resonance venography. *J Vasc Surg*. 2004;40(4):612–619.

83. Ruehm SG, Zimny K, Debatin JF. Direct contrast-enhanced 3D MR venography. *Eur Radiol*. 2001;11(1):102–112.

84. Blomgren L, Engstrom J, Rosfors S. A comparison of magnetic resonance venography findings and venous occlusion plethysmography variables in postthrombotic syndrome. *Vascular*. 2017;25(4):406–411.

85. Rudolphi PB, Recke A, Langan EA, et al. Are sonographically measured vascular haemodynamic parameters reproducible using magnetic resonance imaging? *Eur J Vasc Endovasc*. 2016;52(5):665–672.

86. Kistner RL, Ferris EB, Randhawa G, Kamida C. A method of performing descending venography. *J Vasc Surg*. 1986;4(5):464–468.

87. Neglen P, Raju S. A comparison between descending phlebography and duplex Doppler investigation in the evaluation of reflux in chronic venous insufficiency: a challenge to phlebography as the "gold standard". *J Vasc Surg*. 1992;16(5):687–693.

88. Baker SR, Burnand KG, Sommerville KM, et al. Comparison of venous reflux assessed by duplex scanning and descending phlebography in chronic venous disease. *Lancet*. 1993;341(8842):400–403.

89. Gagne PJ, Tahara RW, Fastabend CP, et al. Venography versus intravascular ultrasound for diagnosing and treating iliofemoral vein obstruction. *J Vasc Surg Venous Lymphat Disord*. 2017;5(5):678–687.

90. Gagne PJ, Gasparis A, Black S, et al. Analysis of threshold stenosis by multiplanar venogram and intravascular ultrasound examination for predicting clinical improvement after iliofemoral vein stenting in the VIDIO trial. *J Vasc Surg Venous Lymphat Disord*. 2018;6(1):48–56.e1.

91. Murphy EH, Johns B, Alias MS, et al. Inadequacies of venographic assessment of anatomic variables in iliocaval disease. *J Vasc Surg*. 2016;63(6). 33S-4S.

92. Raju S, Buck WJ, Crim W, Jayaraj A. Optimal sizing of iliac vein stents. *Phlebology*. 2018;33(7):451–457.

93. Meissner MH. The clinical presentation and natural history of acute deep venous thrombosis. In: Gloviczki P, ed. *Handbook of Venous and Lymphatic Disorders*. Boca Raton: CRC Press; 2017:205–219.

94. Labropoulos N, Manalo D, Patel NP, et al. Uncommon leg ulcers in the lower extremity. *J Vasc Surg*. 2007;45(3):568–573.

95. Kistner R, Eklöf B. Classification and etiology of chronic venous disease. In: Gloviczki P, ed. *Handbook of Venous Disorders*. 3rd ed. London: Hodder Arnold; 2009:37–46.

96. Smith JJ, Guest MG, Greenhalgh RM, Davies AH. Measuring the quality of life in patients with venous ulcers. *J Vasc Surg*. 2000;31(4):642–649.

97. Kahn SR, M'Lan CE, Lamping DL, et al. Relationship between clinical classification of chronic venous disease and patient-reported quality of life: results from an international cohort study. *J Vasc Surg*. 2004;39(4):823–828.

98. Launois R, Reboul-Marty J, Henry B. Construction and validation of a quality of life questionnaire in chronic lower limb venous insufficiency (CIVIQ). *Qual Life Res*. 1996;5(6):539–554.

99. Lamping DL, Schroter S, Kurz X, et al. Evaluation of outcomes in chronic venous disorders of the leg: development of a scientifically rigorous, patient-reported measure of symptoms and quality of life. *J Vasc Surg*. 2003;37(2):410–419.

100. Coleridge-Smith P. Drug treatment of varicose veins, venous edema and ulcers. In: Gloviczki P, ed. *Handbook of Venous Disorders*. 3rd ed. London: Hodder Arnold; 2009:359–365.

101. Eberhardt RT, Raffetto JD. Chronic venous insufficiency. *Circulation*. 2005;111(18):2398–2409.

102. Martinez MJ, Bonfill X, Moreno RM, et al. Phlebotonics for venous insufficiency. *Cochrane Database Syst Rev*. 2005;3:CD003229.

103. Pittler MH, Ernst E. Horse chestnut seed extract for chronic venous insufficiency. *Cochrane Database Syst Rev*. 2006;1:CD003230.

104. Nelson EA, Prescott RJ, Harper DR, et al. A factorial, randomized trial of pentoxifylline or placebo, four-layer or single-layer compression, and knitted viscose or hydrocolloid dressings for venous ulcers. *J Vasc Surg*. 2007;45(1):134–141.

105. Dale JJ, Ruckley CV, Harper DR, et al. Randomised, double blind placebo controlled trial of pentoxifylline in the treatment of venous leg ulcers. *BMJ*. 1999;319(7214):875–878.

106. Falanga V, Fujitani RM, Diaz C, et al. Systemic treatment of venous leg ulcers with high doses of pentoxifylline: efficacy in a randomized, placebo-controlled trial. *Wound Repair Regen*. 1999;7(4):208–213.

107. Hirsh J, Guyatt G, Albers GW, et al. Executive summary: American College of Chest Physicians Evidence-Based Clinical Practice Guidelines (8th Edition). *Chest*. 2008;133(6 Suppl):71S–109S.

108. Coleridge-Smith P, Lok C, Ramelet AA. Venous leg ulcer: a meta-analysis of adjunctive therapy with micronized purified flavonoid fraction. *Eur J Vasc Endovasc Surg*. 2005;30(2):198–208.

109. Moneta G, Partsch B. Compression therapy for venous ulceration. In: Gloviczki P, ed. *Handbook of Venous Disorders*. 3rd ed. London: Hodder Arnold; 2009:348–358.

110. Partsch B, Partsch H. Calf compression pressure required to achieve venous closure from supine to standing positions. *J Vasc Surg*. 2005;42(4):734–738.

111. Ibegbuna V, Delis KT, Nicolaides AN, Aina O. Effect of elastic compression stockings on venous hemodynamics during walking. *J Vasc Surg*. 2003;37(2):420–425.

112. Zajkowski PJ, Proctor MC, Wakefield TW, et al. Compression stockings and venous function. *Arch Surg*. 2002;137(9):1064–1068.

113. Mayberry JC, Moneta GL, Taylor Jr. LM, Porter JM. Fifteen-year results of ambulatory compression therapy for chronic venous ulcers. *Surgery*. 1991;109(5):575–581.

114. Callam MJ, Harper DR, Dale JJ, et al. Lothian and Forth Valley leg ulcer healing trial: part 1. Elastic versus non-elastic bandaging in the treatment of chronic leg ulceration. *Phlebology*. 1992;7(4):136–141.

115. Fletcher A, Cullum N, Sheldon TA. A systematic review of compression treatment for venous leg ulcers. *BMJ*. 1997;315(7108):576–580.

116. Partsch H, Flour M, Smith PC. Indications for compression therapy in venous and lymphatic disease consensus based on experimental data and scientific evidence. Under the auspices of the IUP. *Int Angiol*. 2008;27(3):193–219.

117. Amsler F, Willenberg T, Blattler W. In search of optimal compression therapy for venous leg ulcers: a meta-analysis of studies comparing diverse [corrected] bandages with specifically designed stockings. *J Vasc Surg*. 2009;50(3):668–674.

118. Palfreyman S, Nelson EA, Michaels JA. Dressings for venous leg ulcers: systematic review and meta-analysis. *BMJ*. 2007;335(7613):244.

119. Barwell JR, Davies CE, Deacon J, et al. Comparison of surgery and compression with compression alone in chronic venous ulceration (ESCHAR study): randomised controlled trial. *Lancet*. 2004;363(9424):1854–1859.

120. Gohel MS, Barwell JR, Taylor M, et al. Long term results of compression therapy alone versus compression plus surgery in chronic venous ulceration (ESCHAR): randomised controlled trial. *BMJ*. 2007;335(7610):83.

121. Geerts WH, Bergqvist D, Pineo GF, et al. Prevention of venous thromboembolism: American College of Chest Physicians Evidence-Based Clinical Practice Guidelines (8th Edition). *Chest*. 2008;133(6 Suppl):381S–453S.

122. Scriven JM, Hartshorne T, Thrush AJ, et al. Role of saphenous vein surgery in the treatment of venous ulceration. *Br J Surg*. 1998;85(6):781–784.

123. Criado E, Lujan S, Izquierdo L, et al. Conservative hemodynamic surgery for varicose veins. *Semin Vasc Surg*. 2002;15(1):27–33.

124. Pittaluga P, Chastanet S, Rea B, Barbe R. Midterm results of the surgical treatment of varices by phlebectomy with conservation of a refluxing saphenous vein. *J Vasc Surg.* 2009;50(1):107–118.

125. Passman M. Transilluminated powered phlebectomy in the treatment of varicose veins. *Vascular.* 2007;15(5):262–268.

126. Bergan JJ. Varicose veins: hooks, clamps, and suction. Application of new techniques to enhance varicose vein surgery. *Semin Vasc Surg.* 2002;15(1):21–26.

127. Gay J. *On varicose disease of the lower extremities and other allied disorders: skin discoloration, induration and ulcer. Lettsomian Lectures delivered before the Medical Society of London in 1867.* London: John Churchill and Sons; 1868.

128. Linton RR. The communicating veins of the lower leg and the operative technic for their ligation. *Ann Surg.* 1938;107(4):582–593.

129. Cockett FB. The pathology and treatment of venous ulcers of the leg. *Br J Surg.* 1955;43(179):260–278.

130. Dodd H. The diagnosis and ligation of incompetent ankle perforating veins. *Ann R Coll Surg Engl.* 1964;34:186–196.

131. Homans J. The operative treatment of varicose veins and ulcers, based open a classification of these lesions. *Surg Gynecol Obstet.* 1916;22:143–158.

132. Mendes RR, Marston WA, Farber MA, Keagy BA. Treatment of superficial and perforator venous incompetence without deep venous insufficiency: is routine perforator ligation necessary? *J Vasc Surg.* 2003;38(5):891–895.

133. Stuart WP, Adam DJ, Allan PL, et al. Saphenous surgery does not correct perforator incompetence in the presence of deep venous reflux. *J Vasc Surg.* 1998;28(5):834–838.

134. Mozes G, Gloviczki P, Menawat SS, et al. Surgical anatomy for endoscopic subfascial division of perforating veins. *J Vasc Surg.* 1996;24(5):800–808.

135. Wilkinson Jr. GE, Maclaren IF. Long term review of procedures for venous perforator insufficiency. *Surg Gynecol Obstet.* 1986;163(2):117–120.

136. Negus D, Friedgood A. The effective management of venous ulceration. *Br J Surg.* 1983;70(10):623–627.

137. Pierik EG, van Urk H, Hop WC, Wittens CH. Endoscopic versus open subfascial division of incompetent perforating veins in the treatment of venous leg ulceration: a randomized trial. *J Vasc Surg.* 1997;26(6):1049–1054.

138. Hauer G. Endoscopic subfascial discussion of perforating veins--preliminary report. *VASA Zeitschrift fur Gefasskrankheiten.* 1985;14(1):59–61.

139. O'Donnell TF. Surgical treatment of incompetent communicating veins. In: Bergan JJ, Kistner RL, eds. *Atlas of Venous Surgery.* Philadelphia: W.B. Saunders; 1992:111–124.

140. Gloviczki P, Cambria RA, Rhee RY, et al. Surgical technique and preliminary results of endoscopic subfascial division of perforating veins. *J Vasc Surg.* 1996;23(3):517–523.

141. Conrad P. Endoscopic exploration of the subfascial space of the lower leg with perforator vein interruption using laparoscopic equipment: a preliminary report. *Phlebology.* 1994;9(4):154–157.

142. O'Donnell TF. The role of perforators in chronic venous insufficiency. *Phlebology.* 2010;25(1):3–10.

143. Gloviczki P, Bergan JJ. *Atlas of Endoscopic Perforator Vein Surgery.* London: Springer-Verlag; 1998.

144. Gloviczki P, Bergan JJ, Rhodes JM, et al. Mid-term results of endoscopic perforator vein interruption for chronic venous insufficiency: lessons learned from the North American subfascial endoscopic perforator surgery registry. The North American Study Group. *J Vasc Surg.* 1999;29(3):489–502.

145. Tenbrook Jr. JA, Iafrati MD, O'Donnell Jr. TF, et al. Systematic review of outcomes after surgical management of venous disease incorporating subfascial endoscopic perforator surgery. *J Vasc Surg.* 2004;39(3):583–589.

146. Luebke T, Brunkwall J. Meta-analysis of subfascial endoscopic perforator vein surgery (SEPS) for chronic venous insufficiency. *Phlebology.* 2009;24(1):8–16.

147. Kistner RL. Surgical repair of a venous valve. *Straub Clin Proc.* 1968;34:41–43.

148. Kistner RL. Surgical repair of the incompetent femoral vein valve. *Arch Surg.* 1975;110(11):1336–1342.

149. Raju S. Surgical repair of deep vein valve incompetence. In: Gloviczki P, ed. *Handbook of Venous Disorders.* 3rd ed. London: Hodder Arnold; 2009:472–482.

150. Gloviczki P, Merrell SW, Bower TC. Femoral vein valve repair under direct vision without venotomy: a modified technique with use of angioscopy. *J Vasc Surg.* 1991;14(5):645–648.

151. Raju S, Fountain T, Neglen P, Devidas M. Axial transformation of the profunda femoris vein. *J Vasc Surg.* 1998;27(4):651–659.

152. Lugli M, Guerzoni S, Garofalo M, et al. Neovalve construction in deep venous incompetence. *J Vasc Surg.* 2009;49(1):156–162. 62 e1-2; discussion 62.

153. Meissner MH, Manzo RA, Bergelin RO, et al. Deep venous insufficiency: the relationship between lysis and subsequent reflux. *J Vasc Surg.* 1993;18(4):596–605. discussion 6-8.

154. Ziegler S, Schillinger M, Maca TH, Minar E. Post-thrombotic syndrome after primary event of deep venous thrombosis 10 to 20 years ago. *Thromb Res.* 2001;101(2):23–33.

155. O'Shaughnessy AM, Fitzgerald DE. Natural history of proximal deep vein thrombosis assessed by duplex ultrasound. *Int Angiol.* 1997;16(1):45–49.

156. Gloviczki P, Hollier LH, Dewanjee MK, et al. Experimental replacement of the inferior vena cava: factors affecting patency. *Surgery.* 1984;95(6):657–666.

157. Neglen P. Endovascular reconstruction for chronic iliofemoral vein obstruction. In: Gloviczki P, ed. *Handbook of Venous Disorders.* 3rd ed. London: Hodder Arnold; 2009:491–502.

158. Raju S, Neglen P. Percutaneous recanalization of total occlusions of the iliac vein. *J Vasc Surg.* 2009;50(2):360–368.

159. Garg N, Gloviczki P, Karimi KM, et al. Factors affecting outcome of open and hybrid reconstructions for nonmalignant obstruction of iliofemoral veins and inferior vena cava. *J Vasc Surg.* 2011;53(2):383–393.

160. Jost CJ, Gloviczki P, Cherry Jr. KJ, et al. Surgical reconstruction of iliofemoral veins and the inferior vena cava for nonmalignant occlusive disease. *J Vasc Surg.* 2001;33(2):320–327. discussion 7-8.

161. Hingorani AP, Ascher E, Marks N, et al. Predictive factors of success following radio-frequency stylet (RFS) ablation of incompetent perforating veins (IPV). *J Vasc Surg.* 2009;50(4):844–848.

162. Masuda EM, Kessler DM, Lurie F, et al. The effect of ultrasound-guided sclerotherapy of incompetent perforator veins on venous clinical severity and disability scores. *J Vasc Surg.* 2006;43(3):551–556. discussion 6-7.

163. Proebstle TM, Herdemann S. Early results and feasibility of incompetent perforator vein ablation by endovenous laser treatment. *Dermatol Surg.* 2007;33(2):162–168.

164. Marks N, Hingorani A, Ascher E. New office-based vascular interventions. *Perspect Vasc Surg Endovasc Ther.* 2008;20(4):340–345.

165. Elias S. Percutenous ablation of perforating veins. In: Gloviczki P, ed. *Handbook of Venous Disorders.* 3rd ed. London: Hodder Arnold; 2009:536–544.

166. Dalsing M. Artificial venous valves. In: Gloviczki P, ed. *Handbook of Venous Disorders.* 3rd ed. London: Hodder Arnold; 2009:483–490.

167. Neglen P, Berry MA, Raju S. Endovascular surgery in the treatment of chronic primary and post-thrombotic iliac vein obstruction. *Eur J Vasc Endovasc Surg.* 2000;20(6):560–571.

168. Raju S, Ward Jr. M, Kirk O. A modification of iliac vein stent technique. *Ann Vasc Surg.* 2014;28(6):1485–1492.

169. Neglen P, Tackett Jr. TP, Raju S. Venous stenting across the inguinal ligament. *J Vasc Surg.* 2008;48(5):1255–1261.

170. Murphy EH, Johns B, Varney E, Raju S. Endovascular management of chronic total occlusions of the inferior vena cava and iliac veins. *J Vasc Surg Venous Lymphat Disord.* 2017;5(1):47–59.

171. Raju S. Best management options for chronic iliac vein stenosis and occlusion. *J Vasc Surg.* 2013;57(4):1163–1169.

172. Neglen P, Oglesbee M, Olivier J, Raju S. Stenting of chronically obstructed inferior vena cava filters. *J Vasc Surg.* 2011;54(1):153–161.

173. Raju S, Hollis K, Neglen P. Obstructive lesions of the inferior vena cava: clinical features and endovenous treatment. *J Vasc Surg.* 2006;44(4):820–827.

174. Bjarnason H. Endovascular reconstruction of complex iliocaval venous occlusions. In: Gloviczki P, ed. *Handbook of Venous Disorders*. 3rd ed. London: Hodder Arnold; 2009:503–513.

175. Neglen P, Hollis KC, Olivier J, Raju S. Stenting of the venous outflow in chronic venous disease: long-term stent-related outcome, clinical, and hemodynamic result. *J Vasc Surg*. 2007;46(5):979–990.

176. Delis KT, Bjarnason H, Wennberg PW, et al. Successful iliac vein and inferior vena cava stenting ameliorates venous claudication and improves venous outflow, calf muscle pump function, and clinical status in post-thrombotic syndrome. *Ann Surg*. 2007;245(1):130–139.

177. Kundu S, Lurie F, Millward SF, et al. Recommended reporting standards for endovenous ablation for the treatment of venous insufficiency: joint statement of The American Venous Forum and The Society of Interventional Radiology. *J Vasc Surg*. 2007;46(3):582–589.

178. Perrin M, Allaert FA. Intra- and inter-observer reproducibility of the Recurrent Varicose Veins after Surgery (REVAS) classification. *Eur J Vasc Endovasc Surg*. 2006;32(3):326–332.

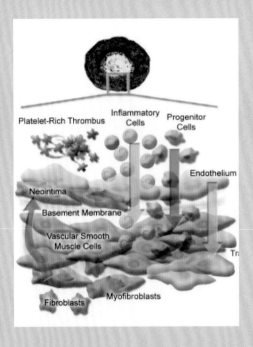

Pulmonary
Hypertension

肺高压

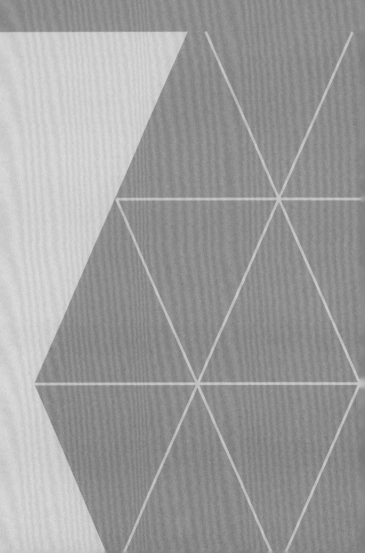

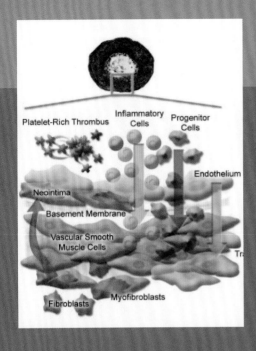

第55章
肺动脉高压

肺动脉高压（pulmonary arterial hypertension，PAH）是一种罕见且复杂的肺血管疾病，据估计全球发病率为0.0015%～0.005%。PAH目前诊断标准为静息状态下平均肺动脉压力≥20 mmHg，肺血管阻力＞3 Wood单位且肺动脉楔压＜15 mmHg，并除外其他可能导致肺高压的因素。虽然近20年PAH的治疗取得了较大进展，但PAH病情进展较快，从诊断PAH到死于右心心力衰竭的中位时间仅为2.8年。PAH的病理改变均发生在外周小的肺动脉（直径100～1000 μm）上，典型特征包括内膜纤维化、血管平滑肌细胞增生及肺动脉闭塞；此外，终末期PAH的标志为血管新内膜的形成，表现为细胞外基质和成纤维细胞的沉积。PAH发生的分子机制主要表现为遗传因素与外源性因子共同作用，造成下游（线粒体代谢、mRNA生物体、PPAR-γ信号、钙通道生物体、炎症等）功能失调，从而导致血管收缩、细胞增殖和血栓形成，造成PAH。PAH的临床病理生理学改变主要为肺血管顺应性下降，随着后负荷（肺动脉压力）增加，右室肥厚扩张，并逐渐出现右心心力衰竭；PAH患者最常见的两个死因为进行性右室功能衰竭和猝死。PAH的诊断需详细询问病史，并结合体格检查、运动测试（6 min步行试验）、胸片、心电图、肺功能测定、超声心动图、心脏MRI、心脏肺栓塞T-CT、动脉血气分析、心导管检查、基因检测等来进行综合判断，并进行风险评估。PAH的治疗包括一般措施（避免剧烈活动、乘坐飞机和妊娠，规律进行流感或肺炎疫苗接种），抗凝治疗，氧疗，针对右心心力衰竭的治疗，肺血管特异性治疗（钙离子通道拮抗剂、PDE5抑制剂、内皮素-1受体拮抗剂、可溶性鸟苷酸环化酶激活剂、前列环素及其类似物等）。对于难治性PAH则可采用房间隔造口术和肺移植。此外，还有一些针对PAH的实验性疗法正处于临床试验阶段，包括使用利妥昔单抗、托珠单抗、NF-κB抑制剂、PDK抑制剂、他克莫司、伊马替尼等。

孙晓刚

Pulmonary Arterial Hypertension

Stephen Y. Chan and Joseph Loscalzo

DEFINITION AND CLASSIFICATION OF PULMONARY ARTERIAL HYPERTENSION

Until 2018, pulmonary arterial hypertension (PAH) was formally defined as a mean pulmonary artery pressure (mPAP) of greater than or equal to 25 mm Hg at rest, accompanied by a pulmonary vascular resistance (PVR) of greater than 3 Wood units with a normal pulmonary artery wedge pressure (<15 mm Hg) in the absence of any known cause of pulmonary hypertension (PH).[1a] A recently revised World Health Organization (WHO) classification system for PAH decreased the upper limit of mPAP from 25 mm Hg to 20 mm Hg. In both prior and revised classification schemes, PAH encompasses the first of the five groups of PH. The pathophysiology and clinical characteristics of Groups 2 through 5 of PH (i.e., PH associated with left-sided heart disease; lung disease/chronic hypoxia; thromboembolic PH; and other groups) are reviewed in Chapter 56. In this chapter, we will focus on WHO Group 1, PAH, which includes idiopathic and hereditary PAH as well as PAH associated with various secondary diseases (Box 55.1). Until improved therapeutic options became available during the past two decades, PAH was considered a rare but rapidly progressive, devastating condition, leading to death from right heart failure by a median of 2.8 years from the time of diagnosis. In recent years, an improved conceptual framework has been developed to better delineate the pathogenesis and clinical presentation of PAH, accompanied by improved directed therapeutic approaches. Nonetheless, PAH still carries a 9% 1-year mortality rate,[2] and current therapeutics have been more effective at slowing illness progression rather than reversing or curing the disease. This chapter will highlight the current molecular understanding of the complex disease, via the still incompletely characterized interplay of genetic and exogenous upstream stimuli with downstream vascular effectors. This framework will then be coupled to the current understanding of the clinical presentation and progression of PAH, and the current and evolving modalities for treatment.

EPIDEMIOLOGY

While PH in general is relatively common, PAH is a rare disease, with recent estimates placing the prevalence at 15 to 50 cases per million worldwide. Of these, idiopathic PAH has been reported with an annual incidence of one to two cases per million persons, and is thought to account for at least 40% of all PAH cases. While diagnoses of heritable causes of PAH are on the rise, the overall prevalence likely accounts for a very small fraction of total PAH prevalence, as reviewed recently.[3] PAH associated with secondary illnesses is thought to account for the remaining cases. For instance, 7% to 12% of patients with systemic sclerosis develop PAH. Moreover, while the prevalence of PAH secondary to human immunodeficiency virus (HIV) infection was originally reported as 0.5%, estimates in sub-Saharan African populations suggest this number may be much higher.[4] PAH associated with the newborn, termed *persistent pulmonary hypertension of the newborn* (PPHN), may occur in 0.2% of live-born term infants.

Overall, however, the exact incidence and prevalence of this disease are difficult to estimate on a global scale, given the difficulty of diagnosing PAH and overall limited access to healthcare worldwide. The disease affects women more frequently than men (1.7:1). This female predominance is exaggerated in the population of African descent (4.3:1), although the overall racial distribution of patients reflects that in the general population. Primary PAH presents most commonly in the fourth decade of life; ages range from 1 to 81 with 9% of the patients older than 60 years of age. Some sources cite a similar gender ratio among children diagnosed with the disease, whereas others note an equal distribution between male and female children. Primary PAH is typically difficult to diagnose, and the average time from the onset of symptoms to diagnosis was 2 years in the NIH Registry, thus resulting in most patients suffering from a more severe stage of disease at initial diagnosis (New York Heart Association [NYHA]/WHO Functional Classes III-IV). More recently, however, owing to improved clinical awareness coupled with more sophisticated invasive and noninvasive techniques for PAP measurements, time to diagnosis has decreased considerably, at least in the developed world.

CELLULAR PATHOGENESIS OF PULMONARY ARTERIAL HYPERTENSION

In humans, the natural history of PAH lesions is unknown, as patients usually present when the disease is advanced. The pathological appearance of severe PAH is similar regardless of the cause and reflects the end stage of a common response to pulmonary vascular injury. Common histologic features in nearly all types of PAH occur at the level of the small peripheral pulmonary arteries (100 to 1000 μm; Fig. 55.1); these include intimal fibrosis, distal localization and proliferation of vascular smooth muscle cells, and pulmonary arterial occlusion. Furthermore, a hallmark of severe, end-stage disease is the formation of a vessel "neointima," characterized by increased deposition of extracellular matrix (ECM) and myofibroblasts. Plexiform lesions can predominate, characterized by overproliferation of endothelial-like cells encroaching upon the vessel lumen.

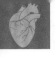

BOX 55.1   Clinical Classification of WHO Group 1 Pulmonary Hypertension

1 Pulmonary arterial hypertension (PAH)
1.1   Idiopathic PAH
1.2   Heritable PAH
1.3   Drug and toxin induced PAH
1.4   PAH associated with
   1.4.1   Connective tissue disease
   1.4.2   HIV infection
   1.4.3   Portal hypertension
   1.4.4   Congenital heart disease
   1.4.5   Schistosomiasis
1.5   PAH with long-term response to calcium channel blockade
1.6   PAH with overt features of pulmonary veno-occlusive disease or pulmonary capillary hemangiomatosis
1.7   Persistent PH of the newborn

Modified from Simonneau G, Montani D, Celermajer D, et al. Haemodynamic definitions and updated clinical classification of pulmonary hypertension. *Eur Respir J.* 2018 [Epub ahead of print].

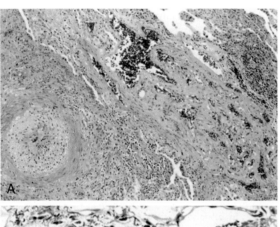

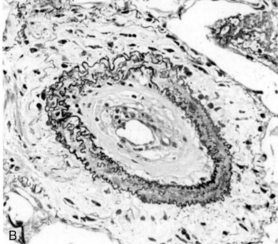

Fig. 55.1 Histopathology of Pulmonary Arterial Hypertension. (A) Hematoxylin and eosin stain of a histologic section of the lungs of an idiopathic pulmonary arterial hypertension (PAH) characteristic vascular lesion: a completely occluded vessel with severe concentric intimal fibrosis and medial thickening *(left)* and a plexiform lesion with multiple lumina *(right)*. (B) Elastin von Gieson stain of internal and external elastic laminae demonstrates the medial hypertrophy and neointimal formation in a small muscular pulmonary artery in a patient with idiopathic PAH. (Courtesy J.L. Faul, MD, Stanford University.)

Multiple cell types in the pulmonary arterial wall and pulmonary arterial circulation contribute to the specific response to injury and the development of vessel remodeling (Fig. 55.2). First, in the endothelium, it is increasingly appreciated that there exists extensive pathogenic reprogramming of pulmonary arterial endothelial cells (PAECs) in PAH, but these programs are complex and poorly understood. Early in the disease, it is thought that the endothelium serves as a central sensor of injurious stimuli, such as hypoxia, shear stress, inflammation, and toxins, leading to cell death and apoptosis. Such PAEC apoptosis has been observed readily in multiple types of animal and human forms of PAH, and plays a causative role particularly early in PAH to trigger pathogenesis.[5-7] Apoptosis may trigger abnormalities in angiogenesis and contribute to the pathophenotype of pulmonary vascular rarefaction that is typical of PAH. Yet, in addition to apoptosis, increased PAEC proliferation also has been noted and linked to PAH pathogenesis.[8] Historically, evidence for proliferation has included the study of plexiform lesions (previously described as "disorganized endothelial proliferation"). Moreover, recent studies[9] have demonstrated that cultured PAECs isolated from human PAH patients demonstrate increased proliferation as compared with nondiseased control PAECs, accompanied by an imbalance of a multitude of downstream secreted vasoactive factors that contribute to overall increases of pulmonary vasomotor tone. Importantly, by modulating either microRNAs[9] or matrix stiffness[10] that consequently affect such endothelial proliferation, PAH manifestations improved in rodent models of PAH, indicating the importance of such proliferation to overall disease development. Other studies have isolated highly proliferative endothelial cells from PAH patients[11] and multiple animal models of PH.[9,12] In total, some investigators believe that endothelial apoptosis early in PAH initiates the selection of apoptosis-resistant endothelial cells that can further proliferate and drive later stages of disease.[13] Yet it is also possible that a single or distinct population of proliferative endothelial cells may exist that continually transforms cellular identity, such as in the endothelial-to-mesenchymal transition that has been observed in PAH.[14,15]

Unlike diseased PAECs where apoptosis and proliferation may contribute in parallel to PAH, pathogenic function of pulmonary artery smooth muscle cells (PASMCs) is characterized by a proproliferative and antiapoptotic phenotype. In these diseased PASMCs, numerous proliferative signaling pathways are dysregulated,[16] accompanied by a profound metabolic shift involving a deregulation of oxidative cellular metabolism in favor of glycolysis. This hyperproliferative, antiapoptotic, and glycolytic phenotype of the vasculature in PH has drawn comparisons to the cellular phenotype (Warburg effect) observed in cancer, collectively contributing to proliferation and resistance to apoptosis. Recently, extrapolation of this "cancer theory of PAH" has led to a reported association of developing PAH with lung cancer.[17] By end-stage disease, such processes result in substantial remodeling and medial arteriolar thickening, leading to a hypercontractile phenotype.

Pulmonary arterial adventitial fibroblasts (PAAFs) also display increased proliferative capacity in PAH and undergo a similar metabolic shift as diseased PASMCs. In response, diseased PAAFs can orchestrate a variety of alterations in the ECM driving profound vascular stiffening. The study of vascular stiffness is an emerging principle in PAH. Stiffness occurs in the proximal and distal pulmonary arterial tree in various forms of PAH,[18,19] and stiffness is an index of disease progression.[20] Vascular ECM remodeling occurs through changes in the balance between collagen and elastin deposition, matrix degradation, and matrix remodeling via collagen crosslinking enzymes such as lysyl oxidase (LOX).[21] Metalloproteinase activation in the ECM can also induce cellular migration and leads to the

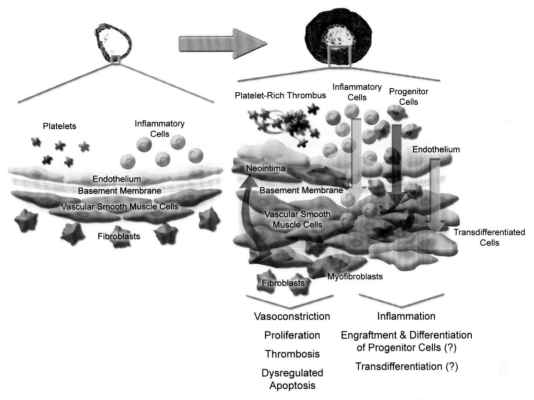

Fig. 55.2 Pulmonary Arterial Pathobiology Involves the Coordinate Action of Multiple Cell Types. The histological progression of the pulmonary vasculature from quiescence to pathogenic activation in pulmonary arterial hypertension involves numerous vascular cell types and phenotypic responses. Initial injury to the endothelium and/or adventitial fibroblasts may initiate pathogenic signaling pathways. These activate an imbalance of secreted vascular mediators that drive the vascular responses of vasoconstriction, proliferation, thrombosis, and dysregulation of apoptosis, leading to the formation of a layer of "neointima." Blood-borne inflammatory cells and platelets also likely play prominent roles in these processes, but their exact mechanistic actions are unclear. Pathophenotypes that may influence disease progression include transdifferentiation of endothelial cells to vascular smooth muscle cells (endothelial-to-mesenchymal transition) and transdifferentiation of fibroblasts and vascular smooth muscle cells to myofibroblasts. Early remodeling of extracellular matrix increases vascular stiffness, which can mechanically activate downstream pathogenic signaling, metabolic dysfunction, and vascular cell-cell crosstalk. Engraftment and differentiation of vascular progenitor cells may contribute as well. (Modified from Chan SY, Loscalzo J. Pathogenic mechanisms of pulmonary arterial hypertension. *J Mol Cell Cardiol.* 2008;44:14–30. Micrographs of pulmonary arteries are courtesy of www.scleroderma.org and Humbert M, Sitbon O, Simonneau G. Treatment of pulmonary arterial hypertension. *N Engl J Med.* 2004;351:1425–1436. Copyright 2004, Massachusetts Medical Society. All rights reserved.)

production of additional mitogenic factors. Recent studies have reported that vascular matrix stiffness is not merely a consequence of long-standing disease but, rather, an early, pervasive driver of PAH. Consequent metabolic and proliferative reprogramming in PAAFs[22] as well as PAECs and PASMCs[23] has been directly linked to mechanoactivation after exposure to stiff matrix[10] as well as inflammatory cell activation.[24]

In addition to the importance of canonical cellular layers of the vascular wall, dysfunction of alternative vascular components may participate in these processes. Multiple lines of evidence now converge to connect immune dysregulation to clinical PAH in humans and animal models. Previous reports suggest altered inflammatory dynamics, such as hematopoietic and myeloid expansion, B- and T-cell dysfunction, mast cell activation, increased cytokine production, circulating autoantibodies, and tertiary lymphoid tissue neogenesis, may initiate or drive PAH.[25] Clinically, there is a well-established causative link between autoimmune connective tissue disorders and PAH. Furthermore, infective agents, such as *Schistosoma mansoni*, HIV, and recently endogenous retrovirus HERV-K,[26] are known to alter the immune cell repertoire and predispose to the development of PAH. Consistent with a significant presence of T and B cells in remodeled vascular lesions in end-stage PAH, lymphocytes have been implicated in a severe inflammatory state in this disease. Athymic nude rats, which lack functioning T cells, display greater sensitivity to PAH. T cell dysregulation may figure prominently, as regulatory T cells (T_{reg}) are increased while $CD8^+$ cytotoxic cells are decreased in idiopathic PAH. An alteration of the helper T cell response (TH1 vs. TH2 vs. TH17) may also factor into the pathogenic response, but these features have not been described fully. Myeloid leukocytes, especially macrophages, are among the primary effectors of inflammation in pulmonary lesions in PH patients. A role of macrophages in aggravating PH pathogenesis has been proposed.[27] A number of soluble chemoattractants and proinflammatory cytokines are upregulated in human and animal models of severe PAH. These include interleukin-1β, interleukin-6, interleukin-8, transforming growth factor-β1, bradykinin, monocyte chemotactic protein-1, fractalkine, RANTES, tumor necrosis factor (TNF)-α, and leukotrienes, among others. In particular, macrophage-derived leukotriene B4 has been implicated in mediating both endothelial[28] and fibroblast[29] dysregulation in PAH. A further mechanistic understanding of the exogenous or endogenous factors that drive immune dysfunction awaits elucidation.

Activated platelets appear to predominate in later stages of PAH, with histological evidence of in situ thrombosis in diseased arterioles of end-stage PAH. Finally, circulating or resident progenitor cells have been proposed to factor significantly in vessel wall injury and repair; dysregulation of these functions may also contribute to PAH. Yet our understanding is still limited regarding the mechanistic role of these cellular populations in disease progression.

MOLECULAR PATHOGENESIS OF PULMONARY ARTERIAL HYPERTENSION

Initiating Molecular Triggers of Pulmonary Arterial Hypertension

Importantly, the WHO classification of PAH refers to distinct patient groups that cluster according to clinical association. In recent years, these clinical associations have been defined by much more precise molecular mechanisms that are now believed to be important in *initiating* or *triggering* this disease.

Genetic Association

An understanding of the mechanism of genetic predisposition to PAH is of paramount importance for the identification of the root pathogenesis

(Fig. 55.3). The familial variety of idiopathic PAH accounts for at least 6% of all cases of PAH. Pedigree analysis has demonstrated an autosomal dominant inheritance but with variable penetrance, as only 10% to 20% of putative genetic carriers develop clinical PAH. Genetic anticipation is present, as each successive generation of affected families is afflicted at a younger age and with greater severity compared with the preceding generation.

Bone morphogenetic receptor 2. Mutations in the transforming growth factor-β receptor (TGF-β receptor) superfamily have been genetically linked to PAH and play a causative role in the development of disease.[30] The most prevalent cohort of hereditary PAH patients carries mutations in the bone morphogenetic protein receptor type 2 (*BMPR2* gene). More than 140 mutations in *BMPR2* have been reported in patients with familial PAH, mainly located in the extracellular ligand-binding domain, in the cytoplasmic serine/threonine kinase domain, or in the long carboxyterminal domain. These account for 70% of all familial pedigrees of PAH and 10% to 30% of idiopathic PAH cases. *BMPR2* loss-of-function mutations have only been found in the heterozygous state. The absence of *BMPR2* mutations in some familial cohorts and in most of the sporadic cases indicates that additional, unidentified genetic mutations can also predispose to development of PAH. Furthermore, the presence of incomplete penetrance (approximately 25% of carriers in affected families develop clinical PAH) and genetic anticipation suggest that *BMPR2* mutations are necessary but alone insufficient to result in clinically significant disease.

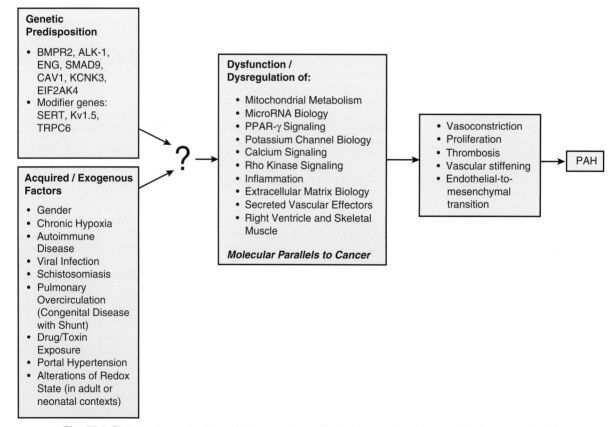

Fig. 55.3 Pathogenic mechanisms that connect genetic and exogenous triggers of pulmonary arterial hypertension *(PAH)* to downstream dysregulated phenotypes are beginning to be explored at the molecular level. Underlying the numerous clinical risk factors that exist in PAH, the complex pathogenic molecular mechanisms that converge upon the pulmonary vasculature and right ventricle continue to be elucidated.

The mechanism of action of BMPR2 is complex, and its role in PAH progression is still unclear (Fig. 55.4A). It functions as a receptor with serine/threonine kinase activity, and it activates a broad and complex range of intracellular signaling pathways.[31] Upon binding one of many possible BMP ligands, BMPR2 forms a heterodimer with one of three type-I receptors. BMPR2 phosphorylates the bound type-I receptor, which, in turn, phosphorylates one of the Smad family of proteins to allow for nuclear translocation, binding to DNA, and regulation of gene transcription. Alternatively, BMPR2 activation can also lead to signaling via the LIM kinase pathway, the p38/MAP kinase/ERK/JNK pathways, or the c-Src pathway, independent of Smad activation.

The cellular effects of BMPR2 activation are multiform and complex. In the adult, BMPR2 is expressed predominantly in the pulmonary endothelium, medial smooth muscle cells, and macrophages. Under normal conditions, BMP ligands bind BMPR2 to suppress the growth of vascular smooth muscle cells. In contrast, binding of BMP2 and BMP7 to BMPR2 in pulmonary endothelium protects against apoptosis. It has been found that selective enhancement of BMPR2 signaling with BMP9 can reverse PAH.[5] Furthermore, BMPR2 signaling has been linked to numerous cellular pathophenotypes important in driving PAH, including metabolic dysfunction,[6] angiogenesis, endothelial-to-mesenchymal transition,[15] cell survival via peroxisome proliferator-activated receptor-gamma (PPAR-γ) signaling,[32] macrophage recruitment,[33] and endothelial migration,[34] among others. These dysfunctional signaling pathways have been corroborated in multiple rodent models of PAH, as well as endothelial cells derived from inducible pluripotent stem cells (iPSCs) of patients carrying pathogenic BMPR2 mutations.[35,36] In correlation, pulmonary levels of BMPR2 are reduced both in familial cases of PAH without any *BMPR2* mutation and in cases of secondary PAH. Thus dysregulation of the BMP signaling pathway may be a common pathogenic finding in multiple types of PAH, due to genetic or exogenous stimuli. However, the comprehensive in vivo effects of these mutations have been difficult to decipher. Specifically, robust PAH has been difficult to reproduce in mouse and rat[14] models harboring specific *BMPR2* heterozygous mutations, again suggesting that dysfunctional BMPR2 is likely insufficient alone to cause disease. As a result, a clear mechanistic explanation of the impact of *BMPR2* mutations on pathogenesis remains elusive.

Additional genetic associations. In addition to mutations of BMPR2, other genetic causes of PAH have been identified in recent years, owing to the advances in genomic sequencing and genome-wide association studies (GWAS).[37] In correlation with the extent of BMPR2 mutations found in hereditary PAH, pathogenic mutations of other BMP/TGF-β superfamily members have been identified in PAH. For instance, a rare group of patients with hereditary hemorrhagic telangiectasia (HHT) and PAH harbor specific mutations in *ALK1* or *endoglin*, genes encoding two such members of the TGF-β receptor superfamily. Other related mutations to BMP/TGF-β signaling include those in the genes *SMAD9* and *caveolin 1*. Rare mutations in the potassium two-pore-domain channel subfamily K member 3 (KCNK3) have been described as pathogenic and thought to control ion channel homeostasis and electrical conduction in diseased PASMCs.[38] By candidate gene strategy approaches, mutations in the gene encoding T-box 4 have been identified in 10% to 30% of pediatric PAH patients, but rarely in adults with PAH. A GWAS identified an association at the CBLN2 locus with PAH[39] but has been difficult to replicate in independent cohorts. Finally, biallelic EIF2AK4 mutations[40] have been identified as a cause of pulmonary veno-occlusive disease (PVOD), a related form of PAH; in some cases, these mutations have been found in PAH patients,[41] either singly or accompanied by BMPR2 mutations.[42] (Additional genes including the water channel AQP1, the ATPase ATP13A3, and more recently Sox17 and HLA-DPA1/DPB1 have been implicated in hereditary PAH.[16a,16b])

Modifier genes. In addition to these primary gene mutations, alternative mechanisms involving complementary "modifier" genes may also contribute to a genetic predisposition to PAH. The most promising data identifying such modifier genes have analyzed the association of particular single nucleotide polymorphisms (SNPs) with the development of PAH. Some analyses of specific SNP variants have suggested certain genes, such as the serotonin transporter (SERT), *Kv1.5*, and the TRP cation channel, subfamily C, member 6 (*TRPC6*).[16] Such associations may not reflect a causal relationship, and thus additional mechanistic data are necessary for proper interpretation.

Acquired/Exogenous Factors

In addition to genetic predisposition, development of PAH likely depends on a variety of physiologic, acquired, and/or exogenous stimuli. Some of these factors have been studied to a sufficient degree to hypothesize a potential pathogenic mechanism(s) (see Fig. 55.3).

Gender predisposition and paradox. In idiopathic PAH, a paradigm of sex predisposition has evolved. Historically, the incidence and prevalence of PAH has been demonstrably higher in females as compared with males in multiple cohort registries. For example, the REVEAL registry, based in the United States, reported a female to male ratio of 4.1:1 in idiopathic PAH patients as compared with a published French registry (1.9:1) and the National Institutes of Health registry (1.7:1).[43–45] A female bias was also reported in other subtypes of Group 1 PAH, including PAH due to congenital heart disease (2.8:1), PAH due to connective tissue disease (9.1:1), and PAH secondary to drugs and toxins (5.4:1).[43] However, a clinical paradox has emerged. Namely, these registries have suggested that when males develop PAH, they tend to present at a much earlier age and have poorer prognosis and survival.[43] Thus increased female susceptibility to disease is balanced by enhanced survival compared with males.

The molecular bases for these observations remain incompletely described. Recent advances have focused on alterations of sex-hormone signaling, mainly in regard to estrogen and its related metabolites. Historically, this concept has been based on observations that PAH has been associated with oral contraceptive (OCP) use. Hormone replacement therapy has also been associated with severe PAH in postmenopausal women. However, a direct mechanistic link between estrogen and PAH has been challenging to prove, given a separate paradoxical finding that many standardized rodent models of PAH are protected from disease with estrogen.[46] Importantly, there are some specialized genetically altered rodent models in which PAH is more prevalent in females. Notably, in rats exposed to both SU5416 (a VEGF2 receptor antagonist) with chronic hypoxia, the aromatase inhibitor anastrozole,[47] an anti–breast cancer drug that prevents the production of estrogen, and metformin,[48] an antidiabetic drug that also inhibits aromatase, both protect against PAH. Clinical trials of anastrazole[49] in PAH are ongoing. Furthermore, recent genetic evidence from mice genetically deficient in both estrogen receptors has indicated that lack of estrogen signaling protects against PAH in BMPR2 mutant mice via reducing the burden of metabolic deficiencies in the pulmonary vasculature.[50] Estrogens may interact with several modifying factors such as serotonin[51–53] and BMPR2[54,55] to enhance potential damaging effects of estrogens on the pulmonary vasculature. Androgens, such as dehydroepiandrosterone, may also contribute but via incompletely described mechanisms. Interestingly, recent data from animal models have proposed a chromosomal explanation for the sex disparity in that the presence of the male Y chromosome can protect against PAH.[56] Currently, it is thought that estrogens or differential sex hormone metabolism influence PAH risk among susceptible subjects in a context-specific manner.[57] Yet it remains unclear why all estrogens and related metabolites do not behave similarly and sometimes paradoxically. Moreover, it is not fully known which factors and pathways may synergize with these hormones to converge on disease manifestation.

901

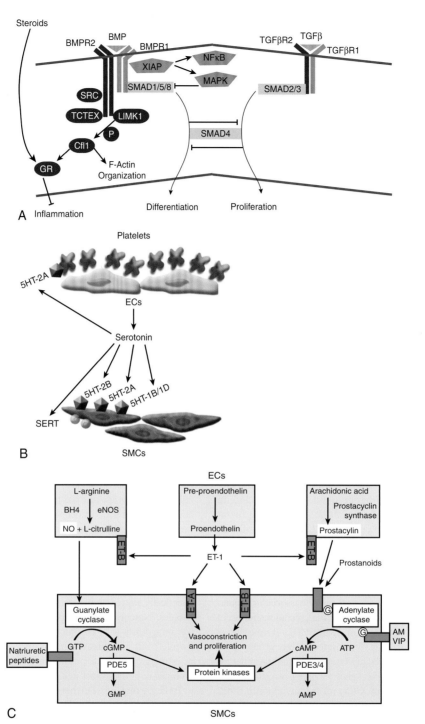

Fig. 55.4 Examples of Molecular Signaling Mechanisms of Pulmonary Arterial Hypertension. (A) BMPR2 signaling in the pulmonary vasculature. Heterozygous loss-of-function mutations in *BMPR2* are found throughout the gene, leading to a complex cascade of dysregulated signaling that predispose to pulmonary arterial hypertension (PAH). When activated by a BMP ligand, BMPR2 heterodimerizes with *BMPR1* to activate *SMAD* transcription factors. SMAD activity can control cellular differentiation, vascular tone, and proliferation, among other functions. BMPR1 can also activate signaling through *XIAP* (X-linked inhibitor of apoptosis), which controls activation of the nuclear factor κB *(NFκB)* and mitogen-activated protein kinase *(MAPK)*, both of which facilitate proinflammatory signaling. BMPR2 also carries a long cytoplasmic tail that binds to numerous intracellular signaling molecules, including *SRC, TCTEX, RACK1* (receptor for activated C-kinase 1), and *LIMK1* (LIM domain kinase 1). LIMK1 can phosphorylate cofilin *(Cfl1)*, which influences F-actin organization and glucocorticoid receptor *(GR)* nuclear translocation, important in inflammation. (B) Serotonin signaling in the pulmonary vasculature. Increased serotonin bioavailability is observed during PAH progression. This stems from increased release by platelets and increased production by endothelial cells. On vascular smooth muscle cells, serotonin receptors *(5HT-2A, 5HT-2B, 5HT-1B/1D)* are activated and induce vasoconstriction and remodeling. Overexpression of the serotonin transporter *(SERT)* enhances the mitogenic effect of serotonin.

(see legend on opposite page)

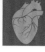

Chronic hypoxia and pseudo-hypoxic HIF-dependent signaling.
The pulmonary vascular response to hypoxia has been well studied in cell culture and in animal models,[58] but its full impact on PAH is unclear. In general, pulmonary vascular responses in acute and chronic hypoxia are thought to drive WHO Group 3 PH due to chronic lung disease. Yet, at least in part, these cellular events in chronic hypoxia overlap with the remodeling events in end-stage PAH. Indeed, various forms of PAH have demonstrated the vascular upregulation of the master transcription factors of hypoxia, HIF-1α and HIF-2α, thus driving the "pseudohypoxic" cellular reprogramming important in disease progression.[59] Recent work with mice carrying conditional genetic deficiencies of these transcription factors have implicated specifically endothelial HIF-2α[60–62] as essential to the development of severe PAH, at least in mouse models of PAH. Acute hypoxia induces vasodilation in systemic vessels but induces vasoconstriction in pulmonary arteries. This acute and reversible effect is mediated in part by upregulation of endothelin-1 (ET-1) and serotonin, and also in part by hypoxia- and redox-sensitive potassium channel activity in pulmonary vascular smooth muscle cells. Coordinately, these events lead to membrane depolarization in smooth muscle cells, increase in cytosolic calcium, and vasoconstriction. In contrast, chronic hypoxia and HIF-activation induce a range of vascular cell reprogramming events. In PASMCs and PAAFs, these events are centered on a profound metabolic shift favoring glycolysis over oxidative metabolism, proliferation, migration; and deposition, remodeling, and crosslinking of ECM.[63] In PAECs, these events influence angiogenesis, elaboration of vasoactive effectors promoting vasoconstriction, and, more recently described, endothelial-to-mesenchymal transition.[62] However, because the histopathology of hypoxic PH does not recapitulate all aspects of PAH, further mechanistic differences in pathogenesis certainly exist but have not yet been fully identified. These are important considerations, especially in the context of interpreting studies of hypoxic PH and extrapolating those findings to the pathogenesis of PAH.

Connective tissue disease. Pulmonary arteriopathy complicates autoimmune diseases, especially in the setting of the CREST variant of limited systemic sclerosis and, to a lesser degree, in mixed connective tissue disease, systemic lupus erythematosus (SLE), and rheumatoid arthritis, as recently reviewed.[64] PAH has been reported in approximately 10% to 30% of patients with mixed connective tissue disease, 5% to 10% of patients with SLE, and more rarely in the settings of rheumatoid arthritis, dermatomyositis, and polymyositis. Sjögren syndrome may rarely be complicated by rapidly progressive PAH. It is particularly important to distinguish between PAH and thromboembolic PH in patients with SLE and antiphospholipid syndrome. The occurrence of PAH in each disease has been associated with the Raynaud phenomenon, suggesting at least some similarities in pathogenesis. The presence of interstitial lung disease and pulmonary fibrosis, seen

at varying frequency in these autoimmune syndromes, may represent a common pathogenic factor in the development of PAH. More recently, significant perivascular inflammation has been hypothesized as a key feature linking various subtypes of PAH, including those associated with autoimmune diseases, which may increase vasoconstriction, proliferation, and vessel remodeling. Murine models of interstitial lung disease and/or autoimmune disease may prove important in further elucidating the pathogenic mechanisms.

Portopulmonary hypertension. Portopulmonary hypertension is defined as PAH associated with portal hypertension (portal pressure > 10 mm Hg), with or without hepatic disease, as reviewed previously.[65] Approximately 9% of patients with severe PAH are reported to have portal hypertension. The diagnosis of PH is usually made 4 to 7 years after the diagnosis of portal hypertension, but it has occasionally been reported to precede the onset of portal hypertension. The correlation between the severity of portal hypertension and the development of PH is debated. The female predominance of primary PAH is not seen in this form of PAH. Because patients with nonhepatic causes of portal hypertension have been reported with this entity, it appears that it is the portal hypertension and not cirrhosis that triggers the development of PAH, yet the molecular mediators of portopulmonary hypertension are unknown. Hypotheses include an inability of the liver to metabolize serotonin and other vasoactive substances. Alternatively, the shear stress from increased pulmonary blood flow may result in endothelial injury, triggering a cascade of events that result in the characteristic adverse remodeling described earlier. The circulating marker macrophage migration inhibitory factor (MIF) has recently been proposed as a specific biomarker of portopulmonary hypertension, but its importance in promoting direct pathogenesis of this form of PAH is unclear.[66] The risk of PH increases with duration of disease and tends to have a much worse prognosis than other forms of PAH. Notably, survival of portopulmonary hypertension patients in the United Kingdom National Pulmonary Hypertension Service was found to be worse than patients with idiopathic PAH, despite the advent of targeted pulmonary vasodilator therapy.[67] Portopulmonary hypertension affects 4% to 6% of patients referred for liver transplantation. Although perioperative mortality in these patients is significantly increased in patients with a mean PAP greater than 35 mm Hg, recent retrospective studies have indicated stabilization and sometimes reversal of portopulmonary hypertension when using a combination of liver transplantation and targeted therapy.[68] However, randomized control trials are lacking in the study of this form of PAH, thus making any treatment recommendations much less definitive.

Drugs/toxins. Exposure to a number of drugs and toxins has been associated with PAH, but not all such toxins have been established as true pathogenic causes.[69,70] Anorexigens have been confirmed as causes for at least two separate outbreaks of PAH. In the 1960s, aminorex

Fig. 55.4, cont'd Furthermore, serotonin receptors on platelets potentiate aggregation. (C) Nitric oxide, endothelin-1, and prostacyclin are dysregulated vasoactive effectors in PAH. In the pulmonary vasculature, nitric oxide *(NO)* is predominantly generated in endothelial cells and is transported to vascular smooth muscle cells; there, it stimulates production of cyclic guanosine monophosphate *(cGMP)* to induce vasorelaxation and to decrease proliferation. Endothelin-1 is also predominantly synthesized and released from endothelial cells. It activates endothelin receptor subtype A *(ET-A)* on smooth muscle cells to induce vasoconstriction and proliferation, while it stimulates nitric oxide and prostacyclin release via endothelin receptor subtype B *(ET-B)* on endothelial cells. Prostacyclin is produced from arachidonic acid and released from endothelial cells. In vascular smooth muscle cells, it activates production of cyclic adenosine monophosphate *(cAMP)* to promote vasorelaxation and inhibit proliferation. In PAH, nitric oxide and prostacyclin levels are significantly reduced while endothelin-1 levels are markedly elevated. This leads to a profound imbalance of these vasoactive effectors and exaggerated vasoconstriction and abnormal vascular smooth muscle proliferation. *AM,* Adrenomedullin; *BH₄,* tetrahydrobiopterin; *PDE,* phosphodiesterase; *VIP,* vasoactive intestinal peptide.(Modified from Archer SL, Weir EK, Wilkins MR. Basic science of pulmonary arterial hypertension for clinicians: new concepts and experimental therapies. *Circulation.* 2010;121:2045–2066.)

fumarate was marketed as an over-the-counter appetite suppressant in Europe, which led to a 10-fold increase of PAH over the next 7 years in Austria, Germany, and Switzerland. Similarly, in 1996, fenfluramine/ phentermine was a combined appetite suppressant approved by the Food and Drug Administration for marketing in the United States. A 23-fold increase of PAH was reported after taking this drug combination for 3 months. While different classes of drugs, these medications may carry similarities in promoting the expression of specific vascular mitogens. In the case of aminorex, its pharmacological effects are thought to be based mainly in the release of catecholamines, which themselves can increase vasoconstriction. In the case of fenfluramine/ phentermine, this drug combination is thought to act as an inhibitor of serotonin reuptake and stimulator of serotonin secretion, thereby leading to increased levels of circulating, free serotonin. Serotonin is both a vasoconstrictor and mitogen that promotes smooth muscle hyperplasia and hypertrophy (see Fig. 55.4B), and many lines of genetic and pharmacologic evidence now point to the dysregulation of serotonin and its signaling and transport pathways as causative for PAH. More recently, stimulants of the central nervous system, such as methamphetamines and cocaine, have become a more prevalent cause of PAH. In particular, methamphetamine-induced PAH is a severe disease subtype and portends a worse prognosis than other forms of PAH.[71] The importance of serotonin release[72] has been suggested in the mechanisms of methamphetamine-induced PAH; however, more recent studies have indicated a more complex yet still undefined pathogenic explanation, implicating endothelial mitochondrial dysregulation and DNA damage[73] and autophagy[74] in disease progression.

Human immunodeficiency virus. HIV infection predisposes to the development of PAH. There are epidemiologic challenges when studying the HIV-PAH population that have led to evolving notions of the exact prevalence of this disease. Originally, prevalence was estimated at 0.5% of HIV-positive individuals.[75] However, echocardiographic evidence indicates that many more HIV-positive individuals suffer from higher pulmonary arterial systolic pressures (PASP) and right ventricle (RV) dysfunction in Africa and in the United States,[76,77] with extrapolations of 1.2 to 3.4 million people in sub-Saharan Africa potentially exhibiting elevated pressures.[4] Importantly, mortality risk in HIV-positive US veterans has been documented to be greater in all persons with higher PASPs.[77] Notably, because echocardiography does not always correlate with invasive pressure measurements, it is unclear if echocardiographic estimates may suggest more subtle or early forms of pulmonary vascular dysfunction rather than overt PAH. However, the global majority of HIV-PAH patients does not have access to invasive hemodynamic study. Thus there is a pressing need to understand the underlying pathogenesis of HIV-PAH in order to design more accurate and noninvasive diagnostics that can track the underlying molecular mechanisms of disease.

Insights into the molecular pathogenesis of HIV-PAH are sparse. Depending on active HIV replication, suppressive antiretroviral therapy (ART) may ameliorate it.[78] Yet ART neither prevents nor cures PAH. Direct HIV infection of the vasculature has not been observed. Contributing mechanisms may include effects of HIV viral proteins such as Nef,[79,80] Tat,[81] and gp120 or the HIV coreceptor CCR5[82]; immune activation induced by HIV or comorbid infections; or risk factors (i.e., drug use[83–85]) in the HIV population. Diastolic left ventricular dysfunction may also contribute, as well.[86] It had been proposed that human herpes virus 8 (HHV-8), the causative agent of Kaposi sarcoma and an opportunistic pathogen highly associated with HIV infection, may play a role in PAH development with progression to plexiform lesions, but that link has not been consistently validated after study of additional populations. Ultimately, HIV-induced PAH likely results from multifactorial effects, and the underlying pathogenesis may involve both direct results of viral infection and indirect consequences of associated pathogens.

Schistosomiasis. Exposure to the parasite *Schistosoma mansoni* accounts for the most frequent cause of PAH in the developing world. While antiparasitic medications and prevention strategies are effective in the treatment of this subtype of PAH, economic, cultural, and political barriers have led to substantial prevalence of this tropical disease. At the molecular level, schistosomiasis-associated PAH is characterized by altered vascular TGF-β signaling, similar to other idiopathic, heritable, and autoimmune-based causes. Recently, the secreted effector thrombospondin-1 (TSP-1) was identified as a key upstream regulator of TGF-β activation and was both necessary and sufficient for developing PAH in Schistosoma-exposed mice. Pharmacologic TSP-1 blockade prevented experimental PAH and thus is being explored as a therapeutic approach for this subtype of PAH and perhaps other TGF-β-dependent vascular diseases.[87]

Congenital heart disease and shunt physiology. Increased flow through the pulmonary circulation has long been associated with development of PAH.[88] Certain types of congenital heart disease with functional systemic-to-pulmonary shunts, such as unrestricted ventricular septal defects (VSDs) and large patent ductus arteriosus (PDA), invariably lead to pulmonary vascular remodeling and the clinical syndrome of PAH during childhood (Eisenmenger syndrome). Approximately one-third of patients with uncorrected VSDs and PDAs die from PAH. The timing of surgical repair greatly influences the outcome. If the shunt is repaired within the first 8 months of life, patients tend to have normal pulmonary pressures regardless of pathologic findings; by contrast, patients operated on after age 2 tend to have persistent PAH. Importantly, when PVR equals or exceeds systemic vascular resistance, surgical correction of a shunt will increase the load on an already overburdened RV, worsen the clinical condition of the patient, and not reverse PAH.

The presence of atrial septal defects (ASDs) with systemic to pulmonary shunts may also lead to PAH over time. Yet, in contrast with cases of unrestricted VSD and PDA, only 10% to 20% of all persons with ASD progress to PAH. This observation may reflect differences in the response of the pulmonary vasculature to pressure overload (as seen in shunts with VSD and PDA) as compared with volume overload (as seen in shunts with ASD). Furthermore, patients with ASD may harbor a specific, unidentified genetic predisposition to the development of PAH that may exacerbate the increased volume load to the pulmonary circulation. Yet data supporting this hypothesis are scarce.

At the molecular level, the physiologic flow patterns of laminar shear stress, turbulent flow, and cyclic strain are all sensed by endothelial cells, leading to transduction of intracellular signals and modulation of a wide variety of phenotypic changes. Significant prior work has focused mainly on the endothelium of the peripheral vasculature, suggesting that laminar flow induces a vasoprotective, quiescent vascular state, while turbulent flow leads to a proinflammatory and thrombogenic state. It is unclear if these flow-dependent phenotypes are recapitulated in the pulmonary vasculature. In part, this stems from the difficulty of directly studying the in vivo or ex vivo flow patterns at the anatomic level of the pulmonary arteriole. Alternatively, studies of large animal models of pulmonary overcirculation have yielded mechanistic insights, implicating dysregulation of endothelial mitochondrial bioenergetics[89] and reactive oxygen species (ROS) secondary to alterations in carnitine metabolism, nitric oxide synthase (NOS),[90] and PPAR-γ.[91,92] Therefore, chronically elevated flow may allow for the selection of cells with dysregulated endothelial cell growth and resulting clonal or polyclonal expansion to plexiform lesions. More recently, pulmonary overcirculation has been identified as a trigger for PASMC hyperproliferation via a decrease of both mitochondrial oxidative metabolism and glycolysis in favor of flux through the pentose phosphate pathway.[93]

Persistent pulmonary hypertension of the newborn. PPHN is characterized by persistent elevation of PVR, right-to-left shunting, and severe hypoxemia.[94] PPHN can occur with pulmonary parenchymal diseases, including sepsis, meconium aspiration, pneumonia, or maladaptation of the pulmonary vascular bed, or without an apparent cause. Persistent PH in newborns may lead to death during the neonatal period, and severe cases may necessitate extracorporeal membrane oxygenation (ECMO). Approximately 14% to 46% of PPHN survivors develop chronic impairments, such as hearing deficits, chronic lung disease, and cerebral palsy, among other neurodevelopmental disabilities. Alterations in redox signaling[95] and inadequate production of nitric oxide (NO)[96] may be important contributors to persistent PPHN. Inhaled NO is useful in treating this disorder. More recently, other targeted pulmonary vasodilators have been studied as effective therapies in this form of PAH.[94] An expert consensus statement has been released regarding best practices for diagnosis and management of pediatric PAH.[97]

Pulmonary veno-occlusive disease. PVOD is a rare form of PAH defined by specific remodeling of pulmonary venules in the absence of histologic alterations in pulmonary arterioles. In the current WHO PH classification, PVOD and pulmonary capillary hemangiomatosis (PCH) are considered to be variants of PAH and common entities thought to reflect separate manifestations of the same root pathogenesis.[98] Clinically, these disease entities offer challenging diagnostic dilemmas, owing to the difficulty in differentiating their presentations from true PAH affecting the pulmonary arterioles. Yet differentiating PVOD from PAH is an important clinical priority, since PVOD carries a worse prognosis, and on occasion fatal pulmonary edema can result from targeted pulmonary vasodilator therapy use in PAH.[99] An accurate diagnostic algorithm for PVOD has been proposed, based on noninvasive testing utilizing specific oxygen parameters, low diffusing capacity for carbon monoxide, and characteristic signs on high-resolution chest computed tomography.[99] Unfortunately, there is a lack of evidence-based recommendations for medical therapy of PVOD. Lung transplantation is the preferred definitive therapy for eligible patients. Molecular pathogenesis is still unclear. Prior studies have implicated the Ets transcription factor Erg and its partner the apelin receptor Aplnr in the pathogenesis of PVOD.[100] Moreover, the recent discovery of biallelic mutations in the *EIF2AK4* gene as a heritable cause of PVOD[40] may spur substantial insight into the origins of this disease subtype in the near future.

Vascular Effectors

Downstream of the genetic and acquired triggers of PAH, the histopathologic processes that predominate later stages of disease include vasoconstriction, cellular proliferation, and thrombosis. These processes are influenced by a complex and dysregulated balance of vascular effectors that serve as signaling messengers for cell-cell crosstalk, controlling vasodilation and vasoconstriction, growth suppressors and growth factors, and pro- versus antithrombotic mediators. Most of these effectors have been described in previous comprehensive reviews and will be described here specifically with regard to their known roles in the pathogenesis of PAH (Table 55.1).

Nitric oxide. Gaseous vasoactive molecules regulate pulmonary vascular homeostasis, and alterations in their endogenous production have been linked to the progression of PAH. NO is the best described of these factors (see Fig. 55.4C). It is a potent pulmonary arterial vasodilator, as well as a direct inhibitor of platelet activation and vascular smooth muscle cell proliferation. NO diffuses into recipient cells (such as vascular muscle), where it activates soluble guanylyl cyclase (sGC) to produce cyclic guanosine monophosphate (cGMP). In turn, cGMP interacts with at least three different groups of effectors: cGMP-dependent protein kinases, cGMP-regulated phosphodiesterase (PDE), and cyclic-nucleotide-gated ion channels. The synthesis of NO is mediated by a family of NOS enzymes. In the pulmonary vasculature, the endothelial isoform (eNOS) figures most prominently and is regulated by a multitude of vasoactive factors and physiologic stimuli, including hypoxia, inflammation, and oxidative stress. Reduced levels and reduced activity of eNOS, reduced NO bioavailability, dysregulated intracellular NO transport via caveolae, and increased degradation of cGMP all aggravate PAH progression in human studies and/or animal models. Dysregulation of NO may also depend on still incompletely characterized processes of NO transport in blood. Specific polymorphisms of NOS have also been associated with PH. Together, these effects indicate a coordinated mechanism of dysregulated vasoconstriction. Correspondingly, murine models that genetically lack eNOS, GTP cyclohydrolase-1 (the rate limiting enzyme for synthesis of an essential cofactor of NOS, tetrahydrobiopterin), or dimethylarginine dimethylaminohydrolase (DDAH, an enzyme important in degradation of NOS inhibitors) all display exaggerated susceptibility to developing PH in response to other endogenous stimuli.[16] Finally, the impact of

	Change in Activity in PAH	Effect on Vasoconstriction	Effect on Cell Proliferation	Effect on Thrombosis
Vascular Effector				
Serotonin	Increased	Increased	Increased	Increased
Nitric oxide	Decreased (increased in plexiform lesions)	Increased	(?) Increased in plexiform lesions	Increased
Thromboxane A2	Increased	Increased	Increased	Increased
Prostacyclin	Decreased	Increased	Increased	Increased
Endothelin-1	Increased	Increased	Increased	(N/A)
Vasoactive intestinal peptide (VIP)	Decreased	Increased	Increased	Increased
Natriuretic peptides	Increased (from cardiomyocyte stretch)	Increased	(?) Decreased	(N/A)
Notch ligands	Increased	(N/A)	Increased	(N/A)

TABLE 55.1   Secreted Vascular Effectors in Pulmonary Arterial Hypertension

PAH, Pulmonary arterial hypertension.

NO has been reflected in its therapeutic role in PAH, such as inhaled NO, NO intermediates such as nitrate and nitrite,[101] and the NO-dependent PDE5 inhibitors (discussed in detail later).

Prostacyclin/thromboxanes. The arachidonic acid metabolites prostacyclin and thromboxane A_2 also play crucial roles in vasoconstriction, thrombosis, and, to a certain degree, cell proliferation in the vessel wall (see Fig. 55.4C). Prostacyclin (prostaglandin I_2) activates cyclic adenosine monophosphate (cAMP)–dependent pathways and serves as a vasodilator, an antiproliferative agent for vascular smooth muscle, and an inhibitor of platelet activation and aggregation. In contrast, thromboxane A_2 increases vasoconstriction and activates platelets. Protein levels of prostacyclin synthase are decreased in small- and medium-sized pulmonary arteries in patients with PAH, particularly with the idiopathic form. Biochemical analysis of urine in patients with PAH has shown decreased levels of a breakdown product of prostacyclin (6-keto-prostacyclin F_2alpha), accompanied by increased levels of a metabolite of thromboxane A_2 (thromboxane B_2). Therefore, it appears that production of these effectors is coordinately regulated with the imbalance toward thromboxane A_2 favored in the development of PAH. The mode of this regulation remains to be characterized. Nonetheless, recognition of this imbalance has led to the success of prostacyclin therapy and improvement of hemodynamics, clinical status, and survival in patients with severe PAH.

Endothelin-1. ET-1 is expressed by pulmonary endothelial cells and has been identified as a significant vascular mediator in PAH (see Fig. 55.4C). It acts as both a potent pulmonary arterial vasoconstrictor and mitogen of pulmonary smooth muscle cells. The vasoconstrictor response relies on binding to the endothelin receptor A (ET-A) on vascular smooth muscle cells, which leads to an increase in intracellular calcium, along with activation of protein kinase C, mitogen-activated protein kinase, and the early growth response genes c-*fos* and c-*jun*. The mitogenic action of ET-1 on pulmonary vascular smooth muscle cells can occur through either the ET-A and/or the ET-B receptor subtype, depending on the anatomic location of cells. ET-A predominantly mediates mitogenesis in the main pulmonary artery, whereas mitogenesis in resistance arteries relies on contributions from both subtypes. The resulting vasoconstriction, mitogenesis, and vascular remodeling are thought to lead to significant hemodynamic changes in the pulmonary vasculature and to PAH. Plasma levels of ET-1 are increased in animal and human subjects suffering from PAH due to a variety of etiologies and correlate with disease severity. Again, improvements in hemodynamics, clinical status, and survival of PAH patients treated with chronic ET receptor antagonists highlight the significance of these effects.

Serotonin. As described previously, serotonin is both a vasoconstrictor and mitogen that promotes smooth muscle hyperplasia and hypertrophy (see Fig. 55.4B). Primarily stored in platelet granules, secreted serotonin binds G-protein-coupled serotonin receptors present on PASMCs. Activation of these receptors leads to a decrease in adenylyl cyclase and cyclic AMP, resulting in an increase in contraction. Furthermore, the cell-surface SERT allows for transport of extracellular serotonin into the cytoplasm of smooth muscle cells, thereby activating cellular proliferation directly through the action of serotonin or indirectly via potential pleiotropic mechanisms.

Numerous observations in idiopathic and familial disease, congenital disease, and environmental exposure have implicated the proliferative effects of serotonin in PAH. In idiopathic PAH, pulmonary expression of serotonin receptors is increased, and plasma levels of serotonin are chronically elevated. A mouse model of hypoxic PH parallels these changes. A positive association has been noted among patients with congenital platelet defects in serotonin uptake (i.e., delta storage pool disease) and development of PAH. As discussed

previously, exposure to anorexigens, such as dexfenfluramine, is associated with levels of circulating serotonin. In mice, these changes are accompanied by increased 5-HT receptor type 2B response and inhibition of SERT responses. In humans, these changes correlate with an increased risk for the development of PAH. In addition, the *L*-allelic variant of SERT is associated with increased expression of the transporter and enhanced smooth muscle proliferation. In some human studies, this variant has been associated with an increased risk of PAH in the homozygous population.

Animal models of PH have also implicated the activated serotonin pathway in disease progression. Treatment with serotonin and chronic hypoxia in a rat model led to worsened hemodynamics and increased vessel remodeling. Exposure to increased serotonin led to worsened PH in a *BMPR2* +/− heterozygote murine model. Similarly, overexpression of *SERT* in mice resulted in spontaneous development of PAH in the absence of hypoxia and exaggeration of PH after an hypoxic stimulus.[102] Conversely, vessel remodeling and hypoxic PH are reduced in a *5-HT1B* receptor-null mouse and are abrogated in a *5-HT2B* receptor-null mouse. As a result, serotonin signaling modulates pulmonary smooth muscle function in both normal and disease states and likely contributes to disease progression of PAH. However, attempts at using selective serotonin reuptake inhibitors (SSRIs) as a therapeutic approach have yielded mixed results[16] to date. Thus the exact contribution of this mechanism in PAH needs further clarification.

Notch ligands. The Notch signaling system comprises a number of ligands and transmembrane receptors that regulate normal embryonic development and vascular homeostasis. In PASMCs, Notch3 signaling has been reported to control proliferation and differentiation state,[103] while Notch1 regulates endothelial proliferation and survival.[104] Recent data have indicated a functional link between BMPR2 and TNF signaling with Notch2 signaling in PAH.[105] Therapeutic interventions may be possible to interrupt these pathogenic signaling axes in PAH, but the complexity as well as the essential nature of this system to normal homeostasis may complicate drug development.

Vasoactive intestinal peptide. Downregulation of vasoactive intestinal peptide (VIP) may also play a pathogenic role. VIP is a pulmonary vasodilator, an inhibitor of proliferation of vascular smooth muscle cells, an inhibitor of platelet aggregation, and free radical scavenger. Decreased concentrations of VIP and VIP receptors have been reported in serum and lung tissue of patients with PAH. *VIP*-null mice suffer from moderate PH. Both pulmonary arterial pressure and PVR in humans decrease after treatment with VIP. There are key questions regarding the mode(s) of regulation of VIP expression and the utility of VIP agonists in PAH. Currently, PB1046, a long-acting form of VIP, is under clinical investigation for its efficacy in PAH (NCT03315507).

Natriuretic peptides. The atrial and brain natriuretic peptides (ANP and BNP) are produced by myocardium in response to stretch. They bind guanylyl cyclase receptors (NPR-A and NPR-B) that induce production of cGMP. Increased plasma concentrations of these peptides in PAH have been used as markers of the extent of RV dysfunction. Genetic inactivation of NPR-A in mice is associated with PH; in contrast, administration of ANP ameliorates PAH in rodent models. In addition, inhibition of the metabolic breakdown of natriuretic peptides via neutral endopeptidase inhibitors has shown promise in animal studies of PAH. Human studies have yet to confirm efficacy.

Other vasoactive effectors. Other released vasoactive factors that likely contribute to PAH pathogenesis include the calcium binding protein S100A4/Mts, galectin-3,[106,107] gremlin 1*,[107a] and the vasodilatory gases carbon monoxide[108] and hydrogen sulfide.[109] These may represent important but yet incompletely described pathogenic contributors and possibly novel diagnostic and therapeutic targets for future development. Furthermore, other mitogenic and angiogenic growth factors such vascular endothelial growth factor (VEGF), platelet derived growth factor (PDGF), basic fibroblast growth factor (FGF2), insulin-like growth factor-1 (IGF1), and epidermal growth factor (EGF) all have been found to play downstream roles in later stages of PAH.

Pathogenic Pathways

While our understanding of the specific actions of released vascular effectors has improved, how they relate to upstream genetic or exogenous triggers of PAH remains unclear. Insight into this topic is offered by the fact that the previously cited effectors are likely subject to upstream, overarching regulatory pathways that modulate the action of multiple pathogenic molecules. Characterization of these regulatory mechanisms may eventually allow for identification of primary molecular triggers of disease and offer novel therapeutic targets for drug development (see Fig. 55.3).

Cancer theory of pulmonary arterial hypertension. The acceleration of discovery of numerous reprogrammed molecular pathways integral to PAH pathogenesis has led the way to comparisons of diseased pulmonary vascular cell transformation to carcinogenesis and cancer progression. Based on in vitro, in vivo, and in situ observations in animal and human models of PAH, there are overarching molecular and cellular similarities in the structural and functional vascular alterations in PAH with tumor formation and growth, particularly when compared with the traditional "hallmarks of cancer," as proposed by Hanahan and Weinberg.[110] These include a profound metabolic shift favoring glycolysis over oxidative mitochondrial metabolism, clonal vascular cell growth and unchecked cell survival at end-stage PAH, alterations in angiogenesis and vasomotor tone, increased DNA damage and genome instability, and activation of inflammation while avoiding immune destruction.[111] Multiple tumor markers, such as survivin, have also been found to be expressed in diseased pulmonary vascular cells such as PASMCs. All appear to contribute substantially to the overall obstructive arterial remodeling characteristic of PAH via synergistic and combinatorial pathways. Interestingly, a recent report has described a connection between lung cancer and the development of PAH.[17]

As in numerous cancers, end stages of PAH are marked by exaggerated expression or activity of multiple growth factors, including PDGF, FGF1, FGF2, EGF, and VEGF. All appear to contribute substantially to the overall obstructive arterial remodeling characteristic of PAH via synergistic and combinatorial pathways. Some of the receptors for these growth factors are transmembrane receptor tyrosine kinases that activate a diverse and overlapping set of intracellular signaling pathways. Inhibition of EGF and PDGF receptors has improved hemodynamics and survival in PAH. Buoyed by case reports of a beneficial effect of adding imatinib (a nonselective tyrosine kinase inhibitor) or sorafenib (a "multikinase inhibitor") to baseline PAH therapy, clinical trials of imatinib in PAH have been pursued. Although improvement of exercise capacity was observed in PAH patients taking imatinib, that benefit was outweighed by adverse events including intracranial bleeding.[112,113] Interestingly, recent data have defined a causative role in PAH for other tyrosine kinase inhibitors such as dasatinib, a drug used in chronic myelogenous leukemia.[114,115] While the pursuit of repurposing chemotherapeutics for PAH continues, lessons regarding both the beneficial and toxic effects of tyrosine kinase inhibitors in PAH should be closely considered. As such, while cancer-like phenotypes alone cannot fully explain PAH, the rapid pace of discovery into cancer pathogenesis suggests that further comparisons among these diseases may yield valuable insights that could usher in a new generation of diagnostics and therapeutics for this condition, as well.

Mitochondrial metabolism and oxidative stress. Over the past 15 years, the profound metabolic and mitochondrial shift observed in both diseased pulmonary vascular cell types and right ventricular (RV) cardiomyocytes in PAH has emerged as a leading candidate in the quest to identify an overarching regulator of pathogenesis. Metabolic alterations in affected vascular and cardiac tissues of PH patients have been observed—notable even during the development of disease rather than just at the end stage.[116] In the setting of hereditary PAH, BMPR2 haploinsufficiency has been linked to metabolic reprogramming.[6] Functional connections have also been reported between such metabolic dysfunction and autoimmune diseases such as scleroderma[117] and HIV infection[118] that predispose to the development of PAH. It is important to emphasize that coupled with these changes in mitochondrial metabolism are alterations of ROS/reactive nitrogen species (RNS), including hydrogen peroxide, superoxide, and peroxynitrite, which increase in PAH relative to antioxidants. These molecules are well-described second messenger molecules that are involved in functional oxidative and nitrosative modification of proteins and have been substantially implicated in the underlying pathophysiology of PAH. These alterations have previously been described in detail[119] and will be discussed as follows in relation to the metabolic reprogramming in which they participate.

In general, multiple diseased vascular cell types and cardiomyocytes preferentially exhibit a downregulation of mitochondrial metabolism with an induction of glycolysis for energy production. Under hypoxic conditions, this so-called Pasteur effect is a normal adaptive event that improves cellular survival by optimizing ATP production while reducing oxygen radicals generated from the mitochondrial electron transport chain. Under normoxic conditions, however, such a shift to glycolysis ("the Warburg effect") is thought to confer inappropriately resistance to apoptosis and is prominently seen in various cancer lineages. Such metabolic changes in the mitochondria are primarily dependent on altered expression of the master transcription factors of hypoxia, HIF-1α and HIF-2α, as previously reviewed.[63] Among the first HIF-responsive genes implicated in the Warburg effect in PH is the mitochondrial enzyme pyruvate dehydrogenase kinase (PDK). This enzyme is well-established as a gatekeeper of oxidative metabolism, and its expression is known to be increased in response to hypoxia and also in PAH.[16] Dichloroacetate (DCA), an inhibitor of PDK developed as a cancer therapeutic, has shown efficacy in improving PAH in a number of animal models of PAH. The beneficial effects of DCA in specific contexts of human PAH lacking specific mutations in the genes *SIRT3* and *UCP2* have recently been reported.[120] Alterations to the tricarboxylic acid (TCA) cycle and its intermediates can also stabilize HIF and modulate PAH, including α-ketoglutarate (α-KG), a cofactor for prolyl hydroxylation and HIF degradation, and the TCA enzyme isocitrate dehydrogenase (IDH), which converts α-KG into isocitrate. Other TCA metabolites can also inhibit prolyl hydroxylation and activate HIF. For example, hypoxia increases the rate at which α-KG is reduced to 2-hydroxyglutarate (2HG), and the *L*- and *D*- enantiomers (L2HG and D2HG) can inhibit prolyl hydroxylation of HIF.[121] In human pulmonary vascular cell types, hypoxia increases L2HG levels, thus controlling glycolysis and oxidative phosphorylation.[122] The influence of TCA cycle intermediates has epigenetic implications, as acetylation and methylation of nuclear histones are regulated by citrate and α-KG, respectively.[121]

Control of iron handling has also emerged as a key metabolic pathway modulating HIF biology, and iron deficiency has previously been reported in PAH populations.[123] Specifically, microRNA-210 (miR-210), a transcriptional target of HIF and key hypoxamir,[123a] was found to downregulate expression of the iron-sulfur (Fe-S) cluster assembly proteins 1 and 2 (ISCU1/2), thus altering mitochondrial electron transport as well as in vivo manifestations of PAH in animal models and a human subject with genetic deficiency in ISCU1/2.[124] PAH has also been reported in infants with a genetic deficiency in NFU1, another Fe-S cluster assembly protein.[125] Iron can also directly regulate the expression of HIF-1α and HIF-2α. Iron-dependent prolyl hydroxylases regulate HIF protein stability, and iron deficiency decreases such hydroxylase activity and promotes HIF stability. In vivo, iron-deficient rats have been found to display HIF upregulation, decreased mitochondrial activity, and pulmonary vascular remodeling; these manifestations of PAH were reversed with iron replacement therapy.[126] Iron deficiency also was found to be associated with elevated hepcidin,[123] which, in turn, can predispose to PAH and could serve as an additional therapeutic target. Furthermore, iron-regulatory proteins such as Irp1 are known to be influenced by both iron levels and hypoxia. Irp1-deficient mice display increased HIF-2α and develop PH.[127]

Beyond the Warburg effect, the proliferative, antiapoptotic, and glycolytic processes seen in the diseased PAH vessels have been linked to additional metabolic processes. Beyond the requisite adenosine triphosphate (ATP) production, sufficient biomass must be generated to support proliferation. Anaplerosis is the replenishing of TCA carbon intermediates via either the glutaminase (GLS1)–mediated deamidation of glutamine or the carboxylation of pyruvate.[128] In multiple subtypes of PAH, it has been reported that two transcriptional coactivators—Yes-associated protein 1 (YAP) and transcriptional coactivator with a PDZ-binding motif (TAZ/WWTR1)—are required for GLS1 upregulation and subsequent glutaminolysis to sustain vascular cell proliferation and migration within stiff pulmonary vessels.[10] TCA cycle and electron transport chain modulations are associated with alterations in ROS, which are known to regulate pulmonary vasodilation or vasoconstriction. The redox-sensitive nuclear factor erythroid 2-related factor 2 (Nrf2) is an example of a transcription factor that decreases ROS generation and subsequent inflammation. A chemical inducer of Nrf2, bardoxolone methyl, is under investigation in a phase II clinical study in PAH patients (NCT02036970).[129] Reviewed in detail previously, ROS dynamics are further influenced in PH by various forms of superoxide dismutase, voltage gated potassium channels (Kv1.5), and L-type voltage gated calcium channels, to name a few.[130]

Alterations of mitochondrial structure and biogenesis, primarily affecting the balance of fission and fusion processes, have been found to drive metabolic alterations in PH. Dynamin-related protein-1 (Drp1) is a GTPase that regulates mitochondrial fission and fragmentation[131] and has been associated with the pro-proliferative vascular state in PH.[132] Decreased levels of mitofusin-2 in PAH have also been implicated in driving mitochondrial fragmentation and an imbalance of proliferation/apoptosis.[133] Pharmacologic inhibition of mitochondrial fission and Drp1 with Mdivi-1[134,135] has been shown to ameliorate both pulmonary vascular and RV dysfunction in animal models of PH. In parallel, decreased activation of peroxisome proliferator-activated receptor-γ coactivator 1α (PGC1α), a transcription factor mediating mitochondrial biogenesis and fission, has been linked to PH.[133] In addition, deficient BMPR2 signaling has been implicated in the control of mitochondrial fission and a proinflammatory state.[6] In combination with PGC1α, Sirtuin 3 (SIRT3), a factor implicated in the control of mitochondrial structure via protein deacetylation, was recently reported to be repressed in rodent PH models, and SIRT3-null mice spontaneously developed PH.[136]

Potassium channel biology. The modulation of voltage-gated potassium channels (Kv) may also represent an overarching pathogenic mechanism of PAH.[16] Kv channels are tetrameric, membrane-spanning channels that selectively conduct potassium ions; in PASMCs, Kv channels aid in the regulation of the resting membrane potential. In response to Kv inhibition or downregulation, depolarization leads to the opening of voltage-gated calcium channels, an increase in intracellular calcium, and the initiation of a number of intracellular signaling cascades promoting vasoconstriction and proliferation and inhibiting apoptosis. Expression array analysis has demonstrated a depletion of Kv1.5 channels in pulmonary tissue derived from PAH patients. It is currently unknown if these Kv channel abnormalities are congenital or acquired; however, a number of polymorphisms in the Kv1.5 channel gene *(KCNA5)* have been described, which may suggest a genetic predisposition to channel depletion. Appetite suppressants, such as dexfenfluramine and aminorex, that are risk factors for development of PAH, can also directly inhibit Kv1.5 and Kv2.1. A variety of transcription factors (HIF-1α, NFAT, and c-Jun) are increased in PAH, with resulting downregulation of the expression of Kv1.5 in PASMCs. The inhibition of these factors consequently increases Kv1.5 expression with resulting improvements in Kv current and, in some cases, improved pulmonary arterial remodeling in hypoxic rodent models of PH. The inhibition of Kv currents in pulmonary smooth muscle cells may be regulated by serotonin, thromboxane A2, and, perhaps, NO. Furthermore, BMP signaling can regulate Kv receptor expression. Taken together, the Kv pathway may represent a common (integrative) point of regulation in pathogenesis. Accordingly, augmentation of Kv activation would be predicted to induce vasodilatation and, perhaps, allow for regression of vessel remodeling. In vivo gene transfer of Kv channels in chronically hypoxic rats has led to improvement of PH and supports its therapeutic potential.

Calcium handling. Contractile and proliferative functions of PASMCs—key cellular actions that promote PAH—depend substantially on intramitochondrial calcium dynamics. Uncoupling protein 2 (UCP2) is a calcium-uniporter that transports calcium from the endoplasmic reticulum (ER) into mitochondria. Genetic studies of UCP2 in cultured PASMCs and PAECs have implicated its function in mitochondrial hyperpolarization, decreased activity of calcium-sensitive mitochondrial enzymes,[137,138] mitophagy, and decreased mitochondrial synthesis.[139] Genetic deficiency of UCP2 in mice increased pulmonary vascular remodeling and promoted the development of PAH.[137,138] In addition, microRNA-dependent impairment of another calcium uniporter—the mitochondrial calcium uniporter complex—resulted in decreased mitochondrial calcium levels and a concomitant PAH phenotype in PASMCs, as well as in PAH rats exposed to monocrotaline.[140] Further downstream, calcium dynamics are dysregulated at the level of the sarco-/endoplasmic reticulum calcium-ATPase (SERCA), a sarcoplasmic reticulum transporter that is downregulated in PAH. Gene transfer of SERCA2a in both rodent and porcine PH models rescued expression of SERCA2 in pulmonary arteries, resulting in decreased PAP and improved RV function.[141,142] Dysregulated calcium homeostasis can also alter electrical dynamics within the cell and mitochondria. Studies have implicated glycolysis in the control of the mitochondrial permeability transition pore, a voltage- and redox-dependent channel that remains closed under hyperpolarized mitochondrial membrane potential and thus promotes cell survival. Calcium sensing receptors (CaSR) can also be activated by alterations in intracellular calcium, promoting the interaction with transient receptor potential cation channels such as TRPC6, further promoting PASMC proliferation and contraction.[143] In general, signaling across multiple TRPC family members has been implicated in calcium-specific alterations in PASMC biology and PAH.[144-146] Finally, the transfer of calcium from the ER to mitochondria, specifically dependent on the protein Nogo-B, has been studied in the pulmonary vasculature and found to be important in the development of PH.[147]

Peroxisome proliferator-activated receptor-gamma signaling. The PPAR-γ may function as an integral factor in PAH.[148] PPARs are ligand-activated nuclear transcription factors that heterodimerize with the retinoid X receptor for subsequent binding to PPAR response elements in the promoters of target genes. PPAR-γ is a direct target of

BMP2 in human PASMCs, leading to stimulation of apolipoprotein E (apoE) synthesis and downstream inhibition of vascular smooth muscle proliferation, as well as dysregulation of WNT signaling in PAECs. Idiopathic PAH patients carry reduced pulmonary transcript levels of PPAR-γ and apoE. A metabolic connection of PPAR-γ with BMP signaling has been suggested via advancing insights into BMPR2 activity in regulating mitochondrial biogenesis and membrane potential, thus promoting a pro-proliferative state.[6] Interestingly, PPAR-γ is a central target of a master microRNA regulator of PAH, the miR-130/301 family, which, in addition to proliferation, can drive vasoconstriction, matrix remodeling, and pulmonary vascular stiffening.[23,149,150] Mice deficient in smooth muscle-specific PPAR-γ are prone to PAH and RV hypertrophy. Similarly, male mice deficient in apoE when fed a high-fat diet develop PAH. This condition is reversed by rosiglitazone, a PPAR-γ agonist. Owing to the increased cardiovascular risk associated with rosiglitazone,[151] clinical testing of PPAR-γ agonists in PAH has been challenging, but this may be changing based on encouraging data in PAH with pioglitazone.[151a]

MicroRNA biology. Over the past decade, our understanding has substantially advanced regarding the pervasive and pleiotropic functions in PAH of an evolutionarily ancient class of molecules called noncoding RNAs (ncRNAs), of which the most widely studied class includes microRNAs (miRNAs).[152] Embedded throughout the human genome, ncRNAs and miRNAs enact widespread transcriptional and post-transcriptional gene regulation. Numerous miRNAs have been studied in cultured pulmonary vascular cells, in various animal models of PH, as well as in human explanted tissues and cells.[152] Relevant to PAH, groups of miRNAs have been found to have convergent actions in controlling relevant molecular signaling pathways, including those involving BMPR2, HIF, PPAR-γ, and estrogen activity. Overlapping miRNAs have also been identified to promote cellular pathophenotypes, including proliferation, mitochondrial metabolism, apoptosis, vasomotor tone, vascular stiffness, and DNA damage. In contrast to these convergent regulatory programs, the targeted pleiotropy of miRNAs has driven the notion that there may exist "master" miRNA regulators of PH that drive pathogenesis via control over numerous, seemingly unrelated, molecular pathways. By combining a computational discovery platform with traditional reductionist biologic examination, miRNAs such as miR-21[153] and the miR-130/301 family[23,149,150,154] have been identified and validated as systems-level regulators of proliferation, vasoconstriction, and matrix remodeling in PAH. Despite the inherent complexity of this system and consequent challenges for drug targeting, this type of systems-level discovery in PH suggests that the divergent activity of specific miRNAs may provide a future opportunity for defining effective diagnostic and therapeutic targets.[155]

Extracellular matrix remodeling. Although the remodeling and stiffening of the pulmonary vascular ECM in PAH has been well known for decades, the study of vascular stiffness as a primary pathogenic driver is an emerging principle in PAH. Stiffness occurs in the proximal and distal pulmonary arterial tree in various forms of PAH,[18,19] and stiffness is an index of disease progression.[20] Vascular ECM remodeling occurs through changes primarily in PAAFs in the balance between collagen and elastin deposition, matrix degradation, and matrix remodeling via collagen crosslinking enzymes such as LOX. Vascular-specific serine elastase activity in the ECM has also been implicated in the pathogenesis of PAH.[156] In pulmonary arterioles, serine elastases are secreted into the extracellular space to activate matrix metalloproteinases (MMPs) and to inhibit tissue inhibitors of MMPs (TIMPs). Both MMPs and elastases degrade most components of the ECM, leading to an upregulation of fibronectin and subsequent enhancement of cellular migration. Matrix degradation also increases integrin signaling with resulting expression of the glycoprotein tenascin C. Tenascin C acts cooperatively with other factors to enhance smooth muscle proliferation.

Increased degradation of elastin has been observed in pulmonary arteries from patients suffering from congenital heart disease and resultant PAH. In pulmonary tissue of PAH patients harboring *BMPR2* mutations and rat models of PAH, increased production and activity of vascular elastases and tenascin C have been reported. This upregulation of elastase function may be induced by a number of vascular effectors implicated in PAH, including NO, serotonin, and, theoretically, the BMP pathway. Elastase inhibitors can induce apoptosis of smooth muscle cells in cell culture and can improve PAH in animal models.

More recently, vascular matrix stiffness has been established as an early, pervasive driver of many types of PAH, controlled by two related transcriptional co-activators, YAP and TAZ/WWTR1, which are members of the overarching Hippo signaling pathway, and downstream induction of the microRNA-130/301 family.[23,150] Importantly, in multiple contexts of human health and disease, YAP and TAZ have been found to be crucial for mechanotransduction, a process that converts extracellular mechanical cues into intracellular signaling[157,158] and is known to regulate proliferation, survival, organ size, and the ECM. Mechanoactivation of YAP/TAZ can promote increased matrix deposition and stiffening, thus propagating vessel stiffness throughout the pulmonary vascular tree in PAH and driving pathogenic vascular crosstalk throughout the vessel wall.[22,23] Independent of YAP/TAZ, pulmonary vessel stiffening has also been driven by a microRNA-dependent process involving the Runt-related transcription factor 2 (Runx2) to promote vascular calcification.[159]

An important intersection of matrix remodeling, metabolic reprogramming, and proliferation has recently been explored. Pulmonary vascular stiffness has been found to induce glutaminase 1 [GLS1] and glutaminolysis, thus replenishing TCA cycle intermediates as described previously (anaplerosis) and providing cellular biomass particularly during glycolysis and driving proliferation in multiple vascular cell types and PAH in vivo.[10] Separately, the activation of metabolic, inflammatory, and proliferative gene regulatory programs has been observed in PAAFs derived from human and bovine (brisket disease) instances of PAH. Notably, these reprogramming events rely heavily on epigenetic alterations via microRNAs, such as miR-124,[160,161] and transcriptional regulators, such as CtBP1.[162] Such molecular advances in our understanding of pulmonary vascular stiffness in PAH present an attractive new cohort of cellular and molecular targets for more precise diagnostic and therapeutic applications in PAH in the future.

Rho kinase signaling. Multiple vascular cell types rely on the rho-kinase signaling pathway for homeostatic function and response to injury.[163] Rho is a guanosine triphosphate (GTP) binding protein that activates its downstream target, rho-kinase, in response to the activation of a variety of G-protein coupled receptors (including those related to BMP/SMAD signaling and serotonin signaling). In vitro activation of these signaling cascades results in the modulation of multiple cellular processes, including enhanced vasoconstriction and proliferation, impaired endothelial response to vasodilators, chronic pulmonary remodeling, and upregulation of vasoactive cytokines via the NF-κB transcription pathway. Rho-kinase activity has also been linked specifically to multiple known effectors of PAH, including ET-1, serotonin, and eNOS, among others. Elevated rho-kinase activity has been demonstrated in animal models of PAH. Furthermore, intravenous fasudil, a selective rho-kinase inhibitor, has induced pulmonary vasodilation and regression of PAH in various animal models, as well as in patients with severe PAH who were otherwise refractory to conventional therapies. Taken together, these data suggest that rho-kinase may control a master molecular "switch" in the pulmonary artery, initiating an activated state in disease from a quiescent state in health. Short-term safety data of fasudil in human PAH are available, but long-term efficacy in PAH has not been assessed.[164]

DNA damage. Recently, genomic instability and DNA damage have been reported in diseased, remodeled vasculature in lungs of both animal and human PAH.[165] Mitochondrial dysfunction, inflammation, and oxidative stress have been shown to play a key role in the development and progression of vascular remodeling and are increasingly being considered as triggers for direct DNA damage. PAH has been linked with decreased breast cancer 1 protein (BRCA1) and DNA topoisomerase 2-binding protein 1 (TopBP1) expression, which are both involved in maintaining genome integrity. An impaired DNA-response mechanism has also been observed in PAH, leading to an increased mutagen sensitivity in PAH patients and perhaps itself driving a pro-proliferative phenotype. These observations correlate well with the cancer model of PAH, while also suggesting the utility of chemotherapeutics in PAH that target DNA damage response pathways.

Right ventricle and skeletal muscle dysfunction. After birth, pulmonary arterial pressures typically decline, leading to involution of the RV to a thin-walled structure in the adult. During pathologic conditions of increased pulmonary arterial pressures in PAH, however, so-called adaptive RV strain and hypertrophy ensue, followed by decompensated RV failure, if left untreated, as recently reviewed.[166] Historically, the molecular pathways governing LV failure, which have been better characterized, had been assumed to play primary roles in RV failure as well. Contemporary evidence suggests there may be distinct molecular and physiological differences between LV and RV failure, which are just beginning to be explored. For example, PDE5, which is expressed in the fetal RV, is selectively upregulated in the hypertrophied RV. Interestingly, the inhibition of PDE5 enhances RV contractility without affecting the LV, where PDE5 expression is absent. However, a key obstacle in understanding this pathophysiology is the lack of a clear definition, both in human and animal examples of PAH, of the physiological and molecular alterations that define adaptive and decompensated changes in the RV.

Unique metabolic changes in the RV have also been reported to drive RV dysfunction. Under nondiseased and baseline activity, fatty acid oxidation (FAO) generates 60% to 90% of energy production in cardiomyocytes, with the remaining 10% to 40% derived from glycolysis and glucose oxidation. A mutually competitive relationship, known as the Randle cycle, exists between these processes. At baseline, increased production of citrate during FAO inhibits phosphofructokinase and leads to an accumulation of glucose-6-phosphate. This metabolite inhibits hexokinase, resulting in a decrease in pyruvate production and further inhibiting glycolysis. Perhaps incited by increased pulmonary arterial pressures and impaired coronary perfusion as a result of advancing RV hypertrophy, initial RV injury in PH is thought to produce an inadequate oxygen supply. Consequently, HIF-1α is activated in cardiomyocytes, thus driving upregulation of glycolytic genes. Via such reprogramming, the RV nearly exclusively relies on glycolysis in PH. AMP-activated protein kinase is activated in RVH, which preserves ATP levels by increasing glucose transport and glycolysis while inhibiting the TCA cycle via repression of acetyl-coenzyme A carboxylase. Furthermore, during RVH, PDK is activated, which also induces a metabolic switch away from oxidative phosphorylation to glycolysis. Inhibition of this process in mice via administration of DCA resulted in increased cardiac output (CO) and function. Targeting the Randle cycle via FAO inhibitors may also be effective, as exhibited by improvement of RV function after administration of FAO inhibitors trimetazidine and ranolazine.[167] FAO inhibitors are under clinical investigation in RV failure and PAH.

Independent of metabolic alterations and RV ischemia, recent data have implicated altered miR-126 activity as a mechanistic cause for failure of both RV cardiomyocytes[168] and skeletal muscle in PAH.[169] Notably, miR-126 is an endothelial-specific, proangiogenic miRNA that when downregulated was found to impair angiogenesis and thus hasten the loss of microcirculation in both muscle types in PAH. It remains to be seen whether other cardiovascular or muscle tissue in other organ systems may be affected by similar processes in PAH, thus suggesting this disease may, in fact, manifest with systemic and syndromic complications rather than simply affect the pulmonary vasculature alone.

CLINICAL PATHOPHYSIOLOGY

The pulmonary vascular bed has a remarkable capacity to dilate and recruit unperfused vessels, adapting easily to large increases in blood flow. In PAH, these properties are lost. RV function is highly afterload dependent and works less efficiently with increases in PVR. With increased afterload, the RV hypertrophies and dilates. In the early stages of PAH, resting PAP remains normal and CO is maintained, but with exercise, PAP becomes abnormally high and the RV is unable to increase CO. With progressive PH, there may eventually be a decrease in the measured PAP due to a decrease in CO, while the PVR remains elevated. Cardiac function is characterized by RV systolic and diastolic overload from tricuspid regurgitation. The left ventricle is not directly affected by pulmonary vascular disease, but when PAP rises to the extent that the RV changes from its normal crescentic shape to expand into the left ventricle recruiting the interventricular septum in the process, it can impair LV filling, increase LV end diastolic pressure, and decrease CO, a phenomenon described as the "reverse Bernheim effect."

The two most frequent causes of death in PAH are progressive RV failure and sudden death. RV failure may be exacerbated by pneumonia, and alveolar hypoxia can cause further vasoconstriction and greater impairment of CO. Sudden death may be caused by arrhythmias that arise in the setting of hypoxemia and acidosis, acute pulmonary emboli, massive pulmonary hemorrhage, and subendocardial RV ischemia.

Diagnostic Evaluation

Initial approach. There is no pathognomonic finding in PAH; thus the diagnosis is one of exclusion. A thorough evaluation must be performed to reveal potentially contributing factors, including causes of secondary forms of PH that require a different treatment approach. It is important to probe for a family history of PH, early unexplained deaths, congenital heart disease, and collagen vascular disease. A complete history should also include all associated risk factors for PH to uncover a possible explanation for the onset of PAH and exclude secondary causes of PH. In addition to a comprehensive history, the diagnostic evaluation should include physical examination, exercise testing (e.g., a 6-minute walk), chest radiograph, electrocardiography, pulmonary function tests (PFTs), arterial blood gas and other blood tests, noninvasive cardiac and pulmonary imaging, and cardiac catheterization with measurement of response to vasodilator administration (Fig. 55.5).

Symptoms. By the time patients develop symptoms, PAH is usually advanced, and CO is often reduced. The nonspecificity of presenting symptoms can cause a long delay in diagnosis in most patients. The most common presenting symptom is dyspnea on exertion, which affects nearly all patients as disease progresses. Other presenting symptoms include fatigue, syncope or near syncope, chest pain, lower extremity edema, and palpitations. Dyspnea may be attributable to impaired oxygen delivery during exercise due to the inability to increase CO to accommodate increased oxygen demand. Syncope occurs when CO is severely limited and inadequate cerebral blood flow with exertion ensues. Chest pain in PAH may be caused by subendocardial RV ischemia.

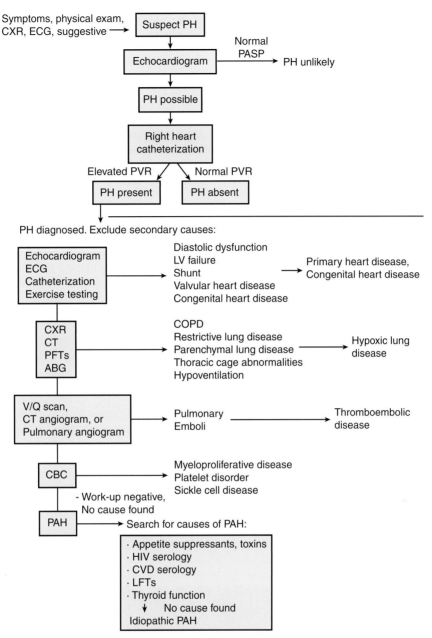

Fig. 55.5 Diagnostic Evaluation for Suspected Pulmonary Arterial Hypertension. Please refer to the subsequent chapter for a discussion of secondary causes of pulmonary hypertension. *ABG*, Arterial blood gas; *CBC*, complete blood count; *COPD*, chronic obstructive pulmonary disease; *CT*, computed tomography scan; *CVD*, collagen vascular disease; *ECG*, electrocardiogram; *HIV*, human immunodeficiency virus; *LFTs*, liver function tests; *LV*, left ventricle; *PAH*, pulmonary arterial hypertension; *PASP*, pulmonary arterial systolic pressure; *PFTs*, pulmonary function tests; *PH*, pulmonary hypertension; *PVR*, pulmonary vascular resistance; *V/Q scan*, ventilation and perfusion nucleotide scan.

Physical findings. Clinical findings in PAH are initially subtle. The first signs of disease may be a right ventricular heave, a loud component of the pulmonic second heart sound, and a right-sided fourth heart sound. Eventually, a right-sided third heart sound and a left parasternal systolic murmur of tricuspid regurgitation may be audible. The findings of jugular venous distension, ascites, and peripheral edema indicate overt right heart failure. Physical examination must include evaluation for signs of specific diseases associated with PAH, including collagen vascular diseases, liver disease, HIV, HHT, thyroid disease, and all secondary causes of PH, including treatable causes such as obstructive sleep apnea (assessed by polysomnography).

Functional class. An overall functional assessment should be made on the basis of the NYHA/WHO functional classification of heart failure. Functional class is an effective predictor of survival.[69,70] Recent studies have reported that worse functional capacity class at presentation is associated with worse 5-year survival,[170] while alterations in functional capacity over time have been correlated positively with survival rates.[171,172] Yet deficiencies have been recognized in relying solely on functional class as a prognostic indicator, given its inherent subjectivity and variability.[173]

Laboratory studies. Secondary causes of PAH should be sought with serology for HIV and connective tissue diseases, liver function tests (LFTs), and toxin exposures. Thyroid function should be evaluated.

Thrombocytopenia may be present in severe PAH and has multiple contributing causes, including platelet activation and aggregation, pulmonary vascular sequestration, hepatosplenomegaly with splenic sequestration of platelets, as well as an autoimmune-mediated syndrome similar to idiopathic thrombocytopenic purpura. Thrombocytopenia may accompany microangiopathic hemolysis when blood flows through fibrin deposits in plexiform lesions with subsequent shearing of red blood cells and activation/deposition of platelets. Thrombocytosis may be present in patients following splenectomy.

In patients with PH, high levels of ANP and BNP or proNT-BNP have paralleled decreased RV function and increased RV strain. Levels of both peptides decrease with targeted pulmonary vasodilator treatment and ensuing hemodynamic improvement. A subsequent increase in plasma BNP has been demonstrated to be an independent predictor of mortality. NT-proBNP may have better prognostic performance than BNP, as reduced levels of NT-proBNP 1 year postdiagnosis have been associated with improvement of 3-[172] and 5-year[174] survival. The search for additional effective, reasonably priced, and accessible prognostic and diagnostic biomarkers for PAH is ongoing.[175]

Radiographic studies. Chest radiographs in PH usually show an enlarged pulmonary trunk and hilar pulmonary arteries, pruning of peripheral vessels, and obliteration of the retrosternal clear space by the enlarged RV (Fig. 55.6). Occasionally, the chest radiograph may appear normal. High-resolution CT is used to evaluate the lung parenchyma for interstitial lung disease. High-resolution CT is also used to evaluate the central pulmonary arteries for the presence of thrombi. Ventilation/perfusion imaging is the preferred modality to rule out chronic pulmonary thromboemboli. In patients with PAH, these scans are normal or show only patchy defects. If inconclusive, a pulmonary angiogram, which will show pruning of peripheral vessels in PAH, must be performed to exclude definitively thromboembolic disease. More recently, CT-determined pulmonary artery diameter:aorta diameter ratios have been used as a noninvasive alternative to diagnose PAH.[176] Moreover, the use of pulmonary magnetic resonance angiography (MRA) to attain automated three-dimensional volumetry has been reported as superior in small cohort studies in identfying PAH as compared with manual measurements on axial images.[177] It remains to

be seen whether such noninvasive tools can be used more extensively in the future to aid diagnosis, particularly in areas of the world that do not have access to invasive hemodynamic testing facilities.

Electrocardiogram. The electrocardiogram (ECG) is not a sensitive nor a specific screening tool in the diagnosis of PAH. In advanced disease, the ECG usually shows signs of right heart strain and enlargement, including right axis deviation and evidence of right ventricular hypertrophy. The presence of a conduction abnormality is not typical of PAH. Electrocardiographic evidence of right heart strain has been associated with decreased survival.

Pulmonary function tests. PFTs are important in excluding secondary causes of PH—particularly chronic obstructive airways disease. Airway obstruction is not typical of PAH, although cases of bronchial obstruction due to enlarged pulmonary arteries have been reported. PAH patients typically demonstrate borderline restrictive physiology, a reduced diffusing capacity for carbon monoxide (D_LCO), and hypoxemia with hypocapnia. The reduction in D_LCO results from the reduced blood volume in the alveolar capillaries. Recent data indicate that low D_LCO, particularly in PAH patients with connective tissue diseases, may portend poor survival.[178]

Echocardiography. Transthoracic echocardiography is a crucial diagnostic tool in evaluating patients for PAH, monitoring efficacy of treatment options, and detecting early or preclinical stages of disease.[179] It can determine the presence of left-sided heart disease, valvular disease, and intracardiac shunts, and it allows for the noninvasive measurement of PAP. A finding of an elevated PAP must be further evaluated with pulmonary artery catheterization. Echocardiography of PAH patients frequently shows RV hypertrophy and dilation, right atrial enlargement, and a decrease in the size of the LV cavity due to bowing of the interventricular septum in advanced disease. The inferior vena cava is typically distended and does not collapse during inspiration in advanced disease. Systolic PAP can be estimated using Doppler measurement of the tricuspid regurgitant flow velocity. The upper limit of normal systolic PAP is generally considered 40 to 50 mm Hg at rest, corresponding to a tricuspid regurgitant velocity of 3 to 3.5 m/s (although this value varies with age, body mass index, and right atrial pressure). Limitations to Doppler measurement of PAP do exist, however, as false-negative

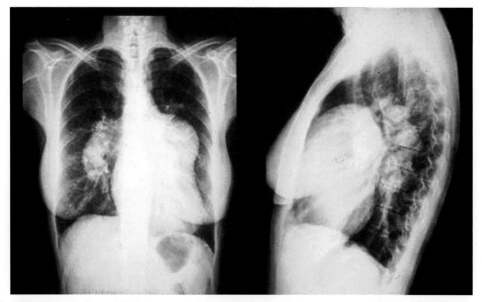

Fig. 55.6 Chest Radiograph in Pulmonary Arterial Hypertension. The pulmonary arteries are highly prominent bilaterally, with abrupt tapering (or "pruning") of vessels due to increased peripheral vascular resistance and diminished flow. There is right atrial and ventricular enlargement. The lung parenchyma is normal.

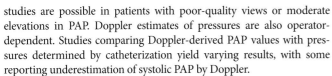

studies are possible in patients with poor-quality views or moderate elevations in PAP. Doppler estimates of pressures are also operator-dependent. Studies comparing Doppler-derived PAP values with pressures determined by catheterization yield varying results, with some reporting underestimation of systolic PAP by Doppler.

Echocardiography is most reliably employed for its negative predictive value, although a number of echocardiographic features of PAH suggest worsened prognosis. These features mostly include echocardiographic markers of RV dysfunction (i.e., right atrial or ventricular size, septal shift toward the left ventricle during diastole, tricuspid annular plane excursion [TAPSE] to approximate RV ejection fraction [RVEF], and right ventricular myocardial index), as well as the presence of pericardial effusion.[173] For example, TAPSE values of <1.8 cm have been associated with reduced 2-year survival rates in PAH. Patients who present with a right atrial area >18 cm^2, either at baseline or follow-up, are considered to be at an increased risk of mortality versus patients with a right atrial area <18 cm^2.[69,70] Pericardial effusion at baseline is a strong predictor of mortality in PAH patients and is an indicator of a high-risk patient.[170] Recent advances in echocardiography to quantify RV size, function, and strain, including three-dimensional echocardiography[180] and two-dimensional strain echocardiography,[181] have been reported to predict long-term adverse outcomes in PAH. However, to date, echocardiography alone is still too imprecise to be used as a single tool for diagnosis and thus should not replace invasive hemodynamic studies.[179]

Cardiac magnetic resonance imaging. Technology has been advancing in magnetic resonance imaging (MRI) for application to diagnosis and prognosis of PAH.[182] Cardiac MRI allows for precise quantification spatial resolution of RVEF, size, strain, and work based on electrocardiographically gated cine images. Dynamics of interventricular septal changes, known to play a critical role in PAH pathophysiology, can be documented in real time. Pulmonary vascular function, alterations in blood flow and velocities, as well as pulmonary artery pulsatility (an index of PA stiffness) can all be measured more readily than resting echocardiography. Delayed enhancement imaging to identify focal myocardial abnormalities as well as RV insertion point enhancement have been found to associate strongly with elevated PA pressures, RV dilation, and RV hypertrophy. Of these parameters, ejection fraction has been studied the most. Poor RVEF (<35%) has been associated with poor survival, independent of PVR, and increases in RVEF after 12 months were associated with improved 6-year survival.[183] Another recent report found that 12 months of targeted vasodilator therapy led to improvement in RVEF.[184] More novel approaches to MRI imaging in PAH include RV T1 mapping to identify diffuse myocardial abnormalities without contrast, RV strain imaging, RV perfusion, and four-dimensional pulmonary artery flow imaging to differentiate the complex flow patterns in normal versus diseased vasculature. The possibility of imaging metabolic derangements in RV tissue via magnetic resonance spectroscopy and cardiac hyperpolarized MR has also been proposed.[185]

Positron emission tomography imaging. The increasing appreciation of the profound metabolic derangement that occurs in both pulmonary vessels and RV tissue in PAH has facilitated the development of positron emission tomography (PET) imaging as a noninvasive method to track the progression of disease by monitoring this metabolic shift.[186] Specifically, the use of 18F-fluorodeoxyglucose (FDG), a tracer that accumulates in tissues avid for glucose, has allowed for quantitative tracking of RV tissue that is progressively more glycolytic as PAH, RV remodeling, and failure advance. Based on recent observations of worsened survival in patients with higher RV FDG accumulation, PET tracer uptake could serve as a novel prognostic factor for PAH.[187] New technologies are promising, to combine PET and MRI imaging as well as to develop other metabolic PET tracers for tracking the PAH disease course noninvasively. However, in contrast to echocardiography, the cost of these studies may preclude wide applicability at this time, particularly in resource-poor patient communities.

Cardiac catheterization. Right heart catheterization (RHC) remains the gold standard for establishing the diagnosis of PAH, defined by mean PAP of greater than or equal to 20 mm Hg at rest, accompanied by a PVR of greater than 3 Wood units with a normal pulmonary artery wedge pressure (≤15 mm Hg) in the absence of any known cause of PH. This procedure can directly measure right heart and PA pressures, as well as pulmonary capillary wedge pressure and CO. It can also be used to assess the vasodilation reserve (discussed later in the section on vasodilator therapy) and is a major determinant in prognosis of PH. In addition, direct measures of right atrial pressure have been associated with poorer survival rates, and low mixed venous oxygen saturation and cardiac index at baseline or over time have been associated with worse outcomes.[174] The optimal frequency of cardiac catheterization to monitor PAH patients is less well established. The 2015 European Society of Cardiology/European Respiratory Society (ESC/ERS) PH guidelines recommend that RHC be considered 3 to 6 months after a change in treatment or for clinical worsening.[69,70] In some centers, yearly screening RHC has been considered; however, in other centers, that frequency has not been feasible either for cost or logistic reasons.

Exercise testing. Exercise testing is recommended as part of the regular and serial assessment of functional capacity of PAH patients. The most widely used, cost-effective, and relatively reproducible exercise test is the 6-minute walk distance (6MWD). This test is usually performed after the diagnosis is confirmed by cardiac catheterization and at regular intervals. The distance walked in 6 minutes has been shown to decrease in proportion to the WHO/New York Heart Association (NYHA) functional class, and is a strong, independent predictor of mortality. Patients with a greater 6MWD demonstrated improved survival rates at 3 years compared with lower 6MWD.[188] In one study, patients with a 6MWD >380 m (median value) at baseline demonstrated improved survival, while the American-based REVEAL registry demonstrated a 6MWD of <165 m was associated with mortality risk.[189] However, perhaps stemming from the inherent variability and relative subjectivity of this test, other studies have reported that alterations of 6MWD from baseline are not associated with long-term outcomes.[173]

Maximal and invasive exercise testing (invasive cardiopulmonary exercise testing or CPET) has been increasingly used in research studies and can be helpful in distinguishing PAH from PH secondary to diastolic heart failure, as well as defining early signs of disease initiation or progression.[190] Additional information available from CPET include any ventilatory inefficiency, peak oxygen uptake (V'_{O_2}), and anaerobic threshold. PAH patients typically carry reduced peak V'_{O_2}, and peak V'_{O_2}, values during exercise have been reported to have the strongest correlation with survival rates,[191] with values <15 mL/min/kg indicating increased risk of death. PAH patients also show ventilatory insufficiency with minute volume (V'_E) to carbon dioxide production (V'_{CO_2}) with slope values >36 being a marker of worsened prognosis.[173] Invasive CPET has also been utilized to diagnose abnormal pulmonary vascular responses to exercise, termed exercise PH.[192] Although the most recent hemodynamic criteria for PAH no longer specify how to interpret such abnormalities with exercise,[1] recent reports have suggested exercise PH as an early marker of disease progression, and targeted pulmonary vasodilators may improve symptoms and outcomes.[193] Exercise echocardiography has also been reported as a more sensitive test for the presence of early PAH.[194] Exercise echocardiography has been studied as a screening tool to identify early PAH in known carriers of pathogenic *BMPR2* mutations,[195] as well as patients with connective tissue diseases who are at risk for developing PAH.

Screening. Screening asymptomatic patients at high risk for PAH is recommended, although the exact population recommended for screening has yet to be precisely defined, as the prevalence of disease is low, even in categories of patients at increased risk. Such patient groups that likely benefit from screening include those with known genetic mutations predisposing to PAH, first-degree relatives in a familial PAH cluster, patients with at-risk connective tissue diseases, those with portal hypertension prior to liver transplantation, and patients with congenital systemic-to-pulmonary shunts. Some patients should be evaluated for PAH only if they present with symptoms suggestive of the disease, including those with connective tissue diseases other than scleroderma, HIV, intravenous (IV) drug use, exposure to appetite-suppressant drugs, and portal hypertension who are not being considered for transplantation. Screening asymptomatic or minimally symptomatic patients should begin with a thorough history and physical examination to elicit symptoms or signs consistent with PH, followed by diagnostic testing if inconclusive. The transthoracic echocardiogram is the best noninvasive test used for screening patients, but exercise testing in the future may prove to be superior in detecting early-stage disease.

Genetic testing. Genetic testing of asymptomatic individuals is not currently advocated as an effective method for diagnosis, considering the low penetrance of disease manifestation, even if a predisposing mutation is present. Furthermore, the risk for disease in first-degree relatives of a patient with PAH is relatively low, which has led to uncertainty in genetic screening of their family members. Advocates suggest that screening asymptomatic patients may enhance knowledge of the prevalence of familial PAH and may shed light on whether early treatment influences the pathogenesis of disease. Screening also allows at-risk individuals to be aware of known risks that theoretically may augment penetrance of the disease; however, the results of genetic testing can be confusing. Even if family members have inherited a predisposing mutation, an approximately 80% chance exists that no discernible disease phenotype will be manifest. Notably, such circumstances may result in detrimental psychological, employment, and insurance effects, and, if pursued, must be supported by appropriate genetic counseling.

Comprehensive assessment and risk scoring. Overall, the diagnostic testing and assessment of the severity of PAH has become complex, necessitating an incorporation of a number of variables to estimate the overall risk of mortality and determine treatment options.[173] Consideration of these variables was based on prior registries of PAH patients that have tracked the course of disease with current targeted therapeutic regimens. Two major observation and prospective registries that have offered the most comprehensive assessments have included the REVEAL registry and the French Pulmonary Hypertension Network (FPHN). Data from the FPHN have led to the development of a French registry risk equation designed to add prognostic information at baseline diagnosis but not necessarily useful for serial assessment. The REVEAL registry data led to the development of a REVEAL risk score, meant for more serial assessments. Both the French registry risk equation and REVEAL risk score have been independently validated.[196] Importantly, both risk assessment tools indicate that no one variable alone can determine overall prognosis, risk of mortality, or response to therapy. Rather, owing to disease complexity, expeditious referral of PAH patients to expert centers that specialize in this disease has been emphasized as an effective tool for improving the clinical trajectory of these individuals. The 2015 ESC/ERS PH guidelines were the first to officially propose a PAH risk assessment approach whereby PAH patients are categorized into low, intermediate, or high risk, with 1-year mortality estimated at <5%, 5% to 10%, and >10%, respectively (Table 55.2). As such, management of PAH can then be guided by a goal of achieving a low risk status, and if that is not achievable, other more aggressive considerations could be made, such as lung transplantation.

TABLE 55.2   Risk Assessment of Patients With Pulmonary Arterial Hypertension

Determinants of Prognosis[a] (estimated 1-year mortality)	Low Risk <5%	Intermediate Risk 5%–10%	High Risk >10%
Clinical signs of right heart failure	Absent	Absent	Present
Progression of symptoms	No	Slow	Rapid
Syncope	No	Occasional syncope[b]	Repeated syncope[c]
WHO functional class	I, II	III	IV
6MWD	>440 m	165–440 m	<165 m
Cardiopulmonary exercise testing	Peak V_{O_2} >15 mL/min/kg (>65% pred) V_E/V_{CO_2} slope <36	Peak V_{O_2} 11–15 mL/min/kg (35–65% pred) V_E/V_{CO_2} slope 36–44.9	Peak V_{O_2} <11 mL/min/kg (<35% pred) V_E/V_{CO_2} slope ≥45
NT-proBNP plasma levels	BNP <50 ng/L NT-proBNP <300 ng/L	BNP 50–300 ng/L NT-proBNP 300–1400 ng/L	BNP >300 ng/L NT-proBNP >1400 ng/L
Imaging (echocardiography, CMR imaging	RA area <18 cm^2 No pericardial effusion	RA area 18–26 cm^2 No or minimal pericardial effusion	RA area >26 cm^2 Pericardial effusion
Hemodynamics	RAP < 8 mm Hg CI ≥ 2.5 L/min/m^2 S_{vo_2} > 65%	RAP 8–14 mm Hg CI 2.0–2.4 L/min/m^2 S_{vo_2} 60%–65%	RAP > 14 mm Hg CI < 2.0 L/min/m^2 S_{vo_2} <60%

[a] Most of the proposed variables and cut-off values are based on expert opinion.

[b] Occasional syncope during brisk or heavy exercise, or occasional orthostatic syncope in an otherwise stable patient.

[c] Repeated episodes of syncope, even with little or regular physical activity.

6MWD, 6-minute walking distance; *BNP*, brain natriuretic peptide; *CI*, cardiac index; *CMR*, cardiac magnetic resonance; *NT-proBNP*, N-terminal pro-brain natriuretic peptide; *RA*, right atrium; *RAP*, right atrial pressure; *Svo2*, mixed venous oxygen saturation; *VE/VCO2*, ventilatory equivalents for carbon dioxide; *VO2*, oxygen uptake; *WHO*, World Health Organization.

From Galiè N, Humbert M, Vachiery JL, et al. 2015 ESC/ERS Guidelines for the diagnosis and treatment of pulmonary hypertension: The Joint Task Force for the Diagnosis and Treatment of Pulmonary Hypertension of the European Society of Cardiology (ESC) and the European Respiratory Society (ERS): Endorsed by: Association for European Paediatric and Congenital Cardiology (AEPC), International Society for Heart and Lung Transplantation (ISHLT). *Eur Heart J*. 2016;37(1):67–119.

Yet, in all of these methods, there are limitations of risk assessment, and good clinical judgment is imperative in determining the appropriate treatment regimen in any given patient.

TREATMENT

There is no known cure for PAH, yet current therapeutic options have dramatically improved the survival and quality of life for patients with the disease. The American College of Chest Physicians has released

consensus recommendations for treatment of PAH.[197] These recommendations can be compared with 2015 ESC/ERS PH guidelines, where a treatment algorithm has been offered and summarized in Fig. 55.7.[69,70] There is considerable overlap among these recommendations, and these points are listed as follows.

General measures. Any behavior that increases oxygen demand or CO can worsen PAH symptoms and RV failure. Heavy physical exertion should be avoided. High altitude and nonpressurized airplane cabins can induce hypoxia and hypoxia-induced PH. Supplemental

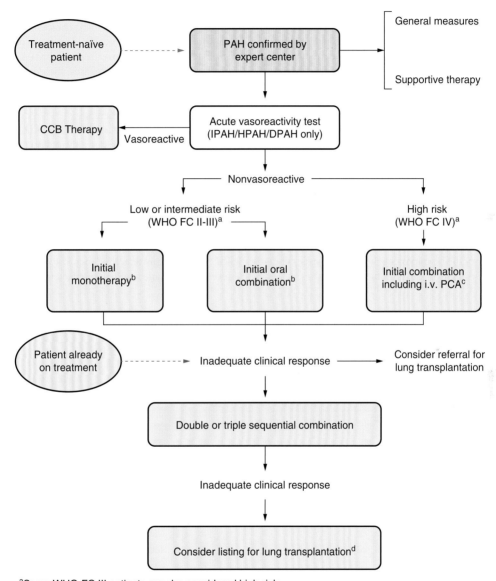

aSome WHO-FC III patients may be considered high-risk.
bInitial combination with ambrisentan plus tadalafil has proven to be superior to initial monotherapy with
  ambrisentan or tadalafil in delaying clinical failure.
cIntravenous epoprostenol should be prioritized as it has reduced the 3 month rate for mortality in
  high-risk PAH patients also as monotherapy.
dConsider also balloon atrial septostomy.

Fig. 55.7 Treatment algorithm of pulmonary arterial hypertension adapted from 2015 ESC/ERS guidelines. *CCB*, Calcium channel blockers; *DPAH*, drug-induced PAH; *HPAH*, heritable PAH; *IPAH*, idiopathic PAH; *i.v.*, intravenous; *PAH*, pulmonary arterial hypertension; *PCA*, prostacyclin analogues; *WHO-FC*, World Health Organization functional class. (Redrawn from Galiè N, Humbert M, Vachiery JL, et al. 2015 ESC/ERS Guidelines for the diagnosis and treatment of pulmonary hypertension: The Joint Task Force for the Diagnosis and Treatment of Pulmonary Hypertension of the European Society of Cardiology [ESC] and the European Respiratory Society [ERS]: Endorsed by: Association for European Paediatric and Congenital Cardiology [AEPC], International Society for Heart and Lung Transplantation [ISHLT]. *Eur Heart J.* 2016;37:67–119.)

oxygen should be used if it is necessary for the patient to be exposed to high altitude. PAH is an absolute contraindication to pregnancy because it may precipitate fatal right heart failure. OCP theoretically can increase the risk of hypercoagulability, leading to thromboembolic events that could exacerbate PAH. Nonetheless, OCPs are often used in nonsmoking women with PAH without a history of thromboembolic disease, owing to the greater risk of pregnancy. Regular influenza and pneumococcal vaccinations are imperative. Regular aerobic exercise training has also been found to be beneficial.[198]

Anticoagulation. Anticoagulation has sometimes been incorporated into the treatment of PAH on the basis of the presence of thrombosis in small PAs, the risk of compounding PAH with a thromboembolic component, and the increased risk of deep venous thrombosis in the setting of a low CO. No controlled trial of anticoagulation in PAH currently exists, but anticoagulation has been used on the basis of the improved survival of patients who received warfarin in historical smaller studies. If used, the usual recommended international normalized ratio is 2 to 2.5. Although prostacyclin inhibits platelet aggregation, additional anticoagulation is typically used in the absence of a contraindication. Since patients with congenital systemic-to-pulmonary shunts are at greater risk for hemoptysis, however, some practitioners do not recommend anticoagulation in those cases. It is also not recommended for scleroderma-associated PAH.

Oxygen therapy. The use of supplemental oxygen therapy should be considered in patients with hypoxemia at rest ($PaO_2 < 55$ mm Hg or $SaO_2 < 88\%$). Shunt-induced hypoxemia in patients with patent foramen ovale or intracardiac shunt is refractory to supplemental oxygen therapy. A controlled trial has not been performed, but oxygen therapy can improve the quality of life by improving dyspnea and exercise capacity, although oxygen equipment can limit mobility.

Treatment of right heart failure. There are no current targeted therapies for the decompensated RV. Diuretics are used to reduce intravascular volume and hepatic congestion. Cautious use of loop and thiazide diuretics may be required for adequate management. Overdiuresis must be avoided, however, as it can impair CO by decreasing RV preload. Digoxin is generally not used in PAH, except for rate control of atrial arrhythmias, which are poorly tolerated.[199] Intravenous inotropes may acutely improve symptoms of right heart failure, although they are not feasible as chronic agents.

Pulmonary vascular specific therapies. In the past 20 years, there has been a substantial acceleration of developing specific targeted therapies for PAH (Table 55.3). The choice of medications is often not straightforward. Importantly, numerous forms of PH outside the realm of true PAH have been overtreated with PAH-specific vasodilator drugs for years. In many such cases, such drugs can be harmful and dangerous. Thus treatment guidelines consistently emphasize the importance of confirming true WHO Group 1 PAH in patients who are being considered for such therapies.[197]

Initial screening for vasodilator reserve. Acute vasoreactivity testing is generally (although not invariably) used as an initial screen to assess for vasodilator reserve and potential response to vasodilator therapy.[69,70] A significant response to vasodilator testing is generally accepted as a decrease in PVR by at least 25% with a decrease in mean PAP to less than 40 mm Hg. Other parameters include a greater than 20% decrease in systolic PAP, a greater than 10 mm Hg drop in mean PAP, or an increase in cardiac index greater than or equal to 30%. The most widely used drugs for acute vasoreactivity testing include inhaled NO and IV prostacyclin (epoprostenol), adenosine, and iloprost, a prostacyclin analog with less effect on the systemic vasculature.

TABLE 55.3	Targeted Drug Development in Pulmonary Arterial Hypertension				
		PH-RELATED MEDICATIONS			
	Calcium Channel Blockers	Prostacyclin Pathway	Endothelin Pathway	Nitric Oxide Pathway	
FDA Approval Date		Prostacyclins	ERAs	PDE5 Inhibitors	sGC Stimulator
N/A	Diltiazem PO (i.e., Cartia, Cardizem), nifedipine PO (i.e., Procardia), amlodipine PO (i.e., Norvasc)				
1995		Epoprostenol IV (Flolan)			
2001			Bosentan PO (Tracleer)		
2002		Treprostinil SC or IV (Remodulin)			
2004		Iloprost Inh (Ventavis)			
2005				Sildenafil PO (Revatio)	
2007			Ambrisentan PO (Letairis)		
2009		Treprostinil Inh (Tyvaso)		Tadalafil PO (Adcirca)	
2010		Epoprostenol new formulation (Veletri)			
2013		Treprostinil PO (Orenitram)	Macitentan PO (Opsumit)		Riociguat PO (Adempas)
2015		Selexepag PO (Uptravi)			

The generic name of the medication is listed along with the route of administration and trade name in parentheses. *ERAs*, Endothelin receptor antagonists; *Inh*, Inhaled therapy; *PDE5*, phosphodiesterase 5; *PH*, pulmonary hypertension; *PO*, oral; *IV*, intravenous; *SC*, continuous parenteral therapy; *sGC*, soluble guanylyl cyclase.
Data from Perrin S, Chaumais MC, O'connell C, et al. New pharmacotherapy options for pulmonary arterial hypertension. *Expert Opin Pharmacother.* 2015;16(14):2113–2131.

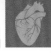

Testing more than one drug offers no advantage. Vasodilator challenge must be performed with care, as drug-induced systemic hypotension (such as with prostacyclin) may reduce RV coronary blood flow and cause RV ischemia. Most studies on PAH report the proportion of responders to vasodilators as between 12% and 25%. There is no particular clinical or disease characteristic that reliably predicts vasodilator response. The lack of response to acute vasodilators predicts the response to oral vasodilator therapy (i.e., nonresponders to inhaled NO do not respond to oral calcium-channel blockers). Response to acute vasodilators, however, does not predict a response to prostacyclin. A trial of long-term calcium-channel blocker therapy is usually recommended as first-line therapy in PAH patients who respond to vasodilator challenge with a decrease in PVR of greater than or equal to 50%

Calcium-channel blockers. Calcium-channel blockers are the oral drugs of choice for patients who have a significant response to acute vasodilators.[69,70] These agents have been shown to improve hemodynamics, RV function, and survival in the subpopulation of PAH patients responding to acute vasoreactivity testing. Empiric therapy without vasodilator testing is not recommended, due to a high rate of treatment failure. Both nifedipine and diltiazem are effective in appropriate patients, and the choice between these two drugs is guided by resting heart rate. The doses of these drugs required to lower PVR are much higher than those used for other indications, which makes systemic side effects a significant problem—particularly hypotension and lower extremity edema. Verapamil is not used because of its greater negative inotropic effects. Acute administration of amlodipine causes pulmonary vasodilation, but its long-term efficacy has not been studied.

Phosphodiesterase 5 inhibitors. Originally marketed for erectile dysfunction, oral PDE5 inhibitors such as sildenafil selectively inhibit the cGMP-specific enzyme PDE5, enabling endogenous NO to exert a more sustained effect.[200] This PDE is highly abundant in the pulmonary vasculature, making such medications relatively selective pulmonary vasodilators. A long-acting PDE5 inhibitor for use in PAH includes tadalafil. In patients with lung fibrosis and PAH, acute administration of sildenafil surpasses the vasodilating effect of NO. The effect is similar to IV epoprostenol, except that sildenafil is more selective for better-ventilated areas of the lung, resulting in improved gas exchange. Clinical efficacy has been reported with the use of sildenafil in patients with primary PAH and PAH associated with congenital shunts, SLE, and HIV. Benefits with treatment include improved symptoms and hemodynamics, and increased 6MWD. In a multicenter, double-blinded, randomized, placebo-controlled study of sildenafil treatment for PAH, significant improvements in exercise ability and quality of life were observed; in the open label follow-up study, 95% survival was measured at 1 year. Major side effects of PDE5 inhibitors include systemic hypotension, especially in the setting of nitroglycerin use. The approved dosing of sildenafil for PAH is three times daily, while tadalafil is typically used once a day. Currently, PDE inhibitors are approved for functional class II to III PAH patients as first-line agents and for class IV patients as second-line agents.

Endothelin-1 receptor antagonists. Presently, three endothelin receptor antagonists (ERAs) are approved for oral use in PAH: bosentan, ambrisentan, and, most recently, macitentan.[201] Bosentan is a nonspecific antagonist recognizing both endothelin receptor subtypes A (ET-A) and B (ET-B), while ambrisentan is specific for ET-A. Macitentan is also a dual ERA, blocking both ET-A and ET-B receptors, but it carries a 50-fold increased selectivity for the ET-A subtype over the ET-B subtype. It is thought that specific inhibition of ET-A may provide more benefit by decreasing the vasoconstrictor effects of ET-A while allowing the vasodilator and ET-1 clearance functions of ET-B receptors. Both bosentan and ambrisentan have been found to improve exercise capacity and hemodynamics in 12- to 16-week clinical trials.

Bosentan has also improved survival in open label studies and comparison with historical control data. Long-term survival data for the selective endothelin inhibitor ambrisentan has appeared favorable in historical studies. More recently, macitentan was approved based on the results of the SERAPHIN study, a randomized, placebo-controlled study of macitentan in PAH patients, comparing 250 patients to placebo, 250 patients to 3 mg daily dose, and 242 patients to 10 mg daily dose. Based on a primary end point of the time of initiation of treatment to a composite end point of death, atrial septostomy (AS), lung transplantation, initiation of treatment with prostanoids, or worsening of PAH, there was a significant reduction of mortality and morbidity, driven primarily by worsening of PAH.[202] Importantly, SERAPHIN was the first study to convincingly demonstrate such an improvement in outcomes by an ERA beyond exercise capacity and hemodynamics.

A major complication of bosentan includes a dose-dependent increase in liver transaminases, which necessitates discontinuation in 2% and dose adjustment in 8% to 12% of patients. Frank hepatic toxicity can also occur. Ambrisentan and macitentan do not appear to increase liver transaminases to the same degree. Teratogenicity is a class effect of these medications. Delayed hemodynamic benefit compared with the immediate effect of prostacyclins should also be expected. Bosentan can alter levels of concurrently dosed OCP, PDE inhibitors, or HIV antiretroviral drugs.

Soluble guanylyl cyclase activators. A specific NO-independent sGC activator has been developed for the treatment of PAH. The principle underlying the development of this drug entails the fact that, in PASMCs, NO binds to sGC and mediates the synthesis of the secondary messenger cGMP, which then attenuates actin–myosin contractility and consequently promotes vasorelaxation. For PAH, riociguat has been studied via a pair of phase III clinical trials. PATENT-1 was a randomized, placebo-controlled study whereby after a 12-week treatment of the drug, exercise capacity was evaluated. Riociguat significantly improved exercise capacity along with secondary efficacy points, such as pulmonary vascular resistance, NT-proBNP levels, WHO functional class, time to clinical worsening, and Borg dyspnea score.[203] Upon completion of PATENT-1, patients were invited to enter PATENT-2, a long-term extension trial. The first interim analysis at 1 year revealed sustained benefits in 6MWD and WHO functional class.[204] Given that both PDE5 inhibition and sGC activation exhibit activity in the same NO pathway, the PATENT PLUS trial was performed to determine the safety and efficacy of using both riociguat and sildenafil in combination.[205] Combination therapy demonstrated little favorable effects and some potentially dangerous safety signals, such as hypotension. Thus the use of riociguat with PDE5 inhibitors is contraindicated.

Prostacyclin and prostacyclin analogs. Prostacyclin is an endogenous prostaglandin (prostaglandin I_2) that causes vasodilation and inhibits platelet aggregation. It also has antiproliferative and weak fibrinolytic activities. Intravenous prostacyclin (epoprostenol or Flolan) was first used to treat PAH in the early 1980s. Multiple trials of epoprostenol since that time demonstrated improved survival, exercise capacity, and hemodynamics in patients with PAH compared with conventional treatment. A chronic, perhaps remodeling, effect of epoprostenol has additionally been suggested by several findings: patients who have no acute response may demonstrate a delayed hemodynamic improvement, hemodynamic improvement increases in patients who show an initial response, and RV dysfunction improves after long-term therapy.

Epoprostenol has an extremely short half-life (approximately 3 to 6 minutes), must be kept cold, and must be administered through a central venous catheter. Thus a major limitation to use of epoprostenol includes the need for permanent central venous access with the associated small risk of catheter-related infection or air embolism and the capacity to handle the catheter and pump. Some clinicians continue the dose escalation until limited by side effects or until there is a plateau in the hemodynamic response. Notably, initiation of epoprostenol can lead to increased CO with LV strain or to isolated pulmonary edema with rapid clinical deterioration. Long-term dose requirements are highly variable among patients, and further dose increases are made in the outpatient setting on the basis of clinical symptoms, exercise testing, and hemodynamic measurements.

The complexities of epoprostenol administration have led investigators to search for alternative agents. Prostacyclin analogs treprostinil, iloprost, and beraprost have been tested in 12-week placebo-controlled trials.[206] All of these agents have demonstrated significant improvements in mean exercise capacity. Treprostinil has a longer half-life (approximately 4 hours) than epoprostenol and can be delivered intravenously or subcutaneously with a pump system similar to that used with subcutaneous insulin. Treprostinil does not require reconstitution nor cold temperature. Pain at the site of subcutaneous infusion is a frequent problem that requires cessation of the drug in 8% to 12% of patients. An implantable pump for treprostinil has been proposed but is not yet available. Iloprost is another chemically stable analog that can be given intravenously and by inhaled routes. Iloprost can be used in a nebulized form that must be administered 6 to 9 times daily for a continuous effect. Treprostinil and iloprost are approved for PAH therapy—both for functional class II to IV. Common side effects of all prostacyclin analogs include jaw pain, headache, diarrhea, flushing, leg pain, nausea, and vomiting. Patients also tend to develop tachyphylaxis to epoprostenol over time.

Most recently, an oral form of treprostinil has been developed for PAH, based on data from the FREEDOM-M trial indicating the efficacy of monotherapy in improving 6MWD compared with placebo. However, both the FREEDOM-C[207] and FREEDOM-C2[208] trials failed to show benefits in 6MWD at week 16 when compared with background ERA and/or PDE5 therapy. Long-term outcomes with oral treprostinil are pending (FREEDOM-EV). Alternatively, selexipag, an agonist of the prostacyclin (IP) receptor, was recently studied in the GRIPHON study, a phase 3 randomized, double-blind, placebo-controlled trial of 1156 patients with PAH treated either with placebo or selexipag in the setting of either background therapy or no additional therapy.[209] Selexipag reduced the risk of the primary composite end point of death or complication of PAH by 40%, but there was no significant difference in mortality. Both oral treprostinil and selexipag have been approved by the US Food and Drug Administration for use in PAH patients with functional class II to IV.

Treatment of Pulmonary Arterial Hypertension Associated With Specific Secondary Diseases

Current treatment guidelines do not distinguish between PAH subgroups in the recommendation for initial therapy. However, most of the provided data supporting vasodilator therapies have originated from patient populations suffering from idiopathic PAH. In addition, vasodilator therapy in PAH patients with collagen vascular diseases has been studied with good evidence for benefit, but with special caveats.[210] As in idiopathic PAH, baseline hemodynamic data do not predict a response to epoprostenol in PAH associated with scleroderma. The acute vasodilator response is present in an even smaller proportion of patients with collagen vascular diseases than with idiopathic PAH. Accordingly, calcium-channel blockers are not beneficial in this group of patients. Nonetheless, prostacyclins can be effective in improving symptoms, hemodynamics, and survival. Skin lesions in patients with scleroderma may also improve substantially with this treatment. There have also been case reports of successful epoprostenol treatment of PAH in patients with SLE; however, treatment in this group has been complicated by severe thrombocytopenia. Patient outcomes with

CREST/scleroderma have also been studied with improved symptoms and hemodynamics after the use of oral ERAs.

The efficacy of such treatment in other PAH subgroups has been studied, but in smaller numbers of patients. Prostacyclin therapy has been shown to improve functional capacity, oxygen saturation, and hemodynamics in a group of adults with Eisenmenger syndrome, in NYHA classes III and IV. Small numbers of adults with repaired or unrepaired congenital heart disease have also been included in clinical trials of endothelin receptor blockers and PDE5 inhibitors that have demonstrated improvement in hemodynamics, exercise capacity, and symptoms. Prostacyclins have also been used successfully in patients with PAH secondary to HIV infection. In patients suffering from portopulmonary hypertension, prostacyclins have facilitated successful liver transplantation. Although liver toxicity had previously been considered a relative contraindication in this patient group, new generation ERAs have been used effectively in PAH patients with hepatic disease,[211] either singly or in combination.[212] There are additional reports of improvement in PAH secondary to portopulmonary hypertension with the use of β-blockers and nitrates, which may also decrease the incidence of variceal bleeding. Yet caveats to PAH treatment exist for this special patient population, such as anticoagulation in these patients, which is controversial owing to the risk of hemorrhage. Finally, although pregnancy in PAH is not recommended, reports are increasing of successful delivery of viable fetuses in patients with PAH. Management recommendations for these particularly challenging patients have been presented, based on expert opinion.[213]

Combination Therapy

Combination therapy using at least two separate classes of PAH medications has been advocated based on the potential for additive or synergistic effects. With the development of larger, longer-term, and more sophisticated PAH trials, the clear benefits of dual and triple combination therapy are finally beginning to emerge.[214]

Historically, improvements with combination therapy were reported in hemodynamics, exercise capacity, and symptoms over 12- to 16- week periods, but these results were inconsistent. More recently, the first clinical trial to demonstrate durable beneficial effects of sequential dual combination therapy was SERAPHIN,[202] where the mortality and morbidity benefit of macitentan was seen in almost two-thirds of patients on background PAH-specific therapy, mostly PDE5 inhibitors. Since then, subsequent substudies and post hoc analyses have reported improvement of PVR and cardiac index, as well as of hospitalizations[215] in patients on background therapy. Furthermore, the GRIPHON study has provided long-term data on the beneficial effects of sequential triple combination therapy with selexipag, indicating that successful combinations of drugs can include more than ERA and PDE5 inhibitors. Nonetheless, not every trial has reported similar success in sequential combination therapies, such as the phase 4 COMPASS-2 trial evaluating bosentan in combination with sildenafil.[216] Although there were limitations to the COMPASS-2 design, results can be interpreted to suggest that only specific combinations of medications may show additive or synergistic benefit.

Alternatively, beyond sequential combination therapy, the first randomized, placebo-controlled study to investigate initial dual combination therapy in PAH was BREATHE-2. In this case, intravenous epoprostenol was combined with bosentan or placebo in a small cohort of patients with severe PAH. A nonstatistically significant improvement in total PVR was observed. This trend was reinforced by additional positive data generated from retrospective observational studies from a small French registry. These historical data served as the basis for the recent AMBITION study, a double-blind trial designed to evaluate the initial combination therapy with ambrisentan and tadalafil versus monotherapy with either agent in 500 newly diagnosed treatment-naïve PAH patients.[217] Importantly, a 50% risk reduction was found in the composite end point of clinical failure events after combination therapy, as compared with pooled monotherapy. This effect was driven primarily by a difference in hospitalization for progressing PAH. Several substudies have demonstrated improvement of hemodynamics with initial combination therapy, and these findings have been replicated in PAH secondary to connective tissue disease.[214] Importantly, when considering these data together, current recommendations now hold that all PAH patients should be offered combination therapy when possible. Prospective studies are now ongoing to determine the effect of initial triple combination therapy in PAH.

Management of Refractory Pulmonary Arterial Hypertension

Failure to demonstrate improvements with targeted PAH medications in symptoms, hemodynamics, and exercise capacity correlates with worse outcomes. In these cases, combination therapy, AS, or lung transplantation should be pursued.[218,219]

Atrial septostomy. The rationale for surgical creation of an interatrial orifice to improve survival is based on the observation that survival in PAH critically depends on right ventricular function, and relieving stress on the RV theoretically improves PAH, in general.[220] For example, PAH patients with a patent foramen ovale or with Eisenmenger syndrome tend to have better cardiac function and survive longer as compared with patients without intracardiac defects. A review of 64 patients who underwent AS prior to contemporary treatment regimens reported improved clinical status in 47 of 50 patients. The median survival of the 54 patients who survived the procedure was 19.5 months (range 2 to 96 months), which represents an improvement as compared with treatments available before targeted vasodilator therapies. However, because of the improved efficacy of the currently available vasodilators, AS is currently only considered as a palliative procedure for patients with severe PAH with clinical deterioration despite maximal medical therapy or as a bridge to transplantation. It should only be attempted in centers with experience in the procedure, as sizing the orifice optimally is a critical determinant of success.

Lung transplantation. Before the introduction of epoprostenol, transplantation was the treatment of choice for severe PAH. It is still the last option in treating severe PAH and the only available cure.[218,219] Patients with persistent NYHA functional class III or IV symptoms, right atrial pressure >15 mm Hg, or cardiac index <2 L/min/m^2 should be considered for lung transplantation. Hemodynamic responses to a 3-month epoprostenol infusion may also aid in identifying a subset of PAH patients who might benefit from being considered earlier for lung transplantation. Poor survival has been noted in patients with NYHA functional classes III and IV who remained in that class or failed to achieve a 30% decrease in PVR after 3 months on continuous IV prostacyclin.

Heart-lung and single- and double-lung transplantations have been successfully performed in patients with PAH. Lung transplantation alone has demonstrated that severe RV dysfunction is reversible, indicating that heart transplantation is not necessary unless the patient has cardiac disease unrelated to PH. The availability of single-lung transplantation is greater, considering the scarcity of donor organs. However, there are disadvantages in marked ventilation-perfusion mismatching and potential for injury. Thus there may be less functional recovery and higher graft-related complications with single-lung transplant. Furthermore, there may be a slightly higher long-term survival rate with double-lung transplantation.

Survival in the early postoperative period is lower for PAH patients as compared with other patients undergoing lung transplantation.

However, the long-term outcome in patients with PAH is similar to that of general transplantation patients. Survival rates at 1, 3, and 5 years after transplantation have been reported as 65%, 55%, and 44%, respectively. PAH has not been reported to recur after transplantation, although a careful examination of those with genetic predisposition has not been performed.

Previously, patients with collagen vascular diseases were excluded from transplantation, but they have recently demonstrated survival rates similar to those of other patient groups. Transplantation can be considered for collagen vascular disease patients in whom extrapulmonary manifestations are not severe. Owing to the high intraoperative and perioperative risks, liver transplantation historically had not been offered to patients with portopulmonary hypertension, but these trends may be changing with contemporary medications. Pulmonary hemodynamics have been reported to improve with liver transplantation, however, and the risk of mortality at surgery is minimal if the mean PAP is less than 35 mm Hg. If the PAP is greater than 35 mm Hg, pretransplantation management with pulmonary vasodilators, such as prostacyclins, may decrease the mortality risk, and has been used as a bridge to transplantation.

Experimental Therapies

Beyond the more established therapies for PAH, additional intriguing, yet still developing, therapeutic approaches are under investigation, as summarized recently.[221] Unlike the current medical therapies that mainly ameliorate disease, there is optimism that regression of pulmonary vascular remodeling and cure for PAH is possible with these evolving treatment paradigms. Possibilities include novel therapies directed at inflammation and immunity. For example, ubenimex is in a phase 2 clinical trial in PAH based on its activity as an inhibitor of the inflammatory effector leukotriene B4. Rituximab is an anti-CD20 monoclonal antibody that targets B cells prevalent in plexiform lesions of diseased PAH vessels; this antibody is being studied for its efficacy in PAH associated with connective tissue diseases. An anti-interleukin-6 antibody, tocilizumab, is being investigated in an open-label phase 2 trial for PAH. Other novel mitochondrial and metabolic therapies are also in development. Bardoxolone methyl is an inhibitor of the inflammatory transcription factor NF-κB that is under clinical investigation, with a phase 3 trial planned. The first human clinical trial data with DCA, an inhibitor of PDK, in PAH have recently been reported.[120] Therapies designed to rescue BMPR2 signaling have also been advancing, including tacrolimus, BMP9 agonists, and ataluren, a drug that permits ribosomal readthrough of premature stop codons that are occasionally found in the BMPR2 gene of hereditary PAH patients.[222] Moreover, given the substantial iron deficiency noted in PAH, iron replacement is being tested as a specific therapy. Despite the disappointing phase 3 trial data with imatinib, a receptor tyrosine kinase inhibitor, in PAH, additional programs are developing to consider other chemotherapeutics for treatment of this "cancer-like" disease.

In addition to the development and repurposing of novel small molecules, antibodies, and chemotherapies, cellular and interventional therapies are being investigated. Progenitor cell infusion with endothelial progenitor cells (EPCs) represents an intriguing, but still nebulous, therapeutic possibility. Two small studies in which adults and children with idiopathic PAH were given a single infusion of autologous mononuclear cells have provided support for the therapeutic potential of such therapy. A recent therapeutic trial suggested reasonable safety and evidence of short-term hemodynamic improvement after administering such cells in patients with PAH.[223] Finally, pulmonary artery denervation, a process by which sympathetic nerve fibers are disrupted, has been reported to improve exercise capacity and hemodynamics in very small proof-of-concept studies.[224]

CONCLUSIONS

PAH refers to a clinical syndrome of vascular diseases with a stereotyped pattern of histopathology and is related to a variety of secondary disease states. It has become increasingly clear that the development of PAH entails a complex, multifactorial pathobiology. Although genetic mutations, exogenous exposures, and acquired disease states can predispose to PAH, no one factor identified thus far is sufficient alone to fully drive the pathogenic process. Similar to carcinogenesis in which a susceptible person with a specific genetic mutation requires additional injuries to manifest disease, a "multiple-hit" hypothesis has emerged to explain the progression to clinical PAH. Better delineated mechanisms of disease have focused on the end-stage condition and the effects of the imbalance of multiple vascular effectors. Some unifying mechanism(s) of disease have become more apparent, linking the regulation of these effectors into a more cohesive model. As a result, effective (often combination) therapeutic approaches have been developed to ameliorate disease and improve survival.

Nonetheless, a comprehensive understanding of these cellular processes is incomplete. In part, this fact stems from the great complexity of overlapping pathogenic mechanisms that drive this unique pathophenotype. In the postgenomic and precision medicine era, it is conceivable that complex clinical syndromes such as PAH can be redefined based on growing genomic, transcriptional, and proteomic data. A "systems-based" network analysis may therefore be helpful in identifying common, overarching pathways of pathogenesis and aid in our understanding of the genetic and mechanistic links among primary disease triggers and end-stage disease.[225] In addition, a challenge of research in PAH is the lack of a comparable small animal model that can be followed and genetically manipulated from initiation through progression to severe disease. There has been some success in the physiologic study of PAH in larger mammals; however, the identification of contributors in the molecular process of pulmonary remodeling has been difficult, owing to incomplete genetic data and tools specific for these models. Conversely, while genetic and molecular studies in the mouse are more tractable, induction of significant PAH in murine models has been challenging. Nonetheless, recent advances have hinted at the possibility of more tractable animal models of PAH, which would be useful for combining genetic study and pathobiologic exposures. Finally, with the decreasing numbers of PAH patients undergoing transplantation, the ability of researchers to obtain human PAH tissue for molecular analysis via traditional routes is dwindling. Nonetheless, with advances in fields such as pulmonary artery catheterization, inducible stem cell biology, and others, the intricate molecular study of even complex human diseased tissue such as in PAH may be much more feasible in the coming years. As a result, the next decade of research will hopefully lead to improvements in the prevention of disease for at-risk individuals, diagnosis of disease at earlier time points, and perhaps identification of specific, precise therapeutic targets useful for the regression of the pathogenic process itself.

REFERENCES

1. Simonneau G, Gatzoulis MA, Adatia I, et al. Updated clinical classification of pulmonary hypertension. *J Am Coll Cardiol.* 2013;62(25 Suppl): D34–D41.

1a. Simonneau G, Montani D, Celermajer D, et al. Haemodynamic definitions and updated clinical classification of pulmonary hypertension. *Eur Respir J.* 2018; [Epub ahead of print].

2. Benza RL, Miller DP, Barst RJ, et al. An evaluation of long-term survival from time of diagnosis in pulmonary arterial hypertension from the REVEAL Registry. *Chest.* 2012;142(2):448–456.

3. Girerd B, Lau E, Montani D, Humbert M. Genetics of pulmonary hypertension in the clinic. *Curr Opin Pulm Med.* 2017;23(5):386–391.

4. Bigna JJ, Sime PS, Koulla-Shiro S. HIV related pulmonary arterial hypertension: epidemiology in Africa, physiopathology, and role of antiretroviral treatment. *AIDS Res Ther.* 2015;12:36.

5. Long L, Ormiston ML, Yang X, et al. Selective enhancement of endothelial BMPR-II with BMP9 reverses pulmonary arterial hypertension. *Nat Med.* 2015;21(7):777–785.

6. Diebold I, Hennigs JK, Miyagawa K, et al. BMPR2 preserves mitochondrial function and DNA during reoxygenation to promote endothelial cell survival and reverse pulmonary hypertension. *Cell Metab.* 2015;21(4):596–608.

7. Goldthorpe H, Jiang JY, Taha M, et al. Occlusive lung arterial lesions in endothelial-targeted, fas-induced apoptosis transgenic mice. *Am J Respir Cell Mol Biol.* 2015;53(5):712–718.

8. Xu W, Erzurum SC. Endothelial cell energy metabolism, proliferation, and apoptosis in pulmonary hypertension. *Compr Physiol.* 2011;1(1):357–372.

9. Kim J, Kang Y, Kojima Y, et al. An endothelial apelin-FGF link mediated by miR-424 and miR-503 is disrupted in pulmonary arterial hypertension. *Nat Med.* 2013;19(1):74–82.

10. Bertero T, Oldham WM, Cottrill KA, et al. Vascular stiffness mechanoactivates YAP/TAZ-dependent glutaminolysis to drive pulmonary hypertension. *J Clin Invest.* 2016;126(9):3313–3335.

11. Duong HT, Comhair SA, Aldred MA, et al. Pulmonary artery endothelium resident endothelial colony-forming cells in pulmonary arterial hypertension. *Pulm Circ.* 2011;1(4):475–486.

12. Antigny F, Hautefort A, Meloche J, et al. Potassium channel subfamily K member 3 (KCNK3) contributes to the development of pulmonary arterial hypertension. *Circulation.* 2016;133(14):1371–1385.

13. Michelakis ED. Spatio-temporal diversity of apoptosis within the vascular wall in pulmonary arterial hypertension: heterogeneous BMP signaling may have therapeutic implications. *Circ Res.* 2006;98(2):172–175.

14. Ranchoux B, Antigny F, Rucker-Martin C, et al. Endothelial-to-mesenchymal transition in pulmonary hypertension. *Circulation.* 2015;131(11):1006–1018.

15. Hopper RK, Moonen JR, Diebold I, et al. In pulmonary arterial hypertension, reduced BMPR2 promotes endothelial-to-mesenchymal transition via HMGA1 and its target slug. *Circulation.* 2016;133(18):1783–1794.

16. Archer SL, Weir EK, Wilkins MR. Basic science of pulmonary arterial hypertension for clinicians: new concepts and experimental therapies. *Circulation.* 2010;121(18):2045–2066.

16a. Graf M, Huter P, Maracci, et al. Visualization of translation termination intermediates trapped by the Apidaecin 137 peptide during RF3-mediated recycling of RF1. *Nat Commun.* 2018;9(1):3053.

16b. Rhodes CJ, Batai K, Bleda M, et al. Genetic determinants of risk in pulmonary arterial hypertension: international genome-wide association studies and meta-analysis. *Lancet Respir Med.* 2018; S2213–2600.

17. Pullamsetti SS, Kojonazarov B, Storn S, et al. Lung cancer-associated pulmonary hypertension: role of microenvironmental inflammation based on tumor cell-immune cell cross-talk. *Sci Transl Med.* 2017;9(416).

18. Wang Z, Chesler NC. Pulmonary vascular wall stiffness: an important contributor to the increased right ventricular afterload with pulmonary hypertension. *Pulm Circ.* 2011;1(2):212–223.

19. Lammers S, Scott D, Hunter K, et al. Mechanics and function of the pulmonary vasculature: implications for pulmonary vascular disease and right ventricular function. *Compr Physiol.* 2012;2(1):295–319.

20. Gan CT, Lankhaar JW, Westerhof N, et al. Noninvasively assessed pulmonary artery stiffness predicts mortality in pulmonary arterial hypertension. *Chest.* 2007;132(6):1906–1912.

21. Schafer M, Werner S. Cancer as an overhealing wound: an old hypothesis revisited. *Nat Rev Mol Cell Biol.* 2008;9(8):628–638.

22. Liu F, Haeger CM, Dieffenbach PB, et al. Distal vessel stiffening is an early and pivotal mechanobiological regulator of vascular remodeling and pulmonary hypertension. *JCI Insight.* 2016;1(8):e86987.

23. Bertero T, Cotrill KA, Lu Y, et al. Matrix remodeling promotes pulmonary hypertension through feedback mechanoactivation of the YAP/TAZ-miR-130/301 circuit. *Cell Rep*. 2015;13(5):1016–1032.

24. Stenmark KR, Tuder RM, El Kasmi KC. Metabolic reprogramming and inflammation act in concert to control vascular remodeling in hypoxic pulmonary hypertension. *J Appl Physiol (1985)*. 2015;119(10):1164–1172.

25. Rabinovitch M, Guignabert C, Humbert M, Nicolls MR. Inflammation and immunity in the pathogenesis of pulmonary arterial hypertension. *Circ Res*. 2014;115(1):165–175.

26. Saito T, Miyagawa K, Chen SY, et al. Upregulation of human endogenous retrovirus-K is linked to immunity and inflammation in pulmonary arterial hypertension. *Circulation*. 2017;136(20):1920–1935.

27. Savai R, Pullamsetti SS, Kolbe J, et al. Immune and inflammatory cell involvement in the pathology of idiopathic pulmonary arterial hypertension. *Am J Respir Crit Care Med*. 2012;186(9):897–908.

28. Tian W, Jiang X, Tamosiuniene R, et al. Blocking macrophage leukotriene b4 prevents endothelial injury and reverses pulmonary hypertension. *Sci Transl Med*. 2013;5(200):200ra117.

29. Qian J, Tian W, Jiang X, et al. Leukotriene B4 activates pulmonary artery adventitial fibroblasts in pulmonary hypertension. *Hypertension*. 2015;66(6):1227–1239.

30. Austin ED, Loyd JE. The genetics of pulmonary arterial hypertension. *Circ Res*. 2014;115(1):189–202.

31. Shi Y, Massagué J. Mechanisms of TGF-beta signaling from cell membrane to nucleus. *Cell*. 2003;113(6):685–700.

32. Alastalo TP, Li M, Perez Vde J, et al. Disruption of PPARgamma/ beta-catenin-mediated regulation of apelin impairs BMP-induced mouse and human pulmonary arterial EC survival. *J Clin Invest*. 2011;121(9):3735–3746.

33. Sawada H, Saito T, Nickel NP, et al. Reduced BMPR2 expression induces GM-CSF translation and macrophage recruitment in humans and mice to exacerbate pulmonary hypertension. *J Exp Med*. 2014;211(2):263–280.

34. Rhodes CJ, Im H, Cao A, et al. RNA sequencing analysis detection of a novel pathway of endothelial dysfunction in pulmonary arterial hypertension. *Am J Respir Crit Care Med*. 2015;192(3):356–366.

35. Sa S, Gu M, Chappell J, et al. Induced pluripotent stem cell model of pulmonary arterial hypertension reveals novel gene expression and patient specificity. *Am J Respir Crit Care Med*. 2017;195(7):930–941.

36. Gu M, Shao NY, Sa S, et al. Patient-specific iPSC-derived endothelial cells uncover pathways that protect against pulmonary hypertension in BMPR2 mutation carriers. *Cell Stem Cell*. 2017;20(4):490–504. e495.

37. Ma L, Chung WK. The role of genetics in pulmonary arterial hypertension. *J Pathol*. 2017;241(2):273–280.

38. Ma L, Roman-Campos D, Austin ED, et al. A novel channelopathy in pulmonary arterial hypertension. *N Engl J Med*. 2013;369(4):351–361.

39. Germain M, Eyries M, Montani D, et al. Genome-wide association analysis identifies a susceptibility locus for pulmonary arterial hypertension. *Nat Genet*. 2013;45(5):518–521.

40. Eyries M, Montani D, Girerd B, et al. EIF2AK4 mutations cause pulmonary veno-occlusive disease, a recessive form of pulmonary hypertension. *Nat Genet*. 2014;46(1):65–69.

41. Hadinnapola C, Bleda M, Haimel M, et al. Phenotypic characterisation of EIF2AK4 mutation carriers in a large cohort of patients diagnosed clinically with pulmonary arterial hypertension. *Circulation*. 2017;136(21):2022–2033.

42. Eichstaedt CA, Song J, Benjamin N, et al. EIF2AK4 mutation as "second hit" in hereditary pulmonary arterial hypertension. *Respir Res*. 2016;17(1):141.

43. Badesch DB, Raskob GE, Elliott CG, et al. Pulmonary arterial hypertension: baseline characteristics from the REVEAL Registry. *Chest*. 2010;137(2):376–387.

44. Humbert M, Sitbon O, Chaouat A, et al. Pulmonary arterial hypertension in France: results from a national registry. *Am J Respir Crit Care Med*. 2006;173(9):1023–1030.

45. Rich S, Dantzker DR, Ayres SM, et al. Primary pulmonary hypertension. A national prospective study. *Ann Intern Med*. 1987;107(2):216–223.

46. Assaggaf H, Felty Q. Gender, estrogen, and obliterative lesions in the lung. *Int J Endocrinol*. 2017;2017:8475701.

47. Mair KM, Wright AF, Duggan N, et al. Sex-dependent influence of endogenous estrogen in pulmonary hypertension. *Am J Respir Crit Care Med*. 2014;190(4):456–467.

48. Dean A, Nilsen M, Loughlin L, et al. Metformin reverses development of pulmonary hypertension via aromatase inhibition. *Hypertension*. 2016;68(2):446–454.

49. Kawut SM, Archer-Chicko CL, DeMichele A, et al. Anastrozole in pulmonary arterial hypertension. a randomized, double-blind, placebo-controlled trial. *Am J Respir Crit Care Med*. 2017;195(3):360–368.

50. Chen X, Austin ED, Talati M, et al. Oestrogen inhibition reverses pulmonary arterial hypertension and associated metabolic defects. *Eur Respir J*. 2017;50(2):1602337.

51. Johansen AK, Dean A, Morecroft I, et al. The serotonin transporter promotes a pathological estrogen metabolic pathway in pulmonary hypertension via cytochrome P450 1B1. *Pulm Circ*. 2016;6(1):82–92.

52. White K, Loughlin L, Maqbool Z, et al. Serotonin transporter, sex, and hypoxia: microarray analysis in the pulmonary arteries of mice identifies genes with relevance to human PAH. *Physiol Genomics*. 2011;43(8):417–437.

53. White K, Dempsie Y, Nilsen M, et al. The serotonin transporter, gender, and 17beta oestradiol in the development of pulmonary arterial hypertension. *Cardiovasc Res*. 2011;90(2):373–382.

54. Mair KM, Yang XD, Long L, et al. Sex affects bone morphogenetic protein type II receptor signaling in pulmonary artery smooth muscle cells. *Am J Respir Crit Care Med*. 2015;191(6):693–703.

55. Chen X, Talati M, Fessel JP, et al. Estrogen metabolite 16alpha-hydroxyestrone exacerbates bone morphogenetic protein receptor type II-associated pulmonary arterial hypertension through microRNA-29-mediated modulation of cellular metabolism. *Circulation*. 2016;133(1):82–97.

56. Umar S, Cunningham CM, Itoh Y, et al. The Y chromosome plays a protective role in experimental hypoxic pulmonary hypertension. *Am J Respir Crit Care Med*. 2018;197(7):952–955.

57. Austin ED, Lahm T, West J, et al. Gender, sex hormones and pulmonary hypertension. *Pulm Circ*. 2013;3(2):294–314.

58. Moudgil R, Michelakis E, Archer S. Hypoxic pulmonary vasoconstriction. *J Appl Physiol*. 2005;98(1):390–403.

59. Boucherat O, Vitry G, Trinh I, et al. The cancer theory of pulmonary arterial hypertension. *Pulm Circ*. 2017;7(2):285–299.

60. Kapitsinou PP, Rajendran G, Astleford L, et al. The endothelial prolyl-4-hydroxylase domain 2/hypoxia-inducible factor 2 axis regulates pulmonary artery pressure in mice. *Mol Cell Biol*. 2016;36(10):1584–1594.

61. Dai Z, Li M, Wharton J, et al. Prolyl-4 hydroxylase 2 (PHD2) deficiency in endothelial cells and hematopoietic cells induces obliterative vascular remodeling and severe pulmonary arterial hypertension in mice and humans through hypoxia-inducible factor-2alpha. *Circulation*. 2016;133(24):2447–2458.

62. Tang H, Babicheva A, McDermott KM, et al. Endothelial HIF-2alpha contributes to severe pulmonary hypertension by inducing endothelial-to-mesenchymal transition. *Am J Physiol Lung Cell Mol Physiol*. 2018;314(2):L256–L275.

63. Cottrill KA, Chan SY. Metabolic dysfunction in pulmonary hypertension: the expanding relevance of the Warburg effect. *Eur J Clin Invest*. 2013;43(8):855–865.

64. Sung YK, Chung L. Connective tissue disease-associated pulmonary arterial hypertension. *Rheum Dis Clin North Am*. 2015;41(2):295–313.

65. Fritz JS, Fallon MB, Kawut SM. Pulmonary vascular complications of liver disease. *Am J Respir Crit Care Med*. 2013;187(2):133–143.

66. DuBrock HM, Rodriguez-Lopez JM, LeVarge BL, et al. Macrophage migration inhibitory factor as a novel biomarker of portopulmonary hypertension. *Pulm Circ*. 2016;6(4):498–507.

67. Sithamparanathan S, Nair A, Thirugnanasothy L, et al. Survival in portopulmonary hypertension: outcomes of the United Kingdom National Pulmonary Arterial Hypertension Registry. *J Heart Lung Transplant*. 2017;36(7):770–779.

68. Savale L, Sattler C, Coilly A, et al. Long-term outcome in liver transplantation candidates with portopulmonary hypertension. *Hepatology*. 2017;65(5):1683–1692.

69. Galie N, Humbert M, Vachiery JL, et al. 2015 ESC/ERS guidelines for the diagnosis and treatment of pulmonary hypertension. *Rev Esp Cardiol (Engl Ed)*. 2016;69(2):177.

70. Galie N, Humbert M, Vachiery JL, et al. 2015 ESC/ERS guidelines for the diagnosis and treatment of pulmonary hypertension: the Joint Task Force for the Diagnosis and Treatment of Pulmonary Hypertension of the European Society of Cardiology (ESC) and the European Respiratory Society (ERS): endorsed by: Association for European Paediatric and Congenital Cardiology (AEPC), International Society for Heart and Lung Transplantation (ISHLT). *Eur Heart J*. 2016;37(1):67–119.

71. Zamanian RT, Hedlin H, Greuenwald P, et al. Features and outcomes of methamphetamine-associated pulmonary arterial hypertension. *Am J Respir Crit Care Med*. 2018;197(6):788–800.

72. Wang Y, Liu M, Wang HM, et al. Involvement of serotonin mechanism in methamphetamine-induced chronic pulmonary toxicity in rats. *Hum Exp Toxicol*. 2013;32(7):736–746.

73. Chen PI, Cao A, Miyagawa K, et al. Amphetamines promote mitochondrial dysfunction and DNA damage in pulmonary hypertension. *JCI Insight*. 2017;2(2):e90427.

74. Orcholski ME, Khurshudyan A, Shamskhou EA, et al. Reduced carboxylesterase 1 is associated with endothelial injury in methamphetamine-induced pulmonary arterial hypertension. *Am J Physiol Lung Cell Mol Physiol*. 2017;313(2):L252–L266.

75. Jarrett H, Barnett C. HIV-associated pulmonary hypertension. *Curr Opin HIV AIDS*. 2017;12(6):566–571.

76. Simon MA, Lacomis CD, George MP, et al. Isolated right ventricular dysfunction in patients with human immunodeficiency virus. *J Card Fail*. 2014;20(6):414–421.

77. Brittain EL, Duncan MS, Chang J, et al. Increased echocardiographic pulmonary pressure in HIV-infected and uninfected individuals in the Veterans Aging Cohort study. *Am J Respir Crit Care Med*. 2018;197(7):923–932.

78. Olalla J, Urdiales D, Pombo M, et al. Pulmonary hypertension in human immunodeficiency virus-infected patients: the role of antiretroviral therapy. *Med Clin (Barc)*. 2014;142(6):248–252.

79. Wang T, Green LA, Gupta SK, et al. Transfer of intracellular HIV Nef to endothelium causes endothelial dysfunction. *PLoS One*. 2014;9(3):e91063.

80. Almodovar S, Hsue PY, Morelli J, et al. Pathogenesis of HIV-associated pulmonary hypertension: potential role of HIV-1 Nef. *Proc Am Thorac Soc*. 2011;8(3):308–312.

81. Cota-Gomez A, Flores AC, Ling XF, et al. HIV-1 Tat increases oxidant burden in the lungs of transgenic mice. *Free Radic Biol Med*. 2011;51(9):1697–1707.

82. Amsellem V, Lipskaia L, Abid S, et al. CCR5 as a treatment target in pulmonary arterial hypertension. *Circulation*. 2014;130(11):880–891.

83. Dhillon NK, Li F, Xue B, et al. Effect of cocaine on human immunodeficiency virus-mediated pulmonary endothelial and smooth muscle dysfunction. *Am J Respir Cell Mol Biol*. 2011;45(1):40–52.

84. Dalvi P, O'Brien-Ladner A, Dhillon NK. Downregulation of bone morphogenetic protein receptor axis during HIV-1 and cocaine-mediated pulmonary smooth muscle hyperplasia: implications for HIV-related pulmonary arterial hypertension. *Arterioscler Thromb Vasc Biol*. 2013;33(11):2585–2595.

85. Dalvi P, Wang K, Mermis J, et al. HIV-1/cocaine induced oxidative stress disrupts tight junction protein-1 in human pulmonary microvascular endothelial cells: role of Ras/ERK1/2 pathway. *PLoS One*. 2014;9(1):e85246.

86. Hsue PY, Hunt PW, Ho JE, et al. Impact of HIV infection on diastolic function and left ventricular mass. *Circ Heart Fail*. 2010;3(1):132–139.

87. Kumar R, Mickael C, Kassa B, et al. TGF-beta activation by bone marrow-derived thrombospondin-1 causes Schistosoma- and hypoxia-induced pulmonary hypertension. *Nat Commun*. 2017;8:15494.

88. Thakkar AN, Chinnadurai P, Lin CH. Adult congenital heart disease: magnitude of the problem. *Curr Opin Cardiol*. 2017;32(5):467–474.

89. Sun X, Sharma S, Fratz S, et al. Disruption of endothelial cell mitochondrial bioenergetics in lambs with increased pulmonary blood flow. *Antioxid Redox Signal*. 2013;18(14):1739–1752.

90. Oishi PE, Wiseman DA, Sharma S, et al. Progressive dysfunction of nitric oxide synthase in a lamb model of chronically increased pulmonary blood flow: a role for oxidative stress. *Am J Physiol Lung Cell Mol Physiol*. 2008;295(5):L756–L766.

91. Sharma S, Barton J, Rafikov R, et al. Chronic inhibition of PPAR-γ signaling induces endothelial dysfunction in the juvenile lamb. *Pulm Pharmacol Ther*. 2013;26(2):271–280.

92. Sharma S, Sun X, Rafikov R, et al. PPAR-γ regulates carnitine homeostasis and mitochondrial function in a lamb model of increased pulmonary blood flow. *PLoS One*. 2012;7(9):e41555.

93. Boehme J, Sun X, Tormos KV, et al. Pulmonary artery smooth muscle cell hyperproliferation and metabolic shift triggered by pulmonary overcirculation. *Am J Physiol Heart Circ Physiol*. 2016;311(4):H944–H957.

94. Mathew B, Lakshminrusimha S. Persistent pulmonary hypertension in the newborn. *Children (Basel)*. 2017;4(8):E63.

95. Sharma M, Afolayan AJ. Redox signaling and persistent pulmonary hypertension of the newborn. *Adv Exp Med Biol*. 2017;967:277–287.

96. Abman SH. Inhaled nitric oxide for the treatment of pulmonary arterial hypertension. *Handb Exp Pharmacol*. 2013;218:257–276.

97. Hansmann G, Apitz C, Abdul-Khaliq H, et al. Executive summary. Expert consensus statement on the diagnosis and treatment of paediatric pulmonary hypertension. The European Paediatric Pulmonary Vascular Disease Network, endorsed by ISHLT and DGPK. *Heart*. 2016;102:86–100. Suppl 2:ii.

98. Montani D, Lau EM, Dorfmuller P, et al. Pulmonary veno-occlusive disease. *Eur Respir J*. 2016;47(5):1518–1534.

99. Chaisson NF, Dodson MW, Elliott CG. Pulmonary capillary hemangiomatosis and pulmonary veno-occlusive disease. *Clin Chest Med*. 2016;37(3):523–534.

100. Lathen C, Zhang Y, Chow J, et al. ERG-APLNR axis controls pulmonary venule endothelial proliferation in pulmonary veno-occlusive disease. *Circulation*. 2014;130(14):1179–1191.

101. Bueno M, Wang J, Mora AL, Gladwin MT. Nitrite signaling in pulmonary hypertension: mechanisms of bioactivation, signaling, and therapeutics. *Antioxid Redox Signal*. 2013;18(14):1797–1809.

102. MacLean M, Deuchar G, Hicks M, et al. Overexpression of the 5-hydroxytryptamine transporter gene: effect on pulmonary hemodynamics and hypoxia-induced pulmonary hypertension. *Circulation*. 2004;109(17):2150–2155.

103. Li X, Zhang X, Leathers R, et al. Notch3 signaling promotes the development of pulmonary arterial hypertension. *Nat Med*. 2009;15(11):1289–1297.

104. Dabral S, Tian X, Kojonazarov B, et al. Notch1 signalling regulates endothelial proliferation and apoptosis in pulmonary arterial hypertension. *Eur Respir J*. 2016;48(4):1137–1149.

105. Hurst LA, Dunmore BJ, Long L, et al. TNFalpha drives pulmonary arterial hypertension by suppressing the BMP type-II receptor and altering NOTCH signalling. *Nat Commun*. 2017;8:14079.

106. Luo H, Liu B, Zhao L, et al. Galectin-3 mediates pulmonary vascular remodeling in hypoxia-induced pulmonary arterial hypertension. *J Am Soc Hypertens*. 2017;11(10):673–683. e673.

107. He J, Li X, Luo H, et al. Galectin-3 mediates the pulmonary arterial hypertension-induced right ventricular remodeling through interacting with NADPH oxidase 4. *J Am Soc Hypertens*. 2017;11(5):275–289. e272.

107a. Cahill E, Costello CM, Rowan SC, et al. Gremlin plays a key role in the pathogenesis of pulmonary hypertension. *Circulation*. 2012;125(7):920–930.

108. Ryter SW, Choi AM. Carbon monoxide: present and future indications for a medical gas. *Korean J Intern Med*. 2013;28(2):123–140.

109. Brampton J, Aaronson PI. Role of hydrogen sulfide in systemic and pulmonary hypertension: cellular mechanisms and therapeutic implications. *Cardiovasc Hematol Agents Med Chem*. 2016;14(1):4–22.

110. Hanahan D, Weinberg RA. Hallmarks of cancer: the next generation. *Cell*. 2011;144(5):646–674.

111. Guignabert C, Tu L, Le Hiress M, et al. Pathogenesis of pulmonary arterial hypertension: lessons from cancer. *Eur Respir Rev*. 2013;22(130):543–551.

112. Hoeper MM, Barst RJ, Bourge RC, et al. Imatinib mesylate as add-on therapy for pulmonary arterial hypertension: results of the randomized IMPRES study. *Circulation.* 2013;127(10):1128–1138.

113. Frost AE, Barst RJ, Hoeper MM, et al. Long-term safety and efficacy of imatinib in pulmonary arterial hypertension. *J Heart Lung Transplant.* 2015;34(11):1366–1375.

114. Guignabert C, Phan C, Seferian A, et al. Dasatinib induces lung vascular toxicity and predisposes to pulmonary hypertension. *J Clin Invest.* 2016;126(9):3207–3218.

115. Weatherald J, Chaumais MC, Savale L, et al. Long-term outcomes of dasatinib-induced pulmonary arterial hypertension: a population-based study. *Eur Respir J.* 2017;50(1):1700217.

116. Saygin D, Highland KB, Farha S, et al. Metabolic and functional evaluation of the heart and lungs in pulmonary hypertension by gated 2-[18F]-fluoro-2-deoxy-D-glucose positron emission tomography. *Pulm Circ.* 2017;7(2):428–438.

117. Perl A. Metabolic control of immune system activation in rheumatic diseases. *Arthritis Rheumatol.* 2017;69(12):2259–2270.

118. Aounallah M, Dagenais-Lussier X, El-Far M, et al. Current topics in HIV pathogenesis, part 2: inflammation drives a Warburg-like effect on the metabolism of HIV-infected subjects. *Cytokine Growth Factor Rev.* 2016;28:1–10.

119. Hansen T, Galougahi KK, Celermajer D, et al. Oxidative and nitrosative signalling in pulmonary arterial hypertension - implications for development of novel therapies. *Pharmacol Ther.* 2016;165:50–62.

120. Michelakis ED, Gurtu V, Webster L, et al. Inhibition of pyruvate dehydrogenase kinase improves pulmonary arterial hypertension in genetically susceptible patients. *Sci Transl Med.* 2017;9(413):eaao4583.

121. Xu W, Yang H, Liu Y, et al. Oncometabolite 2-hydroxyglutarate is a competitive inhibitor of alpha-ketoglutarate-dependent dioxygenases. *Cancer Cell.* 2011;19(1):17–30.

122. Oldham WM, Clish CB, Yang Y, Loscalzo J. Hypoxia-mediated increases in L-2-hydroxyglutarate coordinate the metabolic response to reductive stress. *Cell Metab.* 2015;22(2):291–303.

123. Rhodes CJ, Howard LS, Busbridge M, et al. Iron deficiency and raised hepcidin in idiopathic pulmonary arterial hypertension: clinical prevalence, outcomes, and mechanistic insights. *J Am Coll Cardiol.* 2011;58(3):300–309.

123a. Chan SY, Zhang YY, Hemann C, et al. MicroRNA-210 controls mitochondrial metabolism during hypoxia by repressing the iron-sulfur cluster assembly proteins ISCU1/2. *Cell Metab.* 2009;10(4):273–284.

124. White K, Lu Y, Annis S, et al. Genetic and hypoxic alterations of the microRNA-210-ISCU1/2 axis promote iron-sulfur deficiency and pulmonary hypertension. *EMBO Mol Med.* 2015;7(6):695–713.

125. Navarro-Sastre A, Tort F, Stehling O, et al. A fatal mitochondrial disease is associated with defective NFU1 function in the maturation of a subset of mitochondrial Fe-S proteins. *Am J Hum Genet.* 2011;89(5):656–667.

126. Cotroneo E, Ashek A, Wang L, et al. Iron homeostasis and pulmonary hypertension: iron deficiency leads to pulmonary vascular remodeling in the rat. *Circ Res.* 2015;116(10):1680–1690.

127. Ghosh MC, Zhang DL, Jeong SY, et al. Deletion of iron regulatory protein 1 causes polycythemia and pulmonary hypertension in mice through translational derepression of HIF2alpha. *Cell Metab.* 2013;17(2):271–281.

128. Hensley CT, Wasti AT, DeBerardinis RJ. Glutamine and cancer: cell biology, physiology, and clinical opportunities. *J Clin Invest.* 2013;123(9):3678–3684.

129. Wang YY, Yang YX, Zhe H, et al. Bardoxolone methyl (CDDO-Me) as a therapeutic agent: an update on its pharmacokinetic and pharmacodynamic properties. *Drug Des Devel Ther.* 2014;8:2075–2088.

130. Chan SY, Rubin LJ. Metabolic dysfunction in pulmonary hypertension: from basic science to clinical practice. *Eur Respir Rev.* 2017;26(146):170094.

131. Westermann B. Mitochondrial fusion and fission in cell life and death. *Nat Rev Mol Cell Biol.* 2010;11(12):872–884.

132. Marsboom G, Toth PT, Ryan JJ, et al. Dynamin-related protein 1-mediated mitochondrial mitotic fission permits hyperproliferation of vascular smooth muscle cells and offers a novel therapeutic target in pulmonary hypertension. *Circ Res.* 2012;110(11):1484–1497.

133. Ryan JJ, Marsboom G, Fang YH, et al. PGC1alpha-mediated mitofusin-2 deficiency in female rats and humans with pulmonary arterial hypertension. *Am J Respir Crit Care Med.* 2013;187(8):865–878.

134. Parra V, Bravo-Sagua R, Norambuena-Soto I, et al. Inhibition of mitochondrial fission prevents hypoxia-induced metabolic shift and cellular proliferation of pulmonary arterial smooth muscle cells. *Biochim Biophys Acta.* 2017;1863(11):2891–2903.

135. Tian L, Neuber-Hess M, Mewburn J, et al. Ischemia-induced Drp1 and Fis1-mediated mitochondrial fission and right ventricular dysfunction in pulmonary hypertension. *J Mol Med (Berl).* 2017;95(4):381–393.

136. Paulin R, Dromparis P, Sutendra G, et al. Sirtuin 3 deficiency is associated with inhibited mitochondrial function and pulmonary arterial hypertension in rodents and humans. *Cell Metab.* 2014;20(5):827–839.

137. Pak O, Sommer N, Hoeres T, et al. Mitochondrial hyperpolarization in pulmonary vascular remodeling. Mitochondrial uncoupling protein deficiency as disease model. *Am J Respir Cell Mol Biol.* 2013;49(3):358–367.

138. Dromparis P, Paulin R, Sutendra G, et al. Uncoupling protein 2 deficiency mimics the effects of hypoxia and endoplasmic reticulum stress on mitochondria and triggers pseudo-hypoxic pulmonary vascular remodeling and pulmonary hypertension. *Circ Res.* 2013;113(2):126–136.

139. Haslip M, Dostanic I, Huang Y, et al. Endothelial uncoupling protein 2 regulates mitophagy and pulmonary hypertension during intermittent hypoxia. *Arterioscler Thromb Vasc Biol.* 2015;35(5):1166–1178.

140. Hong Z, Chen KH, DasGupta A, et al. MicroRNA-138 and microRNA-25 down-regulate mitochondrial calcium uniporter, causing the pulmonary arterial hypertension cancer phenotype. *Am J Respir Crit Care Med.* 2017;195(4):515–529.

141. Aguero J, Ishikawa K, Hadri L, et al. Intratracheal gene delivery of SERCA2a ameliorates chronic post-capillary pulmonary hypertension: a large animal model. *J Am Coll Cardiol.* 2016;67(17):2032–2046.

142. Hadri L, Kratlian RG, Benard L, et al. Therapeutic efficacy of AAV1.SERCA2a in monocrotaline-induced pulmonary arterial hypertension. *Circulation.* 2013;128(5):512–523.

143. Tang H, Yamamura A, Yamamura H, et al. Pathogenic role of calcium-sensing receptors in the development and progression of pulmonary hypertension. *Am J Physiol Lung Cell Mol Physiol.* 2016;310(9):L846–L859.

144. Dietrich A, Gudermann T. TRP channels in the cardiopulmonary vasculature. *Adv Exp Med Biol.* 2011;704:781–810.

145. Zhou C, Townsley MI, Alexeyev M, et al. Endothelial hyperpermeability in severe pulmonary arterial hypertension: role of store-operated calcium entry. *Am J Physiol Lung Cell Mol Physiol.* 2016;311(3):L560–L569.

146. Francis M, Xu N, Zhou C, Stevens T. Transient receptor potential channel 4 encodes a vascular permeability defect and high-frequency Ca(2+) transients in severe pulmonary arterial hypertension. *Am J Pathol.* 2016;186(6):1701–1709.

147. Sutendra G, Dromparis P, Wright P, et al. The role of Nogo and the mitochondria-endoplasmic reticulum unit in pulmonary hypertension. *Sci Transl Med.* 2011;3(88):88ra55.

148. Watson G, Oliver E, Zhao L, Wilkins MR. Pulmonary hypertension: old targets revisited (statins, PPARs, beta-blockers). *Handb Exp Pharmacol.* 2013;218:531–548.

149. Bertero T, Cottrill K, Krauszman A, et al. The microRNA-130/301 family controls vasoconstriction in pulmonary hypertension. *J Biol Chem.* 2014;290(4):2069–2085.

150. Bertero T, Lu Y, Annis S, et al. Systems-level regulation of microRNA networks by miR-130/301 promotes pulmonary hypertension. *J Clin Invest.* 2014;124(8):3514–3528.

151. Wang S, Dougherty EJ, Danner RL. PPARgamma signaling and emerging opportunities for improved therapeutics. *Pharmacol Res.* 2016;111:76–85.

151a. Legchenko E, Chouvarine P, Borchert P, et al. PPARγ agonist pioglitazone reverses pulmonary hypertension and prevents right heart failure via fatty acid oxidation. *Sci Transl Med.* 2018;10(438):eaao0303.

152. Chun HJ, Bonnet S, Chan SY. Translating microRNA biology in pulmonary hypertension: it will take more than "miR" words. *Am J Respir Crit Care Med.* 2017;195(2):167–178.

153. Parikh VN, Jin RC, Rabello S, et al. MicroRNA-21 integrates pathogenic signaling to control pulmonary hypertension: results of a network bioinformatics approach. *Circulation.* 2012;125(12):1520–1532.

154. Bertero T, Cottrill KA, Annis S, et al. A YAP/TAZ-miR-130/301 molecular circuit exerts systems-level control of fibrosis in a network of human diseases and physiologic conditions. *Sci Rep.* 2015;5:18277.

155. Negi V, Chan SY. Discerning functional hierarchies of microRNAs in pulmonary hypertension. *JCI Insight.* 2017;2(5):e91327.

156. Rabinovitch M. Molecular pathogenesis of pulmonary arterial hypertension. *J Clin Invest.* 2012;122(12):4306–4313.

157. Dupont S, Morsut L, Aragona M, et al. Role of YAP/TAZ in mechanotransduction. *Nature.* 2011;474(7350):179–183.

158. Piccolo S, Dupont S, Cordenonsi M. The biology of YAP/TAZ: hippo signaling and beyond. *Physiol Rev.* 2014;94(4):1287–1312.

159. Ruffenach G, Chabot S, Tanguay VF, et al. Role for runt-related transcription factor 2 in proliferative and calcified vascular lesions in pulmonary arterial hypertension. *Am J Respir Crit Care Med.* 2016;194(10):1273–1285.

160. Zhang H, Wang D, Li M, et al. The metabolic and proliferative state of vascular adventitial fibroblasts in pulmonary hypertension is regulated through a MiR-124/PTBP1/PKM axis. *Circulation.* 2017;136(25):2468–2485.

161. Caruso P, Dunmore BJ, Schlosser K, et al. Identification of miR-124 as a major regulator of enhanced endothelial cell glycolysis in pulmonary arterial hypertension via PTBP1 and PKM2. *Circulation.* 2017;136(25):2451–2467.

162. Li M, Riddle S, Zhang H, et al. Metabolic reprogramming regulates the proliferative and inflammatory phenotype of adventitial fibroblasts in pulmonary hypertension through the transcriptional corepressor C-terminal binding protein-1. *Circulation.* 2016;134(15):1105–1121.

163. Shimokawa H, Sunamura S, Satoh K. RhoA/Rho-kinase in the cardiovascular system. *Circ Res.* 2016;118(2):352–366.

164. Zhang Y, Wu S. Effects of fasudil on pulmonary hypertension in clinical practice. *Pulm Pharmacol Ther.* 2017;46:54–63.

165. Ranchoux B, Meloche J, Paulin R, et al. DNA damage and pulmonary hypertension. *Int J Mol Sci.* 2016;17(6):E990.

166. van der Bruggen CEE, Tedford RJ, Handoko ML, et al. RV pressure overload: from hypertrophy to failure. *Cardiovasc Res.* 2017;113(12):1423–1432.

167. Fang YH, Piao L, Hong Z, et al. Therapeutic inhibition of fatty acid oxidation in right ventricular hypertrophy: exploiting Randle's cycle. *J Mol Med (Berl).* 2012;90(1):31–43.

168. Potus F, Ruffenach G, Dahou A, et al. Downregulation of microRNA-126 contributes to the failing right ventricle in pulmonary arterial hypertension. *Circulation.* 2015;132(10):932–943.

169. Potus F, Malenfant S, Graydon C, et al. Impaired angiogenesis and peripheral muscle microcirculation loss contribute to exercise intolerance in pulmonary arterial hypertension. *Am J Respir Crit Care Med.* 2014;190(3):318–328.

170. Farber HW, Miller DP, Poms AD, et al. Five-year outcomes of patients enrolled in the REVEAL Registry. *Chest.* 2015;148(4):1043–1054.

171. Barst RJ, Chung L, Zamanian RT, et al. Functional class improvement and 3-year survival outcomes in patients with pulmonary arterial hypertension in the REVEAL Registry. *Chest.* 2013;144(1):160–168.

172. Ghofrani HA, Grimminger F, Grunig E, et al. Predictors of long-term outcomes in patients treated with riociguat for pulmonary arterial hypertension: data from the PATENT-2 open-label, randomised, long-term extension trial. *Lancet Respir Med.* 2016;4(5):361–371.

173. Raina A, Humbert M. Risk assessment in pulmonary arterial hypertension. *Eur Respir Rev.* 2016;25(142):390–398.

174. Nickel N, Golpon H, Greer M, et al. The prognostic impact of follow-up assessments in patients with idiopathic pulmonary arterial hypertension. *Eur Respir J.* 2012;39(3):589–596.

175. Yildiz M, Sahin A, Behnes M, Akin I. An expanding role of biomarkers in pulmonary arterial hypertension. *Curr Pharm Biotechnol.* 2017;18(6):491–494.

176. Shen Y, Wan C, Tian P, et al. CT-base pulmonary artery measurement in the detection of pulmonary hypertension: a meta-analysis and systematic review. *Medicine (Baltimore).* 2014;93(27):e256.

177. Rengier F, Worz S, Melzig C, et al. Automated 3D volumetry of the pulmonary arteries based on magnetic resonance angiography has potential for predicting pulmonary hypertension. *PLoS One.* 2016;11(9):e0162516.

178. Kang KY, Jeon CH, Choi SJ, et al. Survival and prognostic factors in patients with connective tissue disease-associated pulmonary hypertension diagnosed by echocardiography: results from a Korean nationwide registry. *Int J Rheum Dis.* 2017;20(9):1227–1236.

179. D'Alto M, Romeo E, Argiento P, et al. Pulmonary arterial hypertension: the key role of echocardiography. *Echocardiography.* 2015;32(Suppl 1):S23–S37.

180. Addetia K, Maffessanti F, Yamat M, et al. Three-dimensional echocardiography-based analysis of right ventricular shape in pulmonary arterial hypertension. *Eur Heart J Cardiovasc Imaging.* 2016;17(5):564–575.

181. Park JH, Park MM, Farha S, et al. Impaired global right ventricular longitudinal strain predicts long-term adverse outcomes in patients with pulmonary arterial hypertension. *J Cardiovasc Ultrasound.* 2015;23(2):91–99.

182. Freed BH, Collins JD, Francois CJ, et al. MR and CT imaging for the evaluation of pulmonary hypertension. *JACC Cardiovasc Imaging.* 2016;9(6):715–732.

183. van de Veerdonk MC, Kind T, Marcus JT, et al. Progressive right ventricular dysfunction in patients with pulmonary arterial hypertension responding to therapy. *J Am Coll Cardiol.* 2011;58(24):2511–2519.

184. Peacock AJ, Crawley S, McLure L, et al. Changes in right ventricular function measured by cardiac magnetic resonance imaging in patients receiving pulmonary arterial hypertension-targeted therapy: the EURO-MR study. *Circ Cardiovasc Imaging.* 2014;7(1):107–114.

185. Schroeder MA, Lau AZ, Chen AP, et al. Hyperpolarized (13) C magnetic resonance reveals early- and late-onset changes to in vivo pyruvate metabolism in the failing heart. *Eur J Heart Fail.* 2013;15(2):130–140.

186. Ahmadi A, Ohira H, Mielniczuk LM. FDG PET imaging for identifying pulmonary hypertension and right heart failure. *Curr Cardiol Rep.* 2015;17(1):555.

187. Tatebe S, Fukumoto Y, Oikawa-Wakayama M, et al. Enhanced [18F]fluorodeoxyglucose accumulation in the right ventricular free wall predicts long-term prognosis of patients with pulmonary hypertension: a preliminary observational study. *Eur Heart J Cardiovasc Imaging.* 2014;15(6):666–672.

188. Humbert M, Sitbon O, Chaouat A, et al. Survival in patients with idiopathic, familial, and anorexigen-associated pulmonary arterial hypertension in the modern management era. *Circulation.* 2010;122(2):156–163.

189. Farber HW, Miller DP, McGoon MD, et al. Predicting outcomes in pulmonary arterial hypertension based on the 6-minute walk distance. *J Heart Lung Transplant.* 2015;34(3):362–368.

190. Chia EM, Lau EM, Xuan W, et al. Exercise testing can unmask right ventricular dysfunction in systemic sclerosis patients with normal resting pulmonary artery pressure. *Int J Cardiol.* 2016;204:179–186.

191. Blumberg FC, Arzt M, Lange T, et al. Impact of right ventricular reserve on exercise capacity and survival in patients with pulmonary hypertension. *Eur J Heart Fail.* 2013;15(7):771–775.

192. Tolle JJ, Waxman AB, Van Horn TL, et al. Exercise-induced pulmonary arterial hypertension. *Circulation.* 2008;118(21):2183–2189.

193. Park MH, Ramani GV, Kop WJ, et al. Exercise-uncovered pulmonary arterial hypertension and pharmacologic therapy: clinical benefits. *J Heart Lung Transplant.* 2010;29(2):228–229.

194. Suzuki K, Akashi YJ, Manabe M, et al. Simple exercise echocardiography using a Master's two-step test for early detection of pulmonary arterial hypertension. *J Cardiol.* 2013;62(3):176–182.

195. Grunig E, Janssen B, Mereles D, et al. Abnormal pulmonary artery pressure response in asymptomatic carriers of primary pulmonary hypertension gene. *Circulation.* 2000;102(10):1145–1150.

196. Sitbon O, Benza RL, Badesch DB, et al. Validation of two predictive models for survival in pulmonary arterial hypertension. *Eur Respir J.* 2015;46(1):152–164.

197. Taichman DB, Ornelas J, Chung L, et al. Pharmacologic therapy for pulmonary arterial hypertension in adults: CHEST guideline and expert panel report. *Chest.* 2014;146(2):449–475.

198. Arena R, Cahalin LP, Borghi-Silva A, Myers J. The effect of exercise training on the pulmonary arterial system in patients with pulmonary hypertension. *Prog Cardiovasc Dis.* 2015;57(5):480–488.

199. Olsson KM, Nickel NP, Tongers J, Hoeper MM. Atrial flutter and fibrillation in patients with pulmonary hypertension. *Int J Cardiol.* 2013;167(5):2300–2305.

200. Perrin S, Chaumais MC, O'Connell C, et al. New pharmacotherapy options for pulmonary arterial hypertension. *Expert Opin Pharmacother.* 2015;16(14):2113–2131.

201. de Raaf MA, Beekhuijzen M, Guignabert C, et al. Endothelin-1 receptor antagonists in fetal development and pulmonary arterial hypertension. *Reprod Toxicol.* 2015;56:45–51.

202. Pulido T, Adzerikho I, Channick RN, et al. Macitentan and morbidity and mortality in pulmonary arterial hypertension. *N Engl J Med.* 2013;369(9):809–818.

203. Ghofrani HA, Galie N, Grimminger F, et al. Riociguat for the treatment of pulmonary arterial hypertension. *N Engl J Med.* 2013;369(4):330–340.

204. Rubin LJ, Galie N, Grimminger F, et al. Riociguat for the treatment of pulmonary arterial hypertension: a long-term extension study (PATENT-2). *Eur Respir J.* 2015;45(5):1303–1313.

205. Galie N, Muller K, Scalise AV, Grunig E. PATENT PLUS: a blinded, randomised and extension study of riociguat plus sildenafil in pulmonary arterial hypertension. *Eur Respir J.* 2015;45(5):1314–1322.

206. Mubarak KK. A review of prostaglandin analogs in the management of patients with pulmonary arterial hypertension. *Respir Med.* 2010;104(1):9–21.

207. Tapson VF, Torres F, Kermeen F, et al. Oral treprostinil for the treatment of pulmonary arterial hypertension in patients on background endothelin receptor antagonist and/or phosphodiesterase type 5 inhibitor therapy (the FREEDOM-C study): a randomized controlled trial. *Chest.* 2012;142(6):1383–1390.

208. Tapson VF, Jing ZC, Xu KF, et al. Oral treprostinil for the treatment of pulmonary arterial hypertension in patients receiving background endothelin receptor antagonist and phosphodiesterase type 5 inhibitor therapy (the FREEDOM-C2 study): a randomized controlled trial. *Chest.* 2013;144(3):952–958.

209. Sitbon O, Channick R, Chin KM, et al. Selexipag for the treatment of pulmonary arterial hypertension. *N Engl J Med.* 2015;373(26):2522–2533.

210. Sobanski V, Launay D, Hachulla E, Humbert M. Current approaches to the treatment of systemic-sclerosis-associated pulmonary arterial hypertension (SSc-PAH). *Curr Rheumatol Rep.* 2016;18(2):10.

211. Cartin-Ceba R, Swanson K, Iyer V, et al. Safety and efficacy of ambrisentan for the treatment of portopulmonary hypertension. *Chest.* 2011;139(1):109–114.

212. Yamashita Y, Tsujino I, Sato T, et al. Hemodynamic effects of ambrisentan-tadalafil combination therapy on progressive portopulmonary hypertension. *World J Hepatol.* 2014;6(11):825–829.

213. McLaughlin VV, Shah SJ, Souza R, Humbert M. Management of pulmonary arterial hypertension. *J Am Coll Cardiol.* 2015;65(18):1976–1997.

214. Sitbon O, Gaine S. Beyond a single pathway: combination therapy in pulmonary arterial hypertension. *Eur Respir Rev.* 2016;25(142):408–417.

215. Channick RN, Delcroix M, Ghofrani HA, et al. Effect of macitentan on hospitalizations: results from the SERAPHIN trial. *JACC Heart Fail.* 2015;3(1):1–8.

216. McLaughlin V, Channick RN, Ghofrani HA, et al. Bosentan added to sildenafil therapy in patients with pulmonary arterial hypertension. *Eur Respir J.* 2015;46(2):405–413.

217. Galie N, Barbera JA, Frost AE, et al. Initial use of ambrisentan plus tadalafil in pulmonary arterial hypertension. *N Engl J Med.* 2015;373(9):834–844.

218. Corris P, Degano B. Severe pulmonary arterial hypertension: treatment options and the bridge to transplantation. *Eur Respir Rev.* 2014;23(134):488–497.

219. Whitson BA, Hayes Jr D. Indications and outcomes in adult lung transplantation. *J Thorac Dis.* 2014;6(8):1018–1023.

220. Al Maluli H, DeStephan CM, Alvarez Jr RJ, Sandoval J. Atrial septostomy: a contemporary review. *Clin Cardiol.* 2015;38(6):395–400.

221. Simonneau G, Hoeper MM, McLaughlin V, et al. Future perspectives in pulmonary arterial hypertension. *Eur Respir Rev.* 2016;25(142):381–389.

222. Drake KM, Dunmore BJ, McNelly LN, et al. Correction of nonsense BMPR2 and SMAD9 mutations by ataluren in pulmonary arterial hypertension. *Am J Respir Cell Mol Biol.* 2013;49(3):403–409.

223. Granton J, Langleben D, Kutryk MB, et al. Endothelial NO-synthase gene-enhanced progenitor cell therapy for pulmonary arterial hypertension: the PHACeT trial. *Circ Res.* 2015;117(7):645–654.

224. Chen SL, Zhang FF, Xu J, et al. Pulmonary artery denervation to treat pulmonary arterial hypertension: the single-center, prospective, first-in-man PADN-1 study (first-in-man pulmonary artery denervation for treatment of pulmonary artery hypertension). *J Am Coll Cardiol.* 2013;62(12):1092–1100.

225. Newman JH, Rich S, Abman SH, et al. Enhancing insights into pulmonary vascular disease through a precision medicine approach. a joint NHLBI-Cardiovascular Medical Research and Education Fund Workshop report. *Am J Respir Crit Care Med.* 2017;195(12):1661–1670.

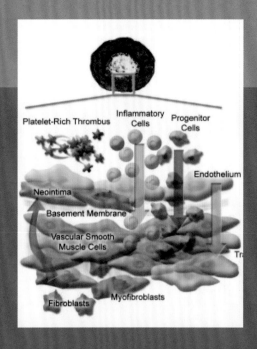

第56章
非肺动脉高压性肺高压

　　肺高压（pulmonary hypertension，PH）是指患者仰卧位时，通过右心导管测量的持续平均肺动脉血压（mean pulmonary arterial pressure，mPAP）≥25 mmHg。其临床综合征包括呼吸困难、活动能力下降和低氧血症。由几种不同的病理生理学和分子机制所介导。在绝大多数患者中，肺高压是由于肺血管收缩、充血或原发性肺、心脏或肺血管血栓栓塞疾病引起肺部血流阻力增高所导致。肺高压的患病率约为1%，在65岁以上的人群中增加到10%。肺高压的发病率、预后、治疗选择和临床发展过程与其原发疾病密切相关。全面的临床评估、放射学、血清学和（或）有创血流动力学监测，用以区分肺动脉高压和非肺动脉高压性肺高压是必要的。导致非肺动脉高压性肺高压的常见疾病包括：①急性或慢性左心心力衰竭及左心瓣膜病；②引起低氧血症的慢性肺部疾病综合征，包括慢性阻塞性肺疾病、间质性肺病等；③以血栓重构导致中央和远端肺动脉腔内闭塞为特征的慢性血栓栓塞性肺动脉高压；④以红细胞结构异常或溶血为特征的血液病，如镰状细胞病等。本章将概述以上导致非肺动脉高压性肺高压的相关疾病的病理生理学、诊断及治疗。

尚玉强

Pulmonary Hypertension in Patients With Nonpulmonary Arterial Hypertension

Bradley A. Maron, George A. Alba, and Joseph Loscalzo

OVERVIEW OF PULMONARY HYPERTENSION

Definition and Nomenclature

Pulmonary hypertension (PH) is defined classically as a sustained mean pulmonary arterial blood pressure (mPAP) $\geq$ 25 mm Hg measured in the supine position by right heart catheterization.[1] The PH clinical syndrome typically includes dyspnea, diminished exercise capacity, and hypoxemia, which may result from several different pathophysiologic and molecular mechanisms. The contemporary PH classification system was created by an international panel of world experts—most recently updated at the Fifth World Symposium on PH in 2013 (Nice, France)—and divides PH patients into five broad groups: pulmonary arterial hypertension (PAH) or PAH-associated conditions (group 1, formerly *primary* PH) and PH occurring in the setting of another cardiopulmonary or systemic disease (groups 2 to 5, formerly *secondary* PH).[2] In the vast majority of patients, PH develops as a consequence of hypoxic pulmonary vasoconstriction; vascular congestion; or impedance to pulmonary blood flow due to primary lung, cardiac, or pulmonary vascular thromboembolic disease. In contrast, PAH, a rare form of PH, results from the interplay between genetic and molecular factors that promotes a proliferative, fibrotic, and plexogenic vasculopathy affecting small- and medium-sized pulmonary arteries in the absence of other cardiopulmonary disease.[3] The hemodynamic profile of PAH is distinguished from other forms of PH by a pulmonary vascular resistance (PVR) of >3 Wood units (240 dynes/s/cm^5) at rest in the setting of a pulmonary artery wedge pressure (PAWP) $\leq$15 mm Hg.[1,2] In PAH, the mPAP is often >40 mm Hg and may reach supra-systemic levels in severe cases; however, this occurs uncommonly in PH from non-PAH etiologies.[4] Thus PAH and PH are distinct pathophysiological and clinical entities. Although symptoms and physical examination signs often overlap between these conditions, the terms are not synonymous.[1] The Sixth World Symposium on PH, held in Nice, France, in 2018, incorporated the latest science to refine the existing classification guidelines.[4a] Recommendations from this symposium suggested expanding the thresholds for mPAP and PVR to >20 mm Hg and >3.0 Wood units, respectively, for patients with pulmonary hypertension not due to left heart disease. Confirming the utility of these updates to clinical practice will require additional time, experience, and research.

Chapter 55 is devoted to a discussion of PAH and PAH-associated conditions, whereas the current chapter provides an overview of the pathophysiology and treatment of disorders associated with secondary forms of PH. Specifically this chapter reviews primary diseases that modulate PH by causing (1) pulmonary venous hypertension, (2) chronic hypoxia, (3) chronic pulmonary thromboembolism, and (4) mechanical disruption of the normal pulmonary vasculature (i.e., WHO PH classification groups 2 to 5, respectively) (Box 56.1).[2] In clinical practice and throughout the published literature, the designation "nonpulmonary arterial hypertension pulmonary hypertension" is often invoked to describe these patients.

Epidemiology, Diagnosis, and Natural History

The prevalence of PH in the general population is not well established; however, a recent review assessing the global burden of PH estimated a prevalence of about 1%, which increased up to 10% in individuals older than 65 years, with lung and left-sided heart diseases being the most frequent etiologies.[5] Recent epidemiologic studies in large referral populations have also provided more granular data on the prevalence of PH and clinical risk. For example, in a community-based study of 2042 patients undergoing echocardiography, of whom 69% had a measurable pulmonary artery systolic pressure (PASP), mortality was significantly increased in those with a PASP of 30 mm Hg or higher compared with others with an estimated PASP of 15 to 23 mm Hg.[6] In a large cohort of Veterans Affairs patients who underwent gold-standard diagnostic testing with right heart catheterization (n = 21,727), 23% had borderline PH (mPAP 19 to 24 mm Hg) and 57% had PH (mPAP $\geq$25 mm Hg). A continuum of risk emerged according to mPAP level when treated as a continuous variable, with the adjusted risk of mortality increasing significantly from 19 mm Hg (hazard ratio 1.183, 95% CI 1.004 to 1.393) (Fig. 56.1).[7]

PH incidence varies substantially according to primary disease subtype. In one report of 455 patients with an elevated left ventricular (LV) end-diastolic pressure (but without left-sided valvular disease), investigators observed that over half had comorbid PH,[8] whereas PH is present in >90% of select patients with chronic obstructive pulmonary disease (COPD).[9,10] Rates of PH also vary significantly within a specific primary disease subpopulation. For example, Handa and colleagues reported a 5% PH prevalence in one cohort of asymptomatic or mildly symptomatic sarcoidosis patients despite abnormal chest radiography, restrictive pattern on pulmonary function testing, and decreased levels of peripheral oxygen saturation. However, if persistent dyspnea is present in sarcoidosis, PH prevalence rates increase to over 50%.[11,12] The likelihood of developing *clinically evident* PH is not well characterized but may be linked to comorbid cardiac or lung disease characteristics. For example, symptomatic PH due to impaired LV diastolic function from chronic systemic hypertension is an indolent process that progresses along with the decline in myocardial compliance.[13] In contrast, severe PH from acute altitude sickness occurs via hypoxic pulmonary vasoconstriction and hyperemia, which may develop independent of pulmonary reserve.[14]

Prognosis, treatment choice, and clinical trajectory in PH are strongly associated with disease subtype. At present, goal-directed medical therapy for the restoration of pulmonary microvascular function with calcium channel blockers, endothelin receptor antagonists (ERAs), nitric oxide–cyclic guanosine monophosphate enhancers, or prostanoid replacement therapy is approved by the US Food and Drug

BOX 56.1 Clinical Classification of Pulmonary Hypertension by Etiology

Pulmonary arterial hypertension (PAH)
- Idiopathic PAH
- Heritable PAH
  - BMPR2
  - ALK-1, ENG, SMAD9, CAV1, KCNK3
  - Unknown
- Drug- and toxin-induced
- PAH-associated diseases
  - Connective tissue disease
  - HIV infection
  - Portal hypertension
  - Congenital heart diseases
  - Schistosomiasis
- 1′ Pulmonary veno-occlusive disease and/or pulmonary capillary hemangiomatosis
- 1″ Persistent pulmonary hypertension of the newborn (PPHN)

Pulmonary hypertension (PH) due to left heart disease
- Left ventricular systolic dysfunction
- Left ventricular diastolic dysfunction
- Valvular disease
- Congenital/acquired left heart inflow/outflow tract obstruction and congenital cardiomyopathies

PH due to lung diseases and/or hypoxia
- Chronic obstructive pulmonary disease (COPD)
- Interstitial lung disease (ILD)
- Other pulmonary diseases of mixed restrictive and obstructive pattern
- Sleep-disordered breathing
- Alveolar hypoventilation disorders
- Chronic exposure to high altitude
- Developmental lung diseases

Chronic thromboembolic pulmonary hypertension (CTEPH)
- Chronic thromboembolic pulmonary hypertension
- Other pulmonary artery obstructions (e.g., angiosarcoma, arteritis)

Pulmonary hypertension with unclear multifactorial mechanisms
- Hematologic disorders: chronic hemolytic anemia, myeloproliferative disorders, splenectomy
- Systemic disorders: sarcoidosis, pulmonary Langerhans histiocytosis, lymphangioleiomyomatosis
- Metabolic disorders: glycogen storage disease, Gaucher disease, thyroid disorders
- Others: tumoral obstruction, fibrosing mediastinitis, chronic renal failure, segmental PH
- Diseases in Groups 2 to 5 are reviewed in the current chapter.

Modified from Simonneau G, Gatzoulis MA, Adatia I, et al. Updated clinical classification of pulmonary hypertension. *J Am Coll Cardiol.* 2013;62(25 suppl):D34–D41.

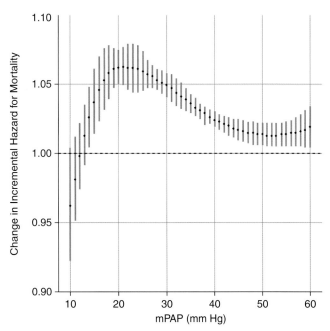

Fig. 56.1 Spline curve demonstrating effect of a unit increase of 1 mm Hg in mean pulmonary arterial pressure *(mPAP)* on hazard of mortality. (Redrawn from Maron BA, Hess E, Maddox TM, et al. Association of borderline pulmonary hypertension with mortality and hospitalization in a large patient cohort: insights from the Veterans Affairs clinical assessment, reporting, and tracking program. *Circulation.* 2016;133:1240–1248.)

Administration (FDA) for use only in PAH patients. As is discussed in greater detail further on, conclusions from small clinical trials have demonstrated a favorable effect of various PAH therapies on pulmonary hemodynamics and exercise tolerance in some WHO class 2 to 5 conditions, and many treatment centers use these medications in select non-PAH patients.[15] For example, a recent study of patients with typical idiopathic PAH (iPAH) (with fewer than three risk factors for left heart disease), atypical iPAH (with three or more risk factors for left heart disease), and PH due to heart failure with preserved ejection fraction (PH-HFpEF) demonstrated that there is a population of patients with precapillary PH and risk factors for HFpEF who benefit from PAH-directed therapy, albeit to a lesser extent than patients with

typical iPAH.[16] Overall, the administration of advanced PAH therapies to non-PAH patients with PH is likely to be ineffective and possibly harmful.[1,8] Therefore the emphasis of contemporary diagnostic algorithms is on distinguishing PAH from non-PAH patients (Fig. 56.2A).[1] Comprehensive clinical, radiographic, serologic, echocardiographic, and/or invasive hemodynamic testing is often necessary to confirm the absence of disease states that predispose to PH prior to making the diagnosis of PAH (see Fig. 56.2B).[9]

PH is underrecognized in clinical practice, and its global burden is only expected to increase.[5,17-19] The initiation of diagnostic testing for PH therefore requires a low index of clinical suspicion among practitioners who must recognize clues that suggest PH pathophysiology, such as familial or genetic risk factors for PAH or comorbid conditions known to promote elevations in PA pressure.

PULMONARY VENOUS HYPERTENSION

Pathophysiology of Pulmonary Hypertension Due to Left-Sided Heart Disease

Acute Left Heart Failure

Among the most common causes of PH is left-sided cardiac disease from LV systolic or diastolic dysfunction, or left-sided valvular disease (Table 56.1). In nonvalvular forms of left-sided heart disease, increased LV end-diastolic filling pressure is transmitted retrograde to the pulmonary venous and arterial circulatory beds. Acute changes to normal LV pressure-volume hemodynamics, as occurs during an acute myocardial infarction or as a consequence of mitral valve leaflet rupture, predispose to sudden and dramatic increases in left atrial (LA) and PA pressure (Fig. 56.3).[20] Owing to the noncompacted and thin-walled architecture of the right ventricle (RV), acute pressure loading is poorly tolerated and results in RV systolic dysfunction, a major determinant of outcome in PH.[21] Acute increases in PA pressure result in a congestive vasculopathy characterized by decreased pulmonary arteriolar compliance and loss of normal autoregulation of pulmonary vasomotor

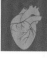

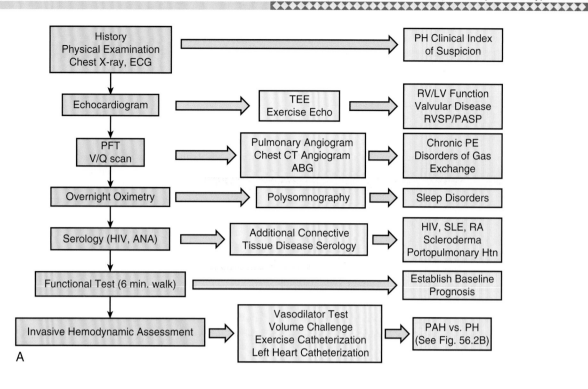

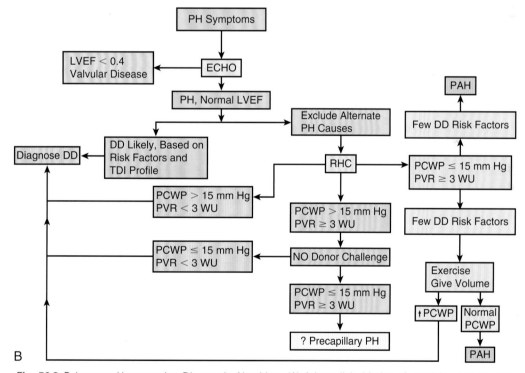

Fig. 56.2 Pulmonary Hypertension Diagnostic Algorithm. (A) A low clinical index of suspicion initiates the clinical evaluation for pulmonary hypertension *(PH)*. Primary test results aid the clinician in establishing a diagnosis of PH and determining the most likely PH classification. Secondary tests are utilized in accordance with the results from primary tests and provide additional information for determining PH etiology. (B) One possible diagnostic algorithm for discriminating pulmonary arterial hypertension (PAH) from PH due to primary left-heart disease. *CT*, Computed tomography; *DD*, diastolic dysfunction; *LV*, left ventricle; *PASP*, pulmonary artery systolic pressure; *PCWP*, pulmonary capillary wedge pressure; *PFT*, pulmonary function test; *RHC*, right heart catheterization; *RV*, right ventricle; *RVSP*, right ventricular systolic pressure; *TEE*, transesophageal echocardiogram; *V/Q*, ventilation/perfusion; *WU*, Wood units. ([A], Modified from McLaughlin VV, Archer SL, Badesch DB, et al. ACCF/AHA 2009 expert consensus document on pulmonary hypertension: a report of the American College of Cardiology Foundation Task Force on Expert Consensus Documents and the American Heart Association developed in collaboration with the American College of Chest Physicians; American Thoracic Society, Inc.; and the Pulmonary Hypertension Association. *J Am Coll Cardiol.* 2009;53:1573–1619. [B], Modified from Hoeper MM, Barbera JA, Channick RN, et al. Diagnosis, assessment, and treatment of non-pulmonary arterial hypertension pulmonary hypertension. *J Am Coll Cardiol.* 2009;54[1 suppl]:S85–S96.)

TABLE 56.1   Cardiovascular Diseases That Predispose to Pulmonary Hypertension

Clinical Feature	Mechanism
Chronic systemic hypertension	↑ LV afterload → LV hypertrophy → ↓ LV compliance → ↑ LV end-diastolic filling pressure → pulmonary venous hypertension
Diabetes mellitus	Intramyocardial microcirculatory and epicardial coronary vascular dysfunction → LV systolic or diastolic dysfunction → pulmonary venous hypertension
Coronary artery disease	Myocardial ischemia → LV systolic or diastolic dysfunction → pulmonary venous hypertension
Atrial fibrillation	Loss of "atrial kick" → ↑ left atrial and pulmonary venous congestion
Impaired diastolic function	↑ End-diastolic filling pressure secondary to restrictive, infiltrative, or genetic cardiomyopathy → pulmonary venous hypertension
Mitral stenosis	↑ Transmitral valve pressure ± atrial fibrillation → ↑ pulmonary venous hypertension
Mitral regurgitation	Chronic LV volume overload → LV cavitary dilation → ↑ LV end-diastolic filling pressure → pulmonary venous hypertension
With elevated mitral regurgitant fraction, PA pressure is elevated secondary to pulmonary circulatory volume and pressure overload, particularly during exercise
Aortic insufficiency	Chronic LV volume overload → LV cavitary dilation → ↑ LV end-diastolic filling pressure → pulmonary venous hypertension

LV, Left ventricle; PA, pulmonary artery.

tone.[22] These pathophysiological changes are generally reversible with pharmacotherapies that promote pulmonary vasodilation, reduce cardiac preload (e.g., NO• donors, particularly nitrate therapy), or directly alleviate pulmonary vascular congestion (e.g., loop diuretics). Pulmonary venous remodeling is increasingly recognized as a contributor to PH in left heart disease in vivo.[23]

Chronic Nonvalvular Left-Sided Heart Failure

In addition to passive pulmonary vascular congestion, circulating levels of the vasoactive peptide endothelin-1 (ET-1) correlate positively with PH severity in chronic left-sided heart failure.[24] Pathophysiological concentrations of ET-1 disrupt normal vasomotor tone by activating $ET_{A/B}$ receptors on vascular smooth muscle cells (VSMCs), thus increasing intracellular $[Ca^{+2}]_i$ levels. ET-1 also promotes the release of neurohumoral factors, such as norepinephrine and aldosterone, that cause pulmonary vascular remodeling.[25-27] Together these processes are linked to pulmonary artery endothelial cell dysfunction and VSMC contraction, which in PH offsets vasodilatory cell signaling pathways to promote pulmonary arterial vasoconstriction and adverse remodeling.

Chronically elevated pulmonary venous pressure induces a cellular environment in pulmonary arterioles characterized by inflammation and increased generation of reactive oxygen species (ROS). Over time, these maladaptive molecular processes are implicated in the development of irreversible pathological changes to normal pulmonary blood vessel architecture, including intimal fibrosis as well as VSMC hypertrophy and proliferation. Chronic RV pressure overload is also linked to the propagation of worsening *left-heart* failure by promoting abnormal changes in RV chamber deformation that adversely influence LV geometry.[28]

Diagnosis, Treatment, and Natural History

The diagnosis of PH from left-sided heart failure is often evident on clinical grounds alone. Complaints of decreased exercise tolerance, dyspnea, and lower extremity edema are common in PH but do not necessarily discriminate right- from left-sided congestive heart failure per se. Therefore echocardiography is utilized to estimate PA systolic pressure and evaluate RV size and function. A recent study of over 66,000 first adult transthoracic echocardiograms found that 18% were suggestive of PH based on an estimated PASP >40 mm Hg; of these, 69% were attributable to left-sided heart disease (37% valvular disease, 20% diastolic heart failure, 8% systolic heart failure, and 5% mixed valvular disease and systolic heart failure).[29] Invasive hemodynamic monitoring with right heart catheterization confirms the diagnosis of PH and excludes alternate etiologies of PH-like symptoms, such as constrictive pericardial disease, in which PVR is usually normal. Importantly, PA pressure, PVR, and RV systolic function are each independent predictors of outcome in patients with chronic left-sided heart failure. In one study of

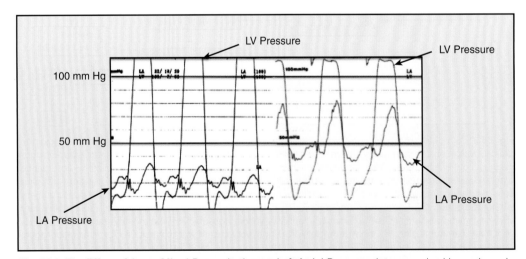

Fig. 56.3 The Effect of Acute Mitral Regurgitation on Left Atrial Pressure. Intraprocedural hemodynamic tracing obtained during a mitral balloon valvotomy captures a dramatic increase in mean left atrial *(LA)* pressure from 20 to 48 mm Hg due to acute mitral insufficiency. Sudden changes in LA or pulmonary pressure are poorly tolerated by the right ventricle and may induce cor pulmonale. (Modified from Ha JW, Chung N, Chang BC, et al. Acute mitral regurgitation due to leaflet tear after balloon valvotomy. *Circulation.* 1998;98:2095–2097.)

377 patients undergoing right heart catheterization with low LV ejection fraction and a history of congestive heart failure, a mPAP >29 mm Hg portended an approximately threefold higher 36-month mortality rate (irrespective of RV function) as compared with a normal mPAP.[30] Interpretation of cardiopulmonary hemodynamics, however, must take into account an individual patient's specific clinical scenario. Typically PA pressure correlates positively with PH severity in chronic left-sided heart failure, but not in all cases. Since the generation of PA pressure is dependent on RV systolic function, abnormally low PA pressure may be observed in severe PH with RV failure. In this scenario, left-sided heart failure–mediated pulmonary vascular congestion results in an increased PVR even if PA pressure is mildly elevated, normal, or even low.[24] Cardiopulmonary hemodynamic indices commonly used in clinical practice are provided in Table 56.2.

Conventional heart failure pharmacotherapy is the cornerstone treatment strategy for PH from nonvalvular left-sided cardiac disease. Angiotensin converting enzyme (ACE) inhibitors, angiotensin-receptor blockers (ARBs), β-adrenergic receptor antagonists, loop diuretics, and vasodilators (e.g., hydralazine) often decrease PVR and PA pressure effectively, thereby promoting favorable responses in RV systolic function. Sufficiently powered randomized clinical trials evaluating the effect of iNO•, prostacyclin replacement, nitric oxide–cyclic guanosine monophosphate enhancers, and ERAs for PH from chronic left-sided heart failure have either failed to demonstrate a beneficial effect on pulmonary vascular hemodynamics or did so but at the cost of significant adverse clinical events, including increased early mortality in one large trial of intravenous epoprostenol.[31] Sildenafil, which promotes vasodilation by inhibiting PDE-5 in lung VSMCs, appears to decrease PA pressure and PVR safely without compromising cardiac output (Fig. 56.4)[32]; however, a randomized clinical trial of sildenafil in patients with PH-HFpEF and modest PH did not result in significant improvement in exercise capacity or clinical status.[33]

TABLE 56.2 Pulmonary Hemodynamic Measurements and Normal Ranges

Measurement	Equation	Normal Range
Mean RAP	Directly measured (PA catheter)	0–8 mm Hg
Pulmonary artery blood pressure	Directly measured (PA catheter)	Systolic (PASP): 15–25 mm Hg
	Directly measured (PA catheter)	Diastolic (PADP): 4–12 mm Hg
	PASP + (2 × PADP)/3	MPAP: 10–20 mm Hg
PA capillary wedge pressure	Directly measured (PA catheter)	6–12 mm Hg
Cardiac output	Heart rate × stroke volume/1000	4–7 L/min
Pulmonary vascular resistance	80 × (MPAP–PAWP)/cardiac output	20–130 dyn/s/cm5 or 0.25–1.6 Wood units
Transpulmonary gradient	MPAP – PAWP	5–8 mm Hg

MPAP, Mean pulmonary artery pressure; *PA,* pulmonary artery; *PADP,* pulmonary artery diastolic pressure; *PASP,* pulmonary artery systolic pressure; *PAWP,* pulmonary artery wedge pressure; *RAP,* right atrial pressure; *SBP,* systolic blood pressure.

Pulmonary Hypertension from Left-sided Valvular Disease

PH from left-sided valvular disease remains the most common cause of group 2 PH and most often occurs from mitral regurgitation (MR) or mitral stenosis and less commonly from severe aortic regurgitation.[29] In aortic stenosis, initial pressure loading–induced LV hypertrophy

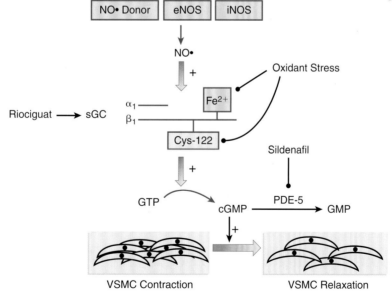

Fig. 56.4 Nitric Oxide–Soluble Guanylyl Cyclase Signaling in Vascular Smooth Muscle Cells. Nitric oxide *(NO•)* generated from nitric oxide synthase(s) or pharmacologic sources (e.g., nitroglycerin or inhaled NO•) activate the heterodimer soluble guanylyl cyclase *(sGC)* to catalyze the conversion of cytosolic GTP to cGMP, which results in the relaxation of vascular smooth muscle cells *(VSMCs)*. In the pulmonary vasculature, phosphodiesterase-5 *(PDE-5)* hydrolyzes cGMP to form GMP, thereby decreasing bioactive levels of cGMP. Sildenafil is a selective PDE-5 inhibitor that increases cGMP levels to promote the dilation of VSMCs. Increases in the formation of pulmonary vascular reactive oxygen species, which occurs in various forms of pulmonary hypertension, may also impair sGC activation via oxidation of the prosthetic heme group or cysteine-122 located in the catalytically active β1 subunit of sGC.

is protective against PH. However, in decompensated aortic stenosis, LV cavitary dilation from volume overload is associated with progressive PH.[34] The final common pathway in the pathophysiology of PH irrespective of the inciting valve lesion is pulmonary venous hypertension. However, PH is a key determinant for the timing of surgical valve therapy only in MR. The American College of Cardiology/American Heart Association (ACC/AHA) guidelines recommend mitral valve surgery (class IIa, level of evidence C) in *asymptomatic* patients with severe MR, preserved LV function, and PH (systolic PA pressure >50 mm Hg).[35] Magne and colleagues reported that in a cohort of 78 asymptomatic patients with at least moderate MR from degenerative mitral valve disease, resting PH (systolic PA pressure >60 mm Hg), and exercise-induced rise in PA pressure were associated with a significantly lower 2-year symptom-free survival rate (36% ± 14% vs. 59% ± 7% and 35% ± 8% vs. 75% ± 7%, respectively). Exercise-induced PH (particularly with systolic PA >56 mm Hg) was also an independent risk factor for the development of symptoms.[36] These data support exercise-induced PH as a potentially useful clinical marker for estimating the timing of surgical intervention for MR.

Considerations for Cardiac Surgery, Orthotopic Heart Transplantation, and Heart-Lung Transplantation in the Patient With Pulmonary Hypertension

In contrast to select end-stage PAH patients for whom bilateral lung transplantation may be indicated, severe preoperative PH in non-PAH patients is associated with an increased rate of adverse outcomes in most cardiopulmonary bypass–requiring cardiac surgery patients.[37] One exception appears to be obstructive hypertrophic cardiomyopathy, in which PH does not affect surgical outcome or complication rate.[38] In the case of orthotopic heart transplant candidates, a transpulmonary gradient >15 mm Hg or PVR >5 Wood units that is unchanged despite preoperative nitric oxide donor or selective PDE-5 inhibitor pharmacotherapy is an absolute contraindication to surgery owing to high rates of postoperative renal failure, premature graft failure, and early mortality.[39]

PH reversibility in response to pulmonary vasodilator therapy appears to improve 30-day posttransplant mortality rates versus patients with "fixed" PH.[40] Although universally accepted pulmonary hemodynamic thresholds do not exist, a target PVR of <2.5 Wood units or a transpulmonary gradient <12 mm Hg is often used in clinical practice to define preoperative optimization for cardiopulmonary bypass–requiring surgery. For patients with fixed PH requiring cardiac transplantation, left ventricular assist device (LVAD) therapy may improve operative candidacy. Zimpfer and colleagues reported that in 35 consecutive cardiac transplant candidates with fixed PH receiving LVAD therapy, PVR decreased from 5.1 Wood units at baseline to 3.2 Wood units 3 days following device implantation, an effect sustained over 6 weeks.[41] Larger clinical trials are necessary to determine the complete risk-benefit profile (including financial costs) of LVAD implantation under these circumstances. The role of right ventricular assist device (RVAD) therapy in improving PH remains under investigation, but a recent study suggests perioperative RVAD support can improve LVAD tolerance in patients with PH and impaired RV function.[42]

PULMONARY HYPERTENSION UNDER CONDITIONS OF HYPOXEMIA

PH is a potential component of most chronic lung disease syndromes that cause hypoxemia. It has long been established that PH severity in COPD, interstitial lung disease, cystic fibrosis, and bronchiectasis is predictive of morbidity and mortality.[1,43] A stronger appreciation has developed over the previous decade regarding the central role of PH in the natural history of sleep-disordered breathing and alveolar hypoventilation disorders.

Hypoxic pulmonary vasoconstriction is the cornerstone pathophysiological process common to lung disease–associated forms of PH. Small and precapillary blood vessel vasoconstriction in response to hypoxia distinguishes the pulmonary from the coronary, cerebral, and skeletal circulations; a drop in alveolar pO_2 to <50 mm Hg results in a 50% increase in PVR.[44,45]

A multitude of cell signaling mechanisms modulated by hypoxia have been implicated in hypoxic pulmonary vasoconstriction, including increased ET-1 production, intracellular $[Ca^{+2}]_i$-mediated activation of oxygen-sensitive Ca^{+2} channels in VSMC, endothelial aldosterone synthesis, and local activation of α-adrenergic receptors. In addition, hypoxia-inducible factor (HIF)-1α, a "master" transcription factor activated in response to hypoxia, may modulate the pathogenesis of PH in chronic lung disease via nuclear factor kappa B (NF-κB)–mediated pulmonary VSMC proliferation, among other pathologic cell signaling pathways that promote negative pulmonary vascular remodeling.[46] Alternatively, suppression of HIF-1α requires iron (Fe[II]), raising speculation that iron supplementation is a potential therapeutic target for the attenuation of pathogenic HIF-1α–dependent cell signaling in PH. For example, Smith and colleagues reported that iron infusion (Fe[III]-hydroxide sucrose) administered to healthy individuals who developed PH following exposure to hypoxic conditions at elevated altitudes decreased PA systolic pressure from a mean of 37 to 31 mm Hg ($P = .01$).[47]

Late-stage findings in hypoxia-mediated PH include arteriolar VSMC hypertrophy and hyperplasia, which lead to medial thickening and may contribute to PH via a reduction in the pulmonary vessel lumen.

Chronic Obstructive Pulmonary Disease

COPD is the most common cause of hypoxemia-induced PH and cor pulmonale, accounting for >80% of cases.[48] A conservative PA systolic pressure cutoff of 20 mm Hg captured 91% of 120 severe emphysema patients in one widely cited retrospective analysis.[10] It is uncommon for PA pressures to exceed 40 mm Hg in patients with COPD.[1]

Diagnosis

The assessment of jugular venous pressure or detection of a loud pulmonic component of the second heart sound may be obscured in COPD patients with PH due to chest hyperinflation. Echocardiography is generally sufficient to screen for PH in COPD patients; however, rotational changes to normal heart anatomy in severely hyperinflated patients may distort acoustic windows and limit detection of the tricuspid regurgitant jet envelope required for PA systolic pressure estimation. In these patients, right heart catheterization is indicated.

Natural History

The progression of PH in COPD patients is indolent, with an average mPAP change of 0.5 mm Hg/year.[49] In one case series of 84 patients undergoing right heart catheterization after initiation of long-term oxygen therapy for severe COPD, the 5-year survival for patients with an initial mPAP >25 mm Hg ($n = 40$) was 36% versus 62% for those with a mPAP ≤25 mm Hg ($n = 44$) ($P < .001$).[50] The identification of COPD patients at risk for RV dysfunction does not, however, necessarily require echocardiography or invasive hemodynamic monitoring. The presence of ≥1 electrocardiographic signs of cor pulmonale in COPD patients is associated with a significantly decreased life span.[51]

Treatment

Supplemental oxygen is the only therapy with proven mortality benefit in patients with PH due to COPD. Two large trials of oxygen in patients with cor pulmonale due to COPD and PaO_2 below 55 mm Hg showed improved mortality and PVR.[52,53] Several trials in patients with COPD

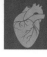

have shown at best mixed effects of PAH-directed therapy on resting and exercise-induced pulmonary hemodynamics and 6-minute walk distance (6MWD), and many have shown worsening oxygenation parameters and quality of life.[54–58]

Interstitial Lung Disease

Interstitial lung diseases (ILDs) are a heterogeneous group of parenchymal lung disorders characterized by impaired gas exchange, patchy collagen fibrosis, and the deposition of fibroblastic foci.[59] Owing to pulmonary blood vessel compression from fibrosis, PH is a potential complication in most forms of ILD. In idiopathic pulmonary fibrosis (IPF), histopathologic findings include adverse vascular remodeling of small muscular pulmonary arteries, destruction of capillary beds, peripulmonary vessel adventitial thickening, and VSMC hypertrophy with increased collagen and elastin accumulation.[60] Together, these changes contribute to low DLCO and the development of PH that are classic features of this condition.

Diagnosis and Treatment

A mean PA diameter >29 mm on computed tomography scan is suspicious for PH; however, echocardiography and right heart catheterization remain the gold-standard diagnostic tests for PH in ILD.[61] Current management emphasizes alleviation of hypoxemia with supplemental oxygen and improvement in alveolar gas exchange (e.g., corticosteroids or novel antifibrotics if appropriate). Several studies have shown limited or no benefit from PAH-directed therapy in patients with PH due to ILD, with some agents demonstrating harm. The best-studied is IPF, where data have been reported for prostacyclin replacement[62]; PDE-5 inhibitors, with best efficacy in patients with RV dysfunction[63,64]; ERAs, with ambrisentan being well described as harmful in ILD[65]; and nitric oxide–cyclic guanosine monophosphate enhancers in the form of riociguat. However, a recent phase II study (RISE-IIP) in patients with idiopathic interstitial pneumonia–associated PH was terminated due to an increase in drug-related adverse events and mortality (clinicaltrials.gov, NCT02138825). Overall, PAH-specific therapy is an ESC/ERS class III indication, implying that these drugs should *not* be used to treat ILD-PH.[66] Although sarcoidosis, pulmonary Langerhans histiocytosis, and lymphangioleiomyomatosis are classified as belonging to group 5 PH, there are isolated case reports and small retrospective case series suggesting that some of these patients may benefit from PAH-directed therapy.[66–70] At this time it is not possible to predict responders.

Pulmonary Hypertension in Obstructive Sleep Apnea

Obstructive sleep apnea (OSA) is a clinical syndrome resulting from involuntary collapse of pharyngeal muscles during sleep. Decreases in PaO_2 and increased sleep arousal and sympathetic tone adversely affect cardiovascular function by increasing LV afterload, systemic blood pressure, and heart rate. The aggregate effect of these pathologic adaptations results in increased rates of OSA-associated ischemic heart disease, congestive heart failure, and arrhythmias. Furthermore, these processes, in turn, promote PH via left-sided heart failure–induced passive pulmonary vascular congestion. Obesity, which is associated with increases in cardiac output compared with lean individuals, correlates positively with PA pressure irrespective of OSA status.[71] This observation suggests that a high cardiac output, perhaps by inducing reactive pulmonary vasoconstriction from increased circulating blood volume, may contribute to elevate rates of PH observed in patients with obesity, OSA, or both.

Continuous positive airway pressure (CPAP), which in OSA patients is associated with improvement in LV diastolic function, decreases PA pressure (~5 mm Hg over 4 months of CPAP use) and is associated with decreased mortality and hospitalization rates in OSA

patients.[71–73] Only case reports describe individual responses to therapy in rarer disorders of ventilation, including kyphoscoliosis and obesity-hypoventilation syndrome.[74]

Chronic High-Altitude Exposure

Over 140 million people live at high altitude (HA) (>2500 m above sea level).[75] A parabolic inverse relationship between PA pressure and peripheral oxygen saturation (SaO_2) exists in populations of native HA dwellers.[75] It is believed that chronic hypoxia-mediated vasoconstriction from low oxygen tension at HA results in several cardiopulmonary adaptations, including RV hypertrophy, VSMC hypertrophy of small and distal pulmonary arterioles, increased oxygen-carrying capacity due to reactive erythrocytosis, and increased heart rate at baseline and with exertion.[75,76] If these protective responses are disrupted, typically from hypoventilation-mediated worsening of hypoxia, a cascade of maladaptive responses may ensue, resulting in chronic mountain sickness syndrome (CMS). Severe PH, cor pulmonale, and excessive polycythemia are hallmark clinical features of CMS. In contrast to acute altitude sickness, pulmonary edema from severe PH is unusual. Descent from altitude is generally required to cure CMS.[77]

PULMONARY HYPERTENSION SECONDARY TO PULMONARY THROMBOEMBOLIC DISEASE

Chronic Thromboembolic Pulmonary Hypertension

Chronic thromboembolic pulmonary hypertension (CTEPH) is characterized by the luminal obliteration of central and distal pulmonary arteries due to thrombotic remodeling, which results in PH and RV failure. The most recent epidemiologic data describing the frequency of CTEPH in the United States, Europe, and Japan suggests that 0.1% to 9% of patients surviving an acute pulmonary embolism are reported to develop this condition.[78] Histopathologic analysis demonstrates intraluminal and in situ thrombus and stenosis from associated fibrous deposition in the walls of pulmonary arteries.[79,80] Pulmonary hypertensive arteriopathy is present in vessels that are distinct from the site of thrombus, suggesting thrombus potentiation of diffuse injury to the pulmonary vasculature.

It is parsimonious to speculate that this syndrome is merely a consequence of incompletely recanalized pulmonary embolism; however, anywhere from 25% to 50% of CTEPH patients had not previously been diagnosed with a pulmonary embolism.[78] Furthermore, a surprisingly strong association between CTEPH and asplenia exists. In one case-controlled analysis of 257 patients, splenectomy was present in 8.5% of CTEPH patients—compared with 2.5% of PAH patients—and in 0.5% of patients with chronic parenchymal lung disease.[81] The precise mechanisms to account for this association remain unknown. Loss of hematopoietic filtering in asplenic patients may generate a prothrombotic environment in vascular tissue owing to elevated circulating levels of platelets and abnormal erythrocytes. Another hypothesis suggests that the platelet-derived vascular effector serotonin, implicated in microthrombus formation and VSMC constriction in PAH-associated conditions, may contribute to PH in asplenic patients. Alternatively, unfiltered, structurally abnormal red blood cells in asplenic patients may function as procoagulant intermediaries owing to expression of the negatively charged phospholipid phosphatidylserine on the outer cell membrane, which interacts with thrombin (see the discussion of hemoglobinopathy, further on).[82,83] Additional risk factors include a history of venous thromboembolism, positive anticardiolipin antibody status, osteomyelitis, a surgically placed ventriculoatrial shunt, inflammatory bowel disease, and malignancy.[84,85]

Diagnosis and Medical Treatment

Akin to other PH subtypes, CTEPH often presents with progressive exertional dyspnea. Late in the disease course, signs and symptoms of decreased right-sided cardiac output—such as exertional chest pain, increased abdominal girth and lower extremity edema, and syncope or near syncope—may be present. A bruit auscultated over the lung fields during a midinspiratory breath hold, present in up to 30% of patients, reflects turbulent flow through partially occluded pulmonary vessels.[86]

In contrast to PAH and most other forms of PH, CTEPH often involves proximal pulmonary arteries. Thus, the presence of one or more ventilation/perfusion (V/Q) mismatched segmental (or larger) defects detected by V/Q scintigraphy is often a key finding distinguishing CTEPH from PAH. Although pulmonary angiography has traditionally been the gold standard diagnostic imaging modality in this condition, multidimensional computed tomography (MDCT) or magnetic resonance angiography is at least equally effective in determining proximal, segmental, and subsegmental clot burden and is superior for detecting alternative PH-associated lung disease (e.g., fibrosing mediastinitis, adenopathy, and tumors of the pulmonary artery) (Fig. 56.5).[87] Nevertheless, pulmonary angiography is recommended to define CTEPH type, which predicts operative success in most pulmonary thromboendarterectomy candidates (see later).

For inoperable CTEPH patients, a systolic PAP >40 mm Hg, elevated PVR (>584 dynes/s/cm^5), and/or elevated right atrial pressure (>12 mm Hg) is associated with a poor prognosis.[88] One study conducted prior to the era of modern PAH pharmacotherapy demonstrated that in CTEPH patients with a mPAP >50 mm Hg treated only with anticoagulation, the 2-year survival rate was below 20%.[89] In contrast, data from contemporary trials in nonoperative CTEPH patients suggest that therapy with PDE-5 inhibitors, ERAs, or prostacyclin replacement therapy improves outcome. For example, one retrospective analysis of 84 inoperable CTEPH patients on maximal medical therapy reported a survival rate of 68% at 5 years.[90] At present, initiation of PAH therapies in CTEPH is generally recommended for poor surgical candidates or those with persistent PH following surgery. Early randomized studies suggested that medical therapy for these patients has hemodynamic and symptomatic benefits. For example, in the BENEFiT trial, 157 patients with inoperable or surgically refractory CTEPH were randomized to receive ERA therapy with the $ET_{A/B}$ receptor antagonist bosentan or placebo. Bosentan was well tolerated and resulted in a statistically significant 24% decrease in PVR from baseline but did not influence exercise tolerance.[91] Subsequently, the soluble guanylyl cyclase stimulator riociguat was studied in a multicenter randomized placebo-controlled trial (CHEST-1) of 261 patients with inoperable CTEPH (189 patients) or persistent PH (72 patients) following pulmonary thromboendarterectomy.[92] Compared with placebo, patients on riociguat had an improved 6MWD and PVR. A follow-up long-term extension study (CHEST-2) reported that prolonged therapy for up to 2 years with riociguat resulted in a similar efficacy and safety profile.[93] Although clinical experience with riociguat is limited, it is the preferred agent for patients with WHO functional class II to III symptoms and inoperable CTEPH; it became the first FDA-approved medical therapy for CTEPH in 2013. Most recently, macitentan was studied in a phase II, double-blind, multicenter, randomized placebo-controlled trial (MERIT-1) in 80 patients with inoperable CTEPH (WHO functional class II to IV, PVR of at least 400 dynes/s/cm^5 and a 6MWD of 150 to 450 m).[94] Patients were randomized to receive oral macitentan (10 mg once a day) or placebo. Investigators found that at week 16, PVR decreased to 73% of baseline in the macitentan group and to 87.2% in the placebo group (geometric means ratio 0.84, 95% CI 0.70 to 0.99, P = .041).

Limited observational data suggest a potential role for percutaneous pulmonary balloon angioplasty (BPA) in selected patients with inoperable CTEPH or with persistent pulmonary artery obstruction after surgery.[95] However, there have been no controlled trials comparing BPA with medical therapy, and the procedure itself carries significant risk of reperfusion injury, cerebral and systemic embolism, and pulmonary artery injury. Further study is needed before it is used outside of highly specialized centers. To help address this question, both the RACE trial (clinicaltrials.gov, NCT02634203) in France and the MR BPA trial (UMIN Clinical Trials Registry, UMIN000019549) in Japan are currently randomizing patients with inoperable CTEPH to riociguat or BPA.

Surgical Treatment

The primary treatment for CTEPH is pulmonary thromboendarterectomy for excision of thromboembolic and fibrotic tissue adherent to the lung vessel wall (Table 56.3 and Fig. 56.6).[96,97] Deep hypothermic

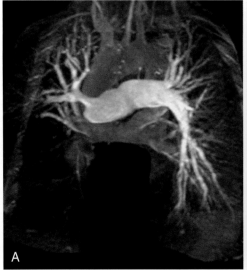
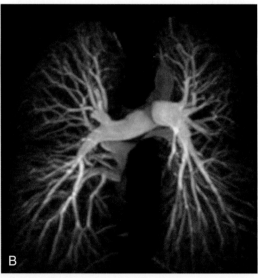

Fig. 56.5 (A) Preoperative pulmonary magnetic resonance angiography in a patient with chronic thromboembolic pulmonary hypertension. (B) Images acquired from the same patient following surgical endarterectomy. (From Hamilton-Craig C, Kermeen F, Dunning JJ, et al. Cardiovascular magnetic resonance prior to surgical treatment of chronic thrombo-embolic pulmonary hypertension. *Eur Heart J.* 2010;31:1040.)

TABLE 56.3   Classification of Chronic Thromboembolic Pulmonary Hypertension According to Intraoperative Findings

Classification	Distribution	Anatomic Involvement	Pathology
Type I	30% of surgical cases	Main or lobar pulmonary arteries	Fresh thrombus Vessel wall disease Clot propagation into primary and secondary pulmonary blood vessels
Type II	60% of surgical cases	Proximal to segmental pulmonary arteries	Intimal thickening Vessel wall fibrosis ± organized thrombus
Type III	10% of surgical cases	Distal segmental and subsegmental pulmonary arteries	Vessel fibrosis Intimal webbing Blood vessel thickening ± organized thrombus
Type IV	<1% of surgical cases	Distal arterioles	Microscopic arteriolar vasculopathy No visible thrombus

Jamieson classification of pulmonary endarterectomy specimens. A higher likelihood of elevated postoperative PA pressure and PVR exists with type III or IV disease.

Data from Jamieson SW. Pulmonary thromboendarterectomy. *Heart.* 1998;79(2):118–120; Thistlethwaite PA, Madani M, Jamieson SW. Pulmonary thromboendarterectomy surgery. *Cardiol Clin.* 2004;22(3):467–478, vii; and Jenkins D, Madani M, Fadel E, et al. Pulmonary endarterectomy in the management of chronic thromboembolic pulmonary hypertension. *Eur Respir Rev.* 2017;26(143).

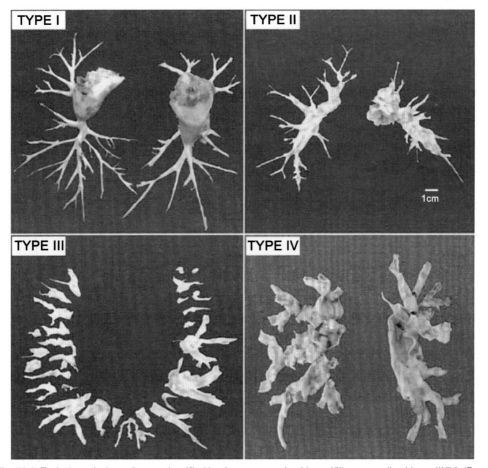

Fig. 56.6 Typical surgical specimens classified by the most proximal (type I/II) to most distal (type III/IV). (From Thistlethwaite PA, Mo M, Madani MM, et al. Operative classification of thromboembolic disease determines outcome after pulmonary endarterectomy. *J Thorac Cardiovasc Surg.* 2002;124:1203–1211.)

circulatory arrest with cardiopulmonary bypass is a strategy utilized to minimize bleeding in the surgical field; at experienced centers this has been met with low neurologic morbidity rates and favorable outcomes.[98] Factors favoring operative success include a proximal clot burden and a decrease in mPAP in response to preoperative iNO• treatment.[99] When successful, surgery results in a substantial reduction in clot burden and PVR (see Fig. 56.5).[100] In one prospective analysis of 181 CTEPH patients, pulmonary thromboendarterectomy compared with nonsurgical treatment was associated with a significantly lower PVR (586 ± 248 vs. 269 ± 201 dyne/s/cm^5) and mPAP, (45 ± 12 vs. 25 ± 11 mm Hg).[101] Lung transplantation should be considered for those with inoperable disease or an incomplete response to thromboendarterectomy.[88] Lifelong anticoagulation is recommended for all patients irrespective of operative candidacy to prevent both recurrent venous thromboembolism and in situ pulmonary artery thrombosis. Warfarin is generally preferred as the anticoagulant of choice, given limited experience with the newer oral anticoagulants that target thrombin or factor X_a (direct oral anticoagulants).

PULMONARY HYPERTENSION AND HEMOGLOBINOPATHIES

PH from primary blood dyscrasias characterized by abnormal erythrocyte structure or hemolysis occurs as a consequence of decreased bioavailable NO•, increased microthrombus formation, and possibly increased vascular endothelial ET-1 synthesis (see later for details of mechanism). Examples include sickle cell disease (SCD), hereditary spherocytosis, β-thalassemia (particularly in patients with splenectomy), and stomatocytosis.

PH is a part of the SCD syndrome in ~40% of patients. The 4-year mortality rate is 40% in SCD patients with PH; when RV systolic pressure >30 mm Hg (corresponding to a likely mPAP >25 mm Hg), there is a 10-fold increase in mortality compared with non-PH SCD patients.[102] Histopathologic findings in SCD and hemolysis-associated PH demonstrate a pulmonary arteriopathy similar to that observed in PAH. Specifically, the presence of pulmonary VSMC hypertrophy, neomuscularization of small- and medium-sized pulmonary arteries, luminal microthrombi, and plexiform lesions are described at autopsy in patients with these various primary disorders of erythrocyte structure (Fig. 56.7).[103]

Potential Mechanisms Linking Pulmonary Hypertension and Sickle Cell Disease
Decreased Bioavailable Nitric Oxide

In the pulmonary vasculature, NO• is a critical intermediary that promotes vasodilation, decreases platelet aggregation, and is a potent antagonist of vascular inflammation. In SCD and hemolytic anemias, erythrocyte deformity or rupture results in the release of free hemoglobin (Hb) into plasma. In the microcirculation, free Hb interacts with NO• to form methemoglobin and nitrate (NO_3^-) [Hb-Fe^{2+} = O_2 + NO• → Hb-Fe^{3+} + NO_3^-], thereby decreasing bioavialable levels of NO•, which increases pulmonary vascular reactivity.

Ischemia-reperfusion injury in small pulmonary arterioles and capillaries is a hallmark feature in the pathophysiology of SCD occlusive crises.[104,105] The downstream molecular effect of these events includes scavenging of bioavailable NO• by O_2^-• in a reaction that generates peroxynitrite anion ($ONOO^-$).[96] Superoxide is generated during ischemia-reperfusion injury via (1) direct activation of ROS-generating enzymes (e.g., xanthine oxidase), (2) increased NADPH oxidase activity modulated by enhanced leukocyte recruitment to the vascular endothelium, (3) uncoupling of eNOS due to enzyme cofactor depletion (e.g., BH_4), and (4) inducible NOS-dependent NO•-mediated ROS formation.[106] In addition to scavenging NO•, O_2^-• is converted to

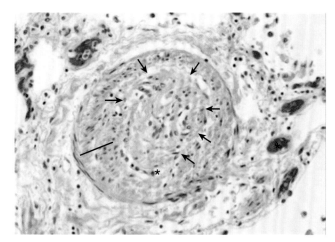

Fig. 56.7 Histopathologic Findings in Pulmonary Hypertension Associated With Sickle Cell Disease. Hematoxylin and eosin preparation of a distal pulmonary blood vessel in a patient with sickle cell anemia reveals vascular smooth muscle cell hypertrophy, intimal thickening *(line)*, and sub-total obliteration of the vessel lumen due to a plexiform lesion *(arrows)*. Microvessel thrombus is also noted *(asterisk)*. (From Machado RF, Gladwin MT. Pulmonary hypertension in hemolytic disorders: pulmonary vascular disease: the global perspective. *Chest.* 2010;137[6 suppl]:30S–38S.)

hydrogen peroxide (H_2O_2), which has been shown in vitro to disrupt endothelium-independent vasodilatory signaling pathways by oxidatively modifiying a key cysteinyl thiol involved in normal NO• sensing by sGC (see Fig. 56.4).[107]

Intracellular levels of arginase, which converts L-arginine to ornithine, are elevated in sickled erythrocytes and released into plasma on hemolysis.[108] It has been postulated, therefore, that since L-arginine is a subtrate for NO• synthesis, this may represent an additional mechanism by which bioavailable NO• is decreased in SCD. Data examining arginine replacement therapy, sildenafil, or iNO• to treat PH in SCD, although encouraging, are limited to case reports or very small patient series.[109] Unfortunately the first placebo-controlled trial (Walk-PHaSST) of sildenafil in SCD patients with echocardiographic evidence of PH was terminated early due to an increase in serious adverse events in the treatment arm, primarily hospitalization for pain crisis.[110] Additionally, a randomized placebo-controlled trial of iNO• to treat vaso-occlusive crises did not improve time to crisis resolution.[111]

The role of arginase in modulating PH in other primary blood dyscrasias has been evaluated. In paroxysmal nocturnal hemoglobinuria (PNH), an *acquired* mutation results in the absence of erythrocyte membrane-bound glycosylphosphatidylinositol-anchored proteins, which predisposes to complement-mediated hemolysis and free Hb scavenging of NO•. Patients with PNH express a low bioactive NO• state in several systems, which is associated with PH, gastrointestinal smooth muscle cell hyperactivity, and erectile dysfunction.[112] Data extracted from patients enrolled in the Transfusion Reduction Efficacy and Safety Clinical Investigation Using Eculizumab in Paroxysmal Nocturnal Hemoglobinuria (TRIUMPH) study demonstrated that plasma arginase activity levels were 10-fold higher compared with the normal range, a finding associated with an approximately 30-fold increase in NO• consumption. Interestingly, by binding to complement C5 and inhibiting the cleavage of C5 by C5 convertase, thereby decreasing erythrocyte hemolysis, eculizumab treatment resulted in a significant decrease in hemolysis, N-terminal pro-brain natriuretic peptide levels, and patient-reported dyspnea.[113]

Less well established mechanisms that may influence NO• bioavailability may involve asymmetric dimethylarginine (ADMA), a nitric

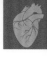

oxide synthase inhibitor, which is present at elevated concentrations in the plasma of SCD patients.[114] In a cohort of 30 children with SCD compared with healthy controls, elevated levels of ADMA correlated with elevated tricuspid regurgitant velocity $\geq 2.5\,\text{m/s}$ ($r = 0.475$).[115]

Hypercoagulable State

In SCD, stroke, veno-occlusive crises, and PH are believed to occur in part from thrombus formation in the cerebral and pulmonary microcirculations. Decreased bioavailable NO• (through loss of platelet aggregation antagonism), increased whole blood tissue factor expression and thrombin formation, and decreased levels of the coagulation pathway inhibitors activated protein C and its cofactor protein S all contribute to a hypercoagulable state. In SCD, β-thalassemia, and/or asplenic patients, abnormal erythrocyte membrane phospholipid disposition results in the abundant exposure of phosphatidylserine on the exterior surface of the bilayer, which is linked to increased erythrocyte-vascular endothelial cell adhesion and thrombin activation.[116] Antiplatelet therapy with aspirin is recommended in select high-risk SCD patients for the primary prevention of ischemic stroke; however, the effect of these agents in modulating a decrease in PA pressure has not been adequately tested.

Despite these observations, the attributable contribution to the pathophysiology of PH by free Hb scavenging of NO• remains unresolved. A surprisingly small difference in reticulocyte count and lactate dehydrogenase (LDH) levels between non-PH and PH patients with SCD; lack of a positive association between extent of hemolysis and PH disease severity; and an absence of extrahematologic clinical signs or symptoms indicative of decreased bioactive NO•, such a esophageal spasm or erectile dysfunction (i.e., impotence but not priapism), has led some to suggest that alternative mechanisms may play an underrecognized role in promoting PH in SCD.[82]

Increased Endothelin-1 Synthesis

A threefold increase in circulating ET-1 levels is observed in patients with SCD compared with age-matched normal controls.[117] This presumably occurs as a consequence of microvascular hypoxia and increased shear stress in SCD that triggers pulmonary vascular endothelial secretion of ET-1. In vitro, exposure of vascular endothelial cells to sickled erythrocytes significantly increases ET-1 gene transcription, suggesting that ET-1 may act as a vasoconstrictor intermediary in SCD.[118] Owing to the central role of ET-1 in the pathophysiology of PAH, investigators have tested the hypothesis that $ET_{A/B}$ receptor antagonism may attenuate PH disease severity in SCD. Early data from small clinical trials demonstrated an ~10% increase in distance performed during a 6-minute walk test in SCD patients with PH treated with bosentan therapy for 6 months. In the same study, a mean drop of 6 mm Hg in estimated systolic PA pressure (by echocardiography) was also observed.[119] Bosentan was subsequently studied in two randomized, placebo-controlled trials in SCD patients with PH; however, the trials were prematurely terminated due to slow patient enrollment. Consequently, efficacy end points were not assessed other than a nonsignificant increase in cardiac output and a nonsignificant decrease in PVR with bosentan observed in both trials.[120]

OTHER SECONDARY CAUSES OF PULMONARY HYPERTENSION

Numerous other, less common disease states are associated with PH by causing direct compression of the pulmonary vasculature via mass effect or vessel wall infiltration. *Fibrosing mediastinitis*, which is associated with granulomatous diseases such as histoplasmosis, is an immunolog-

ically mediated response to caseous nodes. Fibrotic encroachment of large and small pulmonary arteries and veins has been observed at necroscopy of patients when this condition includes severe PH. A similar PH pathophysiology has been implicated in *sarcoidosis*, where impedance to pulmonary blood flow occurs secondary to fibrosis of the pulmonary vasculature in the setting of extensive parenchymal lung disease or direct invasion of the intima and media of the pulmonary arteries with noncaseating granulomas, resulting in blood vessel encroachment.

Primary inflammatory vascular diseases, such as Takayasu arteritis and Behçet disease (see Chapters 39 and 40), are rare causes of PH. An important but increasingly uncommon iatrogenic etiology of PH is that secondary to pulmonary vein stenosis as a complication of pulmonary vein isolation radiofrequency ablation for the treatment of atrial fibrillation. In the previous decade, pulmonary vein stenosis was reported in up to 20% of patients undergoing this procedure. However, improved technology and enhanced awareness among operators appear to have resulted in a substantial downward trend in the frequency of this potentially devastating procedural complication, with contemporary case series reporting event rates of 1% to 3%.[121]

REFERENCES

1. McLaughlin VV, Archer SL, Badesch DB, et al. ACCF/AHA 2009 expert consensus document on pulmonary hypertension a report of the American College of Cardiology Foundation Task Force on Expert Consensus Documents and the American Heart Association developed in collaboration with the American College of Chest Physicians; American Thoracic Society, Inc.; and the Pulmonary Hypertension Association. *J Am Coll Cardiol.* 2009;53(17):1573–1619.
2. Simmoneau G, Gatzoulis MA, Adatia I, et al. Updated clinical classification of pulmonary hypertension. *J Am Coll Cardiol.* 2013;62:D34–D41.
3. Farber HW, Loscalzo J. Pulmonary arterial hypertension. *N Engl J Med.* 2004;351(16):1655–1665.
4. Benza RL, Miller DP, Gomberg-Maitland M, et al. Predicting survival in pulmonary arterial hypertension: insights from the Registry to Evaluate Early and Long-Term Pulmonary Arterial Hypertension Disease Management (REVEAL). *Circulation.* 2010;122(2):164–172.
4a. Simonneau G, Montani D, Celermajer DS, et al. Haemodynamic definitions and updated clinical classification of pulmonary hypertension. *Eur Respir J.* 2019;53(1):pii:1801913.
5. Hoeper MM, Humbert M, Souza R, et al. A global view of pulmonary hypertension. *Lancet Respir Med.* 2016;4(4):306–322.
6. Lam CS, Borlaug BA, Kane GC, et al. Age-associated increases in pulmonary artery systolic pressure in the general population. *Circulation.* 2009;119(20):2663–2670.
7. Maron BA, Hess E, Maddox TM, et al. Association of borderline pulmonary hypertension with mortality and hospitalization in large patient cohort: insights from the Veterans Affairs clinical assessment, reporting, and tracking program. *Circulation.* 2016;133(13):1240–1248.
8. Leung CC, Moondra V, Catherwood E, et al. Prevalence and risk factors of pulmonary hypertension in patients with elevated pulmonary venous pressure and preserved ejection fraction. *Am J Cardiol.* 2010;106(2):284–286.
9. Hoeper MM, Barbera JA, Channick RN, et al. Diagnosis, assessment, and treatment of non-pulmonary arterial hypertension pulmonary hypertension. *J Am Coll Cardiol.* 2009;54(1 Suppl):S85–S96.
10. Scharf SM, Iqbal M, Keller C, et al. Hemodynamic characterization of patients with severe emphysema. *Am J Respir Crit Care Med.* 2002;166(3):314–322.
11. Handa T, Nagai S, Miki S, et al. Incidence of pulmonary hypertension and its clinical relevance in patients with sarcoidosis. *Chest.* 2006;129(5):1246–1252.
12. Baughman RP, Engel PJ, Taylor L, et al. Survival in sarcoidosis associated pulmonary hypertension: the importance of hemodynamic evaluation. *Chest.* 2010;138(5):1078–1085.

13. Damy T, Goode KM, Kallvikbacka-Bennett A, et al. Determinants and prognostic value of pulmonary arterial pressure in patients with chronic heart failure. *Eur Heart J.* 2010;31(18):2280–2290.

14. Maggiorini M, Melot C, Pierre S, et al. High-altitude pulmonary edema is initially caused by an increase in capillary pressure. *Circulation.* 2001;103(16):2078–2083.

15. Trammell AW, Pugh ME, Newman JH, et al. Use of pulmonary arterial hypertension-approved therapy in the treatment of non-group 1 pulmonary hypertension at US referral centers. *Pulm Circ.* 2015;5(2):356–363.

16. Opitz CF, Hoeper MM, Gibs JSR, et al. Pre-capillary, combined, and post-capillary pulmonary hypertension: a pathophysiological continuum. *J Am Coll Cardiol.* 2016;68(4):368–378.

17. Pengo V, Lensing AW, Prins MH, et al. Incidence of chronic thromboembolic pulmonary hypertension after pulmonary embolism. *N Engl J Med.* 2004;350(22):2257–2264.

18. Deaño RC, Glassner-Kolmin C, Rubfenfire M, et al. Referral of patients with pulmonary hypertension diagnoses to tertiary pulmonary hypertension centers: the multicenter RePHerral study. *JAMA Intern Med.* 2013;173(10):887–893.

19. Maron BA, Choudhary G, Khan UA, et al. Clinical profile and underdiagnosis of pulmonary hypertension in US veteran patients. *Circ Heart Fail.* 2013;6(5):906–912.

20. Ha JW, Chung N, Chang BC, et al. Acute mitral regurgitation due to leaflet tear after balloon valvotomy. *Circulation.* 1998;98(19):2095–2097.

21. Zafrir N, Zingerman B, Solodky A, et al. Use of noninvasive tools in primary pulmonary hypertension to assess the correlation of right ventricular function with functional capacity and to predict outcome. *Int J Cardiovasc Imaging.* 2007;23(2):209–215.

22. Hirakawa S, Suzuki T, Gotoh K, et al. Human pulmonary vascular and venous compliances are reduced before and during left-sided heart failure. *J Appl Physiol.* 1995;78(1):323–333.

23. Wallner M, Eaton DM, Berretta RM, et al. A feline HFpEF model with pulmonary hypertension and compromised pulmonary function. *Sci Rep.* 2017;7(1):16587.

24. Moraes DL, Colucci WS, Givertz MM. Secondary pulmonary hypertension in chronic heart failure: the role of the endothelium in pathophysiology and management. *Circulation.* 2000;102(14):1718–1723.

25. Furutani H, Zhang XF, Iwamuro Y, et al. Ca2+ entry channels involved in contractions of rat aorta induced by endothelin-1, noradrenaline, and vasopressin. *J Cardiovasc Pharmacol.* 2002;40(2):265–276.

26. Kaddoura S, Firth JD, Boheler KR, et al. Endothelin-1 is involved in norepinephrine-induced ventricular hypertrophy in vivo. Acute effects of bosentan, an orally active, mixed endothelin ETA and ETB receptor antagonist. *Circulation.* 1996;93(11):2068–2079.

27. Maron BA, Zhang YY, White K, et al. Aldosterone inactivates the endothelin-B receptor via a cysteinyl thiol redox switch to decrease pulmonary endothelial nitric oxide levels and modulate pulmonary arterial hypertension. *Circulation.* 2012;126(8):963–974.

28. Puwanant S, Park M, Popovic ZB, et al. Ventricular geometry, strain, and rotational mechanics in pulmonary hypertension. *Circulation.* 2010;121(2):259–266.

29. Weitsman T, Weisz G, Farkash R, et al. Pulmonary hypertension with left heart disease: prevlance, temporal shifts in etiologies, and outcome. *Am J Med.* 2017;130(11):1272–1279.

30. Ghio S, Gavazzi A, Campana C, et al. Independent and additive prognostic value of right ventricular systolic function and pulmonary artery pressure in patients with chronic heart failure. *J Am Coll Cardiol.* 2001;37(1):183–188.

31. Califf RM, Adams KF, McKenna WJ, et al. A randomized controlled trial of epoprostenol therapy for severe congestive heart failure: the Flolan International Randomized Survival Trial (FIRST). *Am Heart J.* 1997;134(1):44–54.

32. Lewis GD, Shah R, Shahzad K, et al. Sildenafil improves exercise capacity and quality of life in patients with systolic heart failure and secondary pulmonary hypertension. *Circulation.* 2007;116(14):1555–1562.

33. Redfield MM, Chen HH, Borlaug BA, et al. Effect of phosphodiesterase-5 inhibition on exercise capacity and clinical status in heart failure with preserved ejection fraction: a randomized clinical trial. *JAMA.* 2013;309(12):1268–1277.

34. Malouf JF, Enriquez-Sarano M, Pellikka PA, et al. Severe pulmonary hypertension in patients with severe aortic valve stenosis: clinical profile and prognostic implications. *J Am Coll Cardiol.* 2002;40(4):789–795.

35. Nishimura RA, Otto CM, Bonow RO, et al. 2014 AHA/ACC guideline for the management of patients with valvular heart disease: a report of the American College of Cardiology/American Heart Association Task Force on Practice Guidelines. *J Am Coll Cardiol.* 2014;63(22):e57–185.

36. Magne J, Lancellotti P, Pierard LA. Exercise pulmonary hypertension in asymptomatic degenerative mitral regurgitation. *Circulation.* 2010;122(1):33–41.

37. Murali S, Kormos RL, Uretsky BF, et al. Preoperative pulmonary hemodynamics and early mortality after orthotopic cardiac transplantation: the Pittsburgh experience. *Am Heart J.* 1993;126(4):896–904.

38. Covella M, Rowin EJ, Hill NS, et al. Mechanism of progressive heart failure and significance of pulmonary hypertension in obstructive hypertrophic cardiomyopathy. *Circ Heart Fail.* 2017;10(4):e003689.

39. Gorlitzer M, Ankersmit J, Fiegl N, et al. Is the transpulmonary pressure gradient a predictor for mortality after orthotopic cardiac transplantation? *Transpl Int.* 2005;18(4):390–395.

40. Chen JM, Levin HR, Michler RE, et al. Reevaluating the significance of pulmonary hypertension before cardiac transplantation: determination of optimal thresholds and quantification of the effect of reversibility on perioperative mortality. *J Thorac Cardiovasc Surg.* 1997;114(4):627–634.

41. Zimpfer D, Zrunek P, Sandner S, et al. Post-transplant survival after lowering fixed pulmonary hypertension using left ventricular assist devices. *Eur J Cardiothorac Surg.* 2007;31(4):698–702.

42. Deschka H, Holthaus AJ, Sindermann JR, et al. Can perioperative right ventricular support prevent postoperative right heart failure in patients with biventricular dysfunction undergoing left ventricular assist device implantation? *J Cardiothorac Vasc Anesth.* 2016;30(3):619–626.

43. Hopkins N, McLoughlin P. The structural basis of pulmonary hypertension in chronic lung disease: remodelling, rarefaction or angiogenesis? *J Anat.* 2002;201(4):335–348.

44. Harris P, Heath D. Influence of Respiratory Gases. In: Harris P, Heath D, eds. *The Human Pulmonary Circulation.* 2 ed. London: Churchill Livingstone; 1986:456–483.

45. Dumas JP, Bardou M, Goirand F, et al. Hypoxic pulmonary vasoconstriction. *Gen Pharmacol.* 1999;33(4):289–297.

46. Diebold I, Djordjevic T, Hess J, et al. Rac-1 promotes pulmonary artery smooth muscle cell proliferation by upregulation of plasminogen activator inhibitor-1: role of NFkappaB-dependent hypoxia-inducible factor-1alpha transcription. *Thromb Haemost.* 2008;100(6):1021–1028.

47. Smith TG, Talbot NP, Privat C, et al. Effects of iron supplementation and depletion on hypoxic pulmonary hypertension: two randomized controlled trials. *JAMA.* 2009;302(13):1444–1450.

48. George MG, Schieb LJ, Ayala C, et al. Pulmonary hypertension surveillance: United States, 2001 to 2010. *Chest.* 2014;146(2):476–495.

49. Weitzenblum E. Chronic cor pulmonale. *Heart.* 2003;89(2):225–230.

50. Oswald-Mammosser M, Weitzenblum E, Quoix E, et al. Prognostic factors in COPD patients receiving long-term oxygen therapy. Importance of pulmonary artery pressure. *Chest.* 1995;107(5):1193–1198.

51. Incalzi RA, Fuso L, De Rosa M, et al. Electrocardiographic signs of chronic cor pulmonale: a negative prognostic finding in chronic obstructive pulmonary disease. *Circulation.* 1999;99(12):1600–1605.

52. Long term domiciliary oxygen therapy in chronic hypoxic cor pulmonale complicating chronic bronchitis and emphysema. Report of the Medical Research Council Working Party. *Lancet.* 1981;1(8222):681–686.

53. Continuous or nocturnal oxygen therapy in hypoxemic chronic obstructive lung disease: a clinical trial. Nocturnal Oxygen Therapy Trial Group. *Ann Intern Med.* 1980;93(3):391–398.

54. Blanco I, Gimeno E, Munoz PA, et al. Hemodynamic and gas exchange effects of sildenafil in patients with chronic obstructive pulmonary disease and pulmonary hypertension. *Am J Respir Crit Care Med.* 2010;181(3):270–278.

55. Stolz D, Rasch H, Linka A, et al. A randomised, controlled trial of bosentan in severe COPD. *Eur Respir J.* 2008;32(3):619–628.

56. Badesch DB, Feldman J, Keogh A, et al. ARIES-3: ambrisentan therapy in a diverse population of patients with pulmonary hypertension. *Cardiovasc Ther.* 2012;30(2):93–99.

57. Dernaika TA, Beavin M, Kinasewitz GT. Iloprost improves gas exchange and exercise tolerance in patients with pulmonary hypertension and chronic obstructive pulmonary disease. *Respiration.* 2010;79(5):377–382.

58. Ghofrani HA, Staehler G, Grünig E, et al. Acute effects of riociguat in borderline or manifest pulmonary hypertension associated with chronic obstructive pulmonary disease. *Pulm Circ.* 2015;5(2):296–304.

59. Ryu JH, Daniels CE, Hartman TE, et al. Diagnosis of interstitial lung diseases. *Mayo Clin Proc.* 2007;82(8):976–986.

60. Patel NM, Lederer DJ, Borczuk AC, et al. Pulmonary hypertension in idiopathic pulmonary fibrosis. *Chest.* 2007;132(3):998–1006.

61. Tan RT, Kuzo R, Goodman LR, et al. Utility of CT scan evaluation for predicting pulmonary hypertension in patients with parenchymal lung disease. Medical College of Wisconsin Transplant Group. *Chest.* 1998;113(5):1250–1256.

62. Saggar R, Khanna D, Vaidya A, et al. Changes in right heart haemodynamics and echocardiographic function in an advanced phenotype of pulmonary hypertension and right heart dysfunction associated with pulmonary fibrosis. *Thorax.* 2014;69(2):123–129.

63. Han MK, Bach DS, Hagan PG, et al. Sildenafil preserves exercise capacity in patients with idiopathic pulmonary fibrosis and right-sided ventricular dysfunction. *Chest.* 2013;143(6):1699–1708.

64. Zimmermann GS, von Wulffen W, Huppmann P, et al. Haemodynamic changes in pulmonary hypertension in patients with interstitial lung disease treated with PDE-5 inhibitors. *Respirology.* 2014;19(5):700–706.

65. Raghu G, Behr J, Brown KK, et al. Treatment of idiopathic pulmonary fibrosis with ambrisentan: a parallel, randomized trial. *Ann Intern Med.* 2013;158(9):641–649.

66. Galie N, Humbert M, Vachiery JL, et al. 2015 ESC/ERS Guidelines for the diagnosis and treatment of pulmonary hypertension: the Joint Task Force for the Diagnosis and Treatment of Pulmonary Hypertension of the European Society of Cardiology (ESC) and the European Respiratory Society (ERS): endorsed by: Association for European Paediatric and Congenital Cardiology (AEPC), International Society for Heart and Lung Transplantation (ISHLT). *Eur Heart J.* 2016;37(1):67–119.

67. Keir GJ, Walsh SL, Gatzoulis MA, et al. Treatment of sarcoidosis-associated pulmonary hypertension: a single centre retrospective experience using targeted therapies. *Sarcoidosis Vasc Diffuse Lung Dis.* 2014;31(2):82–90.

68. Bonham CA, Oldham JM, Gomberg-Maitland M, et al. Prostacyclin and oral vasodilator therapy in sarcoidosis-associated pulmonary hypertension: a retrospective case series. *Chest.* 2015;148(4):1055–1062.

69. Le Pavec J, Lorillon G, Jaïs X, et al. Pulmonary Langerhans cell histiocytosis-associated pulmonary hypertension: clinical characteristics and impact of pulmonary arterial hypertension therapies. *Chest.* 2012;142(5):1150–1157.

70. Cottin V, Harari S, Humbert M, et al. Pulmonary hypertension in lymphangioleiomyomatosis: characteristics in 20 patients. *Eur Respir J.* 2012;40(3):630–640.

71. McQuillan BM, Picard MH, Leavitt M, et al. Clinical correlates and reference intervals for pulmonary artery systolic pressure among echocardiographically normal subjects. *Circulation.* 2001;104(23):2797–2802.

72. Devaraj A, Wells AU, Meister MG, et al. Detection of pulmonary hypertension with multidetector CT and echocardiography alone and in combination. *Radiology.* 2010;254(2):609–616.

73. Shahar E, Whitney CW, Redline S, et al. Sleep-disordered breathing and cardiovascular disease: cross-sectional results of the Sleep Heart Health Study. *Am J Respir Crit Care Med.* 2001;163(1):19–25.

74. Hosokawa Y, Yamamoto T, Yabuno Y, et al. Inhaled nitric oxide therapy for secondary pulmonary hypertension with hypertrophic obstructive cardiomyopathy and severe kyphoscoliosis. *Int J Cardiol.* 2012;158(1):e20–e21.

75. Penaloza D, Arias-Stella J. The heart and pulmonary circulation at high altitudes: healthy highlanders and chronic mountain sickness. *Circulation.* 2007;115(9):1132–1146.

76. West JB. Physiological effects of chronic hypoxia. *N Engl J Med.* 2017;376(20):1965–1971.

77. Penaloza D, Sime F. Chronic cor pulmonale due to loss of altitude acclimitization (chronic mountain sickness). *Am J Med.* 1971;50(6):728–743.

78. Gall H, Hoeper MM, Richter MJ, et al. An epidemiological analysis of the burden of chronic thromboembolic pulmonary hypertension in the USA, Europe and Japan. *Eur Respir Rev.* 2017;26(143):160121.

79. Hoeper MM, Mayer E, Simonneau G, et al. Chronic thromboembolic pulmonary hypertension. *Circulation.* 2006;113(16):2011–2020.

80. Klepetko W, Mayer E, Sandoval J, et al. Interventional and surgical modalities of treatment for pulmonary arterial hypertension. *J Am Coll Cardiol.* 2004;43(12 Suppl S):73S–80S.

81. Jais X, Ioos V, Jardim C, et al. Splenectomy and chronic thromboembolic pulmonary hypertension. *Thorax.* 2005;60(12):1031–1034.

82. Bunn HF, Nathan DG, Dover GJ, et al. Pulmonary hypertension and nitric oxide depletion in sickle cell disease. *Blood.* 2010;116(5):687–692.

83. Eldor A, Rachmilewitz EA. The hypercoagulable state in thalassemia. *Blood.* 2002;99(1):36–43.

84. Bonderman D, Jakowitsch J, Adlbrecht C, et al. Medical conditions increasing the risk of chronic thromboembolic pulmonary hypertension. *Thromb Haemost.* 2005;93(3):512–516.

85. Sharma S, Lang IM. Current understanding of the pathophysiology of chronic thromboembolic pulmonary hypertension. *Thromb Res.* 2018;164:136–144.

86. Fedullo PF, Auger WR, Kerr KM, et al. Chronic thromboembolic pulmonary hypertension. *N Engl J Med.* 2001;345(20):1465–1472.

87. Tardivon AA, Musset D, Maitre S, et al. Role of CT in chronic pulmonary embolism: comparison with pulmonary angiography. *J Comput Assist Tomogr.* 1993;17(3):345–351.

88. Piazza G, Goldhaber SZ. Chronic thromboembolic pulmonary hypertension. *N Engl J Med.* 2011;364(4):351–360.

89. Riedel M, Stanek V, Widimsky J, et al. Longterm follow-up of patients with pulmonary thromboembolism. Late prognosis and evolution of hemodynamic and respiratory data. *Chest.* 1982;81(2):151–158.

90. Saouti N, de Man F, Westerhof N, et al. Predictors of mortality in inoperable chronic thromboembolic pulmonary hypertension. *Respir Med.* 2009;103(7):1013–1019.

91. Jais X, D'Armini AM, Jansa P, et al. Bosentan for treatment of inoperable chronic thromboembolic pulmonary hypertension: BENEFiT (Bosentan Effects in iNopErable Forms of chronIc Thromboembolic pulmonary hypertension), a randomized, placebo-controlled trial. *J Am Coll Cardiol.* 2008;52(25):2127–2134.

92. Ghofrani HA, D'Armini AM, Grimminger F, et al. Riociguat for the treatment of chronic thromboembolic pulmonary hypertension. *N Engl J Med.* 2013;369(4):319–329.

93. Simonneau G, D'Armini AM, Ghofrani HA, et al. Predictors of long-term outcomes in patients treated with riociguat for chronic thromboembolic pulmonary hypertension: data from the CHEST-2 open-label, randomised, long-term extension trial. *Lancet Respir Med.* 2016;4(5):372–380.

94. Ghofrani HA, Simonneau G, D'Armini AM, et al. Macitentan for the treatment of inoperable chronic thromboembolic pulmonary hypertension (MERIT-1): results from the multicentre, phase 2, randomised, double-blind, placebo-controlled study. *Lancet Respir Med.* 2017;5(10):785–794.

95. Lang I, Meyer BC, Ogo T, et al. Balloon pulmonary angioplasty in chronic thromboembolic pulmonary hypertension. *Eur Respir Rev.* 2017;26(143).

96. Jamieson SW. Pulmonary thromboendarterectomy. *Heart.* 1998;79(2):118–120.

97. Thistlethwaite PA, Madani M, Jamieson SW. Pulmonary thromboendarterectomy surgery. *Cardiol Clin.* 2004;22(3):467–478.

98. Jenkins D, Madani M, Fadel E, et al. Pulmonary endarterectomy in the management of chronic thromboembolic pulmonary hypertension. *Eur Respir Rev.* 2017;26(143).

99. Skoro-Sajer N, Hack N, Sadushi-Kolici R, et al. Pulmonary vascular reactivity and prognosis in patients with chronic thromboembolic pulmonary hypertension: a pilot study. *Circulation.* 2009;119(2):298–305.

100. Hamilton-Craig C, Kermeen F, Dunning JJ, et al. Cardiovascular magnetic resonance prior to surgical treatment of chronic thrombo-embolic pulmonary hypertension. *Eur Heart J.* 2010;31(9):1040.

101. Bonderman D, Skoro-Sajer N, Jakowitsch J, et al. Predictors of outcome in chronic thromboembolic pulmonary hypertension. *Circulation.* 2007;115(16):2153–2158.

102. Gladwin MT, Sachdev V, Jison ML, et al. Pulmonary hypertension as a risk factor for death in patients with sickle cell disease. *N Engl J Med.* 2004;350(9):886–895.

103. Haque AK, Gokhale S, Rampy BA, et al. Pulmonary hypertension in sickle cell hemoglobinopathy: a clinicopathologic study of 20 cases. *Hum Pathol.* 2002;33(10):1037–1043.

104. Gibson WH, Roughton FJ. The kinetics and equilibria of the reactions of nitric oxide with sheep haemoglobin. *J Physiol.* 1957;136(3):507–524.

105. Aslan M, Freeman BA. Redox-dependent impairment of vascular function in sickle cell disease. *Free Radic Biol Med.* 2007;43(11):1469–1483.

106. Hammerman SI, Klings ES, Hendra KP, et al. Farber HW. Endothelial cell nitric oxide production in acute chest syndrome. *Am J Physiol.* 1999;277(4 Pt 2):H1579–H1592.

107. Maron BA, Zhang YY, Handy DE, et al. Aldosterone increases oxidant stress to impair guanylyl cyclase activity by cysteinyl thiol oxidation in vascular smooth muscle cells. *J Biol Chem.* 2009;284(12):7665–7672.

108. Iyamu EW, Cecil R, Parkin L, et al. Modulation of erythrocyte arginase activity in sickle cell disease patients during hydroxyurea therapy. *Br J Haematol.* 2005;131(3):389–394.

109. Morris CR, Morris Jr SM, Hagar W, et al. Arginine therapy: a new treatment for pulmonary hypertension in sickle cell disease? *Am J Respir Crit Care Med.* 2003;168(1):63–69.

110. Machado RF, Barst RJ, Yovetich NA, et al. Hospitalization for pain in patients with sickle cell disease treated with sildenafil for elevated TRV and low exercise capacity. *Blood.* 2011;118(4):855–864.

111. Gladwin MT, Kato GJ, Weiner D, et al. Nitric oxide for inhalation in the acute treatment of sickle cell pain crisis: a randomized controlled trial. *JAMA.* 2011;305(9):893–902.

112. Brodsky RA. Advances in the diagnosis and therapy of paroxysmal nocturnal hemoglobinuria. *Blood Rev.* 2008;22(2):65–74.

113. Hill A, Rother RP, Wang X, et al. Effect of eculizumab on haemolysis-associated nitric oxide depletion, dyspnoea, and measures of pulmonary hypertension in patients with paroxysmal nocturnal haemoglobinuria. *Br J Haematol.* 2010;149(3):414–425.

114. Kato GJ, Wang Z, Machado RF, et al. Endogenous nitric oxide synthase inhibitors in sickle cell disease: abnormal levels and correlations with pulmonary hypertension, desaturation, haemolysis, organ dysfunction and death. *Br J Haematol.* 2009;145(4):506–513.

115. El-Shanshory M, Badraia I, Donia A, et al. Asymmetric dimethylarginine levels in children with sickle cell disease and its correlation to tricuspid regurgitant jet velocity. *Eur J Haematol.* 2013;91(1):55–61.

116. Manodori AB, Barabino GA, Lubin BH, et al. Adherence of phosphatidylserine-exposing erythrocytes to endothelial matrix thrombospondin. *Blood.* 2000;95(4):1293–1300.

117. Werdehoff SG, Moore RB, Hoff CJ, et al. Elevated plasma endothelin-1 levels in sickle cell anemia: relationships to oxygen saturation and left ventricular hypertrophy. *Am J Hematol.* 1998;58(3):195–199.

118. Phelan M, Perrine SP, Brauer M, et al. Sickle erythrocytes, after sickling, regulate the expression of the endothelin-1 gene and protein in human endothelial cells in culture. *J Clin Invest.* 1995;96(2):1145–1151.

119. Minniti CP, Machado RF, Coles WA, et al. Endothelin receptor antagonists for pulmonary hypertension in adult patients with sickle cell disease. *Br J Haematol.* 2009;147(5):737–743.

120. Barst RJ, Mubarak KK, Machado RF, et al. Exercise capacity and haemodynamics in patients with sickle cell disease with pulmonary hypertension treated with bosentan: results of the ASSET studies. *Br J Haematol.* 2010;149(3):426–435.

121. Holmes Jr. DR, Monahan KH, Packer D. Pulmonary vein stenosis complicating ablation for atrial fibrillation: clinical spectrum and interventional considerations. *JACC Cardiovasc Interv.* 2009;2(4):267–276.

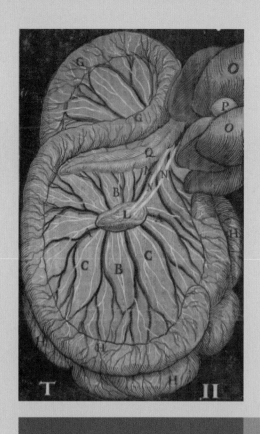

PART XVII

第十七部分

Lymphatic Disorders

淋巴疾病

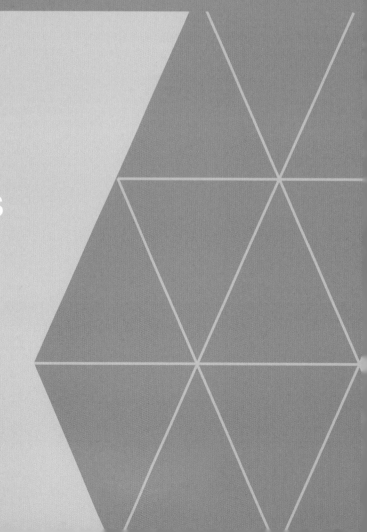

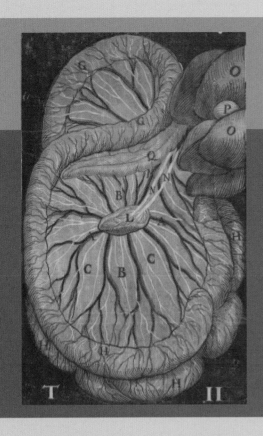

第57章
淋巴系统疾病

　　淋巴系统疾病一般认为与遗传性（原发性）缺陷或获得性（继发性）淋巴结构或功能破坏有关。原发性淋巴系统疾病是由淋巴脉管系统发育不良或内源性功能紊乱引起。不管是哪种机制，这些疾病中的每一种都会导致淋巴转运障碍。继发性淋巴功能障碍最常发生于淋巴通道中断后，通常发生在外伤、感染、肿瘤或手术干预的背景下。在所有形式的淋巴血管功能不全中，当局部淋巴管流量不足以维持组织间液稳态时，就会出现组织液积聚并出现局部肿胀。慢性淋巴瘀滞会伴随着软组织结构的紊乱，且几乎总是以皮下组织内的脂肪肥大为特征。静脉性水肿的存在和组织肥大是淋巴水肿的决定性特征，是淋巴管系统的终末器官衰竭状态。淋巴功能不全出现在内脏时，会导致严重的新陈代谢紊乱。除了在维持体液平衡中起到保存组织液的作用，淋巴循环还负责免疫系统从外周组织到淋巴器官的交通。因此，除了水肿的存在，淋巴血管功能障碍还伴随着区域性和系统性免疫反应的功能损害。淋巴系统疾病的治疗选择相当有限，这也反映了对淋巴水肿病理生理学的不完全理解；然而，近年来在淋巴成像和治疗学及血管生物学方面出现了新见解，从而为获得更明确的治疗方法提供了更多可能。除外各种加压治疗、外科淋巴管重建治疗、姑息性的外科减容减脂治疗，激光治疗等新疗法目前正在研究阶段，分子治疗的未来令人可期。

　　　　　　　　　　　　　　　　　　　　　　　　姜维良

Diseases of the Lymphatic Circulation

Stanley G. Rockson

Diseases of the lymphatic circulation reflect either intrinsic, presumptively heritable (primary) defects or the aftermath of an acquired (secondary) disruption of lymphatic structure or function. Primary lymphatic disorders are thought to arise from faulty development of the lymphatic vasculature or from intrinsic functional derangements. Without regard to the mechanism, each of these disorders results in a disturbance in lymph transit. Secondary lymphatic dysfunction most often occurs following disruption of lymphatic channels, typically in the setting of trauma, infection, neoplasia, or surgical interventions.

In all forms of lymphatic vascular insufficiency, interstitial fluid accumulates and regional swelling ensues when regional lymphatic flow is insufficient to maintain tissue homeostasis. When lymph stasis is chronic, there is accompanying derangement of the soft tissue histological architecture that is nearly always characterized by adipose hypertrophy within the subcutis. The presence of hydrostatic edema and tissue hypertrophy is the defining characteristic of lymphedema, the end-organ failure state of the lymphatic vasculature. Because proliferative pathology of the lymphatic vessels often produces a functionally incompetent vasculature, these conditions are also often typified by the presence of a lymphedema component. When present in the viscera, lymphatic insufficiency can also lead to profound metabolic disturbances. In addition to its role in the preservation of tissue fluid homeostasis, the lymphatic circulation is responsible for immune traffic from the peripheral tissues to the lymphoid organs. Thus, in addition to the presence of edema, lymphatic vascular dysfunction is accompanied by functional compromise of regional and systemic immune responses.

Historically, the rather limited therapeutic options for lymphatic disease have reflected an incomplete understanding of the pathophysiology of lymphedema; nevertheless, recent advances in imaging and therapeutics, as well as insights gained from vascular biology, hold promise for the elaboration of more definitive therapies.

ANATOMY OF THE LYMPHATIC CIRCULATION

It was in the 17th century that Gasparo Aselli recognized the lymphatic vasculature as a distinct anatomic entity.[1] On July 23, 1622, the anatomist undertook a demonstration of the action and innervation of the canine diaphragm.

While I was attempting this, and for that purpose had opened the abdomen and was pulling down with my hand the intestines and stomach…I suddenly beheld a great number of cords, as it were,

exceedingly thin and beautifully white, scattered over the whole of the mesentery and the intestine, and starting from almost innumerable beginnings…. I noticed that the nerves belonging to the intestine were distinct from these cords, and wholly unlike them, and besides, were distributed quite separately from them. Wherefore struck by the novelty of the thing, I stood for some time silent…. When I gathered my wits together for the sake of the experiment, having laid hold of a very sharp scalpel, I pricked one of these cords and indeed one of the largest of them. I had hardly touched it, when I saw a white liquid like milk or cream forthwith gush out. Seeing this, I could hardly restrain my delight.[1]

The chylous return from the intestine of the postprandial dog allowed Aselli to visualize the mesenteric lymphatics; when he repeated the demonstration several days later, no vessels were to be seen. Aselli eventually realized the relation between feedings and the visibility of the mesenteric lymphatics and duplicated the work in several species (Fig. 57.1). Over the following half century, Aselli's work was extended by Pecquet, Bartholinus, and Rudbeck, who defined the gross anatomy of the lymphatic system in toto.[1] By the 18th century, smaller lymphatic channels were visualized by Anton Nuck, using mercury injections. With those techniques, Sappey observed and recorded the human lymphatic system in exquisite detail (Fig. 57.2). Even greater resolution of the anatomy was provided by von Recklinghausen in 1862, with his discovery that the lymphatic endothelium stained darkly with silver nitrate. Using that technique, von Recklinghausen was able to differentiate lymphatic capillaries from the capillaries of the blood vascular system. Most recently, substantial advances in the techniques of immunohistochemistry and transmission electron microscopy have enabled the certain identification of the lymphatic microcirculation and its discrimination from the blood vasculature.[2,3]

It is now well established that the lymphatic capillaries are blind-ended tubular structures formed by a single layer of endothelial cells. These endothelial cells closely resemble those of blood vessels and have a common embryonic origin.[4,5] Like blood vascular endothelium, cultured lymphatic endothelial cells form confluent "cobblestone" monolayers that "sprout" to form tubules. They elaborate many identical histologic markers (von Willebrand factor, F-actin, fibronectin, and Weibel-Palade bodies). Unlike systemic capillaries, the basement membrane of lymphatic capillaries is absent or widely fenestrated, allowing greater entry of interstitial proteins and particles.

The capillaries join to form larger vessels (100 to 200 μm) that are invested with smooth muscle and are capable of intrinsic

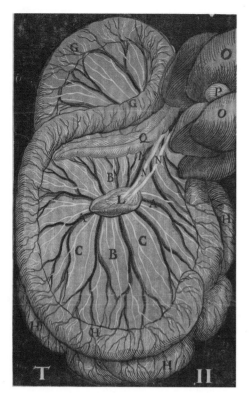

Fig. 57.1 The original anatomic illustration of the visceral lymphatics by Gasparo Aselli. (From the monograph De Lactibus Sive Lacteis Venis, courtesy Harvard Medical Library, Francis A. Countway Library of Medicine.)

vasomotion. These vessels, in turn, merge to form larger collecting conduits composed of three distinct layers: intima, media, and adventitia. The collectors possess intraluminal valves: these, separated by millimeters to centimeters, ensure that lymph flow will be directed centrally.[6,7]

In the lower limbs, the lymphatic collectors aggregate into a system that is divided into superficial and deep components. The superficial component is composed of medial and lateral channels. The medial channel originates on the dorsum of the foot and runs along the course of the saphenous vein. The lateral channel begins on the lateral aspect of the foot and ascends to the midleg, where the tributaries cross anteriorly to the medial side to follow the course of the medial lymphatics up to the inguinal nodes. Deep lymphatics do not usually communicate with the superficial system except through the popliteal and inguinal lymph nodes. The latter originate in the subcutaneous compartment, follow the course of the deep blood vessels, and eventually pass through the inguinal nodes.

Small- and medium-sized lymphatic vessels empty into main channels, of which the thoracic duct is the largest. The duct, approximately 2 mm wide and 45 cm long, ascends from the abdomen through the lower chest just to the right of the vertebral column and anterior to it. At approximately the level of the fifth thoracic vertebra, it crosses to the left of the spine, where it continues to ascend through the superior mediastinum to the base of the neck and eventually empties into the left brachiocephalic vein. Other large right- and left-sided lymphatic ducts may exist, although their arrangement, size, and course are highly variable. Those vessels join with the main thoracic duct or empty directly into great veins; they provide important collateral conduits if the thoracic duct becomes obstructed.

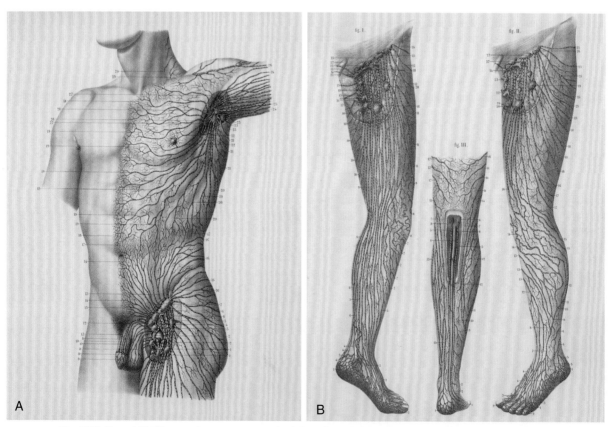

Fig. 57.2 (A and B) Nineteenth-century anatomic delineation of the cutaneous lymphatics. (From the text Anatomi, Physiologie, Pathologie des Vaisseaux Lymphatiques, by PC Sappey [1874], courtesy Harvard Medical Library, Francis A. Countway Library of Medicine.)

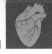

PHYSIOLOGY OF THE LYMPHATIC CIRCULATION

In 1786 William Hunter and two of his pupils, William Cruikshank and William Hewson, published the results of their work, laying the foundation for the physiology of the lymphatic system.[1] They correctly inferred from clinical observations that the lymphatics are involved in the response to infection as well as in the absorption of interstitial fluid. A century later, their theories received experimental support from the physiologic studies of Karl Ludwig and Ernest Starling. Ludwig cannulated lymph vessels, collected and analyzed the lymph, and proposed that it was a filtrate of plasma. Starling elucidated the forces governing fluid transfer from the blood capillaries to the interstitial space and offered evidence that the same forces apply to the lymphatic capillaries. He proposed that an imbalance in those forces could give rise to edema formation:

> In health, therefore, the two processes, lymph production and absorption, are exactly proportional. Dropsy depends on a loss of balance between these two processes—on an excess of lymph-production over lymph-absorption. A scientific investigation of the causation of dropsy will therefore involve, in the first place, an examination of the factors which determine the extent of these two processes and, so far as is possible, the manner in which these processes are carried out.

As first enunciated by Starling, interstitial fluid is largely an ultrafiltrate of blood. Its rate of production reflects the balance between factors that favor filtration out of capillaries (capillary hydrostatic pressure and tissue oncotic pressure) and those that favor reabsorption (interstitial hydrostatic pressure and capillary oncotic pressure). Under normal conditions, filtration exceeds reabsorption at a rate sufficient to create 2 to 4 L of interstitial fluid per day. There is a net filtration of protein (primarily albumin) from the vasculature into the interstitium; approximately 100 g of circulating protein may escape into the interstitial space daily. The interstitial fluid also receives the waste products of cellular metabolism as well as foreign matter or microbes that enter through breaks in the skin or by hematogenous routes.

A more recent revisiting of the Starling relationship suggests that the accumulation of capillary filtrate in the tissue spaces is avoided mainly through lymph drainage and not, as was previously thought, through reabsorption.[8] Direct observations demonstrate that, in most vascular beds, there is net filtration along the entire length of well-perfused capillaries.

Entry of interstitial fluid into the lymphatic capillary is primarily governed by the prevailing interstitial fluid pressure; under steady-state conditions, this is typically subatmospheric.[9] In situations where the pressure drops below the normal value of −6 mm Hg, lymph flow becomes negligible. However, any physical force that increases interstitial fluid pressure will increase lymph flow. According to the Starling equation, *increased capillary hydrostatic pressure, decreased plasma oncotic pressure, increased interstitial oncotic pressure*, or *increased capillary permeability* can each result in an increase in tissue lymph production. Lymph flow becomes maximal when interstitial pressure is slightly higher than the atmospheric pressure. Paradoxically, the average prevailing pressure gradients do not seem to favor fluid entry into the terminal lymphatics,[10] but it has been proposed that *cyclical* changes in the existing pressure gradients provide the dynamic force that favors fluid entry.[11-13] Furthermore, active regulation of transendothelial transport of solutes, lipids, and even water across lymphatic capillaries can occur.[14] These active mechanisms are thought to potentiate rapid control over rates of lymph formation without altering the integrity of the lymphatic vessels.[14]

The volume and the composition of the interstitial fluid are kept in balance by the lymphatic system. The functions of that system include (1) transport of excess fluid, protein, and waste products from the interstitial space to the bloodstream; (2) distribution of immune cells and substances from the lymphoid tissues to the systemic circulation; (3) filtration and removal of foreign material from the interstitial fluid; and (4) in the viscera, to promote the absorption of lipids from the intestinal lumen.

Not surprisingly, the lymphatics require a complex interplay of specific anatomy and function to meet physiological requirements. Several forces drive fluid through the lymphatic system. Once interstitial fluid enters the lymphatic vasculature, its further transport relies on the effects of both intrinsic and extrinsic pumps.[15] The extrinsic pump mechanism reflects the cyclical lymphatic compression and expansion produced by extrinsic tissue forces. These include the physical movement of parts of the body, skeletal muscle, arterial pulsation, and tissue compression by extrinsic forces. In other tissues, such as the splanchnic and cutaneous systems, it is primarily contractions of lymphatic smooth muscle that generate the driving force.[16,17] Normal lymphatic pump function is determined by the intrinsic properties of lymphatic muscle and the regulation of pumping by lymphatic preload, afterload, spontaneous contraction rate, contractility and neural influences.[15] These contractions are increased in frequency and amplitude by elevated filling pressure, sympathetic nerve activity, and shock; they may be modulated by circulating hormones and prostanoids.[18-20] Considerable force can be generated by those contractions; experimentally induced obstruction of the popliteal lymphatic system augments the strength and frequency of contraction, generating pressures of up to 50 mm Hg. Other factors that may contribute to lymphatic flow include intermittent compression from arterial pulsations, and gastrointestinal peristalsis. In addition, it has recently been proposed that the initial lymphatics (the small lymphatic capillaries that begin blindly in the tissues) most likely possess a two-valve system.[21,22] In addition to the classically described secondary intralymphatic valves, the initial lymphatics are thought to possess a primary valve system at the level of the endothelium to ensure unidirectional flow at this level. Once lymph enters the thorax, negative intrathoracic pressure generated during inspiration aspirates fluid into the thoracic duct (the "respiratory pump").

Failure of adequate lymph transport promotes lymphedema and likely contributes to the pathological presentation of a wide variety of lymphatic vascular diseases.

LYMPHATIC INSUFFICIENCY (LYMPHEDEMA)

Pathogenesis of Edema

Edema develops when the production of interstitial fluid (lymph) exceeds the transport capacity of the lymphatic vasculature. Thus either an overproduction of lymph (augmented lymphatic load) or a decreased ability to remove fluid (defective transport) from the interstitium, or both, can promote edema formation. Conditions associated with the overproduction of lymph include elevated venous pressures, increased capillary permeability, and hypoproteinemia. Elevated postcapillary hydrostatic pressure increases capillary filtration (as seen in right-sided congestive heart failure, tricuspid regurgitation, and deep venous thrombosis). Alternately, local inflammation increases capillary permeability, thus accelerating the egress of protein and fluid into the interstitium despite a normal capillary hydrostatic pressure. Lymph production may increase by 10- to 20-fold, exceeding lymphatic transport and resulting in marked edema.[23] Hypoproteinemia may also lead to marked edema, in which case hydrostatic pressure and capillary permeability are normal but capillary oncotic pressure is reduced, favoring net fluid transit to the interstitium. The edema that ensues in these conditions can, strictly speaking, be called lymphedema only when there is objective evidence of impaired lymphatic clearance or physical evidence of consequences of impaired lymphatic function in the skin or subcutaneous tissues.

Pathogenesis of Lymphedema

Lymphedema occurs whenever lymphatic vessels are absent, underdeveloped, or obstructed. Impedance to lymphatic flow may be due to an inborn defect (primary lymphedema) or an acquired loss of lymphatic patency (secondary lymphedema).

Primary Lymphedema

Prevalence estimates for the heritable causes of lymphedema are difficult to ascertain and vary substantially. Primary lymphedema is thought to occur in approximately 1 of every 6 to 10,000 live births. Females are affected 2- to 10-fold more commonly than males.[24] Primary lymphedema represents a heterogeneous group of disorders; therefore its classification schemes are numerous. Affected individuals can be classified by age of onset, functional anatomic attributes, or clinical setting.

Age of Onset

When distinguished by age of clinical onset, primary lymphedema can typically be divided into the following categories[25]:
1. Congenital lymphedema, clinically apparent at or near birth.
2. Lymphedema praecox, with onset after birth and before age 35; *lymphedema praecox*, a term used by Allen in 1934, most typically appears in the peripubertal years.
3. Lymphedema tarda appears after the age of 35.

Anatomic Patterns

An alternative classification scheme relies on an anatomic description of the lymphatic vasculature.[26,27]
1. Aplasia: no collecting vessels identified.
2. Hypoplasia: a diminished number of vessels are seen.
3. Numeric hyperplasia (as defined by Kinmonth): an increased number of vessels are seen.
4. Hyperplasia: in addition to an increase in number, the vessels have valvular incompetence and display tortuosity and dilation (megalymphatics).

Approximately one-third of all cases are secondary to agenesis, hypoplasia, or obstruction of the distal lymphatic vessels, with relatively normal proximal vessels.[28,29] In those cases the swelling is usually bilateral and mild and affects females much more frequently than males. The prognosis in such cases is good. Generally, after the first year of symptoms, there is little extension in the same limb or to uninvolved extremities. Although the extent of involvement is established early in the disease in about 40% of patients, the girth of the limb continues to increase.

In more than half of all cases, the defect primarily involves obstruction of the proximal lymphatics or nodes, with initial lack of involvement of distal lymphatic vessels. Pathologic studies reveal intranodal fibrosis. In those cases the swelling tends to be unilateral and severe; there may be a slight predominance of females in this group. In patients with proximal involvement, the extent and degree of the abnormality is more likely to progress and require surgical intervention. Initially uninvolved distal lymphatic vessels may become obliterated over time.

A minority of patients have a pattern of bilateral hyperplasia of the lymphatic channels or tortuous dilated megalymphatics. In these less common forms of primary lymphedema, there is a slight male predominance. Megalymphatics are associated with a greater extent of involvement and a worse prognosis.

Clinical Characteristics

As a third alternative, the primary lymphedemas can often be characterized by associated clinical anomalies or abnormal phenotype.[27] Although sporadic instances of primary lymphedema are more common, the tendency for congenital lymphedema to cluster in families is significant. The syndrome of a familial predisposition to congenital lymphedema, ultimately described as an autosomal dominant form of inheritance with variable penetrance, was first delineated by Milroy in 1892. He reported "hereditary edema" affecting 22 individuals of one family over six generations. Although Milroy ultimately described praecox and tarda forms as variants of the syndrome, the praecox form of primary lymphedema more often carries the eponym of Meige disease.[30]

In fact, a long list of disorders is associated with heritable forms of lymphedema. Increasingly these disorders have yielded to chromosomal mapping techniques. Lymphedema-cholestasis, or Aagenaes syndrome, has been mapped to chromosome 15q.[31] In several family cohorts of Milroy disease, it has been determined that the disorder reflects missense inactivating mutations in the tyrosine kinase domain of vascular endothelial growth factor receptor 3 (VEGFR3),[28,29] thus underscoring the likelihood that the pathogenesis of this condition likely reflects an inherited defect in lymphatic vasculogenesis. Several additional lymphedema syndromes have recently lent themselves to successful genetic mapping.[27] Lymphedema-distichiasis, an autosomal dominant, dysmorphic syndrome in which the lymphedema presents in association with a supplementary row of eyelashes arising from the meibomian glands, has been linked to truncating mutations in the forkhead-related transcription factor FOXC2[32]; mutations in FOXC2 have subsequently been associated with a broad variety of primary lymphedema presentations.[33] Similarly, a more unusual form of congenital lymphedema, hypotrichosis-lymphedema-telangiectasia, has been ascribed to both recessive and dominant forms of inheritance of mutations in the transcription factor gene SOX18.[34] Most recently, linkage analysis of three affected family cohorts has associated the occurrence of autosomal recessive congenital lymphatic dysplasia (Hennekam syndrome) to the gene CCBE1,[35,36] also identified as critical to lymphangiogenesis in zebrafish.[35] It is altogether plausible that further elucidation of the molecular pathogenesis of these diseases linked to FOXC2, SOX18, and CCBE1 mutations will lead to enhanced insights into mechanisms of normal and abnormal lymphatic development. Furthermore, mutational analysis of families expressing inherited forms of lymphedema have disclosed specific mutations in HGF (which encodes hepatocyte growth factor) and MET (the HGF receptor).[37] GJC2, the gene that encodes connexin 47, has also been implicated in the familial occurrence of lymphedema.[38]

At present, 12 distinct genes have been identified in association with syndromic and nonsyndromic primary lymphedema.[39] In general, autosomal or sex-linked recessive forms of congenital lymphedema occur less commonly than the dominant forms of inheritance. The list of heritable lymphedema-associated syndromes is long and growing (Box 57.1).[39] Primary lymphedema has been described in association with various forms of chromosomal aneuploidy, such as Turner and Klinefelter syndromes, with various dysmorphogenic-genetic anomalies such as Noonan syndrome and neurofibromatosis, and with various as yet unrelated disorders such as yellow nail syndrome, intestinal lymphangiectasia, lymphangiomyomatosis, and arteriovenous malformation.[40] The association of lymphedema with vascular anomalies likely derives from the shared embryological origin of the lymphatic and venous vasculature.

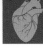

BOX 57.1   Hereditary Conditions Associated With Lymphedema

Chromosomal Aneuploidy

Trisomy 13
Trisomy 18
Trisomy 21
Triploidy
Klinefelter syndrome
Turner syndrome

Dysmorphogenic-Genetic Disturbances

Cantu syndrome
Cardiovaciocutaneous syndrome
CHARGE syndrome
Cholestasis-lymphedema syndrome (Aagenaes syndrome)
CLOVE syndrome
Down syndrome
Emberger syndrome
Fibroadipose hyperplasia
Fabry disease
Frank-Ter Haar syndrome
Hennekam syndrome
Hereditary fibrosing poikiloderma
Hypotrichosis-lymphedema-telangiectasia syndrome
Irons Bianchi syndrome
Klippel-Trénaunay-Weber syndrome
Lymphedema-distichiasis
Lymphedema-hypoparathyroidism syndrome
Lymphedema-microcephaly-chorioretinopathy
Macrocephaly capillary malformation syndrome
Meige lymphedema (lymphedema praecox)
Mucke syndrome
Neurofibromatosis type I (von Recklinghausen)
Noonan syndrome
Noone-Milroy hereditary lymphedema
Oculo-dento-digital syndrome
OL-EDA-ID syndrome
Phelan-McDermid syndrome
Prader-Willi syndrome
Progressive encephalopathy with edema, hypsarrhythmia, optic atrophy
Proteus syndrome
Thrombocytopenia absent radius syndrome
Tuberous sclerosis
Velo-cardio-facial syndrome
Yellow nail syndrome

Secondary Lymphedema

Secondary lymphedema is an acquired condition that can arise after loss or obstruction of previously adequate lymphatic channels. A wide variety of pathologic processes may lead to such lymphatic obliteration.

Infection

Recurrent episodes of bacterial lymphangitis lead to thrombosis and fibrosis of the lymphatic channels and are among the most common causes of lymphedema.[41] The responsible bacteria are almost always streptococci, which tend to enter through breaks in the skin or fissures induced by trichophytosis. Recurrent bacterial lymphangitis is also a frequent complicating factor of lymphedema from any cause.

Filariasis, a nematode infection endemic to regions of South America, Asia, and Africa, is the most common cause of secondary lymphedema in the world. The World Health Organization estimates that more than 130 million people may be affected by filarial infections; in India alone there are up to 14 million symptomatic cases. Common tropical filaria include *Wuchereria bancrofti* and *Brugia malayi* or *timori*. Other *Brugia* species are found in North America and occasionally cause lymphatic obstruction.

The microfilaria are transmitted by a mosquito vector and induce recurrent lymphangitis and eventual fibrosis of lymph nodes. It is unclear whether filaria themselves produce the lymphangitis or simply predispose those afflicted to recurrent episodes of bacterial lymphangitis. The filaria can also be identified in blood specimens of tissue obtained by fine-needle biopsy of the affected areas, and eosinophilia is a common local and systemic feature. Diethylcarbamazine remains the most popular drug for treating filariasis; although side effects are frequent, it is extremely efficacious.[42] Ivermectin is a newer antifilarial agent that may replace diethylcarbamazine; it is less toxic, and a single oral dose (25 µg/kg) appears to be as efficacious as a 2-week course of diethylcarbamazine.[43]

Lymphatic Trauma

Within this category, by far the most common mechanism of lymphedema relates to the surgical excision of lymph nodes.[44] This most often occurs in the setting of cancer staging and therapeutics. Breast cancer–associated lymphedema is the most common form of lymphedema in the United States. Both axillary lymph node dissection and adjuvant radiation therapy, particularly to breast and the axilla, predispose to the development of secondary lymphedema of the upper extremity.[45] In clinical follow-up after periods of up to 13 years following invasive treatment of breast cancer, an aggregate incidence of lymphedema of 14% can be expected in surgically treated patients with adjuvant postoperative irradiation.[46] Even less radical surgery (e.g., lumpectomy) can occasionally be complicated by lymphedema. Despite improvements in surgical and radiotherapeutic techniques, lymphedema remains a potential complication.[47,48] Similarly, edema of the leg may occur after surgery for pelvic or genital cancer, particularly when there has been inguinal and pelvic lymph node dissection or irradiation.[49] Its reported frequency varies between 1% and 47%.[50,51] Pelvic irradiation increases the frequency of leg lymphedema after surgery[52] for such conditions as malignant melanoma, prostate cancer, and gynecologic malignancies.

Lymphedema can also ensue from other mechanisms of lymphatic trauma, among them burns, large or circumferential wounds of the extremity, or other iatrogenic causes.[53]

Malignant Diseases

In addition to cancer therapeutics, various malignancies may induce secondary lymphedema. Tumor cells may obstruct lymphatic vessels, inducing lymphedema directly or by predisposing the patient to bacterial lymphangitis. In males the most common neoplastic etiology is prostate cancer; in females it is lymphoma.

Other Causes

Other conditions leading to or associated with obstruction of lymphatic channels include tuberculosis, contact dermatitis, rheumatoid arthritis, and pregnancy.[54] Autoimmune destruction of the lymphatics remains an interesting but unproven etiology.[55] Factitious lymphedema (*oedema bleu*) also occurs; that condition usually affects the hand, arm, or both; it is unilateral and is induced by the application of tourniquets, self-inflicted cellulitis, or maintenance of the limb in an immobile and dependent state. Chronic subcutaneous injections of drugs (most notably pentazocine hydrochloride) may also lead to lymphatic sclerosis and obstruction.

Pathology of Lymphedema

Early in the natural history of lymphedema there is variable thickening of the epidermis: the skin becomes rough, with hyperkeratosis and accentuation of the skin folds. Organization and fibrosis may lead to the development of papillomatosis. Early on, substantial edema of the dermis may occur. On cut section of gross specimens, the dermis is firm and gray, as is the deep fascia. Usually later in the course, but sometimes quite early, there may be expansion of the subcutaneous adipose tissue, often septated by prominent fibrous strands. In some specimens compression causes lymph to exude from the dermis and subcutaneous tissue, although this is not a prominent feature. Microscopic examination reveals hyperkeratosis with prominent dermal fibrosis as well as variable degrees of dermal edema (Fig. 57.3). Abundant subcutaneous fat with prominent fibrous septa is apparent in all cases. Often, perivascular inflammatory cells (lymphocytes, plasma cells, and occasionally eosinophils) can be seen. The lymphatic vessels are often difficult to visualize and may be obliterated or thrombosed by previous inflammatory episodes or may be congenitally absent or hypoplastic. Dilation of the lymphatics may be seen.

Clinical Presentation

The clinical signs of lymphedema largely depend on the duration and severity of the disease. Initially the interstitial space is expanded by an excess accumulation of relatively protein-rich fluid volume. The swelling produced by that fluid collection is typically soft, is easily displaced with pressure ("pitting edema"), and may substantially decrease with elevation of the limb. In the lower extremities, the edema typically extends to the distal aspects of the feet, resulting in the characteristic "square toes" seen in this condition. Over a period of years, the limb may take on a woody texture as the surrounding tissue becomes indurated and fibrotic (Fig. 57.4). In these later stages, pitting edema is no longer a major component and limb elevation or external compression is much less successful at reducing the girth of the extremity.

Proliferation of subcutaneous connective and adipose tissue leads to thickening of the skin and loss of flexibility; the affected limb is grossly enlarged, and a mossy or "cobblestone" skin texture may develop.

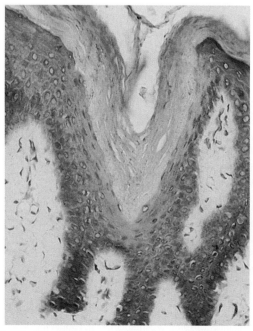

Fig. 57.3 Skin biopsy in chronic lymphedema disclosing characteristic hyperkeratosis and hypercellularity.

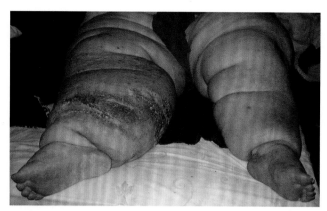

Fig. 57.4 Profound cutaneous and subdermal changes in chronic lower extremity lymphedema.

Correlates of these changes that can be sought on physical examination include the *peau d'orange* that reflects cutaneous and subcutaneous fibrosis as well as the so-called Stemmer sign (inability to tent the skin at the base of the digits), which is considered to be pathognomonic of lymphedema when present in a swollen limb.[56] In many cases of long-standing lymphedema, the deposition of substantial amounts of subcutaneous adipose tissue has been described,[57] hypothetically due to abnormalities of adipogenesis or lipid accumulation that accompany chronic stagnation of lymph.[58] However, the mechanisms of this consequence of chronic lymphatic circulatory insufficiency have not yet been delineated.

Natural History and Differential Diagnosis

The natural history of lymphedema is quite variable and may often encompass a substantial interval of subclinical asymptomatic disease. For example, even 3 years following modified radical mastectomy and axillary lymph node dissection, more than 80% of women remain free of any overt clinical evidence of lymphatic impairment despite the extensive iatrogenic destruction of the lymphatic architecture in these patients. Similarly, in many forms of primary lymphedema, there may be a protracted phase of apparently adequate lymphatic function despite the inherited anatomic or functional pathology. The precipitating factors for the appearance of overt lymphedema are unknown. At the onset of clinical lymphedema, swelling of the involved extremity is typically described as puffy; sometimes, the edematous changes may even be intermittent. With chronicity, the involved structures develop the characteristic features of induration and fibrosis.[59] In many of these patients, the maximal volume increase of the involved limb is determined within the first year after clinical onset unless there are supervening complications such as recurrent cellulitis. The propensity to recurrent soft tissue infection is one of the most troublesome aspects of long-standing lymphedema. In addition to the proinfectious features of accumulated fluid and proteins, the lymphatic dysfunction also impairs local immune responses.[60,61] With recurrent infections, there is progressive damage of lymphatic capillaries.

In rare cases, long-standing, chronic lymphedema may be complicated by the local development of malignant tumors. Although it is unnecessary to burden the patient about the possibility of malignancy, the patient should be alerted to report any changes in the appearance of the limb. Neoplastic transformation of the blood or lymph vessels can develop in long-standing lymphedema of any cause, including primary or secondary lymphedema.[62,63] Angiosarcomas or lymphangiosarcomas are potentially devastating but fortunately uncommon complications of long-standing lymphedema, occurring in less than 1% of cases.[64]

Lymphangiosarcomas can be either sclerotic plaques or multicentric lesions with blue-tinged nodules or bullous changes. Early detection and amputation can be lifesaving, but recognition of the condition is often delayed by a lack of awareness on the part of both the patient and the physician. Other malignancies—including lymphoma, Kaposi sarcoma, squamous cell cancer, and malignant melanoma—have been reported in association with chronic lymphedema.

The hypertrophied limb with thickened skin seen in chronic lymphedema has little similarity to the edematous limb of deep venous insufficiency. In the latter case, a soft pitting edema is prominent and seen in association with stasis dermatitis, hemosiderin deposition, and superficial venous varicosities. The history and examination easily differentiate chronic lymphedema from venous disorders and other causes of limb swelling (see Fig. 57.4). Earlier in the presentation, however, it may be more difficult to distinguish lymphedema from venous disease, reflex sympathetic dystrophy, or other causes of limb swelling.

Myxedema can be characterized by lower extremity edema, which superficially resembles lymphedema. In hypothyroidism, edema arises when abnormal mucinous deposits accumulate in the skin. Hyaluronic acid–rich protein deposition in the dermis produces edema with resulting abnormal structural integrity and reduced skin elasticity. In thyrotoxicosis, this process is localized to the pretibial region. Myxedema is characterized by roughening of the skin of the palms, soles, elbows, and knees; brittle, uneven nails; dull, thinning hair; yellow-orange discoloration of the skin; and reduced sweat production.

Lipedema is a condition that affects women almost exclusively, although it can be seen in men with a feminizing disorder. The edema is caused by the accumulation of subcutaneous adipose tissue in the legs, with sparing of the feet. The prevalence of lipedema is said to be 11% of the female population, according to one estimate,[65] and 10% to 18% of patients referred to a lymphedema clinic have lipedema.[66] Although the pathophysiology of lipedema is uncertain, it does involve an increase of subcutaneous adipocytes with structural alterations in the small vascular structures within the skin. Indeed, regional abnormalities of the circulation may cause the initial accumulation of fat in the affected regions. The characteristic distribution, with sparing of the feet, should suggest the correct diagnosis. The absence of a Stemmer sign is an additional clue. Most often, lipedema arises within 1 to 2 years after the onset of puberty. In addition to the near lifelong history of heavy thighs and hips, affected patients often complain of painful swelling. In addition, these individuals are commonly predisposed to easy bruising, perhaps due to the increased fragility of capillaries within the adipose tissue.

Diagnostic Modalities

Sometimes it is necessary to obtain more information about the nature and degree of lymphatic involvement when (1) the etiology of a swollen limb remains uncertain, (2) the diagnosis is evident but the etiology is unclear, or (3) a surgical procedure is being considered.

Lymphangiography

Human lymphatics were first visualized in vivo by Hudack and McMaster at the Rockefeller Institute in 1933.[1] They used one another as subjects to demonstrate superficial lymphatic plexuses along the forearm and inner thigh, using subcutaneous injection of vital dyes. In 1948 Glenn cannulated a lymphatic vessel in the dog hind limb and injected contrast media to produce a lymphangiogram in the canine leg and groin.[1] Subsequently, Servelle and Deysson visualized the lymphatics in patients with elephantiasis using retrograde injection.[1] Visualization of the dilated lymph channels, however, depended on partial or complete valvular incompetence. Direct contrast lymphangiography was developed by Kinmonth and coworkers[67] in 1952. The technique involves

identification of a distal vessel made visible by an intradermal injection of a vital dye into the metatarsal web spaces. The vessel is isolated and cannulated, and iodinated contrast material is injected. Following the injection, the contrast material is visualized radiographically as it progresses proximally through lymphatic channels.

There are several drawbacks to the procedure, including frequent requirements for surgical exposure in the edematous limb, microsurgical techniques to achieve direct cannulation, and occasionally the need for general anesthesia. Of greater importance is the fact that the irritation caused by the contrast agent resulted in lymphangitis in one-third of the studies, potentially worsening the lymphedema.[68] For these reasons the use of lymphangiography as a diagnostic modality for the edematous limb has largely been abandoned and is contraindicated in patients with lymphedema. Nevertheless, direct lymphangiography is still indicated for the evaluation and interventional treatment of patients with complex lymphatic vascular disorders.[69]

Lymphoscintigraphy

Lymphoscintigraphy involves the injection of radiolabeled macromolecules, such as sulfur colloid or albumin, into the distal subcutaneous tissue of the affected extremity (e.g., the dorsum of the foot). The progress of the radionuclide through the lymphatic system is followed by a radioscintigraphic camera. In primary lymphedema, channels are obliterated or absent; in a small percentage of cases, they are ectatic and incompetent. In secondary lymphedema, often with dilatation of the vascular channels, the level of obstruction can often be determined.[70] In lymphedema of any cause, the proximal progression of the radionuclide is delayed and its accumulation distally in the dilated channels of the dermis is manifested as a "dermal backflow" pattern (Fig. 57.5).

Lymphoscintigraphy is easier to perform than lymphangiography and is not reported to cause lymphangitis. It lacks the spatial resolution of lymphangiography; resolution is maximized by reducing the swelling of the extremity as much as possible before the study (reducing

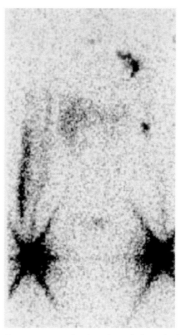

Fig. 57.5 Bilateral upper extremity lymphoscintigraphy is accomplished by subcutaneous interdigital injection of radiolabeled sulfur colloid. The study illustrates the absence of nodal uptake in the right axilla along with prominent "dermal backflow" in the right forearm. These findings confirm the diagnosis of unilateral lymphedema.

dilution of the radionuclide in stagnant lymph). Effective use of lymphoscintigraphy to plan therapeutic interventions requires an understanding of the pathophysiology of lymphedema and the influence of technical factors such as selection of the radiopharmaceutical agent, imaging times after injection, and patient activity on the images after injection.[23] It has been proposed that quantitative analysis of the lymphoscintigraphic mean transit times can be used to distinguish the presence of lymphatic dysfunction.[71] Furthermore, stress lymphoscintigraphy has been proposed as a useful modality to predict responsiveness to treatment interventions.[72]

Computed Tomography

Computed tomography (CT) scans of a lymphedematous limb are characterized by a honeycomb pattern in the affected area.[73] CT cannot directly localize the level of obstruction.[74] This technique can, however, provide insight into volume changes within various compartments visualized on cross-sectional images of the affected limb.[75] The greatest utility of CT is its ability to distinguish some of the causes of secondary lymphedema (e.g., lymphoma, pelvic tumor). Certainly the typical honeycomb pattern of lymphedema can be sought. In addition, elements of the differential diagnosis (venous obstruction, obesity, hematoma, ruptured popliteal cyst) can be further delineated through the CT images.

Magnetic Resonance Imaging

Magnetic resonance imaging (MRI) is an alternative and most likely a superior technique for imaging the soft tissues in edema.[76] With MRI it is possible to visualize cutaneous thickening with a honeycomb pattern in the subdermis, dilated lymphatic channels (when present as a consequence of lymphangioma or lymph reflux), and dermal accumulation of free fluid with surrounding fibrosis. This technique has particular virtue in differentiating lymphedema from lipedema. In addition, more recently, it has been demonstrated that nonenhanced three-dimensional heavily T2-weighted images obtained with two-dimensional prospective acquisition and correction has the capacity to visualize the thoracic duct, cisterna chyli, and lumbar lymphatics, at least in healthy volunteers.[77] More recently, magnetic resonance lymphography for the assessment of lymphedema has been demonstrated to have a specificity and sensitivity superior to that of standard radionuclide lymphoscintigraphy.[78]

Treatment
Medical Therapy

Successful treatment of lymphedema requires close collaboration between patient and physician. To that end, the physician should (1) carefully instruct the patient in the details of the medical program and (2) attend to the psychological impact of the disease. Associated emotional problems are not uncommon and are often neglected by physicians.[30] The need to address the psychological aspects of long-term disfigurement, especially with adolescent patients, cannot be overemphasized. In discussing these issues with the patient, the physician should be realistic about the possibility of progression but should also emphasize the patient's ability to modulate the course of the disease by careful attention to the details of the medical program.

The physiotherapeutic approach to lymphedema has been termed *decongestive lymphatic therapy*. Meticulous attention to control of edema may reduce the likelihood of disease progression and limit the incidence of soft tissue infections.[79] The elements of this therapeutic approach have been designed to accomplish the initial reduction in edematous limb volume, to maintain these therapeutic gains, and ensure optimal health and functional integrity of the skin.[80,81] In addition to the acute reduction in limb volume that is attainable, a well-maintained

therapeutic program has been demonstrated to accelerate lymph transport and to enhance the dispersal of accumulated protein. Decongestive lymphatic therapy integrates elements of meticulous skin care, massage, bandaging, exercise, and the use of compressive elastic garments.

To hydrate and soothe the skin, water-soluble emollients should be applied in a consistent and diligent manner. For excessive hyperkeratosis, these emollients can be supplemented with the application of salicylic acid ointments. Where skin cracking is prominent, meticulous attention to hygiene can be coupled with topical antiseptic agents.

The specialized massage technique for these patients (so-called manual lymphatic drainage or therapy) is an empirically derived technique. Its goal is to enhance lymphatic contractility and augment and redirect lymph flow through the unobstructed cutaneous lymphatics. Manual lymphatic drainage should not be confused with other forms of therapeutic massage that do not share this ability to augment lymphatic contractility and may, in fact, be detrimental to lymphatic function (e.g., athletic massages). The mild tissue compression during manual lymphatic drainage results in enhanced filling of the initial lymphatics and improves transport capacity through cutaneous lymphatic dilatation and the development of accessory lymph collectors.[81] Typically 20 to 30 consecutive daily sessions of manual lymphatic drainage are required to achieve optimal reduction of limb volume in a previously untreated patient.

During this acute approach to volume reduction, nonelastic compressive bandages should be applied in multiple layers after each session of manual lymphatic drainage (Fig. 57.6). These are worn during muscular exertion (which is encouraged) to prevent reaccumulation of fluid and promote lymph flow during exertion. Multilayer bandaging can also help to reverse skin changes, soften the subcutaneous tissues, and reduce lymphorrhea when present. In the maintenance phase of lymphedema care, the use of multilayer bandages is most often supplanted by the daily use of compressive elastic garments.

Elastic support hose should be fitted to the patient's limb after the edema in the extremity has been maximally reduced by compression and elevation.[41] This is an important detail. The stocking or sleeve does not reduce the size of the limb but maintains the circumference

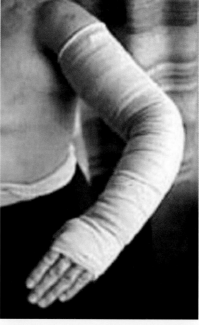

Fig. 57.6 Short-stretch multilayer compression bandaging in secondary lymphedema of the upper extremity.

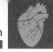

to which it is fitted. However, if the limb is fitted for a stocking while in a swollen state, the limb will be maintained by the stocking in a swollen state. The prescription of compressive garments is a necessary adjunct to all other forms of maintenance lymphedema therapy. Relatively inelastic sleeves, stockings, and underwear that transmit high-grade compression (40 to 80 mm Hg) will prevent reaccumulation of fluid after successful decongestive treatments. Garments must be fitted properly and replaced when they lose their elasticity (every 3 to 6 months). In addition to the standard fitted garments for upper and lower extremities, various additional appliances are now available. They provide the capacity to maintain limb volume during sleep, when the sleeve or stocking is removed, and during various forms of activity.

Without guidance from the physician, some patients become sedentary in response to uncomfortable or heavy sensations in the affected limb. Reduced physical activity at work and at home leads to apathy and malaise; this consequence can be averted by encouraging physical activity with proper support hose. Regular exercise appears to reduce lymphedema as long as elastic support (or hydrostatic pressure) is applied. Swimming is a particularly good physical activity for these patients because the hydrostatic pressure of the surrounding water negates the need for compressive support.

Although the elements of decongestive lymphatic therapy were initially derived empirically, the efficacy of these interventions has now been demonstrated in numerous prospective observations.[82–84] Long-term efficacy is particularly enhanced when attention is focused on patient instruction in the maintenance self-care.[83]

Various adjunctive treatment approaches have been investigated. Of these, perhaps the most useful is intermittent pneumatic compression (IPC). Multichamber pneumatic devices are available that intermittently compress the limb; techniques that employ sequential graduated compression (in which the cuffs are inflated sequentially from distal to proximal sites with a pressure gradient from the most distal cuff to the most proximal) are the most efficacious.[85] Pneumatic compression techniques cannot, however, clear edema fluid from adjacent non-compressed sections of the limb. Consequently, as fluid shifts occur during pneumatic compression, the root of the limb must be decompressed with the manual techniques mentioned previously. In addition, it should be stressed that any form of compressive therapy requires a sufficient arterial blood supply to the limb. In cases where severe peripheral artery disease coexists, any form of sustained compression can further compromise arterial blood flow.

The incorporation of IPC into a multidisciplinary therapeutic approach has been long advocated empirically by some physiotherapeutic schools.[85] Individual reports of complications and lack of efficacy have reduced enthusiasm for the use of pneumatic compression as stand-alone therapy. More recently, it has been demonstrated that when IPC is used adjunctively with the other established elements of decongestive lymphatic therapy, it enhances the therapeutic response, both in the initial and maintenance approaches to the patient. Pneumatic compression is well tolerated and remarkably free of complications.[86,87] In addition, this adjunctive treatment approach has demonstrable benefits for the reduction of both medical resource utilization and healthcare costs.[88–90]

Other physical forms of therapy are under investigation. Low-level laser therapy may be effective in postmastectomy lymphedema: in one small series, subjective improvement accompanied an objective documentation of improved bioimpedance and reduced extracellular and intracellular fluid accumulation.[91] In other hands, such techniques as local hyperthermia or the intraarterial injection of autologous lymphocytes[92] have independently produced favorable results. In the latter approach, it is postulated that regression of edema is linked to the

expression of L-selectin, a lymphocyte-specific adhesion molecule.[92] The observations in these pilot studies must be confirmed in larger controlled trials.

Additional standard treatment approaches are directed toward the prevention and control of infection. Recurrent cellulitis and local infections pose a constant threat of exacerbation. Skin hygiene is essential. In addition to the application of emollients to the skin, trauma must be avoided (when the patient is ambulatory, his or her feet should be covered by slippers or shoes; a podiatrist should attend to nail care as needed). Fungal infections should be aggressively treated with topical antifungal agents. The patient should be instructed to take antibiotics at the earliest sign of cellulitis and should be given a prescription for a course of an oral semisynthetic penicillin, cephalosporin, or (for penicillin-sensitive patients) erythromycin. In lymphedema, acute inflammatory episodes may not elicit typical, clearly demarcated erythematous skin responses or associated systemic evidence of infection. Nevertheless, these more subtle presentations should be treated aggressively with antibiotics. After a course of therapy, the edema once again responds to compressive therapy and the tenderness resolves. Various broad-spectrum oral antibiotics can be used to good effect, particularly with attention to the spectrum of activity against streptococcal and staphylococcal species. For individuals who are prone to repetitive episodes of soft tissue infection, the use of prophylactic antibiotic regimens is safe and is associated with demonstrable reductions in the recurrence, incidence, and time to next episode of infection.[93]

Other than antibiotic therapy where needed, pharmacotherapy has had little role in the management of lymphedema. Diuretics, though widely prescribed for this chronic edematous condition, typically provide only transient benefit and may be deleterious to the long-term outcome. On the other hand, in edema of mixed origin, diuretics often have a beneficial effect through their ability to reduce circulating blood volume and thereby reduce capillary filtration. An understanding of the mechanisms inducing the proliferation of subcutaneous connective tissue and lymphedema may lead to more definitive treatment. Agents might then be designed to alter the relationship between the deposition and lysis of collagen fibers such that lysis is favored, thereby reducing fibrosis.[5,94] Benzopyrones (coumarin, hydroxyethylrutin) represent a class of agents that have been reported to reduce volume in affected limbs, purportedly by stimulating tissue macrophages, which in turn increase interstitial proteolysis. Although initial trials appeared favorable,[95,96] subsequent evaluation suggests that the therapeutic gains are small[97]; furthermore, the utility of coumarin is significantly hampered by the risk of drug-related hepatotoxicity.[98] An important question left unanswered is whether coumarin is additive in its effects to the usual compressive measures. The agent is not yet approved by the FDA for use in the United States. Another experimental therapy is intralymphatic injections of steroids, which may help by inhibiting the proliferation of connective tissue. The development of angiogenic steroids that have some tissue specificity could make this a feasible approach. Alternatively, flavonoids such as hesperidin and diosmin have been employed to beneficial effect. Their use is supported by preclinical experimental investigations suggesting that these agents have the capacity to improve microvascular permeability and augment lymphatic contractile activity. Extract of horse chestnut seed containing escin, a bioflavonoid, has been shown to reduce venular capillary permeability and edema of lymphatic or venous etiology.

More recent investigational studies suggest that the future potential of molecular therapy in lymphedema is promising. Mechanistic investigations of lymphedema in animal models strongly suggest an inflammatory pathogenesis for the disease,[99–102] and targeted antiinflammatory therapy has been demonstrated to reverse both edema and tissue structural changes in experimental lymphedema.[103] Quite recently, there has been an elucidation of the specific role of leukotriene B_4 (LTB_4), an inflammatory prostanoid, in the pathogenesis of the inflammatory cascade that leads to the generation of experimental lymphedema; abrogation of the LTB_4 effect with a specific antagonist restores $VEGF_3$ and Notch signaling, thereby reversing the lymphedema pathology.[104,105] Clinical trials of this approach are under way in human lymphedema.

Surgical Treatment

There is burgeoning interest in the role of microsurgical interventions to ameliorate or reverse lymphedema of the limb.

Direct microsurgical anastomotic procedures are increasingly employed.[106,107] Lymphovenous anastomosis can be established utilizing the lymphatic vasculature and neighboring venous structures distal to a lymphatic obstruction; such anastomoses allow lymph from the obstructed region to flow directly into the venous system. Anastomoses can also be made from the lymph nodes to the adjacent vein. These operations obviously are of no value when the lymphatic obstruction is at the level of the smaller distal vessels. The argument has been made, however, that lymphatic bypass operations should be performed as soon as possible after the onset of obstruction to avoid the cutaneous changes of chronic lymphedema as well as the gradual destruction of the distal lymphatic channels. An appropriate candidate for such surgery would be an individual with a recent onset of lymphedema secondary to trauma and with an otherwise normal lymphatic system proximal and distal to the area of obstruction. A recent review of the published literature suggests substantial symptomatic relief among the recipients of this approach,[108] including patients with primary forms of lymphedema.[109]

An alternative approach, increasingly employed, involves vascularized, surgical transfer of lymph nodes (vascularized lymph node transfer [VLNT]) to orchestrate lymphatic repair and relief of lymphedema symptomatology.[110] Lymph node donor sites for autotransplanted free transfer include superficial groin, submental, supraclavicular, thoracic, and omental areas. Responses to such interventions are favorable but not universal. Imaging techniques to optimize the surgical outcome continue to evolve. An additional evolving approach involves the utilization of biological scaffolds to facilitate lymphatic engraftment of the transplant.[111]

For late-stage lymphedema, which is predominated by bulky overgrowth of cutaneous elements and subcutaneous adipose hypertrophy, it is appropriate to consider palliative reduction procedures. Historically such procedures have required resection of a portion of the skin and subcutaneous tissue and subsequent closure of the wound to reduce the limb diameter. Acute complications include wound infection or necrosis of the skin flaps; late complications include recurrent cellulitis or verrucous hyperplasia of the skin grafts. Swelling of the extremity is more likely to progress if recurrent bouts of cellulitis are not adequately controlled or if adequate compressive support is not provided postoperatively (the procedure does not correct the obstruction to lymph efflux). Of much greater interest is the now widely employed debulking technique that entails suction-assisted lipectomy of the late-stage lymphedema limb. This approach can safely attain a stable, significant reduction of limb volume in both upper and lower limb lymphedema. In one series, an average long-term reduction of edema volume of 106% was observed in 28 patients with an average edema volume of 1845 mL.[57] Liposuction combined with long-term decongestive compression therapy reduces edema volume more successfully than does compression therapy alone. However, the volume reduction is unsuccessful unless compression therapy is maintained after the surgical intervention.[57]

Prospects for Molecular Therapy

Among the mitogenic substances that initiate and regulate the growth of vascular structures, those in the VEGF family play a central role.[112,113] VEGF-C and VEGF-D direct the development and growth of the lymphatic vasculature in embryonic and postnatal life through binding to VEGFR-3 receptors on lymphatic endothelia.[113-115] Exogenous administration of VEGF-C upregulates the VEGFR-3 receptor, leading to a lymphangiogenic response[116] and, in transgenic mice that overexpress VEGF-C, the lymphatic vessels demonstrate a hyperplastic, proliferative response with secondary cutaneous changes.[115]

These molecular observations have shed light on the mechanisms that contribute to disease expression in the most common heritable form of lymphedema, the autosomal dominant condition known as Milroy disease, which has been linked to the FLT4 locus, encoding vascular VEGFR-3.[28] Disease-associated alleles contain missense mutations that produce an inactive tyrosine kinase, thereby preventing downstream gene activation. It is believed that the mutant form of the receptor is excessively stable as well as inactive, so that the normal signaling mechanism is blunted, leading to hypoplastic development of the lymphatic vessels.[117]

The prospects for therapeutic lymphangiogenesis in human lymphedema have been underscored by the description of a mouse model of inherited limb edema based on mutations in the VEGFR-3 signaling mechanism and pathology that resembles human disease.[118] In this model, therapeutic overexpression of VEGF-C using a viral vector induces the generation of new, functional lymphatics and the amelioration of lymphedema. Similarly, in rodent models of acquired postsurgical lymphatic insufficiency (i.e., resembling postmastecomy lymphedema), the exogenous administration of human recombinant VEGF-C restores lymphatic flow (as assessed by lymphoscintigraphy),[119] increases lymphatic vascularity, and reverses the hypercellularity that characterizes the untreated lymphedematous condition (Fig. 57.7).[99,120]

Many barriers remain. Hyperplastic growth can be induced with administration of high doses of VEGF-C or in VEGF-C–overexpressing systems and in collecting vessels, VEGF-C–induced hyperplasia causes malformation of the collecting valves or vessel hyperpermeability.[121] Intensive future investigation is necessary to verify the therapeutic potential of such approaches as well as to establish dose-response relationships and durability of the therapeutic response. As with other

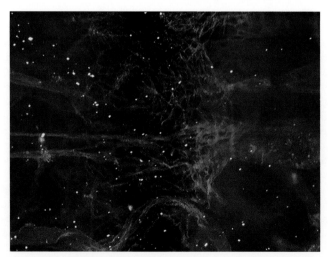

Fig. 57.7 The whole mount section of mouse tail skin demonstrates therapeutic lymphangiogenesis in response to human VEGF-C.

forms of angiogenic therapy, the relative virtues of growth factor (gene product) therapy versus gene therapy must be established.

DISEASES OF THE LYMPHATIC VASCULATURE

Complex Vascular Pathology With Lymphatic Anomalies

There is a broad constellation of developmental anomalies of the arteriovenous circulation that concurrently distort lymphatic anatomy, function, or both. These mixed vascular deformities are best characterized by the dominant vascular anomaly, whether angiomatous, venous, or arteriovenous.[26]

Klippel-Trénaunay Syndrome

Klippel-Trénaunay syndrome (KTS) is the most common congenital venous anomaly to affect the entire limb. It is a congenital disorder in which varicose veins, cutaneous nevi, and limb hypertrophy are observed. Lymphedema is reported in 5% of these patients. It has been suggested that this syndrome reflects a generalized disturbance of mesodermal development, thereby engendering such commonly associated anomalies as bony overgrowth, soft tissue hypertrophy, syndactyly, hypospadias, and lymphatic hypoplasia. Treatment is generally restricted to meticulous skin care (i.e., hydration, protection from trauma); compressive therapy for the associated lymphedema and venous insufficiency; prevention of superficial bleeding from the varicose veins; and prophylaxis against deep venous thrombosis.

More recently, KTS patients, and, in particular those syndromic patients who manifest lymphatic malformations, have been identified to represent part of the disease spectrum associated with activating somatic mutations in the PIK3CA gene.[122] These mutations, observed commonly in human cancers, now provide a potential mechanistic explanation for the overgrowth presentations as well as an opportunity to consider specific therapeutic interventions to impede the overgrowth response.[123]

Maffucci Syndrome

The Maffucci syndrome is described as severe dyschondroplasia in association with multiple lymphangiomata (see later). In this condition, the lymphatic vasculature and nodes are typically hypoplastic.[26]

Parkes Weber Syndrome

This syndrome is characterized by the presence of multiple arteriovenous fistulas with associated enlargement of the girth of a single limb. The condition can be ascribed at least in part to the concomitant dilated, tortuous lymphatics and consequent lymphedema. The pathophysiology of this disorder likely reflects the enormous increase in blood flow consequent to the multiple arteriovenous fistulas; this increase in capillary filtration would then lead to an increase in lymphatic load, producing first vascular dilatation and, ultimately, insufficiency. The lymph reflux in the limb may lead to the appearance of lymph vesicles in the skin, which should be treated conservatively. We have had some initial success with percutaneous and intravascular catheter-based embolization of associated arteriovenous fistulas (unreported observations).

Parkes Weber syndrome belongs to a constellation of vascular malformations collectively known as capillary malformation–arteriovenous malformation. This constellation has recently been identified to be associated with heterozygous mutations in the *RASA1* gene.[124] The gene encodes a protein that acts as a negative regulator of the RAS signal transduction pathway.

Proliferative Growth of Lymphatic Vascular Structures and Neoplasm

Lymphatic Vascular Malformation

These developmental malformations are first detectable in infants. They are not, despite their name, strictly speaking tumors. Rather, these lesions are composed of profuse numbers of dilated, thin-walled, lymphatic vascular structures. They can occur throughout the body but are seen most commonly on the proximal extremities and at the limb girdle. Small clear vesicles are observed in the skin, sometimes with associated cutaneous bleeding. When these lesions are encountered in the setting of dyschondroplasia, the designation of Maffucci syndrome is applied.

Cavernous Lymphangioma and Cystic Hygroma

These hamartomatous lesions appear within the first years of life if not present at birth. Like lymphangiomas, these lesions contain dilated lymphatic vascular structures. The cavernous lesions are typically found in the mouth, in the mesentery, and on the extremities; cystic hygromas present in the neck, axillae, and groin. These lesions are often surgically resected to prevent complications.

Generalized Lymphatic Anomaly

This is a rare developmental condition in which proliferation of lymphatic vascular structures involves dermis, soft tissue, bone, and parenchyma in a diffuse manner. The organs most typically affected are liver, spleen, lung, and pleura. Associated lymphangiectasia can be observed in numerous additional organs, including liver, kidney, testes, lymph nodes, adrenals, and intestines. Involvement of the viscera typically confers a poor prognosis. When chylothorax is present, repeated thoracentesis and pleurodesis is often required. In one small series, all patients died within 6 to 33 months of clinical presentation.[125]

A recent, exciting development in the management of complex vascular malformations, including those that feature lymphatic components, has been the therapeutic application of mTOR inhibition to limit vascular growth. Sirolimus has recently been successfully utilized in a prospective phase II trial in 62 such patients, including patients with generalized lymphatic anomaly, venous lymphatic anomaly, capillary lymphaticovenous malformation, and microcystic lymphatic malformation.[126]

Lymphangiosarcoma

Lymphangiosarcomas, malignant angiosarcomas that develop in association with lymphedema, develop as multicentric lesions that have a high propensity for systemic metastasis. The vast majority of such lesions have been observed in lymphedema patients who are breast cancer survivors with chronic, significant edema. Lymphangiosarcoma is seen only rarely in other forms of lymphedema. Whatever the clinical substrate, the prognosis for survival is poor, even following radical amputation.

Visceral Lymphatic Disorders

Chylous Reflux, Chylothorax, Chylous Ascites

When the lymphatics are incompetent, obstructed, or hypoplastic, fluid has the capacity to reflux. In visceral disease, this fluid can be lymph or chylous lymph. The presence of chylous lymph denotes incompetence of lymphatic flow that extends to the level of the lacteals at the point where they join the preaortic lymphatics and the cisterna chyli. The anatomical substrate of this problem can be either primary or secondary. In the former case, hypoplastic or dilated incompetent lymphatics reflect the inherited defect of lymphatic development; in secondary forms, thoracic duct obstruction occurs through surgical mishap, trauma, malignancy, or the damage created by filariasis.

Lymph or chyle reflux can occur directly into the lower limbs. The abnormal fluid drains directly from vesicles on the surface of the leg or on the genitalia. Variants of this same presentation can produce chylothorax, chylous ascites, chylous arthritis, and chyluria. In general, if chyle is present in the refluxing body fluid, the therapeutic approach should include a fat-restricted diet with supplementation of medium-chain triglycerides; if the response is not satisfactory, complete elimination of chyle from the fluid can be accomplished, at least temporarily, with total parenteral nutrition.

The prognosis for such presentations is not favorable. The natural history of reflux reflects the tendency for the condition to worsen with the passage of time. In some patients, there may be an episodic pattern of leakage with sudden exacerbations; others experience a steadily increasing tendency to lymphorrhea and reflux. In patients with the secondary form, an assiduous search for predisposing malignancy or extrinsic lymphatic obstruction should always be undertaken. In patients with the various forms of visceral involvement, complex surgical interventions are sometimes required to mitigate the functional and symptomatic consequences of reflux into the serous cavities.

Protein-Losing Enteropathy

The presence of visceral lymphatic vascular disease can predispose to a life-threatening form of metabolic insufficiency called protein-losing enteropathy. When chyle refluxes back into the villi as a consequence of the effective blockade of its passage into the central lymphatics, this condition engenders weight loss, diarrhea, and steatorrhea as protein, fat, calcium, and fat-soluble vitamins are malabsorbed. In addition to the secondary forms of lymphatic obstruction (usually malignant), the primary hypoplastic and lymphangiectatic disorders can also predispose to enteropathy[94]; in these cases lymphedema of an extremity often precedes or accompanies the appearance of the enteropathy. As with other forms of reflux, the initial therapeutic strategy should entail supplementation of medium-chain triglycerides with restriction of total dietary fat intake. Where the response to conservative therapy is insufficient, it has been suggested that systemic treatment with octreotide may help to alleviate the severity of the disorder, although the mechanism of benefit is not entirely understood.[127-129]

REFERENCES

1. Kanter MA. The lymphatic system: an historical perspective. *Plast Reconstr Surg*. 1987;79(1):131–139.
2. Rockson S. Preclinical models of lymphatic disease: the potential for growth factor and gene therapy. *Ann N Y Acad Sci*. 2002;979:64–75.
3. Shin WS, Szuba A, Rockson SG. Animal models for the study of lymphatic insufficiency. *Lymphat Res Biol*. 2003;1(2):159–169.
4. Oliver G. Lymphatic vasculature development. *Nat Rev Immunol*. 2004;4(1):35–45.
5. Oliver G, Srinivasan RS. Lymphatic vasculature development: current concepts. *Ann N Y Acad Sci*. 2008;1131:75–81.
6. Baldwin M, Stacker S, Achen M. Molecular control of lymphangiogenesis. *Bioessays*. 2002;24:1030–1040.
7. Gashev A. Physiologic aspects of lymphatic contractile function: current perspectives. *Ann N Y Acad Sci*. 2002;979:178–187.
8. Mortimer PS, Rockson SG. New developments in clinical aspects of lymphatic disease. *J Clin Invest*. 2014;124(3):915–921.
9. Aukland K, Reed RK. Interstitial-lymphatic mechanisms in the control of extracellular fluid volume. *Physiol Rev*. 1993;73(1):1–78.
10. Zawieja DC. Contractile physiology of lymphatics. *Lymphat Res Biol*. 2009;7(2):87–96.
11. Negrini D, Moriondo A, Mukenge S. Transmural pressure during cardiogenic oscillations in rodent diaphragmatic lymphatic vessels. *Lymphat Res Biol*. 2004;2(2):69–81.
12. Moriondo A, Mukenge S, Negrini D. Transmural pressure in rat initial subpleural lymphatics during spontaneous or mechanical ventilation. *Am J Physiol Heart Circ Physiol*. 2005;289(1):H263–H269.
13. Grimaldi A, Moriondo A, Sciacca L, et al. Functional arrangement of rat diaphragmatic initial lymphatic network. *Am J Physiol Heart Circ Physiol*. 2006;291(2):H876–H885.
14. Wiig H, Swartz MA. Interstitial fluid and lymph formation and transport: physiological regulation and roles in inflammation and cancer. *Physiol Rev*. 2012;92(3):1005–1060.
15. Scallan JP, Zawieja SD, Castorena-Gonzalez JA, Davis MJ. Lymphatic pumping: mechanics, mechanisms and malfunction. *J Physiol*. 2016;594:5749–5768.
16. Cotton KD, Hollywood MA, McHale NG, Thornbury KD. Outward currents in smooth muscle cells isolated from sheep mesenteric lymphatics. *J Physiol*. 1997;503(Pt 1):1–11.
17. von der Weid PY, Zawieja DC. Lymphatic smooth muscle: the motor unit of lymph drainage. *Int J Biochem Cell Biol*. 2004;36(7):1147–1153.
18. Gashev AA, Zawieja DC. Physiology of human lymphatic contractility: a historical perspective. *Lymphology*. 2001;34(3):124–134.
19. Muthuchamy M, Gashev A, Boswell N, et al. Molecular and functional analyses of the contractile apparatus in lymphatic muscle. *FASEB J*. 2003;17(8):920–922.
20. McHale NG, Thornbury KD, Hollywood MA. 5-HT inhibits spontaneous contractility of isolated sheep mesenteric lymphatics via activation of 5-HT(4) receptors. *Microvasc Res*. 2000;60(3):261–268.
21. Trzewik J, Mallipattu SK, Artmann GM, et al. Evidence for a second valve system in lymphatics: endothelial microvalves. *FASEB J*. 2001;15(10):1711–1717.
22. Mendoza E, Schmid-Schonbein GW. A model for mechanics of primary lymphatic valves. *J Biomech Eng*. 2003;125(3):407–414.
23. Szuba A, Shin WS, Strauss HW, Rockson S. The third circulation: radionuclide lymphoscintigraphy in the evaluation of lymphedema. *J Nucl Med*. 2003;44(1):43–57.
24. Rockson SG. Lymphedema. *Am J Med*. 2001;110(4):288–295.
25. Szuba A, Rockson SG. Lymphedema: classification, diagnosis and therapy. *Vasc Med*. 1998;3(2):145–156.
26. Kinmonth JB, Taylor GW, Tracy GD, Marsh JD. Primary lymphoedema; clinical and lymphangiographic studies of a series of 107 patients in which the lower limbs were affected. *Br J Surg*. 1957;45(189):1–9.
27. Rockson S. Syndromic lymphedema: keys to the kingdom of lymphatic structure and function? *Lymphat Res Biol*. 2003;1:181–183.
28. Karkkainen MJ, Ferrell RE, Lawrence EC, et al. Missense mutations interfere with VEGFR-3 signalling in primary lymphoedema. *Nat Genet*. 2000;25(2):153–159.
29. Irrthum A, Karkkainen MJ, Devriendt K, et al. Congenital hereditary lymphedema caused by a mutation that inactivates VEGFR3 tyrosine kinase. *Am J Hum Genet*. 2000;67(2):295–301.
30. Smeltzer DM, Stickler GB, Schirger A. Primary lymphedema in children and adolescents: a follow-up study and review. *Pediatrics*. 1985;76(2):206–218.
31. Bull LN, Roche E, Song EJ, et al. Mapping of the locus for cholestasis-lymphedema syndrome (Aagenaes syndrome) to a 6.6-cM interval on chromosome 15q. *Am J Hum Genet*. 2000;67(4):994–999.
32. Fang J, Dagenais SL, Erickson RP, et al. Mutations in FOXC2 (MFH-1), a forkhead family transcription factor, are responsible for the hereditary lymphedema-distichiasis syndrome. *Am J Hum Genet*. 2000;67(6):1382–1388.
33. Finegold DN, Kimak MA, Lawrence EC, et al. Truncating mutations in FOXC2 cause multiple lymphedema syndromes. *Hum Mol Genet*. 2001;10(11):1185–1189.
34. Irrthum A, Devriendt K, Chitayat D, et al. Mutations in the transcription factor gene SOX18 underlie recessive and dominant forms of hypotrichosis-lymphedema-telangiectasia. *Am J Hum Genet*. 2003;72(6):1470–1478.
35. Alders M, Hogan BM, Gjini E, et al. Mutations in CCBE1 cause generalized lymph vessel dysplasia in humans. *Nat Genet*. 2009;41(12):1272–1274.
36. Connell F, Kalidas K, Ostergaard P, et al. Linkage and sequence analysis indicate that CCBE1 is mutated in recessively inherited generalised lymphatic dysplasia. *Hum Genet*. 2010;127(2):231–241.

37. Finegold DN, Schacht V, Kimak MA, et al. HGF and MET mutations in primary and secondary lymphedema. *Lymphat Res Biol.* 2008;6(2):65–68.

38. Ferrell RE, Baty CJ, Kimak MA, et al. GJC2 missense mutations cause human lymphedema. *Am J Hum Genet.* 2010;86(6):943–948.

39. Mortimer PS, Gordon K, Brice G, Mansour S. Hereditary and familial lymphedemas. In: Lee BB, Rockson SG, Bergan J, eds. *Lymphedema: A Concise Compendium of Theory and Practice.* 2nd ed. London: Springer; 2018:29–43.

40. Wheeler ES, Chan V, Wassman R, et al. Familial lymphedema praecox: Meige's disease. *Plast Reconstr Surg.* 1981;67(3):362–364.

41. Schirger A. Lymphedema. *Cardiovasc Clin.* 1983;13(2):293–305.

42. Bockarie M, Tisch D, Kastens W, et al. Mass treatment to eliminate filariasis in Papua New Guinea. *N Engl J Med.* 2002;347:1841–1848.

43. Kumaraswami V, Ottesen EA, Vijayasekaran V, et al. Ivermectin for the treatment of Wuchereria bancrofti filariasis. Efficacy and adverse reactions. *JAMA.* 1988;259(21):3150–3153.

44. Szuba A, Rockson S. Lymphedema: classification, diagnosis and therapy. *Vasc Med.* 1998;3:145–156.

45. Rockson SG. Precipitating factors in lymphedema: myths and realities. *Cancer.* 1998;83(12 Suppl American):2814–2816.

46. Hojris I, Andersen J, Overgaard M, Overgaard J. Late treatment-related morbidity in breast cancer patients randomized to postmastectomy radiotherapy and systemic treatment versus systemic treatment alone. *Acta Oncol.* 2000;39(3):355–372.

47. Tengrup I, Tennvall-Nittby L, Christiansson I, Laurin M. Arm morbidity after breast-conserving therapy for breast cancer. *Acta Oncol.* 2000;39(3):393–397.

48. Petrek JA, Heelan MC. Incidence of breast carcinoma-related lymphedema. *Cancer.* 1998;83(12 Suppl American):2776–2781.

49. Fiorica JV, Roberts WS, Greenberg H, et al. Morbidity and survival patterns in patients after radical hysterectomy and postoperative adjuvant pelvic radiotherapy. *Gynecol Oncol.* 1990;36(3):343–347.

50. Werngren-Elgstrom M, Lidman D. Lymphoedema of the lower extremities after surgery and radiotherapy for cancer of the cervix. *Scand J Plast Reconstr Surg Hand Surg.* 1994;28(4):289–293.

51. Soisson AP, Soper JT, Clarke-Pearson DL, et al. Adjuvant radiotherapy following radical hysterectomy for patients with stage IB and IIA cervical cancer. *Gynecol Oncol.* 1990;37(3):390–395.

52. Lynde CW, Mitchell JC. Unusual complication of allergic contact dermatitis of the hands - recurrent lymphangitis and persistent lymphoedema. *Contact Dermatitis.* 1982;8(4):279–280.

53. Rockson SG, Rivera KK. Estimating the population burden of lymphedema. *Ann N Y Acad Sci.* 2008;1131:147–154.

54. Nagai Y, Aoyama K, Endo Y, Ishikawa O. Lymphedema of the extremities developed as the initial manifestation of rheumatoid arthritis. *Eur J Dermatol.* 2007;17(2):175–176.

55. Majeski J. Lymphedema tarda. *Cutis.* 1986;38(2):105–107.

56. Stemmer R. A clinical symptom for the early and differential diagnosis of lymphedema. *Vasa.* 1976;5(3):261–262.

57. Brorson H, Ohlin K, Olsson G, Karlsson M. Breast cancer-related chronic arm lymphedema is associated with excess adipose and muscle tissue. *Lymphat Res Biol.* 2009;7(1):3–10.

58. Rosen E. The molecular control of adipogenesis, with special reference to lymphatic pathology. *Ann N Y Acad Sci.* 2002;979:143–158.

59. Schirger A, Harrison EG, Janes JM. Idiopathic lymphedema. Review of 131 cases. *JAMA.* 1962;182:124–132.

60. Mallon E, Powell S, Mortimer P, Ryan TJ. Evidence for altered cell-mediated immunity in postmastectomy lymphoedema. *Br J Dermatol.* 1997;137(6):928–933.

61. Beilhack A, Rockson SG. Immune traffic: a functional overview. *Lymphat Res Biol.* 2003;1(3):219–234.

62. Muller R, Hajdu SI, Brennan MF. Lymphangiosarcoma associated with chronic filarial lymphedema. *Cancer.* 1987;59(1):179–183.

63. Benda JA, Aljurf AS, Benson AB. Angiosarcoma of the breast following segmental-mastectomy complicated by lymphedema. *Am J Clin Pathol.* 1987;87(5):651–655.

64. Servelle M. Surgical treatment of lymphedema: a report on 652 cases. *Surgery.* 1987;101(4):485–495.

65. Földi E, Földi M. Das lipödem. In: Földi M, Kubik S, eds. *Lehrbuch der Lymphologie.* 5th Ed. München-Jena: Gustav Fsicher; 2002:449–458.

66. Szolnoky G. Differential diagnosis: lipedema. In: Lee BB, Rockson SG, Bergan J, eds. *Lymphedema: A Concise Compendium of Theory and Practice.* 2nd ed. London: Springer; 2018:239–249.

67. Kinmonth JB, Taylor GW, Harper RK. Lymphangiography; a technique for its clinical use in the lower limb. *Br Med J.* 1955;1(4919):940–942.

68. O'Brien BM, Das SK, Franklin JD, Morrison WA. Effect of lymphangiography on lymphedema. *Plast Reconstr Surg.* 1981;68(6):922–926.

69. Itkin M. Lymphatic intervention is a new frontier of IR. *J Vasc Interv Radiol.* 2014;25(9):1404–1405.

70. Vaqueiro M, Gloviczki P, Fisher J, et al. Lymphoscintigraphy in lymphedema: an aid to microsurgery. *J Nucl Med.* 1986;27(7):1125–1130.

71. Hvidsten S, Toyserkani NM, Sorensen JA, et al. A scintigraphic method for quantitation of lymphatic function in arm lymphedema. *Lymphat Res Biol.* 2018;16(4):353–359.

72. Tartaglione G, Visconti G, Bartoletti R, et al. Stress lymphoscintigraphy for early detection and management of secondary limb lymphedema. *Clin Nucl Med.* 2018;43(3):155–161.

73. Hadjis NS, Carr DH, Banks L, Pflug JJ. The role of CT in the diagnosis of primary lymphedema of the lower limb. *AJR Am J Roentgenol.* 1985;144(2):361–364.

74. Gamba JL, Silverman PM, Ling D, et al. Primary lower extremity lymphedema: CT diagnosis. *Radiology.* 1983;149(1):218.

75. Vaughan BF. CT of swollen legs. *Clin Radiol.* 1990;41(1):24–30.

76. Liu NF, Wang CG. The role of magnetic resonance imaging in diagnosis of peripheral lymphatic disorders. *Lymphology.* 1998;31(3):119–127.

77. Matsushima S, Ichiba N, Hayashi D, Fukuda K. Nonenhanced magnetic resonance lymphoductography: visualization of lymphatic system of the trunk on 3-dimensional heavily T2-weighted image with 2-dimensional prospective acquisition and correction. *J Comput Assist Tomogr.* 2007;31(2):299–302.

78. Bae JS, Yoo RE, Choi SH, et al. Evaluation of lymphedema in upper extremities by MR lymphangiography: comparison with lymphoscintigraphy. *Magn Reson Imaging.* 2018;49:63–70.

79. Gniadecka M. Localization of dermal edema in lipodermatosclerosis, lymphedema, and cardiac insufficiency. High-frequency ultrasound examination of intradermal echogenicity. *J Am Acad Dermatol.* 1996;35(1):37–41.

80. Rockson SG, Miller LT, Senie R, et al. American Cancer Society Lymphedema Workshop. Workgroup III: diagnosis and management of lymphedema. *Cancer.* 1998;83(12 Suppl American):2882–2885.

81. Kubik S. The role of the lateral upper arm bundle and the lymphatic watersheds in the formation of collateral pathways in lymphedema. *Acta Biol Acad Sci Hung.* 1980;31(1-3):191–200.

82. Ko DS, Lerner R, Klose G, Cosimi AB. Effective treatment of lymphedema of the extremities. *Arch Surg.* 1998;133(4):452–458.

83. Szuba A, Cooke JP, Yousuf S, Rockson SG. Decongestive lymphatic therapy for patients with cancer-related or primary lymphedema. *Am J Med.* 2000;109(4):296–300.

84. Badger CM, Peacock JL, Mortimer PS. A randomized, controlled, parallel-group clinical trial comparing multilayer bandaging followed by hosiery versus hosiery alone in the treatment of patients with lymphedema of the limb. *Cancer.* 2000;88(12):2832–2837.

85. Leduc O, Leduc A, Bourgeois P, Belgrado JP. The physical treatment of upper limb edema. *Cancer.* 1998;83(12 Suppl American):2835–2839.

86. Szuba A, Achalu R, Rockson SG. Decongestive lymphatic therapy for patients with breast carcinoma-associated lymphedema. A randomized, prospective study of a role for adjunctive intermittent pneumatic compression. *Cancer.* 2002;95(11):2260–2267.

87. Mayrovitz HN. The standard of care for lymphedema: current concepts and physiological considerations. *Lymphat Res Biol.* 2009;7(2):101–108.

88. Brayton KM, Hirsch AT, O'Brien PJ, et al. Lymphedema prevalence and treatment benefits in cancer: impact of a therapeutic intervention on health outcomes and costs. *PLoS One.* 2014;9(12):e114597.

89. Karaca-Mandic P, Hirsch AT, Rockson SG, Ridner SH. The cutaneous, net clinical, and health economic benefits of advanced pneumatic compression devices in patients with lymphedema. *JAMA Dermatol.* 2015;151(11):1187–1193.

90. Karaca-Mandic P, Hirsch AT, Rockson SG, Ridner SH. A comparison of programmable and nonprogrammable compression devices for treatment of lymphoedema using an administrative health outcomes dataset. *Br J Dermatol.* 2017;177(6):1699–1707.

91. Piller NB, Thelander A. Treatment of chronic postmastectomy lymphedema with low level laser therapy: a 2.5 year follow-up. *Lymphology.* 1998;31(2):74–86.

92. Ogawa Y, Yoshizumi M, Kitagawa T, et al. Investigation of the mechanism of lymphocyte injection therapy in treatment of lymphedema with special emphasis on cell adhesion molecule (L-selectin). *Lymphology.* 1999;32(4):151–156.

93. Dalal A, Eskin-Schwartz M, Mimouni D, et al. Interventions for the prevention of recurrent erysipelas and cellulitis. *Cochrane Database Syst Rev.* 2017;(6):CD009758.

94. Bliss CM, Schroy IP. Primary intestinal lymphangiectasia. *Curr Treat Options Gastroenterol.* 2004;7(1):3–6.

95. Casley-Smith JR, Morgan RG, Piller NB. Treatment of lymphedema of the arms and legs with 5,6-benzo-[a]-pyrone. *N Engl J Med.* 1993;329(16):1158–1163.

96. Casley-Smith JR, Wang CT, Zi-hai C. Treatment of filarial lymphoedema and elephantiasis with 5,6-benzo-alpha-pyrone (coumarin). *BMJ.* 1993;307(6911):1037–1041.

97. Badger C, Preston N, Seers K, Mortimer P. Benzo-pyrones for reducing and controlling lymphoedema of the limbs. *Cochrane Database Syst Rev.* 2004;(2):CD003140.

98. Loprinzi CL, Kugler JW, Sloan JA, et al. Lack of effect of coumarin in women with lymphedema after treatment for breast cancer. *N Engl J Med.* 1999;340(5):346–350.

99. Tabibiazar R, Cheung L, Han J, et al. Inflammatory manifestations of experimental lymphatic insufficiency. *PLoS Med.* 2006;3(7):e254.

100. Avraham T, Daluvoy S, Zampell J, et al. Blockade of transforming growth factor-beta1 accelerates lymphatic regeneration during wound repair. *Am J Pathol.* 2010;177(6):3202–3214.

101. Zampell JC, Yan A, Avraham T, et al. Temporal and spatial patterns of endogenous danger signal expression after wound healing and in response to lymphedema. *Am J Physiol Cell Physiol.* 2011;300(5):C1107–C1121.

102. Gousopoulos E, Proulx ST, Bachmann SB, et al. Regulatory T cell transfer ameliorates lymphedema and promotes lymphatic vessel function. *JCI Insight.* 2016;1(16):e89081.

103. Nakamura K, Radhakrishnan K, Wong YM, Rockson SG. Anti-inflammatory pharmacotherapy with ketoprofen ameliorates experimental lymphatic vascular insufficiency in mice. *PLoS One.* 2009;4(12):e8380.

104. Jiang X, Nicolls MR, Tian W, Rockson SG. Lymphatic dysfunction, leukotrienes, and lymphedema. *Annu Rev Physiol.* 2018;80:49–70.

105. Tian W, Rockson S, Jiang X, et al. Leukotriene B4 antagonism ameliorates experimental lymphedema. *Sci Transl Med.* 2017;9(389):eaal3920.

106. Damstra RJ, Voesten HG, van Schelven WD, van der Lei B. Lymphatic venous anastomosis (LVA) for treatment of secondary arm lymphedema. A prospective study of 11 LVA procedures in 10 patients with breast cancer related lymphedema and a critical review of the literature. *Breast Cancer Res Treat.* 2009;113(2):199–206.

107. Campisi C, Boccardo F. Microsurgical techniques for lymphedema treatment: derivative lymphatic-venous microsurgery. *World J Surg.* 2004;28(6):609–613.

108. Cornelissen AJM, Beugels J, Ewalds L, et al. The effect of lymphaticovenous anastomosis in breast cancer-related lymphedema: a review of the literature. *Lymphat Res Biol.* 2018;16(5):426–434.

109. Lee JH, Chang DW. Surgical treatment of primary lymphedema. *Lymphat Res Biol.* 2017;15(3):220–226.

110. Paek LS, Baylan JM, Becker C, Nguyen DH. Vascularized lymph node transfer for the treatment of lymphedema. In: Lee BB, Rockson SG, Bergan J, eds. *Lymphedema: A Concise Compendium of Theory and Practice.* 2nd ed. London: Springer, pp 638-652.

111. Hadamitzky C, Zaitseva TS, Bazalova-Carter M, et al. Aligned nanofibrillar collagen scaffolds - guiding lymphangiogenesis for treatment of acquired lymphedema. *Biomaterials.* 2016;102:259–267.

112. Olofsson B, Jeltsch M, Eriksson U, Alitalo K. Current biology of VEGF-B and VEGF-C. *Curr Opin Biotechnol.* 1999;10(6):528–535.

113. Veikkola T, Karkkainen M, Claesson-Welsh L, Alitalo K. Regulation of angiogenesis via vascular endothelial growth factor receptors. *Cancer Res.* 2000;60(2):203–212.

114. Kaipainen A, Korhonen J, Mustonen T, et al. Expression of the fms-like tyrosine kinase 4 gene becomes restricted to lymphatic endothelium during development. *Proc Natl Acad Sci U S A.* 1995;92(8):3566–3570.

115. Jeltsch M, Kaipainen A, Joukov V, et al. Hyperplasia of lymphatic vessels in VEGF-C transgenic mice. *Science.* 1997;276(5317):1423–1425.

116. Enholm B, Karpanen T, Jeltsch M, et al. Adenoviral expression of vascular endothelial growth factor-C induces lymphangiogenesis in the skin. *Circ Res.* 2001;88(6):623–629.

117. Karkkainen MJ, Petrova TV. Vascular endothelial growth factor receptors in the regulation of angiogenesis and lymphangiogenesis. *Oncogene.* 2000;19(49):5598–5605.

118. Oh SJ, Jeltsch MM, Birkenhager R, et al. VEGF and VEGF-C: specific induction of angiogenesis and lymphangiogenesis in the differentiated avian chorioallantoic membrane. *Dev Biol.* 1997;188(1):96–109.

119. Szuba A, Skobe M, Karkkainen M, et al. Therapeutic lymphangiogenesis with human recombinant VEGF-C. *FASEB J.* 2002;16:U114–U130.

120. Jin DP, An A, Liu J, et al. Therapeutic responses to exogenous VEGF-C administration in experimental lymphedema: immunohistochemical and molecular characterization. *Lymphat Res Biol.* 2009;7(1):47–57.

121. Guc E, Briquez PS, Foretay D, et al. Local induction of lymphangiogenesis with engineered fibrin-binding VEGF-C promotes wound healing by increasing immune cell trafficking and matrix remodeling. *Biomaterials.* 2017;131:160–175.

122. Luks VL, Kamitaki N, Vivero MP, et al. Lymphatic and other vascular malformative/overgrowth disorders are caused by somatic mutations in PIK3CA. *J Pediatr.* 2015;166(4):1048–1054. e1041-1045.

123. di Blasio L, Puliafito A, Gagliardi PA, et al. PI3K/mTOR inhibition promotes the regression of experimental vascular malformations driven by PIK3CA-activating mutations. *Cell Death Dis.* 2018;9(2):45.

124. Revencu N, Boon LM, Mendola A, et al. RASA1 mutations and associated phenotypes in 68 families with capillary malformation-arteriovenous malformation. *Hum Mutat.* 2013;34(12):1632–1641.

125. Ramani P, Shah A. Lymphangiomatosis. Histologic and immunohistochemical analysis of four cases. *Am J Surg Pathol.* 1993;17(4):329–335.

126. Adams DM, Trenor 3rd CC, Hammill AM, et al. Efficacy and safety of sirolimus in the treatment of complicated vascular anomalies. *Pediatrics.* 2016;137(2):e20153257.

127. Tibballs J, Soto R, Bharucha T. Management of newborn lymphangiectasia and chylothorax after cardiac surgery with octreotide infusion. *Ann Thorac Surg.* 2004;77(6):2213–2215.

128. Makhija S, von der Weid PY, Meddings J, et al. Octreotide in intestinal lymphangiectasia: lack of a clinical response and failure to alter lymphatic function in a guinea pig model. *Can J Gastroenterol.* 2004;18(11):681–685.

129. Lee HL, Han DS, Kim JB, et al. Successful treatment of protein-losing enteropathy induced by intestinal lymphangiectasia in a liver cirrhosis patient with octreotide: a case report. *J Korean Med Sci.* 2004;19(3):466–469.

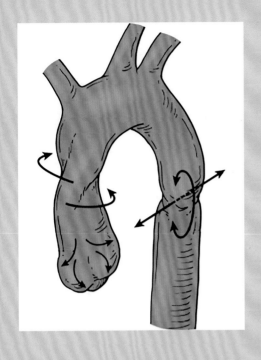

PART XVIII

第十八部分

Miscellaneous

其他杂类血管疾病

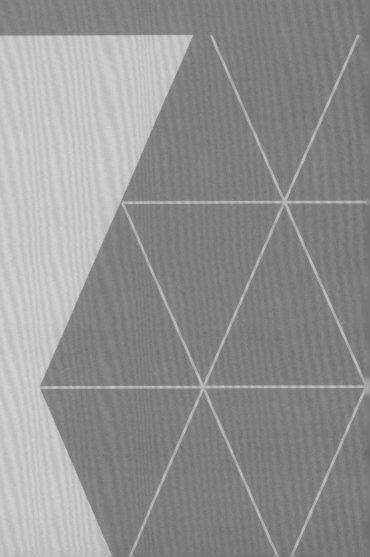

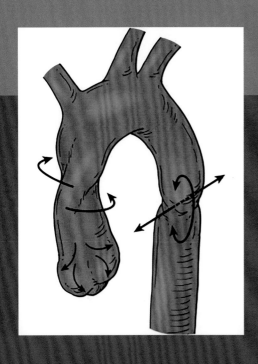

第58章
纤维肌发育不良

　　纤维肌发育不良是一种非动脉粥样硬化性血管疾病，主要累及中等大小动脉，可见于全身各处动脉，尚未见于静脉系统。一般人群患病率尚不清楚，最常见于中年女性，也可见于男性、儿童和老年人。有限的研究提示其有潜在遗传性，吸烟、性激素等可能与之相关，机械力被认为是病因。该疾病的分类最初由Harrison/McCormack基于受累动脉的组织病理学提出，现常采用基于有创或无创影像学的二分类系统（局灶性和多灶性）。纤维肌发育不良的临床表现多样（表58.1），与受累血管、病变类型和严重程度相关，它可导致血管狭窄、闭塞、动脉瘤、夹层、血栓形成或这些症状的结合。多数患者表现出至少一种临床症状/体征，但越来越多无症状患者通过偶然的影像学检查而确诊。经导管血管造影是纤维肌发育不良影像检查的金标准，可见具有特异性的"串珠征"典型征象。该疾病的治疗目标是控制症状、控制血压和预防血管并发症。对于该疾病的认识主要来源于近10年国际注册的临床研究，本章将综合已有文献对纤维肌发育不良的分类、流行病学、遗传学和病因、临床表现、诊断评估及治疗管理进行叙述。

李毅清

Fibromuscular Dysplasia

Khendi T. White Solaru and Heather L. Gornik

Fibromuscular dysplasia (FMD) is a nonatherosclerotic vascular disease that primarily affects medium-sized arteries but can be observed in nearly every artery of the body. It is not known to involve the venous system. Although FMD most commonly presents in middle-aged women, it can affect both sexes, as well as children and the elderly. The clinical manifestations of FMD are variable based upon the type and severity of lesions, as well as the vessels involved. Arterial stenosis, occlusion, aneurysm, and dissection are the mechanisms by which symptoms and vascular complications develop. However, a growing number of asymptomatic patients are diagnosed with FMD incidentally when imaging is performed for another indication. Much knowledge about this poorly understood vascular disease has been learned from clinical studies, especially international registries, performed in the past decade. Specifically, the ongoing United States Registry for FMD, as well as French/Belgian Assessment of Renal and Cervical Artery Dysplasia (ARCADIA) and broader European registries, have improved our understanding of the clinical presentation, diagnostic evaluation, natural history, and therapeutic management of this disease.[1–7]

HISTORICAL PERSPECTIVE

The first description of FMD was by Leadbetter and Burkland of Johns Hopkins Hospital.[8] In their description published in 1938, they reported a case of a 5-year-old African-American boy who underwent nephrectomy for uncontrolled hypertension. Pathology of the right renal artery revealed partial occlusion of the lumen due to a focal thickening of smooth muscle with no evidence of aneurysmal dilation. In 1958, McCormack and colleagues at the Cleveland Clinic introduced the term *fibromuscular dysplasia* and ultimately provided the first pathologic description of the disease.[9,10] In 1964, Palubinskas and Ripley described extrarenal FMD of the iliac, visceral, and internal carotid arteries in a series of nine patients, providing the first suggestion of FMD as a systemic arterial disease rather than a process limited to the renal arteries.[11] Harrison and colleagues at Mayo Clinic and McCormack and colleagues at Cleveland Clinic further developed a classification that correlated histopathology from surgical specimens with renal angiography.[12,13] Angiographically, the stenotic lesions were represented as focal, multifocal, or tubular, and this classification remains similar to the modified classification system currently used.

CLASSIFICATION

The original Harrison/McCormack classification is based on the histopathology of the affected arteries, and an updated version of this system is shown in Table 58.1. FMD was historically classified according to the layer of the arterial wall affected (intima, media, or adventitia) and the composition of the arterial lesions (fibrosis/fibroplasia or hyperplasia). Medial fibroplasia is the most common type of FMD, accounting for 60% to 70% of all cases.[2,5] Intimal fibroplasia accounts for approximately 2% of adult cases of FMD in the US Registry but is more common in European series, where it accounted for 8% of all adult cases.[2,5] Intimal fibroplasia is much more common in the pediatric population, where it is the predominant type of FMD.[14] Perimedial fibroplasia is a rare type of FMD and usually presents in young girls.[15] Both medial hyperplasia and adventitial fibroplasia are believed to be rare and require a histopathological specimen for diagnosis. The term *fibroplasia* refers to a disarray of collagen-thickened areas and thinned media. The most common presentation of medial fibroplasia is narrowing with poststenotic dilation on angiography.[16] Intimal and adventitial fibroplasia may present as tubular or focal lesions. The rare presentation of medial hyperplasia is due primarily to proliferation of smooth muscle cells rather than collagen deposits.[16]

The histopathologic classification of FMD is currently much less relevant because most diagnoses of FMD are made based upon angiography or noninvasive imaging studies. Biopsy is rarely if ever obtained, and surgical pathology is relatively uncommon. A binary classification of FMD was first proposed by Savard and colleagues as representing two distinct clinical phenotypes.[17] Multifocal FMD represents the classical "string of beads" appearance of lesions on angiographic imaging, whereas (uni)focal FMD refers to a focal, smooth stenosis regardless of length. It is possible to have more than one type of FMD in the same patient. A European consensus proposed a classification using multifocal, tubular, and unifocal categories of FMD.[6,7] Similar to this system and that of Savard and colleagues, the current American Heart Association classification uses a binary system which categorizes lesions as multifocal or focal.[2] Angiographic examples of multifocal and focal FMD lesions are shown in Fig. 58.1.

An advantage of the binary angiographic classification system for FMD is that it simplifies efforts to study clinical outcomes according to disease category. In this context, it is important to appreciate that multifocal and focal FMD may actually represent two different vascular disease processes.[18,19] In one study of patients

TABLE 58.1   Classification of Fibromuscular Dysplasia

Histological	Angiographic	
Harrison and McCormack (1971)	European Consensus (2012)	American Heart Association (2014)
Medial	Multifocal	Multifocal
Medial fibroplasia (60%–70%)		
Perimedial fibroplasia (15%–25%)		
Medial hyperplasia (5%–10%)		
Intimal fibroplasia (1%–2%)	Unifocal (<1 cm) Tubular (≥1 cm)	Focal
Adventitial (<1%)		

Modified from Olin JW, Gornik HL, Bacharach JM, et al. Fibromuscular dysplasia: state of the science and critical unanswered questions: a scientific statement from the American Heart Association. *Circulation*. 2014;129:1048–1078. Copyright 2014, American Heart Association, Inc.

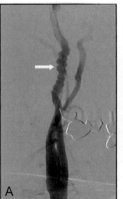
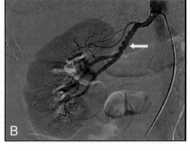
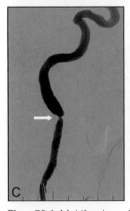
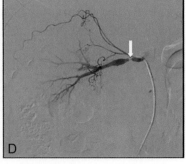

Fig. 58.1 Multifocal and Focal Fibromuscular Dysplasia (FMD). Angiographic presentations of multifocal (A and B) and focal FMD (C and D) in the internal carotid arteries (A and C) and renal arteries (B and D). The multifocal FMD demonstrates the classic string of beads appearance (*arrows* in A and B), whereas the focal FMD has a single, bandlike narrowing in the vessel (*arrows* in C and D). (From Poloskey SL, Olin JW, Mace P, Gornik HL. Fibromuscular dysplasia. *Circulation*. 2012;125:e636–e639. Copyright 2012, American Heart Association, Inc.)

with renal artery FMD, 31% of patients with focal lesions were male compared with 17% male patients among those with multifocal lesions.[17] However, this pattern of sex differences among patients with focal versus multifocal FMD was not reported in the US FMD Registry and may represent a difference in age distribution between the cohorts.[1,14] Pediatric FMD occurs with a more balanced male and female distribution compared with adult FMD. Forty-two percent of patients younger than 18 years were male in the US Registry versus only 6% of those older than 18 years.[14] FMD lesions in children and young adults are more commonly of the focal rather than multifocal type.[14]

EPIDEMIOLOGY

Prevalence of Fibromuscular Dysplasia

The prevalence of FMD in the general population is unknown, though studies of specific populations have been informative. Although FMD has historically been considered a rare disease and is recognized as such by the National Organization for Rare Diseases (as defined by an estimated prevalence of <200,000 US residents), it is likely that FMD is more common than previously thought. Insight into the prevalence of FMD has emerged from studies of living renal transplant donors.[20] In the first reports spanning the 1960s–1980s, there was a 3% to 4% prevalence of FMD among potential kidney donors diagnosed by catheter angiography.[21–23] The most contemporary cohort of healthy renal donor candidates undergoing catheter-based angiography included 716 patients from 1988 to 1998.[24] They found that 47 patients (6.6% of the cohort) had renal FMD, which is the highest rate reported in the donor literature. More recent living donor studies have used noninvasive computed tomographic angiography (CTA) or catheter-based angiography and found similar FMD prevalence rates of 3% to 4%.[25–28] Of note, the presence of FMD is not an absolute contraindication to kidney donation for transplantation, but surgical planning must be modified accordingly. Although providing some data as to the prevalence of renal FMD, potential donor studies may not accurately reflect the general population because they represent a self-selected healthy population that is less likely to have hypertension or chronic kidney disease than the general population. Alternatively, they may possibly enrich for familial FMD given that most potential kidney donors have a family member with severe chronic kidney disease.[29,30] The recent Cardiovascular Outcomes in Renal Atherosclerotic Lesions (CORAL) trial examined the prevalence of FMD in an older population with hypertension and atherosclerosis.[30] They found that the prevalence of FMD in the trial population was 5.8%.[30] This is likely an overestimate of the true frequency given the high prevalence of drug-resistant hypertension in that population, although notable because a known diagnosis of FMD was an exclusion criterion for initial enrollment in CORAL.[30]

Historically, studies have focused primarily on renal artery FMD, although the US Registry has recently shown that cerebrovascular involvement (primarily of the extracranial internal carotid and/or vertebral arteries) occurs nearly as frequently as renal artery FMD.[1] Autopsy and cerebral angiography series provide some data regarding the prevalence of cerebrovascular FMD in select populations. One large retrospective study reviewed 4000 cerebral angiograms performed from 1970 to 1978 and identified 37 patients (0.9%) with cerebrovascular FMD.[31] Another meta-analysis of smaller studies showed that the prevalence of cerebrovascular FMD among patients undergoing cerebral angiography ranges from 0.3% to 3.2%.[32]

The prevalence of FMD on cerebral angiograms is dependent on the characteristics of the patients reported. The largest autopsy series published by the Mayo Clinic reviewed 20,244 consecutive autopsies and found histopathologic internal carotid artery FMD in only four patients (0.02% of the study population).[33]

Demographics of Fibromuscular Dysplasia

Recently, much has been learned about the demographics of FMD from international registries. The US Registry for FMD initially reported on 447 patients at nine tertiary referral centers.[1] The mean patient age was 56 years, and women accounted for 91% of the cohort. Although FMD primarily affects middle-aged women, it has been observed in both sexes and in every age group. The ethnic makeup of the US Registry consisted of 95% Caucasians, 2% Blacks, 2% Hispanics, and 0.5% Asians, and 0.5% self-identified as other.[1] It is unknown if this accurately reflects the racial makeup of the FMD population, because minorities have historically been underrepresented in clinical trials and may not be adequately represented at tertiary referral centers for FMD.[34] The French/Belgian ARCADIA cohort consisted of 84% women and 89% Caucasians, with the remainder ethnic groups not specifically identified.[5] The mean age of diagnosis was 51 years of age for patients with single-site disease and 56 years of age for multisite disease.[5]

GENETICS AND ETIOLOGY

Genetics

The genetics of FMD remains poorly understood. However, family studies and published case reports in twins suggest there is underlying heritability.[35] A pedigree analysis of 20 families with FMD suggested autosomal dominant inheritance with incomplete penetrance; however, the diagnosis of family members was flawed because it was based on nonspecific clinical features (history of hypertension, stroke, etc.) rather than imaging confirmation of a diagnosis of FMD.[36] A study of 104 subjects with angiographically confirmed FMD found that 10.5% had at least one sibling with documented FMD.[37] All familial cases occurred in women, and there were no cases of vertical transmission from mother to child. However, in the US Registry, only 7.3% of FMD patients reported a first- or second-degree relative with a diagnosis of FMD.[1] In contrast, 23.5% of registrants reported a first- or second-degree relative with an aortic or arterial aneurysm. Given overlapping features of FMD with well-characterized vascular connective tissue disorders such as Loeys-Dietz and vascular Ehlers-Danlos syndromes, there has been interest in pursuing genetic testing for known arteriopathies among patients with FMD. In these studies, the yield of currently available genetic testing for connective tissue disorders was low among populations of FMD patients (e.g., Col3A1, TGFβR1/2, fibrillin-1, smooth muscle α-actin 2, SMAD3).[38,39] One study reported increased levels of circulating and fibroblast-secreted levels of TGFβ1/2 among a cohort of 47 patients with multifocal FMD compared with matched controls.[39] The significance of this finding remains unclear and has yet to be replicated in larger series. Another study found an association between the HLA-DRw6 antigen, a class II major histocompatibility complex allele, and an increased risk of developing FMD.[40]

A recent multistage genetic association study found that of approximately 26,000 common variants analyzed in 249 patients with FMD and 689 controls the strongest association for FMD occurred in the rs9349379 variant of the phosphatase and actin regulator 1 (PHACTR1) gene.[41] The presence of the rs9349379 variant of PHACTR1 increased the risk of FMD by 40% compared with controls in a meta-analysis of five patient cohorts. This PHACTR1 A allele has also been previously associated with migraine headache and cervical artery dissection, whereas it may be protective from risk of atherosclerotic coronary artery disease.[41] The PHACTR1 locus (6p24) has been recognized as a noncoding variant involved in the regulation of the expression of endothelin-1, a peptide known to cause vasoconstriction.[42] Further studies must be done to clarify the role of PHACTR1 and to identify other specific genetic mechanisms of FMD.

Other Mechanistic Factors: Tobacco and Sex Hormones

In addition to genetic factors, it is likely that environmental interactions play a role in the development of FMD. Cigarette smoke and estrogen exposure have been associated with FMD anecdotally and in epidemiological studies. Savard and colleagues reported that, in 337 FMD patients matched to controls, there was a significantly higher proportion of current smokers in the FMD group.[43] Smaller studies with angiographically confirmed FMD have shown that nearly 50% of FMD patients were current smokers.[40,44] Smoking has also been associated with earlier disease onset and increased severity of FMD.[44-46]

It is likely that sex hormones play a role in the development of FMD given the heavy female predominance among patients with this disease. In the US Registry, 91% of patients enrolled were women, though men seem to have a more severe phenotype.[46] Although 65% of the women in the US Registry were postmenopausal, there was exposure to either oral contraceptives or hormone replacement therapy in 70% of the women, and 14% of women had received systemic hormone replacement therapy at the time of enrollment in the US Registry.[1] In a case-control study by Sang and colleagues, there was no significant difference in oral contraceptive use, age of menarche, number of pregnancies, spontaneous abortions, gynecological disorders, or hysterectomy between female patients with FMD and unmatched non-FMD controls.[40] Given these data, it is clear that there is much work to be done to determine the role of sex hormones in the development of FMD.

Mechanical Forces

Mechanical force as a consequence of traction, gravity, or trauma have been postulated as an etiology for the development of FMD in susceptible vascular territories. Kaufman and colleagues were the first to show that abnormal kidney hypermobility (renal ptosis) was associated with renal artery FMD in a small cohort of patients.[47] Of the 17 patients with FMD in this cohort, 12 were found to have renal ptosis as a result of hypermobility of the kidney in the retroperitoneal space. Renal ptosis occurs more commonly in women and affects the right kidney more often than the left, as does FMD.[48] It has been hypothesized that the accordion-like action on the renal artery created by repeat ascent and descent of the hypermobile kidney may predispose the renal artery to the formation of multifocal areas of stenosis and dilation, classically seen with FMD.[48]

The carotid and vertebral arteries are presumably not subject to the same forces of traction, but recurrent mechanical trauma could play a role in the vascular changes taking place in the cervical vasculature. Miller and colleagues proposed that once a vessel's integrity has been compromised, as is the case with elongated or tortuous vessels, it is vulnerable to pulsation-induced "kinking."[49] In their small cohort of 14 patients with 24 affected carotid arteries, they found that 96% of vessels demonstrated at least some degree of excessive movement with 100% of movement focally associated with the FMD "beaded" site.[49]

CLINICAL PRESENTATION AND VASCULAR MANIFESTATIONS

The clinical manifestations of FMD are varied and related to the vascular bed(s) affected, nature of the arterial lesions, and the severity of disease. FMD can lead to the development of stenosis, aneurysm, dissection, thrombosis, or a combination of these. In the US Registry, most patients presented with at least one clinical sign or symptom, and only 6% of patients were truly asymptomatic at the time of diagnosis, likely identified on the basis of incidental findings on imaging studies.[1] Typical presenting symptoms of FMD classified by the vasculature affected are shown in Box 58.1. According to data from the US Registry, patients with FMD have involvement of the renal arteries approximately 80% of the time and involvement of the extracranial, cerebrovascular arteries approximately 75% of the time.[1] Multifocal renal artery FMD commonly affects the mid and distal portions of the artery, as opposed to atherosclerotic disease which tends to affect branching points

BOX 58.1 Clinical Manifestations of Fibromuscular Dysplasia (FMD)

Renal Artery FMD
- Hypertension
- Abdominal or flank bruit
- Flank pain
- Renal artery dissection
- Renal artery infection (due to dissection or embolic event)
- Renal artery aneurysm
- Acute or chronic renal insufficiency (uncommon)

Carotid and Vertebral Artery FMD
- Headaches, especially migraine type
- Pulsatile tinnitus or "swooshing" in ears
- Dizziness
- Cervical bruit
- Transient ischemic attack or stroke (due to dissection or embolic event)
- Cervical artery dissection
- Extra- or intracranial aneurysm
- Subarachnoid hemorrhage
- Partial Horner syndrome (usually in association with cervical artery dissection)

Mesenteric Artery FMD
- Abdominal bruit
- Mesenteric angina with anorexia and weight loss
- Mesenteric artery dissection
- Mesenteric artery aneurysm

FMD of the Extremities
- Vascular bruits over the antecubital fossa, femoral arteries, or lower abdomen
- Arm or leg claudication
- Limb or digital ischemia (due to dissection or embolic event)
- Discrepant blood pressures in the arms

Coronary Artery FMD
- Acute coronary syndrome due to spontaneous coronary artery dissection (SCAD)

Aortic FMD
- Middle aortic syndrome (focal FMD)
- Aortic aneurysm

and the ostial and proximal vessel.[50,51] FMD can occur unilaterally or bilaterally within a vascular bed and is often found in multiple vascular beds (multivessel FMD). Multivessel FMD is more common in older patients and patients with multifocal rather than focal disease.[5,13] In the ARCADIA study, systematic angiographic imaging of intraabdominal and cervical/intracranial arteries identified multivessel FMD lesions in 48% of patients.[5] It is important to recognize that the phenotypic presentation of FMD is not just limited to focal and multifocal stenoses.[52] There is a strong association between presence of aneurysms, dissections, and tortuosity in one vascular bed with stenotic FMD lesions in other vascular beds. This occurred in approximately 66.1% of patients in the ARCADIA trial. Arterial tortuosity and redundancy have been recognized as a manifestation of FMD. In the internal carotid artery, such tortuosity often leads to an "S-curve" appearance (Fig. 58.2). In one vascular lab-based series, this feature was present in one-third of all patents with carotid FMD.[53]

Renal Artery Fibromuscular Dysplasia

In the US and ARCADIA Registries, the renal arteries are the most common site of FMD involvement (Fig. 58.3).[1,5] The typical manifestation of renal artery FMD is hypertension, although the severity and age of onset are highly variable.[2] In children and adolescents, FMD of the renal arteries is the most common cause of hypertension, although this may change as childhood obesity becomes more prevalent.[54–55] Among patients enrolled in the US Registry, 79.7% had renal artery involvement and 63.8% initially presented with hypertension.[1] However, the average age of onset of hypertension was 43 years of age, which represents significant overlap with the age of onset of essential hypertension in the general population. In the ARCADIA study, 64.8% patients had renal artery involvement and average age at time of diagnosis of FMD was 53 years.[5] Nevertheless, FMD should be suspected as a potential diagnosis in a woman with early-onset hypertension (i.e., before age 50) or drug-resistant hypertension (i.e., requiring three or more antihypertensive medications including a diuretic). In addition to hypertension being the most common manifestation of FMD, renal artery angioplasty for hypertension is also the most common vascular procedure among patients with FMD (see Chapter 24).[56]

Epigastric and/or flank bruits may be present on physical examination among patients with renal (or mesenteric) artery FMD.[1] According to the US Registry, the sensitivity of an epigastric or flank bruit for identifying renal or mesenteric FMD is 24% with a specificity of 93%.[1] Given the low sensitivity of abdominal bruits for detection

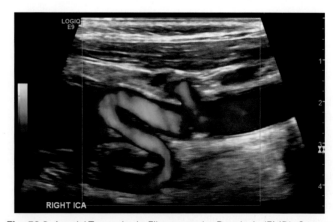

Fig. 58.2 Arterial Tortuosity in Fibromuscular Dysplasia (FMD). S-curve of the right internal carotid artery as demonstrated by color power angiography in a 55-year-old woman with multifocal FMD. The S-curve is due to elongation, redundancy, and tortuosity of the vessels.[53] She also had mild atherosclerotic plaque. This patient also had multifocal FMD of the left renal artery.

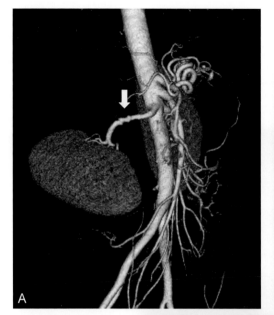
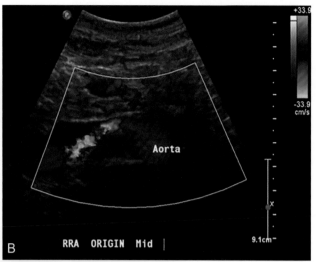
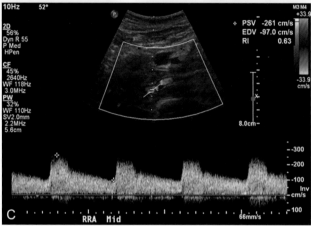

Fig. 58.3 Multifocal Renal Fibromuscular Dysplasia (FMD). Reconstructed three-dimensional computed tomography angiography of the abdomen demonstrates beading *(arrow)* of multifocal FMD in the mid right renal artery of a 45-year-old woman with hypertension (A). Renal duplex ultrasound in the same patient exhibits turbulence on color Doppler (B) and elevated velocities (peak-systolic velocity 261 cm/s) and turbulent flow within the spectral waveform (C).

of FMD, physical examination alone is inadequate, and patients with suspected FMD should undergo an appropriate imaging study.

Flank pain is a less common manifestation of renal artery FMD but can be the sole presenting symptom in some patients and may be related to renal dissection with renal infarction. In one case report the presentation of acute flank pain and microscopic hematuria in a patient without hypertension led to a misdiagnosis of ureteral colic prior to the angiographic discovery of multifocal FMD with acute renal infarction.[57] Flank pain may also be reported among patients with renal FMD even in the absence of dissection or infarct. Renal insufficiency is less common with FMD than with atherosclerotic renal artery stenosis.[58] Although renal insufficiency is very uncommon (1% of patients in the US Registry), renal artery dissection and infarction can rarely lead to chronic kidney disease.[1,59] Progression of FMD to end-stage renal disease is exceedingly rare.

Interestingly, headaches are common among patients with isolated renal artery (without cerebrovascular) FMD.[2] Mechanisms of headache among patients with renal artery FMD have yet to be elucidated but have been hypothesized to be related to increased sympathetic stimulation and hyperactivity of circulating vasoconstrictor agents released by the kidneys as a compensatory response to decreased renal blood flow (e.g., stenosis, dissection, or aneurysm) with subsequent alterations of cerebral blood flow.[60,61] Uncontrolled hypertension among patients with renal FMD can also contribute to the development of headaches.

Cerebrovascular Fibromuscular Dysplasia (Carotid and Vertebral Arteries)

It is currently recognized that cerebrovascular FMD is likely as common as renal artery involvement. Extracranial internal carotid and/or vertebral artery involvement was found in 74.3% of patients in the US Registry.[1] An example of internal carotid artery FMD is shown in Fig. 58.4. The hallmark symptom of cerebrovascular FMD is headache, which is often, but not always, of the migraine type. In the US Registry, 64.1% of patients with FMD experienced significant headaches with approximately one-half of those being of migraine type.[62] A total of 12.5% of FMD patients with headaches reported daily recurrence and 12.5% required suppressive medication(s).[1,62] Those with headaches were diagnosed with FMD at a younger age (49 vs. 57 years), more likely to have tinnitus (either pulsatile or non-pulsatile), and more

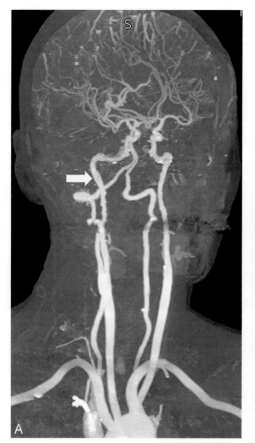
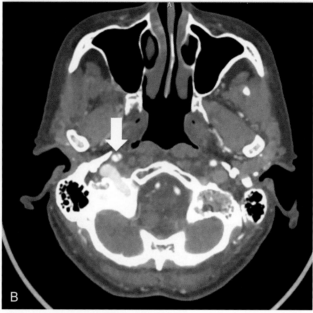

Fig. 58.4 Multifocal Carotid Fibromuscular Dysplasia (FMD). Reconstructed computed tomography angiography of the head and neck of a 66-year-old woman with multifocal FMD of bilateral internal carotid arteries (A). There is a focal dissection of the distal right internal carotid artery *(arrows)* (A and B).

likely to have had a transient ischemic attack (TIA), stroke, cervical dissection, or cerebrovascular aneurysm.[62]

As mentioned earlier, migraine is the most common type of headache among patients with FMD and has been found to be associated with both cervical artery dissection and stroke, although the mechanisms of this association are unknown.[63–65] The etiology of migraine among patients with FMD is not well understood but is likely multifactorial. Proposed mechanisms include turbulence of flow within the cerebrovasculature related to arterial beading, increased dural pain sensitivity, endothelial dysfunction, and vascular reactivity.[65–67] Among patients with FMD, headaches may also be the initial presenting symptoms of a neurologic complication such as a subarachnoid hemorrhage (SAH), large intracranial aneurysm, or cervical artery dissection.[1]

Other signs and symptoms of cerebrovascular FMD include presence of a cervical bruit, neck pain, pulsatile tinnitus, (partial) Horner syndrome, and dizziness.[67,68] An isolated cervical bruit may be the sole manifestation of carotid or vertebral artery involvement. It is the most common bruit among patients with FMD and was present at the time of diagnosis in 22.2% of patients in the US Registry.[1] On physical examination, cervical bruits due to FMD are generally higher in the neck (near the mandible) than those due to atherosclerotic carotid artery stenosis (at the carotid bifurcation). Pulsatile tinnitus is a repetitive sound, often described as a "swooshing" or "whooshing" noise, that coincides with the patient's heartbeat.[69] The prevalence of pulsatile tinnitus is high among patients with FMD, occurring in up to one-third of patients.[1,31,70] As expected, extracranial carotid and or vertebral artery involvement is more common among patients with pulsatile tinnitus as opposed to isolated renal or mesenteric involvement, and

patients with pulsatile tinnitus are also more likely to have multivessel FMD.[70] Nonspecific symptoms of neck pain, nonpulsatile tinnitus, and dizziness are fairly common symptoms of extracranial cerebrovascular FMD. The dizziness is often reported as a lightheadedness and is not a true vertigo.

Stroke and TIA are serious and dreaded complications of cerebrovascular FMD. In the initial report of the US Registry, 13.4% of patients suffered a hemispheric TIA, 9.8% suffered an ischemic stroke, and 5.2% experienced amaurosis fugax (presumed retinal ischemia).[1] Among patients with FMD, an ischemic event may develop due to multiple possible mechanisms, although cervical artery dissection seems to be most common, as this was an initial manifestation of FMD in 12.1% of patients in the US Registry.[1] In addition to TIA or stroke, cervical artery dissection may present with severe and persistent headaches and (partial) Horner syndrome due to the disruption of the neurons in the oculosympathetic pathway.[2] Dissection of the internal carotid artery results in compression of the postganglionic nerves within the carotid sheath resulting in the loss of oculosympathetic tone and the findings of unilateral ptosis and miosis, generally without anhidrosis.[68]

Rupture of a cerebral aneurysm is another dreaded complication of FMD, and its prevention supports the rationale for screening with intracranial imaging. Among patients in the US Registry who underwent imaging of the head, cerebral aneurysm was identified in 12.9% of patients, 42.0% of which were either 5 mm or larger in size or had required repair.[71] Despite this, cerebral aneurysm rupture and SAH are uncommon occurrences among patients with FMD, with the latter reported in only 1.1% of patients enrolled in the US Registry.[1] Optimal surveillance and treatment protocols for cerebral aneurysm among patients with FMD have not yet been defined and currently these aneurysms are managed the same as those among patients without FMD.[72]

Carotid Bulb Diaphragm

Carotid bulb diaphragm (CBD) has been suggested as a possible clinical variant of cerebrovascular FMD. The term corresponds to an isolated, focal linear filling defect usually located on the posterolateral aspect of the carotid bulb that has been found to be associated with embolic stroke.[73,74] It is likely that CBD represents a different disease process altogether because it has primarily been reported in patients of African descent, in contrast to multifocal FMD which seems to have a Caucasian predominance.[74] Further investigation of this entity is needed to determine if and how it is related to FMD.

Mesenteric Artery Fibromuscular Dysplasia

FMD involving the celiac (and its hepatic/splenic branches) and mesenteric arteries has been reported and may present as an incidental finding on an imaging study, or as a visceral artery aneurysm, and/or dissection.[2] Among patients who underwent celiac/mesenteric imaging in the US Registry, 26.3% had evidence of FMD.[1] Involvement of the mesenteric arteries occurs more commonly in children with FMD as opposed to their adult counterparts (38.9% vs. 16.2%) and is generally of the focal type in the pediatric population.[14] Among patients in the US Registry, the celiac and mesenteric arteries accounted for 5.9% of all arterial dissections and 13.0% of all arterial aneurysms.[4] The most common location of visceral artery aneurysms among patients with FMD is the splenic artery.[1] Hepatic artery involvement with FMD is quite rare and may initially present with life threatening intraabdominal bleeding due to aneurysm rupture.[75] Dissection of the celiac and/or mesenteric arteries may be the initial manifestation of FMD and may present with acute abdominal pain without or with bloody diarrhea related to mesenteric ischemia. Mesenteric ischemia in the absence of dissection is uncommon but could occur either due to a thromboembolic event or severe stenosis with a low-flow state. Mesenteric artery FMD may also cause a chronic postprandial abdominal pain syndrome with associated weight loss, although this is uncommon.[2] Mesenteric artery FMD is often misdiagnosed because its presentation can be nearly indistinguishable from other diseases causing stenosis, aneurysm, or dissection of the visceral arteries such as atherosclerotic disease, vasculitis, and segmental arterial mediolysis (SAM) (see Chapter 25).[76–78]

Fibromuscular Dysplasia of the Extremity Arteries

Involvement of the extremity arteries is less common than the renal or cerebrovascular arteries. When present, FMD of the extremities most commonly affects the external iliac arteries of the legs or the brachial arteries of the arm but can also affect the common and internal iliac and common femoral arteries, as well as the subclavian arteries (Figs. 58.5 and 58.6).[79–82] The most common manifestation of external iliac artery involvement is an asymptomatic femoral bruit. When symptomatic, external iliac artery involvement may manifest as lower extremity claudication, arterial dissection, or rarely acute limb ischemia.[80–82] The most common presentation of brachial artery FMD is as an asymptomatic imaging finding, including on arteriography when arterial access is obtained through the upper extremity for a coronary or vascular procedure.[2] There are case reports of hand and digital ischemia due to microembolization from brachial artery FMD.[83–86] Cyanosis or gangrenous digits, hand or finger paresthesias, upper extremity weakness, or a pulsating mass in the arm are rare presenting signs.[87–92] Discrepant blood pressures in the arms or a bruit over the antecubital fossa may be appreciated on physical examination. Subclavian involvement is typically related to focal FMD and may present as subclavian steal syndrome or arm claudication.[93–95] Both lower and upper extremity involvement

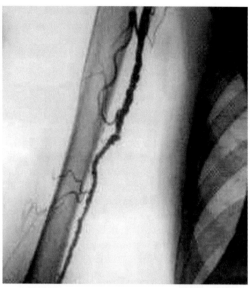

Fig. 58.5 Upper Extremity Fibromuscular Dysplasia (FMD). Catheter angiogram showing multifocal FMD of the right brachial artery. This is the most common location for upper extremity involvement. (Image courtesy John R. Bartholomew, MD, Cleveland Clinic.)

with FMD is generally managed conservatively (i.e., antiplatelet therapy and imaging surveillance) in the absence of severe symptoms.

Coronary Artery Fibromuscular Dysplasia

FMD in the coronary arteries manifests primarily as spontaneous coronary artery dissection (SCAD), which presents as chest pain due to acute coronary syndrome, and typically as ST- or non–ST-segment elevation myocardial infarction. The mechanism of SCAD involves

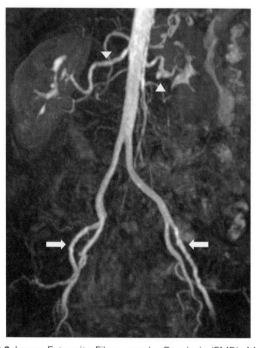

Fig. 58.6 Lower Extremity Fibromuscular Dysplasia (FMD). Magnetic resonance angiography of multifocal FMD in bilateral external iliac arteries (arrows) in a 64-year-old woman with claudication and femoral bruits. She also has bilateral internal carotid artery FMD (not shown) and multifocal right renal FMD with a small left renal artery aneurysm (arrowheads).

spontaneous development of intramural hemorrhage in the presence or absence of an intimal tear with subsequent narrowing of the true coronary artery lumen by the mural hematoma.[99] An angiographic classification system for SCAD has been developed by Saw and colleagues and describes lesions of three varieties based upon presence/absence of a dual lumen and diffuse tapering or focal narrowing of the vessel.[97] Type 1 SCAD is an evident arterial wall stain with the accumulation of contrast dye and presence of dual coronary lumens.[98] Type 2 SCAD, which is the most common presentation, is a smooth, diffuse coronary stenosis of varying severity and length (Fig. 58.7).[98,99] Lastly, type 3 SCAD is focal in nature, mimics atherosclerosis, and often requires optical coherence tomography (OCT) or intravascular ultrasound (IVUS) to confirm the diagnosis.[98] Lesions due to SCAD most commonly involve the mid to distal left anterior descending artery, but all coronary segments can be affected.[97,98]

An association between SCAD and the presence of underlying FMD has currently been well established by case series from Vancouver General Hospital, Mayo Clinic, and other institutions.[98–103] In prospective cohort studies of patients who have survived SCAD, extracoronary FMD, diagnosed by catheter-based angiography or noninvasive imaging, was found to be present in 45% to 72% of patients.[2,4,96,99] Although underlying FMD is present in a significant percentage of patients who have survived SCAD, there is a paradoxical relationship between SCAD and FMD, because the large majority of patients with FMD, such as those in the US Registry, have never had a SCAD event.[2,4,100] Indeed, in the US Registry, only 3% of patients with FMD have had SCAD and less than 7% have had any coronary event.[2,4] Although management of SCAD is beyond the scope of this chapter, most patients are managed with medical therapy (rather than intervention), including antiplatelet agents and β-blockers, allowing time for the dissection to heal.[97,99,102] It is recommended that patients who have suffered SCAD should be evaluated for FMD and other occult vascular abnormalities with brain to pelvis imaging.[102]

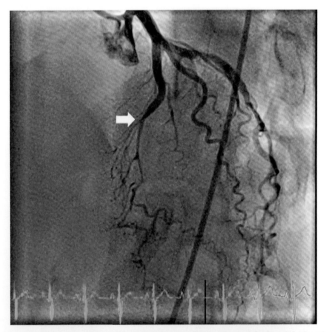

Fig. 58.7 Spontaneous Coronary Artery Dissection (SCAD). SCAD of the left anterior descending (LAD) artery in a 57-year-old woman with unstable angina. The coronary angiogram demonstrates tapering of the LAD *(arrow)* tapering to less than 50% of its original caliber, which persists from the mid to distal vessel consistent with type 2 SCAD. The patient was subsequently found to have subtle changes of multifocal FMD in the right renal artery, carotid tortuosity, and later a vertebral artery dissection.

Other manifestations of coronary FMD have been reported and include marked arterial tortuosity, multifocal or focal stenoses, and coronary ectasia.[99,104–106] Saw and colleagues examined the coronary angiograms of 32 patients with extracoronary multifocal FMD.[99] They found that all patients had at least mild tortuosity present in a coronary artery.[99] A subset of patients underwent OCT, which demonstrated distorted coronary wall architecture in a pattern not typical for atherosclerotic disease and possibly reflective of coronary FMD-related abnormalities, although this was not confirmed by histopathology.[99]

FMD has been associated with sudden cardiac death and sudden infant death syndrome in isolated case reports and case series of autopsies, often due to sinoatrial and/or atrioventricular nodal artery involvement.[107–113] However, these are histopathological findings of unclear significance because histological evidence of FMD of these arteries has uncertain relation to the development of lethal cardiovascular events. Indeed, such FMD-like arterial changes of the conducting system are relatively common on autopsy.[114–117] One report showed findings of nodal artery FMD in a significant number of patients with healthy hearts who suffered traumatic deaths (84% in 100 patients ages 0 to 40 in the study).[114] Sudden cardiac death has not been reported in adults or children being followed in the US Registry, although 15.4% of the adult patients and 11.1% of the pediatric patients report a family history of sudden death among first- or second- degree relatives.[1,14] The clinical significance of coronary FMD, beyond its association with SCAD, is an area in need of further research.

Fibromuscular Dysplasia in Other Locations

Aortic FMD has been reported among pediatric patients with focal FMD. These lesions cause middle-aortic syndrome and can mimic vasculitis.[14] There may be an association of FMD with aortic aneurysm. In the US Registry, aortic aneurysms accounted for 10.0% of all aneurysms, and a single-center case series of a screening CTA of the chest, abdomen, and pelvis for patients with FMD reported aortic findings in 4.0% of patients.[4,118] In the US Registry, 23.5% of patients with FMD reported a family history of aneurysm, including aortic aneurysms.[1] There are single case reports in the literature of FMD affecting other vessels, including the internal mammary arteries.[119]

DIAGNOSTIC EVALUATION OF FIBROMUSCULAR DYSPLASIA

Differential Diagnosis

A thorough and detailed investigation is necessary to differentiate FMD from other artery diseases (Table 58.2). Atherosclerosis is the most common cause of arterial stenosis and can be distinguished from FMD on the basis of differing risk factors and imaging features. Although atherosclerotic lesions can coexist with FMD, particularly in older individuals, one important distinction is that they tend to occur at the ostium or proximal portion of an artery, as opposed to the mid and distal involvement found in renal or cerebrovascular multifocal FMD. The presence of arterial calcification and the lipid-rich plaque of atherosclerotic lesions also distinguishes these from FMD. Focal FMD may be more challenging to distinguish from atherosclerosis than the multifocal form. Standing waves due to catheter- or contrast-induced vasospasm can be mistaken for multifocal FMD on angiography (Fig. 58.8).[120] However, two important differences may be seen with standing waves that are not found in FMD: (1) presence of undulations on angiographic imaging that are *regular* and *without stenosis* or (2) rapid reversal of the abnormality with infusion of a vasodilator or withdrawal of a catheter.[120,121]

TABLE 58.2   Differential Diagnoses of Fibromuscular Dysplasia (FMD)

Diagnosis	Similarity to FMD	Distinguishing Characteristic(s)
Atherosclerosis	Tubular stenosis on imaging	Affects ostium or proximal vessel (near branch points); associated with arterial calcification and lipid-rich plaque, patients usually have CVD risk factors
Standing waves	Multifocal beading on angiography	Presence of undulations that are regular and without stenosis
Vasospasm	Focal or beaded lesion on angiography	May be related to presence of indwelling arterial catheter; rapid reversal of the abnormality with infusion of vasodilator
Large-vessel vasculitis	Focal or tubular stenoses involving the aorta and large branches, similar patient demographics	Inflammatory process associated with constitutional symptoms and elevated acute phase reactants; diffuse and often concentric arterial wall thickening may be appreciated on imaging studies
Primary arterial dissection	Dissection of a single artery or multiple arteries; may have focal or beaded appearance on imaging studies in acute phase or with healing	Dissection flap or dual lumen flow may be visualized; absence of classical beaded lesion in another vascular territory
Segmental arterial mediolysis (SAM)	Dissections, aneurysms, or occlusions of the visceral vessels; also noninflammatory	Highly aggressive, acute presentation. More likely to present with acute hemorrhage/ischemia; male predominance; histology shows vacuolization and destruction of the vessel media[116]
Loeys-Dietz syndrome (LDS)	Aneurysms, dissections, and arterial tortuosity	Family history, autosomal dominant disorder (TGF-β pathway mutations, SMAD3, others) confirmed with genetic testing for one of multiple mutations, may be associated with extensive craniofacial abnormalities or bifid uvula[127]
Ehlers-Danlos syndrome (EDS), type IV or vascular type	Aneurysms, dissections	Aneurysms prone to rupture; associated skin findings and risk of bowel perforation and obstetrical complications; Family history, vascular type is autosomal dominant (COL3A1 mutation), confirmed with genetic test

CVD, Cardiovascular disease; *TGF*, transforming growth factor.

Vasculitis is an inflammatory process consisting of diffuse narrowing and usually presents with constitutional symptoms and elevated acute phase reactants. FMD is a noninflammatory arterial disease, and patients should not have elevated acute phase reactants (unless infarction of the kidney or bowel is present). In some cases of focal FMD, particularly those with aortic and visceral involvement, distinguishing FMD from large vessel vasculitis can be challenging. Primary dissections in the cervical, coronary, renal, or visceral arteries, especially in women, can raise suspicion of FMD, but in the absence of a classical beaded or focal lesion in another vascular territory, the diagnosis of FMD cannot be made. This may be a "form fruste" of FMD. In addition, it may be difficult to distinguish healing dissections from the beading and ectasia of FMD. SAM is a rare vascular disease characterized by spontaneous arterial dissections, occlusions, or aneurysms, often involving multiple vessels simultaneously.[122] SAM most commonly affects the visceral arteries in a skip pattern and can be challenging to distinguish from mesenteric FMD on imaging alone (see Chapter 25). Some authors have proposed that SAM may represent a variant of FMD or a precursor of certain types of FMD, although this theory has not been widely embraced.[122–125] In contrast to FMD, SAM has a slight male predominance and more often presents with hemorrhage (due to artery rupture) and acute mesenteric ischemia.[116] A definitive diagnosis of SAM requires histopathologic examination.[126] Autosomal dominant, inherited disorders such as vascular Ehlers-Danlos syndrome (EDS) and Loeys-Dietz syndrome (LDS) may present with aneurysms or dissections but can be easily differentiated from FMD by a detailed history and appropriate genetic testing (i.e., for mutations of Col 3A1, TGF-β Receptors 1/2, SMAD3, TGFβ2/3, others).[127]

Laboratory Evaluation

There is no blood test for FMD, and tissue specimens for histopathology are rarely procured unless an open surgical procedure is indicated. There is no role for tissue biopsy in the diagnosis of FMD because accurate and noninvasive imaging studies are available, in addition to catheter-based angiography. It is reasonable to obtain blood chemistries, particularly for renal function in all patients in whom FMD is suspected. However, in most cases, renal function will be normal. Unlike with atherosclerotic disease, renal blood flow is relatively preserved with no differences between the glomerular filtration rate of the affected and nonaffected kidney in patients with unilateral renal FMD.[128] Assessment of lipid parameters and acute phase reactants (complete blood count, erythrocyte sedimentation rate, C-reactive protein, and others) can be useful when distinguishing FMD from other clinical entities (i.e., atherosclerosis, vasculitis). Genetic testing may be indicated to rule out arteriopathies (e.g., EDS, LDS) which may overlap with FMD in the setting of multivessel aneurysm or dissection.

IMAGING STUDIES FOR DIAGNOSIS OF FIBROMUSCULAR DYSPLASIA

Although catheter-based angiography remains the "gold standard" for diagnosis of FMD, different noninvasive imaging modalities may be used, namely duplex ultrasound, CTA, and magnetic resonance angiography (MRA). There are sparse comparative accuracy data for the different modalities for diagnosis of FMD, in contrast to atherosclerotic disease for which more data are available. Thus the choice of imaging study depends upon local imaging resources and expertise and location of disease, such as whether it is accessible to scanning by duplex ultrasound. Catheter-based angiography is generally reserved for cases of diagnostic uncertainty on noninvasive studies or when intervention is required.

The objective of imaging, regardless of modality used, is to accurately and reliably detect FMD lesions (focal and multifocal), aneurysms, and dissections and to assess perfusion, if possible. The severity of stenosis associated with multifocal FMD can be challenging to determine via noninvasive means and even with catheter-based angiography.[129,130]

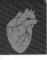

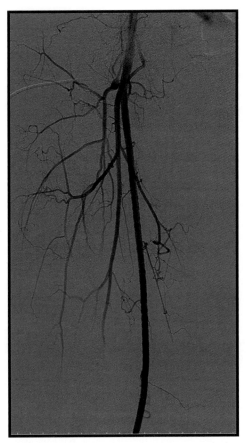

Fig. 58.8 Standing Waves. Standing waves are a physiologic response to arteriography and should not be misdiagnosed as fibromuscular dysplasia (FMD). Shown here are standing waves in the superficial femoral artery. This patient did *not* have FMD. (From Sharma AM, Gornik HL. Standing arterial waves is not fibromuscular dysplasia. *Circ Cardiovasc Interv.* 2012;5:e9–e11. Copyright 2012, American Heart Association, Inc.)

Duplex Ultrasound

When performed in an experienced vascular laboratory, duplex ultrasound, combing gray scale, color Doppler, and spectral Doppler imaging, remains an excellent initial test for both renal artery and carotid artery FMD (also see Chapter 12). Duplex ultrasound has the advantages of being relatively inexpensive, widely available, and accurate when performed and interpreted by experienced personnel and requires neither contrast material nor ionizing radiation.

Duplex ultrasound evaluation of FMD requires sonographer skill encompassing knowledge of the local anatomy, normal waveform physiology, and image optimization. Spectral and color Doppler are used to determine patency and detect flow disturbances that indicate hemodynamically significant lesions. Disturbed, turbulent blood flow associated with elevated velocities within the mid to distal renal or internal carotid arteries are hallmarks of multifocal FMD on duplex ultrasound. Multifocal FMD may exhibit the classic "string of beads" appearance on color Doppler or color power angiography, but areas of FMD may be less classic and difficult to distinguish from atherosclerosis or dissection. In carotid artery evaluation, the absence of atherosclerotic plaque with abnormalities at the mid to distal cervical segment may suggest FMD. It is important to note that specific criteria for determination of severity of stenosis due to FMD have not been validated and diagnostic criteria for atherosclerotic disease of the internal carotid/renal arteries

are often erroneously applied. In the setting of multifocal FMD with its tandem lesions of stenosis and dilatation, these criteria are likely not accurate; thus a correct interpretation should exclude terminology referring to a specific percentage of renal or internal carotid artery stenosis and simply describe elevated velocities, tortuosity, and turbulence consistent with FMD.[2] S-shaped redundancy and tortuosity of the internal carotid arteries has been described on duplex ultrasound among patients with FMD (see Fig. 58.2).[53] Duplex ultrasound has a number of limitations in assessment of FMD, including the inability to assess intracranial vessels or most of the vertebral arteries, limited visualization of renal artery branches or accessory renal arteries, and limited visualization of arterial dissection and aneurysm. However, once the diagnosis of FMD has been established, duplex ultrasound can be an excellent, low-risk modality for routine surveillance of FMD lesions in the renal and internal carotid arteries and other sites, including the mesenteric and extremity arteries.

Computed Tomography Angiography

CTA is an excellent noninvasive modality for visualizing focal and multifocal lesions of FMD throughout the body, as well as for assessing for aneurysm or dissection. Images can be reconstructed in maximal and three-dimensional projections, allowing detailed anatomic visualization that is superior to ultrasound (see Figs. 58.3 and 58.4). High spatial resolution and short acquisition time are the other major advantages of CTA. In addition, CTA has much better temporal resolution than MRA.[2] Two retrospective studies compared CTA with catheter-based angiography for diagnosis of renal artery FMD. In both studies, CTA correctly detected all lesions after review of all CTA reconstructions.[131,132] However, subtle FMD lesions were frequently missed in a single projection. In addition, the diagnostic accuracy of CTA for renal artery FMD may be limited by presence of adjacent or overlapping structures such as renal veins. CTA allows for comprehensive assessment of cerebrovascular FMD by imaging the internal carotid, vertebral, and intracranial arteries. There are no studies comparing CTA to catheter-based angiography for diagnosis of carotid FMD. CTA has a high sensitivity and specificity in detecting cerebrovascular dissections and large aneurysms but is less sensitive at detecting aneurysms <3 mm in size.[133–135] Among patients with cerebrovascular FMD, a dedicated CTA protocol of the chest, abdomen, and pelvis to assess the aorta and its iliac, renal, and celiac/mesenteric branches may allow for detection of new areas of arterial beading, aneurysm, and dissection beyond those known at patient intake suggesting a substantial and incremental diagnostic yield.[135]

Magnetic Resonance Angiography

In experienced centers, MRA provides similar anatomic visualization as CTA and is preferred in patients with an allergy to iodinated contrast or to reduce radiation exposure in younger patients.[2] One study showed that contrast-enhanced MRA has a high sensitivity (95% to 97%) and specificity (93%) for detection of renal FMD compared with catheter-based angiography, although no studies have compared the accuracy of MRA versus catheter-based angiography for the detection of cerebrovascular FMD.[136] Compared with unenhanced two-dimensional time-of-flight MRA, contrast-enhanced MRA measurements had less error, correctly diagnosed FMD more frequently, and identified more accessory renal arteries.[136,137] Head-to-pelvis imaging with MRA or CTA also allows for detection of multisite FMD. Major limitations of MRA include low spatial resolution, inability to use gadolinium-based contrast agents in patients with renal dysfunction, recent concerns regarding gadolinium accumulation, and false-positive "beading" related to motion artifact.[136]

Catheter-Based Angiography

Catheter-based arteriography remains the diagnostic gold standard for renal and cerebrovascular FMD. It has unsurpassed spatial resolution and is the only way to reliably detect branch vessel involvement.[2] It is a minimally invasive procedure and is thus reserved for cases when the diagnosis is uncertain or when subsequent intervention is likely.

Catheter-based renal angiography provides an excellent display of both multifocal and focal FMD lesions (see Fig. 58.1). Expert consensus recommendations addressing assessment for hemodynamically significant FMD lesions have been recently published.[138] A standard protocol for angiography includes a flush aortogram to demonstrate the origin of the main renal arteries and the presence of any accessory renal arteries.[138] Selective catheterization of the renal arteries and branch vessels allows for visualization of FMD multifocal or focal lesions, dissections, or aneurysms. It has been recently recognized that accurate diagnosis of hemodynamically significant multifocal renal FMD depends on the measurement of a translesional pressure gradient because visual assessment alone cannot determine the severity of stenosis.[138] Similar to the technique for assessment of atherosclerotic renal artery stenosis, a pressure gradient in the setting of FMD can be obtained by advancing a pressure wire across cross the renal artery FMD lesion(s).[2,138,139] Fractional flow reserve has recently been proposed to assess the severity of renal artery stenosis for atherosclerotic diseaes.[139-142] The ratio of the renal arterial pressure distal to the lesion (Pd) is compared with the proximal arterial (aortic) pressure (Pa) and a Pd/Pa ratio of less than 0.9 is indicative of hemodynamically significant stenosis.[140, 142] Although mentioning Pd/Pa and a ratio of less than 0.9 as potential threshold for hemodynamic significance, the international consensus statement acknowledges that this parameter requires validation in the context of FMD.[138] In addition to selecting patients for angioplasty, pressure gradient measurements can be made following balloon angioplasty to confirm that lesions have been adequately treated with resolution (or near resolution) of the pressure gradient. In addition to pressure gradient measurements, the use of IVUS for assessment of renal FMD has been described.[129]

Catheter-based cerebrovascular angiography is rarely used solely for diagnosis of FMD given the risk of adverse complications (e.g., stroke) and availability of high-quality noninvasive imaging modalities. Catheter-based angiography is indicated prior to intervention for patients with significant symptoms despite medical therapy, to confirm the diagnosis in equivocal cases, and to assess intracranial aneurysms when their anatomy cannot be adequately determined by noninvasive imaging.[2] Osborn and Anderson initially reported three types of cerebrovascular FMD based on angiographic appearance.[51] Type 1, which was present in 89% of cases, demonstrated the classic "string of beads" appearance, currently known as multifocal FMD.[51] Type 2, present in 7% of cases, consisted of tubular stenosis consistent with focal FMD, and type 3, present in 4% cases, demonstrated an atypical corrugated outpouching that may appear aneurysmal and could represent a pseudoaneurysm from a prior cervical artery dissection.[51] Of note, all types spare the carotid bifurcation, which is an important distinction from carotid atherosclerotic disease and CBD.

MANAGEMENT OF FIBROMUSCULAR DYSPLASIA

Management of FMD includes medical therapy and lifestyle modification, appropriate referral for vascular interventional procedures (if and when indicated), and clinical follow-up. A summary of management for patients with FMD is shown in Box 58.2.

BOX 58.2 Components of Care for Patients With Fibromuscular Dysplasia

- Imaging studies
  - Comprehensive (i.e., brain to pelvis) initial imaging to identify areas affected by FMD and to rule out aneurysms throughout the body
  - Follow-up imaging studies focused on affected areas
- Education for warning signs and symptoms of TIA, stroke, and arterial dissection
- Lifestyle changes
  - Smoking cessation
  - Customized exercise recommendations
  - "Dissection precautions" (e.g., no chiropractic neck manipulation, no contact sports, no roller coaster rides)
  - Assessment of risk of pregnancy (if relevant)
- Medical therapy
  - Antihypertensive therapy
  - Antiplatelet agents
  - Preventive and treatment medications for migraine headaches
  - Management strategies for pulsatile tinnitus (e.g., sound therapy, white noise machine, cognitive behavioral therapy or biofeedback)
- Vascular procedures
  - Balloon angioplasty of renal arteries for hypertension
  - Less common procedures
    - Endovascular treatment (stenting) of severe carotid or vertebral artery dissections
    - Endovascular coiling of brain or other artery aneurysms
    - Surgical clipping of brain aneurysms
    - Surgical bypass for severe arterial stenosis or failure of angioplasty procedures
    - Surgical revascularization of complex renal artery and branch disease (bypass or ex vivo reconstruction)
    - Surgical treatment of renal or other artery aneurysms

FMD, Fibromuscular dysplasia; *TIA,* transient ischemic attack. Modified from Khoury MH, Gornik HL. Fibromuscular dysplasia (FMD). *Vasc Med.* 2017;22(3):248–252. 2017 Society for Vascular Medicine, with permission.

Medical Therapy

The goal of treatment for FMD is to manage symptoms and high blood pressure and to prevent future vascular complications. FMD is a chronic medical condition, and there is no medication or procedure that can cure the disease. The mainstay of medical therapy includes lifestyle changes, antiplatelet agents, and antihypertensive therapy. Although patients with FMD can have a myriad of symptoms, not all complaints can be attributed to the disease. In caring for a patient with this disease, it is important to determine which symptoms are due to FMD and which might be due to other health problems for which a different treatment approach may improve symptoms and quality of life.

Lifestyle Changes

Lifestyle changes are based on general principles of cardiovascular health because there are no specific guidelines for FMD. As for all patients, smoking cessation should be strongly encouraged. It appears that patients with FMD who continue to smoke have a more aggressive course than those who do not smoke.[43-45] Beyond smoking and hypertension, there is no clear association between FMD and other atherosclerotic cardiovascular risk factors (e.g., diabetes, hyperlipidemia).[1,35] Nevertheless, efforts to minimize such risk factors including weight management, regular exercise, moderation of alcohol intake, and adherence to a healthy diet should be implemented. For patients with cerebrovascular involvement, precautions against dissection are recommended such as refraining from certain high-risk activities (e.g., lifting heavy objects, extreme or contact sports, roller coaster rides, and undergoing chiropractic neck manipulations).[143] Although FMD tends to be diagnosed later in life, patients with FMD of childbearing age should discuss risk of pregnancy with their doctors prior to conception.[143] Those patients with prior history of arterial dissection, particularly cervical dissection or SCAD, as well as those with uncontrolled hypertension, should be considered at high-risk for pregnancy due to increased risk of preeclampsia and recurrent dissection.[144,145]

Antiplatelet and Anticoagulant Therapy

Antiplatelet therapy is recommended for patients with cerebrovascular FMD for primary prevention of TIA or stroke, as well as for secondary prevention among patients who have previously experienced an ischemic event, dissection, or undergone angioplasty/intervention. In multisocietal guidelines for Management of Extracranial Carotid and Vertebral Artery Disease, the administration of antiplatelet therapy to patients with FMD, regardless of symptoms, was given a class IIa recommendation.[146] The appropriate agent and dose are unknown, but it is reasonable to use aspirin 75 to 325 mg once daily to reduce the likelihood of platelet adherence to the FMD-related webs and the potential for thromboembolic complications.[2] Clopidogrel monotherapy may be a good alternative for patients with aspirin allergy or intolerance, or significant atherosclerotic comorbidity. In the US Registry, 56.8% of all patients received aspirin alone, 4.6% received clopidogrel alone, and 72.9% patients received any antiplatelet agent.[3] Patients who had a history of coronary artery disease, prior neurological event, or prior interventional procedure had a significantly higher likelihood of receiving dual antiplatelet therapy (DAPT) than aspirin monotherapy, but no significant difference compared with clopidogrel monotherapy.[3] Of note, there are no data regarding the efficacy of different antiplatelet regimens among patients with cerebrovascular FMD, and this is an area in need of future study.

Although there are limited data regarding the use of antiplatelet therapy in renal FMD and FMD at other locations, it is reasonable to prescribe this for patients in the absence of contraindication. The recently published International Consensus recommends antiplatelet therapy as reasonable for patients with FMD, in the absence of contraindication, and regardless of location of disease.[138] Among patients with FMD who have had SCAD, antiplatelet therapy, often with DAPT, is a mainstay of therapy.[96,102,103] Anticoagulation with either heparin, low-molecular-weight heparin (LMWH), or warfarin may be indicated for the initial treatment of an acute arterial dissection. According to recent guidelines, cervical artery dissection is managed with heparin or LMWH followed by oral anticoagulation with warfarin for 3 to 6 months and ultimately antiplatelet therapy (class IIa).[146] However, data have challenged this approach and support the use of antiplatelet therapy alone for selected patients with cervical artery dissection.[147,148] Unfortunately, a definitive trial on this issue was not conclusive.[147] Formal guidelines for management of dissection in other vascular beds do not exist.[2] Anticoagulation can be used to manage renal or visceral artery dissection, but similar to cervical artery dissection, the available literature does not demonstrate a clear benefit of anticoagulation over antiplatelet therapy.[147–151] Following a renal or visceral artery dissection, anticoagulation may be extended to 3 to 6 months after the event, followed by long-term antiplatelet therapy, and patients should

have long-term imaging follow-up because some may develop aneurysmal dilatation of the vessel during its healing, sometimes requiring intervention.[152,153]

Antihypertensive Therapy

Given the high prevalence of hypertension in this population, antihypertensive medications constitute an important treatment modality. Overall, 71.7% of FMD patients in the US Registry received antihypertensive medications.[3,5,6] The median number of medications was one, but 21.5% of patients received three or more antihypertensive medications.[3] In the French and Belgian ARCADIA study, 77.6% of all patients with renal FMD and 54.5% of patients with cerebrovascular FMD patients received antihypertensive medications.[4] Although blood pressure control is important to prevent end-organ damage, there are no current guidelines for specific target blood pressure values in patients with FMD. Thus the current practice is to follow published consensus guidelines for the treatment of hypertension in the general population which have recently been updated by ACC/AHA committees.[154] The most recent guidelines recommend treating systolic/diastolic blood pressure to less than 130/80 mm Hg, which is lower than the previous goal recommended by Joint National Committee 7 (JNC7).[154,155] It has been recommended that first-line antihypertensive therapy among patients with renal FMD is an ACE inhibitor or angiotensin receptor blocker (ARB) given the suppressive effect of these medications on the renin-angiotensin-aldosterone pathway.[3] If a second medication is required, a thiazide diuretic or calcium channel blocker can be considered.[154,155] β-Blockers are recommended for patients with FMD who have a history of SCAD, stable ischemic heart disease, or a history of congestive heart failure with reduced ejection fraction.[96]

Other Medical Therapies

There is little evidence to support the use of statins in patients with FMD; thus the current practice is to administer only to those who meet criteria based on the presence of concomitant atherosclerotic vascular disease or hyperlipidemia per current lipid guidelines.[156]

An individualized risk versus benefit assessment should be performed prior to prescription of oral contraceptive therapy or postmenopausal hormone replacement for patients with FMD. This includes assessment of the extent and severity of disease and vascular bed involvement, blood pressure control, severity of postmenopausal symptoms (for hormone replacement therapy), prior history of coronary or other arterial dissection or other thromboembolic vascular events (including venous thromboembolism), and other elements of the medical history (e.g., personal or family history of breast cancer). In general, those patients who have had a prior history of myocardial infarction, stroke, or venous thromboembolic events should avoid the use of oral contraceptive therapy or postmenopausal hormone replacement.[157,158]

Although headaches, and especially migraines, are common among patients with FMD, little is known about the efficacy of preventive or abortive therapies in this population. There is some concern about the use of triptans as an abortive medication for migraines due to the risk of vasoconstriction leading to stroke or arterial dissection.[29] Nonsteroidal antiinflammatory drugs can be used judiciously in patients with renal FMD, except in those patients with renal insufficiency. There are no evidence-based or consensus recommendations for preventative headache therapy in patients with FMD.

For patients with pulsatile tinnitus, consultation with an ear, nose, and throat physician or audiologist may be helpful.[143] Specific treatment modalities may include sound therapy (e.g., use of white noise machines), cognitive behavioral therapy, and biofeedback.

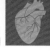

ENDOVASCULAR THERAPY FOR FIBROMUSCULAR DYSPLASIA

Renal Artery Angioplasty

Percutaneous transluminal angioplasty (PTA) of the renal arteries is the most common vascular procedure performed for FMD and can be effective in curing or improving hypertension in well-selected patients (see Chapter 24).[2] The primary goal in treating patients with renal artery FMD is to control blood pressure to treat associated symptoms (e.g., headache), prevent end-organ damage, and potentially reduce the number of medications required long term. Referral for angioplasty for renal artery FMD is driven by symptoms and duration and severity of hypertension and not merely the presence of multifocal or focal renal artery lesions. It is important to recognize that patients with renal FMD may not have hemodynamically significant renal artery stenosis and may simply have essential hypertension, an entity which will not respond to balloon angioplasty. Indications for renal artery revascularization for FMD are listed in Table 58.3. It has been shown that patient factors including age at intervention, duration of hypertension, multifocal versus focal FMD, and renal function may have an impact on the efficacy of PTA for renal artery FMD.[5,159–161] Younger patients, patients with shorter duration of hypertension, those with preserved renal function, those with multifocal (vs. focal) FMD, and those without features of the metabolic syndrome are more

likely to have long-term resolution of hypertension following angioplasty.[159–161] Despite reported technical success rates of ≥90% in case series and meta-analyses, the overall long-term hypertension cure rate after PTA in patients with FMD is between 42% and 50%.[162–164] It is likely that improved patient selection for angioplasty, including confirmation of a hemodynamically significant gradient across a segment of renal FMD prior to angioplasty and hemodynamic confirmation of angiographic success following angioplasty (i.e., complete or near complete obliteration of translesional pressure gradient), will improve long-term outcomes among patients with renal artery FMD referred for revascularization.[2,138]

For renal artery FMD, PTA alone is generally effective and there is rarely a need for stent implantation; this is in contrast to atherosclerotic renal artery stenosis for which stenting is routinely performed. Selected indications for stenting in renal artery FMD include technical failure (e.g., if the gradient cannot be obliterated by angioplasty alone) or to treat a renal artery dissection or perforation.[138] Covered stent placement may also be indicated to treat renal artery aneurysm. It is important to recognize that there may be a residual beaded appearance of the artery even after a successful angioplasty with complete obliteration of the translesional pressure gradient, and this does not constitute a technical failure. Restenosis rate or need for repeat renal angioplasty for FMD has been reported in 18% to 29% of patients in published case series.[159,161] Unfortunately, restenosis rates are higher for lesions that require stenting, and these patients may be better served by surgical revascularization.[165] Stent fracture requiring surgical bypass has been reported in patients with renal FMD and may be related to nephroptosis and mechanical stress on the stent.[165,166] If a stent is required in the setting of renal FMD, placement of the shortest stent length to effectively treat the lesion is advised.

The optimal postrevascularization monitoring schedule following renal angioplasty has not been established, but it is reasonable to obtain duplex ultrasonography at the first office visit after intervention (or prior to hospital discharge) with serial imaging every 6 months for the first 24 months and then annually.[2] The development of significant restenosis when accompanied by worsening hypertension should prompt repeat catheter-based angiography with potential for repeat angioplasty.

Endovascular Therapy for Cerebrovascular Fibromuscular Dysplasia

The endovascular treatment options for patients with cerebrovascular FMD include balloon angioplasty, stenting, and coiling (for aneurysms or pseudoaneurysms). Even more so than for renal FMD, intervention for cerebrovascular FMD is reserved for the few patients who are highly symptomatic on medical therapy or those with cerebral aneurysms. For symptomatic multifocal or focal FMD, angioplasty alone is usually performed, but stenting may be indicated, particularly for treatment of carotid or vertebral artery dissection.

For nonruptured cerebral aneurysms among patients with FMD, early, invasive treatment in asymptomatic patients may be indicated to prevent rupture. Rupture risk is significantly higher with increasing aneurysm size (≥7 mm) and with location in the basilar, posterior, or anterior communicating arteries.[167] Although there are no guidelines specific for management of cerebral aneurysm in patients with FMD, guidelines from the American Association of Neurosurgery suggest that it is reasonable to offer treatment to asymptomatic patients <60 years of age with a cerebral aneurysm >5 mm in size and for all patients <70 years of age with aneurysms >10 mm.[168] Ruptured cerebral aneurysms should be treated with urgent endovascular coil embolization or microsurgical clipping with a craniotomy. A randomized, controlled trial in 2143 patients with ruptured cerebral aneurysm

TABLE 58.3 Indications for Renal Artery Revascularization in Patients With Fibromuscular Dysplasia

European Consensus (2014)	American Heart Association (2014)
Medical treatment failure of HTN (drug resistance or intolerance)	Resistant HTN (failure to reach goal blood pressures in patients on an appropriate three-drug regimen including a diuretic)
First line treatment for HTN of recent onset	HTN of short duration with goal of cure
Renal insufficiency or deterioration of renal function especially after administration of an ACEi, ARB, or renin inhibitor	Renal artery dissection. If intervention is required, stenting is procedure of choice.
Reduction in the size of the kidney >1 cm downstream of the stenosis over ≥ two successive examinations (DUS, CTA, or MRA)	Renal artery aneurysm with surgical resection, endovascular coiling, or placement of a covered stent
	Branch renal artery disease and hypertension
	Preservation of renal function with severe, symptomatic stenosis

ACEi, Angiotensin converting enzyme inhibitor; *ARB*, angiotensin receptor blocker; *CTA*, computed tomography angiography; *DUS*, duplex ultrasound; *HTN*, hypertension; *MRA*, magnetic resonance angiography.
Data from Persu A, Giavarini A, Touzé E, et al. European consensus on the diagnosis and management of fibromuscular dysplasia. J Hypertens. 2014;32(7):1367–1378; and Olin JW, Gornik HL, Bacharach JM, et al. Fibromuscular dysplasia: state of the science and critical unanswered questions: a scientific statement from the American Heart Association. Circulation. 2014;129:1048–1078.

compared coiling versus clipping and found a 7.4% absolute risk reduction in morbidity and mortality that favored coiling, but there were no data reported regarding FMD.[169]

Endovascular Therapy for Fibromuscular Dysplasia at Other Sites

Patients with FMD who present with acute coronary syndrome should undergo diagnostic coronary angiography to establish the diagnosis of SCAD. Patients with SCAD are typically managed with medication alone because patients who receive angioplasty or stents have an increased risk of dissection propagation and other morbid complications with attempted percutaneous coronary intervention.[170] Revascularization is reserved for refractory ischemia or management of high-risk lesions, such as those in the left main coronary artery.[170] Multispecialty scientific statements on the management of SCAD have been recently published and are consistent with a medical therapy–first approach.[102,103] For FMD lesions at other sites, including the mesenteric and limb arteries, the decision to revascularize is guided by symptoms. If patients are highly symptomatic, the first-line treatment is usually PTA.[6,171]

SURGERY FOR FIBROMUSCULAR DYSPLASIA

Surgical intervention is generally considered second-line therapy for FMD because angioplasty and other endovascular techniques are effective for treating most FMD lesions. However, surgery may be preferred in patients with unfavorable anatomy. In renal artery FMD, this includes patients with small renal arteries (<4 mm), branch renal artery disease especially when associated with aneurysm, or extensive intimal or perimedial fibroplasia, particularly in children.[2] For renal FMD, aortorenal bypass may be performed with the hypogastric artery (in pediatric populations) or other reconstructed conduits or with an autogenous saphenous vein, although aneurysmal degeneration of such grafts has been reported (see Chapter 24).[172,173] Blood pressure cure rates appear to be similar to those achieved with PTA.[161,174] For highly complex anatomy, including extensive renal branch–vessel involvement and aneurysmal disease, ex vivo microvascular reconstruction and autotransplantation, generally performed in collaboration between urological and vascular surgery, is a treatment option.[175,176] For children with focal renal artery FMD, and especially those with associated middle aortic syndrome, surgical revascularization is often preferred for durable long-term outcomes.[14] Similarly aortomesenteric bypass may provide a reliable alternative to PTA for pediatric focal FMD.[15] For cerebral aneurysms, especially those with a wide neck or other unfavorable geometric features that may not be amenable to coil embolization, open surgical clipping may be required.[2]

FOLLOW-UP AND PROGNOSIS

Although FMD does not seem to be a progressive disease, it is recommended that patients with FMD receive periodic vascular surveillance and follow-up with a knowledgeable specialist.[138] Our general practice is for all patients to undergo one-time comprehensive imaging ("head to pelvis") with subsequent follow-up studies focused on areas of documented vascular involvement and as indicated following revascularization or for monitoring of aneurysms or dissections. Periodic follow-up visits also allow for discussion of FMD-related symptoms and adequacy of their control (e.g., for headaches), compliance with medical therapy, control of hypertension, and review of warning signs and symptoms of arterial dissection or other vascular events.

REFERENCES

1. Olin JW, Froehlich J, Gu X, et al. The United States registry from fibromuscular dysplasia: results in the first 447 patients. *Circulation*. 2012;125:3182–3190.
2. Olin JW, Gornik HL, Bacharach JM, et al. Fibromuscular dysplasia: state of the science and critical unanswered questions: a scientific statement from the American Heart Association. *Circulation*. 2014;129:1048–1078.
3. Weinberg I, Xiaokui G, Giri J, et al. Anti-platelet and anti-hypertension medication use in patients with fibromuscular dysplasia: results from the United States registry for fibromuscular dysplasia. *Vasc Med*. 2015;20: 447–453.
4. Kadian-Dodov D, Gornik HL, Gu X, et al. Dissection and aneurysm in patients with fibromuscular dysplasia: findings from the U.S. registry for FMD. *J Am Coll Cardiol*. 2016;68:176–185.
5. Plouin P, Baguet J, Thony F, et al. High prevalence of multiple arterial bed lesions in patients with fibromuscular dysplasia. The ARCADIA registry (Assessment of Renal and Cervical Artery Dysplasia). *Hypertension*. 2017;70:652–658.
6. Persu A, Giavarini A, Touzé E, et al. European consensus on the diagnosis and management of fibromuscular dysplasia. *J Hypertens*. 2014;32(7):1367–1378.
7. Persu A, Touzé E, Mousseaux E, et al. Diagnosis and management of fibromuscular dysplasia: an expert consensus. *Eur J Clin Invest*. 2012;42:338–347.
8. Leadbetter W, Burkland L. Hypertension in unilateral renal disease. *J Urol*. 1938;39:611–626.
9. McCormack LJ, Hazard JB, Poutasse EF. Obstructive lesions of the renal artery associated with remediable hypertension. *Am Jr Pathol*. 1958;34:582.
10. McCormack LJ, Poutasse EF, Meaney TF, et al. A pathologic-arteriographic correlation of renal arterial disease. *Am Heart J*. 1966;72:188–198.
11. Palubinskas AJ, Ripley HR. Fibromuscular hyperplasia in extrarenal arteries. *Radiology*. 1964;82:451–455.
12. Harrison EG, Hunt JC, Bernatz PE. Morphology of fibromuscular dysplasia of the renal artery in renovascular hypertension. *Am J Med*. 1967;43:97–112.
13. Harrison EG, McCormack LJ. Pathologic classification of renal arterial disease in renovascular hypertension. *Mayo Clin Proc*. 1971;46:161–167.
14. Green R, Gu X, Kline-Rogers E, et al. Differences between the pediatric and adult presentation of fibromuscular dysplasia: results from the US registry. *Pediatr Nephrol*. 2016;31(4):641–650.
15. Slovut DP, Olin JW. Fibromuscular dysplasia. *N Engl J Med*. 2004; 350:1862–1871.
16. Kincaid OW, Davis GD, Hallermann FJ, Hunt JC. Fibromuscular dysplasia of the renal arteries: arteriographic features, classification, and observations on natural history of the disease. *Am J Roentgenol Radium Ther Nucl Med*. 1968;104:271–282.
17. Savard S, Steichen O, Azarine A, et al. Association between 2 angiographic subtypes of renal artery fibromuscular dysplasia and clinical characteristics. *Circulation*. 2012;125:3182–3190.
18. Olin JW. Is fibromuscular dysplasia a single disease? *Circulation*. 2012;126:2925–2927.
19. Sharma AM, Kline B. The United States registry for fibromuscular dysplasia: new findings and breaking myths. *Tech Vasc Interv Radiol*. 2014;17(4):258–263.
20. Shivapour DM, Erwin P, Kim ES. Epidemiology of fibromuscular dysplasia: a review of the literature. *Vasc Med*. 2016;21:376–381.
21. Cragg AH, Smith TP, Thompson BH, et al. Incidental fibromuscular dysplasia in potential renal donors: long-term clinical follow-up. *Radiology*. 1989;172:145–147.
22. Spring DB, Salvatierra Jr O, Palubinskas AJ, et al. Results and significance of angiography in potential kidney donors. *Radiology*. 1979;133:45–47.
23. Frick MP, Goldberg ME. Uro-and angiographic findings in a 'normal' population: screening of 151 symptom-free potential transplant donors for renal disease. *AJR Am J Roentgenol*. 1980;134:503–505.

24. Neymark E, LaBerge JM, Hirose R, et al. Arteriographic detection of renovascular disease in potential renal donors: incidence and effect on donor surgery. *Radiology*. 2000;214:755–760.

25. Lorenz EC, Vrtiska TJ, Lieske JC, et al. Prevalence of renal artery and kidney abnormalities by computed tomography among healthy adults. *Clin J Am Soc Nephrol*. 2010;5:431–438.

26. Andreoni KA, Weeks SM, Gerber DA, et al. Incidence of donor renal fibromuscular dysplasia: does it justify routine angiography? *Transplantation*. 2002;73:1112–1116.

27. Blondin D, Lanzman R, Schellhammer F, et al. Fibromuscular dysplasia in living renal donors: still a challenge to computed tomographic angiography. *Eur J Radiol*. 2010;74:67–71.

28. McKenzie GA, Oderich GS, Kawashima A, Misra S. Renal artery fibromuscular dysplasia in 2,640 renal donor subjects: a CT angiography analysis. *J Vasc Interv Radiol*. 2013;24:1477–1480.

29. O'Connor SC, Gornik HL. Recent developments in the understanding and management of fibromuscular dysplasia. *J Am Heart Assoc*. 2014;3:e001259.

30. Hendricks NJ, Matsumoto AH, Angle JF, et al. Is fibromuscular dysplasia underdiagnosed? A comparison of the prevalence of FMD seen in CORAL trial participants versus a single institution population of renal donor candidates. *Vasc Med*. 2014;19(5):363–367.

31. Mettinger KL, Ericson K. Fibromuscular dysplasia and the brain. I. Observations on angiographic, clinical, and genetic characteristics. *Stroke*. 1982;13:46–52.

32. Touze E, Oppenheim C, Trystram D, et al. Fibromuscular dysplasia of cervical and intracranial arteries. *Int J Stroke*. 2010;5:296–305.

33. Schievink WI, Bjornsson J. Fibromuscular dysplasia of the internal carotid artery: a clinicopathologic study. *Clin Neuropathol*. 1996;15:2–6.

34. Noah B. The participation of underrepresented minorities in clinical research. *Am J Law Med*. 2003;29:221–245.

35. Bigazzi R, Bianchi S, Quilici N, et al. Bilateral fibromuscular dysplasia in identical twins. *Am J Kidney Dis*. 1998;32:E4.

36. Rushton AR. The genetics of fibromuscular dysplasia. *Arch Intern Med*. 1980;140:233–236.

37. Pannier-Moreau I, Grimbert P, Fiquet-Kempf B, et al. Possible familial origin of multifocal renal artery fibromuscular dysplasia. *J Hypertens*. 1989;14:472–479.

38. Poloskey SL, Kim ES, Sanghani R, et al. Low yield of genetic testing for known vascular connective tissue disorders in patients with fibromuscular dysplasia. *Vasc Med*. 2012;17:371–378.

39. Ganesh SK, Morissette R, Xu Z, et al. Clinical and biochemical profiles suggest fibromuscular dysplasia is a systemic disease with altered TGF-β expression and connective tissue features. *FASEB J*. 2014;28:3313–3324.

40. Sang CN, Whelton PK, Hamper UM, et al. Etiologic factors in renovascular fibromuscular dysplasia. A case-control study. *Hypertension*. 1989;14(5):472–479.

41. Kiando SR, Tucker NR, Castro-Vega LJ, et al. PHACTR1 is a genetic susceptibility locus for fibromuscular dysplasia supporting its complex genetic pattern of inheritance. *PLOS Genet*. 2016;12(10):e1006367.

42. Gupta RM, Hadaya J, Trehan A, et al. A genetic variant associated with five vascular diseases is a distal regulator of endothelin-1 gene expression. *Cell*. 2017;170(3):522–533.

43. Savard S, Azarine A, Jeunemaitre X, et al. Association of smoking with phenotype at diagnosis and vascular interventions in patients with renal artery fibromuscular dysplasia. *Hypertension*. 2013;61:1227–1232.

44. Bofinger A, Hawley C, Fisher P, et al. Increased severity of multifocal renal arterial fibromuscular dysplasia in smokers. *J Hum Hypertens*. 1999;13:517–520.

45. O'Connor S, Gornik HL, Froehlich JB, et al. Smoking and adverse outcomes in fibromuscular dysplasia: U.S. registry report. *J Am Coll Cardiol*. 2016;67(14):1750–1751.

46. Kim ES, Olin JW, Froehlich JB, et al. Clinical manifestations of fibromuscular dysplasia vary by patient sex: a report of the United States registry for fibromuscular dysplasia. *J Am Coll Cardiol*. 2013;62(21):2026–2028.

47. Kaufman JJ, Hanafee W, Maxwell MH. Upright renal arteriography in the study of renal hypertension. *JAMA*. 1964;187:977–980.

48. Kaufman JJ, Maxwell MH. Upright aortography in the study of nephroptosis, stenotic lesions of the renal artery, and hypertension. *Surgery*. 1963;53:736–742.

49. Miller DJ, Marin H, Aho T, et al. Fibromuscular dysplasia unraveled: the pulsation-induced microtrauma and reactive hyperplasia theory. *Med Hypotheses*. 2014;83:21–24.

50. Olin JW, Pierce M. Contemporary management of fibromuscular dysplasia. *Curr Opin Cardiol*. 2008;23:527–536.

51. Osborn AG, Anderson RE. Angiographic spectrum of cervical and intracranial fibromuscular dysplasia. *Stroke*. 1977;8:617–626.

52. Olin JW. Expanding clinical phenotype of fibromuscular dysplasia. *Hypertension*. 2017;70:488–489.

53. Sethi SS, Lau JF, Godbold J, et al. The S curve: a novel morphological finding in the internal carotid artery in patients with fibromuscular dysplasia. *Vasc Med*. 2014;19(5):356–362.

54. Olin JW, Sealove BA. Diagnosis, management, and future developments of fibromuscular dysplasia. *J Vasc Surg*. 2011;53(3):826–836.

55. Fenves AZ, Ram CV. Fibromuscular dysplasia of the renal arteries. *Curr Hypertens Rep*. 1999;1:546–549.

56. Giavarini A, Savard S, Sapoval M, et al. Clinical management of renal artery fibromuscular dysplasia: temporal trends and outcomes. *J Hypertens*. 2014;32:2433–2438.

57. Barbey F, Matthieu C, Nseir G, et al. A young man with a renal colic. *J of Int Med*. 2003;254:605–608.

58. Safian RD, Textor SC. Renal-artery stenosis. *N Engl J Med*. 2001;344:431–442.

59. Shanley PF. The pathology of chronic renal ischemia. *Semin Nephrol*. 1996;16:21–32.

60. Field DK, Kleinig TJ, Thompson PD, Kimber TE. Reversible cerebral vasoconstriction, internal carotid artery dissection and renal artery stenosis. *Cephalalgia*. 2010;30(8):983–986.

61. Burnstock G. Pathophysiology of migraine; a new hypothesis. *Lancet*. 1981;1:1397–1399.

62. Verma R, Gu X, Kline-Rogers E, et al. Understanding patient characteristics and clinical significance of headaches in patients with fibromuscular dysplasia: a report of the United States registry for fibromuscular dysplasia. [Abstract 12390]. *Circulation*. 2013;128:A12390.

63. D'Anglejan-Chatillon J, Ribeiro V, Mas JL, et al. Migraine—a risk factor for dissection of cervical arteries. *Headache*. 1989;29:560–561.

64. Pessini A, Zotto ED, Giossi A, et al. The migraine-ischemic stroke connection: potential pathogenic mechanisms. *Curr Mol Med*. 2009;9:215–226.

65. Rist PM, Diener HC, Kurth T, Schurks M. Migraine, migraine aura, and cervical artery dissection: a systematic review and metaanalysis. *Cephalalgia*. 2011;31:886–896.

66. O'Connor SC, Poria N, Gornik HL. Fibromuscular dysplasia: an update for the headache clinician. *Headache*. 2015;55(5):748–755.

67. Mettinger KL. Fibromuscular dysplasia and the brain. II. Current concept of the disease. *Stroke*. 1982;13(1):53–58.

68. Kasravi N, Leung A, Silver I, Burneo JG. Dissection of the internal carotid artery causing Horner syndrome and palsy of cranial nerve XII. *CMAJ*. 2010;182(9):E373–E377.

69. Kessler MM, Moussa M, Bykowski J, et al. ACR Appropriateness Criteria Tinnitus. *J Am Coll Radiol*. 2017;14:S584–S591.

70. Mahmood RZ, Olin J, Gu X, et al. Unraveling pulsatile tinnitus in FMD: a report of the United States registry for fibromuscular dysplasia. *J Am Coll Cardiol*. 2014;63(12):A2060.

71. Lather HD, Gornik HL, Olin JW, et al. Prevalence of intracranial aneurysm in women with fibromuscular dysplasia: a report from the US registry for fibromuscular dysplasia. *JAMA Neurol*. 2017;74(9):1081–1087.

72. Etminan N, Brown Jr. RD, Beseoglu K, et al. The unruptured intracranial aneurysm treatment score: a multidisciplinary consensus. *Neurology*. 2015;85:881–889.

73. Lenck S, Labeyrie MA, Saint-Maurice JP, et al. Diaphragms of the carotid and vertebral arteries: an under-diagnosed cause of ischaemic stroke. *Eur J Neurol*. 2014;21(4):586–593.

74. Joux J, Boulanger M, Jeannin S, et al. Association between carotid bulb diaphragm and ischemic stroke in young Afro-Caribbean patients. *Stroke.* 2016;47:2641–2644.

75. Jones HJ, Starud R, Williams Jr. RC. Rupture of a hepatic artery aneurysm and renal infarction: 2 complications of fibromuscular dysplasia that mimic vasculitis. *J Rheumatol.* 1998;25(10):2015–2018.

76. Guill CK, Benavides DC, Rees C, et al. Fatal mesenteric fibromuscular dysplasia: a case report and review of the literature. *Arch Intern Med.* 2004;164:1148–1153.

77. Meacham PW, Brantley B. Familial fibromuscular dysplasia of the mesenteric arteries. *South Med J.* 1987;80:1311–1316.

78. Stokes JB, Bonsib SM, McBride JW. Diffuse intimal fibromuscular dysplasia with multiorgan failure. *Arch Intern Med.* 1996;156:2611–2614.

79. Brinza E, Grabinski V, Durga S, et al. Lower extremity fibromuscular dysplasia: clinical manifestations, diagnostic testing, and approach to management. *Angiology.* 2017;68:722–727.

80. Thevenet A, Latil JL, Albat B. Fibromuscular disease of the external iliac artery. *Ann Vasc Surg.* 1992;6:199–204.

81. Walter JF, Stanley JC, Mehigan JT, et al. External iliac artery fibrodysplasia. *AJF Am J Roentgenol.* 1978;131:125–128.

82. Sauer L, Reilly LM, Goldstone J, et al. Clinical spectrum of symptomatic external iliac fibromuscular dysplasia. *J Vasc Surg.* 1990;12:488–495.

83. Suzuki H, Daida H, Sakurai H, Yamaguchi H. Familial fibromuscular dysplasia of bilateral brachial arteries. *Heart.* 1999;82(2):251–252.

84. McCready RA, Pairolero PC, Hollier LH, et al. Fibromuscular dysplasia of the right subclavian artery. *Arch Surg.* 1983;117:1243–1245.

85. Bonardelli S, Vettoretto N, Tiberio GA, et al. Right subclavian artery aneurysm of fibrodysplastic origin: two case reports and review of literature. *J Vasc Surg.* 2001;33:174–177.

86. Cheu HW, Mills JL. Digital artery embolization as a result of fibromuscular dysplasia of the brachial artery. *J Vasc Surg.* 1991;14:225–228.

87. Yoshida T, Ohashi I, Suzuki S, Iwai T. Fibromuscular disease of the brachial artery with digital emboli treated effectively by transluminal angioplasty. *Cardiovasc Intervent Radiol.* 1994;17:99–101.

88. Lin WW, McGee GS, Patterson BK, et al. Fibromuscular dysplasia of the brachial artery: a case report and review of the literature. *J Vasc Surg.* 1992;16:66–70.

89. Dorman Jr. RL, Kaufman JA, LaMuraglia GM. Digital emboli from brachial artery fibromuscular dysplasia. *Cardiovasc Intervent Radiol.* 1994;17:95–98.

90. Nguyen N, Sharma A, West JK, et al. Presentation clinical features, and results of intervention in upper extremity fibromuscular dysplasia. *J Vasc Surg.* 2017;66:554–563.

91. Shin JS, Han EM, Min BZ, et al. Fibromuscular dysplasia of bilateral brachial arteries treated with surgery and consecutive thrombolytic therapy. *Ann Vasc Surg.* 2007;64:138–145.

92. Shipolini AR, Wolfe JH. Fibromuscular dysplasia and aneurysm formation in the brachial artery. *Eur J Vasc Surg.* 1993;7:740–743.

93. Becquemin JP, Lejonc JL, Melliere D, et al. Fibromuscular dysplasia of the right subclavian artery. *Eur J Radiol.* 1983;3:378–379.

94. Chambers JL, Neale ML, Appleber L. Fibromuscular hyperplasia in an abberant subclavian artery and neurogenic thoracic outlet syndrome: an unusual combination. *J Vasc Surg.* 1994;20:834–838.

95. Kiernan PD, Dearani J, Byrne WE, et al. Aneurysm of an aberrant right subclavian artery: case report and review of the literature. *Mayo Clin Proc.* 1993;68:468–474.

96. Saw J, Humphries K, Aymong E, et al. Spontaneous coronary artery dissection: clinical outcomes and risk of recurrence. *J Am Coll Cardiol.* 2017;70(9):1148–1158.

97. Saw J, Aymong E, Sedlak T, et al. Spontaneous coronary artery dissection: association with predisposing arteriopathies and precipitating stressors and cardiovascular outcomes. *Circ Cardiovasc Interv.* 2014;7:645–655.

98. Saw J. Coronary angiogram classification of spontaneous coronary artery dissection. *Cath Cardiovasc Intervent.* 2014;84:1115–1122.

99. Saw J, Bezerra H, Gornik H, et al. Angiographic and intracoronary manifestations of coronary fibromuscular dysplasia. *Circulation.* 2016;133:1548–1559.

100. Tweet MS, Hayes SN, Pitta SR, et al. Clinical features, management, and prognosis of spontaneous coronary artery dissection. *Circulation.* 2012;126:579–588.

101. Saw J, Ricci D, Starovoytov A, et al. Spontaneous coronary artery dissection: prevalence of predisposing conditions including fibromuscular dysplasia in a tertiary center cohort. *JACC Cardiovasc Interv.* 2013;6:44–52.

102. Hayes SN, Kim ESH, Saw J, et al. Spontaneous coronary artery dissection: current state of the science. A scientific statement from the American Heart Association. *Circulation.* 2018;137:e1–e35.

103. Adlam D, Alfonso F, Maas A, et al. European Society of Cardiology, Acute Cardiovascular Care Association, SCAD study group: a position paper on spontaneous coronary artery dissection. *Eur Heart J.* 2018;0:1–21.

104. Lie JT, Berg KK. Isolated fibromuscular dysplasia of the coronary arteries with spontaneous dissection and myocardial infarction. *Hum Pathol.* 1987;18:654–656.

105. Michelis KC, Olin JW, Kadian-Dodov D, et al. Coronary artery manifestations of fibromuscular dysplasia. *J Am Coll Cardiol.* 2014;64:1033–1046.

106. van Twist DJL, de Leeuw PW, Kroon AA. Coronary tortuosity: a clue to the diagnosis of fibromuscular dysplasia? *Am J Hypertens.* 2017;30(8):776–780.

107. Jing HL, Hu BJ. Sudden death caused by stricture of the sinus node artery. *Am J Forensic Med Pathol.* 2002;23:83–89.

108. James TN, Marshall TK. De subitaneis mortibus. XVII. Multifocal stenosis due to fibromuscular dysplasia of the sinus node artery. *Circulation.* 1976;53(4):736–742.

109. Cohle SD, Suarez-Mier MP, Aguilera B. Sudden death resulting from lesions of the cardiac conduction system. *Am J Forensic Med Pathol.* 2002;23:83–89.

110. Zack F, Terpe H, Hammer U, Wegener R. Fibromuscular dysplasia of coronary arteries as a rare cause of death. *Int J Legal Med.* 1996;108:215–218.

111. Iannaccone SF, Farkas D, Ginelliova A, et al. Sudden death due to cystic tumor of the atrioventricular node and fibromuscular dysplasia involving branches of the coronary arteries. *Am J Forensic Med Pathol.* 2017;0:1–4.

112. Ropponen KM, Alafuzoff I. A case of sudden death cause by fibromuscular dysplasia. *J Clin Pathol.* 1999;52:541–542.

113. Hill SF, Shepphard MN. Non-atherosclerotic coronary artery disease associated with sudden cardiac death. *Heart.* 2010;96(14):1119–1125.

114. Zack F, Kutter G, Blaas V, et al. Fibromuscular dysplasia of cardiac conduction system arteries in traumatic and nonnatural sudden death victims aged 0 to 40 years: a histological analysis of 100 cases. *Cardiovascular Pathol.* 2014;23:12–16.

115. Dominguez FE, Tate LG, Robinson MJ. Familial fibromuscular dysplasia presenting as sudden death. *Am J Cardiovasc Pathol.* 1988;2(3):269–272.

116. Paz Suarez-Mier M, Aguilera B. Histopathology of the conduction system in sudden infant death. *Forensic Sci Int.* 1998;93:143–154.

117. Zack F, Kutter G, Blaas V, et al. Fibromuscular dysplasia of cardiac conduction system arteries in traumatic and non-natural sudden death victims aged 0 to 40 years: a histological analysis of 100 cases. *Cardiovas Pathol.* 2014;23:12–16.

118. Bolen MA, Brinza E, Renapurkar RD, et al. Screening CT angiography of the aorta, visceral branch vessels, and pelvic arteries in fibromuscular dysplasia. *JACC Cardiovasc Imaging.* 2017;10(5):554–561.

119. Heidt ST, Ganesh SK, Liu P, et al. Bilateral internal mammary artery fibromuscular dysplasia discovered upon evaluation for reconstructive breast surgery. *Vasc Med.* 2015;20(5):487–488.

120. Sharma AM, Gornik HL. Standing arterial waves is not fibromuscular dysplasia. *Circ Cardiovasc Interv.* 2012;5:e9–e11.

121. Jacobsen JCB, Beierholm U, Mikkelsen R, et al. "Sausage-string" appearance of arteries and arterioles can be caused by instability of the blood vessel wall. *Am J Physiol Regul Integr Comp Physiol.* 2002;283:R1118–R1130.

122. Alhalabi K, Menias C, Hines R, et al. Imaging and clinical findings in segmental arterial mediolysis (SAM). *Abdom Radiol.* 2017;42(2):602–611.

123. Slavin RE, Saeki K, Bhagavan B, Maas AE. Segmental arterial mediolysis: a precursor to fibromuscular dysplasia? *Mod Pathol.* 1995;8(3):287–294.

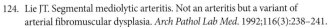

124. Lie JT. Segmental mediolytic arteritis. Not an arteritis but a variant of arterial fibromuscular dysplasia. *Arch Pathol Lab Med.* 1992;116(3):238–241.

125. Kalva SP, Somarouthu B, Jaff MR, Wicky S. Segmental arterial mediolysis: clinical and imaging features at presentation and during follow-up. *J Vasc Interv Radiol.* 2011;22(10):1380–1387.

126. Fillipone EJ, Foy A, Galanis T, Pokuah M, et al. Segmental arterial mediolysis: report of 2 cases and review of the literature. *Am J Kidney Dis.* 2011;58:981–987.

127. Meester JAN, Verstraeten A, Schepers D, et al. Differences in manifestations of Marfan syndrome, Ehlers-Danlos syndrome, and Loeys-Dietz syndrome. *Ann Cardiothorac Surg.* 2017;6(6):582–594.

128. van Twist DJL, Houben AJ, de Haan MW, et al. Renal hemodynamics and renin-angiotensin system activity in humans with multifocal renal artery fibromuscular dysplasia. *J Hypertens.* 2016;34(6):1160–1169.

129. Gowder MS, Loeb AL, Crouse LJ, Kramer PH. Complementary roles of color-flow duplex imaging and intravascular ultrasound in the diagnosis of renal artery fibromuscular dysplasia: should renal arteriography serve as the "gold standard"? *J Am Coll Cardiol.* 2003;56:525–532.

130. White CJ, Olin JW. Diagnosis and management of atherosclerotic renal artery stenosis: improving patient selection and outcomes. *Nat Clin Pract Cardiovasc Med.* 2009;6:176–190.

131. Sabharwal R, Vladica P, Coleman P. Multidetector spiral CT renal angiography in the diagnosis of renal artery fibromuscular dysplasia. *Eur J Radiol.* 2007;61:520–527.

132. Beregi JP, Louvegny S, Gautier C, et al. Fibromuscular dysplasia of the renal arteries: comparison of helical CT angiography and arteriography. *Am J Roentgenol.* 1999;172:27–34.

133. Hanning U, Sporns PB, Schmiedel M, et al. CT versus MR techniques in the detection of cervical artery dissection. *J Neuroimaging.* 2017;27(6):607–612.

134. Lu L, Zhang LJ, Poon CS, et al. Digital subtraction CT angiography for detection of intracranial aneurysms: comparison with three-dimensional digital subtraction angiography. *Radiology.* 2012;262:605–612.

135. Donmez H, Serifov E, Kahriman G, et al. Comparison of 16-row multislice CT angiography with conventional angiography for detection and evaluation of intracranial aneurysms. *Eur J Radiol.* 2011;80:455–461.

136. Willoteaux S, Faivre-Pierret M, Moranne O, et al. Fibromuscular dysplasia of the main renal arteries: comparison of contrast enhanced MR angiography with digital substraction angiography. *Radiology.* 2006;241(3):922–929.

137. Fabegra-Foster KE, Agarwal S, Rastegar N, et al. Efficacy and safety of gadobutrol-enhanced MRA of the renal arteries: results from GRAMS (Gadobutrol-enhanced renal artery MRA study), a prospective, intraindividual multicenter phase 3 blinded study. *J Magn Reson Imaging.* 2018;47(2):572–581.

138. Gornik HL, Persu A, Adlam D, et al. First International Consensus on the diagnosis and management of fibromuscular dysplasia. *Vasc Med.* 2019. [Epub ahead of print]

139. Colyer WR, Cooper CJ, Burket MW, et al. Utility of a "0.014" pressure sensing guidewire to assess renal artery translesional systolic pressure gradients. *Cath Cardiovasc Interv.* 2003;59:372–377.

140. De Bruyne B, Manoharan G, Pijls NH, et al. Assessment of renal artery stenosis severity by pressure gradient measurements. *J Am Coll Cardiol.* 2006;48:1851–1855.

141. Drieghe B, Madaric J, Sarno G, et al. Assessment of renal artery stenosis: side-by-side comparison of angiography and duplex ultrasound with pressure gradient measurements. *Eur Heart J.* 2008;29(4):517–524.

142. Kądziela J, Januszewicz A, Prejbisz A, et al. Prognostic value of renal fractional flow reserve in blood pressure response after renal artery stenting (PREFER study). *Cardiol J.* 2013;20(4):418–422.

143. Khoury MH, Gornik HL. Fibromuscular dysplasia (FMD). *Vasc Med.* 2017;22(3):248–252.

144. Vance CJ, Taylor RN, Craven TE, et al. Increased prevalence of preeclampsia among women undergoing procedural intervention for renal artery fibromuscular dysplasia. *Ann Vasc Surg.* 2015;29(6):1105–1110.

145. Berra E, Dominiczak AF, Touys RM, et al. Management of a pregnant woman with fibromuscular dysplasia. *Hypertension.* 2018;71(4):540–547.

146. Brott TG, Halperin JL, Abbara S, et al. 2011 ASA/AACF/AHA/ ANNN/ AANS/ACR/ASNR/CNS/SAIP/SCAI/SIR/SNIS/SVM/SVS guideline on the management of patients with extracranial carotid and vertebral artery disease: executive summary. *Circulation* 2011;124:489–532.

147. CADISS Trial Investigators, Markus HS, Hayter E, et al. Antiplatelet treatment compared with anticoagulation treatment for cervical artery dissection (CADISS): a randomised trial. *Lancet Neurol.* 2015;14(4):361–367.

148. Georgiadis D, Arnold M, von Buedingen HC, et al. Aspirin vs anticoagulation in carotid artery dissection: a study of 298 patients. *Neurology.* 2009;72:1810–1815.

149. Im C, Park HS, Kim DH, Lee T. Spontaneous renal artery dissection complicated by renal infarction: three case reports. *Vasc Specialist Int.* 2016;32(4):195–200.

150. Ramamoorthy SL, Vasquez JC, Taft PM, et al. Nonoperative management of acute spontaneous renal artery dissection. *Ann Vasc Surg.* 2002;16:157–162.

151. DeCarlo C, Ganguli S, Borges JC, et al. Presentation, treatment, and outcomes in patients with spontaneous isolated celiac and superior mesenteric artery dissection. *Vasc Med.* 2017;22(6):505–511.

152. Galastri FL, Cavalcante RN, Motta-Leal-Filho JM, et al. Evaluation and management of symptomatic isolated spontaneous celiac trunk dissection. *Vasc Med.* 2015;20:358–363.

153. Vaidya S, Dighe M. Spontaneous celiac artery dissection and its management. *J Radiol Case Rep.* 2010;4:30–33.

154. Whelton PK, Carey RM, Aronow WS, et al. ACC/AHA/AAPA/ABC/ ACPM/AGS/APhA/ASH/ASPC/NMA/PCNA Guideline for the Prevention, Detection, Evaluation, and Management of High Blood Pressure in Adults: A Report of the American College of Cardiology/ American Heart Association Task Force on Clinical Practice Guidelines. *Hypertension.* 2018;71(6):e13–e115.

155. Chobanian AV, Bakris GL, Black HR, et al. The Seventh Report of the Joint National Committee on Prevention, Detection, Evaluation, and Treatment of High Blood Pressure: the JNC 7 report. *JAMA.* 2003;289:2560–2572.

156. Grundy SM, Stone NJ, Bailey AL. 2018 AHA/ACC/AACVPR/AAPA/ ABC/ACPM/ADA/AGS/APhA/ASPC/NLA/PCNA guideline on the management of blood cholesterol: a report of the American College of Cardiology/American Heart Association Task Force on Clinical Practice Guidelines. *Circulation.* 2018.

157. Stegeman BH, de Bastos M, Rosendaal FR, et al. Different combined oral contraceptives and the risk of venous thrombosis: systematic review and network meta-analysis. *BMJ.* 2013;347:f5298.

158. Roach RE, Helmerhorst FM, Lijfering WM, et al. Combined oral contraceptives: the risk of myocardial infarction and ischemic stroke. *Cochrane Database Syst Rev.* 2015;8:CD011054.

159. Davies MG, Saad WE, Peden EK, et al. The long term outcomes of percutaneous therapy for renal artery fibromuscular dysplasia. *J Vasc Surg.* 2008;48:865–871.

160. Gavalas MV, Gasparis AP, Tassiopoulos AK, et al. Long-term follow-up for percutaneous transluminal angioplasty in renal artery fibromuscular dysplasia. *Int Angiol.* 2015;34(6):529–537.

161. Trinquart L, Mounier-Vehier C, Sapoval M, et al. Efficacy of revascularization for renal artery stenosis caused by fibromuscular dysplasia: a systematic review and meta-analysis. *Hypertension.* 2010;56:525–532.

162. Ramsay LE, Waller PC. Blood pressure response to percutaneous transluminal angioplasty for renovascular hypertension: an overview of published series. *BMJ.* 1990;300:569–572.

163. Matsumoto AH, Spinosa DJ, Angle F, et al. Evaluation and endovascular therapy for renal artery stenosis. In: Baum S, Pentecost MJ, eds. *Abram's Angiography: Interventional Radiology.* 2nd ed. Philadelphia: Lippincott Williams & Wilkins; 2006:362–397.

164. Mousa AY, Campbell JE, Stone PA, et al. Short- and long-term outcomes of percutaneous transluminal angioplasty/stenting of renal fibromuscular dysplasia over a ten-year period. *J Vasc Surg.* 2012;55:421–427.

165. Barrier P, Julien A, Guillaume C, et al. Technical and clinical results after percutaneous angioplasty in nonmedial fibromuscular dysplasia: outcome after endovascular management of unifocal renal artery stenosis in 30 patients. *Cardiovasc Intervent Radiol.* 2010;33(3):270–277.

166. Raju MG, Bajzer CT, Clair DG, et al. Renal artery stent fracture in patients with fibromuscular dysplasia: a cautionary tale. *Circ Cardiovasc Interv*. 2013;6:e30–e31.

167. van der Kolk NM, Algra A, Rinkel GJ. Risk of aneurysm rupture at intracranial arterial bifurcations. *Cerebrovasc Dis*. 2010;30:29–35.

168. Komotar RJ, Mocco J, Solomon RA. Guidelines for the surgical treatment of unruptured intracranial aneurysms: the first annual. J Lawrence Pool Memorial Research Symposium: controversies in the management of cerebral aneurysms. *Neurosurgery*. 2008;62:183–193.

169. Molyneux A, Kerr R, Stratton I, et al. International Subarachnoid Aneurysm Trial (ISAT) of neurosurgical clipping versus endovascular coiling in 2143 patients with ruptured intracranial aneurysms: a randomised trial. *Lancet*. 2002;360:1267–1274.

170. Tweet MS, Eleid MF, Best PJM, et al. Spontaneous coronary artery dissection: revascularization versus conservative therapy. *Circ Cardiovasc Interv*. 2014;7:777–786.

171. Ketha SS, Bjarnason H, Oderich GS, Misra S. Clinical features and endovascular management of iliac artery fibromuscular dysplasia. *J Vasc Interv Radiol*. 2014;25(6):949–953.

172. Stanley JC, Henke P. Vascular surgery. In: Lumley JS, Hoballab JJ, eds. *Renal Artery Bypass. Springer Surgery Atlas Series*. Berlin, Springer-Verlag; 2009.

173. Lindblad B, Gottsäter A. Renal disease: fibrodysplasia. In: Cronenwett JL, Johnston KW, eds. *Rutherford's Vascular Surgery*. 7th ed.Philadelphia: Elsevier; 2010.

174. Stanley JC, Whitehouse Jr. WM, Zelenock GB, et al. Reoperation for complications of renal artery reconstructive surgery undertaken for treatment of renovasuclar hypertension. *J Vasc Surg*. 1985;2(1):133–144.

175. Novick AC. Microvascular reconstruction of complex branch renal artery disease. *Urol Clin North Am*. 1984;11(3):465–475.

176. Duprey A, Chavent B, Meyer-Bisch V, et al. Editor's choice – Ex vivo renal artery repair with kidney autotransplantation for renal artery branch aneurysms: long-term results of sixty-seven procedures. *Eur J Vasc Endovasc Surg*. 2016;51(6):872–879.

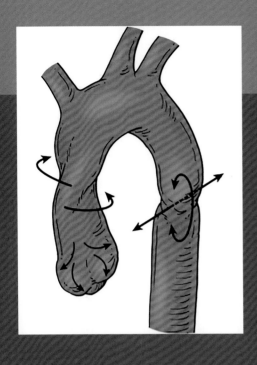

中文导读

第59章
血管感染

　　血管感染至今仍然是难以诊断和面临技术挑战的疾病，常合并其他疾病导致患者营养不良和免疫缺陷。目前已发表的相关文献尚不足，限制了医师的循证医学医疗决策。血管感染包括原发性感染和继发性感染。原发性感染通常是在已有的血管病理基础（如动脉粥样硬化斑块、动脉瘤、动脉夹层或先前的损伤）上菌血症所致。由于人体自身抗感染的免疫机制多样，无血管病理状态或损伤的原发性血管感染是少见的。继发性感染主要见于人工移植物或支架材料被感染原定植，并引起邻近血管结构的感染。继发性感染更为常见，因为较低的细菌滴度即可引起人工移植物感染。从理论上讲，血管感染可以发生在血管结构的任何地方，然而，部分解剖部位发生感染的概率更高。本章将描述较常见的外周血管（动脉和静脉）感染的定义、病理生理学、预防、诊断和治疗，不包括涉及颅内血管或冠状血管的感染。

李毅清

Vascular Infections

Jayer Chung

Vascular infections represent difficult diagnostic and technical challenges for even the most experienced physicians. Multiple comorbidities frequently afflict the patients, resulting in nutritional and immunologic deficiencies. Patients are often near the end of life as well, further complicating the decision-making for the patients, caregivers, and physicians. Moreover, published series regarding vascular infections are underpowered, which limits the ability for physicians to provide data-driven care.

Vascular infections include both primary and secondary infections. Primary infections often result from bacteremia seeding an underlying vascular pathology, such as atherosclerotic plaque, aneurysm, dissection, or prior injury. Due to multiple, redundant mechanisms that exist to prevent vascular infection, primary vascular infections without an underlying vascular pathology or injury are rare. Secondary infections occur when prosthetic graft or stent material becomes seeded, and cause infection of the adjacent vascular structures. Secondary infections are much more common, due to the lower bacterial inoculum required to cause a prosthetic infection. Theoretically, vascular infections can occur wherever a vascular structure becomes infected; however, there are several anatomic locales where infections occur most frequently. This chapter will describe the definitions, pathophysiology, prevention, diagnosis, and management of some of the more commonly encountered vascular infections in the periphery, excluding those involving the intracranial or coronary circulations. Arterial and venous infections are discussed.

PRIMARY ARTERIAL INFECTIONS

Primary arterial infections (PAIs) were first described by Koch, who detailed the case of a patient who presented with a ruptured mycotic superior mesenteric artery (SMA) aneurysm in 1851.[1] Since then, there have been multiple small case series and case reports of PAI in the literature, affecting multiple vascular beds. The definition of PAIs has been difficult, as there are multiple specific etiologies of PAI. Categorization of PAIs did not occur until 1978 when Wilson et al. described six different variants of PAIs (Table 59.1).[2]

Mycotic aneurysms describe areas of previously uninfected artery that are seeded by septic emboli secondary to endocarditis. This segment of artery subsequently undergoes degeneration, and becomes aneurysmal. Mycotic aneurysms tend to occur in areas where a septic focus might lodge, though theoretically, these can occur anywhere in the arterial circulation.[2] *Microbial arteritis* occurs when bacterial seeding of a previously uninfected atherosclerotic plaque occurs without aneurysmal degeneration.[2] *Infected aneurysms* result from seeding of a preexisting aneurysm secondary to bacteremia. Since the thrombus of aneurysms is rarely sent for culture, the true prevalence of infected aneurysms is unknown.[2] *Traumatic infected pseudoaneurysms* occur at a site of focal rupture of the artery secondary to iatrogenic arterial access, intravascular drug abuse, or trauma (blunt or penetrating). The surrounding tissues contain the hemorrhage, such that the wall of the pseudoaneurysm is composed of compressed periarterial connective tissue. The hematoma and pseudoaneurysm are likely seeded at the time of the initial insult.[2]

Contiguous arterial infections occur when an infectious nidus erodes into an adjacent artery, resulting in pseudoaneurysm formation and/or rupture. These often occur in the context of resection for neoplasms. The fields are frequently irradiated, with the patient often having undergone chemotherapy, resulting in complex chronic wounds. When wounds are adjacent to major vascular structures, the contiguous infection may compromise the nearby vasculature.[2] A *primary aortoenteric fistula (AEF)* is thought to form when a mycotic aneurysm gradually enlarges, resulting in repetitive pulsatile pressure upon adjacent gastrointestinal (GI) structures. Over time, iterative pressure and aneurysmal enlargement coupled with weakening of intestinal wall causes a communication between the mycotic aneurysm and GI tract, resulting in an AEF.[2] To limit confusion, and to maintain continuity with prior chapters, the terms *infected aneurysm* and *PAI* will be used interchangeably to generally refer to these six entities (see Table 59.1).

Untreated PAI have several sequelae, the most significant of which is the propensity of arterial rupture and exsanguination. Microbes cause degradation of the arterial wall, resulting in aneurysm and pseudoaneurysm formation. Unchecked, the microbial-mediated destruction of arterial integrity will exceed the ability to contain hemorrhage.[1,2] Second, the site of PAI can serve as a nidus of septic arterial embolus formation, particularly when accompanied by aneurysmal degeneration. Septic emboli can also result in end-organ ischemia, further complicating the management of the PAI.[2] Finally, PAI can serve as a source of bacteremia, resulting in septic complications, and further inoculate previously uninfected sites in the vasculature.[2]

Pathophysiology of Primary Arterial Infections
Destruction of the Aortic Wall

Infected aneurysms are characterized by focal destruction of the arterial wall. They grow more rapidly than their noninfected counterparts, and are considered to have an increased rupture risk.[3] Pathologic specimens of infected aneurysms are infrequently reported. Hsu and Lin[4] showed that 100% of infected aneurysms showed evidence of atherosclerosis. The next most frequent finding was acute suppurative inflammation, found in two-thirds of their specimens. Atherosclerosis and chronic inflammation were found in 15% of their subjects.[4] This suggests that the organisms causing PAI are more likely to be rather virulent, inciting a vigorous acute inflammatory response. This significance of atherosclerosis was affirmed by Miller et al.[5] who found atherosclerosis was present in 75% of their mycotic aneurysm specimens.

Collagenases and elastases appear to play a central role in the development of infected aneurysms. The precise origin of these

TABLE 59.1   Variants of Primary Arterial Infections

Term	Definition
Mycotic aneurysm	Area of previously uninfected artery that is seeded by septic emboli, which subsequently undergoes degeneration and aneurysmal enlargement
Infected aneurysm	Hematogenous seeding of a preexisting aneurysm
Traumatic infected pseudoaneurysm	Area of focal rupture of an artery, which forms a pseudoaneurysm. The associated hematoma becomes infected, likely seeded at the time of injury
Contiguous arterial infection	Erosion of an infectious nidus into an adjacent artery
Primary aortoenteric fistula	Erosion of an aneurysm into an adjacent gastrointestinal structure, most commonly the duodenum
Microbial arteritis	Hematogenous seeding of previously uninfected atherosclerotic plaque

proteases is unclear, however. Buckmaster et al.[3] isolated the bacteria as well as the aortic tissue from four patients undergoing suprarenal mycotic aortic aneurysm repair. The authors concluded that elastases were produced mainly from host neutrophils, rather than the infecting microorganism, or the host macrophages. The exception was *Pseudomonas aeruginosa* which was the only microbe to produce elastin-degrading enzymes.[3]

Conversely, other works have shown that bacteria, such as *Streptococcus mutans, Bacteroides* sp., *Escherichia coli, Staphylococcus aureus,* and *Staphylococcus epidermidis*[6] can produce collagenases. Moreover, many microbes are capable of activating matrix metalloproteinases-1, -8, and -9, which can degrade the aortic wall resulting in infected aneurysms.[7] Since collagen provides much of the tensile strength to the aortic wall, the activation of collagenases and subsequent rapid degradation of the aortic wall is significant. While the precise mechanism of infected aneurysm development is unclear, further investigations will prove illuminating when attempting to understand the pathophysiology, and to design novel therapeutics for the management of PAI. The pathophysiology of PAI is summarized in Fig. 59.1.

Source of Infection and Host Response

The source of bacteria is variable. Infective endocarditis is no longer the most prevalent cause of infected aneurysms.[8] Contiguous spread, bacteremia, and embolization from a septic source represent frequent sources of infection, though many times, the etiology is unclear. Atherosclerotic lesions, areas of preexisting aneurysmal degeneration, and traumatic injury all predispose patients toward the development of infected aneurysms.[4,5]

Some authors posit that infected and uninfected aneurysms may represent either end of the spectrum of the same disease, with the presentation hinging upon the virulence of the organism and the host immunologic response. These authors cite the fact that approximately half of presumably uninfected aneurysms harbor *Chlamydia pneumoniae*.[9] While this opinion is not widely held, the concept emphasizes the role of the host immunologic response in the development of infected aneurysms, which does play a significant role in the destruction of the

vessel wall. Immunodeficiency (chronic immunosuppressive use, malnutrition, diabetes mellitus, malignancy, human immunodeficiency virus [HIV] syndrome, chronic hepatitis) appears necessary in over 50% of cases,[10] which is logical given the prevalence of bacteremia in everyday life, relative to the infrequency of PAI.

Bacteriology of Infected Aneurysms

The microbes responsible vary depending upon the series, era of publication, and location of the infected aneurysm. In the past, grampositive organisms were predominantly found in blood and arterial cultures of patients afflicted with infected aneurysms.[2] More recent series have found gram-negative organisms to occur more frequently than in prior reports,[11] perhaps due to the concomitant increased prevalence of gram-negative bacteremia noted in the elderly population. The bacteriology seems to be continually evolving, though this may reflect publication bias, where only novel microorganisms now merit publication. Other microorganisms recently described include *Streptococcus agalactiae*,[12] methicillin-resistant *S. aureus, E. coli*, and other gramnegative species.[13] *Mycobacterium bovis* and other caseating microorganisms are also being reported.[14] However, the broader distribution of causal organisms in PAI may reflect an increased prevalence of immunocompromised hosts.[14,15] Improvements in culture techniques may also be partly responsible for the increased identification of atypical organisms, such as *Campylobacter, Listeria*, or *Coxiella* sp.[15]

Salmonella infections merit special mention in PAI. This is especially true for primary aortic infections,[4,9] where the prevalence ranges between 17% and 67%. The prevalence of *Salmonella* appears highest among East Asian populations.[4] Within Western populations, *Salmonella* causes a higher percentage of PAI compared to secondary arterial infections (SAIs). However, other microorganisms are more prevalent than *Salmonella* in Western populations. Interestingly, *Salmonella* infections may be associated with a lower risk of mortality relative to infection with other microorganisms.[4] The significance is that a history of an antecedent gastrointestinal illness may help to heighten a physician's suspicion of an infected aneurysm caused by *Salmonella*.

Syphilis was the most common cause of mycotic aneurysms prior to antibiotics. Since the introduction of penicillin, however, the prevalence of cardiovascular manifestations of chronic syphilis has declined to where the description is rare enough to warrant publication as a case report.[16] Previous reports cited that most of these aneurysms occurred in the aortic arch and thoracic aorta.[16] The causal treponemal infection of the vasa vasorum results in significant inflammation which weakens the involved segments of the aorta, resulting ultimately in aneurysmal degeneration.[16] While rare, syphilis must remain in the differential diagnosis, especially in the setting of immunodeficiency and a history of other sexually transmitted diseases.

Common Locations and Presentations of Primary Arterial Infections

Theoretically, PAI can occur anywhere in the arterial tree. Among aortic infections, the suprarenal and thoracic aorta are most common and clinically problematic. Aneurysms of the visceral arteries and carotid arteries are frequently mycotic, and represent significant clinical challenges due to the infrequency of clinical presentation, and the technical challenges associated with repair. Femoral artery pseudoaneurysms, either due to iatrogenic catheterizations or due to intravenous drug abuse, are increasing in prevalence due to the increase in percutaneous coronary and peripheral vascular interventions. Presentations depend upon the location, with infected aneurysms that are more superficial, providing more classic symptoms of hemorrhage, pulsatile mass, overlying erythema, with pain or tenderness to palpation. Conversely,

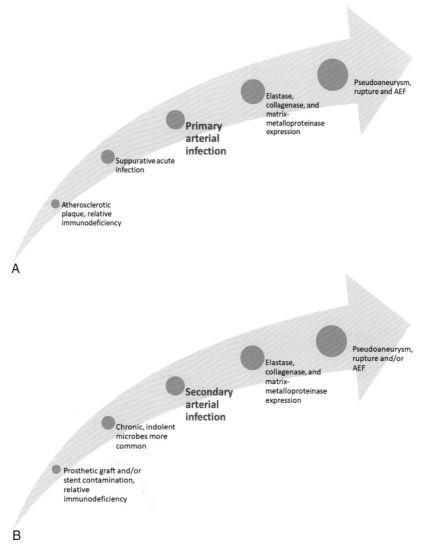

Fig. 59.1 Pathophysiology of primary (A) and secondary (B) arterial infections. The pathophysiology for primary arterial infections is dominated by infection of preexisting atherosclerotic plaque with suppurative microorganisms. Conversely, secondary arterial infections are more commonly caused by indolent microorganisms that contaminate a prosthetic material. The classic microorganism is *Staphylococcus epidermidis. AEF,* aortoenteric fistula.

infected aneurysms occurring more centrally, such as those within the visceral arteries or in the aorta, present more insidiously with a significant amount of symptom overlap with other conditions. Aortic and visceral artery infected aneurysms therefore require a higher index of suspicion from the physician.

Primary Infections of the Aorta

More recent European data suggest that there is no significant predilection of infection in any segment of the aorta.[15] Prior American studies, however, suggest that approximately one-third of PAIs occur in the infrarenal aorta. The remainder are found in the ascending aorta, arch, descending thoracic aorta, or suprarenal aorta.[17,18] The variability in the distribution appears to stem from the variable sample sizes reported in the literature. Mycotic aortic aneurysm comprises approximately 0.7% to 2.6% of all aneurysm diagnoses in the United States.[11]

Symptomatic presentations are common, occurring in up to 84% of patients, with overt rupture exceeding 50%.[15,17,18] Rapid expansion is the norm, occurring in as little as 7 days,[17,18] and likely varies depending upon the virulence of the predominant organisms causing

the infected aneurysm, as well as host factors. Saccular morphologies were found in 94% in the Mayo experience, and echoed in other series.[15,17,18] Symptoms are likely common at presentation due to the indolent course prior to presentation with rupture, AEF, and/or sepsis. Moreover, due to their infrequency, lack of physician suspicion likely results in delays in diagnosis, until the patient symptoms and extremis necessitate and obviate the diagnosis.

Visceral Artery Infected Aneurysms

Visceral mycotic aneurysms include those occurring within the distribution of the celiac axis, SMA, inferior mesenteric artery (IMA), or renal arteries. As a whole, these entities are exceedingly rare. The most frequent arterial distribution for visceral artery infected aneurysms is the SMA, comprising 88% of visceral artery aneurysms in older series.[8] Hence much of the discussion will focus on SMA infected aneurysms.

A recent review of mycotic SMA aneurysms revealed that approximately two-thirds present with epigastric pain, with 60% presenting with fever.[19] Nonspecific malaise, nausea and vomiting, and weight loss also occur in approximately 20% to 25% of patients. The median age is 36 years, with a male predominance of 3:1. An antecedent history of subacute bacterial endocarditis and intravenous drug abuse appear most frequently.[19] Because the symptoms are nonspecific, some have recommended entertaining the diagnosis of infected SMA aneurysms in the differential if patients present with the pentad of abdominal pain, fever of unknown origin, malaise, weight loss, and nausea. The microbiology is somewhat different from mycotic aortic aneurysms, with *Streptococcus* sp. appearing in almost 50% of case reports.[19] *Staphylococcus* sp. occur next in frequency, occurring in almost 30% of reports.[19]

Infected aneurysms of the celiac axis are the next most frequently reported. Symptoms are slightly different, with jaundice and hematemesis accompanying the abdominal pain.[20] Reports of septic embolization and infarction have also been reported with celiac axis–infected aneurysms.[12] Microbiology is similar to SMA mycotic aneurysms.[12,20] Also similar to SMA-infected aneurysms, bacterial endocarditis and intravenous drug abuse histories often precede the discovery of infected celiac axis aneurysms.[12,20]

Mortality from infected visceral artery aneurysms with antibiotic therapy alone has been reported in up to 50%, with rupture-associated mortality approaching 100%.[8,19] Therefore surgical intervention is warranted should the patient be physiologically fit enough to tolerate the required procedure. Specific surgical options will be discussed in the ensuing sections regarding management.

Femoral Artery Infected Pseudoaneurysms

Infected femoral artery pseudoaneurysms due to intravenous drug abuse. Intravenous drug abusers can theoretically damage any vessel used to inject illicit substances. Most frequently, the common femoral and superficial femoral artery in the groin are involved (Fig. 59.2).[21–24] Other less common sites include the axillary and brachial arteries.[21] Iterative puncture without sterile technique results in repetitive intraarterial introduction of microbes. Multiple products are also combined with the illicit substances to augment or dilute the effect, all of which may also be caustic to the artery and the surrounding tissues.[21,24] Symptomatic presentations, including acute hemorrhage,

systemic sepsis, a pulsatile mass, or limb ischemia, are frequent.[21–24] The most common presentation varies depending upon the series and the location of the mycotic pseudoaneurysm. Without appropriate surgical therapy, hemorrhage, limb loss, and/or death ensues rapidly.

Most patients are young, with the majority presenting in their early 30s.[21–24] Reports vary in their description of the predominant gender. Bacteriology of mycotic pseudoaneurysms from drug abuse vary among reports. If single microbial isolates are reported, the most common organisms are *S. aureus* and *S. epidermidis*.[21–24] Methicillin-resistant *S. aureus* may be becoming more prevalent in the United States.[23] However, 18% to 50% of series describe polymicrobial infections,[22,24] which is intuitive given the repeated arterial punctures without adherence to sterile technique. Concurrent infection with hepatitis C and/or HIV is the norm, occurring in as many as 90% and 67%, respectively.[22] A history of prior iliofemoral deep venous thrombosis is also common, occurring in over 70% of subjects in one series.[22]

Iatrogenic infected pseudoaneurysms of the femoral artery. In spite of advances in the medical management of atherosclerosis, the rates of percutaneous coronary intervention remain largely unchanged. Approximately 600,000 to 1,000,000 procedures per annum are performed in the United States.[25] This number underestimates the true figure, however, as peripheral interventions are not included in these studies. Moreover, percutaneous methods of closure are becoming increasingly prevalent following aortic endografting and structural heart procedures. Thus while iatrogenic catheterization-related infected aneurysms are rare, they remain a clinically significant entity simply due to the volume of catheterizations performed annually in the United States.

The rate of infection varies from 0.01% to 0.9%, depending upon the source.[26,27] A recent meta-analysis suggests that infection is three times as likely with a vascular closure device versus manual compression alone.[26] The specific mechanisms of action for the vascular closure device does not seem to impact infection rates, though no study is adequately powered to truly address this question. Likely, however, those that leave more foreign material are more likely to become infected, as the inoculum required to infect foreign material is lower. Risk factors

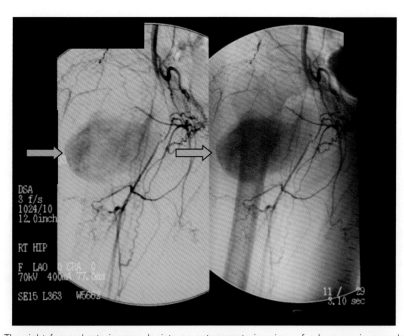

Fig. 59.2 The right femoral arteriogram depicts an anteroposterior view of a large groin pseudoaneurysm *(blue arrows)* secondary to intravenous drug abuse. Note that the chronic injection and the mass effect of the pseudoaneurysm also resulted in the occlusion of the underlying common and profunda femoral arteries.

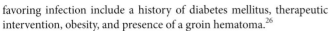

favoring infection include a history of diabetes mellitus, therapeutic intervention, obesity, and presence of a groin hematoma.[26]

Patients often present with pain, tenderness, and a pseudoaneurysm of the common femoral or superficial femoral artery in conjunction with fever and/or chills. Gram-positive organisms, such as *S. aureus* or *S. epidermidis*, predominate, though gram-negative organisms have also been isolated.[27] Due to the predominance of skin flora, periprocedural contamination is the most likely source. Hence periprocedural adherence to antiseptic technique is critical. Symptoms may occur within days to weeks of the initial procedures.[27] While the presentation is often milder than with infected aneurysm from intravenous drug abuse, the patients are frequently older, with atherosclerotic risk factors.

Primary Carotid Artery Infections

Primary infected aneurysms of the extracranial carotid are exceedingly rare. Over 35 years, only 45 cases had been reported in the world literature.[28,29] However, due to the anatomic location and importance of the end-organ that the carotid artery supplies, these entities merit special mention. Typical presentations include an enlarging, painful pulsatile mass in the lateral neck associated with fever, dysphonia, and dysphagia.[28,29] Impingement of nearby nerves can present as palsies of cranial nerves X and XII, Horner syndrome, exophthalmos, or ophthalmoplegia.[29] Untreated, these may result in septic embolization of mural thrombus within the infected aneurysm sac. Alternatively, these may rupture, which may present as oropharyngeal bleeding, airway compromise, and/or stroke.[29]

Frequent responsible microorganisms include *S aureus*. Case reports of multiple other microbes include *Salmonella* sp., *Klebsiella* sp., *E. coli*, *Proteus mirabilis*, *Yersinia* sp., and *Corynebacterium* sp. Prior to the widespread use of antibiotics, *Mycobacterium* sp. and *Treponema* sp. infections were also common.[28] While infrequent, *Mycobacteria* and *Treponema* infection remain important in the differential among immunocompromised patients, or among patients without access to modern medical care. Leukocytosis and/or an elevated sedimentation rate may be present, but are often nonspecific.[30] Blood cultures may aid in the diagnosis, but are negative in up to half of cases.[30] The differential diagnosis includes carotid body tumor, peritonsillar abscess, cervical lymphadenitis, or kinking/redundancy of the extracranial carotid vasculature.[28–30]

Other Primary Infected Aneurysms

The aforementioned sites are the most common sites of PAI. In the lower extremities, there have been infrequent case reports describing primary infected aneurysms of the popliteal, tibial, and pedal vasculature.[31–33] In the lower extremity vasculature, due to the relatively superficial location compared to the abdomen or chest, presentation is relatively consistent, with a painful, pulsatile enlarging mass with fever and erythema overlying the involved artery.[31–33] Signs and symptoms of distal ischemia may also be present. The infected aneurysms of the lower extremity vasculature are classically caused by endocarditis with septic emboli,[32] though hematogenous spread from a noncontiguous source,[33] or from direct puncture (iatrogenic, or due to illicit drug injections) are also prevalent. The true frequency of microorganisms causing infected peripheral aneurysms in the lower extremity is unclear due to publication bias, which likely results in underreporting of the more common infections. Gram-positive organisms are most frequently found in the literature, though cases of *Salmonella* sp. as well as *Candida* sp. have also been reported.[31–33]

Upper extremity infected arterial aneurysms are also rare. The most frequently reported are secondary to illicit drug abuse and iatrogenic puncture.[21] Signs and symptoms are similar to infected aneurysms of other superficial sites, with an enlarging, painful, pulsatile mass with overlying erythema and fevers. Signs of distal ischemia may also be present, such as cyanosis, petechiae, and splinter hemorrhages.[21] The microbiology is similar to that of other peripheral infected aneurysms, with gram-positive organisms predominating, but with a significant minority of gram-negative and mixed infections as well.[21]

SECONDARY ARTERIAL INFECTIONS

Prosthetic conduits have extended the ability of physicians to manage arterial pathologies. Unfortunately, the advent of prosthetic conduits has given rise to the rare, though devastating, complication of SAIs, where the conduit and the adjacent artery become infected. While multiple advances have occurred over the last several decades, SAIs remain a difficult diagnostic challenge, and among the most challenging technical and emotional problems a surgeon may encounter.

Prosthetic graft infections are classified by extent of graft involvement, timing since initial implantation, and severity of graft involvement when associated with surgical site infections. While not widely used clinically, these classifications are helpful when studying SAIs, and ensure equitable outcome comparisons. Bunt described graft infections as cavitary and extracavitary.[34] A P0 infection involves a cavitary (intraabdominal or intrathoracic) graft, or the cavitary portion of a graft. Examples include infections of an aortic tube graft or infections of the aortic portion of an aortobifemoral bypass graft. P1 infections are extracavitary only, such as prosthetic lower extremity bypass graft infections. P2 infections are those that involve the extracavitary portion of a graft that has both intracavitary and extracavitary components. An example is an isolated infection of the femoral limb of an aortobifemoral bypass graft. P3 infections involve prosthetic patches, such as an infected femoral artery patch after a common femoral endarterectomy. Bunt's classifications also include qualifiers for aortoenteric erosions (AEE), and AEF, which he termed graft-enteric erosions and fistulae, respectively.[34] AEE and AEF are similar in that both involve a communication between an enteric structure and infected aortic prosthesis. They differ in that AEE do not involve the suture line between the aorta and the infected prosthetic. Finally, there is a qualifier for an aortic stump infection, where there is an infection of the distal prosthetic stump after ligation and extra-anatomic bypass for a prior aortic graft infection.

Early graft infections are those that occur with 4 weeks of implantation of the prosthetic. When these are associated with surgical site infections, these wounds are classified by the Szilagyi classification, which has since been modified by Samson and colleagues.[35,36] Szilagyi class I and II infections are superficial wound infections, and do not pertain to vascular infection. Szilagyi class III infections are those that involve the vascular graft and native artery.[35] Samson and colleagues further classified those that involve the graft into several categories. Group 3 infections involve the graft, but do not involve the graft-arterial anastomosis. Group 4 infections are complicated by an exposed anastomosis, but do not have bacteremia or bleeding. Group 5 infections are the worst, and involve the anastomosis and are associated with bleeding from the suture line and/or bacteremia.[36] The Szilagyi and Samson classifications are not necessarily named when describing surgical site infections involving vascular prostheses. However, these definitions do aid in risk stratification and clinical decision-making.

Pathophysiology of Secondary Arterial Infections

Immunodeficiency and nutritional deficiency that exist for PAI also occur in the SAI populations, thereby acting as a cofactor for prosthetic graft infections. Infectious sources include intraoperative contamination, hematogenous spread, or spread from a contiguous source.

The role of collagenases and elastases upon the pathogenesis of SAI is similar to PAI, and have been discussed previously. Hence this section will highlight the mechanisms underlying the increased susceptibility to infection with prosthetic materials.

Prosthetic arterial grafts become infected more easily than native arteries, and require a 10,000-fold lower inoculum to become infected.[37] The most common prosthetic materials include polyethylene terephthalate (Dacron) and polytetrafluoroethylene (Gore-Tex).[37] Specific to SAI, there are three separate factors that potentiate SAI: graft factors, ineffective host immune responses, and bacterial biofilm formation. Microbes preferentially adhere to prosthetic graft relative to the host tissue for several reasons. Synthetics are irregularly surface fomites, that create relatively avascular pockets that may harbor microbes.[38] Upon implantation, prosthetic grafts are also coated almost immediately by multiple host proteins, the most notable of which are fibrinogen, fibronectin, and laminin. These each increase the risk of prosthetic infection as they mediate bacterial binding.[38,39] Charged prosthetics, in contrast to electrically neutral materials, also increase the propensity for bacterial adherence.[39] Hydrophilic materials exhibit decreased bacterial adherence relative to hydrophobic materials.[39]

The host response can also paradoxically abrogate immune cells ability to eradicate pathogens. For instance, contact with the prosthetic causes neutrophils and natural killer cells to degranulate. Hence when they do contact bacteria, even if favorably opsonized by complement, these cells are less likely to be bacteriocidal, as they no longer have sufficient respiratory burst to act upon the bacteria.[37] Similarly, phagocytic cells exhibit impaired activity against bacteria in the presence of prosthetic material.[37] Attenuation of the immune cell response is worsened with increased complement activation against the foreign material, which increases inflammation and further attracts phagocytes and neutrophils to the area of implantation.[37] Neointimal formation along the graft is critical to decreasing infection rates, and requires a minimum of 2 weeks to form.[37]

Bacteria have also developed several mechanisms to evade the host immune response, the most notorious of which is the formation of biofilm.[37–39] This occurs after adhesion of the bacteria to the graft, which then begin to form exopolysaccharide matrix, or "slime."[39] The slime improves adherence, and protects the bacteria from immune cells and antibiotics in the serum. Within the biofilm, the metabolic rate is altered via quorum-sensing, or the ability to decrease the metabolic rate when other microbes are in close proximity. Quorum-sensing decreases the ability of host defenses to detect and eradicate microbes.[38,39] Biofilms also serve as a method to more efficiently transport nutrients and waste to and from the colony.[39]

Finally, bacteria may reside within the cells of the host.[37] Certain microorganisms are obligate intracellular organisms. Other microorganisms, however, are traditionally considered extracellular bacteria, but develop the capacity to live within the host cells in the presence of prosthetic materials.[37] When intracellular, the microorganisms dramatically decrease their metabolic rate, and are protected against the immune response by the host cell. These small intracellular colonies can then proliferate slowly over the course of years, until they reach a sufficient density, become extracellular, and infect the prosthesis.[37]

Common Locations and Presentations of Secondary Arterial Infections

SAI can theoretically occur wherever a prosthetic graft, patch, or stent is placed in continuity with the artery. Hence these infections will be localized to where prosthetics are frequently utilized. The presentation depends upon the virulence of the microorganisms, the extent of graft involvement, and anatomic locale involved. These will be described in further detail in the following subheadings. There are three main locations where prosthetic arterial infections occur: the aorta, the lower extremity, and the carotid artery.

Aortic Graft Infections

Aortic graft infections are highly lethal and represent some of the most diagnostically, technically, and emotionally challenging cases that surgeons may face. The inflammation that is frequently encountered with infection is worsened by the scar tissue and adhesions from the prior surgery, which obliterates anatomic dissection planes. Each case requires individualized management that matches the patients' and caregivers' wishes with the anatomic and surgical requirements for appropriate therapy.

While significantly more prevalent than primary aortic infections, aortic graft infections remain underdiagnosed, with significant diagnostic delays translating into treatment delays with markedly diminished chances of successful outcome. Data from the United Kingdom Small Aneurysm Trial suggest that 2% of open aortic reconstructions are complicated by infection.[40] More contemporary registry data, however, portray a lower rate of aortic graft infections, with both open and endovascular aortic graft infections occurring in less than 1%.[41] Large single center cohort data from Baylor College of Medicine also confirm the <1% rate of graft infection after open thoracoabdominal aortic aneurysm repairs.[42] The rates after thoracic endograft placement are difficult to measure, as the series in the literature are significantly smaller than those describing infrarenal aortic endograft infections.[43,44] Logically this follows, since the prevalence of thoracic endograft placement is significantly lower than infrarenal aortic endograft placement. No particular manufacturer or stent graft design is associated with an increased risk of aortic endograft infection.[43,44]

The microbiology of aortic graft infections belies the most likely causes of aortic graft infections, and differs somewhat from that of primary aortic infected aneurysms. *Staphylococcal* and *Streptococcal* sp. are responsible for up to 55% of aortic graft infections.[43–45] These microorganisms are consistent with the theory that intraoperative contamination is responsible for many, and perhaps most, aortic graft infections. Gram-negative organisms and anaerobes are the next most frequent organisms.[45] *Candida* sp. are particularly prevalent with AEF.[45–49] Hence their presence should raise one's suspicion of an AEF. The causal organisms are not cultured many times, due likely to the lack of cultures prior to the institution of antibiotic therapy.[45–49] Moreover, culture techniques are biased against slow-growing organisms so that the prevalence of anaerobes, fungi, and fastidious organisms is likely underrepresented.

Common clinical presentations of aortic graft infections. Since delays in therapy can be catastrophic, recognizing common presentations is essential to minimize diagnostic delays. This is especially true since many of the signs and symptoms overlap significantly with other conditions that occur with greater frequency. Frequently, patients with aortic graft infection present similarly to patients with fever of unknown origin and malaise. Pain in the region of the infection is also common. Laboratory markers of inflammation are usually present, such as an elevated C-reactive protein or erythrocyte sedimentation rate.[45,47] Local signs and symptoms of infection are more difficult to localize when occurring in the intracavitary portions of aortic grafts. The urgency of the presentation and therapy depends upon the severity of sepsis upon presentation. Patients with more severe hypotension and tachycardia unresponsive to resuscitation will require a more urgent intervention.

If a patient has these symptoms and an aortic graft, a history of potential sources of infection should be ascertained as well. Patients with aortic graft infections often have a history of prior or concurrent infection, such as pneumonia or urinary tract infections.[47] Previous gastrointestinal illness may suggest infection with *Salmonella*.[4] A history of any other concurrent infection in the setting of an aortic graft should also raise the physician's suspicion for a possible aortic graft infection.

The majority of patients have a condition that predisposes them to aortic graft infection.[43–49] Patients therefore should also be queried for any condition that may predispose to relative immunocompromise. Diabetes mellitus, concurrent HIV infections, chronic hepatitis, and/ or malnutrition are often found in conjunction with aortic graft infections. Disease states that require immunosuppressive medications also may predispose to prosthetic graft infection. Malignancy has also been associated, independent of chemotherapeutic agents or radiation that are also immunosuppressive. This has been especially true of patients with *Clostridium septicum* infections in the setting of colorectal malignancy.[50] One should also investigate a history of intravenous drug abuse or arterial catheterizations, as these can result in the introduction of bacteremia.

Groin pseudoaneurysms with or without a draining sinus in patients with an aortofemoral bypass should also be assumed to be infected until proven otherwise. Over 60% of femoral pseudoaneurysms associated with aortofemoral bypasses have been found to be infected.[51] A draining sinus is suggestive of increased virulence of the microbes responsible for the infected pseudoaneurysm (Fig. 59.3).

Graft thrombosis may also be associated with an occult graft infection, though most graft thromboses are not infected, making the diagnosis of infection difficult.[52] Coagulated blood is an outstanding culture medium. In addition, the graft itself is much more prone to infection, as described above. It is unclear whether the infection or the thrombosis occurs first.[52] Regardless, a graft thrombosis is not always innocently associated with restenosis. Physician suspicion should be higher for occlusions in the aortoiliac position, where the flow volume and the anastomoses created are very large.

Ureterohydronephrosis is often asymptomatic and discovered incidentally during imaging examinations for other indications. In the setting of a prior aortofemoral bypass, however, the presence of ureteral obstruction should raise the physician's suspicion for a possible

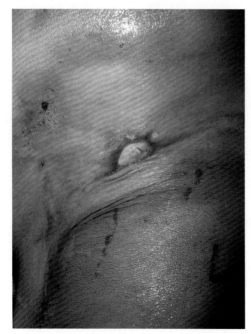

Fig. 59.3 Left groin pseudoaneurysm with overlying fibrinous exudate with a history of prior aortofemoral bypass with an obliquely oriented groin incision.

aortic graft infection.[53] The obstruction results from technical errors while tunneling the graft, or secondary to inflammatory changes in the retroperitoneum in response to an infected aortofemoral limb. Ureterohydronephrosis is associated with four times the risk of an aortic graft infection in the setting of a history of a prior aortofemoral bypass.[53]

Aortoenteric fistula. AEF represent a particularly lethal subset of aortic graft infections. Patients presenting with upper gastrointestinal bleeding and a history of an aortic bypass or endograft placement should be assumed to have an AEF until proven otherwise. While other causes of gastrointestinal bleeding are more common, delays in the diagnosis of AEF can have disastrous consequences. Communications between the aortic graft and the gastrointestinal tract which occur at the anastomosis between the graft and the aorta are termed AEF.[48,49] Communications between the aortic graft and gastrointestinal tract that do not involve the graft-arterial anastomosis are termed AEE.[50] With AEE, bleeding occurs due to mucosal irritation, rather than communication with the aorta itself. This distinction appears mostly academic, as recent series have shown that the outcomes between the two are similar.[49] For the purposes of this chapter, the two entities will be referred to as AEF.

AEF may present with a "herald bleed" in which the patient has an upper gastrointestinal bleeding event that spontaneously, temporarily ceases. The interval of hemostasis is variable, ranging from hours to days in recent series.[47,49] The majority of AEF occur between the 3rd or 4th portion of the duodenum and the aortic graft.[47,49] AEF can occur secondary to either open or endovascular aortic procedures. Rarely, they occur with primary mycotic aortic aneurysms.[4]

Lower Extremity Bypass Graft Infections

Lower extremity prosthetic bypass graft infections represent a unique challenge. Frequently the bypass was placed for limb-threatening ischemia, without viable autogenous conduit to utilize. Hence if infection occurs, maintaining sufficient circulation to the limb is challenging.[54,55] Recent series cite prosthetic graft infection rates ranging between 3.8% and 18%.[54,55] Redo bypass, active concurrent infection in the perioperative period, female gender, and diabetes mellitus all independently predict prosthetic graft infection.[55] Amputation early after graft placement due to revascularization failure and early graft revision are particularly high risk procedures for infecting prosthetic grafts. Both major amputation and early graft revision (within 4 weeks of implant) independently increase the odds of infection of the prosthetic graft by over 11-fold.[54] Graft thrombosis also predicts graft infection.[52,54] The type of graft fabric (Dacron or Gore-Tex) does not impact graft infection rates, nor do prior ipsilateral arterial catheterizations or partial foot/ toe amputations.[55]

Suture line involvement at presentation is common, occurring in almost 80% of lower extremity bypass infections.[55] A draining sinus may not be present, and depends upon the virulence of the microbe primarily responsible for the infection. Approximately 50% of the infections occur within the first 3 months after implantation.[55] Microbes most frequently responsible for lower extremity bypass infection include *S. epidermidis* and *S. aureus,* which account for almost 75% of prosthetic bypass infections.[52,55] Most *S. aureus* infections are methicillin-resistant.[55] Ten percent of prosthetic bypass graft infections are polymicrobial.[55]

Carotid Patch Infections

Carotid patch infections or infections of bypasses involving the carotid artery are very rare, likely due to the excellent vascularity of the subcutaneous tissues of the neck. Systematic review of the world literature has revealed little over 120 carotid patch infections.[56,57] Patients may describe an antecedent history of skin cellulitis or infection of the drain site during the perioperative period prior to presentation with a patch infection.[57] However, most cases do not have any history of antecedent infection.[56–58] Bovine pericardium may be more resistant to infection, though the number of cases are too few to appropriately power comparisons.[56,57] Although fewer cases of bovine pericardial patch infection have been documented, there is a time-lag bias present, in that bovine pericardium has not been available as widely as other prosthetics; hence the potential number of patients that could be infected, and the time that they could have been infected, is significantly less. While the use of a vein patch would markedly reduce the risk of infection, the risk of patch rupture is highest with a vein patch.[59] Moreover, the risk of patch rupture is similar to the risk of infection of the prosthetic patch at <1%.[57–60] Expert opinion suggests that simply trading the risk of one complication for another is without significant benefit for the patient.[56] Finally, use of prosthetic spares the greater saphenous vein for future use as a conduit for bypass.

Timing of infection appears to influence presentation. Those that occur less than 2 months after the initial carotid endarterectomy present mostly with wound infections and abscess. Conversely, those that present after 6 months from the carotid endarterectomy present more frequently with pseudoaneurysms and/or a draining skin sinus.[57] The predominant organisms are commensal microbes, such as *S. aureus* and *Streptococcal* sp., which account for over 90% of all reported carotid patch infections.[57] Untreated, the infection may disrupt the patch anastomosis resulting in hemorrhage with airway compromise and/or stroke.[56,57]

Bare Metal Stent Infections

Bare metal stent infections are exceedingly rare, with only 77 cases reported in the world literature as of 2013.[60–62] They are associated with significant morbidity and mortality, however, due to delays in diagnosis and treatment, the comorbidities and indications dictating the initial stent placement, and the magnitude of the procedures required to extirpate the stent, remove the infection, and restore the circulation.[62] Coronary stent infections are the most frequent, followed by iliac, superficial femoral, and renal artery stent infections.[61] Other sites are rare due to infrequency of bare metal stent placement in these locations, but are theoretically possible wherever a stent is placed. Due to their infrequency a high index of suspicion is required to limit delays in diagnosis. Patients with a history of fevers, chills, bacteremia, and prior stent placement with or without localizing symptoms to the area of stent placement should have stent infection within the differential diagnosis.

Untreated the infections will progressively destroy the contiguous vessel, resulting ultimately in pseudoaneurysm and possibly rupture.[60–62] Risk factors include contemporaneous bacteremia (i.e., other infection, presence of indwelling arterial or venous catheter), breaks in sterile technique during implantation, prolonged indwelling catheter use, nonsterile site of puncture, and hematoma/pseudoaneurysm complicating puncture.[60,61] Organisms are predominantly commensal skin flora, such as *S. aureus* and *S. epidermidis*.[61]

DIAGNOSTIC TESTS TO AID THE DIAGNOSIS OF ARTERIAL INFECTIONS

Unfortunately, despite a high index of clinical suspicion, clinicians are faced with the conundrum of attempting to identify whether primary or SAI is the cause of the patient's symptoms. There is significant symptom overlap with other diagnoses, which increases the imprecision of the history, physical, and laboratory findings. No diagnostic test is perfect, as all tests are variably reliable when identifying infection with less virulent organisms and early graft infections. Nonetheless, it is vital to understand the strengths and weaknesses of several diagnostic tests to improve the ability to diagnose arterial infection, and decrease

clinically significant delays in diagnosis and treatment.[63] Much of the data revolves around the diagnosis of primary and secondary aortic infections. Many of the tenets of aortic infection, however, hold true for other peripheral arterial infections.

Computed Tomographic Angiography: Primary Modality to Diagnose Arterial Infection

Computed tomographic angiography (CTA) has become a mainstay in the diagnostic evaluation of all arterial infections, but especially within the thorax, abdomen, and pelvis. CTA is readily available in most centers, with the necessary equipment, experience, and software capabilities to replicate the results published from experienced centers. Metal artifact can limit visualization, and some patients may have a contrast allergy that limits testing. Ionizing radiation is a theoretical limitation as well.

The main impediment to universal CTA testing is contrast-induced nephropathy. The physician must weigh the risks and benefits of the CTA on behalf of his/her patient. The author favors performing CTA for almost all patients, especially for those with more dangerous presentations, such as suspected AEF or overt sepsis. For these patients, the author considers potential delays in diagnosis to be more detrimental than the risks of contrast-induced nephropathy, even if the patient presents with some acute renal failure.

For aortic infections, findings consistent with infection include perigraft/periaortic air and/or fluid, discontinuity of the aortic wall, and soft tissue attenuation/stranding around the aorta/aortic graft (Fig. 59.4).[18,64] Pseudoaneurysm, focal bowel wall thickening, and ectopic gas may be present in the setting of AEF (Fig. 59.5).[18,64] Ectopic gas is more prevalent in AEF; however, gas may be found without an AEF if gas-forming microbes are responsible for the infection.[64] Extravasation into the bowel lumen is pathognomonic of AEF, though this is rarely found.[64] Oral contrast is typically not recommended, as this would interfere with visualization should an aortic stent graft be necessary. Moreover, oral contrast obscures visualization of extravasation of blood into the bowel lumen.[64] Abscesses or other evidence of infectious foci (i.e., pneumonia) can also be visualized well with CTA.[18] Osteophytes may also be present, suggestive of AEF. For aortic as well as other peripheral arterial infections, CTA is also critical to provide anatomic detail for operative planning.

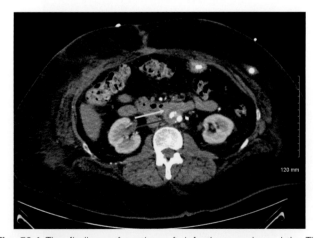

Fig. 59.4 The findings of aortic graft infection can be subtle. The computed tomographic angiography shows effacement of the soft tissue planes between the aorta and the overlying duodenum *(yellow arrow)* with soft tissue stranding, and fluid surrounding the graft *(red arrow)*. Despite the lack of air around the graft the patient was found to have an aortoenteric fistula upon exploration.

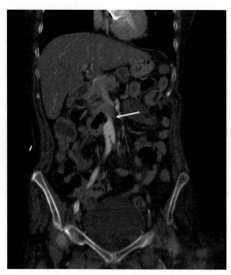

Fig. 59.5 Computed tomographic angiography findings of an aortoenteric fistula, with abundant air surrounding the graft *(yellow arrow)*, the classic finding in an aortoenteric fistula.

The sensitivity (40% to 90%) and specificity (33% to 100%) varies significantly depending upon the virulence of the organism.[65] For SAI, early infections are also significantly more difficult to diagnose.[18,64,65] Less virulent microbes incite a less vigorous immune response. Hence there is less vigorous soft tissue attenuation or stranding, fluid, ectopic gas, or soft tissue thickening. With regard to secondary aortic infections, air may be normally present for up to 2 months.[64] Similarly, a small amount of fluid may be normally present for up to 3 months after the reconstruction.[64]

Magnetic Resonance Imaging

Magnetic resonance imaging (MRI) offers two advantages relative to CTA: (1) there is no ionizing radiation; and (2) contrast is not required, as patency of the arteries can be inferred by T_1- and T_2-imaging (see Chapter 13).[66] Moreover, MRI may be better at distinguishing early graft infections from the perigraft fibrosis found after an aortic graft heals normally.[67,68] Early after graft implantation, recent hematoma will have a higher water content, which results in a low-to-medium signal intensity on T_1-imaging, and a high-intensity signal on T_2-imaging. As healing progresses and fibrosis increases, both T_1- and T_2-signal intensity decreases.[68] Moreover, early on after graft implantation, the solid elements within blood separate from the fluid, resulting in heterogeneous T_1- and T_2-signal intensity in the perigraft regions. Conversely, with time, these perigraft collections become more homogeneous as fibrosis ensues.[68] Finally, MRI may have increased ability to characterize surrounding perigraft changes, and may distinguish between biofilm and normal perigraft inflammation.[67] This feature is particularly salient with respect to biofilms of indolent organisms, which are notoriously difficult to diagnose.[67]

The disadvantages of MRI are that the examinations are prolonged and less widely available than CTA. Also, MRI is contraindicated in the presence of certain metal implants. Finally, the inter- and intraobserver variability is higher with MRI, which limits the external validity of single-center reports touting the abilities of MRI to distinguish infection.[67] Together, these limitations limit more widespread applicability of MRI. In spite of some single-center reports suggesting improved discriminatory ability of MRI, other reports show that MRI is not superior to CTA or other diagnostic modalities, especially with respect to early graft infections or infections with less virulent organisms. Shahidi et al.[66] found the positive predictive value of MRI

was 95%, with a negative predictive value of 80%, which is comparable to that of CTA.

Duplex Ultrasound

Duplex ultrasound (DUS) is advantageous in that it is not invasive and does not utilize contrast or radiation.[67] Moreover, DUS can evaluate in vivo effects of stenoses, which may also complicate an infection, especially in the setting of an SAI. DUS provides the peak systolic velocity, peak systolic arterial ratios, color duplex imaging, and resistivity index, all of which may characterize the in vivo effects of a stenosis (see Chapter 12). These data ultimately inform the surgeon how best to maintain end-organ perfusion after the infected material has been removed.

Unfortunately, DUS is limited significantly by body habitus and overlying bowel gas. Artifacts from prior scarring and metal implants can create significant artifacts that limit visualization. Hence there is significant inter- and intraobserver variability in the performance and interpretation of the examinations.[67,69] In fact, the sensitivity and specificity have yet to be quantified in the literature.[67] DUS is also unable to discriminate between infection and normal postoperative changes early (<3 months) after a prosthetic implant has been placed. Finally, visualization of the adjacent anatomic structures is often inadequate for appropriate surgical planning, necessitating either a CTA or MRI. Nonetheless, ultrasound provides a safe, accurate method to identify superficial PAI and SAI of the extremities or neck.[67,69] DUS findings consistent with infection in the literature include "corrugation" of a carotid patch,[69] a hypoechoic or anechoic "halo" or fluid surrounding a bypass graft,[70] and pseudoaneurysm.[67,70]

Radionuclide-Labeled Imaging

Nuclear medicine imaging techniques were developed to surmount the limitations of other diagnostic modalities to identify infections with low-virulence organisms or early primary and secondary vascular infections. All nuclear imaging techniques rely on the concept that infection will incite a detectable inflammatory response. None of the nuclear imaging techniques have robust data to support their use, as the technologies and techniques are currently evolving rapidly. For all radionuclide scans, specific threshold values for uptake parameters to distinguish infection from normal metabolic activity have not been determined. While all radionuclide scanning techniques are imperfect, understanding the benefits and limitations of these tests is essential to improve detection of occult vascular infections.

Tagged White Blood Cell Scan

Leukocyte scintigraphy, or tagged white blood cell (WBC) scans, use leukocytes that have been labeled with either [111]indium or [99m]technetium.[67,71] Gamma rays are then used to detect and quantify the radionuclide-labeled cells. Leukocyte scintigraphy can be used with concurrent antibiotic therapy. Moreover, tagged WBC scans can be used for both primary and secondary aortic infections.[72] However, it is a time-consuming, labor intensive study, with significant inter- and intraobserver variability.

The test is plagued by false positives due to cross-labeling of platelets, which can therefore misidentify thrombus that surrounds recent graft implants as infection, especially in the early postoperative period.[67,71] Adjacent tissue with a significant number of leukocytes, such as the GI tract, may also create a false positive finding. Intact chemotaxis and a minimum WBC count of 2000 cells/μL is required, which is not always possible in immunocompromised hosts.[71] Due to the aforementioned limitations, sensitivity and specificity vary widely, between 50% and 100%.[71] Because the predictive value is so variable, the author does not rely upon tagged WBC data alone to identify occult vascular infections. As an adjunct to other technologies, however, leukocyte scintigraphy may have a role in the evaluation of vascular infections.

Single Photon Emission Computed Tomography

Single photon emission computed tomography (SPECT) provides three-dimensional data by acquiring two-dimensional gamma photon data from multiple projections. These γ-photons measure the emission of radionuclides that correlate with the concentration of the labeled cells in the area. These data are then interpolated via software algorithms to generate a three-dimensional image.[73] In this fashion, SPECT can provide data to localize the infection further.

Anatomic localization is imperfect with SPECT alone, due to attenuation of the photons from where the radionuclide-labeled cells have accumulated and the gamma photon detector.[73] Hence SPECT has been combined with computed tomography (CT) in order to generate SPECT/CT images that further help to distinguish between areas of infection versus areas of artifact.[73,74] Early experience with SPECT/CT is encouraging and rapidly growing. Erba et al.[74] showed that the fusion of SPECT with CT was able to change the final assignment of the scan from negative to positive for infection in 14 of 57 cases when compared to tagged WBC scanning alone. Similarly, SPECT/CT changed the assignment of the scan from negative to positive for infection in 9 of 57 cases compared to standalone SPECT.[74] In their experience, SPECT/CT had a 100% sensitivity and specificity, which was markedly superior to both ultrasound and CTA.

Future studies may prove SPECT/CT to be an invaluable adjunct to help diagnose indolent or early graft infections. However, SPECT/CT remains rather labor-intensive and lengthy to perform. Furthermore, expertise is not uniform across all centers. Moreover, traditional examinations, such as CTA, MRI, and DUS in the appropriate clinical context, may be sufficient. Hence the author reserves SPECT/CT for cases where CTA, the history, physical, and laboratory examination are inconclusive for the diagnosis of vascular infection.

¹⁸Fluorodeoxyglucose-Positron Emission Tomography

^{18}Fluorodeoxyglucose-positron emission tomography (^{18}FDG-PET) capitalizes upon the increased uptake of radionuclide-labeled glucose in metabolically active cells. The increased uptake results in the ability to localize inflammation associated with infectious processes. ^{18}FDG-PET is unaffected by metallic implants. Generally speaking, ^{18}FDG-PET is less labor-intensive, completed in a shorter time, and is associated with a lower radiation exposure than SPECT.[67] Parameters measured include maximum standardized uptake value (SUV) and the pattern of uptake (focal vs. diffuse). Standalone ^{18}FDG-PET appears better at excluding infection, with a sensitivity, specificity, accuracy, positive predictive value, and negative predictive value of 91%, 64%, 73%, 56%, and 93% respectively.[67]

Similar to SPECT, fusion of ^{18}FDG-PET with CT has helped to improve anatomical localization of infection (Fig. 59.6). This has improved the sensitivity, specificity, and interobserver agreement of ^{18}FDG-PET/CT versus standalone ^{18}FDG-PET.[67,74] Unfortunately, as data have accumulated, not all results are congruent with early smaller series touting the efficacy of ^{18}FDG-PET/CT.[75] The difficulty arises due to the lack of consensus regarding which parameters should be studied. Similar to SPECT/CT, further clarity regarding the appropriate role of ^{18}FDG-PET/CT will be gleaned as experience accumulates. Comparisons between SPECT-CT and ^{18}FDG-PET/CT remain sparse in the literature. Further study will be required to quantify the marginal efficacy of one modality versus the other. The author also reserves ^{18}FDG-PET/CT for cases where traditional methods of diagnosis fail, in spite of a high degree of suspicion from the clinician.

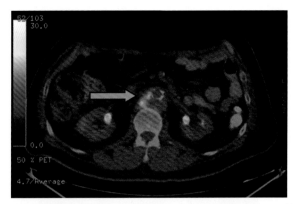

Fig. 59.6 Fluorodeoxyglucose-positron emission tomography combined with computed tomography permits improved anatomic localization of acute inflammation associated with infectious processes *(blue arrow)*.

Additional Diagnostic Adjuncts

Image-guided perigraft aspirates are considered by some to be the gold-standard for the diagnosis of vascular infection.[75] Unfortunately, sufficient fluid is not always present. Moreover, proximity to nearby vascular structures or bowel can preclude safe aspiration. The tissue may also be too viscous or fibrotic to permit aspiration. Moreover, the previously sterile fluid may actually be seeded with microbes due to the diagnostic procedure. For these reasons, the author reserves image-guided perigraft aspiration for the rare patient where the diagnosis cannot be reached by other means and surgical extirpation of the infected material is contraindicated due to other patient comorbidities and/or technical difficulty. Rarely, aspiration can also be used to manage patients with arterial infections, should nonresectional therapy be chosen (see subsequent section regarding Management of Primary and Secondary Arterial Infections: Conservative, Nonresectional Management, and Partial Resectional Strategies).

Diagnostic arteriography is rarely necessary, as advancements in cross-sectional imaging with three-dimensional reconstructions have obviated the need for diagnostic arteriography. In the past, there may have been cases where delineation of the anatomy was necessary for future case planning. Theoretically, bowel filling may be seen in the presence of an occult AEF.[76] Arteriography is unlikely to uncover an occult AEF where current imaging techniques described previously fail to diagnose the AEF. The author limits the application of arteriography only for cases where endovascular interventions to manage arterial infections are deemed necessary.

Esophagogastroduodenoscopy (EGD) is useful to exclude other causes of upper GI bleeding when the clinician is suspicious of an AEF. Approximately 25% of AEF are diagnosed with EGD.[77] While the diagnostic yield is not optimal, the author recommends EGD in hemodynamically stable patients where prior diagnostic evaluation has been inconclusive. Care must be taken not to disrupt thrombus found on EGD in the context of suspected AEF, as this may unleash uncontrollable hemorrhage.

MANAGEMENT OF PRIMARY AND SECONDARY ARTERIAL INFECTIONS

Once the diagnosis is confirmed, PAIs and SAIs are managed similarly. The main determinants of management hinge upon the technical difficulty of the proposed operation, the surgeon's preferences, the patient's comorbidities, and the values of the patient and the patient's caregivers. After obtaining blood cultures, prompt implementation of antibiotics and resuscitation is paramount for all patients. For patients who are hemodynamically stable, evaluation for occult cardiac and pulmonary disease is warranted for perioperative risk stratification and counseling patients.

Conservative, Nonresectional Management, and Partial Resectional Strategies

Advocates of conservative management of aortic grafts consider non-excisional approaches to be ideal for those with significant medical comorbidities and/or infections that exist in locations that incur preclusive morbidity and/or mortality with excision.[78] Lifelong antibiotics are the mainstay of therapy. However, neither intravenous nor oral antibiotics alone are sufficient, with only rare case reports of survivors of aortic infections with standalone antibiotic therapy.[78] Other adjunctive therapies to assist in drainage of abscesses or phlegmon surrounding the infection are required to minimize the infection. Indolent, gram-positive organisms, like *S. epidermidis,* also are more conducive to conservative management.[78,79] After the majority of the infection has been eradicated, lifelong oral antibiotics can be utilized to maintain suppression of the infection. Rifampicin has emerged as a popular choice due to its activity against many of the organisms commonly existing with aortic infections.[78]

There are several conservative adjuncts used for aortic infections: percutaneous drainage, open debridement with continuous irrigation catheters, and muscle and/or omental flaps. These adjuncts have been used either as a bridge to explantation or as destination therapy.[80–83] Percutaneous drainage consists of image-guided catheter placement, which is then used to aspirate the infected material surrounding the infected aorta. This also facilitates identification of the predominant organisms and their sensitivities which can then be used to tailor antibiotic therapy.[80,81] As a bridge to definitive surgery, patients treated with initial drainage prior to definitive explantation had a better survival relative to those who proceeded directly to definitive explantation and revascularization.[80] The improved survival with initial drainage is attributed to the treatment of systemic sepsis and stabilization of the patient prior to surgical removal and restoration of arterial continuity. Gordon et al. report that six of nine patients survived 4 years with initial drainage followed by open surgery.[79]

Open debridement entails exposing the area of infection and removing as much of the infected material and necrotic debris as possible without disrupting vascular continuity.[82] Afterward, catheters are left in place through which antibiotics and saline are continuously irrigated until cultures are negative. The catheters are then removed and the patient placed upon oral antibiotics.[83] Debridement and irrigation resulted in an 80% 1-year survival in small case series.[83]

Muscle and/or omental flaps have also been used in conjunction with open debridement to preserve grafts as well. Most frequently, this has been utilized to treat both early and late infections of lower extremity grafts.[83,84] The most frequently encountered site is the groin, which is also the most difficult to manage.[54,55,83] Graft-preservation begins with a thorough open debridement of infected tissue.[83–85] After debridement and irrigation, vascularized soft tissue is then utilized to cover the graft. In the groin, there are multiple options, including the sartorius, gracilis, rectus femoris, or rectus abdominis muscle flaps.[83,84] The sartorius is popular due to its proximity and surgeon familiarity with the technique. Unfortunately, the sartorius can also be inflamed, atretic, or ischemic due to the severity of infection, as well as a pattern of underlying atherosclerotic disease.[83] The benefit of soft-tissue coverage is to reduce dead space, decrease bacterial burden, improve antibiotic delivery, and physically protect vascular structures from the environment. Following soft-tissue coverage, wound vac application is frequently utilized.[83,84]

Graft, as well as limb salvage, is superior when the wound is free of prosthetic material, though this is not always possible to achieve.[83,84] Graft salvage rates are variable, ranging from 55% to 100%.[84] Limb salvage, however, is more reliable, approaching 90%. Predictors of failure of graft preservation strategies for lower extremity bypass include the presence of exposed graft, especially the suture line. Gram-negative infections, especially with *Pseudomonas* and methicillin-resistant *S. aureus* infections, also have higher failure rates. Patient risk factors, such as malnutrition, diabetes, prolonged operative times, reoperative fields, and chronic renal insufficiency, also reduce success rates.[85] The most dreaded complication of graft-preservation techniques is rupture, due to disruption of the suture line or erosion of the native vessel wall. This complication, while rare, is most common with exposed anastomoses, as well as with *Pseudomonas* infections.[85] Treatment of rupture can require ligation of the common femoral artery, though concurrent revascularization is often difficult due to the emergent nature of cases involving rupture.

Antibiotic polymethylmethacrylate beads may serve to sterilize wound beyond what can currently be achieved with serial debridement and soft-tissue flap coverage.[86] Smaller series have shown that limb-salvage, graft preservation, and wound sterilization can be achieved in over 85% of lower extremity bypass infections. Rarely, these beads may be used for aortic graft infections as well.[87] While rare, erosion into nearby structures can occur with prolonged implantation.[87] Ideally, the beads should be exchanged until both granulation tissue has covered the graft anastomosis and the wound cultures show no further growth.[86] While excellent limb-salvage and graft preservation rates have been achieved, appropriately powered comparisons of soft tissue coverage without antibiotic bead exchanges has not been performed. Hence the marginal benefit of antibiotic polymethylmethacrylate beads is unclear, and will require further study.

Complete resection of an aortobifemoral graft/aortic endograft and revascularization may be too hazardous due to the anatomic location of the graft and patient comorbidities. Hence several authors have advocated resection of only a portion of the graft.[88–90] Theoretically, partial excision should be feasible, as the amount of graft that is infected is frequently disincorporated and culture positive.[90] The sensitivity of disincorporation identifying graft infection is 74%, with a specificity of 97%, yielding an accuracy of 85%.[90] Moreover, reinfection rates after partial resection of aortobifemoral bypass grafts are high, ranging between 36% and 47%, and increase with longer follow-up.[88,89] Infection limited to the infrainguinal locations appears to fare better.[88] With respect to lower extremity bypass grafts, prosthetic remnants appear prone to infection, even when infection appears absent at the time of initial operation.[52] Hence several authors recommend removal of all prosthetic material if it appears clinically uninfected at the time of initial exploration.[52]

The data to guide therapy regarding conservative or partial resectional strategies are very poor. Most series are comprised of small cohorts, limiting statistical power. Moreover, patient comorbidities and infection severity vary significantly between cohorts, rendering equitable comparisons impossible. Given the paucity of data, future appropriately powered multi-institutional studies will be required to measure the efficacy of conservative strategies versus strategies that result in aggressive resection, debridement, and revascularization. This is particularly true for areas where infections occur rarely, such as the carotid artery, and with endovascular stent infections. The author limits conservative or partial-resectional strategies for those with limited life-expectancy due to prohibitive medical comorbidities. Moreover, those that decline aggressive resection and debridement of the infected material with revascularization are offered conservative management. Finally, those with infections in prohibitively difficult places to resect are also offered conservative or partial resectional strategies.

Resection, Debridement, and Revascularization

For all arterial infections, ideal therapy entails resection of the infected and prosthetic material if present. The necrotic and inflamed tissue surrounding the infected vessel also requires debridement. Finally, revascularization ensues to prevent end-organ ischemia, though in isolated cases, ligation of the healthy vessel beyond the area of infection is performed. The bulk of the infections concern the lower extremities and aorta; hence much of the subsequent discussion will focus upon methods of aortic and lower extremity repair. Principles of repair from these locales are extrapolated to other vascular beds. If there are treatments specific to an anatomic bed, special mention will be made in the subsequent sections.

Reconstruction for Primary and Secondary Aortic Infections

Emergent presentations of hemorrhage and sepsis preclude a thorough preoperative evaluation. For patients with less urgent presentations, preoperative evaluation is performed to inform the surgeon, anesthesiologists, patients, and their caregivers regarding the risks of subsequent complications and mortality so that a thoughtful decision can be made regarding the future care of the patient. Treatment of the infection should not be delayed to attempt to optimize underlying cardiac risks, though management strategies may be altered to abrogate the physiologic stress imparted by the procedure. In this context, a 12-lead electrocardiogram and echocardiogram to evaluate for ischemia, valvular dysfunction, and pulmonary hypertension is reasonable to perform.[91] Pulmonary testing is generally avoided unless the patient history and physical suggests the patient's pulmonary function is so poor as to preclude significant pulmonary complications. The author also routinely measures ankle-brachial indices to warn of the potential need to perform a lower extremity revascularization after an aortoiliac reconstruction.[70] Lower extremity vein mapping of the greater saphenous and femoral veins is performed if autogenous veins are being considered for the reconstruction. Femoral veins with evidence of acute or chronic deep venous thrombosis or a diameter less than 6 mm are considered unsuitable for aortoiliac revascularization.[70]

Due to the length of these procedures, and capacity for rapid exsanguination, close collaboration with anesthesia is required to optimize surgical outcomes. Hypothermia is avoided with the use of warming, heated air blankets, warmed intravenous fluids, and increasing the operating room temperature. The surgical bed after resection of infected arteries tends to ooze diffusely despite control of major vascular structures. Blood loss can become significant with prolonged procedures. Hence the authors recommend a lenient threshold for blood transfusion to prevent complications of unintended intraoperative anemia. Coagulopathy can occur due to hemorrhage, prolonged exposure, and hypothermia, in spite of the care team's attempts to mitigate these problems. Hence fresh-frozen plasma, platelets, and cryoprecipitate should be available to transfuse quickly. Broad spectrum antibiotics are maintained at therapeutic levels throughout the case, as culture results are unavailable until later when the specimens are obtained intraoperatively. There is no guideline directing which empiric antibiotic therapy is most efficacious, though the author favors vancomycin and piperacillin/tazobactam to provide coverage for the most common causal organisms.[70]

Excision and debridement is central to removing the infectious nidus.[70] The surgeon must be aggressive to remove all infected artery, surrounding inflamed, infected tissue, and prosthetic to ensure infection, pseudoaneurysmal degeneration, and possible rupture do not persist or recur. Exposure of the aorta can be achieved via a thoracoabdominal, mid-line transabdominal, or retroperitoneal approach, depending upon the extent of infectious involvement, and the preferences of the surgeon. Proximal control of the aorta must be obtained in healthy aorta, away from the area of infection itself. For infrarenal aortic infections, for instance, this mandates suprarenal, or supraceliac control. Distally, control is again achieved in the healthy vessel away from the area of infection. To achieve this after an aortobifemoral graft, for instance, the author recommends an incision lateral to the sartorius muscle to facilitate control of the profunda and superficial femoral arteries distal to areas of scar and/or infection. This can be combined with a more traditional vertical incision directly overlying the femoral bifurcation to aid in dissection. Control can be obtained with either vessel clamps, or an intraaortic balloon.[70] Once proximal and distal control is achieved, the patient is systemically heparinized with 100 units/kg of intravenous heparin, and the proximal and distal clamps are applied. The infected aorta and prosthetic material are then removed in their entirety. Thorough debridement of the retroperitoneum is essential to minimize the amount of devitalized tissue and infectious burden.

Removal of an infected endograft merits special mention. While infection is rare after endograft repair, the increased prevalence of endograft implantation for AAA repair is such that vascular specialists must remain aware of the management of infected aortic endografts. Aortic stents are technically demanding to remove, due to the fixation elements that prevent facile removal without damaging the aortic neck or injuring the surgeon. Multiple techniques have arisen without superiority of a single method. Supraceliac control facilitates removal, especially when the endograft has a suprarenal stent. The author prefers to reconstrain the endograft with a technique similar to that used to reconstrain endografts for back-table modification prior to fenestrated endograft implantation. The assistant loops the endograft with an umbilical tape and constrains the endograft. The surgeon then loops the endograft with another umbilical tape adjacent to where the assistant is looping the endograft and ties the umbilical tape. This process continues proximally and distally until the main body of the endograft is reconstrained. The active fixation elements are then removed from the aortic wall gently by advancing the endograft cephalad slightly. This frees the endograft from the aorta, which can then be removed.[49]

Extra-Anatomic Bypass and Aortic Stump Ligation

Extra-anatomic bypass and aortic stump ligation has been the traditional gold-standard therapy for restoring vascular continuity after resection and debridement of the infected aorta (Fig. 59.7).[92–94] While this technique has been supplanted by in situ methods of reconstruction (see below), extra-anatomic bypass and aortic stump ligation remain important tools to control infection and maintain vascular continuity. This is particularly useful in more emergent settings of overwhelming sepsis and/or hemorrhage where the patient is not physiologically fit to withstand a prolonged in situ reconstruction. Moreover, this is an excellent solution for surgeons that are not comfortable with in situ methods of revascularization.

After removal of the graft and debridement of the retroperitoneum, aortic stump ligation ensues. This is performed in two layers with 2-0 monofilament suture.[92–94] Soft tissue flaps, such as omentum, may then be used to buttress the aortic closure. Axillobifemoral bypass is performed to restore arterial continuity. Bypass can be performed in a staged fashion with the axillobifemoral bypass performed several days prior to the aortic debridement and aortic ligation, if the patient does not present with overwhelming sepsis or hemorrhage. When axillobifemoral bypass is performed several days prior to the aortic debridement, mortality does seem to improve.[92] If performed in this fashion, the duration between the axillobifemoral bypass and aortic procedure should be minimized to prevent competitive flow from causing thrombosis of the axillobifemoral bypass.[92]

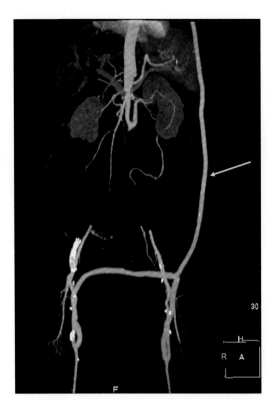

Fig. 59.7 Coronal projection of a computed tomography angiogram depicting an axillobifemoral bypass *(yellow arrow)* performed for prior aortic infection. Note the aortic stump has been ligated with preservation of the left and right renal arteries.

Multiple centers no longer perform axillobifemoral bypass as the primary method of revascularization[46] due to multiple limitations of axillo-bifemoral bypass. Mortality is high, ranging between 18% and 43%, with survivorship higher with staged procedures.[92–94] Aortic stump rupture is a catastrophic complication, which occurs in as high as 32% of patients at 3 months after the initial aortic ligation and debridement (Fig. 59.8).[95] The proximal stump is more commonly associated with rupture, but the distal stump may also bleed (see Fig. 59.8). Moreover, due to the extent of infection, some patients do not have sufficient aorta to perform a proper two-layer closure. Patency is modest, ranging between 64% and 80% at 5 years. Reinfection rates are significantly higher than in situ methods of revascularizations, and have been reported as high as 22%.[92–94]

In Situ Methods of Revascularization

In response to suboptimal outcomes after axillobifemoral bypass, several centers have developed unique methods of reconstructing the aorta to restore anatomic, in-line flow. No individual technique is superior. The data are retrospective and confounded by publication bias, ascertainment bias, and referral bias. Samples sizes are small also, due to the relative rarity of aortic infections. Each method uses a different conduit to restore arterial continuity. When data from in situ methods of reconstruction are aggregated, they support the concept that in situ reconstruction is superior to axillobifemoral bypass.

Rifampin-Soaked and Silver-Impregnated Dacron

Rifampin inhibits *S. epidermidis* and *S. aureus*. Moreover, rifampin bonds well to collagen and gelatin coatings of Dacron grafts.[96] The grafts are soaked in 600 mg of rifampin mixed with 250 mL of normal saline for a minimum of thirty minutes.[46,47] Rifampin-soaked grafts are advantageous, as they are widely available and familiar to most hospitals. Moreover, these are less labor-intensive or costly compared to other conduits.

Theoretically, reinfection rates should be prohibitively high with in situ replacement with a prosthetic, especially since rifampin does not provide antibiotic coverage against all potential organisms that may cause an aortic infection. However, reinfection rates appear reasonable, especially when utilizing contemporaneous omental wrapping. Oderich et al.[47] described the experience at the Mayo Clinic of AEF repairs, which should, theoretically, have the highest reinfection rates due to the enteric contamination with multiple organisms. In their series, however, 5-year outcomes were as follows: survival was 59%; graft patency was 97%; and reinfections occurred in 4%.

Silver-impregnated Dacron is particularly effective against *S. aureus* infections. Silver acts by two mechanisms. First, it disrupts bacterial cell membranes, thereby preventing cell replications. Secondly, it prevents protein transcriptions from messenger ribonucleic acid.[96] In vitro studies in dogs have shown silver to be more effective than rifampin at preventing recurrent infections.[97] Delva et al.[98] found that for AEF, unfortunately, reinfection was high, at 22%. One-year primary patency was 60.5%, with a secondary patency of 89%; 55% of their population were deceased at 1 year. The experience of Delva et al.[98] was different from Oderich et al.[47] in that partial graft excisions were also performed within their experience, which may explain their higher reinfection rates. Regardless, current data do not support superiority of silver-impregnated Dacron versus rifampin-soaked Dacron.

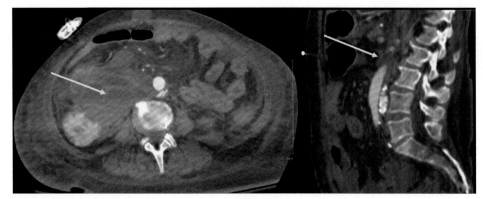

Fig. 59.8 Axial and sagittal computed tomography angiogram showing a distal aortic stump hemorrhage *(yellow arrows)* complicating an axillobifemoral bypass and aortic stump ligation performed for aortic graft infection.

Cryopreserved Allograft

Cadaveric allografts (Fig. 59.9) were first described by Alexis Carrel over 100 years ago. The presumed benefit was that cadaveric tissue would be more resistant to infection.[99] Cadaveric allografts were largely abandoned due to difficulties in procurement and inconsistent preservation techniques. The technique resurfaced in the 1980s. Over the intervening decades, centralization in procurement, preparation, and storage techniques have led to increased availability and consistency of the allografts. Multiple, creative configurations can be constructed to customize the revascularization for specific patients (see Fig. 59.9). Cryopreserved allografts will never be as readily available as Dacron grafts, since they require shipping from centralized centers in Europe or the United States. Moreover, they also require ABO blood antigen cross-matching, and significant preparation time once thawed. Finally, they are costly, with an aortoiliac segment costing approximately US$18,000 in 2011.[47]

Reinfection or persistent infection can still occur with cryopreserved allograft use. Harlander-Locke et al. reviewed the multicenter US experience with cryopreserved allograft, and found that 5-year patency was 97%. One percent of the cohort required subsequent explantation of the newly implanted allograft for recurrent sepsis. In their data, persistent sepsis, recurrent infection, and AEF recurrence occurred in 14% of patients.[48] Similarly, Batt et al. reviewed their experience with AEF reconstructions, for which they used eight allografts. Of these, three became reinfected.[100] Rupture and pseudoaneurysm formation also plague a minority of cryopreserved allografts.[48,100]

Autogenous Femoral Vein

Use of the patient's own femoral vein (Fig. 59.10) to create a neo-aortoiliac surgical reconstruction (NAIS) has several advantages.[45,70] Theoretically, this should be the most resistant to infection. Moreover, it is less costly than cryopreserved allograft. Disadvantages include prolonged procurement time and surgeon unfamiliarity with the

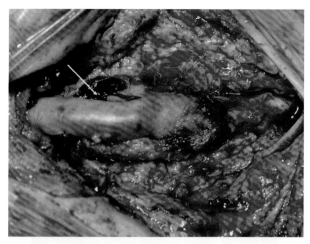

Fig. 59.10 Autogenous femoral vein utilized to treat an infected limb of an aortobifemoral bypass that suffered an isolated infection to the right limb. In this case, a single segment of femoral vein *(yellow arrow)* was used to bypass from the well-incorporated portion of the preexisting, uninfected graft, and bypass to the common femoral artery.

technique. These disadvantages have limited more widespread application of NAIS, particularly for emergent indications. Harvest technique is described in detail elsewhere.[70] Venous congestion is a theoretical pitfall, though it appears to be unfounded. Early in the experience, prophylactic fasciotomies were more frequently performed, so that the perioperative fasciotomy rate was 17%. However, as experience with the technique grew, tolerance for perioperative swelling has accrued, such that perioperative fasciotomies are now almost never performed. Risk factors for perioperative fasciotomy include a preoperative ankle-brachial index ≤0.55, and concurrent harvest of the ipsilateral greater saphenous vein.[101] Late venous insufficiency is common, occurring in up to one-third of patients. Symptoms are mild, however, with no patients presenting with venous ulcerations secondary to venous harvest.[102]

Outcomes appear comparable to other methods of reconstruction, with perioperative mortality ranging between 8% and 10%,[45,103] which is congruent with other methods of arterial reconstruction. Reinfection occurred in 5%, with a primary patency of 81% at 72 months. Limb salvage approaches 100%[105] and primary patency ranges between 81% and 91% at 5 years.[45,103] Late pseudoaneurysmal degeneration of the femoropopliteal vein rarely occurs.[45]

Summary of Alternative Methods of Aortic Reconstruction

The different methods of arterial reconstruction are summarized in Fig. 59.11. Direct comparisons of alternative methods of arterial reconstruction are rare in the literature. Single-center studies do not have sufficiently large study bases to statistically detect potential differences between different methods of arterial reconstruction. One recent study occurring over 14 years confirms no significant difference between extra-anatomic or in situ methods of arterial reconstruction.[104] Of note, however, the authors observed a reinfection rate of 25% occurring at a median of twenty months after reconstruction. This reinfection rate was lowest for prosthetic in situ reconstructions.[104] This is noteworthy, as this contradicts several other studies,[46,49] as well as the surgical mantra that autogenous or cadaveric conduits have the lowest risk of reinfection. Additional appropriately powered studies may help to further clarify which conduit serves to best resist infection.

A systematic review has been performed, evaluating the pooled estimates for major amputations, conduit patency, mortality, and

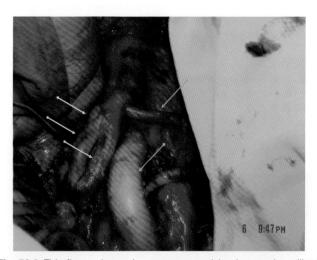

Fig. 59.9 This figure shows the surgeon creativity that can be utilized to customize revascularization options after the aortic infection has been eradicated. The head is oriented superiorly in the picture, with the feet oriented toward the bottom of the picture. The green arrow shows an aortoiliac segment with a femoropopliteal segment sewn on, so that the celiac, superior mesenteric, and right renal arteries could be perfused *(three yellow arrows)*. Additionally, another femoropopliteal segment *(blue arrow)* was sewn onto the aortoiliac segment and sewn behind the thoracic segment that was sewn from the supraceliac aorta to the infrarenal aorta after the infected portion had been resected.

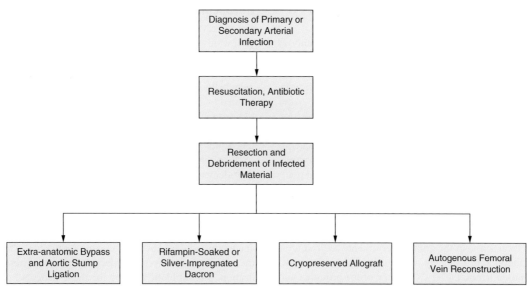

Fig. 59.11 General workflow for the management of primary and secondary aortic infections, and summary of the different revascularization options. While the anatomic considerations may vary, the same principles remain for the management of arterial infections in other vascular beds.

reinfection.[105] The authors confirmed that extra-anatomic bypass and aortic stump ligation has the highest rate of complications. In their analysis, rifampin-soaked prosthetic bypasses performed the best, with a greater than two-fold reduction in postoperative events compared to extra-anatomic bypass and aortic stump ligation.[105] Rifampin-soaked prosthetic bypasses appeared to have the best patency and limb-salvage rates compared to other conduits, with autogenous venous conduits having the worst. Mortality was also the lowest for rifampin-soaked bypasses compared to other methods or revascularization. Reinfection rates were highest, unfortunately, for rifampin-soaked prostheses and lowest for autogenous venous conduits.[105]

Two sub-groups merit attention: AEF and endograft infections. With respect to the management of AEF, the data are conflicting, though the choice of conduit appears to impact outcomes. The largest single center series evaluating AEF management suggest that rifampin-soaked conduits with omental wrapping may perform better, due to the increased mortality after NAIS.[47,49] However, in a recent systematic review, the authors found that among in situ methods of reconstruction, vein grafts had the best AEF related survival.[106] In addition, the management of the enteric defect appears to be particularly impactful.[49,107] Chopra et al.[49] observed that GI complications, namely GI leak from the enteric defect, independently predicted mortality after AEF repair. Intuitively, this would suggest that performance of simple, direct suture repairs of the enteric defect would be associated with an increased risk of GI complications and mortality. However, simple repairs have not been associated with an increased leak rate or mortality in two series.[49,107] Most likely, repairs that adhere to sound surgical principles perform well, regardless of whether simple or complex GI repairs are performed. The principles include aggressive debridement of devitalized, infected tissue, and creation of a tension-free anastomosis with well-vascularized tissue.[49] Additional study regarding the impact of arterial conduit and methods to minimize gastrointestinal complications will be required to further optimize outcomes.

Reconstruction after aortic endografts appears to favor nonprosthetic reconstructions. After endograft explantation, the remaining aorta is often friable, and difficult to sew. Hence using a conduit that is most easy to suture and least prone to suture-line leak would be ideal. In this context, Smeds et al.[44] retrospectively evaluated 206 endograft infections, and found that those repaired with either femoral vein or cadaveric allograft had improved survival (71% at 5 years) relative to rifampin-soaked prosthetic (53% at 5 years). The reason for the survival difference is unknown, and merits further study. Survival after endograft explantation is 51% at 5 years and superior for infrarenal endografts, compared to thoracic endografts.[44]

Role of Endovascular Techniques in Aortic Infection Management

With respect to infrarenal or juxtarenal aortic infections, endovascular aortic repair (EVAR) has been successfully utilized to temporize bleeding AEF, permitting the surgeon to optimize the patient's medical condition prior to definitive open repair.[106] Systematic review suggests that there is an early mortality benefit to endovascular exclusion prior to open repair.[106] Unfortunately, only 98 of 823 patients (11.9%) in the review were treated with endovascular means, which precludes robust conclusions.

There are multiple limitations of endografting for AEF. Endovascular temporization of AEF is not always possible, due to inadequate seal zone. Fenestrated endograft for infection is technically possible, with small series demonstrating short-term success.[108] Unfortunately, subsequent explantation and in situ reconstruction after fenestrated EVAR is a very morbid procedure, with case reports of early perioperative death after explantation.[109]

The early survival benefit of EVAR for AEF appears to be lost over time the longer the endograft remains in place.[106] However, there are emerging data that suggest that definitive endografting with antibiotic therapy and/or drainage may be feasible for primary mycotic aneurysms.[108,110] The benefit appears to be especially true for thoracic aortic infection patients.[108,110] Unfortunately, much of the earlier data suggest that persistent infection and/or recurrent hemorrhage plague endografts performed for aortic infection.[111] Failures for EVAR for primary mycotic aneurysms persist for *Salmonella*-related infections. Hence the author reserves infrarenal/juxtarenal EVAR for two groups of patients. (1) Those with adequate seal zone, and hemorrhagic shock due to AEF. The author performs these with the intent to bridge toward definitive open resection and revascularization. (2) Those with comorbidities that preclude open surgery and a primary mycotic aneurysm.

Reconstruction for Primary and Secondary Lower Extremity Infections

Graft preservation is undertaken frequently in the lower extremity, as described in the previous sections. For those that require explantation, the principles of reconstruction of the lower extremity arterial tree are similar to the aorta. Debridement is key, especially of remnant prosthetic material, which can serve as a nidus for further infection.[52] After debridement and removal of all infected material, the first decision hinges upon whether revascularization is required. Many patients have underlying arterial occlusive disease, and hence have robust collaterals that permit survival of the limb after ligation of the infected portion. This strategy is most frequently utilized in patients with infected pseudoaneurysms secondary to intravenous drug abuse.[21–24] Common femoral artery ligation and serial debridement of these infections evolved from failures of attempted in situ repairs of infected common femoral artery pseudoaneurysms. These failures occurred due to overwhelming systemic and local sepsis in the groin. Intermittent claudication is common, occurring in approximately one-fourth of patients after ligation of the common femoral artery.[24] Patency of the profunda and superficial femoral artery junction is ideal, as many of the collaterals required for limb preservation emanate from the internal iliac artery and course to the profunda femoral artery.[24] Acute limb-threatening ischemia is infrequent, occurring in <2% when the profunda and superficial femoral artery junction is preserved.[24] Amputation markedly increases when each of the femoral vessels require individual ligation.[21–23] Treatment requires individualization, however, as some authors note success when in situ revascularization is performed in the setting of intravenous drug abuse.[23]

Obturator bypass is a useful, though uncommon, method of revascularizing the limb when the common femoral artery requires ligation.[112] This is performed with a variety of conduits in planes uninvolved with infection. The inflow for the bypass is the native common or external iliac artery, or incorporated portion of the aortofemoral limb. The site of the distal anastomosis is chosen in an uninfected area of the distal superficial femoral artery. An opening is made in the ventromedial portion of the obturator foramen, which is placed laterally to the pubis. The foramen in incised and a blunt tunneling device is then passed through the foramen, and tunneled until the desired distal anastomosis site is reached with the tunneler. Recent series describe excellent 30-day outcomes, without evidence of early graft failure, amputation, or mortality.[112] Primary graft patency is modest (65% at 24 months). However, secondary patency is 88% at 24 months. Given the paucity of other options for revascularization, obturator bypass is a safe and reasonable option in the setting of ischemia and common femoral artery infection. Moreover, the principle of tunneling a new graft through an uninfected plane is important to any vascular reconstruction for infection.

Cadaveric vein allografts have been used in the setting of lower extremity infection, to theoretically provide a conduit that is more resistant to infection than prosthetic conduits. Unfortunately, outcomes are suboptimal, with Chang et al. reporting a primary patency of 27% and 17% at 1 and 3 years after implantation.[113] Reintervention does not assist patency significantly, with primary-assisted patency rates of 38% and 18% at 1 and 3 years postoperatively.[113] Other series report a more dismal primary patency, of 17% at 1 year and 9% at 18 months. ABO blood antigen compatibility and systemic anticoagulation with warfarin improves patency.[113,114] Cadaveric allografts are expensive, costing approximately US$7500 per graft. There are no direct comparisons between cadaveric allograft and prosthetic bypasses, but given the poor outcomes and cost, the author reserves the use of cadaveric allograft to the rare case where the patient has either: (a) no conduit, and/or (b) no other alternative to either open or endovascular revascularization.

Revascularization in Other Vascular Beds

Carotid revascularization is best performed with interposition grafting after wide local debridement of all infected material.[56,57] Greater saphenous vein, femoral vein, and cryopreserved allograft may be utilized as a conduit.[58] Ligation is required in a minority of cases, with preoperative balloon-occlusion testing, and intraoperative test clamping performed to evaluate the adequacy of collateral cerebral circulation prior to ligation.[56] Carotid stenting and antibiotic therapy has been utilized in a minority of cases, with case reports of success, though with limited follow-up.[115]

Visceral artery infected aneurysms are also ideally treated with debridement and interposition grafting with autogenous vein. A thorough evaluation of the collateral supply of the mesenteric vessels is required.[19] This knowledge enables the surgeon to decide which infected visceral artery aneurysms can be safely ligated.[19] Endovascular management with coils and/or stents to exclude infected visceral artery aneurysms, followed by long-term antibiotics is also feasible.[20] Because the coils can also become infected, the author reserves coil embolization and antibiotic therapy for those patients in whom technical considerations and patient comorbidities preclude safe resection and vascular reconstruction.

SUPPURATIVE THROMBOPHLEBITIS

Venous infections often are complications of venous thrombosis. These can occur anywhere a vein develops a thrombus, though there are common scenarios in patients. Description of superficial infusion-related suppurative thrombophlebitis and indwelling catheter-related central vein suppurative thrombophlebitis follows. Suppuration can also occur in the central/pelvic veins, portal venous system (pylephlebitis), cavernous sinus, and the jugular vein (Lemierre syndrome).

Superficial Vein Suppurative Thrombophlebitis

Infusion-related thrombophlebitis is common, occurring in up to 70% of patients in some reports.[116] However, suppuration occurs relatively rarely, in up to 2% of all peripheral intravenous (IV) insertions in one study.[117] Diagnosis can be difficult, due to overlapping symptoms with noninfectious, infusion-related thrombophlebitis. Lee et al. defined suppuration by: (1) the presence of purulent drainage, pustules, or boils at the insertion site; (2) cellulitis or abscess diagnosed by physical exam and/or intraoperatively; (3) organisms derived from the site with localized swelling, erythema; (4) at least two of the aforementioned signs or symptoms without other known cause which persist after removal of the intravenous catheter for at least 3 days.[118]

Organisms responsible are commensal skin flora, such as *S. aureus,* and coagulase-negative *Staphylococcus* in approximately 20% of cases. No growth can be observed in approximately 15% of cases.[118] The remainder of organisms are a mix of gram-negative organisms and variety of other organisms. Insertion of the IV in the lower extremity is independently associated with an increased risk of suppurative thrombophlebitis, and increases the risk by more than eightfold.[118] Other independent predictors of suppuration include continuous IV infusion for >24 hours, use of infusion pumps, and hospitalization due to a neurosurgical condition. Other risk factors include a history of IV drug abuse, concomitant steroid therapy, and recent burn injuries.[119] Hence peripheral IVs ideally should be placed in the upper extremities and changed every 72 hours.

Management includes removal of the peripheral IV catheter, and intravenous broad-spectrum antibiotics. For severe cases of suppuration, resection of the infected vein, and debridement of the surrounding tissue is required, similar to necrotizing soft tissue infections. Untreated, suppurative thrombophlebitis may result in septic pulmonary emboli, systemic bacteremia, and sepsis.[118,119] Exploration of the vein should continue proximally until uninfected vein is encountered, with all tributaries and infected segments of vein resected to healthy vein. The wound should then be left to heal by secondary intention. Antibiotics should then be continued for 2 to 3 weeks afterwards.[120]

Central Venous Suppurative Thrombophlebitis

In contrast to superficial venous thrombophlebitis, surgical resection of the offending vein is often not recommended, due to the associated morbidity with the procedure. Hence the mainstay of therapy for all of the deep venous suppurative thrombophlebitis presentations remains IV heparin and antibiotic therapy.[121–124] Failure of nonsurgical therapy should be considered if the patient has not defervesced within 48 hours. Duplex ultrasound, CTA, or MRI are used to confirm the presence of central vein clot. Finally, a thorough history, physical, and relevant imaging should be performed to exclude the presence of another source of sepsis. For these patients, surgical options may provide clinical improvement.[121] In patients with persistent sepsis refractory to nonsurgical therapy, surgical thrombectomy may be performed. Over 90% patency and 84% resolution of sepsis can be achieved with less than 8% rates of wound hematoma.[121] Endovascular solutions also exist, such as thrombolysis, and pharmacomechanical thrombectomy.[123] Endovascular therapies are advantageous, as the patient population is often malnourished, immunocompromised, and/or having other comorbidities that may preclude open surgical thrombectomy. Surgical interventions remain options of last resort and are rarely employed, as experience with surgical or endovascular thrombectomy is limited to case reports and small case series.

Indwelling Central Vein Catheter-Related Thrombophlebitis

The diagnosis of central-line associated septic thrombophlebitis hinges upon a high degree of clinical suspicion. The patients often have a history of malnutrition and immunosuppression in addition to prolonged central venous catheter use.[121,122] The diagnosis may elude physicians, as current imaging techniques have significant limitations in detecting infection, particularly in small veins.[122] Patients that have a history of persistent bacteremia with IV antibiotics and removal of the central venous catheter are at increased risk of having a septic catheter-related thrombophlebitis.[121,122] History, physical examination, and other adjunctive testing are required, however, to rule out other sources of potential fever and bacteremia.[121,122]

The gold standard of management remains removal of the offending catheter, IV antibiotic therapy, and anticoagulation. Systematic review revealed that the addition of heparin to IV antibiotics results in clinical improvement and/or defervescence at a mean of 1.5 to 2.5 days.[122] The goal partial thromboplastin time was 1.5 to 3.0 times normal.[122] IV antibiotics were used for all studies within the systematic review. Overall, mortality with this strategy is less than 2% in the systematic review.[122] Individual case series vary, however, with failure of IV antibiotics and heparin reaching as high as 28%.[122] Common organisms include *S. aureus, Candida albicans,* and gram-negative bacteria.[121]

Lemierre Syndrome, Pelvic Venous Thrombophlebitis, and Pylephlebitis

Suppurative thrombophlebitis of the internal jugular vein can result from catheter-related thrombosis that becomes secondarily infected. However, the classic cases describe presentations where patients suffer oropharyngeal infections, gingivitis, or complications of dental procedures.[122,123] The triad of anaerobic septicemia, internal jugular thrombophlebitis, and metastatic abscesses (commonly the lung, joints, and liver) comprise Lemierre syndrome. Patients classically present with a recent history of pharyngitis, and pain and swelling overlying the

anterior cervical triangle.[124] Rarely, Lemierre syndrome complicates hypercoagulable disorders, such as protein S and/or C deficiency, and hormonal replacement therapy.[123]

Untreated, potential complications include septic pulmonary embolism, systemic sepsis, rupture of the adjacent carotid artery, superior vena cava syndrome, and chylothorax. Transient jugular foramen syndrome may also ensue, resulting in unilateral paresis of the soft palate and larynx.[123] The classic microorganism is *Fusobacterium necrophorum,* which is an anaerobic gram-negative rod that normally inhabits the mouth. Other organisms include anaerobic streptococcal species, and other commensal flora of the mouth.

Pelvic suppurative thrombophlebitis occurs in less than 1% of postpartum women.[125] However, among patients with fever greater than 5-days postpartum while on broad spectrum antibiotics, the prevalence of septic pelvic thrombophlebitis can be as high as 20%.[126] Independent predictors of pelvic suppurative thrombophlebitis include an age less than 20 years, black race, multiple gestation, and preeclampsia. Black race was most strongly associated with an increased risk of pelvic suppurative thrombophlebitis.[125] Other risk factors include prior perinatal infections, wound complications, hysterectomy, caesarean delivery, and blood transfusion.[125] Pelvic thrombophlebitis tends to occur on the right, due to the left-to-right venous flow in the upright state.[126]

Presentations are nonspecific with fever and colicky abdominal pain.[126] On abdominal or pelvic examination, a sausage shaped mass may be palpable, though this is not uniformly identified.[126] Approximately one-third of patients will present with septic pulmonary emboli. Ureteral obstruction may also occur. For patients where the diagnosis is uncertain, CT or MRI can help to visualize inflammation and thrombosis of the ovarian veins.[126] Management includes IV antibiotics and systemic anticoagulation. Modern antibiotic regimens include imipenam or ertapenam for 7 days. The classic antibiotic regimen included clindamycin, ampicillin, and gentamycin for 7 days. In refractory cases, ligation of the septic thrombosed veins has proven effective.[126]

Pylephlebitis consists of thrombosis and infections of the portal venous system, resulting from intraabdominal infections with portal venous drainage. Classically, appendicitis had been the main inciting infection. Early application of broad spectrum antibiotics has decreased the incidence of pylephlebitis such that recent series now cite pancreatitis and diverticulitis as the most prevalent causes.[127] Other causes include inflammatory bowel disease, hypercoagulable states, and iatrogenic complication (i.e., hemorrhoidal banding, lap-band, CT-guided liver biopsy).[127] The main portal veins are affected more commonly than the mesenteric veins.[127] Common organisms include *S. viridans, E. coli,* and *Bacteroides fragilis,* with 50% of cases resulting from polymicrobial infections.[128] *B. fragilis* is the classic microorganism described, due to its ability to augment fibrin cross linking, and its facilitation of the coagulation cascade.[127] Untreated, suppurative mesenteric venous thrombosis can result in venous mesenteric ischemia. Mortality rates as high as 25% have been cited.[127,128] Unfortunately, the diagnosis is often delayed due to the nonspecific symptoms at presentation, such as malaise, fever, nausea, and abdominal tenderness. Often, these symptoms overlap with the preceding inciting intraabdominal infection, which may cause the physician to overlook pylephlebitis as a potential etiology. Jaundice ensues when hepatic involvement because severe.[127]

The initial therapy includes broad spectrum antibiotic therapy for 4 to 6 weeks.[127] Anticoagulation is frequently utilized also, though several case reports have excluded anticoagulant therapy with similar success.[127,128] When utilized, anticoagulation is administered for a median of 3 to 4 months, with repeat imaging utilized to confirm resolution of the infection. Invasive procedures, such as catheter-directed thrombolysis or surgical thrombectomy, have been reported in case reports only. However, there have been several authors that recommend against invasive treatment, due to the morbidity associated with the procedure.[127,128]

SEPTIC CAVERNOUS SINUS THROMBOSIS

Septic cavernous sinus thrombosis is a rare entity in the antibiotic era, with only 88 adult cases reported in the literature.[129] One-third of case reports detail a history of immunosuppression.[129] Infections of regions that drain to the cavernous sinus precede the septic cavernous sinus thrombosis, such as sinus infections, dental infections, and other midface infections, with rare reports of infection originating from distant sites.[129,130] *S. aureus* (both methicillin-sensitive and methicillin-resistant) are frequently reported. Immunocompromised patients frequently had reports of fungal infections, of which *Aspergillus fumigatus* was most commonly reported.

Fever, ptosis, chemosis, and external ophthalmoplegia are frequent physical findings. Headache, papilledema, and periorbital swelling are also common.[129,130] CTA and MRA can be utilized to confirm the diagnosis.

Antibiotics and anticoagulation remain the mainstay of therapy.[129,130] Adjunctive endoscopic sinus drainage has been utilized in some cases with success.[130] Surgery is reserved for refractory cases, with rare reports of subdural abscess drainage and craniotomy with incision and drainage of the sigmoid sinus.[129] Corticosteroids have been used in a minority of cases to theoretically decrease periorbital swelling and cranial nerve compression. Corticosteroids do not appear efficacious, however, with similar outcomes achieved with cases where corticosteroids were not utilized.[129]

CONCLUSIONS

PAIs and SAIs are rare entities, though of these, SAIs are significantly more prevalent. Untreated, both PAIs and SAIs have the propensity to destroy the adjacent arterial wall, resulting in pseudoaneurysms and arterial rupture. Septic arterial emboli and bacterial seeding can both result in synchronous infections in distant sites. A high index of clinical suspicion is required to avoid unnecessary delays in diagnosis and therapy. In addition to a thorough history and physical, CTA is an invaluable tool to aid in the diagnosis. However, for occult infections, other testing may be required, such as [18]FDG-PET and SPECT/CT. More urgent therapy is required for cases where hemorrhagic or septic complications are present, especially AEF. For all arterial cases, source control with debridement and resection of all infected material is ideal. Subsequent arterial reconstruction depends upon the preferences of the surgeon, without clear superiority of one particular method within the literature. Conversely, most venous infections are typically managed with antibiotics and anticoagulation. The exception is superficial suppurative thrombophlebitis, where wide local excision is beneficial. Surgery is utilized sparingly as a last resort for most instances of septic venous thromboses.

REFERENCES

1. Koch L. *Ueber aneurysma der arterial mesenterichae superioris.* Inag Di Erlangen, 1851.
2. Wilson SE, Van Wagenen P, Passaro Jr E. Arterial infection. *Curr Probl Surg.* 1978;15:1–89.
3. Buckmaster MJ, Curci JA, Murray PR, et al. Source of elastin-degrading enzymes in mycotic aortic aneurysms: bacteria or host inflammatory response? *Cardiovasc Surg.* 1999;7:16–26.
4. Hsu RB, Lin FY. Surgical pathology of infected aortic aneurysm and its clinical correlation. *Ann Vasc Surg.* 2007;21:742–748.
5. Miller DV, Oderich GS, Aubry MC, et al. Surgical pathology of infected aneurysms of the descending thoracic and abdominal aorta: clinicopathologic correlations in 29 cases (1976 to 1999). *Hum Pathol.* 2004;35:112–120.
6. McGregor JA, Lawellin D, Franco-Buff A, et al. Protease production by microorganisms associated with reproductive tract infection. *Am J Obstet Gynecol.* 1986;15:109–114.
7. Okamoto T, Akaike T, Suga M, et al. Activation of human matrix metalloproteinases by various bacterial proteinases. *J Biol Chem.* 1997;272:6059–6066.
8. Brown SL, Busuttil RW, Baker JD, et al. Bacteriologic and surgical determinants of survival in patients with mycotic aneurysms. *J Vasc Surg.* 1984;1:541–547.
9. Ailawadi G, Eliason JL, Upchurch GR. Current concepts in the pathogenesis of abdominal aortic aneurysm. *J Vasc Surg.* 2003;38:584–588.
10. Muller BT, Wegener OR, Grabitz K, et al. Mycotic aneurysms of the thoracic and abdominal aorta and iliac arteries: experience with anatomic and extra-anatomic repair in 33 cases. *J Vasc Surg.* 2001;33:106–113.
11. Oderich GS, Panneton JM, Bower TC, et al. Infected aortic aneurysms: aggressive presentation, complicated early outcome, but durable results. *J Vasc Surg.* 2001;34:900–908.
12. Achilli P, Guttadauro A, Bonfanti P, et al. Streptococcus agalactiae infective endocarditis complicated by multiple mycotic hepatic aneurysms and massive splenic infarction: a case report. *BMC Gastroenterol.* 2017;17:170–175.
13. Dubois M, Daenens K, Houthoofd S, et al. Treatment of mycotic aneurysms with involvement of the abdominal aorta: single-centre experience in 44 consecutive cases. *Eur J Vasc Endovasc Surg.* 2010;40:450–456.
14. Psoinos CM, Simons JP, Baril DT, et al. A Mycobacterium bovis mycotic abdominal aortic aneurysm resulting from bladder cancer treatment, resection and reconstructions with cryopreserved aortic graft. *Vasc Endovascular Surg.* 2013;47:61–64.
15. Brosier J, Lesprit P, Marzelle J, et al. New bacteriologic patterns in primary infected aorto-iliac aneurysms: a single-centre experience. *Eur J Vasc Endovasc Surg.* 2010;40:582–588.
16. Chitragari G, Laux AT, Hicks TD, et al. Rare presentation of a syphilitic aneurysm of the infrarenal aorta with contained rupture. *Ann Vasc Surg.* 2018;47(279):e13-279.e17.
17. Leon Jr LR, Mills Sr JL. Diagnosis and management of aortic mycotic aneurysms. *Vasc Endovasc Surg.* 2010;44:5–13.
18. Macedo TA, Stanson AW, Oderich GS, et al. Infected aortic aneurysm: imaging findings. *Radiology.* 2004;231:250–257.
19. Kordzadeh A, Watson J, Panayiotopolous Y. Mycotic aneurysm of the superior and inferior mesenteric artery. *J Vasc Surg.* 2016;63:1638–1646.
20. Chaudhari D, Saleem A, Patel P, et al. Hepatic artery mycotic aneurysm associated with staphylococcal endocarditis with successful treatment: case report with review of the literature. *Case Reports Hepatol.* 2013;610818.
21. Devecioglu M, Settembre N, Samia Z, et al. Treatment of arterial lesions in drug addicts. *Ann Vasc Surg.* 2014;28:184–191.
22. Peirce C, Coffey JC, O'Grady H, et al. The management of mycotic femoral pseudoaneurysms in intravenous drug abusers. *Ann Vasc Surg.* 2009;23:345–349.
23. Jayaraman S, Richardson D, Conrad M, et al. Mycotic pseudoaneurysms due to injection drug abuse: a ten-year experience. *Ann Vasc Surg.* 2012;26:819–824.
24. Hu ZJ, Wang SM, Li XX, et al. Tolerable hemodynamic changes after femoral artery ligation for the treatment of infected femoral artery pseudoaneurysm. *Ann Vasc Surg.* 2010;24:212–218.
25. Epstein AJ, Polsky D, Yang F, et al. Coronary revascularization trends in the United States, 2001-2008. *JAMA.* 2011;305:1769–1776.
26. Biancari F, D'Andrea V, Di Marco C, et al. Meta-analysis of randomized trials on the efficacy of vascular closure devices after diagnostic angiography and angioplasty. *Am Heart J.* 2010;159:518–531.
27. Smilowitz N, Kirtane AJ, Guiry M, et al. Practices and complications of vascular closure devices and manual compression in patients undergoing elective transfemoral coronary procedures. *Am J Cardiol.* 2012;110:177–182.

28. Nader R, Mohr G, Sheiner NM, et al. Mycotic aneurysm of the carotid bifurcation in the neck: case report and review of the literature. *Neurosurgery*. 2001;48:1152–1156.

29. O'Connell JB, Darcy S, Reil T. Extracranial internal carotid artery mycotic aneurysm: case report and review. *Vasc Endovascular Surg*. 2009;43:410–415.

30. Rogers AC, Bourke M, Galbraith AS, et al. Mycotic aneurysm of the extracranial internal carotid artery, resect, ligate, or reconstruct? *Ann Vasc Surg*. 2016;35(203):e5-203.e10.

31. Gabrielli R, Rosati MS, Marcuccio L, Siani A. Mycotic aneurysm of dorsalis pedis artery due to recurrent *Candida albicans* foot infection. *J Vasc Surg*. 2014;59:1707–1708.

32. Larena-Avellaneda A, Debus ES, Daum H, et al. Mycotic aneurysms affecting both lower legs of a patient with *Candida* endocarditis-endovascular therapy and open vascular surgery. *Ann Vasc Surg*. 2004;18:130–133.

33. Ghassani A, Delva JC, Berard X, et al. Stent graft exclusion of a rupture mycotic popliteal pseudoaneurysm complicating sternoclavicular joint infection. *Ann Vasc Surg*. 2012;26:730e.13-730.e15.

34. Bunt TJ. Synthetic vascular infections. *I Graft infections Surgery*. 1983;93:733–746.

35. Szilagyi DE, Smith RF, Elliott JP, Vrandecic MP. Infection in arterial reconstruction with synthetic grafts. *Ann Surg*. 1972;176:321–333.

36. Samson RH, Veith FJ, Janko GS, et al. A modified classification and approach to the management of infections involving peripheral arterial prosthetic grafts. *J Vasc Surg*. 1988;8:147–153.

37. Zimmerli W, Sendi P. Pathogenesis of implant-associated infection: the role of the host. *Semin Immunopath*. 2011;33:295–306.

38. Brunstedt MR, Sapatnekar S, Rubin KR, et al. Bacterial/blood/material interactions. I. Injected and preseeded slime-forming Staphylococcus epidermidis in flowing blood with biomaterials. *J Biomed Mater Res*. 1995;29:455–466.

39. MacKintosh EE, Patel JD, Marchant RE, Anderson JM. Effects of biomaterial surface chemistry on adhesion and biofilm formation of Staphylococcus epidermidis in vitro. *J Biomed Mater Res A*. 2006;78:836–842.

40. United Kingdom Small Aneurysms Trial Participants, Powell JT, Brady AR, et al. Long-term outcomes of immediate repair compared with surveillance of small abdominal aortic aneurysms. *N Engl J Med*. 2002;346:1445–1452.

41. Vogel TR, Symons R, Flum DR. The incidence and factors associated with graft infection after aneurysm repair. *J Vasc Surg*. 2008;47:264–269.

42. Coselli JS, LeMaire SA, Preventza O, et al. Outcomes of 3309 thoracoabcominal aortic aneurysm repairs. *J Thorac Cardiovasc Surg*. 2016;151:1323–1337.

43. Murphy EH, Sveto WY, Herdrich BJ, et al. The management of endograft infections following endovascular thoracic and abdominal aneurysm repair. *J Vasc Surg*. 2013;58:1179–1185.

44. Smeds MR, Duncan AA, Harlander-Locke MP, et al. Treatment and outcomes of aortic endograft infection. *J Vasc Surg*. 2016;63:332–340.

45. Ali AT, Modrall JG, Hocking J, et al. Long-term results of the treatment of aortic graft infection by in situ replacement with femoral popliteal vein graft. *J Vasc Surg*. 2009;50:30–39.

46. Oderich GS, Bower TC, Cherry KJ, et al. Evolution from axillofemoral to in situ prosthetic reconstruction for the treatment of aortic graft infection at a single center. *J Vasc Surg*. 2006;43:1166–1174.

47. Oderich GS, Bower TC, Hofer J, et al. In situ rifampin soaked grafts with omental coverage and antibiotic suppression are durable with low reinfection rates in patients with aortic graft enteric erosion or fistula. *J Vasc Surg*. 2011;53:99–106.

48. Harlander-Locke MP, Harmon LK, Lawrence PF, et al. The use of cryopreserved aortoiliac allograft for aortic reconstruction in the United States. *J Vasc Surg*. 2014;59:669–674.

49. Chopra A, Cieciura L, Modrall JG, et al. Twenty-year experience with aorto-enteric fistula repair: gastrointestinal complications predict mortality. *J Am Coll Surg*. 2017;225:9–18.

50. Alimi Y, Sosin M, Borsinger TM, et al. Implications of Clostridium septicum in vascular surgery: a case report and outcomes literature review. *Ann Vasc Surg*. 2017;43:e5-314.e11.

51. Seabrook GR, Schmitt DD, Bandyk DF, et al. Anastomotic femoral pseudoaneurysm: an investigation of occult infection as an etiologic factor. *J Vasc Surg*. 1990;11:629–634.

52. Marsan BU, Curl GR, Pilai L, et al. The thrombosed prosthetic graft is a risk for infection of an adjacent graft. *Am J Surg*. 1996;172:175–177.

53. Wright DJ, Ernst CB, Evans JR, et al. Ureteral complications and aortoiliac reconstruction. *J Vasc Surg*. 1990;11:29–35.

54. Brothers TE, Robison JE, Elliott BM. Predictors of prosthetic graft infection after infrainguinal bypass. *J Am Coll Surg*. 2009;208:557–561.

55. Siracuse JJ, Nandivada P, Giles KA, et al. Prosthetic graft infections involving the femoral artery. *J Vasc Surg*. 2013;57:700–705.

56. Writing Group for the ESVS, Naylor AR, Ricco JB, et al., ed. Editor's choice - management of atherosclerotic carotid and vertebral artery disease: 2017 clinical practice guidelines of the European Society of Vascular Surgery (ESVS). *Eur J Vasc Endovasc Surg*. 2018;55:3–81.

57. Mann CD, McCarthy M, Nasim A, et al. Management and outcome of prosthetic patch infection after carotid endarterectomy: a single-centre series and systematic review of the literature. *Eur J Vasc Endovasc Surg*. 2012;44:20–26.

58. Naughton PA, Garcia-Toca M, Rodriguez HE, et al. Carotid artery reconstruction for infected carotid patches. *Eur J Vasc Endovasc Surg*. 2010;40:492–498.

59. Riles TS, Lamparello PJ, Giangola G, Imparato AM. Rupture of the vein patch: a rare complication of carotid endarterectomy. *Surgery*. 1990;107:10–12.

60. Bosman WMPF, Borger van der Berg BLS, Schuttevaer HM, et al. Infections of intravascular bare metal stents: a case report and review of literature. *Eur J Vasc Endovasc Surg*. 2014;47:87–99.

61. Hogg ME, Peterson BG, Pearce WH, et al. Bare metal stent infections: case report and review of the literature. *J Vasc Surg*. 2007;46:813–820.

62. Quintas A, Alves G, Aragao de Morais J, et al. Iliac artery reconstruction with femoral vein after bare metal stent infection. *EJVES Short Rep*. 2017;34:28–31.

63. Perera GB, Fujitani RM, Kubaska SM. Aortic graft infection: an update on management and treatment options. *Vasc Endovascular Surg*. 2006;40:1–10.

64. Mathias J, Mathias E, Jausset F, et al. Aorto-enteric fistulas: a physiopathological approach and computed tomography diagnosis. *Diagn Interv Imaging*. 2012;93:840–851.

65. Vu QD, Menias CO, Bhalla S, et al. Aortoenteric fistulas: CT features and potential mimics. *Radiographics*. 2009;109:197–209.

66. Shahidi S, Eskil A, Lundof E, et al. Detection of abdominal aortic graft infection: comparison of magnetic resonance imaging and indium-labeled white blood cell scanning. *Ann Vasc Surg*. 2007;21:586–592.

67. Bruggink JLM, Slart RHJA, Pol JA, et al. Current role of imaging in diagnosing aortic graft infections. *Semin Vasc Surg*. 2011;24:182–190.

68. Spartera C, Morettini G, Petrassi C, et al. Role of magnetic resonance imaging in the evaluation of aortic graft healing, perigraft fluid collection, and graft infection. *Eur J Vasc Surg*. 1990;4:69–73.

69. Lazaris A, Sayers RD, Thompson M, et al. Patch corrugation on duplex ultrasonography may be an early warning of prosthetic patch infection. *Eur J Vasc Endovasc Surg*. 2005;29:91–92.

70. Chung J, Clagett GP. Neoarotoiliac system (NAIS) procedure for the treatment of the infected aortic graft. *Semin Vasc Surg*. 2011;24:220–226.

71. Palestro CJ, Torres MA. Radionuclide imaging of nonosseous infection. *Q J Nucl Med*. 1999;43:46–60.

72. Ryu SW, Allman KC. Native aortic and prosthetic vascular stent infection on 99m-Tc-labeled white blood cell scintigraphy. *J Nucl Med Technol*. 2014;42:120–121.

73. Even-Sapir E, Keidar Z, Bar-Shalom R. Hybrid imaging (SPECT/CT and PET/CT) - improving the diagnostic accuracy of functional/metabolic and anatomic imaging. *Semin Nucl Med*. 2009;39:264–275.

74. Erba PA, Leo G, Sollini M, et al. Radiolabelled leucocyte scintigraphy versus conventional radiological imaging for the management of late, low-grade vascular prosthesis infections. *Eur J Nucl Med Mol Imaging*. 2014;41:357–368.

75. Saleem BR, Berger P, Vaartjes I, et al. Modest utility of quantitative measures in ^{18}F-fluorodeoxyglucose positron emission tomography scanning for the diagnosis of aortic prosthetic graft infection. *J Vasc Surg*. 2015;61:965–971.

76. Thompson WM, Jackson DC, Johnsrude IS. Aortoenteric and paraprosthetic-enteric fistulas: radiologic findings. *AJR Am J Roentgenol.* 1976;127:235–242.

77. Armstrong PA, Back MR, Wilson JS, et al. Improved outcomes in the recent management of secondary aortoenteric fistula. *J Vasc Surg.* 2005;42:660–666.

78. Lawrence PF. Conservative treatment of aortic graft infection. *Semin Vasc Surg.* 2011;24:199–204.

79. Gordon A, Conlon C, Collin J, et al. An eight year experience of conservative management for aortic graft sepsis. *Eur J Vas Surg.* 1994;8:611–616.

80. Belair M, Soulez G, Oliva VL. Aortic infection: the value of percutaneous drainage. *AJR Am J Roentgenol.* 1998;171:119–124.

81. Mueller KH, Rodriguez HE, Kibbe MR, Eskandari MK. Percutaneous drainage and explanation of an infected aortic endoluminal stent graft. *Ann Vasc Surg.* 2003;17:550–553.

82. Morris GE, Friend PA, Vassallo DJ, et al. Conservative treatment of major aortic graft infection. *Eur J Vasc Surg.* 1990;4:63–67.

83. Ali AT, Rueda M, Desikan S, et al. Outcomes after retroflexed gracilis muscle flap for vascular infections in the groin. *J Vasc Surg.* 2016;64:452–457.

84. Herrera FA, Kohanzadeh S, Nasseri Y, et al. Management of vascular graft infections with soft tissue flap coverage: improving limb salvage rates--a Veterans Affairs experience. *Am Surg.* 2009;75:877–881.

85. Tossios P, Karatzopoulos A, Tsagakis K, et al. Treatment of infected thoracic aortic prosthetic grafts with the in situ preservation strategy: a review of its history, surgical technique, and results. *Heart, Lung Circ.* 2014;23:24–31.

86. Poi MJ, Pisimisis G, Barshes NR, et al. Evaluating effectiveness of antibiotic polymethylmethacrylate beads in achieving wound sterilization and graft preservation in patients with early and late vascular graft infections. *Surgery.* 2013;153:673–682.

87. Clarke J, Halhoub J, Das SK. Ceramic gentamicin beads in vascular graft infection--a cautionary note. *Vasc Endovasc Surg.* 2013;47:76–77.

88. Calligaro KD, Vieth FJ, Schwartz ML, et al. Selective preservation of infected prosthetic arterial grafts. Analysis of a 20-year experience with 120 extracavitary-infected grafts. *Ann Surg.* 1994;220:461–471.

89. Crawford JD, Landry GJ, Moneta GL, Mitchell EL. Outcomes of unilateral graft limb excision for infected aortobifemoral graft limb. *J Vasc Surg.* 2016;63:407–413.

90. Padberg FT, Smith SM, Eng RHK. Accuracy of disincorporation for identification of vascular graft infection. *Arch Surg.* 1995;130:183–187.

91. Fleisher LA, Beckman JA, Brown KA, et al. ACC/AHA 2007 guidelines on perioperative cardiovascular evaluation and care for noncardiac surgery: executive summary: a report of the American College of Cardiology/American Heart Association Task Force on Practice Guidelines (Writing Committee to Revise the 2002 Guidelines on Perioperative Cardiovascular Evaluation for Noncardiac Surgery). *Circulation.* 2007;116:e418–e500.

92. Reilly LM, Stoney RJ, Goldstone J, et al. Improved management of aortic graft infection: the influence of operation sequence and staging. *J Vasc Surg.* 1987;5:421–431.

93. Seeger JM, Pretus HA, Welborn MB, et al. Long-term outcome after treatment of aortic graft infection with staged extra-anatomic bypass grafting and aortic graft removal. *J Vasc Surg.* 2000;32:451–459.

94. Yeager RA, Taylor Jr LM, Moneta GL, et al. Improved results with conventional management of infrarenal aortic infection. *J Vasc Surg.* 1999;30:76–83.

95. O'Hara Hertzer NR, Beven EG, Krajewski LP. Surgical management of infected abdominal aortic grafts: review of a 25-year experience. *J Vasc Surg.* 1986;3:725–731.

96. Schneider F, O'Connor S, Becquemin JP. Efficacy of collagen silver-coated polyester and rifampin-soaked vascular grafts to resist infection from MRSA and *Escherichia coli* in a dog model. *Ann Vasc Surg.* 2008;22:815–821.

97. Hardmann S, Cope A, Swann A, et al. An in vitro model to compare the antimicrobial activity of silver-coated versus rifampin-soaked vascular grafts. *Ann Vasc Surg.* 2008;18:308–313.

98. Delva JC, Deglise S, Berard X, et al. In-situ revascularisation for secondary aorto-enteric fistulae: the success of silver-coated Dacron is closely linked to suitable bowel repair. *Eur J Vasc Endovasc Surg.* 2012;44:417–424.

99. Carrel A. Ultimate result of aortic transplantation. *J Exp Med.* 1912;15:389–398.

100. Batt M, Jean-Baptiste E, O'Connor S, et al. Early and late results of contemporary management of 37 secondary aortoenteric fistulae. *Eur J Vasc Endovasc Surg.* 2011;41:748–757.

101. Modrall JG, Sadjadi J, Ali AT, et al. Deep vein harvest: predicting need for fasciotomy. *J Vasc Surg.* 2004;39:387–394.

102. Modrall JG, Hocking JA, Trimaran CH, et al. Late incidence of chronic venous insufficiency after deep vein harvest. *J Vasc Surg.* 2007;46:520–525.

103. Daenens K, Fourneau I, Nevelsteen A. Ten-year experience in autogenous reconstruction with the femoral vein in the treatment of aortofemoral prosthetic infection. *Eur J Vasc Endovasc Surg.* 2003;25:240–245.

104. Charlton-Ouw KM, Sandhu HK, Huang G, et al. Reinfection after resection and revascularization of infected infrarenal abdominal aortic grafts. *J Vasc Surg.* 2014;59:684–692.

105. O'Connor S, Andrew P, Batt M, Becquemin JP. A systematic review and meta-analysis of treatments for aortic graft infection. *J Vasc Surg.* 2006;44:38–45.

106. Kakkos SK, Bicknell CD, Tsolakis IA, et al. Editor's choice--Management of secondary aorto-enteric and other abdominal arterio-enteric fistulas: a review and pooled data analysis. *Eur J Vasc Endovasc Surg.* 2016;52:770–786.

107. Schoell T, Manceau G, Chiche L, et al. Surgery for secondary aorto-enteric fistula or erosions (SAEFFE) complicating aortic graft surgery: a retrospective analysis of 32 patients with particular focus on digestive management. *World J Surg.* 2015;39:283–291.

108. Sorelius K, Wanhainen A, Furebring M, et al. Nationwide study of the treatment of mycotic abdominal aortic aneurysms comparing open and endovascular repair. *Circulation.* 2016;134:1822–1832.

109. Terry C, Houthoofd S, Maleux G, Fourneau I. Explantation of an infected fenestrated abdominal endograft with autologous venous reconstruction. *EJVES Short Rep.* 2017;34:21–23.

110. Sorelius K, Mani K, Bjorck M, et al. Endovascular treatment of mycotic aortic aneurysms: a European multicenter study. *Circulation.* 2014;130:2136–2142.

111. Leonhardt H, Mellander S, Snygg J, et al. Endovascular management of acute bleeding arterioenteric fistulas. *Cardiovasc Intervent Radiol.* 2008;31:542–549.

112. Bath J, Rahimi M, Long B, et al. Clinical outcomes of obturator canal bypass. *J Vasc Surg.* 2017;66:160–166.

113. Chang CK, Scali ST, Feezor RJ, et al. Defining utility and predicting outcome of cadaveric lower extremity bypass grafts in patients with critical limb ischemia. *J Vasc Surg.* 2014;60:1554–1564.

114. Zehr BP, Niblick CJ, Downey H, Ladowski JS. Limb salvage with CryoVein cadaver saphenous vein allografts used for peripheral arterial bypass: role of blood compatibility. *Ann Vasc Surg.* 2011;25:177–181.

115. Naylor AR. Management of prosthetic patch infection after carotid endarterectomy. *J Cardiovasc Surg.* 2016;57:137–144.

116. Di Nisio M, Peinemann F, Porreca E, Rutjes AW. Treatment for superficial infusion thrombophlebitis of the upper extremity. *Cochrane Database Syst Rev.* 2015;11:CD011015.

117. Lee WL, Chen HL, Tsai TY, et al. Risk factors for peripheral intravenous catheter infection in hospitalized patients: a prospective study of 3165 patients. *Am J of Infect Control.* 2009;37:683–686.

118. Lee WL, Liao SF, Lee WC, et al. Soft tissue infections related to peripheral intravenous catheters in hospitalized patients: a case-control study. *J Hosp Infect.* 2010;76:124–129.

119. Pruitt Jr BA, McManus WF, Kim SH, Treat RC. Diagnosis and treatment of cannula-related intravenous sepsis in burn patients. *Ann Surg.* 1980;191:546–554.

120. Villani C, Johnson DH, Cunha BA. Bilateral suppurative thrombophlebitis due to Staphylococcus aureus. *Heart Lung.* 1995;24:342–344.

121. Kim M, Kwon H, Hong SK, et al. Surgical treatment of central venous catheter related septic deep venous thrombosis. *Eur J Vasc Endovasc Surg.* 2015;49:670–675.

122. Falagas ME, Vardakas KZ, Athanasiou S. Intravenous heparin in combination with antibiotics for the treatment of deep vein septic thrombophlebitis: a systematic review. *Eur J Pharmacol.* 2007;557:93–98.

123. Kar S, Webel R. Septic thrombophlebitis: percutaneous mechanical thrombectomy and thrombolytic therapies. *Am J Therap*. 2014;21:131–136.

124. Zhao A, Samannodi M, Tahir M, et al. Lemierre's syndrome: case report and brief literature review. *IDCases*. 2017;10:15–17.

125. Dotters-Katz SK, Smid MC, Grace MR, et al. Risk factors for postpartum septic pelvic thrombophlebitis: a multicenter cohort. *Am J Perinatol*. 2017;34:1148–1151.

126. Garcia J, Aboujaoude R, Apuzzio J, Alvarez JR. Septic pelvic thrombophlebitis: diagnosis and management. *Infect Dis Obstet Gynecol*. 2006;1581461.

127. Choudhry AJ, Baghdadi YM, Amr MA, et al. Pylephlebitis: a review of 95 cases. *J Gastrointest Surg*. 2016;20:656–661.

128. Kannellopoulou T, Alexopoulou A, Theodossiades G, et al. Pylephlebitis: an overview of non-cirrhotic cases and factors related to outcome. *Scand J Infect Dis*. 2010;42:804–811.

129. Weerasinghe D, Lueck CJ. Septic cavernous sinus thrombosis: a case report and review of the literature. *Neuroopthamology*. 2016;40:263–276.

130. Lize F, Verillaud B, Vironneau P, et al. Septic cavernous sinus thrombosis secondary to acute bacterial sinusitis: a retrospective study of seven cases. *Am J Rhinol Allergy*. 2015;29:e7–e12.

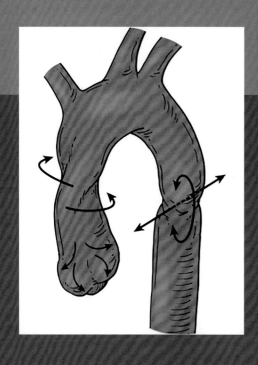

第60章
血管疾病的皮肤表现

　　皮肤的改变是缺血性血管疾病的重要表现，为疾病早期诊断、评估进展、判断预后提供直接的线索。随着影像学技术的不断成熟及血液检查项目的全面优化，现代医学诊断变得更容易。仔细的体格检查对识别慢性血管疾病异常皮肤表现至关重要。准确识别外周动脉疾病的皮肤表现有助于明确诊断及疾病分级和分类，尤其是血管舒缩性疾病，主要靠反复出现的特异性皮肤表现来明确诊断。另外，准确判断血管疾病的皮肤表现可以避免昂贵但不必要的检查，减少潜在有害的放射性操作与医疗成本。本章作者展示了其在临床实践过程中收集的高清、典型的代表性彩图，描述了周围动脉疾病、雷诺现象、手足发绀、红斑性肢痛症、冻疮及冻伤性疾病、网状青斑、混合血管舒缩性疾病、慢性静脉功能不全、淋巴性水肿等血管疾病的典型及非典型的皮肤表现，重点阐述了图片中异常皮损表现及对应诊断，以更加形象、灵活、直接的方式让读者对血管疾病皮肤表现产生深刻的印象。本章内容在准确识别血管疾病皮肤表现方面是非常实用的临床图谱，有助于指导血管外科医师早期识别、准确诊断血管疾病。

戈小虎

Dermatological Manifestations of Vascular Disease

Steven M. Dean

In the modern-day era of medical diagnosis facilitated by sophisticated radiographic imaging and/or comprehensive serological testing, a thorough physical examination remains vital in recognizing the dermatological manifestations of chronic vascular diseases. Accurately identifying cutaneous signs of lymphovenous hypertension and peripheral artery disease (PAD) assists in their diagnosis as well as associated staging and classification. Similarly, the vasomotor diseases are principally diagnosed by their unique and often overlapping cutaneous manifestations. It is important that the vascular specialist consistently recognizes not only classic but also nuanced dermal expressions of lymphatic, venous, arterial, and vasospastic disease. Correct identification of dermatological vascular manifestations obviates expensive and unnecessary testing including potentially deleterious invasive radiological procedures as well as costly consultations. A pictorial review of classic and "not so classic" cutaneous manifestations of vascular diseases is presented with an emphasis on esoteric photographic depictions.

PERIPHERAL ARTERY DISEASE

PAD includes stenotic and occlusive diseases predominantly mediated by atherosclerosis and thromboemboli affecting the aorta and the arteries of the lower extremity (see Chapters 11 and 18).

The arterial vascular examination typically documents weak or absent pulses below the level of arterial stenosis with occasional bruits over stenoses. Although poorly sensitive and nonspecific, the examination in critical limb ischemia often yields thin, dry, shiny, and hairless skin with toenails that are brittle, hypertrophic, and slow growing. Muscle atrophy from inability to exercise may exist. Comparison of color, temperature, and trophic changes between extremities can provide a reasonable assessment of PAD severity unless bilateral disease exists.

Ischemic ulcerations from PAD are typically located on the distal part of the toes and between the digits or at sites of increased focal pressure, such as the metatarsal heads and malleoli. PAD ulcerations are typically severely painful, dry, pale, or black, and punched out with a nongranulating base. Dry gangrene displays a dry, hard texture usually with a clear demarcation between viable and black, necrotic tissue (Fig. 60.1). Wet gangrene is moist and mephitic with blistering and swelling.

While typical PAD-mediated ischemic ulcers are easily identified, correctly diagnosing an *atypical* ischemic ulceration of the lower extremity can be more challenging. Although the dried, pale, or necrotic appearance of the ulcer base is similar in both cases, the location of typical PAD and atypical ischemic limb ulcerations is frequently dissimilar. Specifically, a PAD ischemic ulceration is usually located distally whereas the atypical ischemic ulceration can involve the more proximal portion of the limb like the thighs and buttocks (Fig. 60.2). Additionally, the abdominal wall and breasts can be ulcerated. In

distinct contrast to typical PAD ulcerations, atypical ischemic ulcerations often evolve in the absence of significant large artery occlusive disease and thus the distal pulses are usually easily palpable. Finally, atypical ischemic leg ulcerations may occur with cutaneous abnormalities such as macules, palpable or retiform purpura, petechiae, hemorrhagic bullae, nodules, and/or livedo reticularis (Fig. 60.3). A differential diagnosis of atypical ischemic ulcerations is listed in Box 60.1.[1]

When the atypical ischemic limb ulceration is misdiagnosed as a sequel of PAD, expensive, unnecessary, and potentially injurious radiological investigations are typically ordered. Additionally, unwarranted arterial revascularization may be undertaken and is more likely to occur in the setting of calciphylaxis and atheroembolic disease as both of these disorders usually occur in a background of PAD.

VASOMOTOR DISEASES

Raynaud Phenomenon

Raynaud phenomenon represents an overactive arterial response to cold or stress that results in characteristic well-demarcated digital color changes with sensory symptoms (see Chapter 46).

With a thorough history and physical examination that includes nailfold capillaroscopy and adjunctive testing, Raynaud phenomenon is classified as primary or secondary. Clinical features that suggest a diagnosis of secondary Raynaud phenomenon are outlined in Box 60.2.

Classic Raynaud phenomenon is exemplified by acute onset digital coldness with well-demarcated color changes of vasoconstriction-mediated pallor (Fig. 60.4), followed by cyanosis from tissue hypoxia, and finally reperfusion-associated erythema. However, not all patients display these triphasic color changes nor do they always follow this stereotypical sequence. Attendant symptoms include pain and paresthesias. Both color changes and symptoms should be rapidly and completely reversible in primary Raynaud phenomenon yet can be more severe, protracted, and disabling in the setting of secondary Raynaud phenomenon. The fingers are more likely to be affected than the toes in both primary and secondary Raynaud phenomenon (Fig. 60.5). The index, middle, and ring fingers are the most likely involved digits whereas the thumb is often spared.[2] Thumb involvement suggests a secondary cause for Raynaud phenomenon exists (Fig. 60.6). Raynaud phenomenon can also affect the ears, nose, face, knees, and nipples.

Scleroderma is noteworthy as it is the most common cause of secondary Raynaud phenomenon. Moreover, 58% of scleroderma patients develop at least one digital ulcer at some point in their lifetime and in one-third of cases the ulcers will become chronic.[3] Although classic scleroderma-mediated ulcerations involve the fingertips, some patients will manifest ulcerations along the extensor surfaces of the fingers including the joints (Fig. 60.7). The genesis of extensor ulcerations is thought to be due to a combination of digital ischemia, flexion contractures with increased skin tension, and repetitive microtrauma.[4]

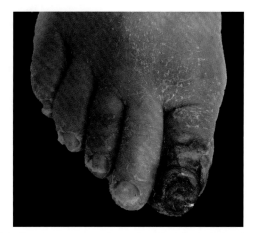

Fig. 60.1 Classic representation of critical limb ischemia with a stereotypical distally located necrotic hallux in the setting of diffusely hairless, dry, scaling skin.

BOX 60.1 Atypical Ischemic Lower Extremity Ulcerations: Differential Diagnosis

Antiphospholipid syndrome
Calciphylaxis
Warfarin skin necrosis
Heparin skin necrosis
Small and medium-sized vasculitis
Atheroembolic disease
Recluse spider bites

Modified from Dean SM. Atypical ischemic lower extremity ulcerations: a differential diagnosis. *Vasc Med.* 2008;13(1):47–54.

BOX 60.2 Clinical Features Suggestive of Secondary Raynaud Phenomenon

Age 40 or older at onset
Male gender
Frequent and severe vasoconstrictive attacks
Asymmetric attacks
Thumb involvement
Fixed digital ischemia (pitting scars, ulcerations, gangrene)
Abnormal nailfold capillaries
Manifestations of an underlying disease
Digital swelling
Ischemic changes proximal to the fingers or toes
Abnormal laboratory parameters

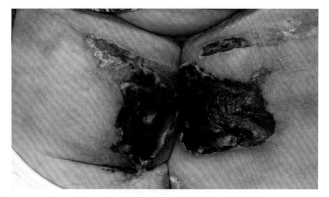

Fig. 60.2 Large Atypically Distributed Ischemic, Necrotic Ulcerations Along the Anterior Proximal Thighs in a Patient With End-Stage Renal Disease–Mediated Calciphylaxis. Faint retiform purpura exists along the upper lateral thighs.

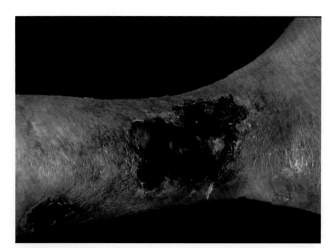

Fig. 60.3 Atypical Ischemic Limb Ulcerations from End-Stage Renal Disease Mediated Calciphylaxis With Dramatic Periulcerative Retiform Purpura With a Characteristic "Puzzle-Piece" Configuration. Unusual cutaneous aberrations such as retiform purpura should not complicate typical ischemic ulcerations of peripheral artery disease.

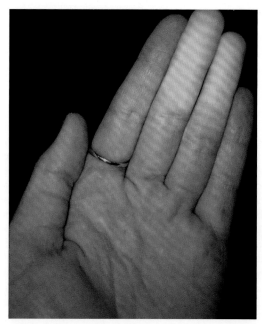

Fig. 60.4 Stereotypical documentation of an acute "white attack" with well-demarcated digital pallor involving the mid and distal aspects of the third and fourth fingers in a young female with primary Raynaud phenomenon.

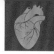

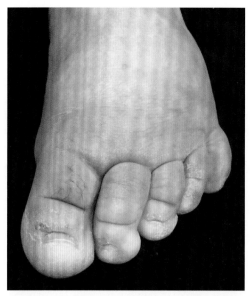

Fig. 60.5 Highly Unusual and Unrelated Coexistence of Primary Raynaud Phenomenon Involving the Toes in the Setting of Long-Standing Primary Lymphedema. Classic Raynaud phenomenon is much more likely to affect the fingers than the toes.

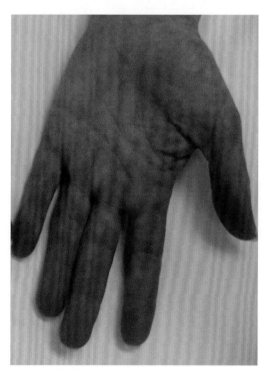

Fig. 60.6 An Acute "Blue Attack" With Characteristic Defined Cyanosis Involving All Fingers Including the Thumb in a Middle-Aged Female With Cold Agglutinin Disease. When the thumb is affected, a secondary cause of Raynaud phenomenon should be suspected.

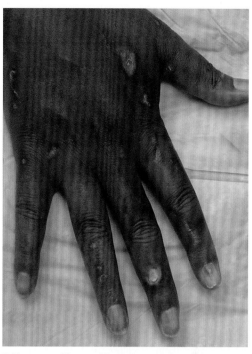

Fig. 60.7 Extensor Finger Ulceration Along the Third Finger in a Patient With Scleroderma-Associated Secondary Raynaud Phenomenon. The combination of hypopigmented scars from healed ulcerations and inflammatory mediated hyperpigmentation (most evident along the proximal third finger) has been referred to as the "salt and pepper" appearance of scleroderma.

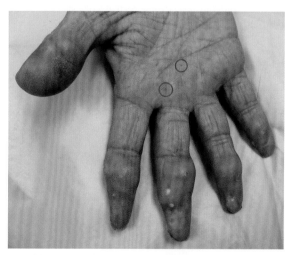

Fig. 60.8 Illustrative Photograph of Diffuse Tumor-Like Nodules from Dystrophic Calcification or "Calcinosis Cutis" Along All of the Distal Fingers in a Patient With Long-Standing Limited Scleroderma. Visible white calcific deposits overlie the third finger. Other noteworthy findings include diffuse tapering of the distal fingers representing acro-osteolysis as well as scattered punctate telangiectasias (red circles).

Limited scleroderma can be complicated by dermal and soft tissue dystrophic calcification or "calcinosis cutis" in 20% to 40% of subjects and is most recognizable in the fingers (Fig. 60.8). Calcinosis can extrude from the skin, ulcerate, and is often quite painful. Lastly, the combination of chronic digital inflammation with active and/or healed ischemic scleroderma ulcerations can yield a characteristic pattern of patchy dermal hyperpigmentation and hypopigmentation referred to as a "salt and pepper" appearance (see Fig. 60.7).

ACROCYANOSIS

Acrocyanosis is a vasomotor condition marked by cool discoloration of different shades of blue in the distal parts of the body (typically involving the hands, feet, and rarely the face) that is usually but not invariably symmetric (see Chapter 47).[5]

Primary acrocyanosis is usually painless and symmetric. Distal pulses are normal in primary disease and there are no skin changes such as fissures or ulcerations. Secondary acrocyanosis is occasionally painful and can be symmetric or asymmetric in distribution. Distal pulses may or may not be palpable and skin changes such as distal ulcerations may occur depending on the underlying disease.

Acrocyanosis always involves the toes and/or fingers. In some cases, the discoloration extends to the feet/hands or even above the level of the ankles/wrists (Fig. 60.9). The color changes are usually persistent and aggravated by cold exposure or limb dependency yet improve with warmth and extremity elevation. Variance in cyanotic hues should be emphasized as acrocyanosis can sometimes exhibit a frequently overlooked lighter erythrocyanotic discoloration (Fig. 60.10). Transient pressure on acrocyanotic skin yields a characteristic blanching with slow and irregular return of blood from the periphery (*not* from beneath the skin) towards the center referred to as Crocq or "iris" sign (Fig. 60.11).[6] The relatively persistent color changes of acrocyanosis should be distinguished from well-demarcated paroxysmal color changes of Raynaud phenomenon. Another useful differentiating clinical feature is that digital pallor only occurs in Raynaud phenomenon.

ERYTHROMELALGIA

Erythromelalgia or "Mitchell disease" is characterized by a classic vasomotor triad of pain, erythema, and heat within the acral portions of the extremities. It is exacerbated by increased temperature and improved with cold (see Chapter 48).

Erythromelalgia is usually classified as primary or secondary. Primary erythromelalgia is most often due to a mutation in voltage-gated sodium channel α-subunit gene SCA9A and is more likely to affect females.[7] Secondary erythromelalgia commonly results from a myeloproliferative syndrome such as polycythemia vera or essential thrombocytosis and is more common in males.

A stereotypical flare of erythromelalgia is exemplified by a complex of paroxysmal acral redness, heat, and burning pain which is frequently complicated by reactive edema (Fig. 60.12). The feet and toes are involved in a sizeable majority of cases whereas the hands and fingers are affected in approximately 25% (Fig. 60.13).[8] Head and neck distribution is distinctly unusual, occurring in 2% of cases. Rarely, the manifestations can extend onto the leg. Erythromelalgia is most often a bilateral and symmetrical phenomenon although unilateral presentations can occur. Provocative factors include ambient heat, exercise, protracted

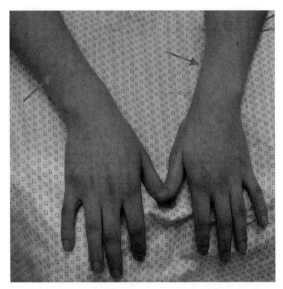

Fig. 60.10 Although acrocyanosis is easily recognized when deeply cyanotic, it can be overlooked when the discoloration displays a lighter erythrocyanotic hue. The arrows demonstrate permanent, palpably cool discoloration proximal to the wrists. Concurrent fine livedo reticularis overlies the dorsal hands.

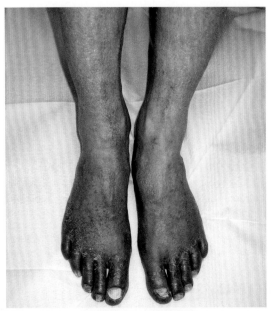

Fig. 60.9 Marked Bipedal Acrocyanosis Extending Above the Level of the Malleoli in a 59-Year-Old Male With Easily Palpable Distal Pulses, a Recent 30-Pound Weight Loss, and Normal Ankle-Brachial Indices. Acrocyanosis is accentuated when the limbs are dependent. He was ultimately diagnosed with paraneoplastic acrocyanosis due to metastatic adenocarcinoma.

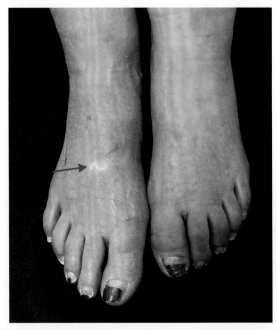

Fig. 60.11 Cutaneous blanching that slowly resolves from the periphery to the center and not rapidly from beneath the skin *(arrow)* exemplifies the Crocq or iris sign in a patient with multiple sclerosis mediated acrocyanosis.

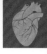

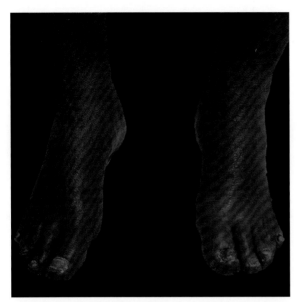

Fig. 60.12 Demonstrably Erythematous, Palpably Hot, Painful Feet in a Patient With Erythromelalgia Secondary to Polycythemia Vera. The extensor tendons cannot be visualized due to associated mild reactive edema that often complicates severe erythromelalgic flares.

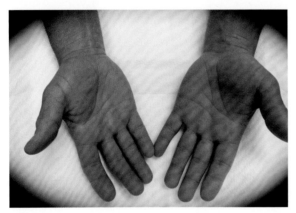

Fig. 60.13 Although less often affected than the feet, hand involvement in erythromelalgia occurs in roughly one in four patients. Mild reactive distal digital edema is present and is most notable in the bilateral second fingers.

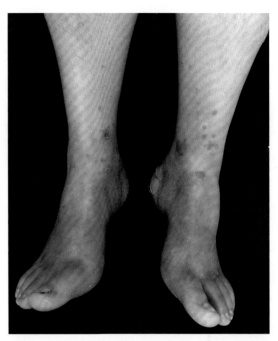

Fig. 60.14 Unusual concurrence of secondary erythromelalgia with cryptogenic cutaneous small vessel vasculitis and associated cutaneous aberrations including purpuric plaques, patches, and ulcerations.

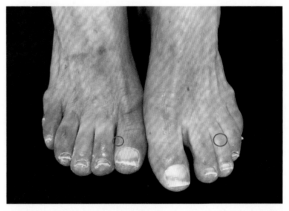

Fig. 60.15 Dramatic Example of Acute Pernio or Chilblains Disease of the Toes of Both Feet With Diffuse Cyanosis and Mild Swelling in the Setting of Palpable Distal Pulses. Stereotypical concurrent perniotic red-purple macules and papules overlie toes and are especially visible on the left side *(red circles)*.

limb dependency, and even alcohol. A typical erythromelalgia episode is intermittent lasting minutes to hours or even days. In rare cases, the manifestations assume a chronic course. Acrocyanosis is frequently noted during symptom-free intervals. Erythromelalgia can be complicated by acral ulcerations in the setting of secondary disease such as myeloproliferative syndrome, chronic venous insufficiency (CVI), or vasculitis (Fig. 60.14), and/or protracted cold-water immersion.

PERNIO/CHILBLAINS DISEASE

Pernio or chilblains disease is an inflammatory acral skin disorder characterized by focal discolored skin changes and swelling after exposure to cold but nonfreezing temperatures (see Chapter 49). Pernio can be primary or secondary although the former is most likely. Although pernio is cold mediated, the exposure temperature is usually *above* freezing. A humid or damp environment increases perniotic susceptibility. Patients frequently relate a multiyear history of annual wintertime outbreaks of the stereotypical lesions.

Within 12 to 24 hours after cold exposure, susceptible patients present with reddish-purple macules, papules, nodules, vesicles, and/or plaques (Fig. 60.15). Perniotic lesions most commonly involve the toes although the feet, fingers, legs, buttocks, and even the face are sometimes involved (Fig. 60.16). In the Mayo Clinic series, 18% of the patients had isolated pernio of the hands/fingers (Fig. 60.17). Nine percent had a combination of both hand and foot involvement.[9] The dorsal portions of the digits are more likely to be affected. The skin manifestations are most commonly painful/tender although up to one in four cases are painless. Less common symptoms include pruritus and burning. Digital swelling often exists and in severe cases, ulcerations can ensue (Fig. 60.18). Blisters and ulcerations may become secondarily infected. The lesions usually heal within 2 to 3 weeks; however, pernio can rarely assume a more protracted or even chronic course. Elderly patients and those with secondary pernio are more likely to suffer from chronic lesions.

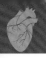

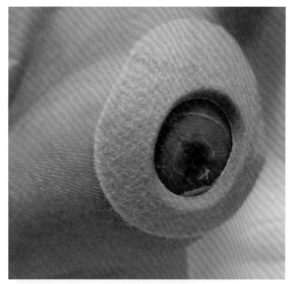

Fig. 60.16 Although pernio typically affects the toes, the heels are rarely affected as well. A healing perniotic ulceration is present along the calcaneus in a 22-year-old male with a hereditary peripheral neuropathy. Note the periulcerative cyanosis.

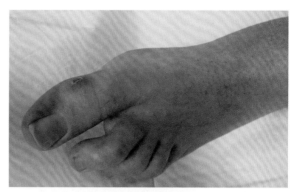

Fig. 60.18 Healing Perniotic Ulceration Along the Medial Hallux of the Previously Mentioned 22-Year-Old Male in Fig. 60.16. Diffuse hammer toes are evident and are a sequela of peripheral neuropathy. Patients with peripheral neuropathy are predisposed to cold-related disorders such as pernio via decreased cold sensation as well as neurogenic vasodysregulation.

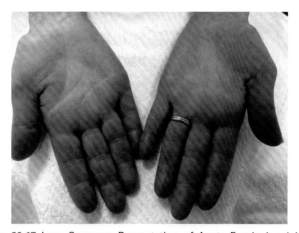

Fig. 60.17 Less Common Presentation of Acute Pernio Involving Only the Fingers of Each Hand. Vivid diffuse digital swelling is evident that even involves the thumbs along with cyanosis and superimposed red-purple macules (most pronounced distal third fingers). In the Mayo Clinic series, approximately one in five patients had isolated pernio of the hands/fingers. (Data from Cappel JA, Wetter DA. Clinical characteristics, etiologic associations, laboratory findings, treatment, and proposal of diagnostic criteria of pernio (chilblains) in a series of 104 patients at Mayo Clinic, 2000 to 2011. *Mayo Clin Proc.* 2014;89:207–215.)

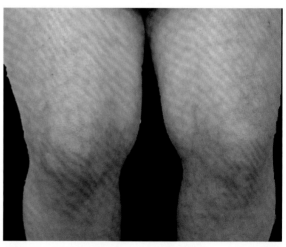

Fig. 60.19 Classic Livedo Reticularis Involving the Lower Extremities With Characteristic Symmetric, Fishnet-Like Erythrocyanotic Mottling That Surrounds a Pallorous Conical Core. In livedo reticularis the discolored cones or rings are relatively regular, symmetrically distributed, and often resolve with limb elevation and/or warming.

LIVEDO RETICULARIS

Livedo reticularis is an ischemic dermopathy characterized by a violaceous reticular or "netlike" mottling that encircles a pallorous central core of skin. It is imperative that the clinician differentiate between the usually but not invariably benign and reversible livedo reticularis and the always pathologic, permanent livedo racemosa.[10] Physiologic arteriolar vasospasm produces the reversible cutaneous mottled discoloration of physiologic or primary livedo reticularis. Protracted arteriolar vasospasm, thrombosis, and/or hyperviscosity underlie the pathologic skin changes of secondary livedo reticularis and livedo racemosa.

In livedo reticularis, a symmetric, fishnet-like red or purple mottling surrounds a pallorous conical core (Fig. 60.19) that is aggravated by cold exposure and may completely dissipate with warming and/or elevation. Livedo is enhanced by limb dependency and lessened by elevation. The skin of the patient with livedo reticularis usually is palpably cool. The livid rings are most pronounced on the lower extremities, yet the upper extremities can be affected as well. When pronounced truncal involvement occurs, a secondary cause should be suspected.

In contradistinction to the symmetric and uniform reticular pattern of livedo reticularis, the discoloration of livedo racemosa is asymmetric, irregular, and "broken" (Fig. 60.20). It does not appreciably improve with warming or limb elevation and is thus permanent. The causative secondary disorder may yield concurrent skin manifestations including purpura, nodules, macules, ulcerations, and/or atrophie blanche type scarring. It is sometimes difficult to distinguish secondary nonreversible livedo reticularis from livedo racemosa. Additionally, retiform purpura is occasionally misdiagnosed as livedo racemosa; however, the reticular discoloration in the latter is morphologically

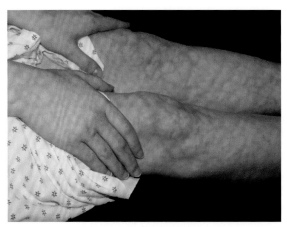

Fig. 60.20 Livedo Racemosa of the Lower and Upper Extremities in a Young Male With the Antiphospholipid Syndrome. In livedo racemosa the discolored cones or rings are "broken" and markedly irregular and do not appreciably improve with limb elevation and/or warming. Livedo racemosa is always due to a secondary, pathologic etiology and may be complicated by other cutaneous pathology including limb ulcerations.

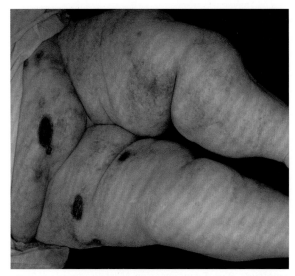

Fig. 60.21 Remarkable Illustration of an Admixture of Both Livedo Racemosa and Retiform Purpura Overlying the Legs and Abdominal Panniculus in an Obese Female Patient With Nonazotemic Calciphylaxis. Concurrent atypical ischemic ulcerations are readily apparent, which exhibit a tropism for fatty regions of the body.

thinner and more angulated than the larger "puzzle-piece" configuration of retiform purpura (see Fig. 60.3). Adding to the diagnostic confusion is the potential for patients to display an admixture of both livedo racemosa and retiform purpura (Fig. 60.21).

HYBRID VASOMOTOR DISEASE

It is not uncommon for the aforementioned vasomotor diseases to coexist. For example, acrocyanosis often manifests concurrent livedo reticularis (Fig. 60.22) and can be complicated by superimposed episodes of Raynaud phenomenon and even pernio (Fig. 60.23). When a patient with erythromelalgia is clinically quiescent, the feet are typically acrocyanotic and livedo reticularis is present. Alternating erythromelalgia and acrocyanosis can be a source of diagnostic confusion to the untrained clinician.

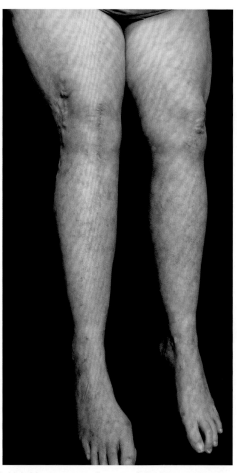

Fig. 60.22 Hybrid vasomotor disease of the bilateral lower extremities exemplified by a compilation of both livedo reticularis and acrocyanosis.

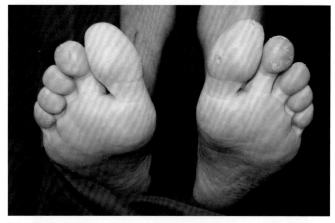

Fig. 60.23 Another Example of Hybrid Vasomotor Disease in a Patient With Resolving Pernio in a Background of Acrocyanosis. Note the stark contrast in discoloration between the acrocyanotic plantar aspect of the feet and the legs.

CHRONIC VENOUS INSUFFICIENCY

The term "chronic venous insufficiency (CVI)" is usually reserved for more advanced signs of venous hypertension such as edema, skin changes, and venous ulcers (see Chapter 54). Although these representative manifestations are typically easily recognized, several less familiar clinical features of CVI warrant additional discussion.

Contemporary consensus documentation and expert opinion exists stating that all peripheral edema represents lymphatic failure[11,12]; thus, the edema of CVI actually represents secondary lymphedema or "phlebolymphedema." Although the concept of all edema representing lymphatic failure is relatively new, the concurrence of combined venous and lymphatic hypertension has been well documented in multiple lymphoscintigraphic studies dating back to the 1990s. In a 2016 study of 12 patients with active unilateral venous stasis ulcerations, all 12 patients exhibited lymphatic dysfunction in their affected limbs via indocyanine green lymphography.[13] Moreover, all contralateral nonulcerated limbs also displayed lymphatic dysfunction in the setting of CEAP classifications (Clinical, Etiological, Anatomical, Pathophysiological) of C4 and C5 disease. Classic phlebolymphedema displays a constellation of characteristic lymphostatic skin changes combined with leg and foot swelling (Fig. 60.24). However, it should be emphasized that foot and toe swelling is *not* required to make the diagnosis of phlebolymphedema.

Although isolated spider and varicose veins are classically associated with early stages (C1 and C2 disease, respectively) of chronic venous disease, corona phlebectatica or "ankle flare" sign represents an exception to this rule. Corona phlebectatica is a fan-shaped confluence of telangiectasias inferior to the medial and/or lateral malleolus and foot and its presence signifies coexistent refluxing perforating veins (Fig. 60.25). Identification of an ankle flare sign is highly relevant as it is the best predictor of subsequent skin changes in patients with initially mild chronic venous disease (C_0 to C_3) and the second-best predictor of eventual stasis ulceration.[14] Thus it is erroneous to classify corona as uncomplicated telangiectasias of the foot or C1 CVD. Interestingly, an ankle flare sign composed of dilated intradermal blue veins is a more reliable predictor of advanced venous hypertension than one comprised of red telangiectasias.

Stasis dermatitis is typically well demarcated, erythematous, dry, and scaly. However, conversion into an acute erythematous, weeping, vesiculobullous allergic or irritant contact dermatitis with attendant burning, stinging, and/or pain can occur. Moreover, contact dermatitis may elicit an acute stasis ulceration (Fig. 60.26). These dermatologic sequelae result from phlebolymphedema-mediated predisposition or "immunocompromised district" to contact sensitization from various lotions, creams, and/or systemic or topical antimicrobials used to treat stasis dermatitis.[15] Chronic pruritus associated with stasis dermatitis can eventuate in a neurodermatitis with associated lichenification and nummular eczema with scarring (Fig. 60.27). Rarely, stasis dermatitis is complicated by an autosensitization dermatitis or "Id" reaction in other body parts such as the trunk.

If long-standing stasis dermatitis with characteristic reddish-brown eczematous scales and patches transforms into violaceous or dark purple plaques and nodules, then a diagnosis of acroangiodermatitis or "pseudo-Kaposi" sarcoma is likely (Fig. 60.28). These associated lesions are sometimes complicated by painful, refractory ulcerations.

Lipodermatosclerosis reflects localized chronic inflammation and fibrosis of the skin and subcutaneous tissues in late stage CVI with strikingly "bound down" or sclerotic skin involving the gaiter region of the calf. In the acute phase, a tender erythematous and edematous plaque develops within the distal anteromedial gaiter distribution. When chronic, progressive dermal and subcutaneous atrophy imparts

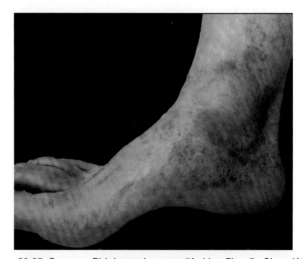

Fig. 60.25 Corona Phlebectatica or "Ankle Flare" Sign With Representative Blue Telangiectasias Most Pronounced Along the Inferior Portion of the Medial Malleolus. Prominent blue spider veins within this specific distribution are a frequent harbinger of advanced venous disease including stasis ulceration.

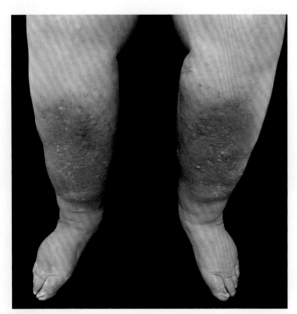

Fig. 60.24 Bilateral chronic venous insufficiency complicated by secondary lymphedema or "phlebolymphedema" as exemplified by the amalgamation of foot and leg swelling combined with hyperpigmented fibrotic papulonodular skin changes within the gaiter distribution.

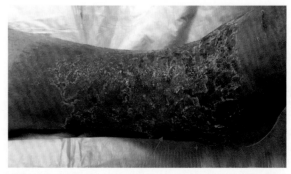

Fig. 60.26 Acute Weeping Eczematous Stasis Dermatitis Along the Distal Right Calf, Ankle, and Foot. Note associated confluent stasis hyperpigmentation and the acute ulceration *(arrow)* triggered by the acute dermatitis.

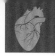

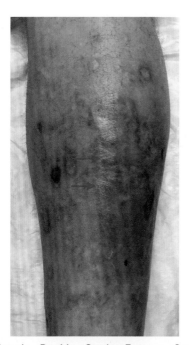

Fig. 60.27 Chronic Pruritic Stasis Eczema Complicated by Neurodermatitis With Associated Nummular or "Coin-Shaped" Hypopigmented Scarring, Discoloration, Plaques, and Traumatic/Stasis Ulcerations. Faint lichenification with exaggerated skin creases overlies the anterior tibial region *(arrows)*.

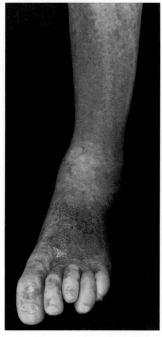

Fig. 60.28 Severe Chronic Venous Insufficiency Complicated by Distinctive Violaceous or Dark Purple Patches and Plaques Along the Dorsal Foot and Toes Consistent With Acroangiodermatitis or "Pseudo-Kaposi" Sarcoma. In contrast, typical stasis hyperpigmentation is brown with a patch morphology and only rarely affects the dorsum of the foot and toes.

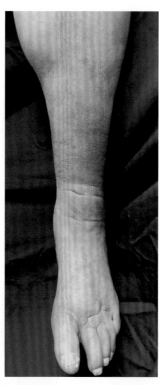

Fig. 60.29 Chronic Lipodermatosclerosis of the Left Calf With a Characteristic Tapered or "Inverted Bowling Pin" Appearance Consistent With Pronounced Subcutaneous Atrophy. Associated foot and toe swelling represents attendant secondary lymphedema that complicates all lipodermatosclerosis.

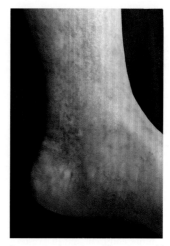

Fig. 60.30 Illustrative case of severe diffuse atrophie blanche scarring along the distal portion of the left calf with associated white atrophic plaques and superimposed capillary stippling.

a concave appearance to the mid/distal calf which resembles an "inverted champagne bottle or bowling pin" (Fig. 60.29).

Atrophie blanche or "white atrophy" is a morphologic term that signifies localized white, atrophic, stellate-shaped plaques and con-

notes advanced CVI. The plaque border is hyperpigmented and sometimes eczematous and dilated, stippled red capillaries are typically interspersed within the avascular, white plaques (Fig. 60.30). The characteristic appearance of atrophie blanche should not be confused with healed stasis ulcer scars as the latter are devoid of capillary stippling.

When a chronic venous stasis ulceration fails to heal despite appropriate therapy and the base begins to manifest highly proliferative, friable granulation tissue, conversion to a squamous cell carcinoma should be considered (Fig. 60.31). In a large-scale epidemiological study, patients

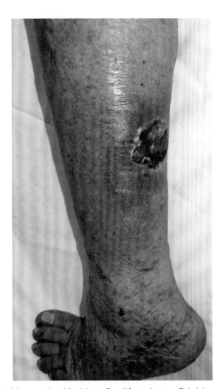

Fig. 60.31 Unusual Highly Proliferative, Friable, Exuberant Granulation Tissue Within the Bed of a Former Chronic Stasis Ulceration That Ultimately Converted to Squamous Cell Carcinoma. The immunocompromised district associated with long-standing phlebolymphedema predisposes patients to various skin cancers. (Data from Ruocco E, Brunetti G, Brancaccio G, et al. Phlebolymphedema: disregarded cause of immunocompromised district. *Clin Dermatol.* 2012;30:541–543.)

with chronic venous stasis ulcerations had a nearly sixfold increased risk of conversion to squamous cell carcinoma.[16] Carcinomatous ulceration conversion represents another sequel of the chronic immunocompromised district associated with phlebolymphedema.[15]

LYMPHEDEMA

Lymphedema is an external manifestation of lymphatic system insufficiency and dysfunctional transport marked by the accumulation of interstitial fluid, protein, cellular debris, and fibroadipose tissue that most commonly affects the limbs (see Chapter 57). Primary lymphedema is genetically determined, more common in females, and lymphedema praecox accounts for 80% of primary cases. Secondary lymphedema is the more common and in Western countries, cancer and its therapies are commonly reported to be the dominant cause. Although underreported, it is likely that a combination of obesity and CVI is equally if not a more likely cause of lower extremity secondary lymphedema (see Fig. 60.24).

The bedside clinical examination is paramount in the diagnosis. Lymphedema usually, although not invariably, begins on the dorsum of the foot (or hand) and progresses proximally. The characteristic dorsal swelling of the foot resembles a "buffalo hump." The toes are usually swollen as well with exaggerated dorsal skin creases (Fig. 60.32). Primary lymphedema is more likely than secondary lymphedema to yield pronounced swelling of the feet and toes (Figs. 60.33 and 60.34). Hypoplastic and concave toenails that are sometimes referred to as "ski-jump" nails are another phenotype of primary lymphedema (Fig. 60.35).[17] In early presentations, the

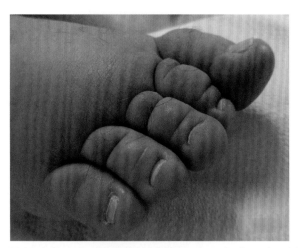

Fig. 60.32 A Singular Example of Primary Lymphedema Involving the Dorsum of the Foot and Toes. Deep digital dorsal skin creases and hypoplastic toenails are also evident.

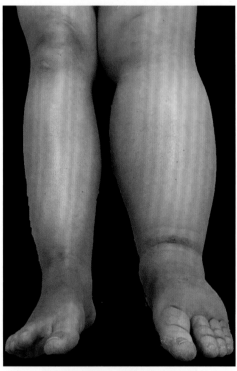

Fig. 60.33 Chronic Primary Lymphedema (Praecox) of the Left Lower Extremity. Note the pronounced foot and toe swelling combined with exaggerated digital dorsal skin creases. Pronounced acral swelling is more likely to occur in primary than secondary lymphedema.

edema typically pits, and the skin along the dorsum of the second toe can be pinched (negative Stemmer sign). However, lymphedema often progresses due to a combination of increased subcutaneous fluid, fibrosis, and significant adipose tissue deposition. In later stages the pitting quality diminishes or even disappears and the skin along the dorsum of the second toe can no longer be pinched (positive Stemmer sign). A multitude of abnormal skin findings can complicate progressive lymphedema including hyperkeratosis, lichenification, peau d'orange ("orange peel") dimpling, confluent papulonodular "cobblestoning," large tumor-like fibrous nodules, and lymphostatic verrucosis where the skin becomes darkened with

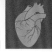

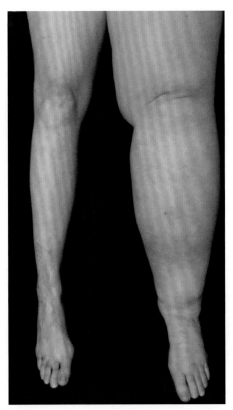

Fig. 60.34 Despite massive postsurgical lymphedema of the left lower extremity from a prior lymph node dissection, the foot is only minimally swollen.

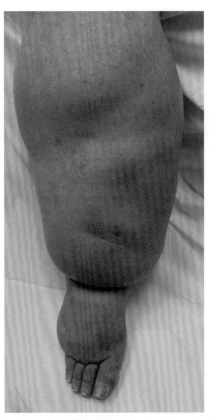

Fig. 60.36 Approximately 50% of the limb volume in this case of primary lymphedema represents secondary fat deposition as chronic lymph stasis is highly adipogenic. Abundant fat deposition in the advanced lymphedematous limb partially explains the lack of pitting as well as failure to significantly reduce the limb girth despite appropriate compression.

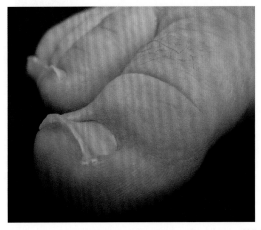

Fig. 60.35 Toenails With Upward Concavity Consistent With "Ski-Jump" Nails of Primary Lymphedema. Recognition of "ski-jump" toenails can be clinically useful for establishing the diagnosis of primary lymphedema in unexplained cases of new-onset leg swelling.

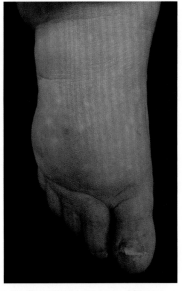

Fig. 60.37 Multiple Physiologic Anemic Macules or "Bier Spots" Overlying the Dorsum of the Foot in a Patient With Primary Lymphedema. Bier spots transiently resolve with pressure (diascopy) or limb elevation and are a benign and often unrecognized manifestation of lymphatic hypertension.

multiple warty projections. Lymphostatic ulcerations with copious lymphorrhea can complicate elephantiasis.

There are several additional clinical features of lymphedema that are not uncommon, yet often unrecognized. For instance, later stages of lymphedema such as elephantiasis are marked by significant local fat deposition which constitutes approximately 50% of the limb volume (Fig. 60.36).[18] Copious fat deposition partially explains the non-pitting nature of advanced lymphedema as well as lack of response to compression. Physiologic anemic macules or "Bier Spots" are not uncommon in the setting of lymphedema (Fig. 60.37).[19] These macules

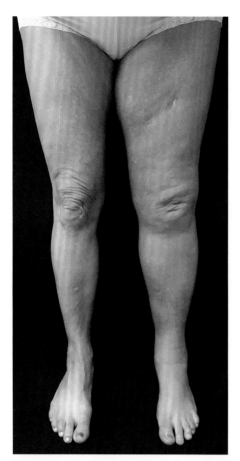

Fig. 60.38 Diffuse Lymphatic Rubor Throughout the Left Leg in a Patient With Post–Lymph-Node Dissection Secondary Lymphedema and No Venous Reflux or Significant Iliac Vein Obstruction. As the limb is typically mildly warm, lymphatic rubor is often mistaken for bacterial cellulitis. However, the diffuse confluent painless discoloration and lack of response to antibiotics is not consistent with cellulitis. The rubor is likely a sequel of chronic lymphatic inflammation with associated increased capillary blood flow.

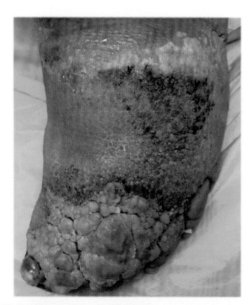

Fig. 60.39 Papillomatosis cutis carcinoides, a squamous cell carcinoma variant, arising in the background of congenital lymphedema complicated by a 5-year history of progressively disfiguring papules and nodules with chronically infected, mephitic lymphostatic ulcerations.

transiently dissipate with pressure (diascopy) or limb elevation and are a benign entity. A curious entity complicating lymphedema that is often mistaken for bacterial cellulitis is lymphatic rubor where the limb displays a uniform pink-reddish hue and sometimes slight increased warmth (Fig. 60.38). The genesis is not well defined but likely represents the chronic inflammatory nature of lymphedema with associated increased flow throughout the capillary beds. As chronic lymphedema represents an immunocompromised district, patients are predisposed to morbid skin cancers including squamous cell carcinoma and its variant "papillomatosis cutis carcinoides" or verrucous carcinoma (Fig. 60.39) as well as deadly lymphangiosarcoma. A low threshold should exist for obtaining a punch biopsy of long-standing lymphedema complicated by either disfiguring, ulcerated verrucous, or purple-appearing nodules.

REFERENCES

1. Dean SM. Atypical ischemic lower extremity ulcerations: a differential diagnosis. *Vasc Med*. 2008;13(1):47–54.
2. Chikura B, Moore TL, Manning JB, et al. Sparing of the thumb in Raynaud's phenomenon. *Rheumatology (Oxford)*. 2008;47:219–221.
3. Doveri M, Della Rossa A, Salvadori S, et al. Systemic sclerosis: outcome and long-term follow-up of 429 patients from a single Italian centre. *Ann Rheum Dis*. 2011;70(Suppl 3):660.
4. Hughes M, Herrick AL. Digital ulcers in systemic sclerosis. *Rheumatology*. 2017;56:14–25.
5. Kurklinsky AK, Miller VM, Rooke TW. Acrocyanosis: the Flying Dutchman. *Vasc Med*. 2011;16(4):288–301.
6. Crocq M. De l' "acrocyanose". *Semaine Med*. 1896;16:298.
7. Han C, Dib-Hajj SD, Lin Z, et al. Early- and late-onset inherited erythromelalgia: genotype-phenotype correlation. *Brain*. 2009;132:1711–1722.
8. Davis MD, O'Fallon WM, Rogers 3rd RS, Rooke TW. Natural history of erythromelalgia: presentation and outcome in 168 patients. *Arch Dermatol*. 2000;136(3):330–336.
9. Cappel JA, Wetter DA. Clinical characteristics, etiologic associations, laboratory findings, treatment, and proposal of diagnostic criteria of pernio (chilblains) in a series of 104 patients at Mayo Clinic, 2000 to 2011. *Mayo Clin Proc*. 2014;89(2):207–215.
10. Dean SM. Livedo reticularis and related disorders. *Curr Treat Options Cardiovasc Med*. 2011;13(2):179–191.
11. Mortimer PS, Rockson SG. New developments in clinical aspects of lymphatic disease. *J Clin Invest*. 2014;124(3):915–921.
12. Lee BB, Andrade M, Antignani PL, et al. Diagnosis and treatment of primary lymphedema. Consensus document of the International Union of Phlebology (IUP)-2013. *Int Angiol*. 2013;32(6):541–574.
13. Rasmussen JC, Aldrich MB, Tan IC. Lymphatic transport in patients with chronic venous insufficiency and venous leg ulcers following sequential pneumatic compression. *J Vasc Surg Venous Lymphat Disord*. 2016;4(1):9–17.
14. Uhl JF, Cornu-Thenard A, Satger B, Carpentier PH. Clinical significance of the corona phlebectatica. *J Vasc Surg*. 2012;55:150–153.
15. Ruocco E, Brunetti G, Brancaccio G, Lo Schiavo A. Phlebolymphedema: disregarded cause of immunocompromised district. *Clin Dermatol*. 2012;30(5):541–543.
16. Baldursson B, Sigurgeirsson B, Lindelöf B. Venous leg ulcers and squamous cell carcinoma: a large-scale epidemiological study. *Br J Dermatol*. 1995;133:571–574.
17. Dean SM. Images in vascular medicine. 'Ski-jump' toenails--a phenotypic manifestation of primary lymphedema. *Vasc Med*. 2015;20(3):268.
18. Harvey NL, Srinivasan RS, Dillard ME, et al. Lymphatic vascular defects promoted by Prox1 haploinsufficiency cause adult-onset obesity. *Nat Genet*. 2005;37(10):1072–1081.
19. Dean SM, Zirwas M. Bier spots are an under-recognized cutaneous manifestation of lower extremity lymphedema: a case series and brief review of the literature. *Ann Vasc Surg*. 2014;28(8). 1935.e13-16.

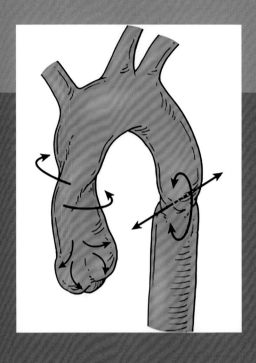

中文导读

第61章
下肢溃疡

　　下肢溃疡在临床上比较常见，西方国家普通人群下肢溃疡的患病率为1%～3.5%，老年人群患病率增加至5%。瑞典的流行病学研究估计每年治疗下肢溃疡的费用约2500万美元。因溃疡愈合所需时间长，复发率高，如不及时治疗，致残率及远期死亡率高，给家庭及社会带来极大的心理创伤及经济负担。下肢溃疡的病理生理学机制复杂，与下肢静脉、动脉，神经病变，感染，足部结构和生物力学异常等因素有关。40%～80%的溃疡由静脉疾病引起，10%～20%由动脉功能不全引起，15%～25%由糖尿病引起，10%～15%的患者存在两种或多种致病因素。本章作者总结大量文献，从生物力学角度分析溃疡病因，探讨病理生理学机制，根据病史、体格检查、有创及无创血管检查，结合经典病例图片及临床表现对溃疡进行全面评估，针对不同原因导致的溃疡，讲述了多学科导向的针对性综合治疗，包括全身性抗感染治疗、采用生物活性药物、生物力学的外科矫正、整形和软组织重建、负压伤口疗法、压力疗法、血运重建、创面护理等，从而提高溃疡愈合成功率并防止复发，具有很好的临床实用价值。

戈小虎

Lower Extremity Ulceration

Bauer E. Sumpio, Peter Blume, and Carlos Mena-Hurtado

Ulceration of the lower extremity is a relatively common condition that causes significant discomfort and disability.[1] An ulcer is defined as a disruption of the skin with erosion of the underlying subcutaneous tissue. This breach may extend further to the contiguous muscle and bone. The pathophysiologic mechanisms underlying ulcer formation are multifactorial and include neuropathy, infection, ischemia, and abnormal foot structure and biomechanics. It is not surprising then that the management of the diabetic foot is a complex clinical problem requiring an interdisciplinary approach.[2,3] Minor trauma, often footwear related, is a frequent inciting event. A chronic ulcer is defined as a full thickness skin defect with no significant re-epithelialization for more than 4 weeks.

Common causes of leg ulcerations are responsible for almost 95% of leg ulcers; about 40% to 80% of ulcers are a result of underlying venous disease, 10% to 20% are caused by arterial insufficiency, 15% to 25% are a consequence of diabetes mellitus, and in 10% to 15% of patients a combination of two or more causes exists. Prolonged pressure and local infection are common causes of leg ulcers with minimal vascular compromise. Rare causes are responsible for less than 5% of all leg ulcers (Box 61.1).[4] The disease entities that usually underlie leg ulceration, such as venous insufficiency, peripheral artery disease, and diabetes mellitus, are associated with significant patient morbidity and mortality. A detailed knowledge of the clinical picture, pathogenesis, relevant diagnostic tests, treatment modalities, and differential diagnosis of leg ulcerations is essential in planning the optimal treatment strategy (Table 61.1). An incorrect or delayed initial diagnosis may harm the patient and increase the risk of serious complications, including permanent disability and amputations.

The exact prevalence of lower extremity ulcers in the United States is unknown. The prevalence of leg ulceration in the general population of Western nations has been reported to be from 1% to 3.5%, with the prevalence increasing to 5% in the geriatric population.[5-8] The data from these studies most likely underestimate the true prevalence because they do not include patients with leg ulcers who are not known to the healthcare system.

The cost of treating leg ulceration is staggering. Epidemiologic studies from Sweden estimated annual costs of treatment of lower extremity ulcers at $25 million. In England, the estimated cost of care for patients with leg ulcers in a population of 250,000 was about $130,000 annually per patient.[9] Items factored into the equation include physician visits, hospital admissions, home healthcare, wound care supplies, rehabilitation, time lost from work, and jobs lost. Adding to the cost is the chronic nature of these wounds, the high rate of recurrence, and the propensity for ulcers to become infected. It is also evident that a true accounting of the cost is difficult because of the unknown prevalence of disease.

The social cost of leg ulcers also becomes a factor as the disease affects a patient's lifestyle and attitude. The ability to work may be temporarily or permanently affected by the condition.[10] Reduction in working capacity adds to the total cost. An estimated 10 million workdays annually are lost in the United States from lower extremity ulcers, and this figure may be low.[11,12] A report in 1994 focused on the financial, social, and psychological implications of lower extremity lesions in 73 patients.[10] Among the study patients, 68% reported feelings of fear, social isolation, anger, depression, and negative self-image because of the ulcers. In addition, 81% of the patients felt that their mobility was adversely affected. Within the younger population that was still actively working, there was a correlation between lower extremity ulceration and adverse effect on finances, time lost from work, and job loss. In addition, there was a strong correlation between time spent on ulcer care and feelings of anger and resentment. These factors combined to have a negative emotional impact on their lives.

BIOMECHANICS OF WALKING AND ULCER FORMATION

An appreciation of the biomechanics required for walking is essential in understanding the etiology of foot ulcers. The foot is a complicated biologic structure containing 26 bones, numerous joints, and a network of ligaments, muscles, and blood vessels. Gait is a complex set of events that requires triplanar foot motion and control of multiple axes for complete bipedal ambulation (Fig. 61.1A).[13] When the heel hits the ground, its outer edge touches first. The foot is in a supinated position, which makes it firm and rigid. The soft tissue structures (muscles, tendons, and ligaments) then relax, allowing the foot to pronate. The foot becomes less rigid and is able to flatten, absorb the shock of touchdown, and adapt to uneven surfaces. During midstance, the heel lies below the ankle joint complex, the front and back of the foot are aligned, and the foot easily bears weight. Toward the end of midstance, the soft tissue structures begin to tighten; the foot resupinates and regains its arch. The foot is again firm, acting as a rigid lever for propulsion. The heel lifts off the ground, it swings slightly to the inside, and the toes push weight off the ground.

Sensory input from the visual and vestibular systems, as well as proprioceptive information from the lower extremities, is necessary to modify learned motor patterns and muscular output to execute the desired action. Various external and internal forces[14] affect foot function. The combination of body weight pushing down and ground reactive force pushing up creates friction and compressive forces—shear results from the bones of the foot sliding parallel to their plane of contact during pronation and supination. Foot deformities or ill-fitting footwear enhance pressure points because they focus the forces

BOX 61.1 Causes of Lower Extremity Ulcers

Vascular

Common

Venous insufficiency

Peripheral artery disease

Rare

Vasculitis

Autoimmune disease (scleroderma)

Hypertension (Martrell ulcer)

Thromboangiitis obliterans (TAO; Buerger disease)

Lymphedema

Hematologic disorders (sickle cell anemia)

Clotting disorders (antiphospholipid syndrome)

Neurotrophic

Diabetes mellitus

Uremia

Acquired immunodeficiency syndrome (AIDS)

Nutritional deficiencies

Biomechanical

Charcot foot

Rheumatoid arthritis (Felty syndrome)

Fracture, dislocations

Others

Infectious diseases

Physical or chemical injury (trauma, pressure ulcers, burns, frostbite)

Metabolic diseases (porphyria, calciphylaxis)

Neoplasms (melanoma, basal cell carcinoma, squamous cell carcinoma, sarcomas)

Drug reactions or side effects (steroids, warfarin)

Ulcerating skin diseases (pyoderma gangrenosum)

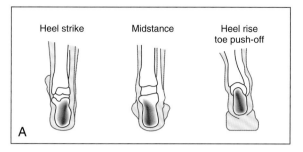

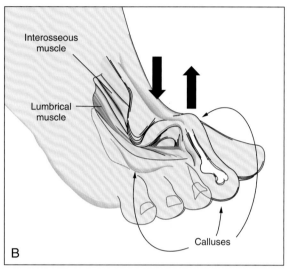

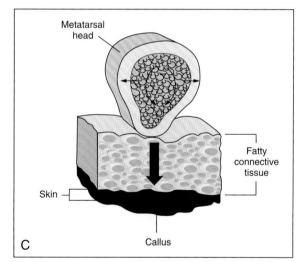

Fig. 61.1 Biomechanics of ulceration.

on a smaller area. When the foot flattens too much or overpronates, the ankle and heel do not align during midstance and some bones are forced to support more weight. The foot strains under the body's weight, causing the muscles to pull harder on these areas, making it more difficult for tendons and ligaments to hold bones and joints in proper alignment. Over time, swelling and pain on the bottom of the foot or near the heel may occur. Bunions can form at the great toe joint, and hammertoe deformities can form at the lesser toes. Abnormal foot biomechanics resulting from limited joint mobility and foot deformities magnify shearing forces, resulting in increased plantar pressure on the foot during ambulation (see Fig. 61.1B and C). This can represent critical causes for tissue breakdown.

TABLE 61.1 Lower Extremity Ulcers Characterized by Etiology

	Site	Skin Appearance	Ulcer Characteristics	Other Findings
Venous	Lower third of leg; malleolar area	Edema, hemosiderin, dermatitis, eczema	"Weeping," irregular borders, painful	Varicose veins, "bottle" leg, ABI normal
Arterial	Most distal areas, toes	Thin, atrophic, dry, "shiny," hair loss	Round, regular borders, no bleeding, dry base, very painful	Weak/absent pulse, poor capillary refill, ABI <0.8
Neurotrophic (diabetes mellitus)	Pressure sites; heel and metatarsal heads	Cellulitis	Round, deep, purulent discharge, painless	Sensory deficit; ABI often >1.3 due to vascular calcification

ABI, Ankle brachial index.

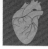

PATHOPHYSIOLOGY OF ULCER FORMATION

Venous Disease

Venous leg ulcers are the most frequently occurring chronic lower extremity wounds (Fig. 61.2A) (also see Chapter 54). The prevalence of lower extremity ulceration secondary to chronic venous disease in European and Western populations is estimated to be 0.5% to 1%. In the United States, it is estimated that between 600,000 and 2.5 million patients have venous ulcerations. Treatment costs in the United States are between $2.5 and $3 billion dollars, with a corresponding loss of 2 million workdays per year.[15] Ten years ago, the annual cost of treatment for venous ulcer patients was almost $40,000 per patient.[16] This cost has risen since then.

The physiology of venous blood flow is straightforward. Blood returns from the lower extremities against gravity to the inferior vena cava, through the deep and superficial venous systems. The deep veins are located within the muscles and deep fascia of the legs. The superficial system consists of the great saphenous vein and the small saphenous vein, and is located within the subcutaneous fat. Valves are present within both systems and prevent retrograde flow of the blood. A portion of blood from the superficial system is directed to the deep system through the communicating perforators. While standing, about 22% of the total blood volume is localized to the lower extremities, and hydrostatic pressure in the foot veins can reach 80 mm Hg. In healthy individuals with competent venous valves, the efficient calf muscle pump can reduce venous pressure by two-thirds during exercise. Venous insufficiency occurs when any of these elements do not function adequately. The pressure in the venous system increases, and most importantly, the ambulatory venous pressure rises during leg exercise. The primary cause of venous hypertension is insufficiency of the valves of the deep venous system and the perforating veins of the leg.

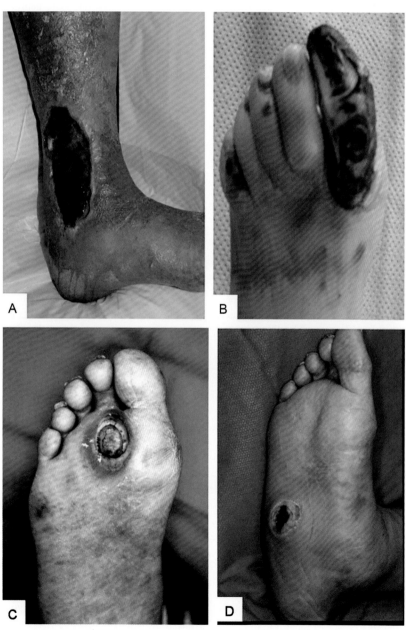

Fig. 61.2 Various Foot Ulcers. (A) Venous stasis. (B) Ischemic. (C) Neurotrophic. (D) Charcot foot.

The exact mechanism by which ulcerations develop in patients with venous insufficiency is not clear. One theory is that ulceration results as a consequence of increased intraluminal pressure within the capillary system of the leg. The capillaries become dilated and elongated. Blood flow is sluggish, resulting in microthrombi formation and frequently leading to occlusion of the capillaries. Fibrin, albumin, and various macromolecules leak into the dermis, where they bind to and trap growth factors, making them unavailable for the tissue repair process.[17] Leakage of fibrinogen through capillary walls results in deposition of pericapillary fibrin cuffs,[18] which has been suggested as a physical barrier impeding the passage of oxygen.[11] Iron deposition, white blood cell accumulation, decreased fibrinolytic activity, and a myriad of inflammatory responses to the vascular damage are all postulated to be the pathways leading to venous ulceration, but it is still not clear whether they are causative factors.

Tissue hypoxia appears to be a major underlying factor for venous ulceration. Unlike ulcers associated with arterial insufficiency, this hypoxic state is not caused by decreased blood flow to the legs; patients with venous insufficiency usually have adequate blood flow to their lower extremities. Direct measurements of transcutaneous oxygen levels on the lower portion of the leg have demonstrated that exercise produces a marked rise in skin oxygen tension in normal legs, but not in those affected by venous insufficiency. Exercise reduces venous pressure in patients with competent valves, thus removing the stimulus for reflex vasoconstriction. In patients with compromised valves, the venous pressure remains high during exercise and reflex vasoconstriction persists.[19]

On the basis of these findings, it is clear that management of lower extremity ulcers caused by venous insufficiency must include measures that improve the abnormal venous blood return from the affected extremity. Leg elevation, compression therapy, local wound care, and surgical correction of selected underlying pathology are all important components of the treatment plan.

Peripheral Artery Disease

The incidence of lower extremity ulcers (see Fig. 61.2B) caused by peripheral artery disease is increasing in Western nations (also see Chapter 16).[8] The general "aging" of the population and better detection techniques provide possible explanations for this observation. Risk factors for the development of atherosclerotic lesions causing leg ischemia include diabetes mellitus, smoking, hyperlipidemia, hypertension, obesity, and age.[3] Lack of perfusion decreases tissue resilience, leads to rapid death of tissue, and impedes wound healing (also see Chapter 17). Wound healing and tissue regeneration depend on an adequate blood supply to the region. Ischemia due to vascular disease impedes healing by reducing the supply of oxygen, nutrients, and soluble mediators that are involved in the repair process.[20]

The Diabetic Foot

Persons with diabetes mellitus are particularly prone to foot ulcers. The "diabetic foot" is a common and serious clinical condition. The American Diabetes Association consensus group found that among persons with diabetes, the risk of foot ulceration was increased in men, in patients who had had diabetes for more than 10 years, and in patients with poor glucose control or cardiovascular, retinal, or renal complications.[21] It is estimated that 15% of US patients with diabetes will develop manifestations of diabetic foot disease in their lifetime.[22,23] In this population, the prevalence of lower extremity ulcers ranges from 4% to 10%, with an annual incidence of 2% to 3%.[24] Although representing only 6% of the population, patients with diabetes account for 46%[24] of the 162,000 hospital admissions for foot ulcers annually. Foot ulcers occur in up to 25% of patients with diabetes and precede more than 8 in 10 nontraumatic amputations. In 2005, approximately 1.6 million people were living with limb loss; this number is expected

to more than double by 2050.[25] Diabetic foot ulcers and their sequelae, amputations, are the major cause of disability, morbidity, mortality, and costs for these patients.[22] Ulceration and infection of lower extremities are also the leading causes of hospitalization in patients with diabetes.[24] Treatment of pedal soft-tissue deficits in the diabetic patient population continues to be a medical and surgical challenge, thereby extending the length of their disability and significantly increasing the cost of medical care. Nearly half of all patients who undergo amputation will develop limb-threatening ischemia in the contralateral limb, and many will ultimately require an amputation of the opposite limb within 5 years. In 2000, the Centers for Disease Control and Prevention (CDC) estimated that 12 million Americans were diagnosed with diabetes, and the estimated annual direct and indirect cost of diabetes treatment in the United States was approximately $174 billion, with one in five diabetes dollars spent on lower extremity care. Preventing ulcerations and/or amputations is critical from both medical and economical standpoints.[2]

Development of diabetic foot disease can be attributed to several primary risk factors, including neuropathy, ischemia, infection, and immune impairment. Four foot-related risk factors have been identified in the genesis of pedal ulceration: altered biomechanics, limited joint mobility, bony deformity, and severe nail pathology.[21]

Neuropathy

Neuropathy is the most common underlying etiology of foot ulceration and frequently involves the somatic and autonomic fibers. Although there are many causes of peripheral neuropathy, diabetes mellitus is by far the most common (see Box 61.1). Neuropathy is present in 42% of diabetic patients after 20 years[26] and is usually a distal symmetric sensorimotor polyneuropathy. The peripheral neuropathy is thought to result from abnormalities in metabolic pathways, of which there are several hypotheses, including deficiencies in sorbitol metabolism via the polyol pathway.[27,28] Neurotrophic ulcers typically form on the plantar aspect of the foot at areas of excessive focal pressures, which are most commonly encountered over the bony prominences of the metatarsal heads and the forefoot region due to the requirements of midstance and heel off during the gait cycle (see Fig. 61.2C). Loss of protective sensation in the foot can rapidly lead to ulceration if patient education and preventive measures are not taken. Diabetic patients are especially prone to development of a neuro-osteoarthropathy, Charcot foot.[29] This condition is thought to involve autonomic-nerve dysfunction resulting in abnormal perfusion to foot bones, which leads to bony fragmentation and collapse (see Fig. 61.2D). The resulting "rocker-bottom foot" is prone to tissue breakdown and ulceration.[22,29]

Several investigators[22,29,30] have demonstrated that there is an increase in both static and dynamic foot pressures when evaluating the neuropathic foot.[31] To date, high pressures alone have not been shown to cause foot ulceration. Rheumatoid patients with high plantar foot pressures but no sensitivity deficit have almost no evidence of foot ulceration.[32] Type-A sensory fibers are responsible for light touch sensation, vibratory sensation, pressure, proprioception, and motor innervation to the intrinsic muscles of the foot. Type-C sensory fibers detect painful stimuli, noxious stimuli, and temperature. When these fibers are affected, protective sensation is lost. This manifests as a distal, symmetric loss of sensation described in a "stocking" distribution and proves to be the primary factor predisposing patients to ulcers and infection.[33] Patients are unable to detect increased loads, repeated trauma, or pain from shearing forces. Injuries such as fractures, ulceration, and foot deformities therefore go unrecognized. Repeat stress to high-pressure areas or bone prominences, which would be interpreted as pain in the nonneuropathic patient, also go unrecognized. Sensory

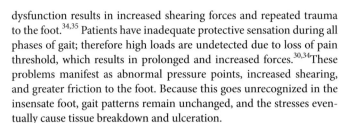

dysfunction results in increased shearing forces and repeated trauma to the foot.[34,35] Patients have inadequate protective sensation during all phases of gait; therefore high loads are undetected due to loss of pain threshold, which results in prolonged and increased forces.[30,34] These problems manifest as abnormal pressure points, increased shearing, and greater friction to the foot. Because this goes unrecognized in the insensate foot, gait patterns remain unchanged, and the stresses eventually cause tissue breakdown and ulceration.

Motor neuropathy is associated with demyelination and motor end-plate damage, which contribute to conduction defects. The distal motor nerves are the most commonly affected, resulting in atrophy of the small intrinsic muscles of the foot. Wasting of the lumbrical and interosseous muscles of the foot results in collapse of the arch and loss of stability of the metatarsal-phalangeal joints during midstance of the gait. Overpowering by extrinsic muscles can lead to depression of the metatarsal heads, digital contractures, and cocked-up toes; equinus deformities of the ankle; or a varus hindfoot.[36]

Autonomic involvement causes an interruption of normal sweating at the epidermal level and causes arteriovenous shunting at the subcutaneous and dermal level. Hypohidrosis leads to a noncompliant epidermis that increases the risk of cracking and fissuring. Arteriovenous shunting diminishes the delivery of nutrients and oxygen to tissue regions, and skin and subcutaneous tissues become more susceptible to breakdown.[37]

Musculoskeletal Deformities

Atrophy of the small muscles within the foot results in nonfunctioning intrinsic foot muscles referred to as an "intrinsic minus foot" (see Fig. 61.1B).[38] The muscles showing early involvement are the flexor digitorum brevis, lumbricales, and interosseous muscles. These groups act to stabilize the proximal phalanx against the metatarsal head preventing dorsiflexion at the metatarsal phalangeal joint (MTPJ) during midstance in the gait cycle. With progression of the neuropathy, these muscles atrophy and fail to function properly. This causes the MTPJs to become unstable, allowing the long flexors (flexor digitorum longus and flexor hallucis longus) and extensors (extensor digitorum longus and extensor hallucis longus) to act unchecked on the digits. Dorsal contractures form along the MTPJs with the development of hammer digit syndrome, also known as *intrinsic minus disease*.

The deformity acts to plantarflex the metatarsals, making the heads more prominent and increasing the plantar pressure created beneath them (see Fig. 61.1B). It also acts to decrease the amount of toe weight bearing during the gait cycle, which also increases pressure on the metatarsal heads. Normal anatomy consists of a metatarsal fat pad located plantar to the MTPJs. This structure helps dissipate pressures on the metatarsal heads from the ground. When the hammer digit deformity occurs, the fat pad migrates distally and becomes nonfunctional. This results in elevated plantar pressures that increase the risk of skin breakdown and ulceration due to shearing forces.[1]

Overpowering by the extrinsic foot muscles also leads to an equinus deformity at the ankle, and a varus hindfoot. A cavovarus foot type can develop, leading to decreased range of motion of the pedal joints, an inability to adapt to terrain, and low tolerance to shock. In essence, a mobile adapter is converted to a rigid lever. Pressure is equal to body weight divided by surface area, thus decreasing surface area below a metatarsal head with concomitant rigid deformities and leading to increased forces or pressure to the sole of the foot. When neuropathic foot disease is associated with congenital foot deformities such as long or short metatarsals, a plantarflexed metatarsal, abnormalities in the metatarsal parabola, or a Charcot foot (see Fig. 61.2D),[29] there is a higher propensity toward breakdown as a result of increased and abnormal plantar foot pressures.

Increasing body weight and decreasing the surface area of contact of the foot components with the ground increases pressure. A low pressure but constant insult over an extended period can have the same ulcerogenic effect as high pressure over a shorter period. This is typical of the effect of tight-fitting shoes. If the magnitude of these forces in a given area is large enough, either skin loss or hypertrophy of the stratum corneum (callus) occurs (see Fig. 61.1C). The presence of callus in patients with neuropathy should raise a red flag because the risk of ulceration in a callused area is increased by two orders of magnitude.

Peripheral Artery Disease

One of the major factors affecting diabetic foot disease is the development of lower extremity peripheral artery disease.[25] Peripheral artery disease is estimated to be two to four times more common in persons with diabetes than in others (see Chaper 18).[22,39] Atherosclerosis occurs at a younger age in persons with diabetes, and its hallmark is the involvement of the tibioperoneal vessels with sparing of the pedal vessels. In addition to being more prevalent in diabetics, atherosclerosis is more accelerated and results in a higher rate of amputations.[40–42] Lesions in persons with diabetes tend to localize to the infracrural region. The relative sparing of the pedal vessels often assists pedal bypass. Occlusive lesions affecting the foot and precluding revascularization are not common in diabetic patients.[22,]

Purely ischemic diabetic foot ulcers are uncommon, representing only 10% to 15% of ulcers in patients with diabetes. More commonly, ulcers have a mixed ischemic and neuropathic origin, representing 33% of diabetic foot ulcers.[22] The initiation of an ischemic ulcer usually requires a precipitating factor such as mechanical stress. Ulcers often develop on the dorsum of the foot, over the first and fifth metatarsal heads. A heel ulcer can develop from constant pressure applied while the heel is in a dependent position or during prolonged immobilization and bed rest. Once formed, the blood supply necessary to allow healing of an ulcer is greater than that needed to maintain intact skin. This leads to chronic ulcer development, unless the blood supply is improved.

Infection

Patients with diabetes appear to be more prone to various infections than their nondiabetic counterparts.[43] Several factors increase the risk of development of diabetic foot infections, including diabetic neuropathy, peripheral artery disease, and immunologic impairment. Several defects in immunologic response relate to increased infection risk in diabetics. Diabetic patients demonstrate a decrease in function of polymorphonuclear leukocytes that can manifest as a decrease in migration, phagocytosis, and decreased intracellular activity. Evidence suggests impaired cellular immune response, as well as abnormalities in complement function.[44,45] Some of the defects appear to improve with control of hyperglycemia.[46]

Undiagnosed clean neuropathic foot ulcers often convert to acute infections with abscess and/or cellulites.[47] Diabetic foot infections can be classified into those that are nonthreatening and those that are life or limb threatening. Non–limb-threatening diabetic foot infections are often mild infections associated with a superficial ulcer. They often have less than 2 cm of surrounding cellulitis and demonstrate no signs of systemic toxicity. These infections have on average 2.1 organisms (Table 61.2).[47] Aerobic gram-positive cocci are the sole pathogens in 42% of these cases, with the most notable organisms being *Staphylococcus aureus*, coagulase-negative *Staphylococcus aureus*, and streptococci. These less-severe infections can often be managed with local wound care, rest, elevation, and oral antibiotics on an outpatient basis. A foot infection in a diabetic patient can present with a more severe, life- or limb-threatening picture. In these patients, there is usually

TABLE 61.2   Percent Frequency of Bacterial Isolates From Diabetic Foot Infection

Organism	INVESTIGATOR (NO. PATIENTS)							
	Louie (20)	Sapico (32)	Gibbons (100)	Wheat (54)	Calhoun (850)	Scher (65)	Grayson (96)	Leichter (55)
Staphylococcus aureus	35	25	54	37	45.9	35.4	56	27.3
Coagulase-negative staphylococci	30	9.3	32	32	22.6	27.7	12.5	40
Enterococcus	45	40.6	32	27	28.7	N/A	29	29
Proteus mirabilis	55	28.1	22	17	26.1	55.8	7.3	12.4
Pseudomonas aeruginosa	20	15.6	14	7	15.9	23.1	7.3	9.1
Bacteroides sp.	85	67	67	33	15.6	84.6	31	9.1

From Frykberg RG, Veves A. Diabetic foot infections. *Diabetes Metab Rev.* 1996;12(3):255–270.

a deeper ulceration or an undrained abscess, gangrene, or necrotizing fasciitis. Methicillin-resistant *Staphylococcus aureus* is an increasingly common isolate.[43] They tend to have greater than 2 cm of surrounding cellulitis, as well as lymphangitis and edema of the affected limb. These more severe cases generally present with fever, leukocytosis, and hyperglycemia.

In contrast to nondiabetic individuals, complex foot infections in diabetic patients usually involve multiple organisms with complex biofilm environments.[48] Studies report an average of five to eight different species per specimen.[49–52] These include a combination of gram-positive and gram-negative, as well as aerobic and anaerobic organisms. The most prevalent organisms identified *are Staphylococcus aureus, coagulase-negative Staphylococcus, group B Streptococcus, Proteus, Escherichia coli, Pseudomonas,* and *Bacteroides.* Recently, methicillin-resistant *Staphylococcus aureus* infection has become more common in diabetic foot ulcers and is associated with previous antibiotic treatment and prolonged time to healing.[43,53,54] Anaerobic infections with *Clostridium* are also not uncommon. These patients require immediate hospitalization, broad-spectrum intravenous antibiotics, and aggressive surgical débridement. Superficial wound cultures are often unreliable, as they may demonstrate organisms responsible for colonization that do not affect the associated infection. Deep wound or bone cultures are the best way to accurately assess the microbiology in a diabetic foot infection and to assess for osteomyelitis.

ASSESSMENT OF THE PATIENT WITH A LOWER EXTREMITY ULCER

Accurate diagnosis of the underlying cause of lower extremity ulceration is essential for successful treatment. The etiology of most leg ulcers can be ascertained quite accurately by careful, problem-focused history taking and physical examination.[31] Diagnostic and laboratory studies are occasionally necessary to establish the diagnosis but are more often performed to guide treatment strategy.[55] A multidisciplinary team is essential to ensure optimum diagnosis and management of these complex patients.[2]

History

Patients with ulcers due to venous insufficiency usually complain of aching and swelling of the legs. They may recount a history of recurrent cellulitis, previous deep vein thrombosis, or previous superficial venous surgery. Symptoms are often worse at the end of the day, exacerbated when the leg is dependent, and relieved by leg elevation.

Arterial insufficiency is suggested by a history of underlying cardiac or cerebrovascular disease, complaints of leg claudication, or rest pain in the foot (see Chapter 18). Patients may complain of pain in the buttocks or calves brought on with activity and relieved with rest

(intermittent claudication) or pain in the forefoot aggravated by elevation and relieved by dependency (rest pain). The presence of an extremity ulcer is an easily recognized but late sign of peripheral arterial insufficiency. Patients with lower extremity ulcers resulting from atherosclerotic disease usually have a risk-factor profile that includes: older age, smoking, diabetes mellitus, hypertension, hypercholesterolemia, and obesity.[22,56] Patients with leg ulcers and multiple atherosclerotic risk factors often have atherosclerosis in other arterial beds.[57]

Up to one-third of patients with diabetes mellitus can have significant atherosclerotic disease, without specific related symptoms. The most common associated complaints are those of neuropathic disease, which include numbness, paresthesias, and burning pain in the lower extremities. Patients also often report previous episodes of foot ulcers and chronic skin infections.

Physical Examination

A complete examination is best performed with the patient supine in an examination gown. The patient's vital signs are recorded and abnormalities noted. The patient's temperature, respiratory rate, heart rate, and blood pressure in both upper extremities should be obtained. Fever may indicate the presence of an infected ulcer, and the presence of tachycardia and tachypnea may support the diagnosis of a septic foot.

A classic look, listen, and feel examination includes inspection of the skin of the extremities, palpation of all peripheral pulses, measurement of ankle-brachial indices, assessment of extremity temperature, auscultation for bruits, and a thorough neurologic examination.[31]

Visual inspection coupled with an accurate history can determine the presence of a chronic vascular condition (Fig. 61.3A). The color of the skin is conferred by the blood in the subpapillary layer and varies with the position of the extremity, temperature of the skin, and degree of blood oxygenation (reduced hemoglobin → blue). Also in chronic arterial insufficiency, the arterioles are maximally dilated as a compensatory response to the chronic ischemia intensifying color changes. In acute arterial occlusion the venules empty, leading to a chalky white appearance regardless of extremity position. When the extremity is at the level of the heart, the pooled blood masks the color imparted by the arterial flow. Elevation of the extremity above the level of the central venous pressure allows the pooled venous blood to drain. The normal extremity remains pink, whereas that with arterial insufficiency becomes pallid. Conversely, allowing the extremity to become dependent causes an intense rubor or cyanosis. The time of return of blood to the dependent extremity is a useful marker of the severity of the deficit (normally <20 seconds). With a diminished nutritional supply to the skin, there is thinning and functional loss of the dermal appendages, evident as dry, shiny, and hairless skin. The nails may become brittle and ridged. Comparison of color and trophic changes between

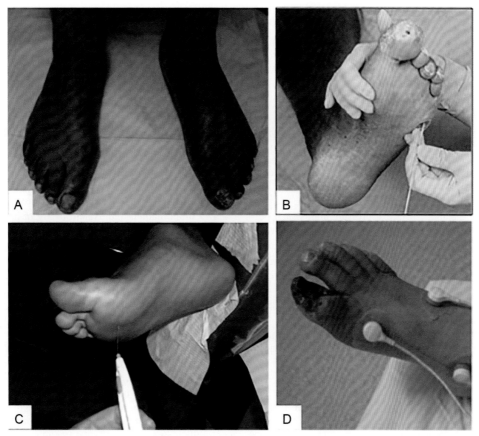

Fig. 61.3 Examination of the Foot. (A) Visual. (B) Probing the wound. (C) Using Semmes-Weinstein monofilament. (D) Transcutaneous oximetry.

extremities gives a good indication of the severity of the process, unless bilateral deficits are present. Skin temperature is a reliable indicator of the blood flow rate in the dermal vessels, though flow is governed primarily by constriction or dilation of the arterioles to maintain a constant core temperature. Nevertheless, the temperature of the skin as a marker of perfusion is useful and can be assessed by lightly palpating the skin with the back of the hand and comparing similar sites from one extremity to the other. An ischemic limb is cool, and demarcation of temperature gives a rough indication of the level of the occlusion. Again, assessment of temperature differences is confounded when both extremities are affected.

In limbs of patients with venous insufficiency, there is evidence of chronic edema. Venous hypertension causes transudation of serous fluid and red blood cells into the subcutaneous tissue. Hemoglobin from the red blood cells breaks down to produce the pigment hemosiderin, leading to hyperpigmentation, especially in the medial paramalleolar areas. Patients with venous insufficiency commonly develop stasis dermatitis. This eczematous process may spread from the area of the medial malleolus and involve the leg circumferentially. The recurrent cellulitis can cause contraction of the subcutaneous tissue in the lower third of the leg, below the knee, and together with the chronic edema can produce a "bottle leg" appearance.

Ulcer Evaluation

A thorough evaluation of ulcers of the lower extremity is critical in ascertaining the etiology and to institute an appropriate treatment strategy. Specific characteristics of the ulcer such as location, size, depth, and appearance should be recorded during the initial evaluation and with each subsequent follow-up visit to determine progress and evaluate the treatment regimen.[58] Ulcers of the foot should be gently examined with a cotton-tipped probe to establish the presence of a sinus tract. The margins of the ulcer should be undermined to evaluate the extent of tissue destruction. Ulcer extension to tendon, bone, or joint should be sought. A positive probe-to-bone finding (see Fig. 61.3B) has a high predictive value for osteomyelitis and is an extremely sensitive and cost-effective screen.[59]

Extremity ulcerations have a characteristic appearance depending on their origin. Ulcerations caused by ischemia are typically located on the tips of the toes (see Fig. 61.2B) and between the digits. The lesions often appear punched out and are painful but exhibit little bleeding. They also occur on the dorsum of the foot and over the first and fifth metatarsal heads. Ischemic ulcers are uncommon on the plantar surface, as the pressure is usually less sustained and the perfusion better. A heel ulcer can develop from constant pressure when the heel is in a dependent position or during prolonged immobilization and bed rest. Once an ulcer is present, the blood supply necessary to heal the wound is greater than that needed to maintain intact skin, resulting in a chronic ulcer unless the blood supply is improved.

Elevated venous pressure due to perforator or deep vein incompetency or venous thrombosis reduces the pressure gradient for perfusion. Venous ulcers rarely occur in the foot and are commonly located in the "gaiter" distribution of the leg, around the medial malleolus, where the venous pressures are highest. These typically are associated with a swollen leg with a distinctive skin appearance (see Fig. 61.2A). Venous ulcerations occur most commonly on the medial aspect of the ankle and are surrounded by areas with induration and brown pigmentation of the surrounding area (brawny induration) and scaling skin. These ulcers are often exquisitely tender and weep copious serous fluid.

The appearance of the extremity in venous insufficiency is distinctive and rarely poses a problem distinguishing between it and arterial insufficiency. It is important to differentiate the rubor associated with venous insufficiency and cellulitis accompanying an infective process. Cellulitic color changes will persist despite extremity elevation. With isolated venous insufficiency, the extremity is warm and variably swollen with the characteristic skin changes described earlier. Acute or chronic arterial vascular insufficiency may be superimposed on the changes of chronic venous insufficiency, impairing the healing of the venous ulcer. In these situations, lower extremity revascularization may be required to assist in healing a venous ulceration that is not responding appropriately to compression therapy. Furthermore, the presence of significant lower extremity swelling or skin changes can complicate arterial reconstructions by altering the surgical approach to distal arterial target sites.

Neuropathic ulcerations typically occur at the heel or over the metatarsal heads on the plantar surface at pressure points (mal perforans ulcer; see Fig. 61.2C) but may also occur in less characteristic locations secondary to trauma. They usually are painless. The sensory neuropathy may limit detection in the diabetic patient and allow the destructive process to go unchecked, with extension into the deep plantar space.

In addition to ulcers, patients may present with varying degrees of tissue loss or frankly gangrenous digits, forefoot, or hindfoot. The presence of dry gangrene is a relatively stable process; however, any progression to an infected wet gangrene requires immediate surgical débridement.

Vascular Examination

A careful physical examination should be performed in patients with leg ulcers to elucidate the underlying cause of leg ulcers (see Chapter 11). The handheld Doppler ultrasound should be used in case of inability to easily palpate a given vessel. These can be supplemented with noninvasive vascular tests (see Chapter 12) and other diagnostic tests as necessary for each clinical situation. An ankle-brachial index is an important tool for assessing perfusion to the foot. Patients with an ankle-brachial index (ABI) less than 0.3 may complain of rest pain; and in patients with tissue loss, the ABI is often less than 0.5.[60] In patients with diabetes and renal failure due to calcification of the vessel, ABI may be falsely elevated and is not reliable to evaluate the level of ischemia.

If the physical examination suggests venous insufficiency, a Trendelenburg test should be performed to assess valve function of the deep venous system and perforators (see Chapter 54). The patient is placed in a supine position and the legs are elevated. After decompression of the superficial veins occurs, a tourniquet is placed around the patient's thigh and the patient is asked to stand. If the varicose veins do not fill within 60 seconds below the tourniquet, the valves in the deep system and perforators are not compromised, and proximal saphenous vein incompetence is likely.

Neurologic Examination

The lower extremity neurologic examination is essential and should include testing for motor strength; deep-tendon reflexes; and vibratory, proprioceptive, and protective sensation.[61] Chronic ischemia can cause varying patterns of sensory loss that is usually within the affected arterial distribution. Neuropathy occurs in 42% of patients with diabetes within 20 years after diagnosis of the disease.[26] The neuropathy alters motor, sensory, and autonomic function, which directly affect the dynamic function of the foot during gait. The gait of the patient should be observed to detect any gross asymmetry or unsteadiness.

Motor neuropathy is associated with demyelinization and motor end-plate damage, which contribute to conduction defects. Atrophy of the small intrinsic muscles of the foot occurs secondary to the distal motor nerve damage. Wasting of the lumbric and interosseous muscles of the foot results in collapse of the arch and loss of stability of metatarsal-phalangeal joints during midstance of the gait.[1] Overpowering by extrinsic muscles can lead to depression of the metatarsal heads, digital contractures, and cocked-up toes. These changes result in abnormal pressure points, increased shearing, and ulcer formation.

Diabetic sensory neuropathy is typically a glove-and-stocking distribution and is associated with a decrement in vibration and two-point discrimination. Loss of protective sensation due to peripheral neuropathy is the most common cause of ulceration in the diabetic population. The use of monofilament gauges (Semmes-Weinstein) is a good objective way of assessing diabetic neuropathy (see Fig. 61.3C).[61] Patients with normal foot sensation usually can feel a 4.17 monofilament (equivalent to 1 g of linear pressure). Patients who cannot detect a 5.07 monofilament when it buckles (equivalent to 10 g of linear pressure) are considered to have lost protective sensation.[62,63] Several cross-sectional studies have indicated that foot ulceration is strongly associated with elevated cutaneous pressure perception thresholds.[61] Magnitudes of association, however, were provided in a case-control study,[64] where an unadjusted sevenfold risk of ulceration was observed in those patients (97% male) with insensitivity to the 5.07 monofilament. Although the nerve conduction test is the gold standard, its expense and limited availability prevent its widespread application as a screening tool for diabetic neuropathy. Use of a Semmes-Weinstein monofilament is a convenient, inexpensive, painless alternative to nerve conduction studies that should be utilized in the initial evaluation of all patients with diabetes mellitus as a screen for peripheral neuropathy. A positive Semmes-Weinstein monofilament test result is a significant predictor of future ulceration and lower extremity amputation, as well in patients with diabetes mellitus.[65] If diabetic patients have positive monofilament results, their chances of ulceration increase 10% to 20%. The relative risk of foot ulceration in patients with a positive monofilament result compared with those with a negative monofilament result ranges from 2.5 to 4.9. In addition, a positive monofilament result in patients with diabetes increases the risks of leg amputation from 5% to 15% compared with those with negative monofilament results. The Semmes-Weinstein monofilament is an important evidence-based tool for determining which patients are at increased risk of complications during follow-up, leading to improved patient selection for early intervention and management. Ultimately, screening with Semmes-Weinstein monofilament may lead to improved clinical outcomes for patients with diabetic foot.[65]

The presence of neuropathy mandates attention to the biomechanics of the foot. There is an important role of the podiatrist or foot surgeon in the evaluation of these patients.[2] Use of a computerized gait analysis system to assess abnormally high-pressure areas has led to greater use of orthotic devices in the prevention of skin breakdown. For example, an F scan system uses an ultrathin Tekscan sensor consisting of 960 sensor cells ($5 mm^2$ each). The sensor is used in a floor mat system designed to measure barefoot or stocking-foot dynamic plantar pressures, indicating those subjects with pressures greater than or equal to 6 kg/cm^2. Abnormal mechanical forces that can result in ulcerations should be addressed with the use of offloading devices or other modalities in order to assist in wound healing.

Particular attention should be paid to a complete neurologic examination on patients who have had a stroke, as much of the rationale for extremity salvage depends on the potential for rehabilitation. The remainder of the physical examination should be undertaken with attention to the presence of comorbidities, which also may influence the decision-making process.

Tests and Imaging Techniques

The use of non–diagnostic-imaging techniques by duplex ultrasound has been covered in depth (see Chapter 12). Other noninvasive imaging methods useful in the assessment of patients with leg ulcers include plain radiography, magnetic resonance imaging (MRI) and angiography (MRA)[66] (see Chapter 13), and computed tomographic angiography (CTA) (see Chapter 14). Imaging techniques can be used to diagnose osteomyelitis and confirm the presence of bony deformities. Plain film radiography is used primarily to exclude bony lesions as a cause of a patient's pain complaints, assess the presence of osteomyelitis beneath an ulcerated foot lesion, and assess the presence of vascular wall calcification. Plain films of the foot are relatively inexpensive and can show soft-tissue swelling, disruption of bone cortex, and periosteal elevation. MRI can provide details of pathologic anatomic features and has a high sensitivity for assessment of deep space infection and the presence of osteomyelitis in the diabetic foot. There is now an increasing recognition of the importance of assessing the microperfusion in the foot,[67] and the role of angiosomes in the strategic revascularization of the foot ulcers.[68]

The assessment of a patient with foot ulcers stemming from peripheral artery disease encompasses a thorough history and physical examination with the adjunctive use of the noninvasive vascular laboratory to confirm, localize, and grade lesions.[60] While multiple noninvasive and invasive methods are available to assess the peripheral vasculature, not every patient requires an exhaustive battery of tests in order to evaluate vascular status. In general, only those tests likely to provide information that alters the course of action should be performed. It is important that flow-limiting arterial lesions are evaluated and reconstructed or bypassed if ischemic foot ulcers are to heal.

MANAGEMENT OF ULCERS

General

Aggressive mechanical débridement, systemic antibiotic therapy, and strict non–weight bearing are the cornerstones for effective wound care.[69] Sharp débridement in the operating room or at the bedside, when applicable, allows for thorough removal of all necrotic material and optimizes the wound environment.[70] All necrotic bone, plus a small portion of the uninvolved bone, soft tissue, and devascularized structures, should be excised, and the degree of penetration of the infection should be established.[70] Curettage of any exposed or remaining cartilage is important to prevent this avascular structure from becoming a nidus of infection. Foot soaks, whirlpool therapy, or enzymatic débridement may be useful but are rarely effective and may lead to further skin maceration or wound breakdown. No prospective randomized studies have demonstrated the superiority of dressing products compared with standard saline wet to dry sterile gauze in establishing a granulation bed. Use of moist dressings in clean, granulating wounds is recommended to enhance the wound environment.[20,71] An "ideal" dressing not only provides protection against further bacterial contamination but also maintains moisture balance, optimizes the wound pH, absorbs fibrinous fluids, and reduces local pain. Various dressings are currently available to target specific characteristics of the wound[72]; however, moist normal-saline dressings are probably sufficient for most wounds. These inexpensive dressings are highly absorptive of exudative drainage and maintain the moist environment.

In the presence of infection and cellulitis, oral antimicrobial therapy should be instituted on the basis of the suspected pathogen and clinical findings. Severe infections should be treated with broad-spectrum intravenous antibiotics,[73] with particular emphasis on the role of biofilms.[48] After bacterial contamination has been controlled, small ulcers can usually be excised and closed immediately. Large open wounds, however, are treated with a staged approach, with frequent débridement and establishment of a granulation base. The clean wounds can then be closed with healthy tissue, with the use of local or free-flap coverage and soft-tissue repair. Meticulous surgical reconstruction of these wounds can help avert the production of inelastic scar tissue over weight-bearing surfaces. Any remaining extrinsic or intrinsic pressures can be reduced with the postoperative use of orthoses.

Surgical correction of biomechanical defects, plastic and soft-tissue reconstruction, and appropriate measures to minimize foot pressure are all essential to enable the patient to walk effectively again. In cases of gross wound infections and rampant cellulitis, use of a silver-containing medication such as Silvadene may be necessary in the initial setting to reduce the bacterial load. Use of bioactive drugs (e.g., Recombinant PDGF, Regranex) or skin substitutes (e.g., Apligraf, Dermagraft) show promising results and have proven useful under specific circumstances. Likewise, the use of negative pressure wound therapy has been a big advance in the care of advanced wounds.[74-76] A clinical practice algorithm for foot ulcers is seen in Fig. 61.4.[77]

Offloading strategies such as total contact casting or removable walkers has resulted in significant decreases in healing times.[78,79] The stresses placed on the foot can be intrinsic, as was previously described with respect to digital contractures, or extrinsic in nature. These external forces can result from inappropriate footwear, traumatic injury, or foreign bodies. Shoes that are too tight or too shallow are a frequent yet preventable component to the development of neuropathic ulcers. Various shoe modifications such as the rocker-sole design and different types of insoles have made it possible to reduce plantar foot pressures, thus decreasing the risks of ulceration.[80-82]

Venous Ulcers

Elevation of the leg is a simple maneuver that can effectively but temporarily eliminate venous hypertension. All patients should be encouraged to elevate the affected leg above the level of the heart for 2 to 3 hours during the day and when lying in bed at night. Compression therapy is also effective in controlling edema and accelerates healing of ulcerations. However, before compression is applied to the limb, significant occlusive arterial disease should be excluded. Compression therapy is generally contraindicated in patients with an ABI less than 0.7 or with other signs and symptoms of compromised blood supply to the leg. Many different types of compression devices are available, including elastic and nonelastic bandages, graduated compression stockings, and compression pumps. The most effective way of delivering compression is decided on an individual basis. Compression should be applied just before arising from bed and removed at bedtime.

Treatment of stasis dermatitis minimizes further trauma to the skin from scratching. Pruritus can be controlled by topically applied corticosteroids or orally administered antihistamines, or both. The goal of local wound care in patients with venous ulcers is to minimize stasis; decrease bacterial contamination of the ulcer; and provide a healthy, moist wound environment that promotes healing. Heavily contaminated venous ulcers with surrounding cellulitis may require systemic antibiotic therapy in addition to local wound control. The predominant organisms cultured from chronic ulcers are gram-positive pathogens like S. aureus and Streptococcus pyogenes. The most common gram-negative bacteria are Pseudomonas aeruginosa, especially in the diabetic population. Various moisture-retentive dressings can be used in conjunction with compression therapy to relieve pain, débride necrotic tissue, and promote granulation tissue formation.

The goal of venous procedures, either by surgical ligation and stripping or endoluminal ablation of the saphenous veins in venous insufficiency is to correct underlying pathology. The long-term outcomes of surgical ligation and stripping and of catheter-based ablation of the

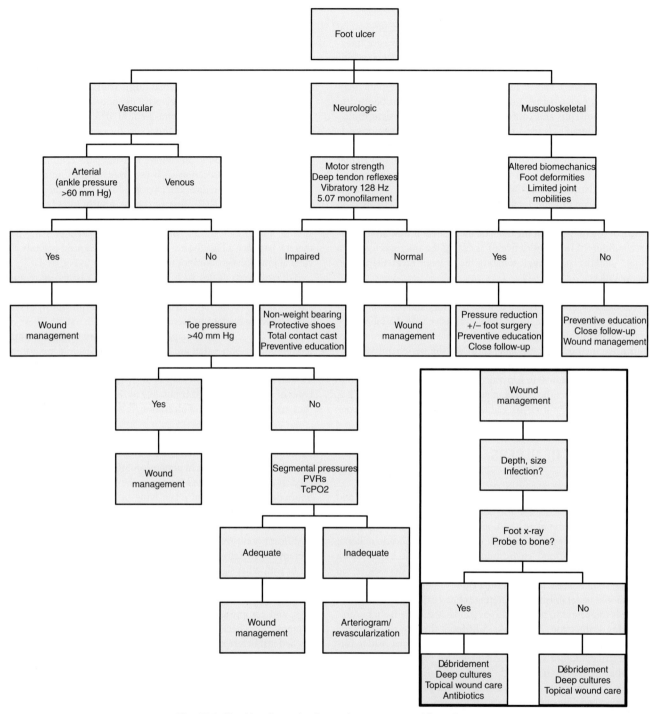

Fig. 61.4 Algorithm for evaluation and management of foot ulcers.

saphenous veins are comparable and excellent if the deep system is not involved. Either intervention can result in healing up to 90% of ulcers and modest long-term results if the diagnostic studies can adequately characterize and localize the incompetent superficial or perforating system valves.[83] Ulcer recurrence is significantly less after superficial venous ablation surgery plus use of compression stockings when compared with compression therapy alone.[84,85] If reflux exists in the deep venous system, interventions on the superficial veins alone have a poor result and high ulcer recurrence rate. Reconstruction of vein valves can be a consideration in some patients.[86,87]

Ischemic Ulcers

The management of ischemic ulcers follows some basic guiding principles. Flow-limiting arterial lesions can be evaluated and reconstructed or bypassed.[88] The optimal strategy is to perform revascularization, if indicated, as soon as possible (see Chapters 20 and 21).[89] Closure of the ulcer by primary healing or secondary reconstructive surgery will then be expedited. If revascularization of an ischemic ulcer is not possible for medical or technical reasons, amputation of the foot or limb may be required. Contraindications to revascularization include nonambulatory patients and a foot phlegmon with sepsis or excessive foot gangrene, precluding a functional foot despite adjunctive plastic surgical procedures such as skin grafts and free flaps.

Diabetic Ulcers

The role of a multidisciplinary group of consultants in the management of diabetic ulcers cannot be overemphasized.[90] Successful management of foot ulcers involves recognition and correction of the underlying etiology, as well as appropriate wound care and prevention of recurrence.[58] Assessment of the ulcer consists of determining the size and depth of the wound and inspection of the surrounding area for local signs of infection or gangrene. Several classification systems have been devised for descriptive purposes and act as prognostic indicators.[91]

The absence of systemic manifestations such as fever, chills, or leukocytosis does not necessarily exclude underlying infection, especially in the immunocompromised diabetic population. The use of plain films to rule out osteomyelitis or deep culture of the wound is frequently necessary.

Neuropathic and Musculoskeletal Management

Reconstructive foot surgery may be considered in order to avoid major amputations in patients with chronic neuropathic wounds. The objectives for management of chronic diabetic foot wounds include prevention of major amputation, prevention of infection, decreased probability of ulceration, maintenance of skin integrity, and improvement of function. Successful outcomes for diabetic foot reconstruction result in less intrinsic pressures via minor amputations, arthroplasties, osteotomies, condylectomies, exostosectomies, tendon procedures, and joint arthrodesis.[90] Open wounds can be treated in one stage and are primarily closed with premorbid tissue using local flap reconstruction and soft tissue repair.[92] Plastic surgical repair of these wounds can avoid the production of inelastic scar tissue over weight-bearing surfaces.[93] Extrinsic and intrinsic pressures can be further neutralized with postoperative accommodative shoe gear.[78,79] Prophylactic diabetic foot surgery is an option to prevent recurrent ulceration and reduce the risk of major amputations.[94,95] Surgical biomechanics, plastic and soft tissue reconstruction, and appropriate offloading are essential to creating a stable platform from which to keep these difficult patients free from tissue breakdown and as functional as possible.

Treatment of these pedal soft tissue wounds in the diabetic population is a medical and surgical challenge. These extend the length of the patient's disability and significantly increase the cost of medical care. Simple closure of these wounds often is difficult because of preexisting bone deformity, tissue inelasticity, location of the defect, and superimposed osteomyelitis. Clinical pathways related to diabetic foot ulcers often involve sharp débridement, expensive wound care products, long-term intravenous antibiotics, total contact casting, total contact casting with tendo-Achilles lengthening, use of skin equivalents, electrical stimulation, multiple offloading orthopedic devices, and even amputation. Newer modalities for accelerating wound healing are being investigated, but their impact is still not established.[96]

Wounds often are allowed to granulate, contract, and heal by secondary intention. Use of negative pressure wound therapy has improved outcomes.[76,90] When these wounds occur on the plantar aspect of the foot, they frequently recur since the resulting scar has decreased extensibility and mobility. Attempted primary wound closure of diabetic pedal defects is often unsuccessful, primarily resulting from inadequate wound assessment, lack of proper evaluation of comorbidities, and an inadequate treatment plan.[97] Reconstructive surgery had traditionally been performed on select patients with severe deformities that cannot be accommodated by custom footwear. More recent considerations emphasize the importance of addressing the underlying

bony pathology in patients with diabetic foot problems, dispelling the unfounded fear of performing surgery on diabetic feet.[92,94,95]

Reconstructive surgery can range from simple metatarsal head resections to subtotal calcanectomies. Local flaps that are often difficult to elevate and inset are more easily mobilized and incised when concomitant bone resection is achieved at the time of flap creation. In addition, a local flap results in greater exposure and direct visualization of the underlying osseous structures compared with a single linear or semielliptical incision. The implementation of local random flaps can eliminate the need for additional incisions often deemed necessary to gain access to a forefoot, midfoot, or rearfoot bony defect. The use of negative pressure wound therapy has greatly enabled the salvage of these complex limb wounds.[76,90]

SUMMARY

Chronic leg ulcers are frequently encountered in clinical practice. Considerable morbidity and mortality are associated with ulcerations of the lower limbs in diabetic and nondiabetic patients. Careful assessment of vascular disease, evaluation and management of biomechanical and metabolic abnormalities, and aggressive treatment of infections are required. A multidisciplinary approach provides a comprehensive treatment protocol and significantly increases the chances of successfully healing the ulcer and preventing recurrence.[90]

REFERENCES

1. Sumpio BE. Foot ulcers. *N Engl J Med.* 2000;343(11):787–793.
2. Sumpio BE, Armstrong DG, Lavery LA, Andros G. The role of interdisciplinary team approach in the management of the diabetic foot: a joint statement from the Society for Vascular Surgery and the American Podiatric Medical Association. *J Vasc Surg.* 2010;51(6):1504–1506.
3. Sumpio BE, Aruny J, Blume PA. The multidisciplinary approach to limb salvage. *Acta Chir Belg.* 2004;104(6):647–653.
4. Mekkes JR, Loots MA, Van Der Wal AC, Bos JD. Causes, investigation and treatment of leg ulceration. *Br J Dermatol.* 2003;148(3):388–401.
5. Beauregard S, Gilchrest B. A survey of skin problems and skin care regiments in the elderly. *Arch Dermatol.* 1987;(123):1638–1643.
6. Clement DL. Venous ulcer reappraisal: insights from an international task force. Veines International Task Force. *J Vasc Res.* 1999;36(Suppl 1):42–47.
7. De Wolfe V. The prevention and management of chronic venous insufficiency. *Prac Cardiol.* 1980;6:187–202.
8. Phillips TJ. Chronic cutaneous ulcers: etiology and epidemiology. *J Invest Dermatol.* 1994;102(6):38S–41S.
9. Ellison DA, Hayes L, Lane C, et al. Evaluating the cost and efficacy of leg ulcer care provided in two large UK health authorities. *J Wound Care.* 2002;11(2):47–51.
10. Phillips T, Stanton B, Provan A. A study of the impact of leg ulcers on quality of life: financial, social, and psychological implications. *J Am Acad Dermatol.* 1994;31:49–53.
11. Browse NL. The etiology of venous ulceration. *World J Surg.* 1986;10(6):938–943.
12. Goldman M, Fronek A. The Alexander House Group: consensus paper on venous leg ulcers. *J Dermatol Surg Oncol.* 1992;18:592.
13. Hutton W, Stokes I. The mechanics of the foot. In: Klenerman L, ed. *The Foot and Its Disorders.* Oxford: Blackwell Scientific; 1991:11.
14. Murray H, Boulton A. The pathophysiology of diabetic foot ulceration. *Clin Podiatric Med Surg.* 1995;12(1):1–17.
15. Phillips TJ. Leg ulcer management. *Dermatol Nurs.* 1996;8(5):333–340. quiz 341-332.
16. O'Donnell Jr TF, Browse NL, Burnand KG, Thomas ML. The socioeconomic effects of an iliofemoral venous thrombosis. *J Surg Res.* 1977;22(5):483–488.
17. Falanga V, Eaglstein WH. The "trap" hypothesis of venous ulceration. *Lancet.* 1993;341(8851):1006–1008.

18. Burnand KG, Clemenson G, Whimpster I, Browse NL. Proceedings: extravascular fibrin deposition in response to venous hypertension—the cause of venous ulcers. *Br J Surg.* 1976;63(8):660–661.

19. Dodd HJ, Gaylarde PM, Sarkany I. Skin oxygen tension in venous insufficiency of the lower leg. *J R Soc Med.* 1985;78(5):373–376.

20. Singer AJ, Clark RA. Cutaneous wound healing. *N Engl J Med.* 1999;341(10):738–746.

21. Mayfield JA, Reiber GE, Sanders LJ, et al. Preventive foot care in people with diabetes [position statement]. *Diabetes Care.* 2003;26(Suppl 1):S78–S79.

22. Knox RC, Dutch W, Blume P, Sumpio BE. Diabetic foot disease. *Int J Angiol.* 2000;9(1):1–6.

23. Reiber GE, Lipsky BA, Gibbons GW. The burden of diabetic foot ulcers. *Am J Surg.* 1998;176(2A Suppl):5S–10S.

24. Boulton AJ. The diabetic foot: a global view. *Diabetes Metab Res Rev.* 2000;16(Suppl 1):S2–S5.

25. Weiss JS, Sumpio BE. Review of prevalence and outcome of vascular disease in patients with diabetes mellitus. *Eur J Vasc Endovasc Surg.* 2006;31(2):143–150.

26. O'Brien IA, Corrall RJ. Epidemiology of diabetes and its complications. *N Engl J Med.* 1988;318(24):1619–1620.

27. Kamal K, Powell RJ, Sumpio BE. The pathobiology of diabetes mellitus: implications for surgeons. *J Am Coll Surg.* 1996;183(3):271–289.

28. Laing P. The development and complications of diabetic foot ulcers. *Am J Surg.* 1998;176(2A Suppl):11S–19S.

29. Lee L, Blume PA, Sumpio B. Charcot joint disease in diabetes mellitus. *Ann Vasc Surg.* 2003;17(5):571–580.

30. Veves A, Fernando D, Walewski P, et al. A study of plantar pressures in a diabetic clinic population. *Foot.* 1991;2:89.

31. Boulton AJ, Armstrong DG, Albert SF, et al. Comprehensive foot examination and risk assessment: a report of the task force of the foot care interest group of the American Diabetes Association, with endorsement by the American Association of Clinical Endocrinologists. *Diabetes Care.* 2008;31(8):1679–1685.

32. Masson E, Hay E, Stockley I, et al. Abnormal foot pressures alone may not cause ulceration. *Diabetic Med.* 1989;6:426–428.

33. Levin ME. Diabetes and peripheral neuropathy. *Diabetes Care.* 1998;21(1):1.

34. Boulton AJ, Hardisty CA, Betts RP, et al. Dynamic foot pressure and other studies as diagnostic and management aids in diabetic neuropathy. *Diabetes Care.* 1983;6(1):26–33.

35. Fernando DJ, Masson EA, Veves A, Boulton AJ. Relationship of limited joint mobility to abnormal foot pressures and diabetic foot ulceration. *Diabetes Care.* 1991;14(1):8–11.

36. Morag E, Pammer S, Boulton A, et al. Structural and functional aspects of the diabetic foot. *Clin Biomech (Bristol, Avon).* 1997;12(3):S9–S10.

37. Saltzman C, Pedowitz W. Diabetic foot infection. *Instr Course Lect.* 1999;48:317–320.

38. Habershaw G, Chzran J. Management of diabetic foot problems. In: *Biomechanical Considerations of the Diabetic Foot.* 2nd ed. Philadelphia: WB Saunders; 1995:53–65.

39. Bullock G, Stavosky J. Surgical wound management of the diabetic foot. *Surg Technol Int.* 2001;(VI):301–310.

40. Bild DE, Selby JV, Sinnock P, et al. Lower-extremity amputation in people with diabetes. Epidemiology and prevention. *Diabetes Care.* 1989;12(1):24–31.

41. Kannel WB, McGee DL. Diabetes and cardiovascular disease. The Framingham study. *JAMA.* 1979;241(19):2035–2038.

42. Melton 3rd LJ, Macken KM, Palumbo PJ, Elveback LR. Incidence and prevalence of clinical peripheral vascular disease in a population-based cohort of diabetic patients. *Diabetes Care.* 1980;3(6):650–654.

43. Dang CN, Prasad YD, Boulton AJ, Jude EB. Methicillin-resistant Staphylococcus aureus in the diabetic foot clinic: a worsening problem. *Diabet Med.* 2003;20(2):159–161.

44. Hostetter MK. Handicaps to host defense. Effects of hyperglycemia on C3 and Candida albicans. *Diabetes.* 1990;39(3):271–275.

45. Hostetter MK, Krueger RA, Schmeling DJ. The biochemistry of opsonization: central role of the reactive thiolester of the third component of complement. *J Infect Dis.* 1984;150(5):653–661.

46. MacRury SM, Gemmell CG, Paterson KR, MacCuish AC. Changes in phagocytic function with glycaemic control in diabetic patients. *J Clin Pathol.* 1989;42(11):1143–1147.

47. Caballero E, Frykberg RG. Diabetic foot infections. *J Foot Ankle Surg.* 1998;37(3):248–255.

48. Davis SC, Martinez L, Kirsner R. The diabetic foot: the importance of biofilms and wound bed preparation. *Curr Diab Rep.* 2006;6(6):439–445.

49. Louie TJ, Bartlett JG, Tally FP, Gorbach SL. Aerobic and anaerobic bacteria in diabetic foot ulcers. *Ann Intern Med.* 1976;85(4):461–463.

50. Sapico FL, Canawati HN, Witte JL, et al. Quantitative aerobic and anaerobic bacteriology of infected diabetic feet. *J Clin Microbiol.* 1980;12(3):413–420.

51. Sapico FL, Witte JL, Canawati HN, et al. The infected foot of the diabetic patient: quantitative microbiology and analysis of clinical features. *Rev Infect Dis.* 1984;6(Suppl 1):S171–S176.

52. Wheat LJ, Allen SD, Henry M, et al. Diabetic foot infections. Bacteriologic analysis. *Arch Intern Med.* 1986;146(10):1935–1940.

53. Day MR, Armstrong DG. Factors associated with methicillin resistance in diabetic foot infections. *J Foot Ankle Surg.* 1997;36(4):322–325. discussion 331.

54. Tentolouris N, Jude EB, Smirnof I, et al. Methicillin-resistant Staphylococcus aureus: an increasing problem in a diabetic foot clinic. *Diabet Med.* 1999;16(9):767–771.

55. Adam DJ, Naik J, Hartshorne T, et al. The diagnosis and management of 689 chronic leg ulcers in a single-visit assessment clinic. *Eur J Vasc Endovasc Surg.* 2003;25(5):462–468.

56. Sumpio B, Pradhan S. Atherosclerosis: biological and surgical considerations. In: Ascher E, Hollier L, Strandness Jr DE, eds. *Haimovici's Vascular Surgery.* Malden, MA: Blackwell Science; 2004:137.

57. Weitz JI, Byrne J, Clagett GP, et al. Diagnosis and treatment of chronic arterial insufficiency of the lower extremities: a critical review. *Circulation.* 1996;94(11):3026–3049.

58. Sumpio BE. Contemporary evaluation and management of the diabetic foot. *Scientifica (Cairo).* 2012;2012:435487.

59. Grayson ML, Gibbons GW, Balogh K, et al. Probing to bone in infected pedal ulcers. A clinical sign of underlying osteomyelitis in diabetic patients. *JAMA.* 1995;273(9):721–723.

60. Collins KA, Sumpio BE. Vascular assessment. *Clin Podiatr Med Surg.* 2000;17(2):171–191.

61. Feng Y, Schlosser FJ, Sumpio BE. The Semmes Weinstein monofilament examination as a screening tool for diabetic peripheral neuropathy. *J Vasc Surg.* 2009;50(3):675–682. 682 e671.

62. Armstrong DG, Lavery LA. Diabetic foot ulcers: prevention, diagnosis and classification. *Am Fam Physician.* 1998;57(6):1325–1332. 1337-1328.

63. Birke J, Sims D. Plantar sensory threshold in the ulcerative foot. *Leprosy Rev.* 1986;57:261.

64. McNeely M, Boyko E, Ahroni J, et al. The independent contributions of diabetic neuropathy and vasculopathy in foot ulceration: how great are the risks? *Diabetes Care.* 1995;18:216–219.

65. Feng Y, Schlösser FJ, Sumpio BE. The Semmes Weinstein monofilament examination is a significant predictor of the risk of foot ulceration and amputation in patients with diabetes mellitus. *J Vasc Surg.* 2011;53(1):220–226. e1-5.

66. Sumpio BE, Lee T, Blume PA. Vascular evaluation and arterial reconstruction of the diabetic foot. *Clin Podiatr Med Surg.* 2003;20(4):689–708.

67. Benitez E, Sumpio BJ, Chin J, Sumpio BE. Contemporary assessment of foot perfusion in patients with critical limb ischemia. *Semin Vasc Surg.* 2014;27(1):3–15.

68. Sumpio BE, Forsythe RO, Ziegler KR, et al. Clinical implications of the angiosome model in peripheral vascular disease. *J Vasc Surg.* 2013;58(3):814–826.

69. Steed DL, Donohoe D, Webster MW, Lindsley L. Effect of extensive debridement and treatment on the healing of diabetic foot ulcers. Diabetic Ulcer Study Group. *J Am Coll Surg.* 1996;183(1):61–64.

70. Granick M, Boykin J, Gamelli R, et al. Toward a common language: surgical wound bed preparation and debridement. *Wound Repair Regen.* 2006;14(Suppl 1):S1–10.

71. Bergstrom N, Bennett M, Carlson C. *Treatment of pressure ulcers*. Rockville, MD: Agency for Healthcare Policy and Research; December 1994.

72. Bello YM, Phillips TJ. Recent advances in wound healing. *JAMA*. 2000;283(6):716–718.

73. Joshi N, Caputo GM, Weitekamp MR, Karchmer AW. Infections in patients with diabetes mellitus. *N Engl J Med*. 1999;341(25):1906–1912.

74. Orgill DP, Manders EK, Sumpio BE, et al. The mechanisms of action of vacuum assisted closure: more to learn. *Surgery*. 2009;146(1):40–51.

75. Sumpio BE, Allie DE, Horvath KA, et al. Role of negative pressure wound therapy in treating peripheral vascular graft infections. *Vascular*. 2008;16(4):194–200.

76. Blume PA, Walters J, Payne W, et al. Comparison of negative pressure wound therapy using vacuum-assisted closure with advanced moist wound therapy in the treatment of diabetic foot ulcers: a multicenter randomized controlled trial. *Diabetes Care*. 2008;31(4):631–636.

77. Frykberg RG, Armstrong DG, Giurini J, et al. Diabetic foot disorders. A clinical practice guideline. For the American College of Foot and Ankle Surgeons and the American College of Foot and Ankle Orthopedics and Medicine. *J Foot Ankle Surg*. 2000;(Suppl):1–60.

78. Bus SA, Valk GD, van Deursen RW, et al. Specific guidelines on footwear and offloading. *Diabetes Metab Res Rev*. 2008;24(Suppl 1):S192–S193.

79. Bus SA, Valk GD, van Deursen RW, et al. The effectiveness of footwear and offloading interventions to prevent and heal foot ulcers and reduce plantar pressure in diabetes: a systematic review. *Diabetes Metab Res Rev*. 2008;24(Suppl 1):S162–S180.

80. Barrow J, Hughes J, Clark P. A study of the effect of wear on the pressure-relieving properties of foot orthosis. *Foot*. 1992;1:195–199.

81. Nawoczenski D, Birke J, Coleman W. Effect of rocker sole design on plantar forefoot pressures. *J Am Podiatr Med Assoc*. 1988;78:455–460.

82. Tang PC, Ravji K, Key JJ, et al. Let them walk! Current prosthesis options for leg and foot amputees. *J Am Coll Surg*. 2008;206(3):548–560.

83. Bello M, Scriven M, Hartshorne T, et al. Role of superficial venous surgery in the treatment of venous ulceration. *Br J Surg*. 1999;86(6):755–759.

84. Barwell JR, Taylor M, Deacon J, et al. Surgical correction of isolated superficial venous reflux reduces long-term recurrence rate in chronic venous leg ulcers. *Eur J Vasc Endovasc Surg*. 2000;20(4):363–368.

85. Ghauri AS, Nyamekye I, Grabs AJ, et al. Influence of a specialised leg ulcer service and venous surgery on the outcome of venous leg ulcers. *Eur J Vasc Endovasc Surg*. 1998;16(3):238–244.

86. Eriksson I. Reconstruction of deep venous valves of the lower extremity. *Surg Annu*. 1992;24(Pt 2):211–229.

87. Plagnol P, Ciostek P, Grimaud JP, Prokopowicz SC. Autogenous valve reconstruction technique for post-thrombotic reflux. *Ann Vasc Surg*. 1999;13(3):339–342.

88. Sarage A, Yui W, Blume P, et al. Aggressive revascularization options using cryoplasty in patients with lower extremity vascular disease. In: Geroulakos G, ed. *Re-do Vascular Surgery*. London: Springer Verlag; 2009:79–84.

89. Chin JA, Sumpio BE. Diabetes mellitus and peripheral vascular disease: diagnosis and management. *Clin Podiatr Med Surg*. 2014;31(1):11–26.

90. Sumpio B, Driver V, Gibbons G, et al. A multidisciplinary approach to limb preservation—the role of VAC therapy. *Wounds*. 2009;Oct Suppl:1–19.

91. Frangos S, Kilaru S, Blume P, et al. Classification of diabetic foot ulcers: improving communication. *Int J Angiol*. 2002;11:158–164.

92. Blume P, Partagas L, Attinger C, Sumpio B. Single stage surgical treatment of noninfected diabetic foot ulcers. *J Plastic Reconst Surg*. 2002;109:601–609.

93. Blume P, Salonga C, Garbalosa J, et al. Predictors for the healing of transmetatarsal amputations: retrospective study of 91 amputations. *Vascular*. 2007;15(3):126–133.

94. Armstrong D, Lavery L, Stern S, Harkless L. Is prophylactic diabetic foot surgery dangerous? *J Foot Ankle Surg*. 1996;35(6):585–589.

95. Catanzariti A, Blitch E, Karlock L. Elective foot and ankle surgery in the diabetic patient. *J Foot Ankle Surg*. 1995;34(1):23–41.

96. Shalaby SY, Blume P, Sumpio BE. New modalities in the chronic ischemic diabetic foot management. *Clin Podiatr Med Surg*. 2014;31(1):27–42.

97. Blume PA, Key JJ, Thakor P, et al. Retrospective evaluation of clinical outcomes in subjects with split-thickness skin graft: comparing V.A.C. therapy and conventional therapy in foot and ankle reconstructive surgeries. *Int Wound J*. 2010;7(6):480–487.

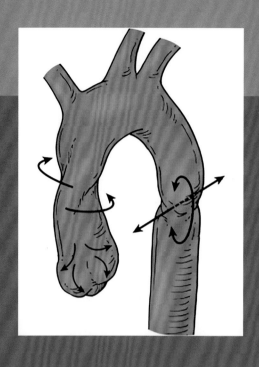

第62章
血管损伤

目前，创伤已成为美国46岁以下人群的主要死亡原因，血管损伤的住院死亡率在12.7%。随着对血管损伤认识的不断深入，诊治技术得到迅速发展，尤其是影像及血管腔内治疗技术的进步，使血管损伤的治疗模式也在不断转变。本章作者通过归纳和总结大量的文献，并结合美国创伤外科协会登记的血管损伤数据，重点讲述了血管损伤的初步评估、损伤类型、损伤机制、损伤征象（硬征和软征）及治疗原则，特别提到治疗上两个值得注意的进展，包括血管损伤院前急救过程中止血带的使用及开放性手术中损伤控制技术的血管内转流管的应用，降低了并发症和死亡率。详细阐述了颈部、胸部、腹部、四肢、内脏和特定部位的血管损伤及医源性、小儿血管损伤的损伤机制、解剖因素及诊治原则。同时，详细讲述了复苏性开胸术、复苏性血管内球囊阻断技术的应用和适应证，探讨损伤控制、缺血再灌注损伤、间隔室综合征的病理生理学机制及治疗原则。本章是非常实用的血管损伤临床诊治指南。

戈小虎

Vascular Trauma

Douglas W. Jones and Alik Farber

Vascular trauma occurs in varying injury patterns, with involved structures ranging from large caliber, high-flow central vessels to small, peripheral extremity vessels. Due to the variability in affected vessels and concomitant injuries, management strategies can vary considerably. Often, evaluation and treatment of vascular trauma occurs concurrently with that of other associated injuries. Therefore, management of vascular trauma requires knowledge of specific techniques for vascular repair throughout the body, but also demands judgment about how and when to implement those techniques.

Current principles of effective management of complex vascular trauma have developed directly out of military experience. During the US Civil War, World War I, and World War II, arterial injuries were seen in a small proportion of battlefield casualties and typically affected the extremities. Such injuries were most frequently treated by arterial ligation and subsequent amputation rates were very high.[1] Arterial reconstruction and limb preservation were rarely attempted and, in fact, discouraged. At the time of the Korean and Vietnam Wars, the rate of recognized vascular injury was higher, and in the Korean War in particular, surgeons in Mobile Army Surgical Hospital (MASH) units began to more regularly attempt vascular reconstruction, leading to vastly improved limb salvage rates.[1,2] More recent data from the Wars in Iraq and Afghanistan suggest that vascular injuries occur in up to 12% of those wounded in combat and still largely affect the extremities.[2] In these more recent conflicts, despite advances in surgical technique, arterial ligation (54%) and reconstruction (46%) were performed in roughly equal proportions.[2]

The increasing rate of diagnosed vascular trauma among military casualties is partially reflective of improved evacuation capabilities that decrease time from injury to medical evaluation. This is supported by the higher observed rates of carotid (7%) and aortic (3%) injuries, which may not have previously been survivable.[2] In addition, improvements in medical imaging have led to increased detection of subtler forms of vascular trauma. This has important implications in civilian vascular trauma, where rapid access to medical care and high-quality imaging is more uniform.

The contemporary relevance of military experience to civilian vascular trauma was recently highlighted by a report from the PROOVIT registry (American Association for the Surgery of Trauma Prospective Vascular Injury Treatment registry) detailing 542 vascular injuries from 14 American trauma centers.[3] The mechanism of injury was blunt trauma in 47% and penetrating trauma in 37% of patients. Similar to recent military reports, injuries were observed throughout the body, frequently involving the head/neck (internal carotid artery involved in 11%), extremities (femoral arteries involved in 11%), and thorax (descending thoracic aorta involved in 7%). Implemented management strategies included nonoperative management, initial open surgical intervention, and initial endovascular therapy in 51%, 38%, and 7%

of patients, respectively. The in-hospital mortality in this registry was 12.7%, illustrating the lethality of vascular trauma, even when patients survive to reach medical care.[3]

Two notable recent developments in the care of patients suffering vascular trauma have been: (1) more widespread use of prehospital tourniquets, which reliably prevent exsanguination from extremity injuries without requiring direct vascular control, and (2) the use of intravascular shunts at the time of initial surgical management to decrease operative time and allow surgeons to address other injuries, prioritizing hemodynamic resuscitation prior to definitive surgical repair.[4] In contemporary practice, PROOVIT reported prehospital tourniquet use in 20% of peripheral arterial injuries and a 2.6% overall rate of temporary shunt use.[3]

This chapter will discuss the initial evaluation of vascular trauma and will describe the management of specific vascular injury patterns. It is important to keep in mind that it is fairly uncommon for these injuries to be discovered in isolation. Furthermore, just as injury patterns have changed over time, treatment techniques continue to evolve, particularly with the advancement of endovascular therapy. Familiarity with the treatment principles outlined as follows is essential for anyone caring for traumatically injured patients. This is increasingly true in recent years, as a 2014 report showed that trauma deaths are occurring more frequently. In fact, trauma has become the leading cause of death in the United States for individuals younger than 46 years.[5]

INITIAL EVALUATION

The initial evaluation of the traumatically injured patient follows the principles of the Advanced Trauma Life Support (ATLS) algorithm with immediate attention initially paid to the patient's airway, breathing, and circulation (ABCs). Typically, the initial physical exam, mechanism of injury, and degree of hemodynamic instability dictate whether the patient will proceed directly to the operating room (OR) for surgical exploration. If this is the case, vascular injuries are explored and managed concurrently with other injuries and ongoing resuscitation. If clinical status permits, trauma workup usually includes at least a chest and pelvis x-ray, and may include ultrasonography and detailed evaluation of blood vessels with computed tomographic angiography (CTA).

TYPES OF VESSEL INJURY

Arterial injuries may affect the different layers of the arterial wall (intima, media, adventitia) to a varying degree (Table 62.1). Focal disruption of the intima may lead to the formation of an intimal flap that has the potential to be flow limiting and can lead to vessel occlusion and subsequent distal ischemia. An intramural hematoma (IMH)

TABLE 62.1   Types of Arterial Injury

Injury Type	Damaged Layers of Arterial Wall	Common Mechanism
Intimal flap	Intima	Blunt > penetrating
Focal dissection/ intramural hematoma	Media (+/− intima)	Blunt > penetrating
Pseudoaneurysm/ arteriovenous fistula[a]	Intima, media	Blunt = penetrating
Partial transection	Intima, media, adventitia	Penetrating > blunt
Complete transection	Intima, media, adventitia	Penetrating > blunt

[a]May also be iatrogenic.

develops when injury leads to a collection of blood within the media. IMH does not necessarily require an intimal injury, though in many cases, an intimal injury may also be present. As the IMH grows, it can propagate along a dissection plane proximally and distally. Such propagation leads to structural weakening of the vessel wall and may increase short-term rupture risk or long-term risk of aneurysmal degeneration. Pseudoaneurysms form when the intima and media are disrupted, leaving the adventitia as the sole layer maintaining vessel wall integrity. This may be referred to as a "contained rupture" since the thin adventitial layer offers little strength, has high risk of fracture, and may lead to free rupture. An arteriovenous fistula (AVF) may form when artery and nearby vein are simultaneously injured, leading to formation of an outflow tract between the artery and vein. Partial and complete transections refer to complete arterial wall disruption, typically associated with a penetrating mechanism of injury. These types of arterial injuries have been formalized into grading systems, commonly used in blunt cerebrovascular and thoracic aortic injuries where they help determine treatment strategy. In the PROOVIT registry, the most common types of injury identified included complete transection (25%), partial transection or flow limiting defect (26%), occlusion (18%), and pseudoaneurysm (9%).[3]

Venous injuries are typically detected at the time of repair of arterial injuries. There is less variation in the presentation of venous injuries, as the vein wall is thinner and, consequently, partial thickness injuries are not typically seen. Venous injuries typically manifest as partial transection, complete transection, vessel thrombosis, or AVF.[6]

MECHANISM: PENETRATING VS. BLUNT TRAUMA

Vascular trauma is usually related to penetrating or blunt mechanism of injury and, accordingly, the resulting injury to the artery and its treatment can vary dramatically.

Penetrating trauma, usually caused by stab or missile wounds, creates varying degrees of injury to the vessel, as previously described, with higher likelihood of partial or complete transection (see Table 62.1). Complete transection of a vessel allows the vessel ends to retract and spasm, which can lead to arterial thrombosis. In this instance, thrombosis can prevent exsanguination. Associated vessel spasm further minimizes bleeding in an under-resuscitated patient. Once the patient has been adequately resuscitated and normal blood pressure and systemic perfusion are restored, bleeding from the transected ends may resume. In contrast, vessels with partial transection may bleed more profusely because of their inability to retract and spasm.

Blunt injuries can be more indolent in their presentation but may result in outcomes just as devastating as those seen in penetrating trauma. Arteries that are tethered at a portion or segments in their course through the body are more susceptible to blunt injury due to the shearing force associated with acceleration and deceleration. These shear forces often cause deformation of the vessel wall that may lead to transmural disruption or dissection. However, unless massive forces are involved, full thickness injury is unlikely.

SIGNS OF VASCULAR INJURY

Certain findings, deemed "hard signs" of vascular trauma, warrant urgent or emergent operative exploration and intervention, particularly in cases of penetrating trauma (Box 62.1).[4] In many instances, such patients present with systemic shock, and resuscitative efforts are best coordinated in the OR. In the PROOVIT registry, nearly one-third of patients presented with a hard sign of vascular injury,[3] illustrating their utility in triaging patients with vascular trauma.

In unusual cases, patients with a blunt injury and hard signs of vascular injury are not immediately explored. For example, distal extremity pulses in a patient with a fracture or dislocation may be absent until the bony injury is reduced at which point the pulses may return. This type of injury would require further imaging workup to formulate a treatment plan but may not require immediate surgical exploration.

Certain findings, deemed "soft signs" of vascular injury (see Box 62.1), require further diagnostic evaluation to plan intervention, if needed. Depending on the hemodynamic status of patients with soft signs of vascular injury, subsequent evaluation should include detailed vascular imaging, typically with CTA.

NECK VASCULAR TRAUMA

Mechanism and Anatomic Considerations

With respect to penetrating injuries to the neck, hemodynamic instability or the presence of hard signs of vascular injury mandate emergent operative exploration prior to detailed axial imaging. In the stable patient, anatomic considerations have traditionally played an important role in determining who should proceed to surgery, based on the anatomic "zones" of the neck, and who should get further diagnostic imaging. When a penetrating injury does not violate the platysma muscle, the risk of occult, deeper injury requiring operative repair is low and therefore no immediate operative exploration is warranted.

However, if the platysma is violated, surgical management has traditionally been dictated by which zone of the neck is affected.

BOX 62.1   Hard and Soft Signs of Vascular Injury

Hard Signs
Rapid external bleeding
Expanding/pulsatile hematoma
Signs of distal ischemia
  Absent pulses
  Pain, pallor, paralysis, cold limb
Thrill/bruit over wound

Soft Signs
History of arterial bleeding
Proximity of wound/blunt injury to a named artery
Nonpulsatile hematoma
Neurologic deficit in injured extremity

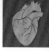

Zone I is the most caudal (classically defined as neck injuries occurring below the level of the clavicles), zone II is the midneck (between the level of the clavicles and the angle of the mandible), and zone III is the most cranial zone of the neck (angle of the mandible to the skull base). A modification of this system describes the uppermost extent of zone I as the cricoid cartilage.[7] These subtle differences in anatomic definitions are unlikely to be clinically meaningful, particularly as the zone-based approach to management is becoming de-emphasized.

Hemodynamically stable patients with zone I or III injuries should undergo additional diagnostic imaging and immediate operative exploration is avoided if possible. Some have advocated for mandatory exploration of all zone II penetrating injuries to avoid missed injuries, especially vascular injuries which can lead to delayed exsanguination and death. However, in recent years, the mandatory exploration of zone II injuries has been challenged as unnecessary, particularly in patients who are asymptomatic.[7,8]

In current practice in the United States, nearly all hemodynamically stable patients undergo additional diagnostic workup with CTA and possible endoscopy or bronchoscopy, regardless of the anatomic zone of injury. Diagnostic angiography is considered in select cases; however, CTA has largely become the diagnostic imaging test of choice. Surgical repair of any involved structures is planned based on such workup. If a patient has significant symptoms associated with a zone II injury (dysphagia, dyspnea, voice changes), even if hemodynamically stable, surgical exploration is usually necessary, but may be preceded by additional diagnostic workup.[7,8]

For blunt cerebrovascular injuries (BCVIs), immediate operative exploration should be similarly pursued in patients with hard signs of vascular injury or hemodynamic instability. In stable patients, the anatomic zone of injury does not guide decision-making, and additional diagnostic imaging is commonly pursued. CTA is indicated in patients with signs/symptoms of BCVI, such as (1) cervical hematoma, (2) cervical bruit, (3) arterial epistaxis, (4) focal neurologic deficit, (5) stroke on CT or magnetic resonance imaging, and/or (6) persistent neurologic deficit inconsistent with head CT.[9] However, because the majority of patients with BCVI are asymptomatic at the time of presentation,[10] a high level of suspicion for BCVI based on associated risk factors should lead to additional imaging. These are generally based on injury mechanism and may include (1) concomitant displaced mid-face fracture, (2) basilar skull fracture/petrous bone fracture, (3) diffuse axonal injury/Glasgow Coma Scale ≤ 8, (4) cervical spine fracture, and/or (5) clothesline type injury or near-hanging.[9,11]

SPECIFIC NECK VASCULAR INJURIES

Carotid and Vertebral Arteries

Penetrating injuries to the carotid artery are typically approached through an incision along the anterior border of the sternocleidomastoid muscle. More proximal injuries may require sternotomy for vascular control whereas more distal injuries may be very difficult to access and, in fact, may be preferentially treated with an endovascular approach. Primary repair of injuries can be performed in some cases, but for extensive injuries or complete transection, interposition grafting with great saphenous vein is usually preferred. Temporary intravascular shunts can be placed in patients who must be further resuscitated and/or have other injuries addressed prior to definitive repair. In rare instances, ligation is performed to prevent exsanguination or if vascular damage is irreparable. Vertebral artery injuries can be difficult to access surgically and are uncommonly repaired with complex surgical reconstruction techniques. Surgeons are more likely to perform

Type/Grade	Radiological/Angiographic Findings and Criteria
I	Vessel wall irregularity or dissection with <25% luminal narrowing
II	Dissection/intramural hematoma with ≥25% luminal narrowing, intraluminal thrombus, or raised intimal flap
III	Pseudoaneurysm
IV	Occlusion
V	Transection with extravasation

TABLE 62.2 Classification of Blunt Carotid Injury

Data from Bromberg WJ, Collier BC, Diebel LN, et al. Blunt cerebrovascular injury practice management guidelines: the Eastern Association for the Surgery of Trauma. *J Trauma.* 2010;68(2):471–477.

proximal ligation or endovascular embolization/occlusion for control of hemorrhage, relying on collateral posterior circulation to prevent cerebral ischemia.[12]

In patients suffering blunt trauma, BCVI is diagnosed with CTA and graded based on a widely accepted injury classification system (Table 62.2), developed to standardize and direct care for different types of vessel injury. Grade I and II injuries typically warrant anticoagulation or antiplatelet therapy as the mainstay of treatment. Pseudoaneurysms (grade III) injury are less likely to resolve with medical therapy and should be considered for repair, either by surgical reconstruction or endovascular treatment using stent grafting or embolization.[13] Occlusions (grade IV) are best managed with anticoagulation with no current role for revascularization. Artery transection with extravasation (grade V) should prompt urgent intervention, whether it be open or endovascular.[11]

The acceptance of endovascular techniques in the management of these injuries has increased, particularly because many are difficult to access surgically. Systematic reviews of patients with blunt or penetrating carotid injury have demonstrated good technical success rates with acceptable perioperative morbidity and promising short-term patency (80% up to 2 years) of carotid stent grafts.[14,15]

Venous Injury

Major cervicothoracic venous injury can pose added complexity to a trauma situation, especially when concomitant arterial injury is present. Venous bleeding can be temporized with direct pressure while repair of concomitant injuries is performed. In the setting of troublesome hemorrhage, the brachiocephalic, internal jugular, or subclavian veins can be ligated with relative impunity. If primary repair can be accomplished without compromising more than 50% of the injured vessel, a lateral venorrhaphy is appropriate. Repair/reconstruction should always be attempted in the presence of obvious venous hypertension or for one of the brachiocephalic or internal jugular veins if bilateral injury is present.

THORACIC VASCULAR TRAUMA

Mechanism and Anatomic Considerations

Penetrating wounds to the thorax have the potential to injure the heart, great vessels, pulmonary vessels, and descending thoracic aorta, in which case exsanguinating hemorrhage can rapidly lead to death. It is typically not possible to determine which structures may have been damaged simply by examining the entry and/or exit wounds. The cardiac "box" overlies the precordium and is bounded by the nipple lines laterally, the clavicles superiorly, and the inferior costal margin inferiorly. When penetrating injuries to the box are discovered, it is assumed that trauma to the heart and other mediastinal structures has occurred until proven otherwise.

Blunt injury to the thorax has potentially catastrophic consequences, with aortic injury and cardiac injury among the most common and fatal. Motor vehicle collisions are the most common mechanism and lead to deceleration and crush injuries. Often, patients will have multiple rib and/or clavicular fractures as evidence of the massive forces involved. It must be kept in mind that some patients may have no external manifestations of injury in the thorax. Mandatory trauma chest x-ray can reveal pneumothorax or hemothorax. Hemorrhage into the chest cavity (whether by blunt or penetrating mechanism) leads to hemothorax, which is initially managed with a tube thoracostomy. Massive hemothorax requires urgent thoracotomy for surgical management of ongoing hemorrhage. Criteria for proceeding to the OR for an exploratory thoracotomy after tube thoracostomy placement are (1) >1500 mL blood output at initial placement of tube thoracostomy, (2) 150 to 200 mL/h of blood output for 2 to 4 hours after tube placement, and (3) persistent blood transfusion requirement to maintain hemodynamic stability.[16]

The Focused Assessment with Sonography for Trauma (FAST) exam has become a standard component of the diagnostic workup of trauma patients. The primary views obtained are pericardial, hepatorenal, perisplenic, and suprapubic (pelvic) views. In addition, a thoracic view can be obtained to evaluate for pneumothorax and/or hemothorax. Of imminently life-threatening problems in the chest, FAST can detect pericardial tamponade and tension pneumothorax, helping to expedite treatment.

Resuscitative Thoracotomy

Hemodynamically unstable patients or those who have lost vital signs en route to the emergency department may be candidates for resuscitative thoracotomy (RT) in the emergency department. Though previously practiced more regularly, the success of this technique is relatively low in certain situations. For patients with penetrating trauma who arrive in shock, success of RT may be as high as 35%. However, for patients with blunt trauma who arrive in shock or have no vital signs, success rates are 2% and 1%, respectively.[17]

In general, patients with penetrating trauma should be considered for RT if profound refractory shock is present (undergoing cardiopulmonary resuscitation [CPR] with signs of life or systolic blood pressure [SBP] <60 mm Hg) or if vital signs have been lost but CPR has been performed for <15 minutes. For patients with blunt trauma, RT should be considered if profound refractory shock is present. It is debated whether RT should be considered at all in blunt trauma patients who are undergoing CPR with no signs of life, though some believe it should be considered if a patient arrives within 10 minutes of initiation of CPR.[17]

An anterolateral left-sided thoracotomy is performed with possible extension across the sternum to the right side (clamshell thoracotomy). The heart is examined and pericardium incised to release tamponade and repair any cardiac injury. If thoracic hemorrhage is encountered, hilar lung bleeding can be controlled with manual compression or clamping. Packing of the apex of the thoracic cavity can help control subclavian vessel bleeding. The descending thoracic aorta is then identified below the left pulmonary hilum and cross-clamped to prevent extrathoracic exsanguination and maximize coronary and cerebral perfusion. Aggressive resuscitation with blood products and defibrillation occurs concurrently with RT. If clinical status permits, the patient is then clinically reassessed and transferred to the OR for definitive operative repair of injuries.

SPECIFIC THORACIC VASCULAR INJURIES

Heart

Penetrating injuries to the heart are suspected based on entry wounds in the cardiac box and possibly by the presence of hemopericardium on FAST exam. If tamponade physiology exists, the hemodynamically unstable patient should be taken immediately to the OR for exploration via sternotomy or left anterolateral thoracotomy. Pericardiocentesis may be performed prior to transfer to the OR. Even in patients with normal hemodynamics, surgical exploration should be expedited if hemopericardium is detected, because tamponade physiology may develop rapidly.

Blunt cardiac injuries may manifest in a variety of ways. The most severe presentation is myocardial rupture which frequently leads to death prior to presentation. Other mechanical injuries to the septum or valves can occur but are uncommon. Blunt cardiac injury may also lead to myocardial infarction, arrhythmia, and/or decreased contractility. The management of these problems is variable but usually supportive.[18]

Thoracic Aorta

Penetrating injuries to the aorta are typically discovered and addressed in the OR at the time of thoracotomy. Open repair may be accomplished either with direct cross-clamping alone or with circulatory assistance (left-sided heart bypass, cardiopulmonary bypass [CPB], or femoral-femoral bypass). Optimal exposure of the thoracic aorta is gained through a posterolateral thoracotomy; however, repair may be required when an anterolateral thoracotomy has already been performed for trauma exploration. The aortic arch may be controlled either with clamping between the left common carotid and left subclavian, or just distal to the left subclavian artery. The descending thoracic aorta is controlled distally immediately beyond the traumatic injury to avert sacrifice of the intercostal arteries. The aorta can then be repaired with direct suturing or graft interposition.[19]

Blunt injury of the thoracic aorta is the second leading cause of death after motor vehicle collisions, with head injury being the first. Further, more than 80% of patients suffering blunt trauma to the aorta will die at the scene of the accident.[19] This makes blunt aortic injury a relatively common but highly fatal problem. The heart and great vessels are thought to be relatively mobile within the chest, compared to the descending aorta which is fixed to the chest wall. As a result, injury is most likely to occur at the isthmus, where a combination of forces converge (Figs. 62.1 and 62.2). Despite this paradigm, injuries may occur at any site in the thoracic aorta.

Of patients who survive to reach medical care, exsanguinating hemorrhage is often contained by one or more layers of the aortic wall. A grading system similar to that described for BCVI has been developed and is also useful in guiding treatment (Table 62.3 and Fig. 62.3). When intimal tears are detected on axial imaging (grade I), blood pressure management and serial imaging are the mainstay of treatment. Patients with IMH or pseudoaneurysm (grades II and III) should be considered for repair, though the management of these abnormalities depends highly on anatomy and concomitant injuries. Repair can often be delayed in these patients so that other injuries can be addressed. Patients with periaortic hematoma ≥15 mm or rupture (grade IV) should undergo emergency repair.[20,21]

Open repair was traditionally the treatment of choice for blunt aortic injury and is still necessary in some cases. However, the emergence of endovascular repair (TEVAR, thoracic endovascular aortic repair) has introduced an alternative to highly morbid open surgical repair (Fig. 62.4). Currently, endovascular repair is favored over open repair of blunt aortic injury in multiple society guidelines[20,21] and in practice.[22] This is based largely on heterogenous data and clinical experience

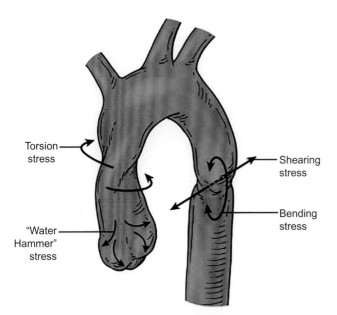

Fig. 62.1 Forces acting on the thoracic aorta during blunt traumatic injury. (Redrawn from Symbas P. *Cardiothoracic Traumas.* London: WB Saunders; 1989. From Azizzadeh A, Shalhub S. Vascular trauma: thoracic. In: Cronenwett JL, Johnston KW, eds. *Rutherford's Vascular Surgery.* 8th ed. Philadelphia: Elsevier; 2014:2451–2465.)

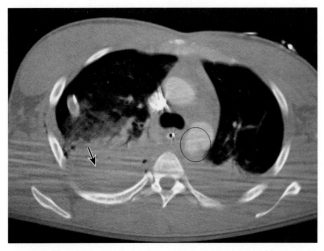

Fig. 62.2 Thoracic Aortic Injury and Associated Nonvascular Injuries. Spiral thoracic computed tomography image demonstrating aortic transection 2 cm distal (*circled*) to subclavian artery origin, with surrounding traumatic thoracic pseudoaneurysm and an intraparenchymal tear of right lung (*arrow*).

suggesting superiority of TEVAR. In a 2011 nonsystematic review, the existing data suggested that TEVAR had lower mortality (10% vs. 26%, $P < .01$) and paralysis rate (0.4% vs. 2.9%, $P < .05$) compared with open repair, though there were limitations to this analysis.[23] Evidence of the safety and effectiveness of TEVAR continues to be reported. In a 2015 report of 74 TEVARs performed for blunt aortic injury (1% grade I, 14% grade II, 74% grade III, 11% grade IV), 30-day mortality was 9% with an estimated 5-year survival of 81%. Reinterventions were required in 16% during the first year, reflecting the need for close surveillance.[24]

A major anatomic factor that should be considered, as it may limit the applicability of TEVAR, is the diameter of the iliac arteries, which must accommodate a relatively large device delivery system (though

TABLE 62.3	Classification of Blunt Aortic Injury
Type/Grade	Radiological/Angiographic Findings and Criteria
I	Intimal tear
II	Intramural hematoma
III	Pseudoaneurysm
IV	Rupture with extravasation

Data from Lee WA, Matsumura JS, Mitchell RS, et al. Endovascular repair of traumatic thoracic aortic injury: clinical practice guidelines of the Society for Vascular Surgery. *J Vasc Surg.* 2011;53(1):187–192.

device profiles have also improved over time). Another important consideration is that traumatically injured patients are often young and underresuscitated; both factors contribute to a small-appearing aorta on axial imaging. The placement of small endografts in these patients may have a higher risk of device complications, including stent graft collapse. Furthermore, the durability of endovascular repair over many decades, if placed in a young patient, is not currently known.

Thoracic Venae Cavae

The superior vena cava is formed by the confluence of the left and right brachiocephalic veins in the superior mediastinum at the level of the right first costal cartilage. It descends 5 to 7 cm to where it enters the posterior aspect of the right atrium at the level of the third costochondral cartilage. The inferior vena cava (IVC) enters the chest at the level of T8 and has a short posterior course to the right atrium. Because of the location and short segments of these structures, the intrathoracic venae cavae rarely suffer traumatic injury. The low-pressure system and distensibility of the vessels make blunt traumatic injury uncommon. Penetrating injury to the chest or iatrogenic injury are more common etiologies. Cardiac tamponade can occur following injury to the thoracic venae cavae, owing to the pericardium's extension and envelopment of the proximal portions of the vessels prior to entering the heart.

Simple isolated injuries to the thoracic venae cavae can be managed with lateral venorrhaphy. Partial-occluding clamps or temporary inflow occlusion can be used in these circumstances to facilitate repair. Complex injuries to the venae cavae or associated injuries to the heart may require CPB and/or interposition grafts for exposure and repair.

Pulmonary Vessels

Trauma to the main right or left pulmonary arteries is extremely rare and almost exclusively found after penetrating traumatic injury. Blunt traumatic injury to the main pulmonary arteries remains exceedingly rare. As with many of the great vessel injuries, cardiac tamponade or hemopericardium is a common presenting finding. Usually the diagnosis is made in the OR during a thoracotomy for hemopericardium. Distal pulmonary vascular injuries beyond the mediastinum can be seen following both blunt and penetrating trauma. Extensive vascular injury or significant injury to the hilar region may necessitate a pneumonectomy.

ABDOMINAL VASCULAR TRAUMA

Mechanism and Anatomic Considerations

Abdominal vascular injury represents roughly 8% of contemporary vascular trauma,[3] but these injuries are often life-threatening, associated with other complex injury patterns, and can be difficult to repair via open or endovascular approaches. Any patient with a penetrating

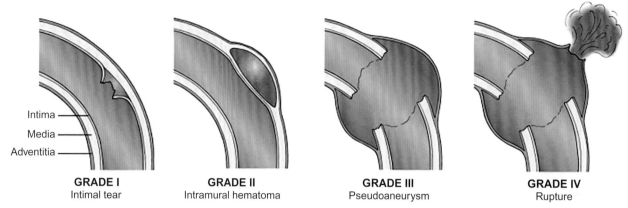

Intima
Media
Adventitia

| GRADE I | GRADE II | GRADE III | GRADE IV |
| Intimal tear | Intramural hematoma | Pseudoaneurysm | Rupture |

Fig. 62.3 Classification of traumatic aortic injury. (From Azizzadeh A, Shalhub S. Vascular trauma: thoracic. In: Cronenwett JL, Johnston KW eds. *Rutherford's Vascular Surgery*. 8th ed. Philadelphia: Elsevier; 2014:2451–2465.)

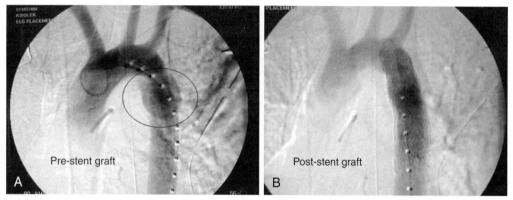

Pre-stent graft

Post-stent graft

A

B

Fig. 62.4 Thoracic Aortic Disruption. (A) Thoracic aortogram illustrating a 4-cm pseudoaneurysm *(circled)* in descending thoracic aorta, 2 cm from subclavian artery. (B) Postdeployment aortogram revealing no endoleak or extravasation.

wound between the nipple line superiorly and the pubic symphysis inferiorly should be considered at risk for intraabdominal injury. Notably, the thoracoabdominal region lies between the nipple line and costal margin, and any penetrating wound in this area has the potential to cause both thoracic and abdominal injury.

Like thoracic trauma, blunt abdominal injury may be caused by rapid deceleration and laceration from sharp bony fractures. However, crushing injury may occur as well, since the abdominal cavity lacks the bony protection of the ribs and sternum. Intraabdominal injuries may be suspected based on abdominal distention or tenderness, but additional imaging with ultrasound or CTA have become essential in determining management.

Ultrasonography is an easy and readily accessible means of acutely assessing for intraperitoneal fluid following trauma to the abdomen and has largely replaced direct peritoneal lavage (DPL) for this purpose. The FAST exam is performed immediately after the primary survey and uses multiple abdominal views (hepatorenal, perisplenic, and suprapubic). In the hemodynamically unstable patient, a positive abdominal FAST exam confirms the need for emergency surgery and focuses the surgeon on planning to perform a laparotomy first (as long as the pericardial and thoracic views are within normal limits).

The FAST exam is particularly useful when a hemodynamically unstable patient with blunt abdominopelvic trauma is being evaluated and there is an urgent need to determine whether to focus initial therapeutic efforts on abdominal or pelvic source of blood loss. A positive

FAST exam for intraperitoneal fluid should direct the patient toward emergency laparotomy with intraoperative assessment of pelvic bleeding. A patient with a negative FAST and complex pelvic fractures is more likely to undergo pelvic stabilization with endovascular embolization of the bleeding source.[25]

In the hemodynamically stable patient, FAST exam is useful, but CTA scanning remains the mainstay for expeditious, reliable imaging. CTA of the abdomen reveals the integrity of solid organs, confirms the presence or absence of free air/fluid, delineates vasculature morphology, and can illustrate traumatic pathology in the retroperitoneum. This means of imaging provides the largest amount of accurate information in the shortest amount of time. In abdominal vascular trauma, diagnostic angiography has a limited role, though endovascular approaches with a therapeutic intent, such as coil embolization of hemorrhage with pelvic fractures, are relatively common.

Resuscitative Endovascular Balloon Occlusion of the Aorta (REBOA)

As discussed in the thoracic trauma section, in certain scenarios, RT may be indicated to address exsanguinating vascular injury. For patients with thoracic vascular injury, thoracotomy also allows for direct assessment of the heart and thoracic aorta. However, for patients with abdominal and pelvic injuries, the primary goal of RT is cross-clamping of the aorta, which may control hemorrhage while improving cerebral and coronary perfusion.

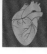

In recent years, there has been great interest in intraaortic balloon occlusion to control hemorrhage in trauma. Resuscitative endovascular balloon occlusion of the aorta (REBOA) is a technique where a balloon is introduced into the aorta through the femoral artery and inflated, resulting in aortic occlusion. This has the potential to provide means for aortic occlusion without requiring a thoracotomy, which can be unnecessarily time-consuming. If widely implemented, REBOA has the potential for application in the prehospital arena as well.[26] However, experience with this technology is still in the early stages. In the most comprehensive study to date, 46 REBOA patients were compared with 68 who underwent RT across 8 trauma centers. Procedures were performed in the emergency room in 74% of cases, and 36% of all cases achieved sustained hemodynamic stability, even though 61% were undergoing CPR at the time of aortic occlusion. In the patients with REBOA, 50% were placed via femoral cutdown and 39% were placed percutaneously. A majority of REBOA balloons were deployed in the thoracic aorta, between the subclavian artery and the celiac artery (79%, "zone 1"). Overall, REBOA was found to be similar to RT in terms of overall mortality (16% vs. 28%, $P = .1$), with few device-related complications.[27] These initial data are encouraging that this technology will continue to be developed for use in trauma.

Early practitioners have begun postulating scenarios in which REBOA might be particularly useful.[26] In patients with thoracic trauma, safe proximal aortic occlusion may not be possible, especially if the thoracic aorta is involved. In these scenarios, RT is the only way to properly assess all possible injuries, when indicated (Table 62.4). For abdominopelvic trauma, however, REBOA has the potential to rapidly control exsanguinating hemorrhage, allowing for transfer to the OR or angiography suite.[26,28]

Damage Control Surgery

For patients requiring emergency exploratory surgery, the systematic approach to the trauma laparotomy allows for identification of all intraabdominal injuries. In an exsanguinating patient, aortic cross-clamping can be a means of obtaining comprehensive proximal control in the face of massive hemorrhage and as an adjunct to resuscitation. Control should be gained at the supraceliac aorta, at the level of the diaphragm. This location is easily accessible and less likely to lead to iatrogenic injury to neighboring structures. If the injury is proximal in the abdominal aorta, control of the aorta may have to be obtained through the chest through a thoracotomy. Cross-clamping the aorta will help control hemorrhage and elevate blood pressure, but causes ischemia to the abdominal viscera and lower extremities. Thus aortic cross-clamping should only be employed in the most extreme circumstances and clamp time should be minimized.

Many patients with abdominal vascular injury who warrant immediate surgery will also face the "trauma triad of death": acidosis, hypothermia, and coagulopathy. Under these conditions, a definitive repair or reconstruction of the injured vessel(s) will delay resuscitation and aggressive physiologic supportive measures. In these circumstances, a damage-control approach is the most appropriate therapeutic management: major venous injuries are ligated, retroperitoneal bleeding/oozing is packed off tightly, and arterial injuries are temporarily shunted. The abdomen is temporarily closed, and the patient is transferred to the intensive care unit for resuscitation. Definitive vascular repair and abdominal closure are deferred until the patient has been adequately resuscitated and his/her condition has stabilized.[29]

SPECIFIC ABDOMINAL VASCULAR INJURIES

Abdominal Aorta and Retroperitoneum

The aorta is the largest artery in the body, and its abdominal portion spans from where it traverses the diaphragm at the level of T12 to where it bifurcates into the iliac arteries at the L4/L5 level. Although traumatic injury to the thoracic aorta is common, particularly with blunt mechanisms, abdominal aortic vascular injury is relatively uncommon. Penetrating abdominal aortic injuries are more common than blunt injuries.[30,31] As in the case of thoracic aortic injuries, this is partly the case because such injuries are rapidly fatal and many patients do not reach the hospital alive. In two large reported series, trauma to the abdominal aorta resulted in a mortality rate of 73% to 79%.[30,31]

Blunt abdominal aortic injury is less common because the abdominal aorta is not subject to the same combination of shearing and torsion forces and may therefore be less vulnerable, despite its relative susceptibility to crush injuries. The Western Trauma Association Multi-Center Trials Group reported injury to the abdominal aorta in only 0.3% of more than 300,000 blunt trauma cases.[32]

Patients with abdominal aortic injury are often diagnosed at the time of exploratory laparotomy because they arrive to the hospital in shock and are emergently taken to the OR. At the time of exploration, the abdomen and retroperitoneum are examined systematically. The retroperitoneum is divided into three main zones of injury: zone 1 is the central/midline retroperitoneum, zone 2 encompasses the perinephric space on either side (lateral), and zone 3 comprises the pelvic retroperitoneum.[25] Of all abdominal vascular injuries, as many as 91%

TABLE 62.4 Management of Hemodynamically Unstable Trauma Patient Incorporating Resuscitative Endovascular Balloon Occlusion of the Aorta

	CPR[a]	SBP <60	SBP 60–80	SBP >80
Thoracic hemorrhage	RT	RT	OR Thoracotomy (vs. RT)	OR Thoracotomy
Abdominal hemorrhage	RT	RT (vs. REBOA)	OR Laparotomy (vs. REBOA)	OR Laparotomy
Pelvic hemorrhage	RT	RT (vs. REBOA)	REBOA	OR Pelvic Packing versus endovascular embolization

[a]With signs of life or without signs of life if CPR <15 min for penetrating trauma, CPR <10 minutes for blunt trauma.
REBOA, Resuscitative Endovascular Balloon Occlusion of the Aorta; *RT,* resuscitative thoracotomy.
Modified from Biffl WL, Fox CJ, Moore EE. The role of REBOA in the control of exsanguinating torso hemorrhage. *J Trauma Acute Care Surg.* 2015;78(5):1054–1058.

will have a retroperitoneal hematoma.[30] Management of retroperitoneal hematomas varies, depending on the anatomical location and mechanism of injury.

Except for certain types of retrohepatic or suprahepatic IVC injury, zone 1 injuries mandate exploration for both penetrating and blunt injury because of the major vascular structures residing in this region. The transverse mesocolon subdivides zone 1 into the central supra- and inframesocolic spaces. Hematomas in the zone 1 supramesocolic space develop behind the lesser omentum and push the stomach forward. These hematomas result from injury to the suprarenal aorta, celiac axis, proximal superior mesenteric artery (SMA), or proximal renal arteries. Zone 1 inframesocolic hematomas present behind the root of the small-bowel mesentery are a consequence of either infrarenal aorta or IVC injury.[33]

Zone 2 retroperitoneal hematomas commonly result from injury to the renal vasculature or parenchyma. Zone 2 hematomas secondary to penetrating trauma necessitate operative exploration because of the risk for vascular injury. On the other hand, stable zone 2 hematomas following blunt trauma are best managed conservatively, as exploration bears a high likelihood of causing further injury to an already damaged kidney.[33] In cases of blunt trauma, zone 2 hematomas are not explored as long as the kidney on the affected side appeared normal on preoperative CT (or angiogram).[33]

Pelvic, zone 3 retroperitoneal hematomas are typically managed nonoperatively or using endovascular methods. Suspicion of iliac vessel injury represents the only true indication for surgical exploration. Iliac injuries are more common following penetrating injury to the pelvis. Pelvic hematomas arising from blunt means typically result from pelvic fractures, where external fixation and angiographic coil embolization are the best treatment modalities.

Abdominal aortic injuries will manifest with a large zone 1 hematoma or free intraabdominal bleeding. In the series by Deree et al., 48% of patients were found to have a retroperitoneal hematoma and 52% were found to have free intraabdominal bleeding, with free intraabdominal hemorrhage acting as a significant predictor of mortality. Of note, 25% had a concomitant IVC injury.[31]

Once a zone 1 injury is encountered, proximal vascular control is obtained at the level of the supraceliac aorta or thoracic aorta, as previously described. The entire length of the abdominal aorta and most of its branches can be exposed by a left medial visceral rotation. The only artery not accessible via this approach is the right renal artery. The left medial visceral rotation is implemented by taking down the lateral peritoneal attachments of the sigmoid and left colon. The left colon, left kidney, and spleen are then swept/mobilized medially toward the midline, exposing the left retroperitoneum and aorta. If the aorta and its branches are intact, the possibility of an IVC injury must be considered. In this case, a right medial visceral rotation is performed for optimal exposure of the IVC. In cases of zone 1 inframesocolic aortic injury, the retroperitoneum can be incised directly over the hematoma to expose the injury, avoiding medial visceral rotation; however, proximal control still often requires a supraceliac aortic clamp.[33]

Once the injury is exposed, it can be repaired with transverse polypropylene sutures if no luminal narrowing results. In situations where large portions of aorta have been damaged, patch aortoplasty with prosthetic material, or aortic replacement with a tube or bifurcated graft may be performed. Every attempt is made to avoid contamination of prosthetic material, since concomitant bowel injuries often occur, and an infected aortic prosthetic is catastrophic. To this end, coverage of the repair with retroperitoneum or omentum is prudent. Redundancy of the aorta may allow for segmental resection of the injured vessel wall with end-to-end anastomosis.

The opportunity for endovascular repair of abdominal aortic trauma is limited, since most injuries are detected at the time of surgical exploration and are therefore repaired with an open approach. However, in blunt trauma patients, axial imaging may reveal injury patterns similar to those seen in thoracic aortic trauma, which may be amenable to an endovascular approach. In the Western Trauma Association series of 113 patients with blunt abdominal aortic trauma, the following injury types were seen: 18% intimal tear, 36% large intimal flap, 16% pseudoaneurysm, and 32% rupture. Of these, 49 patients (43%) underwent primary open repair, commonly for rupture and hemodynamic instability. Seventeen patients (15%) underwent primary endovascular repair, using a variety of stent grafts. Endovascular approaches were mostly used in the infrarenal aorta, where endograft deployment is unlikely to cover major branch vessels. Endovascular approaches were only used to treat intimal tears, large intimal flaps, and pseudoaneurysms, and were not used in cases of free rupture.[32] Currently, endovascular repair has a limited role, and appropriate indications for endovascular therapy are still developing.

Inferior Vena Cava

Though the overall incidence of injury to the IVC is low, it is among the most commonly injured vascular structures in the abdomen and carries a high mortality rate. Penetrating mechanism of injury is much more common than blunt, and additional vascular injuries are often seen.[34] Similar to aortic injury, IVC injuries are often diagnosed at the time of exploratory surgery when a zone 1 retroperitoneal hematoma is discovered. A right medial visceral rotation is performed, providing exposure to the infrarenal vena cava and iliac vessels. The right colon along with the third and fourth portion of duodenum are released from their lateral attachments, then reflected medially and superiorly. This maneuver provides additional exposure to the suprarenal IVC and makes the portal venous system accessible.

IVC hemorrhage is controlled with direct pressure or a side-biting clamp. Primary repair with transverse suture is usually performed. Large prosthetic patches or interposition tube grafts can be placed but are often not necessary, as some degree of IVC narrowing postrepair is well tolerated.[25]

Infrarenal caval ligation can be an acceptable treatment in a young, hemodynamically unstable patient with significant associated traumatic injuries. Ligation above the level of the renal veins is not well tolerated and invariably leads to renal failure. If ligation of the infrarenal IVC is performed, the patient's bilateral lower extremities should be wrapped and elevated so as to prevent morbid lower-extremity edema.[34]

Injuries to the retrohepatic and suprahepatic IVC are very difficult to access and repair and carry high mortality rates. If an injury to these portions of the IVC is suspected in penetrating trauma, it is appropriate to observe the hematoma and choose not to explore it if it is stable and nonpulsatile. Packing of this area may help tamponade any venous injury. Surgical exploration of the retrohepatic and suprahepatic IVC may involve combined entry into the chest and abdomen and extensive mobilization of the liver, atriocaval shunting, total vascular occlusion, or hepatic vascular isolation. In extreme circumstances, direct exposure of the IVC can also be accomplished through division of the liver along the Cantlie line, though it is rarely employed and performed only in the setting of concomitant, significant liver injury.[25]

Visceral and Renal Vessels

In addition to the major axial vessels of the abdomen, the aorta, and IVC, injury to any of several abdominal arterial or venous branches can lead to catastrophic hemorrhage and end-organ ischemia.

Celiac artery injuries are rare and almost always a result of penetrating trauma. In a review of 302 patients with abdominal vascular injuries, the celiac artery was injured in only 3.3% of cases.[30] The celiac axis gives rise to the left gastric, splenic, and common hepatic arteries. Primary repair should be performed whenever possible. If necessary, ligation of the three proximal branches can usually be performed without ischemic sequelae because of the robust collateral circulation of the proximal gastrointestinal tract.

SMA injury presents as either free intraperitoneal hemorrhage, a zone 1 retroperitoneal hematoma, and/or ischemic proximal small bowel. Once an SMA injury is identified, the surgical approach is driven by the location of the injury. Primary repair of injuries to the proximal SMA should be performed whenever possible. Ligation of the artery at this level results in significant small-bowel ischemia and resultant increased mortality. If primary repair cannot be performed, revascularization with autogenous or prosthetic conduits is considered, sometimes necessitating extra-anatomic routes. Concurrent pancreatic injuries are often seen, and postoperative pancreatic leak can have devastating consequences to an adjacent SMA reconstruction. Ligation of the more distal SMA can be performed if primary repair is not possible and usually leads to localized segmental small-bowel ischemia. However, temporary shunt placement can also be employed in the hemodynamically unstable patient, allowing a future opportunity at revascularization. A second-look laparotomy is mandatory to assess the viability and integrity of the small bowel following any surgical manipulation of the SMA.

Superior mesenteric vein (SMV) injuries are infrequent but incur high mortality rates due to the difficulty in obtaining prompt exposure and hemorrhage control. These may coexist with concomitant portal vein injury. Lateral venorrhaphy is the preferred surgical means of repair for an isolated SMV injury, as with other venous injuries. Graft conduits can restore flow, but thrombosis can be a devastating complication. Ligation of the vein is a plausible surgical option, especially in hemodynamically unstable patients,[35] however, carries a risk of venous mesenteric ischemia secondary to splanchnic sequestration. Aggressive resuscitation is vital following venous ligation, and a second-look laparotomy is standard.

Injury to the inferior mesenteric artery (IMA) is typically managed by ligation. In rare cases, collateral circulation to the descending and sigmoid colons and the upper rectum may be inadequate and result in ischemia; however, this is uncommon because of rich collateral flow. Ligation of the inferior mesenteric vein is tolerated much better than that of the SMV.

Renovascular injury (renal artery, renal vein, kidney) is suspected when a hematoma is found in zone 2 of the retroperitoneum. Revascularization of renal vessel injury is performed via primary repair, vein patch angioplasty, interposition grafting, or segmental resection with reanastomosis. In cases of bilateral vascular injury, every attempt at revascularization should be made to preserve renal function. For unilateral injury, a nephrectomy is an accepted option. Renal vein injury can be repaired similarly to the artery. Ligation of the left renal vein near its confluence with the IVC is tolerated due to collateral venous drainage through the left gonadal, left adrenal, and lumbar veins. Attempts to repair the right renal vein should be made, since the absence of adequate venous collateral flow on the right side will lead to loss of the right kidney.

Endovascular approaches to manage mesenteric and renovascular trauma have potential utility, especially in the setting of blunt trauma. Similar to what is seen in other arterial beds, partial-thickness injuries to mesenteric and renal arteries may result in intimal defects or pseudoaneurysms detected on axial imaging. These can be managed with endovascular stents to prevent ischemia or delayed rupture, though observation and serial imaging may be most appropriate in some cases.[36] In cases of parenchymal renal injury with hemorrhage, embolization is increasingly used, though repeated interventions are sometimes necessary.[37]

Portal Vein Injury

The portal vein is made up by the confluence of the superior mesenteric and splenic veins behind the neck of the pancreas, subsequently traveling to the liver in the portal triad. Hematoma or hemorrhage in the portal triad is suggestive of portal vein and/or hepatic artery injury.

Though some portal vein injuries may be repaired without extensive surgical exposure, a right medial visceral rotation may be required. In some circumstances, especially with combined SMV injuries, this exposure may not be adequate, warranting division of the neck of the pancreas. These patients present in such poor condition that complex reconstructions are rarely feasible or advisable. Primary repair, if possible, is the best surgical treatment. Complex reconstructions should only be done in patients with associated hepatic artery injury that is not amenable to repair, as combined absence of blood flow through the portal vein and hepatic artery will lead to liver failure and death. These situations merit revascularization with autogenous saphenous vein graft. Ligation is another option that should be considered for devastating retropancreatic injuries, as long as hepatic artery flow can be preserved.[25,33]

Iliac Vessel Injury

Beneath the bifurcation of the aorta, the common iliac arteries descend into the pelvis, bifurcating again to form the internal and external iliac arteries. The internal branch gives off multiple branches to pelvic structures, while the external branch proceeds under the inguinal ligament and into the leg to become the femoral artery. Injury to the iliac arteries often leads to the development of a pelvic, zone 3, hematoma. The iliac arteries are among the most commonly injured vascular structures in the abdomen.[3,22]

When discovered at the time of exploration for penetrating trauma, zone 3 hematomas should be explored, particularly when iliac artery or vein injury is suspected. The proximity and shared course of the iliac veins make combined arteriovenous injuries a frequent occurrence.[38] Proximal control is gained at the infrarenal aorta, with distal control gained at the external iliac artery at the level of the inguinal ligament. The ascending colon can be reflected medially and superiorly via right medial visceral rotation, exposing the pelvic retroperitoneum. Primary repair is the preferred method of repair for a simple arterial injury. Reconstruction can also be accomplished with end-to-end anastomosis of autogenous saphenous vein or prosthetic grafts.[39] It is important to be cognizant of the fact that prosthetic grafts may be problematic in an environment contaminated by associated small-bowel or colon injury. Iliac injuries are amenable to bailout or damage-control procedures when a patient is critically ill due to other traumatic injuries. Temporary shunt insertion, arterial ligation with delayed extra-anatomical reconstruction, or packing of venous injury may be employed in this situation.

Iliac vein injury can be even more complex with regard to gaining access and control of the vessel. Occasionally, the iliac artery must be divided to allow adequate access to the venous structures, and then reconstructed following venous repair. Concerns of edema and compartment syndrome following prolonged ischemic time or vein ligation merit a low threshold for lower-extremity fasciotomies.

Endovascular techniques have shown utility in selected cases of iliac artery injury. Patients with AVFs, pseudoaneurysms, or major intimal tears may benefit from endovascular stenting and/or coiling, rather than open exploration (Fig. 62.5). In a recent analysis of the National

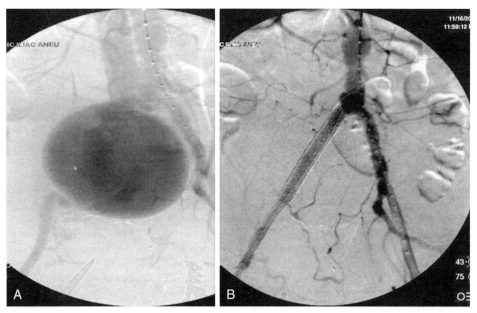

Fig. 62.5 Penetrating Iliac Artery Injury. (A) Arteriogram revealed 10-cm right common iliac artery aneurysm with iliocaval fistulae following gunshot wound to abdomen. (B) Arteriogram following successful deployment and placement of a covered stent.

Trauma Data Bank from 2002 to 2008, the proportion of patients with common/external iliac artery injuries undergoing endovascular repair increased from 0.4% to 20.4% over 6 years ($P < .001$), and for internal iliac artery injuries, this proportion increased from 8.0% to 40.3% ($P < .001$). By comparison, the proportion for thoracic aortic injury, where endovascular treatment may be preferred, increased from 0.5% to 21.9% ($P < .001$).[22] In practice, endovascular treatment of iliac artery injuries is being broadly applied, given the difficulty with surgical exposure (as described previously). These approaches show promise, particularly in patients with blunt injury.

EXTREMITY VASCULAR TRAUMA

Mechanism and Anatomic Considerations

Extremity vascular trauma is one of the most common types of injury encountered, accounting for 79% of contemporary military vascular trauma[2] and 44% to 51% of civilian vascular trauma.[3,22] Penetrating mechanism is more common, outnumbering blunt extremity vascular injury 3:1.[40] Prehospital tourniquet use, adopted from military experience, is now commonly employed in penetrating extremity trauma. Tourniquets were used in 20% of vascular trauma patients in the PROOVIT registry[3] and have been acknowledged as a major step forward in the care of patients with vascular trauma.[4]

Similar to other injury patterns, patients with extremity vascular trauma should proceed immediately to operative exploration if hard signs are present (see Box 62.1). Soft signs of vascular injury may also prompt surgical intervention, but additional diagnostic imaging can be obtained in the hemodynamically stable patient. Duplex ultrasound and CT angiography are particularly useful in this regard.

When assessing for hard signs, it is important to determine whether distal ischemia is present. This is sometimes manifest by absent pulses or the other components of the "6 Ps" (Pain, Pallor, Paralysis, Pulselessness, Paresthesias, Poikilothermia). However, it is also standard to measure the arterial pressure index (API). The API is a ratio of the systolic blood pressure at the extremity distal to an injury, relative to the systolic blood pressure in the unaffected extremity. This is anal-

ogous to an ankle-brachial index (ABI) in lower extremity trauma and wrist-brachial index in upper extremity trauma. An API of less than 0.9 is indicative of vascular disease and, in the setting of trauma, vascular injury.[4] API measurements should be repeated after reduction of bony fracture or dislocation, as they will often normalize. If low API persists, further diagnostic imaging or exploration is warranted.

SPECIFIC EXTREMITY VASCULAR INJURIES

Subclavian-Axillary Injury

Much of the course of the subclavian/axillary artery and vein are covered by the clavicle and overlying pectoralis musculature, making injury to these structures uncommon. Penetrating trauma accounts for the overwhelming majority of cases.[41] Blunt injury to these structures is rare, but clavicle and first rib fractures/dislocations have been associated with blunt vascular injury in multiple studies.

Minimizing prehospital time is key to successful management, as tourniquets are not effective in preventing exsanguination. Upon presentation, acute ischemia of the upper extremity is uncommon, and a palpable pulse may be present in the extremity owing to the rich collateral circulation around the axillary artery. Uncontained hemorrhage can be devastating and result in mortality at the scene. One study demonstrated an overall mortality rate of 39% in a series of 54 consecutive subclavian artery injuries.[41]

If the decision is made for surgical exploration, the standard incision for a proximal axillary or midsubclavian artery injury extends from the jugular notch along the clavicle and then downward in the deltopectoral groove. This incision can be combined with a median sternotomy to gain exposure for proximal subclavian injuries. A trapdoor incision has been described for proximal left subclavian injuries but carries a host of complications that can be avoided with anterolateral thoracotomy. Arterial repair can be accomplished with primary repair, patch angioplasty, or bypass, as described previously for other injury types. Combined arterial and venous injuries are often indicative of extensive trauma and are associated with a threefold increase in mortality compared to isolated arterial injuries.[42]

Endovascular therapy has been used with high success in both blunt and penetrating trauma in selected patients. Those who are hemodynamically stable and found to have traumatic AVFs, false aneurysms, and focal dissections are ideal candidates. It is important to note that lesions in close proximity to the origins of the vertebral and/or right CCAs may preclude safe deployment of an endovascular stent graft without covering the origin, thereby risking cerebral or cerebellar injury. Subclavian and axillary artery injuries may be particularly suited to endovascular approaches due to favorable vessel diameters and the difficulty of surgical exposure in some cases.[40]

Brachial and Forearm Vessel Injury

The brachial artery is commonly injured, representing up to 8% of all vascular trauma.[3] The upper-arm arterial supply is made up by the brachial and deep brachial arteries. The forearm blood supply consists of the radial, ulnar, and interosseous arteries. Penetrating trauma is the most common etiology of injury, and nerve injury is widely accepted as the most important prognostic factor and indicator of function.[43] Concomitant bone, nerve, or venous injury is common.

Expedient repair of all brachial or forearm arterial injuries is vital. Severe ischemia may develop in as short as 4 hours following injury if not repaired.[43] Isolated injury to the radial or ulnar artery can usually tolerate ligation without subsequent ischemia because of the rich collateral circulation of the forearm and hand. However, it is important to remember that only 80% to 85% of the population has an intact palmar arch. Under these circumstances, the patient may require repair to the ulnar or radial artery to prevent hand ischemia. Although compartment syndrome is less commonly seen in the upper extremity than the lower extremity, a fasciotomy should be considered following any vascular injury in the arm.

Femoral Vessels

Injuries to the femoral vessels are among the most common extremity vascular injuries.[3,22] Exsanguination can occur, but the superficial course of the vessel allows for prehospital control of hemorrhage through direct pressure. For more distal superficial femoral artery injuries, tourniquets can be effective. Lower extremity arterial injuries are more likely to occur by blunt mechanisms and are associated with higher mortality and amputation rates (compared with the upper extremity).[44]

When surgical exploration is required, proximal control of the external iliac vessels may be necessary if the injury is at the level of the groin. Otherwise, exposure of the femoral vessels can be gained through a linear incision along the medial edge of the sartorius muscle below the inguinal ligament. Combined vein and arterial injury can prove challenging, with venous bleeding occasionally proving more difficult to control. The contralateral limb great saphenous vein can be harvested, if needed, for repair of the injured artery or vein, either as patch, interposition graft, or bypass. Temporary shunts can be placed if a damage control strategy is being pursued. Ligation is avoided, if at all possible. In the case of small intimal flaps and pseudoaneurysms, observation or endovascular techniques may provide effective therapy, though most repairs are still performed surgically.[40]

Popliteal and Calf Vessel Injury

The popliteal, anterior and posterior tibial, and peroneal arteries reside at the level of the knee or below. Popliteal artery injuries represent some of the most challenging of all vascular extremity injuries to manage. This artery is the second most commonly injured artery in the leg, and more commonly results from penetrating injury. Blunt popliteal injury is commonly seen following posterior knee dislocation, which can have significant orthopedic and neurological consequences.[45]

The outcome from popliteal injury depends significantly on the mode of injury. Amputation rates may reach as high as 20% to 50% following a high-velocity gun or shotgun blast, which may lead to significant soft-tissue injury and septic sequelae. A recent review of 24 published series demonstrated a much lower amputation rate of 11%, indicating the marked improvement in limb salvage in modern civilian series.[45]

The operative approach to popliteal artery injuries is typically through a medial approach. However, focal midpopliteal injuries can be approached posteriorly, with the patient in the prone position. This positioning is often not possible when patients have other traumatic injuries that require repair. However, the posterior approach should be considered in patients with focal, isolated popliteal artery injuries, such as those inadvertently caused at the time of knee replacement.

Popliteal vein injuries should be taken very seriously, with repair or reconstruction performed whenever possible, since the popliteal vein is the primary venous drainage of the lower leg. Because of the significant risk of reperfusion injury and venous congestion, a low threshold should be maintained for fasciotomy in the setting of severe popliteal vessel injury associated with prolonged ischemia or combined arterial/venous injury.

Injury to one of the three infrapopliteal arteries rarely results in limb ischemia in the absence of preexisting occlusive disease. In the setting of isolated hemorrhage from one of these vessels, ligation or embolization is an option. However, when the tibioperoneal truck or two or more of the infrapopliteal arteries are injured, repair or revascularization is vital for limb salvage. Nerve, bone, and soft-tissue damage in this region of the body plays a major role in limb salvage.

ISCHEMIA-REPERFUSION INJURY

Ischemia/reperfusion is a complex pathological process involving intracellular and extracellular processes that result in metabolic, thrombotic, and inflammatory changes in brain, intestine, heart, kidney, and skeletal muscle.[46] A devastating component of ischemia/reperfusion injury is the paradoxical increase in tissue injury associated with restitution of blood flow to ischemic tissues. This is of particular importance in extremity trauma, where revascularization may lead to clinical deterioration if not recognized and managed appropriately.

There are metabolic, thrombotic, and inflammatory components of reperfusion injury. The degree to which reperfusion either restores tissue integrity or exacerbates ischemic injury is dependent primarily on the duration of ischemia. Though extremity skeletal muscle can tolerate longer durations of ischemia than other tissues, this also leads to high risk of reperfusion injury. Familiarity with the mechanism of ischemia-reperfusion injury, and its clinical consequences, is essential in the management of vascular trauma, particularly as prehospital tourniquet use increases. Though this practice has the potential to decrease exsanguinating extremity hemorrhage, it may also increase the proportion of patients with longer periods of ischemic distal tissues.

COMPARTMENT SYNDROME

Acute compartment syndrome is a surgical emergency. Compartment syndrome is seen when increased tissue pressure in a closed myofascial space exceeds tissue perfusion pressure. This results in disturbed microcirculation that leads to irreversible neuromuscular ischemic damage.[47] Acute compartment syndrome commonly occurs following lower-limb trauma. Emergency decompression through open and extensive fasciotomies is the treatment of choice. The cardinal clinical feature is severe pain, greater than would be expected from the original insult. The pain may be exacerbated by passive extension of the tendons crossing the symptomatic compartment or arising from the muscles within it. The need for prompt intervention and the benefits of timely surgical decompression require a high index of suspicion and effective clinical assessment to make the diagnosis.

Clinical assessment may be supported by compartment pressure measurements, in which a needle is inserted into the compartment and pressure monitored using a pressure transducer. The methods for measuring and interpreting compartment pressures vary. Recent studies have focused on measuring a pressure "gradient" (diastolic blood pressure–compartment pressure, or mean arterial pressure–compartment pressure), with a gradient <30 mm Hg suggestive of compartment syndrome.[47] Absolute intracompartmental pressure thresholds have also been described (i.e., absolute intracompartmental pressure >30 mm Hg suggestive of compartment syndrome). In general, compartment pressures must be interpreted in the context of other clinical findings, and no specific thresholds have been agreed upon that mandate fasciotomy.[48]

A single method of fasciotomy is not universally suitable for all indications. However, the investing fascia for all four calf compartments must be widely incised for proper release of pressure. This is typically performed using two incisions in the calf (medial and lateral). In the thigh, two incisions (medial and lateral) are also performed to decompress the three compartments. In the forearm, complex curvilinear incisions are sometimes required to fully release the lateral and volar compartments, and a separate incision along the dorsal aspect of the forearm releases the dorsal compartment. Attempts to minimize skin incisions when performing fasciotomies often lead to higher risk of incomplete fasciotomy and inadequately treated compartment syndrome.[48]

A recent 10-year review of the incidence of compartment syndrome in a level I trauma center indicated that after lower-extremity trauma, 2.8% of patients will require fasciotomy. A majority (94%) of fasciotomies in this series were performed when compartment syndrome was suspected (i.e., therapeutic fasciotomy). Risk factors identified for fasciotomy were presence of vascular injury (arterial, venous, or combined), need for packed red blood cell (RBC) transfusion, male gender, open fracture, elbow or knee dislocation, and age younger than 55. Combined arterial and venous injury resulted in fasciotomy in 42% of patients.[49]

In the setting of vascular injury requiring surgical repair, the decision is often made to perform prophylactic fasciotomies to prevent occurrence of compartment syndrome after vascular repair and reperfusion. Prolonged ischemia time, in particular, is thought to increase the risk of compartment syndrome and often prompts prophylactic fasciotomy.[50] In these cases, early/prophylactic fasciotomy may be associated with lower risk of amputation and shorter hospital stay.[50] Some have advocated screening high-risk trauma patients for compartment syndrome, using a clinical evaluation and compartment pressure checks, to determine who may benefit from early/prophylactic fasciotomy. In a prospective single-center trial, the rate of lower extremity compartment syndrome was 20% in patients who met any of the following criteria: pulmonary-artery catheter-directed shock resuscitation, open or closed tibial shaft fracture, major vascular injury below the aortic bifurcation, abdominal compartment syndrome, or pelvic or lower extremity crush injury. This screening protocol led to aggressive fasciotomy implementation and no amputations. However, the mortality rate of patients with compartment syndrome was found to be 67%, reflecting the lethality of this clinical problem.[47]

IATROGENIC VASCULAR INJURY

An increased incidence of iatrogenic vascular injury has been associated with the development of catheter-based cardiac and peripheral interventions to treat cardiovascular disease. In a recent review of vascular trauma at an English hospital system, iatrogenic injuries outnumbered noniatrogenic injuries 3:1.[51] These findings are highly dependent on local trauma patterns and therefore not generalizable. However, it illustrates that in some hospitals, iatrogenic injuries may make up the majority of vascular trauma encountered.

Iatrogenic pseudoaneurysm due to catheter-based interventions should be suspected when postprocedure physical exam reveals groin hematoma, excessive ecchymosis, or persistent, severe pain at the puncture site. Presence of a bruit and ongoing pulsatile bleeding are highly suggestive of a pseudoaneurysm. Although physical examination alone is not diagnostic for femoral pseudoaneurysm, it can be highly accurate and specific for detecting the presence of an AVF. A to-and-fro holosystolic/diastolic bruit at the puncture site is both diagnostic and pathognomonic for an AVF. When concerning clinical findings are present, duplex ultrasound, which has a sensitivity of >94% in detection of femoral pseudoaneurysms, should be obtained.[52]

For pseudoaneurysms <2 cm that are minimally symptomatic, observation and surveillance with duplex ultrasound may be pursued. In many cases, the pseudoaneurysm will spontaneously thrombose and resolve. Surveillance is essential in case expansion occurs. In patients on systemic anticoagulation, even small pseudoaneurysms are unlikely to thrombose and should be treated. Ultrasound-guided compression was the first treatment developed for access site pseudoaneurysm. In this technique, the ultrasound probe is used to manually compress the pseudoaneurysm, promoting thrombosis. However, ultrasound-guided compression is labor intensive and can be intolerably painful for the patient. As a result, this modality is rarely used.

Ultrasound-guided thrombin injection is currently the preferred treatment method for pseudoaneurysms >2 cm. Thrombin injection is accomplished by inserting a 22-gauge needle under direct ultrasound visualization through the superficial aspect of the pseudoaneurysm. Thrombin (usually 50 to 1000 units) is injected until blood flow ceases on color Doppler ultrasound imaging. Repeat injections may be required, but the ultimate success rate may be as high as 99%.[53] Thrombin injection is contraindicated in the presence of an AVF or a pseudoaneurysm with a very short, broad neck because of the risk of embolizing a thrombin clot into the artery and down the leg.

AVFs can also be detected by duplex ultrasound in patients with clinical findings suggestive of access site complication; however, percutaneous treatment is usually not an option. In some cases, an AVF will result from inadvertent puncture of the superficial femoral artery and adjacent vein. In this scenario, a stent graft can be placed over the site of arterial injury without any threat to the profunda femoris origin or common femoral artery. Up to one-third of iatrogenic AVFs may close within 1 year, so surveillance may be an appropriate initial management strategy.[54]

Urgent repair is indicated in patients with a large hematoma or pseudoaneurysm, resulting in (1) impending skin necrosis, (2) compression of the adjacent nerve or vein, (3) distal ischemia, (4) persistent hypotension, (5) ongoing transfusion requirement, or (6) intractable pain. On rare occasion, especially when the presentation is delayed or there is suspicion of an infectious process, access to the retroperitoneum may be necessary to achieve proximal control of lower-extremity inflow at the level of the iliac vessels. Regardless, exposure should be obtained proximal and distal to the puncture site, and digital control of the bleeding can be obtained. In most cases, the defect in the artery can be repaired primarily. It is essential to check the back wall of the artery to be sure there is not another source of bleeding. Rarely, when significant injury is present in an atherosclerotic artery, a patch may be required to avoid compromising the lumen.

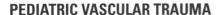

PEDIATRIC VASCULAR TRAUMA

Vascular trauma in the pediatric population is uncommon, occurring in only 0.6% of all pediatric trauma patients. Although less frequent than in adults, penetrating trauma is responsible for a slight majority of pediatric vascular injuries.[55,56] Vascular trauma in children presents a unique challenge based on the characteristics of small, thin-walled vessels with poor tissue support and pronounced tendency for vasospasm in the setting of small intravascular volumes.[56,57] Vessels of the upper extremity are the most commonly injured and are commonly managed nonoperatively, with relatively good outcomes.[58] Injuries of the thoracic aorta and great vessels are rare. Injury to the carotid artery is exceedingly rare but can have devastating morbidity and mortality, if not recognized and managed promptly.[59] Decisions regarding operative management in the pediatric population must take into account vessel size and future growth potential, which may require future vascular revision. Amputations are usually reserved for severely mangled extremities; all attempts should be made for limb salvage. Overall, pediatric patients have an improved adjusted mortality when compared with adults.[60]

REFERENCES

1. Friedman SG. Korea, M*A*S*H, and the accidental pioneers of vascular surgery. *J Vasc Surg.* 2017;66(2):666–670.
2. White JM, Stannard A, Burkhardt GE, et al. The epidemiology of vascular injury in the wars in Iraq and Afghanistan. *Ann Surg.* 2011;253(6):1184–1189.
3. DuBose JJ, Savage SA, Fabian TC, et al. The American Association for the Surgery of Trauma PROspective Observational Vascular Injury Treatment (PROOVIT) registry: multicenter data on modern vascular injury diagnosis, management, and outcomes. *J Trauma Acute Care Surg.* 2015;78(2):215–222. discussion 22-3.
4. Feliciano DV. For the patient—evolution in the management of vascular trauma. *J Trauma Acute Care Surg.* 2017;83(6):1205–1212.
5. Rhee P, Joseph B, Pandit V, et al. Increasing trauma deaths in the United States. *Ann Surg.* 2014;260(1):13–21.
6. Meissner MH, Wakefield TW, Ascher E, et al. Acute venous disease: venous thrombosis and venous trauma. *J Vasc Surg.* 2007;46(Suppl S):25S–53S.
7. Sperry JL, Moore EE, Coimbra R, et al. Western Trauma Association critical decisions in trauma: penetrating neck trauma. *J Trauma Acute Care Surg.* 2013;75(6):936–940.
8. Tisherman SA, Bokhari F, Collier B, et al. Clinical practice guideline: penetrating zone II neck trauma. *J Trauma.* 2008;64(5):1392–1405.
9. Biffl WL, Cothren CC, Moore EE, et al. Western Trauma Association critical decisions in trauma: screening for and treatment of blunt cerebrovascular injuries. *J Trauma.* 2009;67(6):1150–1153.
10. Burlew CC, Biffl WL, Moore EE, et al. Blunt cerebrovascular injuries: redefining screening criteria in the era of noninvasive diagnosis. *J Trauma Acute Care Surg.* 2012;72(2):330–335. discussion 6-7, quiz 539.
11. Bromberg WJ, Collier BC, Diebel LN, et al. Blunt cerebrovascular injury practice management guidelines: the Eastern Association for the Surgery of Trauma. *J Trauma.* 2010;68(2):471–477.
12. Herrera DA, Vargas SA, Dublin AB. Endovascular treatment of traumatic injuries of the vertebral artery. *AJNR Am J Neuroradiol.* 2008;29(8):1585–1589.
13. Magge D, Farber A, Vladimir F, et al. Diagnosis and management of traumatic pseudoaneurysm of the carotid artery: case report and review of the literature. *Vascular.* 2008;16(6):350–355.
14. DuBose J, Recinos G, Teixeira PG, et al. Endovascular stenting for the treatment of traumatic internal carotid injuries: expanding experience. *J Trauma.* 2008;65(6):1561–1566.
15. Spanos K, Karathanos C, Stamoulis K, Giannoukas AD. Endovascular treatment of traumatic internal carotid artery pseudoaneurysm. *Injury.* 2016;47(2):307–312.
16. Mowery NT, Gunter OL, Collier BR, et al. Practice management guidelines for management of hemothorax and occult pneumothorax. *J Trauma.* 2011;70(2):510–518.
17. Burlew CC, Moore EE, Moore FA, et al. Western Trauma Association critical decisions in trauma: resuscitative thoracotomy. *J Trauma Acute Care Surg.* 2012;73(6):1359–1363.
18. Clancy K, Velopulos C, Bilaniuk JW, et al. Screening for blunt cardiac injury: an Eastern Association for the Surgery of Trauma practice management guideline. *J Trauma Acute Care Surg.* 2012;73(5 Suppl 4):S301–S306.
19. Neschis DG, Scalea TM, Flinn WR, Griffith BP. Blunt aortic injury. *N Engl J Med.* 2008;359(16):1708–1716.
20. Lee WA, Matsumura JS, Mitchell RS, et al. Endovascular repair of traumatic thoracic aortic injury: clinical practice guidelines of the Society for Vascular Surgery. *J Vasc Surg.* 2011;53(1):187–192.
21. Writing C, Riambau V, Bockler D, et al. Editor's choice - Management of descending thoracic aorta diseases: clinical practice guidelines of the European Society for Vascular Surgery (ESVS). *Eur J Vasc Endovasc Surg.* 2017;53(1):4–52.
22. Branco BC, DuBose JJ, Zhan LX, et al. Trends and outcomes of endovascular therapy in the management of civilian vascular injuries. *J Vasc Surg.* 2014;60(5):1297–1307. 307 e1.
23. Karmy-Jones R, Ferrigno L, Teso D, et al. Endovascular repair compared with operative repair of traumatic rupture of the thoracic aorta: a nonsystematic review and a plea for trauma-specific reporting guidelines. *J Trauma.* 2011;71(4):1059–1072.
24. Steuer J, Bjorck M, Sonesson B, et al. Editor's choice - Durability of endovascular repair in blunt traumatic thoracic aortic injury: long-term outcome from four tertiary referral centers. *Eur J Vasc Endovasc Surg.* 2015;50(4):460–465.
25. Feliciano DV. Injuries to the great vessels of the abdomen. In: Souba WW, ed. *ACS Surgery: Principles and Practice.* Ontario, Canada: Decker; 2007:1341–1352.
26. Biffl WL, Fox CJ, Moore EE. The role of REBOA in the control of exsanguinating torso hemorrhage. *J Trauma Acute Care Surg.* 2015;78(5):1054–1058.
27. DuBose JJ, Scalea TM, Brenner M, et al. The AAST prospective Aortic Occlusion for Resuscitation in Trauma and Acute Care Surgery (AORTA) registry: data on contemporary utilization and outcomes of aortic occlusion and resuscitative balloon occlusion of the aorta (REBOA). *J Trauma Acute Care Surg.* 2016;81(3):409–419.
28. Brenner ML, Moore LJ, DuBose JJ, et al. A clinical series of resuscitative endovascular balloon occlusion of the aorta for hemorrhage control and resuscitation. *J Trauma Acute Care Surg.* 2013;75(3):506–511.
29. Chovanes J, Cannon JW, Nunez TC. The evolution of damage control surgery. *Surg Clin North Am.* 2012;92(4):859–875. vii-viii.
30. Asensio JA, Chahwan S, Hanpeter D, et al. Operative management and outcome of 302 abdominal vascular injuries. *Am J Surg.* 2000;180(6):528–533. discussion 33-4.
31. Deree J, Shenvi E, Fortlage D, et al. Patient factors and operating room resuscitation predict mortality in traumatic abdominal aortic injury: a 20-year analysis. *J Vasc Surg.* 2007;45(3):493–497.
32. Shalhub S, Starnes BW, Brenner ML, et al. Blunt abdominal aortic injury: a Western Trauma Association multicenter study. *J Trauma Acute Care Surg.* 2014;77(6):879–885. discussion 85.
33. Feliciano DV, Moore EE, Biffl WL. Western Trauma Association Critical Decisions in Trauma: management of abdominal vascular trauma. *J Trauma Acute Care Surg.* 2015;79(6):1079–1088.
34. Sullivan PS, Dente CJ, Patel S, et al. Outcome of ligation of the inferior vena cava in the modern era. *Am J Surg.* 2010;199(4):500–506.
35. Asensio JA, Petrone P, Garcia-Nunez L, et al. Superior mesenteric venous injuries: to ligate or to repair remains the question. *J Trauma.* 2007;62(3):668–675. discussion 75.
36. Tulsyan N, Kashyap VS, Greenberg RK, et al. The endovascular management of visceral artery aneurysms and pseudoaneurysms. *J Vasc Surg.* 2007;45(2):276–283. discussion 83.
37. Hotaling JM, Sorensen MD, Smith 3rd TG, et al. Analysis of diagnostic angiography and angioembolization in the acute management of renal trauma using a national data set. *J Urol.* 2011;185(4):1316–1320.

38. Lauerman MH, Rybin D, Doros G, et al. Characterization and outcomes of iliac vessel injury in the 21st century: a review of the National Trauma Data Bank. *Vasc Endovascular Surg.* 2013;47(5):325–330.

39. Asensio JA, Petrone P, Roldan G, et al. Analysis of 185 iliac vessel injuries: risk factors and predictors of outcome. *Arch Surg.* 2003;138(11):1187–1193. discussion 93-4.

40. Ganapathy A, Khouqeer AF, Todd SR, et al. Endovascular management for peripheral arterial trauma: The new norm? *Injury.* 2017;48(5):1025–1030.

41. Lin PH, Koffron AJ, Guske PJ, et al. Penetrating injuries of the subclavian artery. *Am J Surg.* 2003;185(6):580–584.

42. Kalish J, Nguyen T, Hamburg N, et al. Associated venous injury significantly complicates presentation, management, and outcomes of axillosubclavian arterial trauma. *Int J Angiol.* 2012;21(4):217–222.

43. Fields CE, Latifi R, Ivatury RR. Brachial and forearm vessel injuries. *Surg Clin North Am.* 2002;82(1):105–114.

44. Tan TW, Joglar FL, Hamburg NM, et al. Limb outcome and mortality in lower and upper extremity arterial injury: a comparison using the National Trauma Data Bank. *Vasc Endovascular Surg.* 2011;45(7):592–597.

45. Mullenix PS, Steele SR, Andersen CA, et al. Limb salvage and outcomes among patients with traumatic popliteal vascular injury: an analysis of the National Trauma Data Bank. *J Vasc Surg.* 2006;44(1):94–100.

46. Gillani S, Cao J, Suzuki T, Hak DJ. The effect of ischemia reperfusion injury on skeletal muscle. *Injury.* 2012;43(6):670–675.

47. Kosir R, Moore FA, Selby JH, et al. Acute lower extremity compartment syndrome (ALECS) screening protocol in critically ill trauma patients. *J Trauma.* 2007;63(2):268–275.

48. Modrall JG, Chung J. Compartment syndrome. In: Cronenwett J, Johnston KW, eds. *Rutherford's Vascular Surgery.* 8th ed. Philadelphia: Elsevier; 2014:2544–2554.

49. Branco BC, Inaba K, Barmparas G, et al. Incidence and predictors for the need for fasciotomy after extremity trauma: a 10-year review in a mature level I trauma centre. *Injury.* 2011;42(10):1157–1163.

50. Farber A, Tan TW, Hamburg NM, et al. Early fasciotomy in patients with extremity vascular injury is associated with decreased risk of adverse limb outcomes: a review of the National Trauma Data Bank. *Injury.* 2012;43(9):1486–1491.

51. Bains SK, Vlachou PA, Rayt HS, et al. An observational cohort study of the management and outcomes of vascular trauma. *Surgeon.* 2009;7(6):332–335.

52. Ahmad F, Turner SA, Torrie P, Gibson M. Iatrogenic femoral artery pseudoaneurysms--a review of current methods of diagnosis and treatment. *Clin Radiol.* 2008;63(12):1310–1316.

53. Krueger K, Zaehringer M, Strohe D, et al. Postcatheterization pseudoaneurysm: results of US-guided percutaneous thrombin injection in 240 patients. *Radiology.* 2005;236(3):1104–1110.

54. Kelm M, Perings SM, Jax T, et al. Incidence and clinical outcome of iatrogenic femoral arteriovenous fistulas: implications for risk stratification and treatment. *J Am Coll Cardiol.* 2002;40(2):291–297.

55. Klinkner DB, Arca MJ, Lewis BD, et al. Pediatric vascular injuries: patterns of injury, morbidity, and mortality. *J Pediatr Surg.* 2007;42(1):178–182. discussion 82-3.

56. Shah SR, Wearden PD, Gaines BA. Pediatric peripheral vascular injuries: a review of our experience. *J Surg Res.* 2009;153(1):162–166.

57. Mommsen P, Zeckey C, Hildebrand F, et al. Traumatic extremity arterial injury in children: epidemiology, diagnostics, treatment and prognostic value of Mangled Extremity Severity Score. *J Orthop Surg Res.* 2010;5:25.

58. Tan TW, Rybin D, Doros G, et al. Observation and surgery are associated with low risk of amputation for blunt brachial artery injury in pediatric patients. *J Vasc Surg.* 2014;60(2):443–447.

59. Chamoun RB, Mawad ME, Whitehead WE, et al. Extracranial traumatic carotid artery dissections in children: a review of current diagnosis and treatment options. *J Neurosurg Pediatr.* 2008;2(2):101–108.

60. Barmparas G, Inaba K, Talving P, et al. Pediatric vs adult vascular trauma: a National Trauma Databank review. *J Pediatr Surg.* 2010;45(7):1404–1412.

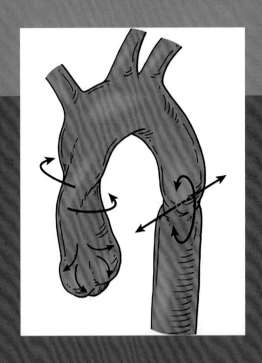

第63章
各类血管压迫综合征

本章主要从解剖学、病理生理学和治疗等方面介绍了常见的血管压迫综合征，包括血管型胸廓出口综合征（thoracic outlet syndrome，TOS）、正中弓状韧带综合征（median arcuate ligament syndrome，MALS）、肾静脉受压综合征、May-Thurner综合征、腘动脉压迫综合征和囊性外膜疾病。胸廓出口综合征是臂丛神经、锁骨下动脉或锁骨下静脉从颈部底部穿过狭窄的胸腔进入上肢时受压引起，可分为神经源性、静脉性和动脉性，静脉性胸廓出口综合征通常表现为先前健康的患者急性单侧上肢肿胀；动脉性胸廓出口综合征患者可出现上肢静息痛。正中弓状韧带综合征是由膈脚和联合脚、正中弓状韧带的纤维弓压迫腹腔干动脉引起，可表现为腹痛或体重减轻，治疗需要分割正中弓状韧带并释放腹腔动脉周围的所有纤维化组织，必要时对腹腔动脉进行血运重建。肾静脉受压综合征是由肠系膜上动脉和主动脉起点压迫左肾静脉引起的临床疾病，症状可能包括血尿、体位性蛋白尿、左侧腰痛、腹痛、左下肢静脉曲张、男性左侧精索静脉曲张和女性盆腔充血综合征，儿童和青少年主要以保守治疗为主。May-Thurner综合征是由右髂总动脉对左髂总静脉的外部压迫引起的临床病症，这种综合征的典型表现包括左下肢肿胀、疼痛或深静脉血栓形成。腘动脉压迫综合征是一种罕见疾病，可导致患者出现间歇性跛行，开放式手术修复是目前首选的治疗。囊性外膜疾病可同时影响动脉和静脉，在外膜中形成黏液性囊肿，导致管腔受压。

李　鑫

Vascular Compression Syndromes

Senthil Jayarajan and Robert Thompson

Vascular compression syndromes are uncommon conditions caused by narrowing or occlusion of vascular structures by adjacent tissues in disparate regions of the body. This chapter will focus on the anatomy, pathophysiology, and management of the more commonly encountered vascular compression syndromes, namely, vascular thoracic outlet syndromes (TOSs), median arcuate ligament syndrome (MALS), nutcracker syndrome, May-Thurner syndrome, popliteal entrapment syndrome, and cystic adventitial disease.

THORACIC OUTLET SYNDROME

TOS represents a group of heterogenous and potentially disabling upper extremity disorders caused by compression of the brachial plexus, subclavian artery, or subclavian vein as they pass through the narrow thoracic aperture from the base of the neck into the upper extremity. Based on the structures involved, TOS is categorized into neurogenic, venous, and arterial. Neurogenic thoracic outlet is the most common (90%), with venous (8%), and arterial (2%) being far less common.

All three forms of TOS are rare but clinically important. If left untreated, they can potentially result in chronic pain syndromes, long-term restrictions to limb use, limb-threatening complications, and significant disability in otherwise relatively young, active, healthy people. This section will review the diagnosis and treatment of venous and arterial TOS.

Venous thoracic outlet syndrome
Clinical Presentation
Paget-Schroetter syndrome (axillosubclavian vein thrombosis or "effort" thrombosis) usually presents with acute unilateral upper extremity swelling in a previously healthy patient, which often prompts urgent medical care. Archetypically, the patient is a young athlete or worker with a component to his or her sport or job that requires prolonged or repetitive stressful positioning of the arm, such as baseball pitchers, swimmers, weight lifters, volleyball players, and mechanics.[1,2]

The involved extremity becomes acutely swollen with varying degrees of discoloration ranging from rubor to cyanosis. Physical examination may reveal the presence of dilated collateral veins around the shoulder and upper arm. The remainder of the physical examination is usually normal. If the condition is ignored, the symptoms may resolve when at rest but can either persist or recur with use of the arm, particularly in a stressed (abducted, externally rotated) position. The collateral channels that develop to allow the swelling to abate when at rest are rarely adequate to accommodate the increased venous return that occurs with activity.[3]

Pathophysiology
The subclavian vein is subject to injury as it passes through the aperture formed between the first rib and clavicle. Anatomical studies have documented positional compression of the subclavian vein by the clavicle, subclavius muscle, and first rib (Fig. 63.1).[4] This can result in intrinsic damage and external scar that contributes to the stenosis and/or occlusion of the subclavian vein.[1]

Diagnosis
History and physical generally suggest the diagnosis due to the sudden spontaneous onset of unilateral upper extremity swelling and discoloration. Duplex ultrasound has been advocated as the first step to diagnose venous TOS. However, duplex ultrasound has a false-negative rate as high as 30%, due to the interference of the clavicle with the acoustic window of the subclavian vein, so it cannot be used to exclude venous TOS.[5]

Contrast-enhanced computed tomography (CT) or magnetic resonance (MR) venography are highly accurate in detecting axillary-subclavian vein occlusion and/or focal stenosis at the level of the first rib (Fig. 63.2).[6] They can be performed with the arms at rest and elevated to determine positional subclavian vein obstruction. They can also identify enlarged collateral veins and the chronicity of any thrombus present. Because these studies provide more anatomical information than venous duplex imaging, CT or MR venography can be used to accurately exclude the diagnosis of venous TOS when ultrasound studies are negative.

The optimal method to both diagnose and initially treat venous TOS is catheter-directed contrast venography. This provides complete anatomical information regarding the site and extent of thrombosis, allows definitive evaluation of the collateral venous pathways, and allows use of thrombolytic therapy. Catheter-based upper extremity venography is the most practical, efficient, and cost-effective approach to evaluating the patient with suspected subclavian vein effort thrombosis.[7]

Treatment
The primary goals of therapy for venous TOS are to return the patient to unrestricted use of the affected extremity with complete symptom relief and freedom from recurrent thrombosis without the need for lifelong anticoagulation. Initial management should be catheter-directed venography and thrombolysis. Pharmacomechanical thrombolysis can reduce the clot burden rapidly, usually within a 1- to 2-hour session.[8] An alternative is continuous infusion of thrombolytic agent over 24 to 48 hours with monitoring in an intensive care unit setting. Balloon angioplasty does not provide a durable benefit and placement of stents is contraindicated due to complications of frequent stent fracture.[9–11] The patient is subsequently maintained on systemic anticoagulation until he undergoes surgery.

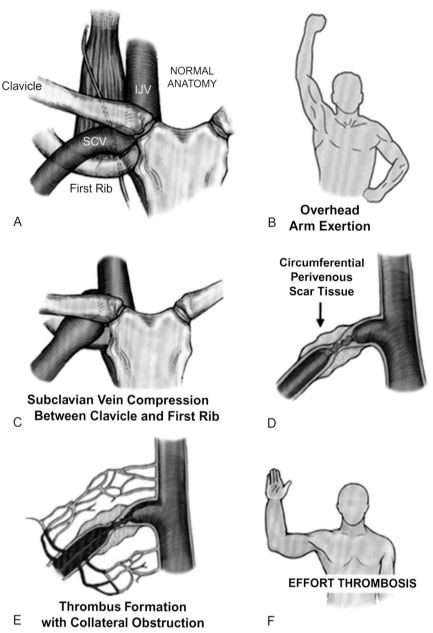

Fig. 63.1 Pathogenesis of Venous Thoracic Outlet Syndrome. (A) Normal anatomy of the thoracic outlet showing the relationship of the internal jugular vein *(IJV)* and subclavian vein *(SCV)* to the clavicle and first rib. (B) Overhead positions of the arm during vigorous activity are associated with the development of venous thoracic outlet syndrome (VTOS). (C) SCV compression between the clavicle and first rib results in focal vein wall injury. (D) Circumferential scar tissue formation around SCV due to repetitive compression injury can lead to severe luminal stenosis. (E) Thrombus formation within the lumen of the constricted SCV causes complete obstruction of the SCV, with extension of thrombus to the axillary vein causing obstruction of collateral veins. (F) Symptomatic presentation of VTOS. (From Melby SJ, Vedantham S, Narra VR, et al. Comprehensive surgical management of the competitive athlete with effort thrombosis of the subclavian vein [Paget-Schroetter syndrome]. *J Vasc Surg.* 2008;47:809–820.e3.)

In patients with a satisfactory result after thrombolysis, surgical treatment is recommended within 4 to 6 weeks after presentation to avoid recurrent thrombosis of the subclavian vein. This time period does allow for some resolution of perivenous inflammation caused by the thrombotic event. Surgery can be safely performed sooner if the patient continues to have marked subclavian vein stenosis or occlusion after lysis.[12,13]

There are several approaches to surgical decompression in venous TOS. However, over a two-decade experience, we have concluded that the paraclavicular approach to venous TOS appears to provide the safest and most effective management of this condition.[5,7,14] All patients with venous TOS undergo surgical treatment using a combination of supraclavicular and infraclavicular incisions. Using the supraclavicular incision, resection of the anterior and middle scalene

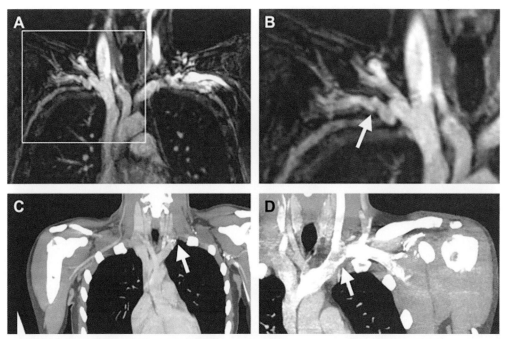

Fig. 63.2 Diagnostic Imaging in Venous Thoracic Outlet Syndrome. (A and B) Contrast-enhanced magnetic resonance imaging shows obstruction of the subclavian vein (SCV) at the level of the first rib *(arrow)*. (C and D) Contrast-enhanced computed tomography in a patient suspected to have left SCV thrombosis, showing central SCV occlusion *(arrows)*. (From Vemuri C, Salehi P, Benarroch-Gampel J, et al. Diagnosis and treatment of effort-induced thrombosis of axillary subclavian vein due to venous thoracic outlet syndrome. *J Vasc Surg Venous Lymphat Disord.* 2016;4:485–500.)

muscles is completed and the posterior first rib is transected at the transverse process. Using the infraclavicular incision, the rib is transected at the edge of the sternum anteriorly and removed. The subclavius muscle is also removed. This facilitates a complete external venolysis from the axillary vein to the junction of the subclavian, internal jugular, and innominate veins via the two incisions. Frequently, external venolysis is sufficient if complete resection of fibrous scar tissue allows the vein to resume its normal diameter and a widely patent subclavian vein with no significant collaterals is seen on venography. Residual vein stenosis or occlusion can be repaired with patch angioplasty or interposition vein bypass.[7] Other approaches include the infraclavicular and transaxillary protocols of treatment of venous TOS. These have been shown to have disadvantages, chiefly relating to the lack of exposure of the vein for a complete venolysis and comprehensive treatment.

Outcomes

A recent review by Vemuri et al. demonstrates the results of surgical management of venous TOS.[7] The paraclavicular approach is associated with greater number of vein bypasses and a longer length of stay. However, satisfactory clinical outcomes were greater with the paraclavicular approach, and the likelihood of remaining on long-term anticoagulation is markedly lower, at less than 5%.

Arterial thoracic outlet syndrome

Clinical Presentation

Arterial TOS is the most rare and varied form of TOS. Compression of the subclavian artery over time leads to progressive inflammation and scarring. This can be associated with poststenotic dilatation, which may progress to aneurysmal degeneration. Patients can present with intermittent claudication or rest pain of the upper extremity.[15] In more severe forms, arterial TOS can be associated with gangrene of the hand

or posterior stroke. Some patients are asymptomatic but have dilation of the subclavian artery noted incidentally during unrelated imaging investigations. A high degree of suspicion is warranted because presentation is so variable.[16,17]

Pathophysiology

Bony abnormalities are typically seen with arterial TOS. Cervical ribs are associated with the majority of these cases. When the cervical rib projects from the transverse process onto the first rib, it displaces the brachial plexus and subclavian artery forward. In this location the subclavian artery is subject to an increased risk for compression or injury (Fig. 63.3). Another common bony anomaly is the presence of an elongated C7 transverse process that acts in a similar fashion. Fibrous bands, if present, from the C7 transverse process to the first rib, can exacerbate compression. Clavicle or first rib fractures are also associated with arterial TOS.[18]

Diagnosis

The diagnosis of arterial TOS can be suggested by the history and physical examination (see Chapter 11). Noninvasive vascular studies can be used to confirm a clinical impression of arterial insufficiency. Diagnostic studies including CT, MR, and catheter-directed arteriography have been used successfully to confirm the presence of arterial TOS.[7,15] Following the diagnosis of arterial TOS, patients are maintained on systemic anticoagulation until surgery.

Treatment

Patients undergo thoracic outlet decompression from a supraclavicular approach. Sometimes, a second infraclavicular incision is also required. During decompression, the bony abnormality is generally encountered and resected. The artery is then inspected. The subsequent management modalities include observation, endarterectomy and patch, or bypass with either vein or Dacron.

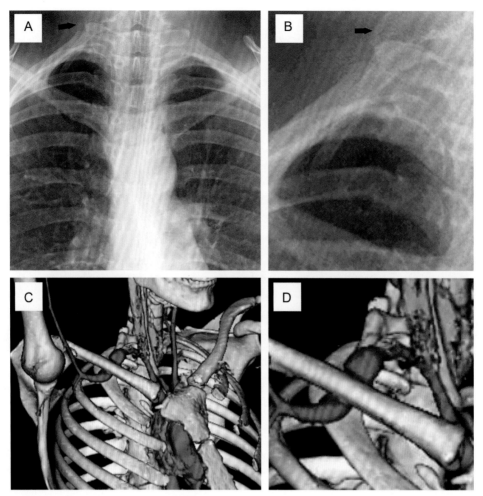

Fig. 63.3 Imaging of Arterial Thoracic Outlet Syndrome. (A and B) Plain chest radiograph illustrates a right cervical rib *(arrows)*. (C and D) Contrast-enhanced computed tomography scan with three-dimensional reconstruction demonstrates a right cervical rib and a poststenotic subclavian artery aneurysm. (From Vemuri C, McLaughlin LN, Abuirgeba AA, et al. Clinical presentation and management of arterial thoracic outlet syndrome. *J Vasc Surg.* 2017;65:1429–1439.)

Outcomes

Arterial TOS is very rare, thus most literature regarding this condition is case reports or series. In the largest series of 40 patients with a follow-up of nearly 5 years, 92% continued to have a patent subclavian artery.[7] There were two reoperations. Chronic symptoms persisted in 15% of patients; these patients had long-standing ischemia prior to intervention. Functionality as measured by the Disabilities of the Arm, Shoulder and Hand (DASH) assessment was improved by nearly 50% in most of the patients. Overall, surgical management of this rare disease entity results in satisfactory outcomes when patients are referred promptly after symptoms ensue.

AXILLARY ARTERY COMPRESSION SYNDROME

Axillary artery compression syndrome is a markedly less frequently encountered syndrome. It manifests primarily in athletes who have repetitive overhead arm movements. These include pitchers, handball players, kayakers, tennis players, and volleyball players.[19] It affects the axillary artery and its branches, such as the circumflex humeral artery. Typical presentation involves digital ischemia due to embolization but can have more subtle findings such as early fatigue of throwing arm or loss of velocity. Repetitive positional compression of the axillary artery

and its branches can lead to intimal hyperplasia, aneurysm formation with mural thrombus, and branch vessel aneurysm.[15] Diagnosis can be confirmed with either a CT arteriogram or catheter-directed arteriogram. Treatment involves a surgical exploration through an upper medial arm incision. The distal axillary artery is exposed and controlled. The lesion is identified by direct palpation and reference to arteriogram. The pectoralis minor muscle rarely needs to be divided. Revascularization can be accomplished via an interposition saphenous vein graft, a patch angioplasty, or an aneurysm excision alone.[20] In the largest series of nine professional baseball players, 89% were able to return to the sport.[15] Duration of symptoms prior to repair appears to be a limiting factor in the recovery process.

MEDIAN ARCUATE LIGAMENT SYNDROME

MALS is also known as the celiac artery compression syndrome, celiac axis syndrome, or Dunbar syndrome. It is caused by the compression of the celiac artery by the diaphragmatic crura and the fibrous arch that unites the crura, the median arcuate ligament.[21] Despite anatomic characterization by Lipshultz in 1917 and description of surgical treatment by Dunbar in 1965, the diagnosis of MALS continues to be controversial.[22]

Clinical Presentation

Many patients experience symptoms for many years prior to recognition of MALS because it is a diagnosis of exclusion.[23–25] The most common presenting symptom is abdominal pain, which can be episodic, postprandial, or constant. Other symptoms can include weight loss and vomiting. On physical exam, epigastric tenderness and a bruit that is amplified by expiration can be present. However, the presence of either tenderness or bruit is not specific for MALS. Abdominal bruits have been noted in 16% of asymptomatic individuals, with only 30% detected in young persons with MALS. It is more prevalent in women (ratio 4:1) aged 30 to 50 years and in those with a thin body habitus. Recently the suggestion that MALS may be a familial syndrome has been raised.

Pathophysiology

The celiac artery is the first abdominal aortic branch that takes off at a 90-degree angle with the aorta. Due to this configuration, it is susceptible to compression by the diaphragmatic crura during thoracic motion, especially with expiration. The median arcuate ligament connects the two crura. In most patients, the stenosis or occlusion caused by the compression is asymptomatic and frequently found incidentally.[26] Manifestation of abdominal pain could be attributed to inadequate collateral flow to the foregut structures via the superior mesenteric artery (SMA) or by compression of neural structures surrounding the celiac artery. Increased flow through the SMA can rarely lead to aneurysm formation or rupture in branches of the SMA.[27–29]

Diagnosis

Due to the high incidence of nonspecific presenting symptoms for MALS, as well as asymptomatic celiac stenosis, thorough evaluation is required to eliminate other possible explanations for their symptoms. Any structural or functional abnormality of the upper abdomen identified should be evaluated and treated first. If other causes of the symptoms have been excluded, celiac artery stenosis or occlusion must be confirmed. Demonstration of variation of the stenosis with respiration is necessary to distinguish from more common causes of celiac artery stenosis such as atherosclerosis. The anatomy can be imaged using catheter angiography (with or without vasodilators), magnetic resonance imaging (MRI), CT, and ultrasound.[21,30–32] When angiography is performed, images should be captured during both inspiration and expiration because the degree of celiac compression is worse during full expiration (Fig. 63.4). However, compression of the celiac axis during expiration can be demonstrated in asymptomatic individuals and further underscores the challenge of establishing this diagnosis.[33] Ultrasound can be advantageous because it provides dynamic information regarding celiac artery flow.

Treatment

The treatment paradigm requires division of the median arcuate ligament and release of all fibrotic tissue surrounding the celiac artery with revascularization of the celiac artery as necessary. Historically, an open approach was used to accomplish both objectives.[34] Recently, laparoscopic surgery is becoming the preferred treatment approach to treat the mechanical compression by skeletonizing the celiac artery.[23] Laparoscopic surgery offers advantages such as smaller incisions, lower perioperative morbidity, and better visualization of surgical field. However, uncontrolled bleeding, potential incomplete release, and injury to aorta due to difficult dissection are potential disadvantages. Robotic surgery and retroperitoneal endoscopic release have also been described for this step.[35–37]

Revascularization of the celiac artery can be accomplished via a second endovascular or surgical operation should it be necessary.[23,38] Because most patients present with varying degrees of celiac stenosis that may not be flow limiting, a widely patent SMA, and symptoms that are not typical of intestinal malperfusion, the decision to

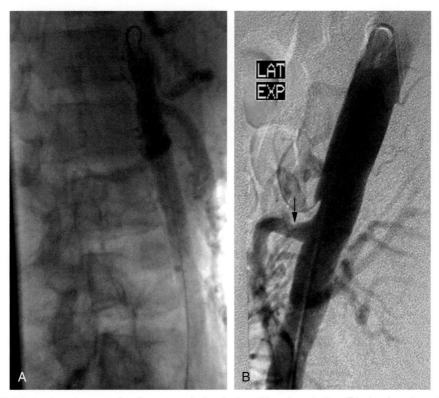

Fig. 63.4 Lateral angiogram of celiac artery in inspiration (A) and expiration (B) showing characteristic compression of artery *(arrow)*.

revascularize is on a case-by-case basis. With the increasing use of laparoscopic techniques to treat MALS, there is a corresponding increase in experience in patients where celiac revascularization is not performed. Some authors advocate decompression alone with minimally invasive techniques, whereas others decompress and revascularize all or most patients immediately via an open approach.

Rupture or aneurysms of gastroduodenal and SMA branches associated with celiac stenosis or occlusion is extremely rare. Patients may present with sudden and severe abdominal pain in hypovolemic shock. Endovascular embolization of this entity is preferred over open surgery because these aneurysms are very difficult to locate and expose surgically.[39,40] Gastroduodenal branches are frequently involved, and definitive open surgery may include a pancreatic resection because of the rich collateral network of arteries in this location.

Outcomes

Patient selection is a key component of obtaining good outcomes for invasive treatment of MALS.[41] Improvement in symptoms is unlikely if the original diagnosis is incorrect. Symptoms can recur even after initial improvement. Minimally invasive approaches to MALS are technically difficult and prone to bleeding complications, requiring conversion to an open procedure. With greater experience of this treatment approach, laparoscopic management of MALS reduces length of stay, significantly decreases recovery time, and reduces conversions to laparotomy.[23]

Regardless of approach and procedures performed, most series show favorable outcomes.[23,34,36,38,41–44] Most patients experience symptom relief and return to normal activity. There is generally limited morbidity and mortality. One report documented that, in a series of six patients with long-term follow-up, all patients would have the surgery again. Contemporary diagnosis and management strategies for this syndrome remain in evolution, but release of median arcuate ligament with or without celiac artery revascularization appears to adequately treat most patients effectively.

NUTCRACKER SYNDROME

Presentation

Nutcracker syndrome is a clinical condition caused by compression of the left renal vein by the origin of the SMA and the aorta. When found radiographically incidentally, it is referred to as *nutcracker phenomenon*. The compression results in venous hypertension of the left renal vein and its branches, which in turn causes the symptomatology of this syndrome. Age of presentation is quite variable but most commonly is young adulthood.[45,46] A slight female preponderance has been noted. There are many reports documenting childhood presentation. Symptoms can include hematuria (microscopic and macroscopic), orthostatic proteinuria, left flank pain, abdominal pain, left lower extremity varicose veins, left varicocele in males, and pelvic congestion syndrome in females.[47,48] Pelvic congestion syndrome symptoms include dyspareunia, dysuria, dysmenorrhea, vulvar varicosities, and vaginal tenderness.[49,50] Younger patients with nutcracker syndrome frequently have associated medical problems that include urolithiasis, Henoch-Schönlein purpura, immunoglobulin A (IgA) nephropathy, hypercalciuria, and familial Mediterranean fever.[51-55]

Pathophysiology

The normal anatomic course of the left renal vein passes under the SMA and over the aorta before emptying into the inferior vena cava (IVC). When the angle between the SMA and aorta is too acute, mechanical compression of the left renal vein can develop (Fig. 63.5).[45,47] Antecedent weight loss with reduced retroperitoneal and mesenteric fat could be a potential contributing factor but is not noted in the

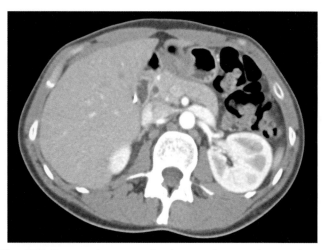

Fig. 63.5 Computed tomography image of nutcracker syndrome anatomy where the left renal vein is compressed between the superior mesenteric artery and aorta with dilation of the proximal renal vein.

majority of patients.[48,56] Renal vein hypertension can cause hematuria and hypertension of the veins that empty into the left renal vein, which include the left gonadal vein. Retroaortic location of the left renal vein is also associated with nutcracker syndrome, with the left renal vein being entrapped between the aorta and the adjacent vertebral body. This is known as *posterior nutcracker syndrome*. A left-sided vena cava can also lead to nutcracker syndrome.

Diagnosis

Left abdominal and pelvic venous hypertension demonstrated on cross-sectional imaging can confirm the diagnosis of nutcracker syndrome. Ultrasound, CT, MRI, and traditional venography with pressure measurements have all been used for this purpose. Typically, demonstration of increased pressures distal to the area of compression is sought before invasive treatment is recommended. Retrograde venography was traditionally used to establish a diagnosis. A renocaval pull back pressure gradient >3 (normal <1) is used as a reference standard for nutcracker syndrome.[46]

Ultrasound is often the first diagnostic investigation, but its range of values for the diagnosis of nutcracker syndrome is variable.[56-58] Cross-sectional imaging such as CT and MR can demonstrate compression of the left renal vein by the SMA and aorta. The narrowing of the left renal vein, as it passes through an acute angle between the SMA and aorta (beak sign), and a left renal vein diameter ratio of greater than 4.9 between the hilum and the aortomesenteric segment are CT findings that demonstrate the greatest diagnostic accuracy. CT has also demonstrated usefulness when patients have a presentation consistent with nutcracker syndrome, where compression of the left renal vein is caused by unusual structures such as the splenic vein, pancreas, duodenum, and the right diaphragmatic crus.[59] MRI has findings that are similar to those found with CT.[60] Recently, MR fast spin echo (FSE) T2-weighted imaging has been explored as an alternative to invasive venography to measure venous pressure gradients.[61]

Treatment

Conservative Management

Conservative management is generally preferred in children and adolescents because symptoms such as hematuria may resolve with further growth. Physical development and increased body mass index may change the positional relationship of the aorta and SMA.[62,63] Angiotensin-converting enzyme (ACE) inhibitors have demonstrated efficacy in pediatric patients for relief of proteinuria.[49,64]

Surgical Management

Open techniques. Multiple open surgical procedures have been described to relieve left renal vein compression. Left renal vein transposition to an area lower on the IVC has been used most frequently with greatest efficacy.[60,65,66] A patch venoplasty with greater saphenous vein can also be performed if there is persistent vein distortion and increased gradient caused by chronic compression. A saphenous vein cuff can be used to create a tension-free anastomosis. Gonadal vein transposition and bypass with saphenous vein or prosthetic can also be used to relieve renal vein hypertension.[67-69] Minimally invasive techniques such as laparoscopic splenorenal venous bypass, laparoscopic placement of an external left renal vein stent using a ringed PTFE graft, laparoscopic left renal vein transposition, and robot-assisted left renal vein transposition have also been performed.[70-73] Renal autotransplantation by both open and laparoscopic approaches represents an uncommon method to treat nutcracker syndrome.[74,75] Nephrectomy is rarely indicated for this condition.

Endovascular techniques. Enthusiasm for endovascular stenting to treat nutcracker syndrome is growing.[76-79] This treatment modality is controversial because many treated patients are very young, and the implanted stent must last for many years. The most common major complication noted with endovascular therapy is stent migration.[80-82]

Outcomes

Due to the rare incidence of nutcracker syndrome, no outcomes from large series have been published. The largest series for open management of nutcracker syndrome is 37 patients from the Mayo Clinic in Rochester,[83] in which the primary, primary assisted with renal stenting or open revision, and secondary patencies were 74%, 97%, and 100%, respectively. Symptom resolution occurred in 87% of patients.

The largest report of endovascular stent placement was in 75 patients over a 10-year period. The median age at stent placement was 27 years. There was a migration rate of 6.9% at a median of 55 months.[80]

Preoperative measurement of vein during a Valsalva maneuver, accurate deployment, and close follow-up with early intervention reduced incidence of stent migration into heart. Another series of 61 patients noted either symptom resolution or marked improvement of 73% at a median follow-up of 66 months.[84]

MAY-THURNER SYNDROME

Presentation

May-Thurner syndrome is the clinical condition caused by extrinsic compression of the left common iliac vein (CIV) by the right common iliac artery (CIA). Typically the presentation of this syndrome involves left lower extremity swelling, pain, or other signs of venous hypertension as a manifestation of deep vein thrombosis (DVT).[85,86] This condition usually manifests in early adulthood, and there is a female predominance. Children can develop May-Thurner syndrome, although this is infrequent.[87,88] Pregnancy can also precipitate DVT in patients with this mechanical finding, likely due to the added compression on the pelvic veins caused by a gravid uterus. Presentation with stroke and pulmonary embolism in patients with patent foramen ovale has also been documented.[89,90] Rupture of the left iliac vein has also been reported as an initial presentation.[91]

Pathophysiology

The right CIA crosses anterior to the left CIV at its confluence with the vena cava. Mechanical compression of the left CIV can occur, with resultant left lower extremity venous hypertension and thrombosis (Fig. 63.6). However, mechanical compression of the left CIV is frequently identified in patients who are asymptomatic, thus calling into question the contribution of mechanical compression in the syndrome.[90,91] Prothrombotic states have been associated in the occurrence of this syndrome, and extrinsic compression after other procedures has also been implicated.[94-97]

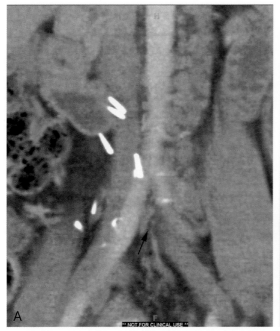
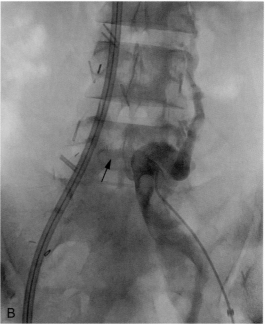

Fig. 63.6 Imaging of May-Thurner Syndrome. (A) Computed tomography venogram demonstrating occlusion of left common iliac vein *(arrow)* as it passes under right common iliac artery. (B) Contrast venogram demonstrates occlusion of left common iliac vein *(arrow)* with flow through collaterals. The catheter marks the inferior vena cava.

Diagnosis

Diagnosis can be delayed until symptoms persist or multiple thrombotic events occur, because CT venography,[98] MR venography,[99] or conventional venography of the pelvis are needed to confirm the presence of May-Thurner syndrome. Lower extremity ultrasound frequently fails to confirm the diagnosis, especially in the setting of extensive iliofemoral DVT.[100] Although quite rare, right-sided and vena cava compression have also been reported.[101,102]

Treatment

Pharmacomechanical thrombolysis is emerging as the most frequent therapy for acute symptomatic extensive iliofemoral DVT in a young low-risk patient.[103,104] If the lytic therapy is successful, completion venography would confirm the diagnosis of May-Thurner syndrome. Two options exist for relief of the mechanical compression: surgery and endovenous stents. The open surgical method involves division of the right CIA and transposing it beneath the left common iliac artery.

Endovenous stents for May-Thurner syndrome have gained increasing popularity to avoid the laparotomy and arterial transection required for the open procedure.[105,106] Stents appear to have the radial force necessary to overcome the compression, and stent fractures from repeated trauma have not been reported. Stents are subject to migration and restenosis that may require reintervention.[107] Stents are frequently deployed in the left CIV and extended into the vena cava. This placement can lead to thrombosis of the right iliac venous system. Endovascular treatment may be preferable when patients presenting with acute complications due to May-Thurner syndrome are also pregnant.[108,109] No randomized trials have been performed to compare endovenous stenting to open surgery, and treatment options are typically individualized for each patient.

Outcomes

Endovascular outcomes have been excellent, with reported initial technical success greater than 90% and an equally high rate of symptom resolution.[110-112] Complications mainly included bleeding, usually related to administration of thrombolytic agents. Over an average of 2 years of follow-up, stent thrombosis occurs in approximately 10% of patients. Most of these stents are reopened using endovascular techniques.

Reports of open surgical procedures for May-Thurner syndrome are scarce. Frequently the results are reported for a mix of clinical presentations including May-Thurner syndrome. The Mayo Clinic has published two reports over multiple years.[113,114] These showed secondary patency rates of 70% at 5-year follow-up.

POPLITEAL ENTRAPMENT SYNDROME

Presentation

Popliteal entrapment is a rare syndrome causing intermittent claudication in younger patients.[115] Patients most commonly present in early adulthood, although the syndrome has been diagnosed in children.[116] Unilateral intermittent claudication is the most frequent symptom. At rest, physical examination is generally normal. However, ankle dorsiflexion, plantar flexion, or knee extension may result in diminished or occluded distal pulses. The presentation may also be bilateral.[117] If the syndrome has been long-standing, patients may present with total occlusion or aneurysmal degeneration of the popliteal artery. Occlusion of the popliteal artery aneurysm may cause significant ischemia. Below-knee DVT may be a presenting symptom as well, if the popliteal vein is involved.[118]

Pathophysiology

The congenital anomalies that disturb the normal relationship between the popliteal artery and the muscular structures within the popliteal fossa cause popliteal entrapment syndrome.[119,120] There are six distinct anatomical presentations of this syndrome (Table 63.1). The most common type (type I), found in approximately 50% of cases, occurs when the popliteal artery passes medial to the normally placed medial head insertion of the gastrocnemius muscle. This configuration results in compression of the artery against the head of the tibia when the muscle contracts (typically during ambulation). One variant also causes entrapment of the popliteal vein either in combination with the artery or in isolation. Type VI is controversial and designated as functional because no anatomic variant has been identified.[121]

Diagnosis

MRI/MRA or CT/CTA are the studies of choice due to visualization of both the soft tissue and arterial anatomy in this region, which facilitate operative planning.[122-125] Ultrasound has been used as an adjunct.[126,127] Catheter-based angiography may also be performed, but forced plantar or dorsiflexion may be required to demonstrate the abnormality because flow may be normal in a neutral position (Fig. 63.7).[117] A medial course of the popliteal artery during angiography also suggests the diagnosis. If the popliteal artery is occluded, angiography may be necessary for operative planning of a distal bypass.

Treatment

Open surgical repair is the current treatment modality of choice. The most common method is that, after prone positioning of the patient, an S-shaped incision is made over the popliteal fossa. A medial approach might also be used; however, it may result in missed abnormality or more likely recurrence. Release of the aberrant muscle segments is tolerated without loss of function. In instances where the entire medial head of the gastrocnemius muscle must be divided, it should be

TABLE 63.1	Types of Popliteal Artery Entrapment	
Type	Anatomic Variation	Embryologic Cause
I	Popliteal artery is medial to normally situated medial head of gastrocnemius muscle head	Popliteal artery completes development before migration of gastrocnemius muscle
II	Popliteal artery is displaced medially by abnormal femoral insertion site of gastrocnemius head	Popliteal artery forms prematurely and partially arrests migration of gastrocnemius muscle
III	A slip of gastrocnemius muscle arises abnormally from medial or lateral femoral condyle	Popliteal artery is found anterior to or originates within embryologic remnants of gastrocnemius muscle
IV	The popliteus muscle passes posterior to the popliteal artery	Persistence of the fetal axial artery as the mature distal popliteal artery
V	Both popliteal artery and vein are involved with any of the variants in types I–IV	Depends on anatomic variation
VI	Functional; no anatomical variation	

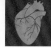

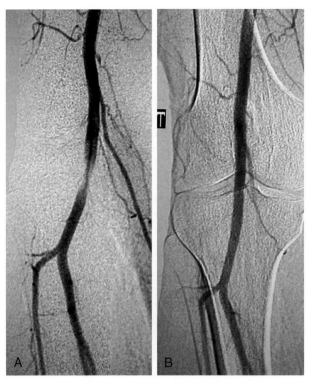

Fig. 63.7 Angiogram of popliteal artery with forced dorsiflexion of foot (A) showing compression of the artery and with relaxation of leg (B), filling of the artery is noted.

relocated and reattached to the tibial condyle. If indicated, arterial reconstruction via either mobilization and end-to-end anastomosis or interposition saphenous vein bypass.[105,128] Endovascular treatment with angioplasty and thrombolysis has also been described; however, long-term results are lacking.[129-131]

Outcomes

Preoperative vascular damage predicts outcomes following intervention for popliteal artery entrapment syndrome. The rarity of the syndrome and the low index of suspicion for arterial insufficiency in this atypical patient population frequently delay diagnosis until significant arterial damage has occurred and signs of advanced ischemia are present. In a meta-analysis of 30 studies, postoperative successful resolution of symptoms was at a median of 77%.[123] One series describes 100% patency at 10 years in 13 limbs but did note two failures subsequent to that.[132]

CYSTIC ADVENTITIAL DISEASE

Presentation

Cystic adventitial disease is a rare entity that can affect both arteries and veins, where mucinous cysts form in the adventitia. These cysts result in vascular compression of the vessel lumen. The cyst is benign but has a tendency to recur. The quality of substance within the cyst is gelatinous. The most common location is the popliteal artery.[133] However, it has been described in external iliac artery, femoral vein and artery, and radial artery.[134-137] The age at presentation is generally younger than those with lower extremity atherosclerosis. It predominantly affects men. Most patients present with intermittent claudication. Few patients report history of trauma.[133,138]

Pathophysiology

The etiology of cystic adventitial disease is unknown. There are multiple theories regarding the origin of this condition. It could be due to direct communication with nearby joint synovium.[139] A more accepted explanation is relocation of adventitial cyst cells from adjacent joint, similar to ganglion cysts.[133,140,141]

Diagnosis

Although ultrasound can reliably be used to identify cystic adventitial disease through compression of vasculature by cystic structures, CT and MRI have the added benefit of defining the anatomical relationships of the artery to external structures as well.[140,142] MRI has been found to be equally diagnostic as catheter angiography.[143] Signs typical of cystic adventitial disease include a scalloped appearance of the artery wall known as a "scimitar" sign or hourglass appearance with normal healthy artery proximal and distal to artery (Fig. 63.8).[144]

Treatment

Treatment involves full resection or enucleation of the cyst with or without revascularization.[138,145,146] Revascularization is typically performed with a saphenous vein interposition graft where appropriate. Despite full resection of the cyst, they are known to recur. Other treatment options include aspiration of the cyst and aspiration combined with introduction of a sclerosing agent into the cyst.[147-149] Endovascular methods have not been successful in treating cystic adventitial disease,[150,151] although angioplasty for treatment of recurrence has been reported.[152]

Outcomes

Determining outcomes of treatment for cystic adventitial disease has been difficult owing to the rarity of this disease process. Recently, a retrospective review at 14 centers was performed with a mean follow-up of 20 months.[138] They identified 47 cases of adventitial cystic disease. Of these, 21 patients underwent resection and interposition graft, 13 cyst resections, 5 cyst resections and bypass, and 2 cyst resections and patch; 18% required reintervention after a mean of 70 days. Those who underwent revascularization during the primary procedure were less likely to require reintervention.

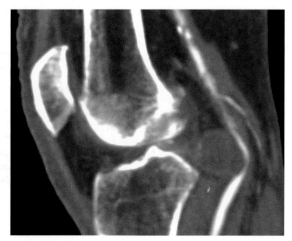

Fig. 63.8 Computed tomography image of adventitial cyst compressing popliteal artery behind the knee, creating the "scimitar sign."

REFERENCES

1. Illig KA, Doyle AJ. A comprehensive review of Paget-Schroetter syndrome. *J Vasc Surg*. 2010;51(6):1538–1547.

2. Alla VM, Natarajan N, Kaushik M, et al. Paget-Schroetter syndrome: review of pathogenesis and treatment of effort thrombosis. *West J Emerg Med*. 2010;11(4):358–362.

3. Sanders RJ, Haug C. Subclavian vein obstruction and thoracic outlet syndrome: a review of etiology and management. *Ann Vasc Surg*. 1990;4(4):397–410.

4. Daskalakis E, Bouhoutsos J. Subclavian and axillary vein compression of musculoskeletal origin. *Br J Surg*. 1980;67(8):573–576.

5. Melby SJ, Vedantham S, Narra VR, et al. Comprehensive surgical management of the competitive athlete with effort thrombosis of the subclavian vein (Paget-Schroetter syndrome). *J Vasc Surg*. 2008;47(4):809–820. discussion 821.

6. Raptis CA, Sridhar S, Thompson RW, et al. Imaging of the patient with thoracic outlet syndrome. *Radiographics*. 2016;36(4):984–1000.

7. Vemuri C, Salehi P, Benarroch-Gampel J, et al. Diagnosis and treatment of effort-induced thrombosis of the axillary subclavian vein due to venous thoracic outlet syndrome. *J Vasc Surg Venous Lymphat Disord*. 2016;4(4):485–500.

8. Schneider DB, Curry TK, Eichler CM, et al. Percutaneous mechanical thrombectomy for the management of venous thoracic outlet syndrome. *J Endovasc Ther*. 2003;10(2):336–340.

9. Guzzo JL, Chang K, Demos J, et al. Preoperative thrombolysis and venoplasty affords no benefit in patency following first rib resection and scalenectomy for subacute and chronic subclavian vein thrombosis. *J Vasc Surg*. 2010;52(3):658–662. discussion 662-663.

10. Rutherford RB. Primary subclavian-axillary vein thrombosis: the relative roles of thrombolysis, percutaneous angioplasty, stents, and surgery. *Semin Vasc Surg*. 1998;11(2):91–95.

11. Urschel HC, Patel AN. Paget-Schroetter syndrome therapy: failure of intravenous stents. *Ann Thorac Surg*. 2003;75(6):1693–1696; discussion 1696.

12. Angle N, Gelabert HA, Farooq MM, et al. Safety and efficacy of early surgical decompression of the thoracic outlet for Paget-Schroetter syndrome. *Ann Vasc Surg*. 2001;15(1):37–42.

13. Caparrelli DJ, Freischlag J. A unified approach to axillosubclavian venous thrombosis in a single hospital admission. *Semin Vasc Surg*. 2005;18(3):153–157.

14. Thompson RW, Schneider PA, Nelken NA, et al. Circumferential venolysis and paraclavicular thoracic outlet decompression for "effort thrombosis" of the subclavian vein. *J Vasc Surg*. 1992;16(5):723–732.

15. Duwayri YM, Emery VB, Driskill MR, et al. Positional compression of the axillary artery causing upper extremity thrombosis and embolism in the elite overhead throwing athlete. *J Vasc Surg*. 2011;53(5):1329–1340.

16. Durham JR, Yao JST, Pearce WH, et al. Arterial injuries in the thoracic outlet syndrome. *J Vasc Surg*. 1995;21(1):57–70.

17. Daniels B, Michaud L, Sease FJ, et al. Arterial thoracic outlet syndrome. *Curr Sports Med Rep*. 2014;13(2):75.

18. Patton GM. Arterial thoracic outlet syndrome. *Hand Clin*. 2004;20(1):107–111. viii.

19. Jackson MR. Upper extremity arterial injuries in athletes. *Semin Vasc Surg*. 2003;16(3):232–239.

20. Schneider K, Kasparyan NG, Altchek DW, et al. An aneurysm involving the axillary artery and its branch vessels in a major league baseball pitcher. A case report and review of the literature. *Am J Sports Med*. 1999;27(3):370–375.

21. Kim EN, Lamb K, Relles D, et al. Median arcuate ligament syndrome-review of this rare disease. *JAMA Surg*. 2016;151(5):471–477.

22. Gloviczki P, Duncan AA. Treatment of celiac artery compression syndrome: does it really exist? *Perspect Vasc Surg Endovasc Ther*. 2007;19(3):259–263.

23. Jimenez JC, Harlander-Locke M, Dutson EP. Open and laparoscopic treatment of median arcuate ligament syndrome. *J Vasc Surg*. 2012;56(3):869–873.

24. Gander S, Mulder DJ, Jones S, et al. Recurrent abdominal pain and weight loss in an adolescent: celiac artery compression syndrome. *Can J Gastroenterol*. 2010;24(2):91–93.

25. Duffy AJ, Panait L, Eisenberg D, et al. Management of median arcuate ligament syndrome: a new paradigm. *Ann Vasc Surg*. 2009;23(6):778–784.

26. Loukas M, Pinyard J, Vaid S, et al. Clinical anatomy of celiac artery compression syndrome: a review. *Clin Anat N Y N*. 2007;20(6):612–617.

27. Armstrong MB, Stadtlander KS, Grove MK. Pancreaticoduodenal artery aneurysm associated with median arcuate ligament syndrome. *Ann Vasc Surg*. 2014;28(3):741.e1-5.

28. Toriumi T, Shirasu T, Akai A, et al. Hemodynamic benefits of celiac artery release for ruptured right gastric artery aneurysm associated with median arcuate ligament syndrome: a case report. *BMC Surg*. 2017;17(1):116.

29. Jimenez JC, Rafidi F, Morris L. True celiac artery aneurysm secondary to median arcuate ligament syndrome. *Vasc Endovascular Surg*. 2011;45(3):288–289.

30. Kopecky KK, Stine SB, Dalsing MC, Gottlieb K. Median arcuate ligament syndrome with multivessel involvement: diagnosis with spiral CT angiography. *Abdom Imaging*. 1997;22(3):318–320.

31. Ozel A, Toksoy G, Ozdogan O, et al. Ultrasonographic diagnosis of median arcuate ligament syndrome: a report of two cases. *Med Ultrason*. 2012;14(2):154–157.

32. Gruber H, Loizides A, Peer S, Gruber I. Ultrasound of the median arcuate ligament syndrome: a new approach to diagnosis. *Med Ultrason*. 2012;14(1):5–9.

33. Skeik N, Cooper LT, Duncan AA, Jabr FI. Median arcuate ligament syndrome: a nonvascular, vascular diagnosis. *Vasc Endovascular Surg*. 2011;45(5):433–437.

34. Duran M, Simon F, Ertas N, et al. Open vascular treatment of median arcuate ligament syndrome. *BMC Surg*. 2017;17(1):95.

35. Do MV, Smith TA, Bazan HA, et al. Laparoscopic versus robot-assisted surgery for median arcuate ligament syndrome. *Surg Endosc*. 2013;27(11):4060–4066.

36. You JS, Cooper M, Nishida S, et al. Treatment of median arcuate ligament syndrome via traditional and robotic techniques. *Hawaii J Med Public Health*. 2013;72(8):279–281.

37. van Petersen AS, Vriens BH, Huisman AB, et al. Retroperitoneal endoscopic release in the management of celiac artery compression syndrome. *J Vasc Surg*. 2009;50(1):140–147.

38. Michalik M, Dowgiałło-Wnukiewicz N, Lech P, et al. Hybrid (laparoscopy + stent) treatment of celiac trunk compression syndrome (Dunbar syndrome, median arcuate ligament syndrome (MALS)). *Wideochir Inne Tech Maloinwazyjne*. 2016;11(4):236–239.

39. Akatsu T, Hayashi S, Yamane T, et al. Emergency embolization of a ruptured pancreaticoduodenal artery aneurysm associated with the median arcuate ligament syndrome. *J Gastroenterol Hepatol*. 2004;19(4):482–483.

40. Ogino H, Sato Y, Banno T, et al. Embolization in a patient with ruptured anterior inferior pancreaticoduodenal arterial aneurysm with median arcuate ligament syndrome. *Cardiovasc Intervent Radiol*. 2002;25(4):318–319.

41. Ho KKF, Walker P, Smithers BM, et al. Outcome predictors in median arcuate ligament syndrome. *J Vasc Surg*. 2017;65(6):1745–1752.

42. Columbo JA, Trus T, Nolan B, et al. Contemporary management of median arcuate ligament syndrome provides early symptom improvement. *J Vasc Surg*. 2015;62(1):151–156.

43. Cienfuegos JA, Estevez MG, Ruiz-Canela M, et al. Laparoscopic treatment of median arcuate ligament syndrome: analysis of long-term outcomes and predictive factors. *J Gastrointest Surg*. 2018;22:713–721.

44. Kohn GP, Bitar RS, Farber MA, et al. Treatment options and outcomes for celiac artery compression syndrome. *Surg Innov*. 2011;18(4):338–343.

45. Copetti R, Copetti E. Renal nutcracker syndrome. *Acta Medica Acad*. 2017;46(1):63–64.

46. Orczyk K, Łabetowicz P, Lodziński S, et al. The nutcracker syndrome. Morphology and clinical aspects of the important vascular variations: a systematic study of 112 cases. *Int Angiol*. 2016;35(1):71–77.

47. Gulleroglu K, Gulleroglu B, Baskin E. Nutcracker syndrome. *World J Nephrol*. 2014;3(4):277–281.

48. Venkatachalam S, Bumpus K, Kapadia SR, et al. The nutcracker syndrome. *Ann Vasc Surg*. 2011;25(8):1154–1164.

49. Kurklinsky AK, Rooke TW. Nutcracker phenomenon and nutcracker syndrome. *Mayo Clin Proc*. 2010;85(6):552–559.

50. Emrecan B, Tastan H, Tanrisever GY, Simsek S. Surgically treated pelvic pain caused by nutcracker syndrome and worsened by Cockett syndrome in a child. *Ann Vasc Surg.* 2017;44:422.e15-422.e17.

51. Altugan FS, Ekim M, Fitöz S, et al. Nutcracker syndrome with urolithiasis. *J Pediatr Urol.* 2010;6:519–521.

52. Shin J, Park J, Shin Y, et al. Superimposition of nutcracker syndrome in a haematuric child with Henoch Schönlein purpura. *Int J Clin Pract.* 2005;59:1472–1475.

53. Shin JI, Park JM, Shin YH, et al. Nutcracker syndrome combined with IgA nephropathy in a child with recurrent hematuria. *Pediatr Int.* 2006;48:324–326.

54. Shin JI, Park JM, Lee JS, et al. Superimposition of nutcracker syndrome in a hematuric child with idiopathic hypercalciuria and urolithiasis. *Int J Urol.* 2006;13:814–816.

55. Ozcan A, Gonul II, Sakallioglu O, et al. Nutcracker syndrome in a child with familial Mediterranean fever (FMF) disease: renal ultrastructural features. *Int Urol Nephrol.* 2009;41:1047–1053.

56. Scultetus AH, Villavicencio JL, Gillespie DL. The nutcracker syndrome: its role in the pelvic venous disorders. *J Vasc Surg.* 2001;34(5):812–819.

57. Park SJ, Lim JW, Ko YT, et al. Diagnosis of pelvic congestion syndrome using transabdominal and transvaginal sonography. *AJR Am J Roentgenol.* 2004;182(3):683–688.

58. Ananthan K, Onida S, Davies AH. Nutcracker syndrome: an update on current diagnostic criteria and management guidelines. *Eur J Vasc Endovasc Surg.* 2017;53(6):886–894.

59. Karaosmanoğlu D, Karcaaltincaba M, Akata D, Ozmen M. Unusual causes of left renal vein compression along its course: MDCT findings in patients with nutcracker and pelvic congestion syndrome. *Surg Radiol Anat.* 2010;32(4):323–327.

60. Said SM, Gloviczki P, Kalra M, et al. Renal nutcracker syndrome: surgical options. *Semin Vasc Surg.* 2013;26(1):35–42.

61. Goldberg A, Halandras PM, Shea S, Cho JS. Utility of magnetic resonance imaging in establishing a venous pressure gradient in a patient with possible nutcracker syndrome. *J Vasc Surg Cases Innov Tech.* 2016;2(3):80–83.

62. Shin JI, Baek SY, Lee JS, Kim MJ. Follow-up and treatment of nutcracker syndrome. *Ann Vasc Surg.* 2007;21(3):402.

63. Tanaka H, Waga S. Spontaneous remission of persistent severe hematuria in an adolescent with nutcracker syndrome: seven years' observation. *Clin Exp Nephrol.* 2004;8(1):68–70.

64. Ha T-S, Lee E-J. ACE inhibition can improve orthostatic proteinuria associated with nutcracker syndrome. *Pediatr Nephrol.* 2006;21(11):1765–1768.

65. Kim JY, Joh JH, Choi HY, et al. Transposition of the left renal vein in nutcracker syndrome. *Eur J Vasc Endovasc Surg.* 2006;31(1):80–82.

66. Reed NR, Kalra M, Bower TC, et al. Left renal vein transposition for nutcracker syndrome. *J Vasc Surg.* 2009;49(2):386–393. discussion 393-394.

67. Benrashid E, Turley RS, Mureebe L, Shortell CK. Gonadal vein transposition in the treatment of nutcracker syndrome. *J Vasc Surg.* 2016;64(3):845.

68. Zhang X, Wang S, Wei J. Prosthetic left renocaval bypass for posterior nutcracker syndrome. *Indian J Surg.* 2015;77(Suppl 1):103–105.

69. Liu Y, Sun Y, Jin X. Left renocaval venous bypass with autologous great saphenous vein for nutcracker syndrome. *J Vasc Surg.* 2012;55(5):1482–1484.

70. Chung BI, Gill IS. Laparoscopic splenorenal venous bypass for nutcracker syndrome. *J Vasc Surg.* 2009;49(5):1319–1323.

71. Hartung O, Azghari A, Barthelemy P, et al. Laparoscopic transposition of the left renal vein into the inferior vena cava for nutcracker syndrome. *J Vasc Surg.* 2010;52(3):738–741.

72. Zhang Q, Zhang Y, Lou S, et al. Laparoscopic extravascular renal vein stent placement for nutcracker syndrome. *J Endourol.* 2010;24(10):1631–1635.

73. Chau AH, Abdul-Muhsin H, Peng X, et al. Robotic-assisted left renal vein transposition as a novel surgical technique for the treatment of renal nutcracker syndrome. *J Vasc Surg Cases Innov Tech.* 2018;4(1):31–34.

74. Salehipour M, Rasekhi A, Shirazi M, et al. The role of renal autotransplantation in treatment of nutcracker syndrome. *Saudi J Kidney Dis Transpl.* 2010;21(2):237–241.

75. Xu D, Liu Y, Gao Y, et al. Management of renal nutcracker syndrome by retroperitoneal laparoscopic nephrectomy with ex vivo autograft repair and autotransplantation: a case report and review of the literature. *J Med Case Reports.* 2009;3:82.

76. Feng K-K, Huang C-Y, Hsiao C-Y, et al. Endovascular stenting for nutcracker syndrome. *J Chin Med Assoc.* 2013;76(6):350–353.

77. Policha A, Lamparello P, Sadek M, et al. Endovascular treatment of nutcracker syndrome. *Ann Vasc Surg.* 2016;36:295.e1-295.e7.

78. Quevedo HC, Arain SA, Abi Rafeh N. Systematic review of endovascular therapy for nutcracker syndrome and case presentation. *Cardiovasc Revasc Med.* 2014;15(5):305–307.

79. Sadek M, Maldonado TS, Policha A, Lamparello PJ. Endovascular treatment of nutcracker syndrome. *J Vasc Surg.* 2015;61(6):71S.

80. Wu Z, Zheng X, He Y, et al. Stent migration after endovascular stenting in patients with nutcracker syndrome. *J Vasc Surg Venous Lymphat Disord.* 2016;4(2):193–199.

81. Rana MA, Oderich GS, Bjarnason H. Endovenous removal of dislodged left renal vein stent in a patient with nutcracker syndrome. *Semin Vasc Surg.* 2013;26(1):43–47.

82. Tian L, Chen S, Zhang G, et al. Extravascular stent management for migration of left renal vein endovascular stent in nutcracker syndrome. *BMC Urol.* 2015;15:73.

83. Erben Y, Gloviczki P, Kalra M, et al. Treatment of nutcracker syndrome with open and endovascular interventions. *J Vasc Surg Venous Lymphat Disord.* 2015;3(4):389–396.

84. Chen S, Zhang H, Shi H, et al. Endovascular stenting for treatment of nutcracker syndrome: report of 61 cases with long-term followup. *J Urol.* 2011;186(2):570–575.

85. Dhillon RK, Stead LG. Acute deep vein thrombus due to May-Thurner syndrome. *Am J Emerg Med.* 2010;28(2):254.e3–254.e4.

86. Kaltenmeier CT, Erben Y, Indes J, et al. Systematic review of May-Thurner syndrome with emphasis on gender differences. *J Vasc Surg Venous Lymphat Disord.* 2018;6(3):399–407.e4.

87. Goldman RE, Arendt VA, Kothary N, et al. Endovascular management of May-Thurner syndrome in adolescents: a single-center experience. *J Vasc Interv Radiol.* 2017;28(1):71–77.

88. Emrecan B, Tastan H, Tanrisever GY, Simsek S. Surgically treated pelvic pain caused by nutcracker syndrome and worsened by Cockett syndrome in a child. *Ann Vasc Surg.* 2017;44:422.e15–422.e17.

89. Kiernan TJ, Yan BP, Cubeddu RJ, et al. May-Thurner syndrome in patients with cryptogenic stroke and patent foramen ovale: an important clinical association. *Stroke.* 2009;40(4):1502–1504.

90. Fasanya AA, LaCapra G. May-Thurner syndrome with pulmonary embolism as the first presentation rather than deep vein thrombosis. *Cureus.* 2016;8(2):e509.

91. Ingram M, Miladore J, Gupta A, et al. Spontaneous iliac vein rupture due to May-Thurner Syndrome and its staged management. *Vasc Endovascular Surg.* 2019;53(4):348–350.

92. Raju S, Neglen P. High prevalence of nonthrombotic iliac vein lesions in chronic venous disease: a permissive role in pathogenicity. *J Vasc Surg.* 2006;44(1):136–143.

93. Kibbe MR, Ujiki M, Goodwin AL, et al. Iliac vein compression in an asymptomatic patient population. *J Vasc Surg.* 2004;39(5):937–943.

94. Sharma R, Joshi W. A case of May-Thurner syndrome with antiphospholipid antibody syndrome. *Conn Med.* 2008;72(9):527–530.

95. Hermany PL, Badheka AO, Mena-Hurtado CI, Attaran RR. A unique case of May-Thurner syndrome: extrinsic compression of the common iliac vein after iliac artery stenting. *JACC Cardiovasc Interv.* 2016;9(5):e39–e41.

96. Pandit AS, Hayes M, Guiney-Borgelt S, Dietzek AM. Iatrogenic May-Thurner syndrome after EVAR. *Ann Vasc Surg.* 2014;28(3):739.e17–20.

97. Murphy EH, Davis CM, Journeycake JM, et al. Symptomatic ileofemoral DVT after onset of oral contraceptive use in women with previously undiagnosed May-Thurner syndrome. *J Vasc Surg.* 2009;49(3):697–703.

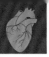

98. Jeon UB, Chung JW, Jae HJ, et al. May-Thurner syndrome complicated by acute iliofemoral vein thrombosis: helical CT venography for evaluation of long-term stent patency and changes in the iliac vein. *AJR Am J Roentgenol.* 2010;195(3):751–757.

99. Gurel K, Gurel S, Karavas E, et al. Direct contrast-enhanced MR venography in the diagnosis of May-Thurner syndrome. *Eur J Radiol.* 2011;80(2):533–536.

100. Oğuzkurt L, Ozkan U, Tercan F, Koç Z. Ultrasonographic diagnosis of iliac vein compression (May-Thurner) syndrome. *Diagn Interv Radiol Ank Turk.* 2007;13(3):152–155.

101. Fretz V, Binkert CA. Compression of the inferior vena cava by the right iliac artery: a rare variant of May-Thurner syndrome. *Cardiovasc Intervent Radiol.* 2010;33(5):1060–1063.

102. Vijayalakshmi IB, Setty HSN, Narasimhan C. Unusual cases of right-sided and left-sided May-Thurner syndrome. *Cardiol Young.* 2015;25(4):797–799.

103. Liew A, Douketis J. Catheter-directed thrombolysis for extensive iliofemoral deep vein thrombosis: review of literature and ongoing trials. *Expert Rev Cardiovasc Ther.* 2016;14(2):189–200.

104. Roy M, Sasson M, Rosales-Velderrain A, et al. Pharmacomechanical thrombolysis for deep vein thrombosis in May-Thurner syndrome. *Innov Phila Pa.* 2017;12(6):466–471.

105. Mousa AY, AbuRahma AF. May-Thurner syndrome: update and review. *Ann Vasc Surg.* 2013;27(7):984–995.

106. Zhang X, Shi X, Gao P, et al. Endovascular Management of May-Thurner syndrome: a case report. *Medicine (Baltimore).* 2016;95(4):e2541.

107. Mullens W, De Keyser J, Van Dorpe A, et al. Migration of two venous stents into the right ventricle in a patient with May-Thurner syndrome. *Int J Cardiol.* 2006;110(1):114–115.

108. DeStephano CC, Werner EF, Holly BP, Lessne ML. Diagnosis and management of iliac vein thrombosis in pregnancy resulting from May-Thurner syndrome. *J Perinatol Off J Calif Perinat Assoc.* 2014;34(7):566–568.

109. Wax JR, Pinette MG, Rausch D, Cartin A. May-Thurner syndrome complicating pregnancy: a report of four cases. *J Reprod Med.* 2014;59(5-6):333–336.

110. Park JY, Ahn JH, Jeon YS, et al. Iliac vein stenting as a durable option for residual stenosis after catheter-directed thrombolysis and angioplasty of iliofemoral deep vein thrombosis secondary to May-Thurner syndrome. *Phlebology.* 2014;29(7):461–470.

111. Moudgill N, Hager E, Gonsalves C, et al. May-Thurner syndrome: case report and review of the literature involving modern endovascular therapy. *Vascular.* 2009;17(6):330–335.

112. Kwak H-S, Han Y-M, Lee Y-S, et al. Stents in common iliac vein obstruction with acute ipsilateral deep venous thrombosis: early and late results. *J Vasc Interv Radiol.* 2005;16(6):815–822.

113. Garg N, Gloviczki P, Karimi KM, et al. Factors affecting outcome of open and hybrid reconstructions for nonmalignant obstruction of iliofemoral veins and inferior vena cava. *J Vasc Surg.* 2011;53(2):383–393.

114. Jost CJ, Gloviczki P, Cherry KJ, et al. Surgical reconstruction of iliofemoral veins and the inferior vena cava for nonmalignant occlusive disease. *J Vasc Surg.* 2001;33(2):320–327. discussion 327-328.

115. Levien LJ. Popliteal artery entrapment syndrome. *Semin Vasc Surg.* 2003;16(3):223–231.

116. Settembre N, Bouziane Z, Bartoli MA, et al. Popliteal artery entrapment syndrome in children: experience with four cases of acute ischaemia and review of the literature. *Eur J Vasc Endovasc Surg.* 2017;53(4):576–582.

117. Levien LJ, Veller MG. Popliteal artery entrapment syndrome: more common than previously recognized. *J Vasc Surg.* 1999;30(4):587–598.

118. Dijkstra ML, Khin NY, Thomas SD, Lane RJ. Popliteal vein compression syndrome pathophysiology and correlation with popliteal compartment pressures. *J Vasc Surg Venous Lymphat Disord.* 2013;1(2):181–186.

119. Aktan Ikiz ZA, Ucerler H, Ozgur Z. Anatomic variations of popliteal artery that may be a reason for entrapment. *Surg Radiol Anat.* 2009;31(9):695–700.

120. Politano AD, Bhamidipati CM, Tracci MC, et al. Anatomic popliteal entrapment syndrome is often a difficult diagnosis. *Vasc Endovascular Surg.* 2012;46(7):542–545.

121. Hislop M, Kennedy D, Cramp B, Dhupelia S. Functional popliteal artery entrapment syndrome: poorly understood and frequently missed? A review of clinical features, appropriate investigations, and treatment options. *J Sports Med (Hindawi Publ Corp).* 2014;2014:105953.

122. Pillai J. A current interpretation of popliteal vascular entrapment. *J Vasc Surg.* 2008;48(6 Suppl). 61S-65S; discussion 65S.

123. Sinha S, Houghton J, Holt PJ, Thompson MM, et al. Popliteal entrapment syndrome. *J Vasc Surg.* 2012;55(1):252-262.e30.

124. Sun X, Liu C, Wang R, et al. Dual source CT angiography in popliteal artery entrapment syndrome. *J Med Imaging Radiat Oncol.* 2013;57(2):156–160.

125. Zhong H, Gan J, Zhao Y, et al. Role of CT angiography in the diagnosis and treatment of popliteal vascular entrapment syndrome. *AJR Am J Roentgenol.* 2011;197(6):W1147–W1154.

126. Altintas U, Helgstrand UVJ, Hansen MA, et al. Popliteal artery entrapment syndrome: ultrasound imaging, intraoperative findings, and clinical outcome. *Vasc Endovascular Surg.* 2013;47(7):513–518.

127. Causey MW, Quan RW, Curry TK, Singh N. Ultrasound is a critical adjunct in the diagnosis and treatment of popliteal entrapment syndrome. *J Vasc Surg.* 2013;57(6):1695–1697.

128. Shen J, Abu-Hamad G, Makaroun MS, Chaer RA. Bilateral asymmetric popliteal entrapment syndrome treated with successful surgical decompression and adjunctive thrombolysis. *Vasc Endovascular Surg.* 2009;43(4):395–398.

129. Wang X, Zhang H, Yan J, Lu Z. Successful endovascular treatment of popliteal artery entrapment syndrome: a case report with 3-years follow-up. *J Thromb Thrombolysis.* 2017;44(1):112–117.

130. Ghotbi R, Deilmann K. Popliteal artery aneurysm: surgical and endovascular therapy. *Chirurg.* 2013;84(3):243–254.

131. Bürger T, Meyer F, Tautenhahn J, et al. Initial experiences with percutaneous endovascular repair of popliteal artery lesions using a new PTFE stent-graft. *J Endovasc Surg.* 1998;5(4):365–372.

132. Yamamoto S, Hoshina K, Hosaka A, et al. Long-term outcomes of surgical treatment in patients with popliteal artery entrapment syndrome. *Vascular.* 2015;23(5):449–454.

133. Desy NM, Spinner RJ. The etiology and management of cystic adventitial disease. *J Vasc Surg.* 2014;60(1). 235-245.e11.

134. Al Shaqsi S, Lesche S, Thomson I. Cystic adventitial disease of the external iliac artery: a rare cause of claudication. *N Z Med J.* 2015;128(1427):61–64.

135. Kim E, Lamb KM, Whisenhunt AK, et al. Venous cystic adventitial disease of the common femoral vein. *J Vasc Surg Venous Lymphat Disord.* 2014;2(2):194–196.

136. Park SJ, Park WS, Min SY, et al. Cystic adventitial disease of the common femoral artery at a previous surgical dissection site. *Ann Vasc Surg.* 2015;29(2):365.e1-365.e3.

137. Scott MF, Gavin T, Levin S. Venous cystic adventitial disease presenting as an enlarging groin mass. *Ann Vasc Surg.* 2014;28(2):489.e15-489.e18.

138. Motaganahalli RL, Smeds MR, Harlander-Locke MP, et al. A multi-institutional experience in adventitial cystic disease. *J Vasc Surg.* 2017;65(1):157–161.

139. Buijsrogge MP, van der Meij S, Korte JH, Fritschy WM. "Intermittent claudication intermittence" as a manifestation of adventitial cystic disease communicating with the knee joint. *Ann Vasc Surg.* 2006;20(5):687–689.

140. Tsilimparis N, Hanack U, Yousefi S, et al. Cystic adventitial disease of the popliteal artery: an argument for the developmental theory. *J Vasc Surg.* 2007;45(6):1249–1252.

141. Spinner RJ, Desy NM, Agarwal G, et al. Evidence to support that adventitial cysts, analogous to intraneural ganglion cysts, are also joint-connected. *Clin Anat N Y N.* 2013;26(2):267–281.

142. Brodmann M, Stark G, Pabst E, et al. Cystic adventitial degeneration of the popliteal artery—the diagnostic value of duplex sonography. *Eur J Radiol.* 2001;38(3):209–212.

143. Peterson JJ, Kransdorf MJ, Bancroft LW, Murphey MD. Imaging characteristics of cystic adventitial disease of the peripheral arteries: presentation as soft-tissue masses. *AJR Am J Roentgenol*. 2003;180(3):621–625.

144. Ali T, Krokidis ME, Winterbottom A. Peripheral non-atherosclerotic arterial disorders: what radiologists need to know. *Acad Radiol*. 2017;24(4):497–505.

145. Hennessy MM, McGreal G, O'Brien GC. Two cases of popliteal cystic adventitial disease treated with excision and primary bypass graft: a review of the literature. *Vasc Endovascular Surg*. 2017;51(7):480–484.

146. Gwon JG, Kwon Y-J, Han YJ, et al. Chronic nonatherosclerotic occlusive popliteal artery disease. *Ann Vasc Surg*. 2018;47:128–133.

147. Yurdakul M, Tola M. Resolution of adventitial cystic disease after unsuccessful attempt at aspiration. *J Vasc Interv Radiol*. 2011;22(3):412–414.

148. Seo H, Fujii H, Aoyama T, Sasako Y. A case of adventitial cystic disease of the popliteal artery progressing rapidly after percutaneous ultrasound-guided aspiration. *Ann Vasc Dis*. 2014;7(4):417–420.

149. Rosiak G, Milczarek K, Cieszanowski A, Rowiński O. Ultrasound-guided percutaneous aspiration of adventitial cysts in the occluded popliteal artery - clinical results and MR findings at 5-year follow-up. *J Ultrason*. 2017;17(70):212–216.

150. Fox RL, Kahn M, Adler J, et al. Adventitial cystic disease of the popliteal artery: failure of percutaneous transluminal angioplasty as a therapeutic modality. *J Vasc Surg*. 1985;2(3):464–467.

151. Khoury M. Failed angioplasty of a popliteal artery stenosis secondary to cystic adventitial disease: a case report. *Vasc Endovascular Surg*. 2004;38(3):277–280.

152. Maged IM, Kron IL, Hagspiel KD. Recurrent cystic adventitial disease of the popliteal artery: successful treatment with percutaneous transluminal angioplasty. *Vasc Endovascular Surg*. 2009;43(4):399–402.

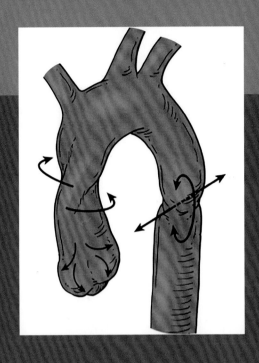

第64章
各类血管发育异常疾病：
血管瘤和血管畸形

　　本章介绍了两类血管异常：增生性的血管（肿）瘤及非增生性的血管畸形。血管瘤是内皮细胞的良性增生，由CD133血管瘤干细胞在子宫内发展而来，肢体血管瘤的解剖分布与胚胎动脉变异相关。典型的血管瘤可以是局灶性、多灶性和（或）节段性的。特别需要注意的是，根据血管瘤不同的临床表现，需要对与其相关的重要临床症状进行评估，其中弥漫性肝血管瘤死亡率高，需尽早干预。目前血管瘤的主要治疗药物为普萘洛尔，根据合并的不同临床表现使用其他药物辅助治疗。血管畸形是由于血管系统发育异常，可能涉及多种类型的血管，极少出现自发性退化。血管畸形可为遗传性，也可散发。遗传性血管畸形为常染色体显性或隐性遗传。治疗上，静脉血管畸形的患者疼痛发作时通常仅采用布洛芬；对于PROS、静脉畸形、淋巴管畸形、Gorham病、PTEN错构瘤综合征、蓝色橡皮疱痣综合征和卡波西型血管内皮瘤（kaposi form hemangioendothelioma，KHE），免疫抑制剂西罗莫司可以取得良好效果。患者需要接受预防性的抗生素治疗并进行血药浓度监测。

李　鑫

Peripheral Vascular Anomalies, Malformations, and Vascular Tumors

Francine Blei

Nonmalignant vascular anomalies can be functionally divided into two groups: vascular tumors and vascular malformations. Unfortunately, this distinction is not universally appreciated, due to "terminologic imprecision."[1,2] Despite efforts by vascular anomalies specialists to publicize the accurate lexicon, the term hemangioma (a vascular tumor) is often incorrectly applied to describe vascular malformations.[3]

The original classification proposed by Mulliken and Glowaki[4] has since been updated to include syndromic vascular anomalies, newly recognized diagnoses, and genetic mutations by The International Society for the Study of Vascular Anomalies (ISSVA) (http://www.issva.org/classification), an international group of vascular anomalies specialists (Table 64.1 and Box 64.1).[5] This group will regularly update the classification as new information emerges.

PROLIFERATIVE VASCULAR ANOMALIES AND TUMORS

Hemangiomas are considered the most common tumors of childhood. They are benign growths of endothelial cells with a unique natural history, characterized by a rapid growth phase usually beginning in the first weeks of life and continuing until 9 to 12 months of age (Fig. 64.1). Most hemangiomas subsequently undergo a spontaneous, gradual, but extensive involution. It is recommended to have infants with hemangiomas evaluated for early therapy to prevent further growth and expedite an earlier, more complete, involution. This will ideally minimize associated morbidities and abrogate the need for surgical intervention in the future.

The precise pathophysiology of hemangioma development is not fully defined; however, it is generally accepted that a CD133 hemangioma stem cell is targeted in utero to develop into a hemangioma postnatally in response to growth factors and environmental conditions. Initially, GLUT1, LYVE-1, and Lewis Y-positive endothelial cells are the predominant phenotype. During involution, apoptosis-related changes occur, dominated by adipocytes and fibrous tissue (Fig. 64.2).[6] One retrospective observational study hypothesized that the anatomic distribution of some extremity hemangiomas correlate with embryonic arterial variants which may cause transient focal intrauterine hypoxia that stimulates hemangioma stem cell proliferation (Fig. 64.3).[7] Less commonly, GLUT-1-positive segmental reticular telangiectatic hemangiomas (usually on the lower and distal extremities) can be associated with minimal cutaneous growth (so-called abortive hemangiomas or infantile hemangiomas with minimal or arrested growth [IH-MAG]) ± soft tissue hypertrophy, and are prone to ulceration.[7–11] Several studies have documented an increased incidence of parenchymal (usually hepatic) hemangiomas when greater than five cutaneous hemangiomas are present.[12] A study of 103 infants with multifocal infantile hemangiomas further categorized the lesions as miliary (small, focal, round, numerous) or nonmiliary (irregular, larger), and found that miliary hemangiomas were more prevalent in premature infants and were more likely to be associated with parenchymal (e.g., hepatic) hemangiomas.[13]

Important exceptions to this growth/regression pattern are the group of rapidly involuting congenital hemangiomas (RICH), which are generally present in full at birth (or even detected prenatally) and spontaneously remit (Fig. 64.4), and noninvoluting congenital hemangiomas (NICH) which do not change size postnatally.[14] Growth curves for these hemangiomas are illustrated in Fig. 64.5. A subset of patients with RICH may have high-flow lesions with prenatal or postnatal high-flow characteristics and/or transient coagulopathy.

"Congenital nonprogressive hemangiomas" have been shown by North and colleagues to be histologically and immunophenotypically distinct from classical hemangiomas of infancy and are speculated to have a differing pathogenesis.[15] NICH-type lesions were found to have high flow clinically (as assessed by Doppler) and inferred histologically (in that small arteries were seen "shunting" into lobular vessels or abnormal veins). Another subtype of hemangiomas are those with "minimal or arrested growth," presenting as areas of telangiectasia with peripheral bulkiness. In one series, most of this type of hemangioma were present on the lower extremities.[8]

"Typical" hemangiomas are known to be most common in females, premature infants, and in the facial region. Several studies have shown an increased incidence in white non-Hispanic infants, multiple gestation, infants born to older mothers, and in association with placenta previa and/or pre-eclampsia.[16] Hemangiomas can be focal, multifocal, and/or segmental. Segmental hemangiomas can be associated with a higher incidence of PHACE(S), visceral hemangiomas, underlying lumbosacral anomalies (e.g., occult spinal dysraphism including lipomyelomeningocele with tethered cord).[17] The PHACE(S) association is an acronym for: **P**osterior fossa structural malformations, **H**emangiomas (segmental), **A**rterial anomalies, **C**ardiac defects, **E**ye abnormalities, (and **S**ternal and other midline deformities).[18] A patient with a facial segmental hemangioma (>5 cm diameter) and one or more of the above criteria has PHACES (Fig. 64.6). Updated consensus-derived criteria for this diagnosis have been reported by Garzon et al.[18] In one series, approximately one-third of patients with facial segmental hemangiomas were found to have PHACES, those at higher risk having large hemangiomas involving more than one anatomical segment, and in the frontonasal or frontotemporal distribution. Of those with PHACES, most (90%) had >1 extracutaneous finding (most commonly central nervous system [CNS] arteriopathy or cardiac anomaly).[19] Similarly, Oza and colleagues observed that patients with large facial segmental cutaneous (Seg1-Seg4) hemangiomas were especially at risk of CNS structural and cerebrovascular anomalies, those with S1 distribution hemangiomas had a higher incidence of ocular anomalies, and those with S3 distribution had airway, ventral, and cardiac anomalies.[20] In this series, all patients with CNS structural

TABLE 64.1   Functional Classification of Vascular Anomalies

VASCULAR TUMORS			VASCULAR MALFORMATIONS	
Benign	**Locally Aggressive**	**Malignant**	**Simple**	**Combined**
Infantile hemangioma	Kaposiform hemangioendothelioma	Angiosarcoma	Capillary malformation (CM)	CVM, CLM
Congenital hemangioma	Retiform hemangioendothelioma	Epithelioid hemangioendothelioma	Lymphatic malformation (LM)	LVM, CLVM
Tufted hemangioma	PILA, Dabska tumor		Venous malformation (VM)	CAVM
Spindle-cell hemangioma	Composite hemangioendothelioma		Arteriovenous malformation (AVM)	CLAVM
Epithelioid hemangioma	Kaposi sarcoma		Arteriovenous fistula	
Pyogenic granuloma				

CAVM, Capillary arteriovenous malformation; *CLAVM,* capillary lymphatic arteriovenous malformation; *CLM,* capillary lymphatic malformation; *CLVM,* capillary lymphatic venous malformation; *CVM,* capillary venous malformation; *LVM,* lymphaticovenous malformation; *PILA,* papillary intralymphatic angioendothelioma.
Modified from International Society for the Study of Vascular Anomalies: ISSVA classification for vascular anomalies; May 2018. http://www.issva. org/classification. Accessed August 3, 2018. Licensed under a Creative Commons Attribution 4.0 International License. https://creativecommons. org/licenses/by/4.0/legalcode.

BOX 64.1   Supplementary Materials: Updated International Society for the Study of Vascular Anomalies Classification of Vascular Anomalies

Vascular Tumors	Vascular Malformations
Infantile hemangiomas	Capillary malformation (CM)
Congenital hemangioma	Port wine stain
Rapidly involuting congenital hemangioma (RICH)	Telangiectasia
	Angiokeratoma
Non-involuting congenital hemangioma (NICH)	Venous malformation (VM)
	Common sporadic VM
Tufted angioma (± Kasabach-Merritt syndrome)	Familial cutaneous and mucosal venous malformation (VMCM)
Kaposiform hemangioendothelioma (± Kasabach-Merritt syndrome)	Glomuvenous malformation (GVM) (glomangioma)
Spindle cell hemangioendothelioma	Blue rubber bleb syndrome
Other, rare hemangioendotheliomas (epithelioid, composite, retiform, polymorphous, Dabska tumor, lymphangioendotheliomatosis, etc.)	Maffucci syndrome
	Lymphatic malformation (LM)
	Fast-flow vascular malformations:
	Arterial malformation (AM)
	Arteriovenous fistula (AVF)
	Arteriovenous malformation (AVM)
Acquired vascular tumors (pyogenic granuloma, targetoid hemangioma, glomeruloid hemangioma, microvenular hemangioma, etc.)	Complex-combined vascular malformations:
	CVM, CLM, LVM, CLVM, AVM-LM, CM-AVM

AV, Arteriovenous; *C,* capillary; *L,* lymphatic; *V,* venous.

Data from International Society for the Study of Vascular Anomalies: ISSVA classification for vascular anomalies; May 2018. http://www. issva.org/classification. Accessed August 3, 2018. Licensed under a Creative Commons Attribution 4.0 International License. https:// creativecommons.org/licenses/by/4.0/legalcode.

anomalies had concomitant CNS arteriopathies. Also identified were supratentorial CNS anomalies (cortical dysgenesis and migration abnormalities). Arteriopathies are most commonly dysplastic vessels with an aberrant course involving the internal cerebral artery and its embryonic branches, ipsilateral to the side of the cutaneous hemangioma. Hypoplasia, agenesis, or absence of normal arteries can also occur and progressive changes can lead to aneurysm formation or moyamoya-type changes, and one group identified RNF213 variants in a PHACE patient who developed moyamoyavasculopathy.[21,22] In one study of 55 PHACE patients, 62% had a nonvascular intracranial anomaly, many of whom had structural brain malformations, pituitary anomalies, and intracranial hemangiomas.[23] Developmental delays and hearing loss may be associated with PHACE syndrome; thus, patients should be monitored closely for age-appropriate neurocognitive milestones.[24,25] Headaches are also more common in patients with PHACE syndrome, and should a patient have a hypoplastic or occlusive cerebral arteriopathy, triptans and other medications that can cause CNS vasoconstriction should be avoided.[26]

Some hemangiomas are small, asymptomatic, and located in areas that are not aesthetically sensitive; these may not require therapy. Hemangioma-associated morbidities include upper airway obstruction, ophthalmologic disturbances, ulceration, bleeding, persistent soft tissue deformity, cerebral vasculopathy, and/or high-output congestive heart failure. Additionally, hemangiomas may be the source of significant psychosocial stress, due to comments by others, and parental fears. Tables 64.2 and 64.3 summarize clinical and therapeutic issues relevant to hemangiomas.

Propranolol (nonselective β-blocker) has become an accepted and well-studied therapy for the treatment of hemangiomas of infancy.[27–29] This has revolutionized the therapy for infantile hemangioma warranting treatment, with numerous publications, the majority documenting its efficacy with high strength of evidence.[16,30] Side effects include cool extremities, sleep disturbances, gastrointestinal symptoms, hypotension, bronchial reactivity, and bradycardia with rare but significant reports of hypoglycemia.[6,16,28,31] Overall, systemic β-blocker therapy is generally well-tolerated, with proper patient selection and parental counseling to prevent undue side effects. Data on neurodevelopment and cognitive function in patients treated with propranolol for hemangiomas of infancy are thus far reassuring.[32–36] Excellent publications reviewing hemangioma management are provided in an Executive Summary by Darrow et al. and a comprehensive systematic review by Chinnadurai et al.[37,38] and reviews in Otolaryngology Clinics of North America (February 2018, Volume 51, Issue 1).

Oral propranolol, a nonselective β-blocker, has supplanted the previously used corticosteroid therapy, based upon a serendipitous observation when an infant with a proliferating infantile hemangioma was treated with this medication due to steroid-related cardiac issues.[39] The mechanism of β blockers on hemangiomas of infancy is under investigation. Studies have demonstrated the following effects: (1) inhibition

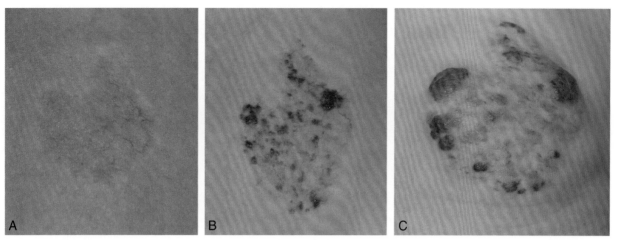

Fig. 64.1 Growth Stages of Infantile Hemangioma. (A) Infant at 6 days of age: note telangiectatic vessels with background pallor. (B) Infant at 5 weeks of age:—note proliferation of vessels. (C) Infant at 6 months of age: note further proliferation of vessels and subcutaneous vascular fullness.

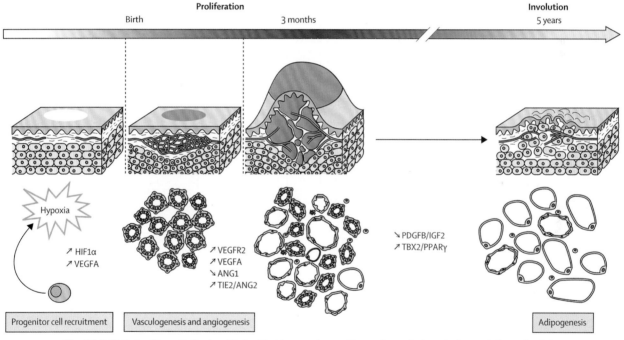

Fig. 64.2 Cellular Growth Cycle of Infantile Hemangioma. Progenitor cells targeted prenatally evolve into proliferative hemangiomas postnatally, with change in environment and growth factor stimuli. Endothelial cells in early proliferation, followed by addition of pericytes and ultimately adipocytes as hemangioma involutes. *ANG*, angiopoietin; *HIF1α*, hypoxic inducible factor 1α; *IGF*, insulin-like growth factor; *PDGF*, platelet-derived growth factor; *PPAR*, peroxisome-proliferator activated receptor; *TBX*, T-box transcription factor; *TIE*, angiopoietin receptor; *VEGF*, vascular endothelial growth factor; *VEGFR*, vascular endothelial growth factor receptor. (From Léauté-Labrèze C, Harper JI, Hoeger PH: Infantile haemangioma. *Lancet.* 2017;390:85–94.)

of proliferation (via G0/G1 cell cycle arrest) and chemotactic mobility and differentiation of cultured endothelial cells, (2) vascular endothelial growth factor (VEGF)-induced phosphorylation of VEGF R-2 and other angiogenesis-related pathways.[40] Several groups have shown the renin-angiotensin system is activated in hemangiomas of infancy, with elevated angiotensin converting enzyme (ACE) and angiotensin receptor 2 (ATII) in proliferating hemangioma cells, as well as serum elevations of ACE, ATII, and renin. Decreases in plasma renin and ATII post treatment downregulates this pathway in hemangiomas.[41–43] Other putative mechanisms involve vasoconstriction resulting from decreased nitric oxide release, cAMP-induced inhibition of VEGF- and

bFGF-induced endothelial cell proliferation, or inducing apoptosis via MAPK induction.[44–46]

Topical β blockers have also been shown to catalyze involution of superficial hemangiomas.[47,48] Systemic absorption of topical therapy is variable, and dependent upon the size and morphology of the hemangioma, application frequency, and technique. For very premature infants, the amount absorbed may be sufficient to cause symptoms.[49,50]

Ulcerated hemangiomas may respond to oral propranolol; however, adjunctive local therapies are often required. Recombinant platelet-derived growth factor has been effective for ulcerated hemangiomas; however, a "Black Box" warning limits its use. Various combinations of

	Area	n	Seg-mental (%)	IH-MAG (%)	Correlation with vascular anatomy
	Arms (total)	38	31 (81.6)	7 (18.4)	
A	Shoulder/ upper arm/ elbow	15	14	1	Superficial or accessory brachial artery
B	Whole arm	1	1	-	Subclavian artery
C	Whole arm (incomplete pattern) or Shoulder/ upper arm plus radial area	2	1	1	Brachioradial artery (either superficial or regular course)
D	Extensor side (covering back of hand), partly plus flexor side	13	11	2	Superficial brachio-ulnar artery or Superficial brachio-ulno-radial artery
E	Medial proximal or distal forearm	7	4	3	Median artery (antebrachial and palmar type)

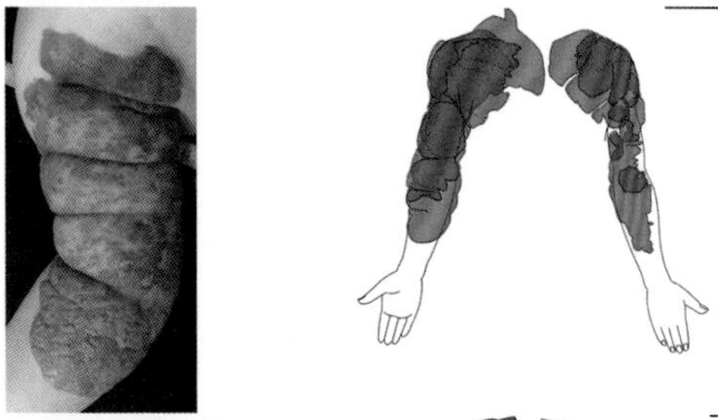

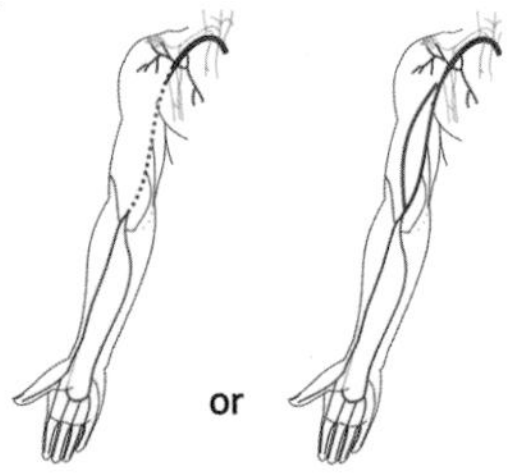

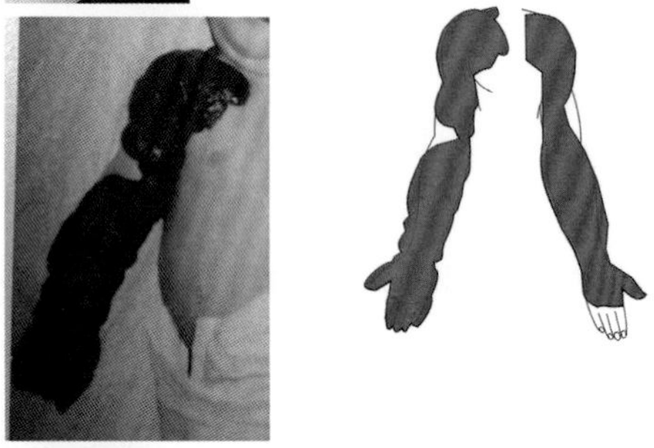

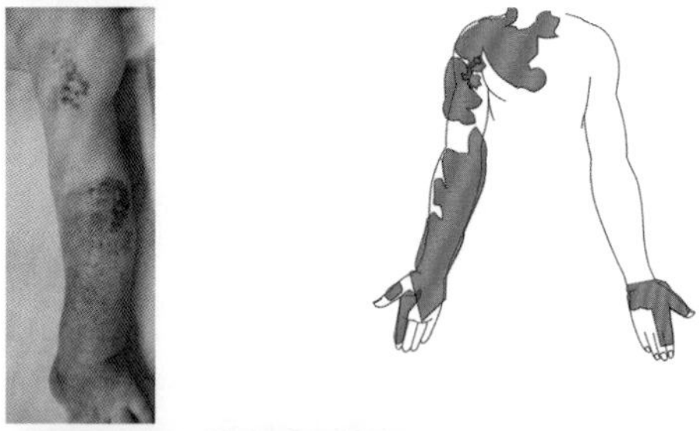

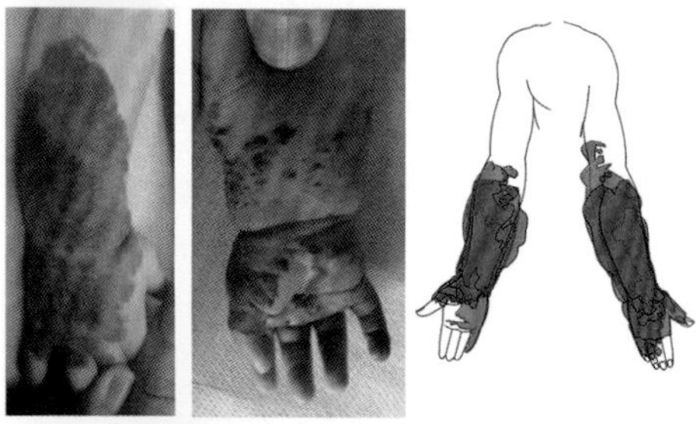

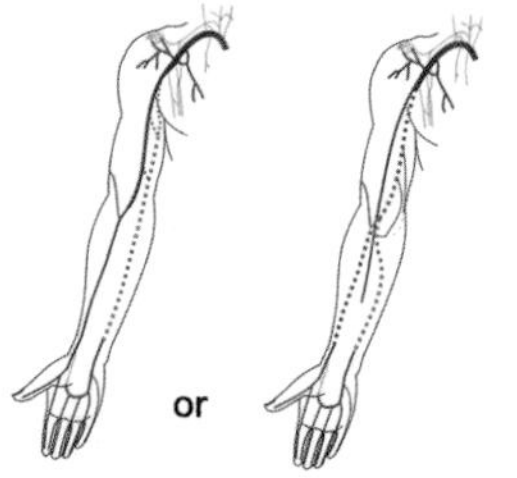

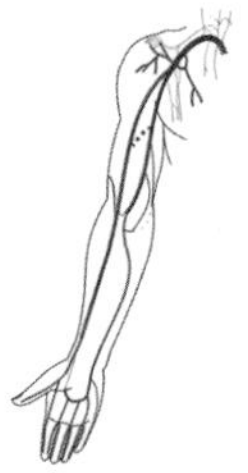

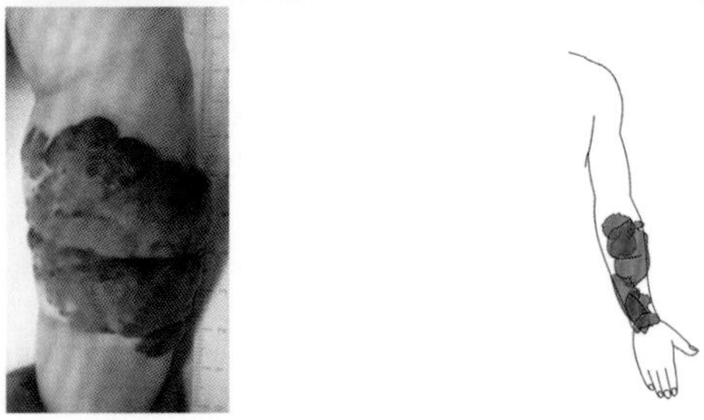

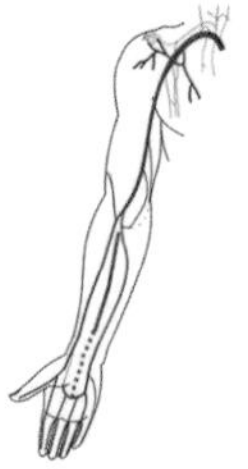

Fig. 64.3 Anatomic Distribution and Types of Extremity Hemangiomas. Areas affected by segmental infantile hemangioma (IH) and IH with minimal or arrested growth (IH-MAG) of the arms (A–E)

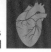

	Area	n	Segmental (%)	IH-MAG (%)		Correlation with vascular anatomy
	Hand-only	*30*	*26 (86.7)*	*4 (13.3)*		
F	Thenar, thumb and index finger	5	5	-	Radialis-sector	Distal radial artery
G	Index finger	6	5	1	Radialis-sector	Radialis index artery
H	Thumb	2	2	-	Radialis-sector	Princeps pollicis artery
I	Distal back of hand and dorsal fingers 2-3	3	2	1	Variations of deep palmar arch	Incomplete palmar arch
J	Back of hand and dorsal fingers	2	2	-	Variations of deep palmar arch	No dorsal net
K	Single fingers with adjacent metacarpal region	10	9	1	Affection of metacarpal and digital arteries	Dorsal metacarpal arteries
L	Little finger	2	1	1	Affection of metacarpal and digital arteries	Proper digital artery V

Fig. 64.3, cont'd and hands (F–L) with correlating arterial supply areas. (From Reimer A, Fliesser M, Hoeger PH. Anatomical patterns of infantile hemangioma (IH) of the extremities (IHE). *J Am Acad Dermatol.* 2016;75:556–563.)

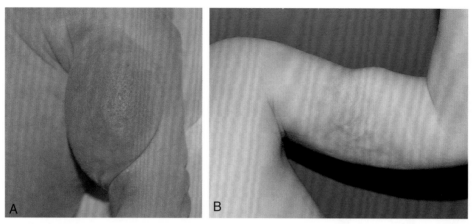

Fig. 64.4 Rapidly Involuting Congenital Hemangioma. (A) 1 week of age: note vascular mass with circumferential pallor. (B) 2 years of age: no treatment; lesion has spontaneously diminished in size, with residual anetoderma, pallor, and residual dilated veins.

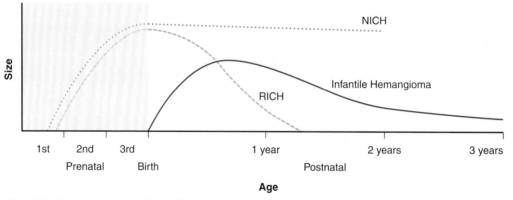

Fig. 64.5 Growth Patterns of Infantile Hemangiomas and Congenital Hemangiomas. Trends of growth for infantile hemangioma, rapidly involuting congenital hemangioma (RICH), and non-involuting congenital hemangioma (NICH). Congenital hemangiomas proliferate in utero and either gradually improve without therapy (RICH) or remain stable (NICH). There is also a subtype that partially involutes. Infantile hemangioma does not proliferate in utero but grows postnatally, then gradually involutes. See text for further details regarding each type of hemangioma. (From Mulliken JB, Enjolras O. Congenital hemangiomas and infantile hemangioma: missing links. *J Am Acad Dermatol.* 2004;50:875–882.)

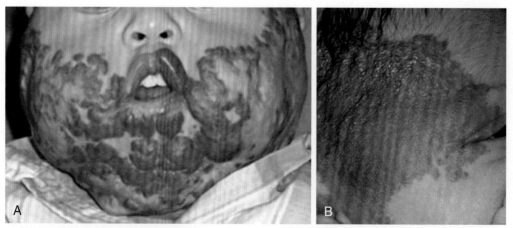

Fig. 64.6 Segmental Hemangiomas. Note "beard distribution" and Seg3 distribution (A). Patient also had subglottic hemangioma. Partial Seg1&2 hemangioma which extended to neck and back (B). Patient was also found to have PHACE arteriopathy.

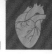

TABLE 64.2 Hemangiomas: Significant Clinical Issues Warranting Evaluation

Clinical Finding	Recommended Evaluation
Hemangiomatosis—multiple, small, cutaneous hemangiomas	Evaluate for parenchymal hemangiomas, especially hepatic/CNS/gastrointestinal
Cutaneous hemangiomas in "beard" distribution	Evaluate for airway hemangioma, especially presenting with stridor
Facial segmental hemangioma involving significant area of face (>5 cm)	Evaluate for PHACES—MRI ± contrast for orbital hemangioma ± posterior fossa malformation MRA brain, neck to thoracic aorta Cardiac, ophthalmologic evaluations supraumbilical raphe, sternal atresia, cleft
Paraspinal midline vascular lesion	Ultrasound (if less than 6 months of age) or MRI to evaluate for occult spinal dysraphism ± underlying vascular lesion
Thrill or bruit, or both, associated with hemangioma	Cardiac evaluation and echo to rule out diastolic reversal of flow of aorta MRI/Doppler of vascular lesion to evaluate flow characteristics
Large hemangioma Hepatic hemangiomas	Ultrasound with Doppler MRI + contrast CBC, metabolic panel, Thyroid function studies, quantitative α fetoprotein
Preferential position (e.g., torticollis)	Consider physical therapy evaluation
Delayed milestones	Consider CNS issues, hearing evaluation

CNS, Central nervous system; *MRA*, magnetic resonance angiography; *MRI*, magnetic resonance imaging.

TABLE 64.3 Clinical Findings and Treatment of Hemangiomas and Vascular Malformations

Clinical Finding	Recommended Treatment
Hemangiomas—severe ulceration/maceration	Encourage cleansing regimen twice daily Sterile saline soaks/air drying/non-stick gauze ± Metronidazole gel/Becaplermin gel ± Flashlamp-pulsed dye laser Oral β blocker Analgesics—topical, oral Surgery
Hemangioma—ophthalmologic sequelae	Patching therapy as directed by ophthalmologist Oral β blocker
Subglottic hemangioma	Laryngoscopy, possible bronchoscopy if not well visualized on laryngoscopy oral β blocker—further intervention depends on response
Kaposiform hemangioendothelioma or tufted angioma with Kasabach-Merritt phenomenon	Sirolimus, corticosteroids, vincristine
Vascular malformation limb-length discrepancy	Shoe insert vs. epiphysiodesis vs. serial observation Orthopedist must follow
Foot size/shoe-size discrepancy	
Vascular malformation—pain	Evaluate for phlebolith, infection, obstruction, or deep venous thrombosis Analgesics Anticoagulation if thrombosis May improve with sirolimus ± Nerve block, ± sclerotherapy (if not thrombosis)
Chylous ascites	Evaluate cause Drainage/low-fat diet/parenteral nutrition/albumin ± Immmunoglobulin replacement Sirolimus if indicated Other medications

local and systemic therapies for ulcerated hemangiomas are included in the reviews noted above. Topical or systemic antibiotics may be warranted for superinfected ulcerated hemangiomas, topical and/or analgesics, as well as hemostatic agents' bleeding.

Hepatic hemangiomas represent a special category. Although many hepatic hemangiomas are asymptomatic, a subset carries a high morbidity and mortality rate. They may be solitary or multiple and may be seen in association with cutaneous hemangiomatosis or be an isolated finding. There are three subtypes—focal, multifocal, and diffuse. The data presented in several recent review articles have demonstrated that focal hepatic hemangiomas are RICH-type hemangiomas, present in utero, and gradually involute without therapy. If symptomatic, highly vascular lesions may require intervention. Multifocal and diffuse hemangiomas are not detected in utero, and grow postnatally, in alignment with the growth curve of hemangiomas of infancy. Multifocal hepatic hemangiomas may transition to diffuse hepatic hemangiomas based on these studies. Diffuse hepatic hemangiomas are uncommon, may be associated with profound consumptive hypothyroidism due to elaboration of type 3-iodothyronine deiodinase and congestive heart failure, and have a high mortality rate. Approximately 50% of patients with diffuse hemangiomas did not have cutaneous hemangiomas.[51-53] Prompt diagnosis and therapy with systemic β blockers may be very effective.

The indications for and timing of surgery for hemangiomas remain controversial. Some surgeons prefer to defer surgery until the hemangioma has undergone substantial involution, with the rationale that the surgery will be less complex and aesthetically more favorable. Other surgeons advocate early intervention, to possibly prevent medical complications, or to avert the psychological stresses on the patient and/or family. In any case, a well-planned strategy with medical, laser, and surgical management decisions discussed among multidisciplinary physicians can provide excellent results. As noted above, as more effective medical therapies have been discovered, the role of surgery for hemangiomas has diminished.[54] Surgical techniques are not discussed in this chapter.

Kasabach-Merritt Phenomenon, Kaposiform Hemangioendothelioma, and Tufted Angioma

Trapping of platelets and other blood elements (Kasabach-Merritt phenomenon) has been known to occur in association with a subset of vascular anomalies since it was first described in 1940.[55] This is an extremely important diagnosis, as early detection and rapid evaluation and treatment (if clinically symptomatic) is essential. Kasabach-Merritt phenomenon is not associated with common hemangiomas of infancy but with Kaposiform hemangioendotheliomas (KHE) or tufted angiomas.[56,57] On examination, the lesion is often edematous, boggy, and ecchymotic (Fig. 64.7). Anatomic predilection is for the chest wall and shoulder, groin extending down the leg, retroperitoneum, or face. The gender distribution tends to be equal. Hematologic features of Kasabach-Merritt phenomenon include thrombocytopenia, hypofibrinogenemia, elevated fibrin degradation products, and elevated D-dimer. Radiologic hallmarks of KHE are cutaneous thickening, diffuse enhancement with ill-defined margins, small feeding/draining vessels, stranding, and hemosiderin deposits. The histologic features

of KHE are spindled endothelial cells resembling Kaposi sarcoma (KS, but not associated with HIV infection), abnormal lymphatic-like vessels, microthrombi, hemosiderin, and decreased mast cells and pericytes (which are often seen in hemangiomas). There may be residual tumor after resolution of hematologic abnormalities, and radiologic studies often demonstrate persistent vascular tumors. Residua of KHE-associated tumors may be "dormant" vascular tumors, rather than "scars." Clinically, as well as histologically, they differ considerably from involuted hemangioma. A subset of patients with KHE do not have an associated coagulopathy.[58] Treatment of KHE is not standardized, and depends on the morbidity, location, and radiologic features. Multimodal therapy may include steroids, chemotherapy (most commonly vincristine), sirolimus, interferon, antifibrinolytic agents, antiplatelet agents, embolization, or radiation. Surgery may be considered for localized lesions; however, excision is often not an option due to diffuse intramuscular involvement.[59,60] Studies are underway to compare different therapies.

Tufted angioma, first described in the late 1980s, is a benign vascular tumor typified by tufts of capillaries in the dermis. The clinical appearance ranges from erythematous, indurated, annular nodules to plaques, with or without hypertrichosis, commonly occurs on the trunk and extremities, and may be associated with Kasabach-Merritt phenomenon. KHE and tufted angioma may represent a continuum.[61] Other vascular diagnoses which may have thrombocytopenia and gastrointestinal bleeding in the neonatal age group include multifocal lymphangioendotheliomatosis with thrombocytopenia (MLT), a rare disorder characterized by multiple red-brown macular lesions with positive lymphatic markers (LYVE-1, D2-40).[62,63] Within the last several years, major research breakthroughs are unraveling potential etiologic factors leading to formation of hemangiomas, detailed in excellent reviews.[6,64-67] As subtypes of hemangiomas with segmental cutaneous distribution and associated visceral anomalies became evident, researchers speculated involvement of neural-crest derived cells, further supported by identification of neural crest cell markers (neurotrophin receptor; p75) in proliferating hemangioma tissue.[68] Several studies demonstrated markers for progenitor mesodermal stem cells (brachyury, GATA), or endothelial and hematopoietic cells (platelet endothelial adhesion molecule-1 (PECAM-1;CD31), intracellular adhesion molecule-2 (ICAM-3), bcl-2 gene expression, KDR+, CD133+, CD34+ endothelial precursor cells, and lymphatic

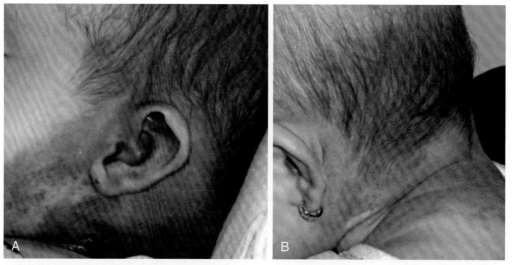

Fig. 64.7 Kaposiform Hemangioendothelioma. (A) Presenting with boggy diffuse mass, thrombocytopenia, and coagulopathy. (B) After several courses of vincristine therapy.

endothelial hyaluronan receptor-1, vWF;Snrk-1) in hemangioma tissue.[68–71] Constitutive activation of the endothelial tie-2 receptor and VEGFR2-related signaling pathways has been identified in human hemangioma of infancy.[64,66,72] Clonality of endothelial cells was demonstrated[73,74] as the potential role of endothelial cells in hemangioma development.[75–77] Bischoff et al. isolated *hemangioma-derived stem cells,* which unlike other precursor cells, grew in vitro and differentiated in vivo into cells with properties of hemangiomas including the eventual presence of adipocytes as seen in involuting hemangiomas.[78] Hemangiomas and placental vessels express common proteins including GLUT-1 (glucose transporter-1).[79] This discovery is of diagnostic utility and spearheaded insights into placenta-based hypotheses. For example, Mihm proposes a "metastatic niche" theory for hemangioma development, suggesting the placenta prepares hemangioma precursor cells which "home" to sites of hemangioma growth.[80] Proliferating hemangiomas have been shown to express VEGF-A as well as genes involved with NF-kappa-B-related pathways.[81,82] More recently, urinary excretion of MicroRNA126 was detected as a possible biomarker for infants with hemangiomas. Levels of this molecule correlated with hemangioma size and proliferative state[83] and VEGF-A isoforms and pericyte expression of DLL4 has been documented.[84] In addition, pro-apoptotic factors and appearance of adipocytes during the involution phase studies support a role for inflammation and immunoregulation in this process.[85] Somatic mutations in GNAQ and GNA11 have been identified in RICH and NICH tissue samples.[86]

Pyogenic Granuloma

Pyogenic granuloma (PG, also termed lobular capillary hemangioma) is an acquired vascular lesion of the skin and mucous membranes seen in pediatric patients. The lesions have a cervicofacial propensity but can also be located on the trunk or extremities. The majority occurs on the skin, and less frequently the mucous membranes (oral cavity and conjunctivae), and they may develop within capillary malformations (port wine stains). These lesions are small, papular, and tend to bleed. Treatment includes: topical β-blocker therapy, excision and linear closure, shave excision, cauterization, cryotherapy, CO_2 or pulsed dye laser, or sclerotherapy.[87] Somatic RAS and BRAF mutations have been identified in PG.[88,89]

Kaposi Sarcoma

KS is a neoplasm commonly but not exclusively seen in patients with AIDS (classic KS vs. AIDS-related KS).[90] Post-transplant KS can occur as a result of immunosuppressive therapy for solid organ or hematopoietic cell transplantation.[91,92] It is an unusual vascular neoplasm originally described in 1872. The clinical appearance begins as violaceous macular patches, which progress to plaques and papules and then nodules, which can extravasate. KS is thought to be multifocal rather than metastatic, with numerous lesions occurring simultaneously at different anatomic locations. Histologic features include spindle cells (derived from mesenchymal precursors), with rare mitotic figures. A novel human herpes virus, known as Kaposi sarcoma-associated herpes virus (KSHV), or human herpes virus type 8 (HHV8), has been identified in KS tissue, supporting a viral etiology. There is evidence that proliferation, inflammation, and angiogenesis occur in KS.[90] One model suggests KSHV contributes to endothelial reinfection by inducing lytic gene expression and interfering with its DNA.[93] Classic KS is more indolent than AIDS-related KS, which can be life-threatening and progress to visceral involvement. Therapies directed against KS include antiviral agents, antiangiogenic drugs, and immunosuppressive agents. Recent studies show the effectiveness of antiretroviral therapy suppressing HIV/AIDS-associated KS growth.[94] Post-transplant KS

has been shown to resolve with immune reconstitution and replacing calcineurin inhibitors with mTOR inhibitors.[90,92]

VASCULAR MALFORMATIONS

Vascular malformations (Tables 64.3 and 64.4) are present at birth and have no propensity to spontaneous involution (with rare exceptions). They are due to developmental anomalies of the vasculature and may involve one or several types of vessels (arteries, veins, capillaries, or lymphatics). They can be isolated lesions or syndromic, occurring in conjunction with other attributes (Fig. 64.8). Vascular malformations are properly described according to the affected anomalous vascular channel and can range from capillary malformations (commonly referred to as port wine stains) (Fig. 64.9) to large, bulky growths that can distort the normal structures of the body and potentially lead to a high output cardiac state (arterial malformations). Vascular malformations can progress with time. Many patients experience symptoms in relation to hormonal changes (e.g., puberty, menstrual cycle), and a subgroup of patients with vascular malformations may have recalcitrant disease (e.g., aggressive arteriovenous malformations [AVMs]). The pathologic basis of vascular malformations is a rich area of basic and genetic research. Several signaling pathways have been identified, leading to new therapies.

It is essential to appreciate the normal development in the vasculature, which has two main components—(1) the closed circulatory system of arteries, veins, and capillaries, and (2) the unidirectional lymphatic system, which drains into the venous system (see Chapter 57). Each vascular branch has specified endothelial cells, designed to perform distinctive properties and functions, with characteristic morphologic features and marker expression. Mesenchyme-derived endothelial progenitor cells differentiate into arterial or venous networks. Lymphatic vessels are derived from venous- and non-venous mesenchymal-derived cells. Complex pathways involving cell-cell interactions modulated by transcription factors, growth factors, and environmental conditions generate the lymphatic and lymphatic vasculature. As vascular and lymphatic cells mature, they express different markers, which are exploited in research studies and clinical diagnosis.[95,96] Disorders of vascular and lymphatic vessel morphogenesis may lead to vascular malformations (capillary, arterial, venous, lymphatic, or combined) lymphangiectasia, lymphatic anomalies with bony involvement (Gorham Stout/generalized lymphatic anomaly), or lymphedema (see Chapter 57).

Vascular malformations can be sporadic or inherited, and genetic mutations have now been identified for many of these (see below). Nonfamilial vascular malformations can be sporadic or due to somatic (post-zygotic) mutations, singularly expressed in a mosaic distribution in affected tissue. Inherited vascular malformations can be transmitted as autosomal recessive or autosomal dominant, or they can be genomic with a second somatic mutation within affected tissues, in which case carriers are unaffected. Inherited disorders can be identified via Sanger sequencing of blood samples, while samples of affected tissue are required to identify the causal mutation in somatic mosaic disorders.[97–100] Happle proposed somatic mosaicism as a mechanism for survival of potentially "lethal genes" (i.e., germline expression would be fatal, thus they can only be conveyed mosaically), and he provides an updated review of this timely topic.[101] Interestingly, most of the causal genes are mutations of TGF-β and phosphatidylinositol 3-kinase signaling pathways, not specific mutations of extracellular matrix or vascular structural proteins, even though the disorders affect specific vessels.[102,103] Several publications summarizing genetic techniques and findings in vascular and lymphatic anomalies are now available.[97,104–109] Studies on patient tissue, zebrafish, and transgenic mice have contributed to

TABLE 64.4   Syndromic Vascular Anomalies and Genetic Information

Name	Features	OMIM
Blue rubber bleb nevus syndrome Bean syndrome TIE2 mutation somatic	Multiple small soft venous malformations on skin, GI tract, elsewhere	112200
CLOVES syndrome PIK3CA somatic	Congenital lipomatous overgrowth, vascular malformations, and epidermal nevi, skeletal/spinal anomalies	612918
Gorham syndrome Gorham Stout syndrome Cystic angiomatosis of bone, diffuse Disappearing bone disease	Lymphangiomatosis, bony destruction	123880
Klippel Trénaunay syndrome PIK3CA somatic	Capillary, venous, ± lymphatic malformation, hypertrophy of the related bones and soft tissues ± Atretic deep venous system of affected extremity	149000
Maffucci syndrome Osteochondromatosis/dyschondroplasia with vascular lesions IDH1, IDH2 somatic	Enchondromatosis and subcutaneous spindle cell hemangioendotheliomas Risk of chondrosarcoma, other malignancies including CNS	166000
Proteus syndrome AKT1 somatic	Gigantism, partial, of hands and feet, nevi, asymmetric and disproportionate overgrowth, hemihypertrophy, macrocephaly, dysregulated adipose tissue, vascular malformations.	176920
Capillary malformation-AVM (Fig. 64.8) **CMAVM1** 5q14.3 RASA-1 loss of function **CMAVM2** 7q22.1 EPHB4 loss of function	Multifocal small macular capillary malformations + AVM	608354
Parkes Weber syndrome 5q14.3 RASA-1 loss of function	AV fistulae of extremity with soft tissue and skeletal hypertrophy	608355
Venous malformations, multiple cutaneous and mucosal; VMCM 9p21 TIE2/TEK gain of function AD Most are sporadic	Focal venous dilation with sparse vascular smooth muscle cells Cutaneous, mucosal, ± underlying areas	600195
Hennekam syndrome 18q21.32 Type 1: CCBE1 Type 3: ADAMTS3	Intestinal lymphangiectasia, severe lymphedema mental retardation	235510
Hypotrichosis-lymphedema-telangiectasia syndrome HLTS 20q13.33 SOX18	Alopecia and/or areas of sparse hair, transparent skin, lymphedema, telangiectasia	607823
Lymphedema-distichiasis syndrome 16q24.3 AD or de novo FOXC2 loss of function	Limb edema and double rows of eyelashes (distichiasis) ± other associated anomalies including cardiac, renal, vascular, CNS gene mutation	153400
Milroy disease 5q35.3 AD, AR, or de novo FLT4 VEGFR3 loss of function	Primary congenital hereditary lymphedema type Ia	153100
Lymphedema praecox Meige disease Late-onset lymphedema	Hereditary lymphedema type II Peri-pubertal onset	153200

(continued)

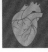

TABLE 64.4 Syndromic Vascular Anomalies and Genetic Information—cont'd

Name	Features	OMIM
Lymphangioleiomyomatosis 16p13.3, 9q34	Pulmonary (and extrapulmonary) lymphangiomyomatosis—female predominance, adult onset	606690
Hereditary hemorrhagic telangiectasia Osler Weber Rendu AD Loss of function *HHT Type I* 9q34.1 Endoglin Part of TGF-β receptor complex *HHT Type 2* 12q11-q14 ALK1/ACVRLK1 Cell-surface receptor for TGF-β superfamily *HHT Type 3* 5q31.3-q32 *HHT Type 4* 7p14 Juvenile polyposis/hereditary hemorrhagic telangiectasia syndrome; JPHT 18q21.1 SMAD4 Tumor suppressor; mutations affect TGF-β signaling	Cutaneous, mucosal, and visceral telangiectasias and AVMs Epistaxis and gastrointestinal bleeding, ± pulmonary AV fistulas, hepatic, CNS, spinal AVM HHT1: cerebral AVMs > pulmonary AVMs HHT2: hepatic AVMs more common	187300 600376 601101 610655 175050
Cutis marmorata telangiectatica congenita CMTC Macrocephaly-cutis marmorata telangiectatica congenita	Cutaneous reticulated mottling, telangiectasia, and phlebectasia, undergrowth or overgrowth of an involved extremity ± other anomalies	219250
Glomuvenous malformation GVM AD 1p22-p21 Glomulin FKBP (FK506 binding proteins)-associated protein, 48-KD; FAP48	Cutaneous venous malformations with glomus cells surrounding distended vein-like channels	138000
PHACES syndrome	**P**osterior fossa brain malformations Segmental facial **H**emangiomas **A**rterial anomalies **C**ardiac anomalies **E**ye abnormalities **S**ternal or midline anomalies	606519
Bannayan-Riley-Ruvalcaba 10q23.31 PTEN gene mutation Tumor suppressor	Macrocephaly, multiple lipomas, vascular anomalies, pigmented macules of the penis	153480
Cowden syndrome 10q23.31 AD PTEN gene mutation Tumor suppressor PTEN hamartoma tumor syndrome (PHTS)	Macrocephaly, multiple hamartomas, cutaneous verrucous lesions, gingival/buccal papules, facial trichilemmomas, risk of breast/thyroid/renal/endometrial malignancies, cerebelloparenchymal disorder VI (Lhermitte-Duclos disease)	158350
Solamen syndrome (type 2 Cowden's) 10q23.31 biallelic AD with ?mosaic PTEN wild-type allelic loss PTEN gene mutation Tumor suppressor Overlap with proteus syndrome phenotype	Segmental overgrowth lipomatosis Arteriovenous malformation Epidermal nevus Cancers—breast, thyroid, ovarian Loss-of-function PTEN activates AKT1	158350

ACVRLK1, Activin A receptor, type II-like kinase 1; *AD,* autosomal dominant; *AVM,* arteriovenous malformation; *CCBE1,* collagen and calcium-binding EGF domain-containing protein 1; *CNS,* central nervous system; *GI,* gastrointestinal; *PTEN,* phosphatase and tensin homolog; *RASA-1,* RAS p21 protein activator 1; *TGF-β,* transforming growth factor-β; *VEGFR3,* vascular endothelial growth factor receptor 3.

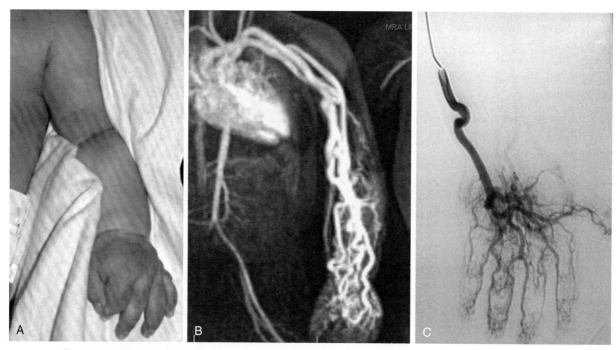

Fig. 64.8 RASA-1 Related Capillary Arteriovenous Malformation. (A) This infant presented with high output cardiac failure, and a thrill and bruit on the left arm. Note the cutaneous macular vascular discoloration. (B) Magnetic resonance image of the patient. (C) Angiogram of the patient. Over time, several new small macular lesions developed. The patient and a parent (who had one cutaneous macular vascular lesion only) harbored the RASA-1 mutation.

vascular and lymphatic vascular biology, providing models for study of specific disorders and potential therapies.[95,110–112]

Several mutations have now been identified in patients with vascular anomalies. Familial vascular anomalies (caused by genomic mutations) include the following: hereditary hemorrhagic telangiectasia, familial mucocutaneous venous malformations, CM-AVM, glomuvenous malformation, PTEN Hamartoma syndrome, and heritable lymphedema syndromes.

Hereditary hemorrhagic telangiectasias (HHT) are caused by mutations in the TGFβ pathway/BMP/SMAD: Eng (endoglin), Alk1 (activin receptor kinase), and SMAD4 (mothers against decapentaplegic homolog 4).[113] Tie-2 venous malformations are caused by activating mutations of the TEK receptor tyrosine kinase, which encodes protein tyrosine kinase Tie2. The ligand for this receptor is angiopoietin-1. Studies by Natynki et al. suggest that mutant TIE2 contributes to the endothelial morphology and coagulopathy seen in venous malformations due to upregulation of the MAPK pathway and plasminogen activator system, respectively.[107] Two types of embryonic stem cells (outside and within the endothelium) have been identified in subcutaneous and intramuscular vascular malformations, with evidence to suggest that the endothelial population arises first, and may be affected by TIE2 mutations.[112] Familial capillary malformation arteriovenous malformation may be associated with RASA1 (CM-AVM1) or EphrinB4 (CM-AVM2).[114,115] RASA 1 mutations have also been identified in patients with Parkes Weber syndrome (OMIM 608355), a condition with multiple arteriovenous fistulas in an extremity, with skeletal and soft tissue hypertrophy.

Glomuvenous malformations (glomulin) are due to germline loss of function mutations in the glomulin gene, expressed in high penetrance.[116] Cowden and Bannayan Riley Ruvalcaba syndromes harbor a germline mutation in the PTEN gene. Heritable lymphedemas may be due to a variety of mutations of genes important in lymphangiogenesis.

Sporadic and syndromic vascular malformations have been shown to be due to somatic mutations in an angiogenesis-related signaling pathway. Somatic mutations of TEK (TIE2) have been identified in sporadic venous malformations and blue rubber bleb nevus syndrome.[117,118] GNAQ somatic mutations have been identified in capillary malformations/Sturge-Weber syndrome and congenital hemangioma.[86,119,120] PI3K-AKT-MTOR-related disorders constitute a wide spectrum, including syndromic vascular anomalies and developmental brain disorders, termed PIK3CA-related overgrowth spectrum (PROS), PTEN mutations, and AKT mutations.[98,105,121,122] Fig. 64.10 illustrates the PI3K-AKT-MTOR pathway. Proteus syndrome, CLOVES (congenital, lipomatous, overgrowth, vascular malformations, epidermal nevi, and spinal/skeletal anomalies and/or scoliosis) syndrome. Klippel Trénaunay syndrome, megalencephaly-capillary malformation (MCAP or M-CM), fibroadipose vascular anomaly as well as other mosaic overgrowth syndromes without vascular malformations are included in the PROS spectrum. Fig. 64.11 delineates the phenotypic criteria and clinical spectrum of PROS (PIK3CA-related overgrowth syndrome) disorders. Proteus syndrome is caused by a somatic AKT mutation, PTEN-related overgrowth syndromes are due to a germline PTEN mutation, and the remainder (CLOVES [congenital, lipomatous, overgrowth, vascular malformations, epidermal nevi, and spinal/skeletal anomalies and/or scoliosis]) syndrome is due to a somatic mutation of PIK3CA. Klippel Trénaunay syndrome, MCAP or M-CM, or fibroadipose vascular anomaly are due to somatic PIK3CA mutations. Recently, Couto et al. identified somatic mutations of mitogen activated protein kinase kinase 1 (MAP2K1) in most tissue samples from patients with extracranial arteriovenous malformations.[123]

Disorders of the lymphatic circulation are common, diverse, and may have complex functional consequences (Fig. 64.12). Clinical issues common to lymphatic anomalies reflect the tendency of these malformations to develop: (1) local (and systemic) infections/cellulitis (infectious and aseptic); (2) leakage (e.g., superficial

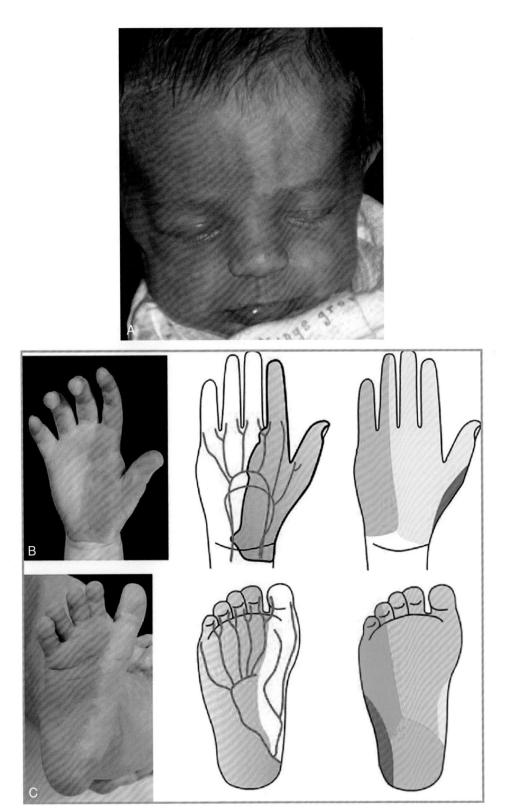

Fig. 64.9 Capillary Malformation in a Patient with Sturge-Weber Syndrome. There is a limb involvement manifest as a port wine stain (A) showing similarity to the vascular distribution in the palm (B) and sole of the feet (C). ([B and C] From Waelchli R, Aylett SE, Robinson K, et al. New vascular classification of port-wine stains: improving prediction of Sturge-Weber risk. *Br J Dermatol.* 2014;171:861–867. Adapted from Gray H, ed. *Anatomy of the Human Body.* 20th ed. Philadelphia: Lea & Febiger; 1918.)

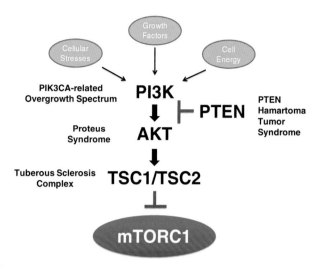

Fig. 64.10 The PI3K-AKT-MTOR Pathway Implicated in the Development of Vascular Malformations. Many vascular malformations are caused by defects in this pathway, targeted pharmacologically with m-TOR inhibitors. (From Nathan N, Keppler-Noreuil KM, Biesecker LG, et al. Mosaic disorders of the PI3K/PTEN/AKT/TSC/mTORC1 signaling pathway. *Dermatol Clin.* 2017;35:51–60.)

blebs, chylous ascites, chylothorax, peritonitis, pleural effusions); (3) malabsorption syndromes with significant metabolic consequences; (4) craniofacial distortion interfering with swallowing, airway, or significant visceral dysfunction; (5) recurrences or complications after surgery; and (6) swelling of the affected anatomy, with functional limitation. More diffuse and aggressive lymphatic lesions may cause osteolysis (Gorham Stout disease), and generalized lymphatic anomaly is associated with multifocal lymphatic malformations ± bony involvement, without loss of cortical bone, as seen in Gorham Stout disease. Clinical and imaging features of Gorham Stout and generalized lymphatic anomalies are reviewed by Lala et al.[124]

SYNDROMIC VASCULAR ANOMALIES

Evaluation of patients with vascular malformations entails a complete history and thorough physical examination. Family history and associated symptoms (e.g., assessment for bleeding, thromboses, pain, airway, neurologic, gastrointestinal, ophthalmologic, or orthopedic issues, head size/macrocephaly, cutaneous abnormalities) are essential to establishing the correct diagnosis. Imaging techniques employed in studying patients with vascular anomalies vary by location and type of vascular anomaly. Ultrasound, magnetic resonance (MR) imaging, MR angiography, MR venography, and lymphoscintigram are utilized, depending on the clinical backdrop. There are several excellent papers reviewing the optimal radiologic assessment of patients with vascular anomalies.[124–128]

There is a spectrum of vascular malformations with dysregulated skeletal/adipose/soft tissue growth. Klippel-Trénaunay syndrome (capillary-lymphatic-venous malformation with ipsilateral limb enlargement or hypoplasia; venous varicosities or developmental anomalies, or both) is one of the most common peripheral vascular malformation syndromes (Fig. 64.13). Males and females are affected in equal proportion, and the lower limb is the most frequent site of the anomaly. In severe cases, there may be an accompanying bleeding diathesis characterized by a normal to slightly decreased platelet count, decrease in fibrinogen, and increased D-dimers and fibrin degradation products (Fig. 64.14).[129]

Patients with Sturge-Weber syndrome have a facial capillary malformation associated with intracranial angiomatosis and dysplasia, seizures, and glaucoma due to dysmorphogenesis of cephalic neuroectoderm. Recent studies have updated the highest risk capillary malformation locations to a large swath of the forehead (medial canthus to helix of ear) correlating with a facial embryonic vascular placode in a somatic mosaic pattern (Fig. 64.15).[130,131] Additionally, patients with lesions with higher surface areas (e.g., bilateral) in the above location had more extensive MRI abnormalities. Two other points of interest in this study also pointed out that (1) capillary malformations of the frontonasal prominence (lower facial placode #1) were associated with Sturge-Weber syndrome, and (2) Sturge-Weber brain abnormalities may also be seen in patients without facial birthmarks (usually with later onset and more attenuated disease).[132] Shirley et al. identified a single nucleotide (c.548G→A, p.Arg183Gln) somatic activating mutation of GNAQ associated with capillary malformations in patients with Sturge-Weber syndrome.[120] Ideally, studies will be able to identify pre-symptomatic high-risk patients and offer preventive treatments.[133]

Other examples of dysmorphic syndromes associated with vascular malformation are Turner and Noonan syndromes, Parkes Weber syndrome, HHT, blue rubber bleb nevus syndrome, Maffucci syndrome, CLOVES syndrome and Proteus syndrome, Bannayan-Riley-Ruvalcaba syndrome, and Cowden syndrome (see Table 64.4). Syndromes noted for CNS vascular anomalies include HHT, von Hippel-Lindau, ataxia-telangiectasia, Sturge-Weber syndrome, and tuberous sclerosis; however, CNS and spinal arterial or venous anomalies are now known to occur in association with a number of vascular anomalies.[23,134–136] Dysmorphic syndromes associated with hemangiomas are predominantly associated with superficial segmental hemangiomas such as PHACES association or sacral and/or genitourinary defects, associated with hemangiomas in the lumbar area.[137]

PTEN-Associated Hamartoma Syndromes

PTEN (phosphatase and tensin homolog protein) is a tumor suppressor gene. Patients with a PTEN mutation are susceptible to cancers and warrant early and regular screening. Some patients with vascular anomalies (arteriovenous, lymphatic, venous) have the PTEN mutation, such as Cowden syndrome and Bannayan-Riley-Ruvalcaba syndromes.[138] A family history or presence of lipomas, thyroid disorders, trichilemmomas, macrocephaly, or penile lentigines should alert the practitioner to a PTEN-related syndrome. Consultation with a geneticist with family screening for mutations is indicated, and early screening for thyroid, breast, brain, gynecologic, and other cancers should be initiated for all individuals with the PTEN mutation.[139] Adipose-rich vascular lesions can be present in patients with PTEN mutations.[140]

Patients with Cowden syndrome have typical skin growths that may resemble small, uniform cutaneous and mucosal warts or skin tags, macrocephaly, and cognitive delay. Malignancies seen in patients with Cowden syndrome include: cancers of the breast, thyroid, gastrointestinal tract, renal structures, or endometrium. Benign tumors include thyroid nodules, breast masses, and a noncancerous brain tumor called Lhermitte-Duclos disease. Often the suspicion of Cowden syndrome begins with a family history of thyroid nodules, lipomas (benign fatty lumps), and/or cancers. If the family history and clinical spectrum (macrocephaly, hamartomas, skin tag-appearing lesions) are present, the patient and family should be referred to a genetics specialist for further discussion and blood testing for the presence of the PTEN mutation. Since not all the mutations are available for testing, more sophisticated tests may be required if the initial test is negative and the patient/family fulfills the criteria for the disorder. Upon the suspicion or diagnosis of Cowden syndrome, individuals should be placed in a

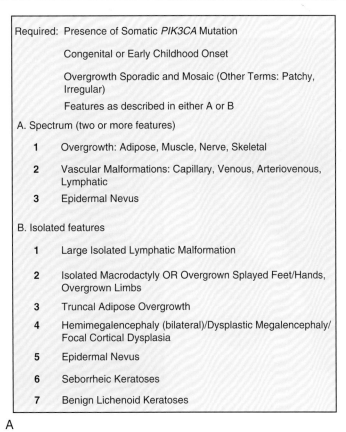

Required: Presence of Somatic *PIK3CA* Mutation

Congenital or Early Childhood Onset

Overgrowth Sporadic and Mosaic (Other Terms: Patchy, Irregular)

Features as described in either A or B

A. Spectrum (two or more features)

1   Overgrowth: Adipose, Muscle, Nerve, Skeletal

2   Vascular Malformations: Capillary, Venous, Arteriovenous, Lymphatic

3   Epidermal Nevus

B. Isolated features

1   Large Isolated Lymphatic Malformation

2   Isolated Macrodactyly OR Overgrown Splayed Feet/Hands, Overgrown Limbs

3   Truncal Adipose Overgrowth

4   Hemimegalencephaly (bilateral)/Dysplastic Megalencephaly/ Focal Cortical Dysplasia

5   Epidermal Nevus

6   Seborrheic Keratoses

7   Benign Lichenoid Keratoses

A

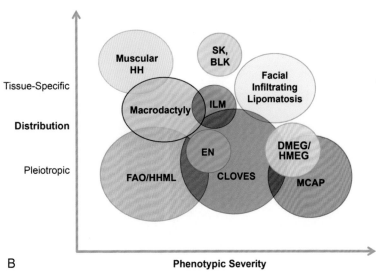

B

Fig. 64.11 Diagnostic criteria (A) and clinical spectrum (B) of PIK3CA-related overgrowth spectrum disorders.

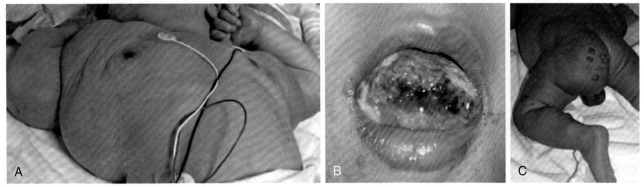

Fig. 64.12 Lymphatic Malformation. Lymphatic malformation of chest wall (A), tongue (B), and buttocks/leg (C).

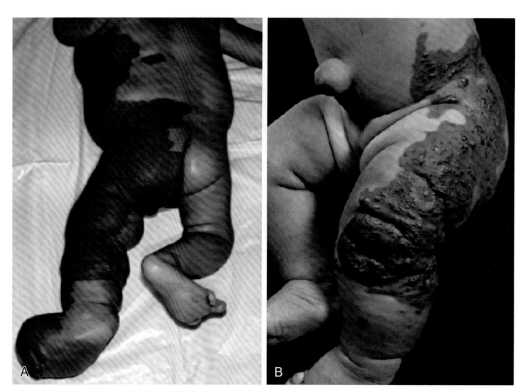

Fig. 64.13 (A) Patient with Klippel-Trénaunay vascular malformation syndrome (capillary, lymphatic, and venous malformation with hypertrophy), complicated by leg-length discrepancy, asymmetric foot size requiring custom orthotics, lymphopenia, and frequent septic episodes due to abnormal lymphatic communications. (B) Patient with Klippel-Trénaunay vascular malformation syndrome, leg length discrepancy, with cutaneous capillary malformation and blebs prone to bleeding.

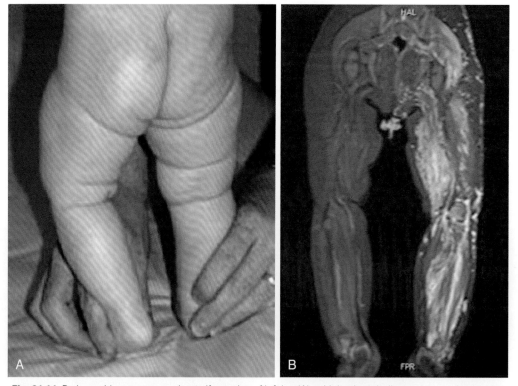

Fig. 64.14 Patient with venous vascular malformation of left leg (A), with leg length discrepancy and extensive involvement as noted on magnetic resonance imaging (B). Patient later developed knee contractures, pain, and coagulopathy.

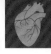

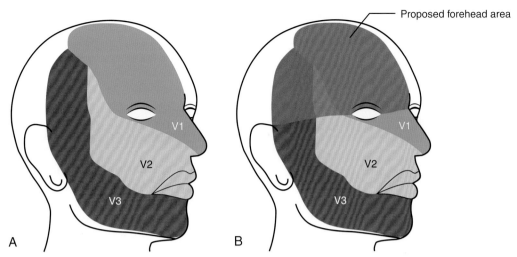

Proposed forehead area

Fig. 64.15 (A and B) Sturge-Weber syndrome. Updated anatomic pattern of distribution (B) delineating patients most at risk of having Sturge-Weber syndrome. (Redrawn from Waelchli R, Aylett SE, Robinson K, et al. New vascular classification of port-wine stains: improving prediction of Sturge-Weber risk. *Br J Dermatol.* 171:861–867.)

cancer surveillance program to facilitate early detection and prompt referral for further evaluation and treatment.

Bannayan-Riley-Ruvalcaba syndrome is characterized by macrocephaly, noncancerous lipomas, vascular malformations, intestinal polyps, thyroid disorders, pectus excavatum, hyperextensible joints, proximal muscle abnormalities, and predisposition to breast and thyroid cancers. Male patients have penile lentigines. Bannayan-Riley-Ruvalcaba syndrome, which is often diagnosed in childhood, is also associated with mutations of the PTEN gene, thus the same guidelines hold true for patients suspected of having this disorder, as well as their family members.

TREATMENT OF VASCULAR MALFORMATIONS
(ALSO SEE TABLE 64.3)

Patients with venous vascular malformations often experience painful episodes—this is often in conjunction with a "phlebolith" or local clot. Therapy with ibuprofen usually suffices. Bleeding from cutaneous blebs may respond to laser cauterization. More severe bleeding from the genitourinary tract may require a combined approach with angiography-guided embolization, laser, or sclerotherapy. Large symptomatic thromboses may require anticoagulation, as might the coagulopathy associated with severe cases.

Sirolimus is increasingly used for patients with vascular malformations. mTOR activation in vascular malformations had been previously demonstrated,[141] and clinical efficacy of sirolimus, an mTOR inhibitor, in patients with lymphangioleiomyomatosis eventually led to clinical trials in patients with vascular malformations. Since the initial study,[142] several case reports and small series have been published, documenting efficacy in a variety of vascular malformations and tumors, especially PROS, venous malformations, lymphatic malformations, Gorham disease, PTEN Hamartoma syndrome, blue rubber bleb nevus syndrome, and KHE.[63,142–148] Additionally, Boscolo et al. demonstrated sirolimus prevented growth of venous malformations in a mouse model harboring the VM-causing TIE2 mutation.[110] Patients treated with sirolimus require frequent blood tests to monitor for toxicity and trough drug levels. Optimal dosing and duration of therapy remains under study. Since this medication is an immunosuppressant, patients should receive prophylactic antibiotics to prevent Pneumocystis pneumonias. Recent fatalities due to

Pneumocystis have been reported in patients who were not receiving this prophylaxis.[149,150] Sirolimus does not seem to be effective for arteriovenous malformations. Microcystic lymphatic malformations and blebs have responded to topical sirolimus.[151] Topical sirolimus in conjunction with laser for capillary malformations is also being studied.[152,153] Clinical trials with oral Miransertib (ARQ 092 [ArQule, Burlington, MA]) are under way for patients with Proteus syndrome and those with PROS-associated vascular malformations.[154,155]

Patients with arterial and venous abnormalities must be cautioned about "triggers." Quiescent vascular anomalies may become more problematic secondary to local trauma, infections, or hormonal fluctuations such as puberty, menstruation, and pregnancy. These changes are usually manifest as increased fullness of the malformation, as well as pain. The etiology of these difficulties is not clearly understood, but in the hormonally mediated settings it is likely related to hormonal stimulation of endothelial cell surface receptors. Use of hormonal birth control can elicit undesirable thromboses and/or pain; thus, alternative means of contraception are advised.

Lymphatic malformations involving the mouth and gastrointestinal tract are prone to infection; therefore, patients with lymphatic malformation in these sites benefit from diligent oral hygiene and occasionally rotating prophylactic antibiotic regimens. Large microcystic lymphatic malformations of the head and neck may respond well to sclerotherapy or surgery, or a combined approach. Lymphatic imaging with intranodal dynamic contrast-enhanced magnetic resonance lymphangiography (DCMRL) is being used to assess lymphatic perfusion in treatment planning for patients with central lymphatic system pathologies.[156–159] Breakthroughs in the embryology and biology of lymphatic vasculature provide insights into the therapeutic potential for lymphangiogenesis with lymphangiogenic growth factors.[126,127,160–162]

Evaluation of patients with lymphedema involves physical examination and radiologic studies including lymphoscintigraphy for extremity involvement (see Chapter 57). Therapy is generally supportive, with hygienic skin care, sclerotherapy when possible, complete decompressive physiotherapy with compression bandaging, and intermittent pneumatic compression therapy. Rockson and Keo provide reviews of evaluation and management of patients with lymphedema.[163–165] Surgical options for lymphedema include liposuction, vascularized lymph node transfer, lymphovenous anas-

TABLE 64.5 Online Resources for Patients and Physicians

Program	Website
Clinical Trials	https://clinicaltrials.gov/
Genetic Testing Registry	https://www.ncbi.nlm.nih.gov/gtr/
Genetics Home Reference	http://ghr.nlm.nih.gov/
HHT Mutation Database	http://www.arup.utah.edu/database/HHT/index.php
Medline Plus	https://medlineplus.gov/
National Organization for Rare Diseases	https://rarediseases.org
Research Studies	https://clinicaltrials.gov/
Vascular Anomaly and Lymphedema Mutation Database	http://www.icp.ucl.ac.be/vikkula/VAdb/home.php

tomosis, and other techniques aimed at restoring lymphatic function.[166,167] Based on preliminary work demonstrating that inhibition of leukotriene B4 (LTB4) was effective in reversing lymphedema in a mouse model, a clinical trial is under way (NCT02700529) assessing the effect of a LTB4 inhibitor (bestatin) for acquired lymphedema.[168]

Tables 64.5 and 64.6 provide helpful resources for healthcare providers, patients, and families who would like to access further information about specific vascular anomalies.

PRENATAL DIAGNOSIS OF VASCULAR ANOMALIES

With the availability of improved techniques in fetal ultrasound and MRI, prenatally diagnosed vascular anomalies are becoming increasingly recognized. Vascular lesions detected prenatally are generally identified by asymmetric limbs and/or highly vascular lesions (e.g., vascular malformations, or high-flow RICH-type lesions). Prenatal genetic diagnosis for inherited vascular malformations is possible when a specific mutation has already been identified (e.g., RASA1).[169] Alternatively, targeted pre-implantation genetic screening of embryos is an option for families with known mutations.

CLINICAL ISSUES (SEE ALSO TABLE 64.4)

Bleeding Associated with Coagulation and Other Abnormalities in Patients with Vascular Anomalies

As noted earlier, bleeding due to Kasabach-Merritt phenomenon (thrombocytopenia, hypofibrinogenemia, and increased fibrinolysis) is often associated with KHE or tufted angioma. In addition to therapy directed toward the primary tumor, antifibrinolytic agents, antiplatelet agents, and heparin are helpful. A transient coagulopathy may be seen in a subgroup of RICH-type lesions.[170] Bleeding may occur with ulcerated hemangiomas. Local hygienic and topical medications can keep the area clean and expedite healing, while oozing that does not halt with mild pressure may respond to topical hemostatic agents. Consensus guidelines have been established for management of HHT, including bleeding problems (e.g., epistaxis).[171] A 6-question Epistaxis Severity Score (available online: https://www2.drexelmed.edu/HHT-ESS/) has been validated for HHT,[172] which may help guide treatment for affected patients. Bleeding is also a predominant feature in patients with MLT.[62]

D-dimer elevation is common in patients with venous malformations. These patients are also prone to thromboses in superficial and/or deep veins.[173] Patients with proteus syndrome and patients with PIK3CA-related overgrowth spectrum are particularly at risk for venous thromboses including pulmonary embolism.[174]

TABLE 64.6 Patient Advocacy Groups

Disorder	Website
CLOVE Syndrome	http://www.clovessyndrome.org/
FAVA Foundation	http://www.thefavafoundation.com/home.html
Hereditary Hemorrhagic Telangiectasia (HHT) Foundation	https://curehht.org/
HEVAS Dutch parents and patients' association for hemangiomas and vascular malformations	https://www.hevas.eu/
Klippel-Trénaunay Support Group	http://www.k-t.org/
Lymphangiomatosis & Gorham's Disease Alliance	https://www.lgdalliance.org/
Lymphatic Disorders	http://littleleakers.com/
Lymphatic Education and Research Network	https://lymphaticnetwork.org/
Lymphatic Malformation Institute	http://www.lmiresearch.org
Macrocephaly-capillary malformation (M-CM)	https://www.m-cm.net/
National Lymphedema Network	http://www.lymphnet.org/
National Organization for Rare Diseases	http://www.rarediseases.org
PHACE Syndrome Community	http://www.phacesyndromecommunity.org/
PTEN Hamartoma Support Group	https://ptenfoundation.org/
Proteus Syndrome Foundation	http://www.proteus-syndrome.org/
Sturge-Weber Foundation	http://sturge-weber.org/
Vascular Anomaly Patient Association (Europe)VASCAPA	http://www.vascapa.org/
Vascular Birthmarks Foundation	https://birthmark.org/

Various foundations provide educational resources, webinars, conferences, advocacy, networking, patient support, research funding.

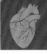

Hemodynamic Sequelae

Rarely, hemangiomas may demonstrate transient high flow, functionally (until they have undergone significant involution) mimicking arteriovenous malformations. Hemangiomas with high flow are most frequently located in the liver. These lesions can lead to significant morbidity, with high output cardiac failure. Nonhepatic hemangiomas, prone to develop a high flow component, include those involving the parotid gland, upper arm, chest wall, scalp, and, rarely, the upper lip. These lesions appear to behave as transiently "arterialized" hemangiomas. During this time, patients may have a failure to thrive-type picture, hyperdynamic precordium, tachycardia, bounding pulses with a widened pulse pressure, and a thrill/bruit over the hemangioma. These findings should alert the treating physician to monitor the hemodynamic status of patients with hemangiomas by careful physical examination and frequent follow-up evaluation. RICH-type hemangiomas may have arterial flow diagnosed pre- or postnatally. Overall, a minority of patients develops high cardiac output states requiring intervention including diuretics, inotropic agents, or an embolization procedure.

Orthopedic Concerns

Orthopedic issues associated with vascular anomalies involve those relating to limb-dimension discrepancies (including limb length/girth discrepancies, hypertrophy, atrophy, macrodactyly, polydactyly, gigantism, scoliosis, intra-articular pathology, scoliosis, and gait disturbances). Serial assessment of limb-length data and bone ages at regular intervals is recommended. Interventions include shoe lifts versus epiphysiodesis (surgical growth plate closure) for more modest discrepancies; however, for discrepancies predicted to be greater than 5 cm, or in patients who have already reached skeletal maturity, limb shortening and lengthening are the only options to equalize limb lengths. Shoeing may be an issue, due to foot size discrepancies, and/or difficulty finding well-fitting shoes.

Options include custom-made shoes, ray or digital resection for macrodactyly of the fingers or toes, debulking procedures, or amputation for severe and otherwise unmanageable cases of hypertrophy. Patients with vascular anomalies can also develop joint contractures. Physical therapy with stretching exercises may be adequate to relieve symptoms; sclerotherapy ± surgery and medical therapy are therapeutic options.[175]

Gynecologic Issues in Patients With Vascular Malformations

Some women with vascular anomalies have such severe menorrhagia that they undergo hysterectomy. Furthermore, pregnancy is not often seen as an option for women with severe vascular anomalies of the lower extremities, due to the exacerbation of leg swelling, pain, and bleeding from the increased pressure of a full uterus. The normal physiologic changes of pregnancy include increased plasma volume and cardiac output, increased venous pressure, leg edema, and venous stasis. Additionally, during pregnancy there is a 5.5 times increased risk of thromboembolism; this risk is augmented in patients with vascular anomalies who already have an increased prothrombotic risk. Increased risk of thrombosis with oral contraceptives limits these patients' choices of contraception. This is also an issue when oral contraceptives are considered to treat dysmenorrhea or other gynecologic problems.[176]

Pregnancy for women with vascular anomalies, especially those in the lower extremities, may cause unique problems due to hormonal changes, as well as compression of venous structures by the enlarging uterus. Preliminary data based on two questionnaire-based studies suggest that the risk of obstetric complications, especially preeclampsia and thromboembolic events, is higher in women with vascular malformations of the lower extremities. Increased postpartum hemorrhage has also been observed. It is recommended that management of pregnancy be under the direction of an obstetrician who is aware of these risks. Therapy with daily injections of low molecular weight heparin during pregnancy may prevent some prothrombotic complications.[176,177] In addition to pregnancy, other hormonal changes, such as those associated with puberty (in males or females) or the menstrual cycle may present an increased risk of thrombosis within vascular lesions, necessitating medical intervention with anticoagulants.

Reproductive counseling should be incorporated into the care plan for patients with vascular anomalies. Family planning options include pregnancy, pre-implantation genetic testing (for genomic mutations), gestational carriers, and adoption. Oocyte retrieval following exogenous hormonal stimulation of ovulation in a female patient with Klippel-Trénaunay syndrome has been reported. Heparin-based anticoagulation was used prior to and after oocyte retrieval to prevent hormone-related thrombosis and to treat an underlying chronic coagulopathy.[178]

Psychosocial Issues

Pathologies affecting the face have been shown to greatly impact quality of life and "induce a significant social penalty."[179,180] Studies using validated instruments to assess quality of life measures, and the burden of disease on the family of infants with hemangiomas, found that hemangiomas in the proliferative stage, located on the head, neck, or viscera (e.g., liver) caused the highest degree of parental stress.[181,182] Early therapy may be considered to prevent morbidity and/or preclude the need for future surgery. In fact, as more effective medical therapies have been discovered, the role of surgery for hemangiomas has diminished. Condition-focused assessment tools have been validated for lymphedema (Lymphedema Life Impact Scale)[183] and vascular malformations, the latter resulting from input by patients, parents, and physicians, in an effort to standardize outcome measures.[184] In one study, depression, anxiety, and posttraumatic stress symptoms were prevalent in respondents to a survey of over 200 adult patients with HHT.[185]

Contact with other families who are going through or have gone through the same experience may decrease feelings of isolation. In this sense, local "family support groups" organized at some medical centers, as well as national support networks and meetings, are increasingly providing the necessary stability for families and patients. The internet has played an enormous role in assisting the exchange of information, as well as enabling families to connect with one another. Many patient advocacy groups provide condition-specific educational materials on their websites and help facilitate access to appropriate medical providers (see Table 64.6). It is now customary to have participation by patient representatives in professional conferences and grant reviews.

Malignancies

Historically, secondary malignancies (thyroid, breast, angiosarcoma) were reported in patients with vascular anomalies due to radiation therapy, an outdated treatment for hemangiomas of infancy. Patients with the PTEN hamartoma syndrome or Maffucci syndrome are prone to malignancies as mentioned above.[139,186–188] Surveillance ultrasound screens for Wilm tumor in infants and young children are becoming standard for patients with CLOVES syndrome and other PIK3CA-related overgrowth syndromes.[189,190] Patients treated with sirolimus need to be monitored for potential skin cancer or lymphoproliferative disorders.

Mimickers of benign vascular lesions include infantile fibrosarcoma, hemangiopericytoma, rhabdomyosarcoma, glioma, neurofibroma, neuroblastoma, leukemia, lymphoma, and others.[191,192] An atypical history and/or physical findings should alert the practitioner to investigate radiologically and obtain a histologic diagnosis.

REFERENCES

1. Hassanein AH, Mulliken JB, Fishman SJ, et al. Evaluation of terminology for vascular anomalies in current literature. *Plast Reconstr Surg.* 2011;127(1):347–351.
2. Greene AK, Liu AS, Mulliken JB, et al. Vascular anomalies in 5,621 patients: guidelines for referral. *J Pediatr Surg.* 2011;46(9):1784–1789.
3. Ahlawat S, Fayad LM, Durand DJ, et al. International Society for the Study of Vascular Anomalies Classification of Soft Tissue Vascular Anomalies: survey-based assessment of musculoskeletal radiologists' use in clinical practice. *Curr Probl Diagn Radiol.* 2019;48(1):10–16.
4. Mulliken JB, Glowacki J. Hemangiomas and vascular malformations in infants and children: a classification based on endothelial characteristics. *Plast Reconstr Surg.* 1982;69(3):412–422.
5. Wassef M, Blei F, Adams D, et al. Vascular anomalies classification: recommendations from the International Society for the Study of Vascular Anomalies. *Pediatrics.* 2015;136(1):e203–e214.
6. Leaute-Labreze C, Harper JI, Hoeger PH. Infantile haemangioma. *Lancet.* 2017;390(10089):85–94.
7. Reimer A, Fliesser M, Hoeger PH. Anatomical patterns of infantile hemangioma (IH) of the extremities (IHE). *J Am Acad Dermatol.* 2016;75(3):556–563.
8. Suh KY, Frieden IJ. Infantile hemangiomas with minimal or arrested growth: a retrospective case series. *Arch Dermatol.* 2010;146(9):971–976.
9. Ma EH, Robertson SJ, Chow CW, et al. Infantile hemangioma with minimal or arrested growth: further observations on clinical and histopathologic findings of this unique but underrecognized entity. *Pediatr Dermatol.* 2017;34(1):64–71.
10. Planas-Ciudad S, Roe Crespo E, Sanchez-Carpintero I, et al. Infantile hemangiomas with minimal or arrested growth associated with soft tissue hypertrophy: a case series of 10 patients. *J Eur Acad Dermatol Venereol.* 2017;31(11):1924–1929.
11. Vega Mata N, Lopez Gutierrez JC, Vivanco Allende B, et al. Different clinical features of acral abortive hemangiomas. *Case Rep Dermatol Med.* 2017;2017.2897617.
12. Horii KA, Drolet BA, Frieden IJ, et al. Prospective study of the frequency of hepatic hemangiomas in infants with multiple cutaneous infantile hemangiomas. *Pediatr Dermatol.* 2011;28(3):245–253.
13. Reimer A, Hoeger PH. Lesion morphology in multifocal infantile hemangiomas. *Pediatr Dermatol.* 2016;33(6):621–626.
14. Mulliken JB, Enjolras O. Congenital hemangiomas and infantile hemangioma: missing links. *J Am Acad Dermatol.* 2004;50(6):875–882.
15. North PE, Waner M, James CA, et al. Congenital nonprogressive hemangioma: a distinct clinicopathologic entity unlike infantile hemangioma. *Arch Dermatol.* 2001;137(12):1607–1620.
16. Smith CJF, Friedlander SF, Guma M, et al. Infantile hemangiomas: an updated review on risk factors, pathogenesis, and treatment. *Birth Defects Res.* 2017;109(11):809–815.
17. Luu M, Frieden IJ. Infantile hemangiomas and structural anomalies: PHACE and LUMBAR syndrome. *Semin Cutan Med Surg.* 2016;35(3):117–123.
18. Garzon MC, Epstein LG, Heyer GL, et al. PHACE syndrome: consensus-derived diagnosis and care recommendations. *J Pediatr.* 2016;178:24–33. e2.
19. Haggstrom AN, Garzon MC, Baselga E, et al. Risk for PHACE syndrome in infants with large facial hemangiomas. *Pediatrics.* 2010;126(2):e418–e426.
20. Oza VS, Wang E, Berenstein A, et al. PHACES association: a neuroradiologic review of 17 patients. *AJNR Am J Neuroradiol.* 2008;29(4):807–813.
21. Heyer GL. PHACE(S) syndrome. *Handb Clin Neurol.* 2015;132:169–183.
22. Schilter KF, Steiner JE, Demos W, et al. RNF213 variants in a child with PHACE syndrome and moyamoya vasculopathy. *Am J Med Genet A.* 2017;173(9):2557–2561.
23. Steiner JE, McCoy GN, Hess CP, et al. Structural malformations of the brain, eye, and pituitary gland in PHACE syndrome. *Am J Med Genet A.* 2018;176(1):48–55.
24. Martin KL, Arvedson JC, Bayer ML, et al. Risk of dysphagia and speech and language delay in PHACE syndrome. *Pediatr Dermatol.* 2015;32(1):64–69.
25. Brosig CL, Siegel DH, Haggstrom AN, et al. Neurodevelopmental outcomes in children with PHACE syndrome. *Pediatr Dermatol.* 2016;33(4):415–423.
26. Yu J, Siegel DH, Drolet BA, et al. Prevalence and clinical characteristics of headaches in PHACE syndrome. *J Child Neurol.* 2016;31(4):468–473.
27. Leaute-Labreze C, Hoeger P, Mazereeuw-Hautier J, et al. A randomized, controlled trial of oral propranolol in infantile hemangioma. *N Engl J Med.* 2015;372(8):735–746.
28. Leaute-Labreze C, Boccara O, Degrugillier-Chopinet C, et al. Safety of oral propranolol for the treatment of infantile hemangioma: a systematic review. *Pediatrics.* 2016;138(4):e20160353.
29. Wedgeworth E, Glover M, Irvine AD, et al. Propranolol in the treatment of infantile haemangiomas: lessons from the European Propranolol In the Treatment of Complicated Haemangiomas (PITCH) Taskforce survey. *Br J Dermatol.* 2016;174(3):594–601.
30. Chinnadurai S, Fonnesbeck C, Snyder KM, et al. Pharmacologic interventions for infantile hemangioma: a meta-analysis. *Pediatrics.* 2016;137(2):e20153896.
31. Cheng CE, Friedlander SF. Infantile hemangiomas, complications and treatments. *Semin Cutan Med Surg.* 2016;35(3):108–116.
32. Labreze C, Voisard JJ, Delarue A, et al. Risk of neurodevelopmental abnormalities in children treated with propranolol. *Br J Dermatol.* 2015;173(6):1562–1564.
33. Moyakine AV, Kerstjens JM, Spillekom-van Koulil S, et al. Propranolol treatment of infantile hemangioma (IH) is not associated with developmental risk or growth impairment at age 4 years. *J Am Acad Dermatol.* 2016;75(1):59–63. e1.
34. Hu L, Zhou B, Huang H, et al. Effects of systemic propranolol treatment on physical growth of patients with infantile hemangiomas. *J Dermatol.* 2016;43(10):1160–1166.
35. Moyakine AV, Spillekom-van Koulil S, van der Vleuten CJM. Propranolol treatment of infantile hemangioma is not associated with psychological problems at 7 years of age. *J Am Acad Dermatol.* 2017;77(1):105–108.
36. Gonzalez-Llorente N, Del Olmo-Benito I, Munoz-Ollero N, et al. Study of cognitive function in children treated with propranolol for infantile hemangioma. *Pediatr Dermatol.* 2017;34(5):554–558.
37. Darrow DH, Greene AK, Mancini AJ, et al. Diagnosis and management of infantile hemangioma: executive summary. *Pediatrics.* 2015;136(4):786–791.
38. Chinnadurai S, Snyder K, Sathe N, et al. *Diagnosis and management of infantile hemangioma. AHRQ comparative effectiveness reviews [Internet].* Report No.: 16-EHC002-EF(168), https://www.ncbi.nlm.nih.gov/pubmed/26889533; 2016.
39. Leaute-Labreze C. Dumas de la Roque E, Hubiche T, et al. Propranolol for severe hemangiomas of infancy. *N Engl J Med.* 2008;358(24):2649–2651.
40. Lamy S, Lachambre MP, Lord-Dufour S, et al. Propranolol suppresses angiogenesis in vitro: inhibition of proliferation, migration, and differentiation of endothelial cells. *Vasc Pharmacol.* 2010;53(5-6):200–208.
41. Itinteang T, Brasch HD, Tan ST, et al. Expression of components of the renin-angiotensin system in proliferating infantile haemangioma may account for the propranolol-induced accelerated involution. *J Plast Reconstr Aesthet Surg.* 2011;64(6):759–765.
42. Dornhoffer JR, Wei T, Zhang H, et al. The expression of renin-angiotensin-aldosterone axis components in infantile hemangioma tissue and the impact of propranolol treatment. *Pediatr Res.* 2017;82(1):155–163.
43. Sulzberger L, Baillie R, Itinteang T, et al. Serum levels of renin, angiotensin-converting enzyme and angiotensin II in patients treated by surgical excision, propranolol and captopril for problematic proliferating infantile haemangioma. *J Plast Reconstr Aesthet Surg.* 2016;69(3):381–386.

44. Storch CH, Hoeger PH. Propranolol for infantile haemangiomas: insights into the molecular mechanisms of action. *Br J Dermatol.* 2010;163(2):269–274.

45. Lee D, Boscolo E, Durham JT, et al. Propranolol targets the contractility of infantile haemangioma-derived pericytes. *Br J Dermatol.* 2014;171(5):1129–1137.

46. Munabi NC, England RW, Edwards AK, et al. Propranolol targets hemangioma stem cells via cAMP and mitogen-activated protein kinase regulation. *Stem Cells Transl Med.* 2016;5(1):45–55.

47. Borok J, Gangar P, Admani S, et al. Safety and efficacy of topical timolol treatment of infantile haemangioma: a prospective trial. *Br J Dermatol.* 2018;178(1):e51–e52.

48. Puttgen K, Lucky A, Adams D, et al. Topical timolol maleate treatment of infantile hemangiomas. *Pediatrics.* 2016;138(3):e20160355.

49. Frommelt P, Juern A, Siegel D, et al. Adverse events in young and preterm infants receiving topical timolol for infantile hemangioma. *Pediatr Dermatol.* 2016;33(4):405–414.

50. Weibel L, Barysch MJ, Scheer HS, et al. Topical timolol for infantile hemangiomas: evidence for efficacy and degree of systemic absorption. *Pediatr Dermatol.* 2016;33(2):184–190.

51. Kulungowski AM, Alomari AI, Chawla A, et al. Lessons from a liver hemangioma registry: subtype classification. *J Pediatr Surg.* 2012;47(1):165–170.

52. Rialon KL, Murillo R, Fevurly RD, et al. Risk factors for mortality in patients with multifocal and diffuse hepatic hemangiomas. *J Pediatr Surg.* 2015;50(5):837–841.

53. Rialon KL, Murillo R, Fevurly RD, et al. Impact of screening for hepatic hemangiomas in patients with multiple cutaneous infantile hemangiomas. *Pediatr Dermatol.* 2015;32(6):808–812.

54. Coulie J, Coyette M, Moniotte S, et al. Has propranolol eradicated the need for surgery in the management of infantile hemangioma? *Plast Reconstr Surg.* 2015;136(4 Suppl):154.

55. Kasabach H, Merritt K. Capillary hemangioma with extensive purpura. *Am J Dis Child.* 1940;59:1063.

56. Sarkar M, Mulliken JB, Kozakewich HP, et al. Thrombocytopenic coagulopathy (Kasabach-Merritt phenomenon) is associated with Kaposiform hemangioendothelioma and not with common infantile hemangioma. *Plast Reconstr Surg.* 1997;100(6):1377–1386.

57. Enjolras O, Wassef M, Mazoyer E, et al. Infants with Kasabach-Merritt syndrome do not have "true" hemangiomas. *J Pediatr.* 1997;130(4):631–640.

58. Gruman A, Liang MG, Mulliken JB, et al. Kaposiform hemangioendothelioma without Kasabach-Merritt phenomenon. *J Am Acad Dermatol.* 2005;52(4):616–622.

59. Liu XH, Li JY, Qu XH, et al. Treatment of kaposiform hemangioendothelioma and tufted angioma. *Int J Cancer.* 2016;139(7):1658–1666.

60. Mahajan P, Margolin J, Iacobas I. Kasabach-Merritt phenomenon: classic presentation and management options. *Clin Med Insights Blood Disord.* 2017;10:1179545X17699849.

61. Croteau SE, Gupta D. The clinical spectrum of kaposiform hemangioendothelioma and tufted angioma. *Semin Cutan Med Surg.* 2016;35(3):147–152.

62. Campbell CM, Beckum KM, Hammers YA, et al. Multiple congenital red-brown macules, thrombocytopenia, and gastrointestinal bleeding. Diagnosis: multifocal lymphangioendotheliomatosis with thrombocytopenia (MLT). *Pediatr Dermatol.* 2010;27(4):395–396.

63. Lanoel A, Torres Huamani AN, Feliu A, et al. Multifocal lymphangioendotheliomatosis with thrombocytopenia: presentation of two cases treated with sirolimus. *Pediatr Dermatol.* 2016;33(4):e235–e239.

64. Arbiser JL, Bonner MY, Berrios RL. Hemangiomas, angiosarcomas, and vascular malformations represent the signaling abnormalities of pathogenic angiogenesis. *Curr Mol Med.* 2009;9(8):929–934.

65. Bischoff J. Progenitor cells in infantile hemangioma. *J Craniofac Surg.* 2009;20(Suppl 1):695–697.

66. Boye E, Olsen BR. Signaling mechanisms in infantile hemangioma. *Curr Opin Hematol.* 2009;16(3):202–208.

67. Greenberger S, Bischoff J. Pathogenesis of infantile haemangioma. *Br J Dermatol.* 2013;169(1):12–19.

68. Itinteang T, Tan ST, Brasch H, et al. Primitive mesodermal cells with a neural crest stem cell phenotype predominate proliferating infantile haemangioma. *J Clin Pathol.* 2010;63(9):771–776.

69. Dadras SS, North PE, Bertoncini J, et al. Infantile hemangiomas are arrested in an early developmental vascular differentiation state. *Mod Pathol.* 2004;17(9):1068–1079.

70. Nguyen VA, Kutzner H, Furhapter C, et al. Infantile hemangioma is a proliferation of LYVE-1-negative blood endothelial cells without lymphatic competence. *Mod Pathol.* 2006;19(2):291–298.

71. Khan ZA, Boscolo E, Picard A, et al. Multipotential stem cells recapitulate human infantile hemangioma in immunodeficient mice. *J Clin Invest.* 2008;118(7):2592–2599.

72. Perry BN, Govindarajan B, Bhandarkar SS, et al. Pharmacologic blockade of angiopoietin-2 is efficacious against model hemangiomas in mice. *J Invest Dermatol.* 2006;126(10):2316–2322.

73. Boye E, Yu Y, Paranya G, et al. Clonality and altered behavior of endothelial cells from hemangiomas. *J Clin Invest.* 2001;107(6):745–752.

74. Walter JW, North PE, Waner M, et al. Somatic mutation of vascular endothelial growth factor receptors in juvenile hemangioma. *Genes Chromosomes Cancer.* 2002;33(3):295–303.

75. Yu Y, Flint AF, Mulliken JB, et al. Endothelial progenitor cells in infantile hemangioma. *Blood.* 2004;103(4):1373–1375.

76. Khan ZA, Melero-Martin JM, Wu X, et al. Endothelial progenitor cells from infantile hemangioma and umbilical cord blood display unique cellular responses to endostatin. *Blood.* 2006;108(3):915–921.

77. Kleinman ME, Blei F, Gurtner GC. Circulating endothelial progenitor cells and vascular anomalies. *Lymphat Res Biol.* 2005;3(4):234–239.

78. Yu Y, Fuhr J, Boye E, et al. Mesenchymal stem cells and adipogenesis in hemangioma involution. *Stem Cells.* 2006;24(6):1605–1612.

79. North PE, Waner M, Mizeracki A, et al. A unique microvascular phenotype shared by juvenile hemangiomas and human placenta. *Arch Dermatol.* 2001;137(5):559–570.

80. Mihm Jr MC, Nelson JS. Hypothesis: the metastatic niche theory can elucidate infantile hemangioma development. *J Cutan Pathol.* 2010;37:83–87.

81. Greenberger S, Adini I, Boscolo E, et al. Targeting NF-kappaB in infantile hemangioma-derived stem cells reduces VEGF-A expression. *Angiogenesis.* 2010;13(4):327–335.

82. Greenberger S, Boscolo E, Adini I, et al. Corticosteroid suppression of VEGF-A in infantile hemangioma-derived stem cells. *N Engl J Med.* 2010;362(11):1005–1013.

83. Biswas A, Pan X, Meyer M, et al. Urinary excretion of microRNA-126 is a biomarker for hemangioma proliferation. *Plast Reconstr Surg.* 2017;139(6):1277e–1284e.

84. Ye X, Abou-Rayyah Y, Bischoff J, et al. Altered ratios of pro- and anti-angiogenic VEGF-A variants and pericyte expression of DLL4 disrupt vascular maturation in infantile haemangioma. *J Pathol.* 2016;239(2):139–151.

85. Sun ZJ, Zhao YF, Zhang WF. Immune response: a possible role in the pathophysiology of hemangioma. *Med Hypotheses.* 2007;68(2):353–355.

86. Ayturk UM, Couto JA, Hann S, et al. Somatic activating mutations in GNAQ and GNA11 are associated with congenital hemangioma. *Am J Hum Genet.* 2016;98(4):789–795.

87. Wollina U, Langner D, Franca K, et al. Pyogenic granuloma - a common benign vascular tumor with variable clinical presentation: new findings and treatment options. *Open Access Maced J Med Sci.* 2017;5(4):423–426.

88. Lim YH, Douglas SR, Ko CJ, et al. Somatic activating RAS mutations cause vascular tumors including pyogenic granuloma. *J Invest Dermatol.* 2015;135(6):1698–1700.

89. Groesser L, Peterhof E, Evert M, et al. BRAF and RAS mutations in sporadic and secondary pyogenic granuloma. *J Invest Dermatol.* 2016;136(2):481–486.

90. Ganem D. KSHV and the pathogenesis of Kaposi sarcoma: listening to human biology and medicine. *J Clin Invest.* 2010;120(4):939–949.

91. Ponticelli C, Cucchiari D, Bencini P. Skin cancer in kidney transplant recipients. *J Nephrol.* 2014;27(4):385–394.

92. Heyrman B, De Becker A, Schots R. A case report of immunosuppression-related Kaposi's sarcoma after autologous stem cell transplantation. *BMC Res Notes*. 2016;9:188.

93. Gramolelli S, Ojala PM. Kaposi's sarcoma herpesvirus-induced endothelial cell reprogramming supports viral persistence and contributes to Kaposi's sarcoma tumorigenesis. *Curr Opin Virol*. 2017;26:156–162.

94. Barbaro G, Barbarini G. HIV infection and cancer in the era of highly active antiretroviral therapy (Review). *Oncol Rep*. 2007;17(5):1121–1126.

95. Aspelund A, Robciuc MR, Karaman S, et al. Lymphatic system in cardiovascular medicine. *Circ Res*. 2016;118(3):515–530.

96. Kazenwadel J, Harvey NL. Morphogenesis of the lymphatic vasculature: a focus on new progenitors and cellular mechanisms important for constructing lymphatic vessels. *Dev Dyn*. 2016;245(3):209–219.

97. Chang F, Liu L, Fang E, et al. Molecular diagnosis of mosaic overgrowth syndromes using a custom-designed next-generation sequencing panel. *J Mol Diagn*. 2017;19(4):613–624.

98. Keppler-Noreuil KM, Rios JJ, Parker VE, et al. PIK3CA-related overgrowth spectrum (PROS): diagnostic and testing eligibility criteria, differential diagnosis, and evaluation. *Am J Med Genet A*. 2015;167A(2):287–295.

99. Keppler-Noreuil KM, Parker VE, Darling TN, Martinez-Agosto JA. Somatic overgrowth disorders of the PI3K/AKT/mTOR pathway & therapeutic strategies. *Am J Med Genet C Semin Med Genet*. 2016;172(4):402–421.

100. Nathan N, Keppler-Noreuil KM, Biesecker LG, et al. Mosaic disorders of the PI3K/PTEN/AKT/TSC/mTORC1 signaling pathway. *Dermatol Clin*. 2017;35(1):51–60.

101. Happle R. The molecular revolution in cutaneous biology: era of mosaicism. *J Invest Dermatol*. 2017;137(5):e73–e77.

102. Wetzel-Strong SE, Detter MR, Marchuk DA. The pathobiology of vascular malformations: insights from human and model organism genetics. *J Pathol*. 2017;241(2):281–293.

103. Potente M, Makinen T. Vascular heterogeneity and specialization in development and disease. *Nat Rev Mol Cell Biol*. 2017;18(8):477–494.

104. Hucthagowder V, Shenoy A, Corliss M, et al. Utility of clinical high-depth next generation sequencing for somatic variant detection in the PIK3CA-related overgrowth spectrum. *Clin Genet*. 2017;91(1):79–85.

105. Akgumus G, Chang F, Li MM. Overgrowth syndromes caused by somatic variants in the phosphatidylinositol 3-kinase/AKT/mammalian target of rapamycin pathway. *J Mol Diagn*. 2017;19(4):487–497.

106. Nguyen HL, Boon LM, Vikkula M. Vascular anomalies caused by abnormal signaling within endothelial cells: targets for novel therapies. *Semin Intervent Radiol*. 2017;34(3):233–238.

107. Natynki M, Kangas J, Miinalainen I, et al. Common and specific effects of TIE2 mutations causing venous malformations. *Hum Mol Genet*. 2015;24(22):6374–6389.

108. Limaye N, Kangas J, Mendola A, et al. Somatic activating PIK3CA mutations cause venous malformation. *Am J Hum Genet*. 2015;97(6):914–921.

109. Siegel DH, Cottrell CE, Streicher JL, et al. Analyzing the genetic spectrum of vascular anomalies with overgrowth via cancer genomics. *J Invest Dermatol*. 2018;138(4):957–967.

110. Boscolo E, Limaye N, Huang L, et al. Rapamycin improves TIE2-mutated venous malformation in murine model and human subjects. *J Clin Invest*. 2015;125(9):3491–3504.

111. Hogan BM, Schulte-Merker S. How to plumb a pisces: understanding vascular development and disease using zebrafish embryos. *Dev Cell*. 2017;42(6):567–583.

112. Tan EMS, Siljee SD, Brasch HD, et al. Embryonic stem cell-like subpopulations in venous malformation. *Front Med (Lausanne)*. 2017;4:162.

113. McDonald J, Wooderchak-Donahue W, VanSant Webb C, et al. Hereditary hemorrhagic telangiectasia: genetics and molecular diagnostics in a new era. *Front Genet*. 2015;6:1.

114. Revencu N, Boon LM, Mendola A, et al. RASA1 mutations and associated phenotypes in 68 families with capillary malformation-arteriovenous malformation. *Hum Mutat*. 2013;34(12):1632–1641.

115. Amyere M, Revencu N, Helaers R, et al. Germline loss-of-function mutations in EPHB4 cause a second form of capillary malformation-arteriovenous malformation (CM-AVM2) deregulating RAS-MAPK signaling. *Circulation*. 2017;136(11):1037–1048.

116. Brouillard P, Boon LM, Revencu N, et al. Genotypes and phenotypes of 162 families with a glomulin mutation. *Mol Syndromol*. 2013;4(4):157–164.

117. Soblet J, Kangas J, Natynki M, et al. Blue rubber bleb nevus (BRBN) syndrome is caused by somatic TEK (TIE2) mutations. *J Invest Dermatol*. 2017;137(1):207–216.

118. Soblet J, Limaye N, Uebelhoer M, et al. Variable somatic TIE2 mutations in half of sporadic venous malformations. *Mol Syndromol*. 2013;4(4): 179–183.

119. Couto JA, Huang L, Vivero MP, et al. Endothelial cells from capillary malformations are enriched for somatic GNAQ mutations. *Plast Reconstr Surg*. 2016;137(1):77e–82e.

120. Shirley MD, Tang H, Gallione CJ, et al. Sturge-Weber syndrome and port-wine stains caused by somatic mutation in GNAQ. *N Engl J Med*. 2013;368(21):1971–1979.

121. Mirzaa G, Timms AE, Conti V, et al. PIK3CA-associated developmental disorders exhibit distinct classes of mutations with variable expression and tissue distribution. *JCI Insight*. 2016;1(9):87623.

122. Loconte DC, Grossi V, Bozzao C, et al. Molecular and functional characterization of three different postzygotic mutations in PIK3CA-related overgrowth spectrum (PROS) patients: effects on PI3K/AKT/mTOR signaling and sensitivity to PIK3 inhibitors. *PLoS One*. 2015;10(4):e0123092.

123. Couto JA, Huang AY, Konczyk DJ, et al. Somatic MAP2K1 mutations are associated with extracranial arteriovenous malformation. *Am J Hum Genet*. 2017;100(3):546–554.

124. Lala S, Mulliken JB, Alomari AI, et al. Gorham-Stout disease and generalized lymphatic anomaly—clinical, radiologic, and histologic differentiation. *Skeletal Radiol*. 2013;42(7):917–924.

125. Mamlouk MD, Nicholson AD, Cooke DL, et al. Tips and tricks to optimize MRI protocols for cutaneous vascular anomalies. *Clin Imaging*. 2017;45:71–80.

126. White CL, Olivieri B, Restrepo R, et al. Low-flow vascular malformation pitfalls: from clinical examination to practical imaging evaluation—part 1, lymphatic malformation mimickers. *AJR Am J Roentgenol*. 2016;206(5):940–951.

127. Steinklein JM, Shatzkes DR. Imaging of vascular lesions of the head and neck. *Otolaryngol Clin North Am*. 2018;51(1):55–76.

128. Johnson CM, Navarro OM. Clinical and sonographic features of pediatric soft-tissue vascular anomalies part 2: vascular malformations. *Pediatr Radiol*. 2017;47(9):1196–1208.

129. Mazoyer E, Enjolras O, Bisdorff A, et al. Coagulation disorders in patients with venous malformation of the limbs and trunk: a case series of 118 patients. *Arch Dermatol*. 2008;144(7):861–867.

130. Waelchli R, Aylett SE, Robinson K, et al. New vascular classification of port-wine stains: improving prediction of Sturge-Weber risk. *Br J Dermatol*. 2014;171(4):861–867.

131. Dutkiewicz AS, Ezzedine K, Mazereeuw-Hautier J, et al. A prospective study of risk for Sturge-Weber syndrome in children with upper facial port-wine stain. *J Am Acad Dermatol*. 2015;72(3):473–480.

132. Dymerska M, Kirkorian AY, Offermann EA, et al. Size of facial port-wine birthmark may predict neurologic outcome in Sturge-Weber syndrome. *J Pediatr*. 2017;188:205–209. e1.

133. Comi AM, Sahin M, Hammill A, et al. Leveraging a Sturge-Weber gene discovery: an agenda for future research. *Pediatr Neurol*. 2016;58:12–24.

134. Hess CP, Fullerton HJ, Metry DW, et al. Cervical and intracranial arterial anomalies in 70 patients with PHACE syndrome. *AJNR Am J Neuroradiol*. 2010;31(10):1980–1986.

135. Thiex R, Mulliken JB, Revencu N, et al. A novel association between RASA1 mutations and spinal arteriovenous anomalies. *AJNR Am J Neuroradiol*. 2010;31(4):775–779.

136. Pascual-Castroviejo I, Alvarez-Linera J, Coya J, et al. Pascual-Castroviejo type II syndrome (P-CIIS). Importance of the presence of persistent embryonic arteries. *Childs Nerv Syst*. 2011;27(4):617–625.

137. Metry DW, Garzon MC, Drolet BA, et al. PHACE syndrome: current knowledge, future directions. *Pediatr Dermatol*. 2009;26(4):381–398.

138. Hobert JA, Eng C. PTEN hamartoma tumor syndrome: an overview. *Genet Med*. 2009;11(10):687–694.

139. Pilarski R, Burt R, Kohlman W, et al. Cowden syndrome and the PTEN hamartoma tumor syndrome: systematic review and revised diagnostic criteria. *J Natl Cancer Inst*. 2013;105(21):1607–1616.

140. Sheybani EF, Eutsler EP, Navarro OM. Fat-containing soft-tissue masses in children. *Pediatr Radiol*. 2016;46(13):1760–1773.

141. Shirazi F, Cohen C, Fried L, et al. Mammalian target of rapamycin (mTOR) is activated in cutaneous vascular malformations in vivo. *Lymphat Res Biol*. 2007;5(4):233–236.

142. Hammill AM, Wentzel M, Gupta A, et al. Sirolimus for the treatment of complicated vascular anomalies in children. *Pediatr Blood Cancer*. 2011;57(6):1018–1024.

143. Adams DM, Trenor 3rd CC, Hammill AM, et al. Efficacy and safety of sirolimus in the treatment of complicated vascular anomalies. *Pediatrics*. 2016;137(2).

144. Boon LM, Hammer J, Seront E, et al. Rapamycin as novel treatment for refractory-to-standard-care slow-flow vascular malformations. *Plast Reconstr Surg*. 2015;136(4 Suppl):38.

145. Nadal M, Giraudeau B, Tavernier E, et al. Efficacy and safety of mammalian target of rapamycin inhibitors in vascular anomalies: a systematic review. *Acta Derm Venereol*. 2016;96(4):448–452.

146. Salloum R, Fox CE, Alvarez-Allende CR, et al. Response of blue rubber bleb nevus syndrome to sirolimus treatment. *Pediatr Blood Cancer*. 2016;63(11):1911–1914.

147. Strychowsky JE, Rahbar R, O'Hare MJ, et al. Sirolimus as treatment for 19 patients with refractory cervicofacial lymphatic malformation. *Laryngoscope*. 2018;128(1):269–276.

148. Triana P, Dore M, Cerezo VN, et al. Sirolimus in the treatment of vascular anomalies. *Eur J Pediatr Surg*. 2017;27(1):86–90.

149. Russell TB, Rinker EK, Dillingham CS, et al. Pneumocystis jirovecii pneumonia during sirolimus therapy for Kaposiform hemangioendothelioma. *Pediatrics*. 2018;141(Suppl 5):S421–S424.

150. Ying H, Qiao C, Yang X, et al. A case report of 2 sirolimus-related deaths among infants with Kaposiform hemangioendotheliomas. *Pediatrics*. 2018;141(Suppl 5):S425–S429.

151. Garcia-Montero P, Del Boz J, Sanchez-Martinez M, et al. Microcystic lymphatic malformation successfully treated with topical rapamycin. *Pediatrics*. 2017;139(5):e20162105.

152. Greveling K, Prens EP, van Doorn MB. Treatment of port wine stains using Pulsed Dye Laser, Erbium YAG Laser, and topical rapamycin (sirolimus)—a randomized controlled trial. *Lasers Surg Med*. 2017;49(1):104–109.

153. Marques L, Nunez-Cordoba JM, Aguado L, et al. Topical rapamycin combined with pulsed dye laser in the treatment of capillary vascular malformations in Sturge-Weber syndrome: phase II, randomized, double-blind, intraindividual placebo-controlled clinical trial. *J Am Acad Dermatol*. 2015;72(1):151–158. e1.

154. Study of ARQ 092 in patients with overgrowth diseases and/or vascular anomalies [Internet]. *US National Library of Medicine*. https://clinicaltrials.gov/ct2/show/NCT03094832; 2018. Accessed May 20, 2018.

155. Dose finding trial of ARQ 092 in children and adults with proteus syndrome [Internet]. *US National Library of Medicine*. https://clinicaltrials.gov/ct2/show/NCT02594215?term=ARQ092&rank=5; 2018. Accessed May 20, 2018.

156. Itkin M. Magnetic resonance lymphangiography and lymphatic embolization in the treatment of pulmonary complication of lymphatic malformation. *Semin Intervent Radiol*. 2017;34(3):294–300.

157. Chavhan GB, Amaral JG, Temple M, et al. MR Lymphangiography in children: technique and potential applications. *Radiographics*. 2017;37(6):1775–1790.

158. Dori Y. Novel lymphatic imaging techniques. *Tech Vasc Interv Radiol*. 2016;19(4):255–261.

159. Itkin M. Lymphatic intervention techniques: look beyond thoracic duct embolization. *J Vasc Interv Radiol*. 2016;27(8):1187–1188.

160. Perkins JA. New frontiers in our understanding of lymphatic malformations of the head and neck: natural history and basic research. *Otolaryngol Clin North Am*. 2018;51(1):147–158.

161. Klosterman T. O TM. The management of vascular malformations of the airway: natural history, investigations, medical, surgical and radiological management. *Otolaryngol Clin North Am*. 2018;51(1):213–223.

162. Sun RW, Tuchin VV, Zharov VP, et al. Current status, pitfalls and future directions in the diagnosis and therapy of lymphatic malformation. *J Biophotonics*. 2018;11(8):e201700124.

163. Rockson SG. Current concepts and future directions in the diagnosis and management of lymphatic vascular disease. *Vasc Med*. 2010;15(3):223–231.

164. Keo HH, Gretener SB, Staub D. Clinical and diagnostic aspects of lymphedema. *Vasa*. 2017;46(4):255–261.

165. O'Donnell Jr TF, Rasmussen JC, Sevick-Muraca EM. New diagnostic modalities in the evaluation of lymphedema. *J Vasc Surg Venous Lymphat Disord*. 2017;5(2):261–273.

166. Scaglioni MF, Fontein DBY, Arvanitakis M, et al. Systematic review of lymphovenous anastomosis (LVA) for the treatment of lymphedema. *Microsurgery*. 2017;37(8):947–953.

167. Gallagher K, Marulanda K, Gray S. Surgical intervention for lymphedema. *Surg Oncol Clin N Am*. 2018;27(1):195–215.

168. Tian W, Rockson SG, Jiang X, et al. Leukotriene B4 antagonism ameliorates experimental lymphedema. *Sci Transl Med*. 2017;9(389):eaal3920.

169. Palmyre A, Eyries M, Senat MV, et al. Prenatal molecular diagnosis in RASA1-related disease. *Prenat Diagn*. 2017;37(12):1261–1264.

170. Baselga E, Cordisco MR, Garzon M, et al. Rapidly involuting congenital haemangioma associated with transient thrombocytopenia and coagulopathy: a case series. *Br J Dermatol*. 2008;158(6):1363–1370.

171. Faughnan ME, Palda VA, Garcia-Tsao G, et al. International guidelines for the diagnosis and management of hereditary haemorrhagic telangiectasia. *J Med Genet*. 2011;48(2):73–87.

172. Hoag JB, Terry P, Mitchell S, et al. An epistaxis severity score for hereditary hemorrhagic telangiectasia. *Laryngoscope*. 2010;120(4):838–843.

173. van Es J, Kappelhof NA, Douma RA, et al. Venous thrombosis and coagulation parameters in patients with pure venous malformations. *Neth J Med*. 2017;75(8):328–334.

174. Keppler-Noreuil KM, Lozier JN, Sapp JC, et al. Characterization of thrombosis in patients with Proteus syndrome. *Am J Med Genet A*. 2017;173(9):2359–2365.

175. Spencer SA, Sorger J. Orthopedic issues in vascular anomalies. *Semin Pediatr Surg*. 2014;23(4):227–232.

176. Rebarber A, Roman AS, Roshan D, et al. Obstetric management of Klippel-Trénaunay syndrome. *Obstet Gynecol*. 2004;104(5 Pt 2):1205–1208.

177. Horbach SE, Lokhorst MM, Oduber CE, et al. Complications of pregnancy and labour in women with Klippel-Trénaunay syndrome: a nationwide cross-sectional study. *BJOG*. 2017;124(11):1780–1788.

178. Martin JR, Pels SG, Paidas M, et al. Assisted reproduction in a patient with Klippel-Trénaunay syndrome: management of thrombophilia and consumptive coagulopathy. *J Assist Reprod Genet*. 2011;28(3):217–219.

179. Dey JK, Ishii LE, Byrne PJ, et al. The social penalty of facial lesions: new evidence supporting high-quality reconstruction. *JAMA Facial Plast Surg*. 2015;17(2):90–96.

180. Dey JK, Ishii LE, Joseph AW, et al. The cost of facial deformity: a health utility and valuation study. *JAMA Facial Plast Surg*. 2016;18(4):241–249.

181. Chamlin SL, Mancini AJ, Lai JS, et al. Development and validation of a quality-of-life instrument for infantile hemangiomas. *J Invest Dermatol*. 2015;135(6):1533–1539.

182. Cazeau C, Blei F, Gonzales Hermosa M, et al. Burden of infantile hemangioma on family: an international observational cross-sectional study. *Pediatr Dermatol*. 2017;34(3):295–302.

183. Weiss J, Daniel T. Validation of the Lymphedema Life Impact Scale (LLIS): a condition-specific measurement tool for persons with lymphedema. *Lymphology*. 2015;48(3):128–138.

184. Horbach SER, van der Horst C, Blei F, et al. Development of an international core outcome set for peripheral vascular malformations: the OVAMA project. *Br J Dermatol*. 2018;178(2):473–481.

185. Chaturvedi S, Clancy M, Schaefer N, et al. Depression and post-traumatic stress disorder in individuals with hereditary hemorrhagic telangiectasia: a cross-sectional survey. *Thromb Res*. 2017;153:14–18.

186. Daly MB, Pilarski R, Axilbund JE, et al. Genetic/familial high-risk assessment: breast and ovarian, version 1.2014. *J Natl Compr Canc Netw.* 2014;12(9):1326–1328.

187. DeLair DF, Soslow RA. Gynecologic manifestations of less commonly encountered hereditary syndromes. *Surg Pathol Clin.* 2016;9(2):269–287.

188. Hirabayashi S, Seki M, Hasegawa D, et al. Constitutional abnormalities of IDH1 combined with secondary mutations predispose a patient with Maffucci syndrome to acute lymphoblastic leukemia. *Pediatr Blood Cancer.* 2017;64(12).

189. Gripp KW, Baker L, Kandula V, et al. Nephroblastomatosis or Wilms tumor in a fourth patient with a somatic PIK3CA mutation. *Am J Med Genet A.* 2016;170(10):2559–2569.

190. Peterman CM, Fevurly RD, Alomari AI, et al. Sonographic screening for Wilms tumor in children with CLOVES syndrome. *Pediatr Blood Cancer.* 2017;64(12).

191. Garzon MC, Weitz N, Powell J. Vascular anomalies: differential diagnosis and mimickers. *Semin Cutan Med Surg.* 2016;35(3):170–176.

192. Brockman RM, Humphrey SR, Moe DC, et al. Mimickers of infantile hemangiomas. *Pediatr Dermatol.* 2017;34(3):331–336.